BONE and JOINT IMAGING

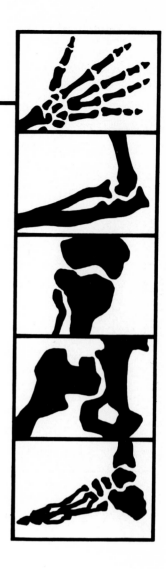

DONALD RESNICK, M.D.

Professor of Radiology
University of California, San Diego
Chief of Radiology Service
Veterans Administration Medical Center
San Diego, California

With the editorial assistance of
Catherine Fix

1989
W. B. SAUNDERS COMPANY
Harcourt Brace Jovanovich, Inc.
Philadelphia   London   Toronto   Montreal   Sydney   Tokyo

W. B. SAUNDERS COMPANY
Harcourt Brace Jovanovich, Inc.

The Curtis Center
Independence Square West
Philadelphia, PA 19106

Library of Congress Cataloging-in-Publication Data

Resnick, Donald

Bone and joint imaging

1. Bones—Imaging.   2. Joints—Imaging.   3. Bones—Diseases—
Diagnosis.   4. Joints—Diseases—Diagnosis.   I. Title.
[DNLM: 1. Bone and Bones.   2. Bone Diseases—diagnosis.
3. Diagnostic Imaging—methods.   4. Joint Diseases—
diagnosis.   5. Joints.   WE 141 R434e]

RC930.5.R47   1989   616.7'107572–dc19   89-5905

ISBN 0-7216-2215-1

Editor: Lisette Bralow
Designer: W. B. Saunders Staff
Production Manager: Bob Butler/Peter Faber
Manuscript Editor: Catherine Fix
Illustration Coordinator: Peg Shaw
Indexer: Catherine Fix
Cover Designer: Brian Preuss

Bone and Joint Imaging   ISBN 0–7216–2215–1

Last digit is the print number: 9   8   7   6   5   4   3   2   1

*To the residents and fellows whose enthusiasm and
quest for knowledge give me purpose.*

Contributors

NAOMI ALAZRAKI, M.D.
Professor of Radiology, Co-Director, Division of Nuclear Medicine, Emory University and Affiliated Hospitals, Atlanta, Georgia

MICHAEL ANDRÉ, Ph.D.
Assistant Adjunct Professor, University of California at San Diego, San Diego, California; Physicist, Veterans Administration Medical Center, La Jolla, California, and UCSD Medical Center, San Diego, California

JOSEPH J. BOOKSTEIN, M.D.
Professor of Radiology, University of California at San Diego, San Diego, California; Chief, Cardiovascular Radiology, Hospital of the University of California, San Diego, California

MURRAY K. DALINKA, M.D.
Professor of Radiology and Orthopedic Surgery, Hospital of the University of Pennsylvania, Philadelphia, Pennsylvania

FRIEDA FELDMAN, M.D.
Professor of Radiology, College of Physicians and Surgeons, Columbia University, New York, New York; Attending Radiologist, Columbia Presbyterian Medical Center, New York, New York

ERICH FISCHER, M.D.
Professor of Radiology, University of Tübingen, Federal Republic of Germany; Robert Bosch Krankenhaus D 7000 Stuttgart, Federal Republic of Germany

HARRY K. GENANT, M.D.
Professor of Radiology, Medicine, and Orthopaedic Surgery, University of California, San Francisco, California

THOMAS G. GOERGEN, M.D.
Associate Clinical Professor of Radiology, University of California at San Diego, San Diego, California; Palomar-Pomerado Hospital District, Escondido, California

AMY BETH GOLDMAN, M.D.
Professor of Clinical Radiology, Cornell Medical School, New York, New York; Attending Physician, Hospital for Special Surgery, New York, New York

GUERDON D. GREENWAY, M.D.
Clinical Assistant Professor of Radiology, University of California, San Diego, California; Clinical Assistant Professor of Orthopedic Surgery, University of Texas Health Science Center, Dallas, Texas; Associate Attending Radiologist, Baylor University Medical Center, Dallas, Texas

PARVIZ HAGHIGHI, M.D.
Clinical Professor, Department of Pathology, University of California at San Diego, San Diego, California; Staff Pathologist, Veterans Administration Medical Center, San Diego, California

VICTOR HAUGHTON, M.D.
Professor, Department of Radiology, Medical College of Wisconsin, Milwaukee, Wisconsin; Radiologist, Froedtert Memorial Lutheran Hospital and Milwaukee County Medical Complex, Milwaukee, Wisconsin

THEODORE E. KEATS, M.D.
Professor and Chairman, Department of Radiology, University of Virginia Hospital, Charlottesville, Virginia; Chief Radiologist, University of Virginia Hospital, Charlottesville, Virginia

MICHAEL KYRIAKOS, M.D.
Professor of Pathology and Surgical Pathology, Washington University School of Medicine, St. Louis, Missouri; Surgical Pathologist, Barnes Hospital, St. Louis, Missouri; Consulting Pathologist, St. Louis Children's Hospital and Shriners Hospital for Crippled Children, St. Louis, Missouri

JOHN E. MADEWELL, M.D.
Professor and Vice Chairman, Department of Radiology, Baylor College of Medicine, Houston, Texas

STAVROS C. MANOLAGAS, M.D., Ph.D.
Associate Professor of Medicine, University of California at San Diego, San Diego, California; Staff Physician, Veterans Administration Medical Center, San Diego, California

WILLIAM H. McALISTER, M.D.
Professor of Radiology and Pediatrics, Washington University School of Medicine, St. Louis, Missouri; Mallinckrodt Institute of Radiology, St. Louis Childrens and Barnes Hospitals, St. Louis, Missouri

WILLIAM A. MURPHY, M.D.
Professor of Radiology, Washington University School of Medicine, St. Louis, Missouri; Co-Director, Musculoskeletal Section and Co-Chairman, Magnetic Resonance Imaging, Mallinckrodt Institute of Radiology, St. Louis, Missouri

LAWRENCE M. NEUSTADTER, D.O.
Hospital of the University of Pennsylvania, Philadelphia, Pennsylvania; Attending Staff, Hospital of the University of Pennsylvania and St. Agnes Medical Center, Philadelphia, Pennsylvania

JOHN A. OGDEN, M.D.
Professor, Department of Orthopaedics, University of South Florida College of Medicine, Tampa, Florida; and Clinical Professor of Surgery (Orthopaedics), Yale University, New Haven, Connecticut; Chief of Staff, Shriners Hospital for Crippled Children, Tampa, Florida; Attending, Tampa General Hospital, University Community Hospital, and Women's Hospital, Tampa, Florida; Consultant, Bay Pines Veterans Hospital and St. Joseph's Hospital, Tampa, Florida

M. B. OZONOFF, M.D.
Professor of Radiology, University of Connecticut School of Medicine, Farmington, Connecticut; Associate Clinical Professor of Radiology, Yale University School of Medicine, New Haven, Connecticut; Director of Radiology, Newington Children's Hospital, Newington, Connecticut; Senior Attending, Hartford Hospital, Hartford, Connecticut

MICHAEL J. PITT, M.D.
Professor of Radiology and (Orthopedic) Surgery, University of Arizona College of Medicine, Tucson, Arizona; University Medical Center, Tucson Veterans Administration Hospital, Tucson, Arizona

DAVID J. SARTORIS, M.D.
Associate Professor of Radiology, University of California at San Diego, School of Medicine, San Diego, California; Attending Staff, University of California San Diego Medical Center and Veterans Administration Medical Center, San Diego, California

WILLIAM SCHEIBLE, M.D.
Department of Radiology, Portland Adventist Medical Center, Portland, Oregon

DONALD E. SWEET, M.D.
Chairman and Registrar, Department of Orthopedic Pathology, Armed Forces Institute of Pathology, Washington, D.C.

BARBARA N. WARREN WEISSMAN, M.D.
Associate Professor of Radiology, Harvard Medical School, Cambridge, Massachusetts; Radiologist and Director, Bone Radiology Service, Brigham and Women's Hospital, Boston, Massachusetts

Preface

Vigorous writing is concise. A sentence should contain no unnecessary words, a paragraph no unnecessary sentences, for the same reason that a drawing should have no unnecessary lines and a machine no unnecessary parts. This requires not that the writer make all his sentences short, or that he avoid all detail and treat his subjects only in outline, but that every word tell.

WILLIAM STRUNK, JR.
The Elements of Style, 1918

This textbook represents the product of a delayed response to a question that has been posed to me on numerous occasions for a number of years by residents and fellows in radiology, orthopedic surgery, and rheumatology: "I like the multivolume book that you and your collaborators have produced" (the question always begins on a positive note), "but could you shorten it a bit" (the precise definition of 'a bit' is rarely specified) "so that I might read it in its entirety during my year(s) of training?" My initial response generally was to explain that musculoskeletal disorders were diverse in nature and that important aspects of their diagnosis required a good deal of text and illustrative material. Furthermore, I explained, radiology was expanding rapidly with the introduction and refinement of numerous imaging methods such as computed tomography and magnetic resonance imaging. Since the question continued to be repeated, however, it became apparent to me that a significant percentage of the persons for whom the original textbook was intended were so intimidated by its size that they had decided not to lift it, let alone read it.

Some months ago, with the permission of my collaborators, I began the process of condensing the information that was contained in our second edition. I anticipated a lengthy and, above all, painful experience (like all authors, I believed that every word and each illustration in that edition were essential to its message). Now the process has been completed, and I can report that it was not as painful as I had expected. That is not to say that the multivolume textbook contained superfluous material, but rather, that the purpose of this current book is quite different. Within these 1300 pages is the information that I believe is *essential* to those physicians who are involved in the interpretation or review of imaging studies of patients with musculoskeletal disorders. Although clinical and pathologic data are presented, it is the imaging abnormalities and their differential diagnoses that are emphasized. The illustrations selected are those that most vividly depict these abnormalities, and tabular material is used, whenever possible, to summarize important concepts or findings in a manner that is easily surveyed and remembered. At the conclusion of each chapter, a limited number of pertinent references have been included, although the interested reader should consult the larger "parent" book for complete bibliographic data.

The current textbook is not meant to be encyclopedic in scope. Rather, it is the essentials alone that are presented. This textbook is directed specifically to residents and fellows in radiology, orthopedic surgery, rheumatology, and related medical fields whose time is limited because of the many responsibilities placed on them during their years of training. It is hoped that between imaging studies, when the surgical duties are completed (or prior to beginning them), or before morning or after evening rounds, a few minutes spent reading these essentials will be both painless and rewarding. Certainly, the multivolume textbook has been "shortened a bit" and, I believe, now can be read in its entirety during the busy but informative years of training.

DONALD RESNICK, M.D.

Acknowledgments

Although this textbook is far shorter than its predecessor, its success is no less dependent on a number of persons who have contributed significantly to it. I wish to acknowledge the assistance of each of the authors, dedicated teachers all, who allowed me to condense their fact-filled chapters in order to provide a version that could be more easily consulted and read in a shorter period of time. I also would like to thank all those who permitted me to use one or more of the cases whose illustrations are contained in this textbook; their contributions are specifically cited in the corresponding legends beneath or beside these illustrations.

I wish to acknowledge the able assistance of many individuals at W.B. Saunders Company, particularly Lisette Bralow, Senior Medical Editor, whose advice and friendship were invaluable, and Robert Butler, the talented production manager. Both of them provided capable assistance not only in the production of this textbook but in that of the parent multivolume textbook as well.

My secretary, Cynde Roche-Williams, and my laboratory assistant, Debra Trudell, once again have given unselfishly of their time and energy, and they must know how deeply I appreciate their efforts. Finally, as in the two previous editions of our larger textbook, I must acknowledge the considerable support provided by Catherine Fix, whose duties included medical writer, copy editor, and indexer. It was she, as before, who kept me focused and on track in this effort, and it is her energy and enthusiasm that provided the framework upon which this textbook was constructed.

To all of these persons, I offer my heartfelt thanks.

Contents

Test Cases

Frequently the radiologist is confronted with radiographic findings that at first seem ambiguous, in that they might be attributed to numerous diseases or pathologic states. In reality, however, careful analysis of the imaging examinations in many instances will reveal a set of features that either are diagnostic of a specific process or make that process the most likely one. On the following pages, fifteen test cases are given, representing three levels of difficulty (1, 2, and 3, with 3 being the most difficult). The reader is invited to choose a diagnosis for each test case. It is emphasized that these are not esoteric or unusual presentations but were selected to illustrate the difficulties radiologists normally encounter in interpreting films.

At the beginning of each section of the book, one of the test cases is repeated. An explanation of the findings and a few selected readings are also given. Each test case number matches the number of the corresponding section—for example, to find the correct diagnosis for Test Case V, turn to Section V.

It is hoped that these cases will be challenging, informative, and entertaining and that they will stimulate the reader to pay increasing attention to patterns and combinations of radiographic findings, as described in this book. Good luck!

CASE I

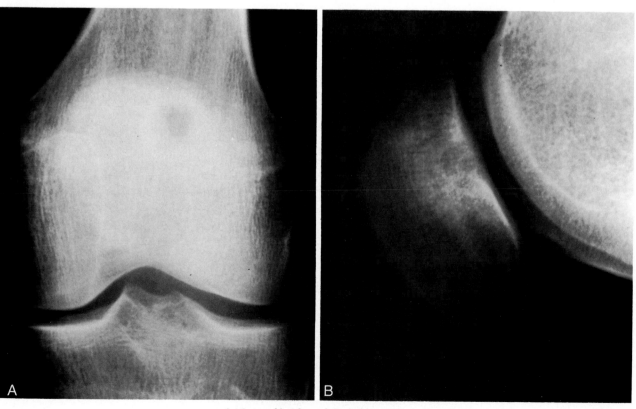

A 16 year old girl complained of knee pain.

CASE II

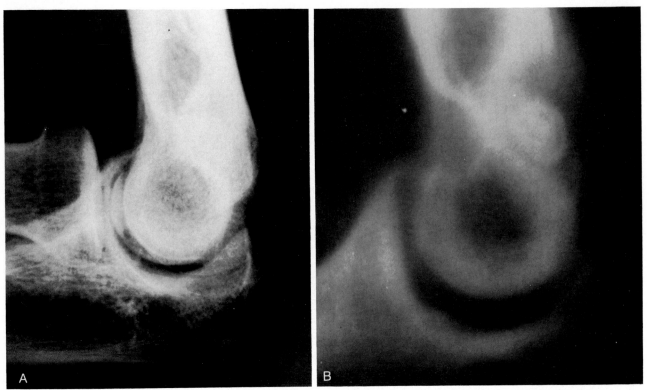

A 20 year old man was examined because of decreased range of motion in his elbow. He had had a previous injury to the elbow.

CASE III

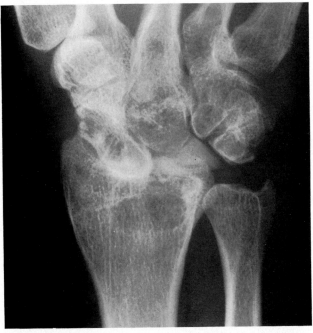

A 30 year old man noted increasing pain, local swelling, and limitation of motion in the wrist. He had had a previous surgical procedure performed on this wrist.

CASE IV

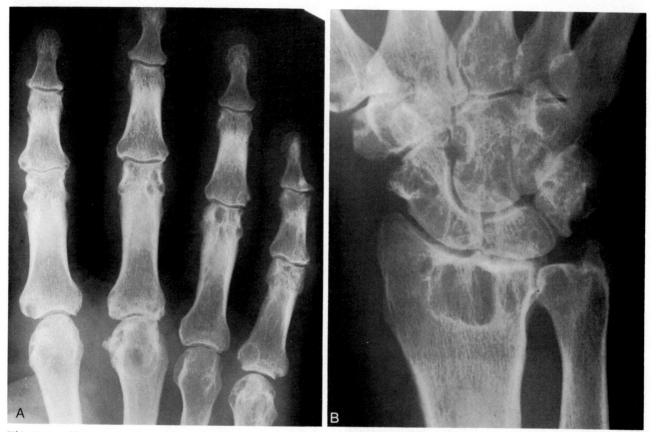

This 66 year old man had a 15 year history of slowly progressive polyarthritis affecting both small and large joints in the upper and lower extremities. Radiographs of the left hand and wrist are shown. The opposite side was similarly involved.

CASE V

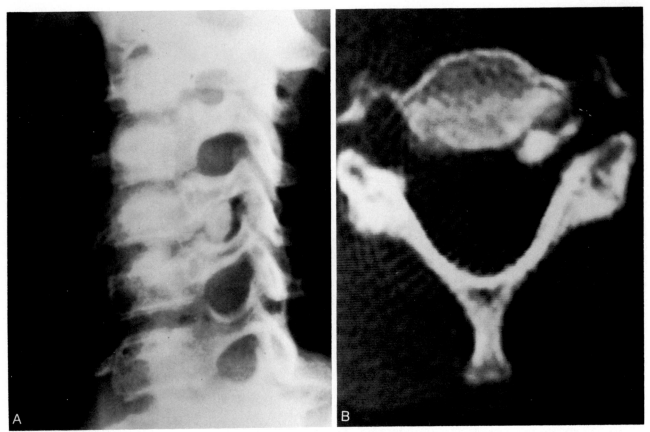

A 9 year old girl had fever, neck stiffness, and torticollis.

CASE VI   *LEVEL OF DIFFICULTY: 2*

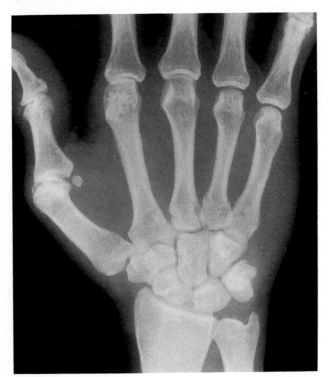

A 70 year old man complained of pain and swelling involving both wrists and the second and third metacarpophalangeal joints in both hands.

CASE VII   LEVEL OF DIFFICULTY: 2

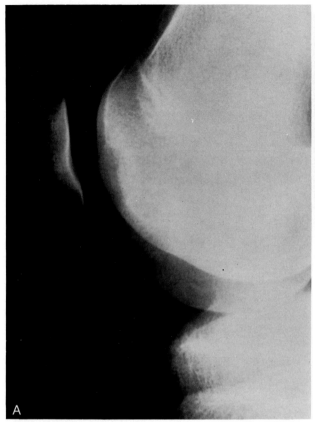

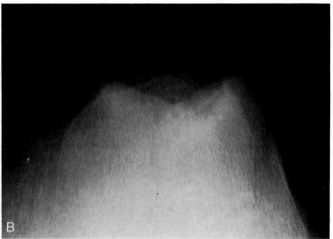

A 15 year old boy developed pain in the anterior aspect of the knee. He had no history of acute injury.

CASE VIII   LEVEL OF DIFFICULTY: 2

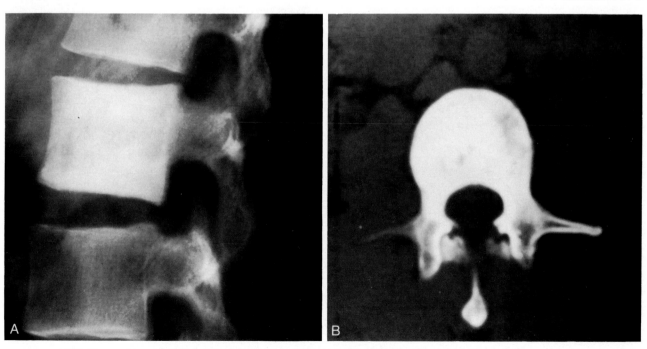

This 37 year old man had back pain. A bone scan (not shown) confirmed that no other skeletal abnormalities were present.

CASE IX

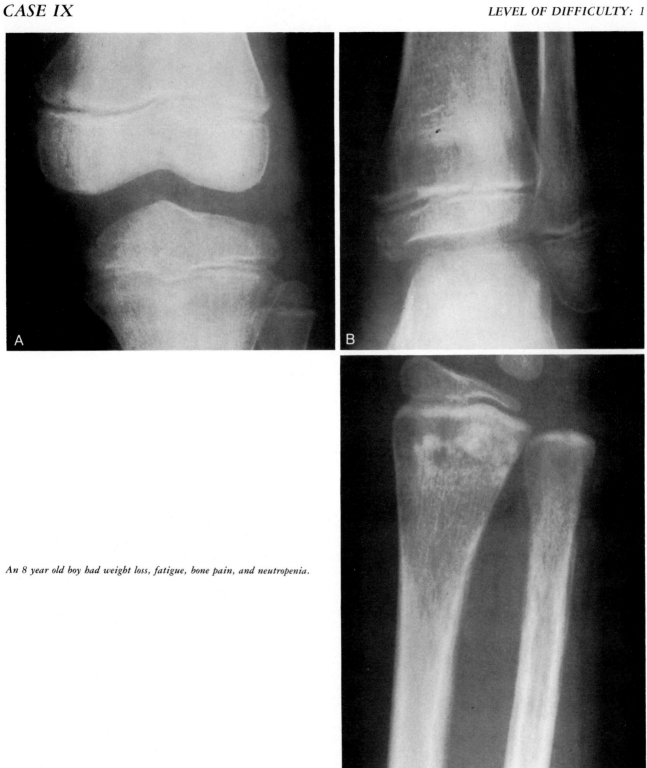

An 8 year old boy had weight loss, fatigue, bone pain, and neutropenia.

CASE X

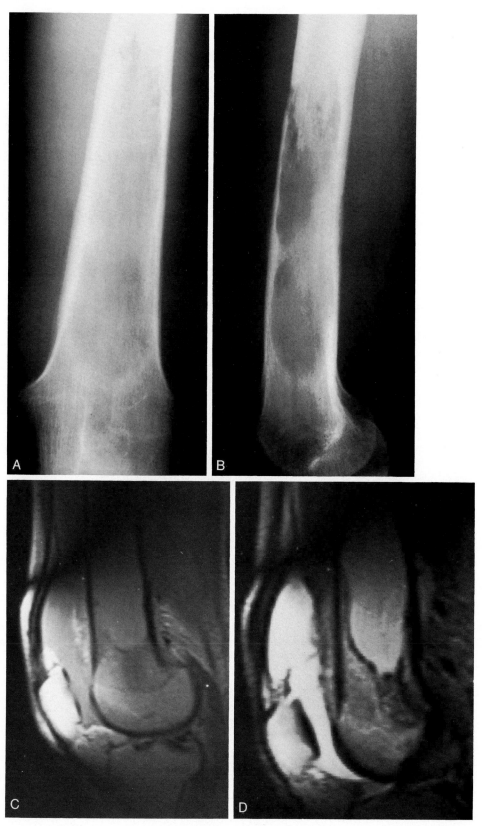

A 23 year old man had a 4 month history of pain in the knee and thigh. On physical examination, an effusion in the knee and a tender, firm mass in the thigh were observed.

CASE XI   LEVEL OF DIFFICULTY: 2

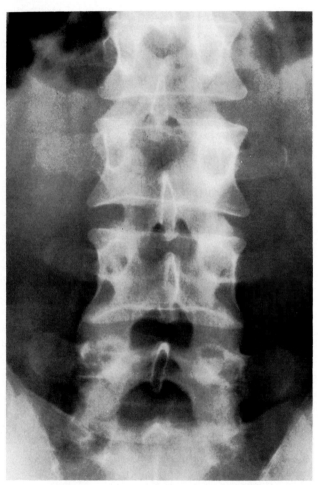

A 37 year old man complained of nonradiating back pain that was exacerbated by prolonged sitting and participation in sporting activities. The pain had been present for 3 years. There was no history of spinal injury.

CASE XII   *LEVEL OF DIFFICULTY: 3*

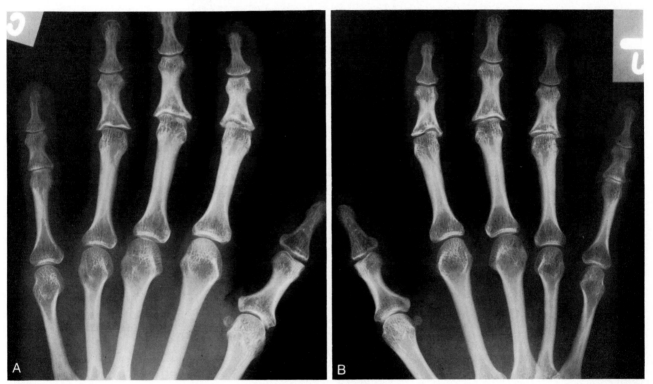

A 34 year old woman had painless swelling about the proximal interphalangeal joints of the hands and deformity of the fingers. She stated that the abnormalities began when she was a teenager. No other skeletal sites were affected.

CASE XIII   LEVEL OF DIFFICULTY: 2

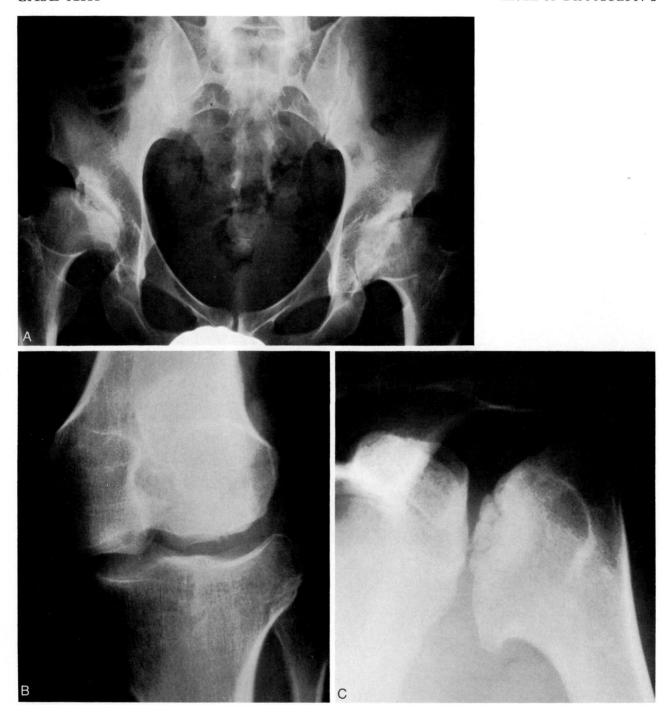

This 26 year old man had pain and restricted motion of multiple joints that had begun in late childhood or adolescence and had progressed in recent years. Physical examination revealed short stature, normal intelligence, and a waddling gait.

CASE XIV

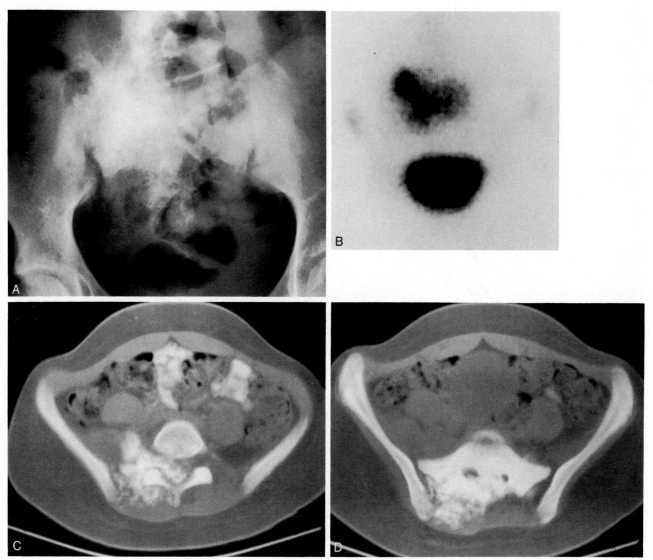

A 13 year old girl developed pain in the right leg and foot that progressed over a period of 2 months.

CASE XV

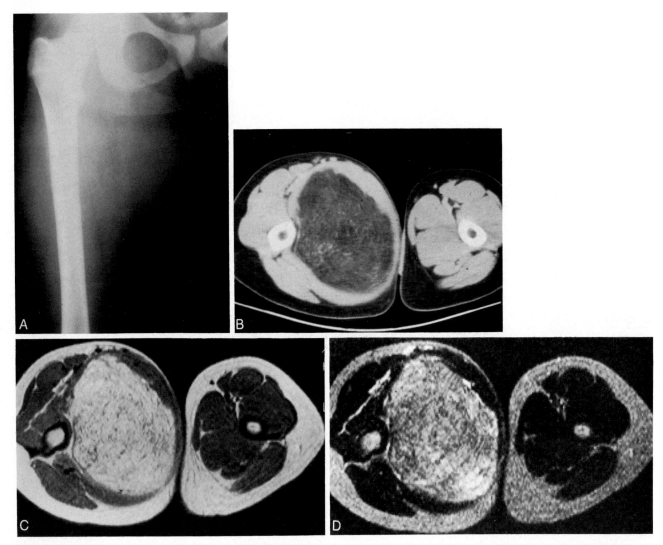

A 12 year old girl had a mass in the medial aspect of the thigh. The mass had been present for several years but had enlarged significantly during the previous few months. It was painless.

Answers to these test cases can be found at the beginning of the related Sections of the book (for example, for Case I, see Section I).

SECTION I

ANATOMY AND PHYSIOLOGY

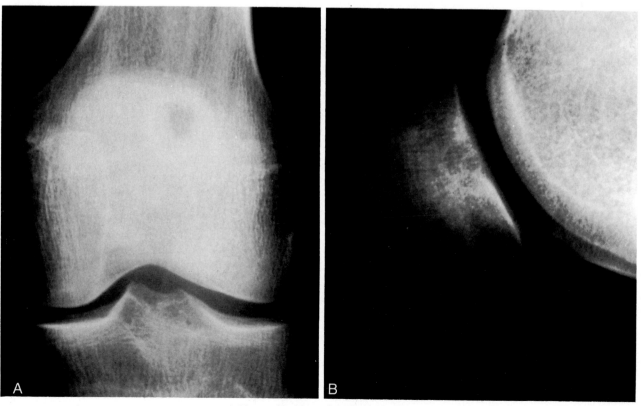

A 16 year old girl complained of knee pain.

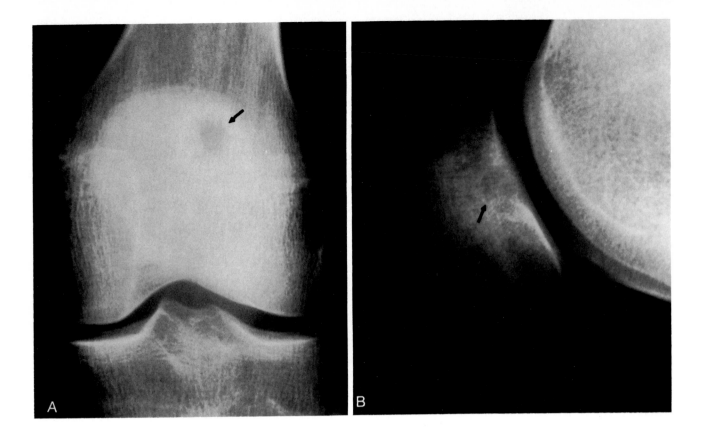

A   B

Anteroposterior and lateral radiographs of the knee (*A* and *B*) reveal a well-defined, ovoid osteolytic lesion (arrows) involving the posterolateral aspect of the patella, extending to the subchondral bone plate. There is a thin sclerotic margin about a portion of the lesion.

Among the tumors and tumor-like processes that may involve the patella are chondroblastoma, osteoblastoma, osteoid osteoma, giant cell tumor, eosinophilic granuloma, aneurysmal bone cyst, intraosseous ganglion, simple bone cyst, and several malignant neoplasms. None of these lesions commonly affects the patella, and their radiographic appearances, with the possible exception of chondroblastoma, would not be expected to resemble that shown in the test case. Although a Brodie's abscess could produce an osteolytic lesion with radiographic features identical to those in Case I, it too is rare in the patella.

Three lesions that characteristically arise in the bone must be given serious diagnostic consideration. The first of these, chondromalacia patellae, typically is confined to the cartilaginous portion of the patella and classically affects the ridge between the medial and the odd facets of the bone. Although osseous abnormalities have been reported in association with chondromalacia patellae, they must be considered an unusual manifestation of the disorder. Therefore, chondromalacia patellae is not a realistic diagnostic choice.

A second process, osteochondritis dissecans, must also be considered in the differential diagnosis of the abnormalities illustrated in Case I. Osteochondritis dissecans of the patella is seen in both male and female patients, usually between the ages of 15 and 20 years. The typical location of the lesion, however, is the medial facet of the patella, in the middle or lower portion of the bone. The process in Case I is located in the superolateral region of the patella, making unlikely the diagnosis of osteochondritis dissecans.

The radiographic abnormalities in the test case are most compatible with the diagnosis of dorsal defect of the patella. This defect is present in approximately 1 per cent of the population, and it may be discovered in children, in adolescents, or, less commonly, in adults. The dorsal defect of the patella is a radiolucent, oval or round lesion that invariably is located in the superolateral aspect of the patella just deep to the cartilaginous surface, precisely the location of the process illustrated in Case I. The dorsal defect may be unilateral or bilateral in distribution, and affected patients may either be asymptomatic or have local pain and tenderness. Arthrography usually reveals intact patellar cartilage in almost all instances, and scintigraphy may show focal accumulation of bone-seeking radiopharmaceutical agents.

The pathogenesis of the dorsal defect of the patella is not clear, although it generally is regarded as an anomaly of patellar ossification. Its predilection for the superolateral aspect of the bone is a feature that also is observed in cases of multipartite patella, suggesting a relationship between these two processes. Indeed, both conditions have been observed in a single patient, and computed tomography in some instances of dorsal defect demonstrates irregularity of the anterior portion of the bone, similar to that which occurs in a multipartite patella. It appears likely that both the dorsal defect of the patella and the multipartite patella are related entities that result from chronic stress provided by the patellar insertion of the vastus lateralis muscle before the bone is fully ossified. This pathogenesis, which is similar to that observed in Sinding-Larsen-Johansson and Osgood-Schlatter syndromes, would explain the occurrence of pain as well as the accumulation of bone-seeking radionuclides in some patients with dorsal defect of the patella.

The lesion illustrated in Case I was excised. A well-defined cystic lesion of the patella was verified surgically. At the base of the lesion, an irregularity of articular cartilage was observed. The histologic findings, which consisted of vascularized fibrous tissue and small fragments of bone, were considered typical of dorsal defect of the patella.

FINAL DIAGNOSIS: Dorsal defect of the patella.

FURTHER READING

Pages 820 and 821 and the following:

1. Goergen TG, Resnick D, Greenway G, Saltzstein SL: Dorsal defect of the patella: A characteristic radiographic lesion. Radiology *130:*333, 1979.
2. van Holsbeeck, M, Vandamme B, Marchal G, Martens M, Victor J, Baert AL: Dorsal defect of the patella: Concept of its origin and relationship with bipartite and multipartite patella. Skel Radiol *16:*304, 1987.

(Case I, courtesy of J. Sokoloff, M.D., San Diego, California.)

Chapter 1

Histogenesis, Anatomy, and Physiology of Bone

Donald Resnick, M.D.
Stavros C. Manolagas, M.D., Ph.D.
Gen Niwayama, M.D.

Bone develops through the processes of endochondral and intramembranous ossification and is subsequently modified and refined by modeling and remodeling to create a structurally and metabolically competent, highly organized architectural marvel. Its cells, including the osteoblasts, osteocytes, and osteoclasts, reside in an organic matrix, and inorganic material is deposited in a form that resembles hydroxyapatite. The process of mineralization is complex and incompletely understood.

Bone is essential in maintaining calcium homeostasis, stabilizing the plasma level of calcium. Its cells are highly responsive to stimuli provided by a number of humoral agents, of which parathyroid hormone, thyrocalcitonin, and 1,25-dihydroxyvitamin D are most important. Synthesis and resorption of bone, which continue normally in a delicate balance throughout life, are mediated by the action of such humoral agents through stimulation of osteoblasts to form bone and of osteoclasts and osteocytes to remove bone. The presence of a variety of diseases results in characteristic alterations that are readily detectable on radiographs or by other imaging methods.

Bone is a remarkable tissue. Although its appearance on the radiograph might be misinterpreted as indicating inactivity, bone is constantly undergoing change, not only in the immature skeleton, in which growth and development are readily apparent, but also in the mature skeleton, through the constant and balanced processes of bone formation and resorption. It is when these processes are modified such that one or the other dominates that a pathologic state may be created. In some instances, the resulting imbalance between bone formation and resorption is easily detectable on the radiograph. In others, a more subtle imbalance exists that may be identified only on the histologic level.

The initial architecture of bone is characterized by an irregular network of collagen, termed woven-fibered bone, which is a temporary material that is either removed to form a marrow cavity or subsequently replaced by a sheet-like arrangement of osseous tissue, termed parallel-fibered or lamellar bone. As a connective tissue, bone is highly specialized, differing from other connective tissues by its rigidity and hardness that relate primarily to the inorganic salts that are deposited in its matrix. These properties are fundamental to a tissue that must maintain the shape of the human body, protect its vital soft tissues, and allow locomotion, transmitting from one region of the body to another the forces generated by the contractions of various muscles. Bone also serves as a reservoir for ions, principally calcium, that are essential to normal fluid regulation and are made available as a response to stimuli produced by a number of hormones, particularly parathyroid hormone, vitamin D, and calcitonin.

HISTOGENESIS
Developing Bone

Bone develops by the process of intramembranous bone formation (by transformation of condensed mesenchymal tissue) or endochondral bone formation (by indirect conversion of an intermediate cartilage model), or both. At some locations, such as the cranial vault, the mandible and maxilla, and the midportion of the clavicle, intramembranous (mesenchymal) ossification is detected; in other locations, such as the bones of the extremities, the vertebral column, the pelvis, and the base of the skull, both endochondral and intramembranous ossification can be identified. The actual sequence of bone formation is essentially the same in both intramembranous and endochondral ossification: (1) osteoblasts differentiate from mesenchymal cells; (2) osteoblasts deposit matrix that is subsequently mineralized; (3) bone is initially deposited as a network of immature (woven) trabeculae, the primary spongiosa; (4) the primary spongiosa is replaced by secondary bone, removed to form bone marrow, or converted into primary cortical bone by filling of spaces between the trabeculae. A variety of congenital disorders may lead to abnormalities in intramembranous or endochondral bone formation, or both.

16

INTRAMEMBRANOUS OSSIFICATION. Intramembranous ossification is initiated by the proliferation of mesenchymal cells about a network of capillaries. At this site, a transformation of mesenchymal cells is accompanied by the appearance of a meshwork of collagen fibers and amorphous ground substance. The primitive cells proliferate, enlarge, and become arranged in groups, becoming osteoblasts that are intimately involved in the formation of an eosinophilic matrix within the collagenous tissue. This initial stage of the ossification process becomes more prominent as the osteoid matrix undergoes calcification with the deposition of calcium phosphate. Some of the osteoblasts on the surface of the osteoid and woven-fibered bone become entrapped as osteocytes within the substance of the matrix in a space called a lacuna. The osteocyte maintains some contact with the precursor cells by sending out elongated processes through canaliculi that extend through the matrix. Embedded osteocytes are devoted primarily to maintaining the integrity of the surrounding matrix and are not directly involved in bone formation. Through the continued transformation of mesenchymal cells into osteoblasts, the elaboration of an osteoid matrix, and the entrapment of osteoblasts within the matrix, the primitive mesenchyme is converted into osseous tissue. The ultimate characteristics of the tissue depend on its location within the bone: In the cancellous areas of the bone, the meshwork of osseous tissue contains intervening vascular connective tissue representing the embryonic precursor of the bone marrow; in the compact areas of the bone, the osseous tissue becomes more condensed, forming cylindrical masses containing a central vascular channel, the haversian system. On the external and internal surfaces of the compact bone, fibrovascular layers develop (periosteum and endosteum) that contain cells which remain osteogenic, giving bone its everchanging quality. In the process of further development, coarse-fibered nonlamellar primitive bone is eventually converted to fine-fibered lamellar mature bone.

ENDOCHONDRAL OSSIFICATION. In endochondral (intracartilaginous) ossification, cartilaginous tissue derived from mesenchyme is replaced with bone (Fig. 1–1). The initial sites of bone formation are called centers of ossification. In the tubular bones, the primary center of ossification is located in the central portion of the cartilaginous model, whereas later-appearing centers of ossification (secondary centers) are located at the ends of the models within epiphyses and apophyses. Vascular mesenchymal tissue or perichondrium, whose deeper layers contain cells with osteogenic potential, surrounds the cartilaginous model.

The initial changes in the primary center of ossification are hypertrophy of cartilage cells, glycogen accumulation, and reduction of intervening matrix. Subsequently, these cells degenerate and become calcified. Simultaneously, the deeper or subperichondrial cells undergo transformation to osteoblasts and, through a process identical to intramembranous ossification, these osteoblasts produce a subperiosteal collar of bone, which encloses the central portions of the cartilaginous tissue. Periosteal tissue is converted into vascular channels, and these channels perforate the shell of bone, entering the degenerating cartilaginous foci. The aggressive vascular tissue disrupts the lacunae of the cartilage cells, creating spaces that fill with embryonic bone marrow. Osteoblasts appear and lay down osteoid tissue in the cartilage matrix. They become

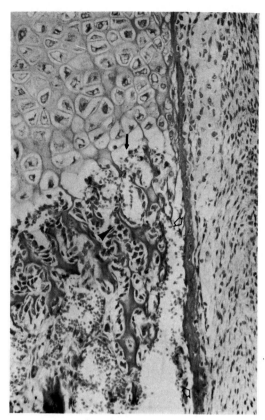

Figure 1–1. Endochondral and intramembranous ossification in a tubular bone: Radius of a 4½ month old fetus. The large and confluent cartilage cell lacunae are being penetrated by vascular channels (solid arrow), thus exposing intervening cores of calcified cartilage matrix. The osteoblasts are depositing osseous tissue on these cartilage matrix cores (arrowhead). Observe subperiosteal bone formation (open arrows).

trapped within the developing bone as osteocytes in a fashion similar to that occurring during intramembranous ossification.

From the center of the tubular bone, ossification proceeds toward the ends of the bone. The periosteal collar likewise spreads toward the ends of the bone. Resorption of some of the initially formed trabeculae creates a marrow space, and through a process of subperiosteal deposition of bone, a cortex becomes evident, grows thicker, and is converted into a system with longitudinally arranged compact bone surrounding vascular channels (haversian system). The frontier of endochondral ossification that is advancing toward the end of the bone becomes better delineated, appearing as a plate of cellular activity. It is this plate that ultimately becomes located between the epiphysis and diaphysis of a tubular bone, forming the growth plate (cartilaginous plate) that is the predominant site of longitudinal growth of the bone. The plate contains clearly demarcated zones: a resting zone of flattened and immature cells on the epiphyseal aspect of the plate, and zones of cell growth and hypertrophy and of transformation with provisional calcification and ossification on the metaphyseal or diaphyseal aspect of the plate.

At the ends of the tubular bones, endochondral bone formation is initiated, creating secondary centers of ossification in the epiphyses. An enlarging ossification nucleus is formed whose peripheral margins contain zones of cell hypertrophy,

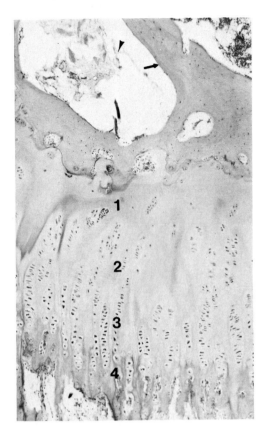

Figure 1–2. Cartilaginous growth plate in a 16 year old patient. Observe the bone (arrow) and marrow (arrowhead) of the epiphysis. The areas of the growth plate include a zone of resting cartilage (1), proliferating cartilage (2), maturing cartilage (3), and calcifying cartilage (4). (86 ×.)

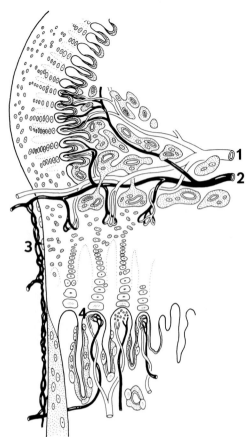

Figure 1–3. Cartilage growth plate and adjacent metaphysis and epiphysis. Note the epiphyseal vein (1) and artery (2), the perichondrial vascular ring (3), the terminal loops of the nutrient artery (4) in the metaphysis, and ongoing endochondral ossification in the physis and epiphysis. (Redrawn from R Warwick, PL Williams (Eds): Gray's Anatomy. 35th British Ed. Philadelphia, WB Saunders Co, 1973, p. 227. Used with permission.)

degeneration, calcification, and ossification. The epiphyseal cartilage is thus converted to bone, although a layer on its articular aspect persists, destined to become the articular cartilage of the neighboring joint. With continued maturation of both the epiphysis and diaphysis, the growth plate is thinned still further (Figs. 1–2 and 1–3). Gradually, cellular activity within the plate diminishes and a layer of bone is applied to its diaphyseal surface. In this fashion, the growth plate disappears, allowing fusion of epiphyseal and diaphyseal ossification centers, followed by cessation of endochondral bone formation deep to the articular cartilage of the epiphysis, with formation of a subchondral bone plate. Although the growth plate has now ceased to function, a band of horizontally oriented trabeculae may persist, marking the previous location of the plate as a transverse radiopaque fusion line.

Abnormalities of endochondral ossification in the physis are well recognized in a number of disorders and are fundamental to the diagnosis of rickets (Fig. 1–4). Transient aberrations of such ossification lead to the development of growth recovery lines.

Developing Joint

An articulation eventually appears in the mesenchyme that is located between the developing ends of the bones. In this interzone, mesenchyme is not converted to cartilage or bone but rather undergoes change that is influenced by the type of articulation destined to be formed. In a fibrous joint, the interzonal mesenchyme is modified to form the fibrous tissue that will connect the adjacent bones; in a synchondrosis it is converted into hyaline cartilage; and in a symphysis it is changed into fibrocartilage. At the site of a synovial joint, the central portion of the mesenchyme becomes loose-meshed and is continuous in its periphery with adjacent mesenchyme that is undergoing vascularization (Figs. 1–5 and 1–6). The synovial mesenchyme that is created will later form the synovial membrane as well as some additional intraarticular structures, whereas the central aspect of the mesenchyme undergoes liquefaction and cavitation, creating the joint space. Condensation of the peripheral mesenchyme leads to joint capsule formation.

Modeling and Remodeling of Bone

Spongy, or woven-fibered bone, gradually becomes converted in the fetus into nonlamellated, parallel-fibered bone termed primary osteons and, subsequently, into typical haversian systems or secondary osteons composed of lamellae of parallel-fibered bone. This transformation continues thereafter throughout life. Although lamellar bone is dominant in the adult, woven bone is prominent in some sites (e.g., lining the tooth sockets) and in some situations (e.g., the repair of

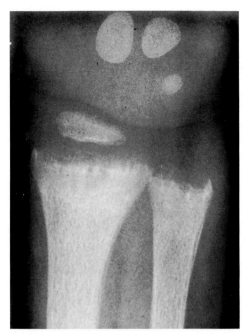

Figure 1–4. Abnormalities of endochondral ossification in the growth plate in rickets. Widening of the physis and irregularity and enlargement of the metaphysis are among the manifestations of this disease.

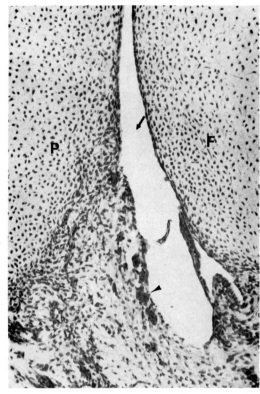

Figure 1–6. Development of the synovial membrane. In the knee joint, a space between the femur (F) and patella (P) can be identified (arrow), which is lined by a synovial membrane. The synovial membrane consists of flat synovial cells and well-formed vascular channels (arrowhead). (215 ×.)

fractures). At any age, bone is constantly undergoing change. Major adjustments in the size and shape of bone, which are prominent in the immature skeleton of the infant, child, and adolescent, are known as modeling; less obvious alterations in the quality of bone are termed remodeling.

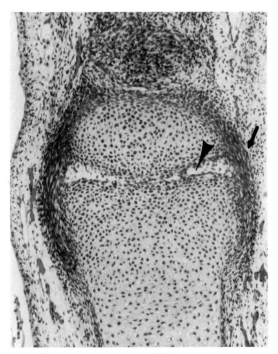

Figure 1–5. Development of a synovial joint. Cavitation (arrowhead) within the interzone between the phalanges of a finger has created the primitive joint cavity. (140 ×.) Condensation at the periphery of the joint (arrow) will lead to capsule formation.

MODELING. Modeling occurs continually throughout the growth period at varying rates and involves all bone surfaces. Classic examples of this process are (1) drifting of the midshaft of a tubular bone; (2) flaring of the ends of a tubular bone; (3) enlargement of the cranial vault and modification of cranial curvature.

The ability of bone to shift or drift eccentrically in a lateral or medial direction to fulfill changing mechanical demands is a prerequisite to the normal development of tubular bones, ribs, and other osseous structures. It is accomplished by both resorption, which dominates in one aspect of a bone, and apposition, which dominates in another. In the long tubular bones of the extremity, resorption is more evident on that side of the bone surface that is nearer the body core and apposition occurs on the opposite surface, accounting for a lateral drift of the entire bone.

The flaring that is normally evident in the end of a long tubular bone is a second example of bone modeling. As the bone grows in length, the wide metaphyseal region is later occupied by a narrow diaphysis, a change that requires close coordination of bone resorption and apposition. Reduction of the metaphysis is accomplished by osteoclastic resorption along its periosteal surface that is coupled with osteoblastic bone formation in the endosteal surface of the metaphyseal cortex. Subsequently, the marrow cavity is enlarged owing to the processes of osteoclastic resorption of trabecular bone and endosteal bone resorption, and the overall diameter of the shaft is increased as a result of periosteal bone formation. A variety of factors may upset this delicate balance of bone

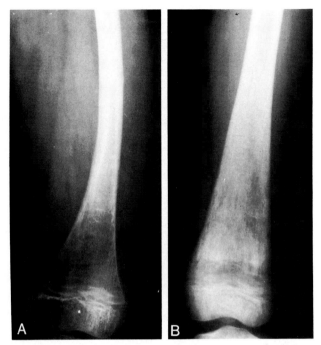

Figure 1–7. Modeling of bone: Abnormalities of tubulation. A Overtubulation. In this child with osteogenesis imperfecta, note the relatively narrow diaphysis compared with the wide appearance of the metaphysis and epiphysis. **B** Undertubulation. In this child with Gaucher's disease, the metaphysis is abnormally wide.

resorption and bone formation. Overtubulation, presumably related to a failure of periosteal deposition of bone, is encountered in osteogenesis imperfecta (Fig. 1–7A), and undertubulation is seen in various bone dysplasias and in certain anemias and storage diseases (Fig. 1–7B).

Some of the constituents of the cranial vault, such as the parietal bone, normally increase in thickness and surface area but also decrease in curvature during growth, becoming less convex. The change in convexity requires periosteal resorption along the internal circumference of the bone and periosteal apposition externally, and it is accompanied by growth at the adjacent sutures.

REMODELING. To maintain biomechanically and metabolically competent tissue, the transformation of woven-type bone to more compact lamellar bone is required. This process of remodeling normally is most prominent in the young but continues at reduced rates throughout life; at any age, when a variety of diseases are present, metabolic stimuli may lead to accentuation of bone remodeling. Remodeling of bone requires the coordinated activity of a group of highly specialized cells, each with a finite life span. These cells plus the altered bone are termed a bone remodeling or basic multicellular unit. The general sequence includes, initially, the activation of progenitor (hematopoietic stem) cells that proliferate into osteoclasts and, later, osteoclastic excavation of a volume of old bone, disappearance of the osteoclasts, smoothing of the resorption space with the production of a reversal zone and the laying down of a cement line, and the appearance of osteoblasts, which produce new bone.

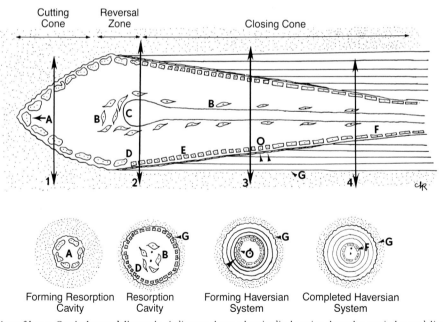

Figure 1–8. Remodeling of bone: Cortical remodeling unit. A diagram shows a longitudinal section through a cortical remodeling unit with corresponding transverse sections below (1–4). A, Multinucleated osteoclasts in Howship's lacunae advancing longitudinally from right to left and radially to enlarge a resorption cavity; B, Perivascular spindle-shaped precursor cells; C, capillary loops; D, mononuclear cells lining reversal zones; E, osteoblasts depositing new bone centripetally; F, flattened cells lining the haversian canal of a complete haversian system.
Transverse sections at different stages of development: 1, Resorption cavities lined with osteoclasts; 2, completed resorption cavities lined by mononuclear cells, the reversal zone; 3, forming haversian system or osteons lined with osteoblasts that had recently formed three lamellae; 4, completed haversian system with flattened bone cells lining canal. G, Cement line; osteoid (arrowheads) is present between osteoblast (O) and mineralized bone.
(Redrawn after Parfitt AM: The action of parathyroid hormone on bone. Relation of bone remodeling and turnover, calcium homeostasis and metabolic bone disease. I. Metabolism 25:809–844, 1976. By permission of author and Grune and Stratton, Inc., Publisher.)

Table 1–1. ADULT BONE SURFACES

Surface	Surface Area ($\times 10^6$ sq mm)
Cortical surfaces	
Periosteal	0.5
Haversian (osteonal)	3.5
Endosteal	0.5
Trabecular surfaces	
Endosteal	7.0
Total surfaces	11.5

Reprinted by permission of the publisher from Jee WSS: The skeletal tissues, *in* L Weiss, L Lansing (Eds): Histology: Cell and Tissue Biology. 5th Ed, p 221. Copyright 1983 by Elsevier Science Publishing Co, Inc. Used with permission.

In the endosteal and periosteal surfaces of the cortex, osteoclastic resorption leads to a tube-shaped tunnel, the resorption canal. The osteoclasts create longitudinally oriented canals, liberate the osteocytes from their lacunae, and displace the vascular channels. When these events are followed by osteoblastic apposition, cylinders of bone are formed about linear vascular channels, representing the basic component of a haversian system or osteon (Fig. 1–8). The primary osteons are later replaced by secondary or tertiary osteons until the creation of the mature haversian system is completed. In trabecular bone, similar events take place on the osseous surfaces rather than within the interior of the bone, as occurs in the cortex.

The processes of resorption and formation predominate on the four types of bone surfaces. Three surfaces are present in the cortical bone: periosteal (outer region of the cortex), haversian or osteonal (within the cortex, along the haversian and Volkmann canals), and endosteal (inner region of the cortex). One surface exists in the trabecular bone, the endosteal surface (at the interface of the marrow and the plates and arches of trabecular bone). At any specific time, these surfaces may be quiescent (free of osteoblasts and osteoclasts), forming bone (containing osteoid and a covering of osteoblasts), or resorbing bone (containing osteoclasts and scalloped cavities

known as Howship's lacunae). The metabolic activity of any particular osseous site depends directly on the surface area of that portion of the bone. Although trabecular bone represents only 20 to 25 per cent of the total skeletal volume, it contributes more than 60 per cent of the total surface area; alternatively, cortical bone is characterized by a relatively small amount of surface area (Table 1–1). Routine radiography is far more sensitive in detecting changes in cortical bone than in trabecular bone. It is this inefficiency that has led to the development of supplementary techniques, such as computed tomography, that can be used in evaluating alterations in the more metabolically active trabecular bone (see Chapter 18).

ANATOMY
General Structure of Bone

The prime ingredients of the mature bone are an outer shell of compact bone (the cortex), which encloses a more loosely appearing meshwork of trabeculae (the cancellous or spongy bone) with its interconnecting spaces containing myeloid or fatty marrow, or both. The cortical bone is clothed by a periosteal membrane, which contains arterioles and capillaries that enter the medullary canal and provide the blood supply to the bone. At sites of attachment to bone, the fibers of tendons and ligaments blend with the periosteum (entheses) (Fig. 1–9). The periosteal membrane is thicker and loosely attached in the infant and child and thinner and more firmly adherent in the adult. These structural characteristics are responsible for the augmented ability of the infant's and child's periosteum to be lifted from the parent bone and to be stimulated to form osseous tissue.

In the cortex (Fig. 1–10) are cylindrical units, called haversian systems or osteons, which consist of a central haversian canal containing neurovascular components, which is surrounded by concentric lamellae of osseous tissue. The haversian canals run in a longitudinal direction, with normal branches connecting each system to neighboring haversian canals. About each haversian canal and contained within the individual lamellae are the osteocytes, each in its own lacuna, which are connected to other osteocytes and to the central canal by radiating canaliculi. Within a single lamella, collagen fiber bundles and hydroxyapatite crystals are oriented in a

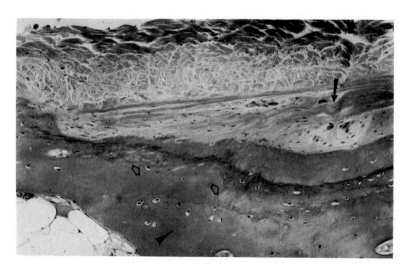

Figure 1–9. Sites of ligament attachment to bone (entheses). The ligament (solid arrow) and the bone (arrowhead) can be identified. Note that the fibers of the ligament are incorporated into the osseous tissue (open arrows). (210 ×.)

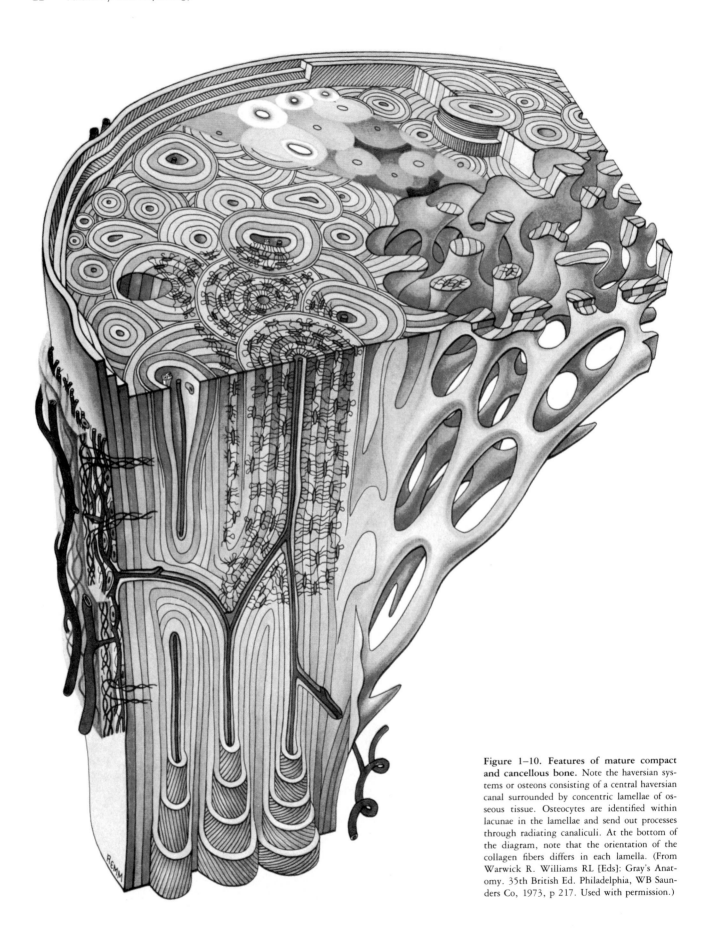

Figure 1–10. Features of mature compact and cancellous bone. Note the haversian systems or osteons consisting of a central haversian canal surrounded by concentric lamellae of osseous tissue. Osteocytes are identified within lacunae in the lamellae and send out processes through radiating canaliculi. At the bottom of the diagram, note that the orientation of the collagen fibers differs in each lamella. (From Warwick R. Williams RL [Eds]: Gray's Anatomy. 35th British Ed. Philadelphia, WB Saunders Co, 1973, p 217. Used with permission.)

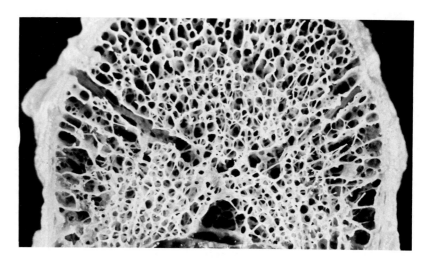

Figure 1–11. Features of mature spongy bone. A transverse section of the midportion of a macerated vertebral body reveals the delicate, honeycomb appearance of the trabeculae. Note a surrounding, thin rim of compact bone and normal vascular channels.

specific and complex fashion, with differing orientation from these substances in adjacent lamellae.

The spongiosa bone differs in structure from the cortical bone. A honeycomb distribution of individual trabeculae can be identified, which divides the marrow space into communicating compartments (Fig. 1–11). The trabeculae often appear most numerous and prominent in areas of normal stress. The major difference, then, between spongy and cortical bone is in the porosity of the osseous tissue.

Cellular Constituents of Bone

Five types of bone cells are found in skeletal tissue: osteoprogenitor cells, osteoblasts, osteocytes, osteoclasts, and bone lining cells.

OSTEOPROGENITOR CELLS. Undifferentiated stromal cells have the capacity to proliferate by mitotic division and develop into osteoblasts, or bone-forming cells. Until recently, it was generally believed that such cells were also able to differentiate into osteoclasts by an identical or similar pathway; it is now known that osteoclasts are derived from a different source, cells of the hematopoietic system.

OSTEOBLASTS. Osteoblasts are derived from cells that are probably components of the stromal system of bone and marrow (Fig. 1–12). The activity of the precursor cells increases when new bone is required, as during the healing of a fracture. Although numerous and large in the developing skeleton, osteoblasts decrease in number and size as the skeleton reaches maturity. A dormant osteoblast, however, is capable of responding to the stimulus produced by a pathologic process. Osteoblasts are fundamental to the process of collagen and mucopolysaccharide production in bone. Their life span as osteoblasts may cease somewhat abruptly with their incorporation into the osseous tissue in the form of a new cell, the osteocyte.

OSTEOCYTES. The osteocytes arise from preosteoblasts and osteoblasts. Initially present at the surface of the bone, the osteoblasts subsequently become entrapped within the osseous tissue as osteocytes (Fig. 1–12). Here, each osteocyte lies in a lacuna and sends out branches through interconnected canaliculi. The osteocyte is concerned with proper maintenance of the bone matrix, a process that is facilitated by the transport of material and fluid via the canaliculi. The osteocyte has the ability to synthesize bone matrix, although this ability is less pronounced than that of the osteoblast. It has been proposed (but not universally accepted) that the osteocyte may also be involved in bone resorption, a process called osteocytic osteolysis.

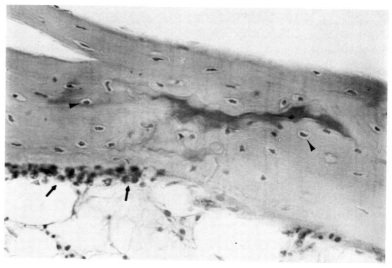

Figure 1–12. Cellular constituents of bone: Osteoblasts and osteocytes. The osteoblasts (arrows) can be identified along the surface of the trabeculae, whereas the osteocytes (arrowheads) are found within the osseous tissue, enclosed in lacunae. An occasional osteoclast is identified. (210×.)

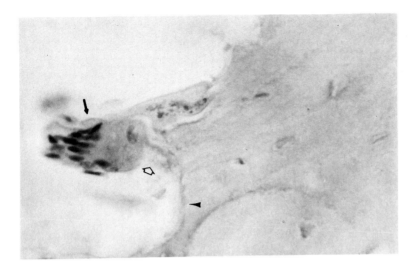

Figure 1–13. Cellular constituents of bone: Osteoclasts. Observe the osteoclast (solid arrow) containing multiple nuclei located within a Howship's lacuna (arrowhead.) A brush-like cellular border is perceptible (open arrow). (840×.)

OSTEOCLASTS. The osteoclast is a multinucleated cell with a short life span that is intimately related to the process of bone resorption (Fig. 1–13). Whereas the osteoblasts are derived from cellular components of the stromal system of bone and marrow (stromal stem cell), the osteoclasts appear to be a product of one of the cell lines of the hematopoietic system, being derived from a hematopoietic stem cell (monocyte-phagocyte line).

Osteoclasts actively engage in bone resorption. The exact manner in which bone resorption takes place about the osteoclast is not entirely known. Bone resorption is associated with the appearance of resorption pits or Howship's lacunae. The osteoclasts within the lacunae often reveal a finely striated brush or ruffled border where they are in contact with the bone. When the erosive process is terminated, the ruffled border is no longer seen, and osteoclasts become less numerous and may even disappear entirely.

Bone-regulating hormones have a dramatic effect on the appearance and function of osteoclasts. Administration of exogenous parathyroid hormone leads to rapid development of ruffled borders, whereas that of calcitonin causes an equally rapid disappearance of these borders. Furthermore, 1,25-dihydroxyvitamin D increases the differentiation of precursor cells into osteoclasts, thereby increasing the number of osteoclasts as well as their activity. As multinucleated osteoclasts originate from the fusion of cells of the mononuclear phagocytic system, it is of considerable interest that blood monocytes can also resorb bone either directly or indirectly through the elaboration of potent bone-resorbing factors, such as prostaglandins and interleukin-1.

BONE LINING CELLS. The precise nature and function of the commonly identified flat and elongated cells with spindle-shaped nuclei that line the surface of the bone are not clear, although they are generally believed to be derived from osteoblasts that have become inactive.

Noncellular Constituents of Bone

The major cellular components account for a very small fraction of the total weight of bone. The other constituents of bone include the remaining organic matrix (collagen and mucopolysaccharides), accounting for approximately 35 per cent of osseous tissue by weight, and the inorganic material, accounting for approximately 65 per cent of osseous tissue by weight.

ORGANIC MATRIX. The organic matrix of bone is composed primarily of protein, glycoprotein, and polysaccharide. Collagen is the major constituent (90 per cent); the collagen is embedded in a gelatinous mucopolysaccharide material (ground substance). Although the mucopolysaccharides represent a minor quantitative part of the structure of osseous tissue, they appear to be very important in the process of bone matrix maturation and mineralization. In the collagen fibers, a characteristic pattern of overlap of adjacent molecules creates a pore or hole zone between the end of one molecule and the beginning of the next; these holes are the sites of earliest deposits of the calcium hydroxyapatite crystals of bone.

INORGANIC MINERAL. The inorganic mineral of bone exists in a crystalline form that resembles calcium hydroxyapatite—$Ca_{10}(PO_4)_6OH_2$—which is distributed regularly along the length of the collagen fibers, surrounded by ground substance. The bone crystals are impure; there also are substantial quantities of carbonate, citrate, sodium, and magnesium in bone mineral.

PHYSIOLOGY
Mineralization of Bone

At present no unified concept of the mechanism of bone mineralization exists. The initial nucleation or deposition of inorganic calcium and phosphate occurs at regular intervals along the longitudinal axis of the collagen fibril. As already stated, it appears likely that these crystals gain access to the substance of the fibril by normal gaps resulting from overlap of linear polymers of collagen. The axes of the deposited crystals are parallel to the axis of the collagen fibril itself. After nucleation has been initiated, further precipitation of calcium and phosphate ions leads to growth of the crystal, which eventually assumes a chemical structure similar to that of calcium hydroxyapatite. The composition of the mineral that is deposited initially, however, is not clear. Certain cellular products, including enzymes such as alkaline phosphatases and inorganic pyrophosphatases, may regulate the process of calcification.

Calcium Homeostasis

The skeleton, containing 99 per cent of the body's calcium, serves as an essential reservoir in the maintenance of stable plasma levels of calcium. The concentration of calcium in the plasma normally is approximately 10 mg/dl. Approximately 70 per cent of the plasma calcium is thought to be maintained by a continuous exchange of calcium ions between bone tissue and extracellular fluid; this interchange occurs between the calcium hydroxyapatite crystals of all bone surfaces and proceeds independently of any change in bone volume (i.e., formation and resorption). Hypocalcemia stimulates a release of calcium ions from the bone mineral into the extracellular fluid and, conversely, hypercalcemia promotes an inward flux of calcium ions from the extracellular fluid to the bone mineral. The remaining 30 per cent of plasma calcium may be mediated by the actions of parathyroid and other hormones.

Important in the transfer of calcium ions between the bone and the plasma fluid compartments is the bone fluid compartment that is intimate with available osseous surfaces, being located between the osteoblasts or bone lining cells, or both, and the endosteal bone surface; and between the osteocytes and their lacunar and canalicular walls. The bone fluid compartment is surrounded by a perivascular fluid compartment that itself surrounds the vascular tissue within the haversian canals, Volkmann canals, bone marrow and other vascular spaces. The transfer of calcium ions between the immediate environment of the tissue and the plasma apparently is accomplished by events transpiring in the bone fluid and the perivascular fluid compartments. Parathyroid hormone represents a key ingredient in the mobilization of calcium from bone and its transfer to the plasma. As there is little evidence to suggest that osteoclasts possess receptors for parathyroid hormone or that osteoclasts respond directly to this hormone, it has been suggested that bone resorption is mediated by the action of parathyroid hormone on osteoblasts. Parathyroid hormone (as well as prostaglandins) induces a change in shape of the osteoblasts that uncovers the bone matrix, exposing it to osteoclast projections.

Bone Resorption and Formation

The processes of resorption and formation occur continuously in normal bone. They are prominent in the immature skeleton; in the mature skeleton these processes are less evident but nonetheless essential for the maintenance of biomechanically competent tissue and calcium homeostasis. Resorption and apposition dominate on the bone surfaces that are present in the cortex (periosteal, haversian or osteonal, and endosteal surfaces) and the spongiosa (endosteal surfaces) (Fig. 1–14).

It is the *coupling* of bone resorption to bone formation that controls the volume of bone present at any particular time. An increase in bone resorption must subsequently be coupled to an increase in bone formation if bone volume is to remain unchanged.

BONE RESORPTION. Although the osteoclast is the principal cell involved in the degradation of the organic bone matrix and the release of bone mineral, a potential (albeit controversial) role for the osteocyte in removing at least a small amount of perilacunar bone has also been suggested. Accumulating evidence has indicated that mononuclear phagocytes, including peripheral blood monocytes and tissue macrophages, are also involved in bone resorption. Mast cells, a virtual storehouse of many potent chemical mediators (prostaglandin and heparin), likewise exert an influence on bone resorption.

Surfaces of bone involved in extensive resorption are sites of accumulation of multinucleated osteoclasts, which reside

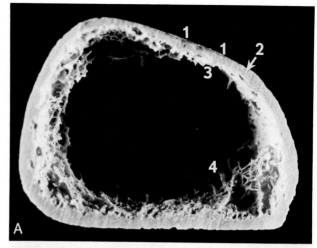

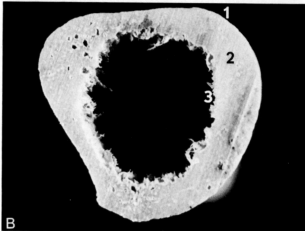

Figure 1–14. Bone resorption and formation: Available bone surfaces. Transverse sections of the metaphysis (**A**) and diaphysis (**B**) of a tubular bone reveal the osseous surfaces that are involved in the processes of resorption and apposition. In the cortex, these are the periosteal (1), haversian or osteonal (2), and endosteal (3) surfaces; in the spongiosa, an endosteal (4) surface is present.

in Howship's lacunae or pits. Among the substances capable of directly or indirectly stimulating existing osteoclasts or increasing the formation of new osteoclasts, or both, are parathyroid hormone, active metabolites of vitamin D, prostaglandin E_2, thyroid hormone, heparin, and interleukin-1; among those substances inhibiting resorption are calcitonin, glucocorticoid, diphosphonates, glucagon, phosphate, and carbonic anhydrase inhibitors.

BONE FORMATION. The principal cell involved in the formation of bone is the osteoblast. The process occurs in two phases, matrix formation and mineralization. Matrix formation precedes mineralization and occurs at the interface between osteoblasts and existing osteoid; mineralization occurs at the junction of osteoid and newly mineralized bone, a region that is designated the mineralization front. The layer of unmineralized matrix, termed the osteoid seam, is approximately 8 to 10 μm wide in adults owing to the usual interval of 10 days between matrix production and mineralization. In certain disease states, such as osteomalacia (Fig. 1–15), the thickness of the osteoid seam is increased.

The major regulators of bone formation can be divided into five groups: (1) calcium-regulating hormones (parathyroid

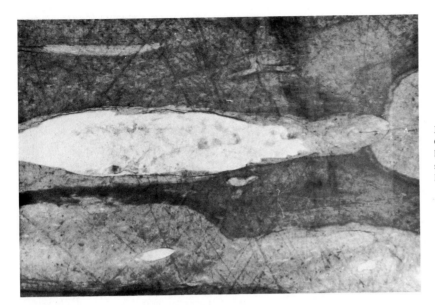

Figure 1–15. Increased thickness of osteoid seams: Osteomalacia. A photomicrograph of undecalcified bone that has been stained for calcium shows a thick, superficial layer of unstained osteoid and adjacent, heavily stained bone. (50×.)

Table 1–2. FACTORS THAT MAY REGULATE BONE GROWTH*

Agent	Effect on Bone Formation	
	Direct	Indirect
Calcium regulatory hormones		
Parathyroid hormone	↓	↑
1,25-Dihydroxyvitamin D	↓	↑
Calcitonin	—	? ↑
Systemic hormones		
Glucocorticoids	↑ ↓ †	↓
Insulin	↑	↑
Thyroxine	?	↑
Sex hormones	—	↑
Growth hormone	—	↑
Growth factors		
Somatomedin (insulin-like growth factor)	↑	↑
Epidermal growth factor	↓	?
Fibroblast growth factor	↓	?
Platelet-derived growth factor	↑	?
Local factors		
Prostaglandin E$_2$	↑ ↓ †	↑
Osteoclast activating factor	↓	?
Bone-derived growth factor(s)	↑	?
Ions		
Calcium	↑	↑
Phosphate	↑	↑

*Agents that have been tested for their direct effects in vitro are listed as increasing (↑), decreasing (↓), or not changing (—) bone formation. When there is evidence for an important indirect effect, mediated through another factor, the dominant direction is indicated.

†Biphasic or dual response, depending on dose or direction of treatment.

Reprinted with permission from Raisz LG, Kream BE: Regulation of bone formation. N Engl J Med 309:29, 1983.

hormone, 1,25-dihydroxyvitamin D, and calcitonin); (2) additional hormones (glucocorticoids, insulin, thyroxine, sex hormones, and growth hormone); (3) growth factors (somatomedin, epidermal growth factor, fibroblast growth factor, platelet-derived growth factor); (4) local factors (prostaglandin E$_2$, interleukins, and bone-derived growth factors); and (5) ions (calcium and phosphate) (Table 1–2).

Humoral Regulation of Bone Metabolism

Bone metabolism and calcium homeostasis are intimately related to the interactions among the skeleton, intestines, and kidneys and to the presence of many chemical factors, of which three hormones—parathyroid hormone, calcitonin, and 1,25-dihydroxyvitamin D—are most important.

PARATHYROID HORMONE. The two main functions of parathyroid hormone are to stimulate and control the rate of bone remodeling and to influence mechanisms governing the control of the plasma level of calcium. This hormone, which is produced by the chief cells of the four parathyroid glands, consists of a single chain polypeptide of 84 amino acids; after secretion into the circulation, the hormone is metabolized to smaller, inactive polypeptide fragments. The synthesis and secretion of parathyroid hormone are closely regulated by the level of ionized calcium in the extracellular fluid, with elevated levels of serum calcium suppressing parathyroid hormone secretion and depressed levels increasing such secretion.

Parathyroid hormone has a direct effect on the bone (enhancing the mobilization of calcium from the skeleton) and on the kidney (stimulating the absorption of calcium from the glomerular fluid) and an indirect effect on the intestines (influencing the rate of calcium absorption). These actions in concert serve to increase the level of calcium in the extracellular fluid.

Osseous Effects. Parathyroid hormone acts directly on bone (Fig. 1–16), and the result of this action may be bone resorption or formation, or both. An immediate action of

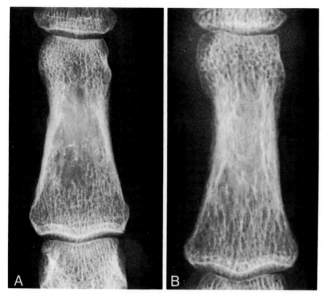

Figure 1–16. Osseous effects of parathyroid hormone: Hyperparathyroidism. Magnification radiographs of the phalanges in a normal person (**A**) and an individual with hyperparathyroidism (**B**) reveal the effects of parathyroid hormone on bone. In **B**, note osteopenia, indistinct trabeculae, and prominent subperiosteal bone resorption.

parathyroid hormone involves the processes of osteoclastic and osteocytic resorption that are fundamental to calcium homeostasis; more prolonged effects of parathyroid hormone influence bone remodeling and are mediated principally by the action of osteoclasts. Thus, at the cellular level, parathyroid hormone influences osteoclasts, osteoblasts, osteocytes, and bone surface cells. Parathyroid hormone, at least indirectly, activates existing osteoclasts or increases the recruitment of new osteoclasts. Morphologic changes in the osteoclasts suggesting increased activity of the cells are also noted. It is also clear that osteoblasts contain receptors for parathyroid hormone and are influenced directly by circulating levels of this hormone. Osteoblast function is decreased initially, leading to a suppression of bone formation. Subsequently, however, stimulation of osteoblasts results in an increase in bone formation.

These known effects of parathyroid hormone reflect the importance of this hormone in maintaining calcium homeostasis. A fall in the serum level of calcium leads to a release of parathyroid hormone and a relatively rapid activation of osteocytes and osteoclasts. These cells promote bone resorption with the mobilization of calcium from the skeleton. As the initial effect of parathyroid hormone on the osteoblast appears to be inhibitory, the mobilized calcium is made available for cellular metabolism. Later, owing to additional effects of parathyroid hormone that occur in the kidney and indirectly in the intestines, supplementary sources of calcium become available to the body, lessening the need for that derived from the skeleton. Stimulation of osteoblasts at this time results in the incorporation of calcium into the skeleton, manifested as an increase in bone synthesis.

Intestinal Effects. An increase in intestinal absorption of calcium that accompanies hyperparathyroidism represents an indirect effect of this hormone that is mediated through regulation of synthesis of 1,25-dihydroxycholecalciferol, a vitamin D metabolite, in the kidney (see Chapter 48).

Renal Effects. The renal excretion of calcium, phosphate, bicarbonate, and other ions is regulated directly by parathyroid hormone. Although calcium reabsorption predominates in the proximal tubules of the kidney, the effect of parathyroid hormone in enhancing reabsorption of calcium from the glomerular fluid appears to occur more distally in the tubules. The inhibition of phosphate resorption in the kidney, the phosphaturic effect, by parathyroid hormone occurs principally in the proximal tubules. Additional renal effects of this hormone include inhibition of bicarbonate reabsorption with alkalinization of the urine and stimulation of the activity of 1-α-hydroxylase enzyme, leading to an increase in the production of 1,25-dihydroxycholecalciferol, the active metabolite of vitamin D.

CALCITONIN. Calcitonin is a peptide consisting of 32 amino acids that is secreted by the parafollicular or C cells of the human thyroid gland. The secretion of calcitonin is controlled by the circulating levels of calcium; as the serum level of calcium rises, calcitonin is released from the thyroid gland with an elevation in its plasma concentration and a fall in the content of calcitonin in the gland itself, owing to depletion of secretory granules from the parafollicular cells. After the release of calcitonin from the thyroid gland, clearance appears to occur in the kidney and, to a lesser extent, in other tissues, including the liver, bones, and thyroid gland.

Calcitonin inhibits bone resorption and may lead to significant hypocalcemia and hypophosphatemia. The importance of calcitonin as a regulator of calcium metabolism in humans, however, is not clear at present. At the cellular level, calcitonin has no direct effect on osteoblasts but rather appears to reduce bone resorption by inactivation of osteoclasts and, perhaps, by decreasing their number. Calcitonin also interferes with the transfer of calcium from bone to extracellular fluid, and its overall effect in producing a decrease in bone resorption is reflected in a reduction in the urinary excretion of hydroxyproline.

VITAMIN D. Vitamin D represents one of the most potent humoral factors involved in the regulation of bone metabolism. Its biochemistry and mechanisms of action are described in detail in Chapter 48.

OTHER HUMORAL FACTORS

Glucocorticoids. Glucocorticoids cause a decrease in intestinal absorption of calcium and phosphate and an increase in their renal excretion, which probably are unrelated to interference in the pathways of vitamin D biosynthesis. As glucocorticoids also inhibit the formation of new bone matrix, wide osteoid seams (osteomalacia) are not apparent. The interactions of glucocorticoids and various calcium-regulating hormones, such as 1,25-dihydroxyvitamin D, calcitonin, and parathyroid hormone, are not clear. Similarly, the direct stimulation of bone resorption by glucocorticoids has not been proved.

Insulin. Although osteopenia with a decrease in bone mass is a recognized manifestation of diabetes mellitus, it is not certain if insulin is directly responsible for this finding, as abnormal levels of calcium-regulating hormones may also be evident in this disease.

Thyroid Hormones. The known association of hyperthyroidism with osteopenia (see Chapter 51) has led to considerable interest in the effects of thyroid hormones on skeletal metabolism. Direct effects of these hormones include stimulation of growth in cartilage and of osteoclastic activity. As thyroid hormones are linked physiologically to other humoral substances such as somatomedin, which is secreted by the liver, it is difficult to define precisely the primary or secondary nature of the skeletal effects of these hormones in patients with hyperthyroidism.

Sex Hormones. The current interest in estrogen as a therapeutic agent in postmenopausal osteoporosis is based primarily on the belief that estrogens, apparently indirectly, inhibit bone resorption, perhaps by increasing the absorption of calcium from the intestines, the synthesis of serum $1,25(OH)_2D$, the secretion of calcitonin, or various combinations of the three. Estrogens, however, appear to have no direct effect on bone.

Growth Hormone. Growth hormone increases bone turnover, the intestinal absorption of calcium, and vitamin D-dependent intestinal calcium-binding protein; the skeletal effects of growth hormone are probably mediated by somatomedins.

Other Agents. Some of the additional humoral factors that affect the skeleton are indicated in Table 1–2.

FURTHER READING

Bonucci E: New knowledge on the origin, function and fate of osteoclasts. Clin Orthop *158:*252, 1981.

Coccia PF: Cells that resorb bone. N Engl J Med *310:*456, 1984.

Jaffe HL: Metabolic, Degenerative, and Inflammatory Diseases of Bones and Joints. Philadelphia, Lea & Febiger, 1972, p. 1.

Jee WSS: The skeletal tissues. *In* L Weiss, L Lansing (Eds): Histology: Cell and Tissue Biology. 5th Ed. New York, Elsevier Biomedical, 1983.

Ledesma-Medina J, Newman B, Oh KS: Disturbances of bone growth and development. Radiol Clin North Am 26:441, 1988.

McKenna MJ, Frame B: The mast cell and bone. Clin Orthop *200:*226, 1985.

Posner AS: The mineral of bone. Clin Orthop *200:*87, 1985.

Raisz LG, Kream BE: Regulation of bone formation. N Engl J Med *309:*29, 1983.

Chapter 2

Articular Anatomy and Histology

Donald Resnick, M.D.
Gen Niwayama, M.D.

An understanding of the structure of joints is essential to proper interpretation of radiographs in numerous diseases. Joints may be classified into three types: fibrous, cartilaginous, and synovial. In addition, supporting structures (tendons, aponeuroses, fasciae, and ligaments) influence the manifestations of articular disorders.

The junctions at which skeletal structures are connected are termed joints or articulations. Joints have been classified according to (1) extent of joint motion, and (2) type of articular histology. On the basis of joint motion, three types of articulations are described:

Synarthroses: Fixed or rigid articulations.

Amphiarthroses: Slightly movable articulations.

Diarthroses: Freely movable articulations.

Any classification based solely upon the extent of joint motion, unfortunately, will group together articulations whose histologic components are very dissimilar.

The classification of joints according to histologic type (Table 2–1) reveals the following categories:

Fibrous articulations: Apposed bone surfaces are fastened together by fibrous connective tissue.

Cartilaginous articulations: Apposed bone surfaces are initially or eventually connected by cartilaginous tissue.

Table 2–1. TYPES OF ARTICULATIONS

Fibrous	
Suture	Skull
Syndesmosis	Distal tibiofibular interosseous membrane
	Radioulnar interosseous membrane
	Sacroiliac interosseous ligament
Gomphosis	Teeth
Cartilaginous	
Symphysis	Symphysis pubis
	Intervertebral disc
	Manubriosternal joint
	Central mandible
Synchondrosis	Physeal plate (growth plate)
	Neurocentral joint
	Sphenooccipital joint
Synovial	
	Large, small joints of extremities
	Sacroiliac joint
	Apophyseal joint
	Costovertebral joint
	Sternoclavicular joint

Synovial articulations: Apposed bone surfaces are separated by an articular cavity that is lined by synovial membrane.

This second method of classification, which is used in this book, also leads to difficulty because joints that are similar histologically may differ considerably in function and degree of allowable motion. Furthermore, some articulations contain admixtures of a variety of tissues, whereas in others, constituent tissues change as they develop.

FIBROUS JOINTS

Suture

Sutures, which are limited to the skull (Fig. 2–1), allow no active motion and exist where broad osseous surfaces are separated only by a zone of connective tissue. Although classically a suture is considered a fibrous articulation, areas of secondary cartilage formation may be observed during the growth period, and in later life sutures may undergo bone union or synostosis. Obliteration of the sutures by bone union varies somewhat in its time of onset and cranial distribution. This obliteration usually occurs at the bregma and subsequently extends into the sagittal, coronal, and lambdoid sutures, in that order. Although normal variations occur in suture development and closure, their assessment is important in the diagnosis of obstructive hydrocephalus as well as of cranial synostosis.

Syndesmosis

A syndesmosis (Fig. 2–2) is a fibrous joint in which adjacent bone surfaces are united by either an interosseous ligament, as in the distal tibiofibular joint, or an interosseous membrane, as at the diaphyses of radius and ulna and of tibia and fibula. An additional example of a syndesmosis is the interosseous ligament between the superior aspect of sacrum and ilium. A syndesmosis may demonstrate minor degrees of motion related to stretching of the interosseous ligament or flexibility of the interosseous membrane.

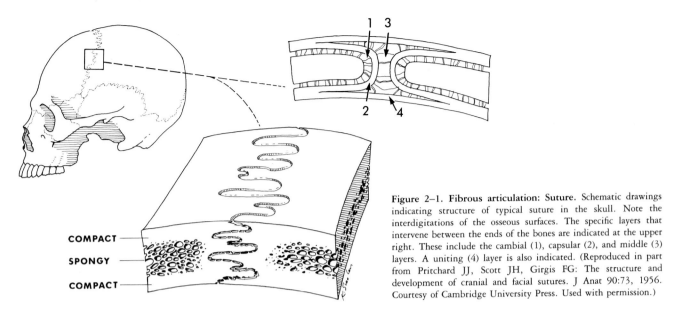

COMPACT

SPONGY

COMPACT

Figure 2–1. Fibrous articulation: Suture. Schematic drawings indicating structure of typical suture in the skull. Note the interdigitations of the osseous surfaces. The specific layers that intervene between the ends of the bones are indicated at the upper right. These include the cambial (1), capsular (2), and middle (3) layers. A uniting (4) layer is also indicated. (Reproduced in part from Pritchard JJ, Scott JH, Girgis FG: The structure and development of cranial and facial sutures. J Anat 90:73, 1956. Courtesy of Cambridge University Press. Used with permission.)

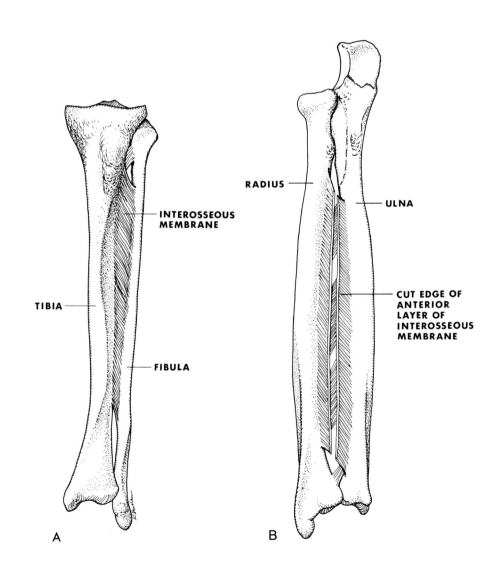

Figure 2–2. Fibrous articulation: Syndesmosis. A An interosseous membrane exists between the lateral border of the tibia and the medial border of the fibula. Note the orientation of its fibers. **B** The interosseous membrane between the medial aspect of the radius and the lateral aspect of the ulna originates approximately 3 cm below the radial tuberosity and extends to the wrist, containing apertures for various interosseous vessels.

INTEROSSEOUS MEMBRANE

TIBIA

FIBULA

RADIUS

ULNA

CUT EDGE OF ANTERIOR LAYER OF INTEROSSEOUS MEMBRANE

A

B

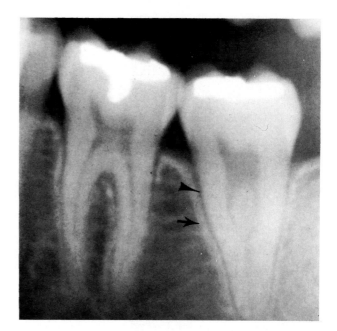

Figure 2–3. Fibrous articulation: Gomphosis. A radiograph reveals the radiolucent periodontal membrane (arrowhead) and the radiopaque lamina dura (arrow).

Gomphosis

A gomphosis, a special type of fibrous articulation (Fig. 2–3), is located between the teeth and maxilla or mandible. At these sites, the joint resembles a peg that fits into a fossa or socket. The intervening membrane between tooth and bone is termed the periodontal ligament. This ligament varies in width from 0.1 to 0.3 mm and decreases in thickness with advancing age.

CARTILAGINOUS JOINTS

There are two types of cartilaginous joints: symphysis and synchondrosis.

Symphysis

In symphyses (Fig. 2–4), adjacent bone surfaces are connected by a cartilaginous disc, which arises from chondrification of intervening mesenchymal tissue. This tissue is composed eventually of fibrocartilaginous or fibrous connective tissue, although a thin layer of hyaline cartilage usually persists, covering the articular surface of the adjacent bone. Symphyses, of which typical examples are the symphysis pubis and the intervertebral disc, allow a small amount of motion, which occurs through compression or deformation of the intervening connective tissue.

Some symphyses, such as the symphysis pubis and manubriosternal joint, reveal a small cleft-like central cavity, which may be demonstrable radiographically owing to the presence of gas (vacuum phenomenon). Symphyses are located within the midsagittal plane of the human body and are permanent structures, unlike synchondroses, which are temporary articulations. Rarely, intraarticular ankylosis or synostosis may obliterate a symphysis, such as occurs at the manubriosternal joint.

Synchondrosis

Synchondroses (Fig. 2–5) are temporary joints that exist during the growing phase of the skeleton and are composed of hyaline cartilage. Typical synchondroses are the cartilaginous growth plate between the epiphysis and metaphysis of a tubular bone, the neurocentral vertebral articulations, and the unossified cartilage in the chondrocranium, the sphenooccipital synchondrosis. With skeletal maturation, synchondroses become thinner and are eventually obliterated by bone union or synostosis.

Figure 2–4. Cartilaginous articulation: Symphysis (symphysis pubis). Note the central fibrocartilage (FC), with a thin layer of hyaline cartilage (HC) adjacent to the osseous surfaces of the pubis.

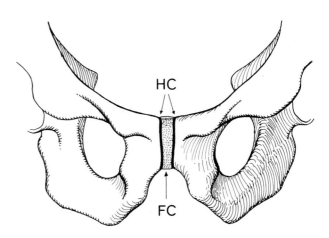

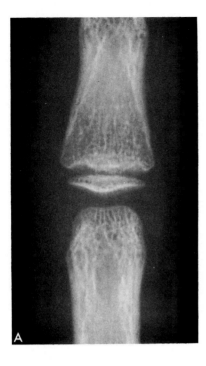

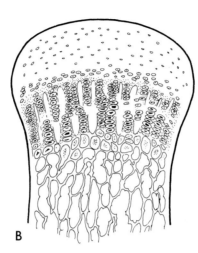

Figure 2–5. Cartilaginous articulation: Synchondrosis. A A radiograph of the phalanges in a growing child demonstrates a typical epiphysis separated from the metaphysis and diaphysis by the radiolucent growth plate. B A schematic drawing of a growth plate between the cartilaginous epiphysis and the ossified diaphysis of a long bone. Note the transition from hyaline cartilage through various cartilaginous zones, including resting cartilage, cell proliferation, cell hypertrophy, cell calcification, and bone formation.

SYNOVIAL JOINTS

A synovial articulation is a specialized type of joint that is located primarily in the appendicular skeleton (Fig. 2–6). The structure of a synovial joint differs fundamentally from that of fibrous and cartilaginous joints; osseous surfaces are bound together by a fibrous capsule, which may be reinforced by accessory ligaments. The inner portion of the articulating surface of the apposing bones is separated by a space, the articular or joint cavity. Articular cartilage covers the ends of both bones; motion between these cartilaginous surfaces is characterized by a low coefficient of friction. The inner aspect of the joint capsule is formed by the synovial membrane, which secretes synovial fluid into the articular cavity. This synovial fluid both lubricates the joint, facilitating motion,

and provides nourishment to the adjacent articular cartilage. In some synovial joints, an intraarticular disc of fibrocartilage partially or completely divides the joint cavity. Additional intraarticular structures, including fat pads and labra, may be noted.

Articular Cartilage

The articulating surfaces of the bone are covered by a layer of glistening connective tissue, the articular cartilage. Its unique properties include transmission and distribution of high loads; maintenance of contact stresses at acceptably low levels; allowing of movement with little friction; and shock absorption. In most synovial joints, the cartilage is hyaline in type; exceptions include the apophyseal joints of the spine,

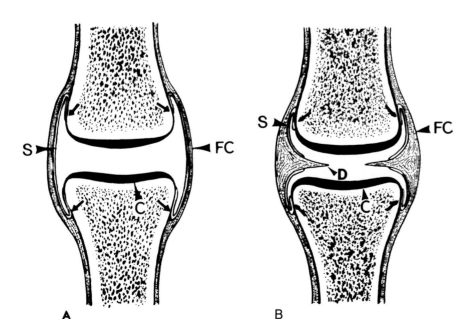

Figure 2–6. Synovial articulation: General features. A Typical synovial joint without an intraarticular disc. A diagram outlines important structures, including fibrous capsule (FC), synovial membrane (S), and articular cartilage (C). Note that there are marginal areas of the articulation where synovial membrane abuts on bone without protective cartilage (arrows). B Typical synovial joint containing an articular disc that partially divides the joint cavity. Diagram reveals fibrous capsule (FC), synovial membrane (S), articular cartilage (C), and articular disc (D). The marginal areas of the joint are again indicated by arrows.

the acromioclavicular and sternoclavicular joints, and the temporomandibular joint.

Articular cartilage is devoid of lymphatic vessels, blood vessels, and nerves. This cartilage largely derives its nutrition from diffusion of fluid from the synovial cavity. A second source of cartilage nourishment is from small blood vessels passing from the subchondral bone plate only into the deepest stratum of cartilage. Additionally, a vascular ring is located within the synovial membrane at the periphery of the cartilage.

Articular cartilage varies in thickness. The cartilage is thicker (1) in large joints than in small joints; (2) in joints or areas of joints in which there is considerable functional pressure or stress, such as those in the lower extremity; (3) at sites of extensive frictional or shearing force; (4) in poorly fitted articulations compared with smoothly fitted ones; and (5) in young and middle-aged individuals. Articular cartilage is thinner in older people, and nonuse of a joint may lead to cartilage thinning.

Subchondral Bone Plate and Tidemark

The subchondral endplate is a layer of osseous tissue of variable thickness located beneath the cartilage. Immediately superficial to the subchondral bone plate is the calcified zone of articular cartilage, termed the tidemark. The tidemark serves a mechanical function; it anchors the collagen fibers of the noncalcified portion of cartilage and is, in turn, anchored to the subchondral bone plate. These strong connections resist disruption by shearing force.

Articular Capsule

The articular capsule is connective tissue that envelops the joint cavity. It is composed of a thick, tough outer layer, the fibrous capsule, and a more delicate thin inner layer, the synovial membrane. At each end of the articulation, the fibrous capsule is firmly adherent to the periosteum of the articulating bones. The fibrous capsule is not of uniform thickness. Ligaments and tendons may attach to it, producing focal areas of increased thickness. Extracapsular accessory ligaments, such as those about the sternoclavicular joint, and intracapsular ligaments, such as the cruciate ligaments of the knee, may also be found. The fibrous capsule is richly supplied with blood and lymphatic vessels and nerves, which may penetrate the capsule and extend down to the synovial membrane.

The synovial membrane is a delicate, highly vascular inner membrane of the articular capsule (Fig. 2–7). It lines the nonarticular portion of the synovial joint and any intraarticular ligaments or tendons. The synovial membrane also covers the intracapsular osseous surfaces, which are clothed by periosteum or perichondrium but are without cartilaginous surfaces. These latter areas frequently occur at the peripheral portion of the articulation and are termed "marginal" or "bare" areas of the joint. Synovial tissue also lines bursae and tendon sheaths. The synovial membrane generally is pink, moist, and smooth, although small finger-like projections, synovial villi, may be apparent on its inner surface. Synovial membrane inflammation or irritation causes excessive villus formation and, in pathologic situations, villous projections may cover the entire inner surface of the synovial membrane.

The synovial membrane varies structurally in different segments of the articulation. In general, there are two synovial

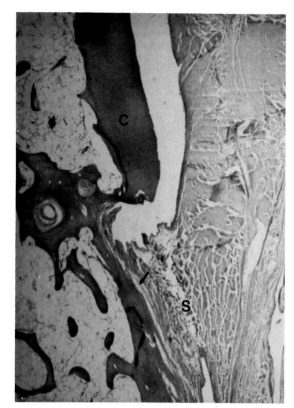

Figure 2–7. Synovial articulation: Synovial membrane. Low power (80 ×) photomicrograph of the chondro-osseous junction about a metacarpophalangeal joint delineates the synovial membrane (S) and articular cartilage (C). The marginal area of the joint at which synovial membrane abuts on bone is well demonstrated (arrow).

layers, a thin cellular surface layer (intima) and a deeper vascular underlying layer (subintima). The subintimal layer merges on its deep surface with the fibrous capsule. In certain locations, the synovial membrane is attenuated and fails to demonstrate two distinct layers. Sites at which the synovial membrane lines intraarticular ligaments or tendons, such as the cruciate ligaments and quadriceps, may not possess a distinct subintima, as the fibrous tissue merges imperceptibly with the adjacent capsule or tendon.

The synovial membrane has several functions. First, it is involved in the secretion of a sticky mucoid substance into the synovial fluid. Second, owing to its inherent flexibility, loose synovial folds, villi, and marginal recesses, the synovium facilitates and accommodates the changing shape of the articular cavity that is required for normal joint motion, an ability that is lost when adhesive capsulitis occurs. In addition, the synovial membrane aids the removal of substances from the articular cavity.

Intraarticular Disc (Meniscus), Labrum, and Fat Pad

A fibrocartilaginous disc or meniscus may be found in some joints, such as the knee, wrist, and temporomandibular, acromioclavicular, sternoclavicular, and costovertebral joints. The peripheral portion of the disc attaches to the fibrous capsule, and most of the articular disc is avascular.

The exact function of intraarticular discs is unknown. Suggested functions include shock absorption, distribution of weight over a large surface, facilitation of various motions (such as rotation) and limitation of others (such as translation), and protection of the articular surface. Intraarticular discs may also play an important role in the effective lubrication of a joint.

Some joints, such as the hip and glenohumeral articulations, contain circumferential cartilaginous folds termed labra. These lips of cartilage are usually triangular in cross section and are attached to the peripheral portion of an articular surface, acting to enlarge or deepen the joint cavity. They may also help increase contact and congruity of adjacent articular surfaces, particularly at the extremes of joint motion.

Fat pads represent additional structures that may be present within a joint. Fat pads may act as cushions, absorbing forces generated across a joint, thus protecting adjacent bone processes. They may also distribute lubricants in the joint cavity.

Synovial Fluid

Minute amounts of clear, colorless to pale yellow, highly viscous fluid of slightly alkaline pH are present in healthy joints. The exact composition, viscosity, volume, and color vary somewhat from joint to joint. Functions of the synovial fluid are nutrition of the adjacent articular cartilage and disc and lubrication of joint surfaces, which decreases friction and increases joint efficiency. The cells within the synovial fluid are important in phagocytosis, removing microorganisms and joint debris.

Synovial Sheaths and Bursae

Synovial tissue is also found about various tendon sheaths and bursae. Tendon sheaths completely or partially cover a portion of the tendon where it passes through fascial slings, osseofibrous tunnels, and ligamentous bands. They function to promote the gliding of tendons and contribute to the nutrition of the intrasheath portion of the tendons.

Bursae represent enclosed flattened sacs consisting of synovial lining and, in some locations, a thin film of synovial fluid, which provides both lubrication and nourishment for the cells of the synovial membrane. Subcutaneous bursae are found between skin and underlying bone prominences, such as the olecranon and patella; subfascial bursae are placed between deep fascia and bone; subtendinous bursae exist where one tendon overlies another tendon; submucosal bursae are located between muscle and bone, tendon, or ligament; interligamentous bursae separate ligaments. When bursae are located near joints, the synovial membrane of the bursa may be continuous with that of the joint cavity, producing communicating bursae. This occurs normally about the hip (iliopsoas bursa) and knee (gastrocnemiosemimembranosus bursa) and abnormally about the glenohumeral joint (subacromial bursa) owing to defects in the rotator cuff. At certain sites where skin is subject to pressure and lateral displacement, adventitious bursae may appear, allowing increased freedom of motion.

Sesamoid Bones

Sesamoids generally are small ovoid nodules embedded in tendons (Fig. 2–8). They are found in two specific situations in the skeleton. First, the sesamoid may be located adjacent to an articulation, with its tendon incorporated into the joint capsule. Examples of this type are the patella and the hallucis and pollicis sesamoids. Second, the sesamoid may be located at sites where tendons are angled about bone surfaces. They are separated from the underlying bone by a synovium-lined

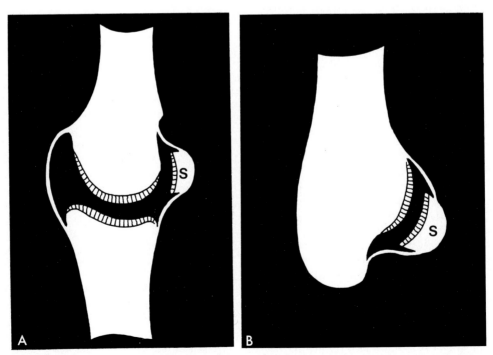

Figure 2–8. Sesamoid bones. There are two types of sesamoids: one **(A)** in which the sesamoid is located adjacent to an articulation, and another **(B)** in which the sesamoid is separated from the underlying bone by a bursa. In both types, the sesamoid is intimately associated with a synovial lining and articular cartilage (hatched areas).

bursa. An example of this type is the sesamoid of the peroneus longus muscle. In both, the arrangement of the sesamoid nodule and surrounding tissue resembles a synovial joint.

In the hand, sesamoid nodules adjacent to joints are most frequently present on the palmar aspect of the metacarpophalangeal joints, particularly the first. Additional sesamoids are most frequent in the second and fifth metacarpophalangeal joints and adjacent to the interphalangeal joint of the thumb. Sesamoid distribution in the foot parallels that in the hand. Two sesamoids are located on the plantar aspect of the first metatarsophalangeal joint in the tendons of the flexor hallucis brevis muscle. Sesamoid nodules may also be present at other metatarsophalangeal joints and the interphalangeal joint of the great toe. Sesamoid bones unassociated with synovial joints are more frequent in the lower extremity than in the upper extremity.

SUPPORTING STRUCTURES
Tendons

Tendons represent a portion of a muscle consisting of collagen fibers that transmit muscle tension to a mobile part of the body. They are flexible cords, white in color, smooth in texture, that can be angulated about bone protuberances, changing the direction of pull of the muscle. Synovial sheaths may surround portions of the tendon. The attachment sites of tendons to bones are termed entheses.

Aponeuroses

Aponeuroses consist of several flat layers or sheets of dense collagen fibers associated with the attachment of a muscle.

Fasciae

Fascia is a general term used to describe a focal collection of connective tissue. Superficial fascia consists of a layer of loose areolar tissue of variable thickness beneath the dermis. Deep fascia resembles an aponeurosis, consisting of regularly arranged, compact collagen fibers. At sites where deep fascia contacts bone, the fascia fuses with the periosteum. It is well suited to transmit the pull of adjacent musculature. Intermuscular septa extend from deep fascia between groups of muscles, producing functional compartments.

Ligaments

Ligaments represent fibrous bands that unite bones. They do not transmit muscle action directly but are essential in the control of posture and the maintenance of joint stability. Histologically and biomechanically, ligaments resemble tendons, and their sites of osseous attachment (entheses) are similar to those of tendons.

VASCULAR, LYMPHATIC, AND NERVE SUPPLY

The blood supply of joints arises from periarticular arterial plexuses that pierce the capsule, break up in the synovial membrane, and form a rich and intricate network of capillaries. A circle of vessels (circulus articuli vasculosus) within the synovial membrane is adjacent to the peripheral margin of articular cartilage.

The lymphatics form a plexus in the subintima of the synovial membrane. Efferent vessels pass toward the flexor aspect of the joint and then along blood vessels to regional deep lymph nodes.

The nerve supply of movable joints generally arises from the same nerves that supply the adjacent musculature. The fibrous capsule and to a lesser extent the synovial membrane are both supplied by nerves. Free nerve endings, numerous at the attachments of fibrous capsule and ligaments, are believed to mediate pain sensation. This would explain the extreme pain that is common after injury to joint ligaments. The synovial membrane itself is relatively insensitive to pain.

FURTHER READING

Barnett CH, Davies DV, MacConaill MA: Synovial Joints; Their Structure and Mechanics. Springfield, Ill, Charles C Thomas, 1961.

Canoso JJ: Bursae, tendons and ligaments. Clin Rheum Dis 7:189, 1981.

Davies DV: The structure and functions of the synovial membrane. Br Med J 1:92, 1950.

Jaffe HL: Metabolic, Degenerative and Inflammatory Diseases of Bones and Joints. Philadelphia, Lea & Febiger, 1972, p. 80.

Resnick D, Niwayama G: Entheses and enthesopathy. Anatomical, pathological, and radiological correlation. Radiology 146:1, 1983.

Resnick D, Niwayama G, Feingold ML: The sesamoid bones of the hands and feet: Participators in arthritis. Radiology 123:57, 1977.

Walmsley R: Joints. In GJ Romanes (Ed): Cunningham's Textbook of Anatomy. 11th Ed. London, Oxford University Press, 1972, p. 207.

Wyke B: The neurology of joints: A review of general principles. Clin Rheum Dis 7:223, 1981.

SECTION II

DIAGNOSTIC TECHNIQUES

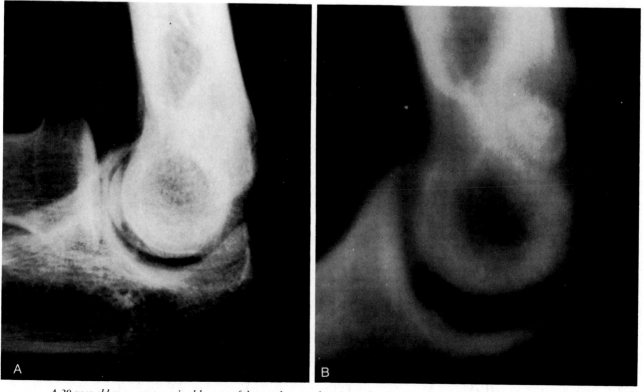

A 20 year old man was examined because of decreased range of motion in his elbow. He had had a previous injury to the elbow.

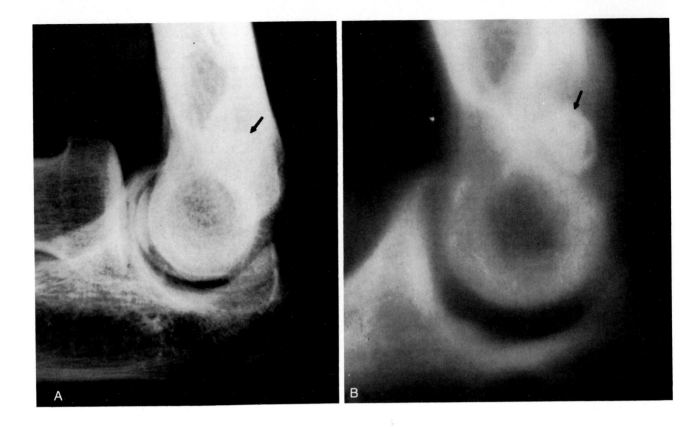

Although the routine lateral radiograph (A) reveals a subtle abnormality (arrow), the precise nature of the abnormality is better demonstrated with conventional tomography (B). On the tomogram, a lamellated ovoid radiodense area (arrow) is evident, lodged within the olecranon fossa in the distal portion of the humerus. The normal coronoid fossa on the anterior surface of the humerus is also evident. The radiographic appearance and location of the radiodense lesion are pathognomonic of an intraarticular osseous body.

Osseous or osteochondral bodies situated within joints can result from a variety of processes, including neuroarthropathy, crystal deposition diseases, rheumatoid arthritis, osteonecrosis, and osteochondritis dissecans or other traumatic lesions. Furthermore, metaplasia of the synovial membrane can lead to idiopathic synovial osteochondromatosis. In this last condition, numerous intraarticular bodies composed of cartilage or cartilage and bone are typical. A single large bone fragment within a joint is rarely observed in idiopathic synovial osteochondromatosis. Although intraarticular calcification can accompany calcium pyrophosphate dihydrate or calcium hydroxyapatite crystal deposition disease, the radiodense area illustrated in Case II is lamellated and ossified, distinguishing it from the calcification that characterizes crystal deposition disorders. Rarely, anomalies of ossification can lead to radiodense bodies that simulate the lesion in the test case.

Osseous or osteochondral bodies may remain at their site of origin or migrate freely within the joint cavity, where they later may become embedded in the synovial membrane. It is not uncommon for intraarticular bodies to lodge within normal recesses or extensions of the joint, examples of which include the subscapular recess in the glenohumeral joint, the acetabular fossa in the hip, and, as in the test case, the humeral fossae in the elbow. In some instances, free intraarticular bodies become located in dependent portions of the joint or extend into adjacent synovial cysts, such as in the popliteal region of the knee. Intraarticular bodies may become smaller or disappear over time or enlarge. A lamellated appearance is characteristic of progressive ossification in such bodies.

The decreased range of elbow motion in the patient illustrated in Case II relates to the location of the osseous body. Lodged within the olecranon fossa, this body will prevent the olecranon process itself from reaching the base of the olecranon fossa during full extension of the elbow.

At the time of arthrotomy of the elbow in this patient, a large ossified body was identified and removed from the olecranon fossa. Two areas of cartilage loss, one in the capitulum and one in the radial head, were seen, although the precise site of origin of the intraarticular body was not clear.

FINAL DIAGNOSIS: Posttraumatic intraarticular osseous body in the olecranon fossa.

FURTHER READING

Pages 817 and 818 and the following:

1. Milgram JW: The classification of loose bodies in human joints. Clin Orthop 124:282, 1977.
2. Milgram JW: The development of loose bodies in human joints. Clin Orthop 124:292, 1977.

(Case II, courtesy of G. Greenway, M.D., Dallas, Texas.)

Chapter 3

Plain Film Radiography: Routine Techniques

David J. Sartoris, M.D.
Donald Resnick, M.D.

Ideally, the radiographic evaluation of a patient will include neither too few nor too many radiographs for correct diagnosis. Careful preliminary clinical evaluation is essential in choosing the best sequence of films. In this chapter, various projections are described, some of which are required for many types of disorders with others being used more specifically. Recommended basic screening examinations for various regions of the body are also given.

Various radiographic projections are available for the evaluation of bones and articulations, a number of which are summarized here. At the end of the chapter, appropriate radiographic surveys for arthritis and other musculoskeletal diseases are discussed. Specialized radiographic procedures and related examinations for investigating patients with bone and joint diseases are discussed in some of the following chapters.

FINGERS AND HAND

Adequate radiographic evaluation of the fingers requires posteroanterior and lateral projections (Fig. 3–1). Placing the hand on a step wedge permits separation of individual fingers in the lateral projection, allowing all digits to be examined on a single radiograph. Because the axis of the thumb differs from that of the other digits, its positioning is unique (Fig. 3–2). Stress views of the first metacarpophalangeal articulation may be required for evaluation of injuries of the ligaments of this joint.

Posteroanterior, oblique, and lateral projections are used to examine the hand (Fig. 3–3). The posteroanterior projection is the best conventional view for demonstrating malalignment, joint space narrowing, and soft tissue abnormalities in early rheumatoid arthritis. Occasionally anteroposterior and lateral flexion radiographs may be useful to further evaluate the dorsum of the hand and the metacarpophalangeal articulations.

WRIST

Routine projections for evaluating the wrist are the frontal and lateral views (Fig. 3–4). In suspected arthritis, oblique projections are also necessary and should include radiographs exposed with the wrist in both a semipronated oblique and a semisupinated oblique position. Radial and ulnar deviation of the wrist helps in visualizing the carpal bones, particularly the scaphoid (ulnar deviation), and in assessing carpal mobility (Fig. 3–5). Similarly, lateral radiographs may be obtained in palmar flexion and dorsiflexion. Specialized projections for the scaphoid may be required to detect fractures. The carpal tunnel view (Fig. 3–5) delineates the osseous structures and soft tissues of the carpal canal, including the hook of the hamate, pisiform, trapezium, trapezoid, and tuberosity of the scaphoid.

RADIUS AND ULNA

Routine radiographic evaluation of the forearm consists of anteroposterior and lateral views, which should include both the elbow and the wrist. The lateral projection is obtained with the elbow joint flexed 60 to 90 degrees and the medial aspect of the elbow and fifth finger placed against the film. Oblique views may be necessary in specific situations, such as fracture assessment in the presence of an internal fixation plate.

ELBOW

Standard examination of the elbow includes anteroposterior and lateral radiographs and, in many cases, an oblique radiograph (Fig. 3–6). The frontal radiographs should be obtained with supination of the hand so that rotation of radius and ulna does not occur. On the oblique radiograph, the coronoid process is well visualized, and the lateral projection, taken in elbow flexion, allows identification of the important fat pads about this articulation. A special radial head—capitulum view has recently proved useful in the evaluation of elbow trauma. Minimally displaced fractures of the radial head, capitulum, and coronoid process are better demonstrated on this view than on traditional radiographs of the elbow.

HUMERUS

Frontal and lateral radiographs of the humerus constitute the basic examination. Both views should include the elbow and articulations of the shoulder, with the elbow manifesting a true lateral configuration in the lateral projection. Under

Text continued on page 48

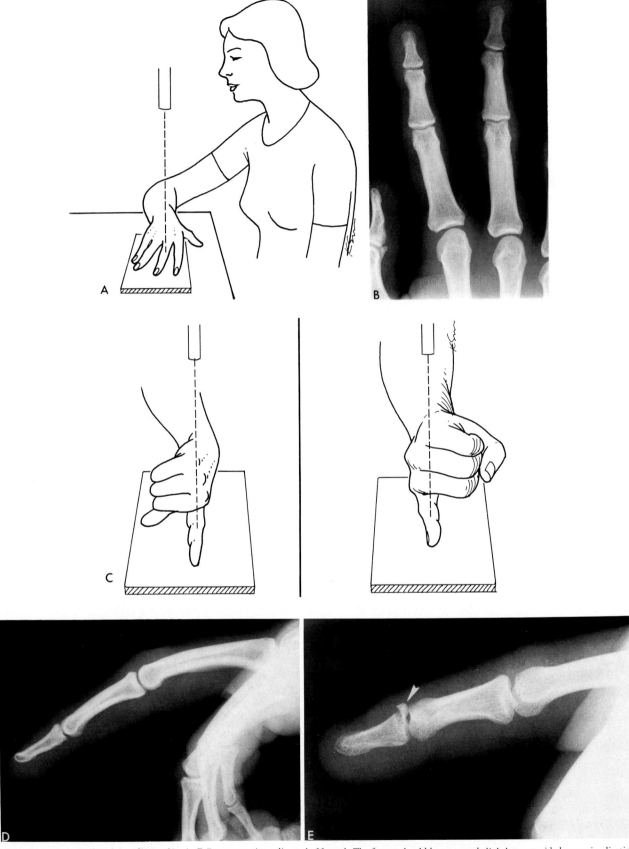

Figure 3–1. Fingers: Routine radiographs. A, B Posteroanterior radiograph: Normal. The fingers should be separated slightly to provide better visualization of the osseous and articular structures. **C, D** Lateral radiograph: Normal. Note that the position of the hand will vary depending on which digit is being examined. The involved finger is extended and the remaining digits are folded into a fist. **E** Lateral radiograph: Dorsal fracture. The intraarticular fracture is well delineated (arrowhead).

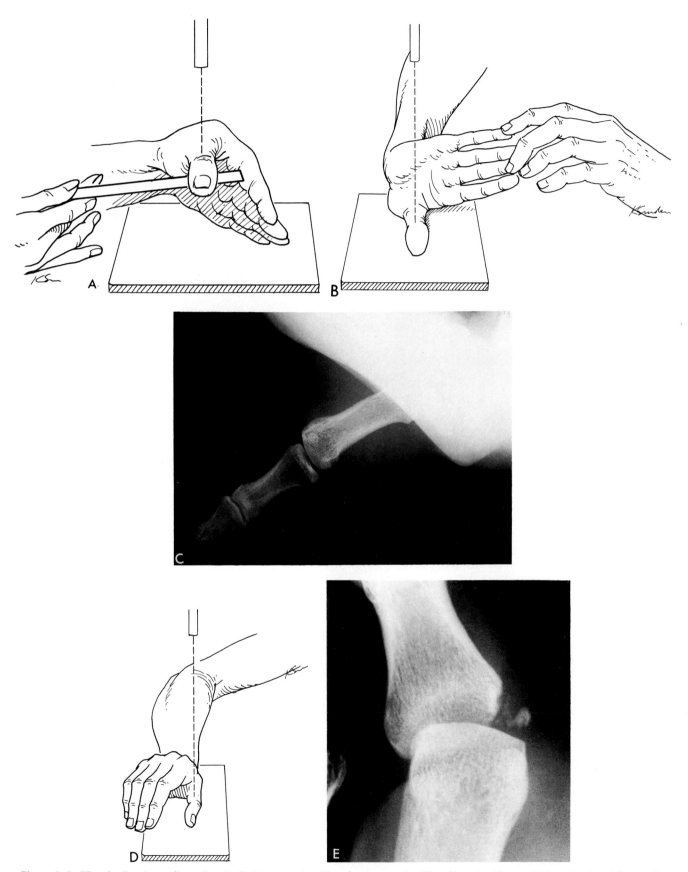

Figure 3–2. Thumb: Routine radiographs. A, B Posteroanterior (**A**) and anteroposterior (**B**) radiographs: Normal. Either view is satisfactory. **C** Anteroposterior radiograph: Normal. **D** Lateral radiograph. **E** Stress radiograph of first metacarpophalangeal joint: Gamekeeper's thumb. With radial stress, laxity of the ulnar aspect of the articulation and avulsion fractures are observed.

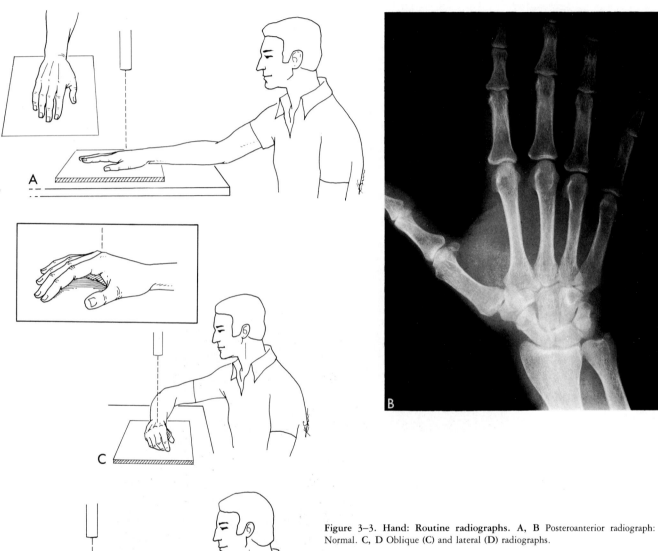

Figure 3–3. Hand: Routine radiographs. A, B Posteroanterior radiograph: Normal. **C, D** Oblique **(C)** and lateral **(D)** radiographs.

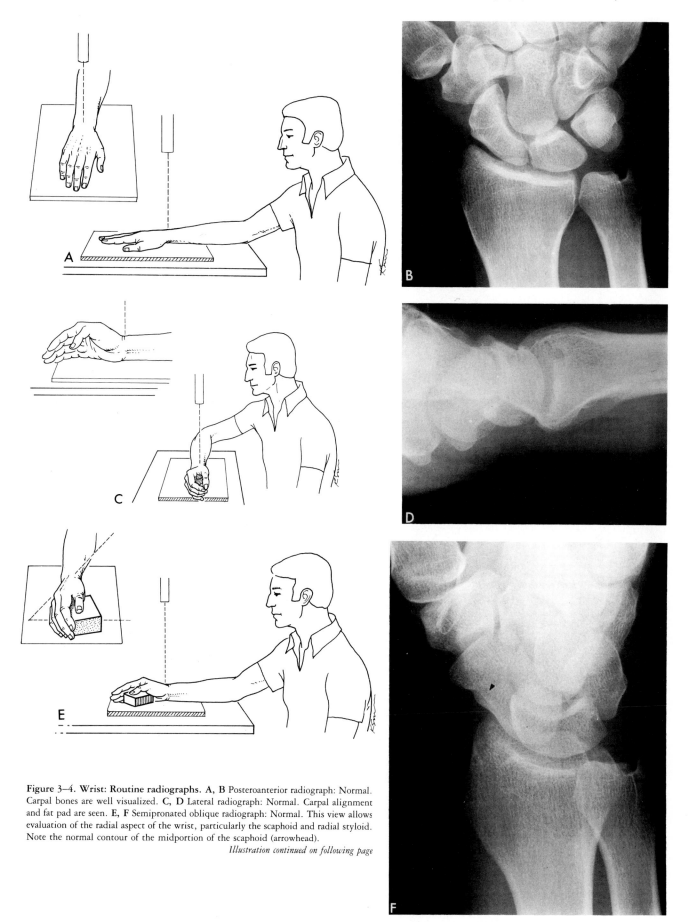

Figure 3–4. Wrist: Routine radiographs. A, B Posteroanterior radiograph: Normal. Carpal bones are well visualized. **C, D** Lateral radiograph: Normal. Carpal alignment and fat pad are seen. **E, F** Semipronated oblique radiograph: Normal. This view allows evaluation of the radial aspect of the wrist, particularly the scaphoid and radial styloid. Note the normal contour of the midportion of the scaphoid (arrowhead).

Illustration continued on following page

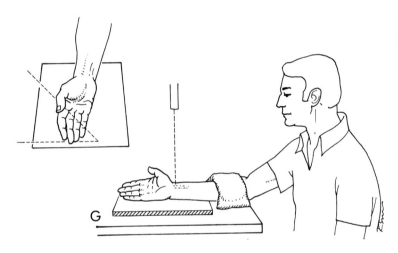

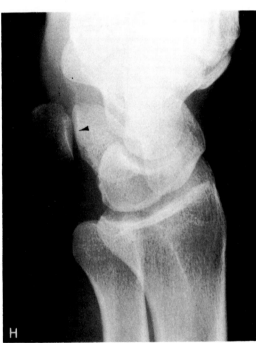

Figure 3–4 *Continued* **G, H** Semisupinated oblique radiograph: Normal. Observe the pisiform bone, which is separated from the remaining carpal bones, and the tangential view of the pisiform-triquetral joint (arrowhead).

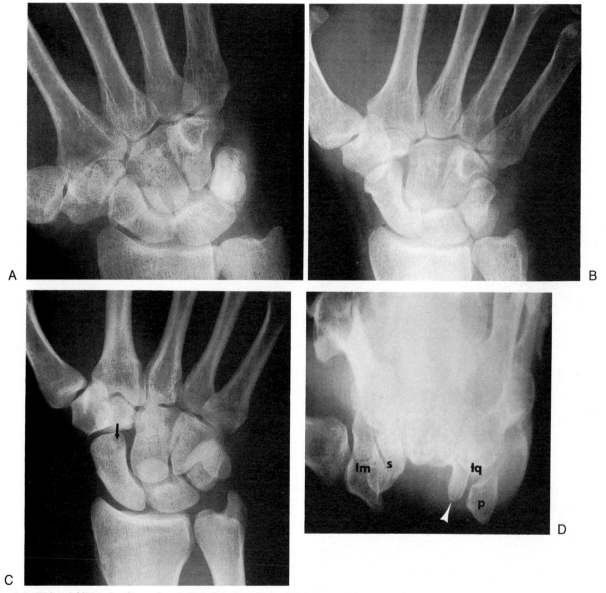

Figure 3–5. Wrist: Additional radiographs. A, B Radial (A) and ulnar (B) deviation. Observe the normal change in alignment of the carpal bones in the two projections. In radial deviation, palmar flexion of the proximal carpal row occurs and the distal scaphoid rotates into the palm; the proximal carpal row moves in an ulnar direction with respect to the distal radius. In ulnar deviation, the scapholunate space may increase slightly and the scaphoid is exposed in full profile. **C** Scaphoid: Specialized view. The hand and wrist are placed horizontally on the film and the central ray is directed 20 degrees toward the elbow. The scaphoid (arrow) is projected free of adjacent osseous structures. **D** Carpal tunnel view. In the normal situation, the trapezium (tm), scaphoid (s), triquetrum (tq), pisiform (p), and hook of the hamate (arrowhead) can be delineated.

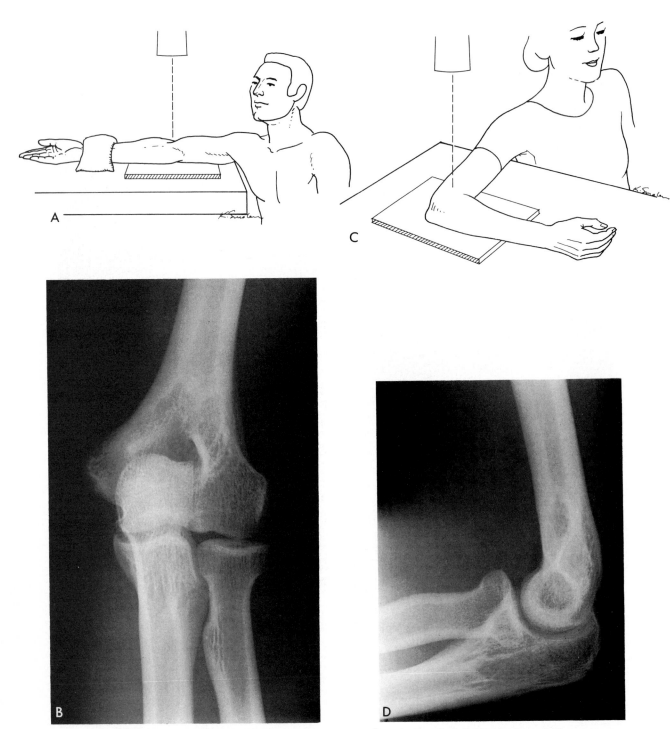

Figure 3–6. Elbow: Routine radiographs. A, B Anteroposterior radiograph: Normal. C, D Lateral radiograph: Normal.

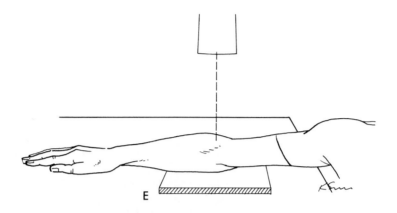

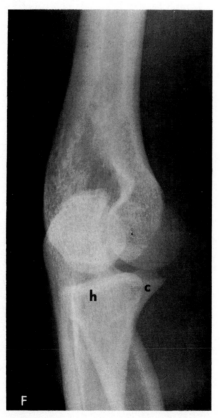

Figure 3–6 *Continued* **E, F** Oblique radiograph: Normal. Observe that the radial head (h) is superimposed on the proximal ulna, and the coronoid process (c) is well visualized.

certain circumstances, oblique views may provide additional information.

GLENOHUMERAL JOINT

Anteroposterior radiographs are obtained in external and internal rotation (Fig. 3–7). The former reveals the greater tuberosity in profile and is useful in detecting calcification in the supraspinatus tendon. A radiolucent area in the greater tuberosity is a normal variation, termed the humeral pseu-

docyst; it is most prominent on radiographs obtained with external rotation of the humerus. As the arm is rotated internally, the greater tuberosity is projected en face over the humerus, and the lesser tuberosity may overlie the glenohumeral joint. In this position, calcification in the infraspinatus and teres minor tendons is seen on the outer aspect of the humerus, and calcification in the subscapularis tendon is seen adjacent to the lesser tuberosity.

It should be recognized that an anteroposterior radiograph of the shoulder is not a true anteroposterior radiograph of the

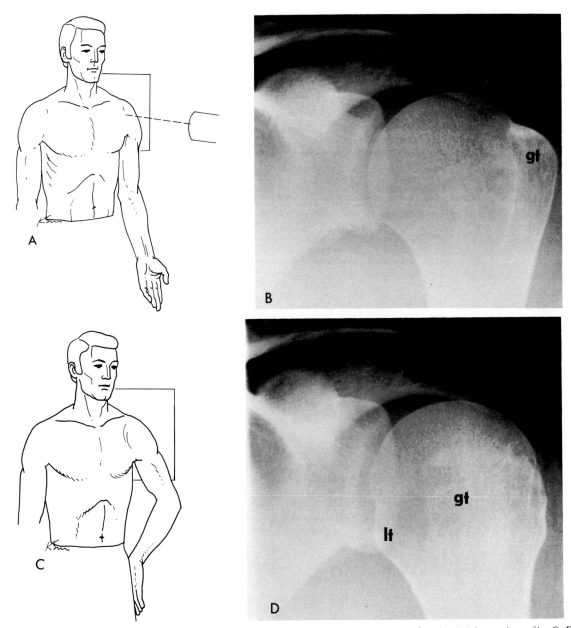

Figure 3–7. Glenohumeral joint: Routine radiographs. A, B External rotation: Normal. The greater tuberosity (gt) is seen in profile. **C, D** Internal rotation. The greater tuberosity (gt) is now projected over the humerus and the lesser tuberosity (lt) is observed on the medial aspect of the humeral head.

scapula, nor does it allow adequate visualization of the gleno-humeral joint space. A true anteroposterior radiograph of the scapula is obtained with the patient in a 40 degree posterior oblique position and is the most favorable projection for visualizing the glenohumeral joint, as this articulation is projected tangentially in this view (Fig. 3–7).

In evaluating the shoulder after trauma, it is mandatory to obtain an additional radiograph at approximately right angles to the frontal radiographs to determine the relative positions of the humeral head and glenoid. This can be accomplished in one of several ways. An axillary projection is particularly useful (Fig. 3–7), although it may be difficult to acquire in patients with fractures and dislocations about the shoulder. A transthoracic projection has been used but it may be difficult to interpret. The most favorable view makes use of a true lateral projection of the scapula (Fig. 3–7), which is acquired with the patient in a 60 degree anterior oblique position.

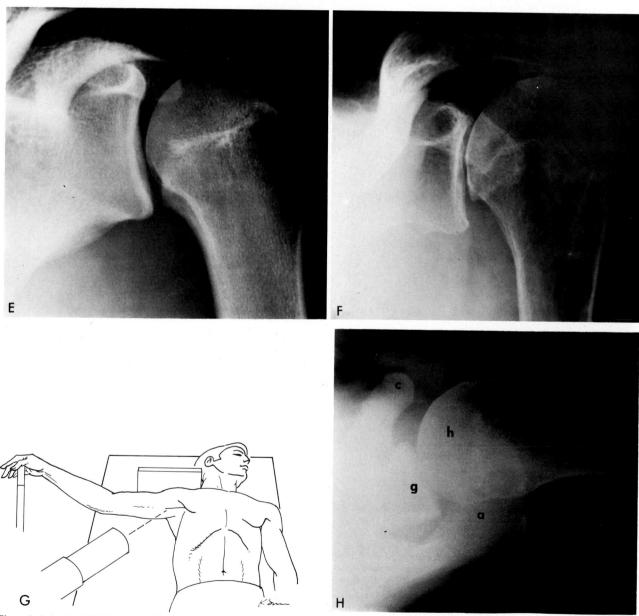

Figure 3–7 *Continued* **E, F** Posterior oblique view. In the normal situation (**E**), the articular surface of the glenoid is seen in profile. In the abnormal situation (**F**), in a patient with a tear of the rotator cuff, the same projection delineates the elevation of the humeral head with respect to the glenoid and the narrowing of the articular space. **G, H** Axillary view: Normal. Visualized structures are the glenoid cavity (g), coracoid process (c), acromion (a), and humeral head (h).

Illustration continued on following page

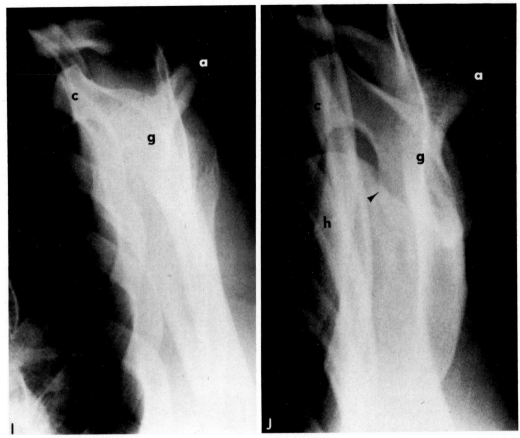

Figure 3–7 *Continued* **I, J** Additional oblique view (lateral scapula view): Normal and abnormal. In the normal situation (I) the humeral head is superimposed on the glenoid (g) between the coracoid process (c) anteriorly and the acromion (a) posteriorly. In an anterior dislocation of the glenohumeral joint (J), the humeral head (h) is projected beneath the coracoid process (c). Observe the Hill-Sachs compression fracture (arrowhead).

Several different radiographic projections have been used to evaluate patients with previous anterior dislocations of the glenohumeral joint and also a typical compression fracture of the posterolateral aspect of the humeral head, the Hill-Sachs lesion, which is associated with such dislocations (Fig. 3–8).

ACROMIOCLAVICULAR JOINT

Although the acromioclavicular articulation is visualized in routine views of the shoulder, it may be superimposed on other osseous structures. Frontal radiographs with the incident beam tilted cephalad approximately 15 degrees are superior in delineating abnormalities of this articulation (Fig. 3–9). Stress radiographs frequently are necessary to diagnose acromioclavicular joint subluxation and dislocation. These are obtained by having the patient hold a 2.3 to 7 kg (5 to 15 lb) mass (weight) in the hand or tying this weight to the wrist. Both acromioclavicular articulations should be viewed on a single film if possible. This allows comparison of the two joints by careful observation of the distance between the coracoid process and clavicle on both sides.

STERNUM AND STERNOCLAVICULAR JOINT

The radiographic evaluation of the sternum requires oblique and lateral projections. Adequate radiographs of the sterno-

clavicular articulations are difficult to obtain. Oblique and frontal radiographs of the sternum frequently are not satisfactory. Many special views have been recommended. The Hobbs view (a superoinferior projection of the sternoclavicular joint) and lordotic projection may both be helpful, particularly in evaluating a patient with a possible dislocation. One additional projection, the Heinig view, can also document dislocation of this joint.

SPINE

The radiographic examination of the spine varies considerably, depending on the vertebral segment being examined and the specific indication for the examination.

Cervical Spine

Although a screening examination of the cervical spine in a patient with widespread articular disease may require only anteroposterior and lateral flexion radiographs, a more complete evaluation may be necessary in a patient with neck pain and is mandatory in a patient who has sustained neck trauma.

The standard examination of the cervical spine consists of multiple views (Fig. 3–10). A frontal radiograph is obtained with the patient either recumbent or erect in an anteroposterior projection with approximately 15 degrees to 20 degrees

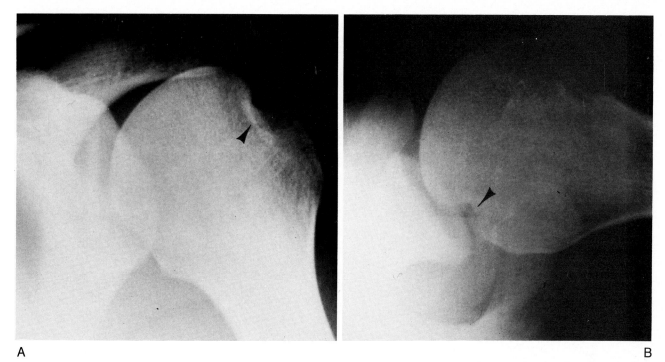

A   B

Figure 3–8. Glenohumeral joint: Evaluation of patients with previous anterior dislocation of glenohumeral joint. Hill-Sachs lesion. In this patient with a previous anterior dislocation of the glenohumeral joint, a Hill-Sachs lesion (arrowheads) is identified in the superolateral aspect of the humeral head in internal rotation (A) and axillary (B) projections.

of cephalad angulation of the tube. The lateral radiograph is usually obtained with the head in neutral position, but it may be supplemented with lateral radiographs obtained with head flexion and extension. Forty-five degree oblique projections are obtained with the patient sitting or standing. An anteroposterior open-mouth projection allows visualization of the atlas and axis. A pillar view for demonstration of the vertebral arches is obtained in an anteroposterior or posteroanterior position with neck extension.

After significant cervical spine trauma, initial radiographs should include cross-table lateral and anteroposterior views,

which may be obtained without disturbing the patient. After this screening examination, additional radiographs can be taken. The complete cervical spine examination in these patients should include those projections that have been noted previously: anteroposterior view with 20 degree caudad angulation of the tube; open-mouth view; right and left 45 degree oblique views; lateral views in neutral position and in flexion and extension; and pillar view. Additionally, shallow oblique radiographs (approximately 20 degrees of obliquity) may be needed.

For some portions of the cervical spine, additional radio-

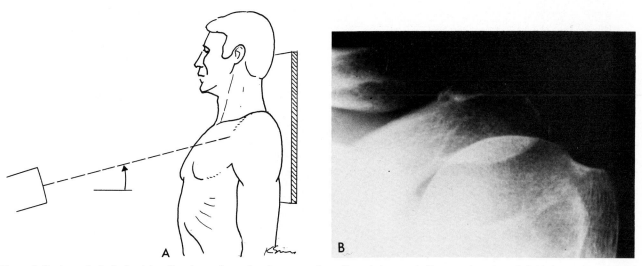

A   B

Figure 3–9. Acromioclavicular joint: Routine radiographs. Anteroposterior radiograph is normal. The central ray is angled 15 degrees in a cephalad direction.

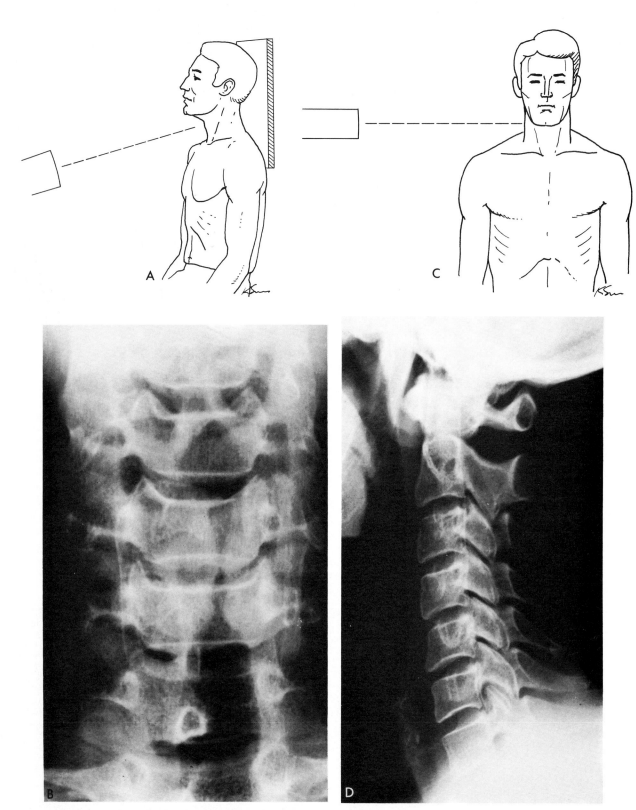

Figure 3–10. Cervical spine: Routine radiographs. A, B Anteroposterior radiograph. Normal. **C, D** Lateral radiograph: Normal.

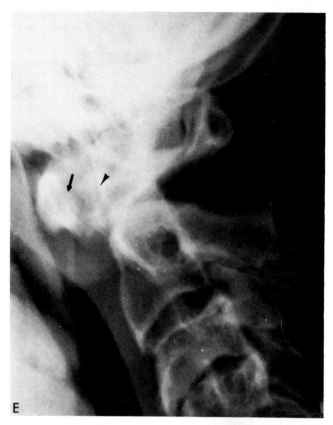

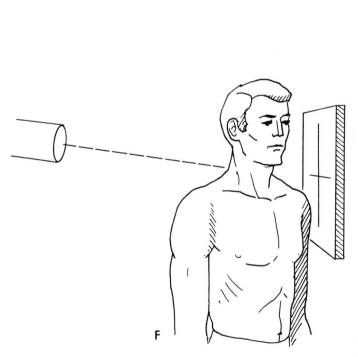

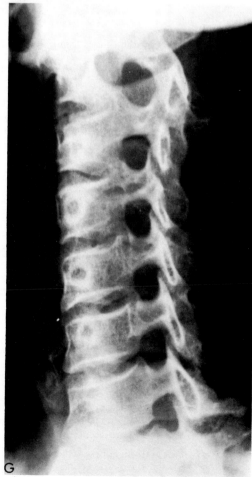

Figure 3–10 *Continued* **E** Lateral radiograph: Atlantoaxial subluxation in rheumatoid arthritis. Note the increased distance between the anterior arch of the atlas (arrow) and the anterior aspect of the odontoid process (arrowhead). **F, G** Oblique radiograph: Normal. The neural foramina are well visualized.

Illustration continued on following page

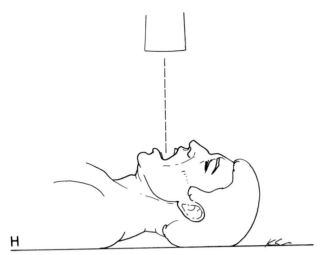

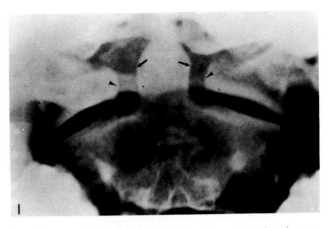

Figure 3–10 *Continued* **H, I** Open-mouth radiograph: Normal. Observe the odontoid process (arrows) symmetrically placed between the lateral masses (arrowheads) of the atlas.

graphs are suggested (Fig. 3–11). For the cervicothoracic region, a recommended view is the swimmer's projection, which is a lateral view with the arms pulled down. To better visualize changes at the atlantoaxial joint, multiple open-mouth views may be necessary. These are obtained with the patient in the frontal position, rotating the head 10 to 15 degrees to either side and tilting it laterally to either side.

Thoracic Spine

A radiographic series of the thoracic spine should include anteroposterior and lateral radiographs and a swimmer's view of the lower cervical and upper thoracic vertebrae (Fig. 3–12). The anteroposterior projection places the spine adjacent to the x-ray film. Because of the normal thoracic kyphosis, diverging incident rays are relatively parallel to the upper and lower aspects of the vertebrae in this position. Certain modifications in the technique may allow more uniform density throughout the entire radiograph.

Lumbar Spine

The frontal radiograph of the lumbar spine can be obtained in the posteroanterior or anteroposterior projection with the patient erect or recumbent (Fig. 3–13). The recumbent anteroposterior radiograph should be taken with the hips and knees flexed, which reduces the lumbar lordosis and better delineates the vertebral bodies and intervertebral discs. The lateral radiograph is also taken with slight flexion of the hips and knees. A coned-down lateral projection of the lumbosacral junction is likewise included. Oblique radiographs allow evaluation of the posterior elements of the lumbar spine. These can be obtained in anteroposterior or posteroanterior positions by turning the patient 45 degrees. An anteroposterior view of the pelvis is generally included in the evaluation of the lumbosacral spine.

Examination of motion of the lumbar spine may provide useful information. To accomplish this, lateral radiographs may be obtained during flexion and extension, and frontal radiographs may be obtained during lateral bending of the spine.

PELVIS

The standard radiographic view of the pelvis is obtained in an anteroposterior position with the patient supine (Fig. 3–14). To overcome the normal anteversion of the femoral necks and to place their longitudinal axes parallel to the film, the feet are rotated internally by approximately 15 degrees.

Various methods have been used to examine the sacroiliac joints (Fig. 3–15); none is ideal, as the normal undulating articular surfaces make evaluation of these joints extremely difficult. Oblique views of this articulation can be obtained in either the supine or the prone position. In either instance, the side of the body being examined is elevated approximately 25 degrees. A better radiographic method for the sacroiliac joints uses the frontal projection (Fig. 3–15). An anteroposterior radiograph can be taken with the tube angulated 25 to 30 degrees in a cephalad direction, or a posteroanterior radiograph can be taken with 25 to 30 degrees of caudal angulation of the tube. In either case, both sacroiliac joints are exposed on a single film, facilitating comparison of the two articulations.

SACRUM AND COCCYX

The radiographic examination of the sacrum and coccyx includes frontal and lateral projections (Fig. 3–16). To visualize the upper sacrum, an anteroposterior radiograph is obtained with 15 degrees of cephalad angulation of the tube. To visualize the lower sacrum, an anteroposterior radiograph without beam angulation is useful. To visualize the coccyx, an anteroposterior radiograph with 10 degrees of caudal angulation of the tube is required. A lateral projection of the sacrum or coccyx is the second required view.

HIP

The most common method of examining the hip joint includes an anteroposterior radiograph of the pelvis and a coned-down anteroposterior radiograph of the hip, both obtained with internal rotation of the foot to elongate the femoral neck, and a frog-leg view obtained with the hip

Text continued on page 63

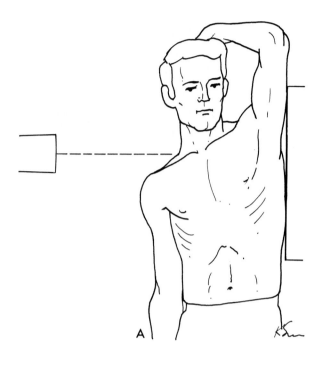

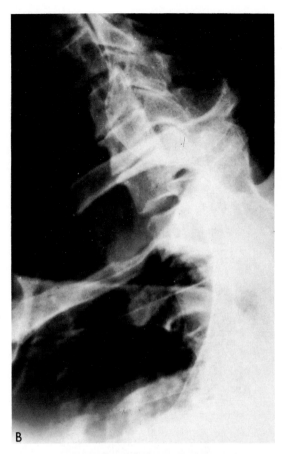

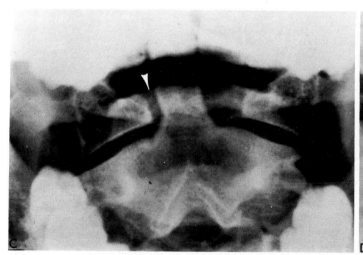

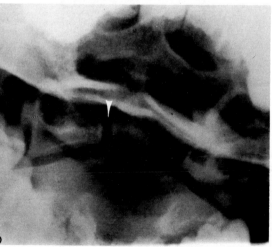

Figure 3–11. Cervical spine: Additional radiographs. A, B Swimmer's projection: Abnormal. The lateral radiograph is obtained with one arm elevated. This allows evaluation of the cervicothoracic junction. Disc space narrowing is apparent. **C, D** Open-mouth views. Rotary fixation of the atlas and axis. These two radiographs were taken with the patient tilting the head. They demonstrate persistent asymmetry at the atlantoaxial junction, with the odontoid associated more closely with the right lateral mass (arrowheads). This indicates rotary fixation at the atlantoaxial junction.

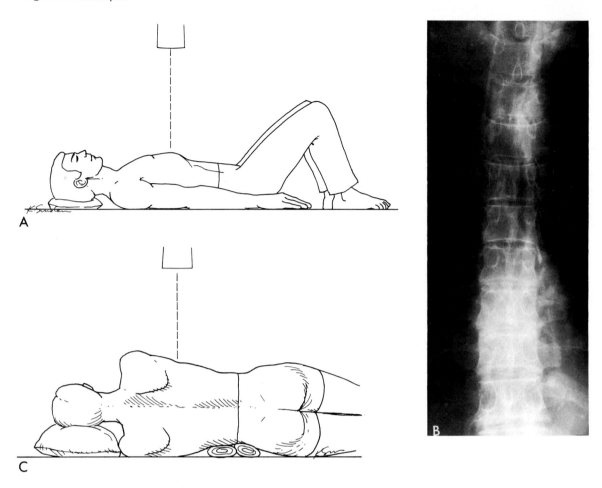

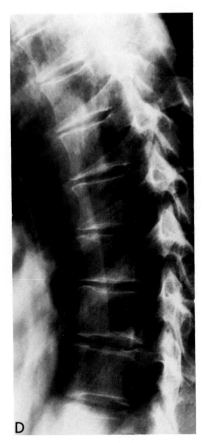

Figure 3–12. Thoracic spine: Routine radiographs. A, B Anteroposterior radiograph: Normal. The flexed position of the knees and hips produces some straightening of the normal thoracic kyphosis. C, D Lateral radiograph: Normal.

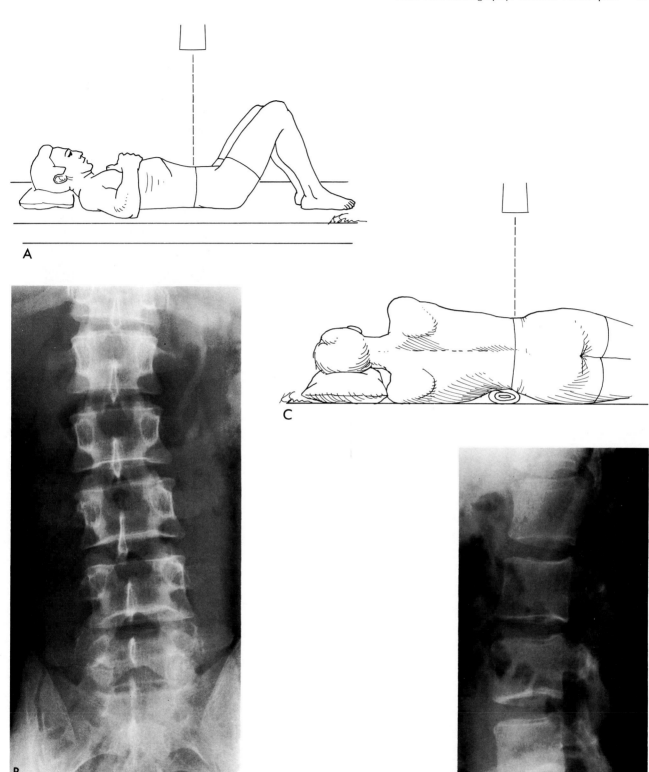

Figure 3–13. Lumbar spine: Routine radiographs. A, B Anteroposterior radiograph: Normal. The knees and hips are flexed to reduce the degree of lumbar lordosis. Mild angulation of the upper spine is seen. **C, D** Lateral radiograph: Normal. The knees and hips are again flexed.

Illustration continued on following page

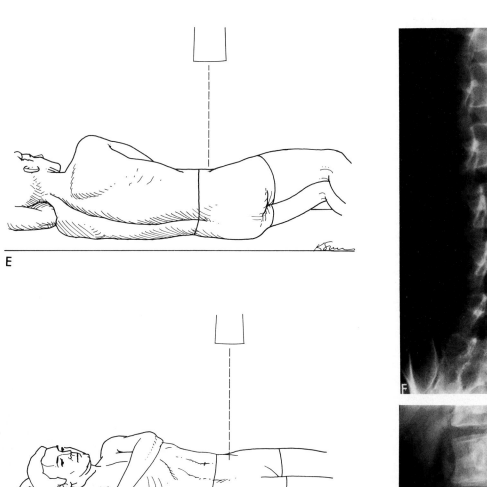

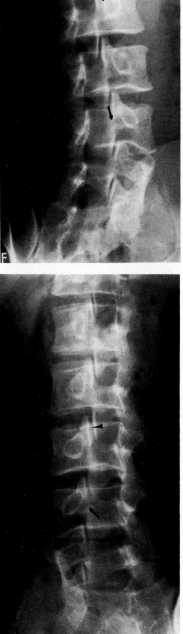

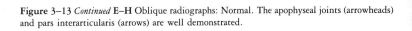

Figure 3–13 *Continued* **E–H** Oblique radiographs: Normal. The apophyseal joints (arrowheads) and pars interarticularis (arrows) are well demonstrated.

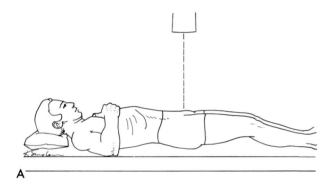

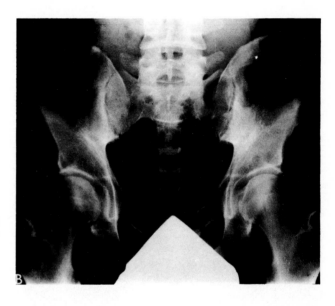

Figure 3–14. Pelvis: Routine radiographs. Anteroposterior radiograph of pelvis: Normal. Internal rotation of the lower legs allows elongation of the femoral necks.

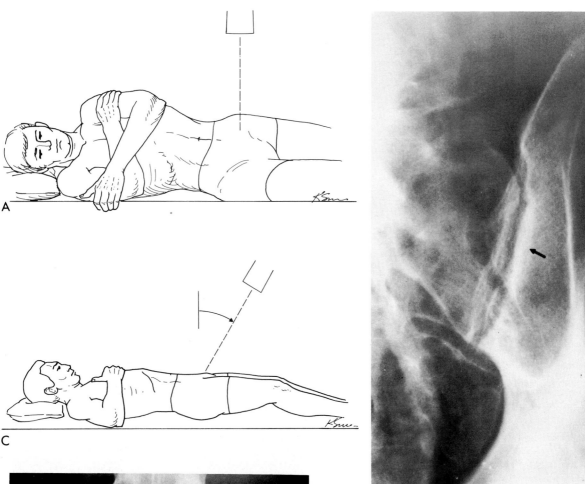

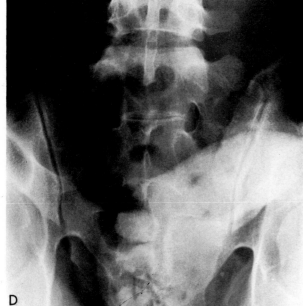

Figure 3–15. Sacroiliac joints: Routine radiographs. A, B Oblique radiograph: Normal. The side of the body being examined is elevated approximately 25 degrees. The sacroiliac joint is demonstrated *(B)* and mild sclerosis on the iliac aspect of the articulation (arrow) represents minimal degenerative joint disease. **C, D** Anteroposterior radiograph with 25 to 30 degrees of cephalad angulation: Normal. Both sacroiliac articulations are projected on a single film.

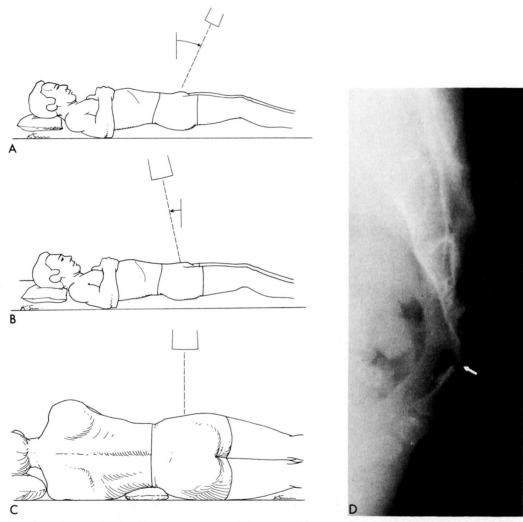

Figure 3–16. Sacrum and coccyx: Routine radiographs. A–C Frontal radiographs of sacrum (**A**) use 15 degrees of cephalad angulation; frontal radiographs of the coccyx (**B**) require 10 degrees of caudal angulation. The lateral radiograph (**C**) is also obtained. **D** Lateral radiograph of sacrum: displaced fracture (arrow).

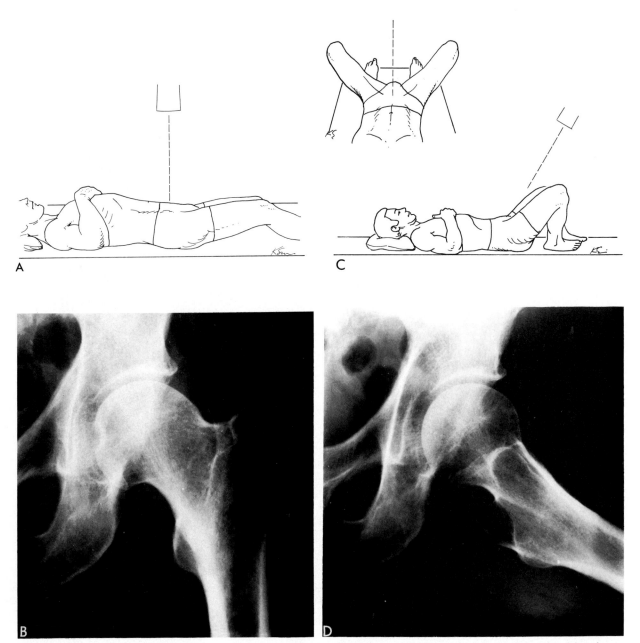

Figure 3–17. Hip: Routine radiographs. A, B Anteroposterior radiograph: Normal. **C, D** Frog-leg view: Normal. The hip is abducted.

abducted (Fig. 3–17). In the evaluation of the hip joint and acetabulum following trauma, 45 degree anterior and posterior oblique projections have been recommended to visualize the anterior and posterior acetabular rims and the bony columns of the pelvis, which are important landmarks (Fig. 3–18).

Radiographs of the hip obtained during traction of 14 to 23 kg (30 to 50 lb) are useful in a variety of articular disorders. This maneuver produces spontaneous intraarticular release of gas, the "vacuum" phenomenon. The pneumoarthrogram is not obtained if the patient has a hip effusion. Traction radiography thus affords an easy and noninvasive means for detecting fluid in the hip joint. In osteonecrosis, gas may be released into the separated fragment of subchondral bone, allowing earlier diagnosis of this condition.

FEMUR

Lateral and anteroposterior radiographs are routine in the evaluation of the femur. Both are obtained with the leg rotated medially about 20 degrees. The hip and knee should be visualized on both views even if this requires two separate exposures with different centering in each projection.

KNEE

An anteroposterior radiograph of the knee is obtained with the beam directed 5 to 7 degrees toward the head, and a lateral radiograph is obtained with the knee flexed 20 to 35 degrees (Fig. 3–19). Although these two views are adequate for the assessment of most disorders of the knee, complete evaluation of patients with knee effusions after acute trauma may require additional views to ensure that occult fractures are not overlooked. Forty-five degree oblique projections are usually necessary in a patient with knee trauma. An angulated frontal view with the knee flexed 40 to 50 degrees, the tunnel view, is used to visualize the intercondylar notch. In patients with knee trauma, a cross-table lateral projection should be added to the examination, allowing demonstration of fat-fluid levels, which are indicative of fractures with release of medullary fat into the articular cavity (Fig. 3–20).

Various techniques have been described for adequate evaluation of the patellofemoral joint (Fig. 3–21). Original descriptions suggested using the prone position with acute knee flexion (the sunrise view). This degree of knee flexion results in the patella's becoming deeply situated within the intercondylar fossa. As most cases of subluxation of the patella occur in lesser degrees of knee flexion, this view is not ideal.

A technique in which the patient is positioned supine with the leg flexed 45 degrees over the end of the table has been proposed (Merchant view). The tube is angulated 30 degrees toward the floor. The direction of the beam also can be reversed and radiographs can be obtained at various degrees of knee flexion, perhaps providing a more accurate appraisal of the patellofemoral area.

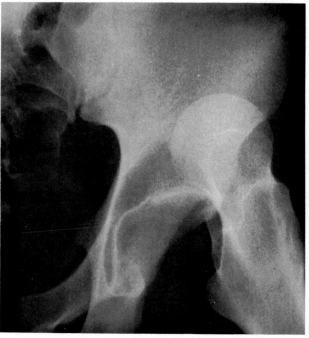
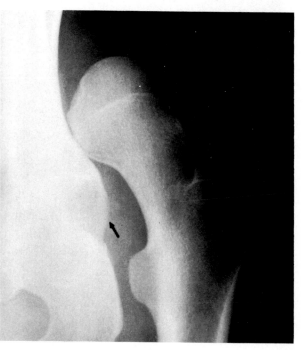

A   B

Figure 3–18. Hip: Additional radiographs. Anteroposterior and oblique radiographs of posterior dislocation of the hip. Although the frontal radiograph **(A)** demonstrates that the femoral head is displaced superiorly, the oblique radiograph **(B)** reveals also its posterior displacement and provides information regarding the posterior acetabular rim (arrow).

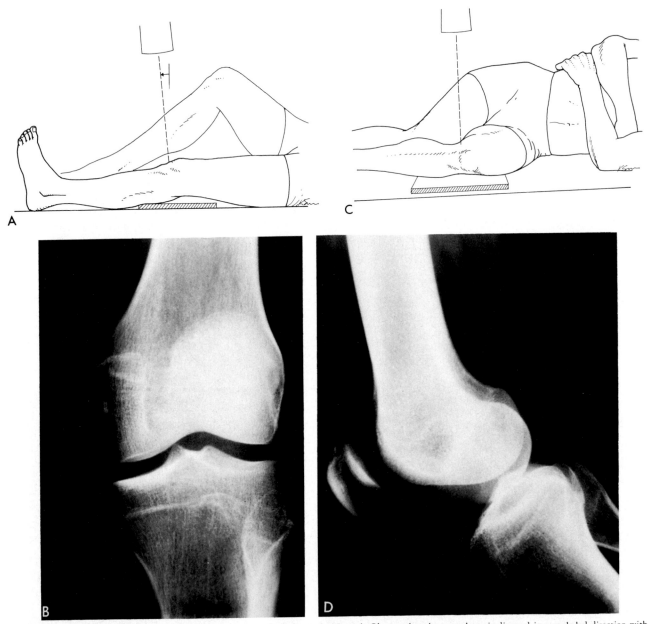

Figure 3–19. Knee: Routine radiographs. A, B Anteroposterior radiograph: Normal. Observe that the central ray is directed in a cephalad direction with an angle of 5 to 7 degrees. **C, D** Lateral radiograph: Normal. The knee is flexed 20 to 35 degrees.

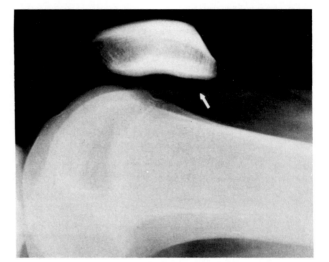

Figure 3–20. Knee: Additional radiograph. Cross-table lateral projection: Fat-fluid level (arrow) in a patient with a tibial plateau fracture. The interface is a sharply delineated horizontal radiodense line. The fat originated in the medullary cavity and was released into the joint following the fracture.

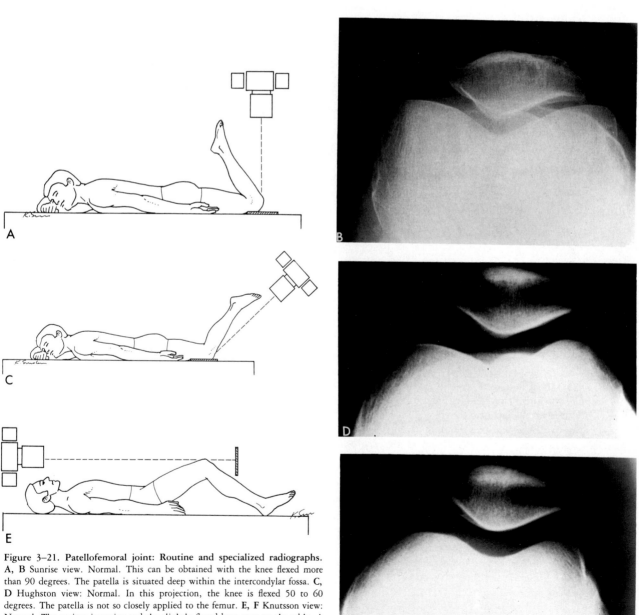

Figure 3–21. Patellofemoral joint: Routine and specialized radiographs. A, B Sunrise view. Normal. This can be obtained with the knee flexed more than 90 degrees. The patella is situated deep within the intercondylar fossa. **C, D** Hughston view: Normal. In this projection, the knee is flexed 50 to 60 degrees. The patella is not so closely applied to the femur. **E, F** Knutsson view: Normal. The patient is supine and the slightly flexed knee rests on the table. A special film holder is necessary.

Illustration continued on following page

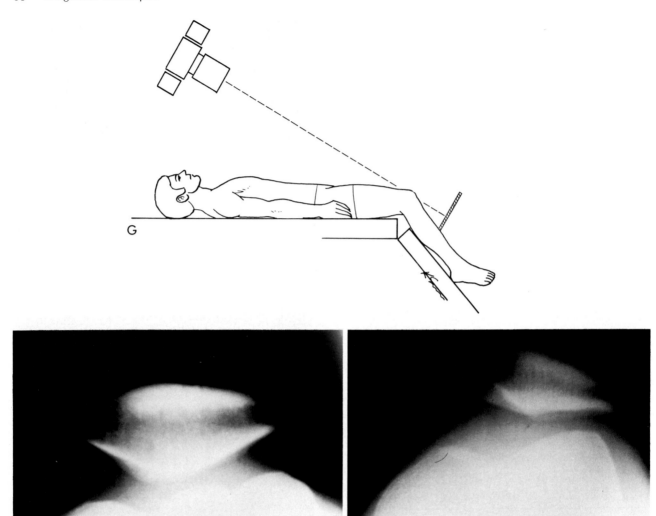

Figure 3–21 *Continued* **G–I,** Merchant view: Normal and abnormal. The patient is placed supine on the table and the knees are flexed 45 degrees over the end of the table (**G**). The central ray is angled 30 degrees from the horizontal in a caudal direction. The normal (**H**) and abnormal (**I**) appearances are illustrated. In **I**, observe the lateral subluxation of the patella.

Weight-bearing radiography of the knee is particularly helpful in evaluating degenerative joint disease, providing a more accurate assessment of the articular space (Fig. 3–22). These views should be obtained on vertically oriented 7 × 17 inch films with the patient standing on the leg being examined. This allows better delineation of the degree of angulation and subluxation at the knee and provides a more reliable indication of the extent of joint space loss.

Radiography performed during varus and valgus stress of the knee allows evaluation of ligament instability.

TIBIA AND FIBULA

The anteroposterior and lateral projections form the standard radiographic assessment of the bones of the lower leg. Supplementary oblique projections may be beneficial in occasional instances.

ANKLE

Anteroposterior and lateral radiographs of the ankle are considered routine (Fig. 3–23). To better evaluate the medial articular space, an anteroposterior radiograph with 15 to 20 degrees of internal rotation of the foot—the mortise view—is optimal to compensate for the approximately 15 to 20 degrees of external rotation of the ankle with reference to the coronal plane of the knee.

FOOT

Anteroposterior, medial oblique, and lateral projections are standard views for evaluation of the foot (Fig. 3–24). For the toes, frontal, oblique, and lateral radiographs are necessary.

Evaluation of the calcaneus can be accomplished by using a lateral projection, similar to that for evaluation of the ankle,

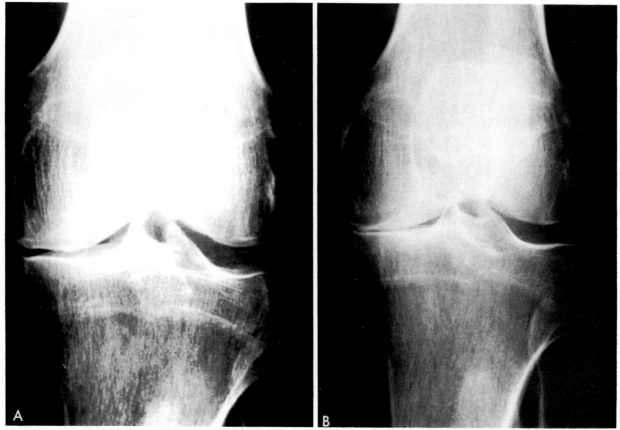

Figure 3–22. Knee: Weight-bearing radiography. Anteroposterior (**A**) and weight-bearing (**B**) radiographs in a patient with degenerative joint disease. With weight-bearing, there is further loss of joint space between the medial femoral condyle and tibia, allowing more accurate appraisal of the articular cartilage.

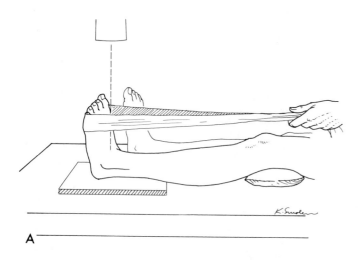

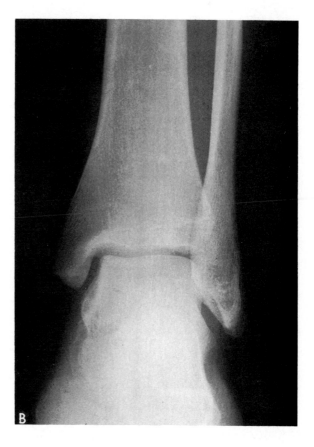

Figure 3–23. Ankle: Routine radiographs. A, B Anteroposterior radiograph: Normal. A sling may be used to provide mild dorsiflexion of the ankle.

Illustration continued on following page

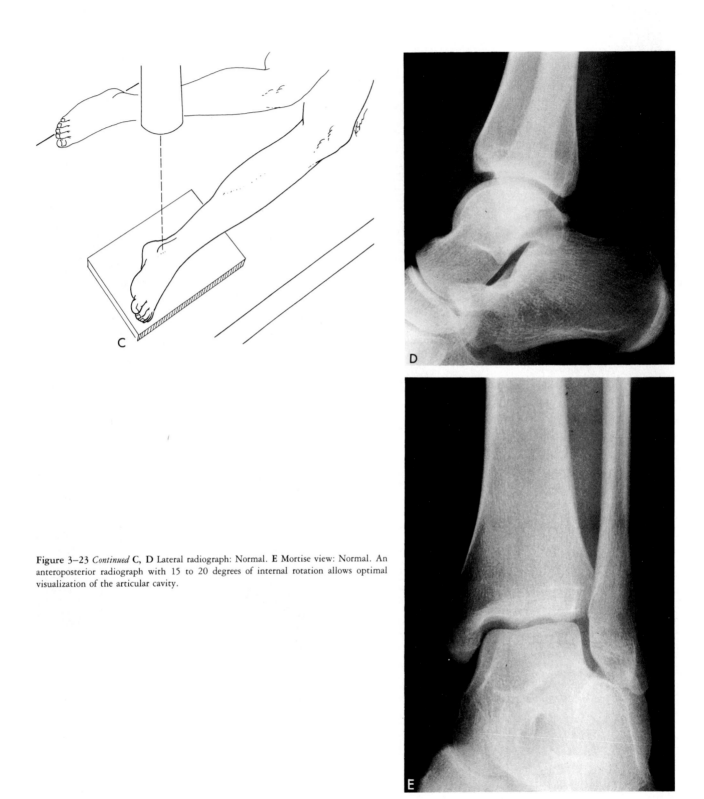

Figure 3–23 *Continued* **C, D** Lateral radiograph: Normal. **E** Mortise view: Normal. An anteroposterior radiograph with 15 to 20 degrees of internal rotation allows optimal visualization of the articular cavity.

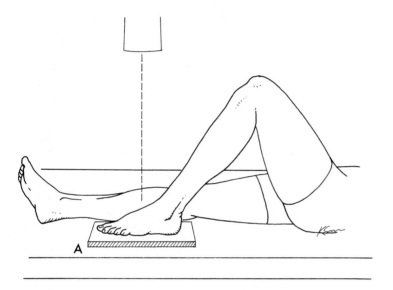

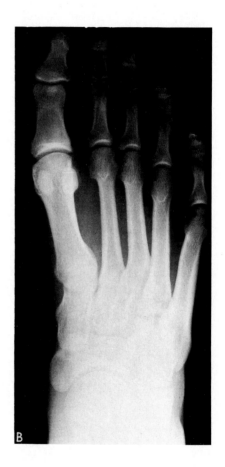

Figure 3–24. Foot: Routine radiographs. A, B Anteroposterior (dorsoplantar) radiograph: Normal.

Illustration continued on following page

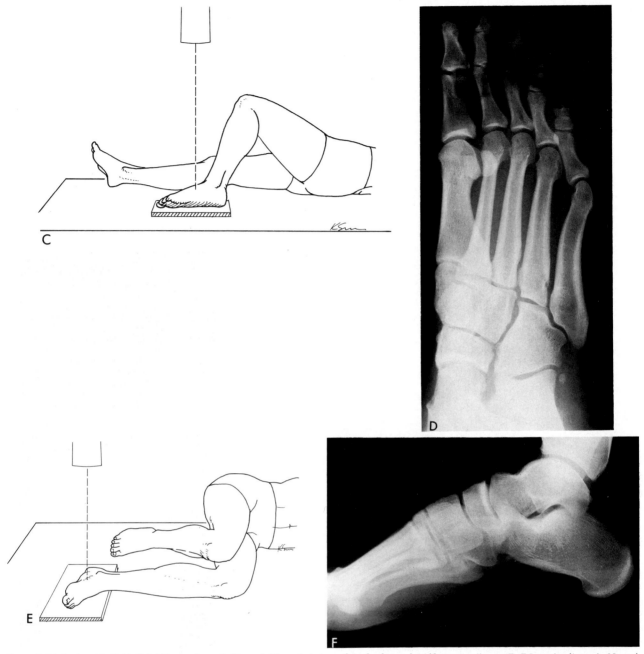

Figure 3–24 *Continued* **C, D** Medial oblique radiograph: Normal. The articulations of the forefoot and midfoot are well seen. **E, F** Lateral radiograph: Normal.

and an angulated frontal view, which can be obtained in an anteroposterior or posteroanterior direction (Fig. 3–25).

The tarsal articulations require special radiographic projections (Fig. 3–26). A penetrated axial view, the Harris-Beath view, is used to demonstrate the subtalar joint and that portion of the talocalcaneonavicular joint about the middle facet of the calcaneus. Medial and lateral oblique views are also helpful in visualizing the subtalar and talocalcaneonavicular joints.

Figure 3–27 summarizes the basic examinations for specific areas of the body.

SURVEY RADIOGRAPHS

Survey radiographs are obtained in the initial evaluation of patients with polyarticular disorders and at various intervals during subsequent examinations. The type of radiographs required will depend in large part on the specific disorder that is suspected clinically and its distribution, as indicated by the patient's symptoms and signs.

Initial survey radiographs in a patient with polyarticular disease must reveal enough information to indicate the type and extent of the disorder without causing either an overuse of the patient's, technician's, and physician's time or involving

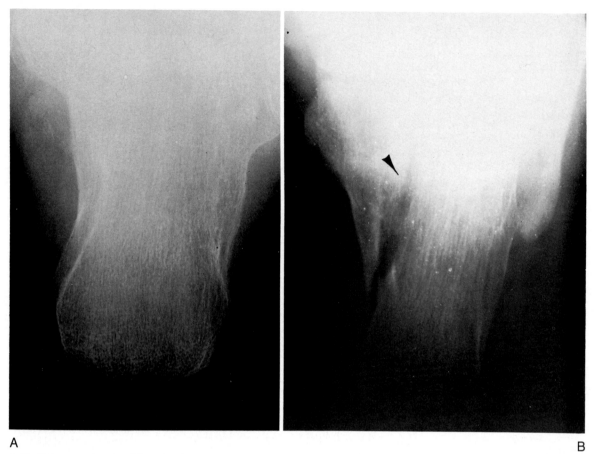

A

B

Figure 3–25. Calcaneus: Angulated frontal radiographs—normal and abnormal. With the patient supine, the central ray is angled at 40 degrees with the long axis of the foot. The normal **A** and abnormal **B** situations are indicated. Observe the calcaneal fracture (arrowhead) extending through the sustentaculum tali.

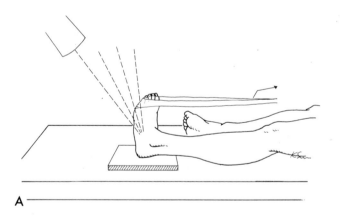

A

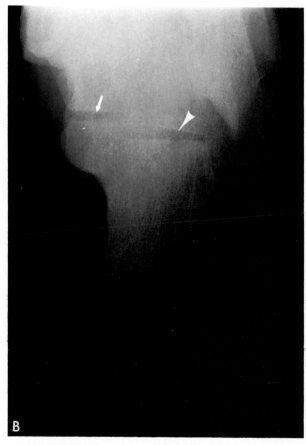

B

Figure 3–26. Tarsal articulations: Normal radiography. A, B Axial (Harris-Beath) view. The central ray can be directed at various angles. The posterior subtalar joint (arrowhead) and talocalcaneal portion of the anterior talocalcaneo-navicular joint (arrow) are demonstrated.

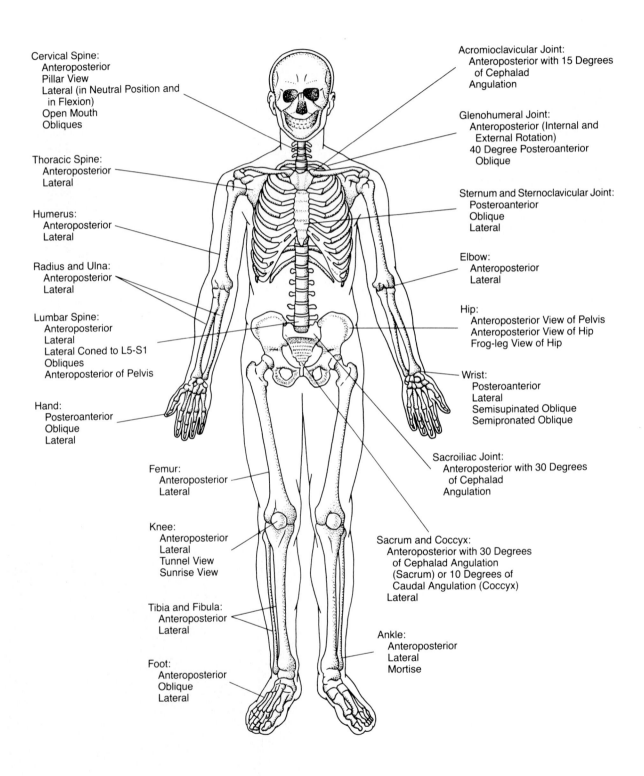

Cervical Spine:
Anteroposterior
Pillar View
Lateral (in Neutral Position and
in Flexion)
Open Mouth
Obliques

Thoracic Spine:
Anteroposterior
Lateral

Humerus:
Anteroposterior
Lateral

Radius and Ulna:
Anteroposterior
Lateral

Lumbar Spine:
Anteroposterior
Lateral
Lateral Coned to L5-S1
Obliques
Anteroposterior of Pelvis

Hand:
Posteroanterior
Oblique
Lateral

Femur:
Anteroposterior
Lateral

Knee:
Anteroposterior
Lateral
Tunnel View
Sunrise View

Tibia and Fibula:
Anteroposterior
Lateral

Foot:
Anteroposterior
Oblique
Lateral

Acromioclavicular Joint:
Anteroposterior with 15 Degrees
of Cephalad
Angulation

Glenohumeral Joint:
Anteroposterior (Internal and
External Rotation)
40 Degree Posteroanterior
Oblique

Sternum and Sternoclavicular Joint:
Posteroanterior
Oblique
Lateral

Elbow:
Anteroposterior
Lateral

Hip:
Anteroposterior View of Pelvis
Anteroposterior View of Hip
Frog-leg View of Hip

Wrist:
Posteroanterior
Lateral
Semisupinated Oblique
Semipronated Oblique

Sacroiliac Joint:
Anteroposterior with 30 Degrees
of Cephalad
Angulation

Sacrum and Coccyx:
Anteroposterior with 30 Degrees
of Cephalad Angulation
(Sacrum) or 10 Degrees of
Caudal Angulation (Coccyx)
Lateral

Ankle:
Anteroposterior
Lateral
Mortise

Table 3–1. SUGGESTED PROTOCOL FOR SURVEY RADIOGRAPHS IN ARTHRITIS

Hands and wrists	Posteroanterior
Shoulders	Anteroposterior, with external rotation
Feet	Anteroposterior
Ankles	Lateral, to include heel
Knees	Anteroposterior, with weight-bearing Lateral
Pelvis	Anteroposterior, to include hips
Cervical spine	Lateral, with neck flexion

excessive radiation exposure. A protocol for examining patients with polyarticular disease is given in Table 3–1.

These guidelines will require modifications depending on the specific diagnosis to be established and the clinical questions to be answered. Follow-up radiographic examinations in patients with widespread articular disorders need not be so extensive as the initial survey. Known target areas of the specific disorder and symptomatic sites should be examined.

Skeletal surveys in patients with neoplastic disease should not be performed before scintigraphic evaluation because of the greater sensitivity of the latter in detecting metastatic foci. Radiographs of only those areas found to be abnormal on bone scans should then be obtained. Exceptions to these rules occur in multiple myeloma, histiocytosis X, and neuroblastoma, which frequently yield false-negative results on radionuclide studies.

FURTHER READING

Clark KC: Positioning in Radiography. 8th Ed. New York, Grune & Stratton, 1964, p. 1.

Merrill V: Atlas of Roentgenographic Positions. Vol 1. 3rd Ed. St Louis, CV Mosby Co, 1967, p. 3.

Meschan I, Farrer-Meschan RMF: Radiographic Positioning and Related Anatomy. Philadelphia, WB Saunders Co, 1968, pp 29, 169.

Chapter 4

Plain Film Radiography: Sources of Diagnostic Errors

Theodore E. Keats, M.D.

Numerous types of anatomic alterations may complicate the interpretation of radiographs. Changes related to normal growth, developmental variations, and positioning artifacts are among the alterations that may simulate disease.

Examples described in this chapter include some of the more common entities and those that have the potential for harm if they are misinterpreted.

The radiographic examination is one of the most important means of diagnosis and differential diagnosis of skeletal disorders. This is particularly true because clinical and laboratory identification of the disease process and its differentiation from other disorders is often still difficult. Therefore, the physician should be aware of the many anatomic variants and radiographic pitfalls that may mislead when assessing the patient with skeletal complaints.

CERVICAL SPINE

Minor variations in configuration of the odontoid process (Fig. 4–1) may sometimes be confused with erosion and destruction of this process, a well-recognized characteristic of a number of inflammatory arthritides. Similarly, the apophyseal joints in the midcervical spine may not be well seen and may give the appearance of fusion, as a result of positioning of the spine and the direction of the x-ray beam (Fig. 4–2). The superior articular surfaces of the fifth to seventh cervical

vertebrae in some normal individuals may show a groove or depression (Fig. 4–3).

CLAVICLE AND RIBS

The point of insertion of the rhomboid ligament at the inferior aspect of the medial portion of the clavicle in some individuals is reflected as a deep and, at times, irregular fossa. The appearance of the normal medial ends of the clavicles in

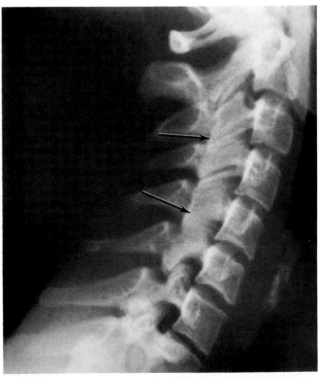

Figure 2–2. Simulated fusion of the posterior cervical elements produced by projection (arrows).

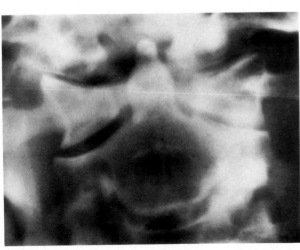

Figure 4–1. Normal pointed configuration of the odontoid tip.

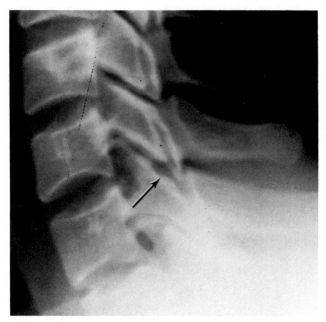

Figure 4–3. Normal notching of the apophyseal joint surface (arrow) of the lower cervical spine. This should not be mistaken for erosion or fracture.

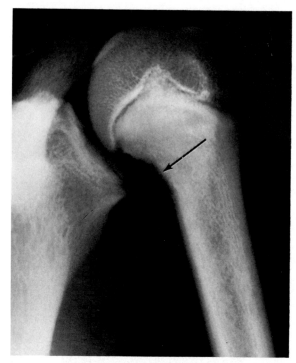

Figure 4–5. Upper humeral notch (arrow) in a 10 year old girl. This is seen between the ages of 10 and 16 years and represents a phase of growth.

adolescence (Fig. 4–4) provides a potential pitfall in the radiologic search for evidence of arthritis.

UPPER EXTREMITY

Notches or shallow grooves in the medial cortex of the metaphysis of the proximal end of the humerus occur as a normal variant in children between the ages of 10 and 16 years (Fig. 4–5). They are asymptomatic and apparently represent a transient event in the growth period. The greater tuberosity of the humerus in some persons contains a large amount of cancellous bone, which projects on the radiograph as a circumscribed area of radiolucency (pseudocyst) that may simulate a destructive lesion (Fig. 4–6). The thin flanges of bone that serve as the attachment of the interosseous membrane in the forearm may be mistaken for abnormal periostitis (Fig. 4–7).

The triangular cartilage of the wrist just distal to the end of the ulna frequently is a site of abnormal calcification. An

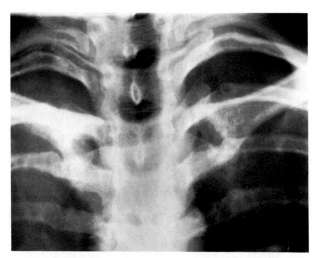

Figure 4–4. Plain film of normal irregularity of the medial ends of the clavicles of an adolescent before development of the secondary ossification centers.

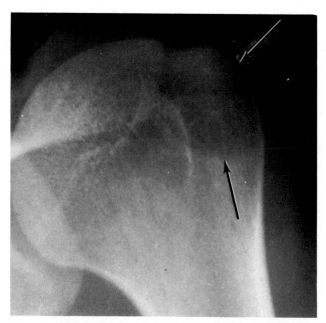

Figure 4–6. Simulated destruction of the greater tuberosity. This normal finding (arrows) appears to represent the fusion line of the lateral portion of the physis.

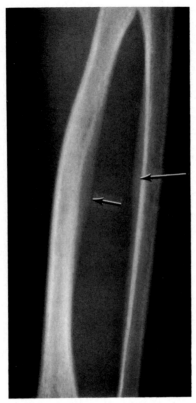

Figure 4–7. Normal bony flanges for the insertion of the interosseous membrane. These may simulate new bone formation (arrows).

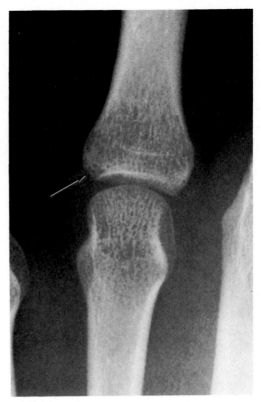

Figure 4–9. Small notches at the bases of the proximal phalanges (arrow). These should not be mistaken for the erosions of inflammatory arthritis, which usually first involve the heads of the metacarpal bones.

accessory bone, the os triangulare, may be found in this position as well (Fig. 4–8).

Common sources of confusion in the early diagnosis of rheumatoid arthritis are apparent small defects in the bases of the proximal phalanges (Fig. 4–9). These can be disre-

garded if there are no associated erosions in the metacarpal heads or disturbances in joint architecture.

The nutrient canals of the distal ends of the proximal phalanges may be quite prominent and cast shadows that simulate areas of intraosseous bone destruction (Fig. 4–10).

The bone ridges and projections seen in the proximal phalanges, which represent areas of insertion of muscles, should not be confused with reactive new bone formation (Fig. 4–11).

PELVIS

The appearance of the sacroiliac joints in adolescents bears a distinct resemblance to the changes of ankylosing spondylitis (Fig. 4–12).

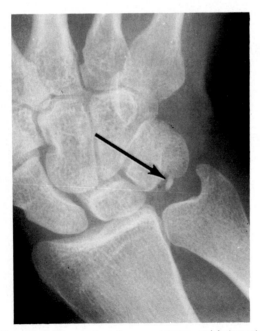

Figure 4–8. The os triangulare, an accessory ossicle (arrow).

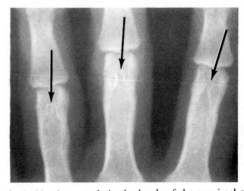

Figure 4–10. Nutrient canals in the heads of the proximal phalanges (arrows).

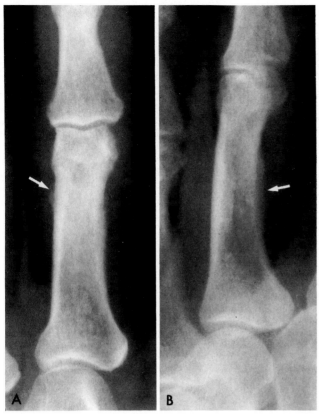

Figure 4–11. Normal ridges and projections on the phalanges associated with muscular insertions. These findings are not to be mistaken for periosteal new bone (arrows).

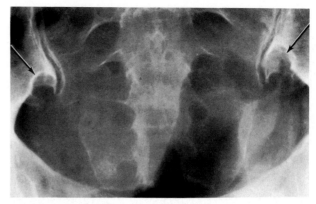

Figure 4–13. Preauricular sulci (arrows). This is a characteristic of the female pelvis and is not necessarily bilaterally symmetric.

The preauricular sulci are anatomic variants evident as fossae in the ilia adjacent to the inferior margins of the sacroiliac joint (Fig. 4–13). They are seen only in women and should not be confused with areas of bone destruction.

In the aged, the bone of the brim of the pelvis often appears laminated and thickened, an appearance that may be confused with Paget's disease (Fig. 4–14).

The normal ischiopubic synchondroses are a source of confusion, as they often appear as swollen, radiolucent areas in young children (Fig. 4–15). This is a normal phenomenon of growth and not evidence of disease.

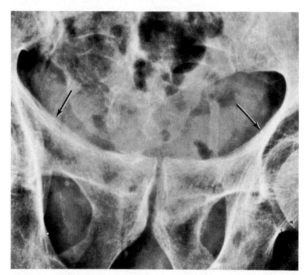

Figure 4–14. Aging changes in the iliopectineal line, which may simulate Paget's disease (arrows).

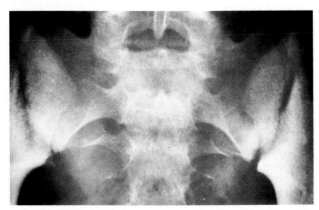

Figure 4–12. Normal sclerosis and irregularity of the sacroiliac joints in a 14 year old boy. These findings resemble the changes of ankylosing spondylitis.

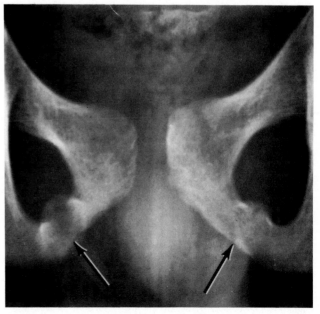

Figure 4–15. Normal ischiopubic synchondroses in a 4 year old boy (arrows).

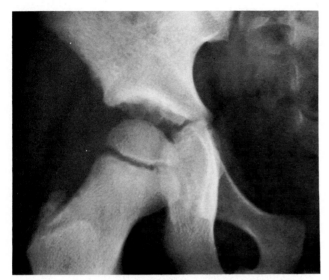

Figure 4–16. Normal irregularity of the acetabular roof in a 5½ year old child.

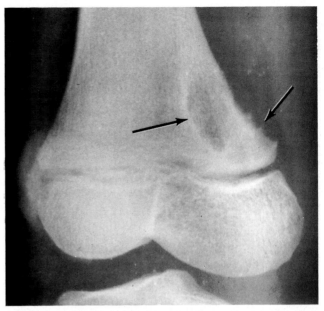

Figure 4–19. Irregularity of the cortex of the medial aspect of the distal femoral metaphysis (arrows). Such irregularity is a common finding between the ages of 12 and 16 years. This is a fibrous lesion, which often demonstrates fine perpendicular spiculation of bone and which may be mistaken for a malignant bone neoplasm.

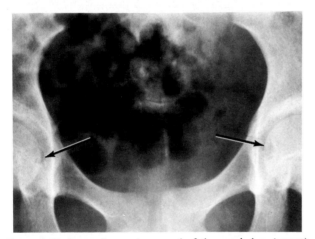

Figure 4–17. Fossae for nutrient vessel of the acetabulum (arrows). This finding may simulate a destructive lesion in the left femoral head owing to overlap of osseous structures.

HIP

The capital femoral epiphysis may ossify from multiple centers rather than from a single center. In like fashion, the roofs of the acetabula in young children are often grossly irregular, representing areas of ossification in the cartilaginous matrix (Fig. 4–16).

The fossae for the nutrient vessels in the acetabulum may be mistaken for a destructive lesion in the femoral head if they are fully superimposed on the head (Fig. 4–17). Additional spurious shadows in the acetabulum may be produced by an undulation in the anterior margin of the acetabulum coupled with superimposition of the shadow of the ischium

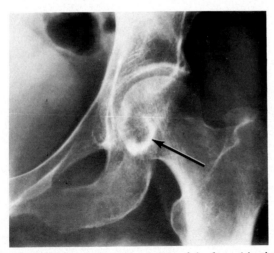

Figure 4–18. Simulated destructive lesions of the femoral head produced by a bony strut in the posterior wall of the acetabulum projected through the femoral head (arrow).

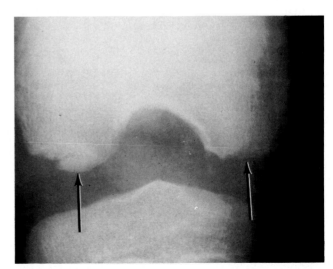

Figure 4–20. Normal irregularity of ossification of the articular surfaces of the distal femur in a 10 year old boy, simulating osteochondritis dissecans (arrows).

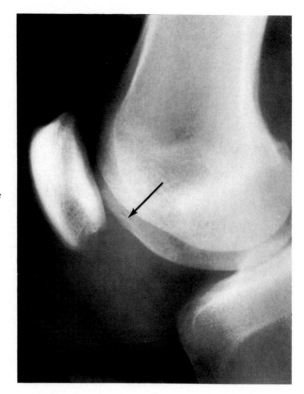

Figure 4–21. Normal depression of the articular surface of the medial condyle of the femur (arrow). A similar groove is evident in the lateral femoral condyle.

or superimposition of bone shadows of the posterior wall of the acetabulum projected through the femoral head (Fig. 4–18).

LOWER EXTREMITY

Several somewhat striking cortical irregularities are seen in the distal femoral metaphysis in adolescent children, which may cause needless concern and investigation. One of these is seen in the lateral projection in the anterior cortex and the others in the posterior cortex on the medial side (Fig. 4–19).

The distal articular surface of the femur in young children is grossly irregular radiologically, representing islands of ossification in the cartilaginous epiphysis (Fig. 4–20). These irregularities are best seen from the ages of 6 to 12 years. They can be differentiated from osteochondritis dissecans by their occurrence in a younger age group and by their appearance in areas of the condyles that are not usually involved in osteochondritis dissecans.

In adults, grooves may be seen in the articular surface of the medial and lateral femoral condyles in the lateral projection of the knee (Fig. 4–21).

A circumscribed radiolucent defect may be seen in the dorsal aspect of the patella in young people, usually as an incidental finding (Fig. 4–22). It is not a manifestation of

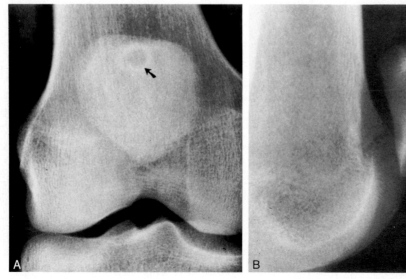

Figure 4–22. The dorsal patellar defect. These radiolucent shadows (arrows) are of no clinical significance and should not be confused with osteochondritis dissecans of the patella.

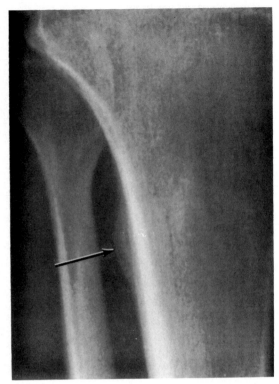

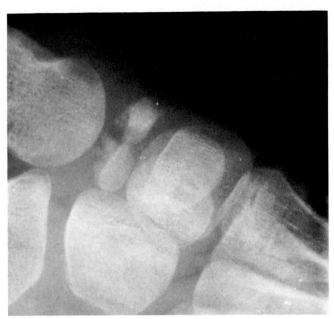

Figure 4–25. Normal developmental irregularity of the tarsal navicular bone in a 6 year old boy.

Figure 4–23. The tibial tubercle simulating laminated periostitis (arrow).

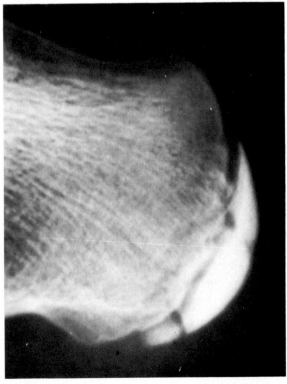

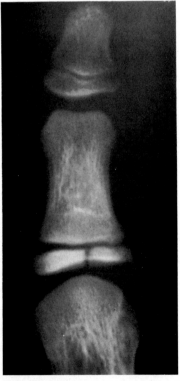

Figure 4–24. Normal density and "fragmentation" of the calcaneal apophysis.

Figure 4–26. Dense ossification center at the base of the proximal phalanx of the great toe. Such a finding, with or without a midline cleft, is a normal variation of growth.

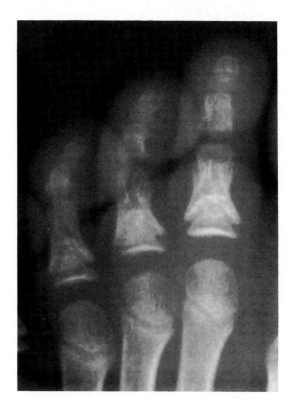

Figure 4–27. Cone-shaped epiphyses at the bases of the proximal phalanges. These may occur in normal children and are unrelated to any skeletal dysplasia or arthropathy.

osteochondritis dissecans of the patella. The lateral aspect of the tibial tubercle in the adult may be seen in the frontal projection as a laminated-appearing mass on the lateral aspect of the tibia and may be confused with a lesion producing new bone (Fig. 4–23).

The ossification of the calcaneal apophysis is associated with two troublesome radiologic aspects. It is normally dense in children who walk, and it also may develop from multiple centers (Fig. 4–24). Neither of these findings should be confused with ischemic necrosis or osteochondritis. Similar irregularities in ossification without increased density may be seen in the tarsal navicular bones (Fig. 4–25). These centers invariably unite and form a single bone. In the stage of

irregular ossification, the lack of sclerosis will differentiate this normal finding from osteochondritis (Köhler's disease).

The ossification center of the base of the proximal phalanx of the great toe is similar to the calcaneal apophysis in that it is usually dense and may occasionally be bifid (Fig. 4–26).

Cone-shaped epiphyses are seen in the proximal phalanges in many normal children and are not necessarily expressions of generalized or local disease (Fig. 4–27).

Many normal individuals do not develop distal interphalangeal joints in their toes. This is most commonly seen in the fifth toe but may also occur in the third and fourth toes.

FURTHER READING

Keats TE: An Atlas of Normal Roentgen Variants that May Simulate Disease. 3rd Ed. Chicago, Year Book Medical Publishers, 1984.
Köhler A, Zimmer EA: Borderlands of the Normal and Early Pathologic in Skeletal Roentgenology. 11th Ed. New York, Grune & Stratton, 1968.

I wish to express my appreciation to the Year Book Medical Publishers for permission to reproduce material from my book, An Atlas of Normal Roentgen Variants that May Simulate Disease. Copyright © 1973, 1978, and 1984 by Year Book Medical Publishers, Inc., Chicago.

Chapter 5

Fluoroscopy

Donald Resnick, M.D.

Fluoroscopy is helpful in the evaluation of a number of musculoskeletal problems. Although the technique commonly is combined with other diagnostic methods, such as arthrography, myelography, and angiography, it also represents an important independent means of supplementing nondiagnostic or equivocal routine radiographs, saving considerable time and effort, and lessening the radiation dose to the patient.

Fluoroscopy is a diagnostic tool that is a fundamental part of many radiologic procedures, including barium studies of the gastrointestinal tract and angiography. Fluoroscopic guidance is a prerequisite for arthrography, tenography, bursography, sinography, myelography, and biopsy procedures (Chapters 13, 14 and 17); consequently it finds considerable application in evaluation of musculoskeletal disorders. A number of orthopedic and neurosurgical procedures, such as insertion of dynamic hip screws, Kuntscher rods, and Ender nails, are best accomplished with fluoroscopic guidance. Additional applications of fluoroscopy to the assessment of musculoskeletal disease are less well known. Many of these are described in appropriate sections of this book, but a few of particular importance are summarized here (Table 5–1).

NORMAL AND ABNORMAL JOINT MOTION

Fluoroscopy with videotaping (or cineradiography) is useful in the evaluation of joint movement. Careful monitoring of vertebral position during flexion, extension, and lateral bending provides information defining the presence and level of spinal instability; abnormal findings include abrupt or "jerky" movement of one vertebra with respect to its neighbors and asymmetric widening of apophyseal joints. The instability is further confirmed by the identification of secondary signs, such as narrowing of the intervertebral disc space, vacuum phenomena, and traction spurs or osteophytes at the discovertebral junction.

The kinematics of the wrist are complex, yet when alterations occur in the normal integrated function of the carpal bones, significant symptoms and signs arise. Conventional plain radiographs, even when obtained as static images in positions of flexion, extension, and radial and ulnar deviation, may not indicate the source of the clinical manifestations. The analysis of wrist motion is better accomplished using either (1) fluoroscopy with spot filming or videotaping, or (2) cineradiography, sometimes in combination with arthrography.

Fluoroscopic monitoring and spot filming while stress is applied by the examiner may provide important diagnostic information in cases of posttraumatic instability in many other sites. Examples include injuries of the cruciate ligaments of the knee, medial and lateral ligaments of the ankle, and acromioclavicular and coracoclavicular ligaments.

FRACTURES

The conventional radiograph remains the most important means of identifying fractures initially after trauma. When the initial radiographs are equivocal, most physicians suggest that additional radiographic projections be used. This approach is time-consuming and commonly unsatisfactory. Fluoroscopy with spot filming represents a more successful approach to this diagnostic problem. The patient can be evaluated in multiple positions until the optimal projection is identified and the findings are recorded on the film.

OSTEOCHONDRITIS DISSECANS

The adequate evaluation of curved and angular bone contours is especially difficult with routine radiography. As these sites are not uncommonly involved in osteochondritis dissecans, it is not surprising that fluoroscopy aids in the assessment of this injury. This technique is particularly important in evaluating osteochondral fractures of the talar dome, as they may not be projected in a tangential fashion on the conventional radiographs (Fig. 5–1).

INTRAARTICULAR OSTEOCHONDRAL BODIES

Fluoroscopy with or without the instillation of contrast material or air into the joint represents an important procedure in identifying intraarticular osteochondral fragments or bodies. The precise position of the radiodense fragment with respect to the articular cavity is evident during the procedure, and additional bodies not seen on the conventional radiographs may be detected.

Table 5–1. SOME INDICATIONS FOR FLUOROSCOPY

Guidance in arthrography, sinography, myelography, and other diagnostic procedures
Assistance in orthopedic and neurosurgical procedures
Evaluation of normal and abnormal joint motion
Assessment of osteochondritis dissecans
Identification of intraarticular osteochondral bodies
Evaluation of shoulder impingement syndrome
Detection of foreign bodies
Assessment of orthopedic appliances

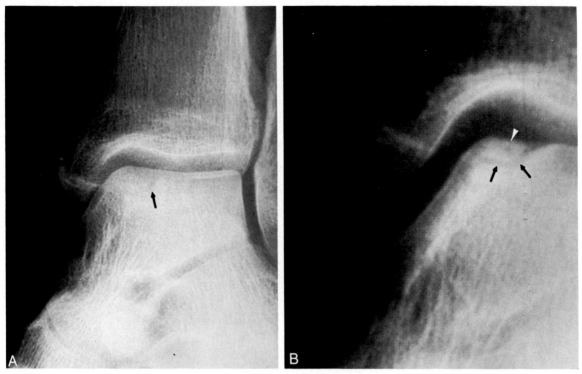

Figure 5–1. Fluoroscopy: Osteochondritis dissecans of the talus. A The initial radiograph shows an area of radiolucency in the superomedial portion of the talus (arrow). **B** A fluoroscopic spot film, accomplished with the patient in an oblique position and with plantar flexion of the foot, reveals a depression of the articular surface (arrows) containing an osseous body (arrowhead).

SHOULDER IMPINGEMENT SYNDROME

The shoulder impingement syndrome is an important source of shoulder pain that occurs when the bone and soft tissue structures of the superior aspect of the shoulder are encroached upon by the coracoacromial ligamentous arch during abduction of the arm. Although the clinical examination commonly is diagnostic, evidence supporting the shoulder impingement syndrome is provided by routine radiography that indicates osseous excrescences (subacromial

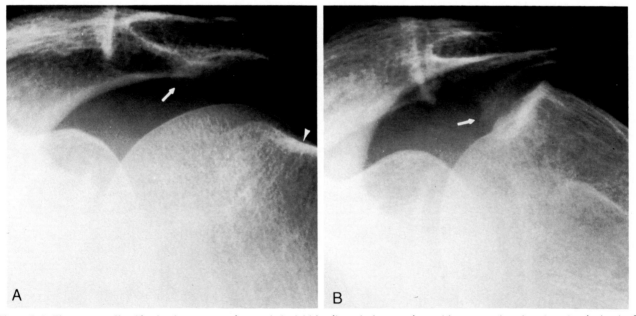

Figure 5–2. Fluoroscopy: Shoulder impingement syndrome. A An initial radiograph shows a subacromial spur or enthesophyte (arrow) and sclerosis of the greater tuberosity (arrowhead). **B** With fluoroscopy, the abnormal contact of the spur (arrow) and the sclerotic and flattened greater tuberosity as the patient abducts the arm is readily apparent.

spurs) arising from the anteroinferior aspect of the acromion and flattening and sclerosis of the greater tuberosity of the humerus. Fluoroscopic examination reveals bone contact between the greater tuberosity and the subacromial spur during abduction of the arm (Fig. 5–2) or close approximation of this tuberosity and the acromion during abduction at a time when the patient experiences typical pain and restriction of motion.

ORTHOPEDIC APPLIANCES

Metal contained in orthopedic appliances creates diagnostic problems during conventional radiography by obscuring adjacent osseous and soft tissue structures. Fluoroscopy allows the examiner to carefully choose an appropriate patient position in which obscurity is less prominent. It also promotes the examination of the orthopedic device itself, defining its relationship to the adjacent bone and joint.

FOREIGN BODIES

Detecting and locating foreign bodies in the soft tissues with conventional radiography can be extremely difficult. Clarifying their presence and location is better accomplished with fluoroscopy.

FURTHER READING

Arkless R: Cineradiography in normal and abnormal wrists. AJR 96:837, 1966.

Choplin RH, Gilula LA, Murphy WA: Fluoroscopic evaluation of skeletal problems. Skel Radiol 7:191, 1981.

Hudson TM: Joint fluoroscopy before arthrography: Detection and evaluation of loose bodies. Skel Radiol 12:199, 1984.

Protas JM, Jackson WT: Evaluating carpal instabilities with fluoroscopy. AJR 135:137, 1980.

Puhl RW, Altman MI, Seto JE, Nelson GA: The use of fluoroscopy in the detection and excision of foreign bodies in the foot. J Am Podiatry Assoc 73:514, 1983.

Chapter 6

Magnification Radiography

Harry K. Genant, M.D.
Donald Resnick, M.D.

For most areas in which magnification (optical or geometric) proves useful, subtle abnormalities of clinical importance are present at bone surfaces or at host-lesion interfaces. This is particularly true for arthritis and metabolic and infectious disorders of bone. In additional instances, serial assessment of the progression of disease or its response to therapy is enhanced by magnification. When gross abnormalities are present, as in most instances of trauma and bone dysplasia, the findings are obvious on conventional radiography, and magnification is not necessary.

Dosimetry measurements show that relatively high radiation doses result from magnification techniques. For this reason and because of the somewhat greater technical difficulty of performing the examination, magnification is recommended as a selective procedure. When employed selectively, magnification radiography may be an important tool in the diagnostic study of skeletal diseases.

Magnification techniques have received increased attention for skeletal radiography and in recent years have been widely applied. High-resolution magnification is achieved by two different techniques. The first is optical magnification of fine-grain films, and the second is direct radiographic magnification. The *optical magnification* technique consists of contact exposures obtained with conventional x-ray equipment and fine-grain industrial films, such as Kodak Type M. The resultant image is viewed with optical enlargement. *Direct radiographic magnification* for skeletal radiography has received less attention. Only with the development of x-ray tubes having small focal spots (100 to 150 μm) and adequate output for clinical examination has this technique become available.

Table 6–1 compares the relative clinical value of magnification with conventional radiography for skeletal applications.

RADIOGRAPHIC TECHNIQUES
Optical Magnification

The standard technique for optical magnification employs Kodak industrial Type M film, which is exposed with approximately 50 to 60 kVp and 500 mA for 0.5 s at 100 cm focus-film distance. A conventional x-ray tube with a 1.2 mm focal spot is used for these contact exposures, and the inherent magnification for thin parts is low (approximately 1.01 to 1.04 times). The industrial film must be developed manually or by means of an industrial processor. The completed industrial radiograph is surveyed without magnification initially, then viewed with a hand lens or a projector for optical magnification (Fig. 6–1). Radiation exposure is high.

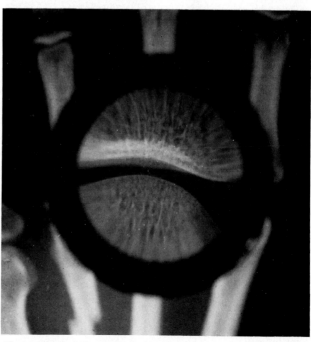

Figure 6–1. Optical magnification. A loupe or hand lens is placed in direct contact with the fine-grain industrial film and the image is viewed at close range.

Table 6–1. RELATIVE VALUE OF MAGNIFICATION

Disorder	Not Helpful	Helpful	Essential
Trauma	X	X	
Dysplasia	X		
Arthritis		X	X
Metabolic Disorders		X	X
Infection		X	X
Neoplasm	X	X	

For this reason, the industrial film with optical magnification should be used selectively in those instances in which delineation of subtle abnormalities in the peripheral skeleton is important.

Radiographic Magnification

For thicker body parts than those of the peripheral skeleton, the optical magnification technique becomes less feasible. The limitations are attributed to the high radiation exposure that is required and the degradation of image quality related to increased geometric unsharpness, blurring by motion, and scattered radiation. Direct radiographic magnification with a microfocus x-ray tube provides a reasonable alternative.

In radiographic magnification, a screen-film system and geometric enlargement of two to four times are employed in conjunction with a microfocus x-ray tube having a nominal focal spot size of 100 μm (Fig. 6–2). This technique may overcome some of the limitations of optical magnification, including the high radiation dose to the patient and the special viewing procedure required.

Technical advantages exist that improve the quality of the radiographic image obtained. The potential disadvantages of radiographic magnification result from the following: (1) the size of the body part examined is limited to small areas; (2) the proper positioning of the area with the lesion may be

difficult; and (3) the skin dose is high compared to that with the conventional screen-film technique, although it is low compared to that with Type M film and optical magnification.

Despite its excellent imaging characteristics, direct radiographic magnification, like optical magnification, should be used selectively because of its potentially high radiation exposure. Magnification results in an approximately fourfold increase in exposure per surface area (skin dose) compared with conventional techniques when recording-system speeds, air-gap, and grid are considered. The size of the field with magnification is significantly reduced, however, which helps lower the total body radiation to a level nearly equivalent to that of conventional techniques.

A variety of experimental and, now, commercially available screen-film systems have been used for direct magnification to help reduce radiation exposure. Most of these consist of rare-earth screen-film systems that have high photon-absorption efficiency and high light-conversion efficiency, thus providing an approximately 50 per cent reduction in exposure compared with conventional calcium-tungstate screens. For thin anatomic parts, single-emulsion, single-screen systems are often used, whereas for thicker anatomic parts, double-screen, double-emulsion systems are used.

CLINICAL APPLICATIONS OF MAGNIFICATION RADIOGRAPHY

Many different categories of clinical disorders have been studied with magnification radiography, among them rheumatoid arthritis, hyperparathyroidism, and infectious disease.

Articular Disorders

RHEUMATOID ARTHRITIS. The largest area of clinical application for high-resolution skeletal radiography has been the assessment of rheumatoid arthritis. The results have demonstrated conclusively that fine-detail radiography is more sensitive than conventional radiography for the detection and evaluation of erosive disease in early rheumatoid arthritis. With magnification techniques, erosive changes are easily identified as a sawtooth or a "dot-dash" appearance in the metacarpal head (Fig. 6–3), and ulnar styloid (Fig. 6–4).

The detection of soft tissue swelling is also improved by the high contrast of fine-detail radiography, primarily because of enhanced visualization of subtle changes such as capsular distention and obliteration of normal fat planes. Such changes are most easily identified at the proximal interphalangeal joints, at the first metacarpophalangeal joint, and over the ulnar styloid process.

OTHER ARTHRITIDES. Magnification radiography may be helpful not only in detecting erosive disease but also in characterizing and differentiating the appearances of various joint afflictions. For example, the erosions seen in psoriatic arthritis, Reiter's syndrome, and the other HLA B-27 associated arthritides are characterized by bone proliferation, producing a fluffy appearance in juxtaarticular regions as well as a linear periosteal new bone response in the adjacent shafts of bones (Fig. 6–5). This appearance is distinct from the typical erosions seen in rheumatoid arthritis. Another form of arthritis, calcium pyrophosphate dihydrate crystal deposition disease, is characterized radiographically by chondrocalcinosis, which corresponds to intraarticular deposition of calcium pyrophosphate dihydrate crystals. When subtle, the

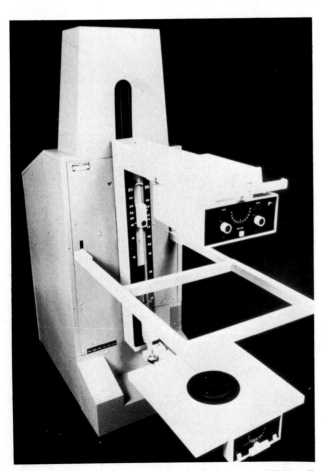

Figure 6–2. The most widely used magnification system, the RSI Mag. II.

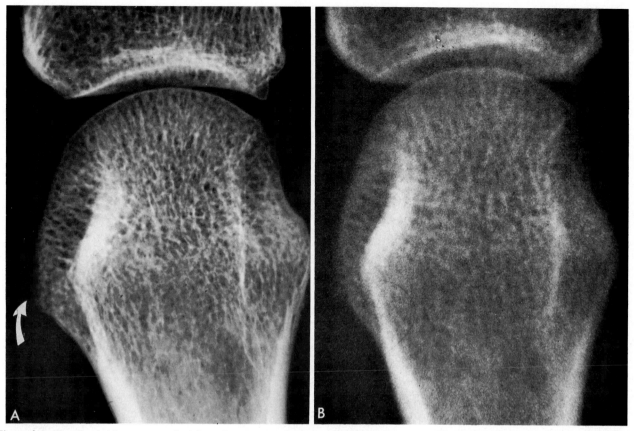

Figure 6–3. The "dot-dash" appearance of subtle surface erosion (arrow) is identified clearly with fine-detail radiography (**A**), but not with conventional radiography (**B**).

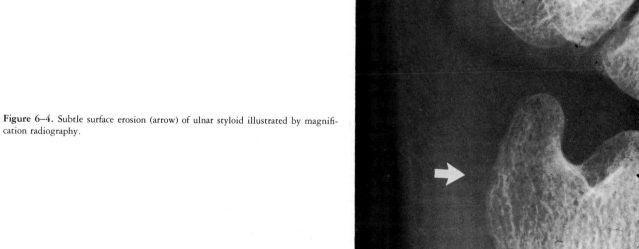

Figure 6–4. Subtle surface erosion (arrow) of ulnar styloid illustrated by magnification radiography.

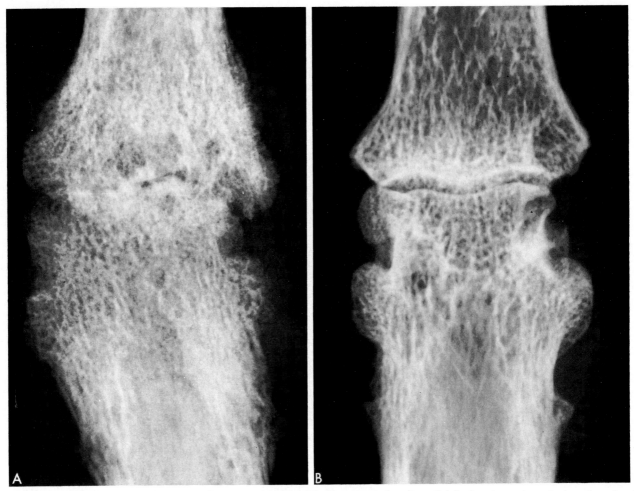

Figure 6–5. Proliferative erosions and periostitis of psoriatic arthritis (**A**) differ in appearance from the well-defined erosions and reactive bone formation of gouty arthritis (**B**).

fine linear and punctate calcifications in the hyaline cartilage and fibrocartilage may be detected only with high resolution magnification techniques (Fig. 6–6). Advanced articular calcification is easily recognized with conventional radiographic techniques.

Metabolic Disorders

HYPERPARATHYROIDISM. The radiographic assessment of osseous changes in hyperparathyroidism has undergone substantial modification in recent years. The classic findings of advanced hyperparathyroid skeletal disease, with striking cortical erosions and cystic brown tumors, are rarely seen today. This change probably reflects the earlier stage of detection and the greater preponderance of benign chemical hyperparathyroidism. Minor degrees of subperiosteal resorption in the phalanges of the hand, therefore, may be the only skeletal indicator of the correct diagnosis. For this reason, high resolution radiographic techniques have been introduced to detect subtle resorptive changes in the peripheral skeleton.

Figure 6–7 shows a phalanx of a hyperparathyroid patient radiographed with fine-detail and conventional techniques. The fine-detail radiograph shows the minute skeletal structure and demonstrates clearly the irregular resorption of the outer cortical margins that is pathognomonic of hyperparathyroidism. Even with high resolution techniques, such *subperiosteal*

bone resorption is being detected uncommonly in primary hyperparathyroidism while being encountered frequently in secondary hyperparathyroidism accompanying renal osteodystrophy (Fig. 6–8). When subperiosteal bone resorption becomes advanced, high resolution radiographic techniques are not necessary for detection. For monitoring the course of the disease or the response to therapy, magnification may be helpful, however.

The second finding in hyperparathyroidism is *cortical striation or tunneling* (Fig. 6–9). It corresponds histologically to widened haversian systems and resorptive spaces that result from excessive bone resorption in the hyperparathyroid state, and it is detected only on fine-detail radiographs unless extremely advanced. Excessive cortical striation on fine-detail radiographs may be considered a sensitive manifestation in the detection of hyperparathyroidism. It is not a specific change, however, because it occurs in a variety of conditions with high bone turnover, such as renal osteodystrophy, thyrotoxicosis, immobilization, reflex sympathetic dystrophy, osteomalacia, and rheumatoid arthritis.

Infectious Disorders

The diagnosis of osteomyelitis or septic arthritis is generally made on the basis of clinical symptoms and findings because conventional radiography demonstrates characteristic features

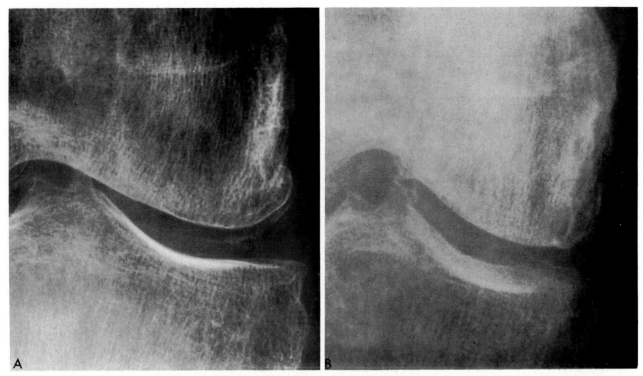

Figure 6–6. Magnification (**A**) and conventional (**B**) views of the knee in a patient with pseudogout. Magnification view clearly shows fine linear calcification of the hyaline cartilage and fibrocartilage, diagnostic of calcium pyrophosphate dihydrate crystal deposition disease. The conventional radiograph fails to reveal definite chondrocalcinosis.

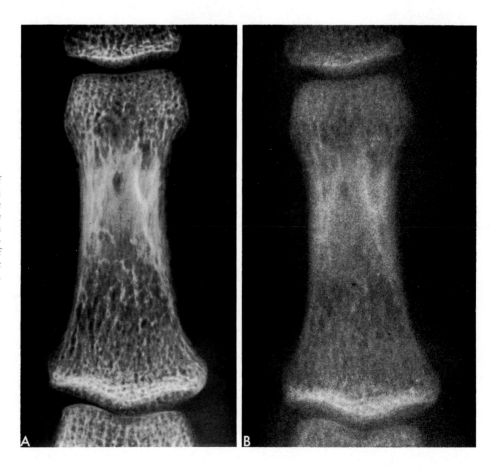

Figure 6–7. Radiograph of a phalanx of a hyperparathyroid patient. Type M film (**A**) shows the irregular resorption of the outer cortical margin not detected in the detail screen-film system (**B**). (From Genant HK, et al: Primary hyperparathyroidism: Comprehensive study of clinical, biochemical and radiographic manifestations. Radiology 109:513, 1973. Used with permission.)

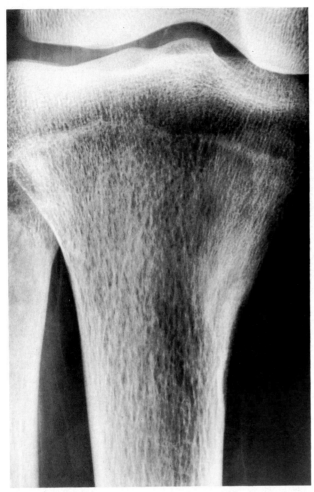

Figure 6–8. Magnification radiograph of a knee of a child with chronic renal disease demonstrates definite subperiosteal resorption of the proximal medial metaphysis of the tibia, as well as mild osteosclerosis of trabecular bone, nearly pathognomonic of renal osteodystrophy.

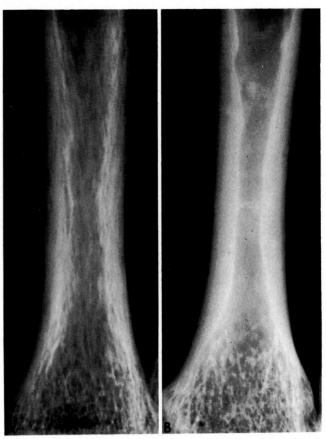

Figure 6–9. Radiographs of metacarpal bones of a hyperparathyroid (**A**) and of a normal (**B**) patient. Intracortical striation is excessive in **A**, compared with solid cortex in **B**. (From Genant HK, et al: Primary hyperparathyroidism: Comprehensive study of clinical, biochemical and radiographic manifestations. Radiology 109:513, 1973. Used with permission.)

only later in the course. Occasionally, however, magnification radiography may reveal subtle cortical destruction or periosteal new bone prior to its demonstration on conventional films. For example, a problem is frequently encountered in an elderly, osteoporotic patient who has ulceration of the soft tissues of the foot related to diabetes mellitus or arterial insufficiency (Fig. 6–10). The diagnostic problem is to determine whether or not there is underlying osteomyelitis. In this setting, conventional radiography often fails to visualize the bone margins adequately owing to the low inherent subject contrast of osteopenic bone. Magnification radiography, however, may clearly delineate the cortical margins and reveal irregular destruction of the outer cortical surfaces, thus permitting a specific diagnosis.

Figure 6–11 demonstrates a radiograph from an elderly man who has had pain in the region of the symphysis pubis for 2 months following a suprapubic prostatectomy. Magnification shows an irregular lysis of the subchondral bone, which indicates the aggressive nature of this process and supports a diagnosis of infectious osteitis pubis.

Neoplastic Disorders

Both primary and metastatic neoplasms of bone have been examined with magnification techniques. These examinations are largely of the thick skeletal parts, such as the ribs, pelvis, hips, spine, and femora, and, therefore, direct radiographic magnification is employed. In some applications, conventional radiographs appear normal or equivocal, and magnification serves to delineate permeative, lytic destruction or subtle periosteal reaction. In other instances, conventional radiography readily demonstrates the presence of the lesion; however, the character or pattern of host response or aggressiveness is best determined by magnification (Fig. 6–12). Frequently, direct magnification is initiated after a positive bone scan and conventional radiographs provide inconclusive results. Serial assessment of the progression of the neoplasm or the response to therapy is also improved by magnification.

Traumatic Disorders

Magnification radiography has had more limited application in the evaluation of trauma because the detection of fractures by conventional radiography generally is adequate. Occasionally, however, magnification radiography may be helpful in delineating and defining subtle fractures, especially in the ribs, carpal scaphoid, and femoral neck.

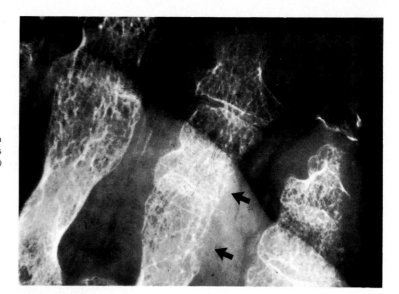

Figure 6–10. Distal aspect of foot of diabetic patient with suspected osteomyelitis. Cortical destruction of the lateral aspects of the middle and proximal phalanges of the fourth digit (arrows) is readily detected with the Type M technique.

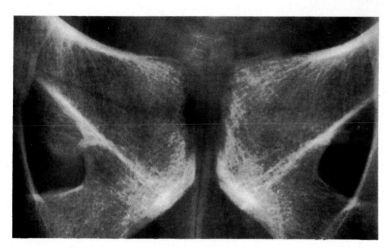

Figure 6–11. The magnification radiograph demonstrates widening of the symphysis pubis. The magnification study, in addition, shows irregular destruction of the subchondral cortical line, producing a ragged, lace-like appearance. These features indicate an aggressive, evolving process and support the diagnosis of infectious osteitis pubis. (From Genant HK, et al: Direct radiographic magnification for skeletal radiology. An assessment of image quality and clinical application. Radiology 123:47, 1977. Used with permission.)

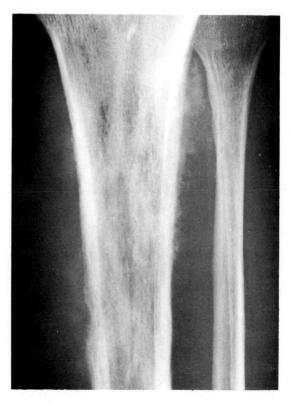

Figure 6–12. Radiograph of the proximal portion of the tibia shows metastatic transitional cell carcinoma of the bladder. The magnification view shows discrete lytic destruction throughout the cortex, with mild reactive sclerosis. Linear periosteal reaction along the medial cortex is seen, as well as cloud-like areas of heterotopic bone formation in the adjacent soft tissues medial and lateral to the tibia. (From Chinn D, et al: Heterotopic bone formation in metastatic tumor from transitional cell carcinoma of the urinary bladder: A case report. J Bone Joint Surg [Am] 58:881, 1976. Used with permission.)

Dysplasias

Magnification techniques have not been found useful in the majority of patients with bone dysplasias. The radiographic findings in these cases are generally advanced and encompass multiple foci and broad anatomic regions.

FURTHER READING

Doi K, Rossmann K: Measurements of optical and noise properties of screen-film systems in radiography. *In* Proceedings of the Symposium on Application of Optical Instrumentation in Medicine. Vol. 56. Bellingham, Washington, Society of Photo-Optical Instrumentation Engineers, 1975, p. 45.

Genant HK, Doi K: High-resolution skeletal radiography: Image quality and clinical applications. Curr Prob Diagn Radiol 7:3, 1978.

Genant HK, Doi K, Mall JC: Optical versus radiographic magnification for fine-detail skeletal radiography. Invest Radiol *10:*160, 1975.

Genant HK, Doi K, Mall JC, Sickles EA: Direct radiographic magnification for skeletal radiology. An assessment of image quality and clinical application. Radiology *123:*47, 1977.

Chapter 7

Low Kilovolt Radiography

Erich Fischer, M.D.

Because of the increase in contrast and resolution obtainable with low kilovolt (kV) radiography, many minute details of bones and soft tissues are clearly perceptible that would otherwise not be visible. These minute details often pertain to different tissues that are situated very close to each other. The number of structures observed is further increased because multiple views are frequently necessary. A magnifying glass is required to analyze the radiographic details in low kV radiography. This limits the field of vision and facilitates a systematic analysis of these detailed radiographic images.

The mammography technique, which uses a molybdenum target and filter and a voltage range between 28 and 35 kilovolts (kV), is also well suited to the extensive diagnostic evaluation of the extremities. The reduced penetration of this low energy x-ray spectrum and the increased radiation exposure restrict this technique to thinner body parts, mainly the hands and feet. Low kV radiography results in greater contrast between fat and water-equivalent tissues and between water-equivalent tissues and bone (calcium). It also allows more specific soft tissue diagnosis and more precise analysis of the margins and thinner portions of the bone. Although it reveals the soft tissues to some extent, conventional radiography lacks sensitivity in this regard.

Low kV radiography of the extremities requires meticulous technique that differs from conventional radiographic methods. For example, as the hand consists of two main parts, the fingers and the wrist, which vary considerably in thickness, delineation of both regions with low kV radiography requires precise radiation exposures as well as comprehensive radiographic projections.

For the hands and sometimes other regions, low kV radiography can be performed with routine mammography equipment. Immersing the hand and forearm (or the forefoot) in 70 per cent ethanol solution improves the resolution of skin and subcutaneous structures because the uniformly deep liquid layer equalizes the differences in thickness of the fingers. Xeroradiography is superior to low kV radiography because of its broad latitude in recording different densities and thicknesses, but important disadvantages of xeroradiography are edge enhancement (which may falsely provide sharp contours to contours that are not sharp) and a halo effect (in which small soft tissue shadows adjacent to bone may disappear).

SYNOPSIS OF SOFT TISSUE CHANGES

In the range of 28 to 35 kV, the following tissues are of "water density": skin, tendons, ligaments, tendon sheaths, joint capsules, muscles, blood vessels, and cartilage. Fatty tissue is interspersed with blood vessels and fine strands of connective tissue. Changes in any of these tissues are produced by numerous disorders.

Thickened Soft Tissues

The skin shows individual variations in thickness that are influenced by occupational stress and abnormal conditions, such as scars, edema, scleroderma, acromegaly, myxedema, Down's syndrome, pachydermoperiostosis, pachydermodactyly, and Fabry's disease. Thickening of tendons and ligaments occurs in rheumatoid arthritis, the seronegative spondyloarthropathies, stress related conditions, lipid storage diseases, gout, calcium hydroxyapatite crystal deposition disease, and amyloidosis.

Dilation of joint capsules may relate to the patient's age and gender, manual work, rheumatoid arthritis, the seronegative spondyloarthropathies, osteoarthritis, gout, amyloidosis, Fabry's disease, multicentric reticulohistiocytosis, and other conditions, such as multiple epiphyseal dysplasia.

Thinned Soft Tissues

Thinning related to atrophy can be demonstrated in the skin and muscles. In some cases, the reduced volume of an entire muscle or a portion of it will be partially compensated for by replacement with fatty tissue. In the metacarpal region, atrophy of muscle indicates long-standing reduced physical activity.

Hazy Soft Tissue Margins

Normally, most soft tissues of water density have distinct contours if they are located adjacent to a fatty layer of adequate thickness. A normal hazy margin results when the fatty layer is too thin or when the skin and the underlying synovial compartments are connected by locally increased strands of connective tissues. This often happens at both sides of the distal interphalangeal joints, the radial side of the second proximal interphalangeal and metacarpophalangeal joints, the medial side of the first metatarsophalangeal joint, the lateral side of the fifth metatarsophalangeal joint, and the outer side of the tendon sheaths along the radial and ulnar styloid processes. A pathologic hazy margin is caused by

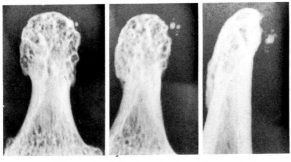

Figure 7–1. Subungual calcifications in the right second finger. The calcifications are better seen in the oblique view (radiograph in the center) and the lateral view (right), because in the posteroanterior view (left) they are covered by the ungual tufts. These subungual calcifications, which were also evident in other fingers, diminished during the following 7 months in this 58 year old woman whose nails were clinically normal. (From Fischer E: Subunguale Verkalkungen. ROFO 137:580, 1982. Used with permission.)

irritation of a synovial compartment or within the enveloping tissue of a tendon.

Increased Number and Thickness of Vessels

The vessels that are recognizable in areolar tissue are, for the most part, veins. Normally, there is marked symmetry in both the width and the number of subcutaneous veins. Inflammation leads to an increased local circulation, and resulting venous alterations can be detected with low kV radiography.

If the venous pattern in an individual finger is augmented, the radiologist should look for subtle changes of synovitis of the joints or tendon sheath of that finger. During acute phases of rheumatoid arthritis and related diseases, the veins about

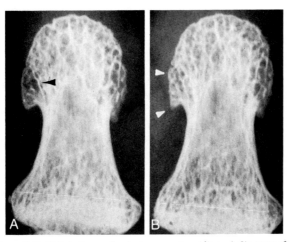

Figure 7–2. Tuftal abnormality in hyperparathyroidism. **A** Six years after the beginning of hemodialysis, note the submarginal localized resorption of trabeculae (arrowhead) and the small calcification at the medial side of the phalangeal base. **B** Three years after **A**, the segment of the ungual tuft between the arrowheads has been resorbed without interruption of the cortical line, and the formerly lost trabeculae in the adjacent area are recalcified. Note the resorption of the calcification at the phalangeal base and the partial loss of the adjacent bone without interruption of the cortical line. (From Fischer E: Die Enstehung von Erosionen am Fingerskelett bei der Auflösung periossärer Verkalkungen. ROFO 141:87, 1984. Used with permission.)

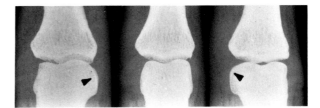

Figure 7–3. Early osteoarthritis. Three views of the right second proximal interphalangeal joint in a 41 year old woman. Shallow sclerotic appositions at the volar margins of the phalangeal head are visible only in the oblique views (left and right, arrowheads). The true posteroanterior view is shown in the center.

the wrist may become greatly dilated and tortuous. Reversal of these abnormal vascular patterns indicates a decrease in the extent of local inflammation.

Changes in Structure of Fine Connective Tissue

Normal fat contains a fine pattern of connective tissue that varies in length, width, direction, and quantity. Edema leads to widening and an increase in the number of thin strands of connective tissue. Furthermore, structures not normally seen will become visible when enlarged owing to edema or bleeding. Edematous fatty tissue increases the distance between

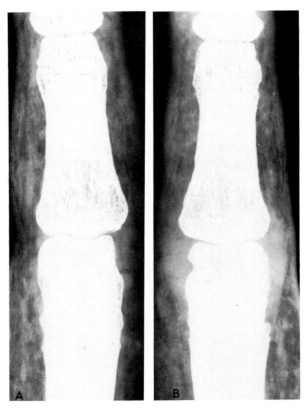

Figure 7–4. Rheumatoid arthritis with subcutaneous edema and moderate thickening of the veins. **A** The left index finger possesses a normal but slightly accentuated subcutaneous venous texture. **B** In the right index finger, moderate thickening of the veins, edema-induced unsharpness of soft tissue contours, and an augmented width of the areolar tissue related to an inflamed and dilated proximal interphalangeal joint capsule are seen. (From Fischer E: Die Weichteilveränderungen der Finger bei der rheumatischen Polyarthritis. Ergebnisse nach Weichstrahlaufnahmen in drei Ebenen. Radiologe 19:119, 1979. Used with permission.)

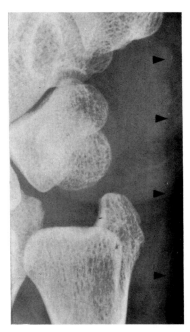

Figure 7–5. Ulnar aspect of the right wrist in rheumatoid arthritis. Substantial thickening of the entire tendon sheath of the extensor carpi ulnaris muscle with globular distention of its distal portion (arrowheads) is present.

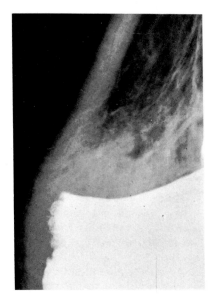

Figure 7–7. Retrocalcaneal bursitis in ankylosing spondylitis; 22 year old woman. Substantial destruction has taken place at the posterior margins of the calcaneal tubercle, and there is marked distention of the bursa proximally and substantial streaky edema proximal to the bursa.

the fascial layers and the muscles or skin, and such tissue becomes water-equivalent in density.

Soft Tissue Masses

Gouty tophi, rheumatoid nodules, and localized sacculations of synovial compartments (analogous to synovial cyst formation) are causes of such masses.

Calcifications and Opaque Foreign Bodies

As a consequence of the technical improvements in low kV radiography, minimal calcifications and opaque foreign bodies are easily recognizable. Beginning in the third decade of life, soft tissue calcifications may be seen; they are frequent, are diverse in shape and size, and, in many cases, may resolve spontaneously. Most often they occur in the ungual tufts, about surrounding joints (especially those of the fingers), and at the volar side of the pisiform bone.

Vascular calcifications are also common. As a rule, arterial calcifications occur at an earlier time in the feet than in the hands. When they occur in the metacarpal region they are usually a sign of severe generalized atherosclerosis.

Embedded foreign bodies, such as glass, wood chips, thorns, and plastic particles, are easily recognizable with low kV radiography because of their contact with fatty tissue.

CLINICAL EXAMPLES OF LOW kV RADIOGRAPHY

Examples of various alterations that are well shown by low kV radiography are illustrated in Figures 7–1 to 7–7.

FURTHER READING

Mäkelä P, Haaslahti JO: Immersion technique in soft tissue radiography. Acta Radiol (Diagn) 19:89, 1977.

Tabár L, Dean PB: Magnification immersion radiography: Better soft tissue visualisation in the hands. ROFO 136:444, 1982.

Tabár L, Dean PB, Mäkelä P, Virtana P: Magnification immersion radiography of the distal extremities. Appl Radiol, 1984, p 99.

Weston WJ, Palmer DG: Soft Tissues of the Extremities. A Radiologic Study of Rheumatic Disease. Berlin, Springer Verlag, 1978, pp. 13, 14.

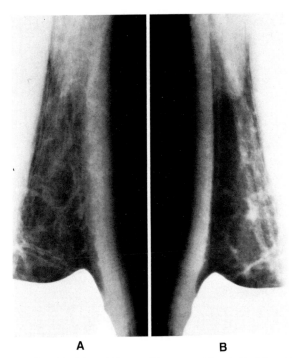

A   **B**

Figure 7–6. Ankle joint of 31 year old woman with painful right ankle after 4 weeks of strenuous gymnastic exercise. A Right ankle: Paratenonitis achillea owing to overstrain. Note moderate thickening and hazy and irregular anterior margin of the Achilles tendon with increased opacity of the preachilles fat pad owing to edema. B Normal left ankle of same patient for comparison. (From Fischer E: Weichteildiagnostic an den peripheren Extremitäten mittels Weichstrahltechnik. Radiologe 14:457, 1974. Used with permission.)

Chapter 8

Xeroradiography

Harry K. Genant, M.D.
Michael André, Ph.D.

The xeroradiographic imaging process differs considerably from conventional screen-film or non-screen radiography, having unique imaging characteristics of edge enhancement, subdued broad area response, and large object latitude. These features make the technique useful in selected cases for imaging low-contrast objects that are defined by sharp edges. Nevertheless, widespread acceptance and usage of xeroradiography for routine musculoskeletal examinations appear unlikely owing to the relatively high radiation exposure required and the comparatively limited availability of the system.

The image produced by xeroradiography is very different from that obtained by conventional film radiography. It is a completely dry process, requires no darkroom, and records the final image on paper. The exposure latitude is very wide compared to that for film; soft tissues and bone may be recorded with the same emphasis; the enhancement of edges gives the appearance of improved resolution; and either a positive or a negative recording mode may be selected.

TECHNICAL CONSIDERATIONS

Semiconductors have the ability to change from a material of high electrical resistance in the resting state to one of relatively low resistance when activated by radiant energy. This constitutes the fundamental principle on which the latent image in xeroradiography is based. The xeroradiographic plate on which the latent image forms has an aluminum base that is coated with a thin photoconductive layer of vitreous selenium. Selenium is a photoconductor that behaves as an insulator until it is exposed to a source of photons (light or x-ray). Although a number of semiconductors are available, selenium has been used most extensively.

Briefly, the steps in image production are as follows: The metal plate is charged to a high positive potential by coronal discharge; then it is placed in a light-tight cassette and used as an image receptor similar to a conventional screen-film system; when the x-rays strike the selenium plate, photoconduction occurs, reducing the electrical charge locally, and resulting in a latent charge image of the object; the latent image is made visible by the use of charged developer particles or toner particles, which are brought into close proximity to the plate; finally, the resultant powder image is transferred to a paper and fused thermally, providing a permanent opaque image.

The operator controls three steps in producing a xeroradiograph: (1) charging of the selenium plate, (2) amount of x-ray exposure, and (3) development of the image. The quality of the final image may be changed considerably by a variation in any of these steps. Two fundamental characteristics of this final image are edge enhancement and broad latitude (broad area contrast suppression). It is important to note that the amount of edge enhancement and the degree of broad area contrast suppression can be manipulated by appropriate selection of the kilovoltage for exposure, the amount of charge potential initially placed on the plate, and the level of back voltage applied during developing. The latter two steps

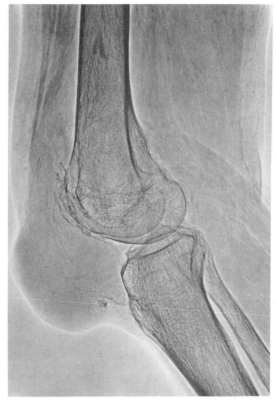

Figure 8–1. Xeroradiograph of the knee, which demonstrates an osteolytic process with a large soft tissue component that has replaced the patella. The edge enhancement and broad latitude of the xeroradiographic system can be appreciated.

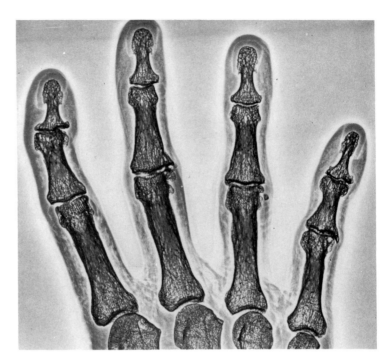

Figure 8–2. Xeroradiograph of the distal portion of the hand of a patient with primary generalized osteoarthritis. Articular and periarticular structures are well shown with the xeroradiographic technique.

provide added recording flexibility, which is not achievable with conventional radiography. Generally, a relatively high kilovoltage exposure (~ 120 kVp) is selected for musculoskeletal applications to increase the recording latitude and to diminish the excessive edge enhancement, which can produce a halo effect or toner deletion at the high contrast interfaces between bone and soft tissue. The sharpness or *spatial resolution* of the xeroradiographic system is high relative to conventional screen-film radiography but is less than that of nonscreen techniques using medical or industrial film. The mottle or *noise* of the xeroradiograph similarly falls between that of a conventional screen-film system and that of a nonscreen-film technique. As a result of these inherent image characteristics, a xeroradiograph may be optically magnified 1.5 to 2 times using a hand lens, and additional useful information may occasionally be derived.

As already noted, the *radiation exposure* required for xeroradiography is relatively high compared to that needed for conventional screen-film radiography, but it is lower than that for nonscreen industrial film. Typically skin doses of 0.3 to 2.0 centigrays (cGy)(rad) are needed for musculoskeletal applications, which generally limits the use of xeroradiography to the thinner body parts.

CLINICAL APPLICATIONS

Xeroradiography has not been widely employed as a recording medium for anatomic parts other than the breast. It appears, however, to have great potential in the depiction of *soft tissue masses* in an extremity or limb girdle (Fig. 8–1). This application, nonetheless, has rapidly been supplanted by computed tomography (see Chapter 10), which has far superior density resolution and the advantage of providing cross-

sectional display. Another area in which xeroradiography has found some success is in the depiction of subtle skeletal abnormalities in patients with early *arthritis* or *metabolic bone disease*. In the former situation the ability to show with a single radiographic exposure both the osseous structures of the joint and the periarticular soft tissues is a potential advantage (Fig. 8–2). It appears, however, that for this application, magnification techniques, either optical or radiographic, are more widely accepted, because they provide superior images. Similarly, in assessing subtle structural changes in the hands or feet in metabolic bone disease, xeroradiography, although superior to conventional screen-film radiography, is inferior to the alternative high-resolution magnification techniques.

In selected cases, xeroradiography has been shown to provide high-quality images of the *cervical spine* and *ribs*. In these cases xeroradiography can record many tissues of different density and thickness; for example, bone, fat, air, and muscle are readily delineated on a single image. Xeroradiography also has had some success in imaging the skeletal structures of an extremity that has been immobilized in a *plaster cast*. In this situation, the superimposition of structures and the broad range of subject density make visualization by conventional radiography difficult.

FURTHER READING

Otto RC, Pouliadis GP, Kumpe DA: The evaluation of pathologic alterations of juxtaosseous soft tissue by xeroradiography. Radiology *120:*297, 1976.

Wolfe JN: Xeroradiography of the bones, joints and soft tissues. Radiology *93:*583, 1969.

Wolfe JN: Xeroradiography: Image content and comparison with film roentgenograms. AJR *117:*690, 1973.

Chapter 9

Conventional Tomography

Donald Resnick, M.D.

Conventional tomography is a useful adjunct to plain film radiography, may compare favorably with computed tomography in the evaluation of certain musculoskeletal problems, *and should be used when standard and specialized views fail to provide needed information for correct diagnosis and adequate treatment.*

Conventional tomography is a technique whereby detailed images are obtained of structures lying in a predetermined tissue plane, at the same time blurring, or eliminating detail of other structures in other planes. This technique, once of significant use in evaluating musculoskeletal disorders, has to a large extent been superseded by computed tomography and magnetic resonance imaging. Nevertheless, important applications remain for the assessment of bone, joint, and soft tissue diseases (Table 9–1).

CLINICAL APPLICATIONS

Although many skeletal structures can be evaluated adequately with routine radiographs, others may be difficult to assess because of their size, their orientation within the body, or the presence of surrounding tissues. The vertebral column,

Table 9–1. SOME INDICATIONS FOR CONVENTIONAL TOMOGRAPHY

Evaluate structures not seen adequately with other methods
Detect and delineate fractures of the vertebral column, tibial plateau, femur, and carpal bones
Identify osteochondral defects
Evaluate fracture healing
Assess intraarticular and periarticular osseous bodies
Identify cortical disruption and sequestra in chronic osteomyelitis
Evaluate bone neoplasms

ribs, sternum, and sella turcica are examples of such structures. Certain joints likewise may be better visualized with conventional tomography, particularly the sternoclavicular (Fig. 9–1), temporomandibular, sacroiliac, costovertebral,

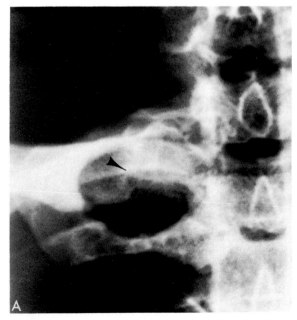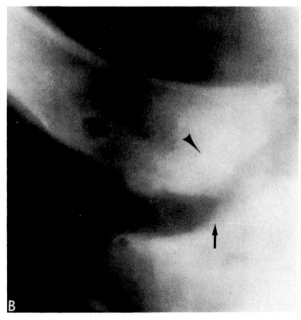

Figure 9–1. Sternoclavicular joint: Osteomyelitis and septic arthritis. A The initial radiograph outlines erosion and eburnation (arrowhead) of the medial aspect of the right clavicle. Sternal alterations are not well delineated. **B** Hypocycloidal tomography reveals considerable osseous erosion of both clavicle (arrowhead) and sternum (arrow). The extensive bony sclerosis, loss of articular space, and superior subluxation of the clavicle are readily apparent. Joint aspiration documented the presence of staphylococci.

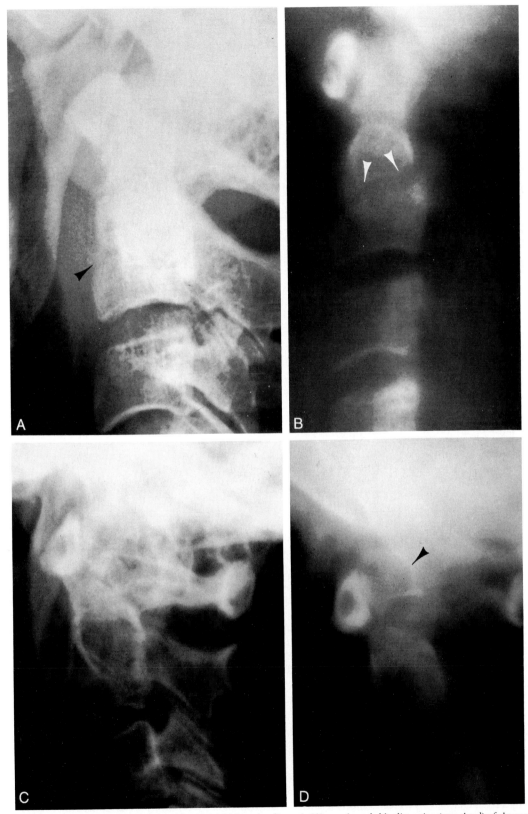

Figure 9–2. Spinal fractures. A, B Fracture of the axis. An initial lateral radiograph (**A**) reveals probable disruption (arrowhead) of the anterior surface of the vertebral body, but the fracture (arrowheads) is much better delineated with conventional tomography (**B**). **C, D** Fracture of the odontoid process (os odontoideum). Although the odontoid process appears abnormal in the routine radiograph (**C**), the characteristics of a separated tip of the odontoid process (arrowhead) and its relationship to the anterior arch of the atlas are better shown with conventional tomography (**D**). This condition results from a previous fracture rather than a congenital abnormality.

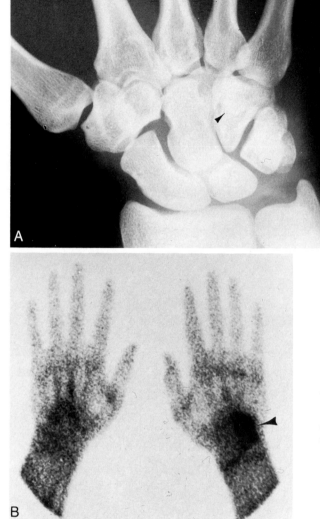

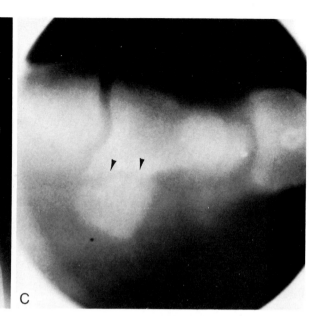

Figure 9–3. Fracture of the hook of the hamate. **A** The initial radiograph is essentially unremarkable. The hook of the hamate can be identified (arrowhead). **B** The bone scan reveals abnormal accumulation of the radionuclide in the region of the hamate (arrowhead). **C** A conventional lateral tomogram reveals the fracture site at the base of the hook of the hamate (arrowheads). Computed tomography is also well suited to the diagnosis of this injury. (Courtesy of V. Vint, M.D., San Diego, California.)

apophyseal, atlantooccipital, atlantoaxial, subtalar, and intertarsal joints.

The optimal patient position during conventional tomography can generally be ascertained from the plain films. In general, a frontal projection is most helpful in visualizing the sacrum and the sacroiliac and sternoclavicular joints; an oblique projection may be beneficial in evaluating the costovertebral and apophyseal joints; and both the frontal and lateral projections may be required to delineate the temporomandibular, atlantooccipital, atlantoaxial, and subtalar joints, as well as the vertebrae and sternum.

Certain problems are evaluated equally well or better with conventional tomography than with the more commonly used computed tomography. As an example, the imaging strategy used in computed tomography of the vertebral column employs transaxial sections, which are not ideal for visualizing alterations that lie in the transverse plane, such as pseudarthrosis after spinal fusion. Even though the computed tomographic image can be reconstructed in a coronal or sagittal

plane, information is lost. Conventional tomography is an important alternative in such instances and also can be used when it is necessary to image a long segment of a bone or bones because the lesion is extensive or because multiple lesions are present. Some clinical situations in which conventional tomography is of value are listed in Table 9–1.

Conventional tomography can be applied to skeletal trauma to detect vertebral column (Fig. 9–2), tibial plateau, and carpal (Fig. 9–3) and femoral fractures; to identify osteochondral defects (Fig. 9–4); and to evaluate fracture healing. Intraarticular or periarticular osseous bodies can be outlined with conventional tomography; intraarticular cartilaginous bodies may require arthrotomography, however. Conventional tomography can also be of benefit in evaluating patients with chronic osteomyelitis by identifying areas of cortical disruption and sequestra, findings that imply active disease. Conventional tomography of bone neoplasms may identify a nidus of an osteoid osteoma, matrix calcification in cartilaginous tumors, and soft tissue extension of malignant disease.

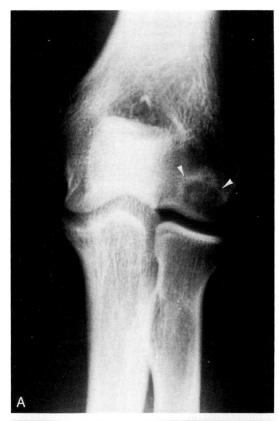

Figure 9–4. **Osteochondral fracture: Capitulum. A** In a 15 year old boy, the initial radiograph shows an osteolytic lesion with a sclerotic margin in the capitulum (arrowheads). **B, C** Frontal and lateral conventional tomograms demonstrate the area of abnormality (arrowheads) and reveal the deformity of the articular surface (arrow). (Courtesy of L. Danzig, M.D., Santa Ana, California.)

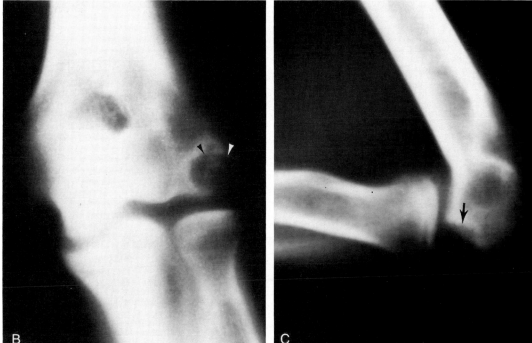

FURTHER READING

Clader TJ, Dawson EG, Bassett LW: The role of tomography in the evaluation of the postoperative spinal fusion. Spine 9:686, 1984.

Morag B, Shahin N: The value of tomography of the sterno-clavicular region. Clin Radiol 26:57, 1975.

Wilkinson M, Meikle JAK: Tomography of the sacro-iliac joint. Ann Rheum Dis 25:433, 1966.

Chapter 10

Computed Tomography

Michael André, Ph.D.
Donald Resnick, M.D.

Cross-sectional display, excellent contrast resolution, and the ability to allow the measurement of specific attenuation values are important characteristics of computed tomography (CT) that make it possible to define soft tissue and bone alterations that may be undetectable with conventional radiography. CT is capable of providing quantitative measures of bone mineral content in the skeleton. Reformation of transaxial images in the coronal or sagittal plane and three-dimensional analysis of image data are significant additional advantages of CT.

Computed tomography (CT) has matured into a reliable and prominent tool for study of the musculoskeletal system. Although both CT and conventional tomography are planar techniques, the images obtained with CT are unhindered by overlying tissue. Contrast resolution is also superior, and CT is capable of providing quantitative measures of bone mineral content of the skeleton. In a dramatic departure from film methods, the CT image is produced in a computer, which allows manipulation of the display. These powerful features may be used improperly, however, causing distortion or masking of structures; for this reason, it is important to understand the limitations of CT scans. Careful attention to the technical details will also improve interpretation of CT scans and enhance their diagnostic and therapeutic utility.

TECHNICAL CONSIDERATIONS

Although general guidelines for CT evaluation of the musculoskeletal system can be given, the ideal examination is one tailored to the diagnostic requirements of the individual patient. The CT approach is best planned after a review of the clinical records and results of other imaging studies, which will clarify the specific indications and clinical questions requiring answers. The development of general CT protocols is a natural consequence of nearly two decades of clinical investigation and experimentation, and the guidelines are certainly useful in the setting of a busy radiology department, in which CT is performed from the early morning hours to late at night. These protocols are also useful at times when a radiologist may not be able to monitor the study closely. Nevertheless, unmonitored examinations using standard protocols are those that are most likely to be technically inadequate.

Availability of Conventional Radiographs and Scan Projection View

As a general rule, it is unwise to perform CT unless preliminary radiographs of the area of the body to be examined have been obtained. Such radiographs will influence the strategy to be employed even when the abnormality itself is not visible. Furthermore, a scan projection view is fundamental to the success of most CT examinations, allowing localization of the region of interest and display of the planned imaging strategy. External radiopaque markers make it easier to locate the area of interest in the projection view and are especially important in patients with palpable but small soft tissue masses that would otherwise be difficult to find.

Scanning Strategy

Theoretically, it is best to obtain initial CT scans in the plane of interest (transaxial, coronal, or sagittal) rather than depend on reformation of image data that were initially acquired in another plane, which would result in the deterioration of image resolution. Practically, the choice of a scanning plane is often severely restricted as a result of anatomic factors. Transverse, or transaxial, scans of the central skeleton (vertebral column and pelvis) in the supine or prone adult patient are mandated by the size and location of the area of interest. In the child, direct sagittal or coronal CT of centrally located structures such as the chest, pelvis, or spine is more feasible. Direct sagittal image acquisition also can be used to evaluate the temporomandibular joint. In more peripheral regions, the choice of image orientation is more flexible. Direct sagittal or coronal imaging of the forearms, elbows, hands, and feet is possible and, in some cases, is indispensable for accurate diagnosis.

The choice of a prone or supine position for the subject during CT commonly is based on patient comfort and convenience. In certain situations it becomes more significant, however. In examination of the lower spine, a supine position and knee flexion produce flattening of the normal lumbar lordosis. Examinations using computed arthrotomography require that the patient be in a precise position for proper distribution of air or radiopaque contrast medium. In addition, certain positions may be contraindicated in acutely injured patients, owing to respiratory problems or fracture location. Last, CT monitoring of biopsy or aspiration procedures requires precise patient positioning for proper placement and advancement of the needle.

Most current CT scanners allow as much as 20 degrees of angulation of the gantry in either direction. Whether or not gantry angulation is necessary in the examination of a specific patient may also need to be addressed. Certain structures, such as the sacrum, are so oriented in the body that true transaxial sections are not possible without gantry angulation. In other locations, such as the hindfoot, limitations in positioning the body part imposed by the gantry itself can be overcome by such angulation, allowing direct coronal scans, which would otherwise be difficult or impossible to obtain.

The choice of slice thickness and table incrementation between slices (overlapping versus contiguous scans) is based on considerations of radiation dosage and examination time, the type, size, and location of the abnormality, the need for image data reformation, and, in many cases, the personal preference of the individual examiner. A commonly employed imaging strategy for soft tissue neoplasms consists of contiguous 1.0 cm thick slices; for bone lesions, contiguous or overlapping 0.5 cm slices are frequently used. Thinner scan slices may be required for the cervical spine, hands, wrists, and feet.

Measurement of Attenuation Coefficient

CT numbers (in the form of Hounsfield units) may be used as absolute values, which allows characterization of the tissue within a lesion (Table 10–1). It has been shown, however, that there are significant differences in absolute CT numbers between most scanners and that the CT numbers are influenced significantly by the location of the body in the scanner and by technical factors used to obtain the scans. The inclusion of a calibration phantom in the field with the patient could minimize some of these errors. Alternatively, the examiner could place less reliance on the ability of attenuation coefficients to predict minor histologic variants in a lesion.

Lesions composed solely or predominantly of fat will usually, but not invariably, produce negative CT numbers allowing a diagnosis of a lipoma (Fig. 10–1). Modifications of these numbers by sarcomatous degeneration in a lipoma are diagnostically useful in some cases. A lesion whose attenuation value is close to that of water is consistent with, but not specific for, a cyst, whereas hematomas characteristically demonstrate inhomogeneous areas with both high

Table 10–1. SAMPLE CT NUMBERS FOR VARIOUS TISSUES

Tissue	CT Number (HU)
Bone	1000
Liver	40 to 60
White matter (brain)	46
Gray matter (brain)	43
Blood	40
Muscle	10 to 40
Kidney	30
Cerebrospinal fluid	15
Water	0
Fat	−50 to −100
Air	−1000

attenuation (approximately 50 HU) and low attenuation (approximately 10 HU) regions in their subacute stage and homogeneous areas with low attenuation (1 to 20 HU) in their chronic stage. The measurement of attenuation values of intraosseous lesions may be more difficult. Replacement of fatty marrow with inflammatory or tumorous tissue possessing higher attenuation values has been used to judge the extent of infective or neoplastic processes, however.

The identification of gas in soft tissue or bone by CT is possible owing to its very low attenuation. This assumes clinical importance when a gas-containing disc fragment is present in the spinal canal. Similarly, gas within a vertebral body is an important sign of ischemic necrosis of bone. Intraosseous gas is also identified in some cases of osteomyelitis and in subchondral cysts ("pneumatocysts").

Administration of Contrast Material

The intravenous, intraspinal, or intradiscal administration of radiopaque contrast material or the intraarticular administration of radiopaque contrast material or air can be a useful adjunct. Intravenous contrast material can aid in identifying a suspected soft tissue mass when initial CT scans are unremarkable, in assessing the vascularity of a soft tissue or osseous lesion when this feature is of diagnostic or therapeutic significance, and in defining the relationship of a tumor and adjacent vascular structures.

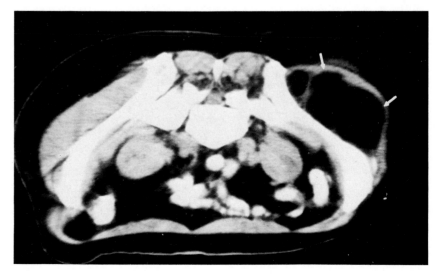

Figure 10–1. Measurement of attenuation values: Negative CT numbers—fat in lipoma. Smooth, homogeneous soft tissue lesions with negative numbers generally represent lipomas. In this case, with the patient in the prone position, a large lipoma in the gluteal region is evident (arrows). Note its internal septation and composition, the latter being identical to that of the subcutaneous fat. (Courtesy of T. Broderick, M.D., Orange, California.)

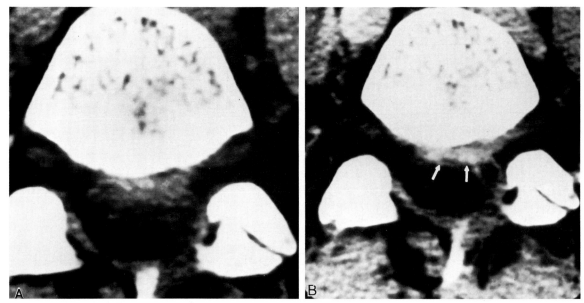

Figure 10–2. Use of contrast material: Intravenous administration for identification of postoperative hypertrophic scar. A, B Preinjection (**A**) and postinjection (**B**) transaxial CT scans reveal contrast enhancement of a soft tissue mass (arrows) behind the vertebral body, consistent with postoperative hypertrophic scar formation. Note strand-like radiodense regions extending from the mass. (Courtesy of J. Mink, M.D., Los Angeles, California.)

Enhancement of a soft tissue mass in the spinal canal after administration of intravenous contrast material is suggested as a reliable way to differentiate by CT between a postoperative hypertrophic scar (which is associated with marked contrast enhancement) and a recurrent herniated intervertebral disc

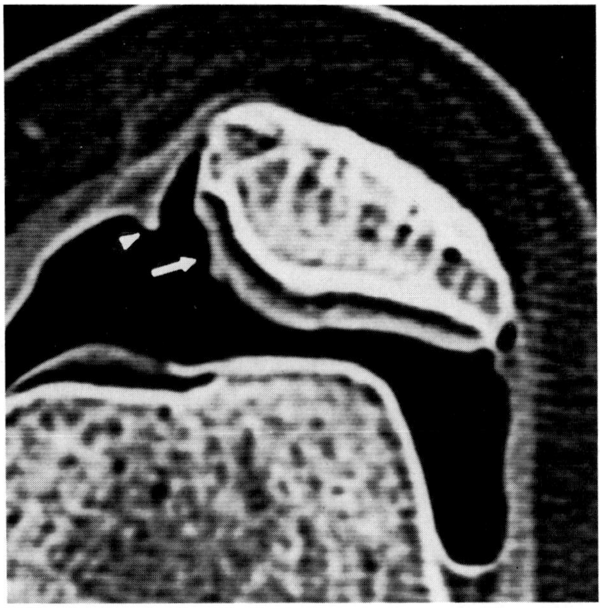

Figure 10–3. Use of contrast material: Intraarticular administration. Chondromalacia and medial synovial plica. Transaxial computed arthrotomography, using both air and radiopaque contrast material, allows identification of chondromalacia of the patella, characterized by cartilage irregularity and imbibition of contrast material (arrow), and a medial plica or synovial fold (arrowhead).

(which is associated with only a thin rim of enhanced tissue) (Fig. 10–2). The value of this sign remains controversial, however.

Contrast enhancement of a joint is useful in defining a periarticular soft tissue mass (e.g., synovial cyst) or intraarticular osteocartilaginous bodies and in evaluating the glenoid labrum, patellar cartilage, synovial plicae and cruciate ligaments of the knee, and osteochondritis dissecans of the talus (Fig. 10–3).

Image Display and Reformation

Although the choice of window width and level is best done at the video console, a near-maximum window width (1000 to 2000 HU) and a relatively high window level (200 to 250 HU) allow good visualization of bones. For soft tissue detail, a window width of 400 to 600 HU and a window level of 0 to 100 HU generally are acceptable.

It is difficult to generalize about the need for reformation of image data in a plane or planes different from those in which such data were acquired (Fig. 10–4). Such decisions are based on, among other factors, the anatomic area and type of abnormality being studied, the plane of the original CT scans, and the personal bias of the examiner. Reformation becomes more important when a particular plane of image display is preferable but unobtainable initially because of the restrictions in patient positioning imposed by the gantry of the CT scanner.

Three-Dimensional Image Display

Three-dimensional display represents a further modification of image data provided by newer computer systems. The clinical applications of this technique are expanding rapidly. Applications to the musculoskeletal system include the analysis of regions of complex anatomy, such as the face, pelvis,

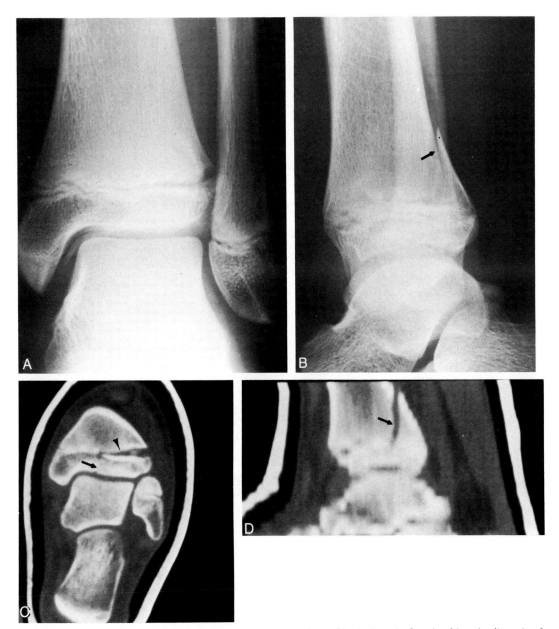

Figure 10–4. Use of reformatted image data: Triplane fracture of the tibia. A, B In the frontal and lateral radiographs of the ankle, the epiphyseal extension of the fracture is not readily apparent. The metaphyseal component (arrow) is seen, suggesting a type II physeal injury. **C** A direct coronal CT scan shows the extent of the physeal widening (arrowhead) and the epiphyseal fracture line (arrow). **D** A sagittal reformatted image reveals the metaphyseal fracture (arrow) and posterior displacement of the epiphysis. Note that the presence of a cast has not significantly interfered with the CT image displays.

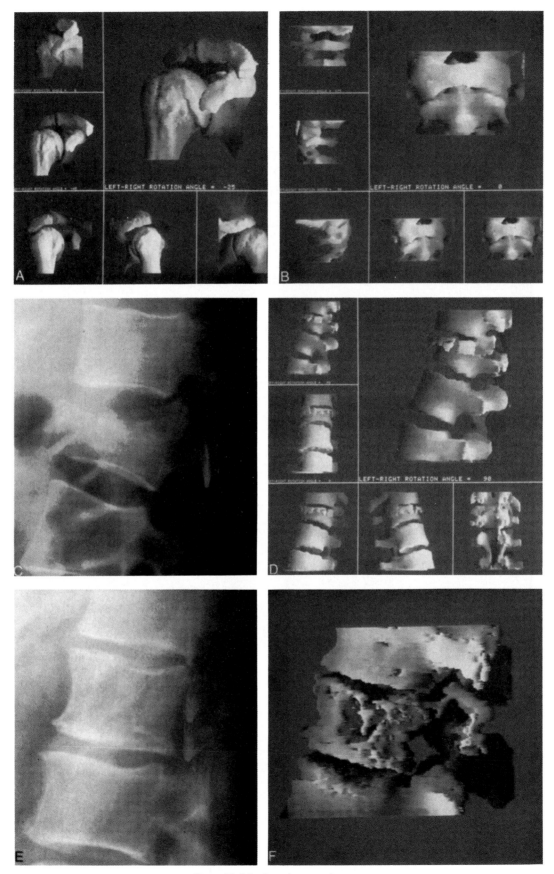

Figure 10–5 See legend on opposite page

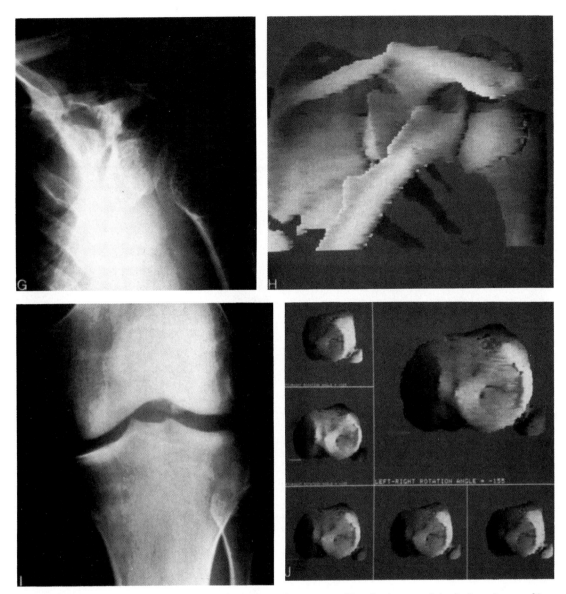

Figure 10–5. Use of three-dimensional image display: Regions of complex anatomy. Note that in some of the displays, the area of interest has been rotated with the rotated images placed about the primary image. A Shoulder: Normal situation. B Cervical spine: Atlantoaxial rotary fixation. The lateral mass of the atlas that is located on the viewer's left has moved forward with respect to the axis, and the opposite mass has moved backward to an equal extent. The odontoid process is located closer to the anteriorly positioned lateral mass of the atlas. C, D Thoracolumbar spine: Complex fracture. E, F Lumbar spine: Plasma cell myeloma. G, H Shoulder: Scapular fracture in osteogenesis imperfecta. I, J Knee: Depressed fracture of the lateral tibial plateau. The degree of osseous depression is well seen on the three-dimensional image, which shows the appearance of the tibial plateau as viewed from above.

spine, shoulder, wrist, knee, midfoot, and hindfoot (Fig. 10–5). It is now possible to devise plastic models of a diseased area based on three-dimensional images, which facilitates operative planning and even allows rehearsal surgery of complex osteotomies or other reconstructive procedures. Plastic models are also useful in the design and manufacture of customized replacements.

CLINICAL APPLICATIONS

CT can be used to evaluate many anatomic regions of the body and a variety of musculoskeletal disorders (Table 10–2).

Anatomic Regions

As a generalization, the more complex the osseous anatomy of a specific region of the body or the more difficult the task of obtaining adequate conventional radiographs, the greater the likelihood that CT will provide additional diagnostic information (Fig. 10–6). CT is a well-established technique in the evaluation of abnormalities of the bony pelvis, hip, sacrum and sacroiliac joint, glenohumeral and sternoclavicular joints, sternum, spine, midfoot and hindfoot, temporomandibular joint, and wrist. The potential applications for CT to assessment of soft tissues are even greater owing to its superior contrast resolution over that of conventional radiography.

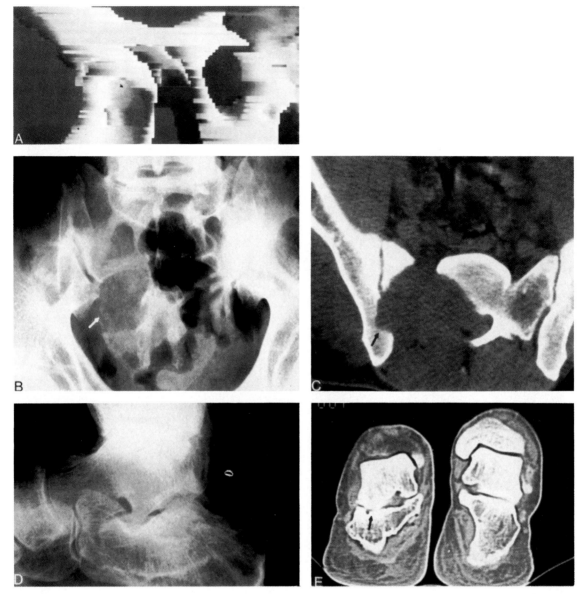

Figure 10–6. Use of CT: Regions of complex anatomy. A Temporomandibular joint: Normal situation. A three-dimensional sagittal CT image shows the normal meniscus of this joint. **B, C** Osseous pelvis: Skeletal metastasis from renal carcinoma. An osteolytic lesion in the sacrum (arrow) is evident in the frontal radiograph (**B**). Its transarticular extension (arrow) is shown with CT (**C**). (Courtesy of G. Greenway, M.D., Dallas, Texas.) **D, E** Hindfoot: Posttraumatic osteoarthritis of the subtalar joint. The lateral radiograph (**D**) reveals an old calcaneal fracture with flattening of Bohler's angle. **E,** The degree of deformity and narrowing of the posterior subtalar joint (arrow) is demonstrated with direct coronal CT imaging. Compare with the opposite (normal) side.

This ability to distinguish between tissues differing only slightly in contrast characteristics explains the benefits of CT in defining the presence, location, and, in some cases, nature of soft tissue masses, which produce nonspecific findings or escape detection altogether on routine radiographs. The superiority of CT over conventional radiography in imaging the soft tissues is not debated; however, magnetic resonance imaging possesses definite advantages over CT, not the least of which is the absence of radiation exposure. In the years ahead, MR imaging will dramatically influence the manner in which CT is used.

Specific Disorders

In the two decades that have passed since the introduction and refinement of CT, the number of its clinical applications

to the musculoskeletal system has increased exponentially. These applications are best considered according to specific categories of disease.

TRAUMA. CT is valuable in skeletal trauma beause of its ability to define the presence and extent of a fracture or dislocation, to delineate intraarticular abnormalities, including cartilage damage and osteocartilaginous bodies, and to assess the adjacent soft tissues.

In the spine, CT has largely replaced conventional tomography as the technique of choice after routine radiography in the evaluation of complex fractures and dislocations. Although considerable information is provided by transaxial CT images, many examiners also emphasize the benefits of coronal or sagittal reformations, or both, especially if the fractures are oriented in a horizontal fashion. The presence of bone frag-

Table 10–2. SOME INDICATIONS FOR COMPUTED TOMOGRAPHY

Trauma:
   Fractures
   Dislocations
   Cartilaginous and ligamentous injuries
Infection:
   Osteomyelitis
   Septic arthritis
Neoplasm:
   Bone
   Soft tissue
Articular disease:
   Sacroiliac joint
Neuromuscular disease
Vascular disease:
   Aneurysms
   Arterial entrapment syndromes
Congenital disease
Metabolic disease
Low back pain

ments in the spinal canal after fractures of the vertebral body is easily overlooked on conventional radiographs but is well shown with CT (Fig. 10–7). Furthermore, CT can be employed after the treatment of such fractures with Harrington instruments, displaying significant information despite some imaging degradation owing to the presence of the metallic rods. Pediculate or laminar fractures and disruption of the capsule about the apophyseal joints are further examples of abnormalities that are well shown with CT. Injuries of the cervical spine that are optimally delineated include Jefferson or burst fractures of the atlas and atlantoaxial rotational fixation.

In the bony pelvis, CT is best used for the evaluation of acute or stress fractures of the sacrum, complex fractures of the pelvic ring, and those fractures that extend into the acetabulum. CT represents an excellent method for demonstrating fracture extent as well as soft tissue injury. It has particular merit in patients with double vertical fractures or subluxations of the hemipelvis or an iliac fracture with extension into the acetabulum. Patients with major injuries of the hemipelvis that are to be treated with open reduction

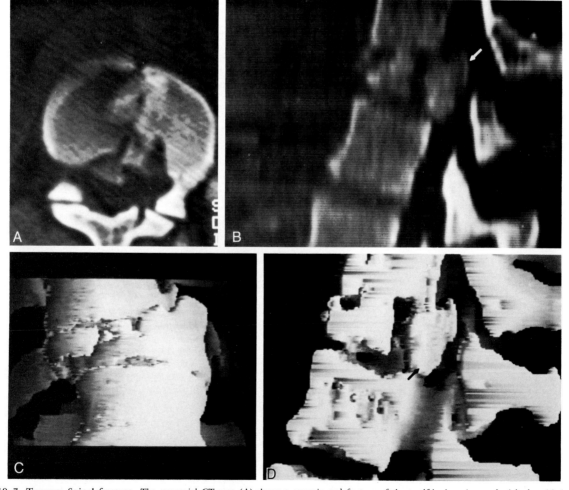

Figure 10–7. Trauma: Spinal fracture. The transaxial CT scan (**A**) shows a comminuted fracture of the twelfth thoracic vertebral body with intraspinal fragments and a fracture of the lamina with subluxation of the ipsilateral apophyseal joint. A sagittal reformatted image (**B**) delineates the complexity of the fracture of the vertebral body and the presence of a large fragment arising from the posterior surface of the vertebral body, displaced into the spinal canal (arrow). A three-dimensional surface display (**C**), viewed from the front, shows the extent of vertebral collapse. A three-dimensional sagittal sectional display (**D**) again documents the presence of an intraspinal fragment (arrow).

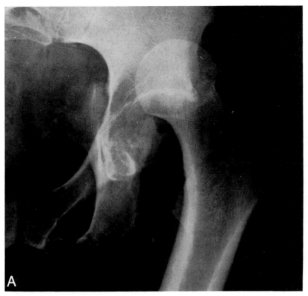
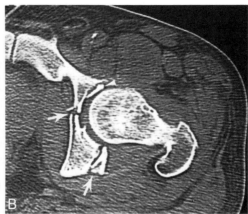

Figure 10–8. Trauma: Fracture-dislocation of the hip. A The initial radiograph reveals a posterior dislocation of the hip with fractures of the medial wall and posterior rim of the acetabulum. B Following reduction of the dislocation, a transaxial CT scan shows the fractures of the acetabulum (arrows) and an intraarticular fragment (arrowhead) with persistent widening of the joint space.

and internal fixation of the posterior part of the pelvic ring are also good candidates for CT. CT identifies occult acetabular fractures that are difficult to visualize with conventional techniques, disruptions of the posterior and anterior acetabular margins that accompany dislocations of the hip, subtle injuries of the femoral head, and intraarticular osteocartilaginous bodies. It provides information about the integrity of the acetabular dome, quadrilateral surface, and iliopubic and ilioischial bone columns. CT can also be used after surgical reduction of pelvic fractures or hip dislocations, to define the adequacy of the reduction, the position of metallic fixation devices, the presence of intraarticular fragments, and, later, the degree of healing and the amount of heterotopic bone formation (Fig. 10–8).

Dislocations of the sternoclavicular joint are extremely difficult to diagnose by conventional imaging techniques, requiring specialized projections. The transaxial plane provided by CT allows immediate documentation of the malpositioned clavicle, showing whether it is located anteriorly or posteriorly with respect to the adjacent sternum, and identifying any soft tissue injury (Fig. 10–9).

Dislocations of the glenohumeral joint are common and are associated with bone or cartilage injuries, or both. When spontaneous relocation occurs, the nature of the injury as well as its propensity to recur may be unclear. Routine radiographs supplemented with special projections have been advocated in these instances to document the presence of osseous and cartilaginous residua of the dislocation, including the Hill-Sachs lesion of the humeral head and the Bankart lesion of the glenoid cavity, which indicate previous anterior dislocation. When the osseous defect in the humeral head or scapula is large, one or both of these lesions will be detected by the conventional studies, but when it is small, CT may be required. When the Bankart lesion is primarily cartilaginous in nature, computed arthrotomography (Fig. 10–10) is the method of choice.

CT is occasionally required in the analysis of fractures or dislocations about the knee, ankle, elbow, and wrist (Fig. 10–11). Examples of specific applications of this technique are subluxations or dislocations of the patella, fractures of the tibial plateau, dislocations of the proximal tibiofibular joint, complex fractures of the distal portions of the tibia and fibula, triplane fractures of the distal segment of the tibia, disruptions of the inferior radioulnar joint, and fractures of the hook of the hamate. CT also is used to analyze extensive fractures of the calcaneus and talus and fractures and dislocations about the tarsometatarsal joints. In any articular location, CT can

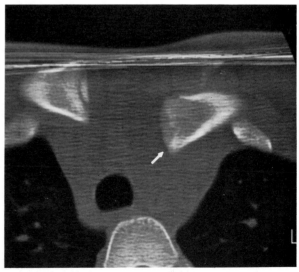

Figure 10–9. Trauma: Posterior dislocation of the sternoclavicular joint. Transaxial CT shows posterior displacement of the left clavicular head (arrow). Note that the adjacent clavicular epiphysis, which normally is seen (as evident on the opposite side), is not identifiable.

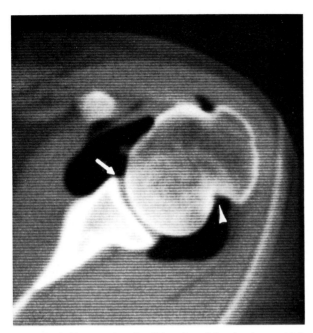

Figure 10–10. Trauma: Anterior dislocation of the glenohumeral joint. Transaxial computed arthrotomography shows loss of the normal anterior portion of the glenoid labrum (arrow), intraarticular cartilaginous debris, and a Hill-Sachs lesion (arrowhead).

further delineate osteochondral fractures and intraarticular osteocartilaginous bodies.

The precise role of CT in the diagnosis of certain intraarticular cartilaginous and ligamentous injuries, especially in the knee and temporomandibular joint, is less well defined; specifically, its advantages over those of other techniques, such as arthrography and magnetic resonance imaging, need further investigation.

INFECTION. The early diagnosis of osteomyelitis is best left to scintigraphy, but defining the intraosseous extent of disease can be accomplished with CT. The negative CT numbers (Hounsfield units) of fat-containing marrow are altered in the presence of osteomyelitis owing to the accumulation of infected tissue. This finding is not specific, being observed in any process that involves the intramedullary portion of the bone. In rare instances, the identification of intraosseous gas allows a more specific diagnosis of infection, as does gas in the soft tissues and fat-fluid levels in osseous or soft tissues.

In chronic osteomyelitis, CT has been used to identify single or multiple sequestra and soft tissue abscesses and sinus tracts. In both chronic and acute osteomyelitis, this technique may guide aspiration or biopsy attempts.

NEOPLASM. Neoplasms of bone and those of soft tissue must be considered separately when considering the role of CT in their assessment. CT has not replaced conventional radiographic techniques in the diagnosis of primary and secondary bone tumors; however, CT is better able to judge the osseous and soft tissue extent of the process. Intraosseous extension of the neoplasm leads to the conversion of fatty marrow, with its negative CT numbers, to marrow containing tumorous tissue, which has higher CT numbers. The ability of CT to delineate the soft tissue extent of a bone neoplasm (as well as of a primary soft tissue neoplasm) is a consequence of its excellent contrast resolution (Fig. 10–12). The relationship between the tumor and major neurovascular bundles can be demonstrated effectively by CT, especially if intravenous contrast material is administered.

These comments indicate that CT is more important in the surgical planning than in the actual diagnosis of primary bone neoplasms; however, in specific instances this technique has definite diagnostic value. By defining the absorption coefficient of the intraosseous process, CT allows differentiation of a cystic and fibrous lesion and the documentation of fat within it (as in an intraosseous lipoma). A CT scan showing a radiolucent region with surrounding bone sclerosis strongly supports the diagnosis of an osteoid osteoma (Fig. 10–13), and a gas-fluid or fluid-fluid level generally indicates a solitary or aneurysmal bone cyst (Fig. 10–14). CT has also been used with variable success to define the thickness of a cartilaginous cap of an osteochondroma, a finding that assumes clinical

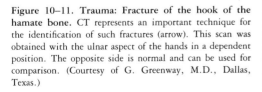

Figure 10–11. Trauma: Fracture of the hook of the hamate bone. CT represents an important technique for the identification of such fractures (arrow). This scan was obtained with the ulnar aspect of the hands in a dependent position. The opposite side is normal and can be used for comparison. (Courtesy of G. Greenway, M.D., Dallas, Texas.)

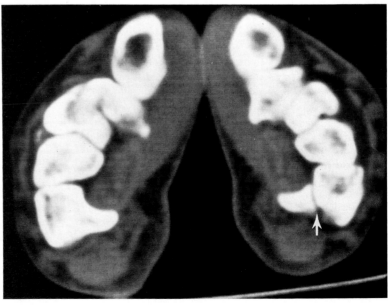

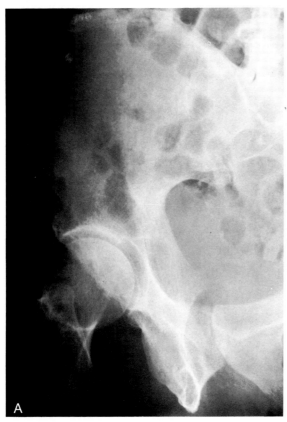

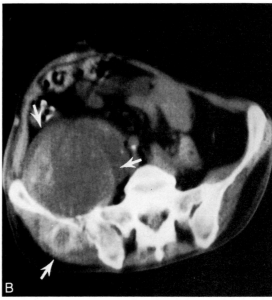

Figure 10–12. Neoplasm: Skeletal metastasis from carcinoma of the colon. It is obvious that compared with routine radiography (A), CT (B) is superior in the delineation of the soft tissue extent of the metastatic lesion (arrows).

importance because thicker cartilage characterizes a chondrosarcoma.

The diagnostic value of CT is more established in patients with primary soft tissue tumors, in which conventional radiography provides little specific information. Low attenuation numbers are characteristic of a lipoma. Liposarcomas may possess areas of both low attenuation and high attenuation, whereas discrete zones of high density indicating lesions of mixed cellularity occur in some cases of angiolipomas and fibrolipomas. Cyst formation, cystic necrosis, and cartilage or bone formation are additional CT characteristics of a soft tissue lesion that are invaluable in defining the nature of the process.

CT is often fundamental to successful aspiration or biopsy of both primary and secondary soft tissue and osseous neoplasms. Furthermore, it represents an excellent technique for monitoring the effects of radiation therapy or chemotherapy on soft tissue and bone neoplasms.

ARTICULAR DISEASE. CT generally is not required in the diagnosis of articular disorders. Occasionally, it will better define the extent of bone involvement in such disorders. The identification of the presence and extent of disease by CT becomes more important in those joints that are difficult to visualize with usual imaging techniques. Such sites include the apophyseal, costovertebral, sternoclavicular, and temporomandibular joints.

The contribution of CT to the diagnosis of sacroiliitis is a subject on which there is no consensus. Furthermore, there is no single opinion regarding the optimal CT technique for evaluating the sacroiliac joints. It is the authors' belief that high-quality radiographs of the sacroiliac articulations, including specialized views, eliminate the need for CT in most patients with sacroiliitis. CT is occasionally useful in the evaluation of patients with septic arthritis (Fig. 10–15) in the sacroiliac joint.

The propensity for rheumatoid arthritis to affect the cervical spine has led to considerable interest in evaluating the extent of such disease with CT. Most attention has been directed toward the occipitoatlantoaxial level owing to its anatomic complexity and the many serious complications of rheumatoid arthritis that occur in this region. The transaxial CT display facilitates evaluation of soft tissue, ligament, and spinal cord involvement.

With regard to joint disease, CT is perhaps best suited to the evaluation of paraarticular soft tissue masses. Synovial cysts (Fig. 10–16) arising adjacent to the glenohumeral joint, hip, knee, and apophyseal joint are well visualized. In hemophilia, hemorrhagic collections in periarticular soft tissues as well as in muscles and bones are identified with CT.

NEUROMUSCULAR DISEASE. Even a glance at a typical transaxial CT scan through virtually any portion of the body would indicate the advantages of this technique over routine radiography for identifying individual muscles and muscle bundles. Although this capability is now well recognized, magnetic resonance imaging will unquestionably alter future imaging strategies devoted to neuromuscular diseases.

Applications of CT to diseases of nerves and muscles include the detection of neurofibromas, schwannomas, and compressive neuropathies, especially those of the sciatic and median nerves, and the evaluation of abscesses, hematomas, tumors,

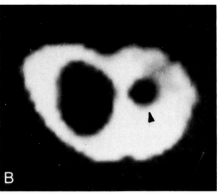

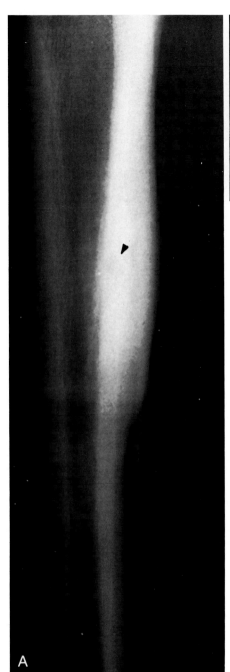

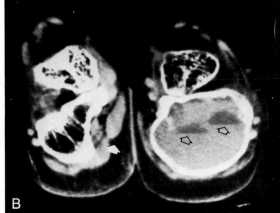

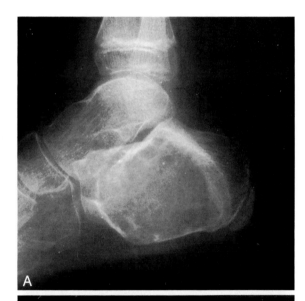

Figure 10–13. Neoplasm: Osteoid osteoma. A The lateral tomogram of the lower leg reveals cortical thickening involving the posterior portion of the tibia. A radiolucent nidus (arrowhead) is also seen. **B** Transaxial CT at the level of the lesion confirms the presence of a nidus (arrowhead) in the thickened tibial cortex. (Courtesy of Mallinckrodt Institute of Radiology, St. Louis, Missouri.)

Figure 10–14. Neoplasm: Aneurysmal bone cyst. A A large, expansile lesion of the calcaneus in this child has a well-defined, partially sclerotic margin and a hazy interior. **B** A coronal CT scan through the lesion documents osseous expansion of the calcaneus and fluid-fluid levels (arrows). (Courtesy of T. Broderick, M.D., Orange, California.).

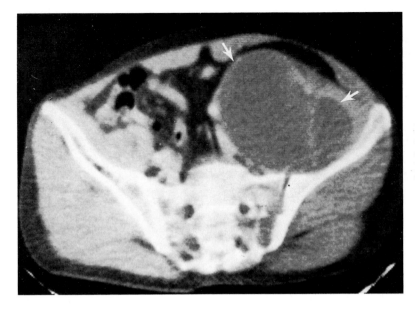

Figure 10–15. Articular disease: Septic arthritis in the sacroiliac joint. A major advantage of transaxial CT is the delineation of the extent of a soft tissue abscess (arrows) in patients with septic arthritis of this joint. Note the osseous destruction in the ilium and sacrum.

muscular dystrophies, and "myositis ossificans." The last-mentioned disorder does not necessarily affect the muscles but leads to a characteristic CT pattern in which a peripheral rim of ossification surrounds a more radiolucent soft tissue area.

VASCULAR DISEASE. CT provides diagnostic information in patients with masses related to aneurysms, pseudoaneurysms, and arterial entrapment syndromes. CT characteristics of an aneurysm are peripheral curvilinear or punctate calcifications on noncontrast scans and partial opacification of its lumen and contrast enhancement of its wall on postcontrast scans.

The early diagnosis of ischemic necrosis of bone is best accomplished with other techniques, such as scintigraphy and magnetic resonance imaging (Fig. 10–17). Cross-sectional CT displays of the femoral head, when combined with sagittal, coronal, and three-dimensional reconstruction of the image data, provide important information in the later stages of ischemic necrosis, when verification of collapse of subchondral bone directly affects operative planning (Fig. 10–17).

CONGENITAL DISEASE. Among the many applications of CT to congenital disorders of the musculoskeletal system, several deserve emphasis. The technique can be used to evaluate the degree of bone deformity, position of the iliopsoas tendon and acetabular labrum, and concentricity of closed reduction in children with congenital dislocation of the hip. CT provides an accurate and reproducible method to measure femoral anteversion, tibial torsion, vertebral rotation in scoliosis, and leg length discrepancy. Congenital tarsal coalition, especially that between the talus and the calcaneus, is well shown by direct coronal CT imaging (Fig. 10–18). In the spine, diastematomyelia, the tethered conus syndrome, anomalies of the posterior osseous structures of the vertebrae, dorsal dysraphism, and meningoceles can be identified with CT, which in some cases should be combined with myelography.

METABOLIC DISEASE. In view of the prevalence of osteoporosis, especially in an elderly population, and its propensity to lead to significant morbidity, mortality, and public health expenditure, it is not surprising that considerable time and effort have been devoted to the development of

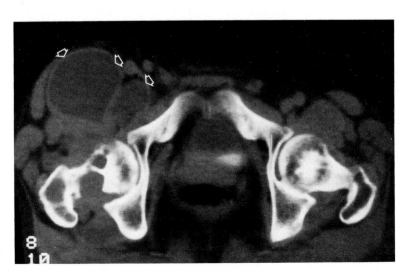

Figure 10–16. Articular disease: Synovial cyst of the hip in rheumatoid arthritis. In this region, a synovial cyst (open arrows) may create a mass that leads to an erroneous diagnosis of an inguinal hernia. Note the destruction of the ipsilateral femoral neck and joint space narrowing.

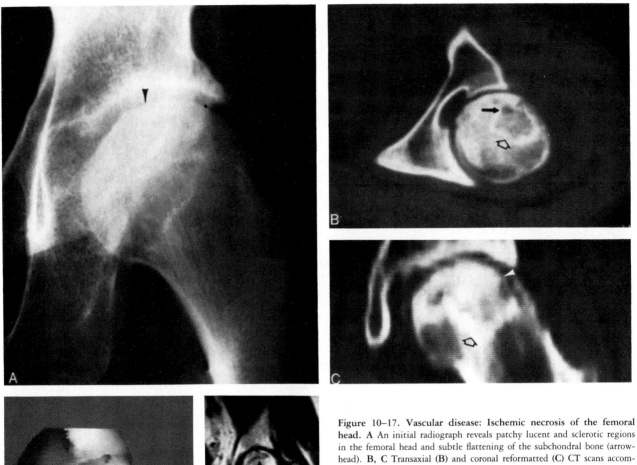

Figure 10–17. **Vascular disease: Ischemic necrosis of the femoral head. A** An initial radiograph reveals patchy lucent and sclerotic regions in the femoral head and subtle flattening of the subchondral bone (arrowhead). **B, C** Transaxial (**B**) and coronal reformatted (**C**) CT scans accomplished somewhat later document fissures in the femoral head (solid arrow), curvilinear osteosclerosis (open arrows), and articular collapse (arrowhead). **D** A three-dimensional display, viewed from the front, of the CT data confirms osseous collapse (arrowhead). **E** In a different patient, a coronal oblique magnetic resonance image documents early ischemic necrosis of the femoral head (solid arrow). (**E**, Courtesy of M. Modic, M.D., Cleveland, Ohio.)

quantitative techniques that allow sensitive and reproducible assessment of bone mineral content. Although all would agree that routine radiographs are remarkably inaccurate in this assessment, the choice of an alternate method has met with less uniformity of opinion. Photon absorptiometry and neutron activation are among the proposed techniques for measuring bone mineral content, and in the last decade, quantitative CT has become an additional established method in this analysis (see Chapter 18).

LOW BACK PAIN. Although a full discussion of the manner in which CT is used to evaluate patients with low back pain and other spinal problems is beyond the scope of this chapter (see Chapters 13 and 36 for further information), a few comments are appropriate here. Without question, CT has profoundly influenced imaging protocols designed for vertebral disorders, owing to both its superior contrast resolution (compared with routine radiography) and its cross-sectional display. CT currently is the imaging method of choice in the evaluation of patients with low back pain. Those who doggedly maintain that myelography alone is diagnos-

tically superior to CT in this clinical setting are becoming fewer in number. The two techniques are not incompatible, however, and the sequential use of myelography followed immediately by CT has definite advantages. Although the results of comparison studies of myelography, CT, and CT combined with myelography have not been uniform, in certain situations, such as extreme lateral discal herniation, CT possesses definite superiority over myelography. In other situations, such as in the evaluation of recurring symptoms and signs after back surgery, a strong argument can be made for using CT and myelography together. The precise place held by magnetic resonance in these imaging strategies is not yet clear, but its remarkable soft tissue contrast resolution and its ability to image the spine directly in the sagittal, coronal, and transaxial planes, and to differentiate between the anulus fibrosus and the nucleus pulposus of the intervertebral disc, underscore the clinical impact that this technique will have in the years ahead (Fig. 10–19).

The CT characteristics of a herniated intervertebral disc need not be discussed in detail here other than to note the

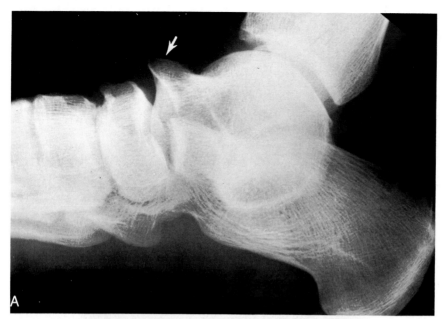

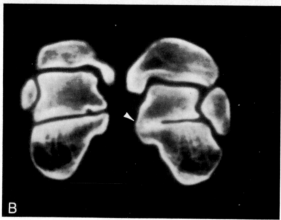

Figure 10–18. Congenital disease: Tarsal coalition. A Findings on a lateral radiograph that suggest the correct diagnosis include the inability to visualize the talocalcaneal articulations and a large talar excrescence, the talar beak (arrow). B A direct coronal CT scan shows a solid bone fusion (arrowhead) between the talus and the calcaneus in the region of the sustentaculum tali. Compare with the opposite (normal) side.

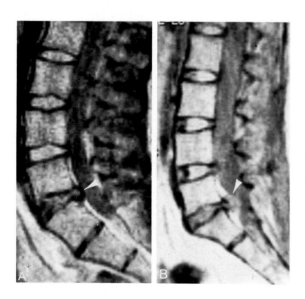

Figure 10–19. Low back pain: Discal herniation. Two examples of use of magnetic resonance imaging are shown in which sagittal images reveal large discal herniations (arrowheads) at the L5-S1 spinal level. In both cases, the main portion of the involved disc has lost signal intensity related to its degeneration (TE, 28 ms; TR, 1.5 s). (Courtesy of M. Solomon, M.D., San Jose, California.)

diagnostic difficulty that may occasionally arise in differentiating a bulging anulus fibrosus and a true discal herniation. With a bulging anulus fibrosus, a general extension of the discal margin beyond that of the vertebral body is seen, whereas with true discal herniation, a focal extension of the intervertebral disc is evident (Fig. 10–20). The extruded (sequestered) intervertebral disc, characterized by discal penetration of the posterior longitudinal ligament, appears on CT as an epidural mass that may either be contiguous with the remaining portions of the intervertebral disc or be separated from them by epidural fat.

The herniated intervertebral disc must be distinguished from other causes of extradural masses, including a dilated nerve root sheath, conjoined nerve roots, and benign and malignant neoplasms (Fig. 10–21). The enlarged nerve root sheath typically produces a rounded mass in the region of the intervertebral foramen that is isodense with the cerebrospinal fluid in the subarachnoid space and that may be accompanied by enlargement of the foramen itself owing to scalloped erosion of the posterolateral aspect of the vertebral body. Conjoined, or composite, nerve roots are identified most commonly at the lumbosacral level in a unilateral distribution. The division of the soft tissue mass into its separate nerve root components allows accurate CT diagnosis in most cases. Benign epidural tumors are usually smoother than discal fragments and may lead to pressure erosion of adjacent bone; malignant epidural tumors may be irregular or smooth, and they too produce bone abnormalities consisting of sclerosis or destruction.

Failure of spinal surgery to alleviate symptoms and signs

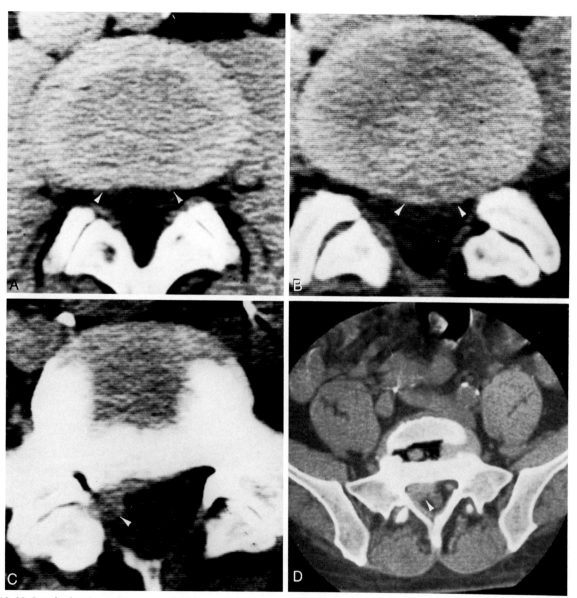

Figure 10–20. Low back pain: Bulging anulus fibrosus versus discal herniation. A Normal situation. The posterior margin of the lumbar intervertebral discs (with the exception of that at L5-S1) is usually concave in configuration (arrowheads). **B** Bulging anulus fibrosus. A general extension of the posterior discal margin is seen (arrowheads). **C** Herniated intervertebral disc. Observe focal extension of discal material (arrowhead) with obliteration of the adjacent nerve root. **D** Herniated intervertebral disc. A similar situation to that in **C** is evident (arrowhead).

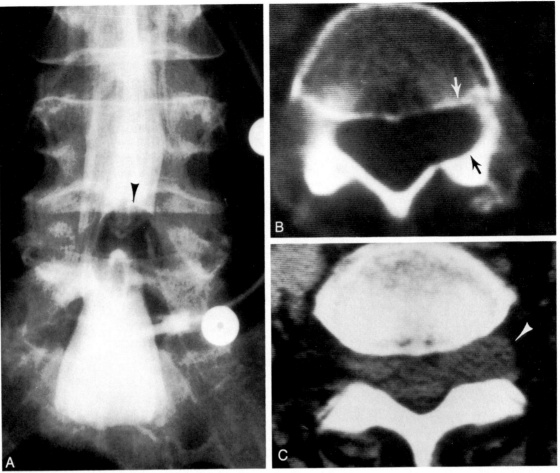

Figure 10–21. Low back pain: Neurofibroma. A A mass at the L4-L5 spinal level has led to a well-defined defect (arrowhead) in the contrast material during myelography. **B, C** Two transaxial CT scans (at different levels and window settings) show the smooth mass (arrowhead) and pressure erosion of neighboring bone (arrows).

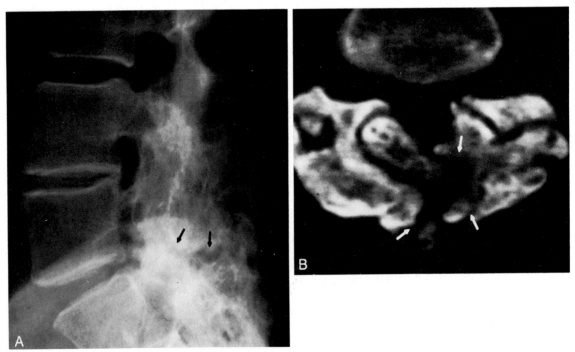

Figure 10–22. Low back pain: Pseudarthrosis following spinal fusion. A In the evaluation of persistent pain following an attempted posterior fusion from the L4 to S1 spinal levels, a lateral radiograph was obtained that reveals an apparent site of nonosseous union (arrows). This abnormality can be further evaluated using bone scintigraphy and radiography obtained with flexion and extension of the patient's spine. **B** Transaxial CT through the abnormal region shows areas of nonosseous fusion (arrows), although the plane of the scan is not ideal and image reconstruction is usually required.

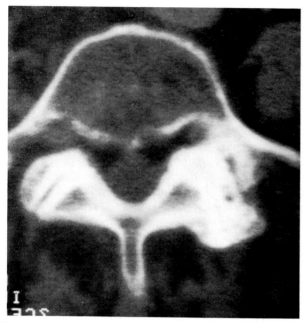

Figure 10–23. Low back pain: Osteoarthritis of the apophyseal joint. Transaxial CT can ideally reveal osteophytosis and bone sclerosis of the apophyseal joints, changes that are indicative of osteoarthritis. In this case, the left apophyseal joint at the L5-S1 spinal level is affected, and involvement has led to distortion of the spinal canal and neural foramen.

and to permit the patient to return to a normal level of physical activity postoperatively is not rare. Causes of this syndrome include inappropriate or inadequate surgery, recurrent discal herniation at the same vertebral level or another level, bone proliferation with spinal stenosis, arachnoiditis, subluxation of the facet joints, infection, and hypertrophic scars. When fusion has also been employed, pseudarthrosis represents an additional cause of new or persistent clinical manifestations (Fig. 10–22).

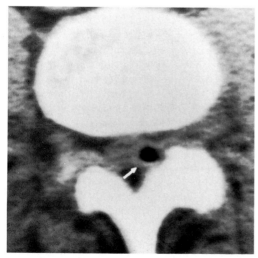

Figure 10–24. Low back pain: Synovial cyst of apophyseal joint. In this example, a mass containing a vacuum phenomenon (arrow) at the level of the left L4-L5 apophyseal joint is evident. The gas arose from the articulation itself.

The extradural scar appears as a soft tissue dense shadow within the spinal canal, usually possessing a higher CT number than the thecal sac and a lower CT number than the intervertebral disc. CT characteristics of the postdiskectomy scar simulate those of a recurrent discal herniation with some minor differences: retraction of the thecal sac toward the soft tissue lesion; mass formation that is contoured around the thecal sac; linear strand-like radiodense shadows; a location that is often above or below the intervertebral disc space; a mass that is not continuous with the intervertebral disc itself; and a CT number of approximately 75 HU, which may increase following the administration of an intravenous contrast material.

The excellent demonstration of the apophyseal joints provided by CT has been welcomed by physicians treating patients with low back pain. CT may provide direct diagnostic information in such patients by demonstrating the osteophytes, bone fragmentation, and spinal stenosis that accompany osteoarthritis (Fig. 10–23) and the extradural mass containing a peripheral rim of calcification or a vacuum phenomenon that characterizes a synovial cyst (Fig. 10–24).

FURTHER READING

Aisen AM, Martel W, Braunstein EM, McMillin KI, Phillips WA, Kling TF: MRI and CT evaluation of primary bone and soft-tissue tumors. AJR 146:749, 1986.

Destouet JM, Gilula LA, Murphy WA, Sagel SS: Computed tomography of the sternoclavicular joint and sternum. Radiology 138:123, 1981.

Deutsch AL, Resnick D, Campbell G: Computed tomography and bone scintigraphy in the evaluation of tarsal coalition. Radiology 144:137, 1982.

Deutsch AL, Resnick D, Berman JL, Mink JH, Cone RO III, Resnick CS, Danzig LA, Guerra J Jr: Computerized and conventional arthrotomography of the glenohumeral joint: Normal anatomy and clinical experience. Radiology 153:603, 1984.

Fishman EK, Drebin B, Magid D, Scott WW Jr, Ney DR, Brooker AF Jr, Riley LH Jr, St. Ville JA, Zerhouni EA, Siegelman SS: Volumetric rendering techniques: Applications for three-dimensional imaging of the hip. Radiology 163:737, 1987.

Heger L, Wulff K, Seddigi MSA: Computed tomography of calcaneal fractures. AJR 145:131, 1985.

Kenney PJ, Gilula LA, Murphy WA: The use of computed tomography to distinguish osteochondroma and chondrosarcoma. Radiology 139:129, 1981.

Kozin F, Carrera GF, Ryan LM, Foley D, Lawson T: Computed tomography in the diagnosis of sacroiliitis. Arthritis Rheum 24:1479, 1981.

Mack JA, Harley JD, Winquist RA: CT of acetabular fractures: Analysis of fracture patterns. AJR 138:407, 1982.

Norman A, Nelson J, Green S: Fractures of the hook of hamate: Radiographic signs. Radiology 154:49, 1985.

Rafii M, Firooznia H, Golimbu C, Minkoff J, Bonamo J: CT arthrography of capsular structures of the shoulder. AJR 146:361, 1986.

Sartoris DJ, Danzig L, Gilula L, Greenway G, Resnick D: Synovial cysts of the hip joint and iliopsoas bursitis: A spectrum of imaging abnormalities. Skel Radiol 14:85, 1985.

Sartoris DJ, Kursunoglu S, Pineda C, Kerr R, Pate D, Resnick D: Detection of intra-articular osteochondral bodies in the knee using computed arthrotomography. Radiology 155:447, 1985.

Schubiger O, Valavanis A: CT differentiation between recurrent disherniation and postoperative scar formation: The value of contrast enhancement. Neuroradiology 22:251, 1982.

Teplick JG, Haskin ME: Intravenous contrast enhanced CT of the postoperative lumbar spine: Improved identification of recurrent disk herniation, scar, arachnoiditis, and diskitis. AJR 143:845, 1984.

Williams AL, Haughton VM, Meyer GH, Ho KC: Computed tomographic appearance of the bulging annulus fibrosus. Radiology 142:403, 1982.

Zimmer WD, Berquist TH, McLeod RA, Sim FH, Pritchard DJ, Shives TC, Wold LE, May GR: Bone tumors: Magnetic resonance imaging versus computed tomography. Radiology 155:709, 1985.

Chapter 11

Magnetic Resonance Imaging

William A. Murphy, M.D.

Magnetic resonance (MR) imaging is an important method for assessing disorders of the musculoskeletal tissues. The images are characterized by great inherent contrast, excellent spatial resolution, and exquisite anatomic display. MR imaging is particularly sensitive to bone marrow alterations and is very effective for detecting and characterizing a wide variety of soft tissue conditions. Advances in surface coil technology will increase the usefulness of MR imaging in the evaluation of articular disease. In addition, chemical shift imaging and spectroscopy will add physiologic information to the anatomic features demonstrated by proton imaging.

In reviewing the history of medical imaging, many investigators cite two major milestones: The first was the discovery by Roentgen of the x-ray at the end of the nineteenth century; the second was the elucidation of the phenomenon termed magnetic resonance (MR) by Block and Purcell in 1946. The advantages of MR imaging over other imaging methods include, foremost, its reliance on the principles of magnetism rather than on the use of ionizing radiation, an ability to provide sectional images of the human body, and the capability of providing physiologic data. The images provided by MR depend on intrinsic tissue parameters that reflect chemical characteristics of that tissue. Although the nuclei of phosphorus, nitrogen, and sodium may also be imaged with MR, it is the distribution of the hydrogen nucleus (proton) that is currently used as the basis of MR imaging. The general attributes that make MR imaging an important diagnostic method for the musculoskeletal system as well as for other human tissues include (1) its great sensitivity to physical differences among tissues and fluids, (2) its ability to display these differences as image contrast, (3) its capacity to emphasize specific physical properties and manipulate them to accentuate tissue contrast, (4) its ability to select an imaging plane to complement the anatomic or pathologic features of interest, (5) its sensitivity to blood flow, which permits visualization of major blood vessels without the need for intravascular contrast agents, and (6) its apparent lack of significant biologic hazard. Although MR imaging is sensitive to some abnormalities, under most circumstances it is not specific with regard to prediction of pathologic conditions. MR images must be interpreted with knowledge of clinical context to achieve diagnostic relevance.

CLINICAL GUIDELINES

A discussion of the physical principles of signal generation with MR and of the various imaging sequences and techniques is beyond the scope of this synopsis, and the interested reader should consult standard textbooks on this method. Several general principles, however, apply to musculoskeletal MR imaging. First, the patient and body part of interest must be positioned correctly. The anatomic region to be studied should be near the center of the external magnetic field. The closer the region of interest is to the center, the better is the field homogeneity and the resultant image. The major axis of the anatomic part to be studied should be parallel to one of the three main orthogonal imaging axes. Second, it is important to select a surface coil that can be positioned as close to the region of interest as possible and that has a size and configuration complementary to anatomic features. The choice directly affects signal intensity, resolution, and magnification. For large parts (e.g., the pelvis), there is little choice but to use the body coil. The pelvis is centered in the field and 10 mm thick slices are obtained. For parts of intermediate size (e.g., hip, thigh, knee, shoulder), smaller coils are more appropriate. Third, once the coil has been chosen to complement the anatomic region, it is important to consider how slice thickness, acquisition magnification, and the number of excitations averaged influence signal intensity and resolution. Generally, a choice of thinner slices and greater magnification results in less available signal but better in-plane resolution. Fourth, tissue contrast (and to some degree signal intensity) is controlled by the pulse sequence that is selected. One or more spin echo sequences have been shown to be effective for imaging nearly all anatomic sites and pathologic conditions. Although every pulse sequence results in an image that is a mixture of the contributions of proton (spin) density, T1 relaxation rate, T2 relaxation rate, and blood flow, the pulse sequence choices have been divided into three general categories on the basis of the combination of repetition time (TR) and echo time (TE). The T1 weighted image combines a short TR (0.5 s or less) with a short TE (40 ms or less). The shorter the TR and TE (e.g., TE, 15 ms; TR, 0.1 s), the greater the T1 weighting. The proton (spin) density weighted image combines a long TR (1.5 s or more) with a short TE (40 ms or less). The T2 weighted image combines a long TR (1.5 s or more) with a long TE (90 ms or more). The longer the TR and TE (e.g., TE, 120 ms; TR, 2.5 s) the greater the T2 weighting. Other combinations provide intermediate mixtures that have less distinct contributions. Finally, many

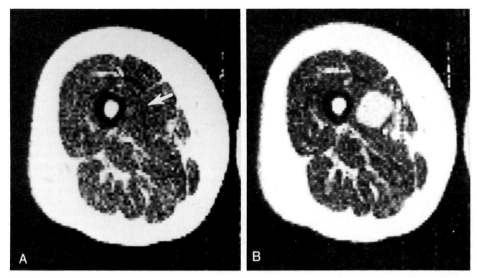

Figure 11–1. Tissue contrast: Influence of pulse sequence selection (intramuscular myxoma). A T1 weighted MR imaging section (TE, 30 ms; TR, 0.3 s) through the thigh shows a region of muscle distortion (arrow), but no contrast difference between the myxoma and the surrounding muscle. **B** Mixed contribution MR imaging section (TE, 60 ms; TR, 0.9 s) at same level as **A** now shows distinct contrast between the myxoma, which is of very high signal intensity, and the surrounding muscle, of much lower signal intensity. (From Murphy WA, Totty WG: Musculoskeletal magnetic resonance imaging. In HY Kressel [Ed]: Magnetic Resonance Annual 1986. New York, Raven Press, 1986, p 4. Used with permission.)

of the choices will be made following consideration of the amount of time necessary to achieve the desired result and complete the examination. Longer repetition times, greater number of excitations averaged, additional imaging planes, and extra pulse sequences all prolong the imaging time.

In MR, as already noted, tissue contrast differences are based on differences of proton (spin) density, T1 relaxation rates, T2 relaxation rates, and blood flow among tissues, all influenced by the particular pulse sequence selected. It has been determined empirically that T1 and T2 weighted images provide the greatest range of contrast. In general, proton density weighting has less diagnostic usefulness in musculoskeletal MR imaging. On T1 weighted images, subcutaneous fat and bone marrow have the brightest signal. Hyaline cartilage is less bright, and muscle is even less bright. Cystic fluid, urine, ligaments, tendons, and bone have little or no signal intensity. On T2 weighted images, cystic fluid and urine have the brightest signal, followed in decreasing order by subcutaneous fat, bone marrow, and muscle. Again, ligaments, tendons, and bone have little or no signal intensity.

Tumors show variation in their appearance on T1 and T2 weighted images depending on their composition. For example, relative to other normal tissues, lipomas have high signal intensity on T1 and T2 weighting. Most other solid tumors have low signal intensity on T1 weighted images (e.g., lower than adjacent muscles) and high signal intensity on T2 weighted images (e.g., higher than fat or bone marrow). The precise characteristics seem to depend on the relative proportions of fat, hydrated tumor cells, and fibrosis.

Blood has special imaging characteristics; it varies in signal intensity depending on the following factors: (1) rate of flow, (2) the character of flow (laminar or turbulent), (3) direction of flow in relation to the slice sequence, (4) existence of a higher signal on even numbered slices in a multislice sequence owing to even echo rephasing, (5) the pulse sequence selected

(e.g., in most sequences the major vessels show no signal because the excited protons exit the section before detection takes place, but in very short TR-TE sequences, the blood can be imaged as a bright signal), and (6) the state of the hemoglobin in areas of hemorrhage.

Because tissue contrast is a function of the combined effect of proton density, T1 relaxation, and T2 relaxation, adjacent normal and pathologic tissues can have identical intensities at a given pulse sequence. It is possible, therefore, that a musculoskeletal lesion will be completely obscured if only a single pulse sequence is employed (Fig. 11–1). Because of this, more than one pulse sequence is obtained in most instances. Choice of an initial pulse sequence depends on the likely location of the anticipated pathologic condition. When the pathologic process is believed to be located in fat, the best first sequence is a T1 weighted examination. Such a choice nearly always results in optimal contrast between the lesion of low signal intensity and the surrounding fat, which is of high signal intensity. Similarly, when the lesion is likely to be located in muscle, the best first sequence is a T2 weighted examination.

The presence of metallic objects, such as ferromagnetic surgical clips, within the human body presents several potential problems for MR imaging. The most important problem is focal loss of signal with or without regional distortion. Metallic objects of any size create "holes" in the image, but ferromagnetic objects cause more distortion. The holes and distortions become greater as field strength increases.

Even when the metallic orthopedic devices are large, however, imaging of nearby tissues is possible. Indeed, images obtained with computed tomography (CT) are more severely degraded by metallic objects than are MR images (Fig. 11–2).

Some indications for MR imaging are summarized in Table 11–1.

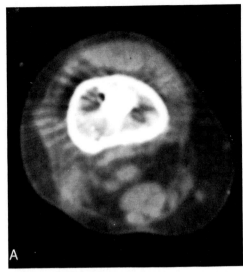
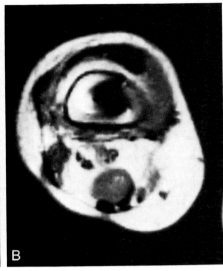

Figure 11–2. Comparison of computed tomographic (CT) and MR imaging artifacts. A Transaxial CT section through the distal end of an intramedullary rod shows radial artifacts throughout most of the image. B Transaxial MR imaging section (TE, 30 ms; TR, 0.5 s) at the same level as the CT section shows that focal loss of signal is restricted to the immediate vicinity of the rod, completely sparing the rest of the section. (From Murphy WA, Totty WG: Musculoskeletal magnetic resonance imaging. In HY Kressel [Ed]: Magnetic Resonance Annual 1986. New York, Raven Press, 1986, p 7. Used with permission.)

BONE MARROW IMAGING

MR imaging is exquisitely sensitive to changes in bone marrow composition. With few exceptions (e.g., aplastic anemia), all conditions that cause infiltration of marrow lengthen the T1 relaxation time locally and are detected by T1 weighted sequences.

Normal Marrow

Normal bone marrow, in comparison to other normal tissues, has high signal intensity on all pulse sequences. The signal presumably results from fat in the marrow; its characteristics are identical to the signal characteristics of subcutaneous fat. The signal from normal bone marrow appears uniform and homogeneous except in specific anatomic locations where there is sufficient trabecular bone (load-bearing trabeculae in metaphyseal locations), cartilage (the physeal plate), or fibrosis (the physeal scar following closure of the growth plate) to cause focally decreased signal intensity. The signal intensity of the marrow varies somewhat from patient to patient but usually is symmetric from one region to another in a given patient. In childhood, epiphyseal (or apophyseal) marrow has a greater signal intensity than metaphyseal or diaphyseal marrow, a pattern that may persist in some young adults (Fig. 11–3).

It is important to recall that marrow comprises two major cell populations, the fat cells and the hematopoietic cells. The proportions of these cells vary according to age, anatomic location, and physiologic stimulation. Infants have marrow that is predominantly hematopoietic (red marrow). With skeletal growth and development, hematopoietic marrow is progressively replaced by fat (yellow marrow), with a proportionately smaller fraction of hematopoietic cells. The epiphyseal and apophyseal growth centers are composed predominantly of yellow marrow throughout life. Hematopoietic marrow tends to be most persistent in the proximal ends of the long tubular bones and in the osseous pelvis, vertebrae, and sternum. Physiologic stresses that require greater hematopoiesis will progressively recruit fatty marrow and convert it back to red marrow. This can be documented in several hematologic diseases and in progressive metastatic disease to bone. Some types of anemias (sickle cell disease, thalassemia) may be associated with hyperplastic red marrow.

The signal patterns of marrow in MR imaging parallel these proportionate changes in yellow and red marrow fractionation and distribution. Fatty (or yellow) marrow has a high signal on T1 weighted sequences owing to the presence of fat protons. Hematopoietic marrow has a much lower signal on T1 weighted sequences owing to the predominance of water protons. Thus, children tend to have a high signal in epiphyses and apophyses because of the large amount of fat and a somewhat lower signal in the metadiaphyseal regions because of the greater amount of hematopoietic tissue. In the mature skeleton, the epiphyses, metaphyses, and diaphyses contain a more homogeneous distribution of cells and have a more homogeneous signal intensity. The signal intensity at any time reflects the balance of yellow and red marrow (Fig. 11–3). With physiologic stresses that cause an increased fraction of hematopoietic marrow, the signal intensity on T1 weighted sequences diminishes (Fig. 11–4).

Table 11–1. SOME INDICATIONS FOR MR IMAGING

Bone Marrow
Neoplasia
Osteomyelitis
Devascularization
Reflex sympathetic dystrophy syndrome

Bones
Neoplasia
Traumatic lesions

Soft Tissues
Neoplasia
Hematomas
Abscesses

Joints
Masses
Arthritis
Ligament and tendon abnormalities
Internal derangements

Muscles
Traumatic lesions
Muscular dystrophy

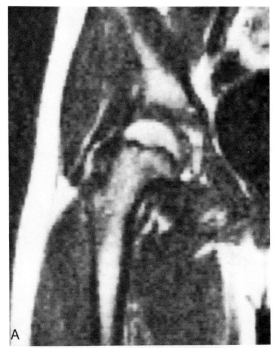

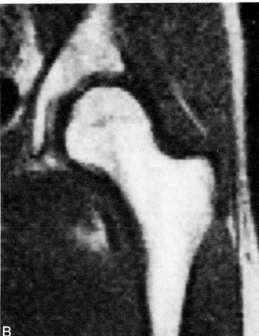

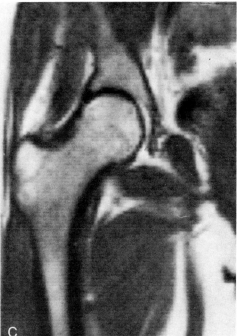

Figure 11–3. Marrow distribution and pattern in the hip. **A** At age 10 years (TE, 35 ms; TR, 0.5 s). The femoral head epiphysis has high signal intensity owing to the predominant fat content, whereas the adjacent metaphysis has much lower signal intensity owing to predominance of hematopoietic tissue. Note the low signal intensity of the physis. **B** At age 30 years (TE, 35 ms; TR, 0.5 s). The proximal portion of the femur has a nearly uniform high fraction of fat cells. The focal areas of lower signal intensity in the femoral head and neck are attributable to trabecular bone and residual physeal scar. **C** At age 32 years (TE, 35 ms; TR, 0.6 s). The femoral head and neck are of nearly homogeneous signal intensity but of a relatively less intensity than in the patient in **B**, owing to the greater fraction of hematopoietic cells. Note that the greater trochanter has high signal intensity owing to the focally increased fat fraction.

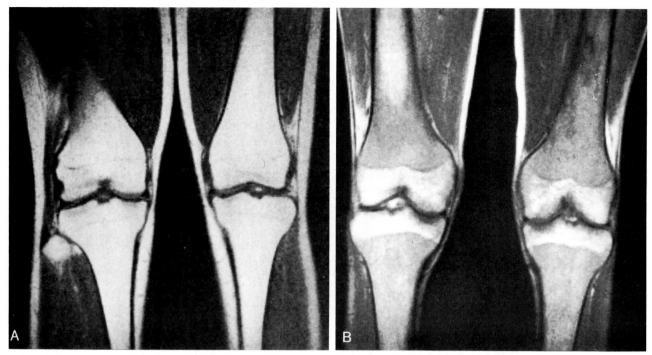

Figure 11–4. Comparison of normal and hyperplastic marrow. A At age 25 years (TE, 30 ms; TR, 0.3 s). Knees of a normal volunteer in a head coil show homogeneous distribution of predominantly fatty (yellow) marrow. Note the lines of low signal intensity from the physeal scars. **B** At age 24 years (TE, 35 ms; TR, 0.5 s). Knees of a patient with sickle cell disease show inhomogeneous but regional signal alterations. Note the predominantly high signal intensity from the epiphyses and the right femoral diaphysis, indicating the high fat fraction in those locations. Note also the low signal intensity of the rest of the marrow, indicating the high fraction of hyperplastic hematopoietic (red) marrow.

Because most pathologic processes cause lengthening of bone marrow T1 times, T1 weighted pulse sequences are recommended to detect bone marrow lesions.

Pathologic Marrow

NEOPLASIA. Metastasis, plasma cell myeloma, leukemia, and lymphoma lead to the replacement of normal bone marrow, resulting in focally decreased marrow signal (Fig. 11–5). These alterations are due primarily to replacement of the fat cells (with short T1 relaxation times) by tumor cells (with long T1 relaxation times), although other mechanisms, including fat necrosis, new bone formation, and fibrosis, contribute to this decrease in signal intensity on T1 weighted pulse sequences. If tumor also involves the subcutaneous fat, T1 weighted sequences are optimal for similar reasons.

It is clear that MR imaging is a very sensitive method for detection of malignant infiltration of bone marrow. MR imaging is not well suited to the evaluation of the entire skeleton, however; when a rapid and effective method is required to survey all regions of the skeleton, scintigraphy using bone-seeking radiopharmaceutical agents is the technique of choice. In the assessment of focal areas of marrow infiltration, MR imaging appears also to be superior to CT for two major reasons: It provides greater contrast resolution between normal bone marrow and tumor, and it allows direct imaging of the long axis of any bone.

Although MR imaging is highly sensitive in the detection of neoplastic involvement of the bone marrow, it must be considered a nonspecific technique. Various neoplastic and non-neoplastic processes that are characterized by marrow infiltration have similar alterations in T1 and T2 values.

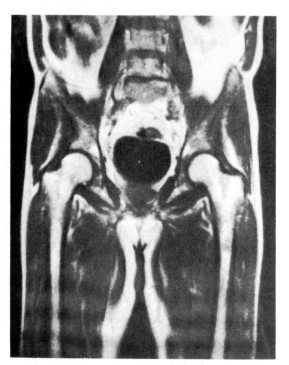

Figure 11–5. Focal marrow replacement by plasma cell myeloma (TE, 35 ms; TR, 0.5 s). Note the focal regions of low signal intensity in the proximal femora. Observe also that the majority of the osseous pelvis shown in this section is of low signal intensity owing to myeloma cell replacement of normal bone marrow.

OSTEOMYELITIS. As with malignant infiltration, osteomyelitis results in replacement of normal marrow by inflammatory cells and fluids that have longer T1 values than those of normal marrow and hence decreased signal intensity on T1 weighted sequences (Fig. 11–6). An MR imaging examination showing only normal marrow is a good indication that there is no infection.

Unfortunately, MR imaging is not a specific method for identifying infection. In addition to osteomyelitis, other processes, such as neoplasms and sterile fluid collections, produce a decreased signal on T1 weighted sequences. The addition of T2 weighted sequences does not improve the specificity of MR imaging for infection. Pyogenic and sterile abscesses and neoplasms all result in prolonged T2 values and increased signal intensity on T2 weighted images.

DEVASCULARIZATION. Devascularization of the bone marrow may result from a variety of insults, including fracture or dislocation, steroid therapy, sickle cell disease, hyperbaric pressure (caisson disease), and cellular infiltration (e.g., Gaucher's disease). Although the causative events may vary, the pathophysiologic processes are similar. Interruption of the blood supply leads to necrosis of trabeculae and marrow elements and is typically followed by a reparative process in which the injured tissue is gradually removed and replaced. The conversion of normal marrow rich in fat to necrotic marrow is characterized on MR imaging by a decrease in signal intensity.

The sensitivity of MR imaging in detecting devascularization of the bone marrow is best documented in processes that involve the femoral head, both in children (Legg-Calvé-

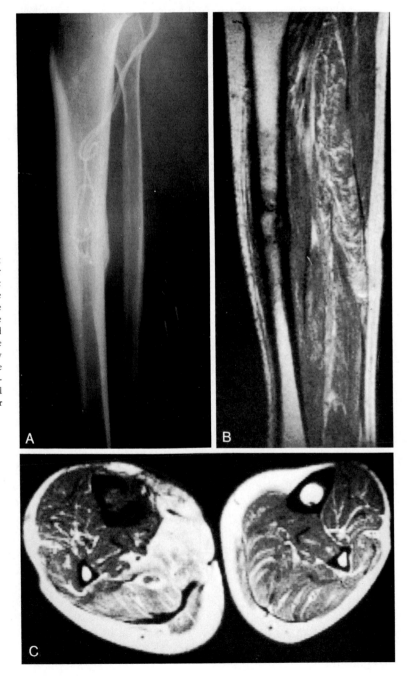

Figure 11–6. Osteomyelitis. **A** Lateral radiograph of the leg of a 37 year old man with chronic tibial osteomyelitis after surgical intervention and placement of a catheter for antibiotic infusion and drainage of the abscess. **B** Parasagittal MR image (head coil; TE, 35 ms; TR, 0.6 s) corresponding to the radiograph in **A** shows extent of marrow involvement of the tibial diaphysis, reactive thickening of the tibial cortex, and alteration of the adjacent soft tissues. **C** Transaxial MR image (head coil; TE, 30 ms; TR, 0.3 s) of both legs shows low signal intensity of the right tibial marrow, destruction of the anteromedial cortex, and atrophy of the soleus and gastrocnemius muscles. Note the normal signal from the left tibial and fibular bone marrow as well as from the right fibular marrow.

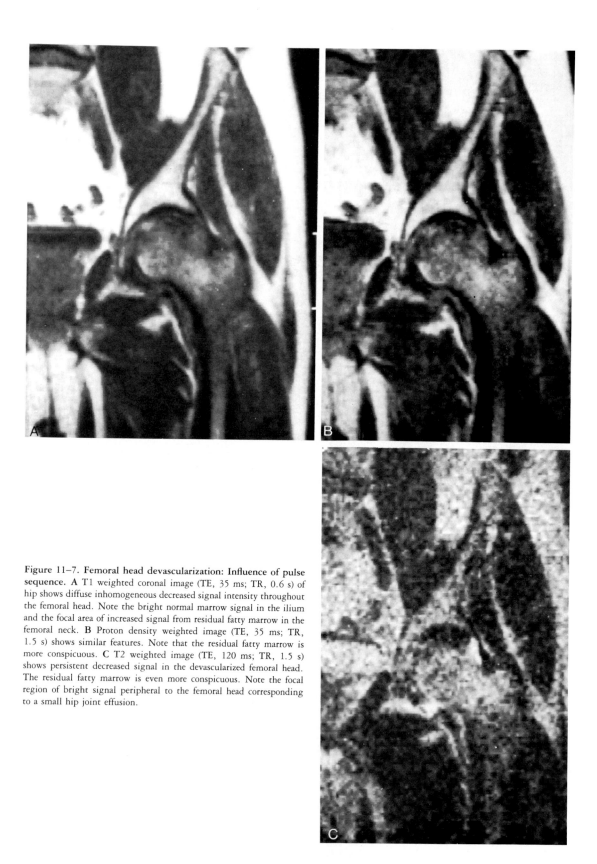

Figure 11–7. Femoral head devascularization: Influence of pulse sequence. A T1 weighted coronal image (TE, 35 ms; TR, 0.6 s) of hip shows diffuse inhomogeneous decreased signal intensity throughout the femoral head. Note the bright normal marrow signal in the ilium and the focal area of increased signal from residual fatty marrow in the femoral neck. **B** Proton density weighted image (TE, 35 ms; TR, 1.5 s) shows similar features. Note that the residual fatty marrow is more conspicuous. **C** T2 weighted image (TE, 120 ms; TR, 1.5 s) shows persistent decreased signal in the devascularized femoral head. The residual fatty marrow is even more conspicuous. Note the focal region of bright signal peripheral to the femoral head corresponding to a small hip joint effusion.

Perthes disease) and in adults. In the femoral head (or in other sites), devascularization leads to areas of low signal intensity that are surrounded by adjacent normal marrow of higher signal intensity. The diminution of signal intensity is independent of the selected pulse sequences, although intraosseous cysts or an adjacent joint effusion may lead to an increase in signal intensity as the TR and TE are prolonged (Fig. 11–7). A T1 weighted sequence in children with Legg-Calvé-Perthes disease reveals focally decreased signal intensity in the epiphyseal ossification center. In adults, four basic patterns of femoral head devascularization (homogeneous, inhomogeneous, band, and ring) have been described.

MR imaging clearly is more sensitive than conventional radiography in detecting femoral head devascularization, and it is at least as sensitive as bone scintigraphy (Fig. 11–8). Furthermore, when radionuclide studies appear normal or when results are indeterminate, MR imaging commonly reveals an abnormality (Fig. 11–9). Under these circumstances, a normal MR imaging examination effectively excludes an abnormality.

Patients with devascularized femoral heads who undergo core decompression procedures may return with persistent or new pain. The ability of MR imaging to distinguish among normal findings, postoperative abnormalities, and ischemic bone marrow in these patients is not shared by conventional radiography or radionuclide studies. Furthermore, MR imaging can sensitively detect devascularization in many other sites of bone marrow, including the humeral head, the bones about the knee, and the carpal bones (Fig. 11–10). Two factors improve the specificity of the MR findings. First, the clinical information and the results of other imaging studies will usually limit the diagnostic possibilities (Fig. 11–11). Second, additional pulse sequences may help distinguish devascularized marrow from that involved by other disease processes. On T2 weighted sequences devascularized marrow remains of low signal intensity whereas more hydrated tissues (as are evident in most neoplastic processes) have increasing signal intensity as the TR and TE are prolonged.

REFLEX SYMPATHETIC DYSTROPHY SYNDROME AND SYNOVITIS. The water content in the bone marrow may be altered by a variety of inflammatory mechanisms. In the reflex sympathetic dystrophy syndrome (and in other forms of transient osteoporosis) or in synovitis, T1 weighted MR sequences show focally decreased signal intensity of the marrow; the T2 weighted sequences reveal reversal of signal intensity, with the abnormal region having a signal intensity equal to or greater than that of normal marrow (Fig. 11–12). Small effusions in the adjacent joint may be evident. These features on MR imaging apparently reflect bone marrow edema as a consequence of hyperemia induced by the reflex sympathetic dystrophy syndrome or synovitis.

BONE TUMORS AND SOFT TISSUE MASSES
Bone Tumors

BENIGN BONE TUMORS. Generally, conventional radiography is adequate to detect and characterize benign bone tumors. MR imaging is similar to or better than CT in detecting and locating benign bone tumors, but as yet it, too, has no real diagnostic advantage. With MR, the signal intensity of the tumor varies according to the composition of the lesion and to the pulse sequence that is employed. Simple

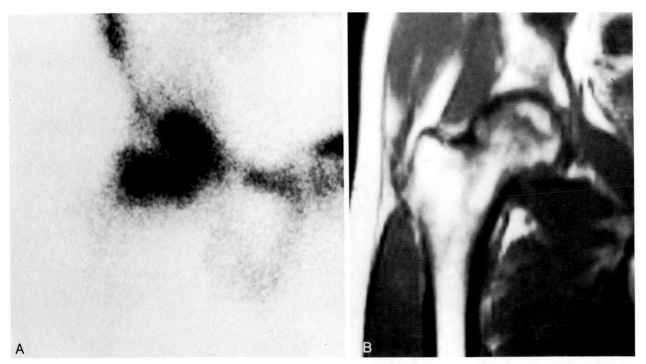

Figure 11–8. Scintigraphically evident ischemic necrosis of the femoral head. A Scintigraphy shows focally increased radionuclide accumulation in the femoral head, characteristic of the healing phase of ischemic necrosis. **B** Coronal MR image (TE, 30 ms; TR, 0.5 s) shows decreased signal intensity of the femoral head, confirming the presence of ischemic necrosis. Note the residual, more normal fatty marrow.

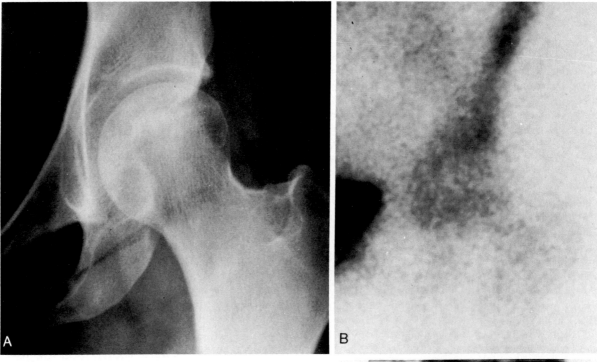

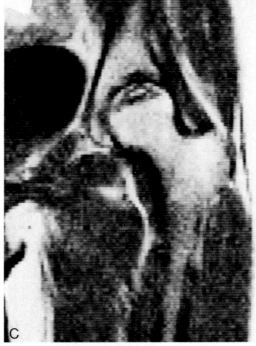

Figure 11–9. **Radiographically and scintigraphically occult ischemic necrosis of the femoral head. A** Anteroposterior radiograph shows no evidence of ischemic necrosis of the femoral head. **B** Scintigraphy likewise shows normal results. **C** Coronal MR image (TE, 30 ms; TR, 0.3 s) confirms the presence of ischemic necrosis of the femoral head, showing the ring pattern.

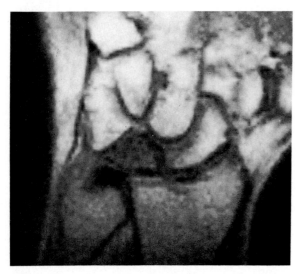

Figure 11–10. **Lunate devascularization.** Surface coil coronal image (TE, 30 ms; TR, 0.6 s) of the carpus shows decreased signal intensity of the lunate bone marrow, indicating lunate devascularization.

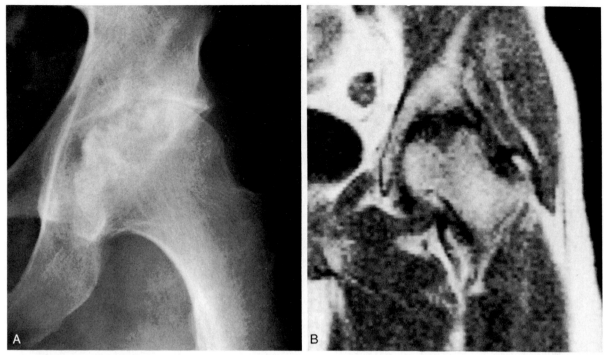

Figure 11–11. Juvenile chronic arthritis A Anteroposterior radiograph of the left hip of a 25 year old man with known arthritis shows cartilage loss, bone erosions, and subchondral cyst formation. **B** Coronal MR image (TE, 30 ms; TR, 0.5 s) reveals findings similar to those of primary bone marrow devascularization. Clinical history and conventional radiography permit a more specific interpretation of the MR imaging examination. (From Murphy WA, Totty WG: Musculoskeletal magnetic resonance imaging. In HY Kressl [Ed]: Magnetic Resonance Annual 1986. New York, Raven Press, 1986, p 17 Used with permission.)

and aneurysmal bone cysts are of low signal intensity on T1 weighted images and may demonstrate fluid levels. Cysts containing blood that is not fresh are of high signal intensity. Bone cysts are also of high signal intensity on T2 weighted examinations. The greater the fraction of water or fibrous tissue in a solid neoplasm, the lower is the signal intensity on T1 weighted images. The greater the amount of water or fat, the higher is the signal intensity on T2 weighted images. If the lesion contains marrow, as exists in portions of osteochondromas, the tumor will have imaging characteristics that are identical to those of the adjacent bone marrow (Fig. 11–13). Calcifications that are detected by conventional radiography will rarely be demonstrated on any MR imaging pulse sequence unless they are large and surrounded by fat.

MALIGNANT BONE TUMORS. As is true of benign bone tumors, the radiologic features of malignant bone tumors are sufficient to allow a specific diagnosis in many cases. MR imaging, however, is at least equal to and often better than CT for combined detection, location, and characterization of the extent of malignant bone tumors. MR imaging, nevertheless, is is often judged superior to CT in the delineation of tumor extent, both within the medullary cavity and in the adjacent soft tissues (Fig. 11–14). Conversely, CT clearly is superior to MR imaging for the detection of calcifications. MR imaging is as effective as CT in documenting cortical involvement by tumor. Endosteal and periosteal new bone formation and cortical infiltration or perforation can therefore be detected (Fig. 11–15).

In the absence of hemorrhage and calcification, malignant bone tumors have long T1 values and low signal intensity on T1 weighted images. They have prolonged T2 values and demonstrate high signal intensity on T2 weighted images.

Subacute and chronic hemorrhage within a tumor leads to short T1 times with a bright signal on T1 weighted images. The greater the amount of tumor calcification, the lower is the signal intensity on T2 weighted images.

Soft Tissue Masses

MR imaging is an effective method for the detection, location, and characterization of soft tissue masses. MR imaging generally is superior to CT because it has better contrast resolution and allows more freedom in the selection of an imaging plane. If clinically the mass is localized to subcutaneous fat, a T1 weighted sequence should be employed first (Fig. 11–16). If the lesion is believed to originate in muscle, a T2 weighted sequence should be used initially (Fig. 11–17).

TUMORS. Because of its great contrast resolution, MR will demonstrate the boundaries of tumors with respect to adjacent fat, muscle, bone, and major blood vessels, especially if a combination of transaxial, coronal, sagittal, and oblique planes is used. The one major disadvantage of MR imaging in the evaluation of soft tissue (as well as osseous) tumors is its inability to detect and characterize any associated calcifications.

Soft tissue tumors have contrast characteristics on MR imaging that depend on their tissue composition. Lipomas have high signal intensity on both T1 and T2 weighted sequences. Solid, cellular tumors or those with a myxoid matrix have low to intermediate signal intensity on T1 weighted sequences and high signal intensity on T2 weighted sequences (Fig. 11–17). Tumors having a high fraction of blood have variable signal characteristics that are dependent on blood flow and the extent and duration of hemorrhage.

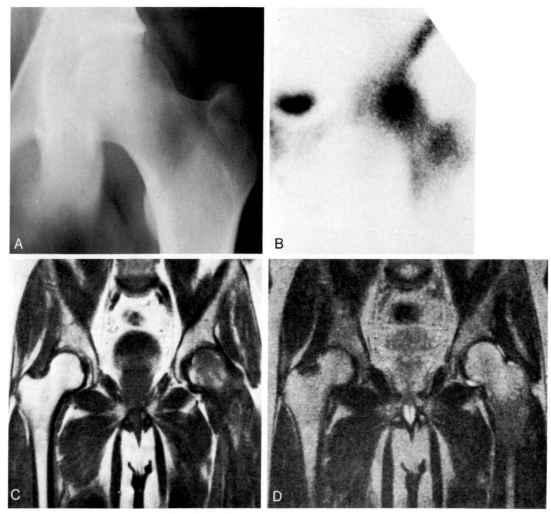

Figure 11–12. Reflex sympathetic dystrophy syndrome. A Conventional tomography of a painful left hip in a 38 year old man shows subtle demineralization of the femoral head. **B** Scintigraphy shows regionally increased radionuclide accumulation. **C** T1 weighted coronal image (TE, 35 ms; TR, 0.6 s) shows decreased signal intensity of the marrow in the proximal portion of the left femur. *D* T2 weighted image (TE, 120 ms; TR, 1.5 s) shows relatively increased signal intensity, presumably confirming the presence of an increased fraction of water protons.

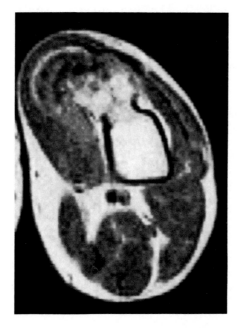

Figure 11–13. Osteochondroma (exostosis). Proton density weighted image (TE, 30 ms; TR, 1.5 s) of the left thigh of a young man shows a large exostosis continuous with the medullary cavity of the femur. Note that the bone marrow in the base of the exostosis is continuous with that in the femur.

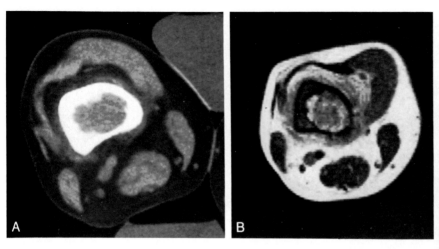

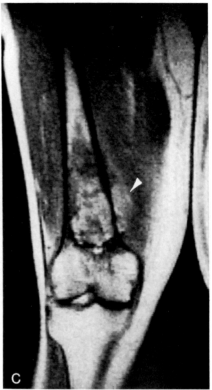

Figure 11–14. Angiosarcoma. A Transaxial computed tomographic scan through the distal portion of the thigh in a 35 year old man shows a tumor in the medullary cavity and infiltration of fat around the femur. B T1 weighted MR transaxial section (TE, 30 ms; TR, 0.5 s) at a similar level as in A shows a tumor in the medullary cavity, penetration of the posteromedial cortex, and more extensive infiltration of surrounding fat. C T1 weighted coronal image (TE, 30 ms; TR, 0.5 s) shows the proximal and distal extent of the tumor, erosion of the medial femoral cortex, and direct extension of the medullary tumor into the medial soft tissues (arrowhead). (Courtesy of M. Kyriakos, M.D., St. Louis, Missouri.)

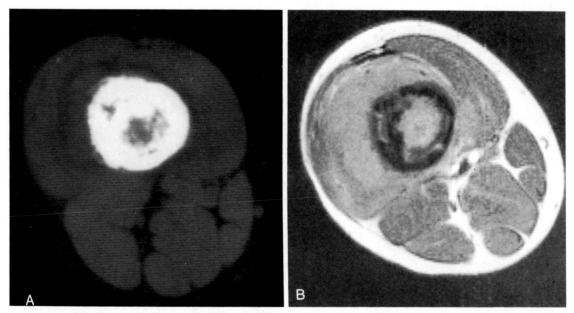

Figure 11–15. Osteosarcoma. A Computed tomographic section through the midfemur of a 15 year old boy shows tumor in the medullary cavity with dense endosteal and periosteal new bone formation. Extraosseous tumor extent is not well delineated at this window setting. B Transaxial T1 weighted section (TE, 30 ms; TR, 0.5 s) at a level similar to that in A shows the medullary tumor and proliferation of endosteal and periosteal bone. In addition, it reveals tumor infiltration of the cortex with extension into the soft tissues surrounding the femur. Note the displacement of the quadriceps muscles and the proximity of the tumor to the femoral blood vessels. (From Murphy WA, Totty WG: Musculoskeletal magnetic resonance imaging. In HY Kressel [Ed]: Magnetic Resonance Annual 1986. New York, Raven Press, 1986, p 26. Used with permission.)

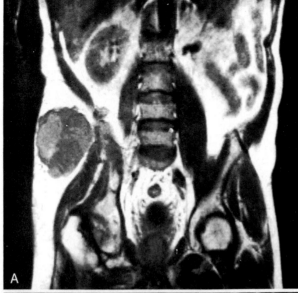

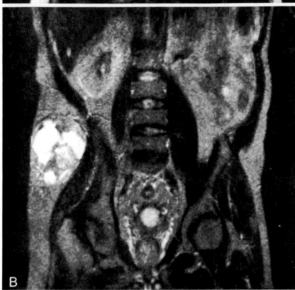

Figure 11–16. **Malignant fibrous histiocytoma. A** T1 weighted coronal section (TE, 35 ms; TR, 0.6 s) of the flank of a 60 year old man shows excellent contrast and spatial resolution of the subcutaneous tumor on the right side. **B** T2 weighted coronal section (TE, 120 ms; TR, 1.5 s) at the same level as in **A** shows the inhomogeneous nature of the tumor. Note how difficult it is to determine the interface between the tumor and the subcutaneous fat with this image sequence.

Lesions with large fractions of fibrous tissue have low signal characteristics on both pulse sequences.

Diagnostically, MR imaging generally is nonspecific. The main exceptions to this rule are lipomas and hemangiomas, which have more characteristic signal behavior (Figs. 11–18 and 11–19). Furthermore, it generally is not possible with MR imaging to distinguish between benign and malignant tumors.

HEMATOMAS. Hemorrhage in soft tissue structures (hematoma) has signal characteristics that change as the blood in the mass ages. Acute hemorrhage has a signal intensity similar to that of muscle on T1 weighted images and a high

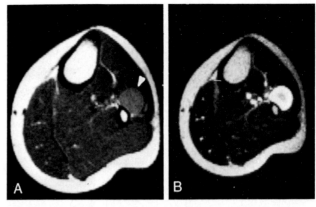

Figure 11–17. **Lipomyxoma. A** T1 weighted transaxial section (TE, 35 ms; TR, 0.6 s) through the calf of a 22 year old woman shows a tumor adjacent to the left fibula (arrowhead). Note the minor difference in contrast between the tumor and the surrounding muscle. **B** T2 weighted section (TE, 90 ms; TR, 1.5 s) at the same level as in **A** shows the tumor to have a very intense signal, whereas the muscle is of very low signal intensity.

signal intensity on T2 weighted images. After approximately 2 days, there is progressive shortening of the T1 relaxation time of the hematoma, and its signal intensity becomes much greater than that of muscle on T1 weighted images. This phenomenon is attributed to sequential changes that occur as the hemoglobin molecules are oxidized to methemoglobin. After several days (subacute) and for many months (chronic), hematomas will have very strong signal intensity on both T1 and T2 weighted pulse sequences, permitting the accurate identification of blood (Fig. 11–20).

ABSCESSES. Abscesses in the soft tissues are readily detected by MR imaging. They appear to be of low signal intensity on T1 weighted images, similar to that of the surrounding muscle, but are of greater signal intensity than muscle on T2 weighted images. They may be homogeneous or inhomogeneous and have smooth or irregular margins.

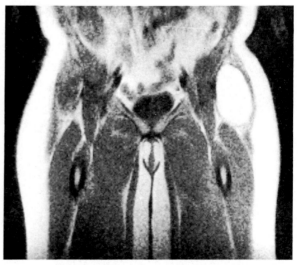

Figure 11–18. **Lipoma.** T1 weighted coronal section (TE, 30 ms; TR, 0.5 s) through the pelvis of a 42 year old woman shows an intermuscular lipoma on the left side. Note that the signal intensity of the lipoma is identical to that of subcutaneous fat.

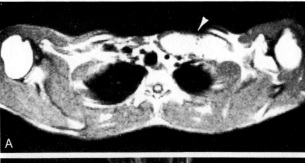

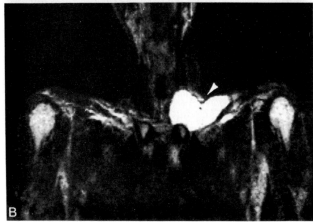

Figure 11–19. **Cavernous hemangioma. A** T1 weighted transaxial section (TE, 30 ms; TR,0.5 s) shows the precise extent of the mass, which has a very high signal intensity (arrowhead). **B** T2 weighted coronal section (TE, 90 ms; TR, 1.5 s) shows the precise extent of the mass, which has a very high signal intensity (arrowhead).

TRAUMATIC ABNORMALITIES
Soft Tissue Injury

Generally, there is little need to obtain MR images of soft tissue injuries except when the injury causes a soft tissue mass or a tear of an important ligament, tendon, or cartilaginous structure.

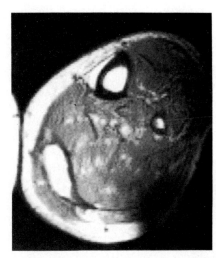

Figure 11–20. **Chronic hematoma.** T1 weighted transaxial image (TE, 30 ms; TR, 0.7 s) of the calf in a 55 year old man shows an oval mass of high signal intensity. This hematoma was many months old.

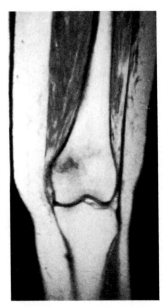

Figure 11–21. **Stress fracture.** T1 weighted coronal image (head coil; TE, 30 ms; TR, 0.6 s) shows a focal area of decreased signal intensity in a transcondylar linear pattern consistent with a stress fracture.

Bone Injury

MR imaging occasionally is useful in defining some of the complications of the acute injury, such as hemorrhage or edema, as well as more chronic changes in the bone marrow resulting from healing. Although scintigraphy is a valuable method in the early identification of stress fractures, MR imaging may also be useful in selected cases because it is very sensitive to alterations in the bone marrow (Fig. 11–21).

ARTICULAR ABNORMALITIES

MR imaging is an effective method for evaluating many types of joint abnormality, including tumors, arthritis, and injuries to ligaments, tendons, and cartilage. It must be emphasized that surface coils should be used routinely to improve the spatial resolution when studying joints.

Masses

Cysts may arise as bursal extensions of the joint and be fluid filled, having low signal intensity on T1 weighted sequences and high signal intensity on T2 weighted sequences. Tumors about joints can be expected to reveal a spectrum of signal behavior determined by their composition.

Arthritis

MR imaging is very sensitive in detecting small amounts of effusion in joints (Fig. 11–22). Periarticular edema also is detected by MR imaging as increased signal on T2 weighted sequences. Bone marrow changes, which include hyperemia and edema, may occur as a response to synovitis.

Ligament and Tendon Abnormalities

As ligaments and tendons are composed of dense collagen fibers with few mobile protons, they have a very short T2 and appear of very low signal intensity on all pulse sequences. Ligament and tendon ruptures are delineated as regions of discontinuity having greater than normal signal intensity with

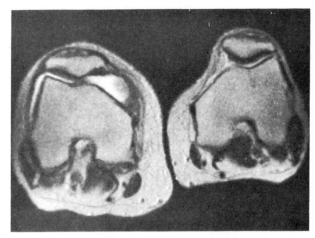

Figure 11–22. **Knee joint effusion:** T2 weighted transaxial image (head coil; TE, 90 ms; TR, 1.5 s) of both knees shows an effusion of high signal intensity within the right knee.

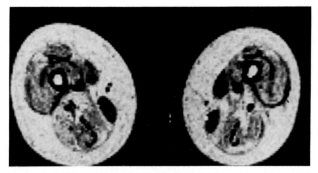

Figure 11–24. **Duchenne muscular dystrophy.** Transaxial MR image (TE, 30 ms; TR, 0.3 s) through the thigh of a 16 year old boy shows extensive fatty replacement of most of the muscles.

associated alterations in signal intensity from adjacent fatty tissues (Fig. 11–23).

Use of surface coils and high field strengths to achieve high resolution has permitted evaluation of meniscal tears in the knee, although the degree of sensitivity of the technique is not yet clear. Hyaline articular cartilage also is well imaged and has a higher signal intensity than that of meniscal cartilage owing to its greater fraction of mobile water protons.

MUSCLE ABNORMALITIES
Normal Muscles

MR imaging is effective for demonstrating normal and diseased muscle. The signal intensity of normal muscle (in all commonly used pulse sequences) is intermediate between those of fat and cortical bone, but it is much less intense than that of fat. The intermuscular fat planes are readily delineated, and muscle groups are identified easily.

Pathologic Muscles

MR imaging can characterize the various types of muscle disease, defining the location and distribution of diseased muscles and the pattern of fatty replacement (Fig. 11–24).

FURTHER READING

Aisen AM, Martel W, Braunstein EM, McMillin KI, Phillips WA, Kling TF: MRI and CT evaluation of primary bone and soft-tissue tumors. AJR 146:749, 1986.

Beltran J, Noto AM, Herman LJ, Mosure JC, Burk JM, Christoforidis AJ: Joint effusions: MR imaging. Radiology 158:133, 1986.

Dooms GC, Fisher MR, Hricak H, Richardson M, Crooks LE, Genant HK: Bone marrow imaging: Magnetic resonance studies related to age and sex. Radiology 155:429, 1985.

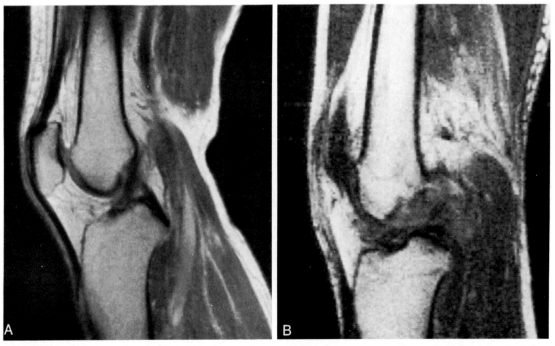

Figure 11–23. **Normal and abnormal cruciate ligaments. A** Proton density weighted sagittal image (head coil; TE, 35 ms; TR, 1.5 s) of a normal knee shows a low signal intensity of the anterior and posterior cruciate ligaments. **B** T1 weighted sagittal image (head coil; TE, 30 ms; TR, 0.3 s) of an abnormal knee shows a joint effusion of low signal intensity and failure to visualize the cruciate ligaments.

Mink JH, Levy T, Cruess JV III: Tears of the anterior cruciate ligament and menisci of the knee: MR imaging evaluation. Radiology 167:769, 1988.

Moon KL Jr, Genant HK, Davis PL, Chafetz NI, Helms CA, Morris JM, Rodrigo JJ, Jergesen HE, Brasch RC, Bovill EG Jr: Nuclear magnetic resonance imaging in orthopaedics: Principles and applications. J Orthop Res 1:101, 1983.

Murphy WA, Totty WG: Musculoskeletal magnetic resonance imaging. In HY Kressel (Ed): Magnetic Resonance Annual 1986. New York, Raven Press, 1986, p 1.

Murphy WA, Totty WG, Carroll JE: MRI of normal and pathologic skeletal muscle. AJR 146:565, 1986.

Reicher MA, Bassett LW, Gold RH: High-resolution magnetic resonance imaging of the knee joint: Pathologic correlations. AJR 145:903, 1985.

Richardson ML, Genant HK, Helms CA, Gillespy T III, Heller M, Jergesen HE, Bovill EG Jr: Magnetic resonance imaging of the musculoskeletal system. Orthop Clin North Am 16:569, 1985.

Shellock FG: MR imaging of metallic implants and materials: A compilation of the literature. AJR 151:811, 1988.

Thickman D, Axel L, Kressel HY, Steinberg M, Chen H, Velchick M, Fallon M, Dalinka M: Magnetic resonance imaging of avascular necrosis of the femoral head. Skel Radiol 15:133, 1986.

Totty WG, Murphy WA, Lee JKT: Soft-tissue tumors: MR imaging. Radiology 160:135, 1986.

Totty WG, Murphy WA, Ganz WI, Kumar B, Daum WJ, Siegel BA: Magnetic resonance imaging of the normal and ischemic femoral head. AJR 143:1273, 1984.

Vogler JB III, Murphy WA: Bone marrow imaging. Radiology 168:679, 1988.

Zimmer WD, Berquist TH, McLeod RA, Sim FH, Pritchard DJ, Shives TC, Wold LE, May GR: Bone tumors: Magnetic resonance imaging versus computed tomography. Radiology 155:709, 1985.

Chapter 12

Diagnostic Ultrasonography

William Scheible, M.D.

The place of diagnostic ultrasonography in clinical imaging is secure. Its role in musculoskeletal disease continues to evolve, but relevant indications have now been defined. Major improvements in resolution and image quality are *unlikely to occur in the near future, but advances in transducer technology may expand its applicability to superficial structures and particularly to intraoperative use.*

Diagnostic ultrasonography has achieved a central role in the evaluation of numerous clinical problems in obstetrics, medicine, and surgery. Although its role in problems related to bone, joint, and soft tissue is limited, there are situations in which the technique offers significant information, usually with less discomfort, risk, cost, and time expenditure than alternative radiographic or isotopic procedures (Table 12–1).

Real-time instruments have come to occupy a central role in clinical ultrasonography; indeed, many examinations are now carried out exclusively with real-time imaging. Real-time can be considered the sonographic equivalent of radiographic fluoroscopy because it entails the observation and recording of dynamic events. The compact size of commercially available units lends itself well to investigation of superficial structures, such as those of the musculoskeletal system. Proper focusing depth can be achieved by simple placement of a water path between the transducer face and the body part; some units have this as a built-in feature. Transducer assemblies can be made quite small and adapted for use in the operating room, where physical access to the area of concern may be limited.

The earliest use of diagnostic ultrasonography was primarily for differentiation of cystic from solid mass lesions that had been detected by clinical or radiographic examinations. Although this is still an important task for sonography, cystic versus solid distinction is only one feature of tissue characterization. Analysis of gray scale patterns can sometimes anticipate the histologic makeup of a given lesion. Fat, for example, tends to be highly echogenic. Deposits of lymphoma, on the other hand, and some neurogenic tumors, although clearly solid, may exhibit features suggestive of cysts. Unfortunately, although experimental work with tissue signatures has been ongoing for years, no truly reliable or practical measurements exist to grant ultrasonography meaningful tissue specificity.

CLINICAL APPLICATIONS

Popliteal Space

The use of ultrasonography for evaluation of various swellings in the popliteal space gained early acceptance. Because fluid-solid distinction was easily accomplished even by early instruments, and because popliteal cysts and popliteal artery aneurysms constitute the majority of masses in this area, sonography has frequently been used in diagnosing these lesions.

Direct comparisons of sonography with contrast arthrography in detection of popliteal cysts generally have shown no distinct advantage for either technique in terms of overall accuracy. Certain circumstances offer potential sources of error for each method. Lack of anatomic continuity between the knee joint and the gastrocnemiosemimembranosus bursa prevents arthrographic or isotopic demonstration of a significant number of cysts. Also, the contrast agent may not fill the entire cyst because of fibrin clots, adhesions, and loculations. Sonography circumvents both of these problems. On the other hand, sonography may fail to detect some ruptured cysts that have decompressed and may miss small cysts. The size threshold for sonographic identification of popliteal cysts should be less than 1 cm, particularly with the use of higher frequency transducers. Variable amounts of septation, debris, or pannus may be seen within the cyst (Fig. 12–1).

Ultrasonography has been recommended as a screening procedure for patients with rheumatoid arthritis who have swelling, painful or asymptomatic, of the popliteal space. Because structural integrity of the knee joint is not an issue in these patients, the risks, discomfort, and costs of arthrography can be avoided. Moreover, ultrasonography is a particularly attractive means of performing serial noninvasive studies to monitor response to various therapeutic endeavors.

Rupture of a popliteal cyst or hemorrhage into the cyst can produce a clinical picture that closely mimics thrombophlebitis. Compression of the popliteal vein by the cyst can also

Table 12–1. SOME INDICATIONS FOR DIAGNOSTIC ULTRASONOGRAPHY

Differentiation of cystic and solid lesions
Evaluation of the popliteal space (popliteal cysts, popliteal artery aneurysms)
Monitoring response to treatment in rheumatoid arthritis
Evaluation of the knee, hip, shoulder, and spine
Evaluation of bone and soft tissue tumors
Detection of infections
Investigation of musculoskeletal trauma
Use during operative procedures
Evaluation of miscellaneous metabolic diseases

136

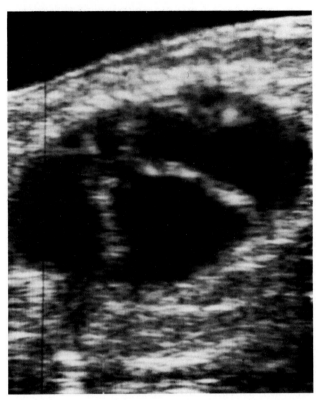

Figure 12–1. Popliteal cyst. High resolution scan using 10 MHz transducer shows a well-demarcated popliteal cyst with internal septation. Frame size is 3 × 4 cm.

produce physical signs resembling thrombophlebitis. The distinction between a popliteal cyst and thrombophlebitis is an important one to make, as anticoagulant therapy is required in the latter instance and is not without hazard. Ultrasonography has been a valuable aid in this clinical setting.

Aneurysms of the popliteal artery are the most frequent of the peripheral arterial aneurysms. Angiography has been the traditional method for diagnosing and evaluating popliteal artery aneurysms. Although it is required to determine the extent of disease and to assess the state of proximal and distal circulation, arteriography suffers from several limitations that are overcome by ultrasonography. Many patients with popliteal artery aneurysms have diffuse vascular disease, and compromised proximal inflow may preclude visualization of the popliteal artery. Thrombus within an aneurysm, easily documented by sonography, is not seen with arteriography, which opacifies only the patent lumen carrying flowing blood. In addition to the ability of sonography to detect aneurysms and thrombus within them, the technique easily accomplishes a survey of the other leg for clinically silent aneurysms.

The ultrasonographic diagnosis of popliteal artery aneurysm is relatively straightforward so long as continuity of the mass with a proximal and distal vessel can be ascertained. This occasionally may be difficult when the popliteal artery is exceedingly tortuous.

Knee

Ultrasonography is capable of measuring the thickness of articular cartilage in the knee and of assessing its surface characteristics. Real-time ultrasonography also is capable of showing the posterior horns of the medial and lateral menisci. This technique has been used to differentiate the normal from the abnormal patellar tendon and to evaluate the closely associated pretibial bursa.

Hip

Ultrasonography can be used as a screening procedure to document the presence of intraarticular fluid in the hip. Sonography can often differentiate among abscesses, hematomas, cellulitis, thrombophlebitis, aneurysm, and lymphadenopathy about the hip, and, if necessary, it affords a convenient method to guide percutaneous aspiration or biopsy of suspicious areas.

Fluid collections within the iliopsoas bursa are often associated with the synovitis that accompanies many arthritides. Sonography aids in establishing this diagnosis, which can be confirmed by subsequent hip arthrography.

A possible role for ultrasonography in congenital hip dysplasia, a relatively common entity, was espoused early on. Articulated arm B-scanners were used, and although the results were encouraging, the technical hurdles encountered in obtaining reproducible images were thought by most radiologists to be considerable. Real-time evaluation with mechanical sector scanners has proved to be a simpler and more easily learned technique. That the femoral head is cartilaginous and does not ossify until about 3 to 6 months after birth is at once a limitation for radiography and an advantage for ultrasonography. The anatomic relationship of the capital femoral epiphysis to the acetabulum can be fairly easily ascertained with sonography. The cartilaginous acetabular labrum is a crucial determinant of these relationships, and only sonography can visualize this structure directly. Importantly, ultrasonic examinations can be carried out during the course of treatment of congenital hip dysplasia, while the child is immobilized in a splint or cast. Sonographic estimation of the percentage of femoral head covered by acetabulum correlates relatively well with standardized radiographic measurements of acetabular indices.

Shoulder

Sonographic diagnosis of shoulder joint effusions is frequently helpful in patients with rheumatoid arthritis who receive steroid therapy. Signs of sepsis can be obscure in this group. Sonography affords a reliable means of diagnosing pyarthrosis and is valuable in assisting percutaneous aspiration of questionably infected joints. Response to therapy can be monitored with serial follow-up sonograms.

Ultrasonography has also proved to be an effective means of evaluating the rotator cuff. Potential sources of interpretive error include calcific tendinitis, fractures, and subluxations, all of which can be predicted by correlative radiographs. The opposite shoulder can be used as a reference standard. Limitations to sonographic visualization of the entire cuff that are imposed by the acromion are minimized by the fact that the majority of tears occur distally, near the insertion of the supraspinatus tendon. Ultrasonography routinely depicts this area.

The overall accuracy of the sonographic diagnosis of rotator cuff tears in patients with arthrographic or surgical confirmation has exceeded 90 per cent. Partial thickness tears

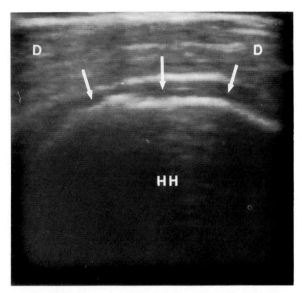

Figure 12–2. Rotator cuff tear. The supraspinatus tendon is absent, only a thin, hypoechoic space being present (arrows). D, Deltoid muscle; HH, humeral head. (Courtesy of L. Mack, M.D., Seattle, Washington.)

missed on standard arthrography can potentially be diagnosed with ultrasonography. The predictive value of a negative sonogram appears to be very high; in other words, false negative interpretations should be rare. Some investigators have concluded that sonography is an effective noninvasive screening procedure and that no further work-up is necessary if results of the examination are normal. Sonographic diagnosis of a cuff tear is made by actual visualization of a defect in the tendon apparatus, or by demonstration of a focally echogenic area within the tendon, thought to be secondary to proliferation of inflammatory tissue (Fig. 12–2).

Evaluation of the biceps tendon is evidently more accurate with sonography than with arthrography. Direct visualization of the tendon itself is possible with ultrasonography, in comparison to the indirect signs on arthrograms, which depend on inconstant filling of the tendon sheath.

Tumors of Bone and Soft Tissue

Modern gray scale methodology has contributed greatly to the depiction of normal and abnormal soft tissues in the trunk and extremities. Although sonography easily separates mass lesions into cystic or solid groupings, little histologic specificity is obtained from sonographic appearances alone. Soft tissue tumors of neural or nerve sheath origin can mimic the findings classically associated with cystic lesions, even though these are solid neoplasms. Fatty tissue is often extremely echogenic and lipomatous tumors can appear quite dense on gray scale sonograms. Neoplasms of lymphatic origin typically contain extensive cystic areas. Highly vascular tumors, such as hemangioma, also can have numerous fluid regions (Fig. 12–3). Once the presence of a lesion is identified, sonography can be employed as a means of monitoring the response of any extraosseous tumor bulk to therapeutic regimens. Enlargement of a tumor mass can be the result of hemorrhage or necrosis rather than tumor growth, a distinction sonography can make. Finally, sonography offers a rapid and accurate

method of localizing a soft tissue mass for percutaneous biopsy.

Infections of Bone and Soft Tissue

Sonographic features of abscesses vary considerably. A typical abscess has an indistinct margin and contains predominantly fluid but often also has debris that is manifested as fine, low-level echoes within the cystic mass. This material sometimes accumulates in the dependent portion of the abscess. Gas-containing abscesses can be quite echogenic on sonograms.

Paravertebral abscesses are present in a significant percentage of patients with infections of the spine. The presence of a paraspinous abscess is often difficult to establish with conventional radiography, and as a rule ultrasonography and computed tomography are more successful (Fig. 12–4).

Musculoskeletal Trauma

Real-time sonography using linear array transducers and a water delay has proved to be helpful in diagnosing intramuscular hematomas and ruptured or torn muscles. Injuries of the Achilles tendon can be evaluated completely by sonography to determine the precise site and extent of the tear and to document the healing response. Although sonography has been used to diagnose the posterior compartment syndrome in the lower leg, its reliability in differentiating simple edema from ischemic muscle necrosis remains to be determined.

Nonradiopaque foreign bodies, such as wood, glass, and plastic, in the soft tissues pose a challenging diagnostic problem that may be solved with sonography.

Miscellaneous Soft Tissue Conditions

Skin thickening is a feature of many dermatologic and nondermatologic conditions. Sonography might be useful for quantitative assessment of the natural history or response to treatment of diseases that affect dermal thickness.

Spine

There are several situations in which diagnostic ultrasonography can be used to advantage in investigating the spinal canal and its contents. Patients with recurrent or persistent symptoms after surgery for spinal cord masses can be challenging subjects for myelography because of adhesions and arachnoiditis. Sonograms can be obtained through laminectomy defects to differentiate tumor recurrence or syrinx formation, which might be approached surgically, from irradiation effects or spinal cord atrophy, for which surgery would be contraindicated.

Children at risk for tethering of the spinal cord can be screened with sonography because in the first year of life, ossification of the posterior elements of the spine is incomplete. This provides a window for scanning from a posterior approach (Fig. 12–5).

Intraoperative Spine Sonography

Considerable advances have been made in neurosurgery of the spinal cord, in part related to the development of intraoperative sonographic techniques. One of the major advantages of sonography is delineation of the extent of a particular problem prior to opening the dura, thus reducing the time and risk of a surgical procedure. Additional appli-

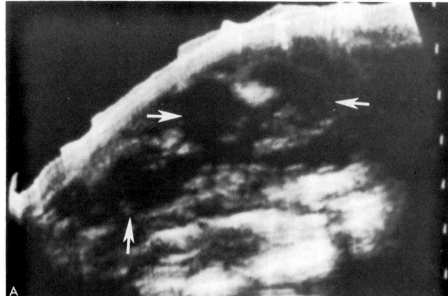

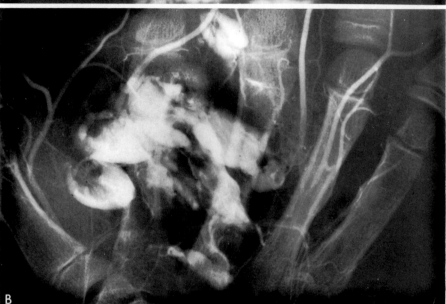

Figure 12–3. Hemangioma. A A superficial lesion of the palm contains many fluid-filled spaces representing dilated vascular channels (arrows). B Arteriography shows the extensive vascular pooling within the cavernous hemangioma.

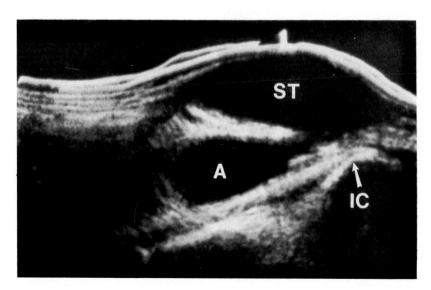

Figure 12–4. Tuberculous psoas abscess. Longitudinal sonogram of the left lower quadrant reveals a psoas abscess *(A)*, which has extended superficially into the subcutaneous tissues (ST). IC, Iliac crest.

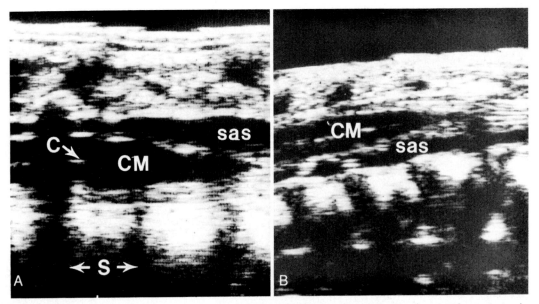

Figure 12–5. Spine sonography. A Normal infant spine. The conus medullaris (CM) lies dependent within the subarachnoid space (sas) and tapers normally in the midlumbar canal. Observe the central canal of the cord (C) and shadowing from the posterior elements (S). **B** Tethered cord. The conus medullaris (CM) is fixed in a dorsal position within the subarachnoid space (sas). On real-time examination, a lack of motion can be documented as well.

cations of intraoperative spine sonography include patients with trauma. Identification of bone fragments, foreign bodies, and cord compression and determination of spinal alignment can be accomplished with sonography. The adequacy of cord decompression and Harrington rod placement can be monitored, and any necessary adjustments can be made instantaneously.

Metabolic Disease

The parathyroid glands are intimately involved in calcium homeostasis and thereby exert considerable influence on bone metabolism. Normal parathyroid glands measure approximately $3 \times 4 \times 5$ mm and, until the advent of high resolution real-time sonography, had by and large evaded all attempts to image them. Owing to technical improvements,

however, if documentation of parathyroid gland enlargement is important for diagnosis and management, ultrasonography is now accepted as the procedure of choice. On sonograms, parathyroid adenomas and hyperplastic glands appear identical, not surprisingly because they have the same appearance histologically as well. The lesions are well circumscribed, often ovoid in shape, and hypoechoic relative to adjacent thyroid glandular tissue.

Somewhat related to parathyroid problems is the significant population undergoing chronic hemodialysis for renal failure. Ultrasonography has potential application in these patients, as it is a rapid and noninvasive means of evaluating vascular access grafts. Complications that confront hemodialysis fistulae include stenosis, thrombosis, aneurysm and pseudoaneurysm, and local infection. Each of these can be identified by ultrasonography.

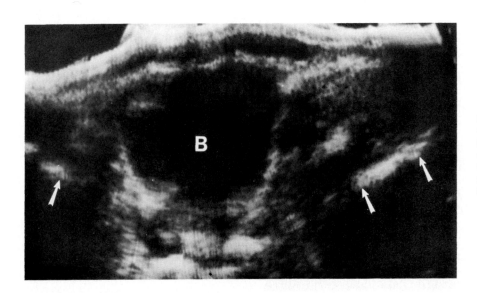

Figure 12–6. Iliopsoas hematoma. Transverse sonogram through the urinary bladder (B) reveals enlargement of the left iliopsoas compartment, with impression on the lateral wall of the distended bladder. The pelvic sidewall is demarcated by the dense reflection from the iliac bones (arrows).

Hemophilia and Altered Coagulability States

The relative ease with which ultrasonography detects fluid collections such as hematomas makes this an attractive method for evaluating patients with altered coagulability states. Sonography has proved efficacious in this clinical problem, both in diagnosing areas of hemorrhage and in following the natural history of the bleeding.

Rectus sheath hematoma is a specific clinical entity that can be evaluated with ultrasonography. Its sonographic appearance is characteristic and consists of an ellipsoid or spindle-shaped fluid collection in the superficial anterior abdominal wall. The tight boundaries of the rectus sheath confine the bleeding, and the process does not cross the midline unless it occurs low, where the posterior portion of the sheath is deficient.

Iliopsoas hematoma is a common complication of hemophilia. A somewhat typical syndrome of pain and nerve deficit occurs with bleeding isolated to the closed iliacus compartment that contains the femoral nerve. The psoas fascia is looser and allows more extensive hemorrhage to take place. Sonography is capable of detecting hemorrhage in both of these muscle compartments (Fig. 12–6).

Depending on the age and chronicity of the hemorrhage, hematomas display a spectrum of appearances on gray scale sonograms. When fresh and composed of liquid blood, a hematoma is homogeneous and appears virtually echo free. Internal echoes appear when a clot begins to organize and then fragment. Liquefaction of a clot may then lead once again to a variable fluid pattern on sonography. This inconstant pattern causes difficulty in attempting to predict the age of a given collection of blood. Considerable overlap exists, with similar features demonstrated by abscesses or tumors, for example.

FURTHER READING

Harcke HT, Grissom LE, Finkelstein MS: Evaluation of the musculoskeletal system with sonography. AJR 150:1253, 1988

Kaftori JK, Rosenberger A, Pollack S, Fish JH: Rectus sheath hematoma: Ultrasonographic diagnosis. AJR 128:283, 1977.

Kottle SP, Gonzalez AC, Macon EJ, Fellner SK: Ultrasonographic evaluation of vascular access complications. Radiology 129:751, 1978.

Little CM, Parker MG, Callowich MC, Sartori JC: The ultrasonic detection of soft tissue foreign bodies. Invest Radiol 21:275, 1986.

Mack LA, Matsen FA, Kilcoyne RF, Davies PK, Sickler ME: US evaluation of the rotator cuff. Radiology 157:205, 1985.

McDonald DG, Leopold GR: Ultrasound B-scanning in the differentiation of Baker's cyst and thrombophlebitis. Br J Radiol 45:729, 1972.

Novick G, Ghelman B, Schneider M: Sonography of the neonatal and infant hip. AJR 141:639, 1983.

Scheible W, James HE, Leopold GR, Hilton SvW: Occult spinal dysraphism in infants: Screening with high-resolution real-time ultrasound. Radiology 146:743, 1983.

Shirkhoda A, Mauro MA, Staab EV, Blatt PM: Soft-tissue hemorrhage in hemophiliac patients: Computed tomography and ultrasound study. Radiology 147:811, 1983.

Silver TM, Washburn RL, Stanley JC, Gross WS: Gray scale ultrasound evaluation of popliteal artery aneurysms. AJR 129:1003, 1977.

Chapter 13

Imaging Techniques in Intraspinal Diseases

Victor Haughton, M.D.

This chapter provides an overview of the more important imaging techniques that are employed in the evaluation of intraspinal diseases. Such methods include routine radiography, computed tomography, magnetic resonance imaging, myelography, and single photon emission computed tomography. The application of these techniques to the analysis of disorders of the facet joints, intervertebral discs, uncovertebral articulations, vertebrae, spinal cord, and meninges is summarized.

This chapter presents an overview of the more important imaging techniques that can be used to evaluate the spine and spinal cord. For a more complete discussion of such techniques, the reader is encouraged to consult other textbooks.

IMAGING TECHNIQUES

The primary diagnostic methods used to evaluate the spine, in addition to routine radiography, are computed tomography, magnetic resonance imaging, conventional tomography, radionuclide scanning, ultrasonography, myelography, and angiography. Each of these methods is considered in the following discussion, with the exception of ultrasonography, which is described in Chapter 12.

Computed Tomography

Computed tomography (CT) is very effective for evaluating any pathologic process that has been localized to a single spinal level. In the investigation of low back pain, CT is the primary imaging method, having greater sensitivity in the diagnosis of discal herniation or facet joint disease than myelography or conventional radiography. For cervical radiculopathy, CT is an efficient and effective alternative to myelography, and it is a complementary study to routine radiography or myelography in the delineation of spinal fractures.

The technical factors that are optimal for a CT examination depend on the precise clinical situation. In the examination of the lumbar spine, sufficient contrast resolution must be available to detect discal fragments (which are slightly more dense than the dural sac), and sufficient spatial resolution is required to demonstrate osseous detail about the facet joints. The orthodox CT techniques for the lumbar spine rely on a sequence of images 5 mm thick for each intervertebral disc level that is to be imaged (Fig. 13–1). In the examination of the cervical (or thoracic) intervertebral discs, a series of 1.5 mm thick images is obtained at, above, and below the level(s)

of interest (Fig. 13–2). In studying a suspected vertebral fracture, thin contiguous CT scans without a change in gantry angle are obtained to facilitate image reformation in a sagittal, coronal, or oblique plane. An aqueous contrast medium can be injected into the subarachnoid space to improve the visualization of intrathecal structures. The intravenous injection of contrast material is a rarely required but potentially effective supplement to the CT examination. The meninges, the nerve root sleeves, and the epidural venous plexuses increase substantially in radiodensity after such intravenous injection (Fig. 13–3).

Magnetic Resonance Imaging

Magnetic resonance (MR) imaging is the best primary diagnostic procedure for spinal intramedullary neoplasms (such as gliomas, lipomas, and hemangioblastomas), cysts, and arteriovenous malformations. It is also the procedure of choice for the evaluation of extradural processes causing myelopathy, such as skeletal metastases. MR imaging is able to detect extramedullary-intradural processes, including a meningioma or neurofibroma, although myelography is still the procedure of choice in the evaluation of these lesions. MR imaging currently is less accurate than CT for demonstrating herniated intervertebral discs and facet joint degeneration, but it is expected that this situation will change in the future.

The choice of an imaging plane is more complex with MR imaging than with CT, as direct sagittal or coronal image acquisition is possible only with MR imaging. In most instances, sagittal MR images of the spine are used, supplemented with transaxial scans at specified levels. For spinal imaging, specially designed small surface receiver coils provide more detailed images by suppressing the signal noise originating from areas outside the region of interest and by displaying a smaller region of interest on the viewing matrix. Both T1 and T2 weighted images are of value in investigations of spinal disorders. With T1 weighting the contours of the spinal cord can be distinguished easily from the surrounding cerebrospinal fluid (CSF). Because bone and CSF are not well

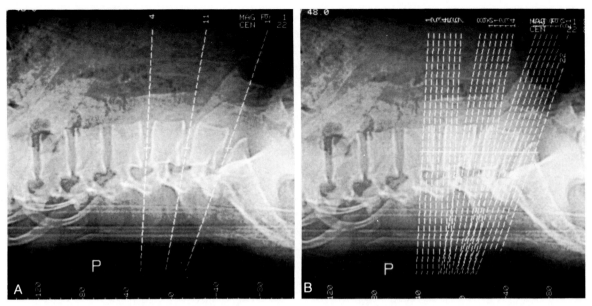

Figure 13–1. Localizer view of the lumbar spine to select the levels of the transaxial slices to be obtained. In **A**, the planes of the lower three lumbar intervertebral discs have been identified. In **B**, a series of slices has been selected, which includes one slice through each of the selected intervertebral discs and slices 5, 10, and 15 mm above and below the center of the disc space. Note that the images completely cover the neural foramina and spine except for small wedges.

distinguished in T1 weighted images, however, osteophytes compressing the subarachnoid space are not easily identified. In T2 weighted images, the high intensity signal of the subarachnoid space contrasts with the lower intensity signal of osseous structures (Fig. 13–4). The spinal cord is demonstrated less effectively in T2 weighted images because of the inferior signal-to-noise ratio and the intense signal from the CSF. For diastematomyelia, syringomyelia, or intramedullary neoplasms, the T1 weighted images are usually definitive.

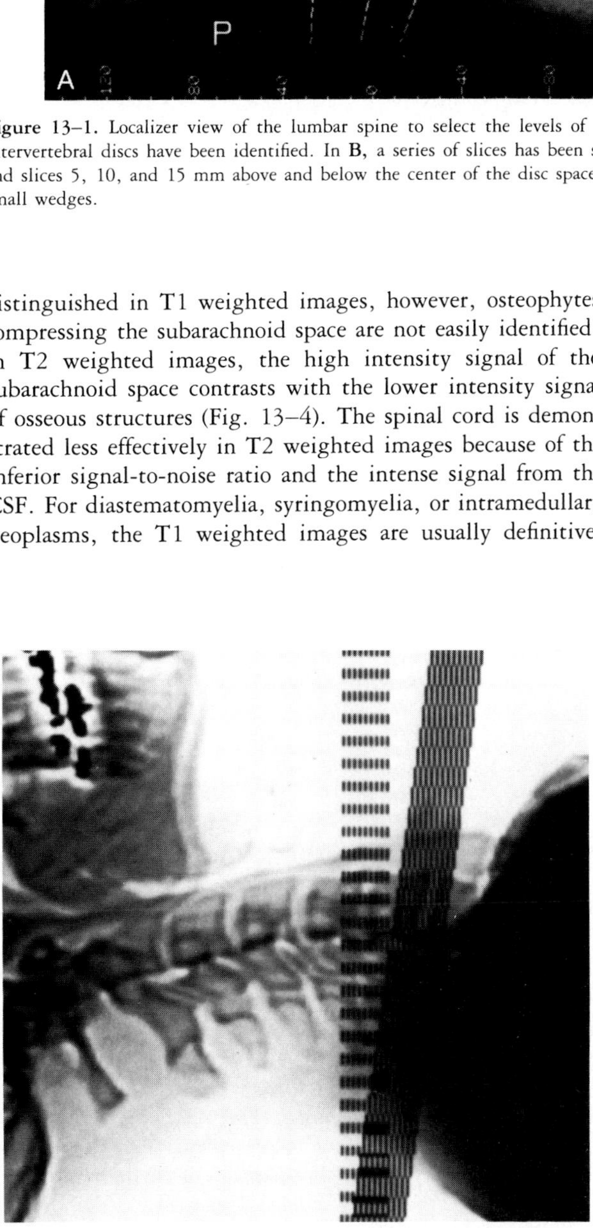

For multiple sclerosis involving the spinal cord or for characterization of some neoplasms, the T2 weighted sequence is useful.

Myelography

Although it is a safe and effective method for demonstrating the subarachnoid space, spinal cord, and nerve root sheaths, myelography is more costly and more invasive than CT or MR imaging. Myelography is indicated in patients with cervical radiculopathy, especially if the results of a cervical CT scan are ambiguous. For evaluation of spinal cord disorders, however, MR imaging is preferred. Myelography is currently indicated in investigations of extramedullary-intradural processes for confirming a complete block of the subarachnoid space. The technique is useful in detecting cysts within the spinal cord or subarachnoid space.

The contrast media for myelography include gas (room air, carbon dioxide, oxygen), water soluble (aqueous) iodinated media (metrizamide, iopamidol, iohexol, iotrol), and oily contrast media (iophendylate). The water soluble media, at present the standard choice for most myelographic studies, have major advantages in that they produce ideal opacification and faithfully demonstrate the subarachnoid space and intrathecal structures. Although iophendylate (Pantopaque) does not produce acute side effects, which are observed with the water soluble media, it does cause arachnoiditis when it remains in the subarachnoid space. Pantopaque is contraindicated if the subarachnoid space contains bloody CSF. Pantopaque also demonstrates the subarachnoid space less effectively because it is immiscible with CSF. Gas is an effective and safe contrast material for studying the spinal cord but requires pluridirectional tomography and special expertise on the part of the examiner. Except when MR imaging is not available or is contraindicated, gas myelography at present has no important indications.

Figure 13–2. Localizer view of the cervical spine to select levels for studying the C5-C6 and C6-C7 intervertebral discs. A series of slices was selected, which includes the intervertebral disc and neural foramina.

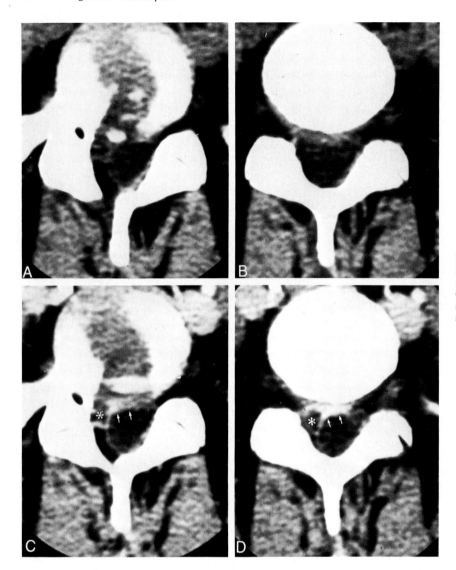

Figure 13–3. CT of the lumbar spine without (**A, B**) and with (**C, D**) intravenous contrast enhancement in a patient with previous laminectomy. Scar (arrows) and a herniated disc fragment (asterisks) are shown. **A** and **C** are at same level; **B** and **D** are at same level.

Single Photon Emission Computed Tomography

There are several skeletal applications for single photon emission computed tomography (SPECT), and it may be used as an appropriate adjunct to conventional bone scanning. In comparison with planar images, SPECT provides increased contrast resolution (because the tomographic technique excludes the noise from tissues outside the plane of imaging) but inferior spatial resolution. SPECT has been used to effectively distinguish between active and inactive processes in the spine and may differentiate a symptomatic and an asymptomatic spondylolysis, the former being associated with increased activity in a pars interarticularis.

Spinal Angiography

The major indications for spinal arteriography are vascular malformations or tumors involving the spinal cord, dura, spine, or subarachnoid space (Fig. 13–5). Spinal angiography may be performed to evaluate the feasibility of embolizing a vascular malformation or a tumor prior to surgery. Some surgeons request spinal arteriography prior to spinal surgery to locate the artery of Adamkiewicz and thereby prevent its injury during the operation. In addition to the general contraindications, a specific contraindication to spinal arteriography is compression of the anterior spinal artery, which might lead to an ascending paralysis if the artery were to be opacified.

Miscellaneous Techniques

DISCOGRAPHY. Discography is not purely an imaging technique because symptoms produced during the test are considered to have as much diagnostic value as the radiographs obtained. The major indication for discography is the further evaluation of neck or low back pain after more routine tests have been nondiagnostic. Duplication of the presenting complaint or entrance of more than 1 ml of fluid into the disc is considered a positive sign of a herniation of the intervertebral disc or other discal pathology. Discography has also been used to document the accurate placement of a needle in the nucleus pulposus prior to the injection of chymopapain.

EPIDURAL VENOGRAPHY. The primary indication for epidural venography has been suspected herniated disc or spinal stenosis that was not detected by myelography. The diagnostic accuracy of the test has varied from poor (because

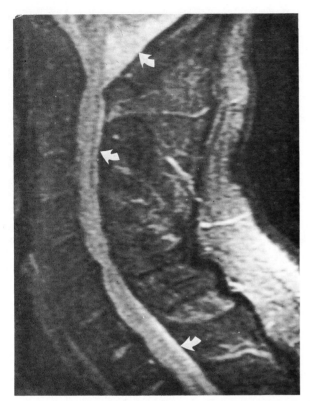

Figure 13–4. T2 weighted (TR, 2.5 s; TE, 25 ms) MR image. Cerebrospinal fluid (arrows) has a high signal intensity.

of technical difficulties in achieving venous filling) to good (when patients were selected carefully and excellent opacification was obtained).

EPIDUROGRAPHY. CT and MR imaging, which provide direct visualization of the epidural space, have essentially replaced epidurography, in which the epidural space is opacified with an aqueous contrast medium.

PLURIDIRECTIONAL TOMOGRAPHY. Although MR imaging and CT have caused a decline in the use of pluridirectional spinal tomography, this technique is indicated when direct sagittal or coronal images of the spinal osseous structures are needed. Trauma is one such indication because vertebral alignment, transverse fractures, and anatomic relationships of the facet joints can be shown effectively.

FACET JOINT DISEASES
Degeneration

Lumbar facet joint degeneration, especially in the later stages, is a significant cause of local or radiating pain. Five stages of degeneration of facet joints have been described: synovitis, joint capsule laxity, articular cartilage destruction, subarticular erosions, and hyperostosis.

SYNOVITIS AND CAPSULAR LAXITY. The first stage, synovitis, is characterized by hyperemia and inflammatory cell infiltration within the synovium and the capsule of the facet joint. Neither CT nor MR imaging has sufficient resolution to detect inflammation confined to the narrow capsule. MR imaging may be used to detect a hydrarthrosis, however, which in T2 weighted images appears as a high intensity signal within this joint space.

The second stage of degeneration is characterized by laxity of the capsule. The vacuum phenomenon (Fig. 13–6) may be the result of this abnormal laxity. In most cases, other evidence of degeneration is found in association with nitrogen within the facet joint.

ARTICULAR CARTILAGE DESTRUCTION. The third stage of degeneration is characterized by thinning of the articular cartilage that lines the superior and inferior articular processes. A narrowed distance between the superior and inferior articular processes in a CT image signifies erosion of the cartilage (Fig. 13–7). Facet joints with articular cartilage thinning (or subarticular bone erosions) are frequently associated with sciatic or low back pain. Injection of the facet joints with an anesthetic agent and steroid preparation is a way of evaluating the association of the facet joints and pain.

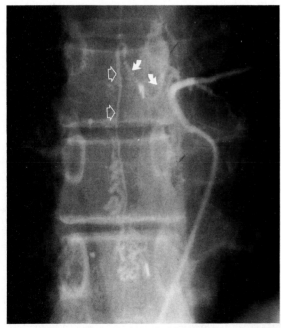

Figure 13–5. Spinal arteriogram demonstrating an arteriovenous malformation. By means of a catheter in an intercostal artery, a radiculomedullary artery (solid arrows) is opacified, which causes filling of the anterior spinal artery (open arrows). The distal tangle of vessels represents the malformation.

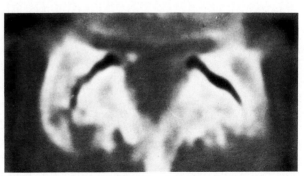

Figure 13–6. Severely degenerated facet joints are accompanied by vacuum phenomena.

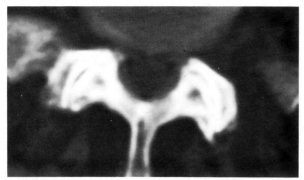

Figure 13–7. Articular cartilage destruction in both apophyseal joints related to osteoarthritis.

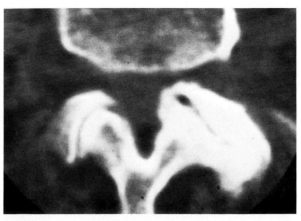

Figure 13–9. Hyperostotic lumbar facet joint. The superior and inferior articular facets on the left side have hypertrophied and caused narrowing of the neural foramen.

Routine radiographic or MR images are poor alternatives to CT for demonstrating facet joint degeneration.

SUBARTICULAR BONE EROSION. The fourth stage of degeneration, subarticular bone erosion, is characterized by changes in the cortical bone adjacent to the facet joint. The CT manifestations of these erosions are irregularities of the articular cortical surfaces or cysts within the adjacent bone (Fig. 13–8). Bone sclerosis frequently accompanies subarticular erosions and, in some cases, obliterates the medullary cavity of the articular processes and even the laminae.

HYPEROSTOSIS. The final stage of degeneration is hyperostosis, which refers both to the transformation of spongy medullary bone into dense bone and to the formation of osteophytes, findings that are well demonstrated with CT (Fig. 13–9). Osteophytes that develop from the medial surface of the articular processes may narrow the spinal canal or the neural foramina and produce sciatic pain by compressing a spinal nerve. Degenerative calcifications in the capsule of the facet joints and the adjacent ligamentum flavum are findings that resemble hyperostosis.

SYNOVIAL CYSTS. Synovial cysts are uncommon lesions of degenerated facet joints, most frequently found at the L4-L5 spinal level. They develop by herniation of synovium and synovial fluid through the joint capsule or by differentiation of synovial cells derived from the degenerating cartilage or the joint capsule, or both. Their clinical manifestations include low back or sciatic pain.

The CT findings of a synovial cyst are usually sufficiently

characteristic that a precise diagnosis can be made (Fig. 13–10). Those synovial cysts that are medial to the ligamentum flavum at the L4-L5 spinal level appear as nearly round structures that displace epidural fat and may indent the dural sac. In 75 per cent of synovial cysts, capsular calcification is present. In some cases the fluid in the cyst is replaced with gas. Intraspinal synovial cysts are almost invariably associated with degeneration in the adjacent apophyseal joint.

Myelography in cases of facet joint degeneration may reveal that the dural sac is deformed, especially along its posterolateral aspect. Except possibly for hydrarthrosis, facet joint disease is not demonstrated effectively by MR imaging.

Ankylosing Spondylitis

In addition to destruction of the facet joints, ankylosing spondylitis may produce a conus medullaris syndrome, related to a meningeal inflammatory process causing dense adhesive arachnoiditis. As a result, the nerve roots become embedded in the thickened arachnoid, and diverticula developing from the dural sac erode the neural arch and vertebral bodies. The CT and myelographic findings in this syndrome are usually diagnostic (Fig. 13–11).

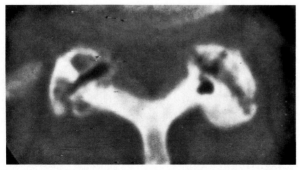

Figure 13–8. An example of subarticular bone erosions demonstrated by CT in the lumbar facet joints. Severe subarticular bone erosions are present, some of which have filled with gas that developed in the adjacent articulations.

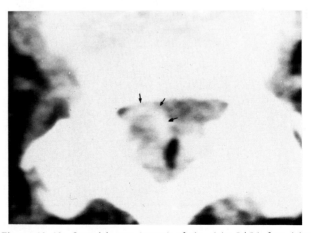

Figure 13–10. Synovial cyst (arrows) of the right L4-L5 facet joint demonstrated by CT. Note that the capsule of the cyst is calcified.

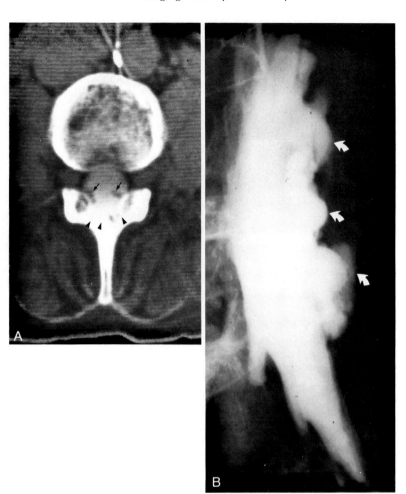

Figure 13–11. Ankylosing spondylitis. The CT examination (**A**), which was enhanced with an intrathecal aqueous contrast medium, demonstrates only a few nerve roots (arrows) because the remainder adhere to the dural sac. The lamina is eroded by diverticula of the dural sac (arrowheads). Myelography (**B**) in the same patient shows the diverticula (arrows) arising from the dural sac.

Trauma

Unstable fractures involving the facet joints or adjacent pars interarticularis, especially in the cervical spine, may be difficult to demonstrate by routine radiographs. When the cervical facet joints are perched, CT shows the superior and inferior articular processes in different transaxial cuts. When the cervical facet joints are locked, the superior articular process can be identified posterior to the inferior articular process (Fig. 13–12).

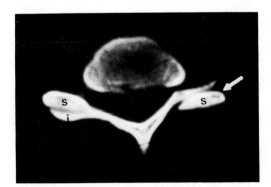

Figure 13–12. Locked cervical facet joints shown by CT. The superior articular process (s) on the left (arrow) lies behind the inferior articular process (i). (From Yetkin Z, et al: Uncovertebral and facet joint dislocations in cervical articular pillar fractures: CT evaluation. AJNR 6:633, 1985. Used with permission.)

INTERVERTEBRAL DISC DISEASES

Degenerative Disease

The degenerative processes that affect the intervertebral disc include lengthening and weakening of the fibers in the anulus fibrosus and loss of water and protein from the nucleus pulposus. If the anular fibers are sufficiently weakened, they rupture, allowing the nucleus pulposus to herniate. Retention of a herniated nucleus pulposus fragment behind the posterior longitudinal ligament is called a subligamentous herniation. A herniated fragment that has penetrated the posterior longitudinal ligament as well is called a sequestered or free fragment. Partial rupture of the anulus fibrosus with escape of nuclear material into the medial rings of the anulus is called a protruded disc. Ninety per cent of herniated intervertebral discs occur at the L4-L5 or L5-S1 disc level and the majority of the remainder at the L3-L4 spinal level. If the nucleus pulposus dehydrates and contracts without rupture of the anular fibers, a bulging anulus fibrosus develops.

HERNIATED DISC. With CT, a subligamentous herniation produces focal, curvilinear extension of the disc margin beyond that of the adjacent vertebral body, with displacement of fat in the epidural space (Fig. 13–13). The nuclear fragment usually has a density similar to that of the intervertebral disc (70 to 110 Hounsfield units [HU]). Calcification or ossification is seen in the margin of the fragment or, less commonly, gas is found within the nuclear fragment (Fig. 13–14).

Discal fragments that are free but still adjacent to the

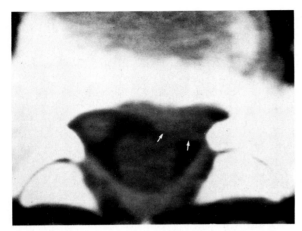

Figure 13–13. Subligamentous herniation at L5-S1. The disc margin has a focal crescentic deformity (arrows), which compresses the left S1 root sheath. The contralateral root sheath is normal.

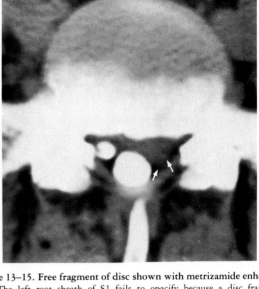

Figure 13–15. Free fragment of disc shown with metrizamide enhanced CT. The left root sheath of S1 fails to opacify because a disc fragment (arrows) compresses it.

intervertebral disc have an irregular contour; when the free fragment has migrated away from the intervertebral disc, the disc margin itself may appear entirely normal. The migrated free fragment may appear as a rounded or irregular mass (Fig. 13–15). A free disc fragment may resemble an epidural neoplasm except that the disc fragment usually has a higher density (70 to 110 HU) than a neoplasm (20 to 60 HU), and the latter is more typically accompanied by bone erosion.

CT has had a great impact in the detection of extreme lateral disc herniations, which occupy a position lateral to the neural foramen and are difficult to delineate with myelography. These nuclear fragments displace fat in and adjacent to the neural foramen and obscure the exiting spinal nerve (Fig. 13–16).

The CT criteria allowing diagnosis of a cervical disc herniation are similar to those used in detecting a herniation of the lumbar spine, although the CT diagnosis can be aided by the use of intrathecal contrast material (Fig. 13–17).

Myelography demonstrates intervertebral disc disease by means of indirect signs, particularly a characteristic change in the contour of the opacified dural sac or root sheath. In the lateral myelographic projection, an angular indentation of the dural sac or a "double density" is a sign of a herniated disc (Fig. 13–18). The most reliable myelographic indication of a herniated disc, however, is shortening and "trumpeting" of a nerve root sheath, in which the nerve root itself appears widened because it is either edematous or compressed and elevated.

Disc herniations can be detected effectively by MR imaging using criteria that are similar to those employed for CT. A focally abnormal disc margin that displaces a spinal nerve and fat in the spinal canal or neural foramen is typical (Fig. 13–19).

Thoracic disc herniations manifested by myelopathy are studied more effectively by MR imaging or myelography, both of which provide a fast way of screening the entire thoracic subarachnoid space, than by CT.

BULGING ANULUS FIBROSUS. With CT, the hallmark of the bulging anulus fibrosus is a disc margin that extends in all directions beyond the adjacent vertebral end-

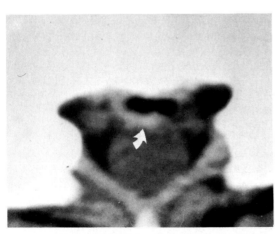

Figure 13–14. Central L5-S1 herniation (arrow) containing gas.

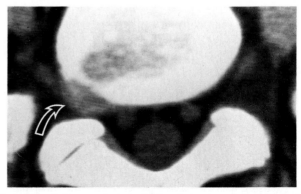

Figure 13–16. Extreme lateral disc herniation (arrow) displaces the fat and right fifth nerve root sheath in the right L5-S1 neural foramen. (From Williams AL, et al: CT recognition of lateral lumbar disk herniation. AJR *139*:345, 1982. Copyright 1982, American Roentgen Ray Society. Used with permission.)

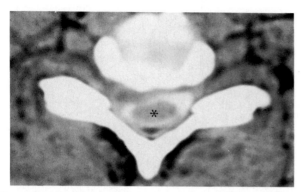

Figure 13–17. Herniated C6-C7 disc using CT with intrathecal enhancement. The spinal cord (asterisk) and subarachnoid space are deformed by the herniation.

plates (Fig. 13–20). The normally straight or concave posterior border of the intervertebral disc either is maintained or becomes convex. The displaced posterior margin of the intervertebral disc leads to narrowing of the spinal canal and the neural foramina. The myelographic appearance of the dural sac in the presence of a bulging anulus fibrosus is also characteristic. In the lateral projection, a curvilinear, thumbprint-like impression on the opacified ventral dural sac, often at multiple levels, is evident. Anteroposterior projections reveal symmetric deformity of the lateral margin of the dural sac. Only rarely do bulging discs displace, compress, or amputate the root sheaths.

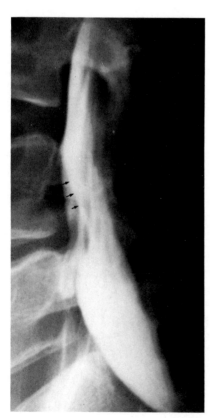

Figure 13–18. Lumbar myelogram with aqueous contrast medium demonstrating an L4-L5 herniated disc. The lateral film shows the double density (arrows) caused by the herniated disc fragment displacing the dural sac asymmetrically.

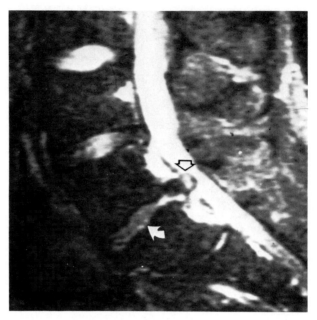

Figure 13–19. Herniated L5-S1 disc (open arrow), demonstrated by a T2 weighted MR image. The diminished signal intensity from the L5-S1 disc (solid arrow) is a nonspecific finding.

SPINAL STENOSIS. Narrowing of the spinal canal may be a complication of many degenerative processes of the spine (see Chapter 36). Osteophytes about the apophyseal joints and thickening of the ligamenta flava are examples of degenerative causes of spinal stenosis. Normally 2 to 3 mm in thickness, the ligamentum flavum exceeds 5 mm in thickness in pathologic cases.

CT, MR imaging, or myelography may be used alone or in combination to evaluate spinal stenosis. These techniques allow assessment of the site and extent of stenosis and identification of any degenerative changes in the facet joints, discs, and ligamentum flavum, as well as developmental abnormalities, such as short pedicles or thick laminae. A

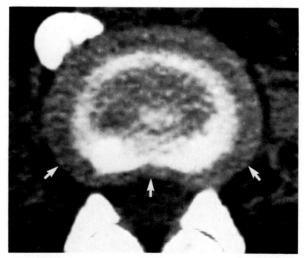

Figure 13–20. Bulging intervertebral disc. The anulus fibrosus (arrows) extends beyond the adjacent vertebral endplate in all directions, although the normal concavity of the posterior disc margin is preserved.

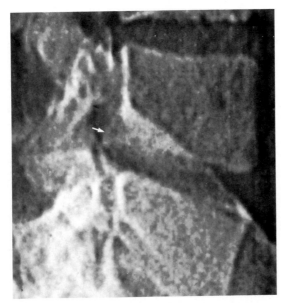

Figure 13–21. Traumatic avulsion of the L4-L5 ring apophysis and rupture of the intervertebral disc. The CT localizer view shows the ring apophysis (arrow) displaced into the spinal canal.

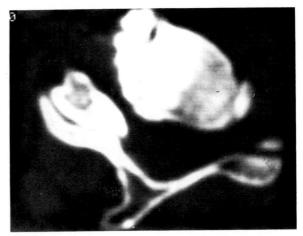

Figure 13–22. Bone erosions and hyperostosis about the right uncovertebral joint of C5-C6.

spinal canal less than 1.5 sq cm in area or a lateral recess less than 3 mm in depth has been considered a sign of stenosis. Obliteration of the epidural fat also is a reliable sign of spinal stenosis on CT or MR images.

Inflammatory Disease

With CT, the characteristic finding of discitis (inflammation of the disc) is multiple erosions of similar size occurring in the osseous endplates on either side of the affected intervertebral disc space at an early stage of the disease. Almost invariably, a soft tissue mass is also seen. An increased signal from the intervertebral disc and adjacent vertebral body in a T2 weighted image and loss of the intranuclear cleft represent MR findings of discitis.

Miscellaneous Disc Abnormalities

CARTILAGINOUS (SCHMORL'S) NODE. The CT appearance of a cartilaginous node includes a defect in the spongy bone, often surrounded by a sclerotic rim of variable thickness.

LIMBUS VERTEBRA. A characteristic defect in the vertebral body, the limbus vertebra, is produced by herniation of a portion of the nucleus pulposus beneath the ring apophysis before its fusion with the vertebral body. The limbus vertebra is thought to result from trauma. CT images show the distorted interface between the intervertebral disc and the adjacent vertebral body.

RUPTURED RING APOPHYSIS. Trauma with compressive loading of the axial spine, especially in young male patients, produces a characteristic type of fracture in which a wedge-shaped fragment of the endplate is dislodged and displaced posteriorly (Fig. 13–21).

UNCOVERTEBRAL JOINT DISEASES
Degeneration

Degenerative changes in the uncovertebral joints can be detected radiographically (see Chapter 36) or with more accuracy by CT. The latter method reveals both the hypertrophic and the destructive changes that accompany degeneration in the uncovertebral joints (Fig. 13–22). As the uncinate process hypertrophies, the neural foramen is narrowed, and compression of the spinal nerves may occur.

Trauma

Although isolated fractures of the uncovertebral joints are rare, the rotation or slippage of one vertebral body on another that may accompany unstable fractures commonly causes a diastasis of the uncovertebral articulations.

OSSEOUS ABNORMALITIES
Neoplasms

CT, angiography, pluridirectional tomography, and MR imaging may be used to visualize the primary osseous tumors that involve the spine. In almost all cases these tumors are detected efficiently by routine radiographic screening prior to imaging with the other techniques, which nevertheless may be useful in characterizing some of these tumors. MR imaging is particularly sensitive for detecting metastatic involvement of the vertebral column, in which the characteristic signal from the bone marrow is replaced by the usually lower signal of the tumor. Invasion of the epidural space can be delineated by displacement of epidural fat.

Trauma

Routine radiographs are the primary diagnostic studies in most cases of spinal trauma. They are, however, insensitive for detecting certain types of fracture, such as undisplaced neural arch fractures, vertically oriented fractures that are nearly perpendicular to the central ray, and atlantoaxial rotatory subluxations. CT is very effective in demonstrating vertically oriented fractures and is sensitive for most fractures through the neural arch and articular pillars and many vertebral body fractures as well. Furthermore, it confirms narrowing of the central spinal canal owing to displacement of fracture fragments (Fig. 13–23). CT also demonstrates soft tissue injuries, such as an epidural hematoma or avulsion of cervical nerve roots.

Pluridirectional tomography is useful for demonstrating transversely oriented fractures as well as the alignment of the

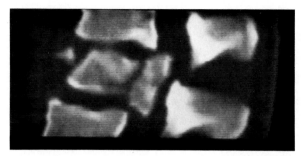

Figure 13–23. Reformatted sagittal CT image of a burst fracture of the L2 vertebral body.

facet joints or the vertebral bodies when plain radiographs have been inconclusive. MR imaging is not an important ancillary diagnostic technique for spinal fractures. Two indications for myelography after trauma are the evaluation of the degree of spinal cord or nerve root compression produced by a fracture or dislocation and the detection of a syringomyelia resulting from a spinal cord injury.

Neural Arch Defects

Neural arch defects include retrosomatic clefts, pars interarticularis defects (spondylolysis), retroisthmic defects, synchondroses, and spina bifida occulta. The retrosomatic cleft, well shown with CT, is a rare defect in the pedicles near their junction with the vertebral body. Although detection of pars interarticularis defects by plain radiographs is efficient, defects are detected in some patients by CT after routine radiographic or myelographic examination yields negative results (Fig. 13–24). The retroisthmic defect is rare and is located posterior to the pars interarticularis (Fig. 13–24).

A synchondrosis may be confused with a neural arch cleft. Synchondroses are evident in the first decade of life and are located anterior to the sites of retrosomatic clefts.

The most common and least significant type of neural arch cleft is spina bifida occulta. It is composed of nonossifying fibrous tissue in the midline between the two halves of the neural arch.

SPINAL CORD AND MENINGEAL DISEASES

Neoplasms and Cysts

By providing sagittal views, MR imaging or myelography screens the spine efficiently in instances of spinal cord or meningeal tumors. The fatty nature of a lipoma is demonstrated by an intense signal in a T1 weighted MR image and, sometimes, by an area of low density (-10 to -40 HU) with CT. Hemorrhage within a tumor provides an MR image appearance characterized by a shortened T1 (i.e., bright signal on short TR, short TE images). The myelographic signs of epidural or vertebral metastases (or other malignant neoplasms) are narrowing or complete obliteration of the subarachnoid space and blocking of the flow of the contrast medium. The ventral, lateral, or dorsal surface of the dura may be affected.

Tumors of the spine are conventionally divided according to location into extradural, extramedullary-intradural, and intramedullary types. Most extradural tumors are malignant in nature, and most involve the osseous vertebral column. The extramedullary-intradural neoplasms typically are benign (neurofibromas and meningiomas). Intramedullary processes include both benign and malignant tumors, cysts, and degenerative changes.

EXTRAMEDULLARY-INTRADURAL LESIONS. Extramedullary-intradural tumors, which enlarge the subarachnoid space by displacing the spinal cord and replacing CSF with solid tissue, have a characteristic myelographic appearance; a cap or meniscus with sharp, smooth, curvilinear borders and displacement of the spinal cord are usually evident. Meningiomas usually occur posterior to the thoracic cord, especially in women; neurofibromas (Fig. 13–25) frequently are found in the neural foramen at any level, often in patients with von Recklinghausen's disease. Calcification sufficient to be detected by CT is uncommon in meningioma and rare in neurofibroma. Pressure erosion involving the pedicles, adjacent vertebral bodies, or neural arches is detected in neurofibromas involving the neural foramen.

Experience with MR imaging in the detection of extramedullary-intradural tumors is fragmentary.

INTRAMEDULLARY LESIONS. The processes that commonly affect the spinal cord include neoplasms, such as an astrocytoma, ependymoma, and, rarely, hemangioblastoma or lipoma; cysts, such as syringomyelia or hydromyelia; and non-neoplastic conditions, such as myelomalacia, multiple sclerosis, arteriovenous malformation, and atrophy. MR im-

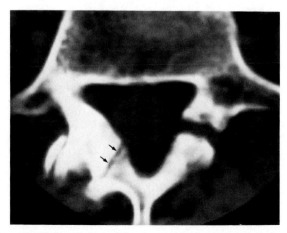

Figure 13–24. Retroisthmic defect (arrows) in the right L5 neural arch. A pars interarticularis defect is present in the left neural arch. (From Johansen JG, et al: The CT appearance of retroisthmic clefts. AJNR 5:835, 1984. Used with permission.)

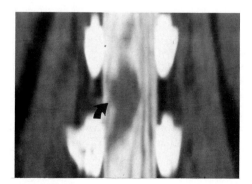

Figure 13–25. Imaging in spinal neurofibroma. A large lobulated neurofibroma (arrow) is identified with a coronal reformatted CT image.

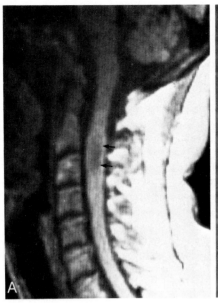
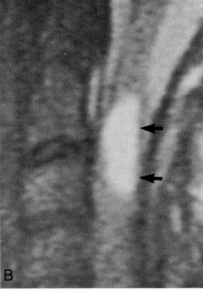

Figure 13–26. T1 (A) and T2 (B) weighted MR images in a cervical ependymoma (arrows). The signal intensity of the tumor differs from that of the cerebrospinal fluid.

aging is the technique of choice for evaluating intramedullary processes, and it detects both changes in cord caliber and changes in signal intensity from within the cord. Neoplasms characteristically enlarge the cord. Gliomas, ependymomas, and hemangioblastomas produce a region of prolonged T1 (darker signal intensity on T1 weighted images) and prolonged T2 (brighter intensity on T2 weighted images) within the cord (Fig. 13–26). In the very vascular tumors, such as hemangioblastoma, abnormal blood vessels may be demonstrated as regions of low signal intensity. Cystic areas in some tumors appear as regions of more prolonged T1 and T2 values. Hemorrhage has a characteristic bright signal in T1 and T2 weighted images.

MR imaging detects syringomyelia or hydromyelia effectively, showing a homogeneous intramedullary process that is sharply demarcated from the spinal cord, with a prolonged T1 and T2 similar to that of CSF (Fig. 13–27). The majority of intramedullary cysts expand the spinal cord. Myelomalacia, demyelination, viral myelitis, and multiple sclerosis may produce a region of prolonged T1 and T2 within the spinal cord. Spinal cord atrophy can be detected by MR imaging, myelography, or contrast-enhanced CT.

Myelography is slightly less sensitive than MR imaging for demonstrating intramedullary lesions. Cysts or tumors may expand the spinal cord, and cysts that communicate freely with the subarachnoid space have a characteristic myelographic appearance because of their opacification. CT is not usually used as a primary diagnostic tool if a spinal cord tumor or cyst is suspected.

Congenital Malformations

CHIARI MALFORMATION. The Chiari II or Arnold-Chiari malformation is characterized by a myelomeningocele and caudal displacement of the cerebellar tonsils and hindbrain. It has many other associated abnormalities.

MR imaging is the procedure of choice for evaluating patients with a suspected Chiari malformation. The sagittal images demonstrate the developmental abnormalities in the posterior fossa (Fig. 13–27) and cerebrum, the anatomic

relationships of the meningocele, spinal cord, filum terminale, and nerve roots, and any associated lipomas or lipomeningoceles. After the administration of intrathecal contrast material, CT may demonstrate the filling defect created by the cerebellar tonsils in the subarachnoid space at the cranial end of the spinal canal and the relationship of the spinal cord, nerve roots, and meningocele in the lumbar spine. Myelography is

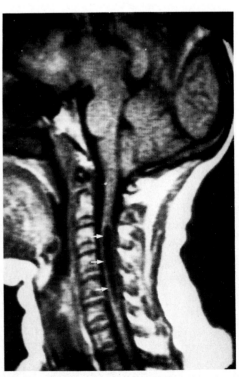

Figure 13–27. MR imaging in hydromyelia. A sagittal T1 weighted image shows a well-defined process (arrows) in the cervical cord at the C3-C5 spinal levels, which is isointense with cerebrospinal fluid. The downward displacement of the cerebellar tonsils and inferior cerebellar vermis indicates an associated Chiari malformation.

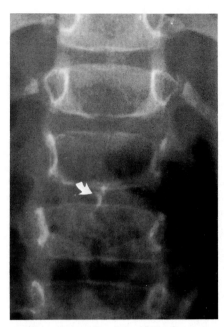

Figure 13–28. Diastematomyelia. A conventional anteroposterior radiograph of the lumbar spine demonstrates widening of the interpediculate distance, a decreased intervertebral disc space between L1 and L2, and a bony spicule overlying the center of the spinal canal (arrow).

sensitive in demonstrating the caudal displacement of the cerebellar tonsils, the meningocele, and the precise position of the spinal cord, but it is less effective in defining the abnormal nerve roots and the frequently associated lipoma involving the filum terminale.

DYSRAPHISM. One type of dysraphism that commonly has associated deformities in the lower extremities is diastematomyelia. Routine radiographic signs of diastematomyelia include scoliosis, narrowing of intervertebral disc spaces, widening of the interpediculate distances, and, in some cases, a bony spur dividing the spinal canal (Fig. 13–28). CT and MR imaging effectively demonstrate the hemicords of dias-

tematomyelia even in the large fraction of cases without osseous abnormalities.

Arachnoiditis

Contrast-enhanced CT is an effective way of demonstrating the changes of arachnoiditis. The subarachnoid space in the intrathecally enhanced images appears devoid of nerve roots because they have been incorporated into the dural sac. With intravenous contrast medium, the thickened dura and epidural fibrosis are enhanced, resulting in increased density. Arachnoiditis also has characteristic myelographic features: a deficiency of nerve roots within the opacified subarachnoid space and the irregular, asymmetric distortions of the dural margin, which lacks an anatomic relationship to the disc space.

FURTHER READING

Carrera GF, Haughton VM, Syvertsen A, Williams AL: Computed tomography of lumbar facet joints. Radiology *134:*145, 1981.

Collier B, Johnson RP, Carrera GF, Meyer GA, Schwab JP, Flatley TJ, Isitman AT, Hellman RS, Zielonka JF, Nobel J: Painful spondylolysis or spondylolisthesis studied by single photon emission computed tomography. Radiology *154:*207, 1985.

Czervionke LF, Daniels DL: Cervical spine anatomy and pathologic processes. Application of new MR imaging techniques. Radiol Clin North Am 26:921, 1988.

Grogan JP, Hemminghytt S, Williams AL, Carrera GF, Haughton VM: Spondylolysis studied with computed tomography. Radiology *145:*737, 1982.

Haughton VM, Williams AL: Computed Tomography of the Spine. St Louis, CV Mosby, 1982.

Hemminghytt S, Daniels DL, Williams AL, Haughton VM: Intraspinal synovial cysts: Natural history and diagnosis by CT. Radiology *145:*375, 1982.

Modic MT, Masaryk TJ, Ross JS, Carter JR: Imaging of degenerative disk disease. Radiology 168:177, 1988.

Modic MT, Pavlicek W, Weinstein MA, Boumphrey F, Ngo F, Hardy R, Duchesneau PM: Magnetic resonance imaging of intervertebral disk disease: Clinical and pulse sequence considerations. Radiology *152:*103, 1984.

Naidich TP, McLone DG, Mutluer S: New understanding of dorsal dysraphism with lipoma (lipomyeloschisis): Radiologic evaluation and surgical correction. AJR *140:*1065, 1983.

Pathria M, Sartoris DJ, Resnick D: Osteoarthritis of the facet joints: Accuracy of oblique radiographic assessment. Radiology 164:227, 1987.

Williams AL, Haughton VM, Daniels DL, Grogan JP: Differential CT diagnosis of extruded nuclear pulposus. Radiology *148:*141, 1983.

Chapter 14

Arthrography

Donald Resnick, M.D.

Arthrographic procedures generally are simple to perform, and the information they provide may be essential for proper diagnosis and treatment. The technique is used alone or in combination with other technologic methods, *such as fluoroscopy, conventional and computed tomography (arthrotomography), and digital radiography. Normal and abnormal arthrographic findings at specific locations in the body are described.*

Radiographic examination of joint cavities after contrast opacification (arthrography) is a useful procedure for evaluation of joints and surrounding tissues. This chapter describes the indications, techniques, and normal and abnormal findings at specific locations in the body. Arthrographic abnormalities in patients with joint prostheses are summarized in Chapter 20.

Although this method originally was used alone, arthrography has been coupled with newer technologic methods, such as fluoroscopy, conventional and computed tomography (arthrotomography), and digital radiography. The contrast agents may be radiolucent (air or carbon dioxide) or radiopaque and are used either alone (single contrast) or in combination (double contrast). Usually the agent is a water-soluble medium such as meglumine diatrizoate (Renografin-M 60) or diatrizoate sodium (Hypaque Sodium 50%). Negative contrast may be obtained by using room air (preferred) or carbon dioxide.

Epinephrine is often administered to improve the quality of the image produced. This agent helps prolong the time during which arthrography or supplementary techniques can be performed by slowing the egress of contrast material from the joint or the entrance of fluid into the joint, or both. Usually 0.2 to 0.3 ml of 1:1000 epinephrine solution is used for large joints (knee, glenohumeral joint), whereas 0.15 ml is used for smaller joints (ankle, elbow).

Film subtraction techniques are sometimes used in evaluation of painful joint prostheses when contrast material is obscured by the radiopacity of the fixation cement.

Best arthrographic results are obtained for some examinations after application of stress or passive or active movement of the joint. Intraarticular pressure may be monitored continuously to determine compliance of the joint capsule and to provide information about the total joint capacity. This is especially useful in diagnosis of adhesive capsulitis of the shoulder, hip, and ankle.

As currently performed, significant complications of arthrography are rare. Hypersensitivity to iodinated contrast material, although it does occur, is also rare.

WRIST

Arthrography of the wrist is performed for a number of reasons (Table 14–1).

Technique

Under fluoroscopic control, a 22 gauge, 1.5 inch long needle is introduced into the wrist from a dorsal approach. The needle is guided under the radial lip and enters the radiocarpal compartment between the scaphoid and the radius. A total of 1.5 to 2.5 ml of 60 per cent meglumine (Renografin) is administered. Fluoroscopic monitoring combined with sequential spot filming, videotaping, or digital technique during the injection of contrast material allows precise delineation of abnormal compartmental communications. Selective injection of the midcarpal compartment, rather than the radiocarpal compartment, has been performed in some patients as a superior method for analysis of the scapholunate and lunate-triquetral ligaments. Indeed, some authorities advocate sequential injections into the radiocarpal, midcarpal, and inferior radioulnar joints as ideal.

Normal Wrist Arthrogram (Fig. 14–1)

Contrast opacification of the radiocarpal compartment reveals a concave sac with smooth synovial surfaces extending between the distal radius and proximal carpal row. The prestyloid recess appears as a finger-like projection that approaches the ulnar styloid process from the ulnar limit of the radiocarpal joint. One or more volar radial recesses are located beneath the distal radius.

Communication between the radiocarpal compartment and other compartments in the wrist during arthrography may be observed in "normal" individuals or cadavers. The radiocarpal compartment may communicate with the midcarpal compartment in 13 to 47 per cent of the population and with the inferior radioulnar compartment in 7 to 35 per cent. The prevalence of these findings increases in older individuals. Communication between the radiocarpal and pisiform-triquetral compartments is observed on arthrography in more than 50 per cent of cases.

Table 14–1. SOME INDICATIONS FOR WRIST ARTHROGRAPHY

Evaluation of:
Presence and extent of synovial inflammation
Injuries to the triangular fibrocartilage, interosseous ligaments, and joint capsule
Soft tissue masses

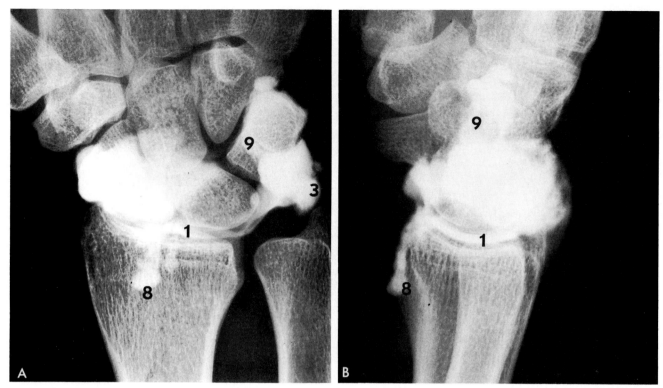

Figure 14–1. Wrist arthrography: Normal arthrogram. A, B Frontal and lateral views. Observe the contrast-filled radiocarpal compartment (1), which is communicating with the pisiform-triquetral compartment (9). Also note the prestyloid recess (3) and volar radial recesses (8).

Rheumatoid Arthritis (Fig. 14–2)

Injection of contrast material into the radiocarpal compartment in patients with rheumatoid arthritis typically reveals corrugated irregularity of the contrast material and opacification of lymphatic vessels. These two findings are not specific for rheumatoid arthritis but are reliable indicators of synovial inflammation. Communication between the radiocarpal compartment and other compartments in the wrist in rheumatoid arthritis is frequent. This communication also lacks specificity as a finding of rheumatoid arthritis because of its common occurrence in normal individuals and in patients with other types of articular disease. The tendon sheaths can be visualized after radiocarpal compartment opacification in approximately 25 per cent of wrists in rheumatoid arthritis, more frequently on the dorsum of the wrist.

Trauma

Arthrographic abnormalities observed most frequently after wrist trauma are compartmental communications, tendon sheath visualization, and mild synovial membrane irregularity. These alterations may follow a single traumatic episode or occur after repeated trauma.

The pattern of compartmental communication depends on the site of trauma. With injuries to the triangular fibrocartilage or ulnar styloid, communication occurs between the radiocarpal and inferior radioulnar compartments (Fig. 14–3). With scaphoid fractures or injuries to the interosseous ligaments between the bones of the proximal carpal row, communication is seen between the radiocarpal and midcarpal compartments (Fig. 14–4). In young individuals,

compartmental communication may provide presumptive evidence of soft tissue injury; however, in older patients, the frequency of such communication in "normal" persons limits the value of wrist arthrography.

Evaluation of Soft Tissue Masses

Arthrography can provide useful information in a patient with a soft tissue mass adjacent to the wrist. Such masses may represent synovial cysts, ganglions, or enlarged tendon sheaths. When evaluating wrist ganglions or synovial cysts (Fig. 14–5), contrast material injected directly into the swelling may fail to opacify the wrist, whereas when contrast material is injected into the wrist it may reveal a communication between the joint cavity and the soft tissue mass.

ELBOW

Arthrography of the elbow is a relatively easy examination that may be used to determine the nature and extent of intraarticular disorders and the cause of adjacent soft tissue masses. Some indications are given in Table 14–2.

Technique

The joint is entered from a lateral approach between the radial head and capitulum. Either 6 to 10 ml of contrast material alone (60 per cent Renografin), 0.5 to 1 ml of contrast material plus 6 to 10 ml of air, or 8 to 12 ml of air alone is used for injection. Use of contrast material alone is particularly good for defining the extent of synovial disorders, capsular integrity, and synovial cysts, whereas the double contrast study or the single contrast study with air alone may

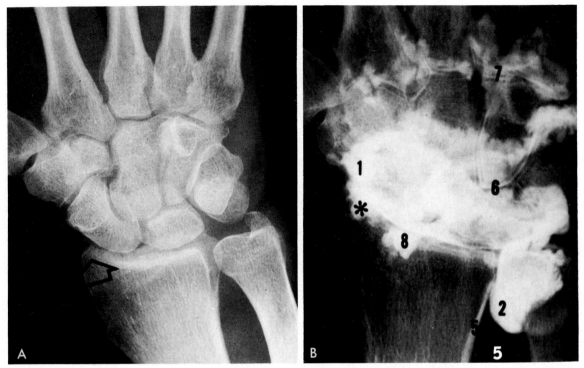

Figure 14–2. Wrist arthrography: Rheumatoid arthritis. A On the initial film, a small erosion of the radial styloid is evident (arrow). **B** Posteroanterior view following arthrography demonstrates severe synovial irregularity or corrugation (asterisk), radiocarpal compartment (1) communication with the inferior radioulnar (2), midcarpal (6), and common carpometacarpal (7) compartments, lymphatic filling (5), and prominent volar radial recesses (8). (From Resnick D: Arthrography in the evaluation of arthritic disorders of the wrist. Radiology 113:331, 1974. Used with permission.)

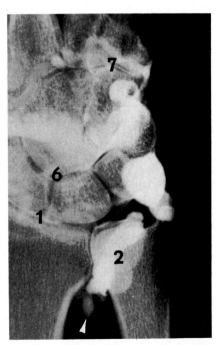

Figure 14–3. Wrist arthrography: Triangular fibrocartilage injury. A wrist arthrogram reveals communication between the radiocarpal compartment (1) and inferior radioulnar compartment (2). The midcarpal (6) and common carpometacarpal (7) compartments are also opacified. Small contrast-filled diverticula near the proximal aspect of the inferior radioulnar joint (arrowhead) may indicate a capsular tear.

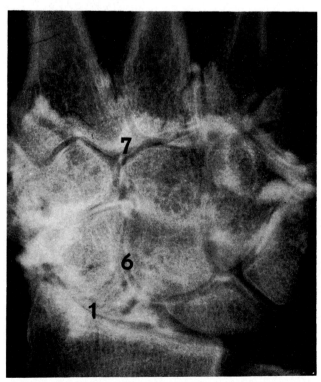

Figure 14–4. Wrist arthrography: Scapholunate dissociation with disruption of the scapholunate ligament. Following arthrography, contrast material has flowed from the radiocarpal compartment (1) into the midcarpal (6) and common carpometacarpal (7) compartments. Contrast material overlies the scapholunate space.

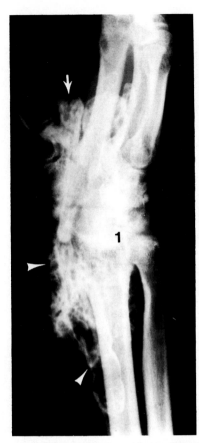

Figure 14–5. Wrist arthrography: Synovial cyst. After injection of the radiocarpal compartment (1) in this patient with rheumatoid arthritis, a large contrast-filled volar synovial cyst can be seen (arrowheads), which communicates with tendon sheaths (arrow). (Courtesy of the late J. Bowerman, M.D., Baltimore, Maryland.)

be superior in demonstrating cartilaginous and osseous defects and intraarticular "loose" bodies. After injection, fluoroscopic spot films and anteroposterior, oblique, and lateral radiographs are obtained, supplemented with tomography when necessary.

Normal Elbow Arthrogram (Fig. 14–6)

On frontal radiographs, a thin layer of contrast material or air is observed between the humerus, radius, and ulna. A periradial prolongation or recess is apparent about the proximal radius, which is indented where the annular ligament surrounds the bone. Proximal extension of contrast material along the anterior surface of the humerus may resemble the ears of a rabbit, the "Bugs Bunny" sign. On a lateral radiograph, the periradial or annular recess is again apparent. In addition, coronoid (anterior) and olecranon (posterior) recesses are seen. Smooth articular cartilage is observed on

Table 14–2. SOME INDICATIONS FOR ELBOW ARTHROGRAPHY

Evaluation of:
    Presence and extent of synovial inflammation
    Intraarticular cartilaginous and osseous bodies
    Soft tissue masses
    Trauma in children

the humerus, radial head, and ulna; it is of uniform thickness except for a portion of the trochlear notch of the ulna, which lacks cartilage.

Abnormal Elbow Arthrogram

RHEUMATOID ARTHRITIS AND OTHER SYNOVIAL DISORDERS. Synovial inflammation with hypertrophy and villous transformation accounts for an irregular outline of contrast material that may be apparent in rheumatoid arthritis (Fig. 14–7) and disorders such as juvenile chronic polyarthritis, ankylosing spondylitis, neuroarthropathy, and septic arthritis. Lymphatic visualization is common and capsular distention, sacculation, and synovial cyst formation are also seen.

Nodular filling defects within the contrast-filled elbow joint may represent hypertrophied synovium, as in rheumatoid arthritis, or synovial masses associated with pigmented villonodular synovitis and idiopathic synovial (osteo)chondromatosis (Fig. 14–8).

TRAUMA. The traumatized elbow joint, particularly after the introduction of air or air and contrast material, may reveal cartilaginous and osseous defects associated with osteochondritis dissecans (transchondral fractures). In these instances, contrast material may dissect beneath the adjacent osseous fragment or reveal loose or embedded bodies elsewhere in the joint cavity. Computed arthrotomography may also be used (Fig. 14–9).

SHOULDER

Contrast opacification of the glenohumeral joint (Table 14–3) is an aid to the diagnosis of rotator cuff tear, adhesive capsulitis, previous dislocation, articular disease, and bicipital tendon abnormalities.

Technique

Both single contrast and double contrast examinations have been advocated for shoulder arthrography. Modifications of these techniques, including conventional and computed arthrotomography, are necessary in certain situations.

SINGLE CONTRAST EXAMINATION. Ten to 15 ml of 60 per cent Renografin is injected into the glenohumeral joint from an anterior approach in the supine patient. A 3 inch, 18 or 20 gauge spinal needle is used. Fluoroscopic spot films, anteroposterior radiographs in internal and external rotation, and axillary and tangential bicipital groove radiographs are obtained. This series of radiographs is repeated following moderate exercise of the shoulder.

DOUBLE CONTRAST EXAMINATION. Double contrast shoulder arthrography is performed with approximately 4 ml of Renografin and 10 ml of air. Following injection and withdrawal of the needle, the patient is placed upright with a 2.3 kg (5 lb) sandbag in his or her hand. Radiographs in internal and external rotation are obtained with or without a spot film device. The patient is then returned to the supine position and internal rotation, external rotation, axillary, and bicipital groove films are made. These radiographs can be repeated after mild exercise of the shoulder. With this technique, the width of the rotator cuff tear and the integrity of cuff tendons can be assessed. Furthermore, the internal structures of the joint, including the glenoid labrum, are better identified.

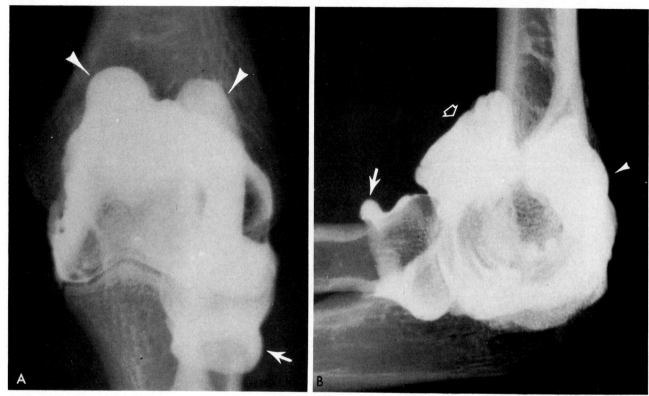

Figure 14–6. Elbow arthrography: Normal arthrogram. A Anteroposterior radiograph. Observe the thin layer of contrast material between humerus and ulna, the proximal extension of material in front of the humerus resembling the ears of a rabbit (arrowheads), and the periradial or annular recess (arrow). **B** Lateral radiograph. Note the periradial or annular recess (arrow), the coronoid or anterior recess (open arrow), and the olecranon or posterior recess (arrowhead).

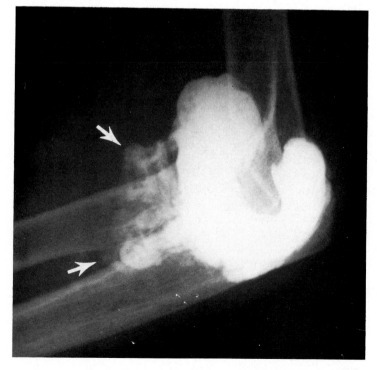

Figure 41–7. Elbow arthrography: Rheumatoid arthritis. An arthrogram from a 50 year old man with rheumatoid arthritis and a periarticular mass due to a synovial cyst. The arthrogram outlines the distal cystic dilatation of the articular cavity with irregular synovium (arrows). (From Ehrlich GE: Antecubital cysts in rheumatoid arthritis—a corollary to popliteal (Baker's) cysts. J Bone Joint Surg [Am] 54:165, 1972. Used with permission.)

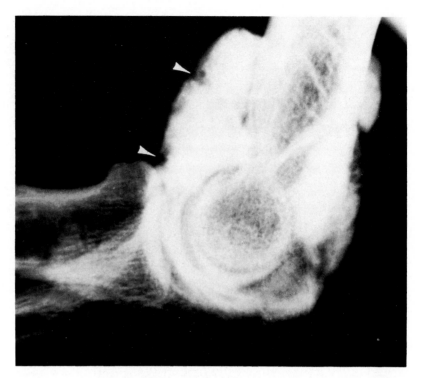

Figure 14–8. Elbow arthrography: Idiopathic synovial (osteo)chondromatosis. A lateral view after arthrography delineates irregular nodular filling defects (arrowheads), which represent cartilaginous foci resulting from synovial metaplasia.

Table 14–3. SOME INDICATIONS FOR GLENOHUMERAL JOINT ARTHROGRAPHY

Evaluation of:
Rotator cuff tears
Adhesive capsulitis
Bicipital tendon abnormalities
Previous dislocations
Presence and extent of synovial inflammation

Normal Glenohumeral Joint Arthrogram (Figs. 14–10 and 14–11)

Contrast material is identified between the humeral head and the glenoid. In external rotation, the contrast substance ends abruptly laterally at the anatomic neck of the humerus. In this view, an axillary pouch may be opacified on the undersurface of the humeral head. In internal rotation, a prominent subscapular recess is observed overlying the glenoid

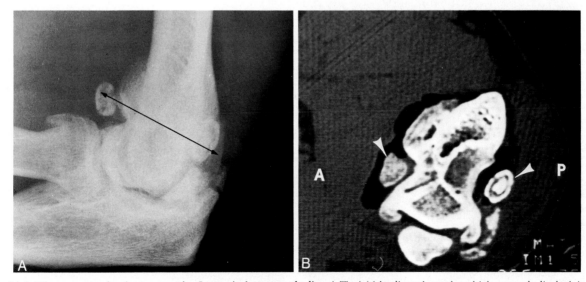

Figure 14–9. Elbow computed arthrotomography: Intraarticular osseous bodies. A The initial radiograph reveals multiple osseous bodies both in front of and behind the distal portion of the humerus. **B** After the introduction of 10 ml of air, a transaxial computed tomographic scan at the approximate level indicated in **A** confirms the intraarticular location of several of the bodies (arrowheads). A, Anterior; P, posterior.

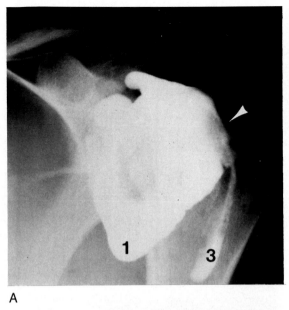

A

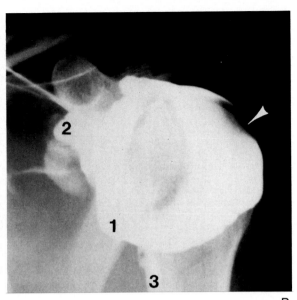

B

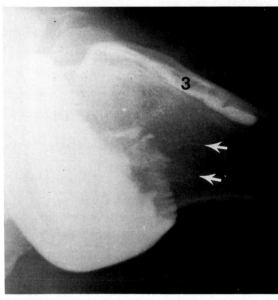

C

Figure 14–10. Glenohumeral joint arthrography: Normal single contrast arthrogram. A Normal arthrogram: External rotation. Visualized structures include the axillary pouch (1) and bicipital tendon sheath (3). Note that the subscapular recess is not well seen and the contrast material ends abruptly laterally at the anatomic neck of the humerus (arrowhead). B Normal arthrogram: Internal rotation. Observe the prominent subscapular recess (2), axillary pouch (1), and bicipital tendon sheath (3). The articular cartilage of the humeral head is well seen (arrowhead). Minimal extravasation of contrast material has occurred in the axilla near the injection site. C Normal arthrogram: Axillary view. Observe the bicipital tendon (3) and the absence of contrast material over the surgical neck of the humerus (arrows).

and lateral scapular region. The tendon of the long head of the biceps is visible as a radiolucent filling defect within the articular cavity and can be traced for a variable distance within the contrast-filled tendon sheath into the bicipital groove and along the metaphysis of the humerus. In the axillary view, contrast material should not overlie the surgical neck of the humerus. The tangential view of the bicipital groove demonstrates an oval filling defect within the contrast-filled sheath, representing the biceps tendon.

Complete and Incomplete Tears of the Rotator Cuff

Tears in the rotator cuff musculature may involve the entire thickness of the cuff (complete tear) or a portion of the cuff (incomplete or partial tear). Their causes and pathogenesis are discussed in Chapter 62. Arthrography remains the most popular technique in the diagnosis of rotator cuff tears despite recent interest in the application of ultrasonography and magnetic resonance imaging to this diagnosis.

COMPLETE TEAR (FIG. 14–12). Abnormal communication exists between the glenohumeral joint cavity and the subacromial (subdeltoid) bursa. Contrast material can be identified within the bursa as a large collection superior and lateral to the greater tuberosity and adjacent to the undersurface of the acromion. Using double contrast shoulder arthrography, the width of the tear and the degree of degeneration of the torn rotator cuff can be recognized.

INCOMPLETE TEAR. A partial tear may involve the deep (inferior) surface of the rotator cuff, the superficial surface, or the interior substance of the tendon. Tears on the inferior surface can be diagnosed on arthrography. In these cases, an irregular circular or linear collection of contrast material may be identified above the opacified joint cavity, near the anatomic neck of the humerus. The intact superficial fibers of the rotator cuff prevent opacification of the subacromial bursa.

Adhesive Capsulitis

Glenohumeral joint arthrography has been used in the diagnosis and treatment of adhesive capsulitis.

DIAGNOSIS (FIG. 14–13). Adhesive capsulitis, which

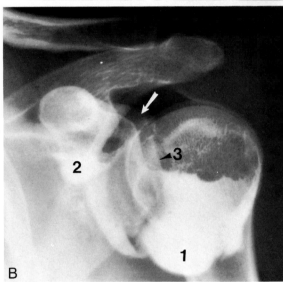

Figure 14–11. Glenohumeral joint arthrography: Normal double contrast arthrogram (upright projections). **A** Normal arthrogram: External rotation. Visualized structures include the axillary pouch (1), bicipital tendon (3), glenoid fibrocartilage (arrow), and articular cartilage of the humeral head. The distended articular cavity (arrowhead) above the bicipital tendon should not be misinterpreted as filling of the subacromial (subdeltoid) bursa. **B** Normal arthrogram: Internal rotation. Visualized structures include the subscapular recess (2), axillary pouch (1), bicipital tendon (3), glenoid fibrocartilage (arrow), and articular cartilage of the humeral head.

prevents normal distention of the glenohumeral joint, generally follows shoulder trauma. Arthrography is a reliable means of detecting its presence. The main arthrographic abnormality in adhesive capsulitis of the glenohumeral articulation is a joint of low capacity evidenced by increased resistance to injection and a "tight" feel. The subscapular and axillary recesses are small or absent. An additional finding is irregularity of the capsular insertion.

TREATMENT. Joint distention during arthrography, the "brisement" procedure, may aid in treatment of this condition. This technique requires slow, intermittent injection of larger and larger volumes of contrast material. This technique has also been applied to the treatment of adhesive capsulitis in other locations, such as the hip.

Abnormalities of the Bicipital Tendon (Fig. 14–14)

Considering the wide variation in the arthrographic appearance of the bicipital tendon and sheath in normal individuals, the radiologist must not rely too heavily on the arthrogram in establishing the existence of a significant abnormality. The arthrographic diagnosis of complete rupture is more accurate in cases of acute tears; findings include distortion of the synovial sheath and absence of the tendon within the opacified sheath. Incomplete tears of the bicipital tendon produce increased width of the tendon and distortion of the synovial sheath. Medial dislocation of the tendon and sheath from their normal positions in the intertubercular groove can be suggested when the positions of these structures do not change on the internal and external rotation radiographs.

Arthrography after Previous Dislocations

Anterior dislocations of the glenohumeral joint are associated with soft tissue damage. As the dislocating humeral head moves anteriorly, it detaches or lifts the articular capsule from the glenoid and neck of the scapula, producing an abnormal recess of variable size between the subscapular and axillary recesses. On arthrography, the abnormal recess fills with contrast material, obscuring the indentation that is normally present between the subscapular and axillary recesses.

Additional findings related to anterior dislocation are in-

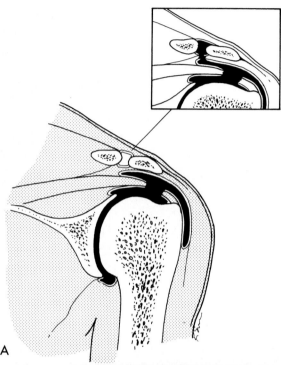

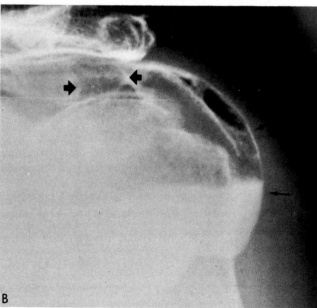

Figure 14–12. Glenohumeral joint arthrography: Complete rotator cuff tear.
A The arthrographic findings of a complete tear of the rotator cuff. Contrast material extends from the glenohumeral joint through the rotator cuff into the subacromial (subdeltoid) bursa. The inset reveals contrast material extending from the glenohumeral joint through the rotator cuff into the subacromial bursa, and from there into the acromioclavicular joint. **B, C** Double contrast arthrography. The external rotation view (**B**) demonstrates that contrast material has extended from the glenohumeral joint into the subacromial (subdeltoid) bursa (thin arrows). The width of the tear of the rotator cuff can be seen (between heavy arrows). In another patient with a rotator cuff tear, an axillary view (**C**) reveals a "saddle-bag" configuration, with contrast material overlying the surgical neck of the humerus (arrowheads). (**B,** Courtesy of J. Mink, M.D., Los Angeles, California.)

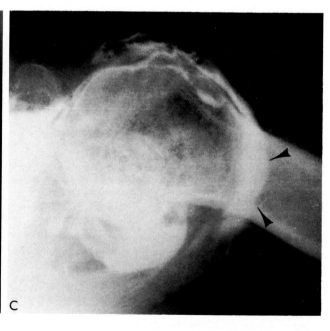

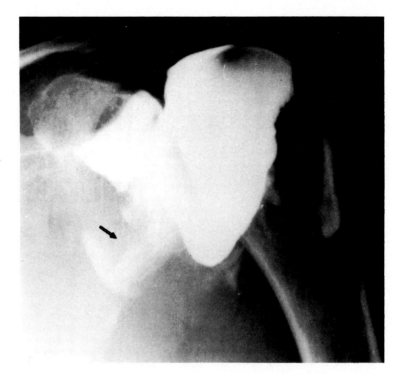

Figure 14–13. Glenohumeral joint arthrography: Diagnosis of adhesive capsulitis. After the introduction of 6 ml of contrast material, the patient complained of pain and there was increased resistance as an additional 4 ml was injected. A radiograph reveals a "tight-looking" articulation with contrast extravasation medially (arrow).

juries of cartilage and bone. The Bankart deformity involves an avulsion or compression defect of the anteroinferior rim of the glenoid and may be purely cartilaginous in nature. The arthrogram, particularly when obtained with double contrast technique, may outline the cartilaginous abnormalities about the glenoid labrum. The second defect associated with previous anterior dislocation is a Hill-Sachs compression deformity on the posterolateral aspect of the humeral head. This finding is generally evident on plain films.

In recent years, the application of conventional and computed arthrotomography to the diagnosis of abnormalities in the unstable shoulder has been emphasized. The latter technique is preferred. Computed arthrotomography is accom-

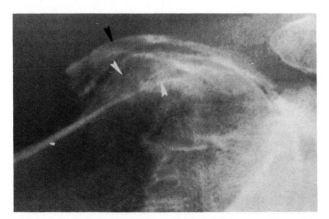

Figure 14–14. Glenohumeral joint arthrography: Abnormalities of the bicipital tendon—dislocation of the tendon. On a modified axillary view of the shoulder, the contrast-filled tendon sheath and tendon (black arrowhead) is displaced from the intertubercular sulcus (white arrowheads). (Courtesy of A. B. Goldman, M.D., New York, New York.)

plished after the injection of 10 to 15 ml of air with or without 1 ml of radiopaque contrast material. The patient is examined in the supine position with arms positioned by the sides and the shoulders in a neutral attitude or in slight internal rotation; to distend the posterior capsule optimally with air, external rotation of the shoulder can be used.

Abnormalities of the glenoid labrum depicted on conventional or computed arthrotomography include foreshortening, thinning, or contrast imbibition along its free margin (Fig. 14–15). The labrum may also be completely detached. An osseous Bankart lesion is typically visualized as an elevation of a small sliver of bone and irregularity of the adjacent glenoid rim. A depression along the posterolateral aspect of the humeral head is indicative of a Hill-Sachs lesion. Additional abnormalities that can be detected include intraarticular osteocartilaginous bodies and subluxation or dislocation of the bicipital tendon.

Rheumatoid Arthritis and Other Synovial Disorders (Fig. 14–16)

Synovial, cartilaginous, osseous, and soft tissue changes of rheumatoid involvement of the glenohumeral joint can be identified on arthrography. These findings include a corrugated, enlarged synovial cavity, nodular filling defects, cartilage loss, contrast filling of osseous erosions, lymphatic filling, enlarging axillary lymph nodes, capsulitis with a restricted joint cavity, and rotator cuff tear. In rheumatoid arthritis and other synovial disorders, synovial cysts about the glenohumeral joint may be documented by arthrography.

Septic arthritis of the glenohumeral joint may lead to synovial irregularity and capsular and rotator cuff rupture, with the formation of soft tissue abscesses. These abscesses appear as irregular contrast-filled cavities on glenohumeral joint arthrography.

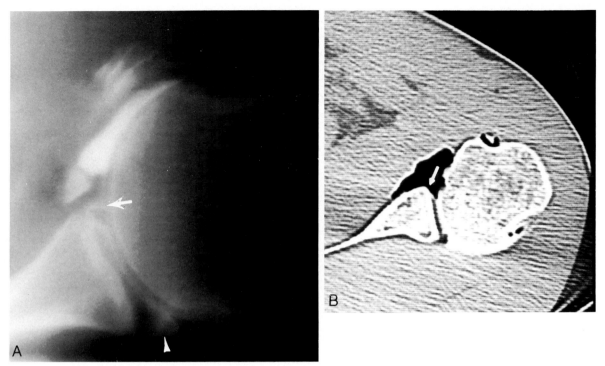

Figure 14–15. Glenohumeral joint arthrography: Glenoid labrum abnormalities. A Conventional arthrotomography delineates a tear of the anterior portion of the glenoid labrum (arrow) and imbibition of contrast material in the posterior portion of the labrum (arrowhead). **B** Computed arthrotomography shows complete detachment of the anterior portion of the glenoid labrum (arrow).

HIP

Although most descriptions of hip arthrography record its application to the investigation of patients with painful prostheses (see Chapter 20), this procedure may also be utilized in patients with congenital, traumatic, and articular disorders (Table 14–4).

Technique

Many techniques exist for puncturing the hip joint. The author uses an anterior approach with the patient supine on the table. The femoral artery is palpated in the groin and a metal marker is placed 2 cm lateral and 2 cm distal to this point. An 18 gauge, 3 inch spinal needle is inserted in a superior direction with fluoroscopic guidance to contact the bone at the junction of the medial aspect of the femoral head and neck. Ten to 15 ml of contrast medium (60 per cent Renografin) is then injected, and the needle is withdrawn. Anteroposterior radiographs in internal and external rotation, a frog-leg view, and true lateral radiographs are obtained before and after mild exercise.

In infants and children, an anterolateral subphyseal plate

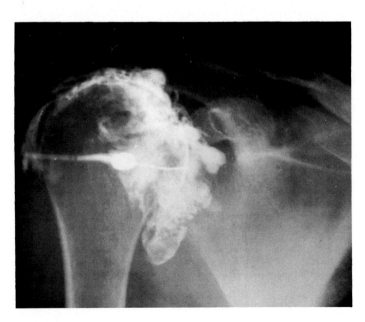

Figure 14–16. Glenohumeral joint arthrography: Rheumatoid arthritis. Contrast opacification of the articular cavity reveals a corrugated synovial pattern with nodular filling defects. The rotator cuff was also abnormal. (Courtesy of J. Mink, M.D., Los Angeles, California.)

Table 14-4. SOME INDICATIONS FOR HIP ARTHROGRAPHY

Evaluation of:
   Congenital dislocation of the hip
   Septic arthritis and osteomyelitis with epiphyseal separation
   Epiphyseal dysplasia and osteonecrosis
   Certain synovial disorders
   Soft tissue masses
   Trauma

site is ideal for contacting the bone. This metaphyseal location is within the joint capsule yet distant from the femoral vessels, cartilaginous femoral head, and growth plate. Approximately 1.5 to 2 ml of contrast agent is injected in infants and 5 to 8 ml in adolescents.

Normal Hip Arthrogram

The normal hip arthrogram in an adult is shown in Figure 14-17.

Congenital Dislocation of the Hip (Fig. 14-18)

In infants with congenital dislocation of the femoral head, the cartilaginous limbus will be apparent as a filling defect beneath the displaced head of the femur. In this situation, the head will deform or compress the limbus and the ligamentum teres will be stretched, leading from the inferior margin of the acetabulum to the fovea of the dislocated femoral head. The capsule will also be stretched around the head, and the opacified hip joint will have an hourglass configuration.

The hip arthrogram may be used to evaluate the adequacy of reduction of a dislocated femoral head, particularly in the older infant or child. In this situation, arthrography may outline an inverted limbus that is interposed between the acetabulum and head, preventing complete reduction.

It should be emphasized that, owing to the unossified nature of the cartilaginous femoral head in the newborn, the differentiation of congenital dislocation of the hip from infectious (see subsequent discussion) and traumatic epiphyseal separation is extremely difficult or impossible by routine radiography. Arthrography will document that the femoral head is situated in the acetabulum in cases of epiphysiolysis and it is, therefore, essential in this differential diagnosis.

Hip arthrography is useful in the clinical setting of neonatal sepsis and an apparent dislocation of the femoral head. In this situation, it is impossible to determine the exact position of the unossified femoral head on initial radiographs. Two possibilities exist: The hip is indeed dislocated, or there is a pathologic epiphyseal separation related to osteomyelitis with a normal relationship between cartilaginous head and acetabulum. A hip arthrogram will allow aspiration of joint contents and documentation of the position of the femoral head. The diagnosis of true dislocation or epiphyseal separation can then be made accurately.

Legg-Calvé-Perthes Disease (Fig. 14-19)

In Legg-Calvé-Perthes disease, one arthrographic finding is an absolute enlargement of the femoral head related to hyperplasia of the epiphyseal cartilage. Using this method to identify the true position of the cartilaginous head may allow the surgeon to determine which position of the hip will be best during treatment of the condition. Arthrography in this disease has also been used to demonstrate the existence of an osteochondral fragment. This uncommon complication relates to the presence of an unhealed necrotic fragment, which appears separate from the remainder of the femoral head.

Trauma

In patients with single or recurrent anterior or posterior dislocations of the femoral head, hip arthrography alone or in

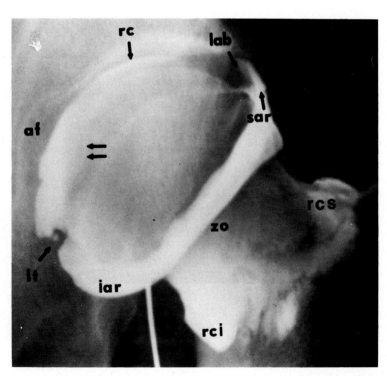

Figure 14-17. Hip arthrography: Normal arthrogram. The recess capitus (rc) is a thin, smooth collection of contrast medium between apposing articular surfaces and is interrupted only where the ligamentum teres femoris (double arrows) enters the fovea centralis of the femoral head. The ligamentum transversum (lt) is seen as a radiolucent defect adjacent to the inferior rim of the acetabulum. The ligamentum teres femoris bridges the acetabular notch and effectively deepens the acetabulum. The inferior articular recess (iar) forms a pouch at the inferior base of the femoral head below the acetabular notch and ligamentum transversum. The superior articular recess (sar) extends cephalad around the acetabular labrum (lab). The acetabular labrum is seen as a triangular radiolucent area adjacent to the superolateral lip of the acetabulum. The zona orbicularis (zo) is a circumferential lucent band around the femoral neck, which changes configuration with rotation of the femur. The recess colli superior (rcs) and recess colli inferior (rci) are poolings of contrast material at the apex and base of the intertrochanteric line and are the most caudal extensions of the synovial membrane. (From Guerra J Jr, et al: The adult hip: An anatomic study. Part II. The soft tissue landmarks. Radiology 128:11, 1978. Used with permission.)

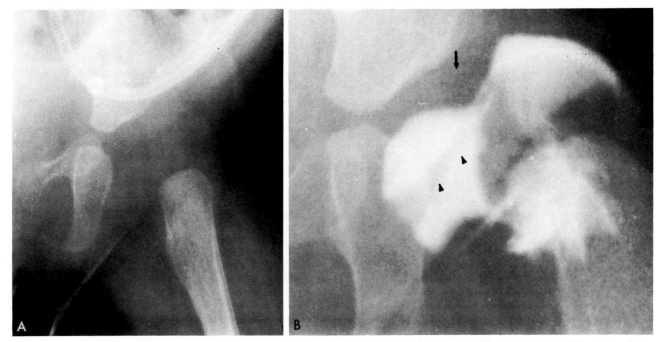

Figure 14–18. Hip arthrography: Congenital dislocation of the hip. A, B A 2 month old infant with hip dislocation. Th initial film (**A**) reveals the lateral position of the femur with respect to the acetabulum. The arthrogram (**B**) obtained in neutral position outlines the radiolucent cartilaginous femoral head, a deformed limbus (arrow) between the displaced femoral head and acetabulum, and a stretched ligamentum teres femoris (arrowheads). Because of the stretched capsule, the opacified hip joint has an hourglass configuration. (From Kaye JJ, et al: Neonatal septic "dislocation" of the hip: True dislocation or pathological epiphyseal separation? Radiology 114:671, 1975. Used with permission.)

combination with computed tomography may outline distortion of or defects in the joint capsule and intraarticular osteocartilaginous bodies. After injury or surgery, or on an idiopathic basis, capsular constriction (adhesive capsulitis) may appear in the hip. In such cases, plain films generally are unremarkable. Accurate diagnosis is accomplished with arthrography, during which a low capacity of the joint cavity is demonstrated. Difficulty in injecting as little as 8 ml of

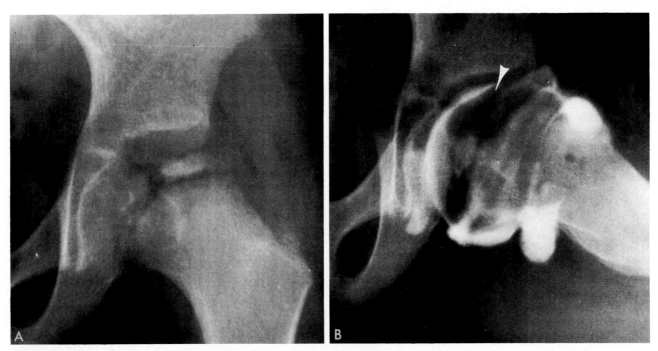

Figure 14–19. Hip arthrography: Legg-Calvé-Perthes disease. A On the initial film, epiphyseal fragmentation and metaphyseal irregularity are apparent. **B** Arthrographic image in hip abduction indicates a relatively smooth radiolucent cartilaginous head (arrowhead), which is well covered by the acetabulum.

contrast material into the hip is encountered, and the normal articular recesses are obliterated.

Articular Disorders

In idiopathic synovial (osteo)chondromatosis or pigmented villonodular synovitis, the extent of synovial and capsular abnormality can be determined with hip arthrography. In patients with septic arthritis, hip arthrography provides a technique for aspiration and culture and also a means of evaluating cartilaginous, osseous, and synovial abnormalities.

Synovial Cysts

Hip arthrography in rheumatoid arthritis and other synovial disorders will reveal the degree of intraarticular alterations and the presence or absence of communicating synovial cysts (Fig. 14–20). Communication of the hip and iliopsoas bursa in the presence of intraarticular diseases such as osteoarthritis, rheumatoid arthritis, pigmented villonodular synovitis, infection, calcium pyrophosphate dihydrate crystal deposition disease, and idiopathic synovial (osteo)chondromatosis may lead to bursal enlargement, producing a mass in the ilioinguinal region that may simulate a hernia and cause obstruction of the femoral vein.

To evaluate suspected synovial cysts about the hip, ultrasonography should be performed after conventional radiography if a probable groin mass or other suggestive clinical manifestations are present. If a nonpulsatile fluid collection without Doppler evidence of flow is demonstrated, diagnostic aspiration of its contents can be accomplished. Fluid analysis should distinguish a synovial cyst or iliopsoas bursitis from a lymphocele, abscess, or hematoma. Subsequent injection of contrast material may opacify the hip joint, confirming the diagnosis; if not, hip arthrography, computed tomography, or magnetic resonance imaging may be desirable for delineation of articular communication if surgery is being contemplated.

KNEE

The role of arthrography is most established for abnormalities of the knee, as it is useful in evaluating this joint in a variety of clinical situations (Table 14–5). The technique of examination has evolved through the years; single contrast examination has been replaced, in large part, by double contrast examination using air and radiopaque contrast material.

Technique

After puncture of the joint and aspiration of joint contents, 2 to 5 ml of contrast material (60 per cent Renografin) and 30 ml of air are injected. The patient then exercises the knee moderately and is placed beneath the fluoroscopic unit. Nine to 18 exposures are made of each meniscus, using slight changes in position and appropriate leg traction. A variety of traction devices have been described to provide appropriate varus and valgus stress during the examination. After fluoroscopy, overhead films or spot films are taken to evaluate articular cartilage and cruciate ligaments and to determine whether a popliteal cyst is present.

Most important to success of the fluoroscopic technique of knee arthrography is the examination of all parts of both menisci. To accomplish this, fluoroscopic spot filming should be begun with the patient in one lateral position and continued through the oblique and frontal positions until the patient is in the opposite lateral attitude. This procedure is then repeated for the other meniscus. The success of knee arthrography also depends on spot films being accomplished with the meniscus projected clear of the femoral and tibial articular surfaces. This is facilitated by raising and lowering the leg. Finally, adequate stress placed on the knee is fundamental to arthrographic success.

To obtain high quality knee arthrograms, it is imperative that most of the intraarticular fluid be aspirated. When considerable fluid is present, contrast coating of the menisci is less than ideal, and subtle tears will be missed. The examination must be performed in a rapid manner, as the contrast coating will deteriorate as time elapses. The addition of intraarticular epinephrine (0.2 ml of 1:1000 solution) may

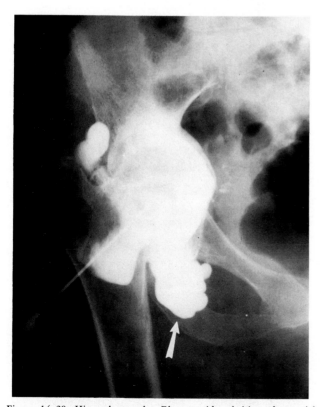

Figure 14–20. Hip arthrography: Rheumatoid arthritis and synovial cyst formation. In this 65 year old woman with rheumatoid arthritis and an apparent "femoral hernia," arthrography indicates that the clinically evident soft tissue mass is related to a synovial cyst (arrow). Observe the sacculation of the articular cavity and a protrusio acetabuli defect.

Table 14–5. SOME INDICATIONS FOR KNEE ARTHROGRAPHY

Evaluation of:
  Meniscal tears, cysts, and ossicles
  Discoid menisci
  Postmeniscectomy syndromes
  Ligamentous injuries
  Transchondral fractures
  Chondromalacia patellae
  Degenerative joint disease
  Intraarticular osseous and cartilaginous bodies
  Synovial disorders
  Blount's disease

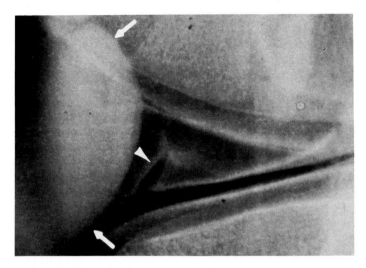

Figure 14–21. **Knee arthrography: Vertical concentric meniscal tear.** Observe the contrast or air-filled linear shadow (arrowhead) in the meniscus. A popliteal cyst is evident (arrows).

enhance meniscal visualization by causing vasoconstriction of synovial vessels, decreasing both the amount of contrast material absorbed from the joint cavity and the amount of intraarticular fluid formed.

Certain overhead films have been recommended after knee arthrography. These are obtained to evaluate the cruciate ligaments, articular cartilage, and synovial cavity.

Normal Knee Arthrogram

The medial meniscus is identified as a sharply defined, soft tissue triangular shadow. Its posterior horn is usually large, averaging 14 mm wide. Its midportion is somewhat smaller, and the anterior horn is usually the smallest portion of the medial meniscus, averaging 6 mm wide. Occasionally the anterior horn may be larger than the midportion. The peripheral surface of the medial meniscus is firmly attached to the medial collateral ligament. Certain normal recesses about the medial meniscus produce focal pouch-like collections of air and contrast material.

The lateral meniscus is more circular in configuration than the medial meniscus. It too is projected as a sharply defined triangular radiodense area surrounded by air and contrast material. It is relatively uniform in width, averaging 10 mm wide. Inferior recesses are frequent beneath both the anterior and the posterior horns. The anterior horn is attached to the lateral ligament, but the posterior horn of the lateral meniscus is separated from this ligament by the synovial sheath of the popliteus tendon. Two delicate bands of connective tissue, termed struts or fascicles, connect the posterior horn of the lateral meniscus to the joint capsule around the popliteal tendon sheath.

Meniscal Abnormalities

MENISCAL TEAR. Arthrography remains a highly accurate technique for the evaluation of a number of meniscal abnormalities, including tears, and is the preferred method of most radiologists despite the recent application of computed tomography, magnetic resonance imaging, and ultrasonography to the assessment of meniscal lesions. Although a system of classification has been devised for meniscal tears, it is often impossible to identify the type during arthrography. The location of the tear is of greater significance. A meniscal tear is more frequent on the medial side, involving particularly

the posterior horn of the medial meniscus. The lateral meniscal tear most commonly involves the anterior horn.

A *vertical concentric tear* (Fig. 14–21) appears as a radiodense line extending through the meniscus. The inner fragment may be displaced, producing a bucket-handle tear, and may lodge in the central portion of the articulation. A *vertical*

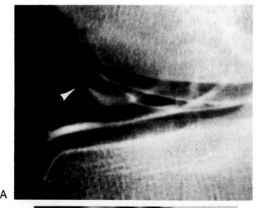

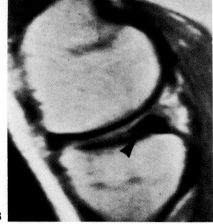

Figure 14–22. **Knee arthrography: Horizontal meniscal tear. A** An arthrogram in a patient with a horizontal tear of the medial meniscus. Note the tear (arrowhead), which is filled with contrast material. **B** A sagittal magnetic resonance image (T1 weighted) reveals a horizontal tear (arrowhead) of the posterior horn of the medial meniscus. (Courtesy of L. Bassett, M.D., Los Angeles, California.)

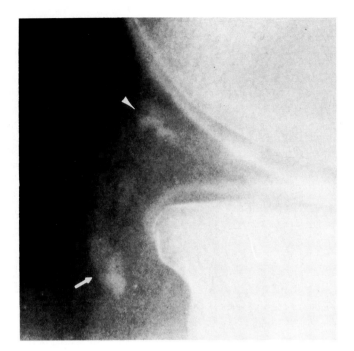

Figure 14–23. Knee arthrography: Meniscal cyst. A cyst of the medial meniscus is opacified (arrow) and associated with a horizontal tear of the meniscus (arrowhead).

radial tear along the inner contour of the meniscus will produce a contrast-coated inner meniscal margin and a blunted meniscal shadow. A *horizontal tear* (Fig. 14–22), which is observed more frequently in older individuals, is seen as a radiopaque line of contrast material overlying the meniscal shadow, extending to the superior or inferior surface.

MENISCAL CYST (FIG. 14–23). Meniscal cysts are multiloculated collections of mucinous material of unknown cause that have predilection for the lateral aspect of the knee. The cysts are generally located at the peripheral meniscal margin. Involved menisci commonly reveal horizontal tears, and tracks may be identified leading from the tear to the cysts.

DISCOID MENISCUS (FIG. 14–24). A discoid meniscus is broad and disc-like rather than semilunar in configuration. The lateral meniscus is much more frequently discoid than is the medial meniscus. The usual age of patients at the time of clinical presentation is between 15 and 35 years, and men are more frequently affected. These patients commonly have symptoms of a torn cartilage.

The pathogenesis of discoid menisci is debated. An embryologic explanation for these menisci has not yet been discovered. The normal sequence of embryologic development of the knee does not contain a stage in which either the medial or the lateral meniscus is discoid in shape; the appearance of such a meniscus in a child or adult therefore cannot occur through persistence of a fetal stage. It has been postulated that the discoid lateral meniscus is acquired after birth as a result of an abnormal attachment of its posterior horn to the tibial plateau. Eventually, a discoid meniscus would be produced owing to repetitive abnormal mediolateral and anteroposterior movement of the meniscus.

Initial plain films in patients with discoid menisci generally are unrewarding. Arthrography reveals the abnormally large and elongated meniscus, frequently extending to the intercondylar notch. An associated meniscal tear frequently is observed.

MENISCAL OSSICLE (FIG. 14–25). Meniscal ossicles, which are rare, represent foci of ossification within the menisci. Patients may be asymptomatic or have local pain

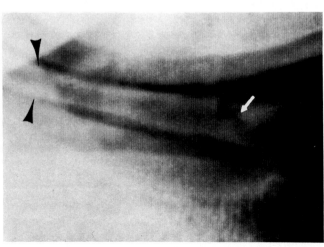

Figure 14–24. Discoid lateral meniscus (slab type) with tear. Observe that the meniscus extends far into the joint cavity (arrowheads). A vertical tear is evident (arrow).

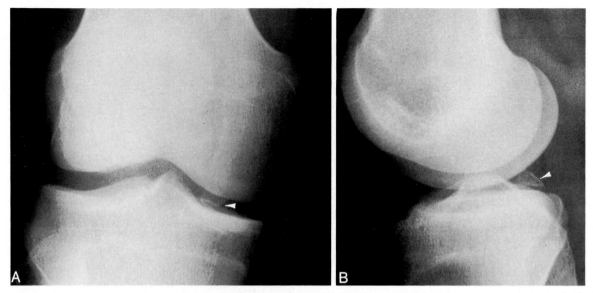

Figure 14–25. Knee arthrography: Meniscal ossicle. The frontal (**A**) and lateral (**B**) radiographs reveal a bone fragment (arrowheads) in the distribution of the posterior horn of the medial meniscus. (Courtesy of G. Greenway, M.D., Dallas, Texas.)

and swelling. Initial films reveal ossification of variable shape in the anterior or posterior portion of either the medial or the lateral meniscus. The most common site is the posterior horn of the medial meniscus. Arthrography confirms the location of the ossification within the meniscus. The meniscus itself may be normal, contain associated tears, or be discoid in shape.

Meniscal ossicles must be differentiated from other causes of articular radiodense areas, particularly intraarticular osteochondral fragments. These latter fragments are not central in location, may move in location from one examination to another, or may appear in the joint recesses.

MENISCECTOMY. A total meniscectomy involves the removal of the entire meniscus from its capsular attachment. In a partial meniscectomy the anterior two thirds of the abnormal meniscus may be removed, leaving the posterior horn in place; or, alternatively, the torn portion of the meniscus may be removed, leaving the remainder of the meniscus intact. After complete meniscectomy, fibrous regeneration of the meniscus occurs within 6 weeks to 3 months. The regenerated meniscus is thinner and narrower than a normal meniscus, with a decreased surface area and diminished mobility. Tears through regenerated menisci are rare.

Arthrographic evaluation following complete or partial meniscectomy may reveal a retained fragment, a regenerated meniscus, or a tear of the opposite meniscus. The retained posterior horn after incomplete meniscectomy will resemble a normal posterior horn, although it may be irregular or contain an obvious tear. Following the removal of the inner fragment of a bucket-handle tear, the retained peripheral fragment will appear as a truncated shadow with rough, irregular surfaces. With regeneration of the meniscus, a small triangular shadow resembling an equilateral or isosceles triangle is observed, varying from 2 to 7 mm in width. It possesses smooth, well-defined margins but is not associated with adjacent normal recesses at the meniscocapsular junction.

Ligamentous Injury

COLLATERAL LIGAMENT TEARS (FIG. 14–26). Injuries of the collateral ligaments may produce plain film radiographic findings, including widening of the joint space during varus or valgus stress and calcification, particularly near the femoral site of attachment of the medial collateral ligament (Pellegrini-Stieda syndrome). Recent tears of the collateral ligaments may be documented by arthrography. Contrast material introduced into the joint space will extravasate into the adjacent soft tissues. This finding is more readily apparent on the medial aspect of the knee, where a linear radiodense region may indicate a contrast-coated outer margin of the medial collateral ligament.

CRUCIATE LIGAMENT INJURIES. Double contrast arthrography is useful in the evaluation of the cruciate ligaments. Two techniques are used: a horizontal cross-table lateral radiograph and fluoroscopic spot films. In both instances, the anterior cruciate ligament is examined while being tensed with a simulated "anterior drawer" maneuver. As an example, for the horizontal cross-table lateral radiograph, the patient sits with the legs flexed between 45 and 75 degrees over the side of the table, and the proximal end of the tibia is pushed anteriorly with respect to the femoral condyles by a firm pillow located behind the calf. Although a properly performed cruciate ligament examination takes only 1 or 2 minutes, it must be done carefully and meticulously. When accomplished by an experienced arthrographer, the accuracy of the technique surpasses 90 per cent.

The fundamental arthrographic criterion of a normal anterior cruciate ligament is an anterior synovial surface that is "ruler-straight." The ligament is considered to be lax but intact if the anterior synovial surface is bowed and concave anteriorly. The arthrographic abnormalities associated with disruption of the anterior cruciate ligament include nonvisualization, a wavy, lumpy, or acutely angulated anterior surface, irregularity of the inferior attachment of the ligament, pooling of the contrast medium in the usual location of the

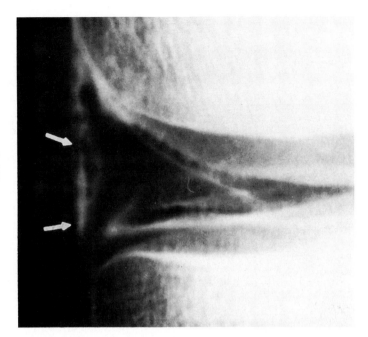

Figure 14–26. Knee arthrography. Collateral ligament injuries. A tear of the medial collateral ligament allows contrast material to pass from the articular cavity into the soft tissues, outlining the lateral aspect of the ligament (arrows).

ligament, and visualization of the plica synovialis infrapatellaris.

An alternative approach to the diagnosis of tears of cruciate ligaments is provided by computed tomography alone or computed tomography combined with arthrography of the knee. There is no uniform agreement regarding the position of the knee in the computed tomography gantry, the necessity for angulation of the gantry, or the benefit of reformatted or even three-dimensional images.

Tears of the anterior and posterior cruciate ligaments and the collateral ligaments also can be identified accurately by magnetic resonance imaging, owing to an altered signal and an abnormal position or configuration of the affected ligament (Fig. 14–27).

Lesions of Articular Cartilage

Contrast material within the joint cavity allows portions of the articular cartilage to be seen. Knee arthrography with conventional tomography may improve visualization of carti-

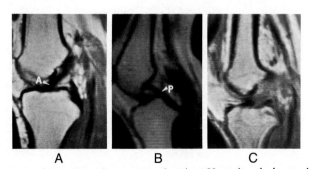

Figure 14–27. Magnetic resonance imaging: Normal and abnormal cruciate ligaments. A, B On sagittal magnetic resonance images in a patient, the normal anterior (A) and posterior (P) cruciate ligaments are visualized. C On this sagittal magnetic resonance image, the anterior cruciate ligament is torn and there is hemorrhage in the joint. (A,C, Courtesy of L. Bassett, M.D., Los Angeles, California.)

laginous surfaces. Abnormalities such as osteochondral fracture (osteochondritis dissecans) and chondromalacia may be identified, although the latter is better studied with computed arthrotomography or magnetic resonance imaging.

OSTEOCHONDRAL FRACTURE (OSTEOCHONDRITIS DISSECANS) (FIG. 14–28). Transchondral fractures occur where tangential shearing forces are applied to the articular surface. In the knee, such fractures are most frequent on the lateral surface of the medial femoral condyle. The fracture fragment may consist of cartilage, cartilage and bone, or bone alone. It may remain in situ with relatively normal overlying cartilage, become depressed with an indentation of the articular surface, or become detached, existing as a loose body in the articular cavity or as an attached body at a distant synovial site.

Arthrography will allow evaluation of the cartilaginous or osseous surface, or both, at the fracture site. Contrast medium may outline a normal, swollen, or depressed cartilaginous surface, or it may dissect beneath the osteochondral fragment. The detection of intraarticular osteochondral bodies accompanying osteochondritis dissecans or other disorders may require the combination of arthrography and conventional or computed tomography (Fig. 14–29).

CHONDROMALACIA PATELLAE. The role of arthrography in the diagnosis of chondromalacia of the patella has been debated. Routine lateral arthrographic projections demonstrate only a small amount of the patellar cartilaginous surface, that near the apex of the ridge. Axial projections increase the cartilaginous area that can be visualized, and oblique projections that are tangential to the medial and lateral facets may further improve this visualization. Computed arthrotomography may also be used (Fig. 14–30). Whether arthrographic diagnosis will ever be more accurate than clinical diagnosis of the disorder, however, remains to be seen.

On arthrography, chondromalacia produces absorption or imbibition of contrast material by the patellar cartilage.

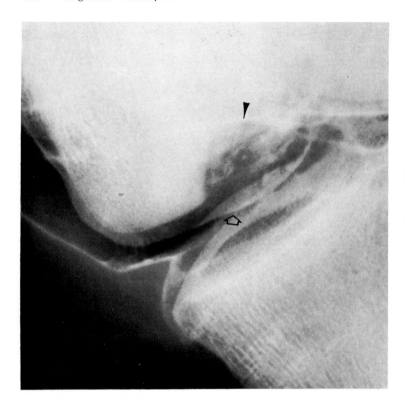

Figure 14–28. Knee arthrography: Osteochondral fracture (arrowhead), evaluated with arthrography. Note swollen articular cartilage over the lesion (open arrow). (From Wershba M, et al: Double contrast knee arthrography in the evaluation of osteochondritis dissecans. Clin Orthop 107:81, 1975. Used with permission.)

Nodular elevation, fissuring, or diminution of the cartilaginous surface may be apparent.

Synovial Plicae

Synovial plicae are remnants of synovial tissue that in early development originally divided the joint into three separate compartments. Such plicae may be found normally in the adult knee. Usually of no consequence, these structures may become pathologically thickened and cause symptoms. The three most commonly encountered plicae are classified according to the partitions from which they took origin—suprapatellar, medial patellar, and infrapatellar. Of these, the infrapatellar plica occurs most frequently, followed by the suprapatellar plica, and then by the medial plica. Each of these septa can be identified by arthrography, computed

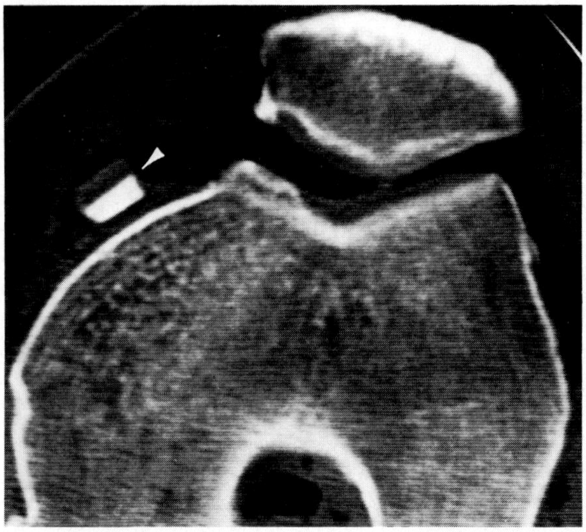

Figure 14–29. Knee arthrography: Osteochondral fragment. After the introduction of air into the knee joint, a transaxial computed tomographic scan reveals the fragment (arrowhead), consisting of cartilage and bone in the medial aspect of the articulation.

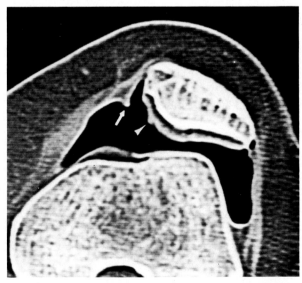

Figure 14–30. Knee arthrography: Chondromalacia patellae. A transaxial image during computed arthrotomography using air and a small amount of radiopaque contrast material shows cartilage fibrillation (arrowhead) and imbibition of contrast material, especially at the junction of the medial and most medial (odd) facets of the patella, consistent with chondromalacia patellae. A small medial plica (arrow) is also evident.

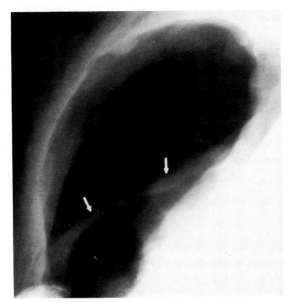

Figure 14–31. Knee arthrography: Suprapatellar plica. An example of the appearance of suprapatellar plicae (arrows) during arthrography.

Table 14–6. SOME CAUSES OF MULTIPLE FILLING DEFECTS ON KNEE ARTHROGRAMS

Rheumatoid arthritis
Pigmented villonodular synovitis
Idiopathic synovial (osteo)chondromatosis
Hemangioma, angioma
Lipoma arborescens

arthrotomography, magnetic resonance imaging, or arthroscopy, depending on its location and size.

The suprapatellar plica, or plica synovialis suprapatellaris, most commonly takes one of three forms: (1) an intact septum completely dividing the suprapatellar pouch from the remainder of the knee; (2) an intact septum except for a variably sized, centrally placed diaphragm known as the porta; or (3) a variably sized, crescent-shaped fold arising medially from the undersurface of the quadriceps tendon above the level of the patella and extending inferiorly to insert along the medial edge of the knee joint (Fig. 14–31).

The medial patellar plica has its origin on the medial wall of the knee joint, near the suprapatellar plica, and courses obliquely downward relative to the patella to insert into the synovium that covers the infrapatellar fat pad (Fig. 14–32).

The infrapatellar plica, or ligamentum mucosum, represents a vestige of the membranous partition that once separated the medial and lateral embryonic compartments of the knee. It descends through the inferior joint space to attach distally to the inferior and medial aspects of the patellar articular cartilage. From there the plica continues as two fringe-like alar folds to cover the infrapatellar fat and separate the synovium from the ligamentum patellae.

Symptomatic plicae are most commonly encountered in what has been referred to as the "plica syndrome." In this syndrome, the medial patellar plica, which normally exists as a fine, thin, flexible fold of synovium of little clinical significance, becomes pathologically thickened and symptomatic. The plica becomes relatively unpliable and no longer glides normally but snaps against the underlying femoral condyle. Repeated irritation and abrasion result in erosive changes of the articular cartilage of the condyle or even the patella.

Articular Disorders (Table 14–6)

DEGENERATIVE JOINT DISEASE (FIG. 14–33). Contrast examination of the knee in patients with degenerative joint disease reveals abnormalities of the articular cartilage and menisci and the presence of intraarticular osseous bodies and popliteal cysts. Arthrography may delineate generalized cartilaginous thinning or localized defects. A rough, irregular surface with imbibition of contrast material may be apparent. Compared with routine and weight-bearing radiographic films, however, arthrography adds little additional information on alterations in the more involved femorotibial compartment. In the less involved (contralateral) compartment, arthrography may reveal information regarding cartilaginous integrity not obtainable by these other examinations.

RHEUMATOID ARTHRITIS. Arthrographic findings include enlargement of the joint cavity or suprapatellar pouch, nodular irregularity or corrugation of the synovial membrane, filling defects within the joint cavity, lymphatic filling, destruction of hyaline cartilage and fibrocartilage, and synovial cyst formation.

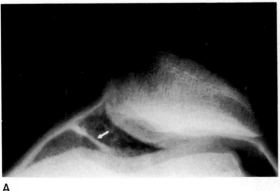

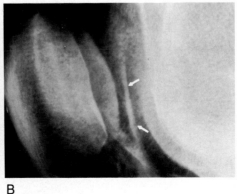

A   B

Figure 14–32. Knee arthrography: Medial patellar plica. A,B, Arthrographic demonstration of a medial patellar plica (arrows) is provided on axial and near-lateral projections.

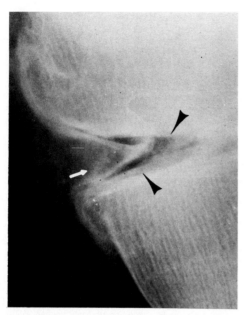

Figure 14–33. Knee arthrography: Degenerative joint disease. In the medial compartment, findings include severe denudation of articular cartilage on both femur and tibia (arrowheads). The medial meniscus is swollen, with an incomplete vertical tear (arrow) and an irregular inner contour.

PIGMENTED VILLONODULAR SYNOVITIS (FIG. 14–34). The knee arthrogram in diffuse pigmented villonodular synovitis reveals an enlarged synovial cavity, irregular synovial outline with "laking" or pooling of contrast material, and nodular filling defects. Arthrographic alterations associated with localized nodular synovitis of the knee may include a mass-like lesion coated with contrast material.

IDIOPATHIC SYNOVIAL (OSTEO)CHONDROMATOSIS (FIG. 14–35). Knee arthrography in idiopathic synovial (osteo)chondromatosis reveals an enlarged synovial cavity and multiple small, sharply defined filling defects. Occasion-

ally larger defects are apparent. The nodular lesions of idiopathic synovial (osteo)chondromatosis are better defined than those of pigmented villonodular synovitis.

Synovial Cysts

Synovial cysts about the knee are most frequent in the popliteal region, where communication between the joint and normal posterior bursae can be identified. The most commonly involved site is the gastrocnemiosemimembranosus bursa, located posterior to the medial femoral condyle between the tendons of the gastrocnemius and semimembranosus muscles. Swelling of this posterior bursa is termed a Baker's cyst. The cause of such cysts is not entirely clear, and various theories have been proposed: (1) herniation of the synovial membrane of the knee through a weak area in the posterior joint capsule; (2) rupture of the posterior joint capsule with extravasation of fluid into the soft tissues and secondary encapsulation; and (3) rupture of the posterior joint capsule, producing communication with a normal posterior bursa.

The presence of a slit between articular cavity and posterior bursa may be responsible for a ball-valve mechanism that has been noted in conjunction with synovial cysts; fluid introduced into a cyst may not enter the joint cavity. Because of this one-way directional flow, arthrography rather than bursography is more accurate in defining the extent of a cyst and its connection with a neighboring joint.

In addition to the gastrocnemiosemimembranosus bursa, other posterior bursae or the proximal tibiofibular joint may communicate with the knee. Occasionally, anterior, medial, and lateral synovial cysts may also be observed. Any of these synovial cysts may enlarge, producing a mass with or without pain. Rupture of a cyst is associated with soft tissue extravasation of fluid contents. Ruptures occurring posteriorly can simulate thrombophlebitis.

Arthrography of the knee is an accurate method of diagnosing synovial cysts, although some investigators also recommend ultrasonic or isotopic examination in this clinical

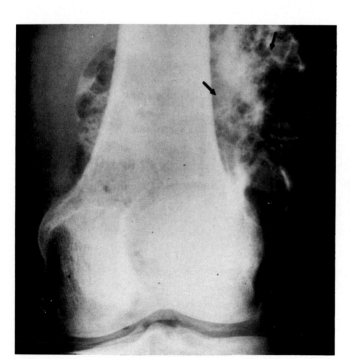

Figure 14–34. Knee arthrography: Diffuse pigmented villonodular synovitis. Observe the irregular distribution and appearance of contrast material (arrows) in the suprapatellar pouch. (From Dalinka MK, et al: Knee arthrography. CRC Crit Rev Radiol Sci 4:1, 1973. Used with permission.)

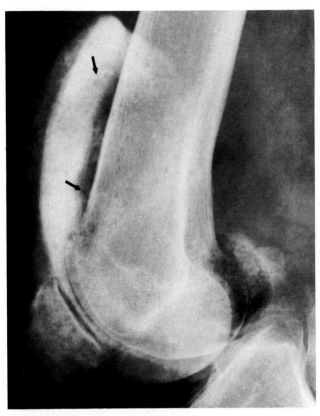

Figure 14–35. Knee arthrography: Idiopathic synovial (osteo)chondromatosis. Observe multiple sharply defined filling defects (arrows) throughout the articular cavity. (From Dalinka MK, et al: Knee arthrography. CRC Crit Rev Radiol Sci 4:1, 1973. Used with permission.)

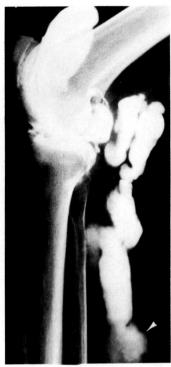

Figure 14–36. Knee arthrography: Synovial cyst formation in rheumatoid arthritis. A typical large popliteal cyst extending into the calf is filled with contrast material. It is slightly irregular in contour, particularly inferiorly (arrowhead), which may reflect synovial inflammation. No free extravasation into the soft tissues is seen.

situation. Magnetic resonance imaging may provide information on the degree of synovial inflammation.

The arthrographic appearance of an abnormal synovial cyst will vary. In most instances, a well-defined, lobulated structure filled with air and radiopaque contrast material will be revealed. It may have an irregular surface related to hypertrophy of its synovial lining and be associated with adjacent lymphatic filling. Alternatively, the entire cyst or a portion of it may rupture, with extravasation of contrast material into soft tissues posteriorly, or less commonly, superiorly or anteriorly.

Any inflammatory, degenerative, traumatic, or neoplastic condition that produces a knee effusion can lead to synovial cyst formation (Fig. 14–36). These conditions include rheumatoid arthritis, degenerative joint disease, gout, pigmented villonodular synovitis, and idiopathic synovial (osteo)chondromatosis, as well as other localized or systemic articular conditions. In the absence of any obvious cause, the radiologist must search diligently for meniscal abnormality.

The differential diagnosis of synovial cysts about the knee includes a variety of neoplasms of soft tissue or bone origin, thrombophlebitis and hematomas, varicose veins, aneurysms, and other conditions.

ANKLE AND FOOT

Arthrography of the ankle is performed for a variety of indications (Table 14–7). Injuries of the ankle are a common problem and may cause considerable disability. Contrast opacification of the ankle allows identification and delineation of ligamentous injuries and can be combined effectively with routine and stress radiography of the ankle.

Technique

Ideally, the examination should be performed within a few days of the acute injury as blood and tissue adhesions about the ligamentous tear may result in false negative examinations if there is a delay.

With the patient recumbent, a 20 gauge, 1.5 inch needle is introduced into the ankle from an anterior approach. Six to 10 ml of 60 per cent Renografin is injected. The needle is withdrawn and radiographs are exposed in anteroposterior, oblique, and lateral projections. Stress radiographs may also be obtained.

Normal Ankle Arthrogram (Fig. 14–37)

Under normal circumstances, ankle arthrography results in opacification of the articular cavity without evidence of

Table 14–7. SOME INDICATIONS FOR ANKLE ARTHROGRAPHY

Evaluation of:
  Ligamentous injuries
  Transchondral fractures
  Intraarticular osseous and cartilaginous bodies
  Adhesive capsulitis

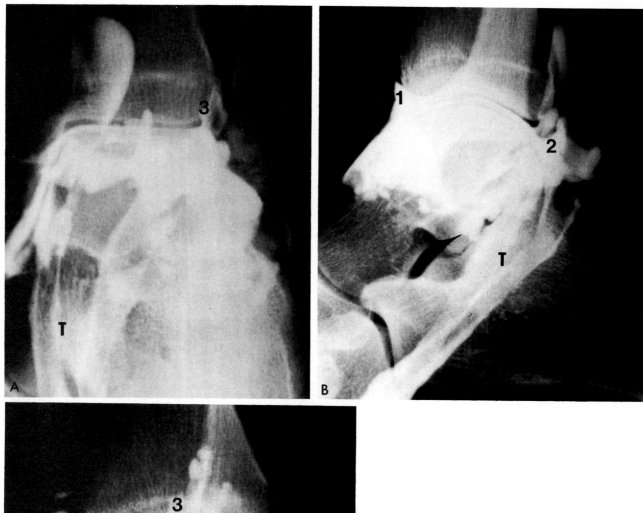

Figure 14–37. Ankle arthrography: Normal arthrogram. A, B Anteroposterior (**A**) and lateral (**B**) views. The tibiotalar joint has been opacified. Note the normal recesses: anterior recess (1), posterior recess (2), and syndesmotic recess (3). Filling of the medial tendon sheaths (T) and posterior subtalar joint (arrowhead) is a normal finding. **C** Lateral veiw from another patient showing prominent (but normal) anterior (1), posterior (2), and syndesmotic (3) recesses.

extraarticular leak except for filling of the tendon sheath of the flexor hallucis longus or the flexor digitorum longus, or both (in about 20 per cent of patients). The posterior subtalar joint will be opacified in approximately 10 per cent of patients. All other patterns of contrast agent extravasation are regarded as abnormal.

Ligamentous Injuries (Fig. 14–38)

ANTERIOR TALOFIBULAR LIGAMENT INJURY. The anterior talofibular ligament extends from the anterior surface of the distal portion of the fibula to the talar neck. It is most susceptible to injury. With tears, contrast material will be seen both inferior and lateral to the distal fibula on frontal radiographs and anterior to the distal fibula on lateral radiographs.

CALCANEOFIBULAR LIGAMENT INJURY. The calcaneofibular ligament, a strong ligament, originates from the posterior aspect of the distal portion of the fibula and inserts on the superior aspect of the calcaneus. When this ligament is torn, contrast material fills the peroneal tendon sheaths as the inner aspect of the sheaths is also torn.

DISTAL ANTERIOR TIBIOFIBULAR LIGAMENT INJURY. This structure extends from the anterior and lateral aspects of the distal portion of the tibia to the adjacent anterior portion of the distal fibula. After injury to this ligament, extravasation of contrast material occurs between distal tibia and fibula, beyond the syndesmotic recess.

DELTOID LIGAMENT INJURY. This ligament originates from the medial malleolus and extends to the talus and calcaneus. With tears of the deltoid ligament, contrast material extravasates beyond the medial confines of the joint.

Any of these ankle injuries may be associated with abnormalities on plain films, including soft tissue swelling and avulsion fractures at the osseous sites of attachment of the specific ligament. Furthermore, stress radiography may indicate ligament weakening by revealing abnormal widening of the joint.

Other Traumatic Disorders

TRANSCHONDRAL FRACTURE. Osteochondral fractures (osteochondritis dissecans) of the talar dome are not infrequent. Arthrography in this situation will outline the integrity of the overlying cartilage and the presence of intraarticular cartilaginous bodies.

ADHESIVE CAPSULITIS (FIG. 14–39). Adhesive capsulitis in the ankle leads to restricted motion following trauma to bone or soft tissue. Arthrography reveals a decrease in the articular capacity, obliteration of normal recesses, opacification of lymphatic vessels, and extravasation of contrast material along the needle tract.

MISCELLANEOUS AREAS
Apophyseal Joints

The facet syndrome, related to abnormalities of the apophyseal joints, leads to pain, which is exacerbated with rotary motion, in the lower back, thighs, buttocks, and legs and to focal tenderness over the affected articulation. Diagnosis and treatment are undertaken with injection of contrast material, anesthetic agent, corticosteroid preparation, or any combination of these into the apophyseal joints of the lumbar spine.

The intrinsically curved lumbar apophyseal joints are less accessible to direct puncture than many of the articulations of the body; however, the puncture technique can be accomplished with fluoroscopy and, occasionally, computed tomography. The patient is first placed prone on the table and, in this position or with only slight rotation of the body into an oblique attitude, the posterior portion of the joint surface is

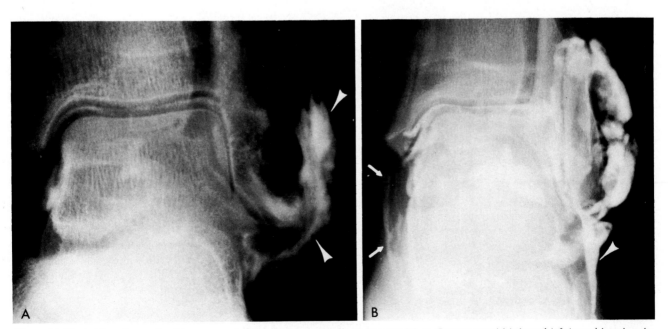

Figure 14–38. Ankle arthrography: Ligamentous injuries. A Anterior talofibular ligament injury. Contrast material is located inferior and lateral to the tip of the fibula (arrowheads). On a lateral view (not shown) the contrast material will be anterior to the distal fibula. **B** Anterior talofibular and calcaneofibular ligament injuries. In addition to extravasation of contrast material lateral to the distal fibula, there is visualization of the peroneal tendon sheaths (arrowhead). Normal filling of the medial tendon sheaths is noted (arrows).

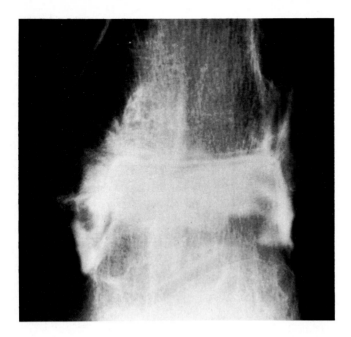

Figure 14–39. Ankle arthrography: Adhesive capsulitis. The oblique view reveals decreased joint volume and irregularities of capsular attachment.

brought into profile. It must be emphasized that minimal rotation of the patient's body generally is adequate. A 20 or 22 gauge spinal needle is directed vertically into the joint space until bone or cartilage is reached (Fig. 14–40). The choice of injection level is based primarily on clinical evidence,

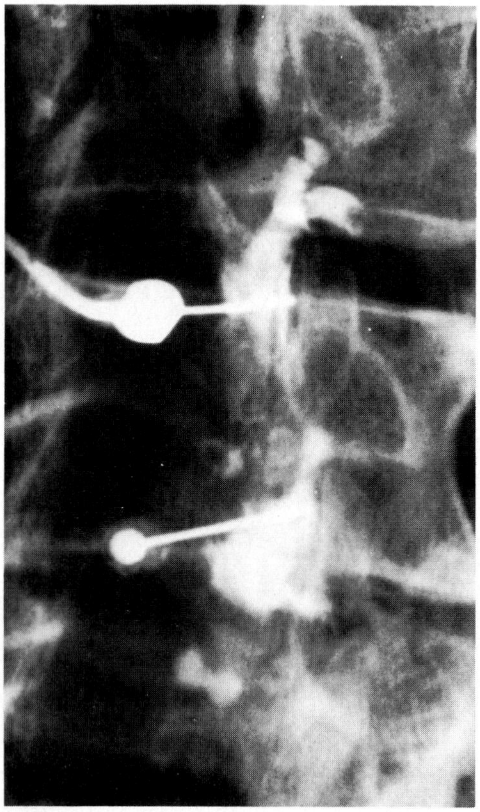

Figure 14–40. Arthrography of the lumbar apophyseal joints. Observe the needle placement in two consecutive apophyseal articulations. Some extravasation of contrast material is evident at the lower level, whereas in the upper joint all of the contrast agent is within the joint.

especially focal tenderness over a joint. Injection of multiple levels on one or both sides of the body is sometimes required.

There is no uniform agreement regarding the amount and the constituents of the solution that should be instilled. It is common practice to initially inject a small amount of radiopaque contrast material (0.5 to 1.5 ml) to confirm the proper placement of the needle, followed by the instillation of approximately 1.0 ml of 0.25 per cent bupivacaine hydrochloride (Marcaine) and 40 mg of methylprednisolone acetate (Depo-Medrol).

The arthrogram itself is used mainly to confirm the intracapsular position of the needle tip, revealing a smooth, oval joint capsule in the frontal projection and an S-shaped configuration in the oblique projection. Arthrographic abnormalities are occasionally seen, including an irregular or nodular appearance in cases of synovial proliferation or synechiae, and a constricted joint in some instances of osteoarthritis. In the presence of spondylolysis, opacification of one lumbar facet joint will outline an abnormal communication with the adjacent facet joint via a tract or channel.

Reports of the therapeutic effects following the intraarticular injection of an anesthetic agent and a corticosteroid preparation have varied, although in the hands of some investigators, the procedure can lead to temporary or permanent relief of the clinical manifestations of the facet syndrome.

Sacroiliac Joints

Arthrography of the sacroiliac joints is indicated only as a sequel to aspiration in cases of suspected infection or crystal deposition disease. Although fluoroscopy can be used to monitor needle placement, computed tomography represents a superior method. Once an aspirate is recovered, opacification of the joint with radiopaque contrast material documents the precise location of the needle tip.

FURTHER READING

Anderson TM Jr: Arthrography. Radiol Clin North Am *19*:215, 1981.
Arndt R-D, Horns JW, Gold RH, Blaschke DD: Clinical Arthrography. Baltimore, Williams & Wilkins, 1981.

Burk DL Jr, Kanal E, Brunberg JA, Johnstone GF, Swenson HE, Wolf GL: 1.5-T surface-coil MRI of the knee. AJR *147:*293, 1986.

Dalinka MK: Arthrography. New York, Springer-Verlag, 1980.

Destouet JM, Gilula LA, Murphy WA, Monsees B: Lumbar facet joint injection: Indication, technique, clinical correlation, and preliminary results. Radiology *145:*321, 1982.

Deutsch AL, Resnick D, Dalinka MK, Gilula L, Danzig L, Guerra J Jr, Dunn FH: Synovial plicae of the knee. Radiology *141:*627, 1981.

Deutsch AL, Resnick D, Mink JH, Berman JL, Cone RO III, Resnick CS, Danzig L, Guerra J Jr: Computed and conventional arthrotomography of the glenohumeral joint: Normal anatomy and clinical experience. Radiology *143:*603, 1984.

Dory MA: Arthrography of the ankle joint in chronic instability. Skeletal Radiol *15:*291, 1986.

El-Khoury GY, Albright JP, Abu Yousef MM, Montgomery WJ, Tuck SL: Arthrotomography of the glenoid labrum. Radiology *131:*333, 1979.

Freiberger RH, Kaye JJ: Arthrography. New York, Appleton-Century-Crofts, 1979.

Freiberger RH, Pavlov H: Knee arthrography. Radiology *166:*489, 1988.

Gilula LA, Reinus WR, Totty WG: Midcarpal wrist arthrography. AJR *146:*645, 1986.

Goldman AB, Ghelman B: The double-contrast shoulder arthrogram. A review of 158 studies. Radiology *127:*655, 1978.

Goldman AB, Dines DM, Warren RF: Shoulder Arthrography. Technique, Diagnosis, and Clinical Correlation. Boston, Little, Brown, 1982.

Goldman AB, Katz MC, Freiberger RH: Post-traumatic adhesive capsulitis of the ankle: Arthrographic diagnosis. AJR *127:*585, 1976.

Hall FM: Arthrography of the discoid lateral meniscus. AJR *128:*993, 1977.

Hendrix RW, Lin P-JP, Kane WJ: Simplified aspiration or injection technique for the sacro-iliac joint. J Bone Joint Surg [Am] *64:*1249, 1982.

Herman LJ, Beltran J: Pitfalls in MR imaging of the knee. Radiology *167:*775, 1988.

Kaye JJ: Knee arthrography today. Radiology *157:*265, 1985.

Kaye JJ, Bohne WHO: A radiographic study of the ligamentous anatomy of the ankle. Radiology *125:*659, 1977.

Killoran PJ, Marcove RC, Freiberger RH: Shoulder arthrography. AJR *103:*658, 1968.

Lequesne M, Becker J, Bard M, Witvoet J, Postel M: Capsular constriction of the hip: Arthrographic and clinical considerations. Skel Radiol *6:*1, 1981.

Lindgren PG, Willen R: Gastrocnemio-semimembranosus bursa and its relation to the knee joint. I. Anatomy and histology. Acta Radiol Diagn *18:*497, 1977.

Middleton WD, Reinus WR, Melson GL, Totty WG, Murphy WA: Pitfalls of rotator cuff sonography. AJR *146:*555, 1986.

Mooney V, Robertson J: The facet syndrome. Clin Orthop *115:*149, 1976.

Murphy WA, Siegel MJ, Gilula LA: Arthrography in the diagnosis of unexplained chronic hip pain with regional osteopenia. AJR *129:*283, 1977.

Newberg AH, Muhn CS, Robbins AH: Complications of arthrography. Radiology *155:*605, 1985.

Nicholas JA, Freiberger RH, Killoran PJ: Double contrast arthrography of the knee. Its value in the management of 225 knee derangements. J Bone Joint Surg [Am] *52:*203, 1970.

Olson RW: Arthrography of the ankle: Its use in the evaluation of ankle sprains. Radiology *92:*1439, 1969.

Pavlov H, Goldman AB: The popliteus bursa: An indicator of subtle pathology. AJR *134:*313, 1980.

Pavlov H, Torg JS: Double contrast arthrographic evaluation of the anterior cruciate ligament. Radiology *126:*661, 1978.

Pavlov H, Ghelman B, Warren RF: Double-contrast arthrography of the elbow. Radiology *130:*87, 1979.

Pavlov H, Hirschy JC, Torg JS: Computed tomography of the cruciate ligaments. Radiology *132:*389, 1979.

Pavlov H, Warren RF, Sherman MF, Cayea PD: The accuracy of double-contrast arthrographic evaluation of the anterior cruciate ligament. A retrospective review of one hundred and sixty-three knees with surgical confirmation. J Bone Joint Surg [Am] *65:*175, 1983.

Rafii M, Firooznia H, Golimbu C, Minkoff J, Bonamo J: CT arthrography of the capsular structures of the shoulder. AJR *146:*361, 1986.

Rauschning W: Anatomy and function of the communication between knee joint and popliteal bursae. Ann Rheum Dis *39:*354, 1980.

Reicher MA, Bassett LW, Gold RH: High-resolution magnetic resonance imaging of the knee joint: Pathologic correlations. AJR *145:*903, 1985.

Resnick D: Rheumatoid arthritis of the wrist. The compartmental approach. Med Radiogr Photogr *52:*50, 1976.

Resnick D, André M, Kerr R, Pineda C, Guerra J Jr, Atkinson D: Digital arthrography of the wrist: A radiographic and pathologic investigation. AJR *142:*1187, 1984.

Ricklin P, Rüttimann A, Del Buono MS: Meniscus Lesions—Practical Problems of Clinical Diagnosis, Arthrography and Therapy. New York, Grune & Stratton, 1971.

Sauser DD, Nelson RC, Lavine MH, Wu CW: Acute injuries of the lateral ligaments of the ankle: Comparison of stress radiography and arthrography. Radiology *148:*653, 1983.

Stoker DJ, Renton P, Fulton A: The value of arthrography in the management of internal derangements of the knee: The first 1000 are the worst. Clin Radiol *32:*557, 1981.

Stoller DW, Martin C, Cruess JV III, Kaplan L, Mink JH: Meniscal tears: Pathologic correlation with MR imaging. Radiology *163:*731, 1987.

Thomas RH, Resnick D, Alazraki NP, Daniel D, Greenfield R: Compartmental evaluation of osteoarthritis of the knee. A comparative study of available diagnostic modalities. Radiology *116:*585, 1975.

Turner DA, Prodromos CC, Petasnick JP, Clark JW: Acute injury of the ligaments of the knee: Magnetic resonance evaluation. Radiology *154:*717, 1985.

Zlatkin MB, Bjorkengren A, Gylys-Morin V, Resnick D, Sartoris DJ: Cross-sectional imaging of the capsular mechanism of the glenohumeral joint. AJR *150:*151, 1988.

Chapter 15

Angiography

Joseph J. Bookstein, M.D.

The role of angiography in the diagnosis and treatment of a variety of musculoskeletal problems includes the documentation of vascular injury following trauma, the control of hemorrhage, visualization of a variety of primary arterial diseases that are associated with or may resemble joint disease, evaluation of the nature and extent of soft tissue masses, visualization of arteritis complicating collagen disorders, and detection of peripheral venous abnormalities, which may simulate articular or periarticular disease.

Although angiography ordinarily is unnecessary, a broad variety of skeletal diseases occasionally require it (Table 15–1). Vascular injury often coexists with musculoskeletal trauma and, if it is suspected, specific arteriographic diagnosis of the nature and extent of arterial injury usually is necessary. Active bleeding at sites not readily amenable to surgical control may be treated effectively by transcatheter hemostasis. In patients with bone tumors, arteriography is sometimes indicated for evaluation of tumor extent and nature, and also to assess any direct invasion or involvement of major arteries. Bone tumors can be palliated by intraarterial chemotherapeutic infusions or by embolization. Angiomatous malformations may be diagnosed and treated through angiographic techniques. Thus, despite the rarity of the foregoing conditions, there is reasonably frequent application of angiographic techniques in patients with skeletal disorders.

TRAUMA

Blunt or penetrating skeletal trauma is one of the most frequent indications for skeletal angiography. Arteriography may demonstrate traumatic aneurysms, intimal dissections, transections, thromboses, and arteriovenous communications (Fig. 15–1). Specific indications include the following:

1. Direct signs of vascular injury, such as pallor and decreased temperature of the injured extremity, loss of distal pulses, or vascular bruit.

2. Fracture with absent or diminished distal pulses.

3. Penetrating trauma proximate to a major artery, regardless of the presence or absence of direct signs of arterial injury.

4. Major pelvic hemorrhage after pelvic trauma, in which case transcatheter embolization is a particularly effective form of treatment.

5. Massive, disproportionate, or progressive limb swelling compatible with arterial or venous hemorrhage or venous thrombosis.

TRANSCATHETER HEMOSTASIS

Hemorrhage may occur in and around bones and joints, most frequently after trauma. Occasionally, control of the hemorrhage via transcatheter embolization may be required.

ANEURYSMS AND OTHER PRIMARY ARTERIAL DISEASES

Aneurysms

Aneurysms not infrequently involve the popliteal artery (Fig. 15–2) and produce a mass in the popliteal space that superficially simulates joint disease or a soft tissue tumor. Although diagnosis is readily confirmed with ultrasonography, arteriography of the aneurysm and adjacent vessels is indicated in planning surgery.

Arterial aneurysms may be associated with osteochondromas about the knee joint (Fig. 15–3). The usual proximity of the popliteal artery to the rough aspect of the osteochondroma and the mechanical trauma secondary to motion of the knee joint combine to produce chronic arterial injury and eventual aneurysm.

Cystic Mucinous Degeneration

Cystic mucinous degeneration may involve the popliteal artery. The usual manifestations are ischemic, secondary to

Table 15–1. SOME INDICATIONS FOR ANGIOGRAPHY

Documentation of vascular injury
Control of hemorrhage
Assessment of primary arterial diseases
   Aneurysm
   Cystic mucinous degeneration
   Popliteal entrapment syndrome
   Hypothenar hammer syndrome
Evaluation of soft tissue masses
Detection of peripheral venous abnormalities
Evaluation of autoimmune diseases
   Rheumatoid arthritis
   Giant cell arteritis
   Polymyalgia rheumatica
   Scleroderma
   Systemic lupus erythematosus
   Polyarteritis nodosa
Assessment of miscellaneous disorders
   Occupational acroosteolysis
   Frostbite
   Reflex sympathetic dystrophy syndrome

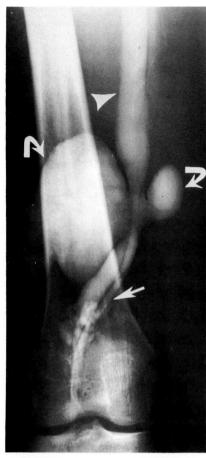

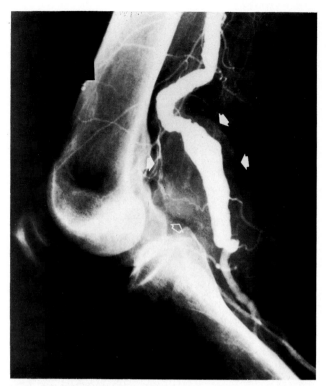

Figure 15–2. Ordinary atherosclerotic aneurysm in a patient with a cool left foot and barely pulsatile mass in left popliteal fossa. Note that much of the aneurysm is filled with nonopacified clot. The margin is demarcated by minimal intimal calcification (open and solid arrows). (Courtesy of L. Wexler, M.D., Stanford, California.)

Figure 15–1. Pulsatile venous aneurysm and arteriovenous fistula after penetrating injury. The arteriogram demonstrates two venous aneurysms at the site of fistula (curved arrows), early venous opacification of a somewhat dilated superficial femoral vein (arrowhead), and delayed flow in the small postfistulous popliteal artery (straight arrow).

arterial obstruction by the cyst. The cause is unknown; a congenital origin is postulated.

Popliteal Entrapment Syndrome

The popliteal entrapment syndrome, leading to intermittent claudication, is produced by compression of the popliteal artery by the medial head of the gastrocnemius muscle. The compression may result from either (1) abnormal position of the popliteal artery medial to the medial head of the gastrocnemius muscle, or (2) compression of a normally situated popliteal artery by an anomalous laterally inserting slip from the medial head of the gastrocnemius.

Hypothenar Hammer Syndrome

The hypothenar hammer syndrome is characterized by thrombosis, spasm, or aneurysm of the ulnar artery secondary to repetitive minor, usually occupational, trauma. Any one finger or combination of fingers may show signs of ischemia. Arteriography demonstrates narrowing, occlusion, or aneurysm of the ulnar artery, usually adjacent to the hook of the hamate.

TUMORS AND OTHER MASSES

Arteriography has been advocated in evaluating the type, extent, and behavioral characteristics of bone tumors; how-

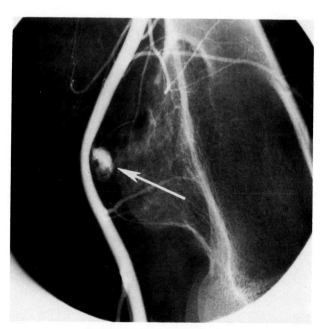

Figure 15–3. Aneurysm secondary to femoral exostosis. Magnification arteriogram in the lateral view shows no pathologic vessels in the region of the exostosis to suggest malignancy. Instead, a pseudoaneurysm is beginning to opacify (arrow) at the site of chronic arterial injury from the exostosis.

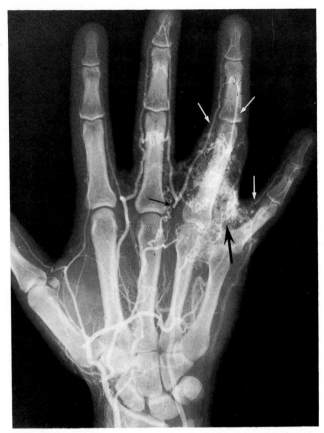

Figure 15–4. Angiography of typical arteriovenous malformation, which persisted after ligation of several feeding arteries. Despite prior surgical occlusion of all of the regional proper digital arteries (small arrows), these arteries as well as the lesion (large arrow) continue to opacify via collateral routes.

ever, biopsy is much more reliable in evaluating behavioral characteristics, and plain films and computed tomography generally are adequate in determining extent.

Transcatheter embolization has been advocated in the palliative management of pain or hemorrhage of bone tumors. Regression of arteriographic features of a bone tumor can play a useful role in evaluating response after chemotherapy.

Arteriography has assumed a larger role in evaluating the nature and extent of soft tissue masses. The procedure is most reliable in the evaluation of arteriovenous malformations or hemangiomas (Fig. 15–4). In some of these vascular masses, extent cannot be well evaluated angiographically because all or portions of the lesion may not opacify, even after pharmacoangiography.

Transcatheter therapy is being applied increasingly in the management of peripheral vascular malformations. Temporary control of pain, swelling, or hemorrhage can usually be achieved by obstructing major vessels leading to the malformation, but symptoms usually recur, owing to development of collateral circulation.

AUTOIMMUNE DISEASES
Rheumatoid Arthritis

Rheumatoid arthritis is expressed predominantly as a disease of synovial membranes, but in a significant percentage of cases vascular disease is also present. Histologic features of

rheumatoid vasculitis include mild perivascular or adventitial inflammation, intimal thickening with little or no cellular reaction, arterial thromboses, and necrotizing arteriolar panarteritis. Corticosteroid therapy has been implicated as a possible etiologic factor in those cases with necrotizing arteritis. Aortitis or aortic valvulitis is also an associated finding. Arteriographic studies have demonstrated arterial stenoses of the digital arteries and nonspecific hyperemia near bony erosions or regions of synovial proliferation.

Giant Cell Arteritis

Giant cell arteritis (also called temporal, cranial, or granulomatous arteritis) is a form of vasculitis characterized histologically by necrosis of the arterial wall and granulomatous vascular reaction with giant cells. Medium-sized arteries, such as the temporal, subclavian, or popliteal arteries, are involved most frequently.

Polymyalgia Rheumatica

Polymyalgia rheumatica is characterized by recurrent rheumatic discomfort involving muscles and joints, particularly of the shoulder and hip girdles, systemic manifestations of fever and malaise, elevated sedimentation rate, and associated arteritis of medium-sized vessels. Arterial biopsy will show arteritis in about 50 per cent of cases; usually giant cells are prominent, and the appearance and distribution of disease are generally indistinguishable from those of giant cell arteritis.

Scleroderma

Scleroderma may be expressed primarily as a disease of small arteries. Intimal arteriolar thickening is the most frequent manifestation, but panarteritis may also occur. Small arteries throughout the body may be involved.

Systemic Lupus Erythematosus

Vascular manifestations of systemic lupus erythematosus generally are confined to the very small arteries, such as the interlobular arteries of the kidney, or renal glomerular capillaries. Histologic changes may vary widely. In advanced disease, necrotizing arteritis can develop.

Polyarteritis Nodosa

Polyarteritis nodosa (Fig. 15–5) is associated with a necrotizing arteritis that may affect arteries anywhere in the body. Arteriography of involved areas may demonstrate small aneurysms, a feature virtually pathognomonic of necrotizing arteritis. Other features include arterial stenoses, occlusions, collateral circulation, marginal irregularities, and evidence of tissue infarction. Renal arteries are involved in a high percentage of cases, and renal arteriography may be the most effective method for reaching a diagnosis.

VENOUS DISEASES

Venography is the most definitive diagnostic procedure in cases of thrombophlebitis. In the presence of thrombosis of lower extremity veins, intraluminal defects due to thrombi are almost always visualized (Fig. 15–6).

MISCELLANEOUS DISORDERS
Occupational Acroosteolysis

Occupational acroosteolysis is characterized primarily by resorption of portions of distal phalangeal tufts, some digital

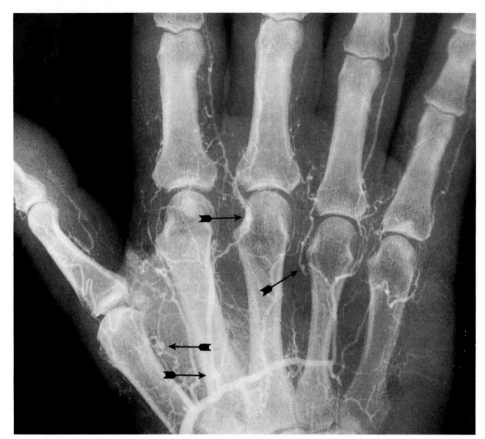

Figure 15–5. Polyarteritis nodosa. Multiple proper digital arteries and the ulnar artery are occluded, a distribution similar to that of scleroderma. However, the presence of a number of small aneurysms (arrows) suggests the possibility of a necrotizing arteritis.

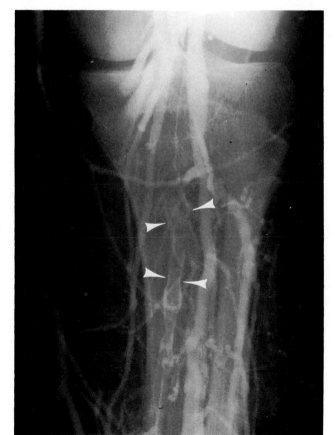

Figure 15–6. Thrombophlebitis producing pain and swelling about the knee joint. Note the thin accumulation of contrast medium between the intraluminal thrombus and the vein wall, confirming the presence of thrombus (arrowheads).

tenderness, and Raynaud's phenomenon. It is observed in workers involved in the manufacture of polyvinylchloride. Arteriography may demonstrate mild hypervascularity adjacent to areas of bone resorption and distal occlusion of the princeps pollicis artery.

Frostbite

The importance of vascular injury in the pathogenesis of frostbite is well recognized. Arteriography will demonstrate marked slowing of blood flow in sizeable branches, probably attributable to spasm and more distal obstruction. As the condition improves, arterial flow improves, but residual occlusions may persist.

Reflex Sympathetic Dystrophy Syndrome

Reflex sympathetic dystrophy syndrome is the currently accepted term for a constellation of symptoms that may follow trauma to the upper or lower extremity (see Chapter 47). Various features of this syndrome have suggested the possibility of vascular disease. The angiographic features are somewhat specific. Blood flow is markedly accelerated on the involved side, with dilation of small veins (particularly of the heel pad) and early venous opacification. These features suggest opening of precapillary arteriovenous shunts.

FURTHER READING

Bookstein JJ: Arteriography. *In* AK Poznanski (Ed): The Hand in Radiologic Diagnosis. 2nd Ed. Philadelphia, WB Saunders Co, 1984, pp 97–112.

Conn J, Bergan JJ, Bell JL: Hypothenar hammer syndrome: Post-traumatic digital ischemia. Surgery 68:1122, 1970.

Gralino BJ, Porter JM, Rösch J: Angiography in the diagnosis and therapy of frostbite. Radiology *119:*301, 1976.

Greenway G, Resnick D, Bookstein JJ: Popliteal pseudoaneurysm as a complication of adjacent osteochondroma: Angiographic diagnosis. AJR *132:*294, 1979.

Hudson TM, Haas G, Enneking WF, Hawkins IF: Angiography in management of musculoskeletal tumors. Surg Gynecol Obstet *141:*11, 1975.

Levin DC, Watson RC, Baltaxe HA: Arteriography in diagnosis and management of acquired peripheral soft-tissue masses. Radiology *104:*53, 1972.

Schlesinger A, Gottesman L: Cystic degeneration of the popliteal artery. AJR *127:*1043, 1976.

Chapter 16

Radionuclide Techniques

Naomi Alazraki, M.D.

During approximately 30 years of experience with bone scanning, broad expansions in the clinical impact of radionuclide imaging on disorders of bones, joints, and soft tissues have occurred. This increased impact had its groundwork laid by advance in radiopharmaceutical agents and instruments that are used for bone imaging. The progression from ^{85}Sr- to ^{99m}Tc-labeled phosphate and phosphonate compounds, coupled with the advance from crude rectilin-

ear scanning techniques to whole body scintillation imaging with large crystal cameras and sophisticated electronics, has encouraged use of radionuclide techniques in the evaluation of musculoskeletal diseases. Many clinical studies have documented the higher degree of sensitivity of the bone scan over that of the radiograph in detecting osseous and articular abnormalities.

With the recognition that radiography is a relatively insensitive technique for evaluating abnormalities of the bone, enthusiasm for a more sensitive imaging approach developed. In 1961, localization of strontium-85 in normal bone with increased uptake of the radionuclide at sites of osseous abnormalities was demonstrated. Since that time, the high sensitivity of the radionuclide bone scan (scintigraphy), particularly after advances in radiopharmaceutical preparations and in imaging instruments, has been well established.

As with most procedures in nuclear medicine, the bone scan is an extremely sensitive but relatively nonspecific method. Any process that disturbs the normal balance of bone production and resorption can produce an abnormality on the bone scan. These abnormalities may be manifested as regions of increased or decreased activity. The large majority of lesions appear as focal areas of increased activity, as the usual response to an insult is osteogenesis. In normal images, however, there are areas in the skeleton that show greater and lesser concentration of the radionuclide, owing to regional differences in bone turnover; for example, in children the epiphyses and metaphyseal growth plates (sites at which bone turnover is most rapid and active) appear as foci of intense tracer activity. In adults, metaphyses of tubular bones may show more activity than diaphyses.

The amount of radiopharmaceutical agent accumulated in any region of bone depends on two major factors: the rate of bone turnover and the integrity of the blood supply. Of these two factors, the intactness of the vascular supply appears to have a more important influence on the bone scan; if there is an absence of blood perfusion to a localized region of bone, the radiopharmaceutical agent cannot be delivered to this area, and a photon-deficient, or "cold," region appears on the scan.

RADIOPHARMACEUTICAL AGENTS

Over the years, a number of radiopharmaceutical preparations have been used for bone scanning. Strontium-85 was the first imageable radionuclide that allowed identification of

abnormalities within bone. Strontium is able to substitute biologically for calcium and be incorporated into the hydroxyapatite crystal of bone as a strontium-hydroxyapatite structure. Strontium is incorporated rapidly into the bones; approximately 30 to 50 per cent of the administered dose is labeled to the bones within 1 hour after its administration. The remainder of the ^{85}Sr is excreted by the kidneys and the gastrointestinal tract. Strontium-85 is a very poor radionuclide for clinical use because of its 65 day physical half-life and unfavorable gamma energy emission of 513 keV. To prevent undue radiation exposure, only small doses of 100 microcuries (μCi) can be used. An ^{85}Sr bone scan takes several hours to perform and results in images of relatively poor quality. Strontium-87m is a more effective radiopharmaceutical agent than ^{85}Sr, as it has a 388 keV gamma ray emission and only a 2.8 hour physical half-life. Its disadvantages are that it is extremely expensive and its short physical half-life requires that imaging be performed 2 to 3 hours after injection, at a time when plasma levels of ^{87m}Sr are still elevated enough to cause an unfavorable bone-to-blood background count ratio.

Fluorine-18 has a 1.9 hour physical half-life and is therefore not widely available; its use is limited to centers with rapid access to a cyclotron or reactor that produces radioisotopes for medical use. Fluorine-18 is a positron emitter; the resulting 511 keV annihilation x-rays can be imaged by the conventional scintillation imaging systems that are available in most institutions. However, a 511 keV photon requires heavy collimation and is inefficiently imaged by the scintillation camera. In contrast to its physical limitations as a bone imaging agent, ^{18}F has superior biologic characteristics. Even when imaging is performed at 2 to 3 hours after intravenous or oral administration of ^{18}F, the bone-to-blood and bone-to-soft tissue background count ratios are very favorable.

Technetium-99m polyphosphate was introduced as a bone imaging agent in 1971. Subsequent work resulted in the discovery of other ^{99m}Tc-labeled phosphate compounds, such as hydroxyethylene diphosphonate (HEDP), PPi (pyrophosphate), and methylene diphosphonate (MDP), compounds that have improved the resolution of bone imaging dramatically. Technetium-99m has a physical half-life of 6 hours and emits a 140 keV gamma ray, which is ideal for imaging with the available scintillation cameras and scanners. The low radiation exposure resulting from this agent permits the use of doses of 15 to 20 mCi for each bone scan. Thus, a whole body, head-to-toe image in an anterior or a posterior projection may be performed in 20 to 35 minutes, and approximately 1 hour is required to produce both posterior and anterior total body images of exceptionally high quality.

Technetium-99m is the most widely used radioisotope in clinical nuclear medicine. After binding to various pharmaceutical agents, it is used for brain, liver, and lung scans, radionuclide angiographic studies, cardiac ejection fraction, and gated cardiac blood pool wall motion studies, as well as bone and bone marrow scans. Bone uptake localization half-times have been measured as 15 to 30 minutes, which is much more rapid than the half-time disappearance from the blood, which has been measured at about 1 hour. The technetium-phosphate complex that is not localized within bone is excreted into the urine. There are slight variations among the various phosphate compounds in the proportion of the administered dose that localizes in the bone and in the rate of excretion of the compound by the kidneys.

The mechanism by which the ^{99m}Tc-labeled phosphate compounds are incorporated into bone is not entirely understood. Because the technetium-phosphate compounds do not carry significant ionic charge, they may be able to diffuse relatively freely across the bone capillary wall, similarly to the behavior of strontium and fluorine. Having arrived at the bone site, therefore, the phosphate compound may chemisorb (chemical and physical processes leading to adsorption) at kink and dislocation sites on the surface of the hydroxyapatite crystal, resulting in a release of tin and ^{99m}Tc, which are hydrolyzed and deposited either separately or together as hydrated tin oxide and technetium dioxide. Sites of rapid bone turnover, such as growth centers and reactive bone lesions, are associated with a large mineral surface that is available for exchange and chemisorption by the ^{99m}Tc-tin-phosphate complex. Although the hypothesis that the ^{99m}Tc-phosphate compounds bind at the bone crystal surface is the current dominant theory, it has also been proposed that such binding predominates at the organic matrix, particularly the immature collagen.

A total body radionuclide bone image in the anterior or posterior projection obtained 2 hours after intravenous injection of 15 mCi of ^{99m}Tc-labeled phosphate compounds will generally take about 30 minutes. This time will vary, depending upon the collimator used, the degree of uptake of the radiopharmaceutical agent in the bones, the amount of renal excretion, the size and build of the patient, the number of millicuries injected, the time elapsed between injection and imaging, and the width of the window setting around the 140 keV photon energy peak of ^{99m}Tc. In most institutions, at least anterior and posterior total body views are obtained, supplemented with spot images of questionably abnormal regions. A 20 per cent window is usually used, limiting the recording of counts to those photons that fall within 20 per cent of the 140 keV peak of activity.

Recently, tomographic imaging instruments capable of displaying multiple planes of selective activity from a single scan of the body have been perfected. These instruments offer a potential similar to that of computed tomographic imaging

devices. This approach can provide more detailed information on the localization of radiopharmaceutical agents in bones and joints. Indeed, there have been several reports indicating the superior ability of SPECT (single photon emission computed tomography) over planar bone imaging in the detection of bone lesions.

CLINICAL APPLICATIONS

A partial list of indications for radionuclide bone imaging is given in Table 16–1.

Neoplasm

SKELETAL METASTASIS AND OTHER MALIGNANT BONE TUMORS. Various studies have documented that approximately 10 to 40 per cent of patients with skeletal metastases have normal radiographs at a time when the bone scan is abnormal, and fewer than 5 per cent of bone scans are normal when radiographs show localized abnormalities. Occasionally, a region may be painful and yet normal on radionuclide bone images. In these cases, evaluation by radiography may show a lytic lesion that apparently has not caused sufficient reactive bone formation on a histologic level to result in increased accumulation of radiopharmaceutical agent. Anaplastic tumors and multiple myeloma are two types of malignant disease that characteristically may not stimulate sufficient osteoblastic reaction for an abnormal focus to be imaged on scan.

The radionuclide bone scan is frequently used to follow the response of neoplasm to irradiation, chemotherapy, or hormone therapy in patients with cancer and bone metastases. It is not uncommon to see dramatic changes in the bone scan after therapy, with resolution of previously abnormal skeletal areas. This therapeutic response does not necessarily mean that no viable tumor cells remain in a region that has converted to normal on the radionuclide images, however. An individual lesion may also show apparent worsening on a bone scan obtained after completion of therapy. In some cases, this response has been identified as a transient flare phenomenon, which may represent repair and healing of the bone rather than progression of disease.

Another scintigraphic pattern that may be associated with widespread metastatic bone disease is the "superscan" seen on whole body imaging. When metastatic bone disease is far

---

Table 16–1. SOME INDICATIONS FOR RADIONUCLIDE BONE SCANNING (SCINTIGRAPHY)

Screen for bone metastases
Localize metastases for diagnostic biopsies
Diagnose osteomyelitis before radiographic changes are evident
Aid in differentiating cellulitis from osteomyelitis
Aid in evaluating painful prostheses for infection and loosening
Detect and evaluate the extent of articular involvement in various forms of arthritis
Aid in the characterization of benign bone lesions
Aid in the workup of compression fractures, particularly when there is a question of the age of the compression fracture
Evaluate bone pain of any cause in the presence of normal radiographs
Aid in diagnosis and management of ischemic necrosis of bone
Aid in management of myositis ossificans
Aid in the prognostic evaluation of microvascular competence required to support healing of soft tissue ulcerations in patients with peripheral vascular disease
Aid in the selection of amputation site or level

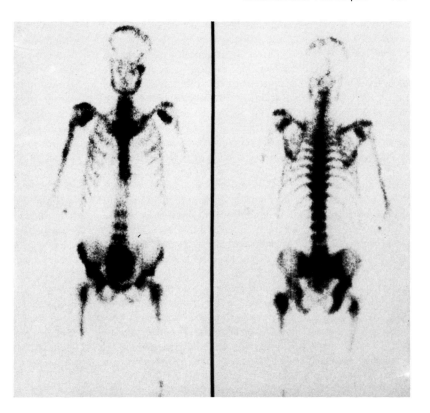

Figure 16–1. "Superscan" in metastatic disease. Anterior and posterior whole body images from a ^{99m}Tc-pyrophosphate scan on a patient with primary cancer of the prostate. The superscan pattern shows absence of activity in the kidneys, low blood background activity, and generalized, uniformly increased uptake by all the bones in the body. Some areas of greater and lesser uptake can be identified on closer examination, particularly in the right humerus, the left distal femur, the right posterior pelvis and iliac bone, the left mandible, the skull, and the ribs.

advanced, the skeletal system may avidly extract the radiopharmaceutical agent from the blood, resulting in greater than 50 per cent bone concentration of the radiopharmaceutical agent and leaving less available radionuclide for excretion by the kidneys (Fig. 16–1). Conversely, one or more photon-deficient or cold areas can represent the scintigraphic response to skeletal metastases (Fig. 16–2).

In about 6 to 8 per cent of patients with skeletal metastases, only a single focal lesion may be seen on the scan. Although approximately 50 per cent of solitary, scintigraphically posi-

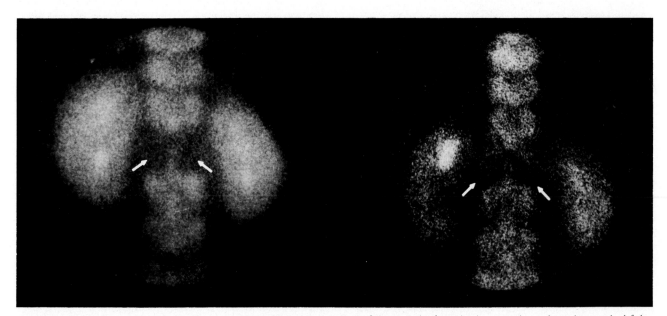

Figure 16–2. Cold focus in metastatic disease. Single scintillation camera views of the upper lumbar spine in two patients; the patient on the left has primary lung cancer, whereas the patient on the right has primary breast cancer. Both patients have metastatic disease involving the bones. The photon-deficient or "cold" region shown in each of these scans is a reflection of metastatic disease in the lumbar vertebral bodies (arrows). Note that the spinous processes of the lumbar vertebrae in both cases appear to be intact. The cold region seen on the scan is postulated to be a secondary effect either of total interruption of blood supply to the vertebral body because of the presence of necrotic tumor that has outgrown its blood supply or of total replacement of the bony structure by tumor, leaving no viable osteoblasts to produce bone that can accrete the radiopharmaceutical agent. Incidentally noted is a dilated calyx in the upper pole of the left kidney in the patient with breast cancer.

tive bone lesions are malignant, 90 per cent of such lesions in the ribs are benign, usually related to trauma or postoperative radiation therapy. Broad scintigraphic characteristics of rib lesions on the basis of their intensity and appearance in serial studies have been described. Fractures are often focal rather than linear, with decreasing intensities over a period of 3 to 6 months, and are aligned so that two or more ribs in the same location are involved (Fig. 16–3).

In contrast to radiographic characteristics that aid in the differentiation between benign and malignant processes, scintigraphic abnormalities can give only a very general indication of the aggressiveness of the lesion. When a single lesion is found on the radiographs, the scan is helpful in confirming the solitary nature of the lesion or in identifying the presence of other bony lesions and in characterizing the lesion as "high grade" or "low grade" in radiopharmaceutical concentration. In general, malignant lesions are hyperemic and, therefore, "hotter" on the scintigraphic image than benign lesions. Additionally, a radionuclide angiogram can be performed with the scintillation camera centered over the radiographically identified abnormality at the time of intravenous injection of the radiopharmaceutical agent; the degree of vascularity of the lesion can be surmised on sequential scintiphotos by comparing the vascularity at the site of abnormality with that of surrounding normal bone.

BENIGN BONE TUMORS AND TUMOR-LIKE LESIONS. Bone scans can be valuable clinically in evaluation of benign bone tumors, particularly in patients with pain in whom radiographs fail to reveal a bone lesion. An osteoid osteoma is a lesion that characteristically is quite "hot" on

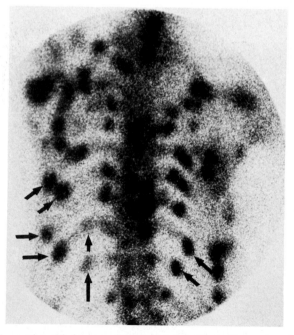

Figure 16–3. Rib fractures. Focal and rounded regions of increased uptake in the ribs correspond to sites of fractures in this patient. Arrows point to fractures that line up from one rib to the next, indicating that they probably occurred at the same time. As the degree of intensity of abnormal radionuclide is influenced by the age of the fracture (younger fractures taking up more radionuclide than older ones), the fractures in the left lower rib cage (vertical arrows) are probably older than most of the others.

the bone scan and yet may be difficult to detect on a radiograph. Closer inspection documents that a "double density" characterizes the region of increased activity on the bone scan in patients with an osteoid osteoma. Autoradiography confirms that the central nidus of the tumor accumulates greater amounts of the radiopharmaceutical agent than the surrounding sclerotic bone, accounting for the double density appearance. Radionuclide techniques have also been used to localize the nidus while the patient is in the operating room or to confirm that the nidus has been removed.

Bone cysts show normal or slightly increased radiopharmaceutical concentration, and a central area of decreased counts may be present. When a fracture complicates a bone cyst, the scan will be "hot."

Bone islands have a variable appearance on the bone scan. When larger than 3 cm in size, they may be manifested as focal regions of increased activity on the bone scan. Generally, bone islands that are less than 3 cm in size show normal uptake of the radiopharmaceutical agent.

Other benign bone tumors and tumor-like lesions, including eosinophilic granuloma, fibrous cortical defect, enchondroma, aneurysmal bone cyst, and osteochondroma, will frequently show increased radiopharmaceutical uptake on the bone scan.

Infection

The role of the radionuclide study in the evaluation of osseous inflammatory disease includes (1) early detection, (2) differentiation of osteomyelitis from cellulitis, and (3) identification of renewed activity in cases of chronic osteomyelitis. Regarding the first, the high degree of sensitivity of the bone scan for identifying the abnormality when radiographs are normal makes the scan important in the workup of patients with possible acute osteomyelitis. Occasionally, very early in the course of osteomyelitis, the lesion will appear on the scan as a "cold," or photon-deficient, focus. This appearance probably can be explained by the interruption of bone blood supply secondary to sludging and thrombosis induced by the inflammatory infiltration of cells. With time, the pattern of a focally increased region of activity will replace the photon-deficient area. Thus, the spectrum of the radionuclide pattern in osteomyelitis varies from areas that are photon-deficient to those that have augmented radionuclide activity (Fig. 16–4). Between these two points, a false-negative scan may result.

As a result of reports of false-negative results ranging in frequency from 5 per cent to as high as 60 per cent, gallium-67 bone imaging has been used as an adjunct to technetium imaging. Gallium-67 citrate images are obtained 6 and 24 hours after the injection of 5 mCi for the diagnosis of osteomyelitis. In many patients, particularly children, the gallium images identify more accurately focal lesions adjacent to growth plates that were masked by adjacent high-intensity uptake on bone scans.

The differentiation between osteomyelitis and cellulitis may be a difficult clinical problem. The three phase or four phase bone scan is widely used for this purpose. At the time of intravenous injection of ^{99m}Tc-MDP, sequential imaging with the scintillation camera centered over the bone in question produces a radionuclide angiogram (phase one) that is followed by an immediate blood pool image (also phase one), disclosing the degree of vascular abnormality of the involved bone. Generally, in either osteomyelitis or cellulitis, increased vas-

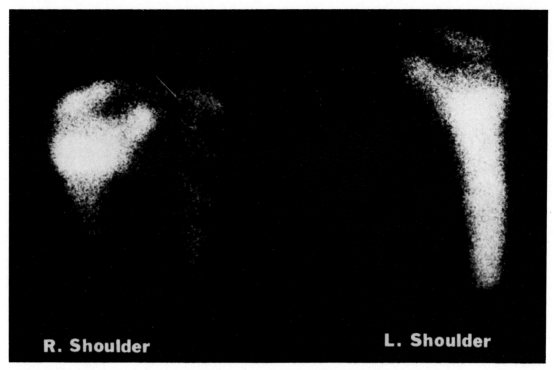

Figure 16–4. Acute osteomyelitis: Scintillation camera views of the shoulders. The left shoulder view shows a markedly increased uptake involving the proximal humerus and extending to the level of midshaft. At a later time, radiographs of this region showed periosteal elevation and other findings consistent with the diagnosis of acute osteomyelitis. The right shoulder is normal.

cularity will be seen. Delayed images are obtained routinely in several projections at about 2 hours after injection (phase two). In either osteomyelitis or cellulitis, focal increased activity may be seen on these images in the region in question. If a second set of delayed images is made at about 5 hours after injection (phase three), the ratio of counts in the region being examined relative to the surrounding normal bone will have increased compared with the ratio at 2 hours in patients with osteomyelitis. The fourth phase is a 24 hour image that further accentuates the increasing count accumulation in regions of osteomyelitis relative to normal bone (Fig. 16–5). In cellulitis, however, just the opposite would be expected: The ratio of counts would slowly decrease over this time period, as most of the activity within the region is due to the hypervascular characteristics of the soft tissue inflammation.

Although ^{67}Ga-citrate and indium-111 labeled leukocytes are widely used in the diagnosis of acute and chronic osteomyelitis, most knowledgeable physicians would probably prefer the three or four phase technetium phosphate bone scan as the initial nuclear imaging procedure, especially in the evaluation of acute osteomyelitis. The high false-negative results of the technetium bone scans in cases of acute osteomyelitis in pediatric patients are perhaps related to a masking effect produced by the normal activity characteristic of the regions of rapid growth in the metaphyses and epiphyses and to the diminished blood flow that is characteristic in the very early stages of osteomyelitis.

In chronic osteomyelitis, comparisons of ^{99m}Tc-phosphate bone imaging and ^{67}Ga-citrate imaging suggest that gallium scans are more accurate in detecting the response or lack of response to therapy. It has been suggested that the clinically important pattern in evaluating this response to therapy is the general direction of the changing scintigraphic findings on serial gallium scans (i.e., toward more normal or more abnormal findings). Bone scans tend to remain positive for longer periods of time than do the gallium scans, even after the infectious process has subsided, probably because of continued bone remodeling and osteogenesis. The gallium scan, on the other hand, tends to remain positive only as long as an active infection continues.

Comparative studies of ^{111}In-leukocyte imaging and ^{99m}Tc-phosphate bone imaging in acute osteomyelitis indicate that white blood cell scans can detect the disease earlier than technetium phosphate bone scans. For detecting renewed activity of infection in patients with chronic osteomyelitis, ^{111}In appears to represent a superior radionuclide agent.

^{99m}Tc-MDP, ^{67}Ga, and ^{111}In-leukocyte imaging all can reveal abnormalities in septic arthritis. These agents may also be used in the evaluation of patients with painful joint prostheses (Fig. 16–6) (see Chapter 20).

Trauma

STRESS INJURIES. Stress fractures may be of two types: *fatigue fractures* and *insufficiency fractures*. Fatigue fractures result from repetitive, perhaps abnormal, muscular stress or torque on normal bones. Insufficiency fractures occur as a result of normal physiologic stresses on abnormal bones having deficient elastic resistance (see Chapter 62). The bone scan has a high degree of sensitivity in detecting stress and insufficiency fractures (Fig. 16–7) and other forms of periosteal injury without fracture, surpassing that of radiography. Scintigraphy in such fractures reveals increased radionuclide uptake that, in a long tubular bone, traverses horizontally across the diaphysis (see Chapter 62). This abnormal pattern can be differentiated from that accompanying another stress injury,

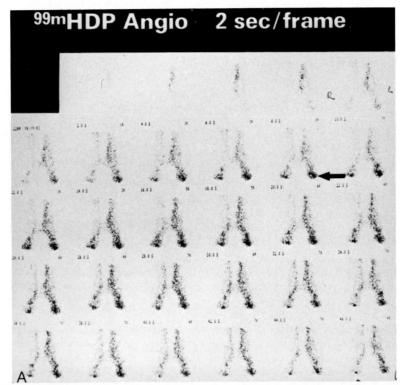

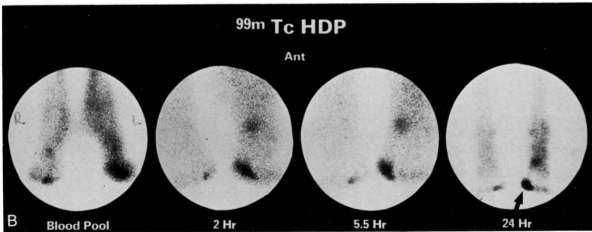

Figure 16–5. Four phase bone scan: Osteomyelitis versus cellulitis. A, Radionuclide angiogram of the feet in a patient with a diabetic ulcer over the left great toe. The sequential 2 s images (left to right) show generalized hypervascularity in the left foot in comparison to the right, with a focus of more intense activity over the left great toe (arrow). **B** Blood pool and delayed images of the 99mTc-HDP bone scan of the feet show that the region of abnormal activity in the left first toe persists (arrow) in comparison to the normal right foot. This pattern of abnormal, persistent uptake of the radionuclide, even at 24 hours, is consistent with the diagnosis of osteomyelitis. Note also that the other bones of the involved foot show generalized increased uptake as well, probably reflecting hypervascularity owing to inflammation.

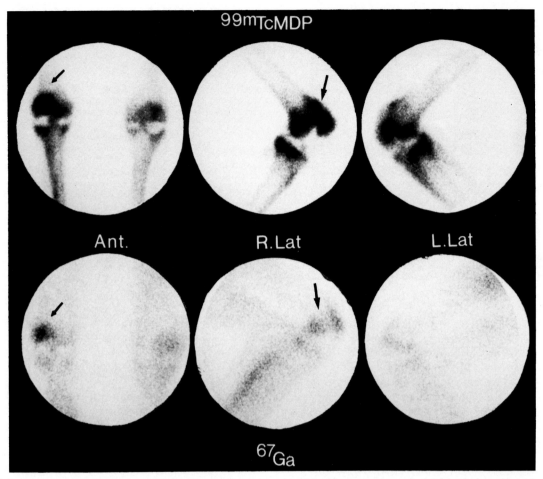

Figure 16–6. Painful prosthesis. Technetium and gallium images in a patient with bilateral knee prostheses and a painful right knee. The right knee shows markedly increased uptake in the femoral component on both technetium and gallium studies (arrows). At surgery, no infection was found; however, there was abundant granulation tissue and loosening of the prosthesis.

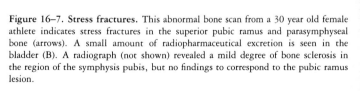

Figure 16–7. Stress fractures. This abnormal bone scan from a 30 year old female athlete indicates stress fractures in the superior pubic ramus and parasymphyseal bone (arrows). A small amount of radiopharmaceutical excretion is seen in the bladder (B). A radiograph (not shown) revealed a mild degree of bone sclerosis in the region of the symphysis pubis, but no findings to correspond to the pubic ramus lesion.

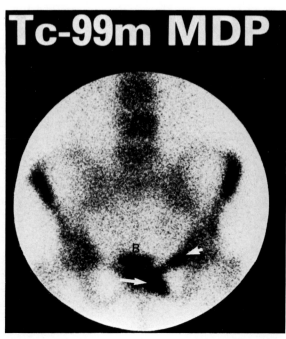

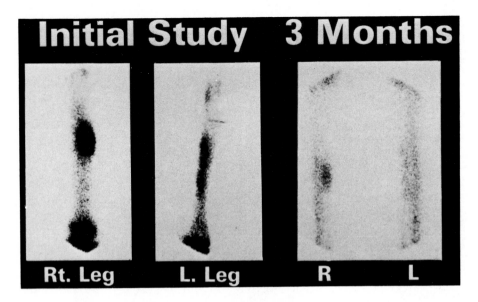

Figure 16–8. Stress fractures and periosteal injury. A 16 year old female runner complaining of shin splints has a true stress fracture (stage V) in the right tibia and periosteal reaction (stage II) in the left tibia. A subsequent examination 3 months later shows rapid resolution of the periosteal reaction on the left with mild residual abnormality at the site of the true stress fracture on the right. (Courtesy of P. Matin, M.D., Roseville, California.)

the shin splint. This term is applied to tightness and aching in the lower legs on exercise, commonly encountered in athletes. Tendinitis, myositis, and periostitis of the anterior or posterior muscle groups of the leg are all probably involved. On bone scan, shin splint pain is associated with periosteal deposition of the radiopharmaceutical agent, with the appearance of a "double stripe" sign, similar to that reported in hypertrophic osteoarthropathy. In these cases, the scan reflects periosteal injury rather than a true stress fracture of bone (Fig. 16–8). Indeed, shin splints represent part of the spectrum of stress injuries, which vary in severity from minimal periosteal reaction (stage I) to a full-thickness stress fracture (stage V).

FRACTURE HEALING. Studies of the pathophysiology of fracture healing show that repair at the fracture site usually begins within 24 hours after the event. Bone scans may show focal abnormalities, perhaps as early as 24 hours after injury, but usually by 3 days. The degree of uptake on the bone scan increases, reaching a maximum within several weeks. This phase is then followed by a decrease in uptake, eventually approaching normal levels (Fig. 16–9).

Although there is some variability in the time of appearance of fractures on scan, in part related to the patient's age, even greater variability exists in the time periods necessary for return of the scan to normal. It is not uncommon to identify abnormal increased focal uptake at a fracture site that is several years old. Generally, recent fractures show intense increased uptake, whereas older fractures show normal or mildly increased uptake.

The bone scan has some potential in assessing fracture healing and nonunion and in predicting which fractures might respond favorably to percutaneous electrical stimulation. Two

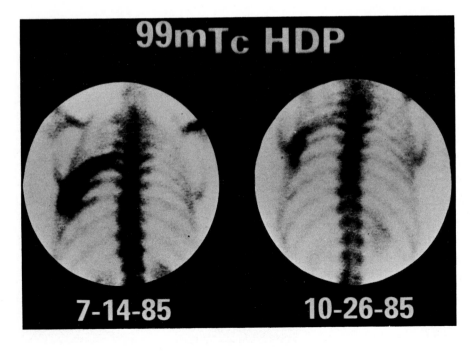

Figure 16–9. Surgical rib trauma. The study in July, 1985, was done within 2 weeks of a thoracotomy and shows markedly abnormal uptake of the radionuclide in those ribs that were injured at the time of surgery. Three months later, the abnormalities on the bone scan are less dramatic.

scintigraphic patterns may be observed in patients with fibrous union: (1) intense activity at the fracture site, which appears quite homogeneous, and (2) a line of decreased activity (negative defect) at the fracture site surrounded by increased uptake on both sides. The first pattern is associated with a good healing response to percutaneous electrical stimulation; the second is associated with a poor response.

CHILD ABUSE. In the evaluation of children suspected of being abused, studies comparing radionuclide bone scans and skeletal radiographic surveys have arrived at conflicting conclusions. Some data support the superiority of bone scanning over radiography in detecting skeletal lesions of child abuse, whereas other results indicate that the bone scan should be a secondary test after complete radiographic skeletal survey when occult fractures are suspected clinically.

Bone scanning has certain limitations in the evaluation of child abuse: Healed fractures may not be evident; epiphyseal and metaphyseal fractures may be difficult to detect because of the normally augmented uptake of the radiopharmaceutical agent in these regions; and technical details such as the use of pinhole collimation and careful positioning of the patient are critical to accurate analysis. False-negative results of bone scanning are most likely to be obtained in the neonate and young child.

Metabolic Bone Disease

Bone scintigraphy is sensitive in detecting focal abnormalities of bone in metabolic disorders. For example, the insufficiency type of stress fracture (pseudofracture) that may appear in osteomalacia can be identified as a focal area of increased uptake on bone scans. Furthermore, the appearance of the bone scan in some patients with osteomalacia is sufficiently different from that in normal persons, with a significantly elevated mean bone-to-soft tissue uptake ratio. In osteomalacia, the most consistent subjective abnormality on bone imaging is an increased uptake of tracer in the long bones, the wrists, the calvarium, and the mandible. These findings have also been noted in other metabolic disorders, such as hyperparathyroidism. Increased activity in the costochondral junctions and the appearance of a "tie sternum" are radionuclide characteristics of some metabolic disorders, as are focal regions of increased uptake at sites of brown tumors in hyperparathyroidism.

In renal osteodystrophy bone scans usually reveal absence of renal images, reflecting poor renal function. Furthermore, focal abnormalities similar to those that occur in primary hyperparathyroidism may be identified. Increased activity may be evident in the ends of the long bones and at the costochondral junctions. Quantitative monitoring shows markedly increased 24 hour retention of the labeled phosphate as well as increased skeletal tracer accumulation relative to that in soft tissue. Similar quantitative findings are observed in osteomalacia.

Scintigraphic patterns in patients with osteoporosis apparently are quite variable; studies may be normal or reveal areas of increased or decreased radiopharmaceutical localization in bones. Whole body retention of labeled phosphates is usually normal. In the reflex sympathetic dystrophy syndrome and in regional migratory osteoporosis, focal abnormalities on bone scan may be seen even before radiographic changes become evident.

Paget's Disease

Bone blood flow and osteogenesis are markedly increased in Paget's disease, and therefore the bone scan shows characteristic intense increased activity in the affected areas. The deformity and the enlargement of the bones that are seen on radiographs are equally characteristic on the radionuclide images.

During the early osteoporotic or lytic phase of the disease, most typically seen in the cranial vault as osteoporosis circumscripta, the bone scan shows markedly increased activity, with greater activity at the advancing margins of the lesion and less increased activity in its central portion (Fig. 16–10). In the later sclerotic phase of the disease, increased osteoblastic and osteoclastic activity may have ceased, and the healed lesions, which are still apparent radiographically, may appear normal on the scan. Thus, the bone scan may be useful in determining true activity of the disease process. In assessing response of pagetic bone to therapy with calcitonin, diphosphonate, or mithramycin, the bone scan may be particularly helpful, and the changing radionuclide pattern may even be quantitated with computer techniques (Fig. 16–11).

Vascular Disease

ISCHEMIC NECROSIS OF BONE. Bone scintigraphy is extremely valuable in the evaluation of ischemic necrosis of

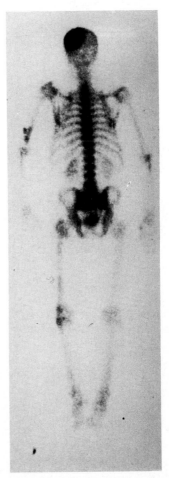

Figure 16–10. Paget's disease: Osteoporosis circumscripta. Total body ^{99m}Tc-MDP bone image in a patient with early Paget's disease involving the skull.

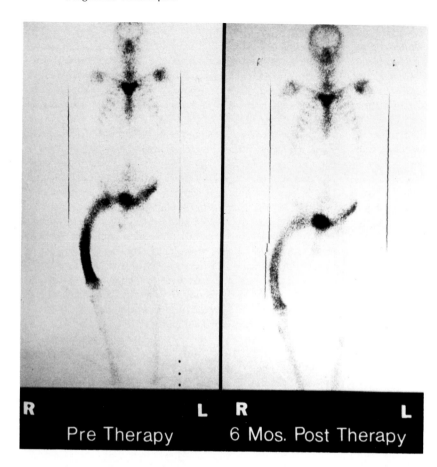

Figure 16–11. Paget's disease: Response to therapy. Two anterior total body bone images 6 months apart after calcitonin therapy in a patient with Paget's disease. The images show a typical pagetic femoral deformity with markedly increased uptake and apparent enlargement and bowing of the bone. After therapy, the degree of increased uptake in the pagetic bone is greatly lessened.

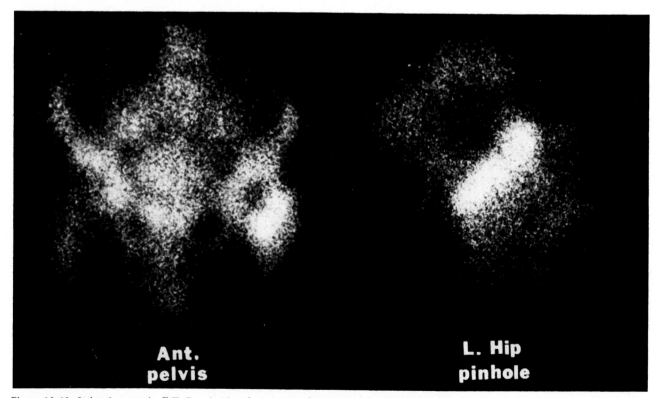

Figure 16–12. Ischemic necrosis. ^{99m}Tc-Pyrophosphate bone images of the pelvis and left hip with pinhole collimator view in a patient with an acute fracture through the femoral neck and secondary ischemic necrosis of the left femoral head. The pinhole view shows that the femoral head is cold and that the linear fracture through the femoral neck is hot.

bone, owing, in part, to greater sensitivity than radiography. Initially, on the bone scan, if a substantial interruption of blood supply has occurred, the radiopharmaceutical agent cannot reach the involved area and there may be decreased activity on the scan. As the bone reacts to the insult with reparative revascularization and reossification, scintigraphy may show increased activity in the involved area. Thus, foci of ischemic necrosis of bone may appear on scintillation images as areas of either decreased or increased radiopharmaceutical uptake. Presumably, as the radionuclide pattern changes between these two states, a period may occur in which uptake is normal. It is therefore important to obtain high resolution images of the affected regions. Either converging or pinhole collimation will be helpful in recognizing focal "cold" defects (Fig. 16–12). This effectiveness may be increased using single photon emission computed tomography.

Another approach, bone marrow imaging, has been used to predict the viability of bone in patients with ischemic necrosis. In general, the absence of radiocolloid uptake in the femoral head and neck on the bone marrow scan indicates vascular impairment, whereas its presence indicates an intact vascular supply through the femoral marrow space. Differentiation between bone infarction and osteomyelitis in patients with sickle cell anemia whose first manifestation is pain is difficult even with the use of bone, bone marrow, and gallium imaging, however.

LEGG-CALVÉ-PERTHES DISEASE. The bone scan has been cited for its superior sensitivity to that of radiography in evaluation of Legg-Calvé-Perthes disease. Characteristically, early in the course of this disease, radionuclide imaging shows a focal region of decreased radiopharmaceutical uptake in the anterolateral aspect of the proximal femoral epiphysis, although the entire epiphysis may be involved in some cases. Revascularization and healing are demonstrated subsequently on the scan as areas of increased activity in the femoral head and adjacent femoral neck. A more accurate assessment of epiphyseal involvement can be obtained if pinhole imaging techniques are used.

Articular Disease

Soon after the introduction of ^{99m}Tc-labeled phosphate compounds for bone imaging, these agents were applied to joint imaging as well. Because diseases affecting the joints also stimulate osteogenesis in the periarticular bone, abnormal uptake of the phosphate-labeled agents may occur in the adjacent bone in joints affected by arthritis. Furthermore, synovial vascularity increases as a result of the joint disease, which also causes increased vascularity in the adjacent bone. The result on imaging, therefore, is focally increased tracer accumulation in the periarticular osseous structures. An additional agent, ^{99m}Tc-pertechnetate, which localizes in the blood pool and extracellular fluid compartments, is used for joint imaging. Comparisons of the ^{99m}Tc-labeled phosphate images with ^{99m}Tc-pertechnetate images have indicated that the phosphate-labeled compounds are far more sensitive in detecting abnormal joints than the pertechnetate.

In most institutions, ^{99m}Tc-labeled phosphate compounds for joint imaging are used in doses similar to those used for bone imaging (i.e., 15 to 20 mCi), with scintigraphy performed approximately 2 hours after the intravenous injection of the material.

DEGENERATIVE JOINT DISEASE. As would be expected, increased accumulation of bone-seeking radiopharmaceutical agents occurs in areas of degenerative joint disease, allowing evaluation of the distribution and extent of the process. Such evaluation is especially useful in osteoarthritis of the knee, guiding the orthopedic surgeon in selection of osteotomy or total joint replacement.

RHEUMATOID ARTHRITIS AND SERONEGATIVE SPONDYLOARTHROPATHIES. The bone scan is considered the most sensitive imaging indicator of active disease in these arthritides. The pattern of abnormal radionuclide activity in rheumatoid arthritis (Fig. 16–13), consisting of symmetric peripheral joint abnormalities, may be distinguishable from that in the seronegative spondyloarthropathies, which tend to have more central skeletal involvement and asymmetric peripheral joint abnormalities. Compared with the radiograph, however, the bone scan is less specific in its ability to distinguish among the clinical entities.

Assessment of sacroiliac joint abnormalities by scintigraphy may be difficult, and quantitative techniques may be required. Studies of quantitative images of the sacroiliac joints using computer-generated ratios of activity over the sacroiliac regions compared with that in the central portion of the sacrum, or profile curves of the changes in uptake across the sacroiliac region, have suggested that separate ratios should be obtained

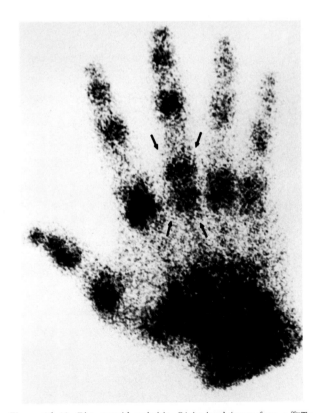

Figure 16–13. Rheumatoid arthritis. Right hand image from a ^{99m}Tc-pyrophosphate bone study in a patient with rheumatoid arthritis. Bands of activity at epiphyseal-metaphyseal areas (arrows) may normally be seen in young patients. In middle-aged individuals, they are abnormal. Multiple joints of the hand and wrist are involved in this patient. (From Weissberg DL, et al: Rheumatoid arthritis and its variants: Analysis of scintiphotographic, radiographic, and clinical examinations. AJR 131:665, 1978. Copyright 1978, American Roentgen Ray Society. Used with permission.)

for each sacroiliac joint and, perhaps, for the superior, middle, and inferior regions of each joint as well. The application of quantitative sacroiliac joint radionuclide examination may prove to be useful in following the course of patients with ankylosing spondylitis and sacroiliitis of psoriatic arthritis or Reiter's syndrome, and in many HLA-B27–positive persons without back pain or radiographic evidence of sacroiliac joint disease.

Several reports have shown that patients with classic ankylosing spondylitis who demonstrated ankylosis of sacroiliac joints on radiography revealed normal or slightly decreased radionuclide activity in the sacroiliac joints on scintigraphy. This probably reflected the inactivity of disease at the time of the scan. Thus, it would appear that the radionuclide examination may offer a means of differentiating active from "burned-out" disease.

Table 16–2. LESIONS AND CONDITIONS THAT HAVE BEEN ASSOCIATED WITH SOFT-TISSUE UPTAKE OF ^{99m}Tc-PHOSPHATE COMPOUNDS

Breast
Lactation
Fat necrosis
Mazoplasia
Gynecomastia
Postmastectomy
Breast prosthesis
Fibrocystic disease and
    mammary dysplasia
Primary breast cancer
Metastatic breast carcinoma

Cardiovascular System
Acute or chronic myocardial
    infarction
Unstable angina
Left ventricular aneurysm
Aortic aneurysm
Myocardial contusion
Mönckeberg's sclerosis
Calcified valves
Calcified coronary arteries
Prosthetic valves
Chemotherapy
Radiotherapy
Amyloidosis
Pericarditis and endocarditis
Chagas' disease
Metastatic calcification
Malignant pericardial effusions
Cardiac metastases
Hemangiopericytoma

Gastrointestinal System
Milk-alkali syndrome
Intestinal infarction
Abdominal aneurysm
Gastric calcification
Necrotizing enterocolitis
Trauma from nasogastric tube
Metastatic calcification
Metastases from rectal
    adenocarcinoma
Mucinous adenocarcinoma of
    the stomach
Malignant ascites
Colorectal metastases

Genitourinary System
Acute tubular necrosis
Chemotherapy
Radiotherapy
Kidney (after radiographic
    contrast)
Iron excess
Thalassemia major
Nephrocalcinosis
Phimosis
Orchitis
Wolman's disease
Leiomyoma of uterus
Chronic renal failure
Kidney in sickle cell anemia
Hypernephroma
Transplant ischemia
Erythroleukemia
Metastatic calcification
Urinoma
Primary renal tumors
Lymphatic lymphosarcoma
Ovarian carcinoma
Metastatic seminoma

Head, Neck, and Neurologic System
Cerebrovascular accident
Brain abscess
Thyroid nodule
Arteriovenous malformation
Cerebritis
Chronic subdural hematoma
Cerebral infarction
Metastatic calcification (thyroid)
Cerebral tumors
Calcified thyroid carcinoma
Brain metastases
Medullary carcinoma
Schwannoma
Neurilemoma
Primary neuroblastoma

Liver
Amyloidosis
Postarteriography
Necrosis
Aluminum excess
Cholangiocarcinoma
Metastases from colon
    carcinoma
Malignant melanoma
Metastases from oat cell
    carcinoma of lung
Neuroblastoma, soft-tissue
    uptake
Metastases from osteosarcoma

Lung
Radiotherapy
Fibrothorax
Sarcoidosis
Interstitial pulmonary
    calcification
Berylliosis
Lung nodules in chronic
    hemodialysis
Metastatic calcification
Bronchogenic carcinoma
Metastases from osteosarcoma
Malignant pleural effusion

Muscle and Periarticular Tissues
Iron dextran injection
Rhabdomyolysis
Polymyositis
Muscle trauma
Overexertion
McArdle's syndrome and
    disorders of glycogenolysis
Muscular dystrophy
Postrevascularization
Myositis ossificans
Precordial electrostimulation
Electric burns
Sickle cell disease
Ischemia
Chemoperfusion
Radiotherapy
Amyloidosis
Synovitis
Calcific tendinitis
Gouty tophi
Calcified myoma
Ipsilateral uptake following
    lumbar sympathectomy
Fibromatosis
Cartilaginous exostosis
Migratory osteolysis
Calcinosis universalis
Dystrophic calcifications
Extravasated calcium gluconate
Rhabdomyosarcoma
Synovioma

Skin and Subcutaneous Tissues
Electrical burns
Precordial electrostimulation
Filariasis
Inflamed breast implant
Pseudoxanthoma elasticum
Amyloidosis
Calcinosis universalis
Tumoral calcinosis
Infiltrated calcium solution
Soft tissue inflammation
Abscess
Surgical incision
Radiotherapy
Hyperhidrosis
Fat necrosis
Spinal cord injury
Drug injection
Urinary contamination
Dermatomyositis
Soft-tissue abscess
Healing wound
Chemoperfusion
Soft tissue irradiation
Folds of fat
Neurofibroma
Metastatic calcification
Angiolipoma
Lipoma
Hematoma
Fibromatosis
Soft tissue sarcoma
Liposarcoma
Malignant fibrous histiocytoma
Ewing's sarcoma of soft parts
Osteosarcoma

Spleen and Hematologic System
G6PD deficiency
Hemosiderosis
Infarction (sickle cell anemia)
Thalassemia major
Uptake in sickle cell disease
Splenic lymphoma
Histiocytic lymphoma
Lymphosarcoma

Other
Filarial infestation
Christmas disease
Lymphoma
Uterine fibroid
Neuroblastoma
Ganglioneuroblastoma

From Alazraki N: *In* JC Harbert, AFG da Rocha (Eds): Textbook of Nuclear Medicine. Vol. 2, Clinical Applications. Philadelphia, Lea & Febiger, 1984. Used with permission.

Diseases of Soft Tissue

A multitude of soft tissue lesions have been reported to concentrate bone-seeking radiopharmaceutical agents (Table 16–2). In identifying a cause for uptake of these agents by soft tissue, it is important to correlate the scan with a radiograph of the affected region, as soft tissue calcification or heterotopic ossification may be evident. Even in the absence of any soft tissue densities on the radiograph, the existence of microscopic foci of calcification or heterotopic bone formation below the limits of resolution of the radiograph cannot be excluded. In addition, certain lesions that do not typically show calcification may concentrate the bone-seeking radiopharmaceutical agents.

The factors that determine the localization of the ^{99m}Tc-labeled phosphate compounds in noncalcified or nonossified soft tissue tumors are not well understood. Increased vascularity, altered capillary permeability or cellular calcium metabolism, presence of immature collagen, and atypical binding of the ^{99m}Tc-phosphate compound to phosphatase enzymes are among the factors that have been considered. In the cases in which calcification or ossification is present in the soft tissue

lesion, the mechanism of ^{99m}Tc-phosphate compound uptake is presumed to be adsorption to the calcific focus similar to the adsorption of ^{99m}Tc-phosphate compound that occurs onto the hydroxyapatite crystal in normal bone.

In patients with heterotopic ossification after paralysis, the bone scan commonly is abnormal before radiographic changes are evident, and it shows an early increase in accumulation of ^{99m}Tc-phosphate in the involved region. Furthermore, bone and bone marrow scanning can effectively assess the maturity of the ectopic bone. If surgical resection is planned to relieve flexion-extension deformity or limitation of motion, it is advisable to be certain that the ectopic bone has matured at the time of surgical intervention, as the likelihood of recurrence will then be minimized. Serial bone scans show that the activity within the ectopic bone tends to decline, reaching a plateau level as the ossification reaches maturity. Bone marrow scanning using ^{99m}Tc-labeled sulfur colloid, which is trapped in the reticuloendothelial cells of the marrow, reveals uptake in the ectopic bone only when bone marrow has been formed. Thus, the presence of bone marrow activity is another indicator of the maturity of the ectopic bone (Fig. 16–14).

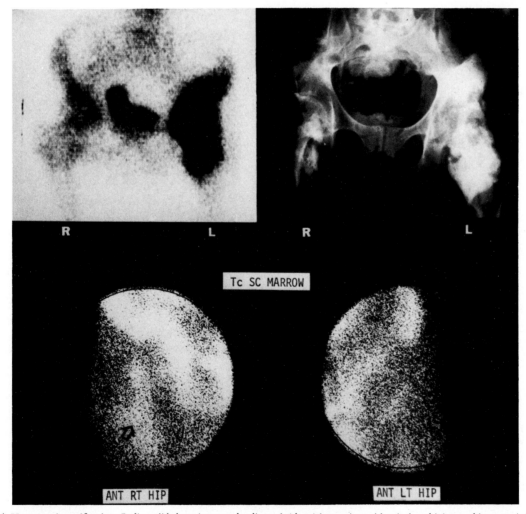

Figure 16–14. Heterotopic ossification. Radionuclide bone image and radiograph (above) in a patient with spinal cord injury and heterotopic bone formation surrounding both hip joints. ^{99m}Tc-Sulfur colloid bone marrow images (below) show uptake of radiopharmaceutical agent in the region of the heterotopic bone (arrow), particularly in the right hip. This indicates the presence of bone marrow formation in the maturing heterotopic bone.

FURTHER READING

Alazraki NP: Soft tissue localization of bone imaging radiopharmaceuticals. *In* BA Siegel (Ed): Nuclear Radiology Syllabus. Chicago, American College of Radiology, 1978.

Alazraki NP, Fierer J, Resnick D: Chronic osteomyelitis: Monitoring by ^{99m}Tc-phosphate and ^{67}Ga-citrate imaging. AJR *145*:767, 1985.

Alazraki N, Dries D, Datz F, Lawrence P, Greenberg E, Taylor A: The value of a 24-hour image (four phase bone scan) in assessing osteomyelitis in patients with peripheral vascular disease. J Nucl Med *26*:711, 1985.

Collier BD, Carrera GF, Johnson RP, Isitman AT, Hellman RS, Knobel J, Finger WA, Gonyo JE, Malloy PJ: Detection of femoral head avascular necrosis in adults by SPECT. J Nucl Med *26*:979, 1985.

Genant HK, Bautovich GJ, Singh M, Lathrop KA, Harper PV: Bone-seeking radionuclides: An in vivo study of factors affecting skeletal uptake. Radiology *113*:373, 1974.

Gilday DL, Paul DJ, Paterson J: Diagnosis of osteomyelitis in children by combined blood pool and bone imaging. Radiology *117*:331, 1975.

Goldberg RP, Genant HK, Shimshak R, Shames D: Applications and limitations of quantitative sacroiliac joint scintigraphy. Radiology *128*:683, 1978.

Goergen TG, Alazraki NP, Halpern SE, et al: "Cold" bone lesions: A newly recognized phenomenon of bone imaging. J Nucl Med *15*:1120, 1973.

Lieberman CM, Hemingway DL: Scintigraphy of shin splints. Clin Nucl Med *5*:31, 1980.

Lisbona R, Rosenthall L: Observations on the sequential use of ^{99m}Tc-phosphate complex and ^{67}Ga imaging in osteomyelitis, cellulitis, and septic arthritis. Radiology *123*:123, 1977.

Mall JC, Bekerman C, Hoffer PB, Gottschalk A: A unified radiological approach to the detection of skeletal metastases. Radiology *118*:323, 1976.

McNeil BJ: Rationale for the use of bone scans in selected metastatic and primary bone tumors. Semin Nucl Med *8*:336, 1978.

Prchal CL, Kahen HL, Blend MJ, Barmada R: Detection of musculoskeletal infection with the indium-III leukocyte scan. Orthopedics *10*:1253, 1987.

Raptopoulos V, Doherty PW, Goss TP, King MA, Johnson K, Gantz NM: Acute osteomyelitis: Advantage of white cell scans in early detection. AJR *139*:1077, 1982.

Roddie ME, Peters AM, Danpure HJ, Osman S, Henderson BL, Lavender JP, Carroll MJ, Neirinckx RD, Kelly JD: Inflammation: Imaging with Tc-99m HMPAO-labeled leukocytes. Radiology *166*:767, 1988.

Rosenthall L, Kaye M: Observations in the mechanism of ^{99m}Tc-labeled phosphate complex uptake in metabolic bone disease. Semin Nucl Med *6*:59, 1976.

Shauwecker DS, Park HM, Mock BH, Burt RW, Kernick CB, Ruoff AC, Sinn HJ, Wellman HN: Evaluation of complicating osteomyelitis with Tc-99m MDP, In-111 granulocytes, and Ga-67 citrate. J Nucl Med *25*:849, 1984.

Shirazi PH, Ryan WG, Fordham EW: Bone scanning in evaluation of Paget's disease of bone. CRC Crit Rev Clin Radiol Nucl Med *5*:523, 1974.

Thomas RH, Resnick D, Alazraki NP, Daniel D, Greenfield R: Compartmental evaluation of osteoarthritis of the knee: A comparative study of available diagnostic modalities. Radiology *116*:585, 1975.

Weissberg DL, Resnick D, Taylor A, Becker M, Alazraki N: Rheumatoid arthritis and its variants: Analysis of scintiphotographic, radiographic, and clinical examinations. AJR *131*:665, 1978.

Chapter 17

Needle Biopsy of Bone

Donald Resnick, M.D.

Open biopsy is an accepted surgical procedure in the diagnosis of a variety of skeletal disorders. Because this procedure requires considerable time and expense, as well as use of general anesthesia in most cases, repeated attempts have been made to devise special instruments for percuta- *neous needle (closed) biopsy of bone. Such procedures are valuable in numerous disorders, including neoplastic, metabolic, and infectious diseases and conditions such as Paget's disease, fibrous dysplasia, eosinophilic granuloma, and sarcoidosis.*

During closed biopsy, the bone specimen can be obtained in one of two ways: an aspiration by needle or a core by trephine. Tissue obtained by needle aspiration is small in quantity and distorted, with loss of cellular configuration; tissue obtained by trephine biopsy is in greater quantity and intact, although this technique requires larger needle size. Needle aspiration is most useful for tissue culture to exclude infection; trephine biopsy is a better technique for histologic diagnosis.

Some of the advantages of closed needle biopsy of bone over open biopsy are obvious: (1) closed needle biopsy can be accomplished quickly, usually within 45 minutes; (2) general anesthesia is not required and, in fact, the technique can be applied as an outpatient procedure; and (3) use of modern fluoroscopic equipment facilitates accurate needle placement. Computed tomography and scintigraphy can be used to further facilitate the procedure.

The major disadvantages of closed needle biopsy are the following:

1. A relatively small amount of material is withdrawn.

2. The biopsy procedure is relatively "blind," so that the ideal area of the lesion may not be biopsied.

3. The success of this procedure requires an experienced pathologist who cooperates closely with the radiologist.

4. Although it is possible that closed biopsy of a tumor could lead to its dissemination in neighboring and distant tissues, this is more theoretical than actual.

INDICATIONS AND CONTRAINDICATIONS

There are many general indications for needle biopsy of bone, some of which are given in Table 17–1.

Table 17–1. SOME INDICATIONS FOR NEEDLE BIOPSY OF BONE

Neoplastic disease
  Skeletal metastasis
  Primary tumors of bone or soft tissue
Metabolic disease
Infectious disease
Miscellaneous disorders
  Paget's disease
  Fibrous dysplasia
  Eosinophilic granuloma
  Sarcoidosis

Neoplastic Disease

With regard to patients with suspected or proved *skeletal metastasis*, potential indications for closed bone biopsy include the following:

1. Patients with a known primary tumor who have a solitary bone lesion detected by conventional radiography, computed tomography, or scintigraphy, or any combination of the three, in whom verification of the nature of the lesion will influence treatment.

2. Patients without a known primary tumor who have solitary or multiple osteolytic or osteoblastic lesions in whom the most probable diagnosis is metastatic disease. In such persons, bone biopsy represents a direct means to quickly establish the cellular characteristics of the metastatic focus. Depending on these characteristics, subsequent decisions regarding the need for and type of further diagnostic evaluation can be made (see Chapter 80).

3. Patients with known multiple primary tumors who have one or more bone lesions.

4. Patients with a primary tumor in whom there is need to determine whether viable tumor cells are present in a radiographically stable metastatic bone lesion (or lesions).

5. Patients with a known primary tumor that is in clinical remission who have developed a new bone lesion (or lesions).

6. Patients who have received radiation therapy for a primary tumor or metastatic bone lesion, or both, who develop bone abnormalities in the irradiated skeleton whose nature is not clear.

7. Patients with a non-neoplastic skeletal problem (e.g., Paget's disease, osteomyelitis) that may predispose to metastatic seeding, who develop a new aggressive lesion at the site of bone involvement whose nature is not clear.

With regard to *primary tumors of bone or soft tissue*, the advantages of closed biopsy over surgical intervention and open biopsy are less clear. Adequate sampling of tissue is fundamental to the success of any closed biopsy procedure in patients with primary osseous or soft tissue neoplasms.

Metabolic Disease

To accurately establish the presence and type of metabolic disease, open wedge resection or percutaneous biopsy of the iliac crest should be accomplished. It is necessary to obtain a full-thickness bone sample with both cortices and medulla to provide adequate material for qualitative and quantitative histologic evaluation.

Infectious Disease

Closed needle biopsy or aspiration can be useful in establishing a diagnosis of osteomyelitis and septic arthritis. Material should be obtained for both histologic diagnosis and appropriate tissue culture.

Miscellaneous Disorders

Closed bone biopsies can provide information in a wide variety of additional diseases, including Paget's disease, fibrous dysplasia, eosinophilic granuloma, and sarcoidosis.

BIOPSY SITES

Use of radionuclide studies in determining appropriate biopsy sites should be emphasized. Scintigraphy may identify additional lesions that are more accessible to closed needle biopsy than the initially detected abnormality. Scintigraphy can also be used to determine the precise entrance point prior to closed (or open) biopsy of lesions that are difficult to visualize fluoroscopically.

The preferred biopsy site is a prominent area of a non–weight-bearing bone. Additional accessible areas for biopsy are the pelvis and extremities. Biopsy of the lumbar spine is performed more easily than biopsy of the thoracic spine. Biopsy of the cranial vault and ribs should be undertaken with appropriate caution.

NEEDLES: TYPES AND TECHNIQUES

Trephine needles are of two basic types: some needles such as the Vim-Silverman and Westerman-Jensen needles contain narrow, paired cutting blades that engage the tissue; other needles, such as the Kormed, Craig, Turkel, Ackermann, and Meunier needles, consist of round tubes with serrated edges that cut the tissue.

The Craig needle is used most frequently (Fig. 17–1). The procedure for using this needle is simple. After administration of local anesthetic, a blunt guide is inserted through the skin down to the biopsy site. A cannula is placed over the guide and held firmly against the bone. The guide is removed, and the cutting needle is then inserted through the cannula. The cutting needle is approximately 2.5 cm longer than the cannula, this distance representing the depth of the biopsy specimen to be taken. With a to-and-fro twisting motion, the cutting needle is driven into the bone. While at its full depth, the needle is moved back and forth to dislodge the specimen. The cutting needle is then removed, and the cannula is left in place. The cannula can subsequently be moved to a different location if a second biopsy specimen is required. The tissue is removed from the cutting needle with a long, thin probe and placed in an appropriate specimen container. The entire procedure should be monitored carefully by fluoroscopy or computed tomography.

With any of the trephine needles, biopsy of a purely osteosclerotic lesion or one surrounded by a thickened cortical surface can require intense physical exertion. Use of a hand drill either to provide a cortical defect in which the biopsy needle can be firmly secured or to form a cortical tunnel to the underlying abnormal medullary canal through which the

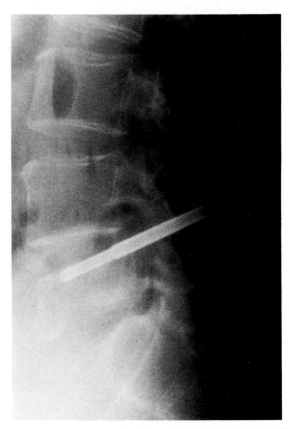

Figure 17–1. Technique of spinal biopsy for the fifth lumbar vertebral body. Observe that the Craig needle has been advanced in an inferior direction, owing to the presence of the iliac crest at a lower level. In this case a biopsy of the upper portion of the vertebral body documented that the cause of an osteolytic area was a cartilaginous node.

needle can be inserted facilitates the procedure in such difficult cases.

Aspiration needles of different sizes are available. For evaluating many lesions, an 18 or 20 gauge needle may be sufficient.

PROCESSING OF THE BIOPSY SPECIMEN

Fluid aspirates should be transferred immediately to culture tubes or delivered rapidly to the laboratory for plating. In cases of suspected articular infection in which no fluid is recovered spontaneously, the instillation of nonbacteriostatic, sterile saline solution should be followed by reaspiration of the joint contents.

Blood that is aspirated from the osseous lesion should not be discarded, as it will frequently provide an accurate diagnosis. The blood is allowed to clot in a syringe or plastic cap, and then it is sent as a tissue specimen in formalin to the laboratory and processed separately from the removed tissue. Smears can also be made from small drops of blood.

Tissue aspirates can be embedded in paraffin for routine histologic analysis or processed for cytologic examination.

COMPLICATIONS

The procedure is usually performed without significant complication. Mild pain and discomfort are common. Hemorrhage can result when biopsy specimens are obtained from patients with vascular tumors or when a venous or arterial structure is injured, particularly in biopsies of the spine. Pneumothorax may complicate spine or rib biopsy, and sinus tracts infrequently may appear after biopsy of a superficial infectious lesion. Additional reported complications include footdrop, pneumonia, pneumoretroperitoneum, meningitis, and even death, but these are extremely rare. In selected patients, therefore, needle biopsy of bone is a safe procedure, which can be accomplished readily in the Radiology Department.

FURTHER READING

Craig FS: Vertebral body biopsy. J Bone Joint Surg [Am] 38:93, 1956.

Debnam JW, Staple TW: Needle biopsy of bone. Radiol Clin North Am 13:157, 1975.

Debnam JW, Staple TW: Trephine bone biopsy by radiologists. Results of 73 procedures. Radiology 116:607, 1975.

Kattapuram SV, Rosenthal DI: Percutaneous biopsy of the cervical spine using CT guidance. AJR 149:539, 1987.

Murphy WA, Destouet JM, Gilula LA: Percutaneous skeletal biopsy 1981: A procedure for radiologists—results, review, and recommendations. Radiology 139:545, 1981.

Ottolenghi CE: Aspiration biopsy of the spine. J Bone Joint Surg [Am] 51:1531, 1969.

Robertson WW Jr, Janssen HF, Pugh JL: The spread of tumor-cell-sized particles after bone biopsy. J Bone Joint Surg [Am] 66:1243, 1984.

Stoker DJ, Kissin CM: Percutaneous vertebral biopsy: A review of 135 cases. Clin Radiol 36:569, 1985.

Tehranzadeh J, Freiberger RH, Ghelman B: Closed skeletal needle biopsy: Review of 120 cases. AJR 140:113, 1983.

Chapter 18

Quantitative Bone Mineral Analysis

David J. Sartoris, M.D.

The ability to measure the mineral content of bone in vivo is becoming an increasingly important and workable technique in diagnostic radiology. Using such determinations, it may be possible to detect early osteoporosis, predict sites of fracture risk, and monitor both the course of disease and its response to therapy. Difficulties arise because most available methods measure the mineral content of specific bones and the results cannot be extrapolated to other regions of the skeleton in the individual patient. Nevertheless, numerous techniques have been developed that are useful under a variety of circumstances.

Routine radiographs are not sufficient to diagnose early bone loss because losses of up to 40 per cent of bone mass may occur before a noticeable radiographic change is detected. Recently, a variety of noninvasive procedures have been developed that permit improved sensitivity in the measurement of bone mineral content (Table 18–1). These methods are useful in the early detection of osteoporosis and prediction of fracture risk.

Fundamental concepts important to an understanding of the relative merits of the various techniques include the following: (1) the total skeleton is composed of approximately 80 per cent cortical bone and 20 per cent trabecular bone; (2) trabecular bone has a turnover rate that is approximately eight times greater than that of cortical bone, which renders it a sensitive component for measuring mineral content that is highly responsive to metabolic stimuli; (3) fractures of greatest epidemiologic importance in osteoporosis occur at sites in the axial skeleton (proximal portion of the femur, spine); (4) the vertebral bodies are an early site of bone loss and fracture in osteoporosis owing to their high trabecular bone content; (5) cross-sectional methods can measure either purely trabecular or purely cortical bone, whereas projectional techniques integrate the cortical and trabecular bone into a single measurement that is the sum of the two components at a given site; and (6) dual energy techniques are able to compensate for variations in soft tissue thickness and bone marrow composition, whereas single energy methods cannot.

An ideal technique for noninvasive bone density assessment would reflect bone mineral content at important sites of fracture as well as in the entire body with (1) high precision, accuracy, and sensitivity; (2) low radiation dose; (3) short examination time; (4) low cost; and (5) minimal patient inconvenience. The methods also should be widely available.

The noninvasive methods currently employed for quantifying bone mineral content are used mainly in patients with those osteopenic conditions in which there is a quantitative decrease in bone mass without a qualitative defect. Hence, the techniques are more appropriate in osteoporosis and less

useful in conditions such as osteomalacia, hyperparathyroidism, and renal osteodystrophy. Measurement of bone mineral content may help differentiate patients who are likely to develop osteoporosis from age-, sex-, and race-matched persons without this tendency.

Current literature dealing with noninvasive bone densitometry is characterized by frequently conflicting results and considerable controversy over which specific method is most accurate in determining bone status at a particular site. Furthermore, the relationship of the measurements of bone mass to the risk of fracture is not clear.

Decreased bone mineral content has been found to be an important determinant of fracture frequency, particularly in the hip. Although femoral strength and likelihood of fracture depend to a significant extent on the integrity of cancellous bone, numerous other factors also are important, including the geometry of the proximal portion of the femur and the supporting influence of adjacent soft tissues, including the bone marrow. Thickness and configuration of compact bone, including the cortex and calcar femorale, also are major determinants of femoral strength and fracture risk; their relative contribution compared with cancellous bone has not been precisely established. Both cortical and trabecular bone loss may predispose to femoral neck fracture, and identification of persons at risk may thus be improved by taking both types of bone deficit into account. A study of women with fractures of the distal portion of the radius has found that measurement of trabecular bone density at this site, or dual photon absorptiometric determinations in the femoral neck, can assist in identifying persons at increased risk of femoral neck fracture.

Measurements of bone mineral content in the appendicular skeleton have been shown to correlate poorly with those in the axial skeleton. In addition, peripheral measurements may be affected by extraneous variables. For example, the distal portion of the radius is influenced by adjacent arthritis, whereas density measurements of the os calcis are affected profoundly by both body weight and physical activity. Both

Table 18–1. COMPARISON OF ESTABLISHED TECHNIQUES FOR MEASURING BONE MINERAL CONTENT

Technique	Precision (per cent)	Accuracy (per cent)	Radiation Exposure	
			Local	*Gonads*
Radiogrammetry			Up to 100 mrad	Negligible
Photon absorptiometry				
Single energy	3–5	1–4	2–5 mrad	Negligible
Dual energy	1–3	4–6	5–15 mrad	2 mrad
Computed tomography				
Single energy	1–3	8	200–250 mrad	Variable: may be as low as 10 mrad
Dual energy	3–5	2–4	Roughly 2 times single energy	Roughly 2 times single energy
Neutron activation analysis	2–3	6	300–5000 mrad	
Dual energy radiography	<1	1	1–2 mrad	Negligible

sites also are subject to especially large measurement errors because of variations in marrow fat and osteoid matrix.

In general, bone density measurements can be performed on either the axial or the appendicular skeleton. Vertebral bone density can be determined by quantitative computed tomography, dual photon absorptiometry, or dual energy radiography. The proximal portion of the femur can also be studied by any of these techniques. Single photon absorptiometry has proved most useful in evaluating the radius and calcaneus, whereas radiogrammetry typically is applied to the metacarpal cortices. Finally, although neutron activation analysis currently is the gold standard for estimation of total body calcium, dual photon absorptiometry and dual energy radiography also can provide such measurements.

RADIOGRAMMETRY

Radiogrammetry measures the thickness of the cortex of metacarpal or other tubular bones on standard anteroposterior radiographs of the hand. From such measurements, various derived indices of the cortical bone volume are calculated. The technique is widely available and simple, requiring the ability only to take reproducible radiographs and to make fine caliber measurements. An individual patient's radiogrammetric data can be compared with those of a large normal population and are usually precise and reproducible. Small changes in the endosteal and periosteal cortices may be found by serial measurements. Radiogrammetry, however, does not reliably reflect absolute bone mineral content and does not measure intracortical bone porosity. Therefore, it provides information only on relative changes in bone volume.

Radiogrammetry involves minimal radiation exposure, with negligible bone marrow or gonadal dose. Although radiogrammetry is useful in measuring bone mineral content of the appendicular skeleton, it is of limited clinical value in assessing the bone status in the axial skeleton, especially in areas with proportionately greater trabecular content, such as the spine.

SINGLE PHOTON ABSORPTIOMETRY

Single photon absorptiometry also measures mineral content in the appendicular skeleton and is usually performed on the radius or calcaneus. A monoenergetic photon source, such as iodine-125, is coupled with a sodium iodide scintillation counter or detector. The difference in photon absorption between bone and soft tissue allows calculation of the total bone mineral content in the scan path, which is inversely related to the measured transmission count rate. Bone mineral content is expressed as grams of bone mineral per square centimeter scanned.

Single photon absorptiometry requires careful positioning of the bone site that is being examined during sequential testing. In addition, the technique requires a uniform soft tissue thickness surrounding the bone and therefore may not accurately predict mineral content in the spine. Single photon absorptiometry involves a 2 mrad to 5 mrad dose to the limb. The total body dose is negligible because there is virtually no radiation scatter.

Over 20 years ago, when single photon absorptiometry was first developed, various skeletal sites were studied in relation to metabolic bone disease. These included the radial shaft, distal portion of the radius, humerus, tibia, and os calcis. Because the distal portion of the radius has slightly elevated trabecular bone content (30 to 50 per cent of the total mass) and the os calcis is largely trabecular (80 to 90 per cent of the total mass), these sites were thought to be potentially sensitive. Despite the fact that reliable (2 per cent error) results could be obtained, the findings reflected overall mineral status no better than did the much simpler method of measuring the radial shaft.

Single photon absorptiometry has since been criticized for its tendency to reflect the status of peripheral long bones, which are composed predominantly of cortical bone, not necessarily the more critical sites of fracture or the entire skeleton. This technique is thus believed by some physicians to be of limited value in individual patient monitoring because of its relative insensitivity to bone changes produced by metabolic stimuli. Cortical bone measurements in the radius have been found to correlate poorly with dual photon absorptiometric determinations in the spine; however, in contrast to the variability and inconsistency reported previously for single photon absorptiometric measurements at the standard "9/10" site on the radius (nine tenths of the measured distance from the ulnar olecranon to the radial styloid process), age-related bone loss as determined at a more distal location, where the radius and ulna are separated by 5 mm, has been found to correlate closely with generalized axial demineralization. It has thus been concluded by some researchers that distal radial density at the latter site can be used in conjunction with midradius density as a preliminary test for both generalized and trabecular bone loss in women. Other investigators, however, maintain that radial density measurements are a poor indication of vertebral bone status and that direct assessment of the particular skeletal site of interest is necessary.

The calcaneus is composed chiefly of trabecular bone and can be evaluated by noninvasive densitometry using both single photon absorptiometry and computed tomography (CT). In some studies, a high correlation has been documented between the bone mineral content of the calcaneus and that of the spine; in other studies, however, changes in the os calcis have been related more poorly to axial osteoporosis than are radiogrammetric measurements. Indeed, complete overlap of os calcis density in fracture patients and age-matched controls has been demonstrated. The poor clinical results obtained at the os calcis have been partially attributed to high intrapopulation variance, and it has been concluded that this site cannot predict bone strength and fracture risk at the osteoporotic fracture sites (spine and proximal portion of the femur).

In normal subjects, measurements of either the os calcis or the distal portion of the radius have been found to predict the area density of the spine or femur with a standard error of estimate (SEE) of about 0.12 g/cm^2; the SEE is usually higher in patients with bone disease (0.15 g/cm^2 to 0.25 g/cm^2).

DUAL PHOTON ABSORPTIOMETRY

Dual photon absorptiometry is a modification of the single energy technique using a radioisotope (gadolinium-153) source that emits photons at two different energy levels. Dual photon measurement eliminates the need for a constant soft tissue thickness across the scan path (allowing its use in areas such as the spine and femur), as the signal produced is independent of variations in the soft tissue that is scanned. The influence of irregular overlying fat distribution also may be corrected during scanning. As with single photon absorptiometry, the method measures total integrated mineral in the path of the beam.

Dual photon absorptiometry does not provide absolute measurement of bone mineral content because the amount of bone scanned differs with the size of the skeleton and must be subsequently normalized. The radiation dose is directed toward the spine or femur and involves a 5 mrad to 15 mrad exposure. The total dose to the ovaries is less than 2 mrad, and the bone marrow dose is less than 0.2 mrad. Routine spinal radiographs for localization may add to the total radiation exposure.

Dual photon absorptiometry can be used to quantify changes in patients with metabolic bone disease or in those who are under treatment with drugs that alter bone mineral content (Fig. 18–1). This technique has been found to have an accuracy error of 4 to 6 per cent. Because this method measures integral bone (both compact and cancellous) its sensitivity as compared with that of quantitative CT (which can selectively measure trabecular bone with its eightfold greater turnover rate) is believed to be low. The presence of osteophytes or vascular calcification may contribute to increased density that falsely elevates dual photon absorptiometric determinations. The accuracy and reproducibility of this technique in the spine also are reduced by vertebral

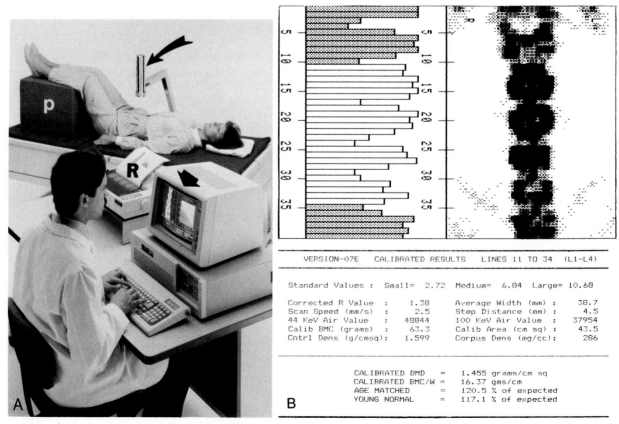

```
VERSION-07E    CALIBRATED RESULTS    LINES 11 TO 34  (L1-L4)


Standard Values :  Small=  2.72  Medium=  6.84  Large= 10.68

Corrected R Value   :      1.38   Average Width (mm)  :     38.7
Scan Speed (mm/s)   :       2.5   Step Distance (mm)  :      4.5
44 KeV Air Value    :     48844   100 KeV Air Value   :    37954
Calib BMC (grams)   :      63.3   Calib Area (cm sq)  :     43.5
Cntrl Dens (g/cmsq):      1.599   Corpus Dens (mg/cc):      286


            CALIBRATED BMD   =   1.455 grams/cm sq
            CALIBRATED BMC/W =  16.37 gms/cm
            AGE MATCHED      = 120.5 % of expected
            YOUNG NORMAL     = 117.1 % of expected
```

Figure 18–1. Dual photon absorptiometry of the lumbar spine. A, Scanning set-up. *P,* Positioning block used to straighten lumbar lordotic curvature; curved arrow, photon detector; straight arrow, computer display of results; *R,* printed report. **B,** Representative scan report. Bone mineral density is expressed as gram per square centimeter and compared with normative data. (Courtesy of Lunar Radiation Corporation, Madison, Wisconsin.)

compression with callus formation, scoliotic deformity, hypertrophy of articular facets, and discogenic sclerosis. Dual photon absorptiometry, however, has desirable characteristics, which include the following: the capability of assessing vertebral, proximal femoral, or total body bone content; independence from effects of marrow fat and other soft tissue; a relatively low radiation dose; and the ability to determine femoral bone density with only a 2 to 3 per cent error of precision and accuracy. Skepticism has been expressed regarding the enhanced discriminatory ability of dual photon absorptiometry of the femur or total body in predicting fracture risk or improving sensitivity in monitoring osteoporosis. Nevertheless, vertebral trabecular bone as measured by CT and total vertebral mineral as determined by dual photon absorptiometry have correlated well. The former technique, however, has been found to be more predictive of vertebral fracture than the latter method. Dual photon absorptiometric measurements in the spine have been shown to correlate poorly with those in the proximal portion of the femur.

Dual photon absorptiometric results from the femur and spine in some patients with femoral neck fractures have been found not to differ significantly from those of age-matched controls. Alternatively, bone density in the region of Ward's triangle in the proximal portion of the femur has been shown to be reduced by 50 per cent among fracture patients compared with age-matched controls and by 70 per cent compared with young normal subjects, and comparable findings have been demonstrated by dual photon absorptiometry in patients with vertebral compression fractures.

QUANTITATIVE COMPUTED TOMOGRAPHY

CT also can be used to measure bone mineral content. A mineral reference standard (such as potassium phosphate [K_2HPO_4] solution) is required for calibration, as is a scout view for localization. Either single or dual energy technique may be used. Data from scans of 3 to 4 cm^3 volumes of the midportion of the vertebral bodies are averaged and used in conjunction with calibration results to calculate mineral equivalent values, expressed in milligrams of K_2HPO_4 per cubic centimeter. Prototype liquid K_2HPO_4 (Picker, Highland Heights, Ohio) or solid calcium hydroxyapatite (Computerized Imaging Reference Systems, Norfolk, Virginia) calibration phantoms that are scanned either before or after the patient also are being tested as potential alternatives to the simultaneously scanned type of phantom, and these offer advantages, including enhanced geometric correction for long-term drift, compensation for bone marrow fat with single energy technique, and ability to obtain densitometric information from CT studies performed for other reasons (Fig. 18–2). The accuracy of single energy CT is variable and depends on the amount of fat in the bone marrow. Dual energy CT affords more accurate determination of bone mineral content, independent of fat and water variation, but at the expense of reduced precision.

The radiation exposure from CT studies of vertebral trabecular bone is significant. Effective studies can be accomplished with radiation doses of 200 to 250 mrad localized to a 10 cm region of the upper abdomen and with a gonadal dose of less than 10 mrad. Some institutions, however, have reported surface radiation doses up to 10 times greater for such studies.

CT can be used to measure cancellous bone, cortical bone, or an integrated sum of both. This capability is advantageous because the selective measurement of trabecular bone rather than integral bone provides a more sensitive means of quantifying changes in metabolic bone disease. The method can identify the absolute mineral content of a specific volume of bone. With technical advances, lower radiation exposure, and a decrease in cost, CT with either a concurrently or a sequentially scanned phantom will become increasingly important in the evaluation of metabolic bone diseases.

Criticisms of single energy CT of the spine, the current mainstay of selective trabecular bone analysis in the axial skeleton, have focused on its tendency to underestimate ash

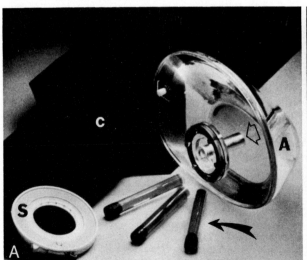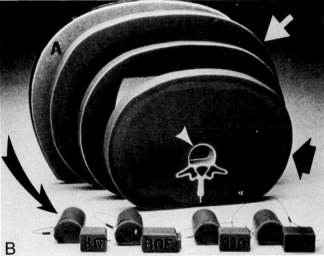

Figure 18–2. Calibration phantoms for quantitative CT of the spine. A, Liquid K_2HPO_4 calibration phantom scanned before or after patient examination. Curved arrow, mineral equivalent inserts; open arrow, insert aperture; c, patient positioning couch; S, data analysis software; A, conical anthropomorphic torso simulator. (Photograph courtesy of Picker, Highland Heights, Ohio.) **B,** Solid calcium hydroxyapatite calibration phantom scanned before or after the patient. Curved arrow, mineral equivalent inserts, one of which (80°F) affords marrow fat correction; straight white arrow, outer fat-equivalent torso simulation rings; straight black arrow, basic torso simulator; arrowhead, insert aperture; A, support base. (Courtesy of Computerized Imaging Reference Systems, Norfolk, Virginia.)

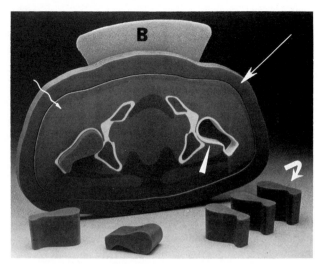

Figure 18–3. Solid calcium hydroxyapatite calibration phantom for quantitative CT of the proximal femur, scanned before or after the patient. Curved arrow, mineral equivalent inserts, one of which affords marrow fat correction; straight white arrow, outer fat-equivalent torso simulation rings; wavy arrow, basic torso simulator; arrowhead, insert aperture; B, support base. (Courtesy of Computerized Imaging Reference Systems, Norfolk, Virginia.)

density as a result of age-related increases in marrow fat. CT measurements may be falsely lowered 20 to 25 per cent in elderly osteoporotic persons because marrow fat concentration increases with age. A 13 mg/cm³ error for a 10 per cent change in fat concentration has been documented, and at 130 kVp, ash density has been shown to be systematically underestimated by about 25 mg/cm³ in men and 40 mg/cm³ in women. This phenomenon may explain the observation that

the apparent loss of vertebral bone with age in men (12 per cent per decade) is greater than the decrease in compact bone of the distal portion of the radius (3 per cent per decade) as determined by single photon absorptiometry. Inaccuracies may be reduced by using age-related regression analysis for calculating mineral content. Accuracy error is reportedly reduced to 6 per cent using dual energy CT, but this entails postprocessing of data and increases the relatively high radiation dose (1000 to 1500 mrad) of the single energy approach. Alternatively, quantitative CT has exhibited great sensitivity and precision in the measurement of alterations in trabecular mineral content at sites including the spine, radius, and tibia. Selective trabecular bone density measurements, as afforded by CT, have been shown to provide much better discrimination between normal and osteoporotic patients than assessment of cortical or total bone mass. CT measurements of trabecular bone in the distal portion of the radius and spine have been shown to correlate only moderately, however. Vertebral CT measurements in both men and women have correlated well with the prevalence of vertebral fracture and have provided an index of fracture risk (fractures are rare above a value of 110 mg/cm³ and may occur below this level).

Quantitative assessment of trabecular bone density in the proximal portion of the femur cannot be performed using the single-slice strategy employed for vertebral mineral determinations by CT because of the inherently complex trabecular architecture and geometry in this region. Three-dimensional histogram analysis overcomes this problem by affording an integral approach to cancellous bone densitometry over a volume encompassing both the femoral neck and the intertrochanteric regions. With calibration by either a concurrently or a sequentially scanned phantom (Fig. 18–3), a frontal localization image is obtained initially. Contiguous 10 mm

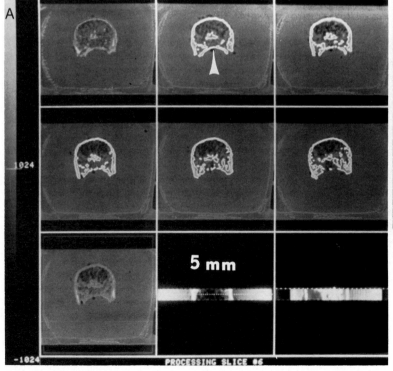

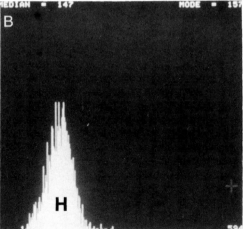

Figure 18–4. Three-dimensional volumetric CT densitometry of the spine. A, Contouring algorithm (white lines, arrowhead) in progress on sequential 5 mm thick slices. Cortical bone and posterior basivertebral venous channels are effectively excluded from trabecular volume of interest. B, Representative data and histogram plot (H) of all pixels included within vertebral trabecular bone volume encompassed by contiguous CT slices. Typical bell-shaped distribution with absence of high density values indicates exclusion of undesired cortical bone by the contouring and editing process.

thick slices are then acquired, beginning at the lateral aspect of the femoral head-neck junction and terminating at the level of the lesser trochanter. Three-dimensional histogram analysis involves contouring each slice independently and obtaining an integral trabecular bone volume as defined by the inner cortical contour using an appropriately low minimum pixel density value. A histogram of all pixels within the known calculated volume of interest is generated, along with mean, standard deviation, median, and mode values. A mineral equivalent value for cancellous bone density in the femoral neck and intertrochanteric region is derived by linear interpolation with data derived from comparable analysis of each chamber of the calibration phantom. Using the same software, histogram analysis of total bone density and cortical bone alone also can be derived for the proximal portion of the femur. Cancellous measurements are most useful in the evaluation of subtle changes in mineral status, whereas cortical and total bone density determinations may more reliably predict femoral strength and potential risk of fracture. Applications of this method to bone densitometry in the spine (Fig. 18–4) and sites of contemplated orthopedic intervention are currently being investigated. Three-dimensional histogram analysis of CT data may be the approach of choice for the assessment of osseous integrity, providing a noninvasive means for estimating bone strength.

NEUTRON ACTIVATION ANALYSIS

Neutron activation analysis uses a source of high-energy neutrons to activate calcium-48 within the body to calcium-49. The subsequent decay back to calcium-48 can be measured with a gamma radiation counter to provide a measurement of total body calcium (Fig. 18–5). Because greater than 98 per cent of total body calcium is located in the skeleton, this technique assesses total bone calcium content. The distribution of calcium within bone, however, may be more important than its total magnitude. Modifications of this method permit the assessment of regional calcium stores.

Total body neutron activation analysis delivers relatively high radiation doses, generally on the order of 300 to 5000 mrad. Partial body neutron activation analysis requires proportionately smaller radiation doses. Neutron activation analysis currently is considered the gold standard for total skeletal calcium measurement but is available only in specialized centers.

DUAL ENERGY PROJECTION RADIOGRAPHY

Dual energy projection radiography of the proximal portions of the femora has been performed in patients for densitometric evaluation. The system consists of a modified General Electric CT/T 8800 scanner, which uses an array of 512 0.7 mm cesium iodide detectors and a stationary fan beam collimated to 1.9 mm thickness. The x-ray generator provides pulses of 85 kVp, 1000 mA, 3.3 msec and 135 kVp, 250 mA, 5.5 msec radiation alternating at 60 cycles/second. These energies do not yield an optimal signal-to-noise ratio but are selected owing to generator restrictions. Spectral overlap reduction is achieved with a synchronized rotating filter composed of erbium and brass for the low and high energy pulses, respectively. As the subject is translated linearly through the fan beam, each pulse produces one line of transmission data. The two resultant low and high energy interlaced images are interpolated by one-half pixel each to ensure perfect registration. The usual scan of a patient covers a 30.0 cm distance, using a table speed of 21 mm/second. Estimated radiation dose is 60 to 120 mrad per examination.

A region of interest of appropriate size and shape is traced on the projected femoral neck on soft tissue cancellation images. The mean attenuation density value per pixel in the irregular region is determined, along with the standard deviation and number of pixels included. Similar determinations are performed for each solution-filled chamber of a calibration phantom included in the image (Fig. 18–6). By linear interpolation, the mean attenuation density reading of each femoral neck is assigned a mineral equivalent value expressed in g/dl of K_2HPO_4.

Dual energy projection radiography provides quantitation of bone density and an estimate of femoral neck strength. Because the method incorporates total cortical and trabecular bone content of the entire femoral neck into a single measurement, it may predict strength more accurately than techniques that assess either component independently. The reliability and accuracy of the method on serial examinations have been documented in specimen studies. A serious limitation is its prototype nature and current availability only in specialized centers, but newer systems of this type are currently under development for use in the spine (Fig. 18–7), femur, and other sites. Preliminary studies using the device developed by Hologic, Inc., of Waltham, Massachusetts, have indicated a number of advantages over dual photon absorptiometry, including a precision of 0.5 per cent or less (versus 2 to 5 per cent), a radiation dose of under 2 mrem (versus 10 to 20 mrem), an image spatial resolution of approximately 2 mm (versus 5 mm), an examination time of 5 minutes (versus 20 to 30 minutes), and 5 year source life (versus 6 to 18 months) without the need for Nuclear Regulatory Commission licensing. In general, results of dual-energy projection radiography correlate well with those derived by dual photon absorptiometry and poorly with quantitative CT measurements of trabecular bone in the spine.

SCANNING SLIT FLUOROGRAPHY

An x-ray videoabsorptiometric technique has been developed for measurement of bone mineral content in vivo. The principal utility of this technique is the precise measurement of commonly fractured bones (such as the femoral neck) that are difficult to measure by other techniques because of problems with repositioning of the patient. Scanning slits reduce scattered radiation and improve linearity of measurements. Heavily filtered, high kVp beams are used to minimize errors from beam hardening, and data renormalization is employed to compensate for spatial nonuniformities of the beam and detector. Linearity of measured bone mineral content over the range 0.8 to 5 g/cm^2 is very good ($r = 0.998$) and compares well with results of single and dual photon absorptiometry. A 1.6 per cent change in measured bone mineral content is observed for a 10 per cent change (approximately 2 cm) in tissue thickness, whereas a 10 per cent change in marrow composition causes a 0.6 to 0.8 per cent change in the bone mineral content measurement.

A technique for accurate determination of bone mineral content using dual energy scanning slit fluorography also is under development. X-ray scatter and veiling glare are sup-

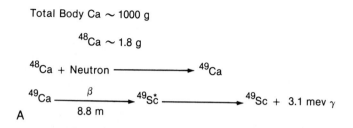

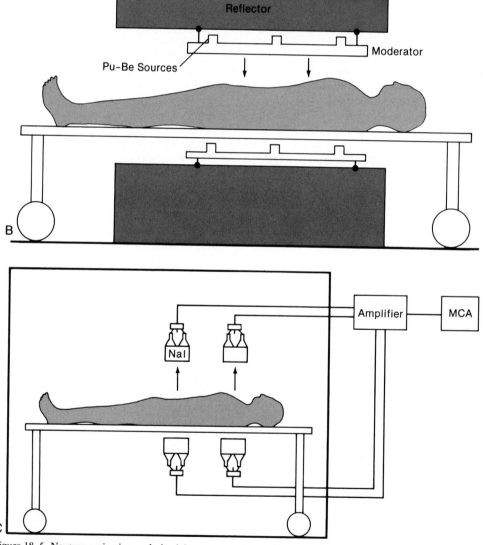

Figure 18–5. Neutron activation analysis. A Isotope proportions and nuclear interactions relevant to neutron activation analysis. **B** Activation phase involves exposure of patient to neutrons derived from plutonium (Pu) and beryllium (Be) sources. **C** Detection phase involves capture of gamma ray photons emitted from patient as part of calcium-49 decay by sodium iodide (NaI) detectors. (Courtesy of Joan E. Harrison, M.D., Toronto, Ontario, Canada.)

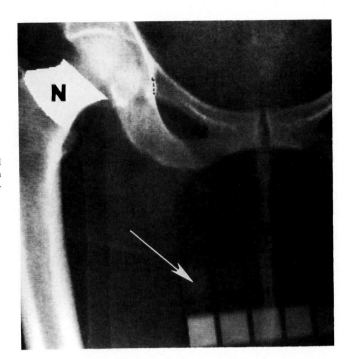

Figure 18–6. Dual-energy projection radiography of the proximal portion of the femur. Representative patient scan image includes an irregular region of interest encompassing the femoral neck (N) and multichambered calibration phantom (arrow).

pressed using a multiple scanning slit device interfaced to a conventional digital subtraction angiography system. The technique employs a pair of calibration step wedges, one tissue-equivalent and one bone-equivalent, that obviate accurate calibration of kVp or the system's response to changes in bone mineral content. Preliminary phantom studies intended to simulate vertebral measurement have indicated that the technique is capable of determining bone mineral content with less than 30 mg/cm² inaccuracy.

COMPTON SCATTERING

Bone density in the distal portion of the radius has been determined by measuring the intensity of the Compton scattered photons, which is proportional to the absolute density of the scatterer (bone) for materials with constant atomic mass : atomic number ratios. A collimated beam from a 500 mCi cesium-137 source is used, with the intensity of the scattered radiation measured at an angle of 90 degrees. A good correlation has been found between density of the radius and the degree of morphologic change in the vertebrae. The density of trabecular bone in the calcaneus also has been measured using such a gamma ray (samarium-153, 103 keV photons) scattering technique. In normal subjects, it has been shown that density can be predicted from body weight and age in both sexes with a standard error of 5.6 per cent. When the calcaneus is subjected to greater than normal mechanical stress by either increased physical activity or excessive body weight, trabecular bone density increments can be documented by this method.

The ratio between the detected coherent and Compton scattered photons from bone can also be used to determine its mineral density. It is generally accepted that a small scatter angle is preferred to ensure adequate counting statistics by favoring the detection of more coherent photons. By increasing the scatter angle, however, smaller changes in the mineral density can be detected, thus improving the sensitivity of the measurement.

This approach has been used for determination of trabecular bone mineral density in the distal portion of the radius. The technique involves measurement of the intensity ratio using an americium-241 radionuclide (59.54 keV photons) as the highly collimated radiation source and a semiconductor crystal (germanium) as the detector. This method affords an accuracy of better than 2 per cent when varying quantities of materials surround the measurement site. A good correlation has been observed between bone ash content and the coherent-to-Compton scattering ratio. Trabecular bone mineral density has correlated well with the mineral density values obtained by single photon absorptiometry, and the technique is reproducible to within 3 per cent.

Conversion of the coherent-to-Compton ratio to bone mineral density requires calibration using bone simulating phantoms. These phantoms are made of bone ash suspended in white petrolatum in varying concentrations. A calibration curve has been established using these phantoms with a range of bone mineral density values from 0 to 347 mg/cm³, for application to calcaneal trabecular bone. The accuracy of the method at this site has been determined to be 5 per cent, whereas its precision is approximately 3 per cent. By this technique, calcaneal trabecular bone mineral density values for healthy men (22 to 77 years) are in the range of 180 to 357 mg/ml, for healthy women (18 to 73 years) are in the range of 160 to 321 mg/ml, and for paraplegic patients are in the range of 90 to 199 mg/ml. Although trabecular bone mineral density may not be uniform within the calcaneus, a region exists in the bone over which the variation is not large. This tissue volume coincides with the midportion of the heel and is the site chosen for application of the coherent-to-Compton scattering ratio technique (Fig. 18–8).

PROTON ACTIVATION ANALYSIS

The feasibility of a new method for in vivo regional bone calcium measurement has been studied in phantoms using a 160 MeV cyclotron. Advantages include the capability of

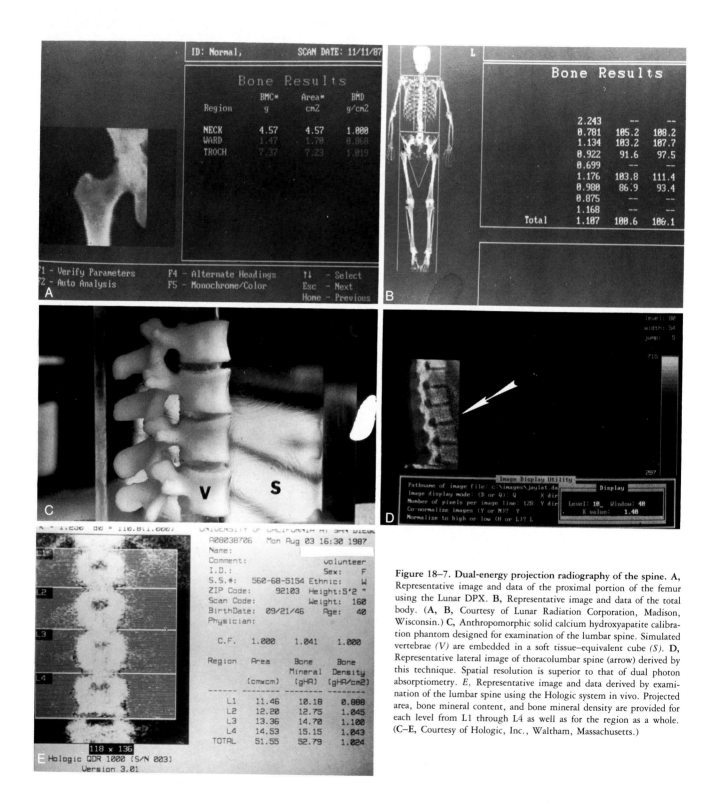

Figure 18–7. Dual-energy projection radiography of the spine. A, Representative image and data of the proximal portion of the femur using the Lunar DPX. **B,** Representative image and data of the total body. (**A, B,** Courtesy of Lunar Radiation Corporation, Madison, Wisconsin.) **C,** Anthropomorphic solid calcium hydroxyapatite calibration phantom designed for examination of the lumbar spine. Simulated vertebrae *(V)* are embedded in a soft tissue–equivalent cube *(S)*. **D,** Representative lateral image of thoracolumbar spine (arrow) derived by this technique. Spatial resolution is superior to that of dual photon absorptiometry. *E,* Representative image and data derived by examination of the lumbar spine using the Hologic system in vivo. Projected area, bone mineral content, and bone mineral density are provided for each level from L1 through L4 as well as for the region as a whole. (C–E, Courtesy of Hologic, Inc., Waltham, Massachusetts.)

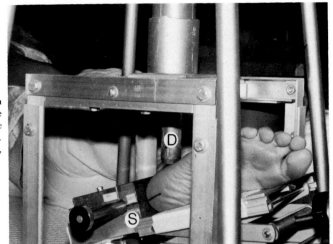

Figure 18–8. Experimental arrangement for measuring the ratio between Compton and coherent scattered photons (CCSR technique) in the calcaneus. The subject's heel is maintained in a lateral position for the examination. *S,* source collimator; *D,* detector collimator. (Courtesy of M. A. Greenfield, Ph.D., J. Craven, Ph.D., and S. Shukla, Ph.D., Los Angeles, California.)

measuring bone calcium directly in a well-defined anatomic site (such as one or several vertebrae or the hand) and restriction of the dose to the immediate region of interest (Fig. 18–9). Proton activation of calcium-40 (97 per cent natural abundance) produces the radionuclide potassium-38, and its 2.17 MeV gamma ray (T 1/2 = 7.71 minutes) is detected by a sodium iodide counter. Phantom studies have shown ^{38}K activity to be highly correlated with calcium content (r = 0.998). Nonlinearities with dose do not appear below the 20 rad level. The precision of phantom measurements at 2.4 rad is 3 per cent and chiefly limited by counting statistics. System reproducibility on phantoms given higher doses has proved better than 0.5 per cent.

High energy proton activation analysis has the ability to achieve very precise localization of the activation volume within a target volume as well as uniform yield for the activation reaction over a predetermined depth in the target. The technique has been applied to measurement of whole body calcium content in animals and to determination of the calcium-to-phosphate molar ratio in small quantities of chemical and biologic samples. Animal experiments have demonstrated the ability to achieve uniform irradiation over a large volume utilizing large sodium iodide crystals with a special chamber for combined detection efficiency, whereas the calcium-to-phosphate molar ratio determination requires a germanium-lithium detector and analysis of the resulting gamma ray spectrum.

QUANTITATIVE MAGNETIC RESONANCE IMAGING

The feasibility of quantitative magnetic resonance imaging of bone marrow has recently been demonstrated. T1 and T2 relaxation times for lumbar vertebral marrow have shown a progressive decrease with age for both sexes, with the exception of the T2 parameter in women, a phenomenon explainable by replacement of hematopoietic marrow by fatty marrow. More rapid and significant loss of bone mineral content may

Figure 18–9. Proton activation analysis for determining calcium content in the hands. A, Alignment radiograph taken before irradiation. A dose of 2.6 rad confined entirely to the hand is given in about 20 seconds. B, Holder used to position the hand for irradiation. Two pins hold the wrist and the clenched configuration is acceptable because of uniform yield over a 10 cm depth in tissue. (Courtesy of J. Sisterson, Ph.D., and A.M. Koehler, Ph.D., Cambridge, Massachusetts.)

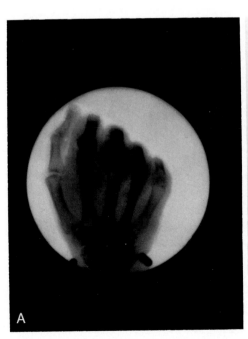

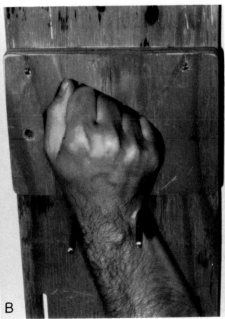

be responsible for the observation that T1 and T2 values are slightly greater among older women than men of comparable age. Because fat deposition within bone marrow tends to vary inversely with trabecular bone density, it is possible that magnetic resonance imaging may be capable of indirectly predicting the latter parameter in the future. The successful implementation of this concept for longitudinal follow-up will ultimately depend on the development of calibration phantoms designed to compensate for variations in magnetic field inhomogeneity and radiofrequency signal sensitivity.

FURTHER READING

Cann CE, Genant HK: Single versus dual energy CT for vertebral mineral quantification. J Comput Assist Tomogr 7:551, 1983.

Genant HK, Cann CE, Ettinger B, Gordan GS, Kolb FO, Reiser V, Arnaud CD: Quantitative computed tomography for spinal mineral assessment: Current status. J Comput Assist Tomogr 9:602, 1985.

Kimmel PL: Radiologic methods to evaluate bone mineral content. Ann Intern Med 100:908, 1984.

Mack LA, Hanson JA, Kilcoyne RF, Ott SM, Gallagher JC, Chesnut CH: Correlation between fracture index and bone densitometry by CT and dual-photon absorptiometry. J Comput Assist Tomogr 9:635, 1985.

Nordin BE, Robertson A, Chatterton BE, Steurer T, Bridges A, Huber T: Comparison of forearm and spinal densitometry in postmenopausal women. J Comput Assist Tomogr 9:628, 1985.

Sambrook PN, Bartlett C, Evans R, Hesp R, Katz D, Reeve J: Measurement of lumbar spine bone mineral: A comparison of dual-photon absorptiometry and computed tomography. Br J Radiol 58:621, 1985.

Wahner HW, Dunn WL, Mazess RB, Towsley M, Lindsay R, Marknard L, Dempster D: Dual-photon (153-Gd) absorptiometry of bone. Radiology 156:203, 1985.

SECTION III
POSTOPERATIVE IMAGING

CASE III   LEVEL OF DIFFICULTY: 3

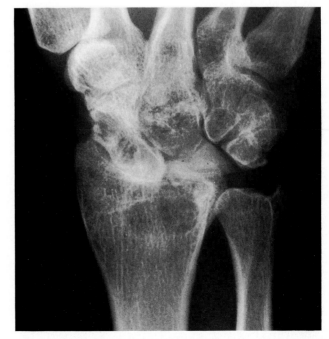

A 30 year old man noted increasing pain, local swelling, and limitation of motion in the wrist. He had had a previous surgical procedure performed on this wrist.

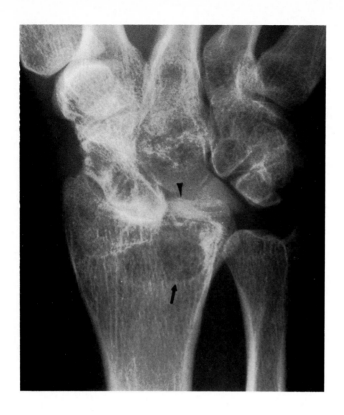

A single posteroanterior radiograph of the wrist (Case III) reveals cystic and erosive lesions within the scaphoid, capitate, hamate, triquetrum, and, especially, distal portion of the radius (arrow). There is joint space loss in the radiocarpal compartment. Although the abnormalities superficially resemble those of rheumatoid arthritis, the correct diagnosis is provided by additional observations. The absence of visible trabeculae within the lunate indicates that the true bone has been replaced with a silicone implant. Furthermore, this implant appears deformed, with loss of height on its radial aspect (arrowhead), and narrowing of the radiolunate and lunate-capitate spaces is seen. The combination of a deformed silicone implant and cystic and erosive abnormalities throughout the wrist is indicative of silicone-induced synovitis. Presumably, the prosthesis had been used for the treatment of Kienböck's disease.

Although flexible silicone implants have been utilized effectively for more than 20 years as replacements for small bones and joints in the hand and foot, synovitis related to a foreign body reaction is recognized as a rare but significant postoperative complication. Silicone implants, which are known for their flexibility and durability, actually may partially disintegrate, and small fragments of the prosthesis become embedded in the synovial membrane, where they lead to synovitis. This complication may occur at variable periods of time after the surgery, although accompanying symptoms and signs may be delayed for more than 1 year after the operative procedure. The resulting foreign body giant cell reaction produces cystic and erosive abnormalities of adjacent bones, which may be combined with deformity of the prosthesis and joint space loss.

Although the differential diagnosis of erosive arthritis of the wrist includes a variety of articular disorders, such as rheumatoid arthritis, gout, pigmented villonodular synovitis, infection, and amyloidosis, recognition of a deformed prosthesis ensures accurate interpretation of the radiographs. Removal of the implant usually reveals a roughened, pitted, and discolored prosthetic surface, and histologic analysis confirms the diagnosis of silicone-induced arthritis.

FINAL DIAGNOSIS: Silicone-induced arthritis of the wrist.

FURTHER READINGS

Pages 238–240 and the following:

1. Smith RJ, Atkinson RE, Jupiter JB: Silicone synovitis of the wrist. J Hand Surg [Am] *10*:47, 1985.
2. Schneider HJ, Weiss MA, Stern PJ: Silicone-induced erosive arthritis: Radiologic features in 7 cases. AJR *148*:923, 1987.

(Case III, courtesy of Naval Hospital, San Diego, California.)

Chapter 19

Imaging After Bone Surgery

Barbara N. Warren Weissman, M.D.

Knowledge of orthopedic devices and techniques is a prerequisite to accurate interpretation of postoperative radiographs. A variety of internal fixation devices, external fixation devices, and polymethylmethacrylate cement are used in fracture fixation. Electrical stimulation may be *used to promote fracture healing, and numerous techniques of bone grafting are described. Resection arthroplasty, arthrodesis, and osteotomy represent additional orthopedic methods.*

This chapter provides a brief description of some of the more commonly encountered orthopedic devices and techniques. Essential principles that are fundamental to the correct interpretation of pertinent imaging studies are provided.

FRACTURE FIXATION

Fixation refers to the maintaining of fracture fragments during healing. Hardware may be placed directly across the fracture site (internal fixation), or the area may be immobilized by casts or by appliances fixed to the adjacent bone (external fixation).

Internal Fixation Devices

Internal fixation devices are usually inserted after open reduction of the fracture fragments. In some cases, however, percutaneous placement of internal fixation devices may follow closed fracture reduction.

Wires, pins, nails, and rods generally are distinguished on the basis of size. Wires (e.g., Kirschner wires) are thinner than pins (e.g., Steinmann pins). Either may be smooth or threaded. Kirschner wires are used for percutaneous or open fixation of fractures involving the small bones of the hands and feet.

INTRAMEDULLARY NAILS AND RODS. Intramedullary rods are used primarily for the treatment of closed transverse or short oblique midshaft fractures of the long bones. Rods should be strong enough to resist angular deformity, but their ability to resist rotation (torque) is limited unless an interlocking mechanism is incorporated into the nail design. Compression can occur at the fracture site with telescoping along the rod. Insertion of an intramedullary rod damages the blood supply to the endosteum; therefore, healing occurs exclusively by periosteal new bone formation and organization of the hematoma at the fracture site. Once healing occurs, the rods are usually removed.

Nails generally are thinner than rods. The *Kuntscher nail* is rigid, clover-leaf shaped in cross section, and split longitudinally for part of its length so that it can expand when bone resorption occurs around it. *Ender nails* are slightly curved, round in cross section, and semi-elastic. These latter nails may be used for the treatment of femoral, humeral, or tibial fractures but are used most often for intertrochanteric fractures (Fig. 19–1).

Complications of intramedullary pins, rods, and nails include splitting of the shaft of the bone; inability to advance or withdraw the nail; separation of fracture fragments; pene-

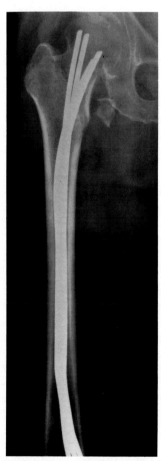

Figure 19–1. Healing intertrochanteric fracture after insertion of Ender nails. Four Ender nails have been threaded across the intertrochanteric fracture site. The nails fill the medullary canal and their proximal tips fan out in the femoral head.

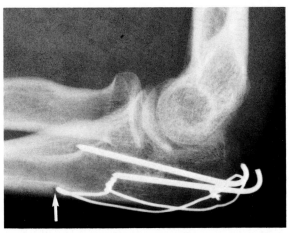

Figure 19–3. Tension band wiring. A lateral radiograph after the treatment of an olecranon fracture shows a tension band wire extending through a drill hole in the ulna distally (arrow) and around Kirschner wires proximally.

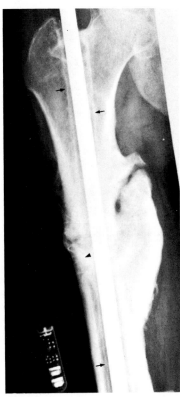

Figure 19–2. Hypertrophic nonunion. Motion of the rod is documented by the radiolucent zones around it (arrows). The fracture has not healed despite the large amount of periosteal reaction medially. An electrical stimulation device with a helical cathode (arrowhead) is present. (From Weissman BN, Sledge CB: Orthopedic Radiology. Philadelphia, WB Saunders Co, 1986. Used with permission.)

tration of the nail into an adjacent joint; pain from a prominent end of the fixation device; inadequate immobilization of the fracture (leading to nonunion) (Fig. 19–2); fracture, bending, or loosening of the rod; migration of the rod; fracture at the site of Ender nail insertion; fat embolization; rod corrosion; and spread of infection along the shaft of the bone. When loosening of an intramedullary nail occurs, periosteal callus formation is abundant and may extend along the entire length of the diaphysis.

WIRES. Wires may be placed around the fracture fragments (cerclage) for compression. This technique, termed tension band wiring, relies on the neutralization of tensile forces on a bone so that compression alone occurs at the fracture site (Fig. 19–3).

SCREWS. Cortical screws are threaded over their entire length. They are primarily used to secure plates or nail-plate devices to bone (Fig. 19–4). Cancellous lag screws are threaded distally and have smooth proximal shafts (Fig. 19–4). The threads are wider than those of cortical screws so that they hold better in cancellous bone. When cancellous screws are used to produce compression across a fracture, the threaded portion of the screw should be completely within the distal fracture fragment, and the screw threads should not cross the fracture line.

The sliding screw plate (e.g., the Richards compression screw) is used primarily in the treatment of intertrochanteric

fractures. This device provides fixation while allowing impaction to occur at the fracture during healing and weight-bearing. It consists of a lag screw and a side plate with a barrel (Fig. 19–5). The threaded portion of the screw is placed in the femoral head, and its shaft is inserted into the barrel of the side plate. The tip of the lag screw should be located centrally within the femoral head and lie about one half inch from the articular surface. The side plate should lie flush with the femoral shaft, and the screws attaching it to the cortex should just penetrate the far cortex. The degree of telescoping of the sliding screw is measured by noting the change in the distance from the end of the barrel to the first screw thread on the initial radiographs in comparison to the most current examination.

Several complications of sliding screw plate fixation occur. "Cutting out" of the nail can be limited by correct placement of the screw (Fig. 19–6). Penetration of the screw into the joint may occur owing to failure of the device to telescope. Bending or breaking of the nail is usually caused by nonunion of the fracture. Occasionally the screw will become disengaged from the barrel. Stress fracture of the femur proximal to the screw, bending or breaking of the side plate, and rotation of the femoral head on the lag screw are additional complications of sliding screw plate fixation.

PLATES. A plate can be used to provide one or more of the following functions: static or dynamic compression, neutralization, and buttressing (Fig. 19–7). Static compression refers to the production of axial compression along cortical fractures, with the potential advantages of more rigid fixation, a smaller fracture gap to be bridged, and reduction in the external immobilization required. Compression can be achieved either by attaching a tension device to a plate at the time of internal fixation or by using a particular type of plate, the dynamic compression plate. This latter type of plate has screw holes with sloped sides that correspond to the slope of the undersurface of the screw. As the screws are tightened, the bone fragment in which the screw is inserted is shifted toward the center of the plate, thus producing compression at the fracture line.

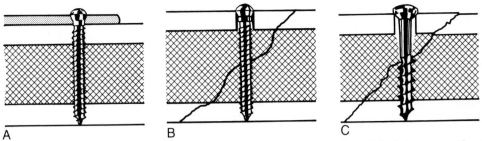

Figure 19–4. Cortical and cancellous screws. A The cortical screw is often used to secure plates to bone. **B** Cortical screws may function as lag screws by overdrilling the proximal cortex so that only the distal threads engage bone. **C** The cancellous (lag) screw has distal threads and a smooth proximal shaft. The threads are more widely spaced than those of a cortical screw.

A neutralization plate bridges a comminuted fracture and transmits bending or torsional forces from the proximal to the distal fragment, protecting the intervening fracture fragments from these forces. Plates used for buttressing support an area of thin cortex or cancellous bone graft, preventing collapse.

The bone under the plate may atrophy, predisposing to fracture and necessitating protection of the extremity after the plate is removed.

External Fixation Devices

External fixation of fractures provides immobilization of fractures while maintaining the potential for adjusting fracture position. External fixators also may be used for compression at sites of attempted fusion (Fig. 19–8) and for distraction during attempted limb lengthening. Several devices are now available that consist of one or more frames anchored to the bone with pins.

Some indications for external fixation of fractures include open fractures in which comminution is present, especially when there is segmental bone loss and soft tissue damage; the presence of major vascular damage requiring repair; severe osteoporosis; and extensive epiphyseal and metaphyseal comminution. External fixators are also used in the treatment of

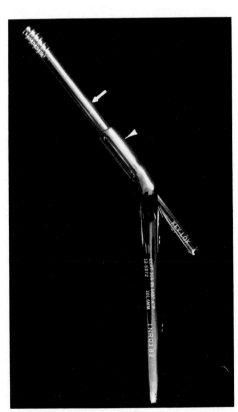

Figure 19–5. Sliding screw plate. The lag screw (arrow) can telescope through the barrel (arrowhead) of the side plate as bone resorption occurs at the fracture site.

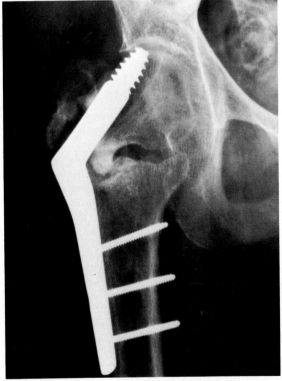

Figure 19–6. Nonunion of intertrochanteric fracture with "cutting out" of compression screw. The compression screw tip was positioned in the lateral half of the femoral head. No compression of the screw could occur because the screw threads are already abutting on the barrel. The cortical screws holding the side plate are unnecessarily long and could cause soft tissue injury. Collapse of the fracture into a varus position and nonunion have occurred, causing the tip of the screw to "cut out" laterally.

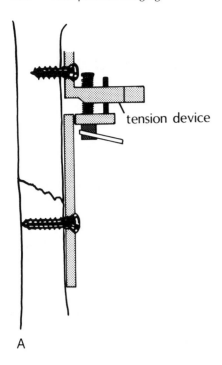

tension device

A

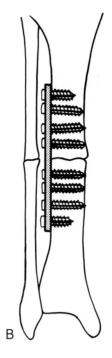

B

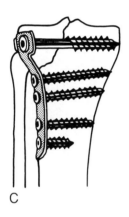

C

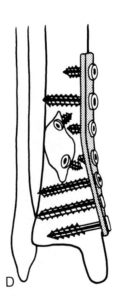

D

Figure 19–7. Functions of plates. A Static compression. **B** Dynamic compression after correction of nonunion with varus deformity. **C** Buttressing. **D** Neutralization. (Redrawn after Muller ME, et al: Manual of Internal Fixation, Technique Recommended by the AO Group. J Schatzker, et al, Transl. New York, Springer-Verlag, 1979. Used with permission.)

infected, nonunited fractures and during healing of free vascularized bone grafts.

Several complications are associated with the use of external fixation. Pin tract infections are most frequent when large amounts of soft tissue are traversed by the pins. Soft tissue damage may lead to pain and contracture. Delayed union or nonunion may result from distraction of fracture fragments and long periods without weight-bearing while the external fixation apparatus is being employed.

Polymethylmethacrylate

In patients with metastatic disease of the long bones or pelvis, polymethylmethacrylate cement has been used as an adjunct to internal fixation so that prompt weight-bearing

and pain relief are achieved. Polymethylmethacrylate instilled into an area of cortical destruction increases the strength of that bone. This substance can be used in the treatment of pathologic fractures, as its presence apparently does not interfere with local radiation therapy.

Cement has also been used to improve fracture fixation in osteoporosis and in spinal fusion.

ELECTRICAL STIMULATION

Bone formation can be stimulated by applying an electrical current; either direct current stimulation or pulsing electromagnetic fields may be used. Direct current stimulation requires placement of the cathode into the fracture or nonunion site. The anode is placed on the skin. Pulsing electro-

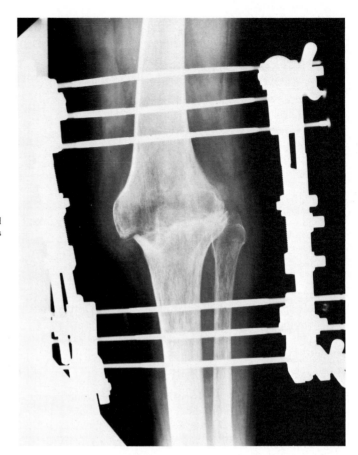

Figure 19–8. External fixation used for compression. An infected prosthesis has been removed. The external fixation (Hoffman) apparatus maintains compression at the site of attempted fusion.

magnetic fields are used by applying an external apparatus over the fracture site. The apparatus is connected to household current for 10 to 12 hours per day.

Fracture healing after electrical stimulation occurs in about 80 per cent of cases, a frequency of healing that is similar to that of bone graft surgery. Contraindications to electrical stimulation include the presence of a pseudarthrosis with a fluid-filled cavity, a large gap at the fracture site, or active infection.

BONE GRAFTS
Terminology

Bone grafts are described according to their origins, the type of bone used for grafting, and the method of graft placement (Table 19–1).

The types of bone used for grafting include cortical bone, cancellous bone, or both cortical and cancellous bone. Cancellous bone grafts are used primarily to promote osteogenesis, whereas cortical bone grafts are used to provide structural stability. When corticocancellous bone grafts are used, they are positioned so that the cancellous surface abuts on the soft tissues to facilitate vascular ingrowth.

Table 19–1. ORIGINS OF BONE GRAFTS

Autografts: The transplanted bone is derived from the same person or animal.
Allografts (homografts): The transplanted material is derived from another person or animal of the same species.
Xenografts (heterografts): The transplanted material is derived from a member of a different species.

Grafts may also be described according to their composition, position, and shape. Onlay grafts consist of cortical bone that is placed across a bony defect (such as a nonunion) and held by screws to a surgically denuded or drilled surface of the host bone. The sliding inlay graft consists of bone cut from the proximal fragment and slid distally across a bony defect. The dowel graft consists of a core of cancellous bone that is inserted into a surgically created channel to stimulate osteogenesis. Muscle pedicle grafts, which are used primarily in the treatment of femoral neck fractures, consist of a segment of bone that includes the insertion of the quadratus femoris muscle. Strut grafts, often composed of a rib or fibula, provide stability and are most often used in the spine.

Indications

Bone grafts generally are used to promote healing or provide stability, or both. Situations in which bone grafting may be used include filling of bony defects; bridging of joints for arthrodesis; and promoting union in cases of delayed union, nonunion, or osteotomy.

Bone Formation After Grafting

Cancellous bone grafts have greater capacity to induce new bone formation than do cortical grafts. If the cancellous graft is immobile, a process of "creeping substitution" takes place, in which new bone is deposited on the scaffold of dead trabeculae. Allografts generally are less satisfactory than autografts in that bone formation is slower and vascular penetration is slower and less dense. Rejection because of sensitization of the host by antigens in the graft is a major

Table 19–2. SOME COMPARISONS BETWEEN CANCELLOUS AND CORTICAL BONE GRAFTS

Cancellous Graft	Cortical Graft
Better survival of osteogenic cells because the structure allows diffusion and early microvascular anastomoses	Dense bone is a barrier to diffusion
Large endosteal surface supplies osteoprogenitor cells	Small endosteal surface
Abundant red marrow supplies many osteoprogenitor cells	Fewer osteoprogenitor cells
Healing by creeping substitution; new bone is deposited on dead trabeculae followed by removal of necrotic matrix	Removal of necrotic matrix from around the central canals of osteons occurs first followed by new bone formation
Relatively weak	Relatively strong

drawback of allografts, although freezing of allograft material may decrease its antigenicity.

A comparison of cancellous and cortical bone grafts is provided in Table 19–2.

Vascularized Bone Grafts

As the incorporation of conventional cortical or cancellous grafts requires necrosis in the graft material followed by ingrowth of granulation tissue, techniques have been developed that allow bone grafts and their associated vasculature to be transplanted so that the grafts remain viable. The relative advantages and disadvantages of this technique are debated. Vascularized bone grafting takes hours to perform, and the procedure is, therefore, usually reserved for cases of massive bone loss, those in which more conventional techniques have failed, or those in which an inadequate soft tissue bed is present.

Donor Sites

The most frequently used donor sites for bone grafting are the iliac crest, tibia, fibula, greater trochanter, distal portion of the radius, and the posterior elements of the spine. Complications at donor graft sites appear to be few. Nonetheless, fracture may occur after cortical graft removal (e.g., from the tibia), and intraoperative bleeding and postoperative pain may follow iliac crest biopsy.

Radiologic Examination

At follow-up examinations, healing of iliac donor sites is seen to occur with sclerosis at the margins of the osseous defects. Graft healing is generally documented by loss of the sharp margins between the graft and the host bone, eventually leading to osseous union with bone continuity across the graft-host junction. Fibrous union is suggested by the persistence of a thin residual radiolucent area between the graft and the host bone. The time required to achieve union depends on the size and the type of graft, the local conditions, and the site of the surgery.

Scintigraphic Examination

In vascularized bone grafts, the accumulation of the bone scanning agent in the area of the graft within the first week after transplantation indicates both an intact vasculature and metabolically viable bone; conversely, the absence of such uptake of the bone scanning agent on serial radionuclide examinations suggests segmental nonviability (Fig. 19–9). Accumulation of the bone-seeking radionuclide after this 1 week period, however, may be due to the laying down of new bone on the surface of dead trabeculae and does not indicate either vascular patency or the presence of viable graft.

Complications

Graft failure may be associated with progressive bone resorption, leading to a decrease in the size and density of the graft and ultimately to its disappearance. Similar graft resorption may be due to recurrent tumor or infection. Stress fractures within cortical grafts are not uncommon.

RESECTION ARTHROPLASTY

Resection arthroplasties consist of the removal of one or both articular surfaces of a joint. Currently these techniques are used primarily as salvage procedures after failed total joint replacement surgery.

Girdlestone Arthroplasty

Although it was developed as a resection arthroplasty for secondarily infected tuberculous hips, the Girdlestone arthroplasty currently is thought of primarily as a salvage procedure, performed when an infected total hip prosthesis is removed. It is also used in some instances of infectious arthritis in preference to hip fusion. Indeed, the term "Girdlestone arthroplasty" is currently applied in a general sense to any hip joint resection.

A Girdlestone arthroplasty may be used in the treatment of an infection after total hip replacement. Various conditions have been reported to be an indication for Girdlestone arthroplasty after total hip replacement (Table 19–3). The results of Girdlestone arthroplasty after removal of an infected hip prosthesis indicate that pain relief and control of infection occur in over 80 per cent of patients. Shortening of the affected extremity, a Trendelenburg gait, and joint instability are invariable sequelae that make walking difficult and tiring, however. Radiographs confirm complete removal of the femoral neck, acetabular rim, and polymethylmethacrylate cement (Fig. 19–10). Although optimally all cement is removed, residual cement does not necessarily result in continued infection.

ARTHRODESIS (JOINT FUSION)

Arthrodesis refers to the surgical stiffening of a joint (derived from the Greek *arthron*, meaning "joint," and *desis*, "a binding together"). Such surgery is usually performed to provide stability or to relieve pain resulting from joint damage owing to prior infection, injury, or failed joint replacement surgery. The bony fusion performed may be intraarticular, extraarticular, or a combination of the two.

Ankle

Ankle arthrodesis remains a valuable procedure for the alleviation of pain due to arthritis, the treatment of paralytic instability, and salvage after a failed total ankle replacement. Results after ankle fusion are surprisingly good. Adequate function after ankle fusion is believed to be attributable to compensatory motion of the small joints of the ipsilateral

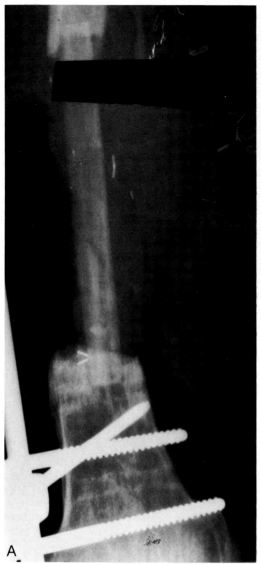

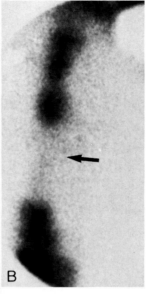

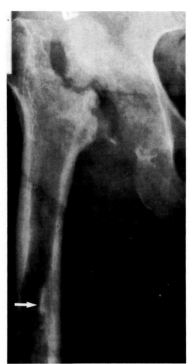

Figure 19–10. Girdlestone arthroplasty. This patient had an infected total hip prosthesis. Some cement remains in the femoral canal (arrow). Infection recurred at the area of retained cement.

Figure 19–9. Absent blood flow to vascularized graft. A A vascularized bone graft was used to bridge a defect created by the removal of a long segment of bone affected with chronic osteomyelitis. B A bone scan shows absent isotope uptake in the graft (arrow), suggesting nonviability.

foot, altered motion of the ankle of the contralateral limb, making gait symmetric, and the use of footwear with an appropriate heel height.

More than 20 techniques for achieving tibiotalar fusion have been developed. The Charnley compression arthrodesis consists of resection of the articular surfaces of the tibia and talus and compression of these surfaces to eliminate shear and maintain bone apposition. Optimal foot position for ankle arthrodesis has been debated, but current studies imply that fusion should be done with the foot in the neutral position in both men and women. Greater than 10 degrees of plantar flexion of the foot may be associated with postoperative pain (Fig. 19–11), and no varus or valgus angulation of the foot should be present.

Radiographically identifiable complications after ankle arthrodesis include pseudarthrosis, malunion, infection, and osteoarthritis of the small joints of the foot.

Hip

Recent reports indicating a high rate of failure after total hip replacement in young persons have sparked renewed interest in hip fusion as a primary procedure and as a salvage procedure after failed total hip replacement. Successful hip

Table 19–3. SOME INDICATIONS FOR GIRDLESTONE ARTHROPLASTY

Presence of virulent, resistant organisms
Presence of gram-negative organisms
Presence of two or more strains of organisms
Unhealthy and edematous soft tissues
Draining sinus
Radiographic evidence of well-established osteomyelitis with bone erosion
Severe loss of bone substance

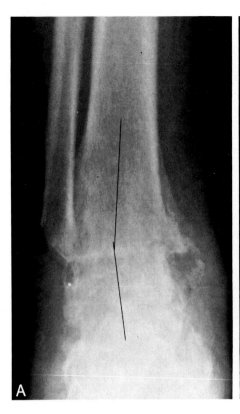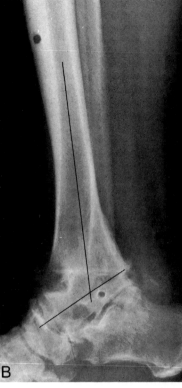

Figure 19–11. Ankle fusion. A The anteroposterior view shows no remaining radiolucency along the tibiotalar surface, indicating healing. There is varus alignment between the long axis of the tibia and that of the talus. **B** On the lateral view, the angle between the long axis of the tibia and the long axis of the talus (through its midportion) has been used to determine the degree of plantar flexion.

arthrodesis results in a painless, stable hip and the ability to engage in strenuous activity. It is, therefore, a procedure to be considered in young patients with incapacitating pain from unilateral hip damage. A large number of techniques have been introduced to achieve intraarticular, combined intra- and extraarticular, or purely extraarticular fusion.

The degree of hip abduction after fusion may be documented on radiographs using a horizontal reference line (along the bottom of the sacroiliac joints or the ischia) and a line drawn along the femoral shaft; similarly, the position of hip flexion may be evaluated on lateral radiographs. It appears that hip flexion of about 30 degrees results in the greatest patient comfort. The appropriate degree of hip abduction depends on the amount of shortening of the leg that is present; when there is no shortening, slight adduction of the fused hip produces the most normal gait. In adults, the leg is usually fused in a position of 5 to 15 degrees of external rotation.

The results of hip fusion are generally good. The major complications relate to the inability to achieve solid fusion and the long-term effect of such surgery on other joints. Malposition, defined as the presence of greater than 15 degrees of adduction or abduction or 60 degrees or more of flexion, may also occur. Back and ipsilateral or contralateral knee pain may be prominent.

Spine

Spinal fusions are performed in a wide variety of circumstances to establish and maintain physiologic alignment, to eliminate abnormal motion, and to avoid the development of fixed deformity after injury.

Fusion may be accomplished anteriorly or posteriorly or by a combination of both procedures (Table 19–4). Anterior fusions involve removal of the intervertebral disc and, in some procedures, the adjacent vertebral endplates or entire vertebral bodies. Bone grafts are usually interposed between the remaining vertebral surfaces, although in unusual circumstances, polymethylmethacrylate and metallic fixation devices may fill this gap (Fig. 19–12). Anterior fusions are used in cases of trauma when it is necessary to remove disc or bone fragments that are encroaching on the spinal cord or nerve roots. Posterior stability is necessary before anterior fusion is performed. In the lumbar region, anterior fusions have definite advantages, enabling the surgeon to avoid sites of previous surgery and decreasing the possibility of nerve root trauma. Disadvantages of anterior fusion include a possible lack of physician familiarity with the anterior surgical approach, a relatively long operative time, the large amount of bone graft that may be needed, and a relatively high rate of pseudarthrosis.

Posterior fusions are used in cases of trauma when there is gross posterior ligament disruption that allows anterior subluxation or dislocation. Bone may be placed between the transverse processes of adjacent vertebrae (intertransverse fusion) (Fig. 19–13). The advantages of intertransverse fusion over a posterior fusion alone include the absence of postoperative bone hypertrophy that may narrow the spinal canal, the absence of postoperative spondylolisthesis because the region of the pars interarticularis is reinforced during fusion, and the presence of resistance to torsional stress.

INSTRUMENTS. Several devices employed during spine arthrodesis provide immediate postoperative stability, but long-term stability depends on the bone fusion established by the solidification of bone grafts.

Harrington distraction rods may be used in cases of trauma when the anterior longitudinal ligament is intact and in

Table 19–4. TECHNIQUES OF SPINAL FUSION

Type of Fusion	Description	Type of Fusion	Description
Cervical			**Thoracic and Lumbar**
Anterior		*Anterior*	Usually not performed as an isolated procedure, but in combination with posterior fusion when anterior access to spinal canal is needed
Smith-Robinson	Removal of the disc and insertion of a slice of iliac crest (bone plug)		
Cloward	The disc and part of the vertebrae are removed and a bone dowel is inserted	*Posterior Lumbar Interbody* (PLIF) (Cloward)	Through a posterior approach, the disc and adjacent cartilage endplates and vertebral cortices are removed and bone grafts are tightly positioned within the created defect
Strut graft	An entire vertebral body is removed and a strut from tibia or iliac bone is notched into the two neighboring vertebral bodies		
Posterior		*Posterior*	
McLauren	The arch of C1 is fused with wires to the spinous process of C2	Intertransverse	Grafts are placed between the transverse processes or along the prepared surfaces of the posterolateral aspects of the facet joints and laminae and the transverse processes
Rogers	One or two wires are sewn or wound around bases of spinous processes; an onlay bone graft is often used		
Sublaminar fusion	The stabilizing wires pass under the laminae and into the epidural space; onlay bone graft can also be placed	Hibbs	The spinous processes are removed, the facet joints excised, and the laminae scraped; fusion is done by interdigitating small bone slivers raised from these areas and then using additional bone graft
Yale fusion	Performed with previous laminectomy; the facets of contiguous vertebrae are wired together		
		Albee	The spinous processes are united by tibial bone graft

From Calenoff L, et al: CRC Crit Rev Diagn Imaging 23:269, 1985, and Weissman BNW, Sledge CB: Orthopedic Radiology. Philadelphia, WB Saunders, 1986. Used with permission.

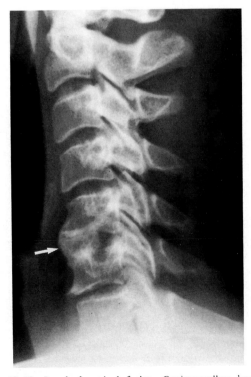

Figure 19–12. Interbody spinal fusion. Corticocancellous bone graft (arrow) has been inserted in the intervertebral disc at the C5–C6 spinal level. The inferior junction between the graft and the C6 vertebral body is blurred, consistent with healing. A thin lucent line remains superiorly.

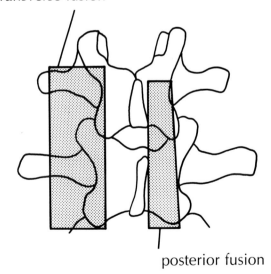

intertransverse fusion

posterior fusion

Figure 19–13. Diagram of areas involved in intertransverse and posterior spinal fusions. The posterior fusion involves the facet joints and laminae. The intertransverse fusion is more extensive and includes the pars interarticularis of the most proximal vertebra. (Redrawn after MacNab I, Dall D: The blood supply of the lumbar spine and its application to the technique of intertransverse lumbar fusion. J Bone Joint Surg [Br] 53:628, 1971. Used with permission.)

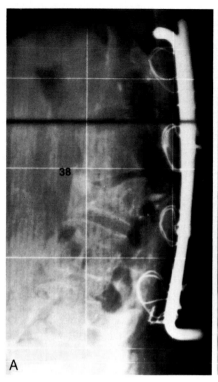
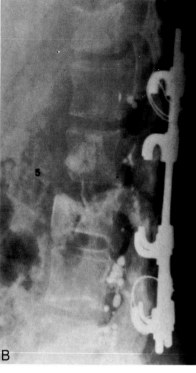

Figure 19–14. Posterior spinal fusion. A Insertion of Luque rods and posterior grafting were done as a revision procedure following trauma with vertebral fracture and kyphosis. A 38 degree kyphosis remains. B Revision surgery with Harrington compression rods and posterior graft led to correction of the kyphosis (which now measures 5 degrees). The deformities of the L2 and L3 vertebrae are visible.

patients with scoliosis. The hooks of the distraction rod are inserted under the laminae of the most superior and most inferior vertebrae to be included in the fusion. Distraction is accomplished by advancing the proximal hook on the ratcheted end of the rod until the hook can no longer be advanced. The rods may be bent to conform to the shape of the spine.

Harrington compression rods (Fig. 19–14) may be used along the convexity of a scoliotic curve and in the treatment of multiple severe anterior compression fractures or severe kyphosis. The hooks are usually placed on the transverse processes of the vertebrae rather than on the laminae.

Weiss springs are compression devices that are hooked to the laminae. *Luque rods* are attached to the spine by a series of wires placed around the laminae (Fig. 19–14). These rods provide considerable stability so that the need for postoperative immobilization is reduced.

A *Dwyer fusion* is a form of anterior spinal fusion that is used in the treatment of patients with severe scoliosis related to paralysis, cerebral palsy, or absence of the posterior osseous elements. The intervertebral discs and vertebral endplates are removed, and bone graft is inserted between the vertebrae. A staple and screw are placed in each vertebral body along the convex side of the spinal curve so that the screw parallels the endplates and penetrates both vertebral cortices (Fig. 19–15). A cable extends through each screw, and tension is applied at each vertebral level.

COMPLICATIONS. Extrusion or displacement of the bone graft and accompanying kyphosis are the most common complications of anterior cervical fusion. Soft tissue complications of this procedure include damage to the great vessels and the esophagus, pneumothorax, vocal cord paralysis, and hematoma with tracheal compression. Complications related to posterior cervical fusion, which are less frequent than those after anterior cervical fusion, include spinal instability, ky-

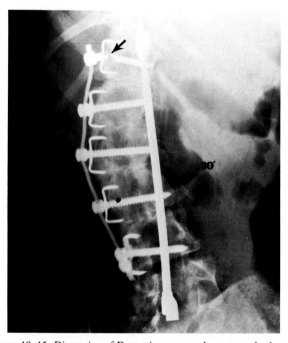

Figure 19–15. Disruption of Dwyer instrument due to pseudarthrosis. Dwyer procedure, Harrington distraction rod insertion, and anterior and posterior fusions had been done for the treatment of scoliosis. The T12-L1 intervertebral disc space remains unfused. The screw in L1 has broken (arrow) as a consequence of a T12-L1 pseudarthrosis. (From Weissman BN, Sledge CB: Orthopedic Radiology. Philadelphia, WB Saunders Co, 1986. Used with permission.)

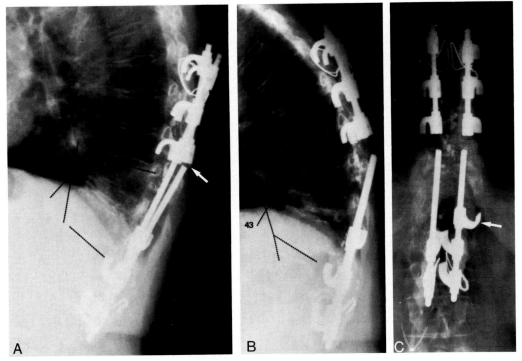

Figure 19–16. Fracture of Harrington rods. A This patient suffered a pathologic fracture of the T11 vertebra. Posterior spinal fusion was done with insertion of Harrington compression rods. A fracture of one of the rods (arrow) is noted. There is 25 degrees of kyphosis. **B** The kyphosis has now increased to 43 degrees, and both rods have fractured and separated. Therefore, the graft must also be disrupted. There is posterior displacement of T11. **C** The frontal view shows the disruption of the rods and the rotation of one of the hooks (arrow) so that it is no longer on the lamina.

phosis, and bowing of sublaminar wires leading to neurologic deficit.

Pseudarthrosis is the most frequent complication of posterior thoracolumbar spinal fusion. It leads to pain and loss of correction or fixation. Approximately 50 per cent of patients with the early onset of postoperative pain have a pseudarthrosis, whereas pain developing later than 18 months after surgery is generally unassociated with this complication. Conventional or computed tomography may be useful in the diagnosis of a pseudarthrosis.

Fracture of a Harrington rod usually occurs at the junction of its solid and ratcheted parts (Fig. 19–16). Although such disruption suggests that a pseudarthrosis is present, this is not always the case.

OSTEOTOMY

The term "osteotomy" refers to the surgical cutting of bone. Osteotomies are usually performed to correct or reduce deformity. In closing wedge osteotomy a triangular wedge of bone is removed from one side and the resection margins are approximated; an opening wedge osteotomy is performed by cutting the bone at an angle, causing one side to open. The defect is then filled with bone graft. A rotational osteotomy consists of rotating the distal fragment on its long axis. A displacement osteotomy involves a shift in the position of the distal fragment with relation to the proximal one.

High Tibial Osteotomy

High tibial osteotomy is usually employed in active patients under 65 years of age with pain in the knee caused by osteoarthritis. The procedure is performed to correct abnormal angulation (e.g., varus deformity) and to shift stress to the less involved femorotibial compartment (e.g., lateral compartment). In patients older than 65 years, total knee replacement is the preferred procedure.

Standing views using 36 inch films that include the leg from hip to ankle are recommended for preoperative evaluation. Under normal circumstances, when points are drawn at the centers of the femoral head, the knee, and the ankle, they all fall on a straight line (the mechanical axis) (Fig. 19–17). This axis is altered in patients with genu varum or genu valgum (Fig. 19–18). A high tibial osteotomy attempts to restore the normal mechanical axis with overcorrection of about 3 to 5 degrees.

The Coventry high tibial osteotomy involves resection of a wedge of bone from the tibial metaphysis between the joint and the tibial tubercle. The thicker part of the wedge to be removed is located laterally (valgus osteotomy) in a patient with genu varum, so that when the bone margins are brought together, an overall valgus alignment of the knee is achieved. Because shortening of the leg is produced by the tibial osteotomy, an osteotomy of the fibular shaft, fibular head excision, or division of the proximal tibiofibular joint is necessary.

A barrel vault osteotomy represents an alternative surgical technique for treatment of the osteoarthritic knee. A curved osteotomy is performed proximal to the tibial tubercle. The fragments are then rotated appropriately.

Distal femoral supracondylar osteotomy is used when osteoarthritis is accompanied by a valgus deformity.

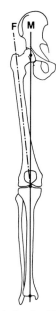

Figure 19–17. The mechanical axis. Normally, a straight line can be drawn from the center of the femoral head through the center of the knee to the center of the ankle. This is the mechanical axis (M). The femoral shaft axis (F) normally deviates from this axis.

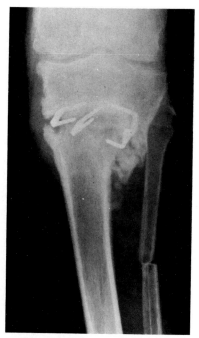

Figure 19–19. Nonunion of high tibial osteotomy. The osteotomy had been performed in a more distal location than usual. Hypertrophic nonunion at the osteotomy site has developed, with marked bone sclerosis and periosteal reaction. A fibular shaft osteotomy had also been done.

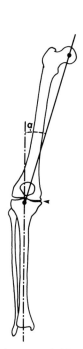

Figure 19–18. Deformity in osteoarthritis. The angle (a) between lines drawn connecting the center of the femoral head, the knee, and the tibial plafond is a measure of the deformity that is present. Medial cartilage space narrowing (arrowhead) with varus deformity is shown. (Redrawn after Maquet P: Treatment of osteoarthritis of the knee by osteotomy. In UH Weil [Ed]: Progress in Orthopedic Surgery, Vol 4. New York, Springer-Verlag, 1980. Used with permission.)

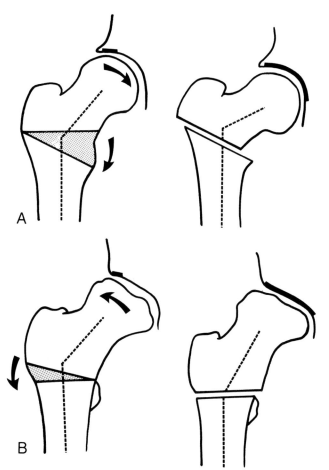

Figure 19–20. Femoral osteotomy. A Varus osteotomy. B Valgus osteotomy. (From Weissman BN, Sledge CB: Orthopedic Radiology. Philadelphia, WB Saunders Co, 1986. Used with permission.)

The average time required for healing of a high tibial osteotomy is 9 weeks. Complications after this procedure are infrequent. Fracture or ischemic necrosis of the proximal tibial fragment may occur, but infection and nonunion (Fig. 19–19) are rare.

Proximal Femoral Osteotomy

Candidates for proximal femoral osteotomy have pain owing to osteoarthritis of the hip and generally are younger than candidates for total hip replacement. Obese persons are not ideal subjects for this osteotomy. Hip flexion of at least 80 degrees and adduction or abduction of 15 degrees or more should be present.

An adduction, or varus, osteotomy (Fig. 19–20) is performed when the femoral head is essentially hemispherical, cartilage loss is evident in the superolateral portion of the joint, and the articulation is more congruent with the hip in abduction. An abduction, or valgus, osteotomy (Fig. 19–20) is considered when the femoral head is not hemispherical and when adduction improves congruency. Patients with insufficient acetabular coverage of the femoral head may undergo correction in more than one plane (i.e., valgus extension osteotomy). Extension and flexion refer to rotation of the femoral head posteriorly (extension) or anteriorly (flexion).

Postoperative radiographs document the degree of correction provided by the osteotomy, the healing of the osteotomy site, and any regression of the preoperative osteoarthritic changes. The osteotomy site heals gradually, with trabecular continuity normally achieved at about 4 months after surgery. Nonunion is indicated by the development of bone sclerosis and irregular bone resorption along the osteotomy surfaces.

FURTHER READING

Bowerman JW, Hughes JL: Radiology of bone grafts. Radiol Clin North Am 13:467, 1975.

Dawson EG, Clader TJ, Bassett LW: A comparison of different methods used to diagnose pseudarthrosis following posterior spinal fusion for scoliosis. J Bone Joint Surg [Am] 67:1153, 1985.

Foley MJ, Calenoff L, Hendrix RW, Schafer MF: Thoracic and lumbar spine fusion: Postoperative radiologic evaluation. AJR 141:373, 1983.

Ford LT: Osteotomies. Nomenclature and uses. Radiol Clin North Am 13:79, 1975.

Harrington KD, Sim FH, Enis JE, Johnston JO, Dick HM, Gristina AG: Methylmethacrylate as an adjunct in internal fixation of pathological fractures. J Bone Joint Surg [Am] 58:1047, 1976.

Heppenstall RB: Bone grafting. In RB Heppenstall: Fracture Treatment and Healing. Philadelphia, WB Saunders Co, 1980, p 89.

Kuntscher GBG: The Kuntscher method of intramedullary fixation. J Bone Joint Surg [Am] 40:17, 1958.

Lipscomb PR, McCaslin FE Jr: Arthrodesis of the hip. Review of 371 cases. J Bone Joint Surg [Am] 43:923, 1961.

Morgan CD, Henke JA, Bailey RW, Kaufer H: Long-term results of tibiotalar arthrodesis. J Bone Joint Surg [Am] 67:546, 1985.

Poss R: Current concepts review. The role of osteotomy in the treatment of osteoarthritis of the hip. J Bone Joint Surg [Am] 66:144, 1984.

Sartoris DJ, Kerr R, Georgen T, Resnick D: Sliding-screw plate fixation of proximal femoral fractures: Radiographic assessment. Skel Radiol 14:104, 1985.

Chapter 20

Imaging After Joint Surgery

Thomas G. Goergen, M.D.

In this chapter a limited but representative group of arthroplasty and related procedures are considered. Modern arthroplasty techniques have received the most attention; they represent the major thrust in reconstructive joint surgery. Radiographic evaluation of such procedures is facilitated by knowledge of material technology, treatment goals, and expected radiographic appearance. Generally, current concepts may be applied in judging the value of newer procedures and prosthetic components as they are developed.

A large variety of arthroplasty procedures are available to the orthopedic surgeon for treatment of pain, joint instability, or decreased range of motion. An understanding of the treatment goals of the various procedures, and of their normal postoperative appearance and the long-term implications is important for the radiologist. Certain principles can then be derived by which newer operations can be evaluated as they appear.

MATERIAL TECHNOLOGY

Metal Arthroplasty Components

Orthopedic metallic implants most commonly consist of one of the following materials: stainless steel, cobalt-chromium-molybdenum alloy, cobalt-chromium-tungsten alloy, tantalum, or titanium. A total joint arthroplasty may consist of a metal component articulating with either another metal (metal-metal) component or a polyethylene (metal-plastic) component. Metal-metal prostheses gradually produce large amounts of metallic wear particles, whereas fewer metallic fragments are generated by metal-plastic implants. These particles are released into the synovial fluid and the periarticular tissues and subsequently pass into the blood stream. Testing has shown metal sensitivity in some patients after placement of metal-metal prostheses. Although less common, allergic reactions may also occur with metal-plastic prostheses. Development of hypersensitivity to metallic wear products has been implicated as a cause of severe local tissue reaction with sterile discharge and bone necrosis, which ultimately may result in prosthesis loosening.

Ultra High Molecular Weight Polyethylene (UHMWP)

A metal component articulating with an ultra high molecular weight polyethylene (UHMWP) component produces the lowest friction and longest wear properties of currently available implants. UHMWP allows some degree of plastic deformity, which improves congruity between sliding surfaces as the load increases, in turn distributing bearing forces more evenly. When hard and soft materials are used as apposing bearing surfaces, the concave surface is made of the softer material, to take advantage of plastic deformity.

The exterior surfaces of plastic components have grooves to improve fixation with bone cement. As UHMWP is radio-lucent, metallic wires may be embedded in the external grooves, serving as locator markers for evaluation of alignment, changes in position, and wear. Occasionally a marker wire may detach from the plastic component. Fixation of plastic hip components to bone is facilitated by drilling holes in the acetabulum, which are filled with bone cement to create a mechanical anchor. Preshaped fine wire mesh cement retainers may be inserted into these sites to restrict extensive entry of acrylic bone cement into the pelvis.

UHMWP components shed wear particles, although there are wide variations in the rate and extent of wear. Hypersensitivity or local tissue reaction to UHMWP is suspected but has not been fully confirmed.

Polymethylmethacrylate (PMM) Bone Cement

An acrylic bone cement consisting of polymethylmethacrylate (PMM) is used to bond various arthroplasty components. Acrylic cement does not act as an adhesive or glue; rather, it forms an accurate cast at the interface between the bone and the prosthetic component, facilitating a more perfect mechanical fit. At the time of surgery, polymerization of the cement results in an exothermic reaction, which causes a temperature increase at the bone-cement interface. Setting of the cement is nearly complete 10 minutes after mixing, although continued hardening occurs over several hours.

Several techniques have been suggested to maximize the longevity of femoral component cement fixation. The major thrust has been to pressure pack the intramedullary bone cement (using an intramedullary restrictor) to uniformly fill the bone interstices, which results in greater shear strength at the bone-cement interface. Currently most bone cement is rendered radiopaque by the addition of 10 per cent barium sulfate during manufacture.

The possibility of allergic reaction to methylmethacrylate has been considered as a cause of local tissue reaction or loosening of prostheses.

Metal-Cement Interface

Although the metal-cement interface exhibits fewer problems than the bone-cement interface, alterations at the metal-cement junction may occasionally lead to failure of the system.

Histologic examination of a small series of radiographically normal femoral prostheses disclosed in each case a thin layer of fibrous tissue interposed between the metal and the cement. Thermal expansion of the metal stem with subsequent contraction, or contraction of the bone cement itself, has been implicated in the generation of this microscopic space. In some cases, an actual gap may be left if bone cement does not fill the entire space around the metal stem.

Bone-Cement Interface

Use of barium-impregnated PMM bone cement allows the relationship of the cement to the adjacent bone to be visualized. Ideally, the radiopaque cement should occupy all the spaces between a prosthetic component and adjacent bone; no gaps or spaces should be noted. A thin radiolucent zone may develop along the bone-cement interface in normal patients during the first 6 months postoperatively. Because radiolucent zones are also noted in patients with prosthetic loosening or infection, radiographic evaluation must consider the time of appearance, length, width, and progression of such zones to differentiate normal phenomena from complications.

Biologic (Cementless) Prostheses

Recently, there has been considerable interest in the development of porous implant surfaces that do not require bone cement and permit biologic fixation by tissue ingrowth. Finishing the prosthesis surface with an irregular material increases the number of points for ingrowth of bone, resulting in distribution of the load over a larger surface area (Fig. 20–1). Such coatings increase the surface area three to four times and provide pores for bone ingrowth.

The irregular metallic coated surfaces of these components are visible radiographically. A thin radiopaque line may be seen within a few millimeters of the bone-implant interface

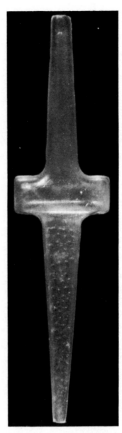

Figure 20–2. Swanson metacarpophalangeal joint prosthesis. Dorsal aspect. The metacarpal stem is longer. A concavity on the volar aspect allows flexion.

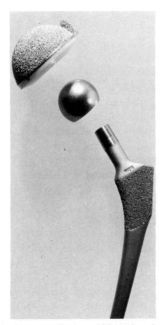

Figure 20–1. Biologic (cementless) total hip arthroplasty. A polyethylene acetabular component is covered with a metallic cap. Note the irregular coated portions of the acetabular and femoral components. The femoral head component is interchangeable, allowing some adjustment in the length of the femoral component.

as healing occurs. Although it has been postulated that this line of bone condensation represents micromotion, it has been seen also when no loosening is demonstrated on direct inspection.

Elastomers

Polydimethylsiloxane (silicone rubber or Silastic)* or polypropylene prostheses have limited application, with use restricted primarily to the wrist, the hand, and the foot. Silicone joint replacements are generally fabricated as single-piece integral hinge prostheses for replacement of the metacarpophalangeal and proximal interphalangeal joints of the fingers and the carpometacarpal joint of the thumb. A single-piece prosthesis with each stem inserted into the intramedullary cavity allows flexion and extension and provides lateral stability. The Swanson type of prosthesis uses the same grade of silicone rubber throughout, whereas the stems of the Niebauer type are coated with a Dacron mesh that is eventually infiltrated by soft tissue (Figs. 20–2 and 20–3). The prosthesis is held in place by periarticular fibrous tissue. The lack of need for fixation simplifies insertion and may help distribute stresses over a wide area. Occasionally, the stems may be fixed in place with suture material or bone cement. Although silicone rubber prostheses are extremely durable, some wear may eventually occur, and a foreign body reaction

---

*Silastic, Dow Corning Corporation, Midland, MI 48640.

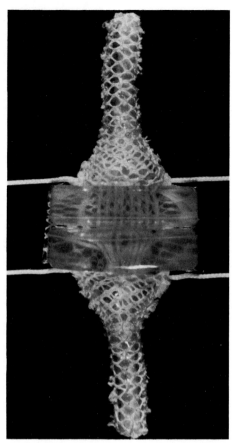

Figure 20–3. Niebauer metacarpophalangeal joint prosthesis. Dorsal aspect. Both stems are covered with Dacron mesh, which is subsequently infiltrated by soft tissue. Sutures are included for fixation.

to silicone wear particles may result in a painful, erosive arthritis.

HIP
Total Hip Replacement Arthroplasty (THA)

The most common indication for THA is primary or secondary osteoarthritis. Rheumatoid and related arthritides constitute additional indications. THA may also be used as a salvage operation for other procedures that have failed, including hip fusion, excision arthroplasty of the proximal femur, cup arthroplasty, failed femoral prosthesis, and osteotomy. Eighty-five to 90 per cent of patients followed for 4 to 5 years have good or excellent results in clinical parameters.

There are two basic types of THA. A metallic acetabular component articulating with a metallic femoral component is represented both by the cemented McKee-Farrar THA (see Fig. 20–8) and by the noncemented Ring prosthesis. The other basic type of THA consists of an UHMWP acetabular component articulating with a metallic femoral component; the Charnley and Charnley-Mueller modifications are the best-known examples (Fig. 20–4).

NORMAL APPEARANCE. Although the normal radiographic appearance of a THA will vary somewhat depending on the type of prosthesis used, principles of radiographic evaluation are similar. When radiopaque acrylic bone cement has been used, it should fill available spaces between the bone

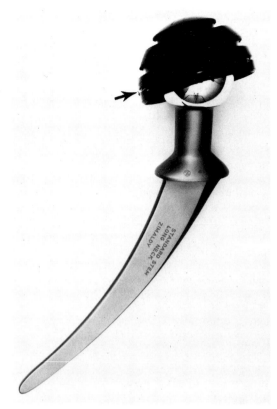

Figure 20–4. Charnley type THA. The ultra high molecular weight polyethylene (UHMWP) grooved acetabular cup articulates with a metallic femoral component. A locater wire is embedded in the groove (arrow).

and prosthesis components without gaps or trapped air bubbles. Cement entering the pelvis should be noted; excessive intrusion into the pelvis may be associated with complications. No loose cement fragments should be present. Both components of the prosthesis should be covered with cement, and bone cement should extend at least 2 cm beyond the tip of the femoral stem.

Orientation of the acetabular cup should be approximately 30 degrees (McKee-Farrar type) or 45 degrees (Charnley type) from the horizontal, and in neutral to slight anteversion (10 degrees). Anteversion is evaluated most easily on lateral radiographs, but the lateral view is not always available, especially in the immediate postoperative period. Acetabular orientation is usually assessed adequately on frontal radiographs by estimation according to the following guides: neutral position (orbital wire appears as a straight line), slight anteversion (wire appears as elongated oval), or increased anteversion (wire assumes a more circular shape). Anteversion may be difficult to evaluate precisely with some of the cementless THA because the acetabular component is completely covered with metal. Less than ideal placement of the acetabular component predisposes the THA to complications of instability, dislocation, or limited range of motion (Fig. 20–5).

The femoral component stem ideally lies in slight valgus position with reference to the femoral shaft or in the central portion of the medullary canal. The flange at the proximal portion of the metallic stem should rest firmly on the resected femoral neck. The head of the femoral prosthesis should lie centrally within the metal or polyethylene acetabular com-

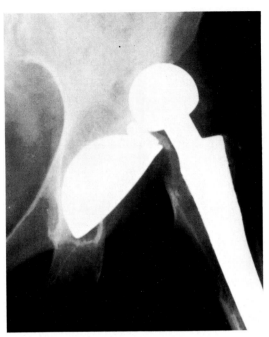

Figure 20–5. Dislocation of femoral component. Note the dislocated biologic arthroplasty; it is difficult to evaluate the degree of acetabular anteversion of this porous coated implant.

ponent, unless an asymmetric acetabular component has been used.

Osteotomy of the greater trochanter may be performed at the time of THA to facilitate exposure of the hip. The trochanter is often reinserted in a more distal and lateral position for improved stability. Fixation of the trochanter is accomplished with heavy wire suture or a trochanteric bolt. Normal bony union of the trochanteric osteotomy occurs in 6 to 12 weeks.

COMPLICATIONS. THA has a high frequency of thromboembolic disease. There also is approximately a 1 per cent risk of deep infection with use of prophylactic antibiotics. Many potential complications may be evaluated radiographically (Table 20–1).

Dislocation. Dislocation is a recognized common complication of THA (0.6 to 7 per cent of cases) and usually appears in the first few weeks after surgery (Fig. 20–5). Significant deviation from the ideal angles of acetabular orientation and anteversion or trochanteric avulsion predisposes to dislocation of the prosthesis. Persistent subluxation in neutral positions should raise the possibility of interposition of material between the prosthetic components: either soft tissue, osseous, cartilaginous, or cement fragments or a piece of wire suture.

Trochanteric Avulsion or Nonunion. It is generally agreed that THA performed without trochanteric osteotomy

Table 20–1. COMPLICATIONS OF TOTAL HIP ARTHROPLASTY

Dislocation
Trochanteric avulsion or nonunion
Heterotopic ossification
Fracture
Cement extrusion and vascular injury
Loosening or infection
Malignancy*

*Not proved.

results in less blood loss, a shorter operation, more rapid recovery, and the absence of complications of nonunion, broken or migrating wires, and trochanteric bursitis. Fibrous union at the osteotomy site is inferred radiographically if there is a lack of bony bridging at 6 months and the wires remain intact, without migration of the trochanter. Breakage of the wire sutures prior to bony or fibrous union may be associated with superolateral migration of the trochanter. Avulsion of the trochanter may also occur without breakage of the wires. Factors implicated in trochanteric detachment include operative error, excessive patient weight, trochanteric fracture, and prosthesis malalignment. Trochanteric avulsion predisposes to chronic recurrent dislocation from lack of abductor muscle support. Loose wire fragments may cause trochanteric bursitis or sciatic neuropathy, or they may migrate to an intraarticular position.

Heterotopic Ossification. Heterotopic paraarticular ossification is a common sequela of THA. Its rate of occurrence varies from 15 to 71 per cent. Two to 5 per cent of patients develop extensive ossification, resulting in limitation of motion (Fig. 20–6). Paraarticular ossification may appear as early as 3 weeks after THA and is always evident by 6 months. Heterotopic bone may show increased uptake on radionuclide bone scanning.

The cause of heterotopic ossification is unknown. Multiple factors have been implicated, including surgical trauma, bone dust, hemorrhage, infection, reoperation, trochanteric osteotomy, and predisposing systemic illnesses (ankylosing spondylitis, diffuse idiopathic skeletal hyperostosis).

Cement Extrusion and Vascular Injury. Extrusion of bone cement into the pelvis during THA is not uncommon; it occurs when the acetabular wall is perforated during surgical preparation. Complications of such extrusion include hematuria, sciatic nerve irritation, small bowel obstruction, bladder fistula, false aneurysm of the external iliac artery, obturator nerve palsy, and dyspareunia.

Serpentine-like bone cement densities have been noted in the veins medial to the femoral component. Bone cement fragments that break away from the cement margins may migrate into the joint, or cement may be introduced directly into the joint during surgery.

Direct vascular trauma at the time of surgery may result in vascular occlusion or perforation.

Fracture. Intraoperative fractures of the femoral shaft are more frequent than pelvic fractures and generally are attributed to one or more factors, including severely osteoporotic bone, excessive or misdirected reaming, and rough handling. Placement of a cortical window for removal of bone cement during prosthetic revision may also be a factor. Such fractures are usually recognized at the time of surgery, either in clinical examination (instability) or radiographically. Postoperative femoral fractures are of two types. First, typical fractures of the distal part of the femur occur after major traumatic events. Second, fractures of the proximal femoral shaft that occur at or just distal to the tip of the femoral stem often are spontaneous or follow minor trauma. Predisposing factors include surgical defects in the femoral cortex and inadequate distribution of bone cement. Recognition of a possible site of femoral weakening prior to or at the time of surgery dictates use of a long-stem prosthesis with additional bone cement. Adequate distribution of bone cement is necessary to prevent concentration of stress forces.

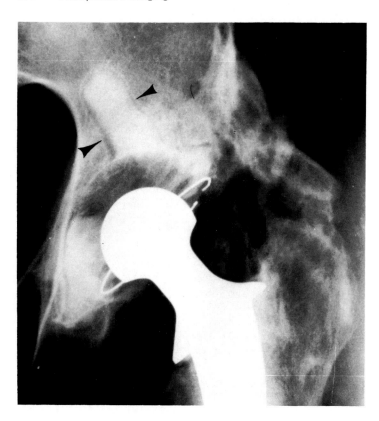

Figure 20–6. Extensive heterotopic bone formation after THA with limitation of motion clinically. A radiolucent zone (1.5 mm in width) is present along the bone-cement interface of the acetabular component (arrowheads); there was no clinical evidence of loosening.

Fractures of the acetabulum after THA may relate to one or more factors: (1) overreaming of the acetabulum, (2) severe protrusio acetabuli with thinning of the available acetabular roof, (3) chronic loosening or infection with increased stresses, (4) perforation of the medial wall of the acetabulum during placement of bone cement anchoring holes, (5) metastatic disease, and (6) large acetabular cysts (Fig. 20–7).

Stress (insufficiency) fractures of the pubic ramus may clinically simulate loosening of a THA. After several weeks with symptoms, patients with stress fractures generally have positive findings on radiographs (Fig. 20–8). Results of radionuclide bone scans may be positive prior to radiographic findings.

Loosening and Infection. The chief long-term complications of THA are loosening and infection. Loosening of a prosthetic component at the bone-cement interface may occur with or without associated infection. Conversely, deep infection is not always associated with component loosening. The likelihood of loosening of the femoral component increases at a fairly constant rate each year; in contrast, acetabular component loosening is rare during the first 5 years but rises markedly after 8 years.

The frequency of deep infection has decreased owing to stringent prophylactic measures, including routine administration of antibiotics. The current frequency rate of deep sepsis is about 1 per cent in large series. Predisposing factors associated with a higher frequency of infection after THA include prior hip surgery or revision of THA, rheumatoid arthritis, steroid therapy, and obesity. Although most latent infections are believed to originate from bacteria introduced at the time of surgery, cases of latent THA infections may occasionally be attributed to hematogenous implantation of bacteria from a distant source in the body. Early detection of deep sepsis, usually before the appearance of radiographic changes, may allow successful treatment with antibiotics alone or antibiotics in conjunction with surgical drainage, leaving the prosthesis in place. When infection is more advanced, removal of the prosthesis, bone cement, and necrotic bone (Girdlestone procedure) is required in addition to appropriate antibiotic therapy.

Prosthetic loosening is defined as visually evident gross movement observed when the prosthesis is stressed manually

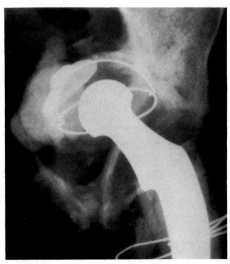

Figure 20–7. Acetabular fracture with protrusion of the acetabular component is evident. There was no evidence of infection at surgery.

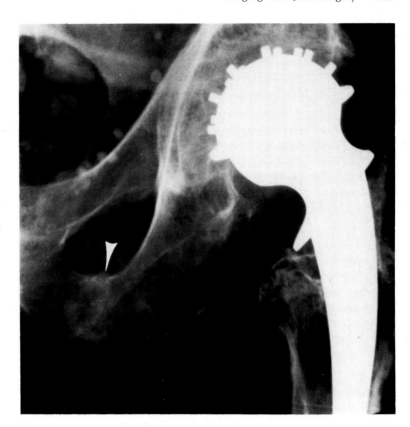

Figure 20–8. Stress fracture of the inferior pubic ramus (arrowhead) following THA (McKee-Farrar type; radiolucent bone cement). This is the typical site of stress fracture after hip surgery.

at surgery. Loose noninfected components may be primarily revised with likelihood of success, whereas infected components are usually removed. Unfortunately, the distinction between loosening and infection may be difficult even with use of multiple techniques, including (1) plain films, (2) radionuclide scanning, (3) hip aspiration, and (4) subtraction arthrography.

Plain Films. On plain radiographs alone, an infected prosthesis is rarely distinguishable from one that is loosened without infection. Development of a radiolucent zone* at the bone-cement interface raises the possibility of loosening. The presence of a zone, however, is not infallible evidence of loosening, as such zones may develop in the normal arthroplasty. Although zones more commonly involve the acetabular component of THA and the tibial component of total knee arthroplasties (TKA), actual loosening is more common in the femoral components of both types of arthroplasties. During the first 6 months postoperatively, zones may initially appear and lengthen or widen on sequential films in normal patients. After 6 months, such phenomena are less likely to be normal (Fig. 20–9). The actual width or appearance of a zone may aid in distinguishing the normal from a loose or infected THA. Zones 2 mm or wider are usually indicative of infection or loosening; zones that extend around the entire bone-cement interface correlate with loosening or infection better than localized zones. Although not every zone represents demonstrable prosthetic loosening, essentially every case of loosening is associated with such a zone.

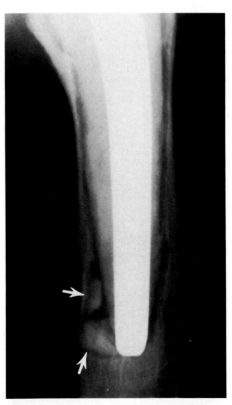

Figure 20–9. Loose femoral component with poor distal coverage of the metallic stem by bone cement (4 years after surgery). Note distal bone-metal contact, radiolucent bone resorption, and cement fragmentation (arrows).

---

*Hereafter in this chapter "zone" refers to a radiolucent line at the bone-cement interface or metal-cement interface.

Several theories have been advocated to explain the appearance of radiolucent zones at the bone-cement interface in normal patients: (1) incomplete removal of acetabular articular cartilage, (2) thermal necrosis of bone from the exothermic bone-cement polymerization reaction, (3) surgical trauma, (4) failure to pack the cement tightly or motion of the prosthetic component prior to setting of cement, (5) interposition of soft tissue or blood, (6) chemical damage from the PMM monomer and free radicals in the cement, and (7) micromotion.

In some cases, a fatigue fracture of the prosthesis stem occurs as the result of increased stresses (Fig. 20–10). In patients with such fractures, the prosthesis is loose but usually not infected, as rigid fixation distally is a prerequisite for increased stress on the stem. Contributing factors implicated in femoral stem failure include (1) patient weight greater than 91 kg, (2) inadequate valgus positioning of the prosthesis, (3) metallurgical failure, (4) increased patient activity, and (5) bilateral arthroplasty.

Fracture of the polyethylene acetabular cup is a rare late complication of THA. Factors implicated in such fractures include areas of thin bone-cement coverage with poor support of the acetabular cup, areas of inherent weakness related to grooves in the acetabular cup, and use of low molecular weight rather than high molecular weight polyethylene to form the acetabular cup. Radiographic clues to these fractures include changes in orientation of the acetabular component,

breakage of localizer wires, protrusion of the prosthetic femoral head, and frank fracture of the acetabular cup.

In recent years, another pattern of osteolytic change has been observed at the bone-cement interface, which is more prominent than that seen with loosening alone (Fig. 20–11). The femoral component is usually affected, and this type of osteolysis typically occurs several years after the arthroplasty. There most often is evidence of component loosening, but infection is rarely present. Histologic examination of the resected tissue in these osteolytic areas shows a foreign body reaction consisting of fibrous stroma with foamy histiocytes and multinucleated giant cells filled with methylmethacrylate particles. Metallic, cement, and polyethylene wear particles have been implicated.

Scintigraphy. Radionuclide bone scanning using various radiopharmaceutical agents, such as [87m]Sr, ^{18}F, and ^{99m}Tc-phosphate complexes, has been employed in the evaluation of patients with painful THA. Normally, increased activity with a diffuse distribution is noted in the first weeks postoperatively; this gradually decreases over a period of 6 to 9 months. A common radionuclide pattern of loosening consists of focal areas of increased uptake, detected more easily on the femoral side, often appearing near the proximal or distal portion of the stem (Fig. 20–12). Another abnormal pattern consists of diffusely increased activity along the prosthesis in patients with either loose or both loose and infected components. Increased activity in the region of the femoral neck and paraarticular soft tissues may be seen in cases of heterotopic bone formation.

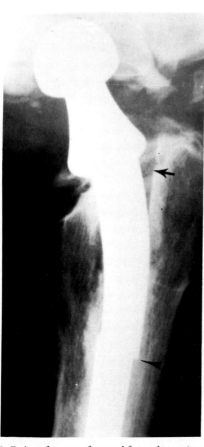

Figure 20–10. Fatigue fracture of a metal femoral stem (arrowhead) with separation at the metal-cement interface proximally (arrow).

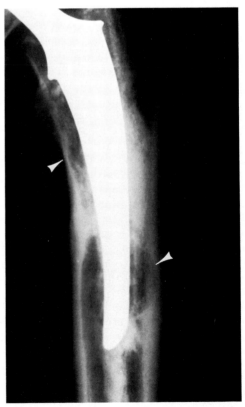

Figure 20–11. Foreign body reaction. Large osteolytic areas of endosteal bone resorption (arrowheads) representing histiocytic foreign body reaction are observed.

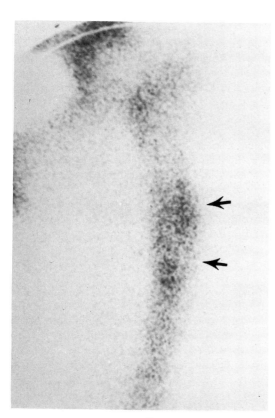

Figure 20–12. Prosthesis loosening. ^{99m}Tc-pyrophosphate scintigram, anterior projection of the left femur in a patient with a painful THA. There is a focal area of increased activity near the tip of the femoral stem (arrows). Loosening of the component was confirmed surgically.

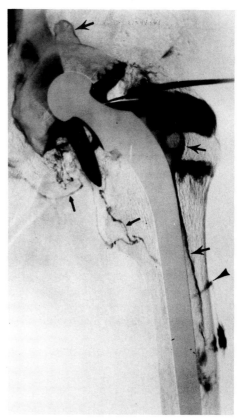

Figure 20–13. Prosthesis loosening. Subtraction arthrogram showing contrast material along the bone-cement interface of the acetabular and femoral components (large arrows). Contrast material is observed tracking through the site of the cortical window into soft tissues (arrowhead). Lymphatic filling is noted (small arrows). (Courtesy of S. Kleiman, M.D., La Jolla, California.)

The radionuclide bone scan seems to have a high sensitivity and specificity for loosening or infection when performed 1 year or more after the surgery. Radionuclide bone scanning, however, cannot differentiate loosening from infection in THA. Even the usefulness of gallium or indium scanning in this differentiation is not clear.

Arthrography. Arthrography of the painful THA is a valuable preoperative diagnostic technique, which may demonstrate a variety of complications (Table 20–2). Aspiration with culture of intraarticular material is performed routinely at the time of arthrography and is of equal importance to performance of the arthrogram itself. Arthrographic demonstration of opaque contrast material along the bone-cement interface is more difficult to delineate when opaque bone cement has been used; subtraction techniques have been developed to improve the detection of radiopaque contrast material adjacent to the opaque bone cement (Fig. 20–13).

During arthrography, contrast material normally fills the irregular pseudocapsule, which may vary considerably in

volume. Lymphatic filling also may be observed (Fig. 20–13). Contrast material penetrating the bone-cement or metal-cement interface clearly indicates a separation or space, although not all areas of communication represent component loosening (Fig. 20–13). The presence of contrast agent penetration around only a portion of a prosthetic component may represent merely a localized separation of the bone and cement without demonstrable loosening of the component at surgery. The greater the extent of contrast material penetration, the more likely it is that the prosthetic component is loose. Conversely, lack of contrast material penetration at the bone-cement interface does not exclude loosening. Granulation or fibrous tissue may obstruct the opening to a potential space. Demonstration of contrast-filled paraarticular cavities or sinus tracts supports a diagnosis of infection. Filling of a single cavity extending over the greater trochanter suggests a trochanteric bursitis.

Other Surgical Procedures

CUP ARTHROPLASTY. After the advent of the THA, cup arthroplasty has been used in joints complicated by sepsis and in patients who have been considered too young for THA. During cup arthroplasty, the affected joint is widened initially by reaming of the acetabulum and the femoral head. A metallic cup is placed over the reamed femoral head, and the hip is reduced. The reparative process after surgery begins with formation of hematoma over the exposed osseous surfaces,

---

Table 20–2. UTILITY OF ARTHROGRAPHY IN TOTAL HIP ARTHROPLASTY

Aspiration for culture
Detection of:
    Presence and extent of loosening
    Sinus tracts, communicating abscess cavities
    Intraarticular material in cases of chronic dislocation
    Trochanteric bursitis
    Nonunion of greater trochanter

which organizes into a fibrous scar. Fibrocartilage on the bone surface underneath the metallic cup also may be evident. After the procedure, radiographs outline a metallic cup that obscures the remaining femoral head and much of the acetabulum. The cup should lie in the axis of the femoral neck and rotate with the femur. In some cases, progressive diminution of acetabular cartilage may be noted, perhaps related to interference of normal chondral nutrition by the cup.

Several complications of this procedure may be noted. The metallic cup may dislocate or sublux, either along with the remaining femoral head or independently (Fig. 20–14). Poor mobility of the cup within the acetabulum may cause fracture of the femoral neck. An infected cup arthroplasty may show bone destruction and periosteal new bone formation. Heterotopic bone formation has been reported in as many as 30 per cent of patients.

FEMORAL HEMIARTHROPLASTY. Proximal femoral replacement in patients with arthritic conditions of the hip that affect the acetabular cartilage has been superseded by THA. Femoral head and neck replacement, however, is currently in use for certain types of femoral neck fractures and, occasionally, in early stages of osteonecrosis of the femoral head.

A new universal proximal femoral hip prosthesis is replacing conventional hemiarthroplasty in some centers. The primary goal of this prosthesis is to reduce the wear and the erosion of the acetabulum that are encountered with the older femoral hemiarthroplasties. A standard femoral stem and head articulate with a high density polyethylene acetabular cup, enclosed within a metallic cup (Fig. 20–15). These prostheses function as a double compound bearing, with movement possible at the articulation of the femoral head and polyethylene cup and of the metallic cup and acetabulum. The prosthesis is designed to promote more motion at the metal femoral head–polyethylene articulation than at the cup–acetabular cartilage articulation, sparing articular cartilage from the degree of wear that is associated with the conventional hemiarthroplasty. Relative motion of the two articulations may be assessed at fluoroscopy.

Normal Appearance. The metallic femoral head should fit snugly in the acetabulum. Subluxation may occur if the selected head is too large. A small head results in increased wear on acetabular articular cartilage. Length of the femoral neck must also be selected properly. The stem is ideally placed in slight valgus position or centrally in the medullary canal with a modest degree of anteversion. Specific designs use varying shapes of the neck, the flange, and the stem. The two most common units are the Austin-Moore and the Thompson prostheses.

Complications. Dislocation is not common and when present is usually related to excessive retroversion or selection of a head size that is too large for the acetabulum. Acetabular protrusion, which may be associated with postoperative pain, may be seen in a significant number of cases (Fig. 20–16). Periarticular heterotopic bone formation after femoral hemiarthroplasty has a significance similar to that in THA. A radiolucent zone at the stem-bone interface exceeding 2 mm is often associated with loosening or infection.

SURFACE REPLACEMENT ARTHROPLASTY. The surface replacement arthroplasty is composed of a polyethylene acetabular component (similar to the component of a THA) and a femoral component consisting of a metallic cup that

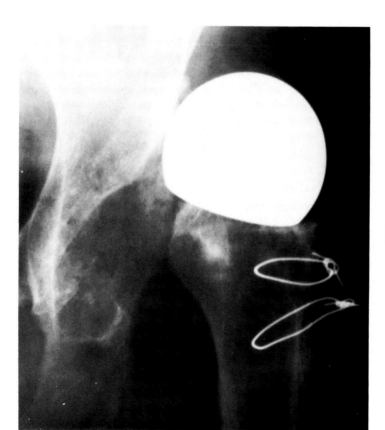

Figure 20–14. **Dislocated cup arthroplasty,** in this case related to acetabular dysplasia.

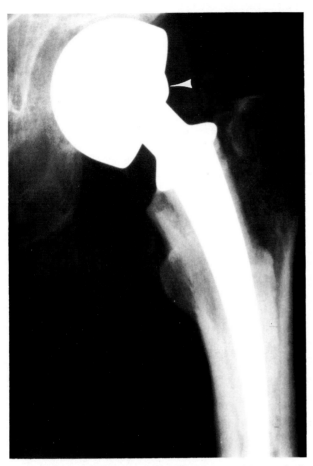

Figure 20–15. Normal universal proximal femoral hip prosthesis, cemented in place. The standard femoral head (arrowhead) articulates with the metal-polyethylene cup.

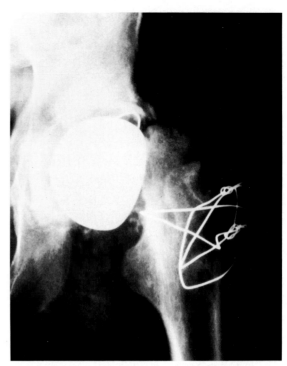

Figure 20–17. Surface replacement arthroplasty with femoral neck fracture. The femoral neck is displaced in a superior direction relative to the metallic cup.

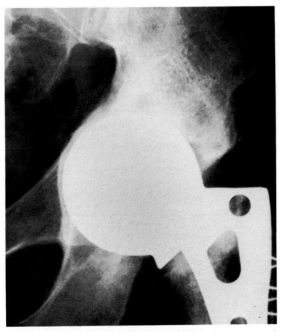

Figure 20–16. Femoral hemiarthroplasty with acetabular protrusion.

covers a surgically reshaped femoral head (similar to what is accomplished during a cup arthroplasty). Both components are fixed to the underlying bone with methylmethacrylate. As in THA, early complications are more common on the femoral side, with acetabular failures noted with longer periods of observation. The cement-bone interface of the femoral component is obscured by the metallic cup, and loosening of this component must be assessed by changes in its position or alignment. Most loose cups shift into varus alignment. Fractures of the femoral neck may occur, under the metallic cup (Fig. 20–17).

KNEE

Total Knee Arthroplasty (TKA)

The primary indication for TKA is pain; instability, deformity, and decreased range of motion are additional criteria. Rheumatoid arthritis and osteoarthritis are the most common preexisting conditions. Infection is a major contraindication to the procedure because of the risk of reactivation. Patients with neuroarthropathy are also unacceptable surgical candidates.

Knee prostheses may be classified by the degree of constraint according to the following scheme: (1) no or minimal constraint; (2) partial constraint; (3) total constraint. For greater degrees of ligament instability, prostheses incorporating design features that impart increasing stability are chosen. Biomechanically, shear forces on the prosthesis increase as constraint increases, resulting in greater stresses on the prosthesis and surrounding bone. Fully constrained prostheses are larger and require more removal of bone, making revision more difficult.

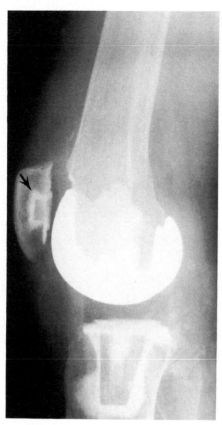

Figure 20–18. Lateral view of total condylar type TKA. Polyethylene patellar resurfacing implant is cemented in place (arrow).

With various modifications, most types of TKA in current use employ metallic femoral components that articulate with polyethylene tibial components, each held in place with radiopaque methylmethacrylate bone cement. The concave polyethylene component(s) are in a dependent position in knee prostheses, in contrast to their location in hip arthroplasties. Thus, metallic wear particles and fragments of bone cement are more likely to pool on the concave surface, leading to increased wear.

The polycentric TKA as developed by Gunston is an example of an unconstrained prosthesis. Partial constraint is provided by the geometric, UCI, and Freeman-Swanson prostheses. Fully constrained knee arthroplasties include the metal-metal Guepar, Walldius, and Shier hinge arthroplasties and the spherocentric metal-polyethylene arthroplasty.

The knee prostheses mentioned previously are not true TKA, as the patellofemoral joint is not replaced. After TKA, postoperative retropatellar pain has been reported in 24 to 58 per cent of patients. The total condylar prosthesis, a typical true TKA, uses a polyethylene button that is implanted in the articular surface of the patella and held in place with bone cement (Fig. 20–18).

NORMAL APPEARANCE. Ideal alignment and position of the prosthetic components vary with the type of unit that is chosen. Normal radiolucent zones at the bone-cement interface appearing during the first 6 months after TKA are much more common about the tibial component than about the femoral component of nonhinged TKA with metal femoral and polyethylene tibial components. Radiolucent zones at the bone-cement interface of the tibial component are best de-

tected on anteroposterior radiographs and at the femoral bone-cement interface on lateral radiographs.

As in THA, radionuclide scanning and joint aspiration with subtraction arthrography may be used in the evaluation of symptomatic knee prostheses. A scintigraphic pattern of focal or unicomponent uptake, especially that which is evident 6 months or longer after surgery, suggests loosening or infection, or both. Subtraction arthrography is performed to enhance detection of contrast-tracking within the bone-cement interface (Fig. 20–19).

COMPLICATIONS. A variety of TKA complications are detectable by radiographic procedures (Table 20–3).

Instability, subluxation, or angulation may be accentuated on weight-bearing or stress views. Synovial cysts may form in the postoperative patient and may appear in unusual locations. As in THA, stress fractures may occur anywhere from the pelvis to the foot owing to increased activity levels after TKA. Fracture and migration of wire locator guides have been noted in some of the tibial components.

The addition of patellar resurfacing has reduced the frequency of patellofemoral pain after TKA, but there are specific complications related to the resurfacing procedure. The frequency of acute or stress patellar fractures after resurfacing varies from 1 to 5 per cent. Factors that have been implicated in these fractures include impairment of the patellar blood supply (with possible ischemic necrosis) and mechanical problems related to overzealous resection or drilling of the patella. Subluxation or dislocation of the patella may occur in patients with and without patellar implants.

Distinguishing prosthetic loosening alone from loosening associated with infection may be difficult. Positive results of cultures, rapid bone resorption or destruction, and draining sinus tracts all support a diagnosis of infection (Fig. 20–20).

HAND, WRIST, ELBOW, AND FOOT
Silicone Arthroplasty

Silicone rubber arthroplasties and implants of the hand, the wrist, the elbow, and the foot do not represent true prostheses. They merely act as spacers, separating bone ends and providing a form for periarticular soft tissues.

NORMAL APPEARANCE. Silicone rubber is less dense radiographically than bone and slightly more dense than the soft tissues. The thicker, hinged portion (midsection) of metacarpophalangeal (MCP) joint prostheses should abut on the adjacent resected margin of the metaphyseal bone. A nonrotated posteroanterior radiograph usually shows a symmetrically located rectangular midsection. On the lateral film, the distal palmar aspect of the midsection is concave, allowing

---

Table 20–3. RADIOGRAPHIC COMPLICATIONS OF TOTAL KNEE ARTHROPLASTY

Intraoperative or postoperative fracture
Stress fracture
Patellar dislocation or locking
Instability
Dislocation or subluxation
Migration of wire marker
Loosening or infection
Implant fracture
Heterotopic bone formation
Postoperative synovial cyst
Patellar pain, degenerative changes

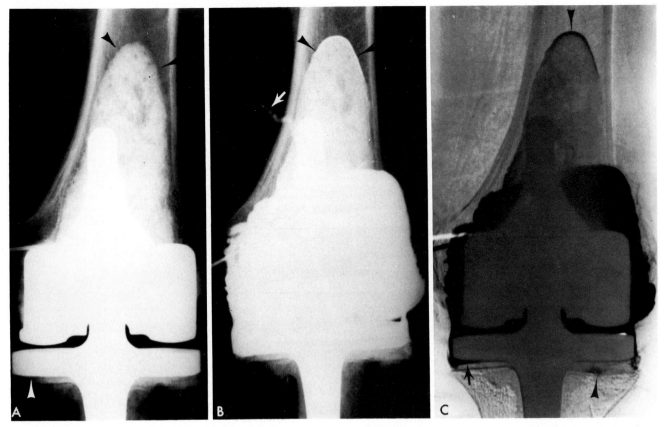

Figure 20–19. Prosthesis loosening. A Radiograph of spherocentric TKA. Narrow (1 mm) radiolucent zones are noted at the bone-cement interface of the femoral component and the metal-cement interface of the tibial component (arrowheads). **B** Arthrogram showing contrast material entering the bone-cement interface of the femoral component (arrowheads) and lymphatic filling (white arrow). Contrast material entering the metal-cement interface along the tibial component is more easily appreciated in the subtraction radiograph (**C**). **C** Subtraction arthrogram demonstrating contrast material entering the metal-cement interface of the tibial component (arrow) as well as the bone-cement interface of both components (arrowheads).

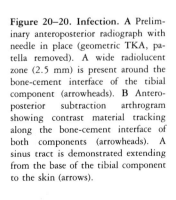

Figure 20–20. Infection. A Preliminary anteroposterior radiograph with needle in place (geometric TKA, patella removed). A wide radiolucent zone (2.5 mm) is present around the bone-cement interface of the tibial component (arrowheads). **B** Anteroposterior subtraction arthrogram showing contrast material tracking along the bone-cement interface of both components (arrowheads). A sinus tract is demonstrated extending from the base of the tibial component to the skin (arrows).

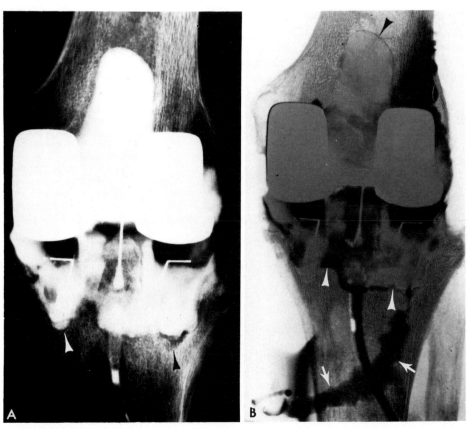

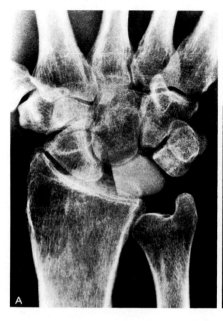 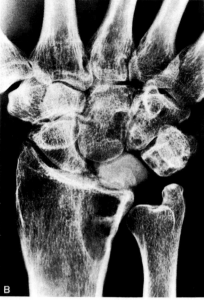

Figure 20–21. Silicone foreign body reaction. A Postoperative radiograph showing the lunate implant. Mild osteoarthritis is evident. **B** Two years later, there are cystic changes of the radius and carpal bones. The implant has decreased slightly in size. (From Telaranta T, et al: Bone cysts containing silicone particles in bones adjacent to a Silastic implant. Skel Radiol *10*:247, 1983. Used with permission.)

flexion but limited hyperextension. It is often difficult to visualize the stem within the medullary canal. In time, a thin sclerotic band of intramedullary bone may form.

COMPLICATIONS. Dislocation of MCP joint implants may occur if a stem slips out of its medullary canal. Radial head, distal ulnar, and carpal bone replacements may sublux or dislocate. Erosion of bone at points of contact between the prosthesis and bone may allow migration of the prosthesis. Fractures, cracking, and fragmentation of the prostheses may be evident. The overall infection rate after MCP joint implants is less than 1 per cent.

Silicone polymers have been thought to be long-lasting and responsible for minimal tissue inflammation. In recent years, however, there have been reports of various complications related to silicone particles, including synovitis with a foreign body giant cell reaction, bone cysts containing silicone particles, and regional lymphadenopathy with silicone debris (Fig. 20–21).

FURTHER READING

Beabout JW: Radiology of total hip arthroplasty. Radiol Clin North Am *13*:3, 1975.

Brooker AF, Bowerman JW, Robinson RA, Riley LH: Ectopic ossification following total hip replacement. Incidence and a method of classification. J Bone Joint Surg [Am] *55*:1629, 1973.

Calenoff L, Stromberg WB: Silicone rubber arthroplasties of the hand. Radiology *107*:29, 1973.

Charnley J: Total hip replacement by low friction arthroplasty. Clin Orthop *72*:7, 1970.

Cheng CL, Gross AE: Loosening of the porous coating in total knee replacement. J Bone Joint Surg [Br] *70*:377, 1988.

Clayton ML, Thirupathi R: Patellar complications after total condylar arthroplasty. Clin Orthop *170*:152, 1982.

Dussault RG, Goldman AB, Ghelman B: Radiologic diagnosis of loosening and infection of hip prostheses. J Can Assoc Radiol *28*:119, 1977.

Elloy MA, Wright JTM, Cavendish ME: The basic requirement and design criteria for total joint prostheses. Acta Orthop Scand *47*:193, 1976.

Gelman MI, Coleman RE, Stevens PM, Davey BW: Radiography, radionuclide imaging, and arthrography in the evaluation of total hip and knee replacement. Radiology *128*:677, 1978.

Head WC: Total articular resurfacing arthroplasty. J Bone Joint Surg [Am] *66*:28, 1984.

Insall J, Ranawat CS, Scott WN, Walker P: Total condylar knee replacement: Preliminary report. Clin Orthop *120*:149, 1976.

Kaplan PA, Montesi SA, Jardon OM, Gregory PR: Bone-ingrowth hip prostheses in asymptomatic patients: Radiographic features. Radiology *169*:221, 1988.

Maus TP, Berquist TH, Bender CE, Rand JA: Arthrographic study of painful total hip arthroplasty: Refined criteria. Radiology *162*:721, 1987.

Morscher EW: Cementless total hip arthroplasty. Clin Orthop *181*:76, 1983.

Ritter MA, Vaughan RB: Ectopic ossification after total hip arthroplasty. Predisposing factors, frequency, and effect on results. J Bone Joint Surg [Am] *59*:345, 1977.

Rosenthal DI, Rosenberg AE, Schiller AL, Smith RJ: Destructive arthritis due to silicone: A foreign-body reaction. Radiology *149*:69, 1983.

Schneider R, Goldman AB, Insall JN: Knee protheses. Semin Roentgenol *21*:29, 1986.

Scott WW, Riley LH, Dorfman HD: Focal lytic lesions associated with femoral stem loosening in total hip prosthesis. AJR *144*:977, 1985.

Swanson AB: Silicone rubber implants for replacement of arthritic or destroyed joints in the hand. Surg Clin North Am *48*:1113, 1968.

Weiss PE, Mall JC, Hoffer PB, Murray WR, Rodrigo JJ, Genant HK: ⁹⁹ᵐTc-methylene diphosphonate bone imaging in the evaluation of total hip prostheses. Radiology *133*:727, 1979.

Weissman BN, Sosman JL, Braunstein EM, Dadkhahipoor H, Kandarpa K, Thornhill TS, Lowell JD, Sledge CB: Intravenous methylmethacrylate after total hip replacement. J Bone Joint Surg [Am] *66*:443, 1984.

SECTION IV

RHEUMATOID ARTHRITIS AND RELATED DISEASES

CASE IV   LEVEL OF DIFFICULTY: 2

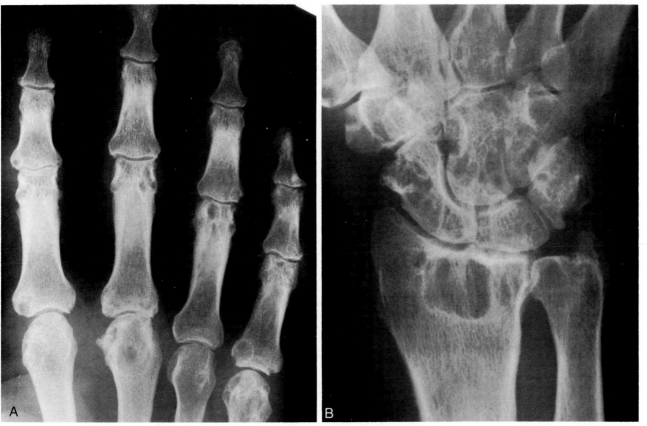

This 66 year old man had a 15 year history of slowly progressive polyarthritis affecting both small and large joints in the upper and lower extremities. Radiographs of the left hand and wrist are shown. The opposite side was similarly involved.

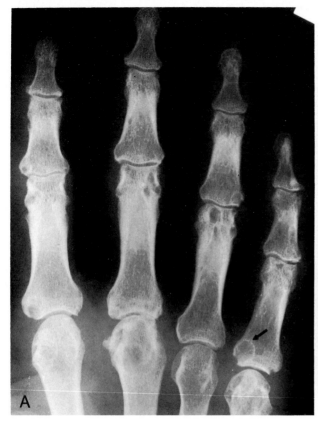 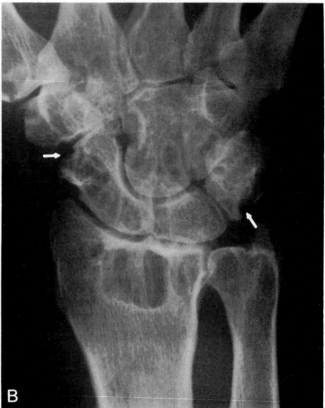

The posteroanterior radiograph of the fingers *(A)* shows abnormalities predominating about the proximal interphalangeal and metacarpophalangeal joints. Periarticular soft tissue prominence is observed, best seen in the second digit. Mild joint space loss in the metacarpophalangeal joints (especially the third) and proximal interphalangeal joints is apparent, although in certain locations, such as the second and fifth metacarpophalangeal joints, relative preservation of joint space is evident. Numerous, sharply circumscribed subchondral cysts and marginal erosions are characterized by a thin rim of sclerosis (arrow). Periarticular osteoporosis is not striking.

The posteroanterior radiograph of the wrist reveals diffuse soft tissue swelling and prominent cystic lesions throughout the carpal bones and in the distal portion of the radius and ulna. Erosions of the surfaces of the scaphoid, triquetrum, and capitate are also seen (arrows). Remarkably, the joint spaces are either normal or minimally narrowed. No chondrocalcinosis is evident.

The radiographic features are those of an articular process which, according to the history, is polyarticular and bilateral in distribution. Such a distribution pattern allows elimination of several diagnoses, such as pigmented villonodular synovitis and infection, which otherwise would be considered owing to the presence of cystic and erosive lesions of periarticular bone. There remain, however, several disease processes that might produce the radiographic abnormalities illustrated in case IV.

Gout commonly involves the joints of the hand and wrist, and this disease can lead to cystic and erosive lesions in the marginal and central portions of the joint. Indeed, sharply circumscribed osseous defects possessing sclerotic margins are characteristic of gout, and relative preservation of joint space is an important diagnostic feature of this disorder. There is no evidence of lobulated soft tissue masses or tophi, however, and the common carpometacarpal compartment of the wrist, located at the bases of the metacarpals, is a typical target site of gout but is unaffected in this patient. Furthermore, the history indicates that similar radiographic alterations were present in the opposite hand and wrist, whereas symmetry is not a usual manifestation of gout.

Calcium pyrophosphate dihydrate crystal deposition disease also can produce cystic lesions of the carpal bones and metacarpal heads. In this disease, however, chondrocalcinosis frequently is present, and marginal erosions of bone are not characteristic. In addition, the radiocarpal compartment of the wrist and the second and third metacarpophalangeal joints usually are narrowed, and prominent changes in the interphalangeal joints typically are absent.

Amyloidosis is a known cause of cystic lesions of bone, and the carpus is a well-recognized site of abnormality. Although multiple joints may be affected, a bilateral and symmetric distribution with abnormalities throughout the hand is not common.

The most likely explanation for the radiographic abnormalities depicted in case IV is cystic rheumatoid arthritis. Indeed, in some patients with rheumatoid arthritis, particularly men, subchondral cystic lesions are the dominant radiographic abnormality, and these lesions may be unaccompanied by joint space loss. This variety of the disease has been termed rheumatoid arthritis of the robust reaction type, as affected individuals may maintain a high level of physical activity.

Presumably, the lesions relate to elevation of intraarticula pressure with resultant intrusion of fluid and granulatio tissue into bone. Although the radiographic abnormalities c cystic rheumatoid arthritis resemble those of gout, bilatera and symmetric alterations and marginal erosions of bone ar important features that generally allow accurate diagnosis.

FINAL DIAGNOSIS: Cystic rheumatoid arthritis.

FURTHER READING

Pages 246 and 247 and the following:

1. DeHaas WHD, DeBoer W, Griffionen F, Oosten-Elst P: Rheumatoid arthritis of the robust reaction type. Ann Rheum Dis 33:81, 1987.
2. Jayson MIV, Rubenstein D, Dixon A St J: Intra-articular pressure and rheumatoid geodes (bone "cysts"). Ann Rheum Dis 29:496, 1970.

(Case IV, courtesy of J. Goobar, M.D., Oestersund, Sweden.)

Chapter 21

Rheumatoid Arthritis and the Seronegative Spondyloarthropathies: Radiographic and Pathologic Concepts

Donald Resnick, M.D.
Gen Niwayama, M.D.

The pathologic and radiographic abnormalities associated with joint involvement in rheumatoid arthritis and the seronegative spondyloarthropathies (ankylosing spondylitis, psoriasis, Reiter's syndrome) are similar in many respects. Involvement of synovial and cartilaginous joints, bursae, tendon sheaths, entheses, tendons, ligaments, soft tissues, and bones can be encountered in any of these disorders. The distribution and extent of abnormalities differ among these diseases, however. In rheumatoid arthritis, alterations in synovium-lined articulations, bursae, and tendon sheaths frequently overshadow those in cartilaginous joints and sites of tendon and ligament attachment to bone. In ankylosing spondylitis, psoriasis, and Reiter's syndrome, abnormalities at cartilaginous articulations, including the discovertebral and manubriosternal joints and symphysis pubis, can be severe. In addition, in these latter conditions, a peculiar enthesopathy produces osseous erosion and proliferation at tendoosseous junctions.

Rheumatoid arthritis and the seronegative spondyloarthropathies (ankylosing spondylitis, psoriasis, and Reiter's syndrome) have in common many radiographic and pathologic characteristics. They affect synovium-lined joints, bursae, and tendon sheaths; cartilaginous articulations; entheses or sites of ligamentous and tendinous attachment to bone; soft tissues; and bones. They lead to inflammation in a variety of tissues, and although the distribution and the extent of abnormalities at specific target areas in the body vary among the disorders, the musculoskeletal effects of this inflammation are fundamentally similar.

RHEUMATOID ARTHRITIS
Overview

The major abnormalities of rheumatoid arthritis appear in synovial joints of the appendicular skeleton, particularly the small joints of the hand and foot, the wrist, the knee, the elbow, and the glenohumeral and acromioclavicular joints. The synovial joints of the axial skeleton may also be affected, especially the apophyseal and atlantoaxial joints of the cervical spine. In most of these synovium-lined cavities, changes are distributed symmetrically in both the right and the left sides

of the body and consist of fusiform soft tissue swelling, regional osteoporosis, diffuse loss of joint space, marginal and central erosions, and fibrous ankylosis. The synovium of bursae and tendon sheaths is also affected. Abnormalities of cartilaginous joints and entheses are less frequent and extensive, with the exception of the discovertebral joints of the cervical spine. Alterations in tendons, ligaments, soft tissues, and vessels complete the radiographic and pathologic picture of musculoskeletal involvement in rheumatoid arthritis.

Synovial Joints (Table 21–1)

SYNOVIAL MEMBRANE. The earliest recognizable pathologic abnormality in rheumatoid arthritis is acute synovitis, which is characterized by congestion and edema of the synovial membrane (Fig. 21–1). Capillary proliferation and abnormal permeability are accompanied by exudation of plasma, which penetrates the loose stroma of the synovial layer, reaching the joint cavity. This exudative phase of rheumatoid arthritis merges into an infiltrative phase. Accumulation of erythrocytes results from altered capillary permeability. Phagocytosis of these cells leads to hemosiderin deposition, with the production of large quantities of synovial

Table 21–1. ABNORMALITIES OF SYNOVIAL JOINTS IN RHEUMATOID ARTHRITIS

Pathologic	Radiologic
Synovial inflammation and production of fluid	Soft tissue swelling and widening of joint space
Hyperemia	Osteoporosis
Pannus destruction of cartilage	Narrowing of joint space
Pannus destruction of "unprotected" bone at margin of joint	Marginal bone erosions
Pannus destruction of subchondral bone	Bone erosions and formation of subchondral cysts
Fibrous and bone ankylosis	Bone ankylosis
Laxity of capsule and ligaments and muscular contraction and spasm	Deformity, subluxation, dislocation, fracture, fragmentation, and sclerosis

iron. Polymorphonuclear leukocytes appear in the acute inflammatory phase. The predominant cells, however, are small lymphocytes. In the superficial portions of the synovium, cellular infiltration occurs diffusely or in small nodular aggregates (Allison-Ghormley nodules). With chronicity, plasma cells and true lymphoid follicles with germinal centers are evident. Distinctive multinucleated giant cells are also found in the synovial membrane in rheumatoid arthritis but are not entirely specific for this disease.

These microscopic abnormalities result in a macroscopically evident thickened and injected synovial membrane. Villous hypertrophy produces papillary fronds of 1 to 2 mm in diameter. Increased amounts of turbid yellow-green synovial fluid of decreased viscosity are produced. The cell content in the synovial fluid frequently is markedly elevated.

These pathologic findings in the early synovial stage of rheumatoid arthritis are accompanied by characteristic radiographic abnormalities (Fig. 21–2). Accumulation of synovial inflammatory tissue within the joint, increase in intraarticular fluid, capsular distention, and surrounding soft tissue edema lead to one early radiographic finding of the disease, soft tissue swelling. The periarticular soft tissue prominence is generally fusiform in configuration. Furthermore, in response to hyperemia provoked by synovial inflammation, regional or periarticular osteoporosis—the second early radiographic sign of rheumatoid arthritis—can be demonstrated. This finding produces thinning and small areas of discontinuity or gaps (dot-dash pattern) in the subchondral bone plate.

ARTICULAR CARTILAGE. After an acute inflammatory episode, the hypertrophied synovial tissue may recede without producing cartilaginous damage. Exacerbations of disease are associated with eventual abnormalities in other articular structures, however, including the cartilage and the bone.

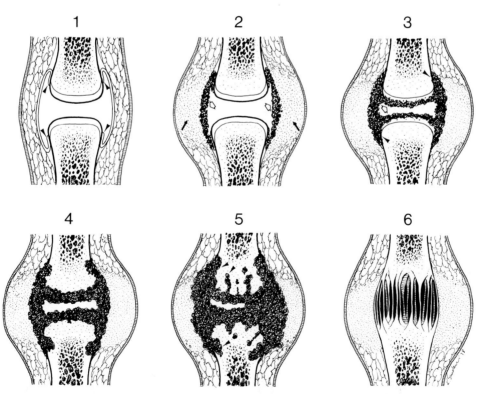

Figure 21–1. Rheumatoid arthritis: Abnormalities of synovial joints. Pathologic overview. In the normal joint (1), observe the articular cartilage and synovial membrane. At the edges of the articulation (arrowheads), synovium abuts on bone that does not possess protective cartilage. The very early abnormalities of rheumatoid arthritis (2) consist of synovial proliferation (open arrows), soft tissue edema (solid arrows), and osteoporosis. At a slightly later stage (3), the inflamed synovial tissue or pannus (open arrow) has extended across the cartilaginous surface, leading to chondral erosion. Capsular distention, soft tissue edema, and osteoporosis are seen. Small osseous erosions at the margins of the joint are appearing (arrowheads). In more advanced stages (4, 5), large marginal and central erosions and "cysts" are noted (arrowheads). In advanced rheumatoid arthritis (6), fibrous ankylosis of the joint is typical.

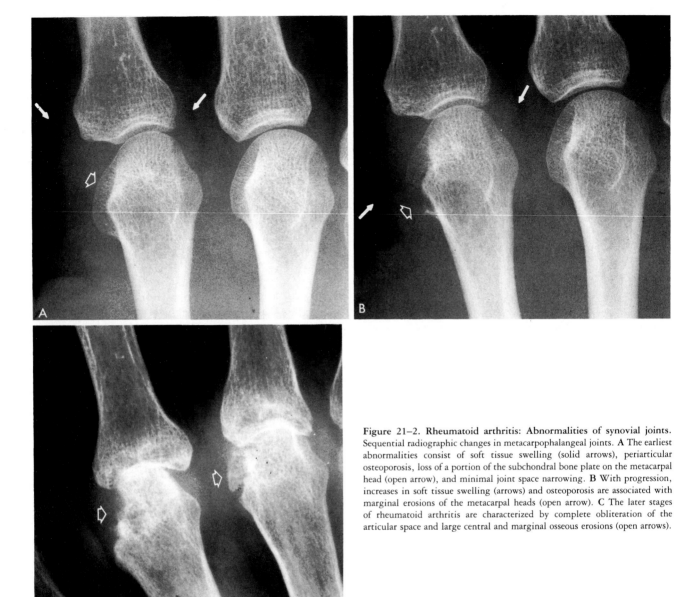

Figure 21–2. Rheumatoid arthritis: Abnormalities of synovial joints. Sequential radiographic changes in metacarpophalangeal joints. **A** The earliest abnormalities consist of soft tissue swelling (solid arrows), periarticular osteoporosis, loss of a portion of the subchondral bone plate on the metacarpal head (open arrow), and minimal joint space narrowing. **B** With progression, increases in soft tissue swelling (arrows) and osteoporosis are associated with marginal erosions of the metacarpal heads (open arrow). **C** The later stages of rheumatoid arthritis are characterized by complete obliteration of the articular space and large central and marginal osseous erosions (open arrows).

The inflamed synovium soon spills from the marginal pockets of the joint and forms an enlarging layer of varying thickness across the surface of the cartilage or extends from the articular recesses through adjacent compact bone into the marrow spaces. The synovial tissue applied to the cartilaginous surface causes morphologic changes owing to enzymatic destruction of cartilage or interference with proper cartilaginous nutrition, or both (Fig. 21–1). In a similar fashion, the synovial tissue within the bone marrow erodes the cartilage from beneath. Cartilage destruction may ultimately become widespread and severe; when the cartilaginous surface on two apposing bones is significantly compromised, granulation tissue may bridge the articular cavity.

The radiographic counterpart of this cartilaginous stage of rheumatoid arthritis is loss of articular space (Fig. 21–2). Along with soft tissue swelling and periarticular osteoporosis, joint space narrowing is one of three early radiographic

characteristics of rheumatoid arthritis (the fourth finding, marginal osseous erosions, is discussed later in this chapter). Loss of the articular space is usually diffuse or widespread, related to the generalized nature of the cartilaginous destruction. This pattern of articular space diminution differs from the focal, segmental, or asymmetric type of joint space loss that occurs in osteoarthritis.

With continuing synovial inflammation and cartilage damage, the articular cavity is partially or completely obliterated by fibrous ankylosis. Although dystrophic calcification and secondary ossification may develop within the inflammatory tissue that fills the articular cavity, producing osseous fusion, these findings are observed less frequently in rheumatoid arthritis than in the seronegative spondyloarthropathies.

SUBCHONDRAL BONE. Two alterations in the subchondral bone that occur in the early stages of rheumatoid arthritis are osteoporosis and marginal erosion. Osteoporosis is initially periarticular in distribution; however, with chronicity of the disease, osteoporosis may extend into the diaphysis. It is related to a combination of disuse of the joint, osteoclastic resorption of the subchondral spongy trabeculae, and steroid-induced osteoporosis.

The initial marginal erosions in rheumatoid arthritis are located in sites of synovial pockets and bare areas that do not possess protective cartilaginous coats (Figs. 21–1 and 21–2). Symmetrically distributed defects appear on both the proximal and the distal bones that constitute the articulation and are usually accompanied by soft tissue swelling, periarticular osteoporosis, and joint space narrowing. Such erosions may be a very early manifestation of the disease, occurring within 1 or 2 years of the onset of joint symptoms.

The radiographic appearance of multiple subchondral lucent areas throughout the joint in patients with more advanced rheumatoid arthritis also is well recognized (Fig. 21–3). The pathogenesis of the cystic lesions (also termed pseudocysts or geodes) is debated. One theory suggests that transchondral extension of superficial pannus or direct extension of subchondral pannus into bone can lead to osseous destruction. Alternatively, such cysts may occur owing to intrusion of synovial fluid through cartilaginous defects or to contusion of bone itself with subsequent osteonecrosis. Finally, cystic defects could be related to true intraosseous rheumatoid nodules.

It has been emphasized that large radiolucent cystic areas may be observed in rheumatoid arthritis patients, particularly men, who have maintained a high level of physical activity. In this peculiar cystic pattern, which has subsequently been termed rheumatoid arthritis of the robust reaction type, lesions have been attributed to the effect of elevated intra-articular pressure forcing synovial fluid or granulation tissue into the bone. In this regard, it is interesting to speculate that cyst formation represents one mechanism of joint decompression (Fig. 21–4). Joint decompression might result from any process allowing fluid to escape from the articulation. Three potential pathways exist for such egress: subchondral cysts, synovial cysts, and fistulae or sinus tracts.

Whatever their pathogenesis, subchondral lucent areas are an important radiographic manifestation in rheumatoid arthritis (Fig. 21–3). They are usually multiple, of small size, and without sclerotic margins. Although joint space narrowing and osteoporosis are frequently encountered as additional findings, subchondral cysts are sometimes observed in the absence of both articular space loss and osteopenia. In these instances, the radiographic manifestations resemble those of gout.

FIBROUS CAPSULE. After prolonged inflammation, capsular contraction can occur. This can aggravate the malalignment and subluxation that are provoked by changes in supporting structures, such as tendons and ligaments, and in periarticular soft tissues (see later discussion). Capsular fibrosis and contraction can be associated with further cartilaginous injury owing to altered mechanical forces across the joint.

SYNOVIAL MEMBRANE, CARTILAGE, AND BONE IN ADVANCED RHEUMATOID ARTHRITIS. In the late stage of rheumatoid arthritis, the total synovial surface area is dramatically increased by the proliferation and hypertrophy of synovial villi, which have occurred during the course of articular inflammation. Once the villi have appeared, they persist even when the synovitis has subsided. Increasing fibrosis of the stroma and accumulations of fibrin within the villous structures are seen. As a terminal event, very elongated

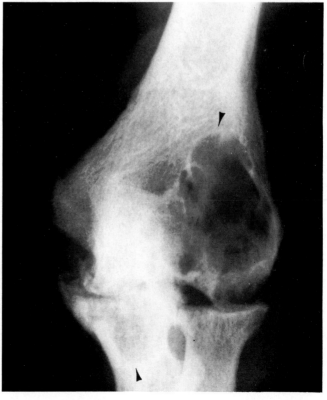

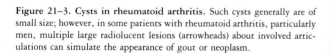

Figure 21–3. Cysts in rheumatoid arthritis. Such cysts generally are of small size; however, in some patients with rheumatoid arthritis, particularly men, multiple large radiolucent lesions (arrowheads) about involved articulations can simulate the appearance of gout or neoplasm.

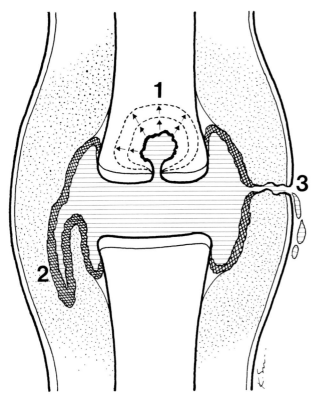

Figure 21–4. Mechanism of decompression of joints with raised intra-articular pressure. The three potential pathways are subchondral cystic lesions (1), synovial cysts (2), and fistulae or sinus tracts (3).

villi may become detached, appearing in the joint cavity as "rice bodies."

In addition to collections of fibrin, fragments of cartilage and bone are found embedded in the synovial tissue (Fig. 21–5). Although the exact pathogenesis of such fragments is unclear, it is probable that they arise from the erosive process that destroys cartilage and bone within the articulation. The fragmentation process can be accentuated by osseous compression, impaction, and fracture produced by the altered mechanics in the involved joint, and it can be further stimulated by the presence of osteoporotic bone and the absence of a protective cartilaginous coat. In some situations, necrotic bone fragments occurring in rheumatoid joints, if numerous and large, may be extruded through the skin. This sequence of events results in fistulous rheumatism (more properly called sinus tract rheumatism).

Osteoarthritis can be a prominent secondary phenomenon in the synovial joints of patients with rheumatoid arthritis. The prerequisites for the development of osteoarthritis in this setting are the subsidence of the inflammation in the synovial membrane, the occurrence of damage to the articular cartilage, and the continued functional use of the joint. When prominent, osteoarthritic abnormalities can obscure the underlying rheumatoid process on both pathologic and radiographic examinations. The possibility of underlying rheumatoid arthritis should be considered whenever radiographs reveal osteoarthritis with unusual features or in unusual sites. Owing to the superimposition of osteoarthritis on rheumatoid arthritis, the diagnosis of the latter disease cannot be eliminated when radiographs demonstrate productive changes (e.g., sclerosis and osteophytes) of bone.

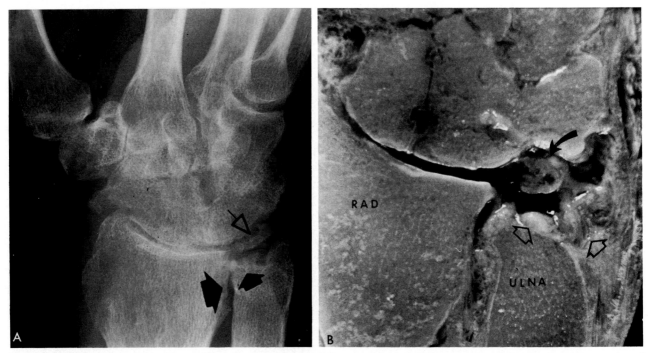

Figure 21–5. Rheumatoid arthritis: Abnormalities of synovial joints. Bone fragmentation. **A** An oblique projection of the wrist demonstrates erosions of the distal portions of the radius and ulna (solid arrows). Carpal fusion, scaphoid erosions with bone production, osteoporosis, and an elongated bone spicule (open arrow) overlying the radiocarpal joint are observed. **B** A coronal section through the wrist reveals the fragment (curved arrow) adjacent to the carpal mass. Abnormal synovium (open arrows) extends across the eroded ulna. The scalloped erosive changes of adjacent portions of the radius (RAD) and ulna are evident. (From Resnick D, Gmelich J: Bone fragmentation in the rheumatoid wrist: Radiographic and pathologic considerations. Radiology *114*:315, 1975. Used with permission.)

Table 21–2. ABNORMALITIES OF BURSAE AND TENDON SHEATHS IN RHEUMATOID ARTHRITIS

Pathologic	Radiologic
Synovial inflammation and production of fluid	Soft tissue swelling
Hyperemia	Osteoporosis
Pannus destruction of subjacent bone	Surface resorption of bone

Table 21–3. ABNORMALITIES OF DISCOVERTEBRAL CARTILAGINOUS JOINTS IN RHEUMATOID ARTHRITIS

Potential Mechanism	Pathogenesis
Synovial Inflammation	"Pannus" is derived from joints of Luschka (cervical region) and costovertebral articulations (thoracic region)
Trauma	Apophyseal joint instability leads to traumatic disruption of discovertebral junction with cartilaginous node formation
Enthesopathy	Inflammation at ligamentous and capsular attachments leads to adjacent osseous erosion

Bursae and Tendon Sheaths (Table 21–2)

Synovial inflammation in rheumatoid arthritis occurs in the synovial lining of tendon sheaths and bursae but is usually of lesser extent than that in the joint. Bursal involvement may occur in the popliteal region of the knee and in the olecranon, subacromial (subdeltoid), and retrocalcaneal bursae, as well as about the wrist and the foot (Fig. 21–6). Tenosynovitis is especially prominent on the dorsum of the hand, the fingers, and the foot.

When inflamed, tendon sheaths and bursae fill with exudate, enlarge, and form clinically detectable soft tissue masses. Acute and chronic inflammatory changes and necrotic foci surrounded by typical palisading cells can be observed histologically. The tendon itself may become affected, leading to a variety of complications, including weakening, subluxation, entrapment, and rupture.

The most common radiographic finding associated with tenosynovitis and bursitis is soft tissue swelling. The swelling is frequently lobulated in outline, simulating the appearance of a gouty tophus. Adjacent soft tissue planes are displaced or obscured by the inflamed mass. Erosion of subjacent bone can be observed, particularly in the posterosuperior aspect of the calcaneus (in relation to retrocalcaneal bursitis), the olecranon process (in relation to olecranon bursitis), and the inferior surface of the acromion and distal end of the clavicle (in relation to subacromial bursitis). In addition, surface resorption of bone beneath inflamed tendon sheaths is characteristic, particularly in the outer aspect of the distal ulna (extensor carpi ulnaris tenosynovitis).

Cartilaginous Joints and Entheses

Although cartilaginous joints (such as the symphysis pubis and manubriosternal and discovertebral articulations) and entheses (such as those related to the spinous processes of the vertebrae, the inferior surface of the calcanei, the iliac wings, the ischial tuberosities, and the femoral trochanters) are involved in rheumatoid arthritis, the frequency and severity of such involvement is far less striking than that which occurs in the seronegative spondyloarthropathies. Furthermore, the pathogenesis of rheumatoid involvement at some cartilaginous and ligamentous sites, such as the discovertebral junction and spinous processes, is controversial.

Of the cartilaginous joints, changes of the discovertebral junction in rheumatoid arthritis have received the most attention (Table 21–3). Such changes predominate in the cervical spine, although their pathogenesis is not agreed on (Figs. 21–7 and 21–8). Various schools of thought have advanced the following suggestions: (1) discovertebral abnormalities occur as a secondary manifestation of synovial inflammation in the adjacent neurocentral articulations (joints of Luschka) in the cervical spine and the neighboring costovertebral articulations in the thoracic spine (the synovial school); (2) discovertebral alterations relate to traumatic insults produced by instability of the posterior elements of the spine (the traumatic school); or (3) discovertebral alterations in rheumatoid arthritis, as in ankylosing spondylitis, are produced by a primary enthesopathy (the enthesopathic school).

Erosion and reactive sclerosis of the spinous processes of the cervical vertebrae appear to be related to two mechanisms. First, an inflammatory process at the sites of ligament attachment to bone is consistent with the enthesopathy that

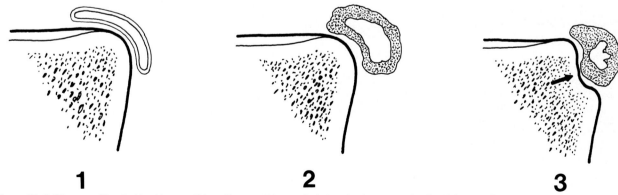

Figure 21–6. Rheumatoid arthritis: Abnormalities of bursae. Diagram depicting the changes associated with bursal inflammation. In the normal situation (1), a collapsed, noninflamed synovial sac is evident. With progressive inflammation (2, 3), hypertrophy of the synovial lining, increased intrabursal fluid, distention, and possible erosion of subjacent bone (arrow) can be seen.

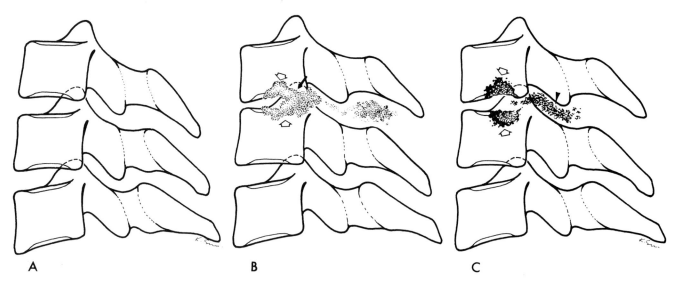

Figure 21–7. Rheumatoid arthritis: Abnormalities of the discovertebral junctions of the cervical spine. The normal situation is depicted in **A**. The proponents of the synovial school of thought suggest that inflammatory tissue in the neurocentral joints of Luschka (solid arrow) spreads across the discovertebral junction (**B**), leading to osseous erosion (open arrows). The proponents of the traumatic school of thought believe that instability of the apophyseal joints owing to synovial inflammation (arrowhead) produces recurrent discovertebral trauma, leading to cartilaginous nodes with surrounding sclerosis (**C**) (open arrows).

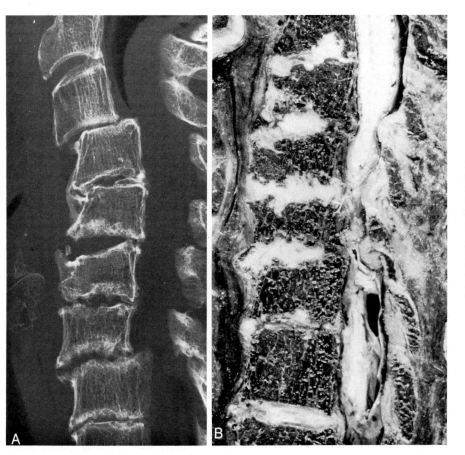

Figure 21–8. Rheumatoid arthritis: Abnormalities of the discovertebral junctions of the cervical spine. A radiograph (**A**) and corresponding photograph (**B**) of a sagittal section of the cervical spine reveal widespread alterations of the discovertebral junctions. Observe narrowing of the intervertebral discs, erosion of the vertebral endplates with intraosseous extension of discal material, multiple subluxations, and only mild osteophyte formation. Spinal cord compression is evident.

is also recognized in ankylosing spondylitis and other seronegative spondyloarthropathies. Second, synovial inflammation in interspinous bursae may contribute to the destructive process in the neighboring bone.

Tendons and Ligaments

Significant abnormalities of tendons and ligaments occur in rheumatoid arthritis. Inflammatory changes and laxity resulting from distortion of these structures by the intraarticular process are seen, contributing to the typical joint deformities that accompany long-standing rheumatoid arthritis.

"Spontaneous" tendon ruptures are a known manifestation of rheumatoid arthritis. They are most frequently encountered in the hand and the wrist, although ruptures of other tendons can occur, including the Achilles, infrapatellar, and rotator cuff tendons. Tendon rupture, which can be provoked by local corticosteroid injection, may be attributable to collagenolysis by abnormal production of proteolytic enzymes that originate from diseased synovium in adjacent structures. Tendon inflammation itself may further enhance the disruption process.

Joint subluxation, malalignment, and deformity in rheumatoid arthritis can be attributed to numerous factors (Fig. 21–9). Inflammatory destruction of intraarticular structures leading to surface incongruity, capsular and ligamentous weakening leading to laxity, tendinitis and tenosynovitis

leading to contracture and rupture, and muscular contraction are all influential in this regard. Articular deformity can become evident in many different sites but is most characteristic at the wrist, the metacarpophalangeal, metatarsophalangeal, and interphalangeal articulations of the hand and the foot, and the atlantoaxial region. On radiographic examination, subluxation is almost invariably combined with typical intraarticular alterations.

Soft Tissues

RHEUMATOID NODULES. The most frequent soft tissue lesion in rheumatoid arthritis is the subcutaneous nodule. Although such nodules were considered virtually diagnostic of rheumatoid arthritis for a period of time, it is now recognized that these or similar nodules are associated with a wide variety of disorders, including rheumatic fever, collagen disorders, sarcoidosis, Weber-Christian disease, gout, dermatologic processes, xanthomatosis, and various infectious disorders, as well as other conditions.

One or more subcutaneous nodules are detectable in approximately 20 per cent of patients with rheumatoid arthritis. They are most commonly located between the skin and an underlying bony prominence. Typical locations include the olecranon, the proximal portion of the ulna, the lateral aspects of the fingers, the gluteal and Achilles tendon regions, and the areas about the femoral trochanters and ischial tuberosities. Similar lesions are encountered in noncutaneous structures,

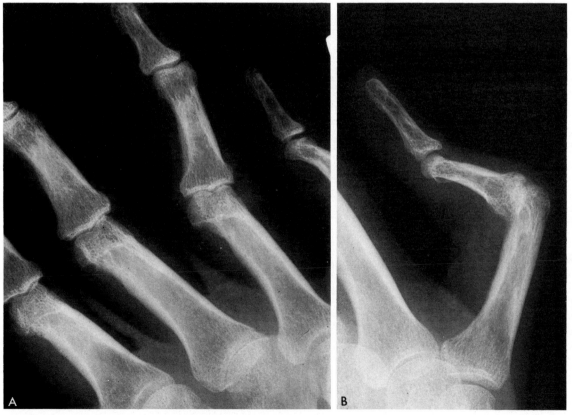

Figure 21–9. Rheumatoid arthritis: Joint malalignment. A, B Typical digital deformities of the hand in rheumatoid arthritis include the swan-neck deformity (hyperextension at proximal interphalangeal joint and flexion at distal interphalangeal joint) **(A)** and boutonnière deformity (flexion at proximal interphalangeal joint and hyperextension at distal interphalangeal joint **(B)**.

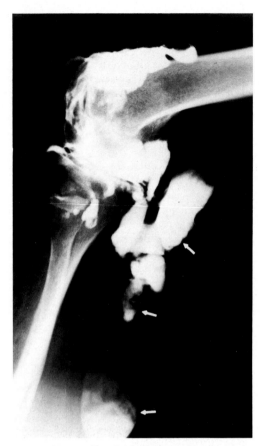

Figure 21–10. Rheumatoid arthritis: Synovial cyst. A typical popliteal cyst (arrows) is demonstrated during knee arthrography. Its margins are somewhat irregular, indicating synovial inflammation.

Radiographically, subcutaneous rheumatoid nodules are associated with lobulated, eccentric soft tissue masses. These masses rarely calcify, a diagnostic point that may be helpful in distinguishing them from gouty tophi, which can contain calcification. In unusual instances, rheumatoid nodules can lead to erosion of subjacent bone, simulating the appearance of a variety of benign soft tissue neoplasms as well as gout, giant cell tumor of a tendon sheath, ganglia, and xanthoma.

An atypical variant of rheumatoid disease, rheumatoid nodulosis, is characterized by the presence of multiple subcutaneous nodules and the absence of significant synovitis or systemic manifestations. Men are usually affected. In addition to nodular soft tissue masses, radiographs may detect intra-articular cystic osseous defects with or without joint space narrowing or osteoporosis. Serologic tests for rheumatoid factor commonly are positive in these persons, and biopsy of the nodules and synovium reveals typical histologic changes of rheumatoid arthritis.

SYNOVIAL CYSTS. Synovial cysts are a well-known manifestation of rheumatoid arthritis (Fig. 21–10). Although some investigators believe synovial cysts arise as rupture of the joint capsule with extravasation of fluid and secondary encapsulation or as herniation of the synovial membrane, most now consider that these lesions represent abnormal distention of various bursae that communicate with the adjacent articulation. These communicating channels frequently possess a valvular mechanism allowing the flow of synovial fluid to proceed in one direction only (from the articulation to the cyst and not from the cyst to the articulation). An optimal way to visualize the cystic mass and its communication with the joint is to inject contrast material directly into the articulation. The contrast-opacified cyst may be smooth or irregular in outline. In some cases, free extravasation of contrast material into the adjacent soft tissue planes indicates cyst rupture. Clinical differentiation of signs and symptoms related to synovial cysts about the knee from those resulting from thrombophlebitis can be difficult.

Arthrography remains the most popular method employed in the diagnosis of synovial cysts, although other techniques, such as ultrasonography, scintigraphy, computed tomography, and magnetic resonance imaging, may be employed.

Although they are most frequently observed in the popliteal region, rheumatoid synovial cysts have been described at other sites, including the calf; the superior, anteromedial, lateral, or retrofemoral aspect of the knee; the ankle; the plantar aspect of the foot; the hip; the hand and wrist; the elbow; and the shoulder.

such as the synovium, the dura mater, the sclera, the retropharyngeal tissue, the lungs, and the heart. Rheumatoid nodules are generally associated with seropositivity for rheumatoid factor. Their presence also suggests a likelihood for severe erosive disease and vasculitis. They may be identified before the clinical onset of arthritis.

Three distinct zones constitute the histologic picture of a rheumatoid nodule. A central area of necrosis is surrounded by a zone of palisading, elongated cells. The outer layer contains granulation tissue, which initially is vascular but later may become fibrotic.

Table 21–4. MECHANISMS AND SITES OF PATHOLOGIC FRACTURES IN RHEUMATOID ARTHRITIS

Mechanism	Typical Sites
Synovial inflammation with erosion of bone	Odontoid process, carpal scaphoid bone, distal portion of ulna
Mechanical erosion of bone	Ribs, articular surfaces of small bones in the hands and feet, medial aspect of the humeral neck
Intraosseous cystic lesions	Proximal portion of ulna, femoral neck, femur and tibia about the knee
Bone deformation	Acetabulum
Generalized osteopenia	Insufficiency fractures of vertebral bodies, sacrum, tubular bones of the lower extremity, small bones of the foot
Ischemic necrosis	Femoral head, vertebral bodies
Osteomyelitis	Variable

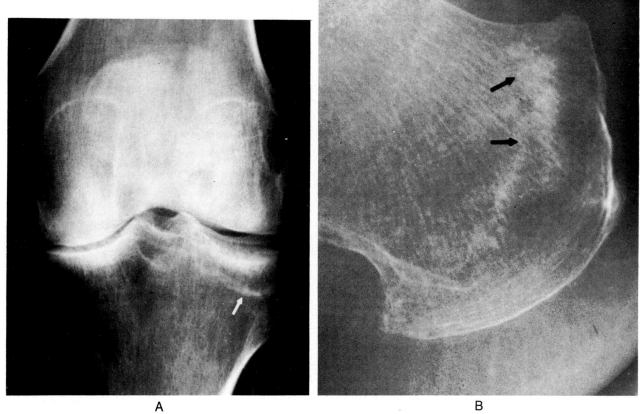

A   B

Figure 21–11. Rheumatoid arthritis: Insufficiency (stress) fractures. A An insufficiency fracture of the lateral tibial plateau (arrow) is seen in this patient with rheumatoid knee involvement. B In another patient with rheumatoid arthritis, a classic insufficiency fracture of the calcaneus (arrows) has produced vertically oriented bone sclerosis.

Bones

Generalized or periarticular osteoporosis is a common manifestation in patients with rheumatoid arthritis. Many factors appear to be important in its pathogenesis, including hypervascularity and disuse. Corticosteroid or salicylate therapy appears to be an additional factor.

Osteoporosis producing osseous weakening contributes to the fractures that are not uncommonly encountered in patients with rheumatoid arthritis (Table 21–4). These may occur after minimal trauma or spontaneously in either spinal sites (compression fractures of vertebral bodies) or extraspinal locations. Indeed, insufficiency or stress fractures of the tubular bones of the lower extremity in rheumatoid arthritis are well recognized (Fig. 21–11); causative factors include osteoporosis, corticosteroid therapy, angular deformity, and flexion contracture. Erosive abnormality of bone related to the rheumatoid process itself can also lead to fracture and deformity (Fig. 21–12). Thus, pathologic fractures through the odontoid or olecranon process and acetabular weakening and fracture leading to protrusion deformity are observed. Other sites of fracture include the scaphoid and humeral neck.

SERONEGATIVE SPONDYLOARTHROPATHIES
Overview

The three major seronegative spondyloarthropathies—ankylosing spondylitis, psoriasis, and Reiter's syndrome—share with rheumatoid arthritis many radiologic and pathologic features. They, too, involve synovial joints and are associated with considerable inflammation of the synovial membrane.

Fundamental differences exist between the spondyloarthropathies and rheumatoid arthritis, however, especially in distribution and morphology of osteoarticular lesions (Table 21–5).

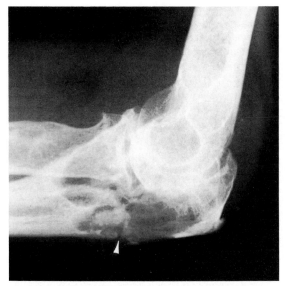

Figure 21–12. Rheumatoid arthritis: Fracture through site of bone erosion—ulnar olecranon. A fracture (arrowhead) through a large cyst is evident.

Table 21–5. RHEUMATOID ARTHRITIS VERSUS THE SERONEGATIVE SPONDYLOARTHROPATHIES

	Rheumatoid Arthritis	Seronegative Spondyloarthropathies
Synovial Joint Involvement	+	+
Soft tissue swelling	+	+
Osteoporosis	+	±
Marginal erosions	+	+
Central erosions and cysts	+	+
Bone ankylosis	±	+
Bone proliferation	−	+
Malalignment and subluxation	+	±
Bursal and Tendon Sheath Involvement	+	+
Soft tissue swelling	+	+
Bone erosions	+	+
Bone proliferation	−	+
Cartilaginous Joint Involvement	±	+
Bone erosions	±	+
Bone proliferation	±	+
Bone ankylosis	±	+
Enthesopathy	±	+
Bone erosions	±	+
Bone proliferation	±	+

+ = Common; ± = less common; − = rare or absent.

All three of these spondyloarthropathic processes produce significant abnormalities of cartilaginous joints and entheses as well as synovial joints. The discovertebral junctions throughout the spine, the symphysis pubis, the manubriosternal joints, and the tendinous and ligamentous attachments in the calcaneus, pelvis, trochanters of the femur, tuberosities of the humerus, and patella are altered to a much greater extent in ankylosing spondylitis, psoriasis, and Reiter's syndrome than in rheumatoid arthritis. When cartilaginous joints and entheses are involved along with the synovial articulations, a characteristic, although not invariable, distribution in each of these seronegative spondyloarthropathies is seen. Ankylosing spondylitis affects primarily the synovial and cartilaginous joints and entheses of the axial skeleton, with less consistent and severe changes in the appendicular skeleton. The distribution of psoriatic arthritis is somewhat variable, although a polyarticular disorder of synovial joints of the appendicular skeleton with prominent involvement of the interphalangeal joints of the hand and foot, combined with changes at the synovial and cartilaginous joints of the axial skeleton and entheses of the axial and appendicular skeleton, is distinctive. In Reiter's syndrome, asymmetric and "spotty" abnormalities of synovial articulations of the lower extremities are frequently coupled with sacroiliitis, spondylitis, and enthesopathy of the inferior surface of the calcaneus.

In addition to these differences in the distribution of articular abnormalities in the various seronegative spondyloarthropathies and rheumatoid arthritis, differences in the morphology of the lesions can also be evident. In this regard, the radiographic and pathologic characteristics of joint involvement in ankylosing spondylitis, psoriasis, and Reiter's syndrome are fundamentally similar and can be distinguished from those in rheumatoid arthritis. In synovial joints, the absence of osteoporosis and the presence of bone proliferation and intraarticular bone ankylosis in the seronegative spondyloarthropathies are most helpful in differentiating the changes from those of rheumatoid arthritis. In cartilaginous joints, the extent of osseous erosion and bone proliferation in the former disorders is also helpful in differential diagnosis. At sites of tendon and ligament attachment to bone, an inflammatory enthesopathy leading to osseous destruction and repair is characteristic of the spondyloarthropathies.

Synovial Joints (Table 21–6)

As in rheumatoid arthritis, the predominant target area in the synovial joints in the seronegative spondyloarthropathies appears to be the synovial membrane (Fig. 21–13). The inflammatory changes in ankylosing spondylitis, psoriasis, and Reiter's syndrome are of less intensity than in rheumatoid arthritis. Fibroplasia, which is followed by cartilaginous metaplasia and chondroossification, can lead to intraarticular bone ankylosis in any of the spondyloarthropathies. Osseous fusion at sites other than the carpal and tarsal areas is relatively unusual in rheumatoid arthritis.

The proclivity to osseous fusion of certain synovial joints, such as the apophyseal and sacroiliac articulations, especially in ankylosing spondylitis, appears to be related, in part, to abnormalities occurring in the capsuloligamentous attachments, perhaps reflecting another manifestation of a generalized enthesopathy. Capsular ossification can lead to interosseous bridging at the periphery of an involved joint (Fig. 21–14). In this fashion, a bone shell can be detected initially that encloses well-preserved articular cartilage.

The central osseous structures (the sites of erosion by superficial or subchondral pannus and, perhaps, of endochon-

Table 21–6. ABNORMALITIES OF SYNOVIAL JOINTS IN THE SERONEGATIVE SPONDYLOARTHROPATHIES

Pathologic	Radiologic
Synovial inflammation and production of fluid	Soft tissue swelling and widening of joint space
Mild to moderate hyperemia	Variable osteoporosis
Pannus destruction of cartilage	Narrowing of joint space
Pannus destruction of "unprotected" bone at margin of joint	Marginal bone erosions
Pannus destruction of subchondral bone	Bone erosions and formation of subchondral cysts
Fibroplasia, cartilaginous metaplasia, chondro-ossification and capsular ossification	Bone ankylosis
Bony proliferation in response to damage	Marginal "whiskering," periostitis, subchondral sclerosis
Noninflammatory proliferation of the periosteum	Cortical atrophy, osteolysis

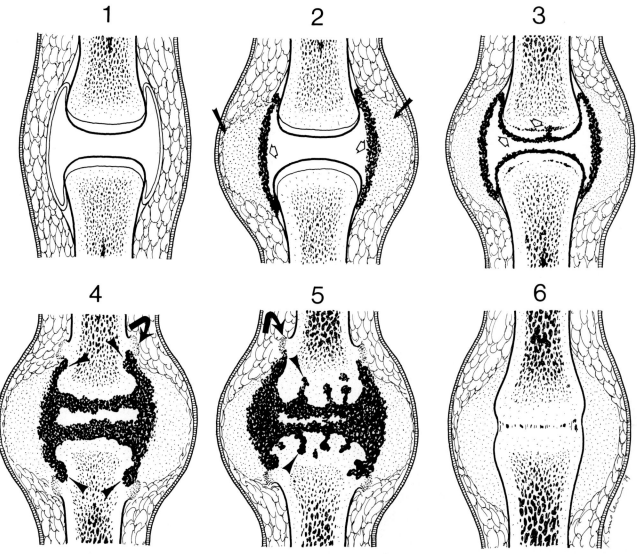

Figure 21–13. Seronegative spondyloarthropathies: Abnormalities of synovial joints—pathologic overview. The normal synovial joint is depicted at the upper left (1). Early changes (2) consist of synovial inflammation (open arrows) and soft tissue edema (solid arrows). Osteoporosis may not be evident. Subsequently (3), synovial inflammatory tissue or pannus extends across and beneath the chondral surface (open arrows), leading to cartilaginous erosion or disruption. At later stages (4, 5), marginal and central osseous erosions develop (arrowheads). Associated bone proliferation (curved arrows) becomes evident. Finally (6), intraarticular bone ankylosis may develop.

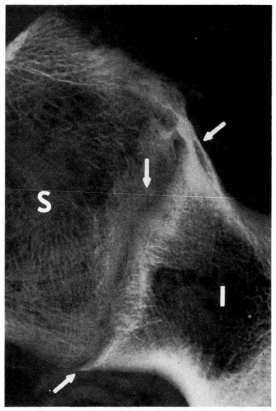

Figure 21–14. Seronegative spondyloarthropathy: Abnormality of synovial joint—radiographic changes of intraarticular bone ankylosis. In a cadaver with ankylosing spondylitis, a radiograph of a coronal section through the sacroiliac joint demonstrates capsular and ligamentous ossification (arrows) producing osseous fusion of the sacrum (S) and ilium (I).

dral ossification) and the peripheral or marginal osseous structures (the sites of destruction by inflamed synovium at the recesses of the joint) respond in a characteristic fashion in the seronegative spondyloarthropathies. Subchondral eburnation, irregular excrescences at the margins of the joint, and periostitis of adjacent diaphyses, particularly in the phalanges, the metacarpal bones, and the metatarsal bones, are distinctive (Fig. 21–15). The exact cause of new bone formation in these disorders is not known.

Osseous erosion in ankylosing spondylitis, psoriasis, and Reiter's syndrome may be superficial and quickly obscured by the profound tendency for bone proliferation. Furthermore, collapse of weakened osteoporotic periarticular bone, a prominent finding in some patients with rheumatoid arthritis, is less frequent and extensive in the seronegative spondyloarthropathies, in which osteoporosis is not commonly a significant finding. Despite this general tendency to less severe erosion and collapse of osseous surfaces, however, some patients, particularly those with psoriasis, can reveal striking osteolysis, which may progress to involve large portions of the supporting bone. Telescoping of one bone into the adjacent one can lead to extensive deformities that can be detected clinically in these circumstances.

Bursae and Tendon Sheaths

The frequency and severity of inflammation in synovium-lined bursae and tendon sheaths in the seronegative spondyloarthropathies may be somewhat less than in rheumatoid arthritis.

Retrocalcaneal bursitis in ankylosing spondylitis, psoriasis, or Reiter's syndrome, however, produces pre-Achilles soft tissue swelling and indistinctness as well as osseous erosion of the subjacent calcaneal surface, findings that are virtually

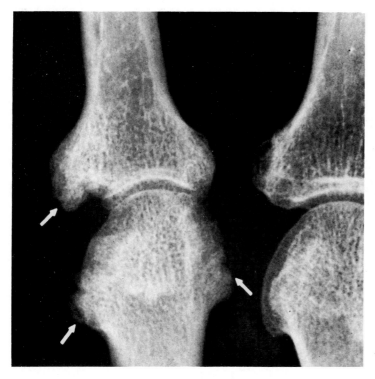

Figure 21–15. Seronegative spondyloarthropathy: Abnormality of synovial joint—radiographic changes of bone proliferation or "whiskering." In a cadaver with ankylosing spondylitis, observe superficial osseous erosion with adjacent bone proliferation (arrows), producing an irregular osseous outline. Osteoporosis is not apparent.

Table 21–7. ABNORMALITIES OF CARTILAGINOUS JOINTS AND ENTHESES IN THE SERONEGATIVE SPONDYLOARTHROPATHIES

Pathologic	Radiologic
Inflammation of subchondral bone	Bone erosion and sclerosis
Bone proliferation	Bone ankylosis
Inflammation of capsular, ligamentous, and tendinous attachments	Bone erosion and sclerosis

indistinguishable from those in rheumatoid arthritis. Similarly, tenosynovitis, a well-known and frequently encountered manifestation of rheumatoid arthritis, has received less attention in ankylosing spondylitis, psoriasis, and Reiter's syndrome, although it may occasionally be a prominent feature in these latter disorders. In fact, periosteal proliferation in the digits in some patients with seronegative spondyloarthropathies can be related to synovitis of adjacent tendon sheaths. Considerable soft tissue swelling in this clinical situation can produce a "sausage-shaped" finger or toe.

Cartilaginous Joints and Entheses (Table 21–7)

The tendency for ankylosing spondylitis, psoriasis, and Reiter's syndrome to affect cartilaginous joints and sites of tendon and ligament attachment to bone is well known. At the manubriosternal joint and symphysis pubis, pathologic observations confirm the presence of chronic inflammatory changes in the subchondral bone, leading to trabecular thickening and intraarticular ossification. Similar abnormalities in

the discovertebral joint produce the "osteitis" of the anterior vertebral margin that is accompanied by erosion and sclerosis of bone and the progressive discal ossification that is associated with syndesmophyte formation (Fig. 21–16).

At each of the cartilaginous joints (the manubriosternal joint, the symphysis pubis, and the discovertebral junction), the changes may relate not only to true chondroosseous inflammation but also to an enthesopathy at the peripheral capsular attachments, indistinguishable from that present at other sites of ligament and tendon attachment to bone. About the intervertebral discs, osseous erosions can be observed at the anterior or anterolateral attachment and, to a lesser extent, the posterior attachment of the outer fibers of the anulus fibrosus to the corners of the vertebral body. At these sites, lymphocytic and plasma cell infiltration can be associated with adjacent reactive bone production.

The pathogenesis of destructive lesions at single or multiple discovertebral junctions during the course of ankylosing spondylitis is not clear. Several mechanisms probably contribute to these lesions, including an increasing enthesopathy, pressure destruction of the intervertebral disc related to kyphosis, cartilage node formation, and pseudarthrosis about a fracture site. The last-mentioned mechanism is expected in long-standing disease in which a rigid vertebral column, caused by widespread bone ankylosis, is predisposed to fracture in a manner similar to that of a long tubular bone. As destructive lesions of intervertebral discs are also observed in early stages of ankylosing spondylitis, other mechanisms must be operational. Inflammation seems a likely cause in these instances.

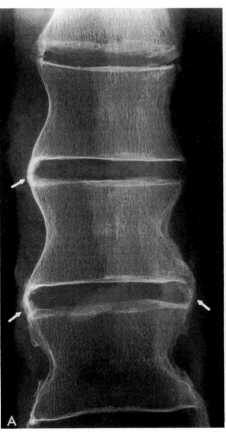 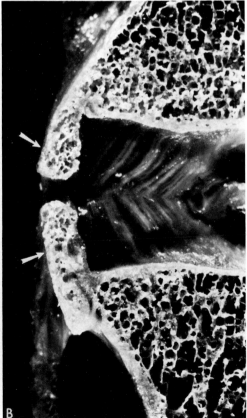

Figure 21–16. Seronegative spondyloarthropathies: Abnormalities of cartilaginous joints of the discovertebral junctions. **A** A radiograph of a coronal section of the spine in a cadaver with ankylosing spondylitis reveals typical syndesmophytes extending as linear osseous bridges from one vertebral body to the next (arrows). **B** On a photograph of a corresponding section from another cadaver with ankylosing spondylitis, the nature of the syndesmophytes is evident (arrows)—they represent chondrification and ossification of the anulus fibrosus.

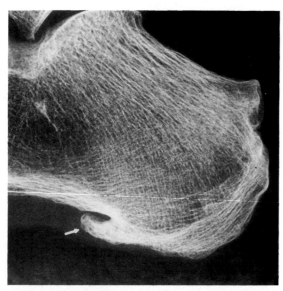

Figure 21–17. Seronegative spondyloarthropathy: Abnormality of attachment of ligament (enthesis). A radiograph of a sagittal section of the calcaneus in a cadaver with ankylosing spondylitis outlines a well-defined osseous excrescence with surrounding proliferation at the ligamentous attachment to the bone (arrow).

An enthesopathy (Fig. 21–17) occurring at other tendinous and ligamentous connections to bone in patients with seronegative spondyloarthropathies is responsible for prominent clinical and radiographic manifestations on the plantar aspect of the calcaneus, the pelvis, the patella, the iliac crest, the ischial and humeral tuberosities, and the femoral trochanters. The enthesopathy leads to osseous erosion that is followed by bone deposition, which leads to a poorly defined or "fluffy" osseous contour.

FURTHER READING

Ball J: Enthesopathy of rheumatoid and ankylosing spondylitis. Ann Rheum Dis. 30:213, 1971.

Bywaters EGL: Rheumatoid and other diseases of the cervical interspinous bursae and changes in the spinous processes. Ann Rheum Dis 41:360, 1982.

Bywaters EGL: Pathology of the spondyloarthropathies. In A Calin (Ed): Spondyloarthropathies. New York, Grune & Stratton, 1984.

Cruickshank B: Pathology of ankylosing spondylitis. Clin Orthop 74:43, 1971.

Fassbender HG: Pathology of Rheumatic Diseases. New York, Springer-Verlag, 1975.

Gardner DL: Pathology of rheumatoid arthritis. In Copeman's Textbook of the Rheumatic Diseases. 5th Ed. Edinburgh, Churchill Livingstone, 1978.

Ginsberg MH, Genant HK, Yu TF, McCarty DJ: Rheumatoid nodulosis. An unusual variant of rheumatoid disease. Arthritis Rheum 18:49, 1975.

Jaffe HL: Metabolic, Degenerative and Inflammatory Diseases of Bones and Joints. Philadelphia, Lea & Febiger, 1972.

Kaye BR, Kaye RL, Bobrove A: Rheumatoid nodules. Review of the spectrum of associated conditions and proposal of a new classification, with a report of four seronegative cases. Am J Med 76:279, 1984.

Martel W: Pathogenesis of cervical discovertebral destruction in rheumatoid arthritis. Arthritis Rheum 20:1217, 1977.

Martel W, Hayes JT, Duff IF: The pattern of bone erosion in the hand and wrist in rheumatoid arthritis. Radiology 84:204, 1965.

Rappoport AS, Sosman JL, Weissman BN: Lesions resembling gout in patients with rheumatoid arthritis. AJR 126:41, 1976.

Rauschning W: Popliteal cysts and their relation to the gastrocnemiosemi-membranosus bursa. Studies on the surgical and functional anatomy. Acta Orthop Scand 179(Suppl):9, 1979.

Resnick D: Radiology of seronegative spondyloarthropathies. Clin Orthop 143:38, 1979.

Resnick D, Cone R: Pathological fractures in rheumatoid arthritis: Sites and mechanisms. RadioGraphics 4:549, 1984.

Resnick D, Niwayama G: On the nature and significance of bony proliferation in "rheumatoid variant" disorders. AJR 129:275, 1977.

Resnick D, Niwayama G, Coutts R: Subchondral cysts (geodes) in arthritic disorders: Pathologic and radiographic appearance of the hip joint. AJR 128:799, 1977.

Resnick D, Feingold ML, Curd J, Niwayama G, Goergen TG: Calcaneal abnormalities in articular disorders. Rheumatoid arthritis, ankylosing spondylitis, psoriatic arthritis and Reiter's syndrome. Radiology 125:355, 1977.

Schneider R, Kaye JJ: Insufficiency and stress fractures of the long bones occurring in patients with rheumatoid arthritis. Radiology 116:595, 1975.

Sokoloff L: The pathology of rheumatoid arthritis and allied disorders. In JL Hollander, DJ McCarty Jr (Eds): Arthritis and Allied Conditions. 8th Ed. Philadelphia, Lea & Febiger, 1972.

Wu PC, Fang D, Ho EKW, Leong JCY: The pathogenesis of extensive discovertebral destruction in anykylosing spondylitis. Clin Orthop 230:154, 1988.

Chapter 22

Rheumatoid Arthritis

Donald Resnick, M.D.
Gen Niwayama, M.D.

Rheumatoid arthritis is a common articular disorder with a characteristic radiographic picture. A symmetric polyarticular disease of the synovial joints of the appendicular skeleton is apparent, with prominent abnormalities of the proximal interphalangeal and metacarpophalangeal joints of the hand, the wrist, the metatarsophalangeal joints of the foot, the posterior and plantar aspects of the calcaneus, the knee, the elbow, the glenohumeral and acromio-clavicular joints, the ankle, and the hip; these abnormalities are commonly combined with changes in the cervical spine. This distribution of synovial joint involvement is sufficiently common to allow accurate diagnosis in most patients with this disorder, especially when the involvement is characterized by fusiform soft tissue swelling, regional or periarticular osteoporosis, marginal and central osseous erosions and cysts, and diffuse loss of interosseous space.

Rheumatoid arthritis is an "everyday" disease whose general clinical, pathologic, and radiologic features are well known to most physicians. An in-depth inspection of the radiographic and pathologic characteristics of rheumatoid arthritis provides a standard by which the other rheumatologic conditions can be measured. Such an inspection must initially consider the basic pathologic and radiologic features of rheumatoid involvement in synovium-lined articulations, bursae, and tendon sheaths, cartilaginous joints, tendinous and ligamentous attachments to bone, and supporting soft tissue structures. This has been accomplished in Chapter 21. From this reference point, an analysis of the changes produced by rheumatoid arthritis in specific locations of the body is appropriate.

DIAGNOSTIC CRITERIA

The accurate diagnosis of rheumatoid arthritis is without difficulty in the patient who reveals a generalized symmetric, peripherally located polyarthritis associated with (1) clinically detectable severe morning stiffness, synovial inflammation, and subcutaneous nodules; (2) radiologic evidence of an erosive articular process; (3) laboratory parameters of the disease, including a positive serologic test for rheumatoid factor and an elevated erythrocyte sedimentation rate; and (4) pathologic documentation of typical rheumatoid lesions of the synovium and the soft tissues. More troublesome, however, is establishing the presence of this disease in the patient who has atypical clinical and radiologic features. Because of this difficulty, basic diagnostic criteria for rheumatoid arthritis have been established. These criteria include the following:

1. Morning stiffness.
2. Pain on motion or tenderness in at least one joint.
3. Soft tissue swelling or fluid accumulation in at least one joint.
4. Swelling of at least one additional joint.
5. Symmetric joint swelling with simultaneous involvement of the same articulation or group of articulations on both sides of the body.

6. Subcutaneous nodules over bone prominences on extensor surfaces or in juxtaarticular regions.
7. Typical radiographic changes in involved joints.
8. Positive sheep cell agglutination test.
9. Poor mucin precipitate from synovial fluid.
10. Characteristic histologic changes in the synovial membrane.
11. Characteristic histologic changes in nodules.

The diagnosis of classic rheumatoid arthritis requires the presence of at least seven of these 11 criteria and of joint symptoms, including swelling, for at least 6 months. The diagnosis of definite rheumatoid arthritis requires the presence of at least five of these criteria and of continuous joint symptoms and signs for at least 6 weeks. Probable rheumatoid arthritis is established when three of the 11 criteria are evident and when joint symptoms and signs have been present for 4 to 6 weeks. Possible rheumatoid arthritis indicates that at least two of the following criteria are evident and that joint symptoms have been apparent for at least 3 weeks: morning stiffness, tenderness or pain on motion, joint swelling, subcutaneous nodules, elevated erythrocyte sedimentation rate or C-reactive protein, and iritis. A number of exceptions or exclusions to these criteria have also been established.

CLINICAL ABNORMALITIES
General Features

Rheumatoid arthritis predominates between the ages of 25 and 55 years. Women are affected more commonly than men, in a ratio of approximately 2 or 3 to 1. An insidious onset is most typical. Various prodromal symptoms, including fatigue, anorexia, weight loss, malaise, and muscular pain and stiffness, can be obscured by prominent articular complaints, which are frequently an early manifestation of the disease. Joint pain and stiffness can initially involve a single joint before more generalized articular findings become manifest. Some patients demonstrate mild clinical manifestations for a long period of time, whereas in others, rapid, severe, and disabling arthritis soon becomes apparent.

Articular Involvement

Articular involvement becomes manifest as pain that is aggravated on motion, swelling, stiffness, and limitation of movement. Periarticular soft tissue swelling is fusiform or spindle-shaped in configuration.

The most typically affected joints are the proximal interphalangeal and metacarpophalangeal joints of the hand, the wrist, the metatarsophalangeal joints of the foot, the knee, the joints of the shoulder, the ankle, and, to a lesser extent, the hip. Symmetry is the hallmark of joint alteration in this disease; there are some exceptions to this rule, however:

1. Although symmetric abnormalities of groups of joints can be seen, the identical digits may not be affected on both sides of the body.

2. Initially, monoarticular or pauciarticular abnormalities can be noted that do not obey the rule of symmetry. The reported frequency of monarthritis in rheumatoid arthritis has varied from approximately 5 to 20 per cent of cases; the knee and the wrist are the two joints that are the most frequent sites of monarthritis.

3. A markedly asymmetric or unilateral distribution in rheumatoid arthritis can be seen in patients with neurologic deficits. Unilateral muscular weakening or paralysis protects the ipsilateral side from the effects of the articular disease. This clinical asymmetry, which can be accompanied by radiographic asymmetry, is not evident when a neurologic deficit develops in a patient already suffering from rheumatoid arthritis.

4. Differences in the distribution of rheumatoid arthritis can occasionally be related to the sex of the patient. In women, a symmetric distribution in the small peripheral joints of the extremities is more typical than in men. In male patients, asymmetric abnormalities in small or large joints can be noted.

5. Atypical cases of rheumatoid arthritis (those that do not meet the necessary criteria for classic or definite disease) are often characterized by asymmetric joint alterations.

Soft Tissue, Muscular, and Vascular Involvement

Subcutaneous nodules are evident in approximately one fourth of patients with rheumatoid arthritis. They appear at pressure points, especially the juxtaarticular regions of the elbow. Other tendinous and soft tissue locations commonly reveal similar nodules, and these lesions may be demonstrated in distant body sites, including the lungs, pleurae, vocal cords, larynx, scalp, sclerae, peritoneum, and abdominal wall.

Muscular weakness and atrophy can be prominent in patients with rheumatoid arthritis. These muscular abnormalities can relate to disuse or inflammatory changes.

A variety of vascular lesions are noted in this disease. Inflammatory and noninflammatory vascular changes lead to peripheral neuropathy, perforation of the bowel, myocardial infarction, Raynaud's phenomenon, gangrene, and pulmonary hypertension.

Systemic Involvement
Felty's Syndrome

The association of rheumatoid arthritis, splenomegaly, and leukopenia represents Felty's syndrome. Additional clinical manifestations of this syndrome include weight loss, anemia, lymphadenopathy, chronic leg ulceration, and abnormal skin pigmentation. Women are affected more frequently than men, and the abnormalities can become severe. Leukopenia probably results from hypersplenism, and the anemia appears to be related to hemolysis.

Metabolic Bone Disorders

Osteopenia is a well-recognized manifestation of rheumatoid arthritis. It usually relates to osteoporosis, the severity of which is influenced by the age and sex of the patient, the duration of the disease, the extent of immobilization, and the administration of corticosteroids. In addition, osteomalacia related to inadequate intake of vitamin D, malabsorption, and lack of sunshine and hypercalcemia with secondary hyperparathyroidism are two additional mechanisms that may contribute to osteopenia.

Sjögren's Syndrome

Sjögren's syndrome is a triad consisting of keratoconjunctivitis sicca, xerostomia, and connective tissue disease (see Chapter 57).

LABORATORY ABNORMALITIES

A moderate normochromic or hypochromic normocytic anemia is common in this disease. The leukocyte count can be normal, elevated, or, rarely, decreased. The erythrocyte sedimentation rate commonly is markedly elevated and tends to parallel the activity of the disease. The C-reactive protein is evident in almost all patients with disease activity. Rheumatoid factors generally are present in high titer in the serum of patients with this disease. They are also evident in a variety of chronic inflammatory conditions but are not detected in great concentration in most other articular disorders.

ABNORMALITIES AT SPECIFIC LOCATIONS
General Distribution

A symmetric arthritis showing predilection for the hands, wrists, feet, knees, shoulders, elbows, ankles, and hips is typical. In the axial skeleton, the joints of the cervical spine are the only sites that are consistently affected. Cartilaginous joints, such as the discovertebral junctions (outside the cervical region), symphysis pubis, and manubriosternal articulations, and tendinous and ligamentous attachments to bone may be involved, but the frequency and severity of changes at these sites are less pronounced in rheumatoid arthritis than in the seronegative spondyloarthropathies (ankylosing spondylitis, psoriasis, and Reiter's syndrome).

Hand
Clinical Abnormalities

The joints of the hand are affected in almost all patients with rheumatoid arthritis. Metacarpophalangeal and proximal interphalangeal joint alterations predominate. Clinical (as well as radiologic) evidence of distal interphalangeal joint disease is less frequent and involvement is rarely severe; however, the diagnosis of rheumatoid arthritis cannot be eliminated by the finding of involvement of the distal interphalangeal joints. In long-standing disease, swan-neck deformities (hyperextension at proximal interphalangeal joints and flexion at distal interphalangeal joints), boutonnière deformities (flexion at proximal interphalangeal joints and hyperextension at distal inter-

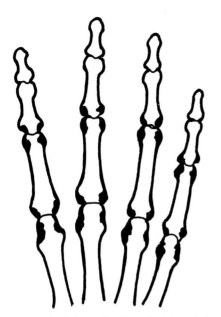

Figure 22–1. Metacarpophalangeal and proximal interphalangeal joints: Target areas. In the four ulnar digits, early osseous erosions may appear at the radial and ulnar aspects of the metacarpophalangeal and proximal interphalangeal joints. The initial changes occur on the radial aspect of the phalanges and metacarpal bones at the second and third metacarpophalangeal joints and on the radial and ulnar aspects of the phalanges at the third proximal interphalangeal joint. Distal interphalangeal joint changes are less constant and less severe.

phalangeal joints), and hitchhiker's or Z-shaped deformity of the thumb (flexion at the metacarpophalangeal joint and hyperextension at the interphalangeal joint) can be observed.

Spontaneous rupture of extensor tendons of the digits is a well-recognized complication of this disease.

Radiographic-Pathologic Correlation

EARLY ABNORMALITIES (FIGS. 22–1 TO 22–4). The second and third metacarpophalangeal joints and the third proximal interphalangeal joint may reveal the earliest abnormalities in rheumatoid arthritis. Indistinctness of osseous outline corresponds in position to the insertion of the capsule on the dorsoradial aspect of the proximal portion of the proximal phalanges of the four medial digits. Soon fusiform soft tissue swelling, periarticular osteoporosis, concentric loss of articular space, and marginal erosions become evident at many or all of the proximal interphalangeal and metacarpophalangeal joints.

The marginal erosions appear at the radial and ulnar aspects of the articulation. At both proximal interphalangeal and metacarpophalangeal joint locations, the erosions are larger on the proximal bone that constitutes the articulation (the metacarpal head at the metacarpophalangeal joint; the proximal phalanx at the proximal interphalangeal joint). At the metacarpophalangeal joints, the radial aspect of the bone is affected more significantly than the ulnar aspect. In the thumb, a characteristic deep erosion may appear at the ulnar side of the volar aspect of the base of the distal phalanx about the interphalangeal joint and at the radial and ulnar sides of the first metacarpophalangeal joint. Marginal erosions about the distal interphalangeal joints generally are small.

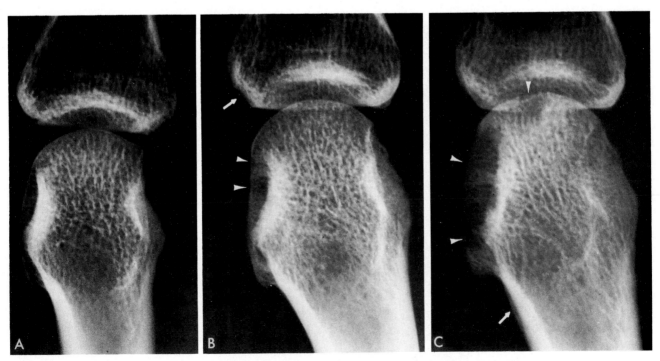

Figure 22–2. Metacarpophalangeal joint abnormalities: Sequential early changes. Initially (A), the bones appear normal, with preservation of the subchondral bone plate on the radial aspect of the metacarpal head. Subsequently (B), small radiolucent areas appear in the metacarpal head, leading to thinning of the bone plate with focal discontinuity or gaps (arrowheads). Tiny erosions and surface irregularity of the proximal phalanx are also evident (arrow). At a later stage (C), obvious osseous defects are seen (arrowheads). Note mild periosteal proliferation (arrow).

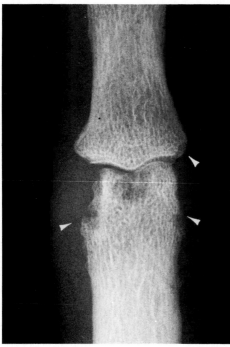

Figure 22–3. Proximal interphalangeal joint abnormalities: Early changes. Initial radiographic changes include soft tissue swelling, joint space narrowing, and marginal erosions (arrowheads).

Table 22–1. TYPES OF BONE EROSION IN THE HAND AND WRIST IN RHEUMATOID ARTHRITIS

Type	Mechanism	Common Sites
Marginal erosion	Pannus destruction of bare areas (without protective cartilage) of bone	Metacarpophalangeal and proximal interphalangeal joints; radial styloid, midportion of scaphoid; triquetrum; capitate; trapezium
Compressive erosion	Collapse of osteoporotic bone by muscular forces	Metacarpophalangeal joints
Surface resorption	Erosion of bone beneath inflamed tendons	Outer aspect of distal ulna; dorsal aspect of first metacarpal bone; proximal phalanx of first digit

In addition to marginal erosions, two other types of bone erosion are evident: compressive (pressure) erosions and superficial surface resorption (Table 22–1). Compressive erosions are related to the effect of muscular forces acting on osteoporotic bones, whereas superficial surface resorption beneath inflamed tendon sheaths can be evident in the diaphyses and metaphyses of the phalanges.

CONTINUED ABNORMALITIES. With further destruction of cartilage and bone, the articular space may be completely obliterated. Erosion of central portions of the joint can lead to apparently enclosed radiolucent defects, cysts, or pseudocysts. Although fibrous ankylosis is the characteristic ultimate fate of severe arthritis of metacarpophalangeal and proximal interphalangeal joints, occasional examples of intraarticular osseous fusion can be seen in these locations.

FINGER DEVIATIONS AND DEFORMITIES. Deviation and deformity of the fingers are common complications of rheumatoid arthritis affecting the hand and the wrist.

Mallet Finger. Although extensive synovial inflammation of the distal interphalangeal joints of the four medial digits

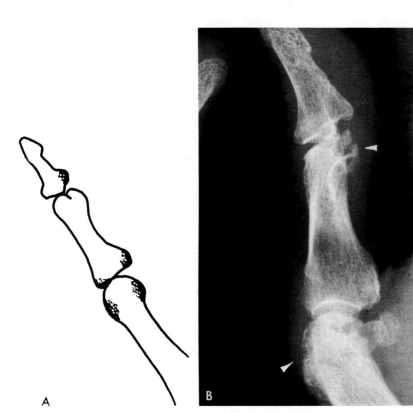

Figure 22–4. Abnormalities of the metacarpophalangeal and interphalangeal joints of the thumb: Early changes. Radial and ulnar erosions at the first metacarpophalangeal joint and ulnar erosion on the volar aspect of the bones at the interphalangeal joint are typical (arrowheads and shaded areas).

A

B

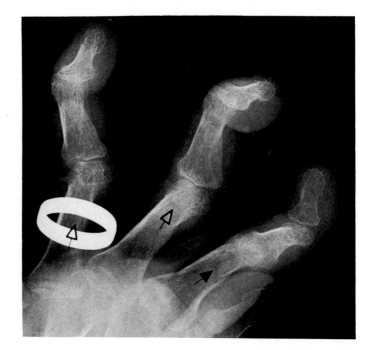

Figure 22–5. **Interphalangeal joint deformities.** Typical swan-neck deformity of the third and fourth digits (open arrows) and a boutonnière deformity of the second digit (closed arrow) are evident in this patient with rheumatoid arthritis.

is relatively uncommon, loosening or disruption of the distal attachment of the extensor tendon to the terminal phalanx may result in the development of a typical mallet or drop finger.

Boutonnière Deformity (Fig. 22–5). In normal situations, the balanced tendon mechanism and ligamentous restriction prevent collapse deformity of the digits, but in rheumatoid arthritis, the vulnerable balance is compromised by the direct effect of this disease on articulations, tendons, and ligaments. Flexion of the proximal interphalangeal joint combined with hyperextension at the distal interphalangeal joint produces the boutonnière deformity of the digit.

Swan-Neck Deformity (Fig. 22–5). Swan-neck deformity consists of hyperextension of the proximal interphalangeal joint and flexion of the distal interphalangeal joint. Its pathogenesis is not fully agreed on. Although synovitis of the proximal interphalangeal joint, hyperextension of the long extensor tendons, deformity of the metacarpophalangeal joint, and carpal collapse may be contributory factors, the primary cause of the deformity is a synovitis of the flexor tendon sheath, which restricts interphalangeal joint flexion.

Deformities of the Metacarpophalangeal Joint (Fig. 22–6). A variety of metacarpophalangeal joint deformities and deviations appear in the rheumatoid hand, including ulnar drift, extensor tendon subluxation, and palmar subluxation and flexion of the joint.

The reported frequency of ulnar deviation at the metacarpophalangeal joints in rheumatoid arthritis varies from approximately 25 to 50 per cent. Its pathogenesis is complex, although inflammatory synovitis of the metacarpophalangeal joint with a rise in intraarticular pressure appears to be the initial factor in the development of this deformity. Instability and ulnar deviation of extensor tendons may be another primary factor. Furthermore, a relationship between radial deviation of the wrist and ulnar deviation at the metacarpophalangeal joints, producing the zigzag deformity of the hand in rheumatoid arthritis, has been noted in many patients.

Thumb Deformities (Fig. 22–7). The malalignments that are encountered most frequently in the thumb in rheumatoid arthritis are collapse deformities (boutonnière deformity) related to disturbance of function at the first metacarpophalangeal joint; swan-neck deformity, related to disturbance of function at the first carpometacarpal joint; and instability,

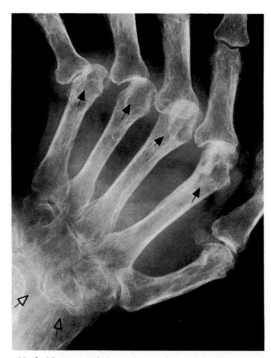

Figure 22–6. **Metacarpophalangeal joint deformities: Ulnar deviation.** The simultaneous occurrence of ulnar deviation at the metacarpophalangeal joints (solid arrows) and radial deviation at the radiocarpal joint of the wrist (open arrows) is well shown in this patient. The resulting appearance is termed the zigzag deformity.

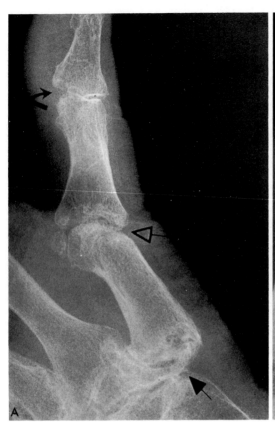
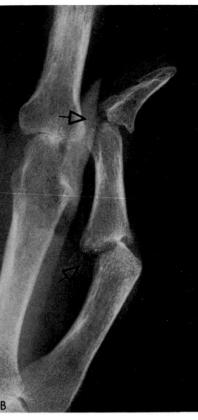

Figure 22–7. Deformities of the thumb. A Swan-neck deformity. Hyperextension at the first metacarpophalangeal joint (open arrow) is seen. Note the severe bone and cartilage destruction at the first carpometacarpal (solid arrow) and first metacarpophalangeal joints, and less dramatic abnormalities at the interphalangeal joint (curved arrow). At this stage, flexion deformity of the interphalangeal joint has not occurred. B Boutonnière deformity. Findings include flexion at the first metacarpophalangeal joint and hyperextension at the interphalangeal joint (open arrows). Associated articular destruction in this and the adjacent digit is evident.

stiffness, or pain of the interphalangeal, metacarpophalangeal, and carpometacarpal joints.

Wrist

Clinical Abnormalities

Wrist involvement is a characteristic feature of rheumatoid arthritis. Clinical findings can relate to synovitis in any of the compartments of the wrist, adjacent tenosynovitis, and attenuation or injury of several soft tissue, tendinous, and ligamentous structures. Soft tissue swelling is common on both the dorsal and volar aspects of the joint. Extensor carpi ulnaris tenosynovitis creates a painless swelling on the ulnar aspect of the wrist, which may appear early in the course of the disease. Subsequent clinical features of the wrist in rheumatoid arthritis relate to dorsal subluxation of the distal portion of the ulna, the carpal tunnel syndrome attributable to synovitis in the carpal tunnel with dysesthesias along the course of the median nerve, rupture of one or more extensor tendons, and various wrist deformities. Furthermore, synovial cysts arising during the disease can create local soft tissue masses.

Radiographic-Pathologic Correlation

EARLY ABNORMALITIES

Distal End and Styloid Process of the Ulna. Erosion and swelling around the distal end of the ulna and the ulnar styloid process are early manifestations of rheumatoid arthritis and are related to abnormality of the prestyloid recess of the radiocarpal compartment, the inferior radioulnar compartment, and the extensor carpi ulnaris tendon and sheath (Fig. 22–8).

The prestyloid recess of the radiocarpal compartment is intimate with the ulnar styloid process and may extend circumferentially around the process or contact only its undersurface. The inflamed synovial tissue within the prestyloid recess in rheumatoid arthritis is in contact with, and may produce erosions of, the tip of the ulnar styloid process. These erosions begin as focal radiolucent areas within the subchondral bone. As erosion progresses, however, the ulnar styloid tip becomes increasingly irregular.

The diseased synovium within the inferior radioulnar compartment extends over the radial and the palmar surfaces of the distal part of the ulna and the adjacent ulnar aspect of the distal end of the radius. Radiographic findings include shallow surface defects, which progress to become extensive scalloped erosions, and sharply angular surfaces on the distal radius and the distal ulna (Fig. 22–9).

Tendinitis and tenosynovitis of the extensor carpi ulnaris tendon and its sheath result in swelling of the soft tissue along the outer aspect of the ulnar head. Subjacent resorption of bone and periostitis occur along the medial margin of the distal part of the ulna beneath the inflamed tendon and sheath (Fig. 22–10).

Radial Styloid Process and Scaphoid. Synovial inflammation within the radiocarpal compartment leads to rheumatoid erosion of the distal end of the radius and the adjacent scaphoid bone (Fig. 22–11). At the former site, there is an unprotected or "bare" area on the surface of the bone adjacent to the radial collateral ligament. Alterations on the lateral midportion of the scaphoid bone are also characteristic; here, too, is a region devoid of cartilage and vulnerable to erosion.

Triquetral and Pisiform Bones. Erosions of the triquetrum and the pisiform are common in early rheumatoid

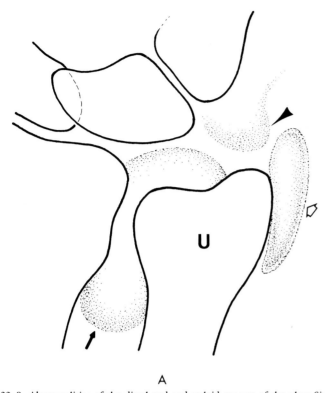

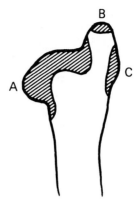

A. EROSIONS RELATED TO INFERIOR RADIOULNAR COMPARTMENT

B. EROSIONS RELATED TO PRESTYLOID RECESS

C. EROSIONS RELATED TO EXTENSOR CARPI ULNARIS TENDON SHEATH

A

B

Figure 22–8. Abnormalities of the distal end and styloid process of the ulna: Sites of early soft tissue swelling and osseous erosion. **A** Soft tissue swelling about the distal end of the ulna (U) may appear as distention of the prestyloid recess of the radiocarpal compartment (arrowhead), of the inferior radioulnar compartment (solid arrow), or of the extensor carpi ulnaris tendon sheath (open arrow). **B** Early osseous erosions appear at three distinct areas in the distal part of the ulna.

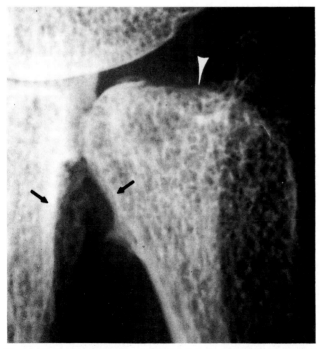

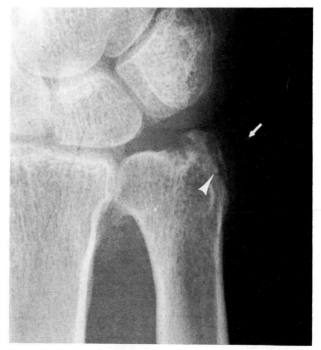

Figure 22–9. Abnormalities of the distal end and styloid process of the ulna: Inferior radioulnar compartment. Magnification radiograph outlines osseous erosion (arrows) of apposing surfaces of distal part of the radius and distal part of the ulna owing to rheumatoid synovitis of the inferior radioulnar compartment. Observe notch-like irregularity of the ulnar end (arrowhead).

Figure 22–10. Abnormalities of the distal end and styloid process of the ulna: Extensor carpi ulnaris tendon and tendon sheath. Wrist of rheumatoid patient showing swelling of soft tissue (arrow) and subjacent resorption of bone with periosteal proliferation (arrowhead). Additional alterations include changes on apposing surfaces of the distal ends of both radius and ulna.

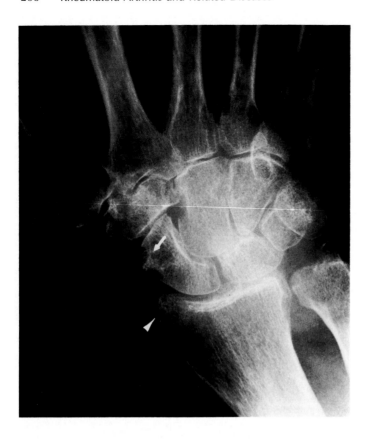

Figure 22–11. Abnormalities of the radial styloid process and scaphoid. Radiograph of rheumatoid wrist showing erosion on radial styloid process (arrowhead) and lateral midportion of the scaphoid bone (arrow), characteristic of rheumatoid arthritis. Widespread abnormalities are present throughout the wrist.

arthritis and occur at three sites: the proximal medial portion of the triquetrum, the distal medial portion of the triquetrum, and the adjacent surfaces of the triquetrum and the pisiform (Fig. 22–12). Initially, a shallow marginal erosion can be seen on the proximal portion of the triquetrum at the medial limit of the radiocarpal compartment (Fig. 22–13). The medial limit of the midcarpal compartment is another site at which marginal erosion of the triquetral bone occurs (Fig. 22–13). An associated marginal erosion of the adjacent hamate bone is frequent.

The pisiform-triquetral compartment is seen tangentially in "reverse" oblique radiographs made with the wrist in a semisupinated position (Fig. 22–14). Plain radiographs may disclose superficial or deep erosion on the palmar surface of the triquetral bone and the dorsal surface of the pisiform bone.

Midcarpal, Carpometacarpal, and Intermetacarpal Compartments. Abnormalities are not uncommon in several other areas of the wrist (Fig. 22–15). Marginal erosion of the trapezium adjacent to the attachment of the radial collateral ligament and on the radial aspect of the capitate bone has been noted. Marginal erosion of the radial aspect of the base of the first metacarpal bone indicates rheumatoid involvement of the first carpometacarpal compartment; scalloped erosion of the base of one or more of the other four metacarpal bones reflects synovial proliferation within the intermetacarpal compartments.

CONTINUED ABNORMALITIES. Continued synovial inflammation within the wrist soon results in significant alteration in all the compartments, characterized by progressive loss and obliteration of the articular space, further osseous erosion, and bone ankylosis (Fig. 22–16). This pancompart-

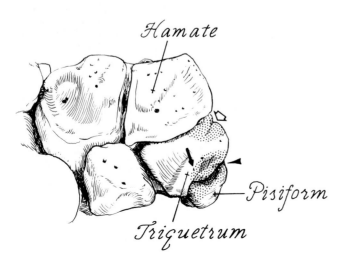

Figure 22–12. Distribution of abnormalities of the triquetrum and the pisiform. Osseous changes occur predominantly at three sites: on the triquetrum at the ulnar limit of the radiocarpal compartment (solid arrow), on the ulnar limit of the midcarpal compartment (open arrow), and on the triquetrum and pisiform related to the pisiform-triquetral compartment (arrowhead).

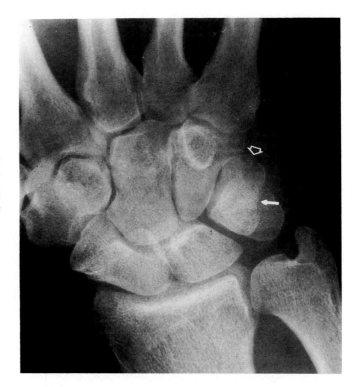

Figure 22–13. Abnormalities of the triquetrum and the pisiform: Radiocarpal and midcarpal compartments. Radiograph of the wrist in a patient with rheumatoid arthritis showing marginal erosions (open and solid arrows) on the triquetrum. The erosions are related to abnormality at the ulnar or medial limit of the midcarpal compartment and, to a lesser extent, the ulnar limit of the radiocarpal compartment.

mental distribution is characteristic of rheumatoid arthritis and allows differentiation from selective compartmental changes that are encountered in a variety of other disease processes affecting the wrist.

Intraarticular osseous fusion can lead to carpal masses of variable size. Most frequently, such ankylosis affects the midcarpal compartment and, to a lesser extent, the common carpometacarpal compartment of the wrist. Radiocarpal compartmental bone ankylosis is unusual; at this site, as elsewhere in the skeleton, fibrous ankylosis is more typical.

WRIST MALALIGNMENT AND DEFORMITY. Incongruity in cartilaginous and osseous surfaces, laxity of the articular capsule and the ligaments, and muscular and tendinous imbalance can cause malalignment of a wrist in rheumatoid arthritis.

Radiocarpal Malalignment. Destruction of the triangular fibrocartilage and dorsal subluxation of the distal end of the ulna disrupt the normal concavity of the radiocarpal compartment. The proximal row of carpal bones migrates in a medial (ulnar) and a palmar direction along the inclined articular surface of the distal radius.

Intercarpal Malalignment (Fig. 22–17). Both palmar flexion instability and dorsiflexion instability occur in the wrist in rheumatoid arthritis. Palmar flexion instability is manifested by medial migration of the proximal row of carpal bones with resulting palmar flexion of the lunate and the scaphoid bones. Dorsiflexion instability is sometimes related to abnormality of the distal attachment of the palmar radiocarpal ligament and disruption of the scapholunate ligament. The scapholunate angle increases, and scapholunate dissocia-

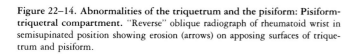

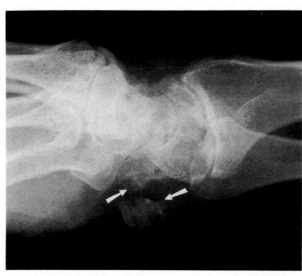

Figure 22–14. Abnormalities of the triquetrum and the pisiform: Pisiform-triquetral compartment. "Reverse" oblique radiograph of rheumatoid wrist in semisupinated position showing erosion (arrows) on apposing surfaces of triquetrum and pisiform.

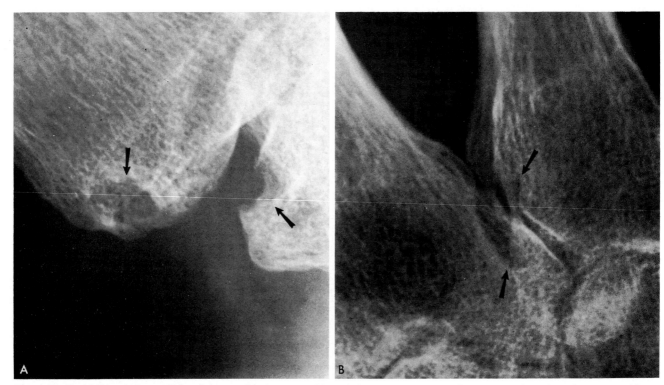

Figure 22–15. Additional abnormalities of the carpal and metacarpal bones. A Marginal erosions are frequent at the base of the first metacarpal bone and adjacent trapezium (arrows). **B** Scalloped osseous erosions (arrows) may appear about the intermetacarpal compartments.

tion becomes apparent. In long-standing disease, disorganization of the carpal bones may be striking.

Inferior Radioulnar and Distal Ulnar Malalignment (Fig. 22–18). Rheumatoid arthritis deformities on the ulnar aspect of the wrist include distal and dorsal subluxation of the ulna and diastasis of the inferior radioulnar compartment. Synovial proliferation in the wrist in rheumatoid arthritis destroys the triangular fibrocartilage, the ulnar collateral ligament, and the articular capsule—the supporting structures of the distal portion of the ulna. In addition, the extensor carpi ulnaris tendon undergoes both palmar and medial subluxation, which impairs its function as a dorsal stabilizer of the distal part of the ulna.

The caput ulnae syndrome, which consists of pain, limited motion, and dorsal prominence of the distal end of the ulna, may be noted in the rheumatoid arthritis patient. The abnormally located, eroded head of the ulna projects into the compartments of the extensor tendons on the dorsum of the wrist and produces fraying of the surfaces of the tendons. Subsequent rupture of the extensor tendons commencing on the ulnar aspect of the wrist can occur.

Elbow

Clinical Abnormalities

The elbow is frequently involved in rheumatoid arthritis. Clinical symptoms and signs are variable but can lead to considerable disability owing to limitation of both flexion and extension of the joint. Additional clinical manifestations include local pain and tenderness, swelling over the lateral aspect of the joint between the radial head and the olecranon, antecubital soft tissue masses related to synovial cysts with

compression of adjacent nerves, and paraolecranon nodules or bursitis.

Olecranon bursitis is seen not only in rheumatoid arthritis but also in gout and in association with trauma or infection. With rheumatoid (or gouty) involvement, palpable nodules within the bursa are noted.

Radiographic-Pathologic Correlation

Synovial inflammation in the elbow with progressive destruction of cartilage and bone produces soft tissue swelling with a positive "fat pad" sign, regional or periarticular osteoporosis, joint space narrowing, and bone erosions. More severe changes are characterized by extensive osteolysis of large portions of the humerus, radius, and ulna, prominent cystic lesions of the olecranon process that can fracture spontaneously, osteophytosis, and rarely bone ankylosis (Fig. 22–19).

Glenohumeral Joint

Clinical Abnormalities

Clinical symptoms of disability related to glenohumeral joint involvement in rheumatoid arthritis are not infrequent. Pain, tenderness, and restricted motion can be evident. Associated subacromial bursitis can result in prominent soft tissue swelling. Synovial rupture of the joint can lead to an acute exacerbation of clinical manifestations.

Radiographic-Pathologic Correlation

Progressive destruction of the chondral surface of the glenoid cavity and humeral head leads to diffuse loss of joint space, which may be accompanied by subchondral cystic

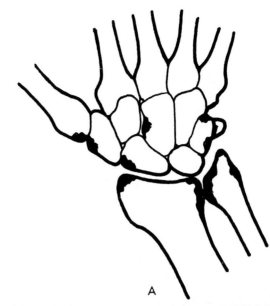

A

Figure 22–16. Pancompartmental abnormalities of the wrist in rheumatoid arthritis. A Some of the typical sites of osseous erosion in rheumatoid arthritis are indicated. Note that all of the compartments in the wrist are soon involved. B A radiograph demonstrates typical pancompartmental osseous erosions of rheumatoid arthritis.

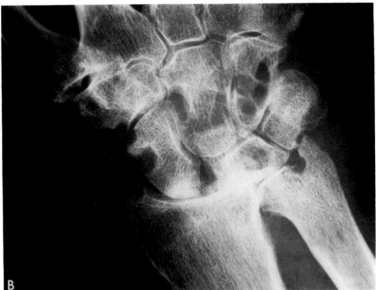

B

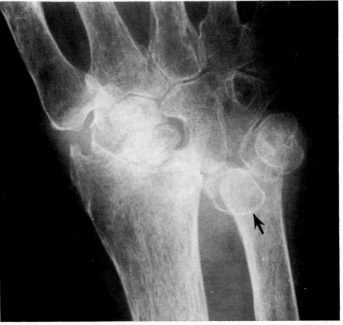

Figure 22–17. Wrist malalignment and deformity: Intercarpal malalignment. In this patient, the lunate (arrow) is located between the radius and ulna.

269

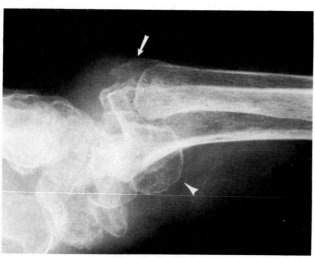

Figure 22–18. Wrist malalignment and deformity: Inferior radioulnar and distal ulnar malalignment. A lateral radiograph reveals severe dorsal subluxation of the distal end of the ulna (arrow) in addition to significant and widespread osseous and articular changes. Note the abnormal position of the lunate (arrowhead) overlying the distal end of the radius.

lesions, osteophytes, and sclerosis. Particularly characteristic are superficial irregularities, deep erosive changes, and cystic changes on the superolateral aspect of the humeral head adjacent to the greater tuberosity (Fig. 22–20). These osseous abnormalities resemble the Hill-Sachs compression fracture occurring after anterior glenohumeral joint dislocation and the marginal erosions of other synovial processes, such as ankylosing spondylitis. Continued destruction leads to extension of the bony erosions so that the entire anatomic neck and greater tuberosity as well as the glenoid cavity become

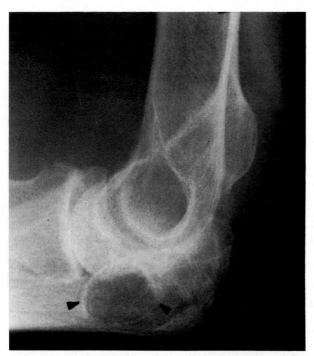

Figure 22–19. Abnormality of the elbow: Articular destruction. Prominent cysts (arrowheads) in the ulnar olecranon may occasionally fracture spontaneously.

altered. Deformity of the articular surfaces can appear. Furthermore, a deep bone erosion may develop on the medial aspect of the surgical neck of the humerus, related to abnormal pressure exerted by the adjacent glenoid margin.

Rotator cuff atrophy or tear is common in long-standing rheumatoid arthritis owing to the damaging effect of the inflamed synovial tissue on the undersurface of the tendons adjacent to the greater tuberosity (Fig. 22–20). This leads to progressive elevation of the humeral head, narrowing of the space between the top of the humerus and the inferior surface of the acromion, sclerosis and cyst formation on adjacent portions of humeral head and acromion, reversal (or concavity) of the normal convex shape of the inferior acromion, and accentuation of cystic and sclerotic changes on the superolateral aspect of the head of the humerus.

In some instances, rheumatoid arthritis can lead to the appearance of one or more synovial cysts in the neighboring soft tissues. Their demonstration is provided by glenohumeral joint arthrography, during which the synovial cysts may be filled and their irregular synovial lining may be outlined.

Acromioclavicular Joint

Pain, tenderness to direct palpation, and local soft tissue swelling can indicate rheumatoid involvement of the acromioclavicular articulation. Bilateral or unilateral abnormalities are observed on radiographs (Fig. 22–21).

Coracoclavicular Joint

An elongated, shallow erosion can be seen along the undersurface of the distal part of the clavicle in rheumatoid arthritis (Fig. 22–22). It usually commences 2 to 4 cm from the distal end of the bone. The pathogenesis of this erosive change is not clear. Subchondral osteoporosis and erosions, predominating on the clavicle, are early findings that may progress to extensive osteolysis of the outer one third of the clavicle.

Sternoclavicular and Manubriosternal Joints

Although clinical evidence of abnormalities in one or both sternoclavicular joints is not uncommon, radiologic evidence of sternoclavicular changes is more difficult to detect because of the inadequacies of routine sternoclavicular joint radiography. Rarely, extensive osteolysis of the medial end of the clavicle with or without associated osteolysis of the distal end of the clavicle can be seen (Fig. 22–23).

Manubriosternal changes in rheumatoid arthritis usually occur after abnormalities become evident in other joints, although, uncommonly, they may appear early in the course of the disease. The pathogenesis of manubriosternal abnormalities is not certain; they may relate to extension of synovial disease from neighboring costochondral joints, traumatic or degenerative processes, primary involvement of cartilaginous joints in the rheumatoid disease process, or transformation of the joint into one with a synovial cavity, with subsequent inflammation.

Rarely, in rheumatoid arthritis, subluxation or dislocation of the manubriosternal joint is evident.

Forefoot
Clinical Abnormalities

Clinical abnormalities of the forefoot are especially common in rheumatoid arthritis (80 to 90 per cent of patients) and

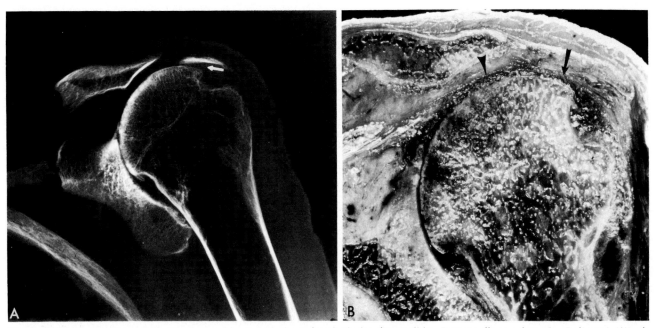

Figure 22–20. Abnormalities of the glenohumeral joint: Articular and periarticular abnormalities. Rotator cuff tear and atrophy. Radiograph (A) and photograph (B) of a coronal section of a rheumatoid glenohumeral joint indicate the presence of severe articular changes and rotator cuff atrophy. Note joint space narrowing and sclerosis, erosion of the superolateral aspect of the humeral head, elevation of the humeral head with respect to the glenoid, and narrowing of the acromiohumeral head distance (arrow). The rotator cuff is atrophic (arrowhead).

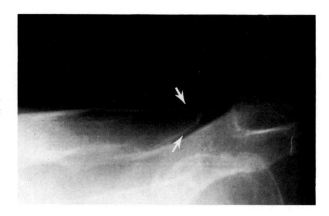

Figure 22–21. Abnormalities of the acromioclavicular joint. On this radiograph observe tapering of the distal end of the clavicle (arrows) with widening of the acromioclavicular joint.

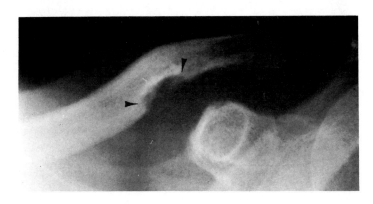

Figure 22–22. Abnormalities of the coracoclavicular joint. An example of scalloped erosion (arrowheads) of the undersurface of the distal clavicle in rheumatoid arthritis.

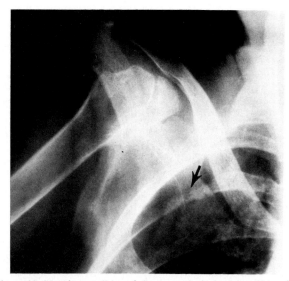

Figure 22–23. Abnormalities of the sternoclavicular joint. This radiograph reveals striking abnormalities of the glenohumeral, acromioclavicular, coracoclavicular, and sternoclavicular joints. Note the resorption of the humeral head, medial and lateral ends of the clavicle, and undersurface of the distal end of the clavicle. In addition, resorption of the superior surface of several ribs can be seen (arrow).

may be the initial manifestation of the disease (10 to 20 per cent of patients). Intermittent or constant pain, tenderness, and soft tissue swelling can be prominent findings, and a shuffling gait and characteristic deformities may appear. These deformities include forefoot spread, hallux valgus, fibular deviation of the digits, hammer toe, and "cock-up" toe. Bursitis and spontaneous sinus tracts can be seen.

Radiographic-Pathologic Correlation

Radiologic abnormalities of the forefoot are also frequent in rheumatoid arthritis. Furthermore, these abnormalities commonly are the initial manifestations of the disease. Earliest alterations appear at the metatarsophalangeal joints, particularly the fifth. With progression, one or more metatarsophalangeal joints are affected in a relatively symmetric fashion in both feet. At these sites, changes predominate on the medial aspect of the metatarsal head with the exception of that in the fifth digit, at which site soft tissue swelling and subjacent osseous erosion on the lateral aspect of the bone can be a very early and important finding of the disease (Fig. 22–24). The interphalangeal joint of the great toe also is commonly and characteristically affected.

Early radiographic alterations at the metatarsophalangeal joints consist of soft tissue swelling, periarticular osteoporosis, concentric joint space narrowing, and marginal and central osseous defects, corresponding to pathologic evidence of synovial inflammation, with resultant cartilage and bone destruction (Fig. 22–24). Some proliferative changes with

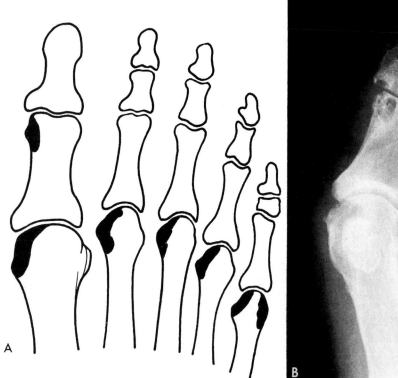

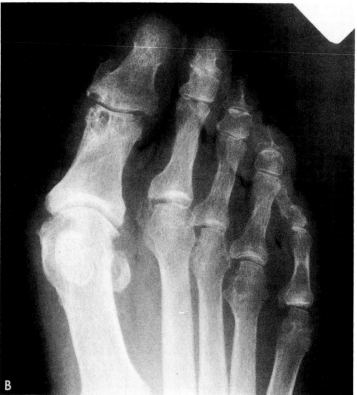

Figure 22–24. Abnormalities of the forefoot: Target areas. A The early osseous erosions of rheumatoid arthritis appear on the medial aspect of the first to fourth metatarsal bones, the medial and lateral aspects of the fifth metatarsal bone, and the medial aspect of the distal portion of the proximal phalanx of the great toe. **B** A radiograph reveals the early erosions. All the metatarsal heads are involved, particularly the medial aspects. Note the prominent changes at the interphalangeal joint of the great toe and the relative absence of findings in other interphalangeal joints.

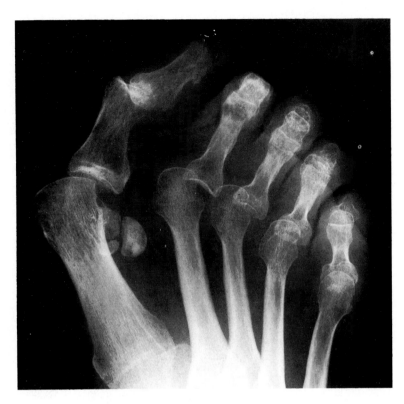

Figure 22–25. Forefoot deformities. Fibular deviation and subluxation of the phalanges typically occur in the first to fourth digits. The relatively mild nature of the osseous erosions in comparison with the degree of deformity that is evident in this patient is somewhat unusual.

sclerosis, osteophytosis, and periostitis of adjacent phalangeal shafts can appear, although they are overshadowed by the presence and degree of osteolysis. Intraarticular bone ankylosis is distinctly unusual at metatarsophalangeal (as well as interphalangeal) joints. In the great toe, the changes in the metatarsal head and the proximal phalanx about the metatarsophalangeal joint are accompanied by osteoporosis, joint space loss, erosions of the adjacent sesamoids, and hallux valgus deformity.

The radiographic characteristics of the deformed forefoot in rheumatoid arthritis include fibular deviation of the toes (with the exception of the fifth digit) and dorsiflexion and lateral subluxation or dislocation of the proximal phalanges at the metatarsophalangeal articulations (Fig. 22–25).

Heel

Clinical Abnormalities

Clinical lesions of the heel that are encountered in rheumatoid arthritis and the seronegative spondyloarthropathies (ankylosing spondylitis, psoriasis, and Reiter's syndrome) are retrocalcaneal bursitis, Achilles tendinitis, and plantar fasciitis. Retrocalcaneal bursitis is characterized by a fluctuating mass that falls to the sides of the Achilles tendon; Achilles tendinitis is associated with pain, local tenderness to palpation, and a thickened or swollen tendinous structure; and plantar fasciitis can lead to redness, swelling, and tenderness of the plantar surface of the calcaneus.

Radiographic-Pathologic Correlation

Synovitis, accumulation of bursal fluid, and surrounding soft tissue edema in association with retrocalcaneal bursitis can produce a soft tissue mass on the posterosuperior aspect of the calcaneus, which obliterates the normal radiolucent region that extends between the top of the bone and the Achilles tendon, and which projects into the inferior portion of the pre-Achilles fat pad (Fig. 22–26). Subjacent erosion of the calcaneus on both its posterior and superior aspects is characteristic.

Achilles tendinitis leads to enlargement and blurring of the tendon, with accompanying soft tissue swelling. The osseous attachments of the Achilles tendon can appear irregular, with spur formation.

Well-defined calcaneal spurs are also observed on the plantar aspect of the bone in patients with rheumatoid arthritis (Fig. 22–26). They are identical to those seen in "normal" individuals, which presumably result from a degenerative process. Poorly marginated plantar outgrowths with adjacent sclerosis, as seen in the seronegative spondyloarthropathies, are rare in rheumatoid arthritis. Although erosions on the undersurface of the calcaneus are seen in this latter disease, they are infrequent and of small size.

Ankle

The frequency of clinical and radiologic abnormalities in the ankle in rheumatoid arthritis is lower than that of the knee and the joints of the hand, wrist, and foot. Synovial hypertrophy in the tibiotalar articulation can lead to radiographically evident masses that are anterior, posterior, or lateral to the joint margin. Continued disease activity leads to cartilaginous and osseous destruction manifested radiographically as joint space loss and marginal and central bone erosions.

Knee

Clinical Abnormalities

The knee is affected frequently in rheumatoid arthritis. The extensive synovial lining at this site reveals inflammation, often at an early stage of the disease. Pain and swelling

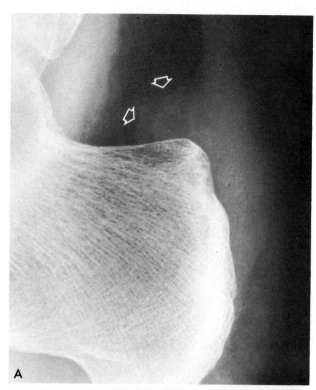

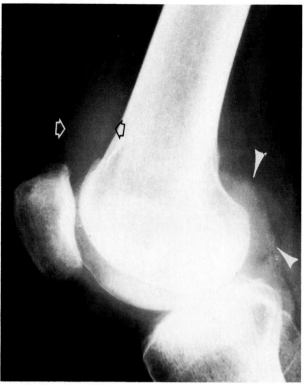

Figure 22–27. Abnormalities of the knee: Synovial effusion. On a lateral radiograph, an effusion is indicated by an enlarged suprapatellar pouch (greater than 10 mm in thickness) (arrows) between two radiolucent fat collections, one above the patella and one anterior to the distal end of the femur, and by increased radiodensity in the posterior recesses (arrowheads).

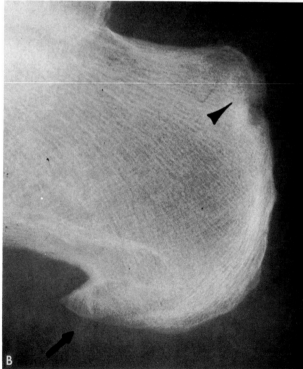

Figure 22–26. Abnormalities of the calcaneus: Posterosuperior and inferior aspects. A A low kV soft tissue radiograph defines a thickened Achilles tendon and a fluid-filled retrocalcaneal bursa (open arrows), which projects into the pre-Achilles fat pad. Focal osteoporosis of the neighboring calcaneus is evident. (Courtesy of J. Weston, M.D., Lower Hutt, New Zealand.) B Observe erosion of the posterosuperior aspect of the calcaneus (arrowhead) and a well-defined plantar calcaneal spur (arrow).

appear. The presence of a joint effusion is documented by careful physical examination and can be further substantiated by radiography accomplished in the lateral projection (Fig. 22–27). Increased fluid accumulation in the joint can be accompanied by small or large synovial cysts, especially on the posterior aspect of the knee. Acute rupture of synovial cysts can lead to clinical findings that simulate those of thrombophlebitis.

Radiographic-Pathologic Correlation

Characteristically, symmetric abnormalities occur in both the medial and the lateral femorotibial compartments (Fig. 22–28) and may be combined with similar changes in the patellofemoral compartment. This bicompartmental or tri-compartmental distribution, which can be depicted on radiography, is an important clue to the correct diagnosis. Small erosions on the medial and lateral margins of the tibia and the femur may be the first radiographic finding. These lesions are occasionally preceded by or soon accompanied by diffuse loss of the interosseous distance between femur and tibia in both the medial and lateral compartments and by the development of subchondral erosions and cysts of variable size.

Although accurate radiographic evaluation of the patellofemoral compartment is difficult, lateral and transaxial radiographs frequently demonstrate joint space loss and subchondral erosions and cysts of the patella (Fig. 22–29).

Subchondral eburnation and, to a lesser extent, osteophytes are observed not infrequently in the knee in rheumatoid

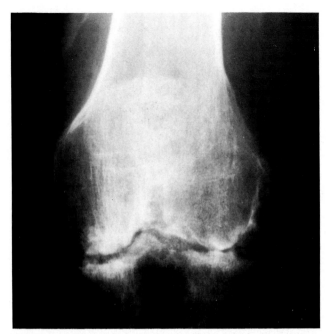

Figure 22–28. Abnormalities of the knee: Femorotibial compartments. Severe femorotibial abnormalities consist of obliteration of the articular space, superficial and deep osseous erosions, and reactive sclerosis in both the medial and lateral compartments.

arthritis, particularly in the distal part of the femur and proximal portion of the tibia. These changes are usually evident in long-standing disease. Furthermore, flexion deformity may complicate the later stages of rheumatoid arthritis. Varus or valgus deformity with or without subluxation can also be evident.

Hip

Clinical Abnormalities

The frequency of abnormalities of the hip is far less than that of knee abnormalities and increases with the duration and the severity of rheumatoid arthritis, especially in those patients receiving corticosteroids. Pain, tenderness, shortening of the limb, gait abnormalities, and decreased range of motion, particularly internal rotation, extension, and abduction, are the observed clinical manifestations. With more chronic and severe involvement, muscle atrophy and a mass in the groin or leg edema related to synovial cyst formation may be encountered.

Radiographic-Pathologic Correlation

Radiographic abnormalities of the hip generally are bilateral and symmetric in distribution. The most typical early abnormality is loss of joint space (Fig. 22–30). In almost all patients, diminution of articular space is concentric, and the femoral head moves inward along the axis of the femoral neck (axial migration).

The degree of articular space loss may increase with progression of the disease. Eventually, this space can be obliterated completely, and the femoral head and acetabulum protrude into the pelvis (Fig. 22–31). Acetabular protrusion, which is defined as inward movement of the acetabular line so that the distance between this line and the laterally located ilioischial line is 3 mm or more in adult men and 6 mm or more in adult women, is particularly characteristic of rheumatoid arthritis. It can also be observed in seronegative spondyloarthropathies, infection, osteoarthritis (with medial migration of the femoral head), osteomalacia, Paget's disease, idiopathic protrusion (Otto pelvis), and additional disorders, however. Protrusio acetabuli has been noted in about 15 per

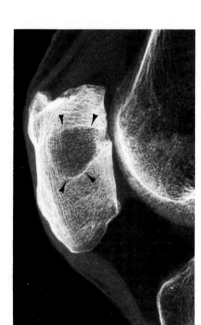

Figure 22–29. Abnormalities of the knee: Patellofemoral compartment. On a radiograph of a sagittal section of a rheumatoid knee, note a large patellar cyst (arrowheads), which is communicating with the patellofemoral compartment.

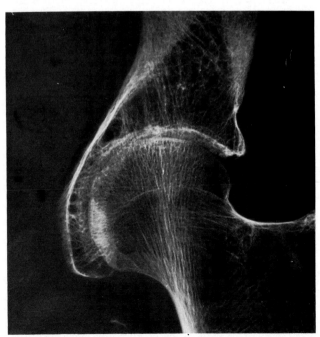

Figure 22–30. Abnormalities of the hip: Early changes. A radiograph of a coronal section of a rheumatoid cadaveric hip indicates diffuse loss of articular space with migration of the femoral head inward or axially along the axis of the femoral neck.

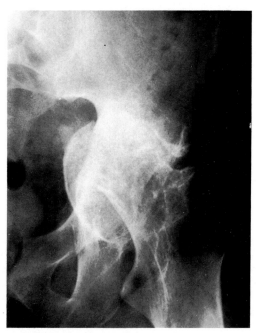

Figure 22–31. Abnormalities of the hip: Late changes with acetabular protrusion. An example of protrusion deformity is shown. Observe the small size of the femoral head.

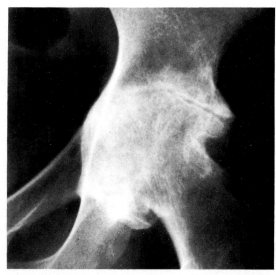

Figure 22–32. Abnormalities of the hip: Sclerosis and osteophytosis. In this rheumatoid arthritis patient, osteophytes on the femoral and acetabular margins are combined with diffuse loss of joint space and subchondral eburnation. Although the resulting radiographic picture resembles that of osteoarthritis alone, the presence of widespread articular space loss suggests that the degenerative abnormalities have been superimposed on an inflammatory arthritis.

cent of rheumatoid arthritis patients with hip disease. The deformity commonly is bilateral and associated with subchondral cystic lesions, osseous collapse of acetabular roof and femoral head, and osteoporosis. In long-standing rheumatoid arthritis, the radiographic appearance of bilaterally protruded acetabula containing small, eroded femoral heads is especially distinctive.

Osseous erosions and cysts are also well-known radiographic and pathologic manifestations of rheumatoid hip disease. Radiographically, the earliest lucent zones appear at the chondroosseous margin of the femoral head near the femoral neck. Additional lesions are observed as surface irregularities throughout the femoral head and, to a lesser degree, the acetabulum. The lesions reflect pannus invasion of bone at the chondroosseous junction and of cartilage and bone in the central articular areas. Rarely, large pseudoneoplastic foci of bone destruction can be seen in either the femoral head or the femoral neck.

Some degree of sclerosis and osteophytosis can appear in the hip after a considerable period of time, presumably related to a reparative response of the diseased bone and cartilage or secondary degenerative joint disease (Fig. 22–32).

Osteonecrosis of the femoral head is not uncommon in rheumatoid arthritis patients being treated with corticosteroids.

Sacroiliac Joint

Asymptomatic radiographic abnormalities of the sacroiliac joint can be present in as many as 25 to 35 per cent of patients with severe, long-standing disease. Abnormalities can be bilateral or unilateral in distribution, but symmetric alterations, which are the rule in ankylosing spondylitis, are not frequent in rheumatoid arthritis. Joint space narrowing varies in severity, although frequently it is mild. Osseous erosions have predilection for the iliac aspect of the joint;

they are superficial and well marginated and are associated with absent or only mild sclerosis.

Ribs

Abnormalities of the thoracic cage in patients with rheumatoid arthritis can include erosions of the superior margin of the posterior aspect of the upper (third, fourth, fifth) ribs (see Fig. 22–23). They are identical to those encountered in other collagen disorders, neurologic processes, and chronic restrictive lung disease. It is probable that rib erosions in rheumatoid arthritis, as well as some other processes, relate to pressure effect from the scapula.

Thoracic and Lumbar Spine

In comparison to the distinctive alterations of the cervical spine, which represent a common and well-known manifestation of rheumatoid arthritis, abnormalities of the thoracic and lumbar spine are relatively infrequent in this disease. Occasionally, destructive lesions of vertebral bodies in the thoracic and lumbar segments are evident. Furthermore, rheumatoid arthritic changes in the apophyseal joints of the thoracic and lumbar spine are reported only rarely.

Alterations at the discovertebral junction of the thoracic and lumbar spine have also been noted. Intervertebral disc space narrowing, irregularity of the subchondral margins of the vertebral bodies, "erosion," and sclerosis can be evident radiographically. Such discovertebral changes could relate to (1) apophyseal joint instability with abnormal motion at the corresponding discovertebral junction, leading to cartilaginous node formation; (2) apophyseal joint synovitis with extension into the vertebral body–intervertebral disc junction; (3) costovertebral joint synovitis (in the thoracic spine) with extension into the vertebral body–intervertebral disc junction; (4) synovial infiltration into fissures within the degenerating nucleus pulposus of the intervertebral disc and subsequent inflammation; (5) neuropathic alterations secondary to analgesic or steroid therapy; and (6) enthesopathy (similar to that occurring in ankylosing spondylitis) resulting in inflammation of ligaments and adjacent areolar tissue, with extension into the vertebral body–intervertebral disc junction.

Cervical Spine

Clinical Abnormalities

Cervical spine involvement in rheumatoid arthritis can lead to severe pain and disability as well as to a variety of neurologic manifestations, although some patients with significant radiographic evidence of disease may be entirely asymptomatic. In rheumatoid arthritis, the cervical spine commonly is affected along with peripheral articular sites, although initial or predominant involvement of the cervical spine can occur without obvious abnormalities at other locations.

Approximately 60 to 70 per cent of rheumatoid arthritis patients develop symptoms and signs related to cervical spine abnormalities at some time during their illness. Pain is most common, although weakness and abnormal mobility can also be evident. Neurologic manifestations include paresthesias, paresis, and muscle wasting; in some instances, quadriplegia and death can occur. Vertebrobasilar vascular insufficiency can lead to transient blindness, nystagmus, vertigo, and loss of consciousness.

Radiographic-Pathologic Correlation

GENERAL FEATURES. The entire cervical spine partakes in the rheumatoid process; changes may be evident as far cephalad as the base of the occiput and as far caudad as the C7-T1 junction. Furthermore, synovial and cartilaginous joints, the joints of Luschka, tendinous and ligamentous attachments, and soft tissues of the cervical region can reveal significant abnormalities in this disease. Recognition of changes in all these sites requires optimal radiography, which must include an open-mouth frontal projection (for the odontoid process) and a lateral view of the flexed neck (for the C1-C2 joints). In those patients who can undergo complete radiographic evaluation, the frequency of radiographic changes of the cervical spine is consistently high (and may reach 85 per cent in patients with classic or definite rheumatoid arthritis). When all radiographic parameters are used, demonstration of abnormalities throughout the cervical spine is frequent, although they usually predominate in the upper cervical region.

OCCIPITOATLANTOAXIAL JOINTS

Atlantoaxial Subluxation (Fig. 22–33). Abnormal separation between the anterior arch of the atlas and the odontoid process (dens) of the axis is a characteristic finding in rheumatoid arthritis, which may be evident in an early stage of the disease. Generally, the interosseous distance between the posterior aspect of the anterior arch of the atlas and the anterior aspect of the odontoid process does not exceed 2.5 mm in adults; a greater distance generally is indicative of atlantoaxial subluxation. An interosseous interval between atlas and odontoid process less than 2.5 mm that changes considerably on flexion and extension can also be abnormal.

A consensus on anterior atlantoaxial subluxation in rheumatoid patients indicates a frequency of 20 to 25 per cent (Fig. 22–34). This frequency rises with increasing severity of the disease. The pathogenesis of this type of atlantoaxial

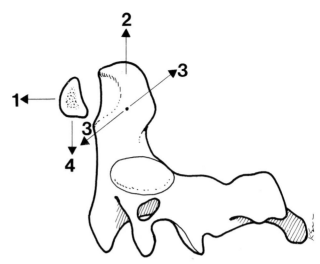

Figure 22–33. Abnormalities of the cervical spine: Directions of atlantoaxial subluxation. Various types of subluxation may occur at the atlantoaxial joints in a rheumatoid arthritis patient. Most typically anterior movement of the atlas with respect to the axis (1) is seen. Vertical translocation of the odontoid process (2) can also occur. Lateral subluxation (3) can be recorded on frontal radiographs as asymmetry becomes apparent between the odontoid process and the lateral masses of the atlas. In addition, the anterior arch of the atlas can move inferiorly (4) with respect to the odontoid process. Finally, in the presence of severe erosion of the odontoid process, the anterior arch can move posteriorly against or over the eroded bone.

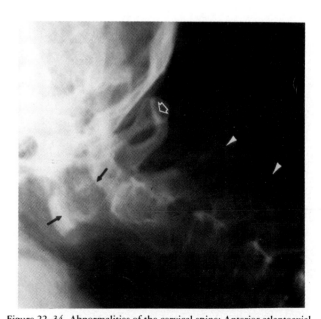

Figure 22–34. Abnormalities of the cervical spine: Anterior atlantoaxial subluxation. Lateral radiograph of the cervical spine obtained during flexion of the neck reveals severe atlantoaxial subluxation. Note the abnormal distance (solid arrows) between the posterior surface of the anterior arch of the atlas and the anterior surface of the odontoid process. The spinolaminar line of the atlas (open arrow) does not align with that of the other cervical vertebrae (arrowheads), confirming the presence of anterior subluxation. (Courtesy of V. Vint, M.D., San Diego, California.)

subluxation relates to the presence of transverse ligament laxity owing to synovial inflammation and hyperemia of the adjacent articulations, especially that between the posterior surface of the odontoid process and the anterior surface of the ligament.

In addition to anterior movement of the atlas with respect to the odontoid process, vertical subluxation at C1-C2 can also be observed in patients with rheumatoid arthritis, which, when extensive, can be fatal (Fig. 22–35). This complication is also referred to as atlantoaxial impaction or cranial settling. As settling progresses, the anterior arch of the atlas gradually assumes a position near the lower portion of the axis. Such settling can be diagnosed on radiographs obtained in a lateral projection or on conventional tomograms obtained in frontal and lateral projections. Cranial settling has been observed in 5 to 22 per cent of patients with rheumatoid arthritis. In general, vertical translocation of the dens results from disruption and collapse of osseous and articular structures between the occiput and the atlas and between the atlas and the axis.

Lateral subluxation of the atlantoaxial joints has also been observed in rheumatoid arthritis patients. In these persons, asymmetry is recorded between the odontoid process (and body of the axis) and the atlas. This complication has been observed in 10 to 20 per cent of rheumatoid arthritis patients. The sequence of events that leads to lateral subluxation of the atlantoaxial joints includes articular space narrowing, bone erosion, disruption of the articular capsules, and, in severe cases, collapse of the lateral masses of the axis, allowing the atlas to shift and tilt laterally (Fig. 22–36). Clinically, patients with lateral subluxation reveal a fixed head tilt toward the side of osseous collapse and rotation of the face toward the opposite side.

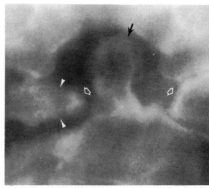

Figure 22–36. Abnormalities of the cervical spine: Lateral atlantoaxial subluxation. A frontal tomogram of the upper portion of the cervical spine demonstrates lateral subluxation of the odontoid process (solid arrow) with respect to the lateral masses of the atlas (open arrows). Note erosion of the base of the odontoid process and severe abnormalities in the occipitoatlantal and lateral atlantoaxial articulations. The right lateral mass of the atlas (arrowheads) as well as the axis is collapsed, and the head is tilted to the right.

The clinical course of patients with atlantoaxial subluxation is variable. In some individuals, only mild symptoms and signs appear, which do not progress. In others, clinical and radiographic deterioration becomes evident, and the patient may develop disabling neurologic abnormalities that require operative intervention to ensure stability.

Odontoid Process Erosion. Odontoid process erosions have been detected in 14 to 35 per cent of patients with rheumatoid arthritis. They occur as the natural consequence

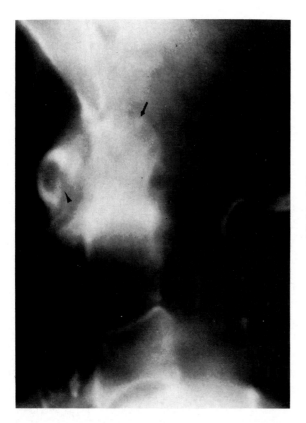

Figure 22–35. Abnormalities of the cervical spine: Vertical translocation of the odontoid process (cranial settling). Conventional tomography of the cervical spine in the lateral projection confirms the presence of this finding. The tip (arrow) of the odontoid process is located in the foramen magnum, and the anterior arch of the atlas (arrowhead) is opposite the lower portion of the odontoid process. (Courtesy of V. Vint, M.D., San Diego, California.)

of synovial inflammation in adjacent joints (Fig. 22–37). Thus, they predominate in the osseous portions that are intimate with the synovium-lined spaces between the anterior arch of C1 and the anterior aspect of the odontoid process, and between the posterior surface of the odontoid process and the transverse ligament. At both sites, early superficial erosions may require conventional tomography for adequate evaluation. Further erosion of the odontoid process, which is usually associated with atlantoaxial subluxation, can lead to considerable osteolysis. In addition, pathologic fracture of the weakened dens can be seen in patients after minimal trauma.

SUBAXIAL JOINTS

Subaxial Subluxation and Dislocation (Fig. 22–38). Subluxation of varying severity is observed at one or more subaxial levels in patients with rheumatoid arthritis. When localized to one area, changes are particularly characteristic at the C3-C4 and C4-C5 levels; however, multilevel subluxations are more typical, producing a "doorstep" or "stepladder" appearance on lateral radiographs.

Apophyseal Joint Abnormalities (Fig. 22–38). In the apophyseal joints of the subaxial region, joint space narrowing and superficial erosions are common. Sclerosis is not characteristic. Generally, fibrous ankylosis is the terminal event; however, bone ankylosis of one or more articulations can be seen.

Discovertebral Joint Abnormalities (Fig. 22–38). At the discovertebral junction of the cervical spine in rheumatoid arthritis, intervertebral disc space narrowing, subchondral osseous irregularity, and adjacent eburnation are the typical findings. Trauma from apophyseal joint instability with intraosseous displacement of discal material and extension of abnormal synovium from the adjacent joints of Luschka are two of the suggested mechanisms to explain these findings.

A characteristic manifestation of rheumatoid discitis is the absence of osteophytosis. Thus, considerable subchondral irregularity and erosion, intervertebral disc space narrowing, and sclerosis can be seen without osteophyte formation. The absence of osteophytes serves to distinguish the cervical spinal

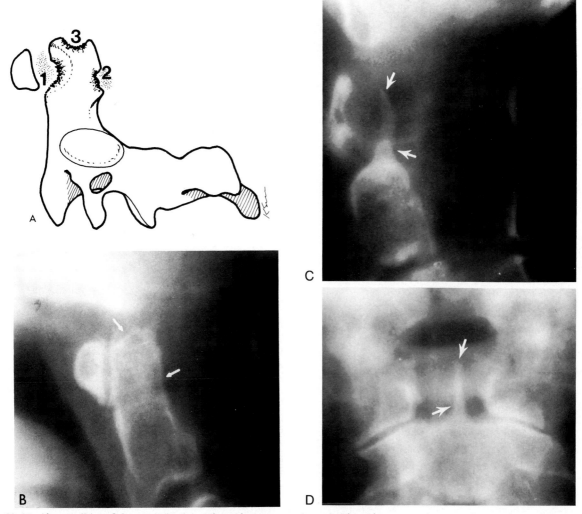

Figure 22–37. Abnormalities of the cervical spine: Odontoid process erosions. A Odontoid process erosions occur in areas that are intimate with the synovial articulations between the anterior arch of the atlas and the dens (1) and between the dens and the transverse ligament of the atlas (2); and in areas that are intimate with the ligamentous attachments (3) at the tip of the odontoid process. **B** A lateral tomogram illustrates osseous erosion at the tip and posterior surface of the dens (arrows) in this rheumatoid arthritis patient. **C, D** Lateral and frontal tomograms reveal severe destruction of the odontoid process (arrows), which has been reduced to an irregular, pointed protuberance.

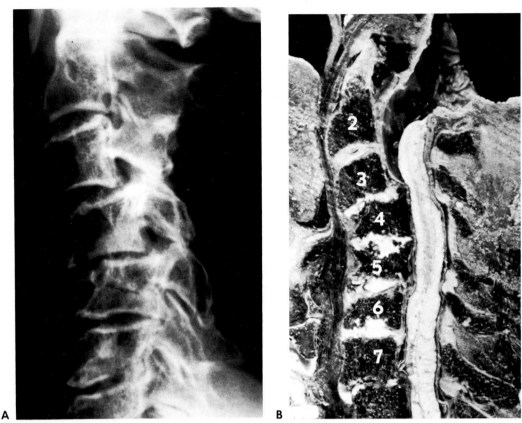

Figure 22–38. Abnormalities of the cervical spine: Subaxial subluxation and apophyseal joint changes. A Note the "stepladder" appearance owing to subluxation at multiple cervical levels associated with narrowing of the intervertebral disc spaces and narrowing, sclerosis, and subluxation of the apophyseal joints. **B** In a photograph of a sagittal section of a rheumatoid spine, subaxial subluxation is most evident in the middle cervical region (vertebral bodies are numbered). Observe compression of the anterior aspect of the spinal cord by the fourth and fifth vertebral bodies and extensive discovertebral irregularity.

abnormalities of rheumatoid arthritis from those of degenerative disc disease.

Spinous Process Erosions. Erosions and destruction of one or more spinous processes are detected in approximately 10 per cent of patients with rheumatoid arthritis. The changes, which are most frequent in the lower cervical spine, can be related to inflammation of the adjacent supraspinous ligaments or neighboring bursae.

DIFFUSE LOCATIONS. Although the foregoing discussion has used a regional approach to cervical spine changes, diffuse involvement of the entire cervical spine is common, particularly in long-standing rheumatoid arthritis (Table 22–

Table 22–2. CERVICAL SPINE ABNORMALITIES IN RHEUMATOID ARTHRITIS

Occipitoatlantoaxial Articulations
  Atlantoaxial subluxation
  Odontoid erosion and fracture
  Apophyseal joint erosion, sclerosis, and fusion

Subaxial Articulations
  Subaxial subluxation
  Apophyseal joint erosion, sclerosis, and fusion
  Intervertebral disc space narrowing
  Erosion and sclerosis of vertebral body margins
  Spinous process erosion
  Osteoporosis

2). The resulting radiographic picture, consisting of atlantoaxial subluxation, odontoid and apophyseal joint erosions, subaxial subluxations, intervertebral disc space narrowing, marginal sclerosis of vertebrae, and spinous process destruction, is virtually pathognomonic of this disease.

Other Joints

Rheumatoid arthritis affects other joints, including the temporomandibular joint, the cricoarytenoid joint, and perhaps even the articulations of the inner ear.

COEXISTENT OSSEOUS AND ARTICULAR DISEASE
Septic Arthritis

Infections are frequent in rheumatoid arthritis patients, especially after the introduction of steroids and immunosuppressive agents. Pulmonary infections (including bronchitis, bronchiectasis, pneumonia, abscess, and empyema), skin infections, osteomyelitis, and septic arthritis have all been noted. The precise cause of the increased susceptibility to infection in rheumatoid arthritis patients is not known.

The reported frequency of suppurative arthritis in patients with rheumatoid disease has varied from less than 1 per cent to 12 per cent. Pyarthrosis is more frequent in elderly rheumatoid arthritis patients with severe disability. Systemic steroid medication had been administered in most reported cases. In the majority of persons, the source of the joint

Table 22–3. RADIOGRAPHIC FEATURES OF SEPTIC ARTHRITIS COMPLICATING RHEUMATOID ARTHRITIS

Monoarticular or polyarticular distribution
Predilection for knee involvement
Asymmetric changes
Progressive soft tissue swelling and joint effusion
Rapid and poorly defined bone erosion

infection is obvious; it may be an ulcerating nodule, an infected prosthesis, a skin infection, or an intraarticular injection. The most frequently reported infecting organism has been *Staphyloccocus aureus*.

Septic arthritis complicating rheumatoid disease frequently affects multiple joints. The knee is the most common site of pyarthrosis. The onset of pyarthrosis in the patient with rheumatoid arthritis may produce only subtle clinical changes, making early diagnosis difficult. Furthermore, on radiographs, cortical destruction and erosive abnormalities are noted but are difficult to distinguish from the underlying rheumatoid alterations (Table 22–3). Radiographic evidence of any rapid deterioration of a joint should be suspected of indicating septic arthritis complicating rheumatoid arthritis. In particular, an enlarging soft tissue mass and a progressive effusion within a joint affected by rheumatoid arthritis in the absence of recent trauma must be viewed with caution. Asymmetric joint disease and poorly defined and rapid destruction of bone are other useful signs of infection in the patient with rheumatoid arthritis.

Gout

The coexistence of rheumatoid arthritis and gout is not common, although it is being reported with increasing frequency. Typically, men are affected, gout is the initial disease, and rheumatoid arthritis develops years later.

Calcium Pyrophosphate Dihydrate (CPPD) Crystal Deposition Disease

The coexistence of rheumatoid arthritis and calcium pyrophosphate dihydrate (CPPD) crystal deposition disease is occasionally encountered. It appears likely that this coexistence is but a chance occurrence; however, accurate diagnosis of both disorders requires evaluation of the radiographs. Bone erosion is not a manifestation of CPPD crystal deposition disease (see Chapter 40) and, when present, should arouse suspicion of a superimposed inflammatory articular process. Similarly, calcification and an arthropathy resembling degenerative disease are not features of rheumatoid arthritis alone, so that the recognition of these atypical features should suggest that a superimposed articular process may be present.

Ankylosing Spondylitis

Rheumatoid arthritis and ankylosing spondylitis may coexist in the same patient (see Chapter 24). In these persons, clinical and radiologic manifestations of rheumatoid arthritis are combined with those of ankylosing spondylitis.

Diffuse Idiopathic Skeletal Hyperostosis

It is not surprising that rheumatoid arthritis and diffuse idiopathic skeletal hyperostosis, both common disorders in middle-aged and elderly patients, may occur together. In

patients with both disorders, atypical clinical features include a high frequency of flexion contractures of the elbows, the ankles, the wrists, or the knees, and atypical radiologic features include the absence of osteoporosis, and the presence of bone sclerosis and proliferation about erosions, osteophytes, and intraarticular bone ankylosis (see Chapter 37).

RADIOLOGIC ASSESSMENT OF DISEASE EXTENT AND PROGRESSION

The importance of an ideal series of radiographs in the evaluation of a patient with suspected rheumatoid arthritis is recognized by radiologists and rheumatologists alike but has led to a great deal of controversy and disagreement. Some investigators recommend a complete joint survey, others a limited survey, and a few are satisfied with one or two radiographs. Most agree that the key to the early and accurate radiographic diagnosis of rheumatoid arthritis lies in the analysis of the hands, wrists, and feet; however, what constitutes the proper projections in each of these anatomic regions is debated.

The limitation of radiography in the evaluation of the patient with rheumatoid arthritis is evident by the difficulty encountered in establishing a grading system that can measure improvement or progression of disease. As osteoporosis, joint space narrowing, and bone erosion are considered characteristic radiographic features of rheumatoid arthritis, most attempts at grading the severity of joint involvement have emphasized one or more of these features. Problems arise as a result of an independence in some cases of one radiographic feature with respect to another (e.g., progression of bone erosion with lack of progression of joint space loss) or of one articulation with respect to another and as a result of the difficulty in defining the changing size of an osseous erosion or the extent of joint space loss.

Existing data confirm an inconstant correlation of disease activity derived from clinical, laboratory, and radiologic parameters. These data also indicate that radiographic abnormalities in rheumatoid arthritis, reflecting bone and cartilage destruction, may progress or become stationary but are largely irreversible. Although radiographic evidence of healing of bone erosions—characterized by a decreased size and a sclerotic margin—has been recorded, it is infrequent and requires a long period of observation, usually a matter of years. Therefore, in planning a radiologic protocol that is appropriate in the patient receiving treatment for rheumatoid arthritis, physicians should use longer intervals between examinations and yet standardize radiographic technique.

OTHER DIAGNOSTIC TECHNIQUES
Fine-Detail Radiography with Magnification

Fine-detail radiography with magnification (see Chapter 6) can identify subtle abnormalities, especially about the small joints of the hand and the foot and about the calcaneus, at a time when conventional radiographs are negative or equivocal.

Low KV Radiography and Xeroradiography

Application of low KV radiography or xeroradiography allows analysis of soft tissues by maximizing the low radiographic contrast between soft tissue structures (see Chapters 7 and 8). In rheumatoid arthritis, this technique delineates capsular distention and periarticular edema at an early stage, before cartilaginous and osseous destruction becomes evident.

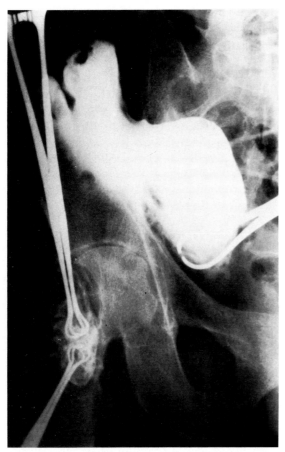

Figure 22–39. Arthrography in rheumatoid arthritis. Intraoperative arthrography in a 50 year old man with rheumatoid arthritis, who had a mass in the groin, confirms the existence of a large synovial cyst arising from an abnormal hip and extending into the pelvis. (Courtesy of J. Scavulli, M.D., San Diego, California.)

Arthrography

In certain situations, arthrography has a definite advantage over routine radiography in patients with rheumatoid arthritis. Rotator cuff disruption, synovial cysts (Fig. 22–39), and sinus tracts are delineated definitively during arthrographic examination.

Scintigraphy

As in other articular disorders, radionuclide examination using bone- or joint-seeking pharmaceutical agents represents a sensitive method for evaluating disease activity in rheumatoid arthritis (see Chapter 16). Technetium pertechnetate and technetium phosphate scans outline joint inflammation, which may antedate clinical activity, and these studies may be used to monitor response to therapy. A typical abnormal radionuclide pattern in rheumatoid arthritis consists of a symmetrically distributed peripheral joint process that can be distinguished from that which is seen in the seronegative spondyloarthropathies.

Computed Tomography

Computed tomography (see Chapter 10) generally is not required in assessing the distribution and the extent of joint involvement in rheumatoid arthritis. Two problems seen in patients with rheumatoid arthritis that can be evaluated with computed tomography are acetabular protrusion (Fig. 22–40) and ischemic necrosis of the femoral head. In the former situation, the degree of displacement and the thickness of the acetabular roof can be determined. In the latter situation, distortion of the trabecular pattern within the femoral head can be diagnostic of ischemic necrosis at a stage when plain

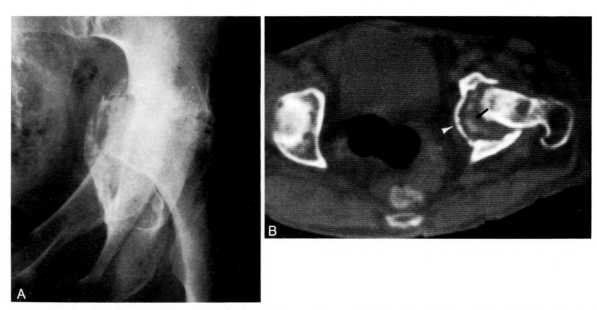

Figure 22–40. Computed tomography in rheumatoid arthritis. This 61 year old woman had a long history of rheumatoid arthritis. Four months prior to admission to the hospital, she fell at home and subsequently developed increasing pain in the hip. **A** The routine radiograph reveals fragmentation of the femoral head and acetabulum, acetabular protrusion, and bone eburnation. **B** On a transaxial section at the level of the hip, computed tomography confirms the presence of a deformed femoral head. Intraarticular bone fragments are seen (arrow). Observe the thin acetabular shell (arrowhead) protruding into the pelvis. The opposite hip, not well shown at this level, was minimally abnormal.

films are normal or equivocally abnormal. It is doubtful, however, that computed tomography will allow the diagnosis of ischemic necrosis of the femoral head at an earlier stage than it can be identified by scintigraphy or magnetic resonance imaging.

Computed tomography is well suited to the evaluation of paraarticular masses, which, in rheumatoid arthritis, commonly are related to synovial cyst formation. The combination of arthrography and computed tomography is ideally applied to outlining synovial cysts in many locations, particularly the hip and shoulder.

Computed tomography has also been advocated as a useful, noninvasive method in the diagnosis and management of cervical spine abnormalities in the rheumatoid arthritis patient. The craniocervical junction and atlantoaxial region are well displayed in the transaxial images obtainable with computed tomography, although multiplanar reconstruction of images is required occasionally.

One additional application of computed tomography is related to the diagnosis and the monitoring of osteopenia, specifically osteoporosis, in the axial skeleton of patients with rheumatoid arthritis and other disorders (see Chapter 18).

Magnetic Resonance Imaging

Preliminary data suggest that magnetic resonance imaging (see Chapter 11), with its dependence on hydrogen proton concentration, is sensitive to changes in water composition and is, therefore, able to detect and localize sites of inflammation (Fig. 22–41). In rheumatoid arthritis, this sensitivity allows the delineation of inflammatory articular effusions and their response to treatment. The technique also allows evaluation of intraarticular structures, such as hyaline cartilage

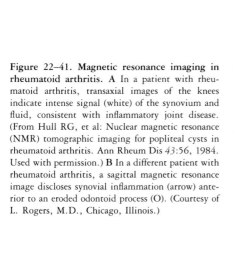

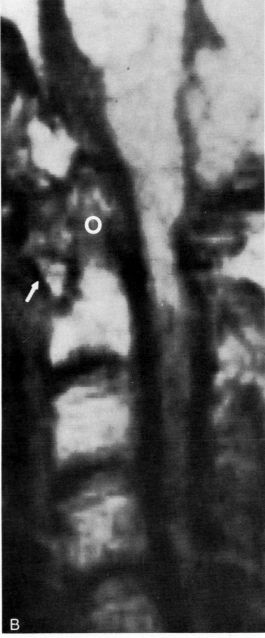

Figure 22–41. Magnetic resonance imaging in rheumatoid arthritis. A In a patient with rheumatoid arthritis, transaxial images of the knees indicate intense signal (white) of the synovium and fluid, consistent with inflammatory joint disease. (From Hull RG, et al: Nuclear magnetic resonance (NMR) tomographic imaging for popliteal cysts in rheumatoid arthritis. Ann Rheum Dis 43:56, 1984. Used with permission.) B In a different patient with rheumatoid arthritis, a sagittal magnetic resonance image discloses synovial inflammation (arrow) anterior to an eroded odontoid process (O). (Courtesy of L. Rogers, M.D., Chicago, Illinois.)

and fibrocartilage, and of adjacent tendons and ligaments. Furthermore, magnetic resonance imaging represents a safe and effective means to outline the extent of synovial cyst formation and the spinal cord; it can be used effectively in the study of the rheumatoid cervical spine.

Finally, the magnetic resonance image is a sensitive indicator of ischemic necrosis of bone, a significant problem in the patient with rheumatoid arthritis who is receiving corticosteroid medication.

DIFFERENTIAL DIAGNOSIS
General Abnormalities

When a radiographic examination reveals a symmetrically distributed articular disorder affecting the proximal interphalangeal and metacarpophalangeal joints of the hands, the wrists, the metatarsophalangeal joints of the feet, the calcanei, the knees, and the elbows, which is characterized by osteoporosis, fusiform soft tissue swelling, concentric joint space loss, and marginal and central erosions, the diagnosis of rheumatoid arthritis is obvious. When the radiographs of rheumatoid arthritis patients disclose some degree of asymmetry, mild or absent osteoporosis, or preservation of joint space, an accurate appraisal is much more difficult. Fortunately, these latter features are not common in the disease, although they are occasionally observed in men with classic rheumatoid arthritis, and in men and women with possible, probable, or definite disease.

Seronegative "Rheumatoid" Arthritis

Many patients with polyarticular inflammatory disease are serologically negative (seronegative) for rheumatoid factor, and the precise nature of their joint abnormality is variable and often not clear. As some of these individuals fulfill other criteria for "definite" disease, they may indeed have rheumatoid arthritis, although some evidence suggests that seronegative "rheumatoid" arthritis is not rheumatoid arthritis at all: (1) there is a disparity in the prognosis of the disease in patients with and without rheumatoid factor; (2) certain clinical features rarely are accompanied by seronegativity; and (3) a family history of disease is more frequent in those patients who are seropositive for rheumatoid factor. Currently, it appears certain that patients who have seronegative "rheumatoid" arthritis can be divided into two major groups of individuals: those with otherwise typical rheumatoid arthritis who are serologically negative for rheumatoid factor and those with some other form of arthritis. With regard to the former group, some of these patients will become seropositive or became seronegative as a result of therapy. With regard to the latter group, it is evident that certain members share clinical and radiologic features that will eventually allow their separation into a more homogeneous disease category.

With respect to radiologic abnormalities, many of the individuals with seronegative "rheumatoid" arthritis have atypical features and, in fact, the observer can often predict such seronegativity when reviewing the radiographs. One such feature is the asymmetry of the articular involvement. Others may include the presence of osteosclerosis, new bone formation, intraarticular bone ankylosis, and predominant carpal involvement, and the relative absence of classic subchondral erosions. The greater the number of such features, the greater is the likelihood of seronegativity.

Spondyloarthropathies

Rheumatoid arthritis characteristically reveals a distribution and morphology of articular lesions that differ from those of the seronegative spondyloarthropathies (ankylosing spondylitis, psoriasis, Reiter's syndrome). Ankylosing spondylitis (which shows predilection for the axial skeleton, although it may also produce appendicular articular disease), psoriasis (which may affect axial and appendicular skeleton as well as distal interphalangeal joints), and Reiter's syndrome (which leads to asymmetric arthritis of the lower extremity with or without sacroiliac and spinal alterations) may each be associated with prominent findings in synovial and cartilaginous joints and entheses. In the synovial joints, the absence of osteoporosis and the presence of bone proliferation and intraarticular osseous fusion are commonly encountered in the seronegative spondyloarthropathies, differing from the features of rheumatoid arthritis. At other sites, prominent erosion and sclerosis of the symphysis pubis, manubriosternal joint, and ligamentous attachments of the pelvis, femur, and calcaneus are typical of seronegative spondyloarthropathies. Widespread spondylitis and sacroiliitis are also characteristic of these latter disorders.

Gout

Gouty arthritis is associated with asymmetric articular disease of the appendicular skeleton characterized by soft tissue masses, eccentric osseous erosions, bone proliferation, preservation of joint space, and absence of osteoporosis. Generally, the features are easily differentiated from those of rheumatoid arthritis, although the radiographic changes in long-standing rheumatoid arthritis and gout can be remarkably similar.

Calcium Pyrophosphate Dihydrate (CPPD) Crystal Deposition Disease

This articular disorder is manifested radiographically as articular and periarticular calcification and pyrophosphate arthropathy. The calcification involves various structures, including cartilage (chondrocalcinosis), and is most prominent in the knees, the wrists, the metacarpophalangeal joints, and the symphysis pubis. Pyrophosphate arthropathy leads to joint space narrowing, eburnation, cyst formation, collapse, and fragmentation. The resulting radiographic picture does not realistically resemble that of rheumatoid arthritis.

Abnormalities at Specific Sites
Hand and Wrist

Symmetric changes at metacarpophalangeal and proximal interphalangeal joints (including the interphalangeal joint of the thumb) are common in rheumatoid arthritis; abnormalities of distal interphalangeal joints are less frequent and are rarely severe. This pattern of distribution differs from that in other disorders. Psoriatic arthritis leads to significant abnormalities of distal interphalangeal joints as well as of more proximal articulations. Osteoarthritis (inflammatory or noninflammatory) most typically affects distal interphalangeal, proximal interphalangeal, and metacarpophalangeal joints. Gouty arthritis can involve any articulation of the hand, including the distal interphalangeal joints. CPPD crystal deposition disease has predilection for the metacarpophalangeal articulations.

Rheumatoid arthritis can initially be manifested as soft tissue swelling, joint space narrowing, and osseous erosions

Table 22–4. COMPARTMENTAL ANALYSIS OF HAND AND WRIST DISEASE*

	DIP Joints	PIP Joints	MCP Joints	Radiocarpal Joint	Inferior Radio-ulnar Joint	Midcarpal Joint	Pisiform-Triquetral Joint	Common Carpo-metacarpal Joint	First Carpo-metacarpal Joint
Rheumatoid arthritis		+	+	+	+	+	+	+	+
Osteoarthritis	+	+	+			+†			+
Inflammatory osteoarthritis	+	+	±			+†			+
Calcium pyrophosphate dihydrate crystal deposition disease			+	+		+†			+
Gouty arthritis	+	+	+	+	+	+		+‡	+
Scleroderma§	+	+			+				+

*Only the *typical* locations for each disease are indicated.
†Has predilection for trapezioscaphoid area of midcarpal joint.
‡Very severe abnormalities may be present in this compartment.
§Some patients have coexistent rheumatoid arthritis.
DIP, Distal interphalangeal; PIP, proximal interphalangeal; MCP, metacarpophalangeal.

in one or two locations of the wrist; radiocarpal, inferior radioulnar, and pisiform-triquetral compartmental changes are especially common. Soon, however, pancompartmental alterations become manifest. The diffuse nature of wrist involvement in rheumatoid arthritis is an important characteristic of this disease (Table 22–4). In patients without a significant history of accidental or occupational trauma, osteoarthritis leads to an articular abnormality that is usually confined to the first carpometacarpal compartment or the trapezioscaphoid space of the midcarpal compartment, or involves both. CPPD crystal deposition disease favors the radiocarpal compartment; scleroderma may selectively involve the first carpometacarpal and inferior radioulnar compartments; and gout produces pancompartmental disease with predominant involvement of the common carpometacarpal compartment.

Glenohumeral Joint

Marginal erosions of the humeral head are seen in rheumatoid arthritis, ankylosing spondylitis, and infection, as well as in other disorders. In ankylosing spondylitis, the size of the defect may be considerably larger than in rheumatoid arthritis. Septic arthritis of the glenohumeral joint is usually monoarticular, differing from the polyarticular nature of rheumatoid arthritis.

Rotator cuff tears may complicate rheumatoid arthritis as well as other synovial processes of the glenohumeral joint, including ankylosing spondylitis and infection. Such tears can also result from trauma and are very common in elderly individuals.

Acromioclavicular Joint

Resorption of the distal clavicle and widening of the acromioclavicular joint are observed in rheumatoid arthritis, ankylosing spondylitis, infection, other collagen disorders, and hyperparathyroidism and after trauma. When the changes are secondary to an articular process, prominent acromial abnormalities may accompany the clavicular alterations. In hyperparathyroidism, subchondral resorption of bone is evident on both the acromial and the clavicular aspects of the joint, but the acromial alterations are relatively mild. Post-traumatic osteolysis of the distal clavicle is accompanied by a pertinent clinical history of injury and frequently by radiographic evidence of fracture and dislocation. Osteolysis predominates in the clavicle, although mild acromial abnormalities may also be seen.

Coracoclavicular Joint

Resorption of the undersurface of the distal clavicle is seen in rheumatoid arthritis, hyperparathyroidism, and ankylosing spondylitis.

Forefoot

The most common sites of articular disease of the forefoot in rheumatoid arthritis are the metatarsophalangeal joints and the interphalangeal joint of the great toe. Although these same articulations are involved in psoriasis, Reiter's syndrome, and gout, extensive abnormality of other interphalangeal joints in one or more digits can be evident in any of these three latter disorders (Table 22–5). Furthermore, forefoot abnormalities are usually symmetric in distribution in rheumatoid arthritis and asymmetric in psoriasis, Reiter's syndrome, and gouty arthritis.

At the interphalangeal joint of the great toe, the changes of rheumatoid arthritis predominate on the medial aspect of

Table 22–5. COMPARTMENTAL ANALYSIS OF FOREFOOT DISEASE*

	Metatarso-phalangeal Joints	Inter-phalangeal Joint of Great Toe	Other Inter-phalangeal Joints
Rheumatoid arthritis	+	+	
Gouty arthritis	+	+	+
Psoriatic arthritis	+	+†	+
Reiter's syndrome	+	+†	+
Osteoarthritis	+‡		

*Only the typical locations of each disease are indicated.
†Severe destructive changes may be observed.
‡Has predilection for the metatarsophalangeal joint of the first digit.

Table 22–6. ABNORMALITIES OF THE HEEL

	Retrocalcaneal Bursitis with Posterosuperior Calcaneal Erosion	Achilles Tendinitis	Spur at Posterior Attachment of Achilles Tendon	Well-defined Plantar Calcaneal Spur	Ill-defined Plantar Calcaneal Spur
Rheumatoid arthritis	+	+	+	+	
Ankylosing spondylitis	+	+	+		+*
Psoriatic arthritis	+	+	+		+*
Reiter's syndrome	+	+			+*
Gouty arthritis	+†	+‡			
Xanthoma	+†	+‡			

*Poorly defined spurs may become better defined with healing.
†Erosion of calcaneus can occur beneath tophus or xanthoma.
‡Nodular thickening of the tendon may be seen.

the joint, especially along the distal portion of the proximal phalanx. Although joint space narrowing and mild subchondral erosions and cysts are encountered in the interphalangeal joint in rheumatoid arthritis, severe destruction usually is not apparent. This latter finding is evident in gout, psoriasis, and Reiter's syndrome.

Midfoot

Diffuse changes with predilection for the talonavicular portion of the talocalcaneonavicular joint characterize midfoot involvement in rheumatoid arthritis. The talonavicular space is also affected in CPPD crystal deposition disease and in neuroarthropathy (especially in diabetic patients), but both of these disorders are associated with bone sclerosis and fragmentation, findings that are not common in rheumatoid arthritis. Midfoot changes are also evident in seronegative spondyloarthropathies and gouty arthritis. In gout, abnormalities may predominate at the tarsometatarsal joints.

Heel

Retrocalcaneal bursitis producing soft tissue swelling and subjacent osseous erosion occurs not only in rheumatoid arthritis but also in ankylosing spondylitis, psoriasis, and Reiter's syndrome (Table 22–6). The changes are virtually indistinguishable in these four disorders, although poorly defined erosions and bone sclerosis are more typical of the seronegative spondyloarthropathies.

Tendon thickening can be seen in any of these four diseases. Nodular prominence of the Achilles tendon can also be encountered in gout (owing to tophi) and hyperlipoproteinemia (owing to xanthoma). Abnormalities on the plantar aspect of the calcaneus in rheumatoid arthritis consist of superficial erosions and well-defined spurs. In the seronegative spondyloarthropathies, prominent erosions, considerable sclerosis, and exuberant, poorly defined excrescences are seen.

Knee

In rheumatoid arthritis, symmetric involvement of the medial femorotibial and lateral femorotibial compartments with or without patellofemoral compartmental changes is seen. In osteoarthritis, asymmetric alterations of the medial and lateral femorotibial compartments (the medial side is more frequently the predominant side of involvement) can be combined with patellofemoral compartmental disease. In CPPD crystal deposition disease, patellofemoral abnormalities

occurring alone or in combination with asymmetric medial and lateral femorotibial alterations are typical. Although any of these three disorders can be associated with varus or valgus angulation of the knee, a varus deformity is especially characteristic of osteoarthritis, whereas valgus deformity is not uncommon in rheumatoid arthritis and CPPD crystal deposition disease.

Marginal erosions of femur and tibia are evident in rheumatoid arthritis, seronegative spondyloarthropathies, gout, and infection, especially tuberculosis.

Popliteal cysts can occur in association with any articular process leading to the accumulation of joint fluid and elevation of intraarticular pressure. Examples of such processes are rheumatoid arthritis, ankylosing spondylitis, psoriasis, gout, infection, juvenile chronic arthritis, and the peripheral arthritis of inflammatory bowel disease. Popliteal cysts can also follow trauma and are frequently associated with meniscal tears or other internal derangements of the knee.

Hip

Symmetric loss of articular space with axial migration of the femoral head with respect to the acetabulum is typical of rheumatoid involvement of the hip. In osteoarthritis, superior or medial migration is more frequent than axial migration, reflecting the asymmetric nature of the cartilaginous destruction. Axial migration of the femoral head can accompany the hip involvement of CPPD crystal deposition disease and ankylosing spondylitis, although both of these disorders are associated with osteophytes and sclerosis. In long-standing rheumatoid arthritis, however, osteophytes may appear as a manifestation of secondary degenerative joint disease.

Acetabular protrusion is a common manifestation of severe rheumatoid hip disease. It is associated with diffuse loss of interosseous space and an eroded and often diminutive femoral

Table 22–7. SOME CAUSES OF PROTRUSIO ACETABULI

Rheumatoid arthritis
Ankylosing spondylitis
Osteoarthritis (medial migration pattern)
Infection
Paget's disease
Osteomalacia
Irradiation
Acetabular trauma

head. Protrusio acetabuli can also be encountered in patients with osteoarthritis, familial or idiopathic protrusion deformities (Otto pelvis), ankylosing spondylitis, infection, osteomalacia, and Paget's disease (Table 22–7).

Sacroiliac Joint

Sacroiliac joint abnormalities are not common or prominent in rheumatoid arthritis. When evident, they are generally asymmetric in distribution and consist of minor subchondral erosions, minimal eburnation, and absent or focal intra-articular bone ankylosis (Table 22–8). These characteristics differ from those of ankylosing spondylitis (bilateral symmetric disease with extensive erosions, sclerosis, and bone fusion), psoriasis and Reiter's syndrome (bilateral symmetric, bilateral asymmetric, or unilateral disease with changes identical to those of ankylosing spondylitis), gout (bilateral or unilateral abnormalities with large erosions), degenerative joint disease (bilateral or unilateral disease with prominent subchondral sclerosis), osteitis condensans ilii (bilateral symmetric alterations of the lower ilium with significant bone eburnation), hyperparathyroidism (bilateral symmetric abnormalities with widening of the interosseous space, erosions, and sclerosis), and infection (unilateral disease with poorly defined osseous defects and reactive sclerosis).

Spine

Unlike ankylosing spondylitis, psoriatic arthritis, and Reiter's syndrome, rheumatoid arthritis produces infrequent abnormalities of the thoracic and lumbar spine. Rheumatoid changes in the cervical spine consisting of apophyseal joint erosion and malalignment, intervertebral disc space narrowing with adjacent eburnation and without osteophytes, and multiple subluxations, including that at the atlantoaxial junction, are virtually diagnostic when they occur as a group. They differ from the cervical alterations of ankylosing spondylitis (widespread apophyseal joint ankylosis and syndesmophytes), psoriatic arthritis (apophyseal joint narrowing and eburnation, and prominent anterior vertebral bone formation), diffuse idiopathic skeletal hyperostosis (flowing ossification and excrescences along the anterior aspect of the spine with preservation of intervertebral disc height), and juvenile chronic arthritis (apophyseal joint ankylosis with hypoplasia of vertebral bodies and intervertebral discs). Atlantoaxial subluxation alone is not a pathognomonic sign of rheumatoid arthritis, however. It is also observed in ankylosing spondylitis, psoriatic arthritis, Reiter's syndrome, and juvenile chronic arthritis, as well as after trauma or local infection. Similarly,

odontoid erosions can be evident in a variety of synovial disorders, and intervertebral disc space narrowing with adjacent osseous irregularity can be apparent after trauma or infection.

FURTHER READING

Adams ME, Li DKB: Magnetic resonance imaging in rheumatology. J Rheumatol 12:1038, 1985.

Berens DL, Lin RK: Roentgen Diagnosis of Rheumatoid Arthritis. Springfield, Ill, Charles C Thomas, 1969.

Braunstein EM, Weissman BN, Seltzer SE, Sosman JL, Wang A-M, Zamani A: Computed tomography and conventional radiographs of the craniocervical region in rheumatoid arthritis. A comparison. Arthritis Rheum 27:26, 1984.

Castillo BA, El Sallab RA, Scott JT: Physical activity, cystic erosions, and osteoporosis in rheumatoid arthritis. Ann Rheum Dis 24:522, 1965.

Currey HLF: Aetiology and pathogenesis of rheumatoid arthritis. In JT Scott (Ed): Copeman's Textbook of the Rheumatic Diseases. 5th Ed. Edinburgh, Churchill Livingstone, 1978.

El-Khoury GY, Larson RK, Kathol MH, Berbaum KS, Furst DE: Seronegative and seropositive rheumatoid arthritis: Radiographic differences. Radiology 168:517, 1988.

El-Khoury GY, Wener MH, Menezes AH, Dolan KD, Kathol MEH: Cranial settling in rheumatoid arthritis. Radiology 137:637, 1980.

Felty AR: Chronic arthritis in the adult associated with splenomegaly and leukopenia. A report of 5 cases of an unusual clinical syndrome. Johns Hopkins Hosp Bull 35:16, 1924.

Fries JF, Bloch DA, Sharp JT, McShane DJ, Spitz P, Bluhm GB, Forrester D, Genant H, Gofton P, Richman S, Weissman B, Wolfe F: Assessment of radiologic progression in rheumatoid arthritis. A randomized controlled trial. Arthritis Rheum 29:1, 1986.

Gelman MI, Ward JR: Septic arthritis: A complication of rheumatoid arthritis. Radiology 122:17, 1977.

Heywood AWB, Meyers OL: Rheumatoid arthritis of the thoracic and lumbar spine. J Bone Joint Surg [Br] 68:362, 1986.

Martel W: The pattern of rheumatoid arthritis in the hand and wrist. Radiol Clin North Am 2:221, 1964.

Martel W: Pathogenesis of cervical discovertebral destruction in rheumatoid arthritis. Arthritis Rheum 20:1217, 1977.

McAfee PC, Bohlman HH, Han JS, Salvagno RT: Comparison of nuclear magnetic resonance imaging and computed tomography in the diagnosis of upper cervical spinal cord compression. Spine 11:295, 1986.

Monsees B, Destouet JM, Murphy WA, Resnick D: Pressure erosions of bone in rheumatoid arthritis: A subject review. Radiology 155:53, 1985.

Park WM, O'Neill M, McCall IW: The radiology of rheumatoid involvement of the cervical spine. Skel Radiol 4:1, 1979.

Resnick D. Patterns of migration of the femoral head in osteoarthritis of the hip: Roentgenographic-pathologic correlation and comparison with rheumatoid arthritis. AJR 124:62, 1975.

Resnick D: Rheumatoid arthritis of the wrist. The compartmental approach. Med Radiogr Photogr 52:50, 1976.

Resnick D, Feingold ML, Curd J, Niwayama G, Goergen TG: Calcaneal abnormalities in articular disorders. Rheumatoid arthritis, ankylosing spondylitis, psoriatic arthritis and Reiter's syndrome. Radiology 125:355, 1977.

Ropes MW, Bennett GA, Cobb S, Jacox R, Jessar RA: Diagnostic criteria for rheumatoid arthritis, 1958 revision. Ann Rheum Dis 18:49, 1959.

Scott JT (Ed): Copeman's Textbook of the Rheumatic Diseases. 5th Ed. Edinburgh, Churchill Livingstone, 1978.

Sharp JT, Young DY, Bluhm GR, Brook A, Brower AC, Corbett M, Decker JL, Genant HK, Gofton JP, Goodman N, Larsen A, Lidsky MD, Pussila P, Weinstein AS, Weissman BN: How many joints in the hands and wrists should be included in a score of radiologic abnormalities used to assess rheumatoid arthritis? Arthritis Rheum 28:1326, 1985.

Swanson AB, Swanson GG: Pathogenesis and pathomechanics of rheumatoid deformities in the hand and wrist. Orthop Clin North Am 4:1039, 1973.

Weissberg D, Resnick D, Taylor A, Becker MA, Alazraki NP: Rheumatoid arthritis and its variants: Analysis of scintiphotographic, radiographic, and clinical examinations. AJR 131:665, 1978.

Weissman BNW, Aliabadi P, Weinfeld MS, Thomas WH, Sosman JL: Prognostic features of atlanto-axial subluxation in rheumatoid arthritis. Radiology 144:745, 1982.

Table 22–8. COMPARISON OF SACROILIAC JOINT ABNORMALITIES IN RHEUMATOID ARTHRITIS AND ANKYLOSING SPONDYLITIS

	Rheumatoid Arthritis	Ankylosing Spondylitis
Distribution	Asymmetric or unilateral	Bilateral and symmetric
Erosions	Superficial	Deep
Sclerosis	Mild or absent	Moderate or severe*
Bone ankylosis	Rare, segmental	Common, diffuse

*Sclerosis may disappear in long-standing disease.

Chapter 23

Juvenile Chronic Arthritis

Donald Resnick, M.D.
Gen Niwayama, M.D.

Juvenile chronic arthritis is composed of a variety of conditions that affect articular structures in children. Several distinct subgroups of patients can be recognized. Although specific radiographic features of juvenile chronic arthritis depend on the subgroup of patients that is being evaluated, certain characteristics are sufficiently common in most patients to allow differentiation of juvenile chronic arthritis from various adult diseases. Loss of articular space and osseous erosions are relatively late manifestations of juvenile disease. Metaphyseal radiolucency, periostitis, in-traarticular bone ankylosis, epiphyseal compression fractures, subluxation or dislocation, and growth disturbances are common. Although changes may be observed in many different skeletal sites, abnormalities of the hand, the wrist, the foot, the knee, the hip, the cervical spine, the mandible, and the temporomandibular joint are especially characteristic.

Differential diagnosis of juvenile chronic arthritis includes hemophilia, idiopathic multicentric osteolysis, mucopolysaccharidoses, epiphyseal dysplasias, and infection.

In 1897, Still, an English pediatrician, detailed an articular condition in 22 children that appeared to be distinct from the adult type of rheumatoid arthritis because of its predilection for large joints rather than small ones, its propensity for producing joint contractures and muscle wasting, and its association with significant extraarticular manifestations, such as splenomegaly, lymphadenopathy, anemia, fever, pleuritis, and pericarditis. Since this report, the designation of Still's disease has frequently been used to describe rheumatoid arthritis in children.

Through the years, there has been a natural tendency to label many articular disorders of children as juvenile rheumatoid arthritis despite variable clinical and radiologic manifestations and an unpredictable disease course. It is now recognized that a number of separate disorders can lead to chronic arthritis in children and that, in many patients, scrutiny of clinical and radiographic features will allow a more precise diagnosis. Currently, there exists no uniformly accepted classification system for juvenile chronic arthritis, however.

CLASSIFICATION

In arriving at a workable classification of articular disease in children, the physician must first exclude certain groups of disorders with characteristic features, such as infection, bleeding diatheses, neoplasms, connective tissue disorders, Sjögren's syndrome, rheumatic fever, and postdysenteric arthritis. The remaining group of diseases is designated juvenile chronic arthritis (or polyarthritis). Within this group are certain disorders, such as ankylosing spondylitis, psoriatic arthritis, and the arthritis associated with inflammatory bowel disease, whose true nature may be revealed only after a variable follow-up period. At the time of their initial presentation, however, it is frequently impossible to classify these children with arthritis into one specific subgroup of juvenile chronic arthritis.

The following subgroups of juvenile chronic arthritis are now recognized (Tables 23–1 and 23–2).

Juvenile-Onset Adult Type (Seropositive) Rheumatoid Arthritis

An articular disease that resembles and behaves like the adult counterpart has been noted in 5 to 10 per cent of children with juvenile chronic arthritis (Fig. 23–1A). It is more frequent in girls than in boys, and it is most common after the age of 10 years. Early involvement of the interphalangeal and metacarpophalangeal joints of the hand, the wrist, the knee, and the metatarsophalangeal and interphalangeal joints of the foot is typical. Severe destructive arthritis is common, and subcutaneous nodules can be detected in approximately 10 to 20 per cent of children. Iridocyclitis is not present.

Radiologic changes include soft tissue swelling, periarticular osteoporosis, and periostitis in the hands and the feet. It is the frequency and the severity of periostitis that constitute a fundamental difference between juvenile-onset and adult-onset disease. Significant osseous erosions are also encountered; these have a marginal distribution and may be unaccompanied

Table 23–1. CLASSIFICATION OF JUVENILE CHRONIC ARTHRITIS

Juvenile-onset adult type (seropositive) rheumatoid arthritis
Seronegative chronic arthritis (Still's disease)
    Classic systemic disease
    Polyarticular disease
    Pauciarticular or monarticular disease
Juvenile-onset ankylosing spondylitis
Psoriatic arthritis
Arthritis of inflammatory bowel disease
Other seronegative spondyloarthropathies
Miscellaneous arthritis

Table 23–2. CLINICAL AND RADIOGRAPHIC FEATURES OF JUVENILE CHRONIC ARTHRITIS

Disorder	Clinical Features	Sites of Articular Involvement	Radiographic Features
Juvenile-onset adult type (seropositive) rheumatoid arthritis	Female predominance > 10 years old Polyarticular involvement ± Subcutaneous nodules ± Vasculitis Seropositive for rheumatoid factor	MCP and IP joints of hand Wrist Knee MTP and IP joints of foot Cervical spine	Soft tissue swelling Osteoporosis Periostitis Erosions ± Joint space loss Atlantoaxial subluxation
Still's disease Systemic disease	Affects males and females equally <5 years old Systemic manifestations Mild articular manifestations	Unusual and mild joint involvement*	
Polyarticular disease	Affects males and females equally Variable age Polyarticular involvement Symmetric	MCP and IP joints of hand Wrist Knee Ankle Intertarsal, MTP, and IP joints of foot Cervical spine	Soft tissue swelling Osteoporosis Periostitis Growth disturbances ± Erosions ± Joint space loss Intraarticular bone ankylosis Apophyseal joint ankylosis with hypoplasia of cervical vertebrae and discs Scoliosis
Pauciarticular or monarticular disease	Female predominance Young age Iridocyclitis ± Systemic manifestations Asymmetric	Knee Ankle Elbow Wrist	Soft tissue swelling Osteoporosis Growth disturbances ± Joint space loss ± Erosions
Juvenile-onset ankylosing spondylitis	Male predominance 10–12 years old Polyarticular or pauciarticular involvement Predilection for the lower extremity Asymmetric ± Back pain ± Iridocyclitis ± Family history HLA-B27 +	Ankle Knee Intertarsal joints Calcaneus Hip ± Sacroiliac joint ± Spine	± Sacroiliitis ± Spondylitis Joint space loss Intraarticular bone ankylosis Erosions Bone proliferation

*When present, findings are similar to those of polyarticular or pauciarticular disease.
MCP, metacarpophalangeal; IP, interphalangeal; MTP, metatarsophalangeal.

by loss of the interosseous space. The appearance of significant erosive abnormality in the absence of joint space loss should be emphasized as a diagnostic sign of juvenile-onset rheumatoid arthritis. Atlantoaxial subluxation is not uncommon.

Seronegative Chronic Arthritis (Still's Disease)

In this largest subgroup (approximately 70 per cent) of juvenile chronic arthritis, children develop systemic or articular (or both) symptoms and signs in the absence of positive serologic test results for rheumatoid factor. Within this subgroup are certain clinical varieties.

CLASSIC SYSTEMIC DISEASE. This pattern, which is usually seen in boys and girls below the age of 5 years and represents approximately 20 per cent of cases of juvenile chronic arthritis, is associated with severe extraarticular clinical manifestations. An acute febrile onset, irritability, listlessness, anorexia, weight loss and a rash may be observed. Generalized lymphadenopathy and hepatosplenomegaly can simulate the findings in leukemia or lymphoma. Pericarditis and myocarditis represent additional serious features of Still's disease. Although joint manifestations are common, they are generally mild in nature. Radiologic findings are unusual, although occasionally chronic and disabling articular changes can become evident. Laboratory features include moderate anemia, elevated erythrocyte sedimentation rate, and leukocytosis.

POLYARTICULAR DISEASE (FIG. 23–1B). Polyarticular arthritis may occur at the onset of Still's disease or as a later complication in a child with systemic manifestations. This pattern is evident in approximately 20 per cent of patients with juvenile chronic arthritis. Some reports indicate boys and girls are affected in equal numbers; others suggest a strong female preponderance. Symmetric involvement of the metacarpophalangeal and proximal interphalangeal joints of the hands, the wrists, the knees, the ankles, and the intertarsal, metatarsophalangeal, and interphalangeal joints of the feet is typical. The cervical spine frequently is a site of early abnormality and characteristically is the only region of the vertebral column that is affected. Accompanying systemic manifestations include rash, splenomegaly, lymphadenopathy, and carditis. Fever and leukocytosis can also be apparent.

Initially, radiographic findings are soft tissue swelling,

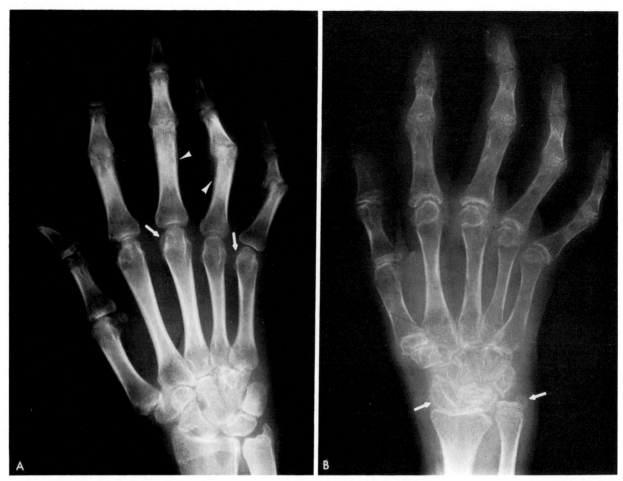

Figure 23–1. Juvenile chronic arthritis: Subgroups of disease. A Juvenile-onset adult type (seropositive) rheumatoid arthritis. An 18 year old girl with seropositive rheumatoid arthritis for approximately 6 years. Observe that the radiographic abnormalities are similar to those seen in adult-onset disease. Involvement occurs in all the compartments of the wrist and in the metacarpophalangeal and proximal interphalangeal joints, with less striking changes in the distal interphalangeal joints. Radiographic changes include soft tissue swelling, periarticular osteoporosis, joint space narrowing, and marginal erosions. At some metacarpophalangeal joints, considerable erosive alterations are not accompanied by severe loss of joint space (arrows). Also note intraarticular osseous fusion at several proximal interphalangeal joints and periostitis of phalangeal shafts (arrowheads). **B** Seronegative chronic arthritis (Still's disease): Polyarticular disease. An 11 year old girl, seronegative for rheumatoid factor, had symmetric articular disease of the hands, wrists, knees, feet, and cervical spine. The radiograph outlines considerable generalized osteoporosis, periarticular soft tissue swelling, superficial erosions of carpal bones and metacarpal heads with irregularity of shape, joint space narrowing, epiphyseal collapse, and enlargement of epiphyses, particularly those of the distal ends of the radius and ulna (arrows). The crenated or "crinkled" appearance of the carpus and metacarpal heads is distinctive. Flexion contractures of several digits are evident.

osteoporosis, and advanced skeletal maturation. In the hands and the feet, abnormalities of shape (squaring) of the carpal and tarsal bones are frequently combined with initial loss of joint space and subsequent intraarticular bone ankylosis. Periostitis of the diaphyses and metaphyses of phalanges and metacarpal and metatarsal bones and premature fusion of the epiphyses of the bones are not uncommon. The epiphyses may appear enlarged, and decrease in bone length is characteristic. Osseous erosion is unusual.

In the larger joints, such as the knee, osteoporosis and epiphyseal overgrowth are more typical than articular space loss and erosive change. Hip involvement is associated with osteoporosis, premature fusion of the femoral neck, coxa valga deformity, hypoplasia of the iliac bones, and protrusio acetabuli.

Apophyseal joint erosions, narrowing, and bone ankylosis predominate in the upper cervical region, particularly at the C2-C3 level. Associated hypoplasia of the vertebral bodies and intervertebral discs is characteristic. Thoracolumbar spinal abnormalities of Still's disease are relatively infrequent.

PAUCIARTICULAR OR MONARTICULAR DISEASE. This pattern, which is observed in young children and may represent 30 to 70 per cent of all cases of juvenile chronic arthritis, generally is confined to large joints, most frequently the knees, the ankles, the elbows, and the wrists. This clinical pattern of arthritis carries with it a serious threat of blindness from iridocyclitis. Additional systemic manifestations are infrequent. Laboratory analysis may be entirely unremarkable.

In monarticular or pauciarticular Still's disease, radiographically demonstrable abnormalities of bone growth may appear at an early stage. Increased size and accelerated maturation of epiphyseal ossification centers, longitudinal overgrowth of bones adjacent to an affected articulation, and regional atrophy and remodeling of bone are observed. Soft tissue swelling and osteoporosis are seen, but bone erosion is a late manifestation.

Juvenile-Onset Ankylosing Spondylitis

Children with this disease, particularly boys, develop sacroiliitis and spondylitis in the presence of the histocompatibility antigen HLA-B27. Although the mean age of onset of disease is 10 to 12 years, there is a wide variation, ranging from 3 to 15 years of age. An asymmetric arthritis is generally observed, and the joints of the lower limbs are affected, particularly the ankle, the knee, and the intertarsal joints. Clinical manifestations may be encountered in the sacroiliac joints, but radiographic changes in these articulations and those of the spine are difficult to interpret in young children. Acute iridocyclitis is not a common presenting feature of the disease but is subsequently apparent in as many as 25 per cent of patients. A family history of ankylosing spondylitis is not infrequent. HLA-B27 may be detected in approximately 90 per cent of individuals.

Radiographic abnormalities in juvenile-onset ankylosing spondylitis simulate those in adult-onset ankylosing spondylitis. Sacroiliac joint alterations may initially be unilateral or asymmetric in distribution, but they soon become bilateral and symmetric. The spinal changes may be seen in the thoracic, the lumbar, and less frequently the cervical regions of the vertebral column. They include osteitis or sclerosis of vertebral corners, squaring of the anterior vertebral surface, syndesmophytosis, and apophyseal joint bone ankylosis.

Radiographic findings in the appendicular skeleton are most common in the hips, the knees, and the shoulders, and include joint space narrowing, erosions, bone proliferation, and even intraarticular osseous fusion. The inferior and posterior aspects of the calcaneus, the ischial tuberosities, and the trochanters of the proximal femur may be affected.

Psoriatic Arthritis

In a small subgroup of children with juvenile chronic arthritis, articular involvement may antedate psoriatic skin disease and can be characterized by severe and progressive joint destruction. Radiographic abnormalities can simulate those in adults with psoriatic arthritis.

Arthritis of Inflammatory Bowel Disease

In this type, spinal, sacroiliac, and peripheral articular findings accompany enteritis and colitis.

Other Seronegative Spondyloarthropathies

In addition to ankylosing spondylitis, psoriatic arthritis, and the arthritis of inflammatory bowel disease, other varieties of seronegative spondyloarthropathy affect children. These include Reiter's syndrome and reactive arthritis.

RADIOGRAPHIC ABNORMALITIES

Although the radiographic abnormalities associated with juvenile chronic arthritis depend on the specific subgroup that is being investigated, certain findings are characteristic in many varieties of the disease.

General Features (Table 23–3) (Fig. 23–2)

SOFT TISSUE SWELLING. Periarticular fusiform soft tissue swelling is a common early manifestation of arthritis. It is variable in extent, although large joint effusions are sometimes apparent.

OSTEOPENIA. Juxtaarticular or diffuse osteoporosis may be encountered. In addition, band-like metaphyseal lucent zones may be seen, particularly in the femur, tibia, radius, and fibula. They are identical to those seen in childhood leukemia. The pathogenesis of this lucent zone in juvenile chronic arthritis may be related to a depression in endochondral bone formation in response to a severe systemic illness or trabecular atrophy due to persistent hyperemia in the vascular metaphyseal regions, or both.

JOINT SPACE ABNORMALITIES. Diminution of the interosseous space in juvenile chronic arthritis is less frequent than in adult-onset rheumatoid arthritis and, when present, is usually a late manifestation of the disease. The combination of osteoporosis and soft tissue swelling without cartilaginous (or osseous) destruction is an important radiographic characteristic of this disease. In later stages of juvenile chronic arthritis, intraarticular bone ankylosis is frequent, especially in the small joints of the hands and the wrists.

BONE EROSION. Destruction of bone is also a relatively late manifestation of juvenile chronic arthritis. The erosive abnormalities may be distributed at the margins of the joint or along the entire articular surface of the bone.

PERIOSTITIS. Periosteal bone formation is a frequent and prominent manifestation of juvenile chronic arthritis. It is most common in periarticular regions of phalanges and metacarpal and metatarsal bones, although periosteal proliferation of metaphyses and diaphyses of long bones may also be observed. Its pathogenesis may include inflammation of the joint capsule and adjacent periosteum and chronic hyperemia, and it is facilitated by the relative ease with which the periosteum of a child is lifted from the underlying bone.

GROWTH DISTURBANCES. Growth disturbances are a remarkable feature of juvenile chronic arthritis. The absence of these abnormalities in adult-onset rheumatoid arthritis is noteworthy.

Table 23–3. GENERAL RADIOGRAPHIC CHARACTERISTICS OF JUVENILE CHRONIC ARTHRITIS VERSUS ADULT-ONSET RHEUMATOID ARTHRITIS*

Finding	Juvenile Chronic Arthritis	Adult-Onset Rheumatoid Arthritis
Soft tissue swelling	Common	Common
Osteoporosis	Common	Common
Joint space loss	Late manifestation	Early manifestation
Bone erosions	Late manifestation	Early manifestation
Intraarticular bone ankylosis	Common	Rare
Periostitis	Common	Rare
Growth disturbances	Common	Absent
Epiphyseal compression fractures	Common	Less common
Joint subluxation	Common	Common
Synovial cysts	Uncommon	Common

*Characteristics will vary depending upon the specific subgroups of juvenile chronic arthritis.

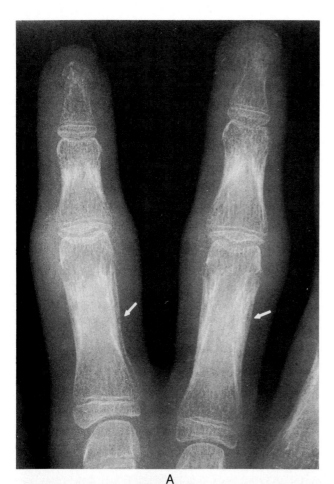

A

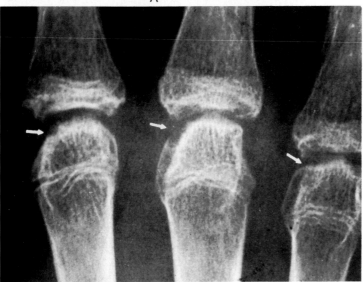

B

Figure 23–2. Juvenile chronic arthritis: General radiographic abnormalities. A Prominent periosteal proliferation of numerous phalanges (arrows) is associated with osteoporosis and periarticular soft tissue swelling. Joint space diminution and erosions are not significant features in this child. **B** The irregular outline of the metacarpal heads (arrows) is produced by compression of weakened osteoporotic bones.

Epiphyseal enlargement owing to accelerated growth stimulated by hyperemia is frequent about small and large joints. This overgrowth is further accentuated by the adjacent constricted appearance of the metaphysis and diaphysis. In addition, relative sparing of the subchondral region of the epiphysis leads to characteristic epiphyseal ballooning. Accelerated osseous growth and maturation in the wrist and the midfoot lead to an increase in the number and the size of the carpal and tarsal bones.

In the diaphyses of tubular bones, atrophy with osteoporosis and reduction in diameter, overgrowth, or undergrowth may be seen. Short, broad phalanges and metacarpal and metatarsal bones simulate the changes in various bone dysplasias. In the lower extremities, leg-length discrepancies are seen.

Typical growth abnormalities in juvenile chronic arthritis are also observed in the mandible and the cervical spine (see discussion later in this chapter).

The pathogenesis of the growth disturbances in this disease

may be multifactorial. Growth accentuation due to hyperemia and growth inhibition due to chronic illness, prolonged steroid therapy, immobilization, and neurogenic factors may be important. Additional factors include inflammation of periarticular connective tissues, epiphyseal destruction, subluxation, muscle spasm and fibrosis, and contracture.

EPIPHYSEAL COMPRESSION FRACTURES. Epiphyseal compression fractures are evident in the weight-bearing epiphyses of the lower extremity as well as in the epiphyses of the hands and the feet. They are produced by abnormal stress acting on weakened osteoporotic bone. Flattening and deformity of the epiphyseal ossification centers are evident.

JOINT SUBLUXATION. Subluxation and dislocation can be observed in any joint but are most common in the hip. These complications result from large intraarticular effusions or ligamentous destruction and muscle foreshortening owing to fibrosis.

SOFT TISSUE CALCIFICATION. Periarticular soft tissue calcific deposits may appear in the joint capsule, the ligaments, or the muscles. The exact cause of periarticular calcification in juvenile chronic arthritis is not known, although an association of this finding with intraarticular corticosteroid therapy has been recorded.

Abnormalities in Specific Locations

HAND (FIGS. 23–1 AND 23–2). Asymmetric abnormalities of both hands are most typical. Swelling and regional osteoporosis can develop about distal interphalangeal, proximal interphalangeal, and metacarpophalangeal joints. Periostitis of metacarpal and phalangeal shafts, preservation of joint space, and absence of significant erosions are most common. Epiphyseal collapse and deformity are also characteristic.

A variety of finger deformities may eventually appear during the course of the disease. Boutonnière deformity and flexion deformity (characterized by flexion at both the proximal interphalangeal and distal interphalangeal joints) appear more frequently than swan-neck deformity. In contrast to the situation in adult-onset rheumatoid arthritis, in which ulnar deviation of the metacarpophalangeal joints frequently is associated with radial deviation of the wrist, radial deviation of the metacarpophalangeal joints in association with ulnar deviation of the wrist is more typical in juvenile-onset disease.

WRIST (FIG. 23–3). Abnormalities of the wrist are extremely common in juvenile chronic arthritis. Soft tissue prominence, osteoporosis, and irregular carpal ossification centers are seen. Marginal erosions may be evident in older children with adult type (seropositive) rheumatoid arthritis.

Intraarticular bone ankylosis of the wrist compartments may be prominent. Generally, at least one of the three major articulations of the wrist (radiocarpal, midcarpal, common carpometacarpal) remains unankylosed, allowing some motion. Investigators have observed a high frequency of bone ankylosis in the common carpometacarpal joint.

Growth disturbances and articular destruction can lead to significant wrist deformities in juvenile chronic arthritis. The ulna may be relatively short compared to the radius, producing ulnar deviation at the wrist.

KNEE (FIG. 23–4). Radiographic abnormalities of the knee in juvenile chronic arthritis include osteoporosis, soft tissue swelling, enlargement with ballooning of the distal femoral and proximal tibial epiphyses, flattening of the femoral condyles, widening of the intercondylar notch, joint space narrowing, and marginal or central osseous erosions. These findings are virtually identical to those in hemophilia. Alterations in patellar shape have also been observed in both

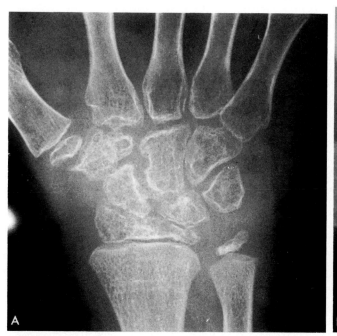
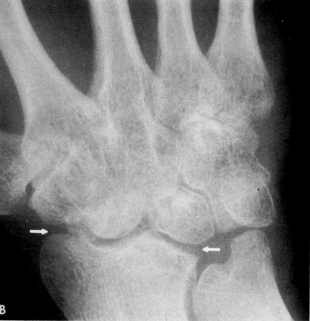

Figure 23–3. Abnormalities of the wrist. A In a young child, erosions of multiple carpal bones have led to crenated osseous contours. There is evidence of joint space narrowing and acceleration of bone maturation in this individual. **B** Observe extensive joint space narrowing and intraarticular bone ankylosis of portions of the midcarpal and common carpometacarpal articulations with relative sparing of the radiocarpal articulation (arrows). At the latter site, deformity of the articular surface of the distal radius is evident. Overgrowth of the ulna and ulnar styloid can also be seen.

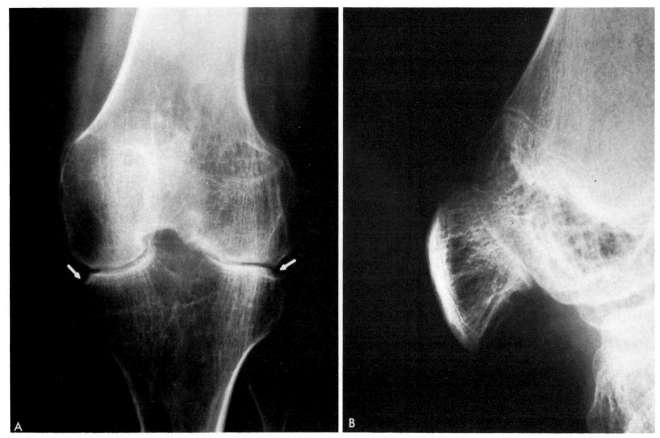

Figure 23–4. Abnormalities of the knee. A The major radiographic abnormalities in this 23 year old woman who had had arthritis for approximately 10 years consist of diffuse joint space narrowing and marginal erosions (arrows), which simulate the findings in adult-onset rheumatoid arthritis, although slight overgrowth of the femoral epiphysis indicates that the disease began at a relatively young age. **B** On a lateral radiograph of a knee, note the flattening of the inferior portion of the patella, resulting in a square configuration of the bone.

juvenile chronic arthritis and hemophilia. These alterations consist of flattening of the inferior pole of the patella, resulting in squaring of the bone.

HIP (FIG. 23–5). The frequency of radiographically evident hip abnormalities in patients with juvenile chronic arthritis is approximately 35 to 45 per cent. The femoral capital epiphysis may be enlarged and irregular in outline, and premature fusion of the growth plate can be evident. Articular space narrowing (diffuse) and osseous erosion may also develop as a joint deteriorates. Restoration of the joint space has been reported in association with vigorous physical therapy and continued ambulation. Protrusio acetabuli is more frequent in older children.

FOOT AND ANKLE. Enlargement and irregularity of the tarsal bones, joint space narrowing, and intraarticular bone ankylosis can be seen. Metatarsophalangeal and interphalangeal joint alterations consist of osteoporosis, epiphyseal enlargement, brachydactyly, and periostitis. At the ankle, tilting or angulation of the distal tibial epiphysis may be encountered.

OTHER ARTICULATIONS OF THE APPENDICULAR SKELETON. Alterations of the humeral head parallel those of the femoral head, with osteoporosis, enlargement, joint space narrowing, erosions, and subluxation. In the elbow, the radial head may become significantly enlarged, a finding that is also seen in hemophilia.

SACROILIAC JOINT (TABLE 23–4). Although children with juvenile-onset ankylosing spondylitis, psoriatic arthritis, and inflammatory bowel disease can reveal significant sacroiliac joint abnormalities, changes in this joint in other varieties of juvenile chronic arthritis are relatively infrequent. Furthermore, documenting the presence of an abnormal sacroiliac joint can be difficult because of the widened articular space and indistinct subchondral bone that characterize the normal sacroiliac joint in the pediatric age group.

CERVICAL SPINE (TABLE 23–4) (FIG. 23–6). Radiographic abnormalities of the cervical spine are a significant feature of juvenile chronic arthritis. Subluxation may develop in any vertebral segment but is most characteristic at the atlantoaxial level. Atlantoaxial subluxation (greater than 4 or 5 mm between the posterior surface of the anterior arch of the first cervical vertebra and the anterior surface of the odontoid process) can be observed in juvenile-onset ankylosing spondylitis and Still's disease but is most characteristic of juvenile-onset adult type (seropositive) rheumatoid arthritis. Atlantoaxial instability in the child is not diagnostic of juvenile chronic arthritis, being observed in trauma and a variety of conditions including those with hypoplasia of the odontoid process and congenital weakening of the surrounding ligaments (such as Down's syndrome), and those associated with inflammation in the neck (Grisel's syndrome).

Erosions of the odontoid process may also be seen in

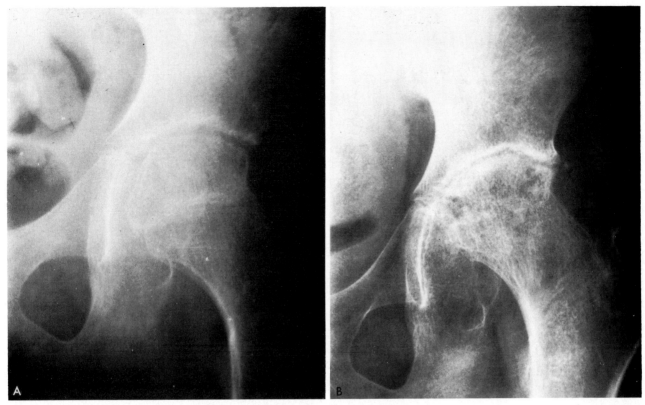

Figure 23–5. Abnormalities of the hip. A, B In a child with juvenile-onset adult type (seropositive) rheumatoid arthritis, the initial radiograph (**A**), obtained at 9 years of age, reveals diffuse joint space narrowing, significant erosions of the femoral head and acetabulum, and osteoporosis. Two years later (**B**), obliteration of the interosseous space can be noted.

juvenile chronic arthritis. Apophyseal joint space narrowing and bone ankylosis in association with subchondral erosions predominate in the upper cervical spine, especially at the C2-C3 and C3-C4 levels; it is distinctly unusual to see significant ankylosis of the lower cervical spine without more proximal involvement.

Growth disturbances consist of decreased vertical and anteroposterior diameters of the vertebral bodies at levels of

apophyseal joint ankylosis. The adjacent intervertebral discs are also diminished in height and may contain calcification. Although apophyseal joint ankylosis can be seen in ankylosing spondylitis, the vertebral bodies are not significantly diminished in size, nor are the intervertebral discs diminutive because the disease onset generally occurs at a more advanced age. Congenital fusion of vertebral bodies (Klippel-Feil deformity) may simulate the changes in juvenile chronic arthri-

Table 23–4. COMPARISON OF RADIOGRAPHIC ABNORMALITIES

	Juvenile Chronic Arthritis*	Adult-Onset Rheumatoid Arthritis	Juvenile-Onset Ankylosing Spondylitis	Adult-Onset Ankylosing Spondylitis
Cervical spine				
C1-C2 subluxation	+	+ +	+	+
Apophyseal joint ankylosis	+ +	±	+ +	+ +
Hypoplasia of vertebral bodies and intervertebral discs	+ +	−	±	−
Thoracolumbar spine				
Apophyseal joint ankylosis	±	−	+ +	+ +
Syndesmophytes	−	−	+ +	+ +
Sacroiliac joints				
Erosions	+	+	+ +	+ +
Ankylosis	±	±	+ +	+ +
Peripheral joints				
Early involvement	+ +	+ +	+ +	±
Erosions	±	+ +	+	+
Joint space narrowing	±	+ +	+	+
Bone proliferation and periostitis	+ +	±	+ +	+ +

*Characteristics of juvenile-onset adult type rheumatoid arthritis and Still's disease.
+ + = very common; + = common; ± = uncommon; − = rare or absent.

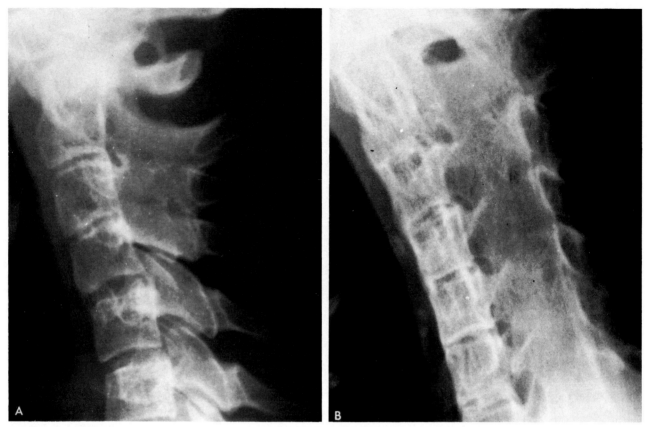

Figure 23–6. Abnormalities of the cervical spine. In two children with Still's disease, apophyseal joint ankylosis is evident. The process is usually first evident in the upper cervical region and progresses to the lower vertebrae. Hypoplasia of vertebral bodies and intervertebral discs is prominent. Atlantoaxial subluxation is also evident in **A**.

tis, although in the former disorder, the spinous processes of several vertebrae may also be involved and elevation of the scapula with an omovertebral bone can be seen.

THORACIC AND LUMBAR SPINE (TABLE 23–4). Compression fractures frequently are evident in the thoracic region in association with osteoporosis. Scoliosis has also been noted in children with long-standing juvenile chronic arthritis.

MANDIBLE, TEMPOROMANDIBULAR JOINT, AND OTHER FACIAL STRUCTURES. Underdevelopment of the jaw (micrognathia) with limitation of bite is not uncommon in patients with juvenile chronic arthritis (approximately 10 to 20 per cent), frequently occurring in association with temporomandibular joint abnormalities. Micrognathia is more typical in those children whose disease begins early in life and in those with systemic or polyarticular disease.

Radiographic abnormalities of the mandible have been observed in as many as 40 per cent of patients with juvenile chronic arthritis. Such changes include shortening of the body and vertical rami of the mandible with widening of the mandibular notches. Both mandibular condyles frequently are flattened and poorly differentiated, although the temporomandibular joints themselves may appear normal. Articular space narrowing, bone erosion, and abnormal joint motion may be encountered in some individuals. Intraarticular osseous fusion has also been noted.

The mechanisms by which micrognathia develops in pa-

tients with juvenile chronic arthritis are not entirely clear. Although a relationship between articular inflammation and mandibular growth is probable, the absence of clinical and radiologic abnormalities of the temporomandibular joint in some children with mandibular hypoplasia should be noted.

Antegonial notching of the mandible has been emphasized as an additional radiographic manifestation of juvenile chronic arthritis. This notching represents a concavity on the undersurface of the mandibular body just anterior to the angular process (gonion). It may appear in a variety of congenital (Treacher Collins syndrome, camptomelic dwarfism, neurofibromatosis) and acquired (temporomandibular joint arthritis or infection, trauma) disorders.

Bird-face, observed in 10 to 30 per cent of patients, has been related to arrested mandibular growth in combination with normal growth of other facial structures, leading to convexity of the facial profile. In some cases, the abrupt appearance of bird-face in this disease may be attributed to acute collapse of osseous structures about the temporomandibular joint.

PATHOLOGIC ABNORMALITIES

Synovial inflammation in juvenile chronic arthritis resembles that in adult-onset rheumatoid arthritis, although the inflammatory process may be less florid in children, with less extensive fibrinous exudate and less proliferation of lining and synovial stroma cells.

Subcutaneous nodules are identified in 10 to 20 per cent

of patients with juvenile chronic arthritis. In children with seropositive disease, the histologic characteristics of the nodule resemble those in the adult variety of disease; in some children, particularly those with seronegative arthritis, the histologic appearance of the nodular lesions may be distinctive. The juvenile type of nodule resembles that which is seen in rheumatic fever.

SPECIAL TYPES OF JUVENILE CHRONIC ARTHRITIS
Adult-Onset Still's Disease (Fig. 23–7)

As a subgroup of children may develop an adult variety of rheumatoid arthritis, it is not surprising that some adults may develop a disorder that is indistinguishable from Still's disease. Adult-onset Still's disease is characterized by a rash, fever, and involvement of the cervical spine and peripheral and sacroiliac joints. Pauciarticular abnormalities predominate, with predilection for the knees, the fingers, and the wrists. The course of the joint disease is mild. Radiographic changes include carpal ankylosis, apophyseal joint fusion in the cervical spine, and patchy sclerosis about the sacroiliac joint. Serologic test results for rheumatoid factor are almost uniformly negative.

A distinctive radiographic pattern of articular disease of the wrist has been noted in affected patients: narrowing of portions of the common carpometacarpal and midcarpal compartments without osseous erosions, which may culminate in bone ankylosis. Selective involvement of the spaces between the second and third metacarpal bones and the adjacent trapezoid and capitate, between the trapezoid and capitate, between the capitate and hamate, and between the capitate and lunate can be identified. More diffuse wrist abnormalities may also be encountered, although the absence of erosive disease is remarkable. The metacarpophalangeal joints characteristically are spared. Intertarsal and tarsometatarsal alterations can also occur.

Similar patterns of ankylosis of the carpal (and tarsal) bones can be observed in children with juvenile chronic arthritis, although such ankylosis appears to be more frequent in children who are 10 years of age or older and in those who have had their disease for at least 2 or 3 years. It thus appears that percapitate bone ankylosis is characteristic of juvenile chronic arthritis no matter what the age of disease onset.

DIFFERENTIAL DIAGNOSIS
Hemophilia

The differential diagnosis of juvenile chronic arthritis and hemophilia can be difficult, particularly when observations are confined to a single articulation. Soft tissue swelling, osteoporosis, subchondral osseous irregularity, interosseous space diminution, and growth disturbances can be evident in both disorders. In the knee, the ankle, or the elbow, the resulting radiographic picture may be identical in the two conditions. Polyarticular disease and significant involvement of the small joints of the hand and the wrist are less frequent in hemophilia than in juvenile chronic arthritis, whereas radiodense joint effusions and multiple subchondral cystic lesions are somewhat more common in hemophilic arthropathy.

Idiopathic Multicentric Osteolysis

Idiopathic multicentric osteolysis is a disorder characterized by multifocal articular destruction beginning in infancy or childhood (see Chapter 84). Because of a remarkable predilection for the carpal and tarsal bones, the disorder is also referred to as carpal and tarsal osteolysis. Radiographic characteristics include osteoporosis, progressive osteolysis, and deformity, findings that may simulate the changes in juvenile chronic arthritis. Clinical features of idiopathic multicentric osteolysis that are helpful in differentiating it from juvenile chronic arthritis are an association of episodes of trauma and

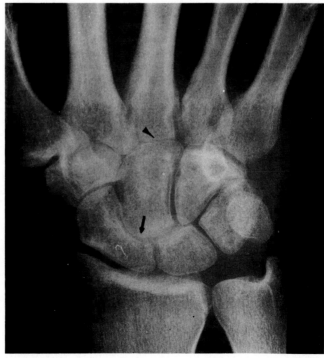

Figure 23–7. Adult-onset Still's disease. This 21 year old man developed classic systemic manifestations of Still's disease and bilateral wrist pain. Narrowing of the midcarpal (arrow) and common carpometacarpal (arrowhead) compartments of the wrists is seen. The radiocarpal compartment is relatively spared. Soft tissue swelling and osteoporosis are evident. (Courtesy of M. Palayew, M.D., Montreal, Quebec, Canada.)

articular symptoms and signs and the absence of both clinical signs of systemic disease and inflammatory changes in biopsy specimens.

Mucopolysaccharidoses and Related Disorders

Articular abnormalities accompanying mucopolysaccharidoses may simulate those in juvenile chronic arthritis, although characteristic findings are noted on skeletal surveys in patients with mucopolysaccharidoses (Morquio, Hurler, Hunter, Sanfilippo, Scheie, and Maroteaux-Lamy syndromes) (see Chapter 74). Joint abnormalities may become particularly prominent in Scheie's syndrome and Farber's syndrome. In addition, Winchester's syndrome can lead to articular changes that may simulate those of juvenile chronic arthritis. An onset in infancy, a pattern of autosomal recessive inheritance, arthralgias, joint stiffening and deformity, coarsened facial features, peripheral corneal opacification, and dwarfism are typical features of this syndrome.

Kniest's syndrome (Swiss cheese cartilage) consists of disproportionate dwarfism, kyphoscoliosis, a peculiar flat and rounded facies, hearing loss, enlarged articular structures, and deformed extremities. In general, the radiographic findings of this syndrome are distinguishable from those of juvenile chronic arthritis (see Chapter 74).

Familial Arthropathy and Congenital Camptodactyly

One or more familial syndromes with flexion deformities of the fingers have been described. Indeed, it appears that several inherited disorders can lead to flexion deformities of the fingers and arthropathy, the patterns of inheritance are not uniform or clear, and the radiographic abnormalities, consisting mainly of osteoporosis and deformity (flattening of the metacarpal and metatarsal heads, coxa vara, and contractures of the fingers, wrists, and elbows), are easily distinguishable from those of juvenile chronic arthritis.

Other Disorders

Multiple epiphyseal dysplasia (and spondyloepiphyseal dysplasia) can lead to irregularity of many epiphyses with secondary degenerative joint abnormalities, which can be confused with the changes of juvenile chronic arthritis (see Chapter 73). Progressive pseudorheumatoid arthritis of childhood is a term applied to a hereditary arthropathy affecting major and minor joints in which findings include restricted articular motion, swelling about interphalangeal joints, platy-

spondyly, and irregularities of vertebral bodies that simulate those in Scheuermann's disease. Infection or synovial hemangiomas can produce abnormalities of single joints, which also simulate the findings of juvenile chronic arthritis. Similarly, neuromuscular disorders may lead to skeletal abnormalities that are indistinguishable from those of juvenile chronic arthritis.

FURTHER READING

Ansell BM: Chronic arthritis in childhood. Ann Rheum Dis 37:107, 1978.

Ansell BM, Kent PA: Radiological changes in juvenile chronic polyarthritis. Skel Radiol 1:129, 1977.

Brill PW, Kim HJ, Beratis NG, Hirschhorn K: Skeletal abnormalities in the Kniest syndrome with mucopolysacchariduria. AJR 125:731, 1975.

Bywaters EGL: Still's disease in the adult. Ann Rheum Dis 30:121, 1971.

Cassidy JT, Levinson JE, Bass JC, Baum J, Brewer EJ Jr, Fink CW, Hanson V, Jacobs JC, Masi AT, Schaller JG, Fries JF, McShane D, Young D: A study of classification criteria for a diagnosis of juvenile rheumatoid arthritis. Arthritis Rheum 29:274, 1986.

Chlosta EM, Kuhns LR, Holt JF: The "patellar ratio" in hemophilia and juvenile rheumatoid arthritis. Radiology 116:137, 1975.

Martel W, Holt JF, Cassidy JT: Roentgenologic manifestations of juvenile rheumatoid arthritis. AJR 88:400, 1962.

Martinez-Lavin M, Buendia A, Delgado E, Reyes P, Amigo M-C, Sabanes J, Zghaib A, Attie F, Salinas L: A familial syndrome of pericarditis, arthritis, and camptodactyly. N Engl J Med 309:224, 1983.

Medsger TA Jr, Christy WC: Carpal arthritis with ankylosis in late onset Still's disease. Arthritis Rheum 19:232, 1976.

Parke WW, Rothman RH, Brown MD: The pharyngovertebral veins: An anatomical rationale for Grisel's syndrome. J Bone Joint Surg [Am] 66:568, 1984.

Poznanski AK, Hernandez RJ, Guire KE, Bereza UL, Garn SM: Carpal length in children—a useful measurement in the diagnosis of rheumatoid arthritis and some congenital malformation syndromes. Radiology 129:661, 1978.

Richardson ML, Helms CA, Vogler JB III, Genant HK: Skeletal changes in neuromuscular disorders mimicking juvenile rheumatoid arthritis and hemophilia. AJR 143:893, 1984.

Schaller J, Wedgwood RJ: Juvenile rheumatoid arthritis: A review. Pediatrics 50:940, 1972.

Spranger J, Albert C, Schilling F, Bartsocas C: Progressive pseudorheumatoid arthropathy of childhood (PPAC): A hereditary disorder simulating juvenile rheumatoid arthritis. Am J Med Genet 14:399, 1983.

Stabrun AE, Larheim TA, Höyeraal HM, Rösler M: Reduced mandibular dimensions and asymmetry in juvenile rheumatoid arthritis. Pathogenetic factors. Arthritis Rheum 31:602, 1988.

Still GF: On a form of chronic joint disease in children. Med Chir Trans 80:47, 1897.

Tyler T, Rosenbaum HD: Idiopathic multicentric osteolysis. AJR 126:23, 1976.

Winchester P, Grossman H, Lim WN, Danes BS: A new acid mucopolysaccharidosis with skeletal deformities simulating rheumatoid arthritis. AJR 106:121, 1969.

Chapter 24

Ankylosing Spondylitis

Donald Resnick, M.D.
Gen Niwayama, M.D.

Ankylosing spondylitis is a disease with widespread musculoskeletal manifestations. Abnormalities are detected at synovial and cartilaginous articulations and at sites of tendinous and ligamentous attachment to bone in spinal and extraspinal locations. The hallmark of the disorder is sacroiliitis, which is typically bilateral and symmetric in distribution. Spondylitis leads to significant abnormalities at the discovertebral junction, apophyseal and costovertebral joints, and posterior ligamentous attachments. Accurate differentiation of ankylosing spondylitis from rheumatoid arthritis is not difficult, although distinguishing the articular abnormalities of ankylosing spondylitis from those in psoriasis and Reiter's syndrome is more troublesome.

Ankylosing spondylitis is a chronic inflammatory disorder of unknown cause that affects principally the axial skeleton, although the appendicular skeleton may also be involved significantly. Alterations occur in synovial and cartilaginous joints and in sites of tendon and ligament attachment to bone.

Although ankylosing spondylitis is now the accepted name for this disease, many synonyms and eponyms have been used in the past, including rhizomelic spondylitis, Marie-Strumpell's disease, and von Bechterew's syndrome. Although the term rheumatoid spondylitis has also been used to describe ankylosing spondylitis, there exists incontrovertible evidence that this disease does not represent rheumatoid arthritis of the spine. Prominent sacroiliac joint abnormalities and spinal ligamentous calcification and ossification are not features of rheumatoid arthritis. Furthermore, rheumatoid arthritis predominates in women (whereas ankylosing spondylitis is more frequent in men) and is associated with rheumatoid nodules and a high frequency of positive serologic test results for rheumatoid factor (whereas this frequency is very low in ankylosing spondylitis). Profound clinical and radiologic dissimilarities exist in the two disorders, and although some pathologic aspects are similar, many differences can be found during the gross and microscopic examination of involved tissues in rheumatoid arthritis and ankylosing spondylitis.

INCIDENCE

Ankylosing spondylitis is a common cause of back pain and disability, especially in young men. It has been estimated that 5 to 10 per cent of military patients with rheumatic symptoms and signs have ankylosing spondylitis. The prevalence of this disease in a general population is more difficult to determine, although a figure of approximately 0.1 per cent is commonly quoted. The prevalence is higher in blacks. The reported ratio of the disease in men compared to women varies from 4 to 1 to 10 to 1. The disease may be more subtle and difficult to diagnose in female patients.

CLINICAL ABNORMALITIES
General Features

The onset of ankylosing spondylitis generally occurs between the ages of 15 and 35 years in both men and women. The disorder in children (juvenile-onset ankylosing spondylitis) is also well recognized (see Chapter 23).

An insidious onset of disease, which occurs in 75 to 80 per cent of patients, can lead to considerable delay in accurate diagnosis. Early clinical manifestations are generally noted in the back (70 to 80 per cent of patients), although they may appear in the peripheral joints (10 to 20 per cent of patients) or in the chest. Sciatic pain may be the initial symptom in 5 to 10 per cent of patients. Constitutional findings include anorexia, weight loss, and low grade fever. With respect to the natural history of the disease, fewer than 20 per cent of patients with adult-onset ankylosing spondylitis progress to a condition of significant disability.

Axial Skeletal Symptoms and Signs

Clinical manifestations related to the spine and the sacroiliac joints are characteristic of ankylosing spondylitis. With evolution of the disease, spread to the higher levels of the vertebral column is frequent. Although the progression may be segmental, beginning in the sacroiliac region and extending first to the lumbar spine and then to the thoracic and cervical regions, symptoms and signs may bypass any level of the spine.

Local pain and tenderness over the sacroiliac joints can be prominent in the early phases of the disease. With ankylosis of these articulations, the clinical manifestations may become mild or disappear completely. In the lumbar spine, paravertebral muscle spasm, straightening of the vertebral column, tenderness to percussion, and muscle atrophy are observed; in the thoracic spine, similar abnormalities may be accompanied by diminished chest expansion and exaggeration of the normal kyphotic curvature. Slight, moderate, or marked limitation of movement can be evident in the cervical spine. The head and neck protrude forward and the patient may eventually be forced to gaze constantly at the floor.

The cauda equina syndrome can be observed in patients with ankylosing spondylitis.

Peripheral Skeletal Symptoms and Signs

Peripheral articular manifestations are apparent initially in approximately 10 to 20 per cent of patients and eventually in as many as 50 per cent of patients. In most persons, the manifestations are mild and transient in nature and are overshadowed by more prominent signs and symptoms in the central skeleton. Pain and swelling can simulate the findings of rheumatoid arthritis, although asymmetry is more frequent and residual deformity is less frequent in ankylosing spondylitis than in rheumatoid arthritis.

Involvement of the proximal or "root" joints (the hips and the shoulders) is particularly characteristic and may lead to severe clinical disability. Pain and tenderness over bony protuberances are elicited in many individuals with ankylosing spondylitis.

Extraskeletal Symptoms and Signs

Iritis occurs in 20 per cent of patients with ankylosing spondylitis and may be the presenting feature of the disease. Spondylitic heart disease can lead to cardiac enlargement, conduction defects, and pericarditis. Aortic insufficiency owing to inflammation of the aortic valve and aorta resembles the finding in syphilitic aortitis. Pulmonary involvement in ankylosing spondylitis can become manifest as peculiar fibrosis and cavitation in the upper lobes, which simulate the findings in tuberculosis.

Additional systemic manifestations of ankylosing spondylitis include an association with inflammatory bowel disease (see Chapter 27) and with amyloidosis.

Laboratory Findings

In general, laboratory parameters are not useful in diagnosing or following patients with ankylosing spondylitis. The erythrocyte sedimentation rate is frequently elevated during the active phase and may become normal in later phases of the disease. Results of serologic tests for rheumatoid and LE factors characteristically are negative. Many patients with ankylosing spondylitis possess the histocompatibility antigen HLA-B27.

RADIOGRAPHIC-PATHOLOGIC CORRELATION
General Distribution

Ankylosing spondylitis affects synovial and cartilaginous joints as well as sites of tendon and ligament attachment to bone (entheses). An overwhelming predilection exists for involvement of the axial skeleton, especially the sacroiliac, apophyseal, discovertebral, and costovertebral articulations (Fig. 24–1).

Classically, changes initially are noted in the sacroiliac joints and next appear at the thoracolumbar and lumbosacral junctions; with disease chronicity, the midlumbar, the upper thoracic, and the cervical vertebrae may become involved. This characteristic pattern of spinal ascent is by no means invariable, however. The disease may become arrested at any stage, although radiographic abnormalities of the sacroiliac joint without vertebral changes are unusual except in the

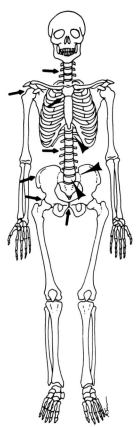

Figure 24–1. Ankylosing spondylitis: Distribution of articular disease. Initial abnormalities are most frequent in the sacroiliac joint and the thoracolumbar and lumbosacral junctions (arrowheads). Subsequent abnormalities are common in the entire vertebral column, the tendinous insertions in the pelvis and proximal femur, the sternal joints, the symphysis pubis, the hips, and the glenohumeral joints (arrows).

early phase of the disorder. Isolated sacroiliac joint abnormalities may be more frequent in women with the disease. Furthermore, in female patients, the combination of sacroiliac joint and cervical spinal abnormalities without significant thoracic or lumbar spinal changes appears more common than in male patients. Spinal alterations without sacroiliac joint changes in either men or women are unusual in classic ankylosing spondylitis, whereas this distribution is more frequent in psoriatic spondylitis.

The frequency of radiographically evident abnormalities in peripheral locations in cases of long-standing ankylosing spondylitis is greater than 50 per cent if all joints are included, approaches 50 per cent if only the hips are excluded, and is approximately 30 per cent if both the hips and the glenohumeral joints are excluded. Although initially only one or two peripheral areas may be involved, the eventual pattern is one of more diffuse articular disease. Radiographic changes predominate in the hips and the glenohumeral joints, followed in descending order of frequency by the knees, the hands, the wrists, and the feet, including the calcaneus. Bilateral symmetric or asymmetric abnormalities are common.

Radiographic abnormalities can also be encountered in the symphysis pubis, the manubriosternal, acromioclavicular, and sternoclavicular articulations, and the temporomandibular joints. Changes are also evident at tendinous and ligamentous attachments to bone, such as the iliac crests, ischial tuberosities, greater and lesser trochanters, spinous processes, and inferior surface of the calcanei.

General Radiographic and Pathologic Abnormalities
Synovial Articulations

The synovitis in ankylosing spondylitis is similar or identical to that in rheumatoid arthritis. In general, however, the inflammatory process in ankylosing spondylitis is more discrete and of lower intensity than in rheumatoid arthritis. The density of the inflammatory cell infiltration and the extent of necrosis are less dramatic. Hyperplastic villi are noted, but severe pannus formation is less frequent. Marked fibroplasia may be followed by cartilaginous metaplasia with chondral ossification. In this manner, intraarticular bone ankylosis can be evident. This ankylotic process in the small joints of the axial skeleton can also result from ossification of the joint capsule. Additional pathologic features occurring in and around the synovial joints in ankylosing spondylitis relate to subchondral bone sclerosis and periosteal elevation.

The basic similarity of pathologic alterations in synovial joints in ankylosing spondylitis and rheumatoid arthritis accounts for the overlap in their radiographic features. Both cause some degree of osteoporosis, joint space narrowing, and osseous erosion. Certain findings are more characteristic of ankylosing spondylitis than of rheumatoid arthritis, however. Prominent periarticular osteoporosis is not common in ankylosing spondylitis. In fact, subchondral eburnation is typical. Periostitis is also observed, resulting in irregular or shaggy periarticular osseous surfaces. Periosteal proliferation can extend into the metaphyses and the diaphyses of the neighboring bones.

Extensive and diffuse joint space narrowing is more frequent in rheumatoid arthritis than in ankylosing spondylitis. In ankylosing spondylitis, intraarticular bone ankylosis is common in the synovial joints of both the axial and the extraaxial skeleton. In adult-onset rheumatoid arthritis, fibrous ankylosis is more characteristic except in the carpal and tarsal areas, at which sites massive osseous fusion may be evident.

The osseous erosions in ankylosing spondylitis typically are smaller and more localized than those of rheumatoid arthritis, although large erosions of metacarpal, metatarsal, and humeral heads can be encountered. Subchondral cyst formation and significant subluxations are two additional features that are more frequent in rheumatoid arthritis than in ankylosing spondylitis.

Cartilaginous Joints (Fig. 24–2)

In the cartilaginous joints of the axial skeleton (the discovertebral junction, the symphysis pubis, and the manubriosternal joint), the fundamental process appears to be inflammatory in nature, as shown by mild to moderate cellular infiltration (plasma cells and lymphocytes) and fibrin accumulation. In the anulus fibrosus, chondroid transformation of the connective tissue, calcification, and ossification produce syndesmophytes that extend from one vertebral body to another. The adjacent bone surface is eroded, with surrounding eburnation. On radiographic examination, findings include erosion and sclerosis of adjacent bone surfaces and osseous bridging.

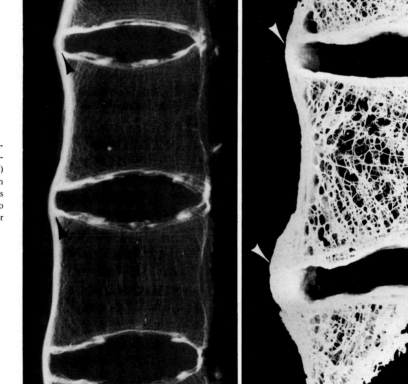

Figure 24–2. Cartilaginous joints: General radiologic and pathologic abnormalities—discovertebral junction. A radiograph (**A**) and photograph (**B**) of a sagittal section of the spine (the left side of each picture is anterior) reveal typical syndesmophytes (arrowheads) extending from one vertebral body to another. Note their vertical direction and thin or slender configuration.

Entheses (Fig. 24–3)

Abnormalities in ligamentous attachments (enthesopathy) are a prominent feature of ankylosing spondylitis and other seronegative spondyloarthropathies. Inflammation is associated with erosion and eburnation of the subligamentous bone. On radiographs, ill-defined erosive abnormalities with surrounding sclerosis are observed. As the lesions heal, the sclerosis decreases, the osseous surface becomes less irregular, and well-defined bone excrescences appear.

Radiographic and Pathologic Abnormalities at Specific Sites
Sacroiliac Joint (Fig. 24–4)

Sacroiliitis is the hallmark of early ankylosing spondylitis. Although an asymmetric or unilateral distribution can be evident on initial radiographic examination, radiographic changes at later stages of the disease are almost invariably bilateral and symmetric in distribution. This symmetry is an important diagnostic clue in this disease.

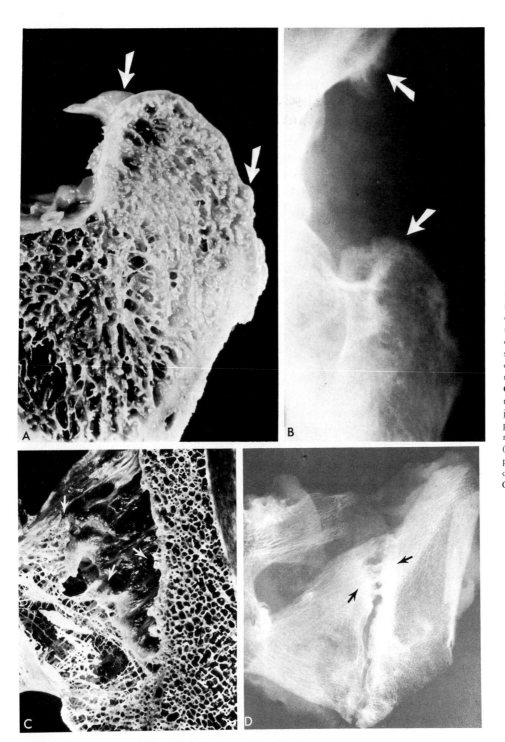

Figure 24–3. Entheses: General radiologic and pathologic abnormalities. Femoral trochanter and sacroiliac joint. A A photograph of a coronal section through the greater trochanter reveals mild osseous excrescences (arrows) related to an enthesopathy. B Radiographic findings include irregular hyperostosis of the trochanter and the iliac crest (arrows). C, D A photograph and radiograph of two coronal sections of the sacroiliac joint show an inflammatory enthesopathy at the sacral and ilial attachments of the interosseous ligament (arrows) above the true synovium-lined portion of the articulation (which itself demonstrates bone ankylosis in C). Osseous proliferation predominates.

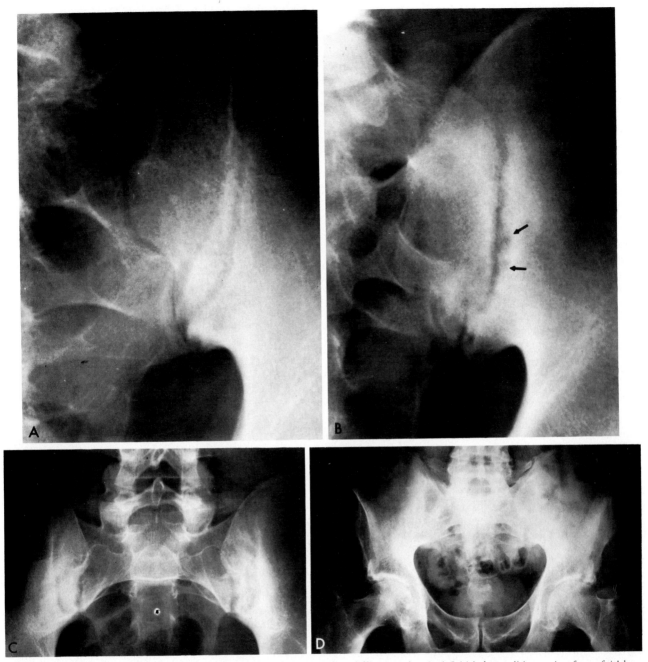

Figure 24–4. Abnormalities of the sacroiliac joint. Radiographic stages (four different patients). A Initial abnormalities consist of superficial bone erosion and eburnation, predominantly on the ilium. **B** At a slightly later stage, note larger erosions (arrows), progressive sclerosis, and focal narrowing of the articular space. **C** At a more advanced stage, bilateral symmetric changes consist of extensive sclerosis and focal ankylosis. **D** Eventually, complete ankylosis of the synovial and ligamentous portions of the sacroiliac space on both sides is evident. Sclerosis has largely disappeared.

Changes in the sacroiliac joint occur in both the synovial and ligamentous (superior) portions. They predominate in the ilium. Initial changes consist of patchy periarticular osteoporosis, particularly about the middle and lower thirds of the joint cavity, and loss of definition, superficial erosion, and focal sclerosis of subchondral bone. A poorly defined subchondral bone plate is an important radiographic sign of sacroiliitis that is not observed in degenerative sacroiliac joint disease. Further erosive changes lead to considerable fraying

of the osseous surface and widening of the interosseous space. This progression of bone destruction is paralleled by increasing eburnation of surrounding osseous tissue. The entire subchondral bone surface may eventually become sclerotic, especially in the ilium. The wide and poorly defined band of sclerosis in this disease differs from the thin and well-defined sclerotic margin typical of degenerative disease and from the localized sclerotic areas characteristic of rheumatoid arthritis.

As proliferative bone changes in the sacroiliac joint become more prominent, irregular bone bridges traverse the articular cavity. Later, complete ankylosis can be observed. Periarticular eburnation can subsequently diminish.

Calcification and ossification of the ligamentous portion of the sacroiliac space are frequent in ankylosing spondylitis. When extensive and combined with intraarticular ankylosis, bone fusion of the entire sacroiliac space (synovial and ligamentous) is seen.

It is difficult to establish the diagnosis of ankylosing spondylitis in the absence of radiographic alerations in the sacroiliac joints. Meticulous radiographic technique is required, however. The complex anatomy and undulating articular surfaces of the sacroiliac joint resist ideal demonstration on routine plain film examination, requiring angulation of the x-ray beam.

Spine (Table 24–1)

Abnormalities of the spine occur in the discovertebral junction, apophyseal joints, costovertebral joints, posterior ligamentous attachments, and atlantoaxial joints.

DISCOVERTEBRAL JUNCTION. Lesions affecting the discovertebral junction include osteitis, syndesmophytosis, erosions, discal calcification, and osteoporosis and discal ballooning.

Osteitis (Fig. 24–5). Focal destructive areas along the anterior margin of the discovertebral junction at the superior and inferior portions of the vertebral body have been termed "Romanus lesions." They are an early and significant feature of ankylosing spondylitis. Osseous erosion (osteitis) of the corners of the vertebral body results in loss of the normal concavity of the anterior vertebral surface, creating a squared or planed-down contour. This change in vertebral configuration is much easier to assess in the lumbar spine and more

Table 24–1. TERMINOLOGY COMMONLY APPLIED TO SPINAL ABNORMALITIES IN ANKYLOSING SPONDYLITIS

Term	Definition
Osteitis	Enthesopathy occurring at discovertebral junction associated with erosion, sclerosis, and syndesmophytosis
"Shiny corner" sign	Increased radiodensity of the corners of the vertebral body related to "osteitis"
Squaring	Straightened or convex anterior margin of the vertebral body related to erosion
Syndesmophyte	Ossification within the anulus fibrosus leading to thin, vertical radiodense areas
Bamboo spine	Undulating vertebral contour owing to extensive syndesmophytosis
Discitis	"Erosive" abnormalities of the discovertebral junction related to several mechanisms (see Table 24–2)
Discal ballooning	Biconvex shape of the intervertebral disc related to osteoporotic deformity of the vertebral body
"Trolley-track" sign	Three vertical radiodense lines on frontal radiographs related to ossification of supraspinous and interspinous ligaments and apophyseal joint capsules
Dagger sign	Single central radiodense line on frontal radiographs related to ossification of supraspinous and interspinous ligaments

difficult to detect in the thoracic spine, at which site the vertebral bodies may normally have a relatively straight configuration. As the erosions heal, reactive sclerosis produces highlighting, "whitening," or a "shiny corner" configuration.

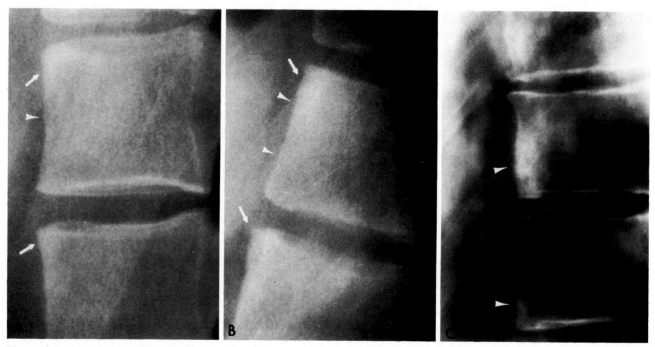

Figure 24–5. Osteitis: Radiographic abnormalities (three different patients). A Osseous erosion and sclerosis have produced whitening of the corners and margins along the anterior surfaces of the vertebrae (arrows). Note the straightening of the vertebral surface (arrowhead). **B** Considerable straightening (arrowheads) and bone formation (arrows) along the anterior vertebral surface are observed. **C** A convex anterior margin (arrowheads) of the vertebral bodies is associated with eburnation.

Syndesmophytosis (Fig. 24–6). The erosive vertebral abnormalities are associated with bone formation, which extends across the margin of the intervertebral disc. Thin vertical outgrowths are termed syndesmophytes and represent ossification of the anulus fibrosus itself. As the syndesmophytes enlarge, ossification can involve the adjacent anterior longitudinal ligament and paravertebral connective tissue. Syndesmophytes predominate on the anterior and lateral aspects of the spine, particularly near the thoracolumbar junction. They eventually bridge the intervertebral disc space, connecting one vertebral body with its neighbor, merging with the vertebral margins on either side. Even in later stages of the disease, the vertical nature of the outgrowths and their connection to the vertebral edges allow their differentiation from spinal osteophytes (which are triangular in shape and arise several millimeters from the discovertebral junction) and the paravertebral ossification of psoriasis and Reiter's syndrome (which begins at a distance from the vertebral body and intervertebral disc). In the later phases of ankylosing spondylitis, extensive syndesmophytes produce the undulating vertebral contour that is termed bamboo spine.

Discovertebral Erosions and Destruction (Table 24–2). Destructive foci that appear throughout the discovertebral junction in ankylosing spondylitis are frequently termed Andersson lesions. These abnormalities have been attributed to various factors, including inflammatory lesions, infections, discal displacements, and fractures with pseudarthroses. The lesions may be localized to a segment of the discovertebral junction or involve the entire intervertebral disc–bone margin;

in addition, they may be observed during early or late phases of disease, and they have occurred in traumatized and nontraumatized spines.

Lesions localized to the central subchondral portions of the discovertebral junction can be observed in ankylosed and nonankylosed spines. In many instances, the cause of these central lesions is cartilaginous node formation. There are three factors in ankylosing spondylitis, which, working independently or together, can contribute to the production of central discovertebral lesions: osteoporosis; abnormalities of the apo-

Table 24–2. TYPES OF DISCOVERTEBRAL EROSIONS IN ANKYLOSING SPONDYLITIS

Type	Probable Mechanism
Localized central lesions	Cartilaginous node formation aggravated by a. Osteoporosis b. Instability due to apophyseal joint disease c. Intraosseous inflammatory changes
Localized peripheral lesions	
1. Anterior	Enthesopathy, cartilaginous node formation, or intervertebral disc changes related to kyphosis
2. Posterior	Enthesopathy or cartilaginous node formation
Extensive central and peripheral lesions	Fracture with pseudarthrosis

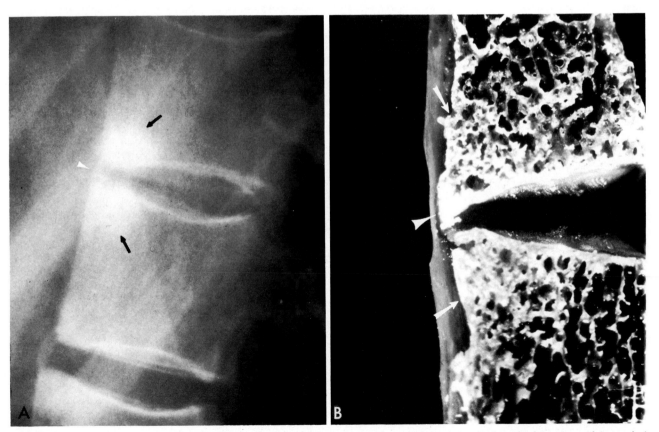

Figure 24–6. Osteitis and syndesmophytosis: Radiographic and pathologic abnormalities. A In association with osteitis of the corners of the vertebral bodies (arrows), early syndesmophyte formation has produced blurring of the margin of the intervertebral disc (arrowhead). **B** A photograph of a sagittal section of two vertebral bodies reveals osteitis (arrows) and syndesmophytosis (arrowhead), representing ossification of the intervertebral disc.

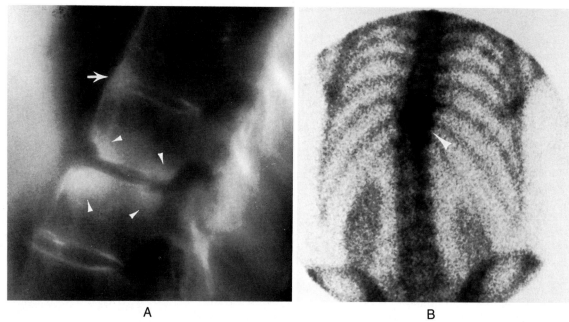

Figure 24–7. Discovertebral erosions and destruction: Localized peripheral lesions. Localized peripheral lesions with bone sclerosis (arrowheads) are observed on a lateral tomogram of the thoracolumbar junction (**A**). Syndesmophytosis (arrow) is also seen. The apophyseal joint at this level is only partially ossified. The bone scan (**B**) demonstrates increased accumulation of the radionuclide at the corresponding level (arrowhead) as well as at adjacent segments. (Courtesy of V. Vint, M.D., San Diego, California.)

physeal joints resulting in instability and recurrent discovertebral trauma; and inflammatory changes in the subchondral bone leading to osseous weakening and discal displacement. Radiographic examination outlines irregularity of the central portion of the superior and inferior vertebral margins, and radiolucent areas with surrounding sclerosis in the vertebral bodies are present.

Similar or additional mechanisms may be important in the production of peripheral discovertebral lesions in ankylosing spondylitis (Fig. 24–7). Progressive kyphosis in spondylitic patients may lead to injury to the anterior fibers of the anulus fibrosus and to invasion and replacement of the discal material by vascular fibrous tissue. Osteoporotic collapse or cartilaginous (Schmorl's) nodes also could be important. Furthermore, inflammation in the outer fibers of the anulus fibrosus related to the spondylitic process may play a role in the development of these lesions.

Destruction of the entire discovertebral junction of two neighboring vertebral bodies occurs almost exclusively in spondylitic patients with advanced ankylosis. Many such patients relate a history of significant trauma, and radiographs (or conventional tomograms) obtained at the time of injury may reveal an associated fracture through the ankylosed apophyseal articulations, the neighboring articular processes, or, rarely, the laminae or spinous process (Fig. 24–8). Subsequently, continued movement at the fracture site leads to nonunion or a pseudarthrosis. The vulnerability of the ankylosed spine in this disease to fracture is well known (Fig. 24–9). The cervical spine is especially susceptible to fracture, and neurologic complications with death may result. Conversely, fractures in the thoracic and lumbar spine in ankylosing spondylitis are often clinically unrecognized, and subsequent motion at the fracture site becomes evident.

The radiographic appearance of a pseudarthrosis of the spine resembles that which is observed in infection or neu-

roarthropathy, although a soft tissue mass is common in infective spondylitis and rare in pseudarthrosis. Detection of bone ankylosis of adjacent vertebral segments and a fracture of the posterior elements ensures accurate diagnosis.

Extensive central and peripheral discovertebral destruction is seen in some patients with ankylosing spondylitis who have not had a spinal fracture. In these persons, uneven or segmental involvement of the vertebral column leads to ankylosed portions separated by a relatively mobile region. Abnormal motion at the latter site creates radiographic alterations that resemble those of a pseudarthrosis.

Discal Calcification (Fig. 24–10). Central or eccentric circular or linear calcific collections may appear within the intervertebral disc at single or multiple sites in the spinal column. These deposits, which are dystrophic in nature, are usually associated with apophyseal joint ankylosis at the same vertebral level and with adjacent syndesmophytes. Calcifications are accentuated by osteoporosis of surrounding vertebral bodies.

APOPHYSEAL JOINTS. Poorly defined erosions of apophyseal joints in the lumbar, thoracic, and cervical segments of the spine are accompanied by reactive subchondral bone formation. These changes can be difficult to detect radiographically in the thoracic and lumbar spine. In the cervical spine, such abnormalities are readily apparent on lateral radiographs and predominate in the upper cervical region.

Apophyseal joint osseous fusion and capsular ossification also are frequent in the lumbar, thoracic, and cervical spine in this disease (Fig. 24–11). These findings, which are less common in psoriatic spondylitis and Reiter's syndrome, can eventually extend throughout the vertebral column. In this situation, frontal radiographs of the thoracic and lumbar segments reveal two vertical radiodense bands representing intra- and extraarticular ossification about the apophyseal joints, which, when combined with a third central band

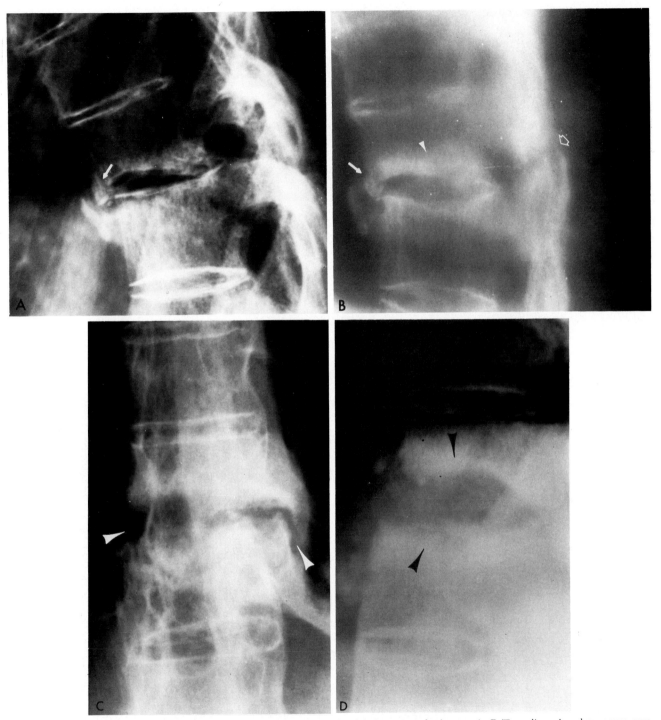

Figure 24–8. Discovertebral erosion and destruction: Central and peripheral lesions—pseudarthroses. A, B The radiograph and tomogram were obtained several weeks after this spondylitic patient suffered a fall. Observe the anterior subluxation (solid arrows) of the superiorly located vertebra, fragmentation, and mild subchondral sclerosis at the discovertebral junction. The subluxation (solid arrow) and sclerosis (arrowhead) are better seen on the tomogram. A fracture through the posterior elements (open arrow) is also evident. **C, D** Frontal and lateral radiographs reveal a typical pseudarthrosis of the lower thoracic spine characterized by extensive osseous resorption and sclerosis (arrowheads). The appearance simulates that of an infection.

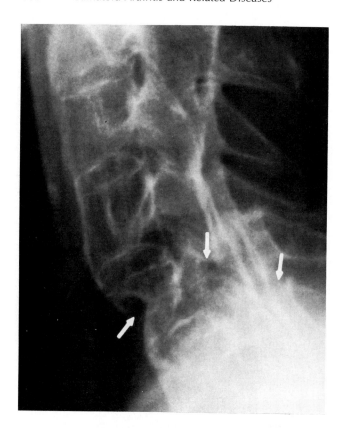

Figure 24–9. Spinal fractures. In a patient with obvious ankylosing spondylitis, an acute fracture through the fifth cervical vertebral body and laminae (arrows) with subluxation is evident.

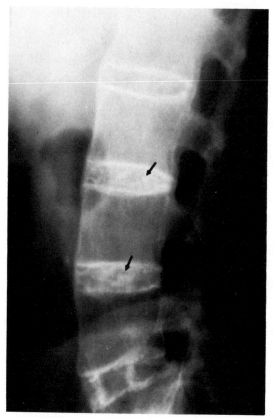

Figure 24–10. Discal calcification and ballooning. Long-standing ankylosing spondylitis is characterized by syndesmophytosis, apophyseal joint ankylosis, discal calcification (arrows), osteoporosis, and ballooning or biconvexity of the intervertebral disc.

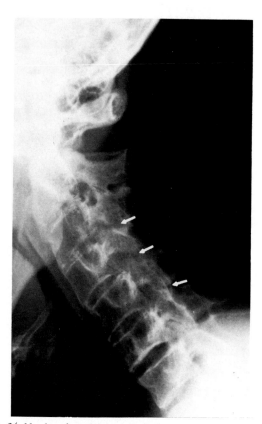

Figure 24–11. Apophyseal joint ankylosis. In the cervical spine, note apophyseal joint narrowing and fusion (arrows) extending from C2 to C7. Syndesmophytes, osteoporosis, and mild subluxation at C4-C5 are seen.

(resulting from ossification of supraspinous and interspinous ligaments), lead to the "trolley-track" sign.

Apophyseal joint ankylosis can be very striking in the cervical spine. Complete obliteration of the articular spaces between the posterior elements of the second through seventh vertebrae results in a true column or pillar of bone. The appearance is reminiscent of that in juvenile chronic arthritis, although hypoplasia of vertebral bodies and intervertebral disc spaces, a prominent finding in juvenile chronic arthritis, is not observed in ankylosing spondylitis.

COSTOVERTEBRAL JOINTS. The costovertebral joints may demonstrate erosion, sclerosis, and ankylosis, although radiographic demonstration of these changes is difficult.

POSTERIOR LIGAMENTOUS ATTACHMENTS. Calcification and ossification of interspinous and supraspinous ligaments represent prominent features of ankylosing spondylitis. In later stages, a central radiodense stripe can be identified on frontal radiographs of the thoracic and lumbar spine, the dagger sign (Fig. 24–12).

Erosion of the tips of spinous processes is encountered most commonly in the lower cervical and upper thoracic regions. A poorly defined and pointed osseous outline becomes evident. A similar appearance can be encountered in rheumatoid arthritis.

ATLANTOAXIAL JOINTS. Synovial tissue surrounds the odontoid process both anteriorly and posteriorly, corresponding to the location of the joint cavity between the anterior arch of the atlas and the anterior surface of the odontoid process (dens) and the joint cavity between the transverse ligament of the atlas and the posterior surface of the odontoid process. Inflammatory changes of the synovial and adjacent ligamentous structures can lead to erosion and resorption of the dens. Similar abnormalities can be evident in rheumatoid arthritis (and psoriatic arthritis).

Although atlantoaxial subluxation can be observed in patients with ankylosing spondylitis (Fig. 24–13), the frequency of this complication appears to be less than that in rheumatoid arthritis. When present, atlantoaxial subluxation generally is observed in the later stages of the disease. Forward subluxation of the atlas with respect to the odontoid process is most typical. Subaxial subluxation in the cervical spine is much less characteristic of ankylosing spondylitis than of rheumatoid arthritis.

COMPLICATIONS OF SPINAL INVOLVEMENT. Neurospinal complications, including spinal cord compression and even death, are a recognized, although infrequent, manifestation of ankylosing spondylitis. Vertebral fractures may be associated with significant morbidity and mortality. Atlantoaxial instability can produce neurologic deficit and may be fatal. Spondylodiscitis has been associated with compression of the cord or nerve roots, especially in the lumbar segment. Spinal stenosis also is being recognized with increasing frequency in patients with ankylosing spondylitis.

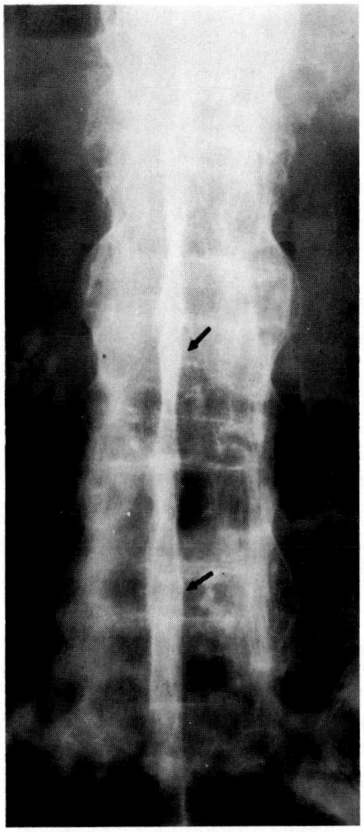

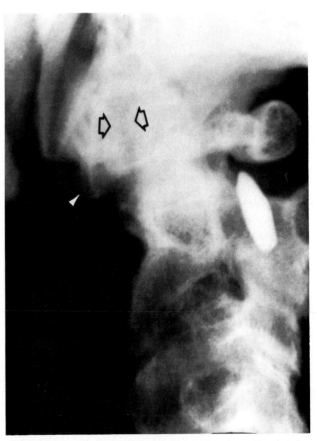

Figure 24–12. Posterior spinal ligamentous ossification. A frontal radiograph of the lumbar spine reveals ossification of the interspinous and supraspinous ligaments, producing a vertical central radiodense shadow (arrows), the dagger sign.

Figure 24–13. Atlantoaxial subluxation. In this patient with ankylosing spondylitis, anterior atlantoaxial subluxation has produced increased distance (between arrows) between the anterior arch of the atlas and the odontoid process. Adjacent hyperostosis (arrowhead) is evident. A previous myelogram had been obtained.

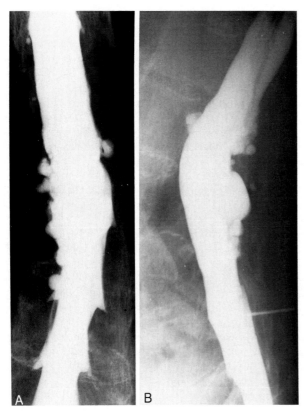

Figure 24–14. Thecal diverticula. An elderly man with ankylosing spondylitis developed a cauda equina syndrome, manifested as loss of sphincter tone and perineal dysesthesia. Frontal (supine) (**A**) and lateral (**B**) radiographs during a myelogram outline multiple arachnoid diverticula. (Courtesy of D. Moody, M.D., Winston-Salem, North Carolina.)

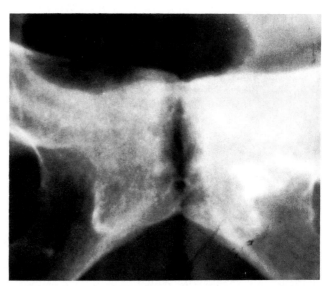

Figure 24–15. Abnormalities of the symphysis pubis. Note narrowing, osseus fusion, and sclerosis of the symphysis pubis.

The cauda equina syndrome is observed in some patients with long-standing ankylosing spondylitis. Widening of the neural canal in the lumbar segment, dilation of the dural sac, and thecal diverticula are the associated pathologic aberrations. Myelography reveals contrast opacification of the saccular diverticula (Fig. 24–14), and computed tomography demonstrates scalloped erosions of the laminae.

Symphysis Pubis (Fig. 24–15)

Alterations of the symphysis pubis occur in approximately 20 per cent of patients with ankylosing spondylitis. Erosion and blurring of the subchondral bone, sclerosis, articular space narrowing, and bone ankylosis may be evident.

Additional Pelvic Sites (Fig. 24–16)

Enthesopathy is especially prominent in certain pelvic sites, such as the ischial tuberosities, the iliac crests, and the sacroiliac spaces above the true synovial joints; similar abnormalities occur at extrapelvic sites, such as the femoral trochanters, humeral tuberosities, inferior clavicular margin at the site of attachment of the coracoclavicular ligament, anterior surface of the patella, and plantar aspect of the calcaneus. Osteoporosis, osseous erosion with poorly defined subchondral bone margins, and reactive sclerosis are the observed radiographic alterations. Although the resulting radiographic picture is reminiscent of that occurring in diffuse

idiopathic skeletal hyperostosis, the degree of sclerosis and surface irregularity is more prominent in ankylosing spondylitis. Similar abnormalities are apparent in psoriatic arthritis, Reiter's syndrome, and inflammatory bowel disorders.

Manubriosternal Joint

Involvement of the manubriosternal articulation can lead to significant clinical findings in patients with ankylosing spondylitis. The radiographic and pathologic changes in the manubriosternal joint are similar to those that are observed at the discovertebral junction and symphysis pubis. Identical abnormalities are evident in other seronegative spondyloarthropathies, particularly psoriatic arthritis.

Hip (Table 24–3)

Clinical and radiologic involvement of the hip is an important feature of ankylosing spondylitis. A bilateral (93 per cent) and symmetric (73 per cent) distribution with concentric joint space narrowing (50 per cent) and osteophytosis (58 per cent) is characteristic.

An early and distinctive abnormality is an osteophyte or "bump" on the lateral aspect of the femoral head (Fig. 24–17). Osteophytes subsequently progress, creating a collar around the femoral neck at the margin of the articular surface. Simultaneously, diffuse or concentric joint space narrowing producing axial migration of the femoral head with respect to the acetabulum is frequently seen (Fig. 24–17). Protrusio acetabuli or intraarticular bone fusion (Fig. 24–18) can eventually occur, and subchondral cysts are not uncommon. The combination of concentric diminution of the articular space and osteophytosis is characteristic of the hip disease in ankylosing spondylitis, although it may also be observed in calcium pyrophosphate dihydrate crystal deposition disease, Paget's disease, and, rarely, uncomplicated osteoarthritis. Although concentric joint space narrowing is also seen in rheumatoid arthritis, osteophytosis is not generally a prominent feature of this disease.

The radiographic course of spondylitic hip disease is vari-

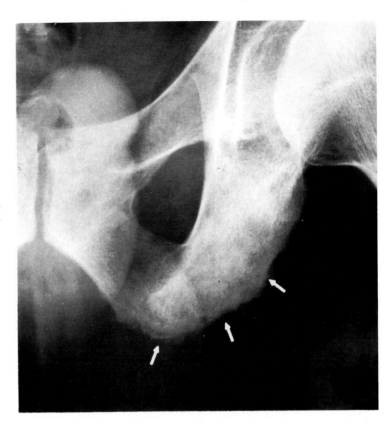

Figure 24–16. Abnormalities of the ischial tuberosity. Observe slight contour irregularity and sclerosis of the ischial tuberosity (arrows).

able. In some cases, however, arthroplasty may be required owing to the presence of considerable hip abnormalities and significant disability. A propensity to develop restricted motion and periarticular bone formation after hip arthroplasty has been observed in some patients with ankylosing spondylitis.

Shoulder

GLENOHUMERAL JOINT. With the exception of the hip, the glenohumeral joint is the most frequently affected peripheral articular site in patients with long-standing ankylosing spondylitis. The abnormalities are more commonly bilateral than unilateral and may appear without changes in any other appendicular skeletal site. Osteoporosis, diffuse joint space narrowing, and erosive changes predominantly in

the superolateral aspect of the humeral head simulate the changes in rheumatoid arthritis (Fig. 24–19). In some spondylitic individuals, the entire outer aspect of the humerus may be destroyed, the "hatchet" sign. Atrophy or disruption of the rotator cuff can lead to elevation of the humeral head with respect to the glenoid cavity.

ACROMIOCLAVICULAR JOINT. Destructive articular changes in this location, which commonly are bilateral in distribution, are identical to those in rheumatoid arthritis.

CORACOCLAVICULAR JOINT. Scalloped clavicular erosion beneath the coracoclavicular ligament occurs not only in ankylosing spondylitis but also in other synovial disorders, as well as in hyperparathyroidism. In ankylosing spondylitis, proliferative alterations may accompany the erosive process, providing a clue to accurate diagnosis.

Table 24–3. DIFFERENTIAL DIAGNOSIS OF HIP INVOLVEMENT

Disease	Typical Distribution	Femoral Head Migration	Osteophytosis	Miscellaneous Findings
Ankylosing spondylitis	Bilateral, symmetric	Axial	Lateral aspect of femur; collar at femoral head–femoral neck junction	Cysts, bone ankylosis, protrusion deformity, postoperative heterotopic ossification
Rheumatoid arthritis	Bilateral, symmetric	Axial	Rare	Osteoporosis, erosions, protrusion deformity
Osteoarthritis	Unilateral or bilateral	Superior or medial	Lateral and medial Femoral and acetabular	Sclerosis, cysts, buttressing
Calcium pyrophosphate dihydrate crystal deposition disease	Bilateral, symmetric, or asymmetric	Axial	Lateral and medial Femoral and acetabular	Sclerosis, cysts, collapse, fragmentation, calcification

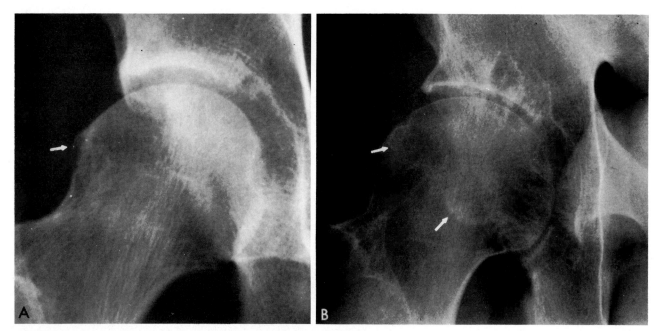

Figure 24–17. Abnormalities of the hip: Osteophytosis and joint space narrowing. A Observe bone formation on the lateral margin of the femoral head (arrow), which has resulted in a bumpy contour. B More extensive osteophyte formation can be seen on the lateral margin of the femoral head with progression over a portion of the femoral neck (arrows). The joint space is diffusely narrowed. (A, B, From Dwosh I, et al: Hip involvement in ankylosing spondylitis. Arthritis Rheum 19:683, 1976. Used with permission.)

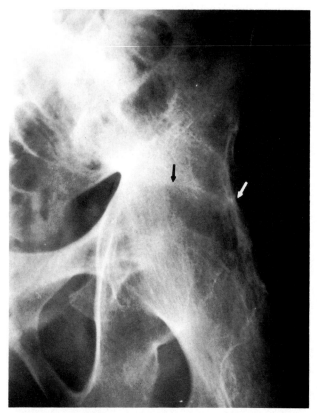

Figure 24–18. Abnormalities of the hip: Intraarticular bone ankylosis. Note the extensive capsular and interior bone ankylosis (arrows). The medial aspect of the articulation is slightly identifiable.

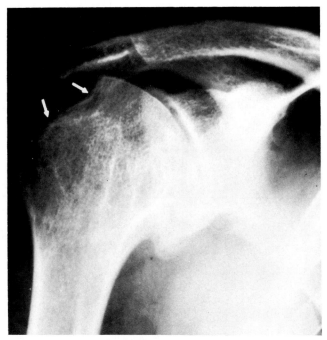

Figure 24–19. Abnormalities of the shoulder. Glenohumeral joint. Observe joint space narrowing, mild osteoporosis, and a large erosive abnormality along the lateral aspect of the humeral head (arrows).

Sternoclavicular Joint

Bilateral or, less commonly, unilateral abnormalities of the sternoclavicular joint in ankylosing spondylitis consist of erosion and sclerosis of the sternum and the medial end of the clavicle. Intraarticular osseous fusion may eventually occur.

Elbow

Radiographic elbow abnormalities are relatively uncommon in ankylosing spondylitis. Effusions, osteoporosis, joint space narrowing, and bone proliferation are detected in a unilateral or bilateral distribution.

Hand and Wrist

Asymmetrically distributed abnormalities of the small joints of the hands and the wrists in ankylosing spondylitis are not infrequent. Periarticular swelling, juxtaarticular osteoporosis, joint space narrowing, and osseous erosions are observed (Fig. 24–20). Metacarpophalangeal, proximal interphalangeal, and distal interphalangeal joints, all the compartments of the wrist, and the ulnar styloid can be affected. In general, erosive abnormalities are less prominent than in rheumatoid arthritis.

Knee

In approximately 30 per cent of patients with ankylosing spondylitis of long duration, radiographic abnormalities appear in the knees. Typically, bilateral and symmetric changes in the three compartments of the knee (medial femorotibial, lateral femorotibial, patellofemoral compartments) include effusions, osteoporosis, and joint space narrowing. Additional manifestations are marginal erosions, subchondral cysts, and juxtaarticular periostitis. Hyperostosis on the anterior aspect of the patella at the quadriceps attachment can be noted. Rarely, in the knee as in other joints, a more aggressive pattern of synovial inflammation is apparent. Extensive soft tissue swelling and a massive synovial effusion simulate the findings of septic arthritis or pigmented villonodular synovitis.

Ankle

Rarely, changes in the ankle can be noted in ankylosing spondylitis. They resemble findings in other joints. Periostitis is particularly characteristic in the distal medial tibia.

Forefoot and Midfoot

Bilateral symmetric or asymmetric abnormalities of the feet show predilection for the metatarsophalangeal and first tarsometatarsal joints and for the interphalangeal joint of the great toe. Soft tissue swelling, diffuse joint space narrowing, erosions with adjacent bone proliferation predominantly on the medial aspect of the metatarsal heads, periostitis of phalangeal and metatarsal shafts, and intraarticular bone ankylosis can be detected. Subluxation at metatarsophalangeal articulations consisting of fibular deviation of the toes is less frequent and severe than in rheumatoid arthritis.

Calcaneus

Although clinically manifest heel abnormalities are infrequent in ankylosing spondylitis, radiographic changes of the calcaneus are common (Fig. 24–21). Bilateral abnormalities predominate. Well-defined plantar or posterior calcaneal spurs, or both, are a common manifestation but are similar in appearance to those in a "normal" population. Retrocalcaneal swelling (related to bursitis), posterior calcaneal erosion, and Achilles tendon thickening are also frequent. Bone

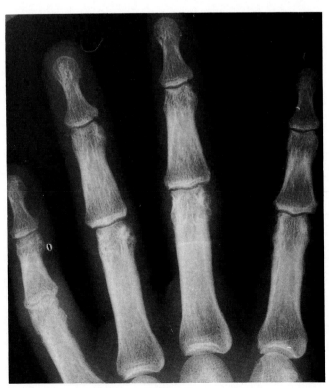

Figure 24–20. Abnormalities of the hand. Note fusiform periarticular soft tissue swelling, mild joint space diminution, and marginal erosion of proximal interphalangeal and distal interphalangeal joints. (From Resnick D: Patterns of peripheral joint disease in ankylosing spondylitis. Radiology 110:523, 1974. Used with permission.)

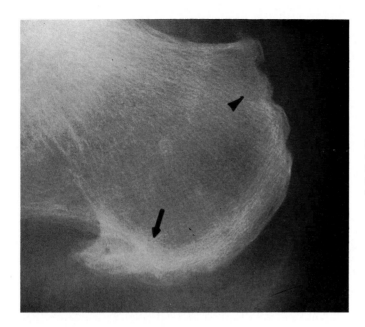

Figure 24–21. Abnormalities of the calcaneus. Findings include erosion of the posterosuperior aspect of the bone (arrowhead), related to retrocalcaneal bursitis, and erosive and proliferative changes of the plantar aspect of the bone (arrow), related to an enthesopathy at the ligamentous attachments.

erosion and proliferation resulting in poorly defined spur formation at the site of ligamentous attachment to bone on the inferior surface of the calcaneus are identical to the findings of psoriatic arthritis and Reiter's syndrome.

Temporomandibular Joint

Clinical and radiographic manifestations resulting from temporomandibular joint arthritis in patients with ankylosing spondylitis have been recorded. Asymmetric or unilateral involvement is frequent. Erosions predominate on the mandibular condyle, either at its anterior margin or superiorly at the junction of its middle and posterior thirds.

COEXISTENCE WITH OTHER DISORDERS
Rheumatoid Arthritis

The concept that ankylosing spondylitis and rheumatoid arthritis are separate and distinct diseases is rarely challenged today. Rarely, both disorders appear to develop in the same individual, however. Typically, a male patient will develop ankylosing spondylitis at a young age and subsequently, at a time when his spondylitic process is largely inactive, he will develop rheumatoid arthritis. In these persons, the diagnosis of rheumatoid arthritis is firmly established by the presence of a high-titer seropositive (for rheumatoid factor), symmetrically distributed erosive arthritis of the joints of the appendicular skeleton, with or without rheumatoid nodules; the diagnosis of ankylosing spondylitis is documented by the presence of typical sacroiliitis and spondylitis in a patient who possesses the histocompatibility antigen HLA-B27.

Diffuse Idiopathic Skeletal Hyperostosis (DISH)

During the radiographic examination of older persons with long-standing ankylosing spondylitis, it is not unusual to document the co-occurrence of DISH. In this situation, widespread intraarticular bone ankylosis of both sacroiliac joints, syndesmophytosis, and apophyseal joint space narrowing or osseous fusion are combined with "flowing" ossification along the anterior aspect of a portion of the spine, particularly

in the thoracic segment. Although there is a natural tendency to attribute all the radiographic findings to one disease, careful analysis ensures the accurate diagnosis of both disorders.

Inflammatory Bowel Disorders

The well-documented association of ankylosing spondylitis and certain inflammatory bowel disorders such as ulcerative colitis and Crohn's disease is discussed in Chapter 27.

Paget's Disease

The difficulty in assessing radiographs of the sacroiliac joints in patients with Paget's disease and the possible association of ankylosing spondylitis and Paget's disease are discussed in Chapter 49.

OTHER DIAGNOSTIC TECHNIQUES
Scintigraphy

Radionuclide techniques have had varying degrees of success in the evaluation of sacroiliac and spinal abnormalities in ankylosing spondylitis. Application of such techniques to the detection of sacroiliitis has been stimulated by the difficulty in recognizing early sacroiliac joint abnormalities on radiographic examination; however, qualitative analysis of the accumulation of bone-seeking radiopharmaceutical preparations in the sacroiliac region is difficult because of the normal radionuclide activity in this location. Quantitative analysis is far superior. It is accomplished by delineating an "area of interest" cursor along a line that encompasses the joints and the sacrum. The ratio of sacroiliac joint to sacral radionuclide activity is calculated and the result is compared to normal values for each individual x-ray department. Generally, ratios greater than 1.3 to 1 or 1.45 to 1 are considered abnormal. Some investigators believe that the sacrum is not an ideal reference point in the assessment of radionuclide activity in the sacroiliac joints as its accumulation of the radiopharmaceutical agent may increase when there is nearby inflammation. Other reference areas, such as the paraspinal soft tissues

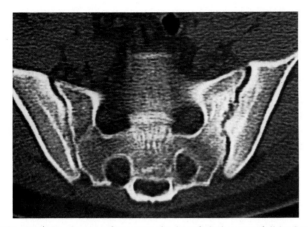

Figure 24–22. Computed tomography in ankylosing spondylitis: Sacroiliitis. A transaxial image through the lower portion of the sacroiliac joint shows bilateral articular abnormalities, greater on the left side, consisting of joint surface irregularity and erosion in both the ilium and the sacrum, with associated new bone formation.

and proximal end of the femur, have been advocated. In patients with advanced disease, radionuclide uptake in the sacroiliac joints (as well as the spine) may not be abnormal. Unilateral alterations are frequently easier to interpret both qualitatively and quantitatively.

Increased accumulation of radionuclide in spinal and peripheral joints can also be observed in patients with ankylosing spondylitis, especially in the presence of active disease. At any location, an abnormal scintigraphic examination is not specific, accurate diagnosis necessitating its correlation with clinical and radiologic investigations. As an example, focal areas of augmented radionuclide accumulation in the spine may indicate the site of an acute fracture or chronic pseudarthrosis.

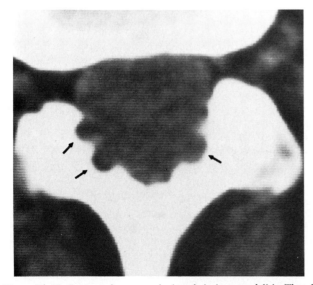

Figure 24–23. Computed tomography in ankylosing spondylitis: Thecal diverticula. In this transaxial image through the lower portion of the lumbar spine, scalloped erosions (arrows) of the laminae are diagnostic of thecal diverticula, a known complication of ankylosing spondylitis. (Courtesy of A. Brower, M.D., Washington, D.C.)

Computed Tomography

Owing to the difficulty in detecting sacroiliitis by conventional radiography and to the controversy regarding the role of scintigraphy in this detection, computed tomography has been employed by some investigators in an effort to delineate early abnormalities of the sacroiliac joint in ankylosing spondylitis. Some reports indicate clear superiority of computed tomography over routine radiography, whereas others question this superiority. In general, computed tomography should be reserved for cases in which the initial radiographs are equivocal or normal, especially in those patients in whom clinical or laboratory parameters indicate a high index of suspicion for sacroiliitis (Fig. 24–22).

Additional indications for computed tomography in patients with ankylosing spondylitis include the detection of spinal fractures, spinal stenosis, thecal diverticula (Fig. 24–23), atlantoaxial instability, and manubriosternal and costovertebral disease. Paraspinal muscle atrophy can also be documented.

ETIOLOGY AND PATHOGENESIS

A strikingly high frequency of the HLA-B27 antigen in patients with ankylosing spondylitis has now been observed all over the world. In most reports, more than 90 per cent of white spondylitic patients possess the B27 gene; the frequency of this gene among whites who do not have ankylosing spondylitis is approximately 6 to 8 per cent. To date, this remains the most significant association between a readily detectable HLA antigen and a well-defined disease, underscoring the importance of genetics in the causation of ankylosing spondylitis. Some studies conclude that ankylosing spondylitis is attributable to an autosomal dominant factor with variable penetrance, although multiple factors may be operational. Of interest, ankylosing spondylitis can develop in the absence of the HLA-B27 antigen.

DIFFERENTIAL DIAGNOSIS
Sacroiliitis

The sacroiliac joint abnormalities in ankylosing spondylitis must be differentiated from those accompanying other disorders (Table 24–4). This can be accomplished by analysis of both distribution and morphology of the articular changes. Classically, a bilateral and symmetric distribution is observed in ankylosing spondylitis. Although a similar pattern can be evident in other seronegative spondyloarthropathies, such as psoriasis and Reiter's syndrome, asymmetric or, rarely, unilateral alterations may accompany these latter disorders (Fig. 24–24). A bilateral and symmetric distribution is also associated with the sacroiliitis of inflammatory bowel disease (ulcerative colitis, Crohn's disease, Whipple's disease), which is identical in every regard to that of classic ankylosing spondylitis. In rheumatoid arthritis, minor sacroiliac articular abnormalities commonly are bilateral but may be asymmetric in appearance. Bilateral and symmetric alterations of the sacroiliac joint are also noted in hyperparathyroidism (and renal osteodystrophy), osteitis condensans ilii, gouty arthritis, and degenerative joint disease, although in the latter two conditions, an asymmetric or unilateral distribution is not uncommon. Unilateral abnormalities are most typical in infection and may accompany contralateral hip disease and ipsilateral paralysis or disuse (cartilage atrophy).

Table 24–4. DISTRIBUTION OF SACROILIAC JOINT ABNORMALITIES IN VARIOUS DISORDERS*

Disorder	Bilateral, Symmetric Distribution	Bilateral, Asymmetric Distribution	Unilateral Distribution
Ankylosing spondylitis	+	−	−
Psoriatic spondylitis	+	+	+
Reiter's syndrome	+	+	+
Sacroiliitis of inflammatory bowel disease	+	−	−
Rheumatoid arthritis	−	+	+
Osteitis condensans ilii	+	−	−
Hyperparathyroidism	+	−	−
Gouty arthritis	+	+	+
Osteoarthritis	+	+	+
Infection	−	−	+

*Only most typical patterns of distribution are indicated.

Poorly-defined erosive abnormality with adjacent sclerosis, particularly in the ilium, and associated joint space narrowing, intraarticular osseous fusion, and ligamentous ossification is the characteristic appearance of sacroiliac joint disease in classic ankylosing spondylitis and in the sacroiliitis of inflammatory bowel disease. In psoriasis and Reiter's syndrome, extensive bone eburnation may be unaccompanied by intraarticular osseous fusion. Sacroiliac joint involvement in rheumatoid arthritis is usually manifested as superficial erosions, minimal sclerosis, and absence of significant bone ankylosis. Subchondral resorption of bone, predominantly in the ilium, in conjunction with primary or secondary hyperparathyroidism leads to irregularity of the osseous surface, adjacent sclerosis, and widening of the interosseous joint space; articular space diminution and bone fusion are not seen. In osteitis condensans ilii, a triangular segment of bone sclerosis is evident in the inferior aspect of the ilium. The joint surface is well defined, and the articular space is not diminished. Sacral alterations are indeed unusual. In chronic tophaceous gouty arthritis, large, gouged-out defects with surrounding sclerosis are observed, whereas in degenerative arthritis, joint space narrowing, bone sclerosis, and anterior osteophytes are associated with a noneroded, smooth subchondral bone margin. Calcification and ossification of the interosseous ligament above the synovial sacroiliac articulation can be encountered in degenerative joint disease, but widespread ossification of this structure, as noted in ankylosing spondylitis, is not common. Cartilage atrophy accompanying paralysis or disuse produces diffuse loss of articular space with surrounding osteoporosis. In some patients with long-standing paralysis, intraarticular osseous fusion is seen, perhaps related to chronic low-grade inflammation.

Spondylitis

Spinal abnormalities in classic ankylosing spondylitis initially appear in the thoracolumbar and lumbosacral junctions and subsequently may extend throughout the thoracic and lumbar spine and into the cervical region. An identical distribution is encountered in the spondylitis of inflammatory bowel disease. Although the entire vertebral column may be altered in psoriasis and Reiter's syndrome, spotty involvement and absence of severe cervical spinal changes are typical of the latter disorder. In some women with classic ankylosing spondylitis, significant sacroiliac joint and cervical spine abnormalities may appear without obvious thoracic and lumbar spinal changes. This same distribution can be encountered in patients with psoriasis. Spondylitis without sacroiliitis is relatively rare in classic ankylosing spondylitis, although it

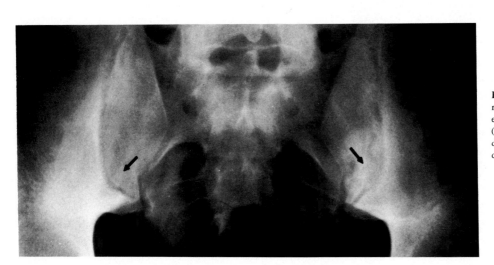

Figure 24–24. Sacroiliac joint abnormalities in Reiter's syndrome. Bilateral asymmetric sacroiliac joint changes (arrows) are more typical of Reiter's syndrome and psoriatic arthritis than of classic ankylosing spondylitis.

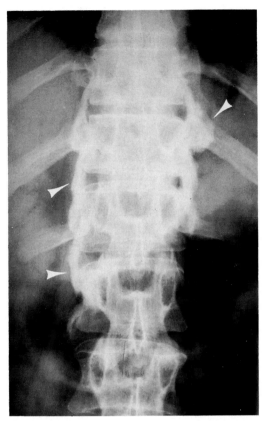

Figure 24–25. Spinal abnormalities in psoriatic spondylitis. Large, bulky irregular, asymmetrically distributed excrescences (arrowheads) are more typical in this disease than in classic ankylosing spondylitis. (Courtesy of E. G. L. Bywaters, M.D., Taplow, Buckinghamshire, England.)

may be observed in both psoriasis and Reiter's syndrome. Spinal involvement in rheumatoid arthritis has predilection for the cervical spine, with relative sparing of the thoracic and lumbar segments.

The thin vertically oriented syndesmophytes that are evident in classic ankylosing spondylitis and the spondylitis of inflammatory bowel disease differ considerably in appearance from the broad asymmetric bone outgrowths of psoriasis and Reiter's syndrome (Fig. 24–25), the triangular outgrowths of spondylosis deformans, and the flowing anterolateral ossification of diffuse idiopathic skeletal hyperostosis (Table 24–5). The bone excrescences accompanying neuroarthropathy, ac-

romegaly, and fluorosis are not realistically confused with the syndesmophytes of ankylosing spondylitis. Syndesmophytes may be seen in patients with alkaptonuria, but additional radiographic manifestations ensure accurate differential diagnosis.

Osteitis with sclerosis and erosion of the anterior corners of the vertebral bodies and squaring are much more commonly encountered in classic ankylosing spondylitis and the spondylitis of inflammatory bowel disease than in psoriasis and Reiter's syndrome. Similarly, apophyseal joint sclerosis and osseous fusion are more typical of classic ankylosing spondylitis and the spondylitis of inflammatory bowel disease than of the other seronegative spondyloarthropathies.

Discovertebral erosions and sclerosis, which are seen in ankylosing spondylitis, are also observed in psoriasis. Similar lesions are evident in the cervical spine in patients with rheumatoid arthritis and throughout the spine in many disorders that are associated with cartilaginous nodes (Schmorl's nodes). When severe, spondylitic erosions can simulate the findings in infection. Spinal pseudarthrosis accompanying ankylosing spondylitis also resembles osteomyelitis.

Odontoid erosion and atlantoaxial subluxation are encountered in ankylosing spondylitis, usually in patients with long-standing disease. Similar findings are observed in psoriasis and, less commonly, in Reiter's syndrome. In rheumatoid arthritis, these findings are combined with other diagnostic features in the cervical spine, such as extensive discovertebral erosions, disc space narrowing, subluxation at subaxial levels, and absence of osteophytes.

In the cervical spine, widespread apophyseal joint ankylosis accompanying ankylosing spondylitis resembles the findings in juvenile chronic arthritis. In this latter disorder, associated hypoplasia of vertebral bodies and intervertebral discs is distinctive. Abnormalities of the cervical spine in other diseases as well can generally be differentiated from those in ankylosing spondylitis (Fig. 24–26).

Abnormalities of Extraspinal Synovial Articulations

The absence of symmetric changes and osteoporosis, and the presence of bone proliferation and intraarticular osseous fusion, are features that are common to all three seronegative spondyloarthropathies (ankylosing spondylitis, psoriasis, and Reiter's syndrome), differing from the characteristics of rheumatoid arthritis (symmetry, osteoporosis, fibrous ankylosis, and absence of bone proliferation) (Table 24–6). Differentiating among the seronegative spondyloarthropathies on the

Table 24–5. BONE OUTGROWTHS OF THE SPINE

Outgrowth	Definition	Representative Disorders	Appearance
Syndesmophyte	Ossification of the anulus fibrosus	Ankylosing spondylitis Alkaptonuria	Vertical outgrowth extending from edge of one vertebral body to the next
Osteophyte	Hyperostosis at attachment of annular fibers	Spondylosis deformans	Triangular outgrowth located several millimeters from edge of the vertebral body
Flowing anterior ossification	Ossification of the intervertebral disc, anterior longitudinal ligament, and paravertebral connective tissue	Diffuse idiopathic skeletal hyperostosis	Undulating outgrowth along the anterior aspect of the spine
Paravertebral ossification	Ossification of paravertebral connective tissue	Psoriatic spondylitis Reiter's syndrome	Poorly- or well-defined outgrowth separated from the edge of the vertebral body and the intervertebral disc

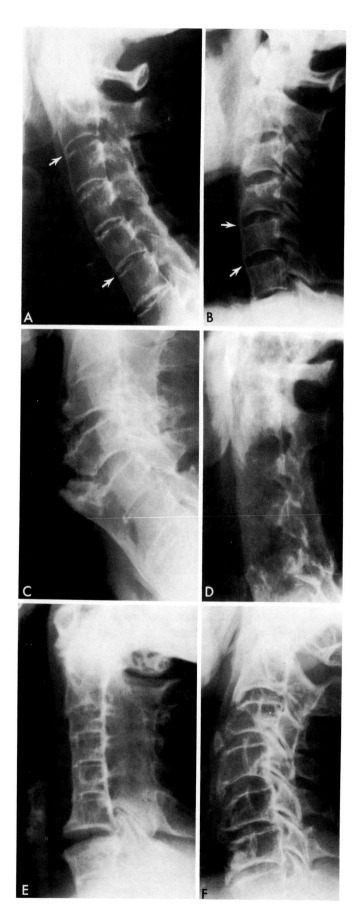

Figure 24–26. Differential diagnosis of cervical spine abnormalities.
A Ankylosing spondylitis is characterized by syndesmophytes (arrows) and apophyseal joint ankylosis. **B** Psoriatic spondylitis leads to bone outgrowths (arrows) that predominate in the lower cervical spine. Apophyseal articulations appear normal. **C** Diffuse idiopathic skeletal hyperostosis is accompanied by extensive bone deposition on the anterior portion of the vertebral column. **D** Sternocostoclavicular hyperostosis is characterized by exuberant bone formation anteriorly and centrally that obliterates the interface between vertebral bodies and intervertebral discs and by apophyseal joint ankylosis. **E** Juvenile chronic arthritis is associated with hypoplasia of the vertebral bodies and intervertebral discs, apophyseal joint ankylosis, and predilection for the upper cervical region. **F** Acromegaly leads to bone deposition that resembles that of spondylosis deformans and an increase in the anteroposterior dimension of the vertebral bodies.

Table 24–6. ABNORMALITIES OF SYNOVIAL ARTICULATIONS

Disease	Symmetric Involvement	Soft Tissue Swelling	Osteoporosis	Joint Space Narrowing	Bone Ankylosis	Erosions, Cysts	Bone Proliferation or "Whiskering"
Ankylosing spondylitis	±	+	±	+	+	+	+
Rheumatoid arthritis	+	+	+	+	±	+	−
Psoriatic arthritis	±	+	−	+	+	+	+
Reiter's syndrome	−	+	±	+	+	+	+
Gouty arthritis	±	+	−	±	−	+	+*
Septic arthritis	−	+	+	+	+	+	+†

*Irregular lips of bone are apparent.
†Ill-defined "fraying" of bone is seen.

basis of abnormalities of synovial joints in the appendicular skeleton can be difficult. Alterations in ankylosing spondylitis are located most commonly in the hip, the glenohumeral joint, and the knee, although changes in the small joints of the hand and the foot can be observed. In psoriasis, predilection for the interphalangeal, metacarpophalangeal, and metatarsophalangeal joints may be marked, whereas in Reiter's syndrome, involvement of the joints of the lower extremities, such as the knee and the metatarsophalangeal and interphalangeal articulations, is noted.

Abnormalities of Extraspinal Cartilaginous Articulations

The seronegative spondyloarthropathies are frequently associated with significant abnormalities of the symphysis pubis and the manubriosternal joint. Although similar changes appear in rheumatoid arthritis, their frequency and severity are less striking.

Enthesopathy

Bone erosion with proliferation at the site of osseous attachment of ligaments and tendons represents a typical lesion of ankylosing spondylitis, psoriasis, and Reiter's syndrome. Abnormalities may be encountered in the iliac crest, the ischial tuberosity, the femoral trochanters, the humeral tuberosities, the plantar aspect of the calcaneus, the malleoli about the ankle, the inferior aspect of the distal clavicle, the spinous processes of the vertebrae, and the patella. In all locations, an irregular frayed surface may be created, which is virtually diagnostic of one of these three conditions.

FURTHER READINGS

Berens DL: Roentgen features of ankylosing spondylitis. Clin Orthop 74:20, 1971.

Cawley MID, Chalmers TM, Kellgren JH, Ball J: Destructive lesions of vertebral bodies in ankylosing spondylitis. Ann Rheum Dis 31:345, 1972.

Cruickshank B: Pathology of ankylosing spondylitis. Bull Rheum Dis 10:211, 1960.

Dwosh IL, Resnick D, Becker MA: Hip involvement in ankylosing spondylitis. Arthritis Rheum 19:683, 1976.

Forestier J, Jacqueline F, Rotes-Querol J: Ankylosing Spondylitis. Springfield, Ill, Charles C Thomas, 1956.

Gelman MI, Umber JS: Fractures of the thoracolumbar spine in ankylosing spondylitis. AJR 130:485, 1978.

Goldberg RP, Genant HK, Shimshak R, Shames D: Applications and limitations of quantitative sacroiliac joint scintigraphy. Radiology 128:683, 1978.

Kozin F, Carrera GF, Ryan LM, Foley D, Lawson T: Computed tomography in the diagnosis of sacroiliitis. Arthritis Rheum 24:1479, 1981.

McEwen C, DiTata D, Longg C, Porini A, Good A, Rankin T: Ankylosing spondylitis and the spondylitis accompanying ulcerative colitis, regional enteritis, psoriasis, and Reiter's disease. A comparative study. Arthritis Rheum 14:291, 1971.

Resnick D, Dwosh IL, Goergen TG, Shapiro RF, D'Ambrosia R: Clinical and radiographic "reankylosis" following hip surgery in ankylosing spondylitis. AJR 126:1181, 1976.

Trent G, Armstrong GWD, O'Neil J: Thoracolumbar fractures in ankylosing spondylitis. High-risk injuries. Clin Orthop 227:61, 1988.

Volger JB III, Brown WH, Helms CA, Genant HK: The normal sacroiliac joint: A CT study of asymptomatic patients. Radiology 151:433, 1984.

Vyas K, Eklem M, Seto H, Bobba VR, Brown P, Haines J, Krishnamurthy GT: Quantitative scintigraphy of sacroiliac joints: Effect of age, gender, and laterality. AJR 136:589, 1981.

Wilkinson M, Bywaters EGL: Clinical features and course of ankylosing spondylitis as seen in a follow up of 222 hospital referred cases. Ann Rheum Dis 17:209, 1958.

Chapter 25

Psoriatic Arthritis

Donald Resnick, M.D.
Gen Niwayama, M.D.

Psoriatic arthritis produces distinctive abnormalities of synovial and cartilaginous joints as well as tendon and ligament attachments to the bone. In most instances, the diagnosis is not difficult and is based on the characteristic radiographic features, which include some degree of asymmetry, progressive intraarticular erosive changes with separation of the subchondral margins of adjacent bones, periosteal proliferation, intraarticular osseous fusion, and absence of osteoporosis in synovial joints; bilateral symmetric or asymmetric sacroiliac joint abnormalities and paravertebral ossification; erosion and sclerosis in cartilaginous joints; erosion and bone proliferation at sites of tendon and ligament attachment to bone; and osteolysis of terminal phalanges.

For many years after the original descriptions of psoriatic arthritis in the late nineteenth century, the joint abnormalities associated with psoriasis were considered to be part of the spectrum of rheumatoid arthritis. Currently, however, the concept that a specific type of arthritis occurs in psoriasis is rarely challenged, but the definition of this arthritis frequently varies from one report to another. This articular disorder has a wide clinical and radiologic spectrum, and placing undue emphasis on any one of its many manifestations may lead to misdiagnosis of others.

INCIDENCE AND SPECTRUM OF PSORIATIC ARTHRITIS

The reported frequency of articular abnormalities in patients with psoriasis has varied from less than 0.5 per cent to greater than 40 per cent. Estimates of the frequency of arthritis in patients with psoriasis in the range of 2 to 6 per cent appear most accurate. Conversely, the reported prevalence of psoriasis among patients with polyarticular arthritis has ranged from 3 to 5 per cent.

Five broad clinical varieties of psoriatic arthritis have been recognized: (1) polyarthritis characterized by distal interphalangeal joint involvement; (2) a deforming type of arthritis characterized by widespread ankylosis and, occasionally, arthritis mutilans; (3) a symmetric seronegative polyarthritis simulating rheumatoid arthritis but without its laboratory parameters; (4) monoarthritis or asymmetric oligoarthritis; and (5) sacroiliitis and spondylitis resembling ankylosing spondylitis (Table 25–1). Although radiographic abnormalities accompany these five types of disease, features in certain groups are much more specific than those in other groups, and in some patients, a single diagnosis of psoriatic arthritis on the basis of radiographic changes cannot be accomplished.

CLINICAL ABNORMALITIES

The age of onset of psoriatic arthritis does not differ significantly from that of rheumatoid arthritis. In most adult patients, a long history of psoriatic skin disease is evident, although in a few individuals, the articular abnormalities coincide with or antedate the appearance of the skin lesions. Articular disease is much more prevalent in patients with moderate or severe skin abnormalities. Furthermore, the severe deforming arthropathy of psoriasis commonly is associated with extensive and exfoliative cutaneous changes. Other than these associations between skin and joint manifestations, it is the nail abnormalities that appear to correlate most closely with articular disease. These nail changes, which include pitting, discoloration, ridging, splintering, erosion, thickening, and detachment, are common at the onset of articular disease and generally are apparent in the same digit in which there is significant distal interphalangeal articular abnormality.

The clinical nature of the articular disease is variable. A monoarticular, pauciarticular, or polyarticular distribution can be encountered, and virtually any joint can be affected, although the small joints of the hands and feet are involved most frequently. In some patients, however, low back complaints predominate, related to involvement of the spine and the sacroiliac joints. The articular symptoms may be acute or insidious in nature. Soft tissue swelling can be prominent, and, indeed, an entire digit may be enlarged (sausage digit). Subcutaneous nodules characteristically are not evident. Additional clinical manifestations may include fatigue, fever, stiffness, and ocular problems, such as conjunctivitis, iritis, and scleritis.

Table 25–1. VARIED PATTERNS OF PSORIATIC ARTHRITIS*

Polyarthritis with distal interphalangeal joint involvement
Symmetric seronegative polyarthritis simulating rheumatoid arthritis
Monoarthritis or asymmetric oligoarthritis
Sacroiliitis and spondylitis
Arthritis mutilans

*In addition, patients with psoriasis may have coincidental rheumatoid arthritis.

Laboratory analysis confirms the absence of serologically detectable rheumatoid factor in the majority of patients. Additional laboratory parameters may include a mild anemia, elevated erythrocyte sedimentation rate, occasionally elevated levels of serum uric acid, and raised concentrations of IgG antiglobulins. The histocompatibility antigen HLA-B27 frequently is present in patients with psoriasis and sacroiliitis.

RADIOGRAPHIC ABNORMALITIES (TABLE 25–2)

In the initial phase of psoriatic arthritis, radiographs may be entirely normal. Early radiographic abnormalities, which may include soft tissue swelling and some degree of osteoporosis, can resolve without any permanent sequelae. With clinical progression of articular problems, more extensive radiographic abnormalities appear, and these may worsen at a variable rate. Significant joint destruction and deformity are more characteristic of psoriatic arthritis than of Reiter's syndrome.

Distribution of Radiographic Abnormalities (Fig. 25–1)

Psoriatic arthritis can affect synovial and cartilaginous joints and sites of tendon and ligament attachment to bone in both the appendicular and the axial skeleton. In this regard, it is similar to Reiter's syndrome and ankylosing spondylitis and differs from rheumatoid arthritis.

Certain characteristics of psoriatic arthritis deserve emphasis. An asymmetric or even unilateral appearance is much more common in psoriatic arthritis than in rheumatoid arthritis. Both upper extremity and lower extremity joints are affected in psoriatic arthritis. This differs from the distribution of Reiter's syndrome, which involves predominantly the joints of the lower extremity. Distal interphalangeal and proximal interphalangeal articulations (as well as metacarpophalangeal and metatarsophalangeal joints) of the hand and the foot are commonly affected. Abnormalities of the phalangeal tufts and calcaneus are also characteristic. In the axial skeleton, sacroiliac joint and spinal abnormalities predominate. Elsewhere in the axial skeleton, the manubriosternal, sternoclavicular, and costovertebral joints, the symphysis pubis, and the tendinous connections of the pelvis may demonstrate significant changes.

General Radiographic Abnormalities (Fig. 25–2)

SOFT TISSUE SWELLING. Fusiform soft tissue swelling is frequently evident, reflecting the presence of synovial effusions and soft tissue edema.

OSTEOPOROSIS. Osteoporosis is not a prominent feature of psoriatic arthritis. This lack of osteoporosis is a reliable sign in the differentiation of psoriatic arthritis from rheuma-

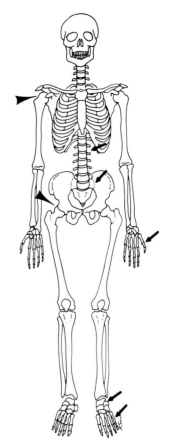

Figure 25–1. Psoriatic arthritis: Distribution of radiographic abnormalities. The most typical sites are the interphalangeal joints of the hand and the foot, the metacarpophalangeal and metatarsophalangeal joints, the calcaneus, the sacroiliac joint, and the spine (arrows). Changes in the knee, ankle, manubriosternal, sternoclavicular, acromioclavicular, and costovertebral joints, symphysis pubis, tendinous connections of the pelvis, elbow, and wrist are not uncommon. Significant alterations of the hip and the glenohumeral joint are relatively unusual (arrowheads).

toid arthritis, although the presence of osteoporosis does not eliminate the diagnosis of psoriatic arthritis.

JOINT SPACE NARROWING AND WIDENING. The articular space may be narrowed or widened. In large joints, diffuse loss of interosseous space is identical to that observed in rheumatoid arthritis. In the small joints of the fingers and toes, severe destruction of marginal and subchondral bone can lead to considerable widening of the articular space.

BONE EROSION. Erosive abnormalities are prominent in psoriatic arthritis. Initially, erosions predominate in the marginal areas of the joint, but as they progress, central areas are also affected. Over a period of time, it appears as if the bones are being gnawed away. In the small articulations of the hands and feet, bone destruction may produce a small blunt osseous surface that projects into the expanded base of a neighboring phalanx, in a pencil-and-cup or cup-and-saucer appearance.

BONE PROLIFERATION. As in the other seronegative spondyloarthropathies, proliferation of bone is a striking feature of psoriatic arthritis. This proliferation about the erosions may create a spiculated, frayed, or "paintbrush" appearance. Osseous erosion in rheumatoid arthritis generally

---

Table 25–2. CHARACTERISTICS OF PSORIATIC ARTHRITIS

Involvement of synovial and cartilaginous joints and entheses
Asymmetric distribution more common than symmetric distribution
Involvement of interphalangeal joints of the hands and feet
Sacroiliitis and spondylitis with paravertebral ossification
Bone erosion with adjacent proliferation
Intra-articular bone ankylosis
Destruction of phalangeal tufts

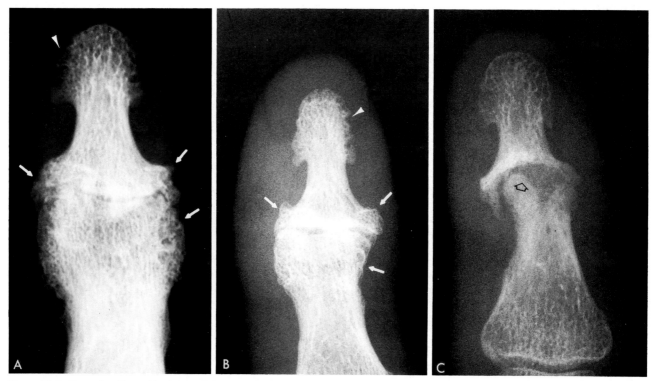

Figure 25–2. General radiographic abnormalities. Classic radiographic changes are depicted about the distal interphalangeal joints in three patients with psoriasis. These changes include soft tissue swelling, lack of osteoporosis, joint space narrowing, osseous erosions with accompanying proliferation (solid arrows), osteolysis with a pencil-and-cup-appearance (open arrow), and tuftal resorption (arrowheads).

is not associated with adjacent bone deposition. Although bone proliferation may accompany erosions in gouty arthritis, the resulting excrescences generally are well defined.

Periostitis in the metaphyses and diaphyses of bones is not uncommon in psoriatic arthritis, particularly in the hands and the feet. This change may appear early in the disease course, associated with soft tissue swelling, before significant abnormalities occur in the adjacent articulations. A similar abnormality accompanies Reiter's syndrome, juvenile chronic arthritis, and infection. Condensation of bone on the periosteal and endosteal surfaces of the cortex and trabecular thickening in the spongiosa can cause an entire phalanx to appear radiodense (the ivory phalanx).

Intraarticular osseous fusion is another manifestation of bone proliferation in psoriatic arthritis. It, too, is particularly prominent in the hands and feet. Although intraarticular osseous fusion is also observed in inflammatory (erosive) osteoarthritis, septic arthritis, and even rheumatoid arthritis (carpal and tarsal areas), it should be stressed as an important radiographic sign of the seronegative spondyloarthropathies (psoriatic arthritis, ankylosing spondylitis, and Reiter's syndrome).

Bone proliferation occurs at sites at which tendons and ligaments insert on bones. These include the posterior and inferior surfaces of the calcaneus, the femoral trochanters, the ischial tuberosities, the medial and lateral malleoli, the ulnar olecranon, the anterior surface of the patella, and the condyles of the distal femur and proximal tibia.

TUFTAL RESORPTION. Resorption of the tufts of the distal phalanges of the hands and feet is characteristic of

psoriatic arthritis. The eroded bone may be smoothly tapered or irregular in outline. Soft tissue swelling and adjacent interphalangeal joint abnormalities are frequent.

MALALIGNMENT AND SUBLUXATION. Deformities of the hands and the feet can be encountered in some patients with psoriatic arthritis. Telescoping of one bone on its neighbor may lead to the "operaglass hand." Ulnar deviation at the metacarpophalangeal joints, fibular deviation at the metatarsophalangeal joints, and boutonnière and swan-neck deformities are not so common in psoriatic arthritis as in rheumatoid arthritis.

Radiographic Abnormalities at Specific Sites

HAND (FIGS. 25–2 AND 25–3). It is the destructive arthritis of distal interphalangeal joints of the hand that is the best-known manifestation of psoriasis. At these sites, bilateral, symmetric or asymmetric, or unilateral changes are observed. Initial erosions occur at the margins of the joint and proceed centrally. The resulting irregular osseous surfaces may become separated from each other. It is this lack of apposition of adjacent bone margins that distinguishes the radiographic picture of psoriatic arthritis from that of osteoarthritis, in which closely applied undulating osseous surfaces are the rule. Adjacent proximal interphalangeal joints frequently are affected, and severe abnormalities may be encountered at the interphalangeal articulation of the thumb. The metacarpophalangeal articulations may be relatively spared.

At any altered interphalangeal site, radiographic findings may include separated and eroded, well-demarcated bone margins, protrusion of a blunted and distorted osseous surface

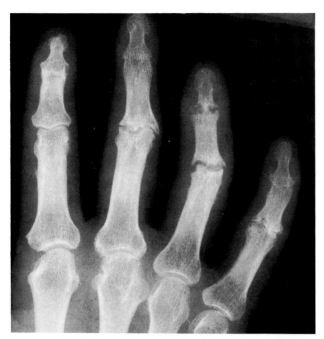

Figure 25–3. **Radiographic abnormalities of the hand.** Interphalangeal joint changes consist of articular space narrowing, intraarticular bone ankylosis, marginal and central erosions, and osteolysis of a phalangeal tuft. Metacarpophalangeal joint abnormalities, although less marked, include joint space narrowing, marginal erosions, and bone proliferation.

into an adjacent expanded one (pencil-and-cup appearance), irregular periosteal bone proliferation (whiskering), and intraarticular osseous fusion.

Tuftal resorption can be evident in one or more terminal phalanges. When severe, tuftal resorption is almost inevitably associated with destructive articular findings. Tuftal resorption simulates that seen in various connective tissue disorders,

particularly scleroderma, or after thermal injuries. Both phalangeal resorption and destructive arthritis of distal interphalangeal joints generally are associated with significant nail changes in the same digit.

WRIST. Abnormalities in the wrist in psoriatic arthritis are not so frequent as those in the fingers and are rarely encountered without more typical distal changes. Any compartment may be altered in one or both wrists.

OTHER UPPER EXTREMITY SITES. Psoriatic arthritis can lead to changes in the elbow, glenohumeral, acromioclavicular, and sternoclavicular joints. As at other sites, findings may vary from minor degrees of osseous erosion to extensive osteolysis.

FOREFOOT (FIG. 25–4). The forefoot is commonly affected in psoriatic arthritis. Bilateral, asymmetric changes predominate in the interphalangeal and metatarsophalangeal articulations and are characterized by the appearance of marginal erosions, bone proliferation, alterations in joint space, and lack of osteoporosis. Extensive destruction of the interphalangeal articulation of the great toe is more characteristic of this articular disorder than of any other disease. Osteolysis of tufts and of phalangeal and metatarsal shafts can be encountered. In the terminal phalanges, extensive new bone formation may lead to increased osseous density of the entire bone, the ivory phalanx.

CALCANEUS (FIG. 25–5). As in other seronegative spondyloarthropathies (Reiter's syndrome, ankylosing spondylitis), erosion and proliferation of the posterior or inferior surface of the calcaneus, or of both surfaces, may be prominent in psoriatic arthritis. Retrocalcaneal bursitis creates a radiodense area adjacent to the posterosuperior aspect of the bone. Subjacent erosion of the calcaneus is associated with surrounding bone proliferation. The neighboring Achilles tendon may be thickened. Inferiorly, erosions of the plantar aspect of the calcaneus frequently evoke extensive sclerosis of the surrounding bone, creating irregular and poorly defined spurs at the attachment sites of the plantar ligaments and aponeurosis.

Figure 25–4. **Radiographic abnormalities of the forefoot.** Findings include joint space narrowing and bone ankylosis of multiple interphalangeal joints and osseous erosion and proliferation, particularly about the interphalangeal joint of the great toe. Note tuftal osteolysis and sclerosis of bone in multiple digits.

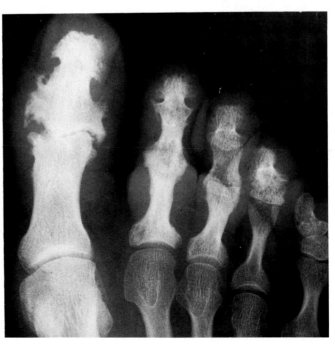

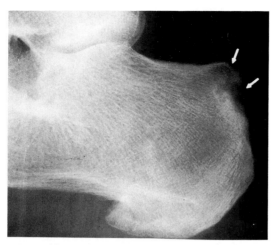

Figure 25–5. Abnormalities of the calcaneus. Retrocalcaneal bursitis is manifested as erosion of the posterosuperior aspect of the calcaneus (arrows). A large plantar calcaneal spur is identified.

OTHER LOWER EXTREMITY SITES (FIG. 25–6). Articular involvement in psoriasis may be apparent in the midfoot or hindfoot, the ankle, or the knee. Abnormality of the hip is relatively unusual.

SACROILIAC JOINT (FIG. 25–7). Ten to 25 per cent of patients with moderate or severe psoriatic skin disease will reveal sacroiliac joint changes on radiographic examination.

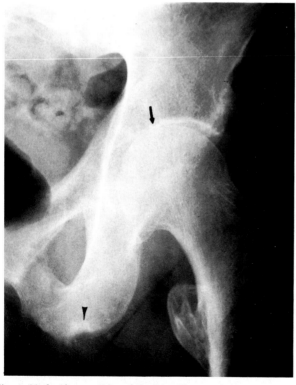

Figure 25–6. Abnormalities of the hip. Observe concentric joint space narrowing of the hip (arrow) associated with erosion and sclerosis of the ischial tuberosity (arrowhead). The sacroiliac joints and spine were also involved. The changes of the lesser trochanter are probably traumatic in origin.

Approximately 30 to 50 per cent of individuals with psoriatic arthritis will develop such changes. Bilateral abnormalities of the sacroiliac joint are much more frequent than unilateral changes in patients with psoriatic arthritis. Although asymmetric findings may be apparent, symmetric abnormalities predominate. Sacroiliitis can appear without spondylitis (in fact, spondylitis may appear without sacroiliitis).

Radiographic sacroiliac joint changes include erosions and sclerosis, predominantly in the ilium, and widening of the articular space. Although significant joint space diminution and bone ankylosis can occur, the frequency of these findings, particularly ankylosis, is less than that in classic ankylosing spondylitis or the spondylitis associated with inflammatory bowel disease. Above the true articulation, interosseous ligament calcification and ossification, as well as hyperostosis with blurring of the adjacent sacrum and ilium, can be noted. Bone proliferation is also apparent in the pelvis at tendoosseous junctions, such as the iliac crest and ischial tuberosities, and may be associated with similar changes of the trochanters and osteitis pubis.

SPINE (FIGS. 25–8 AND 25–9). As in Reiter's syndrome, paravertebral ossification about the lower thoracic and upper lumbar segments can occur in psoriatic arthritis, and it may represent an early manifestation of the disease. Initially, ossification appears as a thick and fluffy or thin and curvilinear radiodense region on one side of the spine, paralleling the lateral surface of the vertebral bodies and the intervertebral discs. Eventually it may produce a large and bulky outgrowth that merges with the underlying osseous and discal tissue. Its greater size, asymmetric distribution, and location farther away from the vertebral column are features that distinguish paravertebral ossification from typical syndesmophytosis of ankylosing spondylitis and of spondylitis in inflammatory bowel disease. Occasionally, however, slender, centrally located, and symmetric spinal outgrowths in psoriasis are identical to the syndesmophytes of ankylosing spondylitis.

In addition to the pattern and distribution of bone outgrowths, there are other features of psoriatic spondylitis that differ from those in classic ankylosing spondylitis. Osteitis and squaring of the anterior surfaces of the vertebral bodies are relatively infrequent in psoriasis. Although apophyseal joint space narrowing, sclerosis, and bone ankylosis may be seen, the frequency of these findings is much less than in ankylosing spondylitis.

Cervical spine abnormalities may become striking in patients with psoriasis. These abnormalities include apophyseal joint space narrowing and sclerosis, osseous irregularity at the discovertebral joint, and extensive proliferation along the anterior surface of the spine. Atlantoaxial subluxation can also be evident. Although anterior subluxation predominates, lateral instability, as observed in rheumatoid arthritis, is also encountered. Associated erosive and sclerotic abnormalities of the odontoid process are frequent in patients demonstrating atlantoaxial subluxation. Rarely, subaxial cervical instability with cord compression is evident in psoriatic spondylitis, resembling changes observed in rheumatoid arthritis.

OTHER SITES. The manubriosternal and sternoclavicular joints can reveal severe alterations, including soft tissue swelling, subchondral erosion, eburnation, and synostosis. The temporomandibular joint can also be affected significantly in psoriatic arthritis.

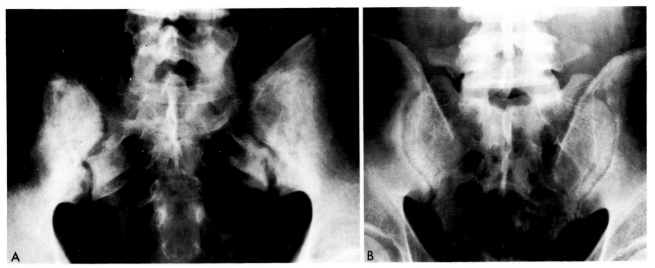

Figure 25–7. Abnormalities of the sacroiliac joint. A Bilateral and symmetric changes consist of erosions and sclerosis, predominantly in the ilium. Intraarticular bone ankylosis is not seen. Spinal alterations are present. **B** In this patient, asymmetric abnormalities are seen. The right sacroiliac articulation reveals joint space narrowing and sclerosis with blurring of the interosseous space above the true joint. Minimal changes are present on the left side.

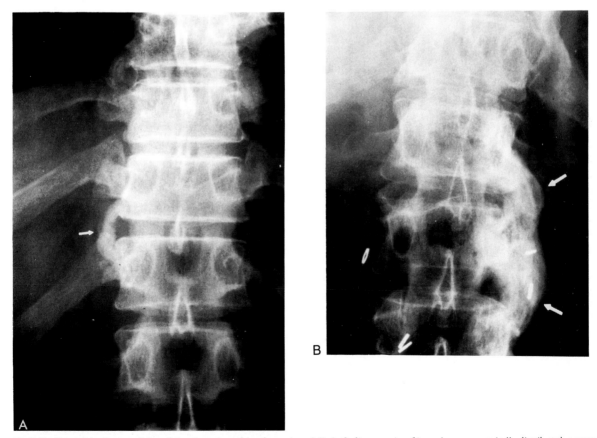

Figure 25–8. Radiographic abnormalities of the thoracic and lumbar spine. A Early findings consist of irregular, asymmetrically distributed, paravertebral bony excrescences (arrow), particularly at the thoracolumbar junction. **B** With progression (in a different patient), bulky outgrowths appear (arrows), which merge with the underlying vertebral bodies and intervertebral discs. Note the asymmetric distribution. Surgical clips are evident.

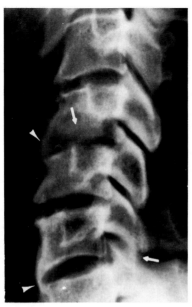

Figure 25–9. Radiographic abnormalities of the cervical spine. Note erosions at the discovertebral junction and apophyseal joints (arrows) and syndesmophytes (arrowheads).

RADIONUCLIDE ABNORMALITIES

Scintigraphy with bone-seeking radiopharmaceutic agents can reveal articular abnormality of psoriatic arthritis prior to its appearance on radiographic examination. Increased radionuclide accumulation predominates at interphalangeal, metacarpophalangeal, and metatarsophalangeal joints of the hands and feet; however, calcaneal, sacroiliac joint, and spinal uptake can be considerable. The asymmetric nature of the scintigraphic alterations in psoriasis will frequently permit its differentiation from rheumatoid arthritis.

PATHOLOGIC ABNORMALITIES

Although the pathologic changes of psoriatic arthritis are basically similar to those of rheumatoid arthritis, there are also some pathologic characteristics of psoriasis that are distinctive. Synovial inflammation is encountered but the degree of cellular infiltration with lymphocytes and plasma cells is much less marked than in rheumatoid arthritis. Early fibrosis of the proliferating synovium is typical of psoriatic arthritis. Inflammatory synovial tissue, or pannus, is prominent only on the surface of the cartilage, whereas in rheumatoid arthritis, hyperplastic synovium is seen in both superficial and deep layers of the cartilage. Bone proliferation is evident in periarticular regions. This may take the form of subchondral trabecular thickening and periosteal bone formation. Fibrous ankylosis of the joint may be noted, as in rheumatoid arthritis. However, in psoriatic arthritis, bony ankylosis is also prominent.

These pathologic aberrations explain some of the more characteristic radiographic features of psoriatic arthritis. The lack of both intense synovial inflammation and severe synovial hyperemia in this disease may account for the absence of significant periarticular osteoporosis. Articular space loss, which is almost universal in rheumatoid arthritis, is much less constant in psoriatic arthritis. In the latter disease, the degree of chondrolysis by the inflamed synovium is variable.

A tendency to new bone formation can be profound. Within the articulation, metaplastic bone can produce partial or complete osseous fusion.

ETIOLOGY AND PATHOGENESIS

Hereditary factors appear to be important in the pathogenesis of uncomplicated psoriasis, but the exact mode of inheritance is not known. Histocompatibility typing among patients with cutaneous disease has revealed an increased frequency of HLA-BW17, HLA-B13, and, more recently, HLA-BW16, indicating that these antigens may be an important genetic marker for the inherited skin manifestations of psoriasis.

The role of heredity in the articular manifestations of this disease has also been emphasized. Histocompatibility typing in patients with psoriatic arthritis has revealed a high frequency (approximately 25 to 60 per cent) of HLA-B27 antigen, particularly in patients with sacroiliitis and spondylitis, but also in those with distal interphalangeal joint involvement. Similarly, elevation of HLA-BW38, CW6, and DR4 has been observed in patients with psoriatic arthritis.

ADDITIONAL DISEASES OF SKIN AND JOINTS

Certain cutaneous disorders are associated with clinical and radiologic findings of arthritis, which in some cases simulate those of psoriasis. *Acne fulminans* is associated with systemic manifestations that include polyarthralgias. Although the joint involvement is usually asymptomatic, sacroiliitis and synovitis in peripheral joints have been observed. In *acne conglobata*, articular disease is seen in adults. Bone erosion about the small joints of the hand, wrist, and foot, periostitis, soft tissue swelling, and osteoporosis are noted. In the axial skeleton, unilateral or bilateral sacroiliitis and syndesmophytosis are the reported manifestations (Fig. 25–10).

Pustular lesions of the skin in the hand and foot (*pustulosis palmaris et plantaris*) are observed in some individuals who develop hyperostosis in the clavicles, upper ribs, and sternum. The syndrome, which is termed sternocostoclavicular hyperostosis, is discussed in Chapter 37.

DIFFERENTIAL DIAGNOSIS (TABLE 25–3)
Other Seronegative Spondyloarthropathies (Ankylosing Spondylitis, Reiter's Syndrome)

The radiographic findings in psoriatic arthritis are fundamentally similar to those in the other two seronegative spondyloarthropathies, ankylosing spondylitis and Reiter's syndrome. In all three disorders, synovial joint involvement is characterized by the absence of osteoporosis and the presence of soft tissue swelling, joint space abnormality, osseous erosion, and bone proliferation. In psoriatic arthritis and ankylosing spondylitis, intraarticular bone ankylosis is not uncommon. In each of these seronegative spondyloarthropathies, abnormalities of cartilaginous joints, consisting of erosion and bone proliferation, may be observed. Similarly, each of these diseases may be associated with abnormalities at tendon and ligament attachments to bone (calcaneus, femoral trochanters, ischial tuberosities).

The distribution of articular abnormalities differs among psoriatic arthritis, Reiter's syndrome, and ankylosing spondylitis. In psoriatic arthritis, an asymmetric polyarticular disorder involving upper and lower extremities with predilection for interphalangeal joints of the hands and metatarso-

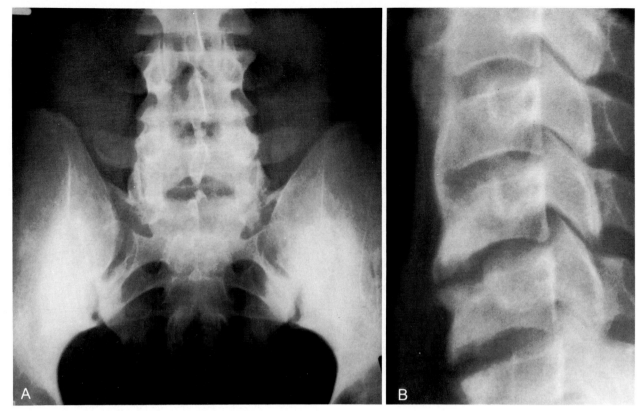

Figure 25–10. Acne conglobata. A In a 20 year old man with acne conglobata, observe bilateral symmetric sacroiliitis. (Courtesy of A. Brower, M.D., Washington, D.C.) B In a different patient with the same disease, bone proliferation involves the anterior surface of the cervical vertebral bodies. Syndesmophytes are seen. The apophyseal joints are normal. (Courtesy of N. Kinnis, M.D., Chicago, Illinois.)

Table 25–3. DIFFERENTIAL DIAGNOSIS OF PSORIATIC ARTHRITIS

	Psoriatic Arthritis	**Reiter's Syndrome**	**Rheumatoid Arthritis**
Types of involved articulations	Synovial Joints	Synovial Joints	Synovial joints*
	Symphyses	Symphyses	
	Entheses	Entheses	
Distribution of arthritis	Appendicular and axial skeleton	Appendicular and axial skeleton	Appendicular and axial skeleton
	Polyarticular or pauciarticular	Polyarticular or pauciarticular	Polyarticular
	Symmetric, asymmetric, or unilateral	Asymmetric	Symmetric
	Upper and lower extremities	Lower extremities	Upper and lower extremities
	Sacroiliac joints and entire spine	Sacroiliac joints and, less commonly, spine	Cervical spine
Nature of lesions†			
Osteoporosis	+	+	+ +
Soft tissue swelling	+ +	+ +	+ +
Joint space narrowing	+	+	+ +
Severe periarticular osteolysis	+ +	+	+.
Intra-articular bone ankylosis	+ +	+ +‡	+
Bone proliferation and periostitis	+ +	+ +	− §
Tuftal resorption	+ +	−	−

*Symphyses and entheses are less commonly and less extensively involved in rheumatoid arthritis than in psoriatic arthritis or Reiter's syndrome.
†− = absent; + = occasionally present; + + = commonly present.
‡Less frequent than in psoriatic arthritis.
§Occasionally seen in male patients with rheumatoid arthritis and in those with both rheumatoid arthritis and diffuse idiopathic skeletal hyperostosis.

phalangeal and interphalangeal joints of the feet is observed. In Reiter's syndrome, asymmetric disease of the articulations of the lower extremity is most characteristic, whereas in ankylosing spondylitis, appendicular skeletal involvement is less prominent than axial skeletal involvement.

Spinal and sacroiliac joint alterations occur in psoriatic arthritis, Reiter's syndrome, and ankylosing spondylitis. In the former two disorders, symmetric or asymmetric abnormalities of the sacroiliac joints and large, broad excrescences of the spine may be seen. In ankylosing spondylitis (as well as in the sacroiliitis and spondylitis of inflammatory bowel disease), bilateral, symmetric sacroiliac joint abnormalities are almost universal, and spinal changes typically consist of thin, linear, and symmetrically distributed outgrowths. In ankylosing spondylitis, apophyseal joint involvement and osteitis with squaring of vertebral bodies are more frequent than in either psoriatic arthritis or Reiter's syndrome.

Rheumatoid Arthritis

In some patients with psoriatic arthritis, the distribution of articular abnormalities in the appendicular skeleton is similar to that in rheumatoid arthritis, whereas in others, asymmetry and extensive distal interphalangeal articular alterations facilitate differentiation from rheumatoid arthritis. In the latter disease, osteoporosis, diffuse joint space narrowing, marginal erosions, and fibrous ankylosis are most characteristic. In psoriatic arthritis, severe marginal and central erosions, bone ankylosis, and the absence of osteoporosis are typical. Furthermore, in psoriatic arthritis, bone proliferation leads to fraying or irregularity of periarticular bone surfaces, a finding not evident in rheumatoid arthritis.

Rheumatoid involvement of the vertebral column is characterized by severe cervical spinal changes. Paravertebral ossification is not observed. Furthermore, sacroiliac joint abnormalities are a minor feature of rheumatoid arthritis.

Other Disorders

Erosive arthritis of distal interphalangeal joints can be observed in many disease processes, including inflammatory (erosive) osteoarthritis, multicentric reticulohistiocytosis, gout, and scleroderma, and after thermal injuries. In most of these disorders, obvious clinical findings allow differentiation from psoriatic arthritis. In addition, in inflammatory (erosive) osteoarthritis, osteophytes are evident, and the erosions may predominate in the central regions of the articulation. In gout, asymmetric soft tissue masses, eccentric erosive changes, preservation of joint space, and osseous proliferation in the form of bone spicules (overhanging edges) are frequent. In scleroderma, soft tissue tuftal calcification is a helpful diagnostic clue. Differentiation of multicentric reticulohistiocytosis and psoriasis on the basis of interphalangeal joint abnormalities can be extremely difficult.

FURTHER READING

Avila R, Pugh D, Slocumb CH, Winkelmann RK: Psoriatic arthritis: A roentgenologic study. Radiology 75:691, 1960.

Forrester DM: The "cocktail sausage" digit. Arthritis Rheum 26:664, 1983.

Hanly JG, Russell ML, Gladman DD: Psoriatic spondyloarthropathy: A long term prospective study. Ann Rheum Dis 47:386, 1988.

Houben HHML, Lemmens JAM, Boerbooms AMT: Sacroiliitis and acne conglobata. Clin Rheumatol 4:86, 1985.

Martel W, Stuck KJ, Dworin AM, Hylland RG: Erosive osteoarthritis and psoriatic arthritis: A radiologic comparison in the hand, wrist, and foot. AJR 134:125, 1980.

Meaney TF, Hays RA: Roentgen manifestations of psoriatic arthritis. Radiology 68:403, 1957.

McEwen C, DiTata D, Lingg C, Porini A, Good A, Rankin T: Ankylosing spondylitis and spondylitis accompanying ulcerative colitis, regional enteritis, psoriasis, and Reiter's disease. Arthritis Rheum 14:291, 1971.

Moll JMH, Wright V: Psoriatic arthritis. Semin Arthritis Rheum 3:55, 1973.

Resnick D, Niwayama G: On the nature and significance of bony proliferation in "rheumatoid variant" disorders. AJR 129:275, 1977.

Sundaram M, Patton JT: Paravertebral ossification in psoriasis and Reiter's disease. Br J Radiol 48:628, 1975.

Chapter 26

Reiter's Syndrome

Donald Resnick, M.D.

Reiter's syndrome has a distinctive radiographic appearance. Synovial and cartilaginous joints as well as sites of tendon and ligament attachment to bone are involved. In the appendicular skeleton, an asymmetric arthritis of the articulations of the lower extremity distal to the hip is most typical. Extensive changes may be observed in the foot. In the axial skeleton, bilateral symmetric or asymmetric (or even unilateral) sacroiliac joint abnormalities are seen. Paravertebral ossification may produce bulky outgrowths.

The classic triad of Reiter's syndrome consists of urethritis, arthritis, and conjunctivitis. The syndrome is named after the investigator who, in 1916, linked this triad with an acute dysenteric illness in a cavalry officer serving on the Balkan front, although he falsely attributed the abnormalities to syphilis. Although currently it is recognized that many patients who apparently have Reiter's syndrome will not demonstrate the entire clinical triad, its place in the spectrum of rheumatic disorders is firmly established. Although radiographic findings may not be an essential part of criteria used to diagnose Reiter's syndrome, few investigators would dispute that radiographs are important in the evaluation of patients with this syndrome.

Reiter's syndrome is accompanied by typical radiographic features, which it shares with other seronegative spondyloarthropathies (psoriatic arthritis and ankylosing spondylitis). It is the distribution of articular abnormalities that allows a firm radiographic diagnosis in many patients with Reiter's syndrome.

CLINICAL ABNORMALITIES

Reiter's syndrome is a relatively uncommon articular disorder. It has greater prevalence in military personnel. It appears likely that the disease can be transmitted in association with either epidemic dysentery or sexual intercourse.

Most patients with Reiter's syndrome are between 15 and 35 years of age. At any age, the disease is much more common in men than in women, the cited ratio of males to females ranging between 5 to 1 and 50 to 1. Reiter's syndrome in female patients is especially common after dysentery and may consist of arthritis, conjunctivitis, and cystitis. The intestinal variety of the disease usually follows bacillary dysentery, although the syndrome may occur after amebic dysentery, shigellosis, and additional gastrointestinal disorders.

General Symptoms and Signs

Urethritis frequently is the initial manifestation of the disease. Although it may be asymptomatic, mucopurulent urethral discharge, dysuria, urinary frequency, and local pain can be associated with an enlarged, soft, and tender prostate gland on physical examination. Circinate balanitis has been noted in 20 to 80 per cent of patients with dysenteric and sexually transmitted forms of Reiter's syndrome. This penile lesion may be the initial mucocutaneous manifestation of the disease.

Early and transient conjunctivitis frequently accompanies the acute attack. Later and more severe ocular involvement may include episcleritis, keratitis, uveitis, iritis, retrobulbar neuritis, corneal ulceration, and intraocular hemorrhage.

The characteristic skin lesion, which occurs in 5 to 30 per cent of patients, is termed keratoderma blenorrhagicum. It is most commonly noted on the soles of the feet and the palms of the hands. Keratosis of the nails may also be observed, simulating the findings of psoriasis. The skin abnormalities frequently are self-limited, persisting for several weeks and then peeling, leaving no residual scar. On the buccal mucosa and the tongue, superficial erythematous ulcerations may be evident in 5 to 10 per cent of patients. Reiter's syndrome may involve other organ systems, including the gastrointestinal tract and the cardiovascular, neurologic, and pulmonary systems.

Additional clinical findings in Reiter's syndrome include fever, weight loss, thrombophlebitis, amyloidosis, and rheumatoid arthritis. Characteristic laboratory findings can include leukocytosis, anemia, and elevation of the erythrocyte sedimentation rate. The serum histocompatibility antigen HLA-B27 may be present in as many as 75 per cent of patients.

Articular Symptoms and Signs

Characteristically, an asymmetric arthritis of the lower extremity becomes evident in Reiter's syndrome. Initially, the most commonly affected joints are the knee and the ankle. Monoarticular arthritis predominates in the early phase of the disease. Subsequently, more widespread articular changes occur, with predilection for the knee, the ankle, the shoulder, the wrist, and the metatarsophalangeal joints, in descending order of frequency.

The occurrence of heel pain and tenderness should be stressed as a common manifestation of Reiter's syndrome. The pain, which may be located posteriorly or inferiorly, can be the initial symptom of the disease, and it can persist for a period of years.

The arthritic attacks of Reiter's syndrome are usually self-limited and of short duration, although recurrences are frequent. Residual disability and deformity occur in approximately 5 per cent of patients.

On joint aspiration, inflammatory synovial fluid is recovered. Occasionally the degree of polymorphonuclear leukocytosis within the fluid is so great as to resemble a purulent arthritis.

RADIOGRAPHIC ABNORMALITIES (TABLE 26–1)

It has been estimated by some observers that 60 to 80 per cent of patients with Reiter's syndrome will develop radiographic alterations. In the early phases of the disease, radiographs may be entirely normal. Acute attacks of arthritis may be accompanied by soft tissue swelling and osteoporosis, but these findings can then disappear completely, without residual abnormalities. With repeated episodes of arthritis, however, permanent radiographic abnormalities are very common.

Distribution of Radiographic Abnormalities

Synovial joints, symphyses, and entheses are affected. Typically, an asymmetric distribution with predilection for articulations of the lower extremity is seen (Fig. 26–1). The most characteristic sites of abnormality are the small joints of the foot, the calcaneus, the ankle, and the knee. Joint alterations in the upper extremity are less frequent, and abnormalities of the hip are uncommon. In the axial skeleton, the sacroiliac joints, the spine, the symphysis pubis, and the manubriosternal joint are frequent target areas.

General Radiographic Abnormalities

The general radiographic characteristics of articular involvement in Reiter's syndrome are similar to those in the other seronegative spondyloarthropathies (ankylosing spondylitis and psoriatic arthritis) and differ from the findings of rheumatoid arthritis (Fig. 26–2).

SOFT TISSUE SWELLING. Soft tissue prominence is related to intraarticular effusion, periarticular edema, and inflammation of bursal and tendinous structures. This finding may result in sausage-like swelling of an entire digit.

OSTEOPOROSIS. Regional or periarticular osteoporosis accompanies acute episodes of arthritis. With recurrent or prolonged bouts of articular disease, osteoporosis may decrease in extent and severity.

JOINT SPACE NARROWING. Loss of the interosseous space is more frequent in the small joints of the foot, hand, and wrist than in the knee and the ankle. Diffuse loss of articular space is more characteristic than is asymmetric joint space diminution.

BONE EROSION. Erosion of articular surfaces may be noted in both the appendicular and the axial skeleton. Erosions initially appear at the joint margins and may later progress to involve the subchondral bone in the central portion of the articulation. Superficial resorption of the osseous surface may

Table 26–1. CHARACTERISTICS OF ARTHRITIS IN REITER'S SYNDROME

Involvement of synovial joints, symphyses, and entheses
Asymmetric arthritis of the lower extremities
Predilection for the small articulations of the foot, the
   calcaneus, the ankle, the knee, and the sacroiliac joint
Bone erosion with adjacent proliferation
Paravertebral ossification

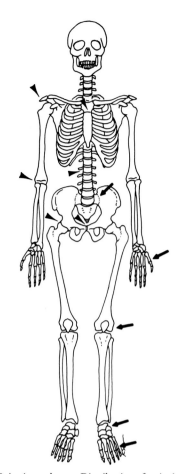

Figure 26–1. Reiter's syndrome: Distribution of articular abnormalities. The most characteristic sites of involvement are the small joints of the foot, calcaneus, ankle, knee, hand, and sacroiliac joint (arrows). Less commonly, the shoulder, elbow, hip, spine, symphysis pubis, and manubriosternal joint are affected (arrowheads).

also occur beneath inflamed bursae and tendon sheaths. The osseous erosions are not distinct in outline. Rather, adjacent bone proliferation produces an irregular osseous surface.

BONE PROLIFERATION. Bone proliferation is particularly characteristic of all three seronegative spondyloarthropathies and is the most helpful radiographic feature in distinguishing these conditions from rheumatoid arthritis. Linear or fluffy periosteal bone proliferation is not uncommon in Reiter's syndrome, especially in the metacarpal, metatarsal, and phalangeal shafts, the malleolar region, and the knee. Periostitis can occur without adjacent articular abnormality.

A second variety of bone proliferation occurs at sites of tendon and ligament attachment to bone. These sites include the plantar aspect of the calcaneus, the ischial tuberosity, the trochanters, and the apposing portions of sacrum and ilium about the true sacroiliac articulation. The osseous surfaces frequently appear poorly defined or frayed.

Intraarticular bone production occurs about sites of osseous erosion. The eroded bone surfaces appear irregular or fuzzy in outline, and the articular bone may be enlarged. Intraarticular bone ankylosis has been recorded in the small joints of the hands and feet in Reiter's syndrome, but this complication is far less frequent in this disease than in ankylosing spondylitis and psoriatic arthritis.

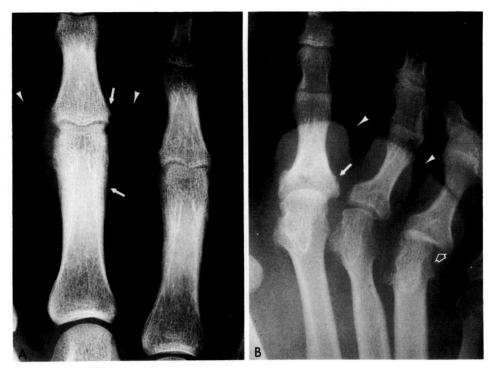

Figure 26–2. General radiographic abnormalities. Note the absence of osteoporosis and the presence of soft tissue swelling (arrowheads), periostitis and "whiskering" (solid arrows), osseous erosions, and subluxation (open arrow).

TENDINOUS CALCIFICATION AND OSSIFICATION. Tendinous calcification and ossification are frequent about the knee in patients with Reiter's syndrome at which site the findings can resemble Pellegrini-Stieda syndrome (posttraumatic calcification of the medial collateral ligament).

Specific Sites of Abnormality

FOREFOOT (FIG. 26–3). Radiographs of the feet frequently reveal asymmetric involvement of the metatarsophalangeal and interphalangeal joints. Selective involvement of the interphalangeal joint of the great toe suggests the diagnosis of Reiter's syndrome or psoriasis. At any location in the foot, osteoporosis, joint space loss, and marginal erosions with adjacent proliferation can be observed as well as periostitis of neighboring diaphyses of metatarsal bones and phalanges. The sesamoid bones can demonstrate significant erosion and proliferation.

Subluxation and deformity of the metatarsophalangeal joints may be evident, an appearance that has been termed Launois's deformity.

CALCANEUS (FIGS. 26–4 AND 26–5). Calcaneal alterations are characteristic of Reiter's syndrome. Both the posterior and the plantar aspects of the bone are affected. Bilateral changes are frequent. Retrocalcaneal bursitis with fluid accumulation creates a radiodense shadow that, on lateral radiographs, obliterates the normal lucent area that exists between the top of the calcaneus and the adjacent Achilles tendon and projects into the preachilles fat pad. Subsequently, poorly defined calcaneal erosions appear on the posterosuperior aspect of the bone. The Achilles tendon frequently is thickened.

On the plantar surface of the bone, osseous erosion, hyperostosis, and poorly defined spurs may develop. The excrescences are similar to those occurring in psoriatic arthritis and ankylosing spondylitis. Initially these spurs appear irreg-

ular in outline, although they may become better defined on follow-up radiographs.

HAND AND WRIST (FIG. 26–6). In the hand, proximal interphalangeal joint abnormalities are more frequent than metacarpophalangeal or distal interphalangeal joint alterations, although the metacarpophalangeal and interphalangeal articulations of the thumb may be affected. Fusiform soft tissue swelling, regional or periarticular osteoporosis, and joint space narrowing can be evident. The erosive changes are accompanied by fluffy new bone formation. Such proliferation can also involve adjacent sesamoids.

Abnormalities may also be apparent in one or both wrists. Involvement is usually asymmetric, although any compartment can be affected.

MANUBRIOSTERNAL JOINT AND SYMPHYSIS PUBIS. Osseous erosion and adjacent bone proliferation at the manubriosternal joint and symphysis pubis are not rare in Reiter's disease. Similar abnormalities occur in the other spondyloarthropathies.

SACROILIAC JOINT (FIG. 26–7). Sacroiliitis is common in Reiter's syndrome. Initially, abnormalities may be detected in 5 to 10 per cent of patients, whereas after several years, the occurrence of sacroiliac joint alterations may reach 40 to 60 per cent. Bilateral symmetric or asymmetric changes are most typical. As opposed to the situation in classic ankylosing spondylitis, however, in which bilateral and symmetric changes are the rule, asymmetric and, less commonly, unilateral sacroiliac joint abnormalities in Reiter's syndrome do occur, particularly early in the disease process.

Osseous erosion and sclerosis on the iliac surface predominate over those on the sacral surface. Early joint space widening may later be replaced by narrowing of the space between sacrum and ilium. Although intraarticular osseous fusion may eventually appear, this finding is less frequent in Reiter's syndrome than in classic ankylosing spondylitis and

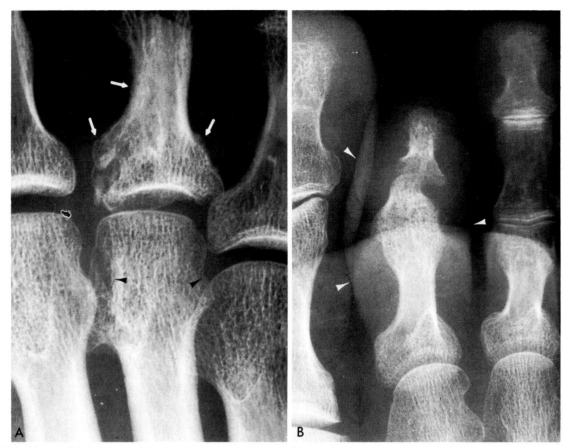

Figure 26–3. Abnormalities of the forefoot. A A magnification radiograph of the third metatarsophalangeal joint outlines erosions of the metatarsal head (arrowheads) and adjacent bone proliferation (arrows). The joint space is not narrowed. **B** A radiograph of the forefoot reveals soft tissue swelling of the second digit (arrowheads), destruction of the distal interphalangeal joint, and intraarticular bone ankylosis of the proximal interphalangeal joint. Note the absence of osteoporosis.

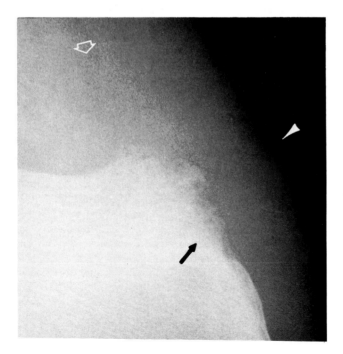

Figure 26–4. Abnormalities of the calcaneus: Posterior aspect. Soft tissue swelling (arrowhead), retrocalcaneal bursitis (open arrow), and irregular osseous erosion and proliferation (solid arrow) are apparent.

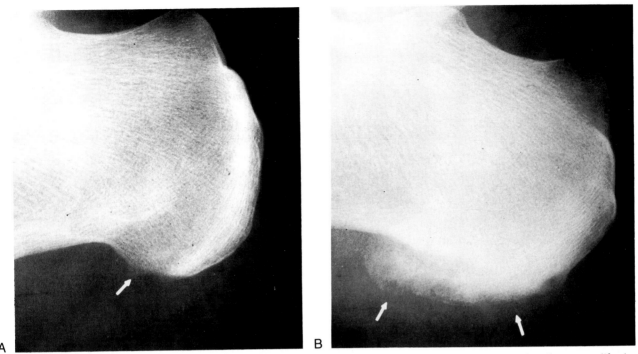

Figure 26–5. Abnormalities of the calcaneus: Plantar aspect. Radiographs obtained 2 years apart reveal striking progression of osseous proliferation (arrows). Note the poor definition of the developing outgrowth.

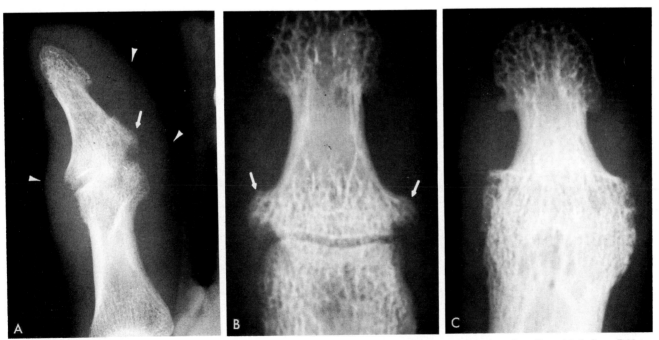

Figure 26–6. Abnormalities of the hand. A Soft tissue swelling (arrowheads), erosion, and bone proliferation (arrow) are the radiographic findings. **B** Note joint space narrowing and irregular excrescences or "whiskers" (arrows) at the margins of the distal interphalangeal joint. **C** In another patient, intraarticular bone ankylosis is evident.

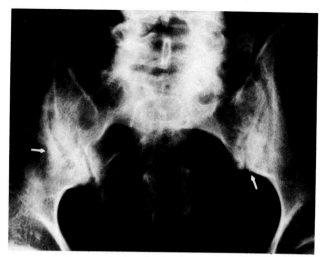

Figure 26–7. Abnormalities of the sacroiliac joint. Bilateral and asymmetric alterations are observed. Erosions and reactive eburnation predominate in the ilium (arrows).

the sacroiliitis of inflammatory bowel disease. A prominent finding in both Reiter's syndrome and psoriasis may be blurring and eburnation of apposing sacral and iliac surfaces above the true joint in the region of the interosseous ligament.

SPINE (FIG. 26–8). Although abnormalities of the spine occur in Reiter's syndrome, their frequency and extent are less than in classic ankylosing spondylitis and psoriatic arthritis. When present, the changes may resemble those of ankylosing spondylitis, although specific radiographic features frequently allow accurate differentiation of the two conditions.

An early finding in Reiter's syndrome (and psoriatic arthritis) is the appearance of paravertebral ossification about the lower three thoracic and upper three lumbar vertebrae.

On frontal radiographs, elongated vertical osseous bridges extend across the intervertebral disc but are separated by a clear space from the lateral margins of both the disc and the vertebral body. The outgrowths may be either well defined and linear or thick and fluffy. Their course is variable, although many of the ossifications eventually fuse with the underlying intervertebral disc and vertebral body, simulating the appearance of bulky osteophytes (spondylosis deformans). Involvement of large segments of the thoracic and lumbar spine as well as the cervical spine may eventually be noted.

The importance of recognizing paravertebral ossification is twofold: The finding may be an initial manifestation of the disease; and the abnormality is diagnostic of Reiter's syndrome or psoriatic arthritis rather than of classic ankylosing spondylitis or the spondylitis associated with inflammatory bowel disease. The asymmetric distribution (right and left sides), the broader or bulkier nature of the radiodense areas, and their relatively distant position from the spine are characteristic of paravertebral ossification. It must be stressed, however, that some patients with Reiter's syndrome and psoriatic arthritis develop typical syndesmophytes of the spine, which may progress to a bamboo spine appearance. In these patients, accurate differentiation among the seronegative spondyloarthropathies cannot be accomplished. Furthermore, apophyseal joint erosion, sclerosis, and osseous fusion may be apparent in Reiter's syndrome, although the frequency of these findings is less than in classic ankylosing spondylitis. Erosion or "osteitis" along the anterior corners of vertebral bodies is also uncommon in Reiter's syndrome.

Cervical spine abnormalities are not frequent in Reiter's syndrome. Occasionally, paravertebral ossification, irregularity at discovertebral junctions and apophyseal joints, atlantoaxial subluxation, and odontoid erosion are evident.

RADIONUCLIDE ABNORMALITIES

Scintigraphy with bone-seeking radiopharmaceutical agents may allow early diagnosis of Reiter's syndrome and provide a more accurate appraisal of the extent of disease. The distribution of abnormal radionuclide accumulation parallels the changes seen on radiographic examination. Asymmetric in-

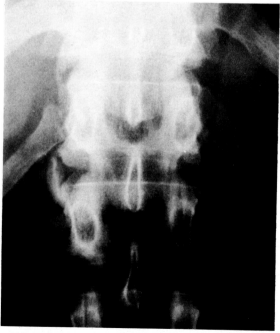

Figure 26–8. Abnormalities of the spine. Paravertebral ossification can be delineated. Note the asymmetric nature and lateral location of the outgrowths.

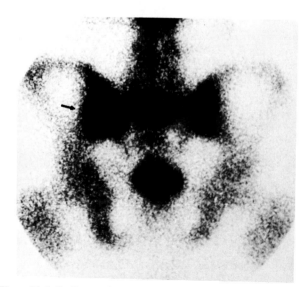

Figure 26–9. Radionuclide abnormalities. Asymmetric sacroiliitis, greater on the right side, is evident on scintigraphy (arrow).

volvement of the joints of the lower extremity is again revealed. Increasing radioactivity related to the plantar and posterior aspects of the calcaneus may be striking. Asymmetric accumulation of the radionuclide about the sacroiliac joints also facilitates the diagnosis of sacroiliitis (Fig. 26–9).

PATHOLOGIC ABNORMALITIES

Synovial biopsy findings confirm the presence of inflammation, although extensive pannus formation is unusual. Bone proliferation results from subchondral osseous hyperplasia and periosteal new bone formation.

ETIOLOGY AND PATHOGENESIS

Of all of the rheumatic diseases, Reiter's syndrome is most suspect for an infectious cause. The syndrome frequently follows an infection of the bowel or lower genitourinary tract, and it seems likely that these sites are the portals of entry for the causative agent. Considerable difficulty has been encountered in attempting to isolate a specific infective agent in Reiter's syndrome, however. To date, no single agent has been definitely incriminated in this disease.

An alternative explanation for the association of Reiter's syndrome and bowel or genitourinary infection is that Reiter's syndrome is related not to purulent arthritis but, rather, to a reaction of a joint (or other target site) to infection elsewhere in the body. The concept of reactive arthritis is discussed in Chapters 27 and 59.

As the clinical expression of disease may be influenced to a great degree by genetic factors, the immunologic nature of Reiter's syndrome has been stressed. The increased frequency of the histocompatibility antigen HLA-B27 in this disorder is well recognized, a frequency that may reach 96 per cent. Possession of this antigen may predispose patients to Reiter's syndrome after exposure to an infectious agent.

DIFFERENTIAL DIAGNOSIS

Other Seronegative Spondyloarthropathies

Although its general features resemble those of the other two seronegative spondyloarthropathies (ankylosing spondylitis and psoriatic arthritis), Reiter's syndrome possesses a sufficiently characteristic articular distribution to allow accurate diagnosis. This syndrome is associated with an asymmetric arthritis of the lower extremity, sacroiliitis, and, less commonly, spondylitis. Ankylosing spondylitis has a similar axial skeletal distribution, but significant peripheral articular changes are less frequent. Psoriatic arthritis may lead to considerable alterations in the articulations of both the appendicular and the axial skeleton. In psoriasis, however, widespread involvement of the upper extremity may be apparent, and distal interphalangeal joint abnormalities are common in both upper and lower extremities.

In all three spondyloarthropathies, the presence of soft tissue swelling, joint space narrowing, erosions, and bone proliferation in synovial joints is typical. In Reiter's syndrome, the frequency of osteoporosis in the acute phase of the disease appears to be greater than in psoriatic arthritis and ankylosing spondylitis, and the frequency of intraarticular bone ankylosis is less than in the other two diseases. In addition, the resolving nature of some of the lesions of Reiter's syndrome is distinctive. Each of the three spondyloarthropathies is associated with abnormalities of cartilaginous joints and of sites of tendon and ligament attachment to bone.

The sacroiliac and spinal changes of Reiter's syndrome are virtually identical to those of psoriasis, although the frequency and severity of these abnormalities and the tendency to involve the cervical spine are greater in psoriasis. Symmetric, asymmetric, or unilateral sacroiliac articular changes and broad asymmetric spinal outgrowths occur in both Reiter's syndrome and psoriatic arthritis. In classic ankylosing spondylitis, symmetric sacroiliac joint changes and symmetric slender bone outgrowths of the spine are typical. Furthermore, vertebral body osteitis, apophyseal joint ankylosis, and intraarticular osseous fusion of the sacroiliac joint are more frequent in ankylosing spondylitis than in Reiter's syndrome or psoriatic arthritis.

Rheumatoid Arthritis

The radiographic features of rheumatoid arthritis differ considerably from those of Reiter's syndrome; in particular, asymmetry and the irregular proliferative erosive changes of the spondyloarthropathies typically are not seen in rheumatoid arthritis.

Septic Arthritis and Osteomyelitis

The early localized abnormalities of Reiter's syndrome may resemble the findings of osseous and articular infection. Soft tissue swelling, osteoporosis, bone and cartilage destruction, and periostitis are evident in both Reiter's syndrome and infectious disease. Eventually, the polyarticular nature of Reiter's syndrome will allow its accurate differentiation from infectious disease.

FURTHER READING

Keat A: Reiter's syndrome and reactive arthritis in perspective. N Engl J Med 309:1606, 1983.

Martel W, Braunstein EM, Borlaza G, Good AE, Griffin PE Jr: Radiologic features of Reiter's disease. Radiology 132:1, 1979.

McEwen C, DiTata D, Lingg C, Porini A, Good A, Rankin T: Ankylosing spondylitis and spondylitis accompanying ulcerative colitis, regional enteritis, psoriasis and Reiter's disease. Arthritis Rheum 14:291, 1971.

Peterson CC Jr, Silbiger ML: Reiter's syndrome and psoriatic arthritis. Their roentgen spectra and some interesting similarities. AJR 101:860, 1967.

Resnick D, Feingold ML, Curd J, Niwayama G, Goergen TG: Calcaneal abnormalities in articular disorders. Rheumatoid arthritis, ankylosing spondylitis, psoriatic arthritis and Reiter's syndrome. Radiology 125:355, 1977.

Sholkoff SD, Glickman MG, Steinback HL: Roentgenology of Reiter's syndrome. Radiology 97:497, 1970.

Sundaram M, Patton JT: Paravertebral ossification in psoriasis and Reiter's disease. Br J Radiol 48:628, 1975.

Weinberger HW, Ropes MW, Kulka JP, Bauer W: Reiter's syndrome: Clinical and pathological observations—a long term study of 16 cases. Medicine 41:35, 1962.

Weldon WV, Scalettar R: Roentgen changes in Reiter's syndrome. AJR 86:344, 1961.

Chapter 27

Enteropathic Arthropathies

Donald Resnick, M.D.

Musculoskeletal manifestations are frequently associated with disorders of the gastrointestinal system. Peripheral joint arthralgias and arthritis accompany ulcerative colitis, Crohn's disease, and Whipple's disease, although radiographic findings generally are minimal and nonspecific. In addition, these three disorders may be associated with sacroiliac and spinal abnormalities that are identical to those of classic ankylosing spondylitis. Intestinal infections related to Salmonella, Shigella, and Yersinia organisms can lead to polyarthritis and, in rare circumstances, sacroiliitis and spondylitis. Intestinal bypass surgery may provoke a similar response in articulations of the appendicular and axial skeleton. In biliary cirrhosis, xanthomas and a peculiar type of erosive arthritis can be evident. Pancreatic disorders may become manifest as subcutaneous nodules, skin lesions, and polyarthritis, probably related to fat necrosis; epiphyseal and diametaphyseal infarction; and skeletal metastasis.

The appearance of musculoskeletal abnormalities in patients with gastrointestinal disorders has been recognized with increasing frequency in recent years. These abnormalities have been designated enteropathic arthropathies because of the close association of articular and intestinal findings (Table 27–1). Ulcerative colitis, Crohn's disease (regional enteritis), and Whipple's disease are three intestinal disorders whose rheumatologic manifestations are now well known. In addition, musculoskeletal abnormalities can occur after certain intestinal infections, specifically those associated with Salmonella, Shigella, or Yersinia organisms, after intestinal bypass surgery, and as a complication of extraintestinal disorders, including Laennec's and biliary cirrhoses, hepatitis, and pancreatic disease.

Several theoretical possibilities exist to explain the relationship between inflammatory intestinal diseases and arthritis. Organisms originating in the gut could secondarily invade articular tissue, or both gastrointestinal tract and joint may be infected simultaneously. The arthritis complicating Salmonella, Shigella, or Yersinia enterocolitis is consistent with this etiologic basis. A second proposed cause implicates immune mechanisms. Cellular or humoral immune responses may be mounted against a tissue antigen shared by the bowel and the joint; or, alternatively, immune complexes formed by the breakdown of the normal intestinal mucosal barrier may incidentally injure the joint as they circulate in the body. This mechanism may be important in the arthritis of ulcerative colitis, Crohn's disease, and intestinal bypass operations. Recent evidence has also indicated that genetic factors play an important role in the development of enteropathic arthropathies. Approximately 90 per cent of patients with ulcerative colitis and Crohn's disease who develop spondylitis or sacroiliitis demonstrate the genetically determined histocompatibility antigen HLA-B27 on their cells. This antigen may enhance the individual's susceptibility to an infectious process, or it may be linked to an immune response gene that controls the generation of a particular pathogenetic immune response.

ULCERATIVE COLITIS
General Abnormalities

Ulcerative colitis is a chronic inflammatory disease of unknown cause with predilection for young adults, which involves predominantly the mucosa and submucosa of the colon. Musculoskeletal abnormalities are the most common extraintestinal manifestation of the disease. The arthritis of ulcerative colitis is a distinct entity whose manifestations have been variously termed colitic arthritis, intestinal arthritis, enteropathic arthritis, and acute toxic arthritis. The type of articular disease can be categorized as peripheral joint arthralgias and arthritis (50 to 60 per cent), sacroiliitis and spondylitis (20 to 30 per cent), and miscellaneous abnormalities (10 to 20 per cent).

Peripheral Joint Arthralgia and Arthritis

The reported frequency of abnormalities of the peripheral joints in ulcerative colitis has varied from 0 to 25 per cent. Adults are usually affected. Although bowel disease usually is evident clinically prior to the onset of arthritis, articular abnormalities may appear before intestinal abnormalities in 10 to 15 per cent of patients. There is a close temporal association between exacerbations of intestinal and of joint findings. Furthermore, articular manifestations appear more commonly with severe and widespread intestinal involvement; they are less frequent with intestinal alterations confined to the descending colon and rectosigmoid area.

The articular findings can be categorized as an acute synovitis that is predominantly monoarticular in distribution. The knees are involved most commonly, followed by the ankles, the elbows, the wrists, the shoulders, and the small joints of the hands and feet. Asymmetric inflammation of the proximal interphalangeal joints of the toes is suggestive of "colitic arthritis." Inflammation in one joint may subside at the same time that other joints are being affected. The attacks are usually self-limited. Permanent joint abnormalities are

Table 27–1. RADIOGRAPHIC MANIFESTATIONS OF ENTEROPATHIC ARTHROPATHIES*

Disorders	Sacroiliitis	Spondylitis	Peripheral Joints	Other Manifestations
Ulcerative colitis	+	+	Soft tissue swelling Osteoporosis Joint space narrowing (r) Erosions, cysts (r)	Periostitis (r)
Crohn's disease	+	+	Soft tissue swelling Osteoporosis Joint space narrowing (r) Erosions, cysts (r) Septic arthritis (r)	Periostitis (r) Osseous granulomas (r) Osteomyelitis (r)
Whipple's disease	+	+	Soft tissue swelling Osteoporosis Joint space narrowing (r) Erosions, cysts (r)	Subcutaneous nodules (r)
Salmonella, Shigella, and Yersinia infections	+	+	Soft tissue swelling Osteoporosis Septic arthritis	
Intestinal bypass surgery	+	+	Soft tissue swelling Osteoporosis Gout (r)	Osteomalacia (r)
Laennec's cirrhosis			Soft tissue swelling Osteoporosis	Soft tissue calcification (r)
Biliary cirrhosis			Soft tissue swelling Joint space narrowing Erosions Destruction Chondrocalcinosis (r)	Osteomalacia Xanthoma Periostitis (r)
Viral hepatitis			Soft tissue swelling (r)	Subcutaneous nodules
Pancreatic disease			Soft tissue swelling (r) Osteoporosis Erosions, cysts (r) Osteonecrosis	Osteolysis Periostitis Metastasis

*+ = present; r = rare.

infrequent even in the setting of recurrent clinical attacks of arthritis.

The radiographic analysis is nonspecific. Soft tissue swelling and periarticular osteoporosis are the two most typical characteristics. Radiographic evidence of osseous and cartilaginous destruction is indeed unusual, although when present, the findings can simulate those of rheumatoid arthritis.

The cause and pathogenesis of peripheral joint disease in ulcerative colitis are not known.

Sacroiliitis and Spondylitis

The reported frequency of ankylosing spondylitis in patients with ulcerative colitis has varied from 1 to 26 per cent. Spondylitis in ulcerative colitis is poorly correlated with activity of the bowel disease. Furthermore, spinal abnormalities may become manifest prior to, at the same time as, or after the onset of intestinal changes. In fact, spondylitis most commonly precedes the onset of colitis and may progress relentlessly without relation to exacerbation, remission, or treatment of the bowel disease.

The clinical features of ankylosing spondylitis in patients with ulcerative colitis are identical to those of classic ankylosing spondylitis. Peripheral joint abnormalities are detected in 50 to 70 per cent of patients, particularly in the hips and shoulders. In these instances, the radiographic features in the appendicular skeleton are those that are typical for ankylosing spondylitis, including the presence of joint space narrowing, osseous erosions, cysts, and bone proliferation, and the absence of osteoporosis (Fig. 27–1).

Laboratory evaluation outlines the presence of a nonreactive serum rheumatoid factor and an increased frequency of the histocompatibility antigen HLA-B27. This antigen is not commonly detected in patients with inflammatory bowel disease with or without peripheral joint disease who do not have spine or sacroiliac joint alterations. The detection of HLA-B27 antigen indicates an increased risk for the development of spondylitis and iritis in patients with inflammatory bowel disorders.

On radiographic examination, spinal and sacroiliac joint abnormalities in ulcerative colitis are virtually indistinguishable from those in classic ankylosing spondylitis. Sacroiliac joint involvement is usually bilateral and symmetric in distribution (Fig. 27–2). Additional pelvic abnormalities include bone erosion and sclerosis about the symphysis pubis and bone erosion and proliferation at the ischial tuberosities and iliac crests. In the spine, vertebral body erosions with alterations of vertebral shape (squaring) are seen. Typical syndesmophytes are also evident. Eventually, a bamboo spine may be seen. In the apophyseal joints, articular space narrowing, erosion, sclerosis, and bone ankylosis are identical to

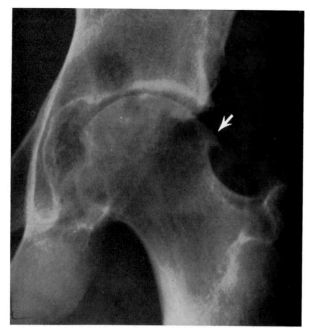

Figure 27–1. Ulcerative colitis and ankylosing spondylitis: Monoarthritis of the hip. Observe diffuse loss of joint space, cystic changes, and osteophytosis, especially on the lateral aspect of the femoral head (arrow). (Courtesy of M. Lequesne, M. D., Paris, France.)

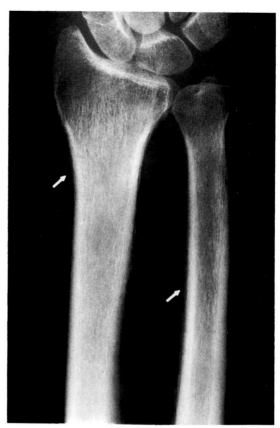

Figure 27–3. Ulcerative colitis: Hypertrophic osteoarthropathy. Note periostitis (arrows) of the diaphyses and metaphyses of the radius and ulna.

changes in classic ankylosing spondylitis. In the hip and glenohumeral articulations, typical joint manifestations of ankylosing spondylitis may appear.

The sacroiliitis and spondylitis of classic ankylosing spondylitis and of ulcerative colitis are readily differentiated from the sacroiliitis and spondylitis of psoriatic arthritis and of Reiter's syndrome. Bilateral symmetric sacroiliac joint changes with eventual intraarticular bone ankylosis are more common in classic ankylosing spondylitis and colitic disease than in psoriasis and Reiter's syndrome. In the spine, vertical syndesmophytes, significant apophyseal joint abnormalities, and vertebral squaring are also more typical of classic ankylosing spondylitis and colitic disorders than of psoriasis and Reiter's syndrome.

Miscellaneous Abnormalities

Clubbing of the fingers is a recognized complication of ulcerative colitis. On rare occasions, hypertrophic osteoarthropathy may also be apparent, leading to periosteal bone formation in the tibia, fibula, radius, and ulna (Fig. 27–3).

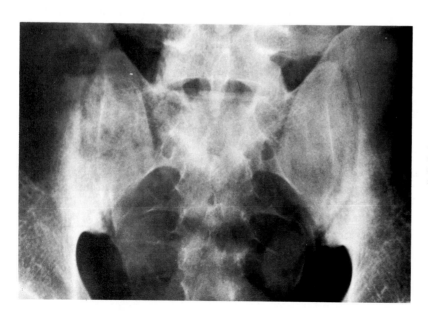

Figure 27–2. Ulcerative colitis and ankylosing spondylitis: Sacroiliac joint abnormalities. Bilateral and symmetric abnormalities are characterized by erosion and sclerosis, predominantly in the ilium.

Differential Diagnosis

Radiographic features (soft tissue swelling and osteoporosis) of peripheral joint arthritis in patients with ulcerative colitis are not specific. Although the appearance of joint space narrowing, erosions, and cysts can simulate changes in rheumatoid arthritis, these abnormalities are not frequent in the arthritis of ulcerative colitis.

Spondylitis and sacroiliitis in ulcerative colitis are identical to the changes in classic ankylosing spondylitis. Bilateral and symmetric sacroiliac joint involvement and syndesmophytosis are seen in both disorders. These same changes are also evident in Crohn's disease. In psoriasis and Reiter's syndrome, sacroiliac joint abnormalities may be asymmetric or even unilateral in distribution, whereas spinal alterations include broad asymmetric bone excrescences that differ in appearance from typical syndesmophytes.

CROHN'S DISEASE

General Abnormalities

Crohn's disease is a chronic and recurrent granulomatous process of unknown cause that involves principally the terminal ileum and proximal portion of the colon, although it may localize in any segment of the gastrointestinal tract from esophagus to rectum. Additional systemic manifestations are ocular inflammation, erythema nodosum, and musculoskeletal abnormalities. The musculoskeletal manifestations in Crohn's disease can take several forms: peripheral joint arthralgias and arthritis; sacroiliitis and spondylitis; and miscellaneous abnormalities.

Peripheral Joint Arthralgia and Arthritis

Enteropathic arthritis has been reported in 1 to 22 per cent of patients with Crohn's disease, especially those with colonic involvement. Its precise cause is unknown. Peripheral joint abnormalities in Crohn's disease are equally frequent in men and women. The pattern of articular involvement most typically is a mild, migratory synovitis of one or several joints, involving the lower extremity more frequently than the upper extremity. The knee is the most common site of abnormality, followed by the ankle, the shoulder, the wrist, the elbow, and the small joints of the hands and feet. Clinical findings generally are self-limited, although they may recur. Arthritis occurs simultaneously with the onset of bowel disease or at any time during its course. Rarely, it may precede intestinal alterations. The recrudescence of arthritis is commonly associated with an exacerbation of intestinal disease. Tests for serum rheumatoid factor yield negative results.

Radiographic abnormalities usually consist of soft tissue swelling and regional osteoporosis. Permanent cartilaginous and osseous changes are rarely present.

Sacroiliitis and Spondylitis

A significant number (3 to 16 per cent) of patients with Crohn's disease develop sacroiliac joint and spinal changes. Men and women are affected with equal frequency. Symptoms and signs may antedate or follow the onset of bowel disease, and exacerbation of clinical findings does not appear to be related to the activity of bowel disease, nor does the treatment of the intestinal disorder influence the progress of the arthritis. Axial skeletal joint alterations are equally frequent in patients with either large or small bowel involvement. Laboratory evaluation demonstrates the presence of HLA-B27 antigen in many patients with Crohn's disease and sacroiliitis or spondylitis.

The radiographic features of spinal and sacroiliac joint abnormalities in Crohn's disease are identical to those of classic ankylosing spondylitis. Bilateral sacroiliac joint narrowing and erosion and sclerosis of ilium and sacrum are evident (Fig. 27–4). Syndesmophytosis, vertebral erosion, sclerosis, and squaring, and apophyseal joint erosion, sclerosis, and narrowing can be noted in the spine. Progressive alterations can lead to a bamboo spine. In those instances in which

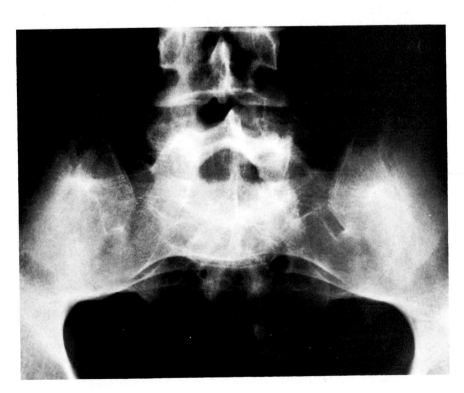

Figure 27–4. Crohn's disease and ankylosing spondylitis: Sacroiliac joint abnormalities. Bilateral symmetric changes are characterized by extreme joint space narrowing and partial ankylosis, as well as sclerosis, predominantly of the ilium.

peripheral joint disease occurs during the course of sacroiliitis and spondylitis, findings are typical of ankylosing spondylitis.

The cause and pathogenesis of axial skeletal involvement in Crohn's disease are unclear, although it is generally assumed that factors similar to those in ulcerative colitis are responsible for the joint involvement. Evidence that documents a relationship between the spondylitis and sacroiliitis of Crohn's disease and the presence of HLA-B27 antigen supports the importance of genetic factors.

Miscellaneous Abnormalities

Digital clubbing has been detected in as many as 40 per cent of patients with Crohn's disease. Bilateral symmetric periostitis is an extremely rare complication of Crohn's disease (Fig. 27–5). Granulomatous and infectious processes of bone also have been reported in association with Crohn's disease. Furthermore, osteomyelitis and septic arthritis in the hip and hemipelvis and psoas abscesses have been recorded in individuals with Crohn's disease, perhaps related to spread of infection from a diseased gut.

In children and adolescents, both Crohn's disease and ulcerative colitis can lead to retarded skeletal maturation and decreased linear growth. Furthermore, skeletal osteopenia can be seen in patients with chronic inflammatory bowel disease, perhaps related to malnutrition, malabsorption, chronic inflammation, and administration of corticosteroids.

Differential Diagnosis

The radiographic abnormalities in the peripheral joints in patients with Crohn's disease lack specificity. Thus, the

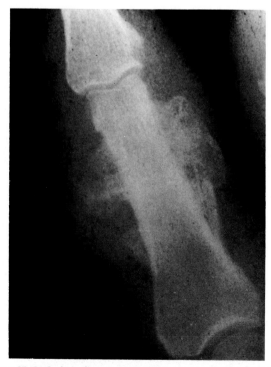

Figure 27–5. Crohn's disease: Hypertrophic osteoarthropathy. Striking periostitis and soft tissue swelling can be noted in the diaphyses of the proximal and middle phalanges of the second finger. The bones in other digits as well as the forearms and lower portions of the legs were affected. (Courtesy of M. Dalinka, M.D., Philadelphia, Pennsylvania.)

findings can simulate the early changes of rheumatoid arthritis. The axial skeletal abnormalities in this disease cannot be differentiated from those of classic ankylosing spondylitis or the spondylitis of ulcerative colitis. The presence of bilateral and symmetric sacroiliac joint changes and syndesmophytosis of the spine is typical of these disorders. Asymmetric or unilateral sacroiliac joint alterations and broad asymmetric spinal outgrowths are not features of enteropathic spondylitis but are apparent in psoriasis and Reiter's syndrome.

WHIPPLE'S DISEASE
General Abnormalities

Whipple's disease (intestinal lipodystrophy) is a rare progressive disorder affecting predominantly men in the fourth and fifth decades of life and leading to fever, weight loss, lymphadenopathy, peripheral edema, hypotension, brown pigmentation of the skin, polyserositis, and polyarthritis. Pathologically, the major feature is the accumulation of periodic acid–Schiff (PAS)-positive inclusions in the macrophages of the lamina propria of the small intestine, lymph nodes, and other tissues. The cause of the disease appears to be related to a bacterial organism, although the specific bacterium has not been identified.

Musculoskeletal manifestations are an important feature of the disease. These manifestations can be divided into arthralgia and arthritis; sacroiliitis and spondylitis; and miscellaneous abnormalities.

Arthralgia and Arthritis

Acute migratory episodic arthralgia and arthritis are apparent in 60 to 90 per cent of patients with Whipple's disease and may antedate other changes by 1 year to as many as 35 years. Articular abnormalities are usually transient, and residual joint deformities are rare. Characteristically, the ankles, the knees, the shoulders, and the wrists are affected. Polyarthritis is more frequent than monoarthritis.

Clinical findings include mild to severe joint pain, swelling, warmth, and restrictive motion. Examination of the synovial membrane may demonstrate a mild nonspecific synovitis, although histiocytic infiltration within the membrane and PAS-positive granules may be apparent. Synovial biopsy therefore has the potential to provide early and accurate diagnosis of Whipple's disease.

Radiographic examination of involved peripheral joints may be entirely normal. Soft tissue swelling, osteoporosis, and joint space narrowing are occasionally evident. These findings are most common in the metacarpophalangeal and metatarsophalangeal joints, the wrist, the ankle, the hip, and the knee.

Sacroiliitis and Spondylitis

Sacroiliitis and spondylitis have been described in patients with Whipple's disease (Fig. 27–6), although the exact frequency of these abnormalities is not known. In most cases, spinal and sacroiliac joint alterations resemble those of classic ankylosing spondylitis.

Miscellaneous Abnormalities

Subcutaneous nodules, particularly on extensor surfaces of the extremities, have been evident in some patients with joint symptoms.

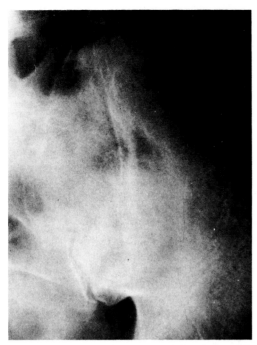

Figure 27-6. Whipple's disease: Sacroiliac joint abnormalities. This man had a 10 year history of polyarthralgias and a 1 year history of steatorrhea. Lymph node and gastric biopsy confirmed the diagnosis of Whipple's disease. The sacroiliac joint reveals narrowing and sclerosis, predominantly in the ilium. The opposite side was affected similarly.

Differential Diagnosis

The peripheral joint abnormalities in Whipple's disease are entirely nonspecific on radiographic evaluation. In the axial skeleton, sacroiliac joint and spinal changes, when present, are identical to those of classic ankylosing spondylitis and the spondylitis of ulcerative colitis and Crohn's disease.

INTESTINAL INFECTIONS AND REACTIVE ARTHRITIS

A variety of infectious agents can initiate or trigger a synovial reaction at one or more sites distant from the area of infection. The phenomenon, which is unrelated to direct contamination of the joint, is referred to as reactive arthritis and is a well-known occurrence in acute rheumatic fever. The term reactive arthritis can also be applied to the articular manifestations in some patients with Reiter's syndrome and in patients with enteropathic arthritis complicating ulcerative colitis and Crohn's disease. Certain genetic factors, such as the presence of HLA-B27 antigen, appear to impart a susceptibility to reactive arthritis in some individuals. Indeed, several distinct mechanisms by which an infectious agent can initiate or perpetuate articular inflammation can be identified (Table 27-2).

General clinical characteristics of reactive arthritis include a symptom-free interval between the initiation of infection and the rheumatic reaction; a self-limited clinical course, usually associated with the acute onset of a migratory polyarthritis and fever; a tendency in some patients toward involvement of the heart; and a negative serologic test for rheumatoid factor. Although the location of the inciting infection varies, three portals of entry are most typical: the

Table 27-2. MECHANISMS OF INFECTION-INDUCED ARTHRITIS

Mechanism	Example
Direct penetration and subsequent multiplication of viable organisms	Bacterial arthritis
"Reactive" arthritis as a response to a distant infection	Rheumatic fever
Immune-mediated response to an antigen in the joint or blood	Hepatitis
Direct toxin released by the infectious agent	?

Modified from Goldenberg DL: "Postinfectious" arthritis. New look at an old concept with particular attention to disseminated gonococcal infection. Am J Med 74:625, 1983. Used with permission.

oronasopharynx (e.g., tonsillitis, dental infection), the urogenital tract (e.g., urethritis), and the intestinal tract.

Seronegative sterile arthritis may follow intestinal infections related to Salmonella, Shigella, Yersinia, or Campylobacter organisms. These enteric pathogens share the features of mucosal involvement and, with the exception of Shigella, lymph node involvement and bacteremia. The frequency of the arthritis in patients after Salmonella or Shigella infection is 1 to 2 per cent; that following Yersinia infection may be as high as 30 per cent. It is to be expected that additional infective processes can be associated with reactive arthritis.

The various forms of sterile arthritis can be associated with soft tissue swelling and joint effusions, but other radiographic features generally are lacking. After bowel disease due to Yersinia, sacroiliitis and spondylitis have been noted. It is significant that approximately 90 per cent of patients in whom sterile arthritis develops after bowel infection with Salmonella, Shigella, or Yersinia organisms have the HLA-B27 antigen.

A true septic arthritis is a definite and serious complication after Salmonella infection, particularly in children. *Yersinia enterocolitica* infection has also been associated with septic arthritis as well as osteomyelitis and psoas muscle abscess.

ARTHROPATHY AFTER INTESTINAL BYPASS SURGERY

Intestinal bypass surgery has been performed for many years for the treatment of intractable obesity. Rheumatologic manifestations in the postoperative period occur in 20 to 30 per cent of patients and include polymyalgia, polyarthralgia, acute or subacute arthritis, and tenosynovitis. The cause and pathogenesis of these manifestations are not clear. They generally develop within 2 years after surgical intervention and resolve within 1 to 2 years. If severe, clinical manifestations of articular involvement may require that the normal anatomic sequence of the gut be restored surgically, a procedure that can relieve the arthritic complaints.

Symmetric polyarthritis is the rule. Articular involvement is most frequent in the knees, the ankles, the fingers, and the wrists. Radiographic evaluation demonstrates soft tissue swelling and osteoporosis. Sacroiliitis and spondylitis have been observed in patients undergoing jejunocolic type bypass procedures who were followed for a long period of time.

PRIMARY BILIARY CIRRHOSIS

General Abnormalities

Primary biliary cirrhosis is a rare disorder of unknown cause affecting women almost exclusively. Clinical findings include the insidious onset of jaundice, pruritus, hepatomegaly, and abnormal liver function. The diagnosis is confirmed by the presence of antimitochondrial antibodies and characteristic findings on liver biopsy. Primary biliary cirrhosis has been associated with a number of other autoimmune diseases, including scleroderma.

Rheumatologic Manifestations

Osteomalacia and osteoporosis in this disorder are probably attributable to a combination of steatorrhea, cholestasis, and hepatic dysfunction. Hypercholesterolemia can lead to xanthoma formation. An erosive arthritis of the hands and wrists has also been noted in patients with primary biliary cirrhosis (Fig. 27–7). Erosions are distributed predominantly in an asymmetric fashion in distal interphalangeal and proximal interphalangeal joints. The pathogenesis of these erosive changes is not known. Furthermore, a destructive arthropathy has also been reported in some patients with primary biliary cirrhosis. Fragmentation, collapse, and disintegration of bone in the hips and glenohumeral joints resemble the findings of osteonecrosis.

PANCREATIC DISEASE

Fat Necrosis

Pancreatic disorders can be complicated by fat necrosis at multiple distant sites, resulting in subcutaneous nodular skin lesions, polyarthritis, and medullary fat necrosis. These manifestations appear most frequently in older men in association with carcinoma of the pancreas, although they can also occur with acute pancreatitis owing to either abdominal trauma (including that related to the abused child syndrome) or alcohol abuse, pancreatic pseudocysts, and pancreatic duct calculi. The temporal relationship between the onset of articular findings and development of subcutaneous nodules and the onset of abdominal complaints is variable.

The skin lesions resemble those of erythema nodosum. Articular abnormalities are characterized by a symmetric or asymmetric polyarthritis. Fat globules may be apparent in the synovial fluid or the periarticular tissue. Radiographic findings related to joint disease are absent or minimal; osteoporosis and soft tissue swelling can be seen, but joint space narrowing and osseous erosion are rarely observed.

Bone involvement can occur simultaneously with subcutaneous nodules and polyarthritis, or it can represent an isolated phenomenon. Osteolytic lesions with motheaten bone destruction and periostitis of the tubular bones of the extremities resemble findings of osteomyelitis or osteonecrosis (Fig. 27–8). These changes occur in the long bones of the extremities or in the small bones of the hands and feet. The lesions may heal, although residual periosteal reaction has been noted.

Although the exact pathogenesis of the articular and osseous findings associated with pancreatic disorders has not been

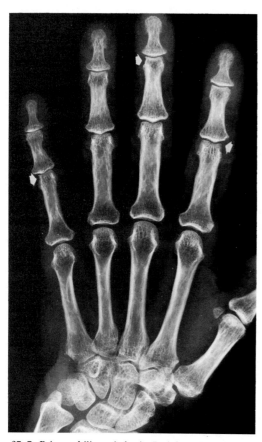

Figure 27–7. Primary biliary cirrhosis: Peripheral joint abnormalities. Note the small marginal erosions in the proximal interphalangeal and distal interphalangeal joints (arrows). (From O'Connell DJ, Marx WJ: Hand changes in primary biliary cirrhosis. Radiology 129:31, 1978. Used with permission.)

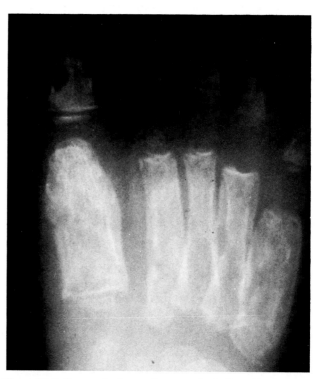

Figure 27–8. Pancreatic disease: Fat necrosis. Radiographic abnormalities. A 3 year old child fell off a moving truck and sustained a skull fracture and back trauma. Observe lytic defects of the phalanges and metatarsals with associated periostitis. (Courtesy of A. Brower, M.D., Washington, D.C.)

delineated accurately, it appears probable that widespread fat necrosis is responsible for these abnormalities. Obstruction of pancreatic ducts by edema, calculi, or tumor or hormonal hypersecretion by acinar cell carcinomas and functioning metastases can lead to release of excess circulating lipase into the bloodstream, which results in autodigestion of fat deposits at distant sites.

Osteonecrosis

Osteonecrosis is a recognized manifestation of pancreatic disease. This complication is associated most frequently with chronic or inactive pancreatitis. Abnormalities of the femoral and humeral heads are typical, although diaphyseal and metaphyseal infarction in long tubular bones can simulate the changes in caisson workers (Fig. 27–9). Radiographically, epiphyseal involvement is characterized by mottled lysis and sclerosis, subchondral radiolucent areas, and partial or complete collapse of bone; diaphyseal and metaphyseal involvement, which is most frequent in the distal end of the femur and proximal end of the tibia, is associated with radiolucency, calcification, and periosteal bone formation. Osteonecrosis can also be encountered in the small bones of the hands and feet.

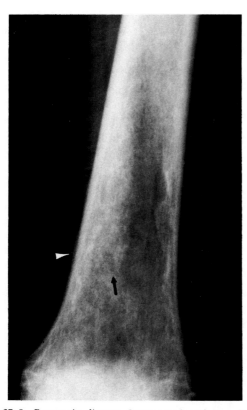

Figure 27–9. Pancreatic disease: Osteonecrosis. Obvious diaphyseal infarction of the distal femur is associated with calcification (arrow) and periostitis (arrowhead).

Skeletal Metastasis

Osteolytic or osteoblastic lesions can occur in patients with skeletal metastasis from adenocarcinoma of the pancreas. The reported frequency of these changes has varied from 6 to 21 per cent. Changes are most common in the vertebral column. Frequent involvement of the upper lumbar spine could conceivably indicate direct invasion of neoplasm rather than hematogenous spread in some patients with pancreatic carcinoma.

Differential Diagnosis

The osseous changes of fat necrosis in patients with pancreatic disease simulate those of osteomyelitis and osteonecrosis. Lytic lesions and periostitis on radiographic examination and areas of increased radionuclide uptake on scintigraphic examination are common manifestations of these disorders. The combination of osteolysis, periosteal bone formation, calcification of medullary bone, and epiphyseal osteonecrosis should stimulate a clinical investigation to exclude a pancreatic origin of these findings.

FURTHER READING

Arlart IP, Maier W, Leupold D, Wolf A: Massive periosteal new bone formation in ulcerative colitis. Radiology 144:507, 1982.

Baron M, Paltiel H, Lander P: Aseptic necrosis of the talus and calcaneal insufficiency fractures in a patient with pancreatitis, subcutaneous fat necrosis, and arthritis. Arthritis Rheum 27:1309, 1984.

Björkengren AG, Resnick D, Sartoris DJ: Enteropathic arthropathies. Radiol Clin N Amer 25:189, 1987.

Clark RL, Muhletaler CA, Margulies SI: Colitic arthritis. Clinical and radiographic manifestations. Radiology 101:585, 1971.

Genant HK, Mall JC, Wagonfeld JB, Vander Horst J, Lanz LH: Skeletal demineralization and growth retardation in inflammatory bowel disease. Invest Radiol 11:541, 1976.

Goldenberg DL: "Postinfectious" arthritis. New look at an old concept with particular attention to disseminated gonococcal infection. Am J Med 74:925, 1983.

Joffe N, Antonioli DA: Osteoblastic bone metastases secondary to adenocarcinoma of the pancreas. Clin Radiol 29:41, 1978.

Khan MA: Axial arthropathy in Whipple's disease. J Rheumatol 9:928, 1982.

McEwen C, DiTata D, Lingg C, Porini A, Good A, Rankin T: Ankylosing spondylitis and spondylitis accompanying ulcerative colitis, regional enteritis, psoriasis and Reiter's disease. Arthritis Rheum 14:291, 1971.

Mueller CE, Seeger JF, Martel W: Ankylosing spondylitis and regional enteritis. Radiology 112:579, 1974.

O'Connell DJ, Marx WJ: Hand changes in primary biliary cirrhosis. Radiology 129:31, 1978.

Radin DR, Colletti PM, Forrester DM, Tang WW: Pancreatic acinar carcinoma with subcutaneous and intraosseous fat necrosis. Radiology 158:67, 1986.

Slovis TL, Berdon WE, Haller JO, Baker DH, Rosen L: Pancreatitis and the battered child syndrome: Report of 2 cases with skeletal involvement. AJR 125:456, 1975.

Stein HB, Schlappner OLA, Boyko W, Gourlay RH, Reeve CE: The intestinal bypass arthritis-dermatitis syndrome. Arthritis Rheum 24:684, 1981.

Chapter 28

Periodic, Relapsing, and Recurrent Disorders

Donald Resnick, M.D.

Familial Mediterranean fever, relapsing polychondritis, and Behçet's syndrome represent three uncommon disorders that may be associated with periodic, relapsing, or recurrent clinical manifestations. In each disease, synovitis can occasionally lead to soft tissue swelling and periarticular *osteoporosis, and in rare instances cartilaginous and osseous destruction can become evident. Furthermore, each of these three disorders has been associated with sacroiliitis, although this association is not frequent, nor is it without controversy in some cases.*

Included in this chapter are three diseases (familial Mediterranean fever, relapsing polychondritis, and Behçet's syndrome) that are characterized clinically by intermittent periods of activity separated by disease-free intercritical periods. These three diseases are relatively uncommon and are associated with nonspecific or unremarkable radiographic findings.

FAMILIAL MEDITERRANEAN FEVER
Clinical Abnormalities

Familial Mediterranean fever (familial recurrent polyserositis) is an uncommon disease that affects predominantly Sephardic (non-Ashkenazic) Jews, Armenians, and Arabs. It is inherited as an autosomal recessive trait with complete penetrance. Men are affected more commonly than women. Symptoms and signs of the disorder usually appear in childhood or adolescence and subsequently recur throughout the remainder of life. The typical manifestations include episodes of fever with abdominal, thoracic, or joint pain owing to inflammation of the peritoneum, pleura, and synovial membrane. Amyloidosis is a recognized common complication of the disease, which can produce the nephrotic syndrome and renal failure, resulting in early death.

Musculoskeletal manifestations can occur in 60 to 70 per cent of patients. Asymmetric arthritis in the larger joints of the lower extremity is most typical. Joint attacks vary in severity, reach a peak in 1 to 2 days, and generally resolve in 1 to 2 weeks. After repeated bouts, a chronic destructive arthritis may develop, especially in the hip.

Radiographic Abnormalities

Osteoporosis can develop rapidly and become profound. In children, hyperemia can lead to epiphyseal overgrowth that, when combined with soft tissue swelling and an effusion, can simulate the findings in juvenile chronic arthritis or hemophilia. Chronicity leads to joint space narrowing and juxtaarticular erosions. Rarely, bone ankylosis, productive osseous changes with sclerosis and osteophytosis, and osteonecrosis are observed, especially in the hip and knee.

Sacroiliac joint abnormalities have also been described in 2 to 15 per cent of patients with familial Mediterranean fever (Table 28–1). Widening of the articular space, loss of the normal subchondral bone definition, sclerosis with or without erosions, predominantly on the ilium, and bone ankylosis can appear in one or both sacroiliac articulations; asymmetric abnormalities predominate (Fig. 28–1). The absence of HLA-B27 antigen in patients with familial Mediterranean fever and sacroiliitis may indicate that the pathogenesis of the articular changes is different from that in classic ankylosing spondylitis.

Differential Diagnosis

The radiographic findings in familial Mediterranean fever are not diagnostic. In children, soft tissue swelling, osteoporosis, and epiphyseal overgrowth are evident in other articular disorders, such as juvenile chronic arthritis and hemophilia. In children and adults, joint space narrowing and osseous erosion can simulate the findings of rheumatoid arthritis and septic arthritis. Sacroiliitis in familial Mediterranean fever simulates that of ankylosing spondylitis and other seronegative spondyloarthropathies.

RELAPSING POLYCHONDRITIS
Clinical Abnormalities

Relapsing polychondritis is an uncommon disorder of unknown cause characterized by episodic inflammation of

Table 28–1. SACROILIAC JOINT ABNORMALITIES

Disorder	Distribution		
	Bilateral Symmetric	Bilateral Asymmetric	Unilateral
Familial Mediterranean fever	×	×*	×
Relapsing polychondritis	×	×*	×
Behçet's syndrome†	×	×	×

*Probably the predominant pattern of involvement.
†Questionable association with sacroiliitis.

344

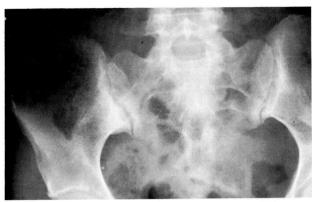

Figure 28–1. Familial Mediterranean fever: Sacroiliitis. Bilateral asymmetric sacroiliac joint disease is characterized by osseous erosions and reactive sclerosis, predominantly in the ilium. (From Brodey PA, Wolff SM: Radiographic changes in the sacroiliac joints in familial Mediterranean fever. Radiology 114:331, 1975. Used with permission.)

cartilaginous tissue and special sense organs; abnormalities are especially prominent in the external ear, nose, trachea, larynx, sclera, ribs, and articular cartilage. Relapsing polychondritis appears in all age groups, with a maximal frequency in the fourth decade of life. Men and women are affected in equal numbers. The initial clinical findings usually are auricular chondritis and arthritis; less typically, respiratory tract involvement, nasal chondritis, and ocular involvement are evident at the outset of the disease.

Arthralgia and arthritis generally affect more than one joint, including the hips, knees, manubriosternal and sternoclavicular joints, costochondral junctions, and small and large joints of the upper extremity. Migratory polyarthritis can simulate rheumatoid arthritis or a seronegative spondyloarthropathy, although occasionally monoarticular arthritis appears that mimics infection or crystal-induced arthritis. Although commonly nonerosive in type, the arthritis may produce considerable deformity and mutilation in some patients. Tendinitis can develop.

Respiratory tract involvement is a potentially serious manifestation of the disease that may require tracheostomy. Laryngeal and tracheal tenderness, cough, hoarseness, and dyspnea secondary to collapse of the tracheal rings, edema, or granulomatous tissue proliferation within the respiratory tree can be evident. Additional manifestations include back pain owing to spinal alterations, chest pain related to costochondritis, hearing loss attributable to obstruction of the external auditory meatus, fever, anorexia and weight loss, and cardiovascular abnormalities. Laboratory findings are not specific. Anemia, leukocytosis, elevated erythrocyte sedimentation rate, and moderate serum protein alterations may be detected.

Radiographic Abnormalities

In most cases, radiographic features of joint involvement in relapsing polychondritis are not striking, although there may be extraarticular findings, such as tracheal narrowing or stenosis, calcification of the auricular cartilage, and aortic alterations after repeated attacks. Periarticular osteoporosis may or may not be evident. Typically, a nonerosive, nondeforming arthropathy appears.

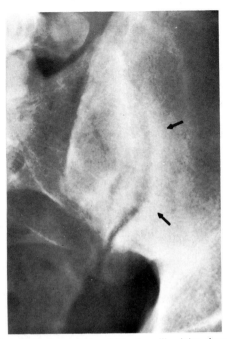

Figure 28–2. Relapsing polychondritis: Sacroiliac joint abnormalities. Moderate osseous erosions and reactive sclerosis are seen (arrows). (From Braunstein EM, et al: Radiological aspects of the arthropathy of relapsing polychondritis. Clin Radiol 30:441, 1979. Used with permission.)

Sacroiliitis has been evident in some patients with relapsing polychondritis, although the frequency probably is not high (Table 28–1). Unilateral or bilateral abnormalities characterized by the presence of joint space loss, erosion, and eburnation, and the absence of spinal alterations, predominate (Fig. 28–2).

Differential Diagnosis

The radiographic features of articular involvement in this disease lack specificity. Periarticular osteoporosis and soft tissue swelling about synovial articulations simulate changes in a variety of disorders. Sacroiliitis in relapsing polychondritis is similar to that in ankylosing spondylitis or other seronegative spondyloarthropathies. Calcification of ear cartilage is seen not only in relapsing polychondritis but also in adrenal insufficiency, acromegaly, alkaptonuria, hyperparathyroidism, and diabetes mellitus and after injury.

BEHÇET'S SYNDROME
Clinical Abnormalities

The classic triad of Behçet's syndrome consists of painful, recurrent oral and genital ulcerations and ocular inflammation. Many additional systems can be affected, however, including the skin, joints, and cardiovascular, neurologic, and gastrointestinal organs. Original cases of Behçet's syndrome were evident in Mediterranean countries, but the disorder has also been noted in individuals throughout Europe, the Middle East and Far East, and the United States. The age of onset varies from 5 to 70 years, with a mean age of approximately 25 to 30 years; men are affected more commonly than women. The cause of the disease is not known.

Over 90 per cent of patients reveal ulcerations in portions of the mouth or pharynx. Ophthalmic lesions are evident in

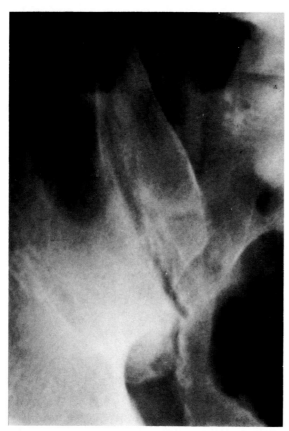

Figure 28–3. Behçet's syndrome: Sacroiliitis. In this patient, unilateral sacroiliitis is characterized by subchondral erosions and reactive sclerosis, predominantly in the ilium. (Courtesy of A. Brower, M.D., Washington, D.C.)

inates, affecting principally the knees. With affliction in the feet, pseudopodagra can develop. The sacroiliac and manubriosternal articulations may also be involved. An insidious onset, a variable duration, and recurrence after disappearance of the findings typify the bouts of arthralgia or arthritis. Joint effusion, stiffness, warmth, and tenderness are observed, but permanent changes are rare.

Laboratory analysis may reveal an elevated erythrocyte sedimentation rate, a strongly positive C-reactive protein, elevation of alpha-2 globulins, anemia, and mild leukocytosis. Many patients reveal high titers of serum antibodies directed against human oral mucosa.

Radiographic Abnormalities

Radiographic findings in the skeleton are usually mild. Osteoporosis and soft tissue swelling can be seen, but joint space narrowing and osseous erosions are encountered only rarely. Spontaneous atlantoaxial subluxation has also been described. Some reports have indicated the occurence of sacroiliitis in Behçet's syndrome (Table 28–1, Fig. 28–3).

Differential Diagnosis

When evident, radiologic alterations of joints in Behçet's syndrome may resemble those of rheumatoid arthritis or related disorders. Sacroiliitis can simulate the changes in ankylosing spondylitis or other seronegative spondyloarthropathies.

FURTHER READING

Ben-Dov I, Zimmerman J: Deforming arthritis of the hands in Behçet's disease. J Rheumatol 9:617, 1982.

Braunstein EM, Martel W, Stillwill E, Kay D: Radiological aspects of the arthropathy of relapsing polychondritis. Clin Radiol 30:441, 1979.

Brodey PA, Wolff SM: Radiographic changes in the sacroiliac joints in familial Mediterranean fever. Radiology 114:331, 1975.

Chajek T, Fairnaru M: Behçet's disease. Report of 41 cases and review of the literature. Medicine 54:179, 1975.

Johnson TH, Mital N, Rodnan GP, Wilson RJ: Relapsing polychondritis. Radiology 106:313, 1973.

Koss JC, Dalinka MK: Atlantoaxial subluxation in Behçet's syndrome. AJR 134:392, 1980.

McAdam LP, O'Hanlan MA, Bluestone R, Pearson CM: Relapsing polychondritis: Prospective study of 23 patients and a review of the literature. Medicine 55:193, 1976.

O'Hanlan M, McAdam LP, Bluestone R, Pearson CM: The arthropathy of relapsing polychondritis. Arthritis Rheum 19:191, 1976.

Schwabe AD, Peters RS: Familial Mediterranean fever in Armenians. Analysis of 100 cases. Medicine 53:453, 1974.

Shahin N, Sohar E, Dalith F: Roentgenologic findings in familial Mediterranean fever. AJR 84:269, 1960.

Sohar E, Gafni J, Pras M, Heller H: Familial Mediterranean fever. A survey of 470 cases and review of the literature. Am J Med 43:227, 1967.

Yazici H, Tuzlaci M, Yurdakul S: A controlled survey of sacroiliitis in Behçet's disease. Ann Rheum Dis 40:558, 1981.

approximately 80 per cent of patients. Typically, iritis is seen, although episcleritis, conjunctivitis, keratitis, iridocyclitis, retinothrombophlebitis, optic neuritis and atrophy, and papilledema can be encountered. Late complications include glaucoma, cataracts, and blindness. Genital lesions appear in approximately 60 per cent of cases. Skin lesions may be observed in approximately 75 per cent of cases, consisting of pyoderma with pustules of varying size and erythema nodosum-like abnormalities of the lower extremity. Additional manifestations include venous thrombosis and thrombophlebitis; gastrointestinal inflammation leading to abdominal pain, distention, and diarrhea; and central nervous system findings. Myositis has also been noted.

Articular alterations appear in more than 50 per cent of patients. Monoarticular or oligoarticular involvement predom-

Chapter 29

Systemic Lupus Erythematosus

Donald Resnick, M.D.

Musculoskeletal abnormalities represent a significant part of the clinical and radiologic picture of systemic lupus erythematosus. These abnormalities include myositis, symmetric polyarthritis, deforming nonerosive arthropathy, spontaneous rupture of tendons, osteonecrosis, soft tissue calcification, osteomyelitis and septic arthritis, and terminal phalangeal sclerosis and erosion. Many of these abnormalities are imitated by changes occurring in other collagen disorders and rheumatoid arthritis.

Systemic lupus erythematosus is a relatively common connective tissue disorder characterized by involvement of multiple organ systems. The musculoskeletal system is frequently affected, leading to a variety of clinical, pathologic, and radiologic findings. Yet, early reports considered lupus erythematosus to be an insignificant disorder of the skin. It is now recognized that the condition is a chronic disease associated with acute exacerbations and a variable outlook. Furthermore, it is known that abnormalities in the immune mechanism are fundamental in the pathogenesis of this disorder; patients produce many autoantibodies that participate in tissue injury throughout the body. Although the exact cause of systemic lupus erythematosus remains unknown, a variety of precipitating events appear to be important, including genetic and infectious factors. In addition, exposure to sunlight or ultraviolet rays or to certain drugs or foreign proteins may lead to exacerbations of this disease.

GENERAL CLINICAL ABNORMALITIES

Systemic lupus erythematosus is much more common in women than in men, and in blacks than in whites. Its familial nature is also well recognized. Although it may have its onset at any age, the disease is most frequent in women during the childbearing years. Children may be affected and, in general, the pattern of disease and its prognosis in childhood are similar to those in adults. The disease is rare in persons over the age of 45 years.

Symptoms and signs are variable, related to the distribution and the extent of systemic alterations. In some individuals, one or two organ systems are affected, whereas in others, multiple systems are involved. Initial clinical manifestations most frequently include constitutional symptoms and signs and articular and cutaneous findings. Subsequently, major clinical abnormalities may relate to the musculoskeletal, cutaneous, neurologic, renal, pulmonary, and cardiac systems. Additional clinical abnormalities may relate to the gastrointestinal system, the reticuloendothelial system, and the peripheral vasculature. Patients with systemic lupus erythematosus also may develop infections, perhaps related to lowered complement levels, impaired delayed hypersensitivity, and defective phagocytosis.

Laboratory analysis can reveal anemia, leukopenia, and abnormalities of plasma proteins (hyperglobulinemia, hypoalbuminemia, false-positive serologic test results for syphilis, positive results for serum rheumatoid factor, positive Coombs' reaction, cryoglobulinemia, lowered serum complement activity, autoagglutination of red blood cells, and the formation of LE cells and other antinuclear factors).

MUSCULOSKELETAL ABNORMALITIES

Characteristic and significant musculoskeletal abnormalities are encountered in patients with systemic lupus erythematosus (Table 29–1).

Myositis

Clinical features suggesting muscle involvement (myositis and myopathy) have been observed in 30 to 50 per cent of patients with systemic lupus erythematosus. Myositis may be associated with diffuse muscular tenderness, weakness, and atrophy and elevation of serum levels of muscle enzymes.

Symmetric Polyarthritis

Articular symptoms and signs of variable severity are present in 75 to 90 per cent of patients. The articular findings most frequently are bilateral and symmetric in distribution,

Table 29–1. MUSCULOSKELETAL MANIFESTATIONS OF SYSTEMIC LUPUS ERYTHEMATOSUS

Myositis
Polyarthritis
Deforming nonerosive arthropathy
Tendon weakening and rupture
Osteonecrosis
Soft tissue calcification
Osteomyelitis and septic arthritis
Acrosclerosis
Tuftal resorption

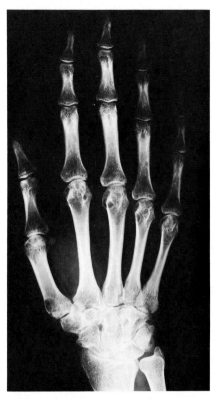

Figure 29–1. Polyarthritis: Radiographic abnormalities. Note multiple well-defined subchondral cysts. (From Leskinen RH, et al: Bone lesions in systemic lupus erythematosus. Radiology 153:349, 1984. Used with permission.)

involving particularly the small joints of the hand, the knee, the wrist, and the shoulder. Joint effusions are detected but are not large. Analysis of synovial fluid reveals less intense inflammation compared with that in rheumatoid arthritis. Synovial membrane biopsy may document synovial inflammation.

Radiographic abnormalities accompanying uncomplicated synovitis in systemic lupus erythematosus consist of soft tissue swelling and periarticular osteoporosis, simulating the abnormalities of rheumatoid arthritis. Although well-defined lytic lesions in periarticular bone have occasionally been recorded in patients with systemic lupus erythematosus, usually they do not resemble the marginal erosions of rheumatoid arthritis (Fig. 29–1). In addition, the joint space generally is not narrowed.

Deforming Nonerosive Arthropathy

A deforming nonerosive arthropathy may be evident in as many as 5 to 40 per cent of patients with systemic lupus erythematosus who have articular abnormalities, particularly those with long-standing disease. Characteristically, the deformities cause little functional disability and are completely reducible; in fact, they may disappear when the hand is placed firmly on the cassette during radiography. In some instances, chronic fixed deformities can appear.

The Jaccoud-like arthropathy has a variable appearance (Fig. 29–2). Symmetric involvement of interphalangeal joints of multiple digits of the hand is most typical. Hyperextension at the proximal interphalangeal joints and flexion at the distal interphalangeal joints create swan-neck deformities. Bouton-

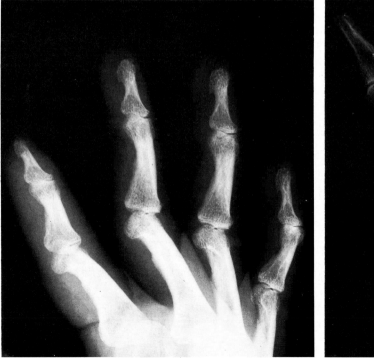
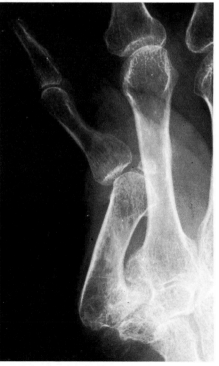

A   B

Figure 29–2. Lupus arthropathy: Appearance of deformities. A Severe (and reversible) swan-neck deformities of all the digits are characterized by hyperextension at the proximal interphalangeal joints and flexion at the distal interphalangeal articulations. **B** In the first ray, observe the considerable subluxation and flexion of the carpometacarpal joint associated with joint space narrowing, sclerosis, and osteophytosis and hyperextension of the metacarpophalangeal joint.

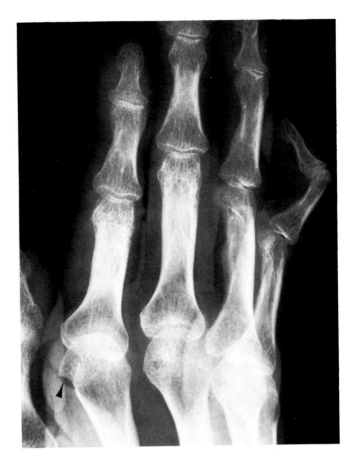

Figure 29–3. Lupus arthropathy: Hook erosions. An oblique radiograph outlines ulnar deviation of metacarpophalangeal joints. Note the flexion deformity of the distal interphalangeal joint of the fifth finger. Observe the hook-like erosion (arrowhead) on the radial and volar aspect of the second metacarpal head. This appearance and location are typical.

nière deformities, with flexion at the proximal interphalangeal joints and hyperextension at the distal interphalangeal joints, can also be seen. Hyperextension at the interphalangeal articulation of the thumb is characteristic. Additional deformities include subluxation with ulnar drift at the metacarpophalangeal joints and subluxation at the first carpometacarpal joint. Associated abnormalities in the foot have been described.

It is important to stress that joint space narrowing and osseous erosion are not prominent in this deforming arthropathy, serving to distinguish it from the articular abnormalities of rheumatoid arthritis. Rarely, cartilaginous and osseous alterations do become evident in lupus arthropathy and may take several forms. Diminution of cartilage may be related either to atrophy of disuse or to pressure erosion from apposing bones in subluxed articulations. Bilateral or unilateral "hook" erosions on the metacarpal heads are occasionally evident (Fig. 29–3). The erosions are probably produced by capsular pressure and deformity. Osteoporosis and cyst formation within the subchondral bone also can occur in lupus arthropathy (Fig. 29–1).

The articular deformities of lupus arthropathy are related to capsular and ligamentous laxity and contracture and to muscular imbalance, perhaps occurring as a response to prolonged, recurrent low grade inflammation of intraarticular and periarticular structures. Similar abnormalities occur in other deforming nonerosive arthropathies, particularly that which is apparent in patients with rheumatic fever. The alterations are distinct from those of rheumatoid arthritis, in which severe intraarticular inflammatory changes produce permanent cartilaginous and osseous destruction, leading to instability and subluxation.

Spontaneous Tendon Weakening and Rupture

Spontaneous rupture of tendons is observed in patients with systemic lupus erythematosus, almost invariably in association with systemically or locally administered steroids. Because such tendon rupture may also occur in patients receiving steroids who do not have systemic lupus erythematosus, it is difficult to ascertain the role of this disease in the attenuation of tendons. Single or multiple tendons at various sites may be torn in systemic lupus erythematosus. In general, tendons in weight-bearing locations are affected.

Osteonecrosis

The appearance of bone necrosis in patients with systemic lupus erythematosus is well documented, the most commonly reported frequency being approximately 5 to 6 per cent, with estimates as high as 40 per cent. Although the femoral head is the most typical site of abnormality, involvement of other and multiple sites has been confirmed, including the humeral head, the femoral condyles, the tibial plateaus, and the talus, and even the small bones of the hand, the wrist, and the foot. Osteonecrosis in systemic lupus erythematosus has been associated with Raynaud's phenomenon and other signs of vasculitis, as well as physical activity.

The pathogenesis of osteonecrosis in this disease has not been fully delineated. Most of the affected patients have

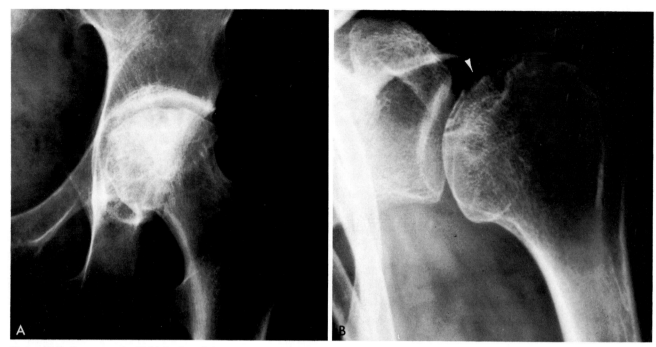

Figure 29–4. Osteonecrosis: Multiple sites. A In the hip, typical changes in the femoral head are characterized by sclerosis, cyst formation, and collapse of the subchondral bone. The opposite side was also involved. B Observe the fragmentation of the humeral head with depression of the subchondral bone (arrowhead).

received corticosteroid medications, although, infrequently, patients with lupus erythematosus who have not received such medication may develop necrosis of bone. Various studies have appeared attributing osteonecrosis in patients with lupus erythematosus to duration, total dose, or initial dose of corticosteroid therapy.

The radiographic and pathologic features of osteonecrosis in patients with systemic lupus erythematosus are identical to those in patients who do not have this disease (Fig. 29–4). The occasional occurrence of bone necrosis in unusual sites, such as the metacarpal heads, carpal bones, tarsus, and metatarsal heads, however, should suggest systemic lupus erythematosus as a potential diagnosis.

Soft Tissue Calcification

Soft tissue calcification is occasionally observed in systemic lupus erythematosus (Fig. 29–5). Several patterns are described: diffuse linear, streaky, or nodular calcification in the subcutaneous and deeper tissues, particularly in the lower extremities; focal or localized plaque-like calcification; periarticular calcification; and arterial calcification. Juxtaarticular calcifications appear as single or multiple deposits of varying size with or without adjacent joint disease; these deposits are usually located in the soft tissues or, more rarely, the joint capsule.

Osteomyelitis and Septic Arthritis

An unusually high frequency of bacterial and mycotic infections exists in patients with systemic lupus erythematosus. Two major factors contribute to this susceptibility to infection—steroid administration and renal disease. The respiratory tract, the urinary tract, the skin, and the soft tissues are the commonly infected sites. Bone and joint infections are less frequent in systemic lupus erythematosus (Fig. 29–

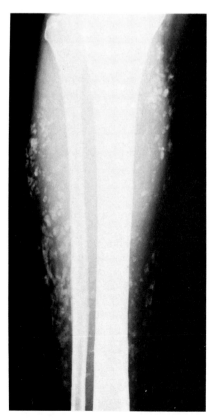

Figure 29–5. Soft tissue calcification. Widespread soft tissue calcification is evident in the lower leg.

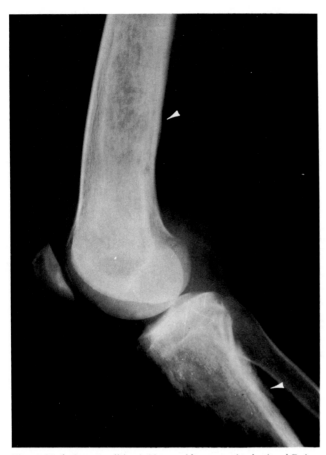

Figure 29–6. Osteomyelitis. A 22 year old woman who developed Escherichia coli septicemia and osteomyelitis of multiple sites. In the distal part of the femur and proximal part of the tibia, changes include a motheaten pattern of bone destruction and periostitis (arrowheads).

6). Implicated organisms have included *Neisseria gonorrheae, Neisseria meningitidis, Staphylococcus aureus*, gram-negative bacilli, atypical mycobacteria, *Mycobacterium tuberculosis*, and *Salmonella typhimurium*.

Sacroiliitis

Rarely, in systemic lupus erythematosus, imaging studies reveal alterations about the sacroiliac joints. On plain films, such abnormalities have included joint space narrowing, bone erosions, and reactive sclerosis in a unilateral or bilateral distribution. These changes are similar to those seen in osteoarthritis.

Miscellaneous Abnormalities

Reported alterations of the terminal tufts of the phalanges in systemic lupus erythematosus have included osteosclerosis and resorption (Fig. 29–7). The appearance of sclerosis at this site (acral sclerosis) must be evaluated with caution, as focal sclerotic lesions of one or several phalanges may be an incidental finding. The detection of diffuse sclerosis of multiple digits may be more significant; this abnormality has been seen in a variety of collagen disorders, including rheumatoid arthritis, and in sarcoidosis. The pattern of resorption of the phalangeal tufts in this disease is identical to that in scleroderma.

The occurrence of clinical and radiologic features of systemic lupus erythematosus in patients with other collagen diseases has been documented in various overlap syndromes, as well as in mixed connective tissue disease (see Chapter 33). In both mixed connective tissue disease and overlap syndromes, musculoskeletal manifestations of systemic lupus erythematosus may be combined with those of scleroderma, dermatomyositis, or rheumatoid arthritis.

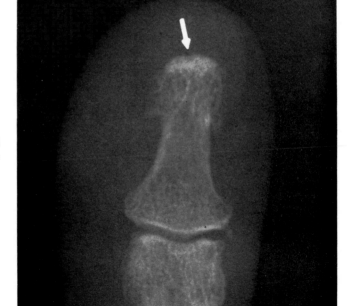

Figure 29–7. Tuftal sclerosis and resorption. Focal bone sclerosis and resorption are evident in the tuft (arrow). (Courtesy of A. Brower, M.D., Washington, D.C.)

Table 29–2. DIFFERENTIAL DIAGNOSIS OF RADIOGRAPHIC ABNORMALITIES IN THE HAND

Diagnosis	Distribution*	Deformities	Erosions	Joint Space Narrowing
Lupus arthropathy	MCP and IP articulations of all the digits; prominent abnormalities of the thumb	Initially reversible; subsequently may become fixed	Hook erosions on radial and volar aspects of metacarpal heads (uncommon)	Cartilage atrophy and pressure erosion in subluxed articulations (uncommon)
Classic Jaccoud's arthropathy	MCP and IP articulations of ulnar digits, particularly the fourth and fifth fingers	Initially reversible; subsequently may become fixed	Hook erosions on radial and volar aspects of metacarpal heads (uncommon)	Cartilage atrophy and pressure erosion in subluxed articulations (uncommon)
Rheumatoid arthritis	MCP and PIP articulations of all the digits; prominent abnormalities	Progressive	Widespread marginal and central erosions at involved sites (common)	"Pannus" destruction of cartilage in subluxed and nonsubluxed articulations (common)

*MCP, Metacarpophalangeal; IP, interphalangeal; PIP, proximal interphalangeal.

DIFFERENTIAL DIAGNOSIS

The symmetric polyarthritis that is associated with systemic lupus erythematosus produces nonspecific radiographic findings, including soft tissue swelling and osteoporosis. These same findings are encountered in other disorders that are characterized by synovial inflammation, such as rheumatoid arthritis.

The deforming nonerosive arthropathy of the hands and wrists (and less commonly the feet) in systemic lupus erythematosus is similar to Jaccoud's arthropathy, which most typically follows rheumatic fever (Table 29–2). In the classic descriptions of Jaccoud's arthropathy, involvement of the ulnar digits (fourth and fifth fingers) is stressed, although a more extensive distribution may be encountered; in the arthropathy of systemic lupus erythematosus, all the digits, including the thumb, are frequently affected, although a more limited distribution may be evident. In rheumatoid arthritis, joint space narrowing and bone erosion are characteristic, although, occasionally, digital deformity may occur in the absence of cartilaginous and osseous abnormalities. In these instances, accurate differentiation of the joint disease of systemic lupus erythematosus from that of rheumatoid arthritis is difficult.

The thumb deformities in systemic lupus erythematosus can be extensive; hyperextension of the interphalangeal joint and subluxation at the first carpometacarpal joint are particularly characteristic. Significant thumb deformity is evident in other collagen disorders, however, such as scleroderma, as well as in Ehlers-Danlos syndrome.

Spontaneous tendon rupture, which has been noted in patients with systemic lupus erythematosus, also occurs without an obvious precipitating event in hyperparathyroidism and in patients who have received steroid medication for any reason.

Osteonecrosis complicating systemic lupus erythematosus generally cannot be differentiated from that accompanying a variety of disease processes. Involvement of the metacarpal and metatarsal heads and the tarsal and carpal bones, however, appears to be especially characteristic of systemic lupus erythematosus.

Soft tissue calcification, which is observed in systemic lupus erythematosus, accompanies other collagen disorders, particularly scleroderma and dermatomyositis. Differentiation among these disorders on the basis of the appearance of soft tissue calcific deposits is extremely difficult. Furthermore, phalangeal tuftal resorption or sclerosis has been identified in many collagen diseases as well as in sarcoidosis.

FURTHER READING

Budin JA, Feldman F: Soft tissue calcifications in systemic lupus erythematosus. AJR 124:358, 1975.

Bywaters EGL: Jaccoud's syndrome. A sequel to the joint involvement in systemic lupus erythematosus. Clin Rheum Dis 1:125, 1975.

Fishel B, Eventov I, Avrahami E, Yaron M: Multiple osteonecrotic lesions in systemic lupus erythematosus. J Rheumatol 14:601, 1987.

Khan MA, Ballou SP: Tendon rupture in systemic lupus erythematosus. J Rheumatol 8:308, 1981.

Klipper AR, Stevens MB, Zizic TM, Hungerford DS: Ischemic necrosis of bone in systemic lupus erythematosus. Medicine 55:251, 1976.

Leskinen RH, Skrifvars BV, Laasonen LS, Edgren KJ: Bone lesions in systemic lupus erythematosus. Radiology 153:349, 1984.

Leventhal GH, Dorfman HD: Aseptic necrosis of bone in systemic lupus erythematosus. Semin Arthritis Rheum 4:73, 1974.

Weissman BN, Rappoport AS, Sosman JL, Schur PH: Radiographic findings in the hands in patients with systemic lupus erythematosus. Radiology 126:313, 1978.

Chapter 30

Scleroderma (Progressive Systemic Sclerosis)

Donald Resnick, M.D.

Scleroderma (progressive systemic sclerosis) leads to characteristic musculoskeletal abnormalities owing to involvement of skin, subcutaneous tissues, muscles, bones, and joints. Many of the diverse clinical manifestations in this disease are represented on radiographs as soft tissue atrophy and calcification and bone resorption. Changes frequently predominate in the phalanges of the hand, although diffuse subcutaneous calcification, widespread periarticular calci- *fication, and bone resorption at other sites, such as the mandible, the ribs, and the clavicles, are encountered. Major articular alterations consist of an erosive arthritis, particularly in the distal interphalangeal, proximal interphalangeal, metacarpophalangeal, first carpometacarpal, and inferior radioulnar joints, and intraarticular calcific collections.*

Scleroderma is an uncommon generalized disorder of connective tissue that affects various organ systems, principally the skin, the lungs, the gastrointestinal tract, the heart, the kidneys, and the musculoskeletal system. Its pathologic characteristics include severe fibrosis and alterations of small blood vessels. The cause and pathogenesis of scleroderma are not known, although three potential mechanisms have been implicated: an abnormality of collagen metabolism, a vascular abnormality, and an immunologic process.

NOMENCLATURE

The many reports of scleroderma and the difficulty in differentiating it from other disorders associated with induration of the skin have led to a variety of descriptive terms and classification systems for the disease. Nomenclature that is commonly encountered includes the following:

Raynaud's Phenomenon or Disease: Paroxysmal occlusion of the digital arteries that is precipitated by cold or emotional stress and relieved by heat. The disorder is termed Raynaud's *disease* when it is primary or idiopathic and Raynaud's *phenomenon* when it is secondary to another condition. Local pallor, cyanosis, pain, burning, numbness, swelling, and hyperhidrosis are the predominant features. Diseases associated with Raynaud's phenomenon include collagen disorders (progressive systemic sclerosis, systemic lupus erythematosus, rheumatoid arthritis, Sjögren's syndrome, dermatomyositis, and mixed connective tissue disease), other vasculitides (cryoglobulinemia, hepatitis B, and paroxysmal nocturnal hemoglobinuria), obstructive arterial disorders (arteriosclerosis, thromboses, and Buerger's disease), drug intoxications (ergot alkaloids, vinyl chloride, cytotoxic drugs, and heavy metals), neurologic and neoplastic processes, and thermal or occupational trauma (frostbite, physical injury, and vibration syndrome).

Acrosclerosis: Sclerosis of facial structures and fingers that is associated with Raynaud's phenomenon.

Diffuse Systemic Sclerosis: Involvement of the skin of the trunk that is commonly associated with systemic abnormalities and that may be associated with peripheral skin involvement.

CRST Syndrome: The association of subcutaneous calcinosis, Raynaud's phenomenon, sclerodactyly, and telangiectasia.

CREST Syndrome: The association of CRST syndrome with esophageal abnormalities.

Thibierge-Weissenbach Syndrome: The combination of calcinosis and digital ischemia.

Scleroderma Circumscriptum, Scleroderma Diffusum, Scleroderma Morphoea, Scleroderma en Bande: Dermatologic variants of the disease.

Shulman Syndrome: Scleroderma-like syndrome with eosinophilia and hypergammaglobulinemia but without systemic or vascular involvement. This syndrome, which is also called eosinophilic fasciitis, may occur after an episode of physical exertion and is associated with painful swelling and induration of the skin and soft tissues, followed by joint contracture.

CLINICAL ABNORMALITIES
General Features

Scleroderma affects women more frequently than men and usually becomes apparent in the third to fifth decades of life. A common presenting manifestation is intermittent pallor of the digits (fingers or toes) on exposure to cold (Raynaud's phenomenon). Additionally, initial symptoms may include gradual thickening and edema of the skin and pain and stiffness in the small joints of the hands and in the knees. In some persons, the onset of scleroderma is characterized by severe muscular weakness or visceral involvement (dysphagia) without involvement of the skin.

As the disease advances, skin changes frequently represent its most characteristic clinical feature. Edema is replaced by rigidity and thickening of the skin, which may become widespread in distribution. Melanotic hyperpigmentation, vitiligo, and telangiectasis can be observed. Calcific collections develop in subcutaneous tissue. Nodular lesions may ulcerate, extruding calcific material on the surface of the skin. Secondary infection of the ulcerated lesions is common.

Systemic involvement in scleroderma can lead to a variety of symptoms and signs, depending on the site of abnormality. Gastrointestinal, pulmonary, renal, and cardiac abnormalities may become prominent.

Rheumatologic Features

Articular involvement is evident initially in 10 to 65 per cent of patients with scleroderma and eventually in as many as 95 per cent of patients. The fingers, the wrists, and the ankles are commonly affected. When symmetric in distribution, manifestations resemble those of rheumatoid arthritis. Tendon and tendon sheath involvement also is seen frequently. Flexion contractures are not uncommon, particularly in the digits of the hand, in the wrist, and in the elbow. Muscle involvement occurs in the majority of patients with scleroderma.

Laboratory analysis may indicate elevation of the erythrocyte sedimentation rate, positive serologic test results for rheumatoid factor, and the presence of antinuclear antibodies.

Overlap Syndromes

Some patients with scleroderma demonstrate clinical patterns that suggest the presence of more than one collagen disease; findings may indicate an overlap condition, consisting of scleroderma and dermatomyositis or scleroderma and systemic lupus erythematosus. Furthermore, the demonstration of serum antibody to an extractable nuclear antigen (ENA) in patients with scleroderma-like clinical findings indicates the presence of mixed connective tissue disease (see Chapter 33).

RADIOGRAPHIC ABNORMALITIES
Bone and Soft Tissue Involvement

HAND AND WRIST (FIG. 30–1). Abnormalities of the hand are characterized by resorption of soft tissue, subcutaneous calcification, and osseous destruction.

Soft tissue resorption of the fingertips is a common finding

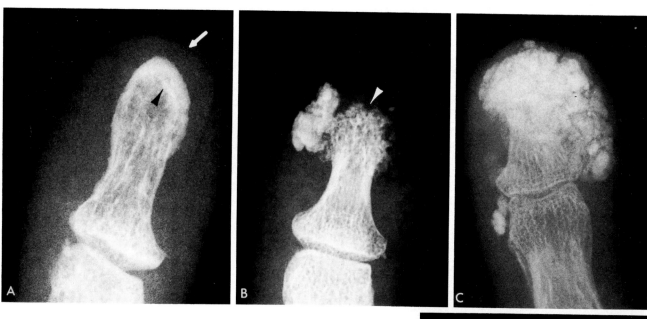

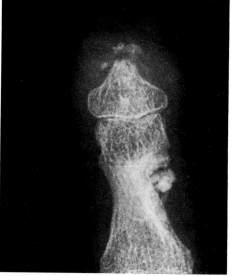

Figure 30–1. Bone and soft tissue abnormalities: Digits of the hand. A Observe atrophy of the soft tissue (arrow) and hyperostosis of the phalangeal tuft (arrowhead). B In this digit, findings include resorption of the tuft (arrowhead) and adjacent calcification. C More extensive calcification is evident in another patient. D Soft tissue swelling, tuftal resorption, and calcification are seen. Note the deformity of the nail.

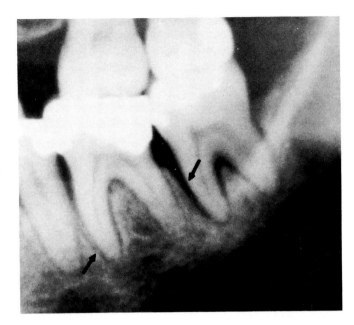

Figure 30–2. **Bone and soft tissue abnormalities: Mandible.** Observe the exaggerated radiolucent area between the teeth and the mandible (arrows) corresponding to the location of a thickened periodontal membrane.

in scleroderma. Its reported frequency has varied from 15 to 80 per cent. Resorption of soft tissue produces a conical shape of the tips of the fingers. Any digit of the hand, including the thumb, may be affected. It is frequently accompanied by adjacent calcific deposits and bone abnormalities.

Amorphous calcification is common in patients with scleroderma. The hand is affected most frequently; digital calcification may appear as small punctate deposits at the phalangeal tip, more extensive conglomerate deposits, and sheetlike or curvilinear collections. The precise mechanism of soft tissue calcification is not clear.

Bone erosion of the phalanges in the hand occurs in 40 to 80 per cent of patients with scleroderma. It commences on the tuft, particularly on the palmar aspect of the bone. Continued resorption leads to "penciling" or sharpening of the phalanx. In severe cases, much or all of the distal phalanx can be destroyed.

Extradigital involvement of the hand and wrist may consist of soft tissue calcification and destruction of portions of the carpus, radius, and ulna.

FOOT. The abnormalities in the foot resemble those in the hand, but they are less frequent and less pronounced.

MANDIBLE (FIG. 30–2). A relatively specific dental sign of scleroderma is thickening of the periodontal membrane. The enlarged membrane creates an exaggerated radiolucent area between the tooth and the mandibular bone. This mandibular alteration may lead to loss of the lamina dura and loosening of the teeth. More extensive mandibular bone resorption also has been noted in this disease.

RIBS (FIG. 30–3). Symmetrically distributed erosions predominate along the posterosuperior aspects of the third to sixth ribs and may occur in the absence of bone resorption at other sites. Some evidence suggests that rib resorption in scleroderma is related to intercostal muscle atrophy with resultant loss of mechanical stress to the cortical bone at the muscle insertions, leading to osseous resorption. Identical changes occur in other disorders associated with muscle atrophy owing either to chest wall restriction or to loss of innervation, such as rheumatoid arthritis, other collagen diseases, poliomyelitis, and restrictive lung disease.

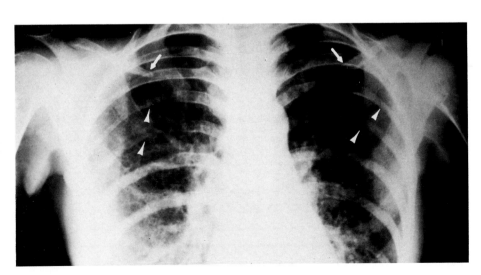

Figure 30–3. **Bone and soft tissue abnormalities: Ribs and clavicle.** Observe resorption of the clavicles (arrows) and ribs (arrowheads) and also abnormalities in the lower lobes of the lungs. (Courtesy of P. Kline, M.D., San Antonio, Texas.)

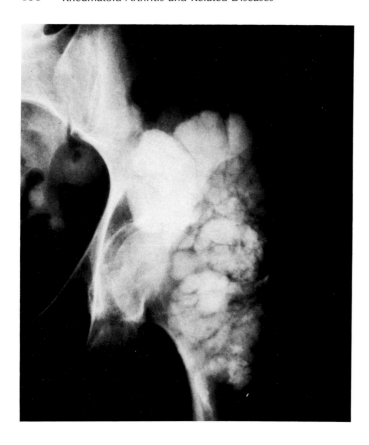

Figure 30–4. Bone and soft tissue abnormalities: Periarticular calcification. Periarticular deposits are evident about the hip.

OTHER SITES AND MANIFESTATIONS (FIG. 30–4). Soft tissue calcification in scleroderma occurs not only in the digits but also in the face, the axilla, the forearms, the lower legs, and pressure areas such as the ischial tuberosities. In addition, periarticular "tumoral" collections can appear at single or multiple sites, simulating the findings in milk-alkali syndrome, hypervitaminosis D, and renal osteodystrophy.

Bone resorption in scleroderma may also be apparent at other sites, including portions of the acromion, radius, and ulna, distal clavicle, humerus, and cervical spine (Table 30–1).

Articular Involvement

In addition to the "articular" abnormalities that result from primary osseous resorption in scleroderma, several other articular manifestations occur in this disease (Table 30–2).

DISTAL INTERPHALANGEAL JOINTS (FIG. 30–5). Alterations at distal interphalangeal joints are usually confined to regional or periarticular osteoporosis and swelling and

thickening of adjacent soft tissues without evidence of joint space narrowing or osseous erosion. Rarely, mild to severe bilateral erosive abnormalities of distal interphalangeal and proximal interphalangeal joints, characterized by articular space narrowing, marginal and central osseous erosions, bone production with osteophytes, and intraarticular bone ankylosis, are seen. The findings resemble changes in psoriasis or inflammatory (erosive) osteoarthritis; unlike rheumatoid arthritis, the metacarpophalangeal and wrist articulations are relatively spared.

PROXIMAL INTERPHALANGEAL AND METACARPOPHALANGEAL JOINTS. An unusual pattern of focal resorption or erosion localized to the dorsal aspect of the metacarpal and proximal phalangeal heads has been described in patients with scleroderma. The abnormalities are best detected on steep oblique or lateral radiographic projections of the digits and are combined with erosions on the volar aspect of the bones. They lack specificity, being observed in some patients with rheumatoid arthritis. The pathogenesis of such peculiar osseous abnormalities is not clear.

FIRST CARPOMETACARPAL JOINTS (FIG. 30–6). Selective involvement of the first carpometacarpal joint can

Table 30–1. SITES OF OSTEOLYSIS IN SCLERODERMA

Phalanges of hand and foot
Carpal bones
Distal ends of the radius and ulna
Mandible
Ribs
Clavicle
Humerus
Acromion
Cervical spine

Table 30–2. SITES OF EROSIVE ARTICULAR DISEASE IN SCLERODERMA

Metacarpophalangeal joints
Proximal and distal interphalangeal joints
First carpometacarpal joint
Inferior radioulnar joint
Metatarsophalangeal joints

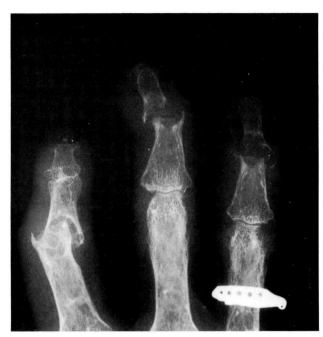

Figure 30–5. Articular involvement: Interphalangeal joints. Extensive bone erosion about distal interphalangeal and proximal interphalangeal joints can be observed. Note the separation of the osseous margins and the sharply demarcated irregular surfaces. Subluxation is also apparent. The findings are reminiscent of psoriatic arthritis.

be apparent in scleroderma. Distinctive bilateral resorption of the trapezium and adjacent metacarpal bone is observed with varying degrees of radial subluxation of the metacarpal base. Associated findings may include intraarticular calcification (discussed later in this chapter) and erosions at additional joints. The other joints of the wrist generally are spared, however.

The pathogenesis of the arthropathy is unknown. Its association with skin tightening, muscle atrophy of the hand and wrist, and contracture of the thumb in adduction may indicate that muscle and tendon imbalance produces joint subluxation at the first carpometacarpal joint, with subsequent pressure erosion of bone. In this regard, a similar arthropathy may be apparent in other disorders that alter muscle and tendon balance, such as systemic lupus erythematosus, Jaccoud's arthropathy, dermatomyositis, and Ehlers-Danlos syndrome.

OTHER SITES AND MANIFESTATIONS (FIG. 30–7). In addition to soft tissue and periarticular calcific deposition, intraarticular (free or intrasynovial) calcification can also become evident in scleroderma (Fig. 30–6). Radiographs reveal cloud-like radiodense regions conforming to a portion of the joint or the entire articulation. Intraarticular calcification is most frequent in the elbow, the inferior radioulnar and first carpometacarpal joints of the wrist, the metacarpophalangeal and metatarsophalangeal joints, the knee, and the hip. Additional radiographic findings in the involved joint include periarticular calcification and osseous resorption. Aspiration of joint contents documents chalky joint effusions containing hydroxyapatite crystals, the same substance found in the periarticular calcific deposits in this disease.

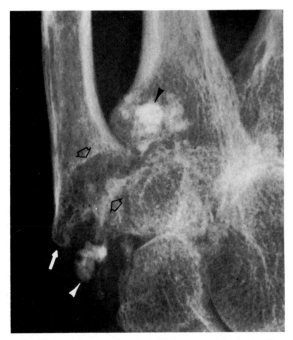

Figure 30–6. Articular involvement: Wrist. Note selective involvement of the first carpometacarpal joint in scleroderma. Observe scalloped erosions of the trapezium and base of the metacarpal (open arrows), radial and proximal subluxation of the metacarpal base (solid arrow) and intraarticular calcification (arrowheads). (From Resnick D, et al: Selective involvement of the first carpometacarpal joint in scleroderma. AJR 131:283, 1978. Copyright 1978, American Roentgen Ray Society. Used with permission.)

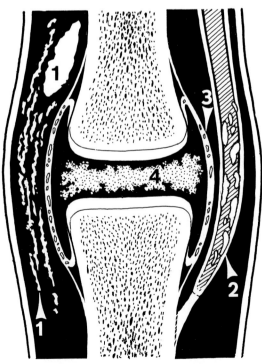

Figure 30–7. Sites of calcification in scleroderma. Deposits may occur in the soft tissues (1), tendons and tendon sheaths (2), and capsule (3), as well as within the joint (4).

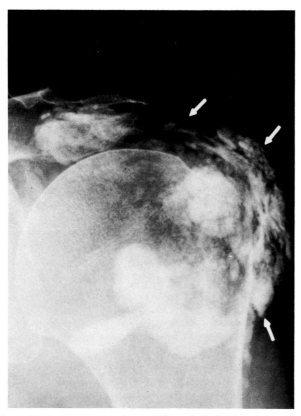

Figure 30–8. Articular involvement: Bursal calcification. Subacromial (subdeltoid) bursal calcification is obvious (arrows).

Synovial calcification may also be apparent within tendon sheaths or bursae in scleroderma (Fig. 30–8), most frequently about the heel, the elbow, the knee, and the shoulder.

A deforming nonerosive articular disease (Jaccoud's arthropathy) identical to that occurring after rheumatic fever occasionally is observed in patients with scleroderma.

Vascular Involvement

Arteriography confirms the presence of vascular abnormalities in patients with Raynaud's phenomenon. Vasospasm, narrowing, and obstructive lesions of digital arteries are observed, although the extent and severity of the occlusive lesions do not always correlate with the clinical severity of digital ischemia. Additional arteriographic findings have included incomplete, poorly formed, or absent palmar arterial arches and ulnar artery.

PATHOLOGIC ABNORMALITIES

The pathologic changes in the skin of patients with scleroderma consist of a low grade inflammatory reaction. Subsequently, progressive increase in compact collagen fibers in the dermis, thinning of the overlying epidermis, and atrophy of dermal appendages are evident. A decrease in thickness of skin in clinically affected areas has been documented by ultrasonography and radiographic techniques. Subcutaneous nodules may develop. Degenerative changes of muscle cells and accumulation of inflammatory cells indicate the presence of myositis.

Abnormalities of the synovial membrane consist of inflammatory changes characterized by hyperemia, cellular infiltration with lymphocytes and plasma cells, vascular sclerosis,

and surface fibrin deposition. The abnormalities resemble those of early rheumatoid arthritis.

ADDITIONAL SYNDROMES AND CONDITIONS ASSOCIATED WITH SCLERODERMA
Chemically Induced Scleroderma-like Conditions

Certain chemicals, including vinyl chloride, pentazocine, and bleomycin, can induce cutaneous abnormalities simulating those of scleroderma. Workers who clean reactor vessels and are exposed to the polymerizing agent vinyl chloride develop Raynaud's phenomenon and pulmonary fibrosis along with a distinctive pattern of acroosteolysis (see Chapter 84).

Scleroderma-like changes are also observed with other chemical agents, including solvents (trichloroethylene, benzene, toluene, xylene), paraffin and silicone implants, and cocaine. Furthermore, a toxic epidemic syndrome leading to scleroderma-like skin involvement has been associated with the consumption of adulterated rapeseed oil, illegally marketed and sold cheaply as a cooking oil.

Eosinophilic Fasciitis

Eosinophilic fasciitis, also known as Shulman's syndrome, is seen predominantly in adults and is associated with inflammation and induration of the skin and subcutaneous tissues of the hands, forearms, feet, and legs, in most cases occurring after an episode of physical exertion. Polyarthralgia, polyarthritis, muscle atrophy, and the carpal tunnel syndrome have been observed. The disorder is associated with peripheral blood eosinophilia, hypergammaglobulinemia, and an elevated erythrocyte sedimentation rate. Raynaud's phenomenon and visceral manifestations of progressive systemic sclerosis are conspicuously absent. Improvement in clinical and laboratory parameters follows the systemic administration of corticosteroids, so that a complete or nearly complete recovery is expected in a period of a few years. Radiographic abnormalities generally are confined to osteopenia.

The cause of eosinophilic fasciitis is unknown. It most resembles scleroderma and, in the minds of some investigators, may not be a separate disorder at all. Although it generally is self-limited and without systemic manifestations, these features too are not uniform.

Graft-Versus-Host Disease

Graft-versus-host disease occurs when immunologically competent cells engrafted onto a foreign host attack the tissues of that host. In current practice, this disease usually appears after allogeneic bone marrow transplantation. The specific prerequisites for identifying graft-versus-host disease are the following: the graft must contain immunocompetent cells; the host must be sufficiently different genetically from the graft to be perceived as antigenically foreign; and the host must be unable to reject the graft effectively.

Graft-versus-host disease occurs in either an acute or a chronic form, the former appearing before 100 days after the transplantation and the latter generally after 100 days. It is the chronic pattern, which develops in 10 to 30 per cent of patients undergoing bone marrow transplantation, that resembles a collagen disease, specifically scleroderma. This pattern is associated with more extensive abnormalities affecting the skin, gastrointestinal tract, liver, salivary glands, lymph nodes, mouth, eyes, lungs, and musculoskeletal system. In untreated cases, tightly bound skin, contractures, and tissue wasting are observed. Laboratory aberrations include anemia, leukopenia, thrombocytopenia, eosinophilia, elevated serum levels of immunoglobulins, and the presence of circulating autoantibodies.

DIFFERENTIAL DIAGNOSIS

Bone Abnormalities

Generalized resorption of the terminal phalanges of the hand or foot, or both, in scleroderma is characterized by "penciling" of the tuft (Fig. 30–9). A similar finding can be seen in other disorders, such as Raynaud's disease without scleroderma, thermal injuries, trauma, other collagen diseases, neuropathic disease (congenital indifference to pain, leprosy, diabetes mellitus, meningomyelocele), articular disorders (psoriasis, Lesch-Nyhan syndrome), hyperparathyroidism, progeria, and epidermolysis bullosa. In most of these diseases, the distribution of changes and the presence of additional abnormalities usually allow accurate diagnosis (Table 30–3). For example, sparing of the first digit in frostbite, destructive articular changes in psoriasis and Lesch-Nyhan syndrome, and subperiosteal resorption of phalanges in hyperparathyroidism are characteristic. Furthermore, the association of tuftal resorption, skin atrophy, and soft tissue calcification in scleroderma is of great diagnostic significance.

Tuftal resorption in scleroderma should not be confused with congenital disorders associated with hypoplasia of terminal phalanges. In these latter disorders, a small but otherwise normal bone is apparent. In addition, the type of bone resorption in scleroderma is usually easily differentiated from disorders characterized by band-like resorption of the distal phalangeal shafts (polyvinyl chloride acroosteolysis, familial acroosteolysis, and hyperparathyroidism) and from those characterized by intraosseous or eccentric destruction of the terminal phalanx (inclusion cyst, glomus tumor, enchondroma, osteomyelitis, and skeletal metastasis). The combination of tuftal resorption and erosive arthritis of the distal interphalangeal joints may be apparent in scleroderma as well as in hyperparathyroidism, psoriasis, thermal injuries, and multicentric reticulohistiocytosis.

Table 30–3. CHARACTERISTIC SITES OF DISTAL PHALANGEAL RESORPTION IN VARIOUS DISORDERS*

Disorder	Site		
	Tuft	Midportion or Waist	Periarticular
Scleroderma	+		+
Hyperparathyroidism	+	+	+
Thermal injury	+		+
Psoriasis	+		+
Epidermolysis bullosa	+		
Polyvinyl chloride acro-osteolysis		+	
Multicentric reticulo-histiocytosis	+		+
Inflammatory (erosive) osteoarthritis			+
Lesch-Nyhan syndrome	+		
Progeria	+		

*Only the characteristic sites of bone resorption are indicated, although in any single disease, considerable variability in these sites may exist.

Soft Tissue Abnormalities

Atrophy of the distal phalangeal soft tissue is a finding of scleroderma that can be observed in association with other collagen diseases, thermal injuries, vascular disorders, Raynaud's phenomenon, and epidermolysis bullosa, as well as additional conditions. Furthermore, as already outlined, scleroderma-like skin changes can also be evident in graft-versus-host disease after allogeneic bone marrow transplantation, in eosinophilic fasciitis, and after exposure to certain chemicals.

Widespread subcutaneous or periarticular calcification, a finding of scleroderma, may be apparent in other collagen diseases, renal osteodystrophy, hypoparathyroidism, pseudohypoparathyroidism, pseudopseudohypoparathyroidism, fat necrosis, hypervitaminosis D, idiopathic hypercalcemia, milk-

Figure 30–9. Phalangeal resorption: Differential diagnosis. The normal situation is depicted in diagram 1. Resorption of the tuft (2) can be seen in scleroderma, other collagen disorders, thermal injuries, hyperparathyroidism, psoriasis, and epidermolysis bullosa. Band-like resorption of the terminal phalanx (3) is seen in familial and occupational acroosteolysis, collagen disorders, and hyperparathyroidism. Erosions about the distal interphalangeal articulation (4) can be noted in psoriasis, multicentric reticulohistiocytosis, gout, thermal injuries, scleroderma, and hyperparathyroidism.

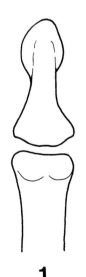

1

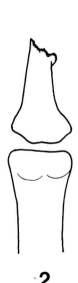

2

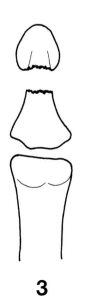

3

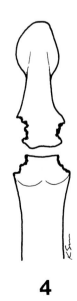

4

alkali syndrome, parasitic infections, Ehlers-Danlos syndrome, sarcoidosis, idiopathic calcium hydroxyapatite crystal deposition disease, Werner's syndrome, and idiopathic tumoral calcinosis.

Articular Abnormalities

An erosive arthritis of distal interphalangeal joints accompanies scleroderma, inflammatory (erosive) osteoarthritis, psoriasis, multicentric reticulohistiocytosis, gout, and thermal injuries.

Scalloped erosions of the first carpometacarpal joint can be seen in a variety of articular disorders, including scleroderma, dermatomyositis, Ehlers-Danlos syndrome, systemic lupus erythematosus, and rheumatoid arthritis. Isolated or predominant involvement of this joint without changes in the other wrist compartments eliminates rheumatoid arthritis as a diagnostic consideration. In scleroderma, the associated phalangeal abnormalities and the presence of intra- and extraarticular calcification at the first carpometacarpal joint allow a precise diagnosis.

Intraarticular cloud-like calcification in scleroderma differs in radiographic appearance from that of calcium pyrophosphate dihydrate crystal deposition disease, idiopathic calcium hydroxyapatite crystal deposition disease, idiopathic synovial osteochondromatosis, intraarticular osseous bodies, gout, and synovioma or hemangioma, although these other disorders are associated with calcific and ossific dense areas in and around joints.

FURTHER READING

Barnett AJ: Scleroderma (Progressive Systemic Sclerosis). Springfield, Ill, Charles C Thomas, 1974.

Bassett LW, Blocka KLN, Furst DE, Clements PJ, Gold RH: Skeletal findings in progressive systemic sclerosis (scleroderma). AJR 136:1121, 1981.

Keats TE: Rib erosions in scleroderma. AJR 100:530, 1967.

Lakhanpal S, Ginsburg WW, Michet CJ, Doyle JA, Moore SB: Eosinophilic fasciitis: Clinical spectrum and therapeutic response in 52 cases. Semin Arthritis Rheum 17:221, 1988.

Monsees B, Murphy WA: Distal phalangeal erosive lesions. Arthritis Rheum 27:449, 1984.

Moore TL, Zuckner J: Eosinophilic fasciitis. Semin Arthritis Rheum 9:228, 1980.

Rabinowitz JG, Twersky J, Guttadauria M: Similar bone manifestations of scleroderma and rheumatoid arthritis. AJR 121:35, 1974.

Resnick D, Greenway G, Vint VC, Robinson CA, Piper S: Selective involvement of the first carpometacarpal joint in scleroderma. AJR 131:283, 1978.

Resnick D, Scavulli JF, Goergen TG, Genant HK, Niwayama G: Intraarticular calcification in scleroderma. Radiology 124:685, 1977.

Rocco VK, Hurd ER: Scleroderma and scleroderma-like disorders. Semin Arthritis Rheum 16:22, 1986.

Rush PJ, Bell MJ, Fam AG: Toxic oil syndrome (Spanish oil disease) and chemically induced scleroderma-like conditions. J Rheumatol 11:262, 1984.

Spielvogel RL, Goltz RW, Kersey JH: Scleroderma-like changes in chronic graft vs host disease. Arch Dermatol 113:1424, 1977.

Chapter 31

Dermatomyositis and Polymyositis

Donald Resnick, M.D.

Dermatomyositis and polymyositis are disorders of unknown cause characterized by inflammation and degeneration of muscle. A variety of clinical patterns may be observed in both children and adults affected by these disorders. The radiographic features of musculoskeletal involvement consist of soft tissue edema, atrophy, contracture, and calcification; bone resorption (phalangeal tufts); and, possibly, articular erosion and subluxation. These features most resemble abnormalities accompanying other collagen diseases, including scleroderma and systemic lupus erythematosus.

Dermatomyositis and polymyositis are disorders of striated muscle characterized by diffuse, nonsuppurative inflammation and degeneration. In dermatomyositis, both the skeletal muscle and the skin are involved, whereas in polymyositis, the skeletal muscle alone is affected. The disorders are of unknown cause and affect patients of all ages, although they are most frequent in middle-aged women. Dermatomyositis and polymyositis are grouped with other collagen diseases because of similar clinical, pathologic, and radiologic features.

NOMENCLATURE AND CLASSIFICATION

The variability in clinical and laboratory features of dermatomyositis and polymyositis has caused difficulty in classification of these diseases. To better define and classify these disorders, five diagnostic criteria have been proposed: (1) proximal symmetric muscle weakness that progresses over a period of weeks to months; (2) elevated serum levels of muscle enzymes or an elevated level of urinary creatinine excretion; (3) an abnormal electromyogram; (4) abnormal muscle biopsy findings that are consistent with myositis; and (5) the presence of cutaneous disease typical of dermatomyositis. Although strict application of these criteria is not without difficulty, the criteria are useful in excluding other causes of myopathy.

Type I: Typical Polymyositis

Type I is the most common type, constituting approximately 35 per cent of cases. It is most frequent in the third, fourth, and fifth decades of life and affects women more often than men, in a ratio of approximately 2 to 1. Cases generally are sporadic. Polymyositis is characterized by gradually increasing muscle weakness, first appearing in the musculature of the thighs and pelvic girdle and later affecting the upper extremity and the laryngeal and pharyngeal muscles. Dermal manifestations are inconstant. Joint manifestations include arthralgias and arthritis, which may be accompanied by a joint effusion and positive results in serologic tests for rheumatoid factor.

Type II: Typical Dermatomyositis

Present in approximately 25 per cent of patients, more frequently women, type II is characterized by muscular weakness and a diffuse erythematous skin rash on the face, the neck, the chest, the shoulders, and the arms. Adults in the fifth or sixth decade typically are affected.

Type III: Typical Dermatomyositis with Malignancy

In patients over the age of 40 years, particularly men, type III dermatomyositis is characterized by the presence of skin rash, muscular weakness, and malignancy. Previous reports suggest that malignancy becomes evident in approximately 15 to 25 per cent of patients. Most commonly, muscular and dermal manifestations antedate the appearance of malignancy by months to years. The neoplasm may originate from almost any site, although the most commonly associated tumors arise from the lungs, the prostate, the female pelvic organs, the breast, and the gastrointestinal tract.

Type IV: Childhood Dermatomyositis

Dermatomyositis or polymyositis affects children or adolescents in approximately 20 per cent of cases. Dermal and muscular alterations appear at any age in childhood, although they are most frequent between the ages of 5 and 10 years. Girls are affected more commonly than boys. Proximal muscle weakness may either progress rapidly, leading to swallowing, phonation, and respiratory difficulties, or fluctuate, with periods of remission and exacerbation. Additional characteristics of childhood dermatomyositis are fever, extensive edema and calcification of skin and subcutaneous tissues, vasculitis, and joint contractures. Dermatomyositis in childhood may be associated with other disorders, including hypogammaglobulinemia and leukemia.

The severity of dermatomyositis in children should be stressed; although the mortality rate in this disease is approximately the same in children and adults, the interval between the onset of myositis and death is shorter, and the degree of soft tissue calcification is more extensive in childhood dermatomyositis.

Type V: Acute Myolysis

Type V disease, which is present in approximately 3 per cent of patients, is characterized by the sudden onset of myolysis, particularly in patients in the first or second decade of life. Intermittent attacks are associated with diffuse muscular weakness, myoglobinuria, and elevation of serum muscle enzymes. A fatal outcome is not infrequent.

Type VI: Polymyositis in Sjögren's Syndrome and Other Connective Tissue Diseases

In about 10 per cent of patients with Sjögren's syndrome progressive weakness of proximal musculature is evident. Myositis accompanies other connective tissue diseases as well, including scleroderma, systemic lupus erythematosus, rheumatoid arthritis, and overlap syndromes.

CLINICAL ABNORMALITIES

The most constant clinical finding is muscular weakness; this manifestation is the presenting symptom in approximately 50 per cent of patients. Symmetric involvement of proximal muscles is most characteristic. Involvement of respiratory muscles may lead to the patient's demise.

Skin rashes are evident eventually in 40 to 60 per cent of patients and are an initial manifestation of the disease in 20 to 25 per cent. Skin abnormalities are frequent about the face, the knuckles, the elbows, the knees, the ankles, the neck, the chest, and the shoulders. Raynaud's phenomenon occurs in about one third of patients with polymyositis.

Arthralgias and arthritis are present in 20 to 50 per cent of patients. In some patients, serologic tests for rheumatoid factor yield positive results. Typically, the wrists, the knees, and the small joints of the fingers are affected symmetrically. Permanent joint damage is unusual.

Clinical manifestations of visceral involvement in dermatomyositis and polymyositis include cardiac, pulmonary, gastrointestinal, renal, neurologic, and ocular abnormalities.

The association of neoplasm and dermatomyositis (and to a lesser extent, polymyositis) is well known. The tumor most commonly is a carcinoma, although myeloma, leukemia, lymphoma, thymoma, and reticulosis have also been recorded. The clinical features associated with myositis in patients with coexistent neoplasm are generally severe, whereas those associated with the neoplasm itself are usually mild.

Laboratory tests reveal characteristic abnormalities in many patients with dermatomyositis and polymyositis. Serum levels of creatine kinase are usually elevated during periods of active myositis. Serum glutamic-oxaloacetic transaminase (SGOT), serum glutamic-pyruvic transaminase (SGPT), and serum aldolase levels may also be elevated.

RADIOGRAPHIC ABNORMALITIES
Soft Tissue Abnormalities

Although soft tissue abnormalities occur in both children and adults, the frequency and severity of the findings are greater in the younger age groups.

The initial soft tissue manifestation is edema of the subcutaneous tissue and muscle, producing increased muscular

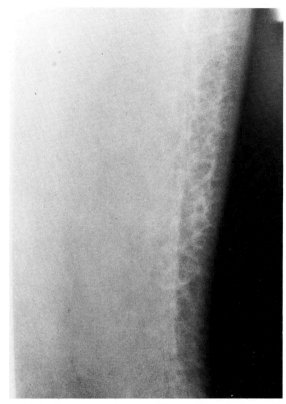

Figure 31–1. Dermatomyositis and polymyositis: Soft tissue edema. Observe extensive edema of the subcutaneous tissue septa. (From Ozonoff MB, Flynn FJ Jr: Roentgenologic features of dermatomyositis of childhood. AJR 118:206, 1973. Copyright 1973, American Roentgen Ray Society. Used with permission.)

bulk and radiodensity, thickening of subcutaneous septa, and poor delineation of the subcutaneous tissue-muscular interface (Fig. 31–1). The changes are more prominent in the proximal musculature, the axillae, the chest wall, the forearms, the thighs, and the calves. After effective treatment, tissue edema can decrease or disappear entirely, although in many patients, fibrosis and muscle atrophy and contracture become apparent.

The most characteristic soft tissue abnormality in dermatomyositis and polymyositis is soft tissue calcification. The frequency of this finding in children is high. The extent of calcification, particularly that within musculature, appears to increase with the severity of the disease. Small or large calcareous intermuscular fascial plane calcification is distinctive (Fig. 31–2), although it may not be so common as subcutaneous calcification. The favored sites of intermuscular calcification are the large muscles in the proximal portion of the limbs. The appearance and distribution of subcutaneous calcification in dermatomyositis and polymyositis simulate those in scleroderma; linear and curvilinear deposits demonstrate predilection for the knees, the elbows, and the fingers (Fig. 31–3). Subcutaneous calcification may be accompanied by cutaneous ulceration and soft tissue infection.

Soft tissue calcification may progress with increasing duration of the disease. Occasionally, spontaneous regression and resolution of calcinosis become apparent at puberty. On rare occasions, soft tissue ossification rather than calcification has been observed.

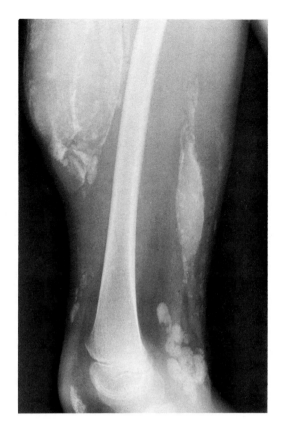

Figure 31–2. Dermatomyositis and polymyositis: Intermuscular fascial plane calcification. In a 10 year old boy with disease of 4 years' duration, large calcareous muscular masses have produced deformity of the overlying skin. Note the "tumoral" nature of the calcifications. (From Ozonoff MB, Flynn FJ Jr: Roentgenologic features of dermatomyositis of childhood. AJR 118:206, 1973. Copyright 1973, American Roentgen Ray Society. Used with permission.)

Articular Abnormalities

The arthralgia and arthritis of dermatomyositis and polymyositis usually are unaccompanied by radiographic abnormalities or are associated with transient soft tissue swelling and periarticular osteoporosis. Destructive joint changes have occasionally been noted. Reported radiographic changes have included soft tissue swelling (particularly in the metacarpophalangeal and interphalangeal joints), periosteal and soft tissue calcification, bone erosions, and alignment abnormalities (Fig. 31–4). Particularly characteristic has been radial

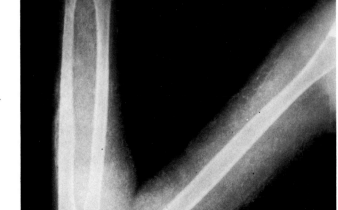

Figure 31–3. Dermatomyositis and polymyositis: Subcutaneous calcification. Diffuse linear subcutaneous calcinosis is evident.

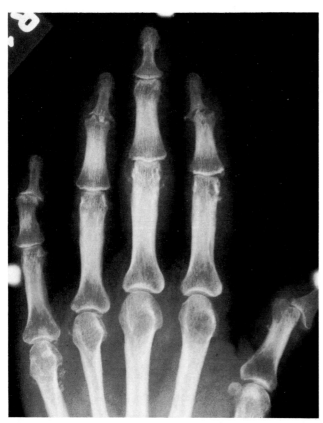

Figure 31–4. Dermatomyositis and polymyositis: Destructive articular abnormalities. The alterations consist of erosions of multiple distal interphalangeal joints, periarticular calcifications, and subluxation of the interphalangeal joint of the right thumb.

subluxation or dislocation at the interphalangeal joint of the thumb ("floppy thumb"sign).

SCINTIGRAPHIC ABNORMALITIES

The role of radionuclide examination in the detection and grading of muscular inflammation is not clear. Technetium polyphosphate and similar agents may accumulate in abnormal muscle in patients with dermatomyositis and polymyositis. This abnormal accumulation demonstrates some correlation with the severity of muscle weakness and may improve after corticosteroid therapy. Gallium may also be used in this clinical situation.

PATHOLOGIC ABNORMALITIES

The microscopic aberrations in involved musculature include focal or extensive degeneration of muscle fibers, regenerative activity, muscle necrosis, infiltration with chronic inflammatory cells, interstitial fibrosis, phagocytosis of ne-

crotic fibers, and variation in cross-sectional diameter of adjacent muscle fibers.

ETIOLOGY AND PATHOGENESIS

Although the cause of dermatomyositis and polymyositis is unknown, there is considerable evidence that a cell-mediated immune mechanism is responsible for muscle damage by affecting either the muscle or the adjacent blood vessels. A genetic predisposition to such immunologic mechanisms has been suggested. An infectious cause is also plausible. The association of dermatomyositis and neoplasm has raised the additional possibility that tumor may precipitate inflammatory muscle disease.

DIFFERENTIAL DIAGNOSIS

Soft Tissue Abnormalities

Soft tissue calcification is a common feature of various collagen diseases, particularly dermatomyositis (polymyositis) and scleroderma. In dermatomyositis and polymyositis, calcific deposits may appear in intermuscular fascial planes, a finding that is seen more rarely in other collagen diseases. A second pattern of calcification in dermatomyositis and polymyositis relates to deposition in subcutaneous tissue. Subcutaneous calcification can also be evident in scleroderma, systemic lupus erythematosus, mixed collagen vascular disease, and overlap syndromes.

Articular Abnormalities

Severe deformity of the interphalangeal joint of the thumb may be apparent not only in polymyositis but also in other collagen disorders, especially systemic lupus erythematosus. Interphalangeal joint erosions may also occur in scleroderma, rheumatoid arthritis, psoriasis, multicentric reticulohistiocytosis, and gout and after thermal injuries.

FURTHER READING

Banker BQ, Victor M: Dermatomyositis (systemic angiopathy) of childhood. Medicine 45:261, 1966.

Black KA, Zilko PJ, Dawkins RL, Armstrong BK, Mastaglia GL: Cancer in connective tissue disease. Arthritis Rheum 25:1130, 1982.

Blane CE, White SJ, Braunstein EM, Bowyer SL, Sullivan DB: Patterns of calcification in childhood dermatomyositis. AJR 142:397, 1984.

Bunch TW, O'Duffy JD, McLeod RA: Deforming arthritis of the hands in polymyositis. Arthritis Rheum 19:243, 1976.

Greenway G, Weisman MH, Resnick D, Zvaifler NJ, Guerra J Jr: Deforming arthritis of the hands: An unusual manifestation of polymyositis. AJR 136:611, 1981.

Ozonoff MB, Flynn FJ Jr: Roentgenologic features of dermatomyositis of childhood. AJR 118:206, 1973.

Schumacher HR, Schimmer B, Gordon GV, Bookspan MA, Brogadir S, Dorwart BB: Articular manifestations of polymyositis and dermatomyositis. Am J Med 67:287, 1979.

Steiner RM, Glassman L, Schwartz MW, Vanace P: The radiological findings in dermatomyositis of childhood. Radiology 111:385, 1974.

Steinfeld JR, Thorne NA, Kennedy TF: Positive 99mTc pyrophosphate bone scan in polymyositis. Radiology 122:168, 1977.

Chapter 32

Polyarteritis Nodosa and Other Vasculitides

Donald Resnick, M.D.

Vasculitis occurs in a number of disorders and may be associated with musculoskeletal manifestations. Although arteriography can reveal characteristic alterations in these disorders, plain film radiographic abnormalities are unimpressive. In polyarteritis nodosa, periosteal bone formation may be seen, particularly in the lower extremity. Articular abnormalities in giant cell (temporal) arteritis relate to its association with polymyalgia rheumatica and include soft tissue swelling and osteoporosis. In Henoch-Schönlein purpura and erythema nodosum, joint effusions are the only characteristic radiographic abnormality. Cryoglobulinemia is occasionally accompanied by cystic and erosive lesions of bone in both the axial and the appendicular skeleton.

A variety of disorders are characterized by inflammation of blood vessels. Clinical symptoms and signs in these disorders are protean, depending on the distribution, the extent, and the severity of the vascular lesions. Although musculoskeletal abnormalities may be encountered, these are usually overshadowed by findings related to involvement of other organ systems. Characteristic radiographic features are detected most reliably by arteriography (see Chapter 15).

The limitations of all classification systems for the vasculitides have become obvious in the last quarter of a century because of the enlarging spectrum of these disorders. Inflammatory vascular complications are now well known in rheumatoid arthritis and systemic lupus erythematosus. Wegener's granulomatosis, a disease that is associated with necrotizing granulomas of the respiratory tract, generalized necrotizing vasculitis, and focal glomerulonephritis, is also well recognized. Less inflammatory types of systemic vascular diseases have also been identified, such as a nonspecific arteritis of the aorta and its branches (Takayasu's disease) and the vascular changes that accompany scleroderma.

The histologic characteristics of the vascular lesions can be used as guidelines for classifying the various systemic vascular disorders despite overlapping of certain clinical and pathologic characteristics. Three groups of diseases are recognized: (1) inflammatory vascular lesions (necrotizing angiitis), including polyarteritis nodosa, hypersensitivity angiitis, granulomatous angiitis, and Wegener's granulomatosis; (2) vasculitides accompanied by granuloma formation, including granulomatous angiitis, Wegener's granulomatosis, temporal arteritis, and Takayasu's disease; and (3) vasculitides associated with intimal hyperplasia, necrosis of the media and elastic lamina, and varying degrees of inflammation in the adventitia and vasa vasorum, including temporal arteritis, Takayasu's disease, and scleroderma.

Guidelines for classification of the vasculitides can be based also on the combination of pathologic characteristics and size of the affected vessels. In this system, three major groups are identified: polyarteritis nodosa group, small vessel vasculitides, and giant cell arteritides. Characteristics of the polyarteritis nodosa group are involvement of medium-sized and, to a lesser extent, small-sized arteries, the presence of micro-aneurysms, the sequential initiation of the arterial damage, and histologic findings varying from acute inflammation to necrosis to scarring. Included in the polyarteritis nodosa group are generalized or classic disease, localized (to pulmonary, mesenteric, or other vessels) disease, and Kawasaki's disease (with prominent coronary artery involvement). Small vessel vasculitides, the second group, are characterized by involvement of arterioles and venules and, commonly, by prominent skin involvement. Disorders in this group may produce granulomatous reaction (Churg-Strauss syndrome, Wegener's granulomatosis). Giant cell arteritides affect large arteries and consist principally of two diseases: cranial (temporal) arteritis and Takayasu's disease, which affects the aorta.

Classification of vascular disorders not on histopathology but on pathogenesis is also possible. Hypersensitivity appears to be important in the development of disorders in the necrotizing angiitis group. The pathogenesis of granulomatous lesions and disorders characterized by intimal hypertrophy is unknown.

POLYARTERITIS NODOSA

Polyarteritis nodosa is a disorder of unknown cause characterized by inflammation and necrosis in the walls of medium-sized and small arteries. It affects men more frequently than women and occurs predominantly in young and middle-aged adults (20 to 50 years of age).

Clinical Abnormalities

The clinical manifestations of polyarteritis nodosa, relate to the distribution and extent of the vascular lesions. The spectrum of disease varies from a mild and limited form to a fulminating and rapidly fatal process. Fever, weight loss, tachycardia, anemia, and leukocytosis are frequent. Renal involvement can lead to blood and protein in the urine, hypertension, and uremia. Acute vascular episodes may involve other abdominal viscera, and cardiac manifestations include myocardial infarction, arrhythmia, and congestive heart failure. Peripheral vascular involvement can lead to gangrene. Vascular changes in the lungs, skin, muscles, and peripheral or central nervous system can lead to additional clinical manifestations.

The most prominent articular manifestation in polyarteritis nodosa is migratory polyarthralgia. Larger joints in the lower extremity typically are affected. Actual synovitis with joint effusion is rare, and synovial fluid analysis reveals findings indicative of mild inflammation.

An association between polyarteritis and rheumatoid arthritis also has been emphasized in recent years.

Radiographic Abnormalities

Plain film radiographic manifestations of polyarteritis nodosa are unusual. Soft tissue swelling may accompany arthritis, but cartilaginous and osseous destruction is not apparent.

Some patients with this disease exhibit periosteal bone formation, which has predilection for men and for the lower extremities, particularly the tibia and fibula. It is associated with pain and swelling, elevated erythrocyte sedimentation rate, and cutaneous abnormalities (Fig. 32–1). Digital clubbing is unusual. Upper extremity involvement also is unusual (Fig. 32–2).

Periostitis in this disease generally is identical to that in hypertrophic osteoarthropathy. A symmetric distribution, frequent involvement of the lower legs, diaphyseal predilection, and regular or irregular bone formation are typical.

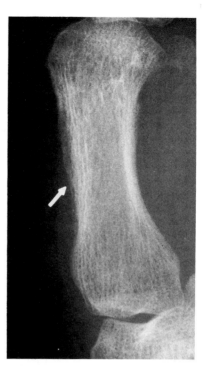

Figure 32–2. Polyarteritis nodosa: Periostitis in upper extremity. In this patient with diffuse vasculitis and prominent clinical findings in the thenar eminence, note periosteal new bone formation along the diaphyseal portion of the first metacarpal bone (arrow).

Pathologic Abnormalities

Medium and small caliber arteries from involved tissues reveal characteristic abnormalities. Initial changes are most common in the tunica media, with subsequent extension into the intima and adventitia and disruption of the internal elastic lamina. Necrosis, fibrinoid change, and cellular infiltration are observed. Weakening of the vessel wall can lead to aneurysm formation, rupture, and hemorrhage. Abnormalities in later stages of the disease include intimal proliferation leading to thrombosis and infarction, recanalization, dissection, and scarring.

GIANT CELL (TEMPORAL) ARTERITIS AND POLYMYALGIA RHEUMATICA

Giant cell (temporal) arteritis is characterized by granulomatous inflammation of large arteries, particularly the internal and the external carotid, the occipital, the temporal, and the ophthalmic arteries. Typically, patients over the age of 50 years are affected. The arteritis is more frequent in women than in men. Constitutional symptoms, such as fatigue, anorexia, and weight loss, may dominate the initial clinical manifestations. Clinical findings include painful swelling of the temporal arteries, headaches, visual disturbances, and peripheral neuropathy. The diagnosis is established by characteristic findings on temporal artery biopsy or angiogram.

Synovitis is detected in approximately 15 per cent of biopsy-proved cases of giant cell arteritis. Clinical findings related to articular involvement usually are confined to soft tissue swelling. Coexistent rheumatoid arthritis has also been documented.

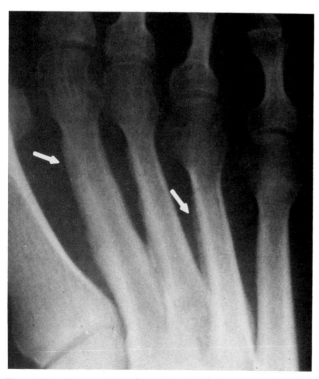

Figure 32–1. Polyarteritis nodosa: Periostitis in lower extremity. Observe periosteal new bone formation, predominating on the medial aspect of multiple metatarsal bones (arrows). (Courtesy of M. Dalinka, M.D., Philadelphia, Pennsylvania.)

An association has been suggested between giant cell arteritis and polymyalgia rheumatica (PMR). This latter condition is encountered most frequently in elderly patients, particularly women, and is associated with progressive pain in the back, the thighs, the neck, and the shoulders. Morning stiffness without joint swelling is particularly characteristic of PMR. A transient synovitis of the knee, shoulder, hip, wrist, and small joints of the fingers can result in soft tissue swelling and osteoporosis on radiographs. A carpal tunnel syndrome, resulting from compression of the median nerve by adjacent synovial tissue, is seen. Significant cartilage and bone abnormalities generally are not found.

Approximately 50 per cent of patients with giant cell arteritis demonstrate a prodromal phase with features of PMR, and approximately 30 per cent of patients with PMR reveal symptoms and signs of giant cell arteritis. In fact, giant cell arteritis may occur in some patients with PMR in the absence of symptoms referable to the temporal artery. In these patients, blind biopsy of the proximal portion of the temporal artery can reveal such clinically silent disease. A normal biopsy specimen in this situation, however, does not exclude arteritis.

HENOCH-SCHÖNLEIN (ANAPHYLACTOID) PURPURA

This syndrome, which consists of nonthrombocytopenic purpura, arthralgia or arthritis, abdominal pain, and renal disease, is related to a generalized angiitis involving arterioles

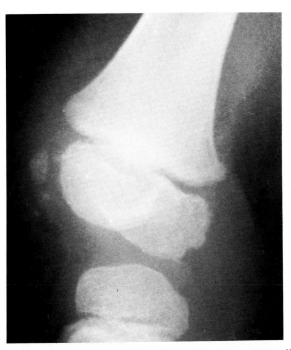

Figure 32–3. Henoch-Schönlein (anaphylactoid) purpura: Joint effusion. In this 4 year old child, observe soft tissue swelling and joint effusion of the knee.

and capillaries. Increased vascular permeability is associated with edema and hemorrhage. The disease is more frequent in children than in adults.

The classic triad of findings, observed in 70 to 80 per cent of cases, consists of purpura, abdominal pain, and arthritis. Soft tissue edema may be evident. The joints involved most commonly are the knees, the ankles, the hips, the wrists, and the small joints of the hand. Periarticular soft tissue swelling, the only radiographic abnormality, is related to synovial effusion (Fig. 32–3). Complete resolution of clinical and radiographic joint abnormalities is characteristic.

CRYOGLOBULINEMIA

Essential cryoglobulinemia is a distinct type of disease that is manifested as arthralgia or arthritis; the skin, lungs, kidneys, nervous system, and gastrointestinal tract are involved. The disorder may follow a chronic course, with minimal symptoms or result in death owing to renal abnormalities. The joints involved most commonly are those in the hands, knees, ankles, and elbows. Although the radiographic features in these locations are not dramatic, well-defined subchondral cystic lesions have been identified. Bone erosions and cyst formation in the articular facets of the cervical spine and vertebral bodies, which are evident in this disease, appear to lack specificity.

ERYTHEMA NODOSUM

Erythema nodosum is a disorder characterized by red, tender, and warm nodular cutaneous lesions (particularly on the lower legs), which, on biopsy, demonstrate vasculitis and cellular infiltration. Erythema nodosum occurs in some patients with ulcerative colitis, Crohn's disease, sarcoidosis, and Behçet's syndrome.

Approximately three fourths of patients with erythema nodosum develop recurrent episodes of arthralgia and arthritis, with predilection for the knees, the ankles, the elbows, the wrists, and the small joints of the hands. Soft tissue swelling related to a joint effusion is the only prominent radiographic abnormality.

FURTHER READING

Alarcón-Segovia D: Classification of the necrotizing vasculitides in man. Clin Rheum Dis 6:223, 1980.

Albert DA, Rimon D, Silverstein MD: The diagnosis of polyarteritis nodosa. Arthritis Rheum 31:1117, 1988.

Fauchald P, Rygvold O, Oystese B: Temporal arteritis and polymyalgia rheumatica—clinical and biopsy findings. Ann Intern Med 77:845, 1972.

Moncada R, Baker D, Rubinstein H, Shah D, Love L: Selective temporal arteriography and biopsy in giant cell arteritis: Polymyalgia rheumatica. AJR 122:580, 1974.

Truelove LH: Articular manifestations of erythema nodosum. Ann Rheum Dis 19:174, 1960.

Weinberger A, Berliner S, Pinkhas J: Articular manifestations of essential cryoglobulinemia. Semin Arthritis Rheum 10:224, 1981.

Woodward AH, Andreini PH: Periosteal new bone formation in polyarteritis nodosa. A syndrome involving the lower extremities. Arthritis Rheum 17:1017, 1974.

Zvaifler NJ: Vasculitides: Classification and pathogenesis. Aust NZ J Med (Suppl 1)8:134, 1978.

Chapter 33

Mixed Connective Tissue Disease and Collagen Overlap Syndromes

Donald Resnick, M.D.

Mixed connective tissue disease (MCTD) is a recently described overlap syndrome defined serologically by the presence of a ribonuclease-sensitive extractable nuclear antigen. It demonstrates clinical features of several collagen diseases, including systemic lupus erythematosus, scleroderma, dermatomyositis, and rheumatoid arthritis, and, in fact, patients with this syndrome may fulfill diagnostic criteria for any or all of these disorders.

The radiographic characteristics of MCTD also under-score the mixed character of the disease. Changes compatible with rheumatoid arthritis (articular erosion, joint space narrowing, periarticular osteoporosis), scleroderma (tuftal resorption, soft tissue calcification), and systemic lupus erythematosus (deforming nonerosive arthropathy) can be observed. The detection on radiographs of skeletal abnormalities characteristic of more than one collagen disease should raise the possibility of MCTD, although other overlap syndromes may reveal similar findings.

The diagnosis of the collagen disorders that are described in Chapters 29 to 32 is based on the composite evaluation of clinical, laboratory, radiologic, and pathologic data and the application of a variety of selective and nonselective disease criteria. In some patients, however, difficulty is encountered because the manifestations of the disease process appear incompatible with a single diagnosis using traditional classification systems. Some examples of this diagnostic dilemma are provided by the patient with rheumatoid arthritis who also demonstrates antinuclear antibodies and positive serologic test results for LE cells or who may develop the skin alterations of scleroderma; or the individual with lupus erythematosus who also has sclerodactyly. These patients, as well as many others, appear to have more than one collagen disease, and the diagnosis of an overlap syndrome is offered as an explanation for the diversity of the clinical, radiologic, and laboratory aberrations. In these situations, it is generally unclear whether classic definitions of the "pure" collagen diseases are too limited, two or more pure collagen disorders coexist at the same time, or a new and distinct clinical entity has emerged. Proponents of the last possibility offer mixed connective tissue disease as evidence of a new disorder that can be effectively segregated from the other collagen diseases primarily on the basis of laboratory data.

MIXED CONNECTIVE TISSUE DISEASE

Mixed connective tissue disease (MCTD), first described in 1972, is characterized by clinical features that suggest an overlap of systemic lupus erythematosus, scleroderma, dermatomyositis, and, more recently, rheumatoid arthritis. The initially described unifying laboratory feature of MCTD was the presence of antibodies to a saline-soluble extractable nuclear antigen (ENA), which was ribonuclease (RNase) sensitive. Subsequently, it has been resolved that ENA consists of two distinct substances: a soluble ribonucleoprotein (RNP) and a glycoprotein termed Sm antigen. Ribonuclease-sensitive ENA is synonymous with RNP. The presence of antibodies to RNP is fundamental to the diagnosis of MCTD, although the antibodies may also be found in a small percentage of patients with systemic lupus erythematosus or scleroderma.

The existence of MCTD as a definite entity is not universally accepted. Rather, it has been suggested that MCTD represents systemic lupus erythematosus that has been altered or modified by the presence of RNP antibodies.

Clinical Abnormalities

MCTD is characterized by overlapping clinical features of scleroderma, systemic lupus erythematosus, dermatomyositis, and rheumatoid arthritis and by the presence in the serum of high titers of antibodies to RNP. Adults or children can be affected. The clinical abnormalities of any one or a combination of these collagen diseases may predominate. The variable clinical alterations of MCTD include fatigue, weight loss, fever, myalgia and myositis, sclerodactyly, digital swelling, Raynaud's phenomenon, dyspnea, dysphagia, diarrhea, skin rash, and neuralgia. The prognosis of the disease is regarded as good, although serious gastrointestinal, neurologic, or renal manifestations can become apparent.

Clinically detectable joint abnormalities indicative of arthralgia or arthritis are common in MCTD. Involvement of the small joints of the hand and foot as well as the wrist is most typical. Knee, elbow, shoulder, and ankle abnormalities are also relatively common. Synovitis of joints, tendon sheaths, and bursae can be detected on clinical examination, and subcutaneous and peritendinous nodules can also be evident. Joint deformities simulating those of rheumatoid arthritis can appear in MCTD. In addition to the presence of RNP antibodies in the serum, patients may reveal positive serologic test results for rheumatoid factor, elevation of erythrocyte sedimentation rate, and anemia.

Radiographic Abnormalities

On radiographs, osseous, articular, and soft tissue abnormalities confirm the overlapping nature of MCTD. Radiographic alterations are most frequent in the hands, wrists, and feet and include the following characteristics (Figs. 33–1 to 33–3).

JOINT DISTRIBUTION. Radiographic abnormalities are most common in the proximal interphalangeal and metacarpophalangeal joints of the hands, midcarpal and radiocarpal compartments of the wrist, and metatarsophalangeal and interphalangeal joints of the feet. A symmetric or asymmetric distribution of abnormalities has been reported.

OSTEOPOROSIS. Diffuse or periarticular osteoporosis is commonly seen. The findings simulate those of rheumatoid arthritis.

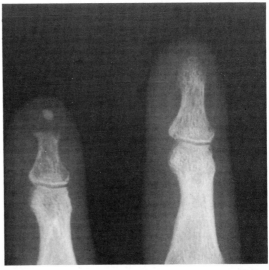

Figure 33–2. Mixed connective tissue disease: Phalangeal tuftal resorption. Observe osteolysis of the terminal phalangeal tuft of the second finger and, to a lesser extent, the third finger. Punctate calcification is evident in the second digit. (Courtesy of D. Alarcón-Segovia, M.D., Mexico City, Mexico.)

SOFT TISSUE SWELLING. Symmetric soft tissue swelling is common about involved joints. Diffuse swelling of the hand is also apparent, related to widespread edema.

JOINT SPACE NARROWING. Diffuse narrowing of the articular space is common. Intraarticular bone ankylosis has also been noted.

EROSIONS. The marginal osseous erosions in MCTD are similar to those in rheumatoid arthritis. Erosions of distal interphalangeal joints of the fingers, however, can be observed

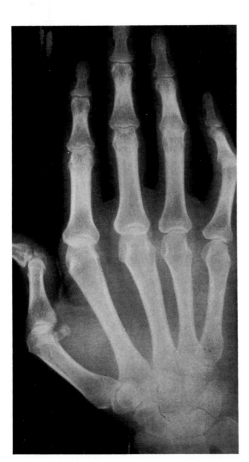

Figure 33–1. Mixed connective tissue disease: Deforming nonerosive arthropathy. Observe flexion at the first metacarpophalangeal joint and hyperextension of the interphalangeal joint of the same digit. Also note radial deviation at the wrist, ulnar deviation and flexion at the metacarpophalangeal joints, and flexion at the proximal interphalangeal joints. (Courtesy of M. Dalinka, M.D., Philadelphia, Pennsylvania.)

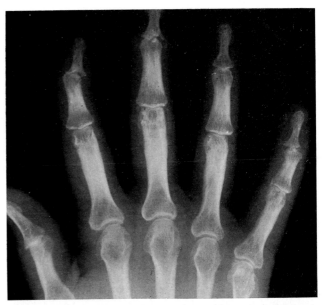

Figure 33–3. Mixed connective tissue disease: Distal interphalangeal joint erosions. The frontal radiograph outlines periarticular osteoporosis, capsular calcification, and a destructive arthritis of multiple distal interphalangeal joints. (Courtesy of M. Dalinka, M.D., Philadelphia, Pennsylvania.)

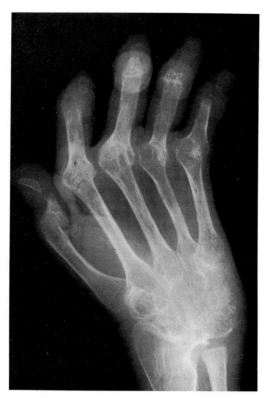

Figure 33–4. Mixed connective tissue disease: Arthritis mutilans. Severe destructive arthropathy involving multiple locations in the hand and wrist resembles psoriatic arthritis. (From Alarcón-Segovia, D., and Uribe-Uribe, O.: Mutilans-like arthropathy in mixed connective tissue disease. Arthritis Rheum 22:1013, 1979. Used with permission.)

mon, radiographic changes in these locations are rarely recorded. Periarticular osteoporosis and calcification may be seen about the knee, the elbow, or the hip (Fig. 33–5). Osteonecrosis has been found in MCTD, perhaps related to corticosteroid administration.

Thus, in MCTD, radiographic features of scleroderma, rheumatoid arthritis, systemic lupus erythematosus, and even dermatomyositis are encountered (Table 33–1). The severity of any one group of radiographic abnormalities varies, just as the clinical similarities to any one collagen disease may vary.

The erosive arthritis of MCTD generally is indistinguishable from rheumatoid arthritis. Although some investigators stress an asymmetric distribution and sharply marginated defects as findings allowing accurate diagnosis of MCTD, these abnormalities are not constant. The soft tissue calcifications that are detected in patients with MCTD generally are indistinguishable from those in scleroderma. Although some investigators suggest that linear calcification overlying or within the joint capsule is of diagnostic significance in MCTD, similar calcification can appear in scleroderma and other collagen diseases, as well as in hyperparathyroidism and calcium pyrophosphate dihydrate crystal deposition disease. Soft tissue swelling in periarticular locations in MCTD is also nonspecific. Diffuse swelling in the hands corresponding to edema is a sign that is suggestive of MCTD.

The diagnosis of MCTD can be suggested when radiographic examination of the skeleton reveals features typical of more than one collagen disease. A variety of overlap syndromes can have a similar radiographic appearance, however (see following discussion).

OVERLAP SYNDROMES

As indicated previously, the clinical features in many patients with collagen disorders cannot be classified precisely as those of a specific disease but rather are consistent with more than one disease. Such overlap syndromes include dermatomyositis and scleroderma; rheumatoid arthritis and scleroderma; systemic lupus erythematosus and dermatomyositis; rheumatoid arthritis and systemic lupus erythematosus; scleroderma and systemic lupus erythematosus; and scleroderma and Sjögren's syndrome. MCTD is but one of the overlap syndromes, which is differentiated from the remainder by the presence of RNP antibodies.

in MCTD. In addition, severe destructive arthritis (Fig. 33–4) in MCTD can simulate the appearance of psoriatic arthritis.

CHANGES IN THE PHALANGEAL TIPS. Soft tissue atrophy, soft tissue calcification, and resorption of the terminal tufts of the phalanges simulate the findings of scleroderma.

SUBLUXATION. When present, joint subluxation is identical to that in rheumatoid arthritis or systemic lupus erythematosus.

Although clinical involvement of other joints is not uncom-

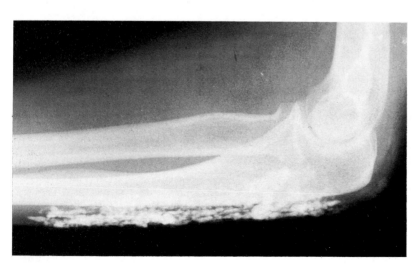

Figure 33–5. Mixed connective tissue disease: Periarticular calcification. Observe extensive linear collections of calcification about the elbow. (Courtesy of M. Dalinka, M.D., Philadelphia, Pennsylvania.)

Table 33–1. RADIOGRAPHIC FEATURES OF MIXED CONNECTIVE TISSUE DISEASE (MCTD)

Scleroderma-like Features	Lupus Erythematosus–like Features	Rheumatoid Arthritis–like Features	Dermatomyositis-like Features
Soft tissue atrophy	Deforming nonerosive arthropathy	Symmetric soft tissue swelling	Soft tissue calcification
Soft tissue or capsular calcification	Osteonecrosis	Periarticular osteoporosis	
Phalangeal tuftal erosion		Diffuse joint space narrowing	
Distal interphalangeal joint erosion		Marginal erosion	
		Soft tissue nodule	

Clinical and radiographic features of other overlap syndromes simulate the findings of MCTD. As in MCTD, the diagnosis of an overlap syndrome rests on the identification of features of more than one collagen disease.

FURTHER READING

Alarcón-Segovia D, Uribe-Uribe O: Mutilans-like arthropathy in mixed connective tissue disease. Arthritis Rheum 22:1013, 1979.

Baron M, Srolovitz H, Lander P, Kapusta M: The coexistence of rheumatoid arthritis and scleroderma: A case report and review of the literature. J Rheumatol 9:947, 1982.

Cohen MG, Webb J: Concurrence of rheumatoid arthritis and systemic lupus erythematosus: report of 11 cases. Ann Rheum Dis 46:853, 1987.

Fischman AS, Abeles M, Zanetti M, Weinstein A, Rothfield NF: The coexistence of rheumatoid arthritis and systemic lupus erythematosus. A case report and review of the literature. J Rheumatol 8:405, 1981.

LeRoy EC: Overlap features of connective tissue disease. Arthritis Rheum 25:889, 1982.

Ramos-Niembro F, Alarcón-Segovia D, Hernandez-Ortiz J: Articular manifestations of mixed connective tissue disease. Arthritis Rheum 22:43, 1979.

Sharp GC, Irvin WS, Tan EM, Gould RG, Holman HR: Mixed connective tissue disease—an apparently distinct rheumatic disease syndrome associated with a specific antibody to an extractable nuclear antigen (ENA). Am J Med 52:148, 1972.

Silver TM, Farber SJ, Bole GG, Martel W: Radiological features of mixed connective tissue disease and scleroderma-systemic lupus erythematosus overlap. Radiology 120:269, 1976.

Udoff EJ, Genant HK, Kozin F, Ginsberg M: Mixed connective tissue disease: The spectrum of radiographic manifestations. Radiology 124:613, 1977.

Chapter 34

Rheumatic Fever

Donald Resnick, M.D.

Articular involvement in rheumatic fever typically appears as polyarthritis and as Jaccoud's arthropathy. Polyarthritis is associated with nonspecific radiographic features. Jaccoud's arthropathy is characterized by typical radiographic abnormalities, which are best classified as deforming non-erosive articular changes. The hand abnormalities, which resemble changes in systemic lupus erythematosus and other collagen diseases, can usually be differentiated from rheumatoid arthritis, in which early and significant cartilaginous and osseous destruction is apparent.

Rheumatic fever is a disorder characterized clinically by fever, carditis, and polyarthritis; historically there usually has been a previous episode of group A beta-hemolytic streptococcal infection. Rheumatic fever affects many tissues of the body, but it is its cardiac involvement that is most significant to the patient. Although rheumatic fever also can involve joints, the resulting abnormalities should not be viewed as those of rheumatoid arthritis. Indeed, certain types of rheumatic fever are associated with a chronic rheumatic syndrome that can be distinguished from rheumatoid arthritis, whereas certain types of rheumatoid arthritis are associated with cardiac lesions that are different from those of rheumatic fever.

A report of post–rheumatic fever arthropathy first appeared in 1867 when Jaccoud described a young man with rheumatic fever who developed a chronic deforming arthropathy. The arthropathy was characterized by muscle atrophy, ulnar deviation with flexion and subluxation at multiple metacarpophalangeal joints, and hyperextension of distal interphalangeal joints. Subsequent reports of Jaccoud's arthropathy have indicated that it may also involve the feet, that it is initially correctable but later may become fixed, and that it is not confined to patients with rheumatic fever but may appear also in patients with collagen disorders.

ARTICULAR ABNORMALITIES

Classically, an attack of rheumatic fever occurs from several days to several weeks after a streptococcal throat infection. Symptoms and signs of the clinical attack are variable; an acute onset may be characterized by fever, night sweats, headaches, and joint pains, whereas an insidious onset may be accompanied by pallor, fatigue, anorexia, weight loss, and muscular pain.

Polyarthritis

Joint involvement of variable severity is the most common clinical manifestation of rheumatic fever (approximately 75 per cent of patients) and frequently appears early during the course of a rheumatic attack. Multiple joints usually are affected, particularly large articulations. Without treatment, joint inflammation may persist from several days to a week, subsequently diminishing and eventually disappearing completely. Radiographs reveal mild osteoporosis and soft tissue swelling without evidence of cartilaginous or osseous destruction. Pathologic characteristics in the acute polyarticular phase of rheumatic fever confirm the mild nature of the synovitis. In a few patients, swelling and stiffness of the metacarpophalangeal and proximal interphalangeal joints persist up to 6 months. In these individuals, interosseous muscle wasting and osteoporosis can be prominent.

Deforming Nonerosive (Jaccoud's) Arthropathy

The deforming arthropathy that may appear after repeated attacks of arthritis in patients with rheumatic fever is also referred to as Jaccoud's syndrome. Although its pathogenesis is not clear, Jaccoud's arthropathy appears to result from capsular inflammation and fibrosis, and it is not confined to patients with rheumatic fever but may also occur in association with systemic lupus erythematosus and scleroderma. The clinical findings are characteristic. A history of previous attacks of rheumatic fever is combined with symptoms and signs of residual heart lesions. Symptomless and reversible joint deformities appear, particularly in the hands, but also in the feet. Typically, ulnar deviation and flexion deformities are evident at the metacarpophalangeal joints, predominantly in the fourth and fifth digits, and may be combined with hyperextension at interphalangeal joints. In the foot, fibular deviation and subluxation at metatarsophalangeal joints can be observed. In the hands and feet, the reversible nature of the articular deformity is striking. On physical examination, the clinician may easily reduce the joint subluxations. During radiography, pressing the hand against the cassette may result in an entirely normal posteroanterior radiograph; placing the hand in an oblique projection with the fingers lifted from the cassette will reveal the striking deformities (Fig. 34–1). Eventually, fixed deformities may appear.

Specific criteria that are necessary for the diagnosis of Jaccoud's arthropathy are as follows:

1. A history of recurrent attacks of acute rheumatic fever.

2. A delayed recovery after joint inflammation with initial stiffness and subsequent deformity, particularly in the metacarpophalangeal joints.

3. A characteristic articular deformity that is associated with periarticular, fascial, and tendon fibrosis rather than synovitis, which consists of flexion and ulnar deviation at the

372

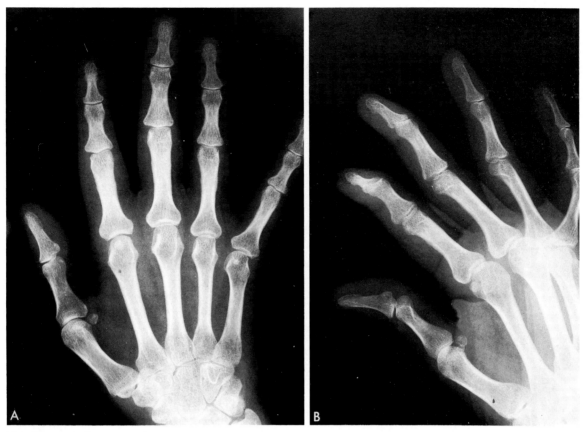

Figure 34–1. Rheumatic fever: Jaccoud's arthropathy. Radiographic abnormalities. A On a posteroanterior radiograph with the hand pressed firmly against the cassette, the only striking deformity is ulnar deviation of the fifth finger at the metacarpophalangeal joint. Mild periarticular osteoporosis is seen. There is no evidence of osseous erosion. **B** On the oblique radiograph, the hand has been lifted from the cassette. Boutonnière and swan-neck deformities of all the digits can be seen.

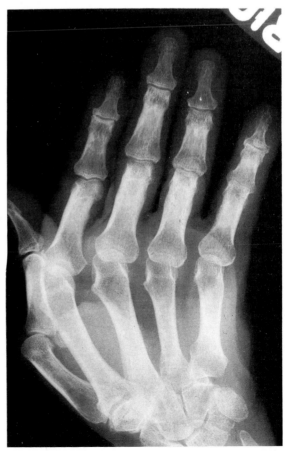

Figure 34–2. Rheumatic fever: Jaccoud's arthropathy. Radiographic abnormalities. The frontal radiograph reveals typical deformities, particularly flexion and ulnar deviation at the metacarpophalangeal joints. Note periarticular osteoporosis and the absence of osseous erosions.

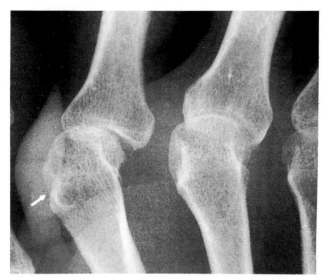

Figure 34–3. Jaccoud's arthropathy—joint space narrowing and osseous erosion. A frontal radiograph reveals ulnar deviation of the second to fourth metacarpophalangeal joints with articular space narrowing. A cystic lesion (arrow) can be seen on the radial aspect of the second metacarpal head. Associated soft tissue swelling and osteoporosis are evident.

metacarpophalangeal joints, particularly in the fourth and fifth digits, in association with soft tissue swelling.

4. Tendon crepitus.

5. Joint disease that generally is asymptomatic, with little evidence of active synovitis and with good functional capacity.

On radiographic evaluation, joint deformities may be apparent (Fig. 34–2) (Table 34–1). In most patients, articular space narrowing and osseous erosions are not evident. Occasionally, however, articular space diminution is encountered, probably representing cartilaginous atrophy owing to disuse and cartilaginous erosion attributable to closely applied subluxed osseous surfaces (Fig. 34–3). Furthermore, hook erosions on the radial and palmar aspects of the metacarpal heads can appear in Jaccoud's arthropathy and superficially resemble the marginal erosions of rheumatoid arthritis.

The arthropathy is not related to synovitis. Rather, capsular and periarticular fibrosis is important in the evolution of the joint disease, and the fibrotic lesion is similar to that occurring in the heart in patients with rheumatic fever. The hook erosion of the metacarpal heads may be produced by pressure erosion beneath the distorted capsule in the deformed articulations. It is not surprising that Jaccoud's arthropathy is often misdiagnosed as rheumatoid arthritis on the basis of the hand and foot deformities. Confusion between the two entities is accentuated by the occasional occurrence of soft tissue nodules in patients with rheumatic fever.

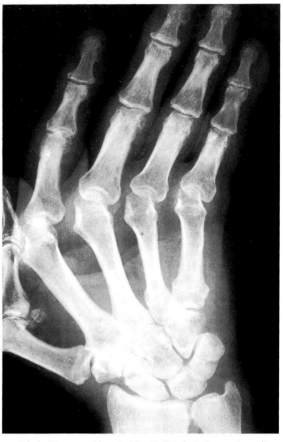

Figure 34–4. Rheumatoid arthritis. Radial deviation at the radiocarpal joint and ulnar deviation at the metacarpophalangeal joints have occurred without significant osseous erosion. Periarticular osteoporosis can be noted.

DIFFERENTIAL DIAGNOSIS

Jaccoud's deforming arthropathy is not diagnostic of rheumatic fever (Table 34–2). The deforming nonerosive arthropathy of rheumatic fever is similar to that of systemic lupus erythematosus and, more rarely, other collagen diseases. Although classically the ulnar digits are affected more commonly in rheumatic fever and all the digits, including the thumb, are affected in systemic lupus erythematosus, the patterns of distribution are variable. Deforming nonerosive arthropathies may also be encountered in agammaglobulinemia (hypogammaglobulinemia), Ehlers-Danlos syndrome, and, rarely, rheumatoid arthritis (Fig. 34–4).

The deformities that occur in association with Jaccoud's arthropathy resemble those in rheumatoid arthritis. In some patients with Jaccoud's arthropathy, the appearance of joint space narrowing and osseous erosion complicates the differ-

---

Table 34–1. RADIOGRAPHIC CHARACTERISTICS OF JACCOUD'S ARTHROPATHY

Flexion and ulnar deviation of metacarpophalangeal joints, particularly fourth and fifth
Flexion and fibular deviation of metatarsophalangeal joints
Periarticular osteoporosis
Joint space narrowing (rare)
Hook erosions on radial and palmar aspect of metacarpal heads (rare)

Table 34–2. DISEASES THAT MAY LEAD TO DEFORMING NONEROSIVE ARTHROPATHY

Rheumatic fever
Collagen disorders, particularly systemic lupus erythematosus
Rheumatoid arthritis (rare)
Agammaglobulinemia (rare)
Ehlers-Danlos syndrome (rare)

entiation between these two disorders. The distribution and extent of articular space loss are less widespread and severe in Jaccoud's arthropathy than in rheumatoid arthritis, however. In addition, diminution of joint space is an early manifestation of rheumatoid arthritis, and, when present, a late manifestation of Jaccoud's arthropathy. The hook erosions of this latter disorder also differ in appearance from erosions in rheumatoid arthritis. They involve the volar and radial aspects of the metacarpal heads, are located farther from the articular margin, and are usually unassociated with joint space narrowing or erosive changes on the ulnar aspect.

FURTHER READING

Bywaters EGL: The relation between heart and joint disease including "rheumatoid heart disease" and chronic post-rheumatic arthritis (type Jaccoud). Br Heart J *12*:101, 1950.

Jaccoud S: Leçons de Clinique Medicale faites a l'Hôpital de la Charité. Vingt-troisième leçon, sur une forme de rhumatisme chronique. Paris, Adrien Delahaye, 1867, p 598.

Murphy WA, Staple TW: Jaccoud's arthropathy reviewed. AJR *118*:300, 1973.

Pastershank SP, Resnick D: "Hook" erosions in Jaccoud's arthropathy. J Can Assoc Radiol *31*:174, 1980.

Zvaifler NJ: Chronic postrheumatic-fever (Jaccoud's) arthritis. N Engl J Med *267*:10, 1962.

SECTION V

DEGENERATIVE DISEASES

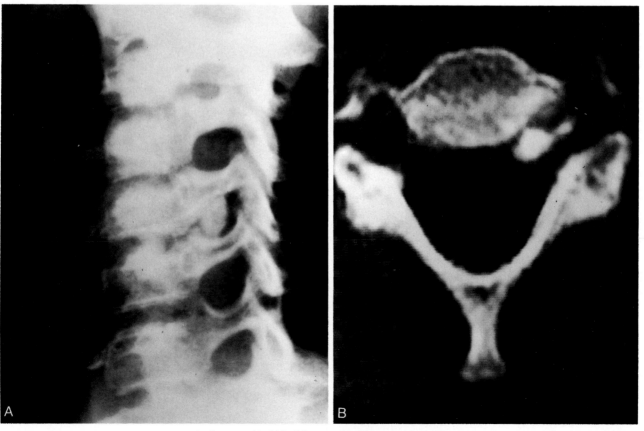

A nine year old girl had fever, neck stiffness, and torticollis.

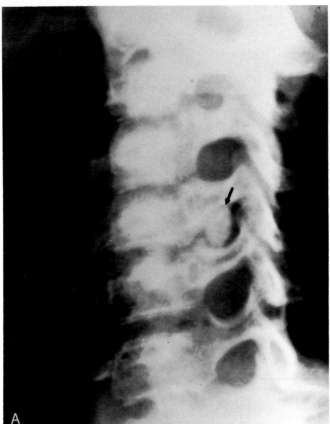

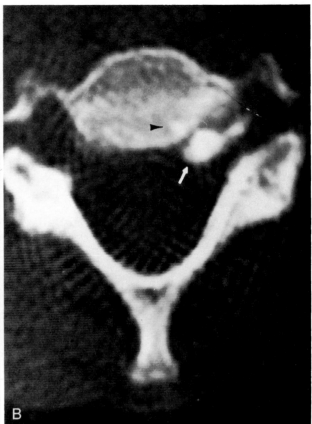

An oblique radiograph (A) and a transaxial computed tomogram (B) reveal a calcific collection (arrows) lying within the medial portion of the left neural foramen between the fifth and sixth cervical vertebrae. Smaller calcific collections are present in the adjacent intervertebral disc (arrowhead), although these discal calcifications were better seen on a slightly lower transaxial image. Although initial consideration might be given to a neoplastic origin for the calcification, the constellation of imaging abnormalities is diagnostic of protrusion of a calcified disc.

Calcification of an intervertebral disc in a child is most commonly observed between the ages of 6 and 10 years and occurs with approximately equal frequency in boys and girls. Discal calcification involving a single level is more typical than multilevel involvement, and the cervical spine is the predominant spinal region affected. Approximately 75 per cent of children with such calcification have significant clinical manifestations, which, in the cervical spine, include pain, stiffness, limitation of motion, torticollis, and fever; laboratory evaluation may reveal leukocytosis and elevation of the erythrocyte sedimentation rate.

Radiographs typically show a single globular region of calcification involving principally the nucleus pulposus of the intervertebral disc. The disc space itself may be normal in height, and the adjacent vertebral bodies are unaltered. Inflammatory changes in the intervertebral disc about the site of calcification may be confirmed on histologic examination.

Both the clinical and the radiographic manifestations usually are transient in nature; pain resolves in a period of days to weeks, and the calcifications generally disappear in a period of weeks to months. Uncommonly, the calcific collection may extrude into the adjacent soft tissues, the spinal canal, the vertebral body, or, as in Case V, the neural foramen, leading to more significant symptoms and signs.

The precise cause of discal calcification in the child is not clear, although inflammatory or traumatic events have been implicated as etiologic factors by some investigators. Although the clinical manifestations resemble those of discitis, another condition of the spine that occurs in children, the relationship of the two disorders is not established.

Of importance, the occurrence of discal calcification in the child should be distinguished from that which is seen in adults. Single or multiple calcifications in the anulus fibrosus or nucleus pulposus, or both, are frequently observed in adults. The collections are generally without clinical significance and presumably occur on a degenerative basis. Calcification of multiple intervertebral discs in an adult, however, also may be a manifestation of a variety of diseases, including alkaptonuria and calcium pyrophosphate dihydrate crystal deposition disease.

FINAL DIAGNOSIS: Idiopathic discal calcification with discal extrusion.

FURTHER READINGS

Pages 434 and 435 and the following:

1. Young LW, Faucher PG, Bowen A: Cervical disc calcification in childhood. Am J Dis Child 134:701, 1980.
2. Blomquist HK, Lindqvist M, Mattson S: Calcification of intervertebral discs in childhood. Pediatr Radiol 8:23, 1979.

(Case V, Courtesy of M. Alcaraz, M.D., Madrid, Spain.)

Chapter 35

Degenerative Diseases of Extraspinal Locations

Donald Resnick, M.D.
Gen Niwayama, M.D.

Degenerative joint disease is widespread and common. In synovial joints, the process is termed osteoarthritis. At these sites, abnormalities predominate in the cartilaginous and osseous tissues, whereas alterations in the synovial membrane generally are mild. Typical findings include joint space loss, eburnation, cyst formation, and osteophytosis. Subluxation, malalignment, fibrous ankylosis, and intra-articular osseous and cartilaginous bodies may complicate osteoarthritis.

The most common sites of extraspinal osteoarthritis are the interphalangeal and metacarpophalangeal joints of the hands, the first carpometacarpal and trapezioscaphoid areas of the wrist, the acromioclavicular and sternoclavicular joints, the hip, the knee, and the tarsometatarsal and metatarsophalangeal joints of the great toe.

Two special varieties of osteoarthritis have been described, although their existence as discrete entities is not universally accepted. Generalized osteoarthritis may be a particular form of degenerative joint disease in which multiple articulations are affected. Inflammatory (erosive) osteoarthritis is associated with clinical and pathologic features of joint inflammation.

Degenerative joint disease is the most frequent articular affliction. Despite its common occurrence, degenerative arthritis was not regarded as a distinct entity until the early twentieth century, at which time it was clearly differentiated from rheumatoid arthritis. Even after this time, degenerative joint disease did not receive a great deal of attention, as many researchers considered this disorder to be the dull and inevitable accompaniment of advancing age. In more recent years, a new curiosity and enthusiasm about degenerative arthritis have finally stimulated the considerable investigation that this common and significant condition deserves.

TERMINOLOGY AND CLASSIFICATION

Degenerative joint disease is the best general phrase to describe degenerative alterations in any type of joint. These alterations may appear in fibrous, cartilaginous, or synovial articulations. The terms osteoarthrosis and osteoarthritis are reserved for degenerative disease of synovial joints. Although in most of these joints, inflammatory changes are not pronounced (and therefore the suffix "-osis" appears more appropriate than "-itis"), the term osteoarthritis rather than osteoarthrosis is widely accepted in the United States.

Traditionally, degenerative joint disease has been further classified into primary (idiopathic) and secondary types. Primary degenerative joint disease has been regarded as a process in which articular degeneration occurs in the absence of any obvious underlying abnormality, whereas secondary degenerative joint disease has been regarded as articular degeneration that is produced by alterations from a preexisting affliction. This classification into primary and secondary degenerative joint disease is misleading. Careful evaluation of many examples of primary degenerative joint disease will disclose some mechanical deviation in the involved articulation that has led to secondary degeneration of the joint. It appears likely, therefore, that primary degenerative joint disease does not truly exist, and use of such a designation seems only to underscore diagnostic limitations.

Articular degeneration may result from either an abnormal concentration of force across a joint with normal articular cartilage matrix or a normal concentration of force across an abnormal joint (one with cartilaginous or subchondral osseous alterations) (Table 35–1). Eventually, of course, abnormalities of force and articular structure will appear together. This classification is useful as it emphasizes that there are many potential causes of secondary degenerative joint disease and that these causes may lead to articular degeneration by increasing the amount of stress on cartilaginous and osseous structures or by directly affecting the cartilage or subchondral bone itself.

ETIOLOGY

Many diverse factors appear to be important in the causation of degenerative joint disease (Table 35–2).

Systemic Factors
Genetics

Although genetic patterns have been recognized in some forms of degenerative joint disease, they are not identifiable in most varieties of the disease. The influence of hereditary factors in the development of joint degeneration is most

Table 35–1. CLASSIFICATION OF DEGENERATIVE JOINT DISEASE

A. Abnormal concentration of force on normal articulation
  1. Intraarticular malalignment
    a. Epiphyseal injuries
    b. Epiphyseal dysplasia
    c. Neuromuscular imbalance
  2. Extraarticular malalignment
    a. Inequality of leg length
    b. Congenital and acquired varus or valgus deformities
    c. Malunited fractures
    d. Ligamentous abnormalities
  3. Loss of protective sensory feedback
    a. Neuroarthropathy
    b. Intraarticular injection of steroids
  4. Miscellaneous
    a. Obesity
    b. Occupational
B. Normal concentration of force on abnormal articulation
  1. Normal concentration of force on abnormal cartilage
    a. Transchondral fractures
    b. Meniscal tears and discoid menisci
    c. Loose bodies
    d. Preexisting arthritis
    e. Metabolic abnormalities (gout, calcium pyrophosphate dihydrate crystal deposition disease, acromegaly, alkaptonuria, mucopolysaccharidoses)
  2. Normal concentration of force on normal cartilage supported by weakened subchondral bone
    a. Osteonecrosis
    b. Osteoporosis
    c. Osteomalacia
    d. Osteitis fibrosa cystica (hyperparathyroidism)
    e. Neoplasm
  3. Normal concentration of force on normal cartilage supported by stiffened subchondral bone
    a. Osteopetrosis
    b. Paget's disease

obvious with respect to Heberden's nodes. It has been suggested that Heberden's nodes are transmitted as a simple autosomal dominant genetic error in women, and as a recessive one in men. A genetic predisposition to polyarticular osteoarthritis has also been defined, a predisposition that may account for involvement of non–weight-bearing sites, particularly those in the upper extremities. Also, a number of hereditary disorders, such as the epiphyseal dysplasias and mucopolysaccharidoses, are accompanied by alterations in the connective tissues that contribute to subsequent articular deterioration.

Obesity

The role of obesity in the development of articular degeneration remains controversial. Although it appears logical that excessive body weight should accentuate stresses across weight-bearing joints, extreme obesity may lead to patient immobility and decreased active joint motion, thereby diminishing the risks of developing degenerative joint alterations.

Age and Sex

There is strong evidence that degenerative joint disease occurs with increasing frequency in older persons, perhaps related to a diminished capacity of aging cartilage to resist mechanical stress owing to changing physical and biochemical cartilaginous properties. The correlation with advancing age is not linear; rather, degenerative joint disease appears to increase exponentially after the age of 50 or 60 years.

The pattern of degenerative joint disease is also influenced by the patient's sex. Although the frequency of the disease is approximately equal in both sexes, men are affected more commonly under the age of 45 years and women more commonly after this age. In addition, women are more often afflicted with primary generalized osteoarthritis, Heberden's nodes, and inflammatory osteoarthritis.

Activity and Occupation (Fig. 35–1)

It is generally assumed that either inactivity or excessive activity leads to articular degeneration. Certain occupations that involve chronic and repetitive articular abuse have reportedly been associated with degenerative joint disease at specific locations. The ankles and feet of ballet dancers, the joints of the lower extremities in soccer and football players, and the articulations of the upper extremities in boxers, wrestlers, and baseball players are thought to be prone to degeneration. The best examples of joint (and bone) damage

Table 35–2. MAIN ETIOLOGIC FACTORS ACCORDING TO LOCATION OF OSTEOARTHRITIS

	Intrinsic Factors					Extrinsic Factors		
	Age	Female Sex	Heredity	Obesity	Inflammation	Trauma	Minor Mechanical Disturbances	Dysplasia or Angulation
Fingers: DIP and nodal generalized osteoarthritis	+	+ +	+ +					
Fingers: PIP and non-nodal generalized osteoarthritis	+			+	+ +			
First carpometacarpal	+	+						
First metatarsophalangeal	(+)						+	
Hip	(+)							+ +
Knee	(+)	+		+			+	+ +
Shoulder	(+)					+	+	
Ankle						+		
Wrist						+		

From Peyron JG: Epidemiologic and etiologic approach of osteoarthritis. Semin Arthritis Rheum 8:288–306, 1979. Used with permission. DIP, Distal interphalangeal joints; PIP, proximal interphalangeal joints.

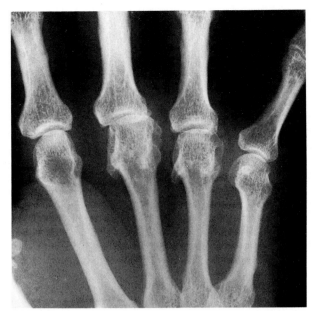

Figure 35–1. **Occupation-induced degenerative joint disease.** This professional boxer developed progressive pain and swelling about the metacarpophalangeal joints of his dominant hand. Observe narrowing of the interosseous space in the third and fourth digits and prominent osteophytes on the radial aspects of the metacarpal heads. (Courtesy of A. Brower, M.D., Washington, D.C.)

from excessive repetitive impulse loading are perhaps the reports of joint abnormality in workers using vibrating tools.

Nutritional and Metabolic Status

The recognition of degenerative joint abnormalities in Kashin-Beck disease has stimulated interest in the role of nutritional factors in the development of articular degeneration. In this disease, which is endemic in Siberia and other parts of the Far East, defective growth and maturation of epiphyses are associated with osteonecrosis and the appearance of osteoarthritis-like aberrations. Although the exact cause of Kashin-Beck disease is not known, it has been attributed to the toxic effects of fungus-contaminated grain, to chronic ingestion of excessive quantities of iron, and to defective mineral content of the grain.

An increased frequency of degenerative joint disease has been described in patients with a variety of endocrine disorders, such as diabetes mellitus and acromegaly. Conversely, it has been suggested that estrogens may afford some protection against such joint disease. Exogenous or endogenous hypercortisolism can lead to osteonecrosis with subsequent degenerative articular changes. Degenerative joint disease can also complicate various metabolic disorders, including Paget's disease, alkaptonuria, hemochromatosis, Wilson's disease, gout, and idiopathic calcium pyrophosphate dihydrate crystal deposition disease.

Osteoporosis

Although osteoporosis and degenerative joint disease are both common in older individuals, increasing evidence supports an inverse correlation between the two findings. Any relationship between the two disorders is a complicated one and probably dependent on multiple factors, although a

reduction in bone mass in subchondral locations may lead to an increase in the tissue's ability to absorb stress and a decrease in degenerative abnormalities.

Local Factors
Trauma

Major or minor traumatic episodes appear to be important in producing abnormal stress across a joint, leading to its degeneration. Repetitive trauma is significant in athletic and occupation-induced degenerative joint disease. It is also implicated in the appearance of joint degeneration in association with ligament laxity (Ehlers-Danlos syndrome, Marfan's syndrome, homocystinuria), loss of protective sensory feedback (neuroarthropathy, intraarticular steroid arthropathy), extraarticular malalignment (inequality of leg length, malunited fractures, congenital and acquired varus and valgus deformities), and intraarticular malalignment (epiphyseal injury or slipping, dysplasias, osteonecrosis, discoid menisci, meniscectomy, neuromuscular imbalance, loose intraarticular osseous and cartilaginous bodies). Single episodes of trauma can also lead to incongruity of apposing articular surfaces, with resultant degenerative joint disease. Traumatic factors may explain the presence of more severe articular degeneration in the upper extremity on the dominant side than on the nondominant side, the lesser frequency of osteoarthritis in joints that are located ipsilateral to and immediately above the site of amputation of a portion of the leg, and the absence of significant joint degeneration in an immobilized or paralyzed limb.

Preexisting Articular Disease or Deformity

Degenerative changes in cartilage and bone may be superimposed on any primary articular process that has led to incongruity and abnormal stress of the joint surfaces. Thus, degenerative arthritis may follow inflammatory joint disease, alterations of synovial fluid, or changes in periarticular supporting structures. Similarly, degenerative joint abnormalities may accompany hemophilia and other bleeding disorders, crystal-induced arthropathy, osteonecrosis, and congenital disorders.

PATHOGENESIS

It is apparent from the previous discussion that numerous factors, in one way or another, create a situation in which the intraarticular structures can no longer resist the physical forces that are being applied to the joint. In some instances, it is the force itself that is abnormal, whereas in other instances, weakened cartilage or subchondral bone is unable to combat the normal forces across the articulation.

Traditionally it has been held that degenerative alterations begin in the articular cartilage. Physical forces apparently disrupt the cartilage matrix and adversely affect the chondrocytes. The alterations in the matrix are almost certainly related to enzymatic destruction. Progressive cartilaginous abnormalities will eventually expose the subchondral bone to increased stress, initiating osseous degenerative alterations.

An alternative theory emphasizes the initial role of subchondral bone abnormalities in the pathogenesis of degenerative joint disease. According to this theory, overload produces microfractures in the subchondral bone trabeculae. Repair of these fractures subsequently leads to increased stiffness of the bone, a reduction in its shock-absorbing efficiency, and exposure of overlying cartilage to increased force. This theory gains support from the clinical observations that some patients with osteoarthritis demonstrate increased bone density, that persons with disorders characterized by increased bone density (Paget's disease, osteopetrosis) may reveal degeneration of neighboring joints, and that patients with osteoporosis of the femoral head may have a lower rate of occurrence of osteoarthritis of the hip.

There is no convincing evidence to suggest that alterations in the synovial membrane and joint lubrication play important roles in the initiation of degenerative joint disease.

After the appearance of degeneration in the cartilage or subchondral bone, a vicious cycle of events occurs, which aggravates the articular insult, resulting in progression of disease. In synovium-lined joints, damage confined to cartilage generally shows poor reparative response whereas that extending to subchondral bone is accompanied by the appearance of cartilaginous tissue formed by vascular invasion. This tissue is not as ideal mechanically in comparison to the original hyaline surface, resembles fibrocartilage, and accounts for such events as restoration of joint space, disappearance of bone eburnation and cysts, and improved joint congruity.

RADIOGRAPHIC-PATHOLOGIC CORRELATION
Synovial Joints
General Considerations (Table 35–3)

Although the concept that excessive wear and tear initiate articular degeneration in the stressed (pressure) areas of a joint is a valuable one, changes also are common in the nonstressed (nonpressure) segments. It is apparent that either excess or diminished pressure is deleterious to cartilage. In normal circumstances, cartilage derives its nutrition from two sources: Intermittent intrusion of synovial fluid occurs during alternating periods of pressure and rest; and vessels in the subchondral bone allow material to pass into the basal layer of cartilage, a process that is increased with normal joint

function. Both sources become defective in the presence of excessive or diminished stress, leading to degenerative changes in the joint.

In general, the type and severity of cartilaginous and osseous abnormalities are different in the stressed and non-stressed segments of the joint. In the stressed segment, pathologically evident thinning and denudation of the cartilaginous surface and vascular invasion, infarction, and necrosis of the subchondral trabeculae account for joint space loss, bone sclerosis, and cyst formation that are apparent on the radiographs; in the nonstressed segment, pathologically evident hypervascularity of marrow and cartilage leads to radiographically detectable osteophytosis. These findings emphasize the simultaneous occurrence of both destructive and reparative processes in this disease.

Cartilaginous Abnormalities (Fig. 35–2)

Cartilage in degenerating joints appears discolored, thinned, and roughened. Irregular crevices, ulcerations, and larger areas of erosion later become evident. The subchondral bone is denuded. In areas of eroded cartilage where bones are not closely apposed, the denuded surface may become covered by connective tissue and fibrocartilage.

It is this progressive loss of cartilage that accounts for one fundamental radiographic sign of degenerative joint disease: loss of joint space. Characteristically, the diminution is located predominantly in the area of the joint that has been subject to excessive pressure. Thus, joint space narrowing is apparent in the superolateral aspect of an osteoarthritic hip and in the medial femorotibial space of an osteoarthritic knee. In certain sites, articular space diminution may be more diffuse; in osteoarthritis of the interphalangeal or metacarpophalangeal joints of the hand, the sacroiliac joint, and the ankle, joint space loss may involve the entire articulation. With these few exceptions, however, it is the focal nature of the cartilaginous destruction and resulting loss of the interosseous space that allows differentiation of osteoarthritis from processes that lead to diffuse chondral alterations such as rheumatoid arthritis.

Subchondral Bone Abnormalities

Subchondral bone abnormalities accompanying degenerative joint disease can be divided into a destructive phase (regressive remodeling) and a productive phase (progressive remodeling), both phases occurring simultaneously. Charac-

Table 35–3. DEGENERATIVE JOINT DISEASE OF SYNOVIAL ARTICULATIONS (OSTEOARTHRITIS): RADIOGRAPHIC–PATHOLOGIC CORRELATION

Pathologic Abnormalities	Radiographic Abnormalities
Cartilaginous fibrillation and erosion	Localized loss of joint space
Increased cellularity and hypervascularity of subchondral bone	Bone eburnation
Synovial fluid intrusion or bone contusion	Subchondral cysts
Revascularization of remaining cartilage and capsular traction	Osteophytes
Periosteal and synovial membrane stimulation	Osteophytes and buttressing
Compression of weakened and deformed trabeculae	Bone collapse
Fragmentation of osteochondral surface	Intraarticular osseous bodies
Disruption and distortion of capsular and ligamentous structures	Deformity and malalignment

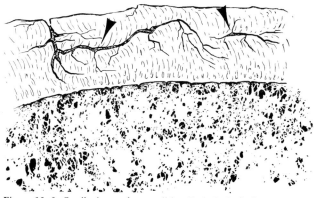

Figure 35–2. Cartilaginous abnormalities: Pathologic findings. Drawing depicts the irregular cracks or crevices (arrowheads) that may appear in the chondral surface.

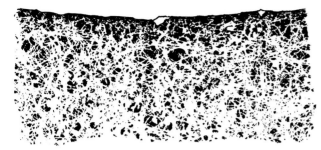

Figure 35–3. Subchondral bone eburnation: Pathologic findings. Drawing depicts the denudation of the cartilaginous surface and trabecular thickening or sclerosis of the subchondral bone.

teristics of the destructive phase are bone eburnation, cyst formation, flattening, and deformity, which predominate in the stressed segment of the joint; characteristics of the productive phase are osteophytes, which predominate in the nonstressed segment of the joint.

EBURNATION (FIG. 35–3). Following cartilage loss, bone eburnation becomes evident in the closely applied osseous surfaces, apparently related to deposition of new bone on preexisting trabeculae and to trabecular compression and fracture with callus formation. The weakened hyperemic subchondral bone in the stressed segment of the joint is vulnerable to collapse and further deformity.

Generally, radiographic evidence of loss of joint space is present before significant eburnation becomes apparent. With progressive obliteration of this space, sclerosis becomes more prominent, extending vertically into deeper regions of the subchondral bone and horizontally into adjacent osseous segments. Although the resulting radiodense area may initially be uniform in appearance, radiolucent lesions of varying size eventually appear, reflecting subchondral cyst formation.

CYST FORMATION (FIG. 35–4). Cysts are an important and prominent finding in osteoarthritis as well as in other articular disorders. These lesions have been variously termed synovial cysts, subchondral cysts, subarticular pseudocysts, necrotic pseudocysts, and geodes.

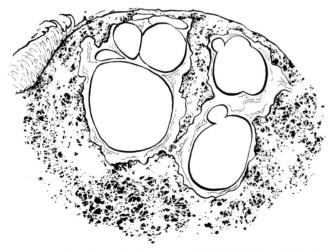

Figure 35–4. Subchondral bone cysts: Pathologic findings. A drawing reveals typical appearance of multiple subchondral cysts of varying size in areas of cartilaginous degeneration or disappearance. They are surrounded by sclerotic bone.

Within the stressed segment of the subchondral bone in osteoarthritis, cystic spaces appear between thickened trabeculae. These cysts commonly are multiple, of variable size (approximately 2 to 20 mm in diameter), and pyriform in shape. Cysts that are single or larger than 20 mm in diameter are unusual. On pathologic examination, some are noncavitary, containing myxoid and adipose tissue mixed with loose fibrous elements; others possess central cavitation containing proteinaceous material, are surrounded by fibrous tissue, and are well demarcated by adjacent eburnated bone. Two types of cartilage may be apparent in these lesions: small fragments of articular cartilage in the central portion; and foci of metaplastic cartilage within the wall. On radiographic examination, cysts appear in association with joint space loss and bone eburnation. Communication with the articular space may or may not be identifiable. Occasionally, radiolucent lesions may be demonstrated farther from the articular surface.

The cystic lesions of degenerative joint disease must be differentiated from the subchondral lucent lesions that may accompany other disorders (Table 35–4). In rheumatoid arthritis, cysts occur initially at chondroosseous junctions as a result of erosion of cartilage-free bone by inflammatory synovial tissue or pannus and are accompanied by early loss of articular space. They frequently are multiple, without sclerotic margins, and subsequently extend over large segments of the joint surface. In calcium pyrophosphate dihydrate crystal deposition disease, multiple large and widespread cystic lesions are characteristic. They resemble the cysts in degenerative joint disease, possessing sclerotic margins and being accompanied by joint space loss and bone eburnation. In calcium pyrophosphate dihydrate crystal deposition disease, however, the cysts are larger, more numerous, and associated more frequently with disruption, collapse, and fragmentation of the subchondral bone plate. In osteonecrosis, cysts appear within the stressed segment of the joint as a result of osteoclastic resorption of necrotic trabeculae, with fibrous replacement of bone. Collapse of the subchondral bone plate and preservation of joint space are additional characteristic features of osteonecrosis.

Subchondral cyst formation occasionally is a sequela of bone injury. A radiolucent lesion of variable size becomes evident over a period of months after the traumatic episode. The lesion, which is observed most commonly about the ankle, knee, or hip, is well marginated by a rim of bone sclerosis and may communicate with the articular cavity (Fig. 35–5). It resembles a degenerative cyst, although its larger size and the relatively normal appearance of the joint itself are useful diagnostic features.

An *intraosseous ganglion* is another subchondral radiolucent lesion that may simulate a degenerative cyst (Fig. 35–6). This lesion, which commonly is encountered in middle-aged adults, is characterized by mild, localized pain and the absence of a significant history of trauma. The ganglion generally is solitary, 0.6 to 6 cm in size, and located in the epiphysis of a long bone (particularly the medial malleolus and femoral head), a carpal bone, or a subarticular region of a flat bone (particularly the acetabulum). An intraosseous ganglion usually is a well-demarcated, sharply circumscribed lytic lesion with a sclerotic margin, which may be apparent in non–weight-bearing segments of a joint and which generally does not demonstrate communication with the joint on radiographic and pathologic examination. An adjacent soft tissue

Table 35–4. DIFFERENTIAL DIAGNOSIS OF SUBCHONDRAL CYSTIC LESIONS

Disorder	Probable Mechanism of Cyst Formation	Radiographic Appearance

Osteoarthritis	Synovial fluid intrusion
	Bone contusion
		Multiple radiolucent lesions
		  within the pressure segment of the joint
		Surrounding sclerotic margin
		Accompanying joint space narrowing
		  and bone sclerosis

Rheumatoid arthritis	Pannus invasion of bone	Multiple radiolucent lesions begin at
		  chondroosseous junction and become
		  widespread
		No surrounding sclerotic margin
		Accompanying joint space narrowing and
		  osteoporosis

Calcium pyrophosphate dihydrate
  crystal deposition disease
	Synovial intrusion
	Bone contusion
		Widespread radiolucent lesions,
		  frequently large
		Surrounding sclerotic margin
		Accompanying joint space narrowing,
		  bone sclerosis, collapse, and
		  fragmentation

Osteonecrosis	Osteoclastic resorption of
	  necrotic trabeculae
		Single or multiple radiolucent lesions
		  within the pressure segment of the joint
		Accompanying bone sclerosis, collapse,
		  and fragmentation

Intraosseous ganglion	Intraosseous penetration of a
	  soft tissue ganglion
	Primary intraosseous process,
	  perhaps related to synovial
	  intrusion, synovial rests, or
	  intramedullary mucoid degeneration
	  due to vascular insufficiency
	  resulting from trauma
		Single or loculated radiolucent
		  lesion in pressure or nonpressure
		  segment of joint
		Surrounding sclerotic margin
		Accompanying soft tissue mass

Neoplastic disorders:
  Chondroblastoma
  Giant cell tumor
  Skeletal metastasis
	Neoplastic proliferation with
	  destruction and displacement
	  of trabeculae
		Variable, depending on the nature
		  of the neoplasm

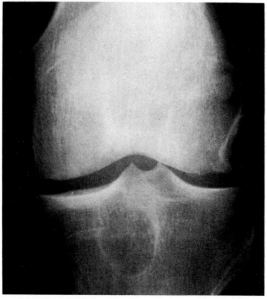

Figure 35–5. Posttraumatic subchondral cyst. This man developed knee pain and swelling after a fall. An anteroposterior radiograph reveals a well-circumscribed radiolucent area in the proximal portion of the tibia.

mass representing a soft tissue ganglion may be observed. Pathologic characteristics include a unilocular or multilocular cystic structure containing whitish or yellowish gelatinous material, which is surrounded by a fibrous lining.

Subchondral cysts in degenerative joint disease must also be distinguished from a variety of primary and secondary neoplasms of bone. These include chondroblastoma (10 to 30 year old age group, solitary lesion), giant cell tumor (20 to 40 year old age group, solitary eccentric trabeculated lesion), and skeletal metastasis (older patients, single or multiple lesions of variable appearance).

OSTEOPHYTOSIS. Osteophytes develop in areas of a degenerating joint that are subjected to low stress; they may be marginal (peripheral) in distribution, although they may become apparent at additional locations (Table 35–5). Most typically, osteophytes arise as a revitalization or reparative response by remaining cartilage, but they may also develop from periosteal or synovial tissue. The features of conversion of cartilage to bone in osteoarthritis resemble those accompanying normal endochondral ossification, with vascular invasion and erosion of the subchondral bone plate and calcified cartilage followed by deposition or accumulation of osseous tissue on the eroded surfaces.

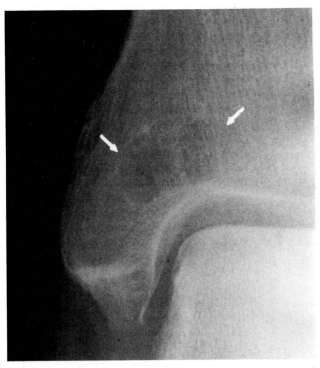

Figure 35–6. Intraosseous ganglion. An intraosseous ganglion is located adjacent to the ankle near the medial malleolus (arrows). It is lucent, surrounded by a thin rim of sclerosis, and apparently does not communicate with the articular cavity.

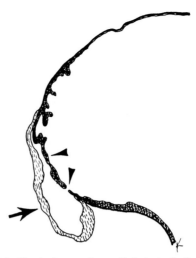

Figure 35–7. Marginal osteophytes: Pathologic findings. A diagram indicates the nature of the marginal osteophyte. It develops as a lip of bone (arrow) as a result of vascularization of the subchondral marrow with the inception of endochondral ossification. As it grows, it leaves behind a remnant of the original calcified cartilage (arrowheads).

Marginal Osteophytes (Fig. 35–7). At the peripheral portions of involved joints, at which sites articular cartilage is continuous with synovial membrane and periosteum, characteristic outgrowths develop in degenerative joint disease. Vascularization of the subchondral bone marrow in this region produces calcification of the adjacent cartilage and the inception of endochondral ossification. The developing outgrowth extends into the "free" articular space, along the path of least resistance. As it grows, it leaves behind remnants of the original calcified cartilage (and subchondral bone plate) as a telltale indicator of the location of the original joint surface. These remnants can be identified not only histologically but also radiographically as a zone of increased density.

Radiographically, marginal osteophytes appear as lips of new bone around the edges of the joint and are of variable size. The excrescences frequently predominate in one side of the joint. Marginal osteophytes develop initially in areas of relatively normal joint space and usually are unassociated with significant adjacent sclerosis or cyst formation.

Marginal excrescences in degenerative joint disease are readily differentiated from osteochondromas, which typically are seen in the metaphyses of young patients. Epiphyseal osteochondromas (dysplasia epiphysealis hemimelica; tarso-epiphyseal aclasis; Trevor's disease), which may exist in childhood, particularly in the lower extremity, do not realistically enter into the differential diagnosis of marginal osteophytes.

Central (Interior Joint) Osteophytes (Fig. 35–8). In central areas in which remnants of articular cartilage still exist, hypervascularity of subchondral bone stimulates endochondral ossification. The resulting excrescences, which are most prominent in the hip and knee, are button-like or flat in configuration and often are demarcated at their bases by remnants of the original calcified cartilage.

Central osteophytes frequently lead to a bumpy articular contour on radiographic examination. The small excrescences can be misinterpreted as evidence of intraarticular osseous (loose) bodies (Fig. 35–9) or cartilage calcification (chondrocalcinosis). The presence of continuity between the osteophyte and the underlying bone and of ossification rather than calcification should lead to correct analysis of the radiographs.

Periosteal and Synovial Osteophytes (Fig. 35–10). In certain joints, bone may develop from cartilaginous stimulation by the periosteum or synovial membrane. This phenomenon is most characteristic in the femoral neck, where it is

Table 35–5. TYPES OF OSTEOPHYTES

Type	Mechanism	Radiographic Appearance
Marginal	Endochondral ossification owing to vascularization of subchondral bone marrow	Outgrowth at the margins (nonpressure segments) of the joint, producing lips of bone
Central	Endochondral ossification owing to vascularization of subchondral bone marrow	Outgrowth at the central areas of the joint, producing bumpy contour
Periosteal (synovial)	Intramembranous type of ossification owing to stimulation of periosteal (synovial) membrane with appositional bone formation	Thickening of intraarticular "cortices" producing buttressing
Capsular	Capsular traction	Lips of bone extending along the direction of capsular pull

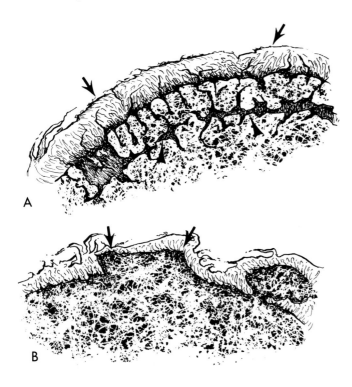

Figure 35–8. Central osteophytes: Pathologic findings. A Reduplication of cartilage and bone. In the central portions of the joint, hypervascularity of subchondral bone can lead to stimulation of remnants of cartilage, producing endochondral ossification. The flat outgrowths that develop (arrows) are frequently demarcated by the original zone of calcified cartilage (arrowheads). B Shifting of cartilage and bone border. In this situation, the osteophyte develops (arrows) without leaving behind a zone of calcified cartilage.

termed buttressing. In the degenerative hip joint, buttressing predominates on the medial aspect of the femoral neck, perhaps related to changes in mechanical stress across the joint. On radiographs, a radiodense line of variable thickness extends along a part of or the entire femoral neck. Associated excrescences may project circumferentially, producing a radiodense line across the neck that simulates a fracture.

Buttressing is observed most commonly in osteoarthritis, although it is also apparent in osteonecrosis, congenital

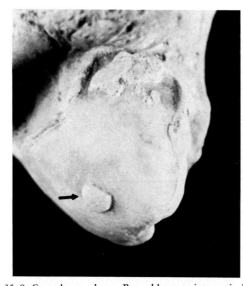

Figure 35–9. Central osteophytes: Resemblance to intra-articular osseous bodies. A photograph of the distal femoral articular surface reveals a button-like bone excrescence (arrow) representing a central osteophyte. Such an outgrowth can be misinterpreted as an intraarticular body during radiographic examination. Marginal osteophytes are also apparent.

subluxation of the hip, rheumatoid arthritis, and ankylosing spondylitis, and even with an adjacent osteoid osteoma.

Capsular Osteophytes (Fig. 35–11). Osteophytes accompanying degenerative joint disease may develop at the site of bone attachment of the joint capsule (and articular ligaments). This phenomenon is particularly characteristic in the interphalangeal joints, in which capsular traction may lead to outgrowths of considerable size. Osteophytes (enthesophytes) may also develop where intraarticular ligaments attach to bone (e.g., cruciate ligaments of knee).

OSTEONECROSIS. Bone necrosis may be apparent on histologic examination of the eburnated surface in the stressed segment of the degenerating joint. The changes of necrosis become more exaggerated as the disease process becomes more advanced; however, bone necrosis generally is a localized microscopic process in osteoarthritis. It cannot usually be detected on radiographic examination. Bone eburnation and cyst formation related to the degenerative process obscure the abnormalities of bone necrosis. Furthermore, flattening and collapse may be apparent in osteoarthritis without indicating the presence of significant osteonecrosis. Indeed, the radiographic (and pathologic) differentiation of osteoarthritis (with or without osteonecrosis) from osteonecrosis with secondary joint degeneration can be extremely difficult (Fig. 35–12).

Synovial Membrane Abnormalities

Synovial membrane alterations are not prominent in most cases of osteoarthritis. In initial stages of the disease, this tissue may be normal or exhibit mild congestion and villous hypertrophy. With increasing severity of cartilaginous and osseous alterations, the changes in the synovial membrane may become more prominent. Cartilaginous and osseous debris that has originated from the articular surfaces may become embedded in the synovial membrane, acting as a local irritant and producing proliferative changes.

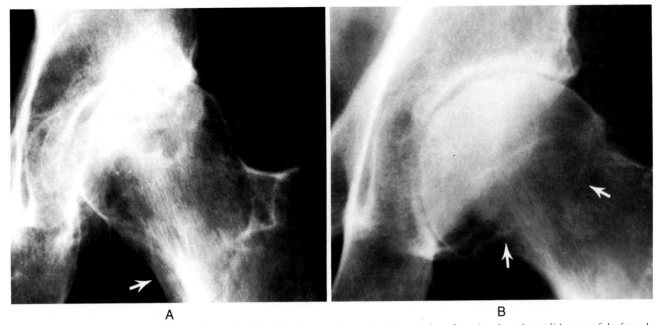

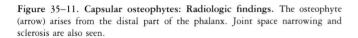

Figure 35–10. **Periosteal and synovial osteophytes: Radiologic findings. A** Buttressing. Note the bone formation along the medial aspect of the femoral neck (arrow) in addition to other changes of osteoarthritis, including joint space narrowing, sclerosis, and cyst formation. **B** Osteophytes have produced radiodense lines (arrows) across the femoral neck, which simulate the appearance of an impacted fracture.

Rarely, synovial abnormalities in osteoarthritis may become so severe that they resemble the changes of rheumatoid arthritis. In the interphalangeal joints of the fingers, such synovial inflammation is present in inflammatory (erosive) osteoarthritis (see discussion later in this chapter).

Synovial effusions may be encountered in osteoarthritis. These generally are of small volume unless they follow a traumatic episode or rapid bone collapse. Sizeable joint effusions that occur in the absence of trauma or osseous collapse should stimulate an investigation to exclude a super-imposed articular process, such as infection or crystal deposition disease.

Abnormalities of Other Articular Structures

Certain joints (knee, wrist, sternoclavicular, acromioclavicular, and temporomandibular joints) possess fibrocartilaginous discs or menisci, which may show considerable degeneration, particularly in older persons or after significant trauma. Degeneration and calcification may also appear in the fibrocartilaginous labrum of the hip and glenohumeral joint.

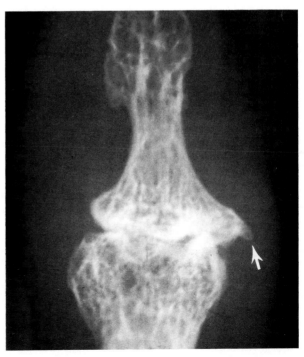

Figure 35–11. **Capsular osteophytes: Radiologic findings.** The osteophyte (arrow) arises from the distal part of the phalanx. Joint space narrowing and sclerosis are also seen.

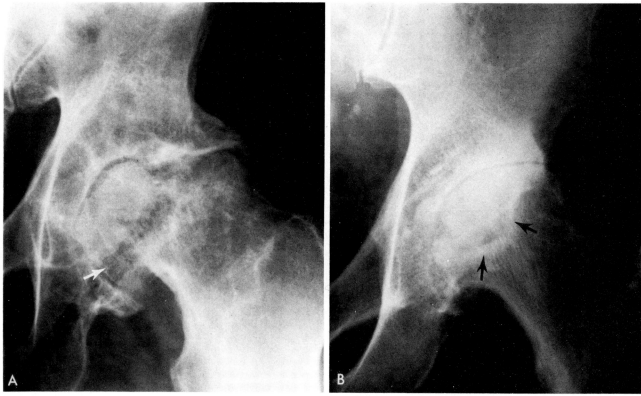

Figure 35–12. Osteoarthritis versus osteonecrosis. A Osteoarthritis with collapse and fragmentation. In this patient with long-standing disease, considerable collapse of the weight-bearing surface of the femoral head is evident. Note superior or upward migration of the femoral head with respect to the acetabulum, a large medial osteophyte (arrow), acetabular osteophytes, and buttressing. The changes are those of osteoarthritis, and the extent of bone collapse, although perhaps indicating secondary osteonecrosis, should not lead to an erroneous diagnosis of primary osteonecrosis. **B** Osteonecrosis with secondary cartilaginous destruction. In this patient, segmental collapse of the femoral head (arrows) is evident. Note symmetric loss of joint space, related either to secondary osteoarthritis or to chondrolysis. Although sclerosis and buttressing are evident, the findings do not resemble those of primary osteoarthritis.

Differential Diagnosis (Table 35–6)

In rheumatoid arthritis, joint effusion, osteoporosis, and uniform joint space loss are characteristic. Erosions occur initially at the chondroosseous junction at the margins of the joint. Bone eburnation and osteophytosis are not prominent.

In ankylosing spondylitis, psoriasis, and Reiter's syndrome (seronegative spondyloarthropathies), bone formation may be seen but it does not resemble the well-defined subchondral sclerosis or osteophytosis of osteoarthritis. Rather, in these disorders, poorly defined proliferation and intraarticular bone ankylosis can be noted. Furthermore, in these latter conditions, marginal erosions are characteristic, and joint space narrowing, when present, frequently is uniform.

In gouty arthritis, bulky asymmetric masses, eccentric well-circumscribed osseous erosions, and preservation of joint space are common. Bone proliferation in the later stages of the disease may lead to enlargement of the epiphyses and osteophytosis, which, when combined with joint space narrowing, can resemble osteoarthritis.

In calcium pyrophosphate dihydrate crystal deposition disease, findings are very similar to those of osteoarthritis. Of diagnostic aid in the former disorder are intraarticular and extraarticular calcification, involvement of unusual joints, large tumor-like cystic lesions, progressive abnormalities with fragmentation and collapse, and absence of osteophytosis.

Osteonecrosis may produce considerable collapse of sub-chondral bone at a time when the joint space is maintained. This combination is not evident in osteoarthritis.

Neuroarthropathy is characterized by severe fragmentation and collapse of the articular surfaces, extensive bone sclerosis, multiple cartilaginous and osseous intraarticular bodies, large joint effusions, subluxation, and malalignment.

Articular manifestations in alkaptonuria, acromegaly, Paget's disease, hemophilia, multiple epiphyseal dysplasia, and spondyloepiphyseal dysplasia include secondary degenerative abnormalities that resemble the findings of "primary" osteoarthritis. In all of these disorders, additional clinical and radiologic manifestations allow accurate diagnosis.

Cartilaginous Joints

In the two major extraspinal symphyses, the symphysis pubis and manubriosternal joints, degenerative changes may occur, particularly in older persons. In both locations, degeneration of cartilage and sclerosis of subchondral bone may be detected. The resulting radiographic picture simulates that of infection and inflammation associated with spondyloarthropathies.

Syndesmoses and Entheses

Degeneration of tendons, interosseous ligaments, and interosseous membranes is common in older persons, particularly near the sites of attachment of these structures to bone.

Table 35–6. DIFFERENTIAL DIAGNOSIS OF OSTEOARTHRITIS

	Osteo-porosis	Joint Space Narrowing	Osseous Erosions	Osseous Cysts	Sclerosis	Osteo-phytosis	Bone "Whiskering"	Intraarticular Osseous Fusion	Osseous Fragmentation, Collapse	Typical Location
Osteoarthritis	−	Asymmetric	−	+	+	+	−	−	In large joints	DIP, PIP, MCP joints of hand; first CMC and trapezio-scaphoid joints of wrist; first MTP, TMT joints of foot; knee; hip; apophyseal joints of spine
Inflammatory osteoarthritis	−	Asymmetric	+	+	+	+	−	DIP, PIP joints	−	DIP, PIP, MCP joints of hand; first CMC and trapezio-scaphoid joints of wrist
Rheumatoid arthritis	+	Symmetric	+	+	−	−	−	Carpal, tarsal areas	Rare	PIP, MCP joints of hand; wrist; MTP joints of foot; knee; elbow; glenohumeral joint; cervical spine
Gouty arthritis	−	May be absent	+	+	+	+	−	Rare	±	MTP, IP joints of foot; DIP, PIP, MCP joints of hand; wrist; elbow; knee
Pyrophosphate arthropathy	−	Symmetric	−	+	+	±	−	−	+	MCP joints of hand; radio-carpal joint of wrist; knee
Seronegative spondylo-arthropathies	±	Symmetric	+	+	+	−	+	+	−	Spine; sacroiliac joint; various articulations of the appendicular skeleton
Osteonecrosis	−	Absent until late	−	+	+	−	−	−	+	Hip; glenohumeral joint; knee; sites of trauma
Neuroarthropathy	−	Variable	−	±	+	±	−	−	+	Sites depend on underlying disorder

DIP, PIP, Distal and proximal interphalangeal; MCP, metacarpophalangeal; CMC, carpometacarpal; MTP, metatarsophalangeal; TMT, tarsometatarsal; IP, interphalangeal.

At syndesmoses (tibiofibular and radioulnar interosseous membrane and ligament), fibrous degeneration and bone proliferation may become apparent. At osseous sites of tendon attachment, a degenerative enthesopathy becomes evident, with hyperostosis of the osseous tissue (Fig. 35–13). The degree of bone proliferation may be considerable, resulting in radiographically detectable excrescences (ischial tuberosity, trochanters) and spurs (calcaneus, ulnar olecranon, patella). These are properly called enthesophytes. Tendon and ligament calcification may also be noted (sacrospinous, sacrotuberous ligaments). These changes are accelerated in the presence of trauma or chronic stress and may be generalized in diffuse idiopathic skeletal hyperostosis.

Enthesopathies are not confined to degenerative disorders. Inflammatory enthesopathies are common in ankylosing spondylitis and other spondyloarthropathies (see Chapter 21). In the latter disorders, the extent of bone formation and the degree of irregularity may be greater than those in degenerative diseases.

COMPLICATIONS OF DEGENERATIVE JOINT DISEASE
Malalignment and Subluxation

In some degenerating joints, malalignment and subluxation of bone may become prominent. Angular deformity in osteoarthritis is not unexpected in view of the nonuniform nature of the joint involvement. Asymmetric loss of joint space is characteristic and may produce, for example, varus (and less commonly valgus) deformity of the knee. Progressive subluxation may ensue, examples of which are lateral displacement of the tibia on the femur, lateral displacement of the femoral head in the acetabulum, and radial and proximal displacement of the first metacarpal base on the trapezium.

Fibrous and Bone Ankylosis

Although fibrous ankylosis may be prominent at some sites of osteoarthritis (sacroiliac joint), bone ankylosis is indeed unusual. An exception to this is the occasional appearance of intraarticular bone ankylosis in association with inflammatory (erosive) osteoarthritis of interphalangeal joints of the hand. In the absence of this clinical situation, bone ankylosis of synovial joints should stimulate a search for more likely causes, including septic arthritis and ankylosing spondylitis.

Bone bridging may accompany traumatic and degenerative alterations in symphyses. At these sites, such bridging may also be a normal aging process.

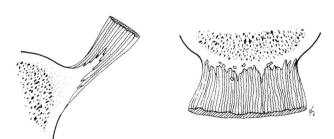

Figure 35–13. Degenerative enthesopathy. Drawings depict the irregular osseous proliferation that can occur at sites of tendon and ligament attachment to bone. One such site is the plantar aspect of the calcaneus.

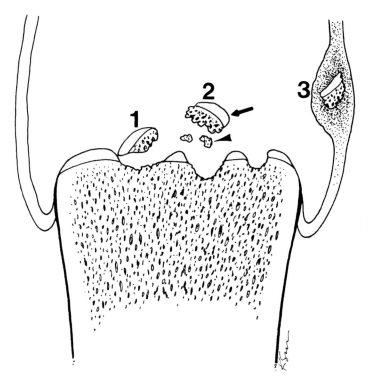

Figure 35–14. Complications of degenerative joint disease: Intraarticular osteocartilaginous bodies. In osteoarthritis, fragmentation of the cartilaginous or osseous surface, or both, can produce intraarticular bodies that remain on the joint surface (1), become dislodged or loose in the joint cavity (2), or become embedded in the synovial membrane at a distant site, evoking a local inflammatory response (3). Fragments can consist of degenerative cartilage and subchondral bone (arrow) or subchondral bone alone (arrowhead).

Intraarticular Cartilaginous and Osseous Bodies ("Joint Mice") (Fig. 35–14)

Osteocartilaginous bodies within a joint can arise from several sources: transchondral fractures, disintegration of the articular surface, and synovial metaplasia. Fragmentation of the joint surface can accompany a variety of disease processes, including osteoarthritis. In this latter disease, cartilaginous and osseous debris may remain on the joint surface or become dislodged or loose in the joint cavity. Debris may subsequently become embedded at a distant synovial site, eliciting a local inflammatory response.

On radiographs, the radiodense areas can increase or decrease in size, disappear, or remain unchanged. In a search for such areas, the physician must carefully evaluate all recesses of the joint, such as the acetabular fossa of the hip, olecranon fossa of the elbow, proximal tibiofibular area of the knee, and subscapular recess of the glenohumeral joint. In certain situations, osteochondral bodies may pass from the cavity into a neighboring communicating synovial cyst. They must be differentiated from other causes of intraarticular and periarticular dense lesions that accompany osteoarthritis, such as central (interior joint) osteophytes and fibrocartilaginous (meniscal) calcification and ossification, or other disease processes, such as idiopathic synovial osteochondromatosis and transchondral fractures (osteochondritis dissecans). Differentiation usually is not difficult in those cases in which osseous or cartilaginous dense lesions are seen in joints that do not reveal any manifestations of osteoarthritis (idiopathic synovial osteochondromatosis, osteochondritis dissecans). Furthermore, idiopathic synovial osteochondromatosis commonly is associated with a large number of cartilaginous or osteocartilaginous bodies of approximately equal size, whereas secondary synovial osteochondromatosis (as is evident in osteoarthritis) leads to fewer bodies (generally less than 10) of varying size.

DEGENERATIVE JOINT DISEASE IN SPECIFIC LOCATIONS (FIG. 35–15)

Interphalangeal Joints of the Hand

Clinical Abnormalities

Osteoarthritis of distal interphalangeal and proximal interphalangeal joints of the hand (including the interphalangeal joint of the thumb) is extremely common, particularly in middle-aged, postmenopausal women. Clinically detectable bone outgrowths about the distal interphalangeal joints are usually designated Heberden's nodes. Similar alterations at proximal interphalangeal joints are termed Bouchard's nodes. Involvement of multiple digits of both hands is characteristic. The altered digits may reveal malalignment such as flexion deformity and radial or ulnar deviation at the distal interphalangeal articulations. Symptoms are not prominent.

The clinical differentiation of osteoarthritis and rheumatoid arthritis in the hand usually is not difficult. The finger deformities in the former disease are characterized by horizontal instability (medial-lateral), whereas in rheumatoid arthritis, vertical subluxations (swan-neck and boutonnière deformities) are apparent.

Radiographic-Pathologic Correlation (Fig. 35–16)

Distal interphalangeal and proximal interphalangeal joints frequently are affected simultaneously and symmetrically; however, extensive alterations at distal interphalangeal joints may occur in the absence of proximal interphalangeal joint abnormalities and, less commonly, isolated abnormalities of proximal interphalangeal joints may be evident. On pathologic examination, apron-like marginal osteophytes may be found to extend around the involved phalanx. At the tips of the osteophytes, separate fragments or ossicles are identified occasionally.

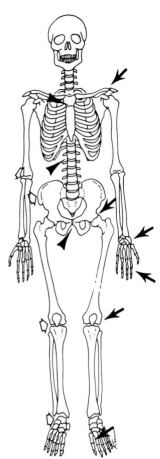

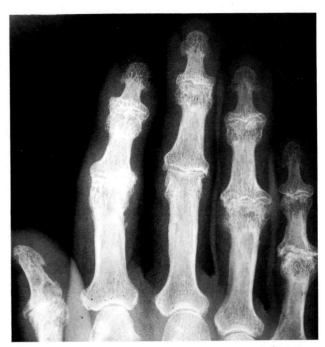

Figure 35–16. Osteoarthritis of the interphalangeal joints of the hand. The typical distribution of osteoarthritis is illustrated here. Findings are apparent in distal interphalangeal, proximal interphalangeal, and, to a lesser extent, metacarpophalangeal joints. The interphalangeal joint of the thumb is also affected.

Figure 35–15. Distribution of degenerative joint disease. The most characteristic sites of synovial joint degeneration (osteoarthritis) are the distal interphalangeal and proximal interphalangeal joints of the hand, the first carpometacarpal (trapeziometacarpal) and trapezioscaphoid areas of the wrist, the acromioclavicular joint, the hip, the knee, and the joints of the first ray of the foot (solid arrows). The most typical sites of degeneration of cartilaginous joints are the intervertebral disc, symphysis pubis, and manubriosternal joint (arrowheads). Degenerative enthesopathy is most common on the plantar aspect of the calcaneus, the pelvis, the ulnar olecranon, and the anterior surface of the patella (open arrows).

Radiographs reveal prominent osteophytes and joint space narrowing, providing close apposition of adjacent enlarged osseous surfaces. It is the closely applied, undulating articular surfaces that produce the diagnostic radiographic appearance of the disease, allowing its differentiation from erosive disorders, which produce separation of the involved bones. In osteoarthritis, the wavy contour of the base of the distal phalanx resembles the wings of a bird, the seagull sign. The involved digits frequently reveal mild to moderate radial and ulnar subluxation at distal interphalangeal or proximal interphalangeal joints, producing a zigzag contour. At the margins of the affected joint, focal radiodense lesions or ossicles are apparent overlying the joint capsule; they resemble intraarticular osseous bodies or fractured osteophytes.

Differential Diagnosis

The diagnosis of digital osteoarthritis usually is obvious. Occasionally, the undulating, irregularly enlarged subchon-

dral bone margins may contain small pockets that may be misinterpreted as osseous erosion, leading to an erroneous diagnosis of inflammatory (erosive) osteoarthritis. Erosive abnormalities of interphalangeal joints accompany various other disorders, including psoriasis, gout, multicentric reticulohistiocytosis, thermal injuries, hyperparathyroidism, and rheumatoid arthritis.

Metacarpophalangeal Joints

Metacarpophalangeal joint involvement in osteoarthritis is almost invariably associated with more prominent abnormalities at distal interphalangeal and proximal interphalangeal joints. Uniform narrowing of one or more metacarpophalangeal interosseous spaces is most characteristic (Fig. 35–16), and cystic lesions and osteophytes may also be apparent. Erosions are absent.

The metacarpophalangeal joint abnormalities in osteoarthritis can usually be differentiated from those accompanying other articular disorders such as rheumatoid arthritis (periarticular osteoporosis, marginal erosions, subluxations, lack of osteophytosis); idiopathic calcium pyrophosphate dihydrate crystal deposition disease or hemochromatosis (large cystic lesions, collapse and fragmentation of the metacarpal heads, prominent hook-like osteophytes, intraarticular and periarticular calcification and debris); gouty arthritis (asymmetric masses, eccentric erosions, preservation of interosseous space); and Wilson's disease (peculiar brush-like spiculation). The metacarpophalangeal joint changes in osteoarthritis are identical to those accompanying inflammatory osteoarthritis (see discussion later in this chapter).

Additional diagnostic help is provided by the distribution of the articular abnormalities. In osteoarthritis, metacarpophalangeal joint abnormalities are invariably accompanied by changes in the distal interphalangeal and proximal interphalangeal joints. This distribution differs from that in rheumatoid arthritis (in which involvement of metacarpophalangeal and proximal interphalangeal joints is common, with relative sparing of distal interphalangeal articulations) and idiopathic calcium pyrophosphate dihydrate crystal deposition disease or hemochromatosis (metacarpophalangeal joint alterations may be a predominant or isolated phenomenon). Thus, "degenerative-like" abnormalities isolated to the metacarpophalangeal joints should stimulate a search for disorders other than osteoarthritis. The one exception to this statement occurs in the first digit, in which alterations at the first metacarpophalangeal joint can be a prominent manifestation of osteoarthritis.

Wrist

The radial distribution of osteoarthritis of the wrist is well known. In the absence of significant accidental or occupational trauma, changes are usually confined to the trapeziometacarpal (first carpometacarpal) joint and trapezioscaphoid space of the midcarpal joint.

Trapeziometacarpal (First Carpometacarpal) Joint

Involvement of the trapeziometacarpal joint can lead to prominent clinical abnormalities. These include pain, restricted movement, crepitus, and instability.

The radiographic features of degenerative joint disease in this location are characteristic (Fig. 35–17). Radial subluxation of the metacarpal base, narrowing of the interosseous space, sclerosis and cystic changes in the subchondral bone, osteophytosis, and bone fragmentation become apparent.

Trapezioscaphoid Space

Osteoarthritis of the trapezioscaphoid space (as well as of the trapezoid-scaphoid space) of the midcarpal compartment of the wrist frequently is combined with degenerative changes at the trapeziometacarpal joint (Fig. 35–17). Isolated abnormalities at this space are also reported, but predominant and severe changes resembling those of degenerative joint disease at this articulation can indicate the presence of other disease processes, including generalized osteoarthritis, calcium pyrophosphate dihydrate crystal deposition disease, and rheumatoid arthritis. Pain and tenderness may accompany osteoarthritis of the trapezioscaphoid space and may be associated with restricted motion and adjacent soft tissue swelling. The soft tissue changes are sometimes related to adjacent ganglia.

Typical radiographic features of osteoarthritis are apparent in a unilateral or bilateral distribution, including joint space narrowing and sclerosis of apposing surfaces of trapezium, trapezoid, and scaphoid.

Other Joints

Osteoarthritis localized to other compartments of the wrist is distinctly unusual in the absence of a history of trauma. Without such a history, joint space narrowing, sclerosis, osteophytes, and subchondral cysts about the radiocarpal, inferior radioulnar, and common carpometacarpal joints as well as the remainder of the midcarpal compartment may be initial radiographic clues to the presence of crystal-induced

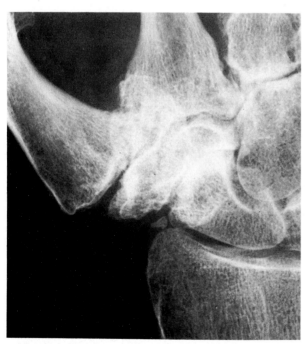

Figure 35–17. Osteoarthritis of the trapeziometacarpal (first carpometacarpal) joint. This radiograph illustrates pantrapezial osteoarthritis with degenerative changes in the trapezium–first metacarpal, trapezioscaphoid, trapeziotrapezoid, and trapezium–second metacarpal spaces. Observe joint space narrowing, eburnation, osteophytes, and radial subluxation of the base of the metacarpal. The additional alterations of the common carpometacarpal compartment at the bases of the second and third metacarpals can be accepted as osteoarthritis in the presence of extensive disease along the radial aspect of the wrist.

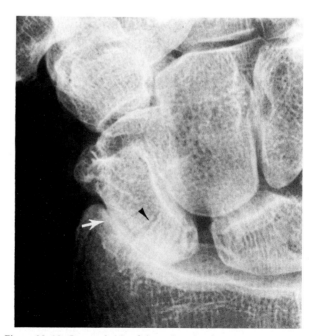

Figure 35–18. Osteoarthritis of the wrist related to trauma. Joint space narrowing between the scaphoid and radius (arrow) and bone eburnation represent osteoarthritis secondary to a previous scaphoid fracture (arrowhead). The proximal pole of the scaphoid is diminutive and eburnated, indicating prior osteonecrosis. Scapholunate separation or dissociation has resulted from posttraumatic disruption of the interosseous ligament.

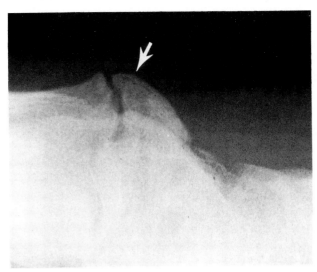

Figure 35–19. Os styloideum. On this lateral radiograph of the hand, note the "osteophytic" appearance of the extra ossification center (arrow.) Clinically, a painless soft tissue lump frequently is evident.

(calcium pyrophosphate dihydrate crystal deposition disease, gout) or occupation-induced articular disease. Fracture, subluxation, dislocation, or osteonecrosis about the wrist can lead to altered joint motion, however, resulting in secondary osteoarthritis (Fig. 35–18). Typical examples include degenerative disease of the radiocarpal and midcarpal compartments after scaphoid injuries; degenerative joint disease of the radiocarpal and inferior radioulnar compartments after osteonecrosis of the lunate (Kienböck's disease); and degenerative joint disease of the inferior radioulnar compartment after subluxation of the distal part of the ulna. Furthermore, a dorsal lip of bone is not infrequent at the common carpometacarpal compartment. In this area, an accessory ossicle, the os styloideum, may fuse with the second or third metacarpal, or both. The resulting soft tissue and osseous prominence is called the "hunchback" carpal bone or carpe bossu (Fig. 35–19). It is probably traumatic in origin, related to either a previous fracture or recurrent stress.

Arthrosis of the lunate-capitate space, leading to interosseous narrowing, sclerosis, and cyst formation, has been emphasized as an additional posttraumatic degenerative condition. This abnormality usually is combined with scapholunate separation, or dissociation, and narrowing of the radioscaphoid space. The resulting radiographic changes are termed the scapholunate advanced collapse pattern, or SLAC wrist, and are virtually identical to alterations accompanying the arthropathy of calcium pyrophosphate dihydrate crystal deposition disease.

Elbow

Osteoarthritis of the elbow is not common. When present, it usually follows accidental or occupational trauma (particularly in miners and drillers). Osteoarthritis of the elbow manifests typical radiographic findings, which include joint space narrowing, sclerosis, cysts, and osteophytes. Olecranon spurs at the attachment of the triceps tendon may accompany these alterations.

Shoulder

Significant osteoarthritis of the glenohumeral joint generally has been regarded as unusual in the absence of local trauma; indeed, the detection of degenerative-like alterations at this site has been believed to require a search for other disorders, such as alkaptonuria, acromegaly, epiphyseal dysplasia, calcium pyrophosphate dihydrate crystal deposition disease, and hemophilia. Although any of these conditions can lead to a degenerative-like process in the glenohumeral joint, it has become increasingly apparent that osteoarthritis does affect this joint, even in patients without prior physical injury.

The most frequent abnormality accompanying osteoarthritis in this site is the formation of *osteophytes* along the articular margin of the humeral head and the line of attachment of the labrum to the glenoid fossa. These osteophytes predominate in the anterior and inferior aspects of the joint margin (Fig. 35–20). A second abnormality is focal or global *eburnation* of the articular surface of the superior and middle portions of the humeral head, manifested radiographically as subchondral sclerosis.

Bone proliferation at adjacent sites accompanies these degenerative alterations. Osseous excrescences with occasional areas of cystic change are observed in the anatomic neck of the humerus, greater and lesser tuberosities, and bicipital groove (Fig. 35–21). Those abnormalities in the tuberosities are indicative, in part, of pathologic alterations in the musculotendinous rotator cuff. Osteophytes commonly are evident in and around the bicipital groove as well.

Deterioration and disruption of the rotator cuff are common, especially in elderly persons (Fig. 35–22). This results in characteristic abnormalities on both plain film radiography (elevation of the humeral head with respect to the glenoid cavity, narrowing of the acromiohumeral space, eburnation

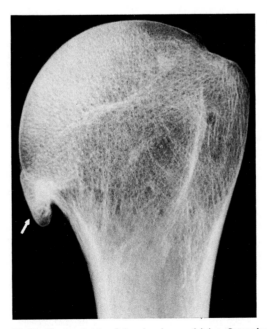

Figure 35–20. Osteoarthritis of the glenohumeral joint: Osteophytosis of the humeral head. A radiograph of a humeral specimen in external rotation documents the presence of osteophytes (arrow) arising at the articular margin.

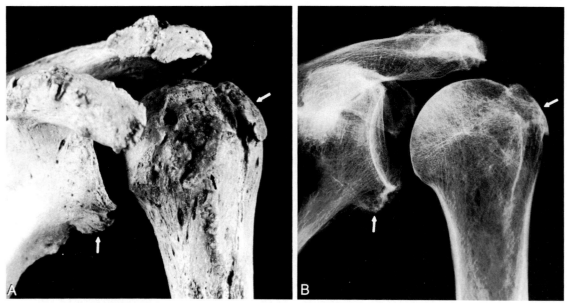

Figure 35–21. Degenerative disease of the shoulder: Enthesopathy. Photograph. (A) and radiograph (B) of matched specimens reveal bone excrescences in the anatomic neck, greater and lesser tuberosities, and glenoid region (arrows).

and cysts of apposing bone surfaces of humeral head and acromion, cystic and notch-like defects in the humeral surface near the bicipital groove, and reversal of the normal inferior convexity of the acromion) and glenohumeral joint arthrography (communication between the articular cavity and the subacromial bursa). It should be emphasized, however, that in young patients, acute tears of the cuff commonly are unassociated with plain film radiographic aberrations, and accurate assessment requires arthrographic (or sonographic) examination. Furthermore, in young and old individuals,

narrowing of the acromiohumeral space, a characteristic alteration of cuff disruption, can be simulated by faulty position of the patient during radiography and can accompany atrophy of the cuff in the absence of a full-thickness tear.

There appears to be a significant association between osteoarthritis of the glenohumeral joint and rotator cuff degeneration. It is not clear, however, if these represent independent and somewhat frequent phenomena of aging or if a common pathogenetic mechanism connects them. Two such mechanisms have been proposed. The first, termed *cuff-*

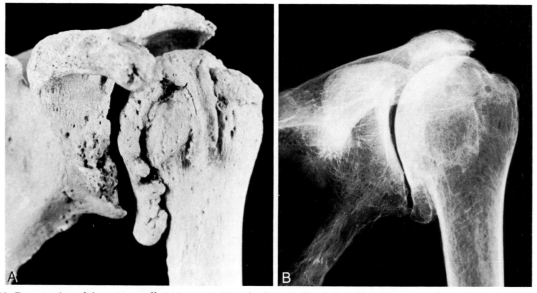

Figure 35–22. Degeneration of the rotator cuff. A photograph (A) and radiograph (B) of matched specimens reveal abnormalities associated with chronic atrophy or disruption of the rotator cuff as well as those associated with osteoarthritis of the glenohumeral joint. With regard to rotator cuff deterioration, observe narrowing of the acromiohumeral space, reversal of the normal convexity of the inferior surface of the acromion, and eburnation and cyst formation of acromion, humeral head, and greater tuberosity. With regard to osteoarthritis of the glenohumeral joint, note interosseous space narrowing and exuberant osteophytosis in the humeral head and glenoid region. Bone proliferation about the bicipital groove with the creation of a bicipital sleeve is also evident.

tear arthropathy, emphasizes initial injury of the rotator cuff with progressive superior migration of the humeral head that produces instability, increasing wear of cartilaginous surfaces, and osteoarthritis. The second mechanism emphasizes (1) abnormal accumulation of calcium hydroxyapatite crystals, with release of these crystals into the synovial fluid together with their tissue matrix to form microspheroids, (2) an assimilation of these particles by the fixed macrophage-like synovial cells, inducing the release of collagenase and neutral protease, and (3) an attack on the periarticular tissues, including the rotator cuff, by the released enzymes, resulting in cuff degeneration. A progressive cycle of events continues, and the eventual arthropathy, which is termed the *"Milwaukee shoulder,"* resembles rheumatoid arthritis or neuroarthropathy.

One additional condition that commonly affects the glenohumeral joint is the *shoulder impingement syndrome*. Impingement exists when there is encroachment on the subacromial space with loss of the normal gliding mechanism between the superior periarticular soft tissues about the glenohumeral joint and the coracoacromial arch. Entrapment of the soft tissue structures between this arch and the greater tuberosity of the proximal portion of the humerus during abduction or elevation of the arm results in subacromial bursitis and tendinitis of the rotator cuff, with eventual progression to cuff fibrosis and rupture. Clinically, the impingement syndrome is seen in two main groups of patients: in young athletic individuals involved in sporting activities and in older persons in whom symptoms appear spontaneously or follow physical exercise.

Although the diagnosis of the impingement syndrome generally is provided by careful physical examination, various imaging studies occasionally are required. Plain film alterations include bone proliferation, eburnation, and cystic change

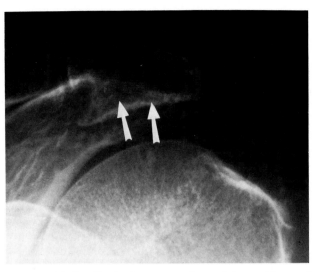

Figure 35–24. Shoulder impingement syndrome: Subacromial spur. A subacromial spur (arrows) is present on the standard anteroposterior radiograph. (From Cone RO, et al: Shoulder impingement syndrome: Radiographic evaluation. Radiology 150:29, 1984. Used with permission.)

in the greater tuberosity (Fig. 35–23). The tuberosity may appear flattened and sclerotic. A well-defined osseous excrescence, termed a subacromial spur, that is evident in some patients with this syndrome (Fig. 35–24) extends from the anteroinferior aspect of the acromion and is best visualized on an anteroposterior radiograph with 30 degrees of caudal angulation of the x-ray beam. The excrescence arises at the site of osseous attachment of the coracoacromial ligament. Fluoroscopy can be used to document the correlation of the patient's pain and restricted motion with the approximation of the greater tuberosity and undersurface of the acromion process (see Chapter 5). Arthrography of the glenohumeral joint is useful to document the presence of a full-thickness tear of the rotator cuff, which, along with bicipital tendinitis and subacromial bursitis, represents a significant complication of the impingement syndrome. Magnetic resonance imaging also may be used to evaluate the impingement syndrome.

Acromioclavicular Joint

Degenerative changes in this synovial joint are almost universal in elderly persons. Although such changes may be the cause of obscure shoulder pain and tenderness, their precise relationship to these and other symptoms and signs is not clear. Radiographic examination of the degenerating acromioclavicular joint reveals joint space diminution, sclerosis of apposing osseous surfaces, marginal osteophytes, hypertrophy and inferior subluxation of the acromial end of the clavicle, and osseous proliferation on the superior surface of the acromion.

Sternoclavicular Joint

Osteoarthritis of the sternoclavicular joint is not uncommon. Its clinical manifestations include pain, tenderness, and palpable enlargement of the articulating bone. Radiographic findings include unilateral or bilateral joint space narrowing, sclerosis, and osteophytosis.

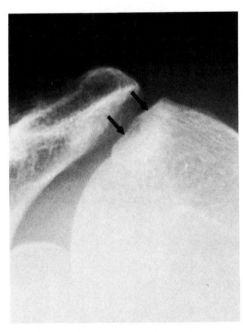

Figure 35–23. Shoulder impingement syndrome: Abnormalities of the greater tuberosity. In this patient with surgically documented impingement syndrome, observe prominent flattening and sclerosis of the greater tuberosity of the humerus (arrows). (From Cone RO, et al: Shoulder impingement syndrome: Radiographic evaluation. Radiology 150:29, 1984. Used with permission.)

Sacroiliac Joint

Pathologic abnormalities in the sacroiliac joint that are consistent with degenerative disease are frequent in specimens derived from middle-aged and elderly persons. Cartilage fibrillation and erosion, denudation of cartilaginous surfaces, partial or complete fibrous ankylosis of the joint cavity, subchondral eburnation, and osteophytes are observed. Changes may be unilateral or bilateral and associated with significant clinical findings, including pain and tenderness.

Radiographic manifestations accompany the pathologic aberrations. After the age of 40 years, most patients reveal focal or diffuse loss of joint space. The subchondral bone of the ilium may become closely applied to that of the sacrum (Fig. 35–25). Condensation of subchondral bone produces either a radiodense line or focal areas of sclerosis. These latter radiodense areas are frequent on the superior and inferior articulating portions of the ilium and, because of the obliquity of the joint, may overlie the articular cavity. Erosion of subchondral bone is infrequent in degenerative disease of the sacroiliac joint. Furthermore, subchondral cystic lesions are also extremely rare.

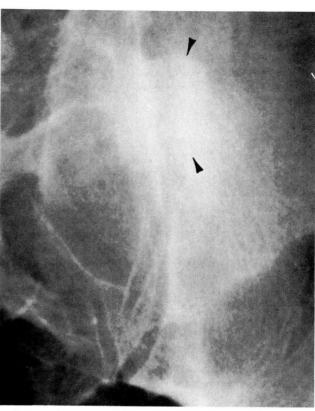

Figure 35–26. Degenerative disease of the sacroiliac joint. Anterosuperior osteophytosis. Note localized radiodense areas overlying the articular space (arrowheads).

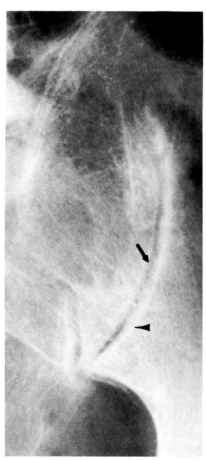

Figure 35–25. Degenerative disease of the sacroiliac joint: Joint space narrowing and bone sclerosis. The joint space is uniformly narrowed (arrow) with linear condensation of bone in the ilium (arrowhead). Note the sharp definition of the subchondral bone. A vacuum phenomenon is apparent within the inferior aspect of the joint. (From Resnick D, et al: Comparison of radiographic abnormalities of the sacroiliac joint in degenerative disease and ankylosing spondylitis. AJR 128:189, 1977. Copyright 1977, American Roentgen Ray Society. Used with permission.)

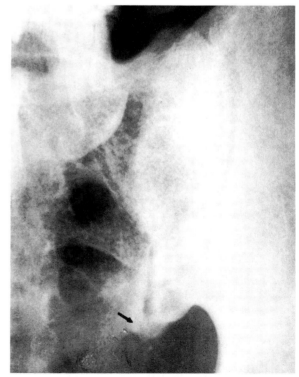

Figure 35–27. Degenerative disease of the sacroiliac joint: Anteroinferior osteophytosis. An inferior osteophyte (arrow) bridges the joint space. (From Resnick D, et al: Comparison of radiographic abnormalities of the sacroiliac joint in degenerative joint disease and ankylosing spondylitis. AJR 128:189, 1977. Copyright 1977, American Roentgen Ray Society. Used with permission.)

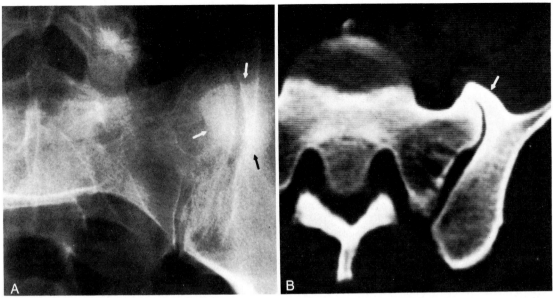

Figure 35–28. Degenerative disease of the sacroiliac joint: Value of computed tomography. A Frontal radiograph demonstrates a radiodense lesion (arrows) overlying the superior aspect of the synovium-lined portion of the sacroiliac joint. B With computed tomography, which provided a transaxial section through this lesion, it is apparent that bone sclerosis and a bridging osteophyte (arrow) are the cause of the abnormal density seen in the plain film. (Courtesy of J. Scavulli, M.D., San Diego, California.)

Osteophytosis is a prominent radiographic characteristic of osteoarthritis of the sacroiliac joint. Osteophytes can occur at any level in the joint but are most characteristic at the anterosuperior (Fig. 35–26) and anteroinferior (Fig. 35–27) limits of the articular cavity. They may produce prominent focal radiopaque lesions, which can simulate the appearance of osteoblastic skeletal metastasis. With further growth, osteophytic outgrowths extend across the anterior aspect of the articular cavity, creating periarticular bone ankylosis that may simulate intraarticular bone ankylosis. The radiologist may erroneously interpret the radiographic findings as those of ankylosing spondylitis. On oblique radiographs or conventional or computed tomograms, the periarticular nature of the ankylosis becomes apparent, facilitating accurate diagnosis (Fig. 35–28).

Focal calcification and ossification are occasionally observed in the iliolumbar and interosseous ligaments above the sacroiliac joint. These degenerative changes usually are associated with radiographic and pathologic evidence of osteoarthritis.

The radiologic characteristics of degenerative disease of the sacroiliac joint may be confused with those of ankylosing spondylitis (Table 35–7). Joint space narrowing occurs in both diseases. When it accompanies degenerative disease, it may be focal in appearance and asymmetric or symmetric in distribution. The adjacent subchondral bone is usually well defined. Joint space diminution in ankylosing spondylitis commonly is widespread and symmetric. The surrounding bone is frayed or irregular in outline. Bone ankylosis may be present in both degenerative disease and ankylosing spondylitis. In degenerative disease, such ankylosis results from periarticular bridging osteophytes, whereas in ankylosing spondylitis true intraarticular ankylosis is characteristic. Subchondral erosions, a prominent feature of ankylosing spondylitis, are infrequent and superficial in osteoarthritis.

Localized areas of increased density in degenerative sacroiliac joints superficially resemble alterations in other disorders. Osteitis condensans ilii, noted primarily in young, multiparous women, is associated with increased bone density, generally confined to a triangular area along the inferior aspect of the ilium adjacent to the sacroiliac joint (Table 35–7). This condition commonly is bilateral and symmetric, and sacroiliac joint abnormality and sacral involvement are rarely

Table 35–7. DIFFERENTIAL DIAGNOSIS OF DEGENERATIVE DISEASE OF THE SACROILIAC JOINT

	Osteoarthritis	Ankylosing Spondylitis	Osteitis Condensans Ilii
Age	Older patients	Younger patients	Younger patients
Sex	Men and women	Men > women	Women > men
Distribution	Bilateral or unilateral	Bilateral, symmetric	Bilateral, symmetric
Sclerosis	Iliac Mild, focal	Iliac May be extensive	Iliac Triangular in shape
Erosions	Absent	Common	Absent
Intraarticular bone ankylosis	Rare	Common	Absent
Paraarticular osteophytosis	Common	Rare	Rare
Ligamentous ossification	Less common	Common	Absent

apparent. The alterations may resolve partially or completely. Degenerative joint disease affects both men and women, may be unilateral or bilateral in distribution, is associated with joint space narrowing and osteophytes, and does not resolve spontaneously.

In certain circumstances, prominent degenerative changes of the sacroiliac joint may have a unilateral distribution owing to altered stress confined to one side of the pelvis. Precipitating factors may include scoliosis and articular disorders or arthrodesis of the contralateral hip joint.

Hip
General Clinical Abnormalities

Osteoarthritis of the hip may produce significant clinical symptoms and signs and lead to considerable disability. Pain can be confined to the hip region or referred to other sites, such as the knee, the buttock, the thigh, the groin, or the region of the greater trochanter. Factors contributing to pain accompanying osteoarthritis in the hip may include fracture of subchondral bone, venous congestion, and low grade synovitis. Restriction of motion also is common.

Radiographic-Pathologic Correlation

Osteoarthritis of the hip is invariably associated with joint space narrowing. With the onset of this narrowing, the femoral head moves toward the acetabulum (Fig. 35–29). Three basic patterns of migration can be observed: superior migration, in which articular space loss is most prominent on the upper aspect of the joint and the femoral head moves in a vertical or upward direction; medial migration, in which

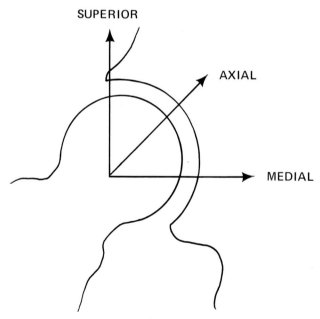

Figure 35–29. Patterns of migration of the femoral head with respect to the acetabulum for the right hip. Three directions can be identified. When superior joint space loss predominates, the femoral head moves in an upward or superior direction with respect to the acetabulum. When joint space loss is confined to the inner one third of the joint, a medial migration pattern is evident. With diffuse loss of articular space, the femoral head migrates axially along the axis of the femoral neck. (Redrawn after Graham J, Harris WH: Paget's disease involving the hip. J Bone Joint Surg [Br] 53:651, 1971. Used with permission.)

joint space loss is most marked on the inner aspect of the articulation and the femoral head moves in a medial direction; and axial migration, in which joint space loss occurs throughout the articular cavity and the femoral head moves inward along the axis of the femoral neck. It should be emphasized that this classification system relies on changes on the frontal radiograph; anterior and posterior patterns of migration, as evident on lateral radiographs or computed tomograms, may accompany these changes.

SUPERIOR MIGRATION PATTERN. The most common location of joint space loss in osteoarthritis is the superior aspect of the articulation, resulting in superior migration of the femoral head with respect to the acetabulum. This pattern can be further classified into a superolateral pattern and a superomedial pattern or tilt deformity.

Superolateral migration of the femoral head is more frequent in women and is usually unilateral or asymmetric in distribution (Fig. 35–30). This pattern may be identified in 15 to 50 per cent of patients with osteoarthritis of the hip. Superolateral migration has been attributed to acetabular dysplasia. Without serial radiographs, however, it is difficult to discern whether acetabular flattening antedates the appearance of osteoarthritis or whether the shallowness of the acetabulum is related to collapse and flattening of the outer aspect of the bone.

On radiography, the femoral head moves superiorly in conjunction with diminution of the interosseous space. Sclerosis and subchondral cystic lesions predominate on the outer aspect of the femoral head and the acetabulum. Flattening of the lateral aspect of the femoral head can be accompanied by substantial lateral displacement with widening of the inferomedial portion of the joint space. Osteophytes occur on the lateral aspect of the femoral head and acetabulum in association with thickening or buttressing of the cortex in the femoral neck, particularly on its medial side.

Superomedial migration (tilt deformity) of the femoral head, which may be detected in 35 to 50 per cent of patients with osteoarthritis, is more frequent in men than in women and commonly is bilateral in distribution (Fig. 35–31). Patients with this pattern of disease may become symptomatic at a relatively young age. Its cause is unknown.

Early radiologic abnormalities consist of superior displacement of the femoral head associated with joint space narrowing in the outer one third of the articular cavity. Progressive joint space loss results in close apposition of the superior and middle surfaces of the femoral head and acetabulum; at this stage, the medial space frequently appears widened. With continued deformity along the outer one third of the femoral head, osteophytosis on its medial and inferior surface is seen. These osteophytes fill in the free space on the medial aspect of the joint cavity. Careful observation of radiographs often reveals the presence of a curvilinear radiodense area on the inner aspect of the femoral head. This represents the original calcified zone of articular cartilage, allowing accurate appraisal of the position of the femoral head before its remodeling.

The tilt deformity resulting from remodeling in the osteoarthritic hip can be differentiated from a similar deformity accompanying epiphysiolysis with secondary degeneration. In the latter case, because of true slipping of the femoral head in relation to the femoral neck, the original zone of calcified cartilage along with the remainder of the head becomes displaced posteromedially.

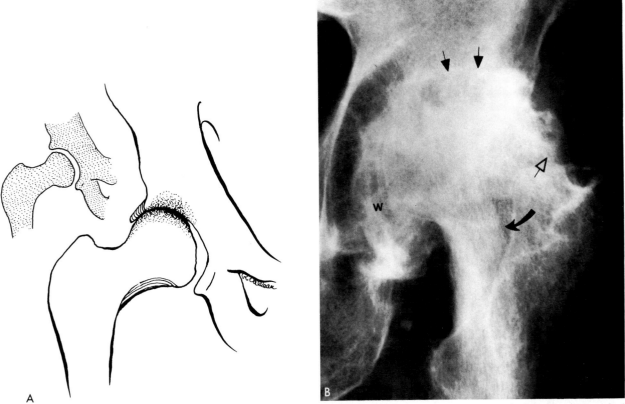

Figure 35–30. Osteoarthritis of the hip: Superolateral migration pattern. A Progressive narrowing of the outer one third of the joint space results in upward migration of the femoral head with respect to the acetabulum. Associated findings include eburnation, lateral acetabular osteophytes, and medial femoral buttressing. **B** Joint space narrowing and sclerosis (solid straight arrows) along the superior articulating surface are associated with subchondral collapse of the adjacent femoral head. A lateral osteophyte (open arrow), widened inferomedial joint space (W), and medial femoral neck buttressing (curved arrow) are noted. (From Resnick D: Patterns of migration of the femoral head in osteoarthritis of the hip. AJR 124:62, 1975. Copyright 1975, American Roentgen Ray Society. Used with permission.)

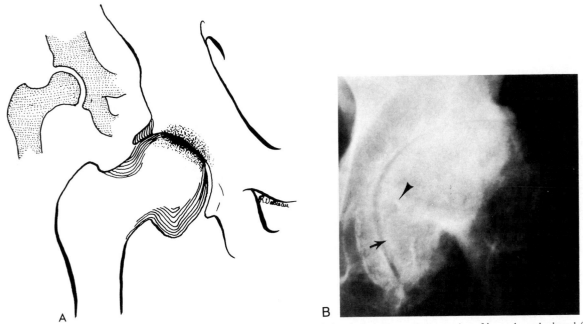

Figure 35–31. Osteoarthritis of the hip: Superomedial migration pattern (tilt deformity). A Progressive resorption of bone along the lateral femoral head and deposition along its medial aspect result in a tilt deformity. **B** A hip radiograph demonstrates superior and middle joint space loss and subchondral sclerosis, medial femoral neck buttressing, and small lateral acetabular and massive medial femoral osteophytes (arrow). The original calcified cartilaginous zone (arrowhead) is faintly visible. (From Resnick D: Patterns of migration of the femoral head in osteoarthritis of the hip. AJR 124:62, 1975. Copyright 1975, American Roentgen Ray Society. Used with permission.)

MEDIAL MIGRATION PATTERN. In 10 to 35 per cent of patients with osteoarthritis of the hip, a pattern of medial migration of the femoral head is evident (Fig. 35–32). This pattern commonly is bilateral and symmetric in distribution and is more frequent in women. Some authors regard this type of osteoarthritis as idiopathic, although others describe underlying deviations from normal acetabular anatomy. The appearance of this pattern of osteoarthritis in other disorders such as Paget's disease suggests that changes in the structure of the proximal femur (varus deformity) can produce osteoarthritis with medial migration of the femoral head.

Radiographic analysis indicates medial displacement of the femoral head with narrowing of the medial joint space and associated widening of the lateral joint space. Mild to moderate protrusio acetabuli deformities may become evident with increased bone density of the central and the inferior aspects of the acetabulum. Osteophyte formation occurs on both the acetabulum and the femur. Buttressing may be detected in the femoral neck, particularly medially. With computed tomography, an asymmetric placement of the femoral head in the anteroposterior plane may be evident (Fig. 35–33).

AXIAL MIGRATION PATTERN. Axial migration of the femoral head due to diffuse or concentric loss of joint space is very infrequent. When radiographs reveal an articular disease resembling a degenerative type associated with symmetric loss of joint space, other primary diagnoses must be considered (see subsequent discussion) prior to attributing the abnormalities to osteoarthritis.

OTHER RADIOGRAPHIC AND PATHOLOGIC CHARACTERISTICS. It is apparent from the previous description that although the pattern of movement of the femoral head with respect to the acetabulum may be variable in osteoarthritis, influencing the distribution of the morphologic changes, the basic radiographic and pathologic abnormalities are similar. These include joint space narrowing, osteophytosis, buttressing, sclerosis, and cyst formation. The cysts can be single or multiple, of varying size, and located on either the femoral or the acetabular side of the joint, or on both sides. Large cystic lesions in the acetabulum occasionally are encountered (Fig. 35–34).

Progressive and asymmetric joint space loss is a fundamental radiographic and pathologic characteristic of this disease. Recovery or restoration of the joint space has been described during the course of osteoarthritis, however. Generally, this

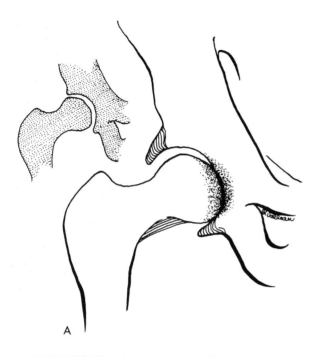

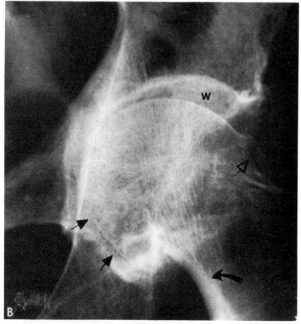

Figure 35–32. Osteoarthritis of the hip: Medial migration pattern.
A As the femoral head migrates medially, joint space narrowing and sclerosis of the inferomedial aspect of the articular surface result, and the superior joint space widens. **B** Medial joint space loss (solid arrows) and a widened lateral joint space (W) have resulted from this pattern of migration. A lateral femoral osteophyte (open arrow) and medial femoral neck buttressing (curved arrow) are evident. Mild protrusion deformity is seen. (From Resnick D: Patterns of femoral head migration in osteoarthritis of the hip. AJR 124:62, 1975. Copyright 1975, American Roentgen Ray Society. Used with permission.)

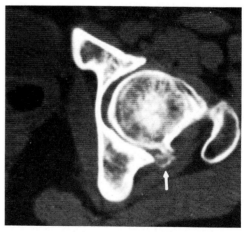

Figure 35–33. Osteoarthritis of the hip: Medial migration pattern. A transaxial section obtained with computed tomography shows that the femoral head is closely applied to the posterior surface of the acetabulum and possesses a prominent posterior osteophyte (arrow). On frontal radiographs (not shown), a typical medial migration pattern was evident. (Courtesy of D. Haselwood, M.D., Sacramento, California.)

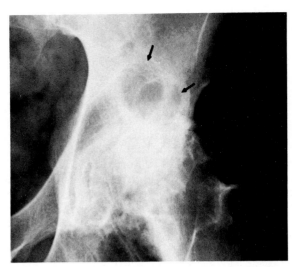

Figure 35–34. Osteoarthritis of the hip: Cysts. The frontal radiograph documents considerable degenerative abnormalities, including a large acetabular cyst (arrows).

phenomenon has been noted after treatment with osteotomy. When present, the restored joint space is characterized histologically by fibrous tissue and fibrocartilage on the osseous surfaces.

Although synovial membrane alterations generally are mild, considerable osseous and cartilaginous debris may become embedded in the synovium of osteoarthritic hips, particularly in the recesses associated with the capsular reflection on the femoral neck. Hypertrophied synovium containing detritus may become prominent in these areas.

Other Diagnostic Methods

Arthrography has occasionally been advocated in the preoperative evaluation of osteoarthritis of the hip. Although this technique does outline the location and extent of cartilaginous loss, similar abnormalities can be detected on routine radiography, obviating the need for arthrography in most patients with degenerative hip disease.

Arteriography has been used to elucidate the vascular abnormalities of osteoarthritis of the hip. Prominent vascularity is manifested as increase in number, length, and width of periarticular and intraosseous vessels.

Intraosseous venography may be used to identify a deviation in the normal pattern of venous drainage from the femoral head and neck that has been observed in osteoarthritis. Initially increased flow occurs via the femoral shaft; subsequently pooling of injected contrast material with decreased or absent venous outflow is seen. It has been suggested that venous congestion and obstruction, which may themselves lead to pain, are caused by capsular fibrosis, muscle spasm, muscle contraction, and cyst formation.

Radionuclide examination with bone-seeking agents demonstrates increased uptake in periarticular osseous tissue. The scintigraphic pattern may outline the presence and extent of disease prior to the appearance of radiographic abnormalities, although the findings are not specific.

Computed tomography is not required in the diagnostic evaluation of most patients with osteoarthritis of the hip. Intraarticular osteocartilaginous debris is identified with computed tomography or arthrotomography, and computed to-

mography can also delineate the degree of anteversion of the femoral neck, a factor that reportedly influences the pattern of osteoarthritis. Similarly, *magnetic resonance imaging* is rarely used in the evaluation of the osteoarthritic hip.

Differential Diagnosis

PATTERNS OF MIGRATION (TABLE 35–8). Osteoarthritis is associated with superior or, less commonly, medial migration of the femoral head with respect to the acetabulum. Axial migration is distinctly unusual. Thus, the appearance of diffuse joint space loss with axial migration usually indicates another disease process, such as rheumatoid arthritis, infection, or cartilage atrophy owing to disuse or immobilization. In all of these diseases, osteophytosis and sclerosis usually are not prominent. If axial migration of the femoral head is accompanied by sclerosis and osteophyte formation, additional diseases should be considered before the diagnosis of osteoarthritis (primary) is accepted; these diseases include ankylosing spondylitis, calcium pyrophosphate dihydrate crystal deposition disease, and alkaptonuria. Furthermore, secondary degenerative joint disease superimposed on another primary process can lead to symmetric loss of joint space, osteophytosis, and eburnation; these processes include trauma with acetabular fracture, synovial disorders such as rheumatoid arthritis, Paget's disease, chondrolysis, epiphyseal dysplasia, and osteonecrosis.

Superior migration of the femoral head in association with sclerosis, cysts, and osteophytes usually ensures the diagnosis of osteoarthritis. Medial migration of the femoral head is observed in "primary" osteoarthritis but also in degenerative joint disease superimposed on other disorders, such as Paget's disease and osteomalacia (Fig. 35–35).

SCLEROSIS, CYST FORMATION, AND OSTEO-PHYTOSIS. Although these radiographic and pathologic findings are most typical of osteoarthritis, they can be observed in other disease processes. Calcium pyrophosphate dihydrate crystal deposition disease can be accompanied by significant sclerosis and prominent cyst formation. Osteophytes may or may not be evident. In this disease, fragmentation and collapse of the femoral head are more prominent than in osteoarthritis. Neuroarthropathy leads to severe bone eburnation; however, the findings of considerable collapse and fragmentation with or without exuberant osteophytes provide helpful clues to its proper diagnosis. The hip disease of ankylosing spondylitis is

Table 35–8. DIFFERENTIAL DIAGNOSIS OF PATTERNS OF FEMORAL HEAD MIGRATION*

	Superior	Axial	Medial
Osteoarthritis	+	Rare	+
Rheumatoid arthritis	Rare	+	
Ankylosing spondylitis	Rare	+	
Calcium pyrophosphate dihydrate crystal deposition disease	Rare	+	
Chondrolysis		+	
Paget's disease with secondary joint degeneration	+	+	+
Osteonecrosis with secondary cartilage loss	+	+	

* + = Common.

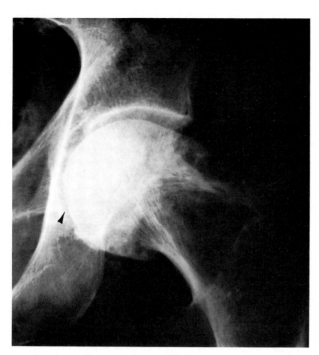

Figure 35–35. Paget's disease with medial migration of the femoral head. Observe the coarse trabecular pattern within the femoral head and femoral neck and narrowing of the medial joint space (arrowhead). The axial and lateral spaces appear relatively normal.

associated with the presence of a characteristic lateral femoral osteophyte, which subsequently extends across the femoral head–femoral neck junction; symmetric loss of joint space is typical of this disease. Osteonecrosis is accompanied by prominent cysts and sclerosis of the femoral head but is usually associated with maintenance of joint space until late in the course of the disease. Acromegaly leads to large osteophytes, but the interosseous space is usually preserved or even widened until secondary cartilage degeneration supervenes. Alkaptonuria and hemophilia can produce joint space narrowing, sclerosis, cysts, and osteophytes, but clinical findings usually allow identification of these disorders.

BUTTRESSING. Thickening of bone along the femoral neck, particularly medially, is characteristic of osteoarthritis. It can be observed in other articular disorders leading to altered stress at the hip joint, however, such as osteonecrosis.

ACETABULAR PROTRUSION. Acetabular protrusion in osteoarthritis is mild and most typically associated with medial migration of the femoral head. Moderate to severe acetabular protrusion, which is accompanied by symmetric loss of articular space (axial migration), can be observed in a variety of disorders, such as rheumatoid arthritis, ankylosing spondylitis, other processes such as Paget's disease, and infection. It may also be apparent as a familial disorder or after acetabular destruction related to neoplasm, irradiation, or trauma.

Knee

There are many factors that contribute to osteoarthritis in the knee. Previous surgery or trauma, angular deformity, osteonecrosis, osteochondritis dissecans, and obesity are but a few of the cited contributing events. All of these factors lead to an increased stress or force per unit area in the knee. In normal circumstances, with the patient standing, the line of weight-bearing passes from the center of the femoral head through the centers of both the knee and the ankle. In the presence of genu varus, the weight-bearing forces pass through the medial side of the joint, and with genu valgus, these forces pass through the lateral side of the knee. Therefore, any condition leading to angular deformity will result in a shift of stress to one compartment of the joint and can predispose to the development of osteoarthritis. Incongruity of articular surfaces, which may result from a fracture, osteochondritis dissecans, or ischemic necrosis, is a second factor leading to increased stress in one or more segments of the joint. A flexion deformity of the knee diminishes the surface area of the articulation, resulting in exaggerated stress as the load is supported by a smaller surface area.

The role of meniscal abnormality or removal in the appearance and progression of osteoarthritis of the knee has received a great deal of emphasis. In view of the important responsibility of the menisci in cushioning forces at the knee joint, it would appear that meniscal changes might lead to degeneration of articular cartilage. Clinical results, however, have been inconclusive, leading to conflicting opinions regarding the advisability and timing of surgery to remove damaged or torn menisci. In addition, there is no uniform agreement regarding the possible effect of meniscal removal on the adjacent articular cartilage.

The relationship of osteoarthritis of the knee to spontaneous osteonecrosis of the femoral condyle has also received emphasis (see Chapter 70). This condition, which appears in middle-aged and elderly persons, leads to collapse of the weight-bearing articular surface of the distal femoral condyles, particularly medially. Ultimately, patients with spontaneous osteonecrosis may develop secondary degeneration of the overlying articular cartilage.

Osteoarthritis of the knee may also be related to abnormality of adjacent joints (hip, ankle), unequal leg length, and weakening or paralysis of the contralateral extremity.

General Clinical Abnormalities

Pain is usually the presenting symptom of osteoarthritis of the knee. This symptom is aggravated by walking or exercise. Stiffness, tenderness, swelling, and warmth may also be recorded. Synovitis with its symptoms and signs is generally less striking in osteoarthritis than in rheumatoid arthritis. Angular deformity (usually varus), instability, and soft tissue atrophy are late manifestations of the disease.

Radiographic-Pathologic Correlation

COMPARTMENTAL DISTRIBUTION. It is useful to regard the joint as consisting of three compartments or spaces: the medial femorotibial, the lateral femorotibial, and the patellofemoral compartments (Fig. 35–36). Radiographic abnormalities usually predominate in one or two of the three compartments, although pathologic aberrations are evident in all three areas. Typical histologic changes include cartilage fibrillation and denudation of the osseous surfaces, eburnation, subchondral cystic lesions, and osteophytosis.

The ability of the radiograph to detect the pathologic abnormalities depends on the method of examination. Routine

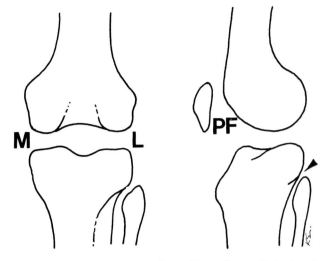

Figure 35–36. Compartmental analysis of knee disease. Evaluation of the medial femorotibial (M), lateral femorotibial (L), and patellofemoral (PF) compartments should be accomplished on all knee radiographs. A fourth area, the proximal tibiofibular joint, may also be affected (arrowhead).

techniques (which include frontal and lateral radiographs) are limited in their sensitivity to delineate early alterations, although some degree of joint space narrowing, sclerosis, cysts, and osteophytes are usually detected in the more involved weight-bearing compartment (medial or lateral femorotibial compartment). "Tunnel" projections obtained during knee flexion may occasionally reveal cartilaginous and osseous lesions that are not evident on the routine films. Films obtained during stress or weight-bearing should be used to supplement the radiographic examination (Fig. 35–37). This latter technique provides a better assessment of cartilage loss as the joint space collapses under the body weight. It also allows more accurate delineation of subluxation of the femur and tibia and of varus or valgus angulation. Even with the addition of the weight-bearing radiograph to the routine examination, the degree of abnormality in the less involved femorotibial compartment is difficult to determine, and it may be better judged with arthrography or radionuclide techniques (see discussion later in this chapter). Patellofemoral compartmental analysis requires special radiographic projections, including tangential and oblique views.

FEMOROTIBIAL COMPARTMENTS. Bilateral (left and right sides) or unilateral alterations may be evident. Radiographic findings are usually more prominent on the medial aspect of the joint (Fig. 35–38). Unicompartmental

Figure 35–37. Osteoarthritis of the knee: Usefulness of standing view. A The non–weight-bearing anteroposterior radiograph reveals irregularity and sclerosis of the articular surfaces. B With weight-bearing, collapse of the medial femorotibial compartment and varus angulation are apparent.

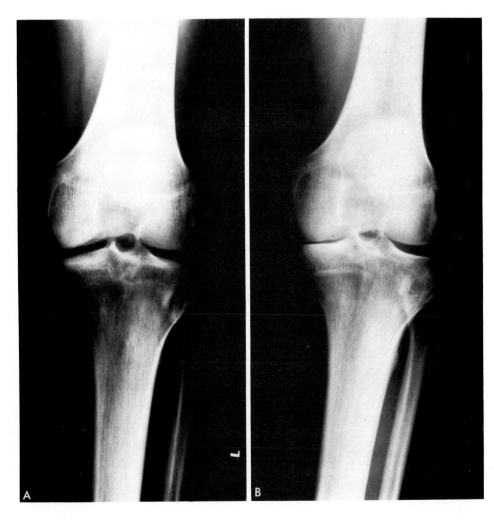

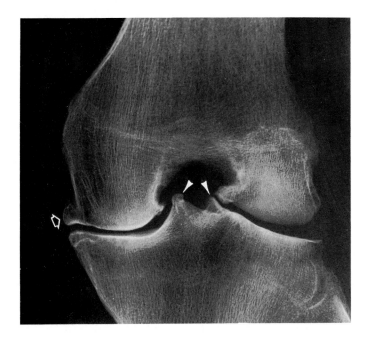

Figure 35–38. Osteoarthritis of the knee: Femorotibial compartmental abnormalities. A radiograph of a coronal section of a cadaveric bone indicates changes of osteoarthritis more prominent in the medial femorotibial compartment. Findings include joint space narrowing related to cartilage erosion, subchondral bone sclerosis, osteophytosis (open arrow), and sharpening of the tibial spines (arrowheads).

(medial or less frequently lateral femorotibial compartment) or bicompartmental (medial femorotibial and patellofemoral compartments or, not as commonly, lateral femorotibial and patellofemoral compartments) involvement is more typical than tricompartmental involvement (medial femorotibial, lateral femorotibial, and patellofemoral compartments) in patients with osteoarthritis. This compartmental distribution provides an important clue to accurate diagnosis. The discovery of alterations confined to or predominating in the medial

femorotibial compartment is most consistent with osteoarthritis. Similar abnormalities in the lateral femorotibial compartment are compatible with this disease, but this pattern requires that rheumatoid arthritis and calcium pyrophosphate dihydrate crystal deposition disease be given careful consideration as alternative diagnoses. Symmetric changes in both the medial and the lateral femorotibial compartments generally indicate a disorder other than osteoarthritis.

Joint space narrowing varies from mild to severe (Fig. 35–

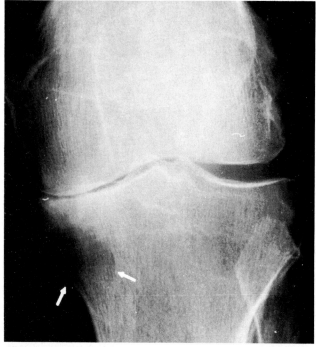

Figure 35–39. Osteoarthritis of the knee: Femorotibial compartmental abnormalities. In addition to obliteration of the medial femorotibial compartmental space, observe an unusually large cyst of the proximal tibia (arrows) in association with bone eburnation.

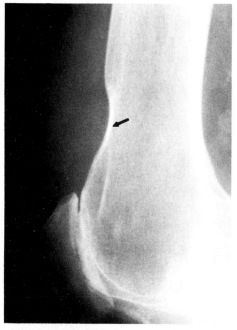

Figure 35–40. Osteoarthritis of the knee: Patellofemoral compartmental abnormalities—anterior femoral scalloping. A lateral radiograph of the knee indicates extensive narrowing of the patellofemoral space with eburnation of both patella and femur. Note the scalloped defect on the anterior aspect of the distal femur (arrow) resulting from mechanical attrition from contact with the diseased patella.

39). Sclerosis of subchondral bone is more frequent in the proximal portion of the tibia. Subchondral cysts are less frequent in the knee than in the hip. In the knee, they are usually apparent in the proximal portion of the tibia, are small in size, and are associated with joint space loss and eburnation. Osteophytes predominate at the margins of the articulation on both femur and tibia. Occasionally, intraarticular surface irregularity as well as sharpening of the tibial spines is noted (Fig. 35–38).

Additional radiographic abnormalities of the femorotibial compartments in osteoarthritis include vacuum phenomena within the articular space or within a diseased meniscus and meniscal calcification.

PATELLOFEMORAL COMPARTMENT. The patellofemoral compartment frequently is affected in osteoarthritis. Detection of abnormalities in this area requires specialized techniques, the most important of which is examination in axial projections. On radiographs, patellofemoral compartmental alterations are usually combined with abnormalities of the femorotibial compartments. Most typically, the medial femorotibial compartment is altered, although occasionally both lateral femorotibial and patellofemoral compartmental changes occur together. Although abnormalities isolated to the patellofemoral area may rarely be observed in osteoarthri-

tis, the radiographic detection of such isolated alterations should lead to a search for another disease process, such as calcium pyrophosphate dihydrate crystal deposition disease or hyperparathyroidism.

Radiographic features of patellofemoral osteoarthritis include joint space narrowing, sclerosis, and osteophytes, particularly on the patellar side of the space. Loss of articular space can be difficult to detect on lateral views alone but is readily apparent on axial radiographs. Osteophytes at the superior and inferior limits of the posterior aspect of the patella may become extremely large. Associated scalloped defects of the anterior cortex of the femur may become prominent (Fig. 35–40). This finding is usually accompanied by severe narrowing of the patellofemoral space. It appears to arise from pressure erosion of the femoral cortex, generally by the adjacent patella; the femoral defect is located at the level that the patella assumes in full extension of the knee.

An additional degenerative phenomenon occurs on the anterior surface of the patella and consists of bone proliferation at the site of osseous attachment of the quadriceps apparatus. This is an enthesopathic alteration probably related to abnormal stress on the ligamentous connection to the bone (Fig. 35–41). It produces hyperostosis of the anterior patellar surface, termed the "tooth" sign.

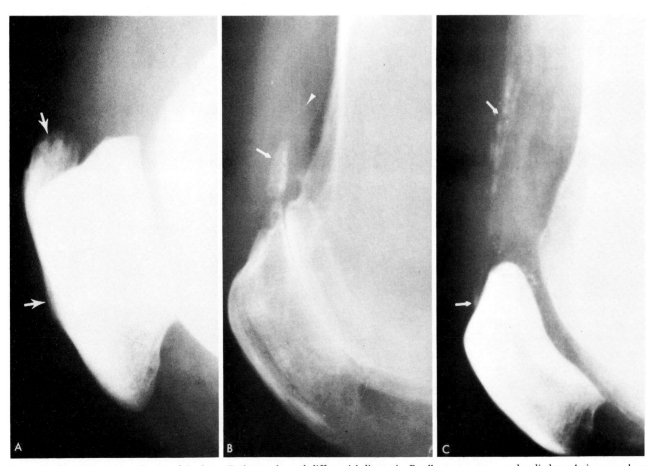

Figure 35–41. Degenerative disease of the knee: Enthesopathy and differential diagnosis. Patellar excrescences and radiodense lesions may have several causes. A Enthesopathy. Typical osseous excrescences are developing at the quadriceps attachment to the anterior surface of the patella (arrows). This is not a manifestation of osteoarthritis. **B Osteoarthritis.** Osteophytes are evident (arrow) at the superior articular surface of the patella. Note patellofemoral compartmental narrowing and an effusion (arrowhead). **C Calcific tendinitis.** Linear radiodense areas (arrows) in the tendon are related to calcific tendinitis. Calcium hydroxyapatite or calcium pyrophosphate dihydrate crystal deposition can create this appearance.

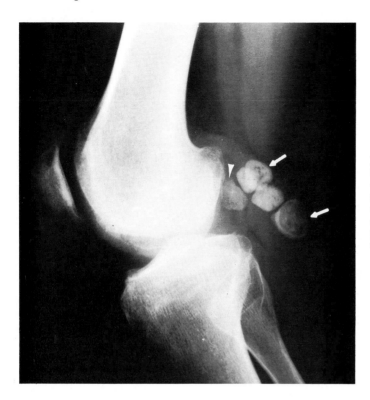

Figure 35–42. Osteoarthritis of the knee: Intraarticular and intrabursal osseous bodies. Numerous radiodense lesions are grouped together (arrows) posterior to the knee joint. This is the typical appearance of osteocartilaginous bodies within a synovial (popliteal) cyst. The presence of one of the radiodense lesions (arrowhead) within the joint itself and osteoarthritis of the patellofemoral articulation probably indicate that the bodies arose from a degenerative knee joint and passed into the synovial cyst.

ANGULATION AND SUBLUXATION. Angulation and subluxation at the knee joint are best determined on a film exposed with the patient standing on the involved leg. Varus angulation is more frequent than valgus angulation. The contralateral femorotibial compartment widens as the ipsilateral (on the concave side of the deformity) femorotibial compartment narrows. Translation or subluxation of the tibia on the femur laterally with varus angulation and medially with valgus angulation is typical.

SYNOVITIS, SYNOVIAL CYST FORMATION, AND INTRAARTICULAR OSTEOCARTILAGINOUS BODIES. Joint effusions are generally small in osteoarthritis of the knee. Synovial cysts are unusual and, when present, generally are small in size.

Cartilaginous and osseous debris arises from the disintegrating articular surfaces of the femur, the tibia, and the patella in osteoarthritis of the knee. Such debris may exist as loose bodies or "joint mice" prior to its incorporation into the synovial membrane. On radiographs, the osseous radiodense lesions must be distinguished from prominent tibial spurs, central osteophytes, and normal sesamoid bones (Fig. 35–42). Specialized techniques, including arthrography and conventional or computed tomography, occasionally are required in the identification and the characterization of intraarticular osteocartilaginous bodies in the knee.

SESAMOID INVOLVEMENT. In osteoarthritis of the knee, cartilaginous fibrillation and erosion and osseous proliferation can be observed in the fabella. On radiographs, the anterior surface of the fabella may reveal flattening and sclerosis. The peroneal nerve may be injured by the enlarged fabella.

Other Diagnostic Methods

The proper surgical treatment of osteoarthritis of the knee necessitates an accurate appraisal of the presence and severity of changes not only in the more involved femorotibial compartment but also in the less affected compartment. Although the most accurate appraisal of the compartmental distribution of the disease can be obtained by direct inspection during surgery or arthrotomy, less invasive diagnostic techniques are also required. Radiography performed during weight-bearing or stress provides information that is superior to that obtained by routine techniques, but it is by no means ideal. Initial results using ultrasonography in the evaluation of the thickness of the femoral cartilage have been promising, but the technique requires further investigation. Arthrography, scintigraphy, magnetic resonance imaging, and computed tomography represent additional methods that are available to evaluate compartmental distribution of osteoarthritis of the knee.

Chondromalacia Patellae and Other Patellar Syndromes

Chondromalacia patellae is a term applied to a syndrome of pain and crepitus over the anterior aspect of the knee, especially in flexion, which is observed in adolescents and young adults. Chondromalacia should be regarded as an alteration confined to cartilage in the posterior surface of the patella.

The patella consists of three facets: the lateral facet, the medial facet, and a more medially located odd facet (Fig. 35–43). Classically, the medial facet of the patella is the typical site of chondromalacia, particularly about the ridge that separates the medial and odd facets of the bone. The cartilaginous changes on the medial facet have been attributed to various etiologic factors, the most popular of which is excessive stress or trauma. The pathologic findings accompanying chondromalacia of the medial facet of the patella consist of swelling and edema of the cartilaginous surface. Cellular

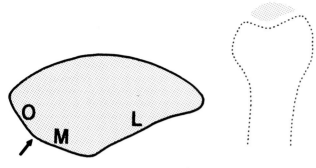

Figure 35–43. Chondromalacia patellae: Distribution of abnormalities. The lateral facet (L), medial facet (M), and odd facet (O) of the patella are indicated on this illustration of the tangential appearance of the bone. Classically chondromalacia is located on the osseous ridge (arrow) that separates the medial and odd facets. In the global pattern of chondromalacia, cartilaginous changes are apparent on the medial and lateral facets. A similar distribution is seen in osteoarthritis. Surface degeneration of cartilage on the odd facet has also been observed.

hyperactivity and disorganized collagen are also observed. Attempts at repair may be evidenced by the presence of immature fibrous tissue. The changes are indeed limited in severity and rarely progress to such an extent that the subchondral bone is exposed.

It is not surprising, therefore, that plain film radiography plays a small role in accurate diagnosis of classic varieties of chondromalacia. Although osteopenia occasionally is evident, other radiographic changes are lacking. The application of angular measurements to the analysis of the radiograph may reveal subtle alterations in patellar position. An association between chondromalacia and an elevated position of the patella (patella alta) has been observed, suggesting that an abnormally high position of the bone might lead to increased patellofem-

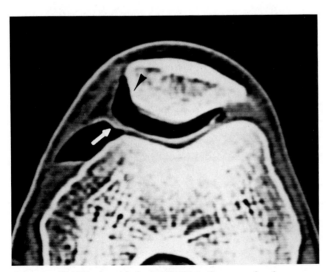

Figure 35–44. Chondromalacia patella: Use of computed arthrotomography. A transaxial image at the level of the midpatella, obtained with computed tomography after the introduction of a large amount of air into the joint, reveals cartilage thinning (arrowhead) in both the odd facet and the ridge that separates the odd and medial facets of the patella. Observe a synovial fold, the medial plica (arrow).

oral incongruence, with resulting damage to the articular cartilage. It is recognized also that an elevated patellar position can lead to recurrent dislocation of the patella or progressive patellofemoral osteoarthritis.

A more direct assessment of cartilage integrity is provided by computed tomography after the introduction of air alone or both air and iodinated contrast agent. Surface irregularities, cartilage thinning, imbibition of contrast material, and increased radiodensity of the chondral coat are the observed abnormalities (Fig. 35–44). Magnetic resonance imaging also can be used to evaluate the patellar cartilage.

The possible relationship of chondromalacia patellae and osteoarthritis of the patellofemoral compartment has not been defined.

Differential Diagnosis

COMPARTMENTAL ANALYSIS (TABLE 35–9). Osteoarthritis does not involve the three compartments of the knee to an equal extent. Most typically, radiographic changes predominate in one of the two femorotibial compartments, usually the medial one. These changes may be combined with significant abnormalities of the patellofemoral compartment. Symmetric medial and lateral femorotibial compartmental disease and isolated patellofemoral compartmental disease are unusual manifestations of osteoarthritis.

The medial and lateral femorotibial compartments are commonly affected to the same degree in rheumatoid arthritis (and other disorders characterized by significant synovial inflammation, such as ankylosing spondylitis and infection). Symmetric joint space loss is characteristic of these disorders. In rheumatoid arthritis (and related disorders), the patellofemoral compartment may also be altered, resulting in tricompartmental disease of the knee.

Isolated patellofemoral compartmental abnormalities are encountered in calcium pyrophosphate dihydrate crystal deposition disease and hyperparathyroidism. Rarely, such changes are noted in osteoarthritis, perhaps related to occupational or accidental trauma or to progressive changes of "chondromalacia patellae." When findings resembling those of degenerative joint disease are confined to the patellofemoral compartment, however, clinical evaluation to exclude other disorders must be accomplished prior to assigning the changes to osteoarthritis.

SCLEROSIS, CYST FORMATION, AND OSTEOPHYTOSIS. Although these changes are characteristic of osteoarthritis, they are also seen in other articular disorders. Crystal-induced arthropathies (gout or calcium pyrophosphate dihydrate crystal deposition disease) can be associated with sclerosis, cysts, and osteophytes; however, the presence of osseous erosions and the absence of articular space loss are typical of gout, whereas extreme sclerosis, large cystic lesions, and considerable fragmentation and deformity are observed in calcium pyrophosphate dihydrate crystal deposition disease. In osteonecrosis, the joint space is maintained, and depression and fragmentation of the osseous surface are recognized in association with sclerosis and cyst formation.

OTHER FINDINGS. Varus deformity is more frequent than valgus deformity in osteoarthritis of the knee, especially in men. The appearance of severe valgus angulation is not uncommon in calcium pyrophosphate dihydrate crystal deposition disease and in rheumatoid arthritis.

Table 35–9. COMPARTMENTAL ANALYSIS OF KNEE DISEASE

	Femorotibial Compartments	Patellofemoral Compartment
Osteoarthritis	medial > lateral	Commonly involved in conjunction with medial or lateral femorotibial disease
Rheumatoid arthritis	medial = lateral	Commonly involved in conjunction with medial and lateral femorotibial disease
Calcium pyrophosphate dihydrate crystal deposition disease	medial > lateral	Commonly involved alone or in conjunction with medial or lateral femorotibial disease
Hyperparathyroidism	*	Involved owing to subchondral resorption, crystal-induced arthropathies, or unknown mechanism

*Subchondral resorption can produce collapse of bone in the medial or lateral femorotibial compartment or both.

The detection of a large synovial cyst is uncommon in uncomplicated osteoarthritis. It is more frequent in rheumatoid arthritis and other inflammatory synovial disorders.

Ankle

In the absence of significant trauma, osteoarthritis of the ankle is infrequent. It may occur after fracture of the neighboring bones, particularly when the ankle mortise is disrupted (Fig. 35–45). Degeneration of the ankle also may develop whenever the talocalcaneal joints are altered, as may occur after congenital or surgical fusion. In addition to joint space narrowing and sclerosis, osteophytes may appear about the degenerating ankle joint. Capsular traction can produce a talar beak on the dorsal aspect of the bone, which, although reminiscent of the beak that accompanies tarsal coalition, is distinctive in appearance.

Tarsal Joints

Significant degenerative changes may develop at the first tarsometatarsal joint. In this location, joint space narrowing

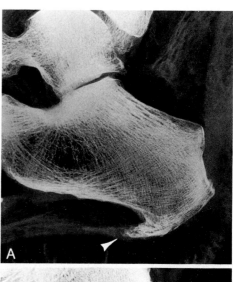

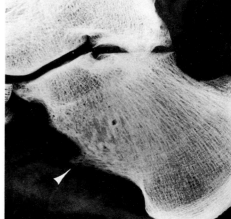

Figure 35–45. Osteoarthritis of the ankle. An anteroposterior radiograph delineates joint space narrowing, sclerosis, fragmentation, and osteophytosis. Note the tilting of the talus with respect to the tibia.

Figure 35–46. Degenerative enthesopathy: Calcaneus. Observe the well-defined osseous excrescences occurring at two typical sites on the plantar aspect of the bone. **A** Site of attachment of the plantar aponeurosis (arrowhead). **B** Site of attachment of the long plantar ligament (arrowhead).

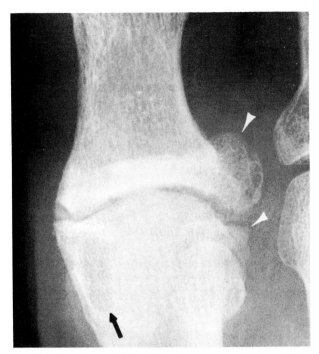

Figure 35–47. Osteoarthritis of the first metatarsophalangeal joint: Hallux rigidus. A frontal radiograph reveals considerable joint space narrowing, sclerosis, and osteophytosis (arrowheads) about the first metatarsophalangeal joint. Observe the flattening of the metatarsal head and a large metatarsal cyst (arrow).

and sclerosis owing to osteoarthritis simulate the findings of gouty arthritis. Alterations at additional tarsal locations may develop after trauma or, rarely, spontaneously. One such site is the talonavicular portion of the anterior talocalcaneonavicular joint. Small osteophytes arise along the dorsal aspect of apposing surfaces of the talus and navicular bones.

Persistent hindfoot pain after a calcaneal fracture is a potential complication of osteoarthritis in one or both subtalar joints. Plain films are commonly inadequate in delineating the degenerative abnormalities, whereas computed tomogra-

phy provides much greater information. Findings include narrowing of the joint space(s), irregularity and depression of the articular surfaces, bone sclerosis and cyst formation, and osteophytes.

Plantar and posterior calcaneal spurs are frequent radiologic findings that can be unassociated with clinical abnormalities. These excrescences develop at the osseous sites of attachment of the Achilles tendon, plantar aponeurosis, and long plantar ligament (Fig. 35–46). When well defined and sharply marginated, they usually represent no more than an incidental degenerative abnormality related to ligamentous or tendinous traction on bone. Alternatively, a poorly defined or fluffy plantar calcaneal bone outgrowth can be an important radiographic finding of ankylosing spondylitis, psoriasis, and Reiter's syndrome.

Metatarsophalangeal and Interphalangeal Joints

Osteoarthritis of the first metatarsophalangeal joint (hallux rigidus) is very common (Fig. 35–47). It may be detected in adolescents or young adults and lead to painful restriction of dorsiflexion of the great toe. The cause of hallux rigidus is unknown.

An additional common lesion of the first metatarsophalangeal joint is termed hallux valgus (Fig. 35–48). Although principally apparent in people who wear shoes, it does occasionally occur in the unshod. The early and essential intrinsic lesion of this condition may be stretching of the ligaments about the metatarsophalangeal joint that attach the medial sesamoid and basal phalanx to the metatarsal, with erosion of the ridge that separates the grooves for the sesamoids on the metatarsal head. Potential anatomic variations that contribute to the deformity include a rounded metatarsal head, a curved or oblique setting of the metatarsal-cuneiform joint, and a lateral facet on the basal lateral aspect of the first metatarsal. On radiographs, valgus angulation frequently is associated with pronation of the great toe and bone hypertrophy or osteophytosis, particularly on the medial aspect of the metatarsal head. The enlarged and irregular medial portion of the metatarsal may contain cystic lesions and thickened trabeculae, findings that can simulate those of gout. The first

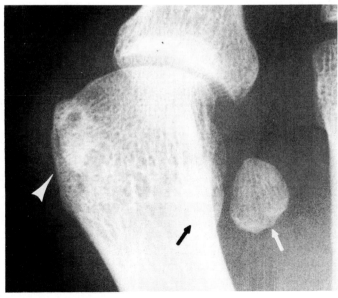

Figure 35–48. Hallux valgus. Abnormalities consist of soft tissue swelling, lateral displacement and rotation of the proximal phalanx and sesamoids (arrows), and bone hypertrophy (arrowhead) on the medial aspect of the metatarsal.

tarsometatarsal joint may be obliquely oriented (metatarsus varus) in patients with hallux valgus; it is not clear which abnormality (valgus alignment at the metatarsophalangeal joint or varus alignment at the tarsometatarsal joint) is the primary change. Changes in the other metatarsophalangeal joints may also become apparent, including subluxation or dislocation.

Osteoarthritis of interphalangeal joints of the toes may be detected as an incidental finding on the radiograph.

SPECIAL TYPES OF DEGENERATIVE JOINT DISEASE
Generalized Osteoarthritis

The concept of a generalized or polyarticular form of osteoarthritis is not universally accepted, despite numerous descriptions of patients with osteoarthritis in multiple locations, including the joints of the hands, wrists, spine, knees, and hips. When radiographs reveal evidence of degenerative changes in multiple sites, diagnoses other than generalized osteoarthritis must be considered. Multiple epiphyseal dysplasia, spondyloepiphyseal dysplasia, osteonecrosis, alkaptonuria, Paget's disease, acromegaly, occupation-induced articular disorders, calcium pyrophosphate dihydrate crystal deposition disease, gout, hemophilia, and inflammatory arthritides may all lead to similar changes at multiple articular locations. In some of these disorders (osteonecrosis, gout, hemophilia, inflammatory arthritides), secondary degenerative abnormalities owing to altered joint mechanics can obscure the more diagnostic radiographic findings, whereas in others (calcium pyrophosphate dihydrate crystal deposition disease, alkaptonuria), abnormalities resembling those of degenerative joint disease are part of the basic disease process.

Inflammatory (Erosive) Osteoarthritis

A peculiar form of interphalangeal osteoarthritis, characterized by acute inflammatory episodes with eventual ankylosis of some joints, has been described in middle-aged and elderly women. Although some reports have used the term *erosive osteoarthritis* to emphasize the juxtaarticular and intraarticular erosions that are evident on radiographic examination of these patients, *inflammatory osteoarthritis* is a preferable term, as patients with typical clinical findings of inflammatory osteoarthritis may not reveal erosive alterations on radiographs of the digits.

Clinical Abnormalities

The onset of the disease may be abrupt. Painful nodules of the distal interphalangeal and proximal interphalangeal joints of the fingers are associated with edema and redness of the overlying skin, and tenderness and restricted motion of joints. Morning stiffness may also develop.

The distribution of the disease is remarkably symmetric. Interphalangeal articulations are affected most commonly, although abnormalities of the metacarpophalangeal and carpometacarpal joints, the trapezioscaphoid area of the midcarpal joints, the knees, and the hips may become apparent. Laboratory analysis generally is unrewarding. Results of serologic tests for rheumatoid factor are nonreactive or, less commonly, positive in low titer dilutions.

The course of the disease is variable. In some patients, the inflammatory signs subside with conservative therapeutic measures after a period of months to years. In others, the inflammatory signs progress and the clinical manifestations resemble or become identical to those of rheumatoid arthritis (see discussion later in this chapter).

Radiologic Abnormalities

The radiologic changes are often characterized by a combination of bone proliferation and erosion. It must be emphasized, however, that proliferative changes may occur in the absence of any erosive abnormalities. Typically, osteophytosis resembles that in noninflammatory osteoarthritis, predominating in the distal and proximal interphalangeal joints. Joint space narrowing is common, with associated subchondral sclerosis.

In some involved joints, erosions may become prominent. They are particularly frequent in interphalangeal articulations (Fig. 35–49), although they may be observed in the first carpometacarpal joint or trapezioscaphoid space. The erosions commonly begin at the central portion of the joint in the form of sharply marginated, etched defects. This central location is characteristic, differing from the marginal location of erosions in rheumatoid arthritis and related disorders. Hence, the erosions in inflammatory osteoarthritis may be related to collapse of subchondral bone rather than to synovial inflammation.

Intraarticular bone ankylosis is also evident in many of the patients with inflammatory osteoarthritis. This finding is virtually confined to one or several interphalangeal joints.

In the wrist, joint space narrowing and sclerosis occur on the radial aspect between the trapezium and base of the first metacarpal and between the trapezium and scaphoid; rarely, erosions are seen in these locations. The findings are identical to those in noninflammatory osteoarthritis. Uncommonly, changes may become evident in the metatarsophalangeal and interphalangeal joints of the feet, the knees, the hips, and the apophyseal joints of the cervical spine.

Pathologic Abnormalities

Synovial biopsies have revealed tissue that may be mildly to severely inflamed, resembling findings in rheumatoid arthritis. In other cases, synovial, cartilaginous, and osseous changes are identical to those of noninflammatory osteoarthritis.

Relationship to Other Articular Disorders

RHEUMATOID ARTHRITIS. In approximately 10 to 15 per cent of cases of inflammatory osteoarthritis, superimposition of clinical, laboratory, and radiologic findings of rheumatoid arthritis may be seen. Typical rheumatoid-like deformities appear, and even rheumatoid nodules and positive serologic test results for rheumatoid arthritis become evident. Indeed, the radiographic findings in these cases are those of rheumatoid arthritis itself. The exact relationship of the two diseases is not certain, however.

OSTEOARTHRITIS. The relationship of inflammatory and noninflammatory osteoarthritis likewise is not clear. The distribution of affected joints in both diseases is almost identical. The major differences between the inflammatory and noninflammatory diseases are the clinical signs of joint inflammation and the radiographic findings of bone erosion and ankylosis in the former disorder. Inflammatory osteoarthritis may represent one extreme in the spectrum of degen-

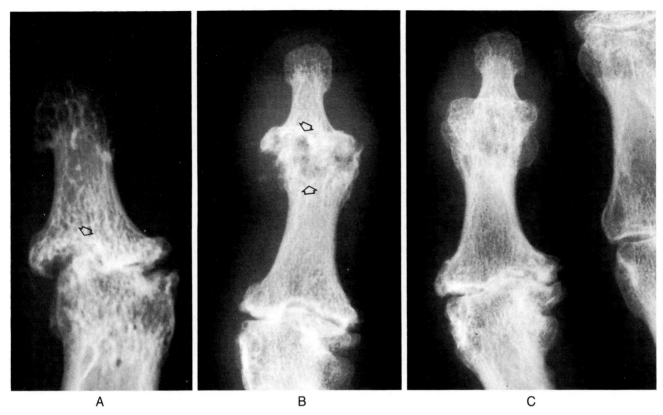

A   B   C

Figure 35–49. Inflammatory (erosive) osteoarthritis: Interphalangeal joint abnormalities. A Early abnormalities consist of "crumbling" of the central articular surface of the bone (open arrow). The other manifestations resemble noninflammatory osteoarthritis with osteophytosis and sclerosis. **B** In a more advanced case, disruption of the entire central aspect of the joint (open arrows) is typical. Note the changes in the proximal interphalangeal joint, which are identical to those of noninflammatory osteoarthritis. **C** The eventual result may be intraarticular osseous fusion, as seen in the distal interphalangeal joint.

erative joint disease, however, rather than being a separate entity.

CALCIUM HYDROXYAPATITE CRYSTAL DEPOSITION DISEASE. In recent years, abnormal accumulation of hydroxyapatite crystals in intraarticular locations has been emphasized. One site of involvement is the interphalangeal joints of the hand, where cloudlike radiodense lesions are delineated on radiographic examination. This pattern of calcification can occur in the absence of additional radiologic alterations, although, in some cases, it arises in a joint that is already the site of osteoarthritis. In these latter instances, the intimate relationship of interphalangeal joint calcification and bone erosion encourages speculation that the two findings share a common pathogenesis.

Differential Diagnosis

Inflammatory osteoarthritis is associated with proliferative and erosive abnormalities of interphalangeal joints. If proliferative changes predominate (such as osteophytosis and sclerosis), the resulting radiographic appearance is identical to that of noninflammatory osteoarthritis. In the presence of erosions or bone ankylosis, the differentiation of inflammatory from noninflammatory osteoarthritis is facilitated.

The erosions of inflammatory osteoarthritis frequently predominate in the central portion of the joint. This central localization differs from the marginal localization that is associated with rheumatoid arthritis, psoriasis, multicentric reticulohistiocytosis, and gout. The most difficult aspect of

the differential diagnosis is distinguishing inflammatory osteoarthritis and psoriatic arthritis. In addition to the central location of the erosions, the widespread and symmetric distribution that characterizes inflammatory osteoarthritis differs from the situation of psoriatic arthritis, in which marginal erosions and poorly defined bone proliferation may be distributed in an asymmetric, unilateral, or even ray-like pattern. The bone erosions accompanying inflammatory osteoarthritis also resemble those reported in a few cases of scleroderma.

Intraarticular bone ankylosis that accompanies inflammatory osteoarthritis may also be evident in psoriasis and, less commonly, in rheumatoid arthritis. Intraarticular osseous fusion is not regarded as a characteristic manifestation of noninflammatory osteoarthritis, gout, or multicentric reticulohistiocytosis.

In both inflammatory and noninflammatory osteoarthritis, medial and lateral subluxations at interphalangeal joints can produce a wavy contour in the involved digit. In rheumatoid arthritis, dorsal and volar subluxations are more typical.

FURTHER READINGS

Arnoldi CC, Linderholm H, Mussbichler H: Venous engorgement and intraosseous hypertension in osteoarthritis of the hip. J Bone Joint Surg [Br] 54:409, 1972.

Burke MJ, Fear EC, Wright V: Bone and joint changes in pneumatic drillers. Ann Rheum Dis 36:276, 1977.

Conway WF, Destouet JM, Gilula LA, Bellinghausen HW, Weeks PM: The carpal boss: An overview of radiographic evaluation. Radiology 156:29, 1985.

Crain DC: Interphalangeal osteoarthritis characterized by painful inflammatory episodes resulting in deformity of the proximal and distal articulations. JAMA 175:1049, 1961.

DePalma AF: Degenerative Changes in Sternoclavicular and Acromioclavicular Joints in Various Decades. Springfield, Ill, Charles C Thomas, 1957.

Ehrlich GE: Inflammatory osteoarthritis. II. The superimposition of rheumatoid arthritis. J Chronic Dis 25:635, 1972.

Feldman F, Johnston A: Intra-osseous ganglion. AJR 118:328, 1973.

Ficat RP, Hungerford DS: Disorders of the Patello-Femoral Joint. Baltimore, Williams & Wilkins, 1977.

Jaffe HL: Metabolic, Degenerative and Inflammatory Diseases of Bones and Joints. Philadelphia, Lea & Febiger, 1972.

Kellgren JH, Moore R: Generalized osteoarthritis and Heberden's nodes. Br Med J 1:181, 1952.

Mankin HJ: The reaction of articular cartilage to injury and osteoarthritis. Part 1. N Engl J Med 291:1285, 1974.

Mankin HJ: The reaction of articular cartilage to injury and osteoarthritis. Part 2. N Engl J Med 291:1335, 1974.

Martel W, Braunstein EM: The diagnostic value of buttressing of the femoral neck. Arthritis Rheum 21:161, 1978.

Martel W, Stuck KJ, Dworin AM, Hylland RG: Erosive osteoarthritis and psoriatic arthritis: A radiologic comparison in the hand, wrist, and foot. AJR 134:125, 1980.

Martel W, Snarr JW, Horn JR: The metacarpophalangeal joints in interphalangeal osteoarthritis. Radiology 108:1, 1973.

McCarty DJ, Halverson PB, Carrera GF, Brewer BJ, Kozin F: "Milwaukee shoulder"—association of microspheroids containing hydroxyapatite crystals, active collagenase, and neutral protease with rotator cuff defects. I. Clinical aspects. Arthritis Rheum 24:464, 1983.

Milgram JW: The development of loose bodies in human joints. Clin Orthop 124:292, 1977.

Neer CS: Anterior acromioplasty for the chronic impingement syndrome in the shoulder. J Bone Joint Surg [Am] 54:41, 1972.

Radin E: Chondromalacia of the patella. Bull Rheum Dis 34:1, 1984.

Resnick D: Patterns of migration of the femoral head in osteoarthritis of the hip. Roentgenographic-pathologic correlation and comparison with rheumatoid arthritis. AJR 124:62, 1975.

Resnick D, Niwayama G: Entheses and enthesopathy. Anatomical, pathological, and radiological correlation. Radiology 146:1, 1983.

Resnick D, Niwayama G, Coutts RD: Subchondral cysts (geodes) in arthritic disorders: Pathologic and radiographic appearance of the hip joint. AJR 128:799, 1977.

Resnick D, Niwayama G, Goergen TG: Comparison of radiographic abnormalities of the sacroiliac joint in degenerative disease and ankylosing spondylitis. AJR 128:189, 1977.

Rose CP, Cockshott WP: Anterior femoral erosion and patello-femoral osteoarthritis. J Can Assoc Radiol 33:32, 1982.

Sokoloff L: Kashin-Beck disease. Rheum Dis Clin North Am 13:101, 1987.

Thomas RH, Resnick D, Alazraki NP, Daniel D, Greenfield R: Compartmental evaluation of osteoarthritis of the knee. A comparative study of available diagnostic modalities. Radiology 116:585, 1975.

Trueta J: Studies of the Development and Decay of the Human Frame. Philadelphia, WB Saunders Co, 1968.

Watson HK, Ballet FL: The SLAC wrist: Scapholunate advanced collapse pattern of degenerative arthritis. J Hand Surg [Am] 9:358, 1984.

Table 36–2. DEGENERATIVE DISORDERS OF THE SPINE

	Intervertebral (Osteo)Chondrosis	Spondylosis Deformans	Osteoarthritis
Major site of abnormality	Nucleus pulposus	Anulus fibrosus	Apophyseal joints; costovertebral joints
Intervertebral disc	Moderate to severe decrease in height; vacuum phenomena	Normal or slight decrease in height	Normal
Vertebral body	Sclerosis of superior and inferior surfaces; cartilaginous nodes	Osteophytosis	Normal
Apophyseal and costovertebral joints	Normal	Normal	Joint space narrowing; sclerosis

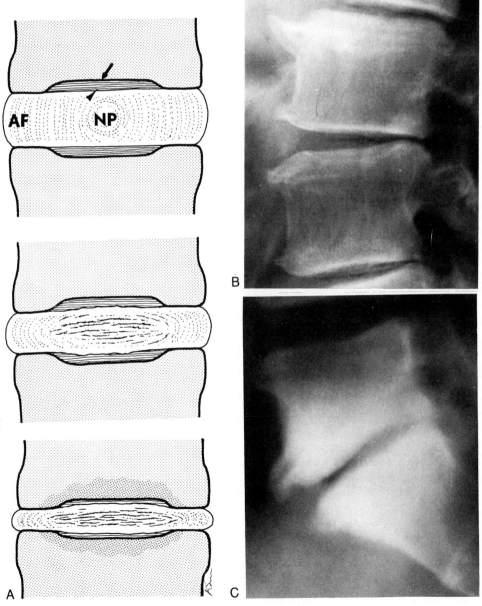

Figure 36–2. Intervertebral (osteo)-chondrosis. A Progressive stages of intervertebral (osteo)chondrosis. The normal situation is depicted in the top drawing. In the middle drawing, the early abnormalities of intervertebral (osteo)chondrosis consist of enlarging clefts within the nucleus pulposus, degeneration of the cartilaginous endplate, and loss of intervertebral disc height. In the bottom drawing, clefts appear in both the nucleus pulposus and anulus fibrosus, the degenerative changes of the cartilaginous endplate have progressed, and further disc space loss is apparent. Reactive sclerosis of adjacent vertebral bodies can be seen. AF, Anulus fibrosus; NP, nucleus pulposus. **B, C** Radiographic abnormalities. In two clinical examples, observe vacuum phenomena, disc space loss, reactive sclerosis, and osteophytosis. In C, conventional tomography indicates the severity of the bone eburnation that may accompany this process.

Table 36–3. INTERVERTEBRAL DISC SPACE LOSS AND ADJACENT SCLEROSIS

Disease	Mechanism	Radiographic Findings
Intervertebral (osteo)chondrosis	Degeneration of the nucleus pulposus and cartilaginous endplate Cartilaginous nodes	Disc space narrowing Vacuum phenomena Well-defined sclerotic vertebral margins
Infection	Osteomyelitis and "discitis"	Disc space narrowing Poorly defined sclerotic vertebral margins Soft tissue mass
Trauma	Discal injury and degeneration Cartilaginous nodes	Disc space narrowing Well-defined sclerotic vertebral margins Fracture Soft tissue mass
Neuroarthropathy	Loss of sensation and proprioception with repetitive trauma	Disc space narrowing Extensive sclerosis of vertebrae Osteophytosis Fragmentation Malalignment
Rheumatoid arthritis*	Apophyseal joint instability with recurrent discovertebral trauma or Inflammatory tissue extending from neighboring articulations	Disc space narrowing Poorly or well-defined sclerotic vertebral margins Subluxation Apophyseal joint abnormalities
Calcium pyrophosphate dihydrate crystal deposition disease	Crystal deposition in cartilaginous endplate and intervertebral disc with degeneration	Disc space narrowing Calcification Poorly or well-defined sclerotic vertebral margins Fragmentation Subluxation
Alkaptonuria	Crystal deposition in cartilaginous endplate and intervertebral disc with degeneration	Disc space narrowing Vacuum phenomena Well-defined sclerotic vertebral margins Calcification

*Usually involves cervical spine.

neuroarthropathy, and renal osteodystrophy. In ankylosing spondylitis, inflammatory changes at the discovertebral junction are associated with loss of disc height and erosions and eburnation of adjacent vertebral bodies.

The vacuum phenomenon deserves special emphasis. In intervertebral (osteo)chondrosis, these phenomena predominate in the nucleus pulposus of the disc. The vacuum phenomenon may appear centrally in the intervertebral disc or be located close to the subchondral bone plate. As the clefts enlarge, the radiolucent areas are observed in the anulus fibrosus as well.

Vacuum phenomena isolated in the outer portions of the anulus fibrosus have a different significance. In some instances, they correspond in position to anular defects seen in spondylosis deformans (see subsequent discussion). Similar gaseous collections have been noted in the discs of the cervical spine after trauma, presumably related to the defect created by avulsion of peripheral disc fibers from the vertebral rim and cartilaginous endplate.

Displacement of portions of a degenerating intervertebral disc into the spinal canal can be associated with gas formation in both the disc and the canal, a finding that is readily apparent with the use of computed tomography (Fig. 36–3). In some cases, the vacuum phenomenon is located within the displaced disc, whereas in others it may be present in the

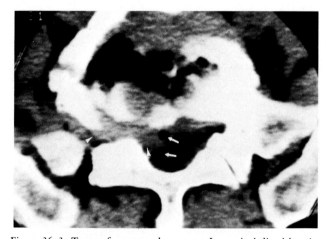

Figure 36–3. Types of vacuum phenomena: Intraspinal discal herniation. A transaxial image obtained with computed tomography at the level of the L5-S1 intervertebral disc shows an intradiscal vacuum phenomenon with two radiolucent collections (arrows) within the spinal canal. The anterior radiolucent focus is present within a large soft tissue mass (arrowheads), indicating discal herniation; the posterior collection may be present in the epidural space.

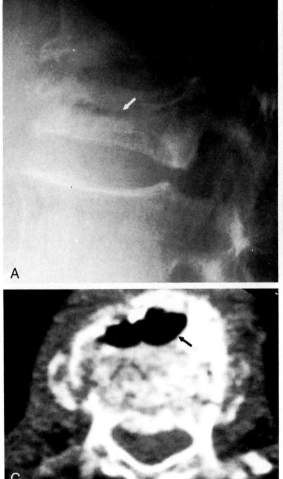

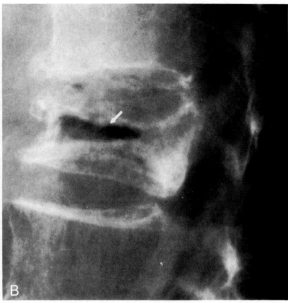

Figure 36–4. Types of vacuum phenomena: Vacuum vertebral body. **A** The initial lateral radiograph, obtained with the patient in a neutral position, reveals a subtle radiolucent collection (arrow) within a collapsed vertebral body. **B** With the patient's back extended, the intraosseous vacuum (arrow) is accentuated. **C** A computed tomographic transaxial image through the collapsed vertebra reveals the vacuum phenomenon (-485 Hounsfield units) in the fragmented vertebral body (arrow). The findings are virtually diagnostic of non-neoplastic, noninfectious vertebral collapse, presumably related to ischemic necrosis. (**A**, Courtesy of G. Greenway, M.D., Dallas, Texas; **B, C**, from Resnick D: Degenerative diseases of the vertebral column. Radiology 156:3, 1985. Used with permission.)

epidural space. In either situation, the observation of gas overlying the spinal canal adjacent to a degenerative intervertebral disc strongly supports the diagnosis of discal herniation.

Intraosseous disc displacement may accompany vertebral collapse, leading to vacuum phenomena within the displaced discal material in the bone. This situation should be differentiated from gaseous collections originating within the collapsed vertebral body itself (Fig. 36–4). Fracture and fragmentation of vertebrae with *intraosseous* vacuum phenomena have been described in cases of ischemic necrosis, particularly in patients on steroid medication. The crescent sign that is produced related to a radiolucent region at the site of a linear subchondral fracture is virtually pathognomonic of bone necrosis and is reminiscent of that which accompanies ischemic necrosis of the femoral or humeral head.

It is apparent from this discussion that vacuum phenomena are a frequent finding in the vertebral column and can be localized to the intervertebral disc or, less commonly, the spinal canal, apophyseal joints, soft tissues, and vertebral bodies (Table 36–4). In all locations, they limit the number of differential diagnostic possibilities. The presence of radiolucent collections within an intervertebral disc or vertebra militates against the diagnosis of infection. Although reports document the occurrence of radiolucent collections in cases of

vertebral osteomyelitis due to gas-forming organisms, such findings are distinctly unusual. Furthermore, when a radiolucent discal collection arises from infection, it represents gas formation by the organisms themselves, a mechanism quite different from the vacuum phenomena of disc degeneration. The finding of a vacuum vertebral body, which virtually excludes the possibility of infection, also makes highly unlikely the presence of tumor.

Table 36–4. TYPES OF SPINAL VACUUM PHENOMENA

Disease or Condition	Location of Vacuum Phenomenon
Intervertebral (osteo)chondrosis	Nucleus pulposus, anulus fibrosus
Spondylosis deformans	Anulus fibrosus
Cartilaginous node	Intervertebral disc within vertebral body
Intraspinal discal herniation	Intervertebral disc within spinal canal or epidural space
Osteoarthritis	Apophyseal joint
Ischemic necrosis	Vertebral body

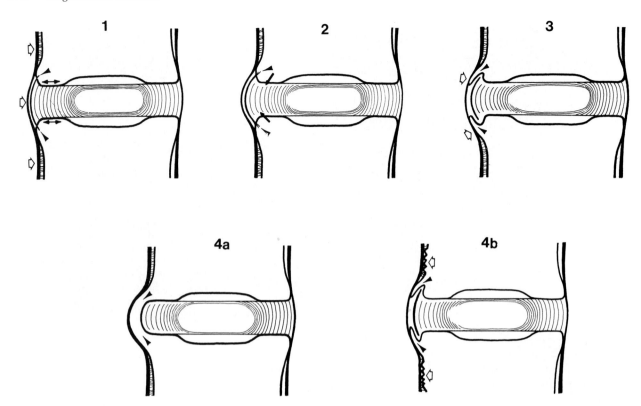

Figure 36–5. Spondylosis deformans: Modified concept of its pathogenesis. Progressive stages of spondylosis deformans. The normal situation is depicted in 1. The anulus fibrosus is attached to the vertebral rim by calcified cartilage (double-ended arrows) and to the anterior vertebral surface by Sharpey's fibers (arrowheads). The anterior longitudinal ligament (open arrows) is connected to the anterior vertebral surface. In 2, breakdown in the sites of attachment of anulus fibrosus to vertebral rim is evident (arrows), although Sharpey's fibers (arrowheads) are intact. Mild anterior discal displacement is seen. With progression of disease, as shown in 3, osteophytes (arrowheads) develop at the site of attachment of Sharpey's fibers to the anterior vertebral surface. The anterior longitudinal ligament (open arrows) is stretched by the displaced intervertebral disc. With still further progression, as in 4a, an osteophyte that bridges the intervertebral disc is seen (arrowheads). Alternatively, as in 4b, continued traction on the anterior longitudinal ligament may lead to proliferative enthesopathy, with the production of new bone (open arrows) at its site of attachment to the anterior vertebral surface, combined with more typical osteophytes (arrowheads). (3, From Resnick D: Degenerative diseases of the vertebral column. Radiology 156:3, 1985. Used with permission.)

SPONDYLOSIS DEFORMANS. The most obvious pathologic and radiographic degenerative disease of the spine is spondylosis deformans, which leads to vertebral outgrowths termed osteophytes. Spinal osteophytosis is extremely common. By the age of 50 years, approximately 60 per cent of women and 80 per cent of men demonstrate such excrescences. Bone outgrowths are more frequent in men than in women and in the older population. Any segment of the vertebral column may be affected; in the thoracic spine, right-sided outgrowths predominate, presumably related to the pulsations of the descending aorta on the left side that inhibit bone production.

It is Schmorl's concept of the pathogenesis of spondylosis deformans that, with some modification, is generally accepted today (Fig. 36–5). This concept emphasizes disruption of the peripheral fibers of the anulus fibrosus as the initiating factor in this disorder. Once disruption occurs in the attachment of portions of the anulus fibrosus to the vertebral rim, minor degrees of anterior and anterolateral discal displacement are possible and may lead to traction at the site of osseous attachment of the outermost fibers of the anulus fibrosus or short perivertebral ligaments to the vertebral surfaces. Osteophytes develop at this location, several millimeters from the discovertebral junction (Fig. 36–6).

The cause of degeneration of the peripheral fibers of the anulus fibrosus has not been determined. In some cases, trauma appears to be an important factor; after a single traumatic episode, localized osteophytes may develop in 1 to 3 months. The duration of time necessary for the development of osteophytes in cases of generalized spondylosis deformans is difficult to determine, however. In general, a period of 1 to 3 years is required before initial outgrowths enlarge to such an extent that they are recognizable on radiographic examination.

The type and severity of clinical manifestations related to spinal osteophytes are also difficult to delineate. These manifestations depend on the size and location of the outgrowths and on their relationship to adjacent soft tissue and neurologic structures. Dysphagia, stiffness, restricted motion, and even pain can probably be attributed to spinal osteophytes in some patients. Neurologic deficits produced by bone impingement on the spinal cord are unusual, a fact that can be explained by the relative infrequency of osteophyte formation on the posterior aspect of the vertebral body even in the presence of massive anterior bone outgrowths.

Spinal osteophytes accompanying spondylosis deformans must be differentiated from other bone outgrowths of the vertebral column (Fig. 36–7). Small triangular osteophytes

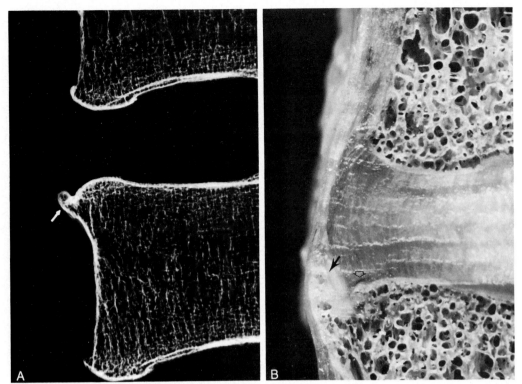

Figure 36–6. Spondylosis deformans. Radiographic-pathologic correlation. A, B A radiograph and photograph of a macerated sagittal section of a lumbar spine reveal the characteristics of an osteophyte (solid arrows). Note that it develops several millimeters from the vertebral rim and extends first in a horizontal direction and then in a vertical one. Observe minor disruption of the outer anular fibers (open arrow). (**A,** From Resnick D: Degenerative diseases of the vertebral column. Radiology 156:3, 1985. Used with permission.)

are encountered in intervertebral (osteo)chondrosis. In this condition, enlarging tears of the nucleus pulposus may extend into the anulus fibrosus and eventually lead to the disruption of anular attachments to bone. Diffuse idiopathic skeletal hyperostosis (DISH) is associated with extensive ossification along the anterior and lateral aspects of the vertebral column that resembles the features of severe spondylosis deformans. It is not clear if this condition represents a separate entity (see Chapter 37).

Ankylosing spondylitis is characterized by ossification within the outer portion of the anulus fibrosus, resulting in outgrowths that are termed syndesmophytes. These outgrowths are typically thin and vertically oriented as they extend from one vertebral body to the next. Ossific collections may eventually involve intervertebral discs and surrounding ligamentous and soft tissue structures, leading to an appearance that resembles that of spondylosis deformans. Attention to other sites, such as the sacroiliac, apophyseal, and costovertebral articulations, allows accurate differentiation of the two disorders. Bone outgrowths in psoriasis and Reiter's syndrome may resemble typical syndesmophytes of ankylosing spondylitis or appear as distinct paravertebral ossifications. In the latter circumstance, they are separated from the vertebral surface and, initially, possess a poorly defined or irregular contour.

Osseous excrescences of the spine accompanying neuroarthropathy and ochronosis do not resemble the outgrowths of spondylosis deformans. Spinal infection or trauma can produce outgrowths that are identical to those of spondylosis deformans; however, they are usually localized to one or two sites.

Fluorosis leads to osteophytosis identical to that in spondylosis deformans, but additional radiographic findings (such as increased osseous density and ligamentous ossification) allow accurate diagnosis.

UNCOVERTEBRAL (NEUROCENTRAL) JOINT ARTHROSIS. The five lowest cervical vertebral bodies (C3 to C7) contain bone ridges extending from each side, the uncinate or lunate processes. Between the superior process of the lower vertebral body and the upper vertebral body exists an articulation, termed the uncovertebral or neurocentral joint or the joint of Luschka. These articulations are difficult to classify according to type as they have anatomic features of both cartilaginous and synovial articulations.

With increasing degeneration of intervertebral disc tissue, there is progressive loss of height of the disc space, and the bone protuberances about the uncovertebral joints approach each other. With further disc deterioration, the articular processes are pressed firmly together, and the intervening articulation degenerates. Osteophytes produce hump-like or pointed outgrowths, which enlarge the articular surface. They project from the posterior edge of the vertebral body into the disc space and into the intervertebral foramina. At the latter site, they compromise the adjacent nerve roots; at the foramen costotransversarium, they may impinge on the vertebral artery.

The radiographic diagnosis of arthrosis in the joints of Luschka generally is not difficult. On frontal projections, the rounded uncinate processes and the narrowed joint space are readily apparent. Similar findings can be seen on oblique and lateral radiographs, although, in the lateral projection, a

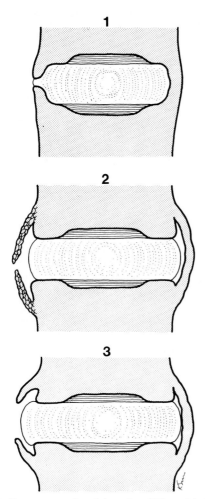

Figure 36–7. Bone outgrowths of the spine: Differential diagnosis. A variety of conditions can lead to development of outgrowths. Illustrated here are ankylosing spondylitis (1), psoriasis or Reiter's syndrome (2), and spondylosis deformans (3). In each drawing, the early appearance of the outgrowth is depicted on the left and the later appearance on the right. In ankylosing spondylitis, ossification occurs within the anulus fibrosus in the form of a syndesmophyte, which may eventually bridge the intervertebral disc space. Observe the vertical configuration of the syndesmophyte. In psoriasis and Reiter's syndrome, paravertebral ossification forms in the connective tissue at some distance from the spine. Initial irregular or poorly defined outgrowths may subsequently become better defined and merge with the vertebral bodies. In spondylosis deformans, the osteophytes begin as triangular outgrowths located several millimeters from the edge of the vertebral body. These, too, may eventually bridge the intervertebral disc space.

radiolucent line extending in an anteroposterior direction, overlying the vertebral body, is easily misinterpreted as a fracture. The lucent shadow is seen most commonly in the midcervical region and is related to the osteophytes that are developing about the uncinate processes and vertebral body (Fig. 36–8).

Synovial Joints

APOPHYSEAL JOINT OSTEOARTHRITIS (OSTEO- ARTHROSIS) (FIG. 36–9). The apophyseal joints of the vertebral column are a frequent site of degenerative joint disease. Although any level may be affected, changes com-

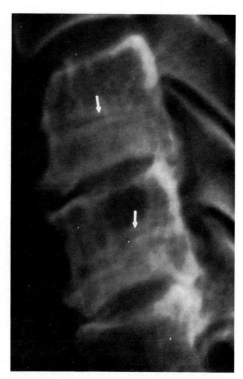

Figure 36–8. Uncovertebral (neurocentral) joint arthrosis. Simulation of a fracture. On a lateral radiograph of the cervical spine, radiolucent lines extending across the midportion of the vertebral bodies (arrows) are located immediately above osteophytes about the uncinate processes. (From Resnick D: Degenerative diseases of the vertebral column. Radiology 156:3, 1985. Used with permission.)

monly predominate in the middle and lower cervical spine, the upper thoracic and midthoracic spine, and the lower lumbar spine. The degenerative changes are induced by abnormal stress across the joint.

The pathologic and radiologic characteristics of osteoarthritis of the apophyseal joints are similar to those accompanying degenerative disease of other synovial joints. Fibrillation, erosion, and denudation of articular cartilage are accompanied by radiographically detectable joint space narrowing. Bone eburnation and osteophytes are frequent and may be associated with intraarticular osseous and cartilaginous bodies. Capsular laxity allows subluxation of one vertebral body on another, a process that has been termed degenerative or pseudospondylolisthesis (see discussion later in this chapter). Occasionally, especially at one or two levels in the cervical spine, intraarticular bone ankylosis can result, simulating the appearance of ankylosing spondylitis or juvenile chronic arthritis.

Computed tomography, with its cross-sectional display, is ideal in delineating osseous and soft tissue alterations of degenerative disease of the apophyseal joints. The relationship of bone proliferation to the central spinal canal, lateral recesses, and neural foramina can be defined. Adjacent soft tissue prominence and mass formation are observed occasionally, which, in some instances, are related to a synovial cyst. Such cysts are reported most frequently about the apophyseal joints between the fourth and fifth lumbar vertebrae, where they produce a well-defined cystic structure with calcification

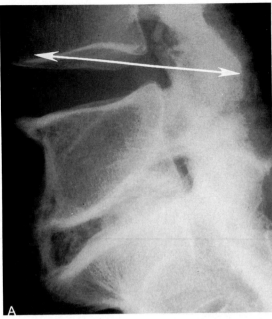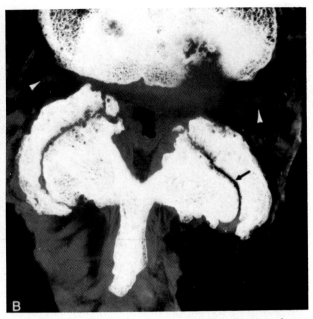

Figure 36–9. Apophyseal joint osteoarthritis: Lumbar spine. A A lateral radiograph of a cadaveric spine shows considerable alterations of osteoarthritis involving the apophyseal articulations between the fourth and fifth lumbar vertebrae and between the fifth lumbar vertebra and sacrum. Joint space narrowing, bone sclerosis, and osteophytes are apparent. **B** A radiograph of a transverse section at the approximate level indicated by the double-headed arrow in **A** reveals the osteoarthritic changes to better advantage. Findings include joint space narrowing, a vacuum phenomenon (arrow), and bone fragmentation in the articular processes. Although the neural foramina are narrowed, there is no impingement on the nerve roots (arrowheads), which have passed through the foramina at a higher level. (**B,** From Resnick D: Degenerative diseases of the vertebral column. Radiology 156:3, 1985. Used with permission.)

in the cyst wall. Rarely, accumulation of gas, derived from the adjacent joint, is noted within the cyst.

Prominent clinical symptoms and signs may accompany osteoarthritis of the apophyseal joints. The capsules and ligaments of these articulations are richly supplied with nerves, which may explain the common, although controversial, occurrence of pain in patients with degenerative joint disease at these sites. In addition, osteoarthritis in this articulation, alone or in combination with degeneration of the intervertebral disc, produces various types of spinal stenosis with resultant spinal cord and nerve root compression.

COSTOVERTEBRAL JOINT OSTEOARTHRITIS (OSTEOARTHROSIS). The costovertebral joints exist between the heads of the ribs and the vertebral bodies and between the necks and tubercles of the ribs and the transverse processes of the vertebrae (costotransverse joints). Degenerative changes predominate in the joints of the eleventh and twelfth ribs, although radiographic demonstration of these changes is difficult because of the adjacent osseous shadows of the vertebral bodies and ribs.

OSTEOARTHRITIS (OSTEOARTHROSIS) OF TRANSITIONAL LUMBOSACRAL ARTICULATIONS (FIG. 36–10). Congenital variations at the lumbosacral junction are frequent. Newly formed joints may exist between the enlarged transverse process of the involved vertebra and the wings of the sacrum (or rarely the ilium). These have a bilateral or unilateral distribution. The joints vary in type and appearance, although they may possess synovium. Osteoarthritis can result from abnormal stress and movement at the various joints. The relationship of back pain to congenital transitional vertebrae at the lumbosacral junction is not clear, and the

relationship between transitional lumbosacral joints and discal herniation is also debated.

Fibrous Joints and Entheses

LIGAMENTOUS DEGENERATION. Degenerative abnormalities may become evident in the anterior longitudinal ligament, posterior longitudinal ligament, ligamenta flava, interspinous, supraspinous, and intertransverse ligaments, ligamentum nuchae, and iliolumbar ligaments. As ligaments contain a rich supply of nerves, these processes are associated with pain and tenderness.

Calcification and ossification within the anterior longitudinal ligament are characteristic of diffuse idiopathic skeletal hyperostosis (DISH); ossification of the posterior longitudinal ligament (OPLL) and at the sites of attachment of the ligamenta flava are also well recognized (see Chapters 37 and 38).

Supraspinous and interspinous ligament abnormalities frequently coexist. Excessive lordosis or extensive disc space loss leads to close approximation and contact of spinous processes and to degeneration of intervening ligaments. The "kissing spines" develop reactive eburnation (Baastrup's disease) and may be associated with considerable pain. The diagnosis of Baastrup's disease requires lateral radiographs of the flexed and extended lumbar spine. Abnormal contact of apposing spinous processes, when combined with sclerosis in the superior and inferior portions of adjacent processes, is the characteristic radiologic abnormality. The spinous processes may appear enlarged (Fig. 36–11).

The ligamentum nuchae, the most posterior of the ligaments of the cervical spine, appears as a midline fibrous

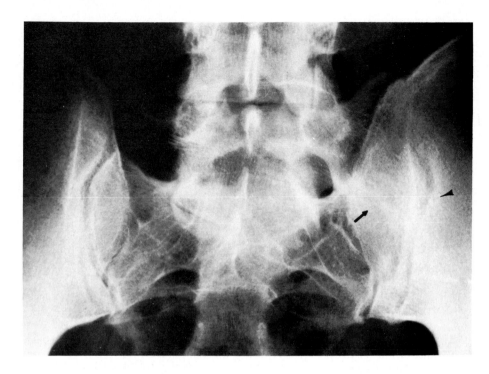

Figure 36–10. Osteoarthritis of transitional lumbosacral joint. A transitional vertebra at the lumbosacral junction possesses a unilateral joint (with osseous bridging) (arrow) with the sacrum and minor adjacent degenerative changes of the sacroiliac joint (arrowhead).

septum that is attached to the spinous processes and paracervical muscles. Ossification of varying degree within the ligamentum nuchae is common and has no clinical significance.

The iliolumbar ligament, extending from the tip of the transverse process of the lowest lumbar vertebra to the iliac crest, not infrequently calcifies or ossifies (Fig. 36–12). Such ossification is of unknown pathogenesis and significance. It is particularly common in patients with diffuse idiopathic skeletal hyperostosis and may also be associated with calcification in the sacrotuberous, sacrospinous (Fig. 36–12) and interosseous sacroiliac ligaments.

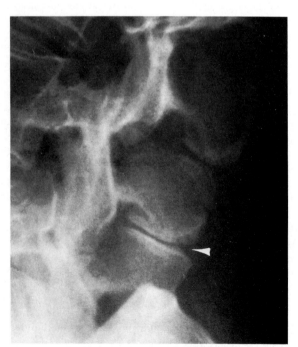

Figure 36–11. Baastrup's disease. Lateral radiograph of the lumbar spine in the extended position shows enlarged spinous processes that are flattened and sclerotic in their inferior and superior portions. Abnormal contact of spinous processes is evident (arrowhead).

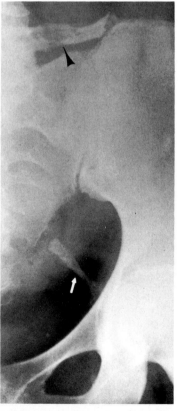

Figure 36–12. Ligamentous degeneration: Pelvic ligaments. Observe ossification in the sacrospinous (arrow) and iliolumbar (arrowhead) ligaments.

DEGENERATIVE DISEASES OF SPECIFIC SEGMENTS OF THE SPINE

Cervical Spine (Fig. 36–13)

Degenerative changes of the intervertebral discs of the cervical spine are common after the age of 40 years and affect more than 70 per cent of patients over the age of 70 years. Both men and women have a similar frequency of abnormality.

Multiple levels are usually altered, and changes predominate in the lower cervical spine. The site involved most commonly is the intervertebral disc at the C5-C6 level, followed by the C6-C7 level. Associated changes in the joints of Luschka show predilection for these same levels, particularly the C5-C6 intervertebral disc space. Osteoarthritis of the apophyseal articulations is also most common in the middle and lower cervical spine.

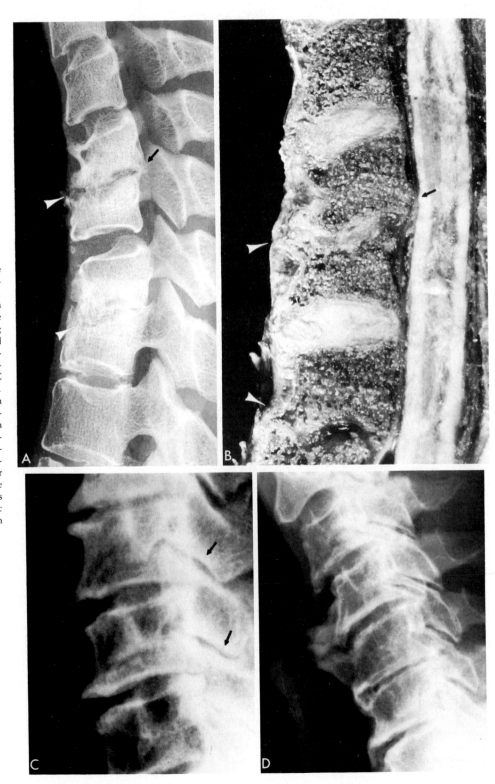

Figure 36–13. Degenerative disease of the cervical spine. A, B Intervertebral (osteo)chondrosis (after trauma). A radiograph and photograph of a sagittal section of the cervical spine reveal extensive disc space narrowing and reactive sclerosis at the C4-C5 and C6-C7 levels (arrowheads). Observe osteophytes, subluxation, and impingement on the spinal cord (arrows). C Osteoarthritis of apophyseal joints. Considerable joint space diminution and sclerosis can be seen in the apophyseal joints of the midcervical region (arrows) in association with intervertebral (osteo)chondrosis and spondylosis deformans. D Spondylosis deformans. Observe the prominent anterior osteophyte formation in the middle and lower cervical spine, which is associated, in this patient, with disc space narrowing and bone eburnation (intervertebral [osteo]chondrosis).

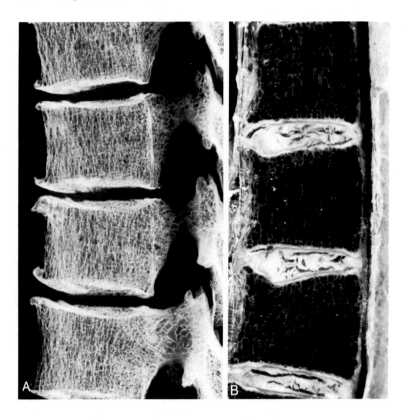

Figure 36–14. Degenerative disease of the thoracic spine: Intervertebral (osteo)chondrosis and spondylosis deformans. A radiograph (**A**) and photograph (**B**) of a sagittal section of the midthoracic region show fissures within both the nucleus pulposus and the anulus fibrosus associated with narrowing of the intervertebral disc and vertebral osteophytes.

Thoracic Spine (Fig. 36–14)

Spondylosis deformans predominates in the middle and lower thoracic region, whereas intervertebral (osteo)chondrosis has predilection for the midthoracic area. Disc protrusions into the spinal canal are also encountered in the thoracic spine, although their rate of occurrence is far less than that of lumbar disc protrusions. Obviously, costovertebral osteoarthritis is confined to the thoracic region.

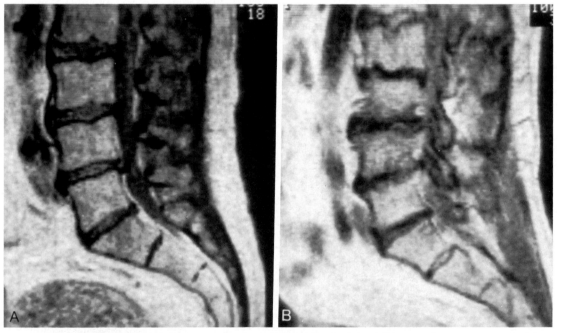

Figure 36–15. Degenerative disease of the lumbar spine: Intervertebral (osteo)chondrosis. **A** With magnetic resonance, a sagittal image reveals a decrease in signal intensity in all of the intervertebral discs, associated with loss of discal height and mild anterior and posterior bulging of discal material, particularly at the L4-L5 level. (TR, 1.5 s; TE, 28 ms.) **B** In a different patient, more severe abnormalities are apparent on a sagittal view with magnetic resonance imaging. The loss of signal intensity at all discal levels is seen. The intervertebral discs are narrowed. (TR, 1.5 s; TE, 28 ms.) (Courtesy of M. Solomon, M.D., San Jose, California.)

Lumbar Spine (Fig. 36–15)

Degenerative changes in the lumbar spine are frequent. These changes predominate in the lower lumbar region, particularly between the fourth lumbar and first sacral segments. Although it is generally assumed that degenerative processes of the lumbar spine may be associated with back symptoms and signs, the results of numerous investigations have been conflicting, and the relationship between lumbar spine degeneration and clinical manifestations remains unclear.

COMPLICATIONS OF DEGENERATIVE DISEASES OF THE SPINE

Alignment Abnormalities

SEGMENTAL INSTABILITY. Assessment of the degree and pattern of motion in the lumbar spine is possible using appropriate radiographs, although the task is made difficult because of the complexity of such motion. In general, lateral radiographs obtained in the neutral position and during spinal flexion and extension are used. Although accurate appraisal of minor aberrations in movement requires calculations of relationships among numerous osseous landmarks on each of the radiographs, less subtle changes are also indicative of abnormal spinal movement. General radiologic findings suggestive of instability include the presence of gas within the intervertebral disc, osteophytes on adjacent vertebral bodies below the rims of the endplate (traction spurs), and evidence of a radial fissure in the intervertebral disc during discography. Lateral radiographs obtained in flexion and in extension should be regarded as positive when they reveal forward or backward displacement of one vertebra on another, an abrupt change in the length of the pedicles, narrowing of the intervertebral foramina, and loss of height of an intervertebral disc. On frontal radiographs obtained with the patient bending first in one direction and then in the other, additional abnormalities include asymmetry in the person's ability to bend in both directions, loss of normal vertebral rotation and tilt, an abnormal degree of disc closure or opening, malalignment of spinous processes and pedicles, and lateral translation of one vertebra on another owing to an abnormal degree of rotation.

Of these radiographic signs of instability, it is the traction spur that has received particular attention (Fig. 36–16). This osseous excrescence arises on the anterior surface of the vertebral body, several millimeters from the discovertebral junction, and extends in a horizontal direction. It has been suggested that the traction spur develops at the site of attachment of the strong outermost fibers of the anulus

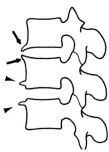

Figure 36–16. Segmental instability: Traction versus claw spur. The traction spur (arrowheads) develops 2 to 3 mm from the edge of the intervertebral disc and projects in a horizontal direction. The claw spur (arrows) develops closer to the discal margin and has a sweeping configuration. (Modified with permission from Macnab I: The traction spur. An indicator of segmental instability. J Bone Joint Surg [Am] 53:663, 1971.)

fibrosus to the vertebral surface when abnormal movement of the vertebrae exists, producing traction in these fibers. Differentiation between the common claw spur and a traction spur usually is not possible, however, limiting the usefulness of its detection as a sign of spinal instability.

DEGENERATIVE SPONDYLOLISTHESIS (TABLE 36–5). The term *spondylolysis* refers to an interruption of the pars interarticularis of the vertebra. Most investigators now believe that spondylolysis is an acquired abnormality characterized by a mechanical failure of bone related to abnormal vertebral stress (see Chapter 62). The term *spondylolisthesis* refers to displacement of one vertebra on another. Formally, spondylolisthesis was recognized as a phenomenon that occurred only when defects existed in the vertebral arch (spondylolysis) (Fig. 36–17), except in rare instances in which development of the posterior elements was defective. It now is known that spondylolisthesis can occur with an intact neural arch and that it commonly is associated with degenerative diseases of the spine (Fig. 36–18).

Degenerative spondylolisthesis accompanying osteoarthritis of the apophyseal joints occurs in approximately 4 per cent of elderly patients and predominates at the interspace between the fourth and fifth lumbar vertebrae in older women. The predilection for this spinal level has been attributed to developmental or acquired alterations in the neural arch that lead to instability and abnormal stress. Unlike the fifth lumbar vertebra, with its broad and strong posterior elements and its firm support provided by the iliac crest and iliolumbar ligaments, the fourth lumbar vertebra at the apex of the lumbar curve has relatively small transverse processes, less

Table 36–5. SPONDYLOLISTHESIS

Type	Initial Cause of Abnormality	Initial Site of Abnormality	Direction of Slippage
Spondylolisthesis with spondylolysis	Trauma (? congenital predisposition)	Pars interarticularis	Anterior slippage of involved vertebra
Spondylolisthesis without spondylolysis:			
Degenerative spondylolisthesis	Osteoarthritis	Apophyseal joints	Anterior slippage of upper vertebra
Retrolisthesis	Intervertebral (osteo)chondrosis	Intervertebral disc	Posterior slippage of upper vertebra

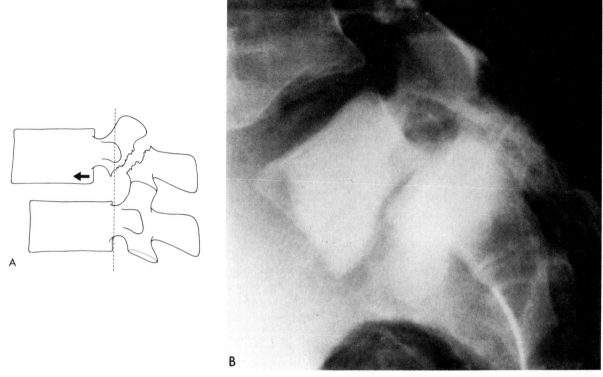

Figure 36–17. Spondylolisthesis with spondylolysis. A Bilateral defects through the pars interarticularis allow anterior displacement of the vertebral body on its neighbor. The alignment of the apophyseal joints is normal. **B** Observe anterior spondylolisthesis of the fifth lumbar vertebral body on the sacrum. The pars defects are not well delineated. Note the considerable intervertebral disc space narrowing, sclerosis, and fragmentation of the osseous surfaces.

ligamentous support, and more mobility. The facets at the L4-L5 level are oriented more sagittally than those at the L5-S1 level and therefore are more able to allow anterior movement. In the presence of degenerative joint changes, the check of one facet lying behind the other becomes deficient, and the inferior facets of the fourth lumbar vertebra gradually erode between the superior facets of the fifth lumbar vertebra, producing forward displacement of L4. The fourth lumbar vertebral body carries with it the intact neural arch so that the spinous process can travel as far forward as the vertebral body. In most cases, the degree of forward slipping is between 10 and 25 per cent of the anteroposterior diameter of the fifth lumbar vertebral body. Rotational abnormalities commonly accompany vertebral slippage.

Clinical patterns associated with degenerative spondylolisthesis include backache with or without leg pain, sciatica with or without backache but with signs of nerve root compression, and intermittent claudication of the cauda equina. Many patients with degenerative spondylolisthesis are symptom-free, however.

Radiographic findings of degenerative spondylolisthesis include osteoarthritis of apophyseal joints (joint space narrowing, sclerosis, and osteophytes), forward slipping of the superior vertebra on the inferior one, and, in some instances, intervertebral (osteo)chondrosis (vacuum phenomena, disc space narrowing, vertebral body sclerosis). Abnormal motion between the malaligned vertebrae is best detected on radiographs obtained with the spine in flexion and extension and bent laterally to each side. Myelography documents incomplete or complete interruption of the flow of contrast material.

Computed tomography ideally displays the pathologic alterations in the apophyseal joints, as well as the location and degree of spinal stenosis.

RETROLISTHESIS. Another pattern of spondylolisthesis without spondylolysis that is degenerative in type (degenerative spondylolisthesis) is associated with intervertebral (osteo)chondrosis. In this pattern, posterior displacement of the vertebra is characteristic, leading to the designation retrolisthesis (Fig. 36–19). Intervertebral (osteo)chondrosis results in decrease in height of the involved discal space, closer approximation of adjacent vertebral bodies, and gliding or telescoping of the corresponding articular processes. Because of the normal oblique inclination of the superior articular processes, they move in an inferoposterior direction, leading to posterior displacement of the superior vertebra relative to the inferior vertebra.

Retrolisthesis is most frequent in mobile portions of the spine, particularly the cervical and lumbar spine. In the lumbar segment, L2 and L1 are commonly affected. Radiographic findings include typical changes of intervertebral (osteo)chondrosis and apophyseal joint instability and subluxation. In the posterior joints, the initial radiographic appearance is characterized by asymmetry of joint space and tilting of one articular process on another; subsequently, joint displacement is observed, and the inferior articular processes of the superior vertebra extend below the articular surfaces of the superior processes.

Clinical findings include pain, an inability or unwillingness to bend forward or backward, rigidity, and neurologic abnormalities related to spinal cord compression.

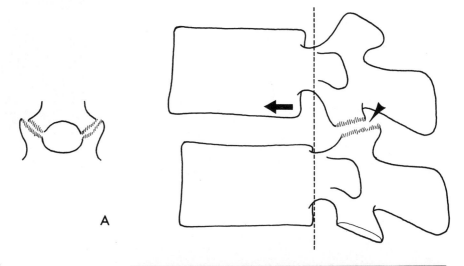

A

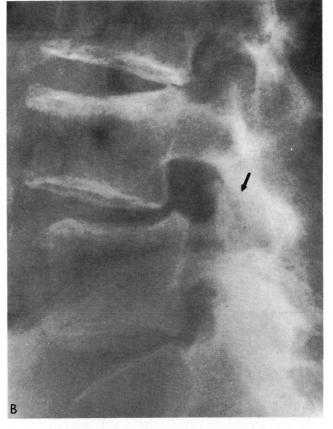

B

Figure 36–18. Spondylolisthesis without spondylolysis: Degenerative spondylolisthesis. A Apophyseal joint osteoarthritis (arrowhead) allows the inferior articular processes to move anteriorly, producing forward subluxation of the superior vertebra on the inferior vertebra. The inset demonstrates the manner in which the abnormal apophyseal joints may allow anterior subluxation. **B** Osteoarthritis of the apophyseal joints between the fourth and fifth lumbar vertebrae (arrow) has led to anterior displacement of the upper vertebra with respect to the lower. (**B,** From Resnick D: Degenerative diseases of the vertebral column. Radiology 156:3, 1985. Used with permission.)

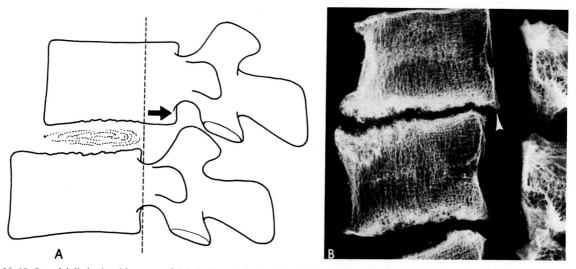

Figure 36–19. Spondylolisthesis without spondylolysis: Retrolisthesis. A As the intervertebral disc space narrows owing to intervertebral (osteo)chondrosis, telescoping of the apophyseal joints allows backward displacement of the upper lumbar vertebra on the lower one. **B** Retrolisthesis of L2 in relationship to L3 (arrowhead) is related to severe intervertebral (osteo)chondrosis in the intervening intervertebral disc. **(B,** From Resnick D: Degenerative diseases of the vertebral column. Radiology 156:3, 1985. Used with permission.)

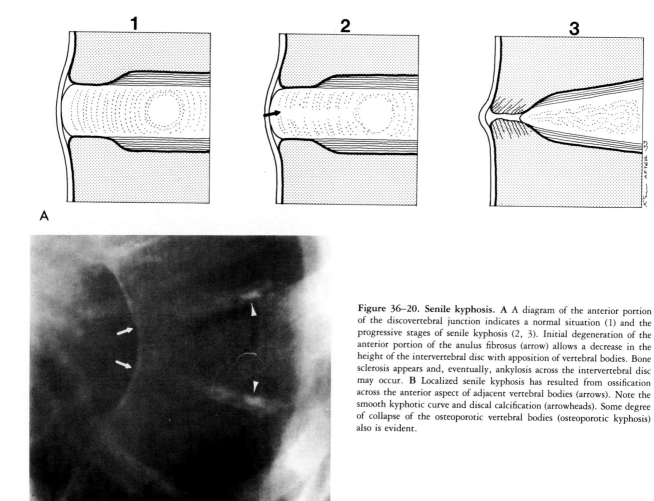

Figure 36–20. Senile kyphosis. A A diagram of the anterior portion of the discovertebral junction indicates a normal situation (1) and the progressive stages of senile kyphosis (2, 3). Initial degeneration of the anterior portion of the anulus fibrosus (arrow) allows a decrease in the height of the intervertebral disc with apposition of vertebral bodies. Bone sclerosis appears and, eventually, ankylosis across the intervertebral disc may occur. **B** Localized senile kyphosis has resulted from ossification across the anterior aspect of adjacent vertebral bodies (arrows). Note the smooth kyphotic curve and discal calcification (arrowheads). Some degree of collapse of the osteoporotic vertebral bodies (osteoporotic kyphosis) also is evident.

Table 36–6. SENILE VERSUS OSTEOPOROTIC KYPHOSIS

	Age Group	Initial Site of Abnormality	Radiographic Abnormalities
Senile kyphosis	Elderly	Anterior aspect of intervertebral disc	Disc space loss Vertebral body sclerosis Ankylosis of intervertebral disc
Osteoporotic kyphosis	Elderly	Anterior aspect of vertebral body	Osteoporosis Wedge-shaped vertebrae

SENILE KYPHOSIS (FIG. 36–20). Exaggerated thoracic kyphosis is a common finding in older persons. This deformity may be related to one of two processes: kyphosis secondary to vertebral osteoporosis (osteoporotic kyphosis), and kyphosis secondary to degeneration of the anulus fibrosus (senile kyphosis). Kyphosis accompanying osteoporosis (see Chapter 47) is noted in the middle and upper thoracic spine. Wedging of the weakened anterior vertebral surface is encountered, particularly at the level of the sixth and seventh thoracic vertebral bodies.

Senile kyphosis appears in older persons, particularly men, who do not have significant vertebral osteoporosis. As the intervertebral disc tissue deteriorates in these patients, the resistant anterior edges of the vertebral bodies may accelerate the degenerative processes in the adjacent fibers of the anulus fibrosus. Gradually, fibrosis and osseous tissue appear within the intervertebral disc, and the anterior part of the disc is transformed into bone. The radiographic features of senile kyphosis resemble those of intervertebral (osteo)chondrosis,

although the disc space narrowing and reactive sclerosis are located in a more anterior position in senile kyphosis. Prior to osseous fusion of vertebral bodies, osteophytosis on the anterior surface of the vertebrae is common; after osseous fusion, the osteophytes may be resorbed.

It is apparent that senile kyphosis and osteoporotic kyphosis are similar in many ways: Both occur in older patients; both involve the anterior aspect of the thoracic spine; and both produce progressive kyphosis (Table 36–6). Both processes are related to mechanical failure of vertebral structures: In senile kyphosis the failure occurs in the anterior aspect of the intervertebral disc, and in osteoporotic kyphosis the failure occurs in the weakened vertebral bodies. Either process alone or both processes together can lead to thoracic kyphosis that is greater than that accepted as normal.

SCOLIOSIS (FIG. 36–21). Several reports have emphasized the occurrence of scoliosis in the lumbar spine of elderly persons. This scoliosis may progress, generally at a slow rate, although occasionally it develops in a rapid fashion. Its relationship to significant symptoms and signs is debated.

The precise cause of the initial presentation or deterioration of scoliosis in the aged is not clear. Typically, degenerative diseases of the spine do not lead to the development of scoliosis, although they may appear during the course of scoliosis and aggravate the condition. Intervertebral (osteo)chondrosis, spondylosis deformans, and osteoarthritis all predominate along the concave aspect of the curve.

Intervertebral Disc Displacement

Normally, the intervertebral disc is a load-bearing structure with hydrostatic properties related to its high content of water. The anatomic arrangement of a centrally located nucleus pulposus surrounded by concentric lamellae of the anulus fibrosus allows the conversion of axial loading forces to tensile strains on the anular fibers and cartilaginous endplates. As the nucleus is subjected to elevated pressure, it attempts to prolapse from its confined space. The direction of this prolapse is variable; the intervertebral disc may be displaced anteriorly and laterally (spondylosis deformans), posteriorly (intraspinal herniation), or superiorly and inferiorly (cartilaginous nodes) (Table 36–7) (Fig. 36–22).

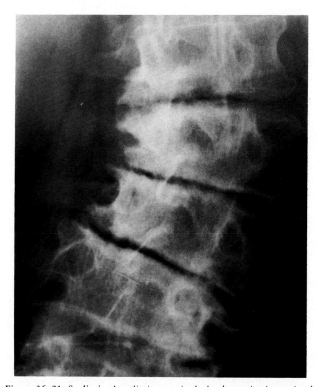

Figure 36–21. Scoliosis. A scoliotic curve in the lumbar region is associated with intervertebral (osteo)chondrosis (vacuum phenomena, disc space narrowing, sclerosis), and spondylosis deformans (osteophytes). Both processes are more exaggerated on the concave aspect of the curve.

Table 36–7. DISCAL DISPLACEMENT

Direction	Resulting Abnormality
Anterior displacement	Spondylosis deformans
Posterior displacement	Intraspinal herniation
Superior displacement	Cartilaginous (Schmorl's) node
Inferior displacement	Cartilaginous (Schmorl's) node

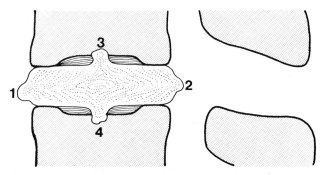

Figure 36–22. Intervertebral disc displacement: Direction of prolapse. A drawing of a sagittal section of the spine indicates the possible directions of discal displacement. Anterior displacement (1) leads to spondylolysis deformans; posterior displacement (2) may produce spinal cord compression; and superior (3) or inferior (4) displacement is associated with cartilaginous node formation.

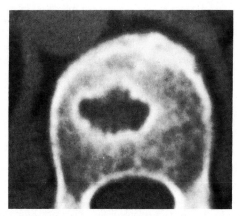

Figure 36–24. Intervertebral disc displacement: Cartilaginous nodes. Computed tomography. On a transaxial image, the typical lesion is radiolucent with a rim of bone sclerosis.

ANTEROLATERAL DISCAL DISPLACEMENT. Displacement of intervertebral disc material after degeneration of Sharpey's fibers of the anulus fibrosus produces the pathologic and radiographic features of spondylosis deformans. Usually, the stretched anterior longitudinal ligament prevents complete displacement of discal contents, although accompanying tears in this ligamentous structure occasionally permit further anterior and lateral protrusion of portions of the intervertebral disc, with possible migration in a cephalad or caudad direction.

SUPERIOR AND INFERIOR DISCAL DISPLACEMENT (FIGS. 36–23 AND 36–24). The appearance of intravertebral discal displacement (cartilaginous nodes) in intervertebral (osteo)chondrosis has already been discussed. Cartilaginous nodes are also apparent in other disease processes that weaken or disrupt the endplate or subchondral bone (Table 36–8).

Although the distribution of cartilaginous nodes is dependent on the precise causative factor, their radiographic and pathologic appearance is fundamentally similar no matter what the specific cause. A radiolucent lesion within the vertebral body surrounded by helmet-shaped sclerosis that borders on the intervertebral disc corresponds to a site of discal displacement contained within eburnated or thickened bone trabeculae. In the presence of intervertebral (osteo)chondrosis, degenerative clefts and collapse of the nucleus pulposus are evident, producing vacuum phenomena and considerable disc space narrowing; the displaced disc material may not extend deeply into the vertebral body.

A distinct type of cartilaginous node formation is characterized by intraosseous penetration of disc material at the junction of the cartilaginous endplate and the bone rim. This abnormality is observed in children in whom the developing apophyses have not yet fused with the remaining portion of the vertebral body. Displaced pieces of the intervertebral disc extend along an oblique course toward the outer surface of the vertebral body, isolating a small segment of bone (Fig. 36–25). The resulting abnormality, which has been termed a *limbus vertebra*, is most common at the anterosuperior corner of a single lumbar vertebral body. The adjacent intervertebral disc commonly demonstrates fissures extending from the nucleus pulposus into the separated cleft.

POSTERIOR DISCAL DISPLACEMENT. Displacement of disc material in a posterior or posterolateral direction is of great clinical significance because of the intimate relationship between the intervertebral disc and important neurologic structures. Anatomic features predisposing to such discal displacement include the somewhat posterior position of the

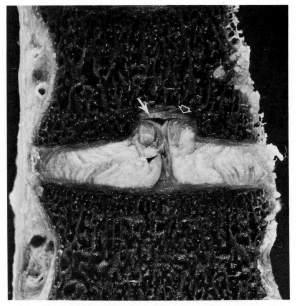

Figure 36–23. Intervertebral disc displacement: Cartilaginous nodes. Pathology. On this photograph of a sagittal section of the spine, a cartilaginous node (open arrow) is evident. The displaced nucleus pulposus contains vertical (arrowhead) and horizontal (solid arrow) fissures. (From Resnick D, et al: Spinal vacuum phenomena: Anatomical study and review. Radiology 139:341, 1981. Used with permission.)

Table 36–8. SOME CONDITIONS ASSOCIATED WITH CARTILAGINOUS (SCHMORL'S) NODES

Intervertebral (osteo)chondrosis
Scheuermann's disease (juvenile kyphosis)
Trauma
Hyperparathyroidism
Osteoporosis
Infection
Neoplasm

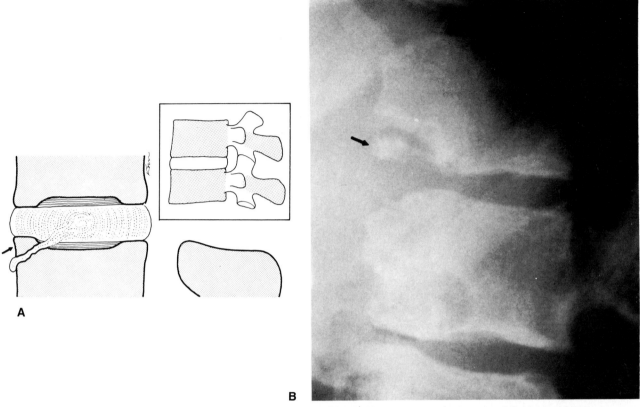

Figure 36–25. Intervertebral disc displacement: Cartilaginous nodes. Limbus vertebra. A Anterior displacement of discal material in the immature skeleton can isolate a small segment of the vertebral rim (arrow), creating a limbus vertebra. **B** In this young patient, observe the discal displacement that has isolated a segment of the vertebral rim (arrow). Irregularity of the anterior surfaces of the vertebral bodies is a common associated finding.

normal nucleus pulposus, the existence of fewer and weaker anular fibers in this region, and a posterior longitudinal ligament that is not so strong as the anterior longitudinal ligament (Fig. 36–26). The herniated discal material may contain not only a portion of the nucleus pulposus but also pieces of the anulus fibrosus and the cartilaginous endplate.

Certain terms are used to indicate the extent of displacement of the intervertebral disc (Fig. 36–27).

Anular bulge: The anular fibers remain intact but protrude in a localized or diffuse fashion into the spinal canal.

Discal prolapse (protrusion): The displaced nucleus pulposus

extends through some of the fibers of the anulus fibrosus but is still confined by the intact outermost fibers.

Discal extrusion: The displaced nucleus pulposus penetrates all of the fibers of the anulus fibrosus and lies under the posterior longitudinal ligament.

Discal sequestration: The displaced nucleus pulposus penetrates or extends around the posterior longitudinal ligament and lies within the epidural space; or the displaced nucleus pulposus, although not extending through this ligament, migrates for a considerable distance in a cephalad or caudad direction as a fragment that is separate from the remaining portion of the intervertebral disc.

If discal herniation is defined as a situation in which the nucleus pulposus extends through some or all of the fibers of the anulus fibrosus, discal prolapse, extrusion, and sequestration are all forms of herniation (Fig. 36–28).

Although the diagnosis of posterior displacement of portions of the intervertebral disc may occasionally be established in routine radiography by the presence of calcification, generally other imaging methods are required, especially various contrast examinations (myelography, lumbar venography, discography), computed tomography, or magnetic resonance imaging. The advantage of one technique over another is related, in part, to which region of the spine is being examined, the precise direction of discal displacement, and the personal experience, expertise, and preference of the examiner. In fact, various combinations of techniques have been suggested.

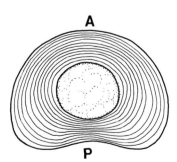

Figure 36–26. Posterior discal displacement: Anatomic basis. A drawing of a transaxial section of the intervertebral disc shows that there are fewer annular fibers posteriorly and that the nucleus pulposus is in a somewhat posterior position. A, Anterior; P, posterior. See also Figure 36–1.

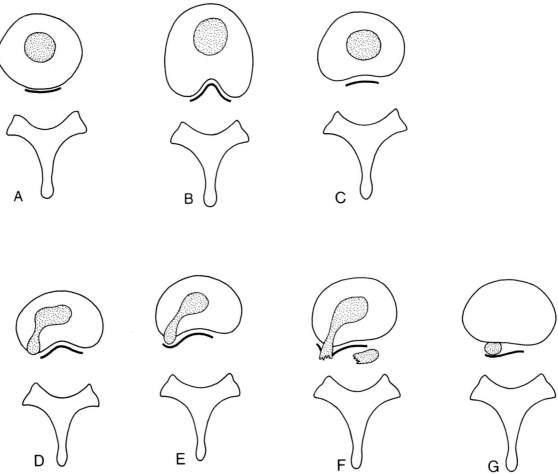

Figure 36–27. Posterior discal displacement: Degree of disc displacement. A-C Annular bulge. Three different patterns are illustrated. **D** Discal prolapse (protrusion). The displaced nucleus pulposus is still confined by the outermost annular fibers. **E** Discal extrusion. The displaced nucleus pulposus has violated the outer fibers of the anulus fibrosus but is still confined by the posterior longitudinal ligament. **F** Discal sequestration. The displaced nucleus pulposus has penetrated the posterior longitudinal ligament and lies within the epidural space. **G,** Discal sequestration. A fragment of the displaced disc has migrated beneath the posterior longitudinal ligament in a cephalad or caudad direction and is separated from the remaining portion of the intervertebral disc.

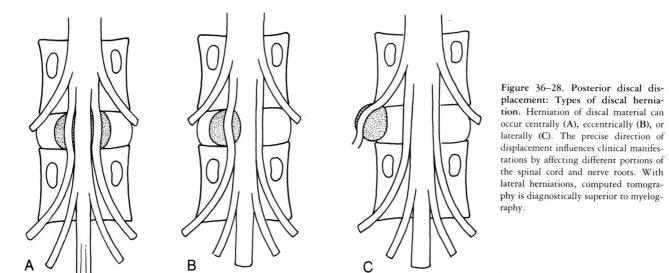

Figure 36–28. Posterior discal displacement: Types of discal herniation. Herniation of discal material can occur centrally **(A)**, eccentrically **(B)**, or laterally **(C)**. The precise direction of displacement influences clinical manifestations by affecting different portions of the spinal cord and nerve roots. With lateral herniations, computed tomography is diagnostically superior to myelography.

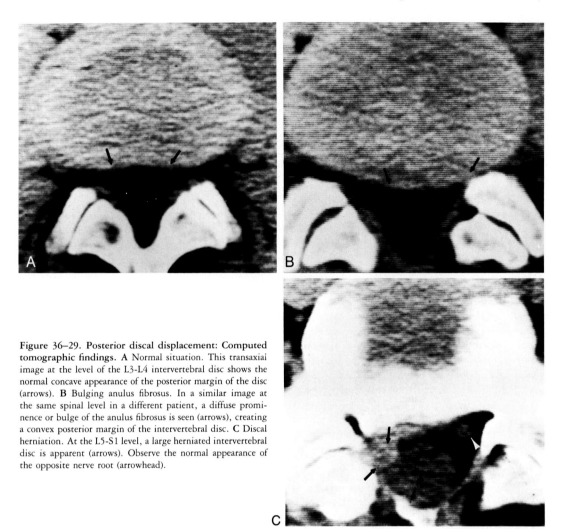

Figure 36–29. Posterior discal displacement: Computed tomographic findings. **A** Normal situation. This transaxial image at the level of the L3-L4 intervertebral disc shows the normal concave appearance of the posterior margin of the disc (arrows). **B** Bulging anulus fibrosus. In a similar image at the same spinal level in a different patient, a diffuse prominence or bulge of the anulus fibrosus is seen (arrows), creating a convex posterior margin of the intervertebral disc. **C** Discal herniation. At the L5-S1 level, a large herniated intervertebral disc is apparent (arrows). Observe the normal appearance of the opposite nerve root (arrowhead).

The differentiation of a bulging anulus fibrosus and discal herniation can be difficult with any imaging method. Myelographic criteria of the bulging anulus include a rounded and symmetric extradural deformity that does not extend above or below the intervertebral disc space and nerve roots that are uniform in caliber and normal in size; myelographic findings of discal herniation include an angular extradural deformity that may extend in a cephalad or caudad direction from the discal level and nerve roots that appear widened. With computed tomography, bulging of the anulus fibrosus typically is found to be associated with generalized extension of the discal contour beyond the margins of the vertebral body in a symmetric and uniform fashion, whereas a focal extension is more typical of a herniated nucleus pulposus (Fig. 36–29). With computed tomography, centrally located herniated discs that lie beneath the posterior longitudinal ligament produce a smooth, focal radiodense area that deforms or displaces the dural sac. When nuclear material penetrates this ligament or extends around it, a soft tissue mass is evident within the epidural fat (Fig. 36–30). Inferior migration of the sequestered fragment is slightly more common than superior migration.

Extreme lateral herniations, which represent approximately 12 per cent of all herniations, present a diagnostic challenge. If the site of such herniation is within the neural foramen or lateral to it, myelographic examinations commonly are nondiagnostic. Computed tomography in these cases is far superior, demonstrating focal protrusion of the disc margin near or in the intervertebral foramen, displacement of epidural fat,

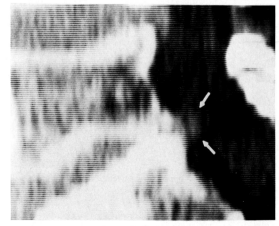

Figure 36–30. Posterior discal displacement: Discal sequestration. A sagittal reformatted computed tomographic image documents the presence of a small sequestered discal fragment (arrows).

absence of dural sac deformity, and a soft tissue mass lateral to the foramen.

Ancillary computed tomographic findings of discal herniation in any location are swelling or dilatation of nerve roots, calcification or gas within the displaced discal material and, if intravenous contrast material is administered in conjunction with computed tomography, enhancement of tissue at the margins of the herniated intervertebral disc.

Additional disorders that lead to myelographic or computed tomographic findings resembling those of a herniated disc include postsurgical fibrosis, osteophytosis, synovial cysts, various neoplasms, infection, cystic dilatation of the nerve root sleeve, and conjoined nerve roots. As a general rule, erosion of bone favors many of these alternative diagnoses.

Segmental Sclerosis of Vertebral Bodies (Fig. 36–31)

The appearance of sclerosis involving that portion of the vertebral body that is adjacent to the intervertebral disc is a recognized manifestation of intervertebral (osteo)chondrosis and cartilaginous node formation. Although vertebral sclerosis can be observed in patients with infection, tumor, and metabolic diseases (Paget's disease, renal osteodystrophy), accurate diagnosis generally is not difficult. There remains, however, a group of patients who develop increased radiodensity of peridiscal vertebral bone, in whom a specific cause cannot be identified. Terms applied to this finding have

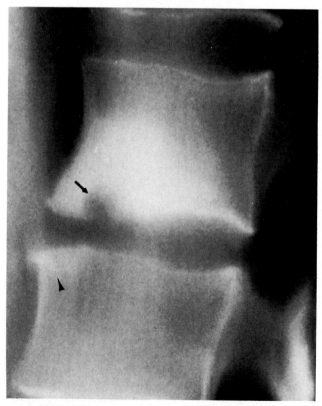

Figure 36–31. Segmental sclerosis of vertebral body. A lateral tomogram reveals bone sclerosis involving the anteroinferior portion of the second lumbar vertebral body with a small osteolytic focus (arrow). Minimal involvement of the adjacent vertebral body is seen (arrowhead), and the intervertebral disc is slightly narrowed. (Courtesy of L. Danzig, M.D., Orange County, California.)

included non-neoplastic sclerosis of the vertebral body, pseudoinfection of the intervertebral disc, traumatic lesions of the discovertebral junction, hemispherical spondylosclerosis, and idiopathic segmental sclerosis of the vertebral bodies.

Idiopathic segmental sclerosis of the vertebral body predominates in the lumbar spine in young and middle-aged women. A history of trauma or back pain has been evident in some of the patients. One, two, or, more rarely, several vertebral bodies are affected.

Radiologic features include bone lysis, bone sclerosis, or both. With regard to the sclerotic lesions, selective involvement of the anteroinferior portion of the vertebral body, especially of L4 and, less frequently, L3, has been observed. A hemispheric band of sclerosis extends for a variable distance from the anterior and inferior margins of the vertebral body to its central portion. The increased bone density commonly is well defined, and the bone may be uniformly dense or possess small osteolytic foci. Narrowing of the intervertebral disc space and involvement of the adjacent vertebral body are evident in some instances. Pathologic findings do not support an infectious or neoplastic process, although the precise cause of the condition is not clear.

The importance of idiopathic segmental sclerosis of the vertebral body lies in its differentiation from other patterns of vertebral sclerosis (Fig. 36–32), including the ivory vertebral body of metastasis or Hodgkin's disease, the rugger-jersey vertebral body of renal osteodystrophy, the picture-frame vertebral body of Paget's disease, marginal condensation of bone in intervertebral (osteo)chondrosis, and focal radiodense lesions with thorny radiations that are characteristic of bone islands (enostoses).

Intervertebral Disc Calcification

Many systemic disorders are associated with discal calcification, including alkaptonuria, hemochromatosis, calcium pyrophosphate dihydrate crystal deposition disease, hyperparathyroidism, poliomyelitis, acromegaly, and amyloidosis. The location, appearance, and chemical nature of the calcific deposits vary from one disorder to the next, although in most of these conditions, multiple intervertebral discs are involved. Calcification of discs may also appear after surgical fusion or spontaneous ankylosis (e.g., juvenile chronic arthritis, ankylosing spondylitis, diffuse idiopathic skeletal hyperostosis) of the adjacent vertebral structures.

Calcification localized to one or two discal levels is encountered in two broad clinical situations. In adults, chronic degenerative calcific deposits may occur in the anulus fibrosus, nucleus pulposus, or cartilaginous endplates, particularly in older men and in the midthoracic and upper lumbar spine. It is not clear how frequently this type of degenerative calcification is symptomatic.

The second situation associated with discal calcification is observed in children (Fig. 36–33). Such calcification is most common between 6 and 10 years of age. It affects boys and girls with equal frequency, and multiple intervertebral discs may be involved. The cervical spine is most commonly affected. Symptoms include pain, stiffness, limitation of motion, and torticollis. Fever, leukocytosis, and elevation of the erythrocyte sedimentation rate can be apparent. On radiographs, calcification involves predominantly the nucleus pulposus, producing single or multiple, oval or flat dense

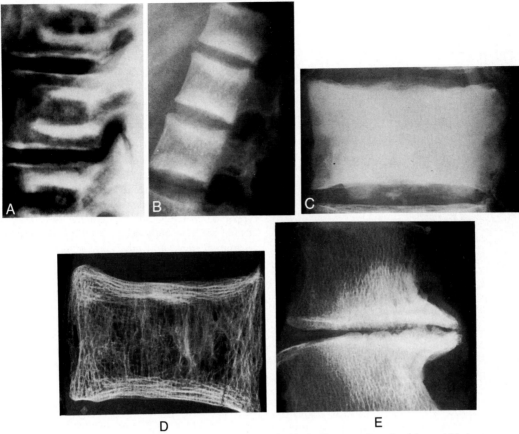

Figure 36–32. Patterns of sclerosis of the vertebral body. A Sandwich vertebral body: Osteopetrosis tarda. A bone-within-bone appearance is created by well-defined radiodense bands. (Courtesy of P. Kaplan, M.D., Omaha, Nebraska.) **B** Rugger-jersey vertebral body: Renal osteodystrophy. Bands of increased radiodensity are evident at the top and bottom of each vertebral body. **C** Ivory vertebral body: Skeletal metastasis (carcinoma of the prostate). The entire vertebral body is radiodense. **D** Picture-frame vertebral body: Paget's disease. The peripheral portions of the vertebral body are radiodense in comparison to the central portion. **E** Marginal condensation: Intervertebral (osteo)chondrosis. Triangular-shaped sclerosis borders on a narrowed intervertebral disc.

areas. Rupture of these calcific collections into the vertebral bodies or adjacent soft tissues may be evident.

The prognosis of discal calcification in children is excellent. In most cases, pain and calcification resolve spontaneously. The cause of discal calcification in children is not known. The clinical findings associated with it resemble those in "discitis," an apparently inflammatory condition associated rarely with ossification of the intervertebral disc.

Spinal Stenosis

A narrow spinal canal may be present at birth. This stenosis can later be accentuated by developmental narrowing produced by postnatal growth abnormalities and by acquired narrowing associated with various disease processes. Degenerative disorders of the vertebral column (osteoarthritis) lead to hypertrophic alterations about involved joints, which may compromise spinal contents. Clinical manifestations vary according to the location and the severity of the stenosis, as well as its cause. Although symptoms and signs occasionally are encountered in the young, they are far more frequent in middle-aged and elderly persons. Stenosis in the cervical region may lead to impingement of the cord or, less prominently, of the nerve roots. In the lumbar segment, clinical findings associated with stenosis include low back pain, sciatica, and a cauda equina syndrome.

The limitations of the plain film radiographic examination in evaluating spinal stenosis must be emphasized; osseous alterations may be outlined, but soft tissue abnormalities escape radiographic detection. Myelography and computed tomography represent more sensitive diagnostic techniques in the evaluation of spinal stenosis.

CERVICAL SPINAL STENOSIS. Radiographic measurement of sagittal diameters of the spine (measured from the posterior surface of the vertebral body to the spinolaminar line) may be used for detecting stenosis of the cervical canal: Cord compression may occur in adults if this diameter is 10 mm or less and is unlikely to occur if this diameter is 13 mm or more. Measurement between these osseous landmarks on radiography does not always provide an accurate appraisal of the width of the spinal cord, however. This method is not useful in instances in which discal protrusion or ligamentous hypertrophy is the cause of the stenosis.

Although cervical spinal stenosis can be related to many congenital factors (anomalies, dysplasias, malformations, subluxations), it can also be acquired in traumatic, infectious, neoplastic, and metabolic disorders. Cervical spinal stenosis also develops in degenerative articular diseases, such as spondylosis deformans and osteoarthritis, as well as in ossification of the posterior longitudinal ligament (see Chapter 38). Osteophytes commonly encroach on the spinal canal (as well

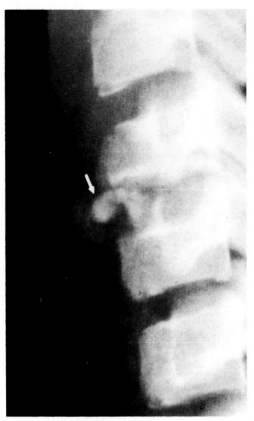

Figure 36–33. Intervertebral disc calcification: Children. Observe the calcified and extruded intervertebral disc (arrow) with adjacent soft tissue swelling. (Courtesy of M. Dalinka, M.D., Philadelphia, Pennsylvania.)

as the neural foramina) in the midcervical region. These bone excrescences may extend from discal or apophyseal joints as well as from the joints of Luschka. Spinal stenosis is accentuated by even minor degrees of degenerative spondylolisthesis or retrolisthesis.

THORACIC SPINAL STENOSIS. Significant spinal stenosis in the thoracic segment related to degenerative joint processes is much less frequent than stenosis in the cervical or lumbar segments.

LUMBAR SPINAL STENOSIS (FIG. 36–34). As in the cervical spine, congenital and developmental factors may lead to a narrowed lumbar spinal canal, which can be further compromised by acquired alterations. With developmental stenosis, characteristic alterations include narrowing of the anteroposterior and interpediculate diameters of the lower two or three lumbar vertebrae, vertical orientation of the laminae, and extreme diminution of the interlaminar space. These osseous abnormalities can be detected radiographically by measuring the anteroposterior (midsagittal) diameter (the distance from the posterior surface of the vertebral body to the base of the superior portion of the spinous process) and the transverse diameter (the distance between the inner aspect of the pedicles) of the spinal canal. The lower limit of normal of the five lumbar vertebrae in men and women for the midsagittal diameter is 15 mm and for the transverse diameter is 20 mm; measurements below these values indicate the presence of lumbar spinal canal stenosis. The midsagittal diameter can be difficult to determine because of the inability

to define a definite dorsal or posterior limit of the bone canal on the standard lateral view, however. Most investigators consider that an anteroposterior spinal diameter less than 12 mm is unequivocally pathologic. On computed tomography, anteroposterior diameters of less than 11.5 mm, interpediculate distances of less than 16 mm, and canal cross-sectional areas of less than 1.45 sq cm are considered small.

Degenerative processes contribute to stenosis of the lumbar spinal canal. Ventral osteophytes, prolapse of the intervertebral disc material, hypertrophy and subluxation of the articular facets, enlargement of laminae, and hyperplasia or ossification of the ligamenta flava lead to further encroachment on the canal and may produce clinical symptoms and signs in a patient whose spine has already been compromised by developmental stenosis. Although these alterations usually are apparent on plain film radiography, their exact location and extent are more fully delineated with computed tomography.

Spinal stenosis in the lumbar segment can be further divided into three groups on the basis of its anatomic location: stenosis of the central canal, stenosis of the subarticular or lateral recesses, and stenosis of the neural foramina.

The central canal normally is round or slightly oval in cross section. Computed tomographic findings of central canal stenosis include distortion of its normal configuration, compression of the thecal sac in an anteroposterior direction, and obliteration of the adjacent epidural fat. Causes of such stenosis are developmental narrowing of the interpediculate distance (as in achondroplasia), hypertrophic changes related to osteoarthritis in the apophyseal articulations, thickening of the ligamentum flavum, ligamentous calcification or ossification, diffuse bone overgrowth (as in Paget's disease), osteophytes in the vertebral body and, in the postoperative period, hypertrophy of bone grafts and fibrosis (Fig. 36–35).

The subarticular or lateral recess lies immediately ventral to the superior articular process and pars interarticularis and is bordered laterally by the medial margin of the pedicle, and anteriorly by the posterior surface of the vertebral body. Its anteroposterior dimension varies, although a measurement equal to or less than 3 mm is definitely abnormal, and one between 3 and 5 mm is highly suggestive of lateral recess stenosis. As the narrowest portion of the recess is situated at the superior or rostral border of the pedicle, close to the superior articular facet, bone hypertrophy about the apophyseal joint is a leading cause of encroachment on the neural elements in this region. Clinical manifestations of lateral recess syndrome include unilateral or bilateral leg pain initiated or aggravated by standing and walking and completely relieved by sitting or squatting.

The intervertebral foramen (Fig. 36–36) is bordered above and below by ipsilateral pedicles at adjacent vertebral levels, anteriorly by the posterior portion of the vertebral body and intervertebral disc, and posteriorly by the pars interarticularis and the superior articular process. As the lumbar nerve passes laterally just below the pedicle of the upper vertebra, it is this portion of the neural foramen in which narrowing has more significance. Causes of foraminal narrowing include discal herniation, osteophytosis involving the vertebral body or articular processes, focal inflammatory diseases, tumors, synovial cysts, proximal placement of the dorsal root ganglia, and postoperative fibrosis. Furthermore, spondylolisthesis commonly is associated with distortion of the foramen and may lead to compromise of the exiting nerve.

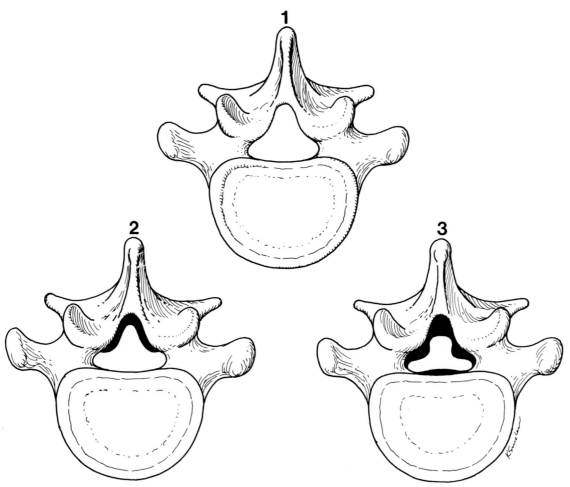

Figure 36–34. Lumbar spinal stenosis. Patterns of spinal stenosis. The normal situation is indicated in 1. Observe stenosis owing to laminal thickening (2) and owing to both anterior and posterior bony overgrowth (3), a situation called the trefoil or fleur-de-lis appearance.

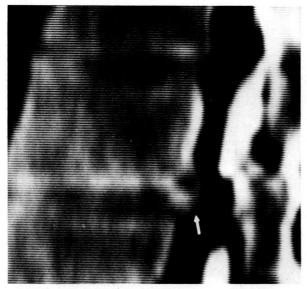

Figure 36–35. Stenosis of the central canal. A reformatted sagittal computed tomographic image after myelography in a young patient with a previous fracture of the third lumbar vertebral body reveals narrowing of the central canal, related, in part, to an osteophyte (arrow).

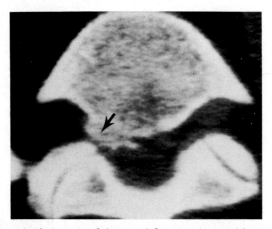

Figure 36–36. Stenosis of the neural foramen. A transaxial computed tomographic scan at the L4-L5 spinal level reveals an osteophyte (arrow) arising from the right posteroinferior margin of the fourth lumbar vertebral body. Although the neural foramen is narrowed, the L4 nerve root has already exited through the foramen above this osteophyte.

IATROGENIC DEGENERATIVE DISEASES OF THE SPINE

Chemonucleolysis

The nonoperative chemical removal of disc material, especially in the lumbar spine, has been used as a therapeutic technique in patients with low back pain and sciatica. Of the various agents that have been studied, chymopapain, a proteolytic enzyme that is extracted from the latex of the Carica papaya tree, is used most widely.

The injection of chymopapain into an intervertebral disc is accomplished under general or local anesthesia with fluoroscopic monitoring. Results of chymopapain injection have been encouraging in those patients who have evidence of a herniated lumbar nucleus pulposus with radiculitis that has not responded after 6 weeks of conservative care; absolute and relative contraindications for the procedure include a proved allergy to chymopapain, paresis or paralysis of the bowel or bladder, calcification within the displaced discal fragment, discal sequestration, pregnancy, diabetes mellitus with peripheral neuropathy, spinal stenosis, a complete spinal block demonstrated by myelography, a transitional lumbosacral junction, and some types of spondylolisthesis. The major complication of the procedure is an allergic response, which has been reported in 0.2 to 1.5 per cent of cases. Other complications of chymopapain injection include rash or urticaria, muscle spasm, back pain, and aseptic or septic discitis. Paraplegia, in some instances related to transverse myelitis, has also followed use of chymopapain.

Chymopapain acts predominantly on the nucleus pulposus, having a dramatic effect on its proteoglycans and possibly matrix proteins. This action is associated with loss of the water-binding capacity of the disc, leading to discal collapse, which may be apparent on the radiographs or computed tomograms. Restoration of normal disc height over a period of time after chymopapain injection has been observed.

Laminectomy and Spinal Fusion

Fusion of the posterior spinal elements is associated with subsequent abnormalities in those intervertebral discs located both within the ankylosed segment and adjacent to it. A direct effect on the nutrition of the intervertebral discs within the area of fusion can be expected, and discal degeneration ensues, which may be apparent radiographically as loss of disc height and calcification.

The effect of anterior or posterior spinal fusion on adjacent unfused segments is a controversial subject, with reports suggesting either a low or a high frequency of discal herniation in such segments. Alterations in spinal motion above, below, and between ankylosed regions of the vertebral column are observed by means of fluoroscopy and cineradiography. Radiographic abnormalities after surgical fusion, especially in the cervical spine, include the presence of osteophytes in the vertebral body and disc space loss as well as osteoarthritis of apophyseal joints adjacent to the areas of ankylosis.

Laminectomy, when extensive, can lead to subsequent mechanical derangement, especially in the cervical spine. Progressive subluxation produces an angular kyphosis, the swan-neck deformity. The abnormality in alignment relates to loss of integrity of supporting ligamentous and osseous tissue.

ADDITIONAL DIAGNOSTIC TECHNIQUES IN DEGENERATIVE DISEASES OF THE SPINE

Myelography, discography, and, more recently, computed tomography and magnetic resonance imaging are important procedures in diagnosing degenerative spinal diseases and their complications. The cross-sectional display of computed tomography is ideally suited to these problems, and the addition of contrast material in the spinal canal or, more rarely, in the intervertebral disc can clarify any diagnostic dilemma that may be encountered. In the postoperative period, the rapid intravenous infusion of contrast agent has been used to differentiate postsurgical fibrosis, which is associated with tissue enhancement, and recurrent discal herniation, which is not associated with such enhancement.

Areas of abnormal accumulation of bone-seeking radiopharmaceutical agents indicate sites of active bone turnover. Such accumulation is more typical of intervertebral (os-

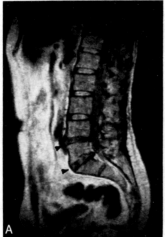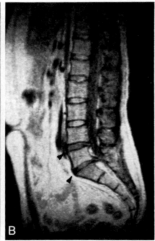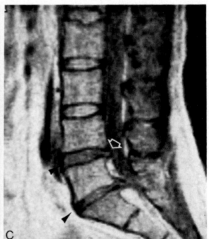

Figure 36–37. Magnetic resonance imaging: Discal degeneration and displacement in spine. A Intervertebral (osteo)chondrosis. Note the decrease in signal intensity at both the L4-L5 and L5-S1 discal levels (arrowheads) with bulging of the posterior discal contours. (TR, 1.5 s; TE, 28 ms.) **B, C** Intervertebral (osteo)chondrosis. A decrease in signal intensity at the L4-L5 and L5-S1 discal levels (arrowheads) is observed. Posterior displacement of the former disc is seen (open arrow). (TR, 1.5 s; TE, 28 ms.) (Courtesy of M. Solomon, M.D., San Jose, California.)

teo)chondrosis and osteoarthritis than of spondylosis deformans. Scintigraphy is not useful in the diagnosis of discal herniation. As is well known, abnormal radionuclide activity in the spine related to degenerative disorders is difficult to differentiate from that associated with other skeletal diseases, particularly metastasis.

Thermography has been used to investigate patients with degenerative disc disease. Increased accumulation of heat manifested as a positive thermogram in patients with a herniated intervertebral disc may be related to muscular spasm adjacent to a compressed nerve.

Magnetic resonance imaging (Fig. 36–37) can be applied successfully to the evaluation of various disorders of the spine and spinal cord, including degenerative processes. Whereas the normal nucleus pulposus is clearly discernible from the surrounding anulus fibrosus, appearing as an area of higher signal intensity (on T2 weighted images), nuclear degeneration is associated with an isodense image of the intervertebral disc. Changes in the subchondral vertebral bone and marrow, which include osteosclerosis and accumulation of fat, lead to additional characteristic abnormalities with magnetic resonance imaging in patients with degenerative alterations in the intervertebral disc. Identification of a herniated nucleus pulposus is likewise possible with magnetic resonance imaging.

Magnetic resonance imaging has also been used to identify sites and patterns of spinal stenosis. Because of the faint signal derived from cortical bone during magnetic resonance imaging, this method may be inferior to computed tomography in differentiating between bone and soft tissue causes of impingement. Postoperative fibrosis is characterized by an increased signal intensity compared with that seen in recurrent discal herniation, which is associated with a decreased signal intensity.

FURTHER READING

Bick EM: Vertebral osteophytosis. Pathologic basis of its roentgenology. AJR 73:979, 1955.

DePalma A, Rothman R: The Intervertebral Disc. Philadelphia, WB Saunders 1970.

Dorwart RH, Vogler JB, Helms CA: Computed tomography of spinal stenosis. Radiol Clin North Am 21:301, 1983.

Edelman RR, Shoukimas GM, Stark DD, Davis KR, New PFJ, Saini S, Rosenthal DI, Wismer GL, Brady TJ: High-resolution surface-coil imaging of lumbar disk disease. AJR 144:1123, 1985.

Epstein JA, Epstein BS, Jones MD: Symptomatic lumbar scoliosis with degenerative changes in the elderly. Spine 4:542, 1979.

Francois RJ: Ligament insertions into the human lumbar vertebral body. Acta Anat 91:467, 1975.

Hadley LA: Anatomico-roentgenographic Studies of the Spine. 2nd Ed. Springfield, Ill, Charles C Thomas, 1973.

Hemminghytt S, Daniels DL, Williams AL, Haughton VM: Intraspinal synovial cysts: Natural history and diagnosis by CT. Radiology 145:375, 1982.

Jacobson HG, Tausend ME, Shapiro JH, Poppel MH: The "swayback" syndrome. AJR 79:677, 1958.

Jones RAC, Thomson JLG: The narrow lumbar canal. A clinical and radiological review. J Bone Joint Surg [Br] 50:595, 1968.

Kirkaldy-Willis WH, Wedge JH, Yong-Hing K, Reilly J: Pathology and pathogenesis of lumbar spondylosis and stenosis. Spine 3:319, 1978.

Knutsson F: The vacuum phenomenon in the intervertebral discs. Acta Radiol 23:173, 1942.

Macnab I: Spondylolisthesis with an intact neural arch—the so-called pseudospondylolisthesis. J Bone Joint Surg [Br] 32:325, 1950.

Macnab I: The traction spur. An indicator of segmental instability. J Bone Joint Surg [Am] 53:663, 1971.

Maldague BE, Noel HM, Malghem JJ: The intravertebral vacuum cleft: A sign of ischemic vertebral collapse. Radiology 129:23, 1978.

Martel W, Seeger JF, Wicks JD, Washburn RL: Traumatic lesions of the discovertebral junction in the lumbar spine. AJR 127:457, 1976.

McCullough JA: Chemonucleolysis: Experience with 2000 cases. Clin Orthop 145:138, 1980.

Modic MT, Masaryk T, Boumphrey F, Goormastic M, Bell G: Lumbar herniated disk disease and canal stenosis: Prospective evaluation by surface coil MR, CT, and myelography. AJR 147:757, 1986.

Pech P, Haughton VM: Lumbar intervertebral disk: Correlative MR and anatomic study. Radiology 156:699, 1985.

Resnick D, Niwayama G: Intervertebral disc herniations: Cartilaginous (Schmorl's) nodes. Radiology 126:57, 1978.

Resnick D, Niwayama G, Guerra J, Vint V, Usselman J: Spinal vacuum phenomena: Anatomical study and review. Radiology 139:341, 1981.

Schmorl G, Junghanns H: The Human Spine in Health and Disease. 2nd Ed. Translated by EF Besemann. New York, Grune & Stratton, 1971.

Silverman FN: Calcification of intervertebral disks in childhood. Radiology 62:801, 1954.

Williams AL, Haugton VM, Daniels DL, Grogan JP: Differential CT diagnosis of extruded nucleus pulposus. Radiology 148:141, 1983.

Chapter 37

Diffuse Idiopathic Skeletal Hyperostosis (DISH)

Donald Resnick, M.D.
Gen Niwayama, M.D.

Diffuse idiopathic skeletal hyperostosis (DISH) appears to be a distinct skeletal disorder that can be distinguished clinically, radiographically, and pathologically from certain other disorders. It is also possible, however, that DISH may represent not a disease per se but rather a vulnerable state in which extensive ossification results from an exaggerated response of the body in some patients to stimuli that produce only modest new bone formation in others. As such, DISH would represent an ossifying diathesis that causes excessive bone formation at skeletal sites subject to normal or abnormal stresses. These sites generally are where tendons and ligaments attach to bone, in both the axial and the extraaxial skeleton. Such bone production predominates in the spine, but similar bone formation may occasionally predominate or even be isolated in extraspinal sites. Further evidence that an ossifying diathesis or bone-forming tendency is present in patients with DISH includes the propensity of these individuals to develop ossification after surgery or in response to skeletal alterations accompanying coexistent diseases, such as rheumatoid arthritis.

Diffuse idiopathic skeletal hyperostosis (DISH) is the proposed name for a skeletal disorder producing characteristic alterations in both spinal and extraspinal structures. DISH has been described previously in the literature under a variety of names (Table 37–1). Although one of the most popular terms has been ankylosing hyperostosis of the spine, this name has certain inadequacies: Vertebral ankylosis, although apparent radiographically, may not be found on pathologic examination, and extraspinal manifestations are common and may be more extensive than spinal alterations. Furthermore, extraspinal changes can exist without vertebral abnormality. As it emphasizes the widespread nature of this disorder, diffuse idiopathic skeletal hyperostosis (DISH) is the most appropriate designation for this disease.

DIAGNOSTIC CRITERIA

There are three criteria for spinal involvement in DISH:

1. The presence of flowing calcification and ossification along the anterolateral aspect of at least four contiguous vertebral bodies with or without associated localized pointed excrescences at the intervening vertebral body-intervertebral disc junctions.

2. The presence of relative preservation of intervertebral disc height in the involved vertebral segment and the absence of extensive radiographic changes of "degenerative" disc disease, including vacuum phenomena and vertebral body marginal sclerosis.

3. The absence of apophyseal joint bone ankylosis and sacroiliac joint erosion, sclerosis, or intraarticular osseous fusion.

All three radiographic criteria must be fulfilled to establish a definitive diagnosis of DISH. Each has been chosen to eliminate other spinal disorders, which potentially could be confused with DISH: The first criterion is helpful in separating this condition from typical spondylosis deformans; the second criterion distinguishes DISH from intervertebral (osteo)chondrosis; the third criterion eliminates patients with ankylosing spondylitis.

Three other points regarding these criteria must be stressed. The choice of four contiguous vertebral bodies as the least extensive ossification that is compatible with the diagnosis of DISH is arbitrary. The decision to use four contiguous vertebral bodies was based on a desire to separate this entity from typical spondylosis deformans, although separation of spondylosis deformans and DISH in this manner may not be correct or even useful (see discussion later in this chapter).

Second, DISH is a disorder of middle-aged and elderly patients, persons in whom some degree of degeneration of the intervertebral disc (intervertebral [osteo]chondrosis) is usually apparent. Although the second criterion insists on relative preservation of disc height and absence of extensive radiographic changes of intervertebral (osteo)chondrosis, it ob-

Table 37–1. DIFFUSE IDIOPATHIC SKELETAL HYPEROSTOSIS (ADDITIONAL SYNONYMS)

Spondylitis ossificans ligamentosa
Spondylosis hyperostotica
Physiologic vertebral ligamentous calcification
Generalized juxtaarticular ossification of vertebral ligaments
(Senile) Ankylosing hyperostosis of the spine
Forestier's disease
Spondylosis deformans
Vertebral osteophytosis

viously eliminates from consideration some patients who have both DISH and "degenerative" disc disease.

Third, as will be discussed subsequently, sacroiliac joint abnormalities do occur in DISH. These abnormalities, which consist of osteophytosis and coexistent osteoarthritis, are associated with sacroiliac joint space narrowing and paraarticular bone bridging. These sacroiliac joint changes should not be confused with those in ankylosing spondylitis, as osseous erosions and intraarticular bone ankylosis are not evident. Furthermore, apophyseal joint space narrowing and sclerosis, particularly in the lumbosacral area, occur in DISH, but bone ankylosis of these joints, which is seen in ankylosing spondylitis, is not observed.

CLINICAL ABNORMALITIES

DISH has long been regarded as a radiographic entity whose clinical manifestations are minor and of little significance. In general, this is true; however, as DISH is not uncommon, many patients with this entity are seen by a rheumatologist or orthopedic surgeon for coexistent rheumatic disorders, and symptoms and signs related to DISH are frequently obscured by the clinical manifestations of the associated diseases. A variety of clinical abnormalities do occur in DISH. Although most appear minor compared with the remarkable alterations apparent on routine radiographs in this disease, some appear to be as specific as the associated radiographic findings.

DISH is a disease of older persons. In reality, the advanced age of these patients with DISH reflects not that the disorder begins in elderly patients but rather that a lengthy period of time is necessary before the spinal abnormalities progress to such a degree that they fulfill specific radiographic criteria. In many patients, musculoskeletal complaints have been noted for many years. DISH predominates in men.

A majority of patients with DISH have symptoms and signs (Table 37–2). The principal musculoskeletal complaints in patients with DISH are spinal stiffness and mild middle to lower back pain, which usually become evident in middle age and may persist for many years. These complaints are initially apparent in the thoracolumbar spine and are characterized as mild intermittent and nonradiating discomfort. Within several years of onset, thoracolumbar spinal stiffness and pain can progress, with involvement of lumbar and cervical segments. Spinal discomfort has been relieved by mild analgesics, such as aspirin or acetaminophen, and local heat.

Cervical dysphagia may be an additional prominent symptom in patients with DISH. Dysphagia is related directly to the presence of prominent cervical osteophytes, particularly those that are located adjacent to areas of normal esophageal fixation, such as at the level of the cricoid cartilage. Cervical dysphagia may improve with conservative therapy; however, if this fails, operative intervention may be necessary.

In general, physical examination reveals little change in normal spinal mechanics, although an occasional slight decrease in lumbar lordosis and a small increase in dorsal kyphosis, as well as mild distortion of spinal mobility in the lower dorsal area, are seen. Uncommon or exceptional findings have been lateral deviation or scoliosis, severe spinal rigidity, and significant restriction of thoracic cage motion.

Clinical abnormalities in the peripheral skeleton occur in approximately 30 per cent of patients with DISH. In those patients with prominent peripheral musculoskeletal symptoms, the shoulders, the knees, the elbows, and the heels are the regions affected most commonly. The pattern of musculoskeletal symptoms in these locations generally is noninflammatory. Tendinitis (particularly appearing as Achilles tendinitis and "tennis elbow") with elbow and heel pain, swelling, erythema, and bone spurs is not uncommon and may require surgical intervention. Close clinical-radiographic correlation is evident; patients with clinically apparent tendinous and osseous problems about bone prominences frequently reveal local osseous proliferation or spurs when examined radiographically.

RADIOGRAPHIC ABNORMALITIES
Spinal Abnormalities

THORACIC SPINE. Radiographic abnormalities of DISH are encountered most commonly in the thoracic spine (Fig. 37–1). They are most frequently apparent between the seventh and eleventh thoracic vertebral bodies and generally decrease in frequency in a craniad direction in the thoracic spine. Laminated calcification and ossification appear along the anterolateral aspect of the vertebral bodies and continue across the intervertebral disc spaces. The deposited bone varies considerably in thickness; when broad, it appears as a radiodense shield in front of the vertebral column. Although ossification may extend to involve both the right and the left lateral aspects of the vertebral column, it is more common and exuberant on the right side, presumably related to an inhibiting effect on ossification by a left-sided, pulsating descending thoracic aorta. Posterior deposition of bone in the thoracic spine is rare. The contour of the involved thoracic spine generally is irregular and bumpy; occasionally examples of a smooth "pseudospondylitic" pattern of ossification may be seen. The bumpy spinal contour is particularly prominent at the level of the intervertebral discs as a result of two processes: increased deposition of bone at the disc space frequently merging with bone excrescences on the superior and inferior margins of the vertebra, and a more anterior position of the deposited bone at the level of the intervertebral disc.

Radiolucent areas within the ossified mass, which are common at the level of the intervertebral discs, correspond to anterolateral extension of disc material. An additional radiolucent lesion in the form of a linear defect is present between the newly deposited bone and the subjacent vertebral body. This radiolucent area may not be apparent at each thoracic level but is usually observed at some level. In some persons, an exaggerated concavity along the anterior aspect of the vertebral body produces a semicircular rather than a linear radiolucent lesion. Thoracic disc space narrowing is generally

Table 37–2. CLINICAL FEATURES FOUND IN SOME PATIENTS WITH DISH

Recurrent Achilles tendinitis
Recurrent "tennis elbow"
Progressive restriction of range of motion
Palpable calcaneal spurs
Palpable olecranon spurs
Nodular masses adherent to quadriceps-patellar tendon
Dysphagia
Restricted motion after total joint replacement

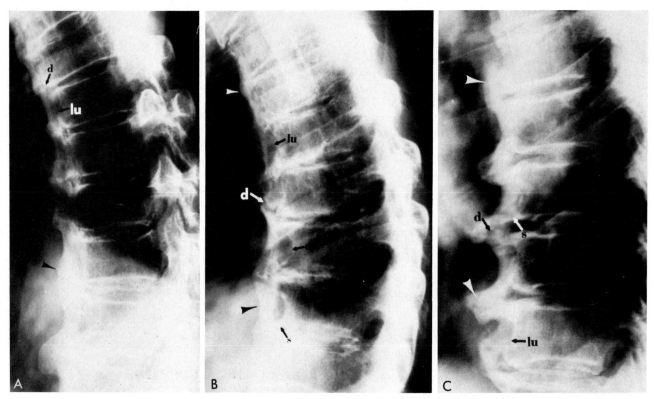

Figure 37–1. Thoracic spine abnormalities in DISH. A Findings include flowing anterior ossification (arrowhead) with a bumpy spinal contour, radiolucent disc extensions (d), and a radiolucent area between the deposited bone and underlying vertebral bodies (lu). **B** Note anterior spinal ossification (arrowheads), radiolucent disc extensions (d), radiolucent areas between deposited bone and subjacent vertebrae (lu), exaggerated anterior vertebral concavity (c), and horizontal bony struts (s). **C** Bumpy spinal contour (arrowheads) reflects anterior hyperostosis with radiolucent disc extensions (d), linear radiolucent areas (lu), and horizontal struts of bone (s). (**A, B,** From Resnick D, et al: Diffuse idiopathic skeletal hyperostosis (DISH) (ankylosing hyperostosis of Forestier and Rotes-Querol). Semin Arthritis Rheum 7:153, 1978; **C,** From Resnick D, Niwayama G: Radiographic and pathologic features of spinal involvement in diffuse idiopathic skeletal hyperostosis (DISH). Radiology 119:559, 1976. Used with permission.)

mild or absent. In fact, the largest amount of bone deposition frequently occurs at levels associated with the smallest degree of disc space loss. Calcification of intervertebral discs and elongation and hyperostosis of spinous processes, with ossification connecting adjacent processes, may also be seen.

CERVICAL SPINE. Cervical spine alterations (Fig. 37–2) are also frequent in DISH. Abnormalities are more common in the lower cervical region (between the fourth and seventh cervical vertebral bodies) than they are in the upper cervical region. Bone excrescences in this area vary from 1 to 12 mm in thickness. The initial finding is hyperostosis of the cortex along the anterior surface of the vertebral body. Gradually, elongated bone outgrowths appear at the anterior margin of the vertebra and extend across the intervertebral disc space. These outgrowths are observed most commonly at the inferior lip of the vertebral body and extend downward. Progressive bone deposition can be either smooth and homogeneous or bumpy and irregular. A flowing pattern of ossification may result, but this ossification frequently is interrupted by radiolucent disc extensions at the level of the intervertebral disc. These disc extensions may isolate a small triangular piece of bone (ossicle) in front of the intervertebral disc space. Radiolucent areas between the deposited bone and underlying vertebral body are less frequent in the cervical spine than in the thoracic spine.

The predilection for anterior deposition of bone in the

cervical spine follows the general distribution of ossification throughout the vertebral column. In the cervical region, however, posterior vertebral abnormalities are not infrequent. These include hyperostosis of the posterior aspect of the vertebral body, posterior spinal osteophytosis, and posterior longitudinal ligament calcification and ossification (see discussion later in this chapter).

LUMBAR SPINE. Lumbar spine abnormalities in DISH are almost as frequent as thoracic spine abnormalities (Fig. 37–3). These findings usually are observed in the upper lumbar region, particularly between the first and third lumbar vertebral bodies. Lumbar changes resemble cervical spine alterations. The deposited bone may vary from 1 to 20 mm in thickness. Additional findings include radiolucent anterior disc extension, occasional radiolucent areas between the deposited bone and the subjacent vertebral body, and the rare occurrence of posterior outgrowths. The predilection for right-sided involvement that is apparent in the thoracic spine is not so obvious in the lumbar region. Close apposition of spinous processes or ossification of interspinous ligaments may also be noted.

Extraspinal Abnormalities (Table 37–3)

Extraspinal radiographic manifestations of DISH are not only frequent but also distinctive, allowing accurate diagnosis of this disorder even in the absence of appropriate spinal

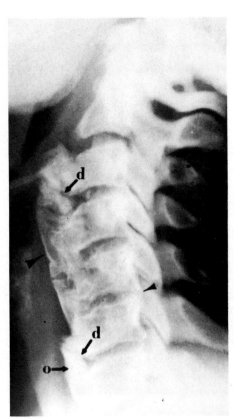

Figure 37–2. Cervical spine abnormalities in DISH. A bony shield (large arrowhead) is evident along the cervical spine. Note also radiolucent disc extensions (d), bone ossicle (o) in front of the intervertebral disc, small posterior osteophytes (small arrowhead), and relatively intact apophyseal joints. (From Resnick D, Niwayama G: Radiographic and pathologic features of spinal involvement in diffuse idiopathic skeletal hyperostosis. Radiology 119:559, 1976. Used with permission.)

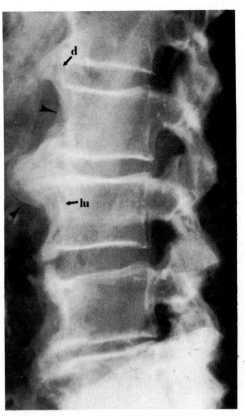

Figure 37–3. Lumbar spine abnormalities in DISH. Severe abnormalities include anterior linear ossification (arrowheads) and radiolucent areas, both beneath the deposited bone (lu) and at the level of the intervertebral disc (d). (From Resnick D, et al: Diffuse idiopathic skeletal hyperostosis (DISH) (ankylosing hyperostosis of Forestier and Rotes-Querol). Semin Arthritis Rheum 7:153, 1978. Used with permission.)

radiographs. Such manifestations can occur at virtually any skeletal site, although they are most characteristic in certain locations. Typically, they have a bilateral and symmetric distribution.

PELVIS (FIG. 37–4). Pelvic abnormalities are common in DISH and consist of bone proliferation or "whiskering," ligament calcification and ossification, and paraarticular osteophytes. Proliferation (whiskering) is seen at sites of ligament and tendon attachment to bone, particularly the iliac crest, ischial tuberosity, and trochanters, and is not unlike that occurring in ankylosing spondylitis, although, in the latter disease, bone erosion and poorly defined bone deposition are more characteristic. Ligament calcification and ossification occur in the iliolumbar and sacrotuberous ligaments. Paraarticular osteophytes are noted along the inferior aspect of the

Table 37–3. COMMON SITES OF EXTRASPINAL ABNORMALITY IN DISH*

Pelvis
Heel
Foot
Elbow
Hand, wrist
Knee

*In order of decreasing frequency.

sacroiliac joint, lateral acetabulum, and superior pubic margins, where they may restrict motion and produce paraarticular osseous bridging.

HEEL (FIG. 37–5). Enthesophytes on the posterior and inferior surfaces of the calcaneus are frequent in patients with DISH. They are of variable size, although frequently they are large; multiple spurs on either or both aspects of the calcaneus may be observed. These spurs are well demarcated and irregular in outline. They are apparent at the sites of calcaneal attachment of the Achilles tendon and plantar aponeurosis. The cortex of the posterior and inferior surfaces of the calcaneus may appear diffusely thickened.

FOOT. Bone excrescences of the foot in patients with DISH show predilection for the dorsal surface of the talus, dorsal and medial portions of the tarsal navicular bone, and lateral and plantar aspects of the cuboid and base of the fifth metatarsal bone. Hyperostosis on the talus may result in a talar beak reminiscent of outgrowths occurring at the same site in patients with tarsal coalition or athletic injuries. Phalangeal changes may take the form of irregular periostitis and tuftal enlargement of the terminal phalanges, simulating the changes in acromegaly.

PATELLA AND KNEE (FIG. 37–6). Patellar and peripatellar alterations occur in DISH. These include ligamentous ossification within the quadriceps mechanism with anterior patellar hyperostosis and irregularities of the tibial tuberosity. Furthermore, prominence of the tibial spines has been reported as a very frequent finding of DISH.

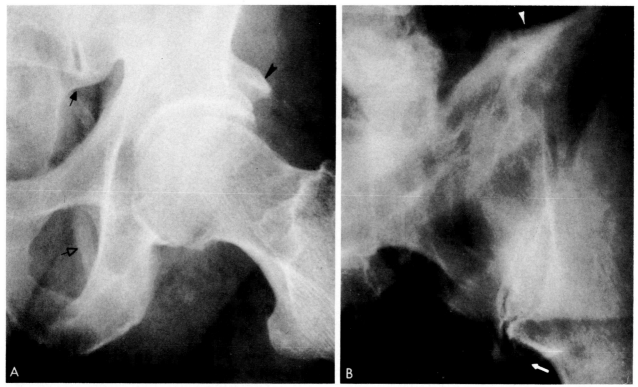

Figure 37–4. Pelvic abnormalities in DISH. A Note sacrotuberous ligament ossification (open arrow), paraarticular sacroiliac joint osteophytes (solid arrow), and irregular bone excrescences above the acetabulum (arrowhead). **B** Radiographic abnormalities include paraarticular osteophytes about the sacroiliac joint (arrow) and iliolumbar ligament ossification (arrowhead). (**A, B,** From Resnick D, et al: Diffuse idiopathic skeletal hyperostosis (DISH) (ankylosing hyperostosis of Forestier and Rotes-Querol). Semin Arthritis Rheum 7:153, 1978. Used with permission.)

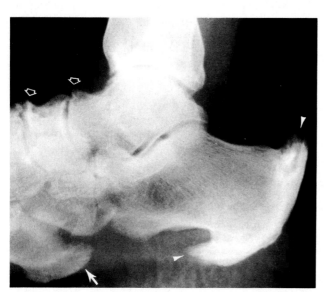

Figure 37–5. Heel abnormalities in DISH. Peculiar osseous excrescences (arrowheads) project from the plantar and posterior aspects of the calcaneus and are associated with dorsal bone outgrowths (open arrows) and irregularity and enlargement of the base of the fifth metatarsal bone (solid arrow). (Courtesy of G. Greenway, M.D., Dallas, Texas.)

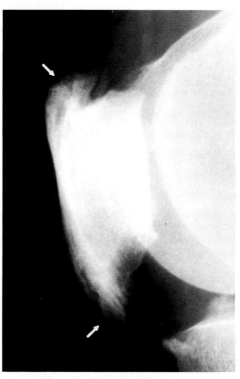

Figure 37–6. Patella abnormalities in DISH. Osseous proliferation has resulted in thickening of the anterior patellar surface with excrescences extending from its superior and inferior margins into the adjacent ligaments (arrows).

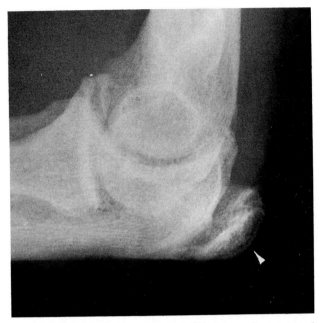

Figure 37–7. Elbow abnormalities in DISH. A large olecranon spur is evident (arrowhead). (From Resnick D, et al: Diffuse idiopathic skeletal hyperostosis (DISH) (ankylosing hyperostosis of Forestier and Rotes-Querol). Semin Arthritis Rheum 7:153, 1978. Used with permission.)

ADDITIONAL LOWER EXTREMITY SITES. Additional sites of hyperostosis in the lower extremity are evident in DISH. Findings include bone formation along the posterior or medial aspect of the femur, osseous bridging between the lateral proximal tibia and fibular head, bone protuberances along apposing surfaces of the tibia and fibula at the site of attachment of the interosseous membrane, and hyperostosis in the proximal medial tibia and about the ankle.

ELBOW (FIG. 37–7). Olecranon spurs are frequent, well defined, and occasionally of considerable size.

SHOULDER AND HUMERUS. Findings in these locations may include prominence and exaggerated bone irregularity along the deltoid tuberosity and greater tuberosity, medial humeral shaft, inferior glenoid, inferior distal clavicle, and osseous attachments of the coracoclavicular ligament.

HAND AND WRIST. Broadening of the distal phalangeal tufts, increased cortical width of tubular bones, enlarged sesamoid bones, hyperostosis along the distal end of the radius and the metacarpal and phalangeal heads, and bone formation in the articular capsule are seen. Although the changes resemble those of acromegaly, soft tissue and cartilage hypertrophy are not evident in DISH but are characteristic of acromegaly.

ADDITIONAL UPPER EXTREMITY SITES. Irregularities at the site of attachment of the interosseous membrane along apposing surfaces of radius and ulna may be evident.

SKULL. Hyperostosis frontalis interna is observed occasionally.

PATHOLOGIC ABNORMALITIES
Thoracic Spine Abnormalities

The pathologic aberrations of thoracic spine involvement in DISH can be separated conveniently into three types, which occur simultaneously.

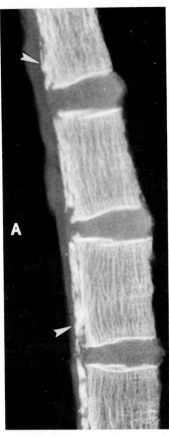

Figure 37–8. Pathologic abnormalities of the thoracic spine in DISH, type I changes. On a radiograph of a sagittal section of a thoracic spine, note ribbon-like calcification (arrowheads) along the anterior (A) surface of the vertebral bodies. This represents calcific deposits within the anterior longitudinal ligament (arrowheads). (From Resnick D, Niwayama G: Radiographic and pathologic features of spinal involvement in diffuse idiopathic skeletal hyperostosis (DISH). Radiology 119:559, 1976. Used with permission.)

TYPE I ABNORMALITIES. These changes are purely ligamentous in nature and do not depend on discogenic abnormalities (Fig. 37–8). Initially, shaggy, ribbon-like calcification or ossification within the anterior longitudinal ligament is noted adjacent to the anterior aspect of the vertebral body. These calcified collections enlarge and extend across the intervertebral disc space. A radiolucent area generally is recognized between the calcified and ossified deposits and the underlying vertebral body. This lucent region, which reflects unossified portions of the anterior longitudinal ligament, eventually may be obliterated segmentally as the ossified ligament fuses with the subjacent vertebral body.

TYPE II ABNORMALITIES. These changes, which are identical to those of spondylosis deformans (see Chapter 36), are associated with intervertebral disc alterations, particularly within the anulus fibrosus. Discoloration, fissures, and tears appear in this area and are associated with anterior expansion of disc material. These disc extensions create radiolucent areas within the ossified mass.

TYPE III ABNORMALITIES. New bone formation in the midanterior portion of the vertebral body is seen (Fig. 37–9). This site represents the enthesis at which the anterior longitudinal ligament is attached to bone. Ossification pro-

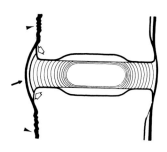

A

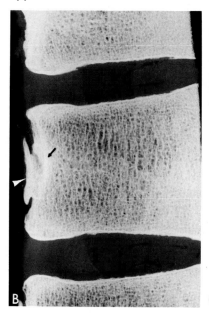

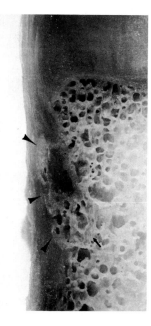

B   C

Figure 37–9. Pathologic abnormalities of the thoracic spine in DISH, type III abnormalities—sagittal sections. **A** Bone formation occurs in the middle of the anterior surface of the vertebral body (arrowheads) where the anterior longitudinal ligament (solid arrow) is attached to the vertebral surface. Open arrows indicate Sharpey's fibers. **B, C** Early stage. Osseous proliferation (arrowheads) in the anterior surface of the vertebral body is seen. Mild sclerosis (arrows) in the vertebral body is also apparent.

gresses within the ligament and eventually sweeps across the intervertebral disc.

Lumbar Spine Abnormalities

In the lumbar spine (and presumably in the cervical spine) pathologic changes most resemble spondylosis deformans. Anulus defects, protrusion of disc material, elevation of the outer anular fibers, and traction osteophytes are sequential abnormalities.

Late Thoracolumbar Spinal Abnormalities

The appearance of a spine that is severely involved is striking. A shell of bone extends across the anterior surface of the vertebral column. In the thoracic spine it predominates on the right side, and in the lumbar spine, both right and left sides of the vertebral body may be involved equally.

The bumpy spinal contour in DISH reflects the increased thickness of deposited bone at the level of the intervertebral disc and, to a lesser extent, the varying thickness of periosteal bone formation at each vertebral level. The radiolucent areas at the level of the intervertebral discs reflect unossified protruded portions of disc material, primarily anulus fibrosus. The radiolucent linear shadows beneath the deposited bone indicate that the deeper portion of the anterior longitudinal ligament is not completely ossified.

Extraspinal Abnormalities

Findings in the peripheral skeleton include hyperostosis at sites of tendon and ligament attachment to bone (pelvis,

trochanters, calcaneus, olecranon, patella, dorsum of the foot), paraarticular osteophytes (sacroiliac joint, acetabulum, symphysis pubis), and ligament ossification (sacrotuberous, iliolumbar). Tendons reveal fraying and irregularity, perhaps related to repetitive stress or trauma. Tendon necrosis with dystrophic calcification is apparent. Enthesophytes arising at the site of osseous attachment of the tendon are more prominent than true calcification of the tendon itself.

CLINICAL AND RADIOGRAPHIC COMPLICATIONS
Postoperative Heterotopic Ossification (Fig. 37–10)

Heterotopic ossification has been reported to occur after hip and knee surgery in patients with DISH, although the finding remains controversial. Postoperative heterotopic ossification may represent one additional indication of a boneforming tendency in patients with DISH, although local environmental factors, including infection and hemorrhage, may be important in initiating such ossification. A similar tendency for heterotopic bone formation in the postoperative period has been noted in patients with ankylosing spondylitis, another disorder characterized by deposition of bone in the vertebral column.

Rheumatoid Arthritis

Rheumatoid arthritis and DISH may not be causally related, but they are both common disorders and can coexist in the same patient. Although the articular distribution of radiographic abnormalities in such patients is typical for rheumatoid arthritis, atypical radiographic features of rheu-

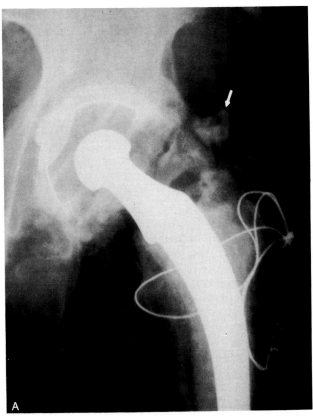

Figure 37–10. Heterotopic ossification in DISH. After a total hip arthroplasty, extensive ossification is seen lateral to the femoral prosthesis (arrow). (From Resnick D, et al: Diffuse idiopathic skeletal hyperostosis (DISH) (ankylosing hyperostosis of Forestier and Rotes-Querol). Semin Arthritis Rheum 7:153, 1978. Used with permission.)

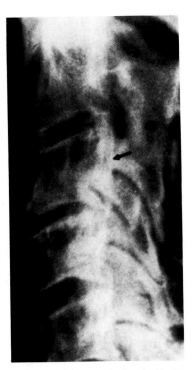

Figure 37–11. Ossification of the posterior longitudinal ligament (OPLL) and DISH. Note calcification and ossification of the posterior longitudinal ligament in the cervical spine (arrow). (B, From Resnick D, et al: Association of diffuse idiopathic skeletal hyperostosis (DISH) and calcification and ossification of the posterior longitudinal ligament. AJR 131:1049, 1978. Copyright 1978, American Roentgen Ray Society. Used with permission.)

matoid arthritis may be encountered, including the absence of osteoporosis and the presence of bone sclerosis and proliferation about erosions, osteophytes, and intraarticular bone ankylosis. Hyperostosis and other atypical radiographic features of rheumatoid arthritis may be observed in patients without spinal excrescences; however, it appears reasonable to speculate that bone production might occur about involved articulations in patients with both rheumatoid arthritis and DISH, as DISH is characterized by bone proliferation at sites of stress.

Ossification of the Posterior Longitudinal Ligament (OPLL) (Fig. 37–11)

Ossification of the posterior longitudinal ligament, which is discussed in detail in Chapter 38, occurs with increased frequency in patients with DISH. In almost all instances, it is the cervical spine that is affected. The association of OPLL and DISH may explain, in part, the occasional appearance of neurologic findings in patients with DISH.

Spinal Stenosis

Some reports have indicated the occurrence of spinal cord compression in patients with DISH. The level and the cause of such compression vary. Compromise of the cord in the cervical region can relate to hyperostosis or ossification of spinal ligaments, whereas such compromise in the thoracic and lumbar regions may be secondary to hypertrophy of the ligamentum flavum or bone proliferation about the apophyseal articulations.

Fracture (Fig. 37–12)

Ankylosing diseases of the spine theoretically predispose the vertebral column to acute fracture and possible pseudarthrosis. These complications are well recognized in ankylosing

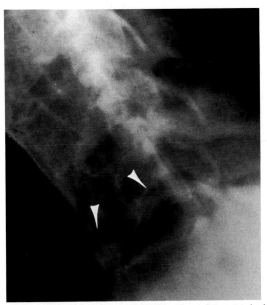

Figure 37–12. Spinal fractures and DISH. After a fall on his back and head, this 59 year old man developed considerable pain. A transverse fracture (arrowheads) through the ankylosed cervical spine is evident. (Courtesy of K. Kattan, M.D., Dayton, Ohio.)

spondylitis. Available reports indicate that fractures also occur in moderate to severe cases of DISH in which osseous fusion of long segments of the spine is present. The ankylosed region is vulnerable to fracture, even with relatively minor trauma; transverse fractures are typical, resembling those in the tubular bones of the extremities. The cervical and thoracic segments appear more susceptible than the lumbar segment. Significant neurologic complications, including quadriplegia, are related, in part, to spinal instability and delay in both diagnosis and treatment.

Apparently there are differences in the appearance of spinal fractures in ankylosing spondylitis and DISH, which are related to their patterns of ossification. In ankylosing spondylitis, the fracture line commonly traverses the intervertebral disc, rather than the vertebral body, as the slender, vertically oriented syndesmophytes represent the weakest portion of the fused spine. In DISH, it is the midportion of the vertebral body that is disrupted, as the thinnest or least dense region of the hyperostosis commonly occurs in this area.

ETIOLOGY

The cause of DISH is unknown. One common factor in patients with DISH is advanced age. Some patients relate a history of spinal trauma or occupational stress; others have no history of significant accidental or occupational trauma.

Because the spinal outgrowths in DISH are similar in appearance to those in a variety of other disorders, it seems attractive to relate these abnormalities of DISH to those in other disorders. Bone hyperostosis of the spine accompanies endocrine diseases such as acromegaly, hypoparathyroidism, and diabetes mellitus. There is no strong evidence, however, to support a link between any of these diseases and DISH. Alterations in glucose metabolism are frequent in DISH, and many patients with DISH have laboratory evidence of diabetes mellitus. This association, however, may be related to a chance occurrence of both disorders in older patients. The occurrence of spinal and extraspinal hyperostosis resembling that of DISH has been reported in association with the administration of a vitamin A derivative (13-cis-retinoic acid) to patients with cutaneous disorders; however, no convincing evidence connecting hyperostosis in DISH with hypervitaminosis A has yet been accumulated. Thus, at the present time, the cause of DISH remains unknown.

DIFFERENTIAL DIAGNOSIS

Although clinical and radiographic features of DISH are characteristic (Tables 37–2 and 37–4), certain other disorders enter into the differential diagnosis of this condition.

Table 37–4. RADIOGRAPHIC ABNORMALITIES IN DISH

Spinal
  Anterolateral flowing ossification
  Bumpy spinal contour
  Radiolucent disc extension
  Radiolucent area beneath deposited bone

Extraspinal
  Bone proliferation
  Ligament calcification, ossification
  Paraarticular osteophytes

Table 37–5. SOME CONDITIONS ASSOCIATED WITH OR CAUSING BONE OUTGROWTHS OF THE SPINE

DISH
Spondylosis deformans
Ankylosing spondylitis
Other seronegative spondyloarthropathies
Acromegaly
Hypoparathyroidism
Fluorosis
Ochronosis
Neuroarthropathy
Trauma
Sternocostoclavicular hyperostosis

Spinal Abnormalities

DISH must obviously be distinguished from other disorders of the vertebral column associated with hyperostosis (Tables 37–5 and 37–6).

INTERVERTEBRAL (OSTEO)CHONDROSIS. The changes of intervertebral (osteo)chondrosis (vacuum phenomena, disc space narrowing, reactive bone sclerosis, and cartilaginous nodes) (see Chapter 36) differ considerably from those of DISH.

SPONDYLOSIS DEFORMANS. Type II thoracic spine alterations in DISH include findings consistent with spondylosis deformans (see Chapter 36). Cleft-like defects in the anulus fibrosus, prolapse of the intervertebral disc material, and pointed bone excrescences at the vertebral body–intervertebral disc junction are present in both DISH and spondylosis deformans. The degree of disc prolapse, the size and number of osteophytes, the presence of ligamentous calcification or ossification, and the occurrence of a proliferative enthesopathy distinguish DISH from typical spondylosis deformans.

ANKYLOSING SPONDYLITIS (FIG. 37–13). The clinical, radiographic, and pathologic features of ankylosing spondylitis differ from those of DISH (see Chapter 24). Ankylosing spondylitis affects predominantly young adults, producing considerable signs and symptoms; DISH affects middle-aged and elderly patients and may be asymptomatic or associated with mild to moderate restriction of motion. In ankylosing spondylitis, syndesmophytes are thin, vertical osseous bridges that extend from one vertebral body to the next. They represent ossification within the peripheral portion of the anulus fibrosus. Ossification of the anterior longitudinal ligament and adjacent connective tissue generally is not apparent. DISH produces exuberant bone formation encompassing anulus, anterior longitudinal ligament, and connective tissue. Outgrowths are broad and irregular, with an anterior distribution. Furthermore, ankylosing spondylitis is characterized by vertebral body osteitis, producing erosion and reactive sclerosis along the anterior corners of the vertebra; sacroiliac joint erosion, sclerosis, and intraarticular bone ankylosis; and apophyseal joint ankylosis. These manifestations are absent in DISH.

OTHER SERONEGATIVE SPONDYLOARTHROPATHIES (FIG. 37–14). Psoriasis, Reiter's syndrome, and bowel disorders such as ulcerative colitis, regional enteritis, and Whipple's disease are associated with bone abnormalities of the vertebral column (see Chapters 25 to 27). In psoriasis and, to a lesser extent, in Reiter's syndrome, such abnormalities consist of (1) outgrowths that may resemble typical

Table 37–6. DIFFERENTIAL DIAGNOSIS OF RADIOGRAPHIC FINDINGS IN DISH, ANKYLOSING SPONDYLITIS, AND INTERVERTEBRAL (OSTEO)CHONDROSIS

Site	DISH	Ankylosing Spondylitis	Intervertebral (Osteo)chondrosis
Vertebral bodies	Flowing ossification and hyperostosis; large osteophytes; bone ankylosis frequent radiographically, less frequent pathologically	Thin syndesmophytes; osteitis with "squaring"; extensive bone ankylosis radiographically and pathologically	Sclerosis of superior and inferior surfaces
Intervertebral discs	Normal or mild decrease in height	Normal or convex in shape	Moderate to severe decrease in height; vacuum phenomena
Apophyseal joints	Normal or mild sclerosis; occasional osteophytes	Erosions; sclerosis; bone ankylosis	Normal
Sacroiliac joints	Paraarticular osteophytes	Erosions; sclerosis; bone ankylosis	Normal
Peripheral skeleton	"Whiskering"; paraarticular osteophytes; ligament calcification and ossification; hyperostosis	"Whiskering"; arthritis	Normal

syndesmophytes of ankylosing spondylitis, (2) asymmetric osteophytes, or (3) paravertebral ossification. In some instances bone formation in these two disorders may resemble DISH, although an anterior linear pattern of ossification usually is not apparent. In general, outgrowths in psoriasis and Reiter's syndrome are better demonstrated on frontal radiographs rather than on lateral radiographs. Also, paravertebral ossification in these two disorders generally is farther from the vertebral surface than the new bone formation in DISH. In bowel disorders, spinal alterations resemble typical syndes-

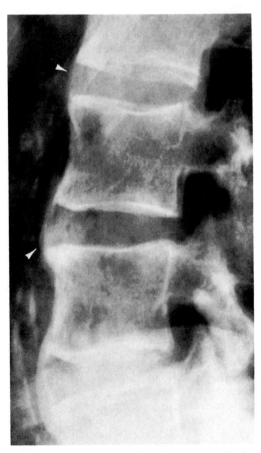

Figure 37–13. Ankylosing spondylitis. Classic radiographic features include squaring of vertebral bodies, osteitis or "whitening" of the vertebral corners, and syndesmophytes (arrowheads). (From Resnick D, et al: Diffuse idiopathic skeletal hyperostosis (DISH) (ankylosing hyperostosis of Forestier and Rotes-Querol). Semin Arthritis Rheum 7:153, 1978. Used with permission.)

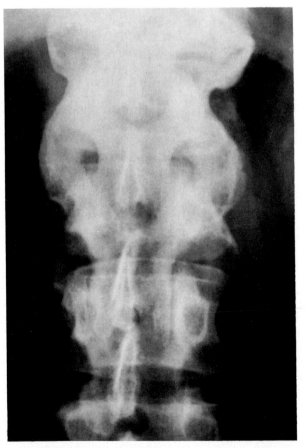

Figure 37–14. Psoriatic arthritis. Spinal involvement is characterized by bulky ossification about multiple lumbar intervertebral discs. (From Resnick D, et al: Diffuse idiopathic skeletal hyperostosis (DISH) (ankylosing hyperostosis of Forestier and Rotes-Querol). Semin Arthritis Rheum 7:153, 1978. Used with permission.)

mophytes and are more slender and delicate than abnormal bone formation in DISH. In psoriasis, Reiter's syndrome, and bowel disorders, sacroiliitis, and apophyseal joint alterations allow proper distinction from DISH.

ACROMEGALY. Acromegaly may be associated with osseous outgrowths of the spine (see Chapter 50). Periosteal new bone formation occurs on the anterior and lateral aspects of the vertebral body, producing apparent flattening of the vertebra related to increased anteroposterior diameter. Osteophytes may bridge the intervertebral disc space. Additional spinal findings in acromegaly are posterior concavity or scalloping of the vertebral body and increased intervertebral disc space height. Patients with DISH lack both typical peripheral skeletal manifestations of acromegaly (such as soft tissue hypertrophy and joint space enlargement) and typical clinical features of acromegaly.

HYPOPARATHYROIDISM. Hypoparathyroidism may be associated with spur formation in the presence of a normal intervertebral disc space as well as ossification of muscle and ligamentous insertions (see Chapter 52). Patients with DISH have no history of tetany or convulsions, and serum levels of calcium, phosphorus, alkaline phosphatase, magnesium, and parathyroid hormone are normal.

FLUOROSIS. Fluorosis is associated with severe osteophytosis of the spine and ligament ossification, particularly of the sacrotuberous ligament (see Chapter 65). These findings may resemble those of DISH, a similarity that is further accentuated by the appearance of calcification in paraarticular ligaments, musculotendinous attachments, and interosseous membranes in fluorosis. Bone sclerosis, which in fluorosis is distinctive, is not apparent in DISH. Clinically, patients with chronic fluoride intoxication have vague, poorly localized pains with subsequent involvement of large joints and vertebral column. In addition, patients complain of hyperesthesias of arms and legs, anorexia, and constipation. Advanced physical findings may include severe restriction of axial skeletal mobility.

OCHRONOSIS. This rare disorder is associated with characteristic spinal changes, which include osteophytosis and anterior disc ossification (see Chapter 43). The presence of extensive discal calcification and vertebral body osteoporosis allows accurate diagnosis. Clinically patients with ochronosis complain of stiffness of the spine and large joints. Frequently, distinctive findings include pigmentation of the sclera and cartilage of the ear and nose.

AXIAL NEUROARTHROPATHY. Axial neuroarthropathy can be noted in syphilis, diabetes mellitus, and syringomyelia (see Chapter 69). Initial radiographic findings may simulate intervertebral (osteo)chondrosis with loss of intervertebral disc space and vertebral body marginal sclerosis. Progressive alterations are increasing sclerosis, subluxation, fragmentation, and bizarre osteophytosis. The presence of disc space loss, extreme sclerosis, and subluxation creates a disorganized look, which differs considerably from the findings of DISH.

STERNOCOSTOCLAVICULAR   HYPEROSTOSIS (FIG. 37–15). This rare syndrome can lead to spinal alterations very similar to those of DISH (see Chapter 83). At other spinal locations, the vertebral changes closely resemble the findings of ankylosing spondylitis. In the cervical spine, unique abnormalities consisting of massive new bone formation are identified occasionally. In sternocostoclavicular hy-

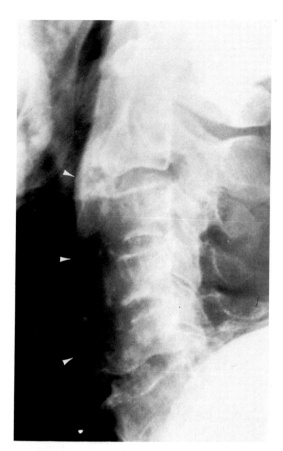

Figure 37–15. Sternocostoclavicular hyperostosis. Exuberant new bone (arrowheads) has developed on the anterior surfaces of the vertebral bodies and intervertebral discs. Note that this obscures the anterior vertebral margins.

perostosis, ossification also affects the medial end of the clavicles, upper ribs, and sternum, and pustular skin lesions are common in the palms and soles.

Extraspinal Abnormalities

Extraspinal manifestations in DISH, such as ligament ossification, paraarticular osteophytes, and hyperostosis, must be distinguished from a variety of other conditions. The importance of making this distinction is twofold:

1. Initial clinical manifestations of DISH may occur in the peripheral skeleton. In such instances radiographs of the axial skeleton are not available, and changes in extraspinal sites must be properly distinguished from abnormalities accompanying other skeletal disorders.

2. It is probable that DISH can involve the extraspinal skeleton without involving the spine.

Ankylosing Spondylitis and Other Seronegative Spondyloarthropathies. These diseases produce abnormalities at sites of tendon and ligament attachment to bone, particularly about the pelvis and proximal femurs. In ankylosing spondylitis and related disorders, osseous erosion and sclerosis are more prominent, and the newly formed bone is poorly defined and irregular. In DISH, proliferative changes frequently are sharply demarcated, without signs of erosion or underlying bone sclerosis.

Acromegaly. Acromegaly alters the peripheral skeleton. Paraarticular osteophytes and bone hyperostosis may be observed in acromegaly, and tuftal enlargement is particularly characteristic; similar alterations occur in DISH. True articular abnormalities, which do not occur in DISH, are noted in acromegaly.

Hypertrophic Osteoarthropathy. Hypertrophic osteoarthropathy is characterized by symmetric periostitis, particularly of the radius, the ulna, the tibia, and the fibula, with lesser involvement of the femur, the humerus, the metacarpal and the metatarsal bones, and the phalanges (see Chapter 83). This disorder frequently is associated with pulmonary and pleural processes, although its occurrence in patients with chronic liver, renal, gastrointestinal, and cardiac diseases and nasopharyngeal tumors is well documented. Although occasionally patients with DISH demonstrate diaphyseal periostitis, particularly in the femur, the humerus, and the metacarpal bones, which simulates hypertrophic osteoarthropathy, this finding usually is not prominent in DISH. The more commonly observed well-defined paraarticular osteophytes and hyperostosis at sites of tendon attachments in DISH are easily distinguished from the periostitis of hypertrophic osteoarthropathy.

Pachydermoperiostosis. Pachydermoperiostosis, a familial disorder, is characterized by the insidious development of digital clubbing, soft tissue thickening of the legs and forearms, thickening and greasiness of the skin, particularly of the face, excessive sweating, and radiographic evidence of symmetric irregular periosteal new bone formation, showing predilection for the radius, the ulna, the tibia, and the fibula (see Chapter 83). Some of the features in this syndrome simulate those occurring in acromegaly, including thickening of the skin, coarsening of facial structures, and tuftal enlargement. These clinical features are not noted in DISH, nor are the radiographic abnormalities of pachydermoperiostosis strikingly similar to those observed in DISH.

Hypervitaminosis A. Although vitamin A intoxication may be associated with extensive bone formation in cats, it generally does not produce changes in humans that resemble DISH (see Chapter 66). Chronic poisoning may lead to periosteal reaction and no other abnormality of bone. These changes, evident in infants and children, may be associated with permanent deformity of long bones. Of interest, prolonged therapy with retinoid drugs (which are similar chemically to vitamin A) in patients with dermatologic disorders has been associated with skeletal hyperostosis in both the axial skeleton (especially the cervical spine) and the appendicular skeleton (see Chapter 66). No difficulty in differential diagnosis between hypervitaminosis A and DISH is anticipated.

Calcium Pyrophosphate Dihydrate Crystal Deposition Disease. Calcium pyrophosphate dihydrate crystal deposition disease is a common disorder, which may coexist with DISH. One of its radiographic features, tendon calcification, super-ficially resembles the findings of DISH. In DISH, mild to moderate calcification and ossification within the tendon substance are more frequent than widespread tendon calcification, as is observed in calcium pyrophosphate dihydrate crystal deposition disease. Other findings of this crystal deposition disease are characteristic, allowing accurate diagnosis (see Chapter 40).

X-Linked Hypophosphatemic Osteomalacia. This disorder, which is characterized by hypophosphatemia, impaired renal tubular reabsorption of phosphate, and defective calcification of cartilage and bone (see Chapter 48), is associated with an enthesopathy in which exuberant calcification of joint capsules and tendinous and ligamentous insertions becomes evident. Commonly involved sites include the hands and sacroiliac joints, and histologic evaluation documents intratendinous lamellar bone without inflammatory cellular infiltration. Changes in the spine are infrequent and mild.

FURTHER READING

Abiteboul M, Arlet J: Retinol-related hyperostosis. AJR *144*:435, 1985.

Blasinghame JP, Resnick D, Coutts RD, Danzig LA: Extensive spinal osteophytosis as a risk factor for heterotopic bone formation after total hip replacement. Clin Orth *161*:191, 1981.

Bundrick TJ, Cook DE, Resnik CS: Heterotopic bone formation in patients with DISH following total hip replacement. Radiology *155*:595, 1985.

DiGiovanna JJ, Helfgott RK, Gerber LH, Peck GL: Extraspinal tendon and ligament calcification associated with long-term therapy with etretinate. N Engl J Med *315*:1177, 1986.

Forestier J, Rotes-Querol J: Senile ankylosing hyperostosis of the spine. Ann Rheum Dis *9*:321, 1950.

Francois RJ: Vertebral ankylosing hyperostosis: What new bone, where and why? J Rheumatol *10*:837, 1983.

Lee SH, Coleman PE, Hahn FJ: Magnetic resonance imaging of degenerative disk disease of the spine. Radiol Clin North Am *26*:949, 1988.

Littlejohn GO, Urowitz MB, Smythe HA, Keystone EC: Radiographic features of the hand in diffuse idiopathic skeletal hyperostosis (DISH). Comparison with normal subjects and acromegalic patients. Radiology *140*:623, 1981.

Polisson RP, Martinez S, Khoury M, Harrell M, Lyles KW, Friedman N, Harrelson JM, Reisner E, Drezner MK: Calcification of entheses associated with X-linked hypophosphatemic osteomalacia. N Engl J Med *313*:1, 1985.

Resnick D, Niwayama G: Radiographic and pathologic features of spinal involvement in diffuse idiopathic skeletal hyperostosis (DISH). Radiology *119*:559, 1976.

Resnick D, Linovitz RJ, Feingold ML: Postoperative heterotopic ossification in patients with ankylosing hyperostosis of the spine (Forestier's disease). J Rheumatol *3*:313, 1976.

Resnick D, Shaul SR, Robins JM: Diffuse idiopathic skeletal hyperostosis (DISH): Forestier's disease with extraspinal manifestations. Radiology *115*:513, 1975.

Resnick D, Curd J, Shapiro RF, Wiesner KB: Radiographic abnormalities of rheumatoid arthritis in patients with diffuse idiopathic skeletal hyperostosis. Arthritis Rheum *21*:1, 1978.

Resnick D, Guerra J Jr, Robinson CA, Vint VC: Association of diffuse idiopathic skeletal hyperostosis (DISH) and calcification and ossification of the posterior longitudinal ligament. AJR *131*:1049, 1978.

Chapter 38

Calcification and Ossification of the Posterior Spinal Ligaments and Tissues

Donald Resnick, M.D.

Calcification and ossification affect a variety of posterior spinal ligaments and tissues. Ossification of the posterior longitudinal ligament (OPLL) is a characteristic disorder of the spine that may be associated with significant neurologic findings. Its radiographic appearance is diagnostic, consisting of a linear band of ossification along the posterior margin of vertebral bodies and intervertebral discs, particularly in the cervical spine. Arachnoiditis ossificans is a rare condition leading to extensive ossification in the arachnoid membrane, especially in the thoracic spine, and producing significant symptoms and signs in some cases.

Osseous proliferation at the cephalad and caudad attachments of the ligamentum flavum is a frequent finding, which generally is of no significance. When extensive,

however, such ossification in the thoracic spine leads to neurologic manifestations and is accompanied by involvement of nearby tissues and ligaments and, in some cases, diffuse idiopathic skeletal hyperostosis. Calcification in the ligamentum flavum is usually observed in the cervical spine and relates to calcium hydroxyapatite crystal deposition or, more rarely, calcium pyrophosphate dihydrate crystal accumulation. A nodular radiodense collection is the typical radiographic abnormality.

Hyperostosis at the osseous site of attachment of the supraspinous ligament, calcification in the interspinous ligament, and ossification of the ligamentum nuchae are additional abnormalities of the posterior spinal tissues.

Diffuse idiopathic skeletal hyperostosis is a disease that is characterized, in part, by calcification and ossification in the anterior longitudinal ligament of the spine. Although such changes are most frequent in this ligament, other spinal ligaments may calcify or ossify (Table 38–1).

ANATOMIC CONSIDERATIONS (FIG. 38–1)

The posterior longitudinal ligament extends from the axis and membrana tectoria above to the sacrum below, within the vertebral canal. It is attached to the intervertebral discs and the margins of the vertebral bodies and is strung like a

bow over the central, concave portion of the vertebral body. The posterior longitudinal ligament is broad in both the cervical and the thoracic segments; in the lumbar spine, it is relatively thin when related to the vertebral surface but becomes broader at the discal levels. Here, the ligament fuses with the outer fibers of the anulus fibrosus.

The ligamenta flava are attached to the articular capsule of the apophyseal joints and the laminae. The ligaments from each side approximate each other at the base of the spinous process, where small clefts exist, allowing passage of veins. The ligamenta flava are thickest in the lumbar segment,

Table 38–1. CALCIFICATION AND OSSIFICATION OF POSTERIOR SPINAL LIGAMENTS AND TISSUES

Condition	Most Common Spinal Location	Clinical Manifestations	Associated Conditions
Ossification of posterior longitudinal ligament (OPLL)	Cervical	May be present	DISH, OLF
Arachnoiditis ossificans	Thoracic	May be present	
Enthesopathy of ligamenta flava	Thoracic	Absent	
Calcification of ligamenta flava	Cervical	May be present	CPPD crystal deposition disease
Ossification of ligamenta flava (OLF)	Thoracic	May be present	OPLL, DISH
Ossification of ligamentum nuchae	Cervical	Absent	DISH
Enthesopathy of supraspinous ligament	Lumbar	May be present	Baastrup's disease, DISH

DISH, Diffuse idiopathic skeletal hyperostosis; CPPD, calcium pyrophosphate dihydrate.

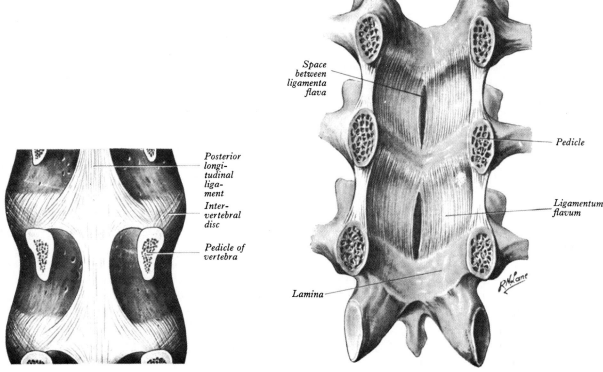

Figure 38–1. Posterior spinal ligaments: Anatomic considerations. A Posterior longitudinal ligament: Lumbar spine. A drawing of the posterior aspect of the vertebral bodies and intervertebral discs shows the position and appearance of the posterior longitudinal ligament. Note that it is narrow at the level of the vertebral bodies and broad at the level of the intervertebral discs. **B** Ligamenta flava: Lumbar spine. A drawing of the anterior aspect of the vertebral arches reveals the position of the paired ligamenta flava. At the bases of the spinous processes, spaces exist between the ligaments allowing the passage of veins. (From Williams PL, Warwick R: Gray's Anatomy. 36th British Ed. Philadelphia, WB Saunders Co, 1980, p 444).

somewhat thinner in the thoracic spine, and thinnest in the cervical region. Composed of yellow elastic tissue, the ligaments allow separation of the laminae during spinal flexion.

The interspinous ligaments extend from the root to the apex of each spinous process, connecting adjoining processes. They meet the ligamenta flava anteriorly and the supraspinous ligament posteriorly. The latter is a strong fibrous structure connecting the apices of the spinous processes from the level of the seventh cervical vertebra to the sacrum. Above this cervical attachment, the ligament expands to form the ligamentum nuchae, which extends cephalad to the external occipital protuberance.

The intertransverse ligaments are located between the transverse processes of the vertebrae.

OSSIFICATION OF THE POSTERIOR LONGITUDINAL LIGAMENT

The association of chronic cervical myelopathy and extensive ossification of the posterior longitudinal ligament (OPLL) was first recorded in Japan in 1960. Subsequent to this report, numerous other patients with OPLL have been discovered, emphasizing that OPLL is both common and widely distributed in the world.

Clinical Abnormalities

OPLL is more frequent in men than in women. The diagnosis of the disorder is usually established in the fifth to seventh decades of life. Although persons with OPLL may be entirely asymptomatic, a variety of clinical manifestations have been associated with this disorder.

Symptoms are initiated by trauma in approximately 20 per cent of cases. Paresthesias may vary from intermittent sensations, including numbness or tingling, to extensive anesthesia of the trunk and lower extremity. Motor disturbances, such as weakness, incoordination, and instability, may be encountered in the upper and lower extremities. Additional symptoms include head and neck pain and stiffness, urinary and rectal incontinence and dysfunction, and loss of libido. On physical examination, patients may reveal muscle atrophy, fasciculations, hyperreflexia, and sensory loss. Laboratory evaluation is usually unrewarding.

Both conservative and surgical methods of treatment have their advocates. The choice of therapy is made difficult by some inconsistency in the relationship between the neurologic manifestations and the degree of ligamentous ossification and by reports of postoperative progression of such ossification.

Radiographic Abnormalities

The diagnosis of OPLL is established by its characteristic radiographic appearance (Figs. 38–2 and 38–3). In the cervical spine, a dense, ossified plaque of variable thickness (1 to 5 mm) is evident along the posterior margins of the vertebral bodies and the intervertebral discs. It is most common in the midcervical region (C3 to C5), although any cervical level may be affected. The ossified ligament may be confined to one or several vertebral bodies, without involve-

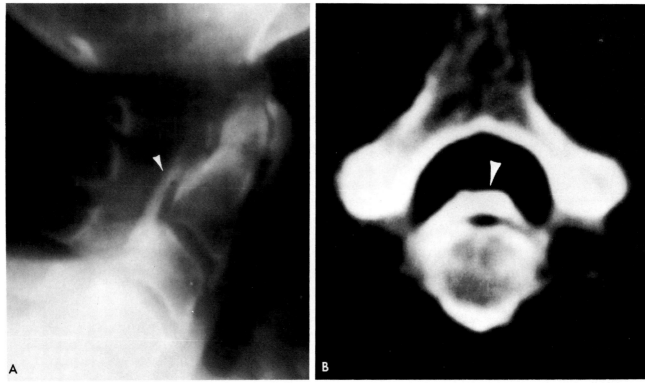

Figure 38–2. Ossification of the posterior longitudinal ligament: Radiographic abnormalities. A A lateral tomogram of the neck outlines characteristic linear ossification of the posterior longitudinal ligament (arrowhead), separated from the vertebral body by a radiolucent area. Proliferative changes on the anterior aspect of several vertebrae, including the first, and possible ossification of the transverse ligament of the atlas are evident. **B** Computed tomography of the neck with the patient prone indicates ossification (arrowhead) posterior to one of the cervical vertebral bodies. A lucent area beneath the ossified ligament is apparent. (Courtesy of J. Mink, M.D., Los Angeles, California.)

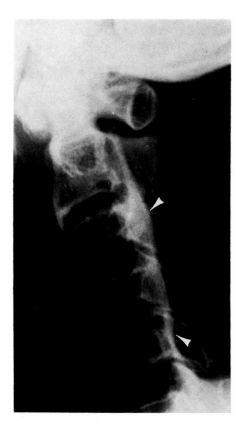

Figure 38–3. Ossification of the posterior longitudinal ligament: Radiographic abnormalities. OPLL extends from the first through sixth cervical vertebral bodies (arrowheads). (From Ono K, et al: Ossified posterior longitudinal ligament. Spine 2:126, 1977. Used with permission.)

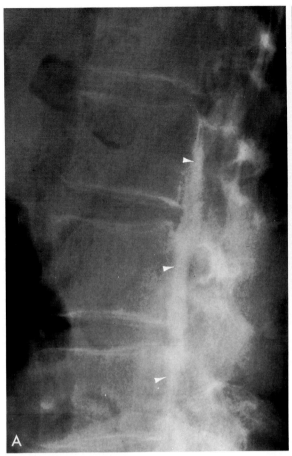

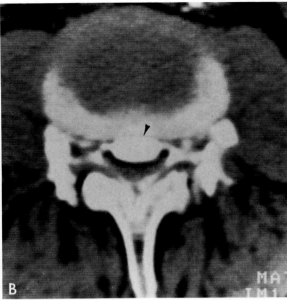

Figure 38–4. Ossification of the posterior longitudinal ligament: Involvement of other ligaments and tissues. **A** The lateral radiograph reveals extensive ossification of the posterior longitudinal ligament (arrowhead) in the lumbar spine. **B** A transaxial computed tomographic image indicates that, in addition to the posterior longitudinal ligament (arrowhead), the dura mater and ligamenta flava are involved.

ment of intervening intervertebral discs (segmental distribution), or extend in an uninterrupted fashion for several vertebrae (continuous distribution). It may be separated from the vertebral body by a thin radiolucent zone. Anterior vertebral osteophytes frequently are identifiable.

OPLL may involve the thoracic and lumbar segments as well. Clinical manifestations related to thoracolumbar ossification may be more severe than those associated with cervical involvement. Often, OPLL in the thoracic and lumbar areas is accompanied by changes in the cervical spine, although isolated involvement in thoracic or lumbar region is common. In the thoracic spine, OPLL is most common in the fourth to seventh thoracic vertebral levels. Involvement in the lumbar spine can be apparent at any level, although changes predominate in the L1 to L2 region (Fig. 38–4). Ossification can also involve the ligamenta flava, capsules of the apophyseal joints, and dura mater. In addition, extensive calcification and ossification along the anterior aspect of the vertebral column may appear.

Pathologic Abnormalities

Bone outgrowth along the posterior aspect of the cervical vertebral bodies predominates in the midline. The adjacent spinal cord exhibits marked flattening owing to compression by the protruded ossified posterior ligament. In places, the ossified mass is attached firmly to the posterior aspect of the vertebral body and intervertebral disc, whereas elsewhere it is separated from these structures by intervening connective tissue.

Etiology and Pathogenesis

The cause of OPLL is not known precisely. In the past, an infectious cause has been suggested but is not proved. Although trauma may lead to formation of spinal osteophytes, an association of OPLL and trauma has not been substantiated. Additional proposed causative factors for OPLL have included fluoride intoxication, diabetes mellitus, localized intervertebral disc abnormality, and an immunologic disorder.

The observation that OPLL is frequent in patients with diffuse idiopathic skeletal hyperostosis (DISH) suggests a common cause and pathogenesis for these conditions. OPLL may be apparent in as many as 50 per cent of cases of DISH; conversely, DISH has been observed in over 20 per cent of cases of OPLL (Fig. 38–5). Both of these disorders are characterized by ligamentous abnormalities that may result in calcification or ossification. In addition, DISH is associated with hyperostosis, bone excrescences, and osteophytosis at multiple skeletal sites, suggesting the presence of an underlying ossifying diathesis.

The association of OPLL with other forms of spinal hyperostosis is also recorded. Ossification of the ligamenta flava can accompany OPLL, and the coexistence of OPLL, DISH (with both spinal and extraspinal manifestations), and ossification of the ligamenta flava is not rare. Ankylosing spondylitis has been seen in approximately 2 per cent of patients with OPLL.

Differential Diagnosis

In spondylosis deformans, osteophytes are most common along the anterolateral aspect of the vertebral column; poste-

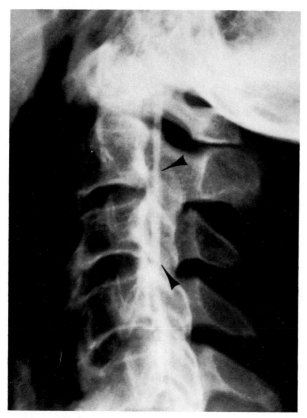

Figure 38–5. Coexistent ossification of the posterior longitudinal ligament and diffuse idiopathic skeletal hyperostosis. Extensive posterior ligamentous ossification (arrowheads) is combined with anterior vertebral changes typical of diffuse idiopathic skeletal hyperostosis.

rior excrescences are absent or of small size. In addition, osteophytes are usually triangular in shape, arising adjacent to the vertebral edge and extending in a horizontal direction. Their appearance, therefore, differs from the linear vertical ossification in OPLL.

In ankylosing spondylitis, syndesmophytes initially form in the outer fibers of the anulus fibrosus. They are vertical in orientation and extend from one vertebral body to the next. Although they may involve the posterior portion of the disc, syndesmophytes are more prominent at anterior and lateral discal margins. Progression of spinal changes in ankylosing spondylitis is associated with extension of ossification into adjacent ligaments and soft tissue; however, linear ossification of the posterior longitudinal ligament generally is not apparent.

In psoriatic (and Reiter's) spondylitis, larger areas of ossification are apparent about the vertebral column, but unlike OPLL, these are most readily apparent on frontal radiographs as asymmetric radiodense areas adjacent to the lateral margins of the vertebrae and intervertebral discs. Similarly, the ossification in DISH bears no resemblance to that of OPLL, although both conditions can occur simultaneously (Fig. 38–5).

Ossification of the transverse ligament of the atlas has been described. A radiodense region is apparent behind the midportion of the odontoid process, which could simulate early stages of OPLL. Additional causes of radiodense areas projected over the spinal canal, such as a protruded calcified

intervertebral disc and calcification within spinal neoplasms or hematomas, do not realistically enter into the different diagnosis of OPLL.

ARACHNOIDITIS OSSIFICANS

Arachnoiditis is an inflammatory process affecting the pia-arachnoid membrane. It is usually observed after spinal surgery or injection of contrast material. Occasionally osseous metaplasia is evident in the dense proliferative collagenous layer, a process called arachnoiditis ossificans.

Arachnoiditis ossificans is seen most commonly in one or more regions of the thoracic spine. Symptoms and signs are variable, although patients with the disorder can be entirely asymptomatic. Plain films may demonstrate linear calcifications and ossifications within the spinal canal; computed tomography demonstrates the plaque-like ossification in the arachnoid membrane.

CALCIFICATION OR OSSIFICATION OF THE LIGAMENTUM FLAVUM

Anatomic studies have verified that osseous proliferation (enthesopathy) in both the cephalad and the caudad attachments of the ligamentum flavum is frequent and, generally, of no clinical significance (Fig. 38–6). At both sites, out-

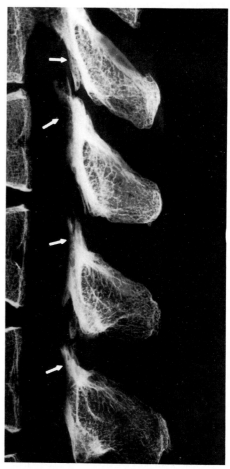

Figure 38–6. Enthesopathy and ossification in the ligamentum flavum. A radiograph of a lateral section of the thoracolumbar segment of the spine delineates osseous proliferation (arrows) at the cephalad and caudad attachments of the ligamenta flava.

growths are small and usually difficult to delineate on plain films and, to a lesser extent, on computed tomograms. The ossifications develop at approximately 20 years of age, remain unchanged for long periods of time, and may diminish in size and frequency in women over the age of 50 years. They appear unrelated to clinical manifestations or the presence of OPLL or DISH.

Extensive calcification or ossification in hypertrophied ligamenta flava has been reported in association with myelopathy or radiculopathy in the cervical, thoracic, and lumbar regions. In the cervical spine, calcification (usually calcium hydroxyapatite in nature) typically occurs in elderly patients, particularly women; the middle cervical region (C3 to C6) is the most common site of involvement. A nodular radiodense collection is the characteristic radiographic abnormality. Myelography may reveal generalized hypertrophy of the ligamentum flavum. The prognosis after surgical removal of the calcific mass is good. In general, the condition is unassociated with calcification or ossification of other spinal ligaments.

In the thoracic spine, ossification (rather than calcification) of the ligamentum flavum predominates. Both men and women are affected, typically in the fifth and sixth decades of life. Neurologic manifestations include decreased sensation, paresis, and even neurogenic bladder. Ossification generally is observed in the lower third of the thoracic spine. Additional ossific deposits frequently are recognized in the posterior longitudinal ligament and, less commonly, in the capsules of the costovertebral and apophyseal articulations, the dura mater, and the interspinous and anterior longitudinal ligaments. Diagnosis is best established by computed tomography.

CPPD crystal deposition disease is a recognized cause of calcification in the ligamentum flavum as well as in other posterior spinal structures, such as the posterior longitudinal ligament, interspinous and supraspinous ligaments, and apophyseal joints (see Chapter 40).

CALCIFICATION OR OSSIFICATION OF OTHER POSTERIOR SPINAL LIGAMENTS

Hyperostosis at the site of attachment of the supraspinous ligament and calcification and ossification within this ligament occur as isolated abnormalities or in association with DISH. Calcification within the interspinous ligament is seen in CPPD crystal deposition disease. Ossification in the ligamentum nuchae is an incidental and frequent radiographic finding that is also seen in DISH.

FURTHER READING

Barthelemy CR: Arachnoiditis ossificans. J Comput Assist Tomogr 6:809, 1982.

Kudo S, Ono M, Russell WJ: Ossification of thoracic ligamenta flava. AJR 141:117, 1983.

Minagi H, Gronner AT: Calcification of the posterior longitudinal ligament: A cause of cervical myelopathy. AJR 105:365, 1969.

Ono K, Ota H, Tada K, Hamada H, Takaoka K: Ossified posterior longitudinal ligament. Spine 2:126, 1977.

Ono M, Russell WJ, Kudo S, Kuroiwa Y, Takamori M, Motomura S, Murakami J: Ossification of the thoracic posterior longitudinal ligament in a fixed population. Radiological and neurological manifestations. Radiology 143:469, 1982.

Resnick D, Pineda C: Vertebral involvement in calcium pyrophosphate dihydrate crystal deposition disease. Radiographic-pathologic correlation. Radiology 153:55, 1984.

Resnick D, Guerra J Jr, Robinson CA, Vint VC: Association of diffuse idiopathic skeletal hyperostosis (DISH) and calcification and ossification of the posterior longitudinal ligament. AJR 131:1049, 1978.

Williams DM, Gabrielsen TO, Latack JT, Martel W, Knake JE: Ossification in the cephalic attachment of the ligamentum flavum. An anatomical and CT study. Radiology 150:423, 1984.

SECTION VI

CRYSTAL-INDUCED AND RELATED DISEASES

CASE VI — LEVEL OF DIFFICULTY: 2

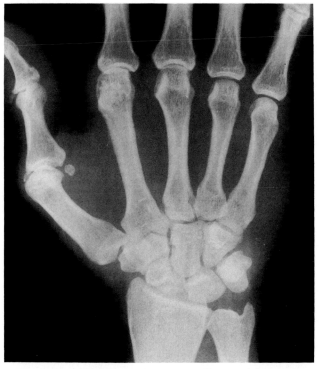

A 70 year old man complained of pain and swelling involving both wrists and the second and third metacarpophalangeal joints in both hands.

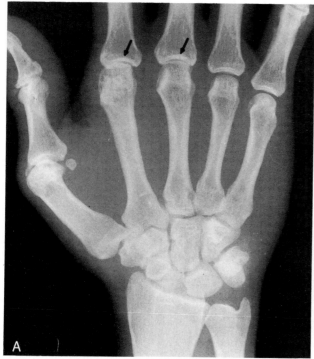 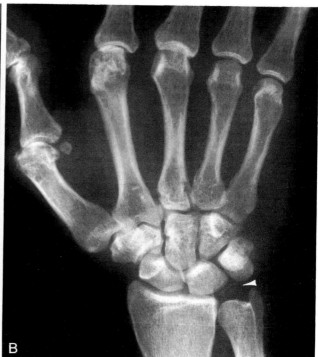

The frontal radiograph of the hand and wrist (A) shows narrowing of the second and third metacarpophalangeal joints (arrows) and, to a lesser extent, the first metacarpophalangeal joint and interphalangeal joint of the thumb. Small cystic areas are evident in the second metacarpal head. Periarticular osteoporosis, marginal erosions of bone, and osteophytes are not seen.

The principal radiographic diagnoses include rheumatoid arthritis, osteoarthritis, gout, and calcium pyrophosphate dihydrate (CPPD) crystal deposition disease. The first of these, rheumatoid arthritis, can be eliminated quickly owing to the absence of osseous erosions about the affected metacarpophalangeal joints. Furthermore, the wrist appears normal, with no evidence of soft tissue swelling about the outer aspect of the ulnar styloid process.

Although osteoarthritis can lead to narrowing of one or more metacarpophalangeal joints, this disorder is more frequent in women, and the diagnosis cannot be established without evidence of articular space narrowing and osteophytes about proximal or distal interphalangeal joints. Similarly, the classic features of gouty arthritis, consisting of lobulated soft tissue swelling, eccentric well-defined osseous erosions, and relative preservation of joint space, are not apparent.

CPPD crystal deposition disease represents the most likely cause of the abnormalities depicted in A. This disorder predominates in middle-aged and elderly men and women, and it commonly affects the hand and wrist. Although abnormal calcification, including cartilage calcification or chondrocalcinosis, represents an important radiographic clue to the diagnosis of this disorder, it is not uniformly evident. Structural abnormalities of the joint, termed pyrophosphate

arthropathy, may occur in the absence of radiographically visible chondrocalcinosis. Such abnormalities predominate in the second and third metacarpophalangeal joints as well as the wrist and knee, and they typically are bilateral and relatively symmetric in distribution. Pyrophosphate arthropathy leads to joint space narrowing that may be accompanied by subchondral cysts and, eventually, bone fragmentation and osteophytosis.

Hemochromatosis may be associated with CPPD crystal deposition and metacarpophalangeal joint abnormalities similar to those shown in A. In hemochromatosis, however, the fourth and fifth metacarpophalangeal articulations also are frequently affected.

A radiograph obtained 9 years later (B) reveals further loss of space in the metacarpophalangeal joints as well as mild ulnar subluxation of the proximal phalanges in the second and third digits. Of interest, abnormal calcification (arrowhead) in the triangular fibrocartilage of the wrist is now evident, confirming the diagnosis.

FINAL DIAGNOSIS: CPPD crystal deposition disease.

FURTHER READING

Pages 477 to 496 and the following:

1. Martel W, Champion CK, Thompson GR, Carter TL: A roentgenologically distinctive arthropathy in some patients with the pseudogout syndrome. AJR 190:587, 1970.
2. Resnick D, Niwayama G, Goergen TG, Utsinger PV, Shapiro RF, Haselwood BH, Wiesner KB: Clinical, radiographic and pathologic abnormalities in calcium pyrophosphate dihydrate deposition disease (CPPD): Pseudogout. Radiology 122:1, 1977.

Chapter 39

Monosodium Urate Crystal Deposition Disease (Gout)

Donald Resnick, M.D.
Gen Niwayama, M.D.

Gouty arthritis, which produces asymmetric polyarticular involvement, affects predominantly the feet, hands, wrists, elbows, and knees. Radiographic manifestations occur late in the course of the disease and include lobulated eccentric soft tissue masses, intraarticular and extraarticular bone erosions, relative preservation of the interosseous joint space, *subperiosteal apposition of bone, intraosseous calcification, and secondary degenerative alterations. Osteoporosis generally is lacking. These radiographic features are, in most instances, readily differentiated from those of other articular disorders.*

Famous and influential people have suffered from the ravages of gout throughout history. The radiographic manifestations of gouty arthritis are well known and are summarized in this chapter.

CLINICAL FEATURES

The biochemical hallmark of the disease is hyperuricemia, which may develop owing to an excessive rate of production of uric acid, a decrease in renal excretion of uric acid, or a combination of the two. Traditionally gout has been classified into two types: (1) *primary gout*, in which the underlying hyperuricemia is the result of an inborn error of metabolism, and (2) *secondary gout*, in which hyperuricemia is a consequence of any of a number of other disorders. More recently it has been observed that a variety of metabolic defects account for hyperuricemia and clinical disease among patients with so-called primary gout. Therefore, it has been suggested that a more meaningful classification system would separate patients with idiopathic gout, which includes the vast majority of persons with the disease, from those in whom the disease is associated with known disorders or enzymatic defects (Table 39–1).

Idiopathic gout occurs far more frequently in men than in women (~20 to 1). The first attack of arthritis most frequently occurs during the fifth decade of life in men and in the postmenopausal period in women. A much higher frequency of disease is found among inhabitants of the Mariana Islands and the Maori of New Zealand. Gout is relatively infrequent in black patients. The hereditary nature of hyperuricemia and gout is well known, the reported familial incidence varying from 6 to 80 per cent.

Idiopathic gout may be divided into several stages.

Asymptomatic Hyperuricemia

Many individuals have hyperuricemia for prolonged periods of time with no symptoms or signs. Urolithiasis or articular attacks of gout mark the end of this phase of the disease.

Table 39–1. CLASSIFICATION OF HYPERURICEMIA AND GOUT*

I. Idiopathic gout
II. Gout associated with other clinical disorders
  A. Hereditary diseases
    1. With excess purine synthesis
      a. Glycogen storage disease, type I (glucose-6-phosphatase deficiency)
      b. X-linked uric aciduria (hypoxanthine-guanine phosphoribosyltransferase [PRT] deficiency)
        1. Lesch-Nyhan syndrome with virtually complete PRT deficiency
        2. Gout with incomplete PRT deficiency
      c. Possible phosphoribosylpyrophosphate amidotransferase deficiency
      d. Mental retardation with autistic behavior
      e. Encephalopathy
    2. With diminished renal clearance of uric acid
      a. Hereditary nephropathy
      b. Glycogen storage disease, type I
    3. Undetermined
      a. Down's syndrome
      b. Vasopressin-resistant nephrogenic diabetes insipidus
  B. Hematologic disorders
    1. Hemolytic disease
    2. Myeloproliferative disease
  C. Endocrine abnormalities
    1. Hypothyroidism
    2. Hypoparathyroidism
    3. Hyperparathyroidism
  D. Vascular disease
    1. Hypertension
    2. Myocardial infarction
  E. Renal disease
    1. Glomerulonephritis and pyelonephritis
    2. Lead poisoning as late effect
  F. Miscellaneous disorders—obesity, starvation, psoriasis, idiopathic hypercalciuria
III. Drug-induced gout

*From Seegmiller JE: Diseases of purine and pyrimidine metabolism. *In* PK Bondy, LE Rosenberg (Eds): Metabolic Control and Disease. 8th Ed. Philadelphia, WB Saunders Co, 1979, p 780. Used with permission.

Acute Gouty Arthritis

Early in the course of gouty arthritis the disorder is usually monoarticular or oligoarticular. Gout has predilection for the joints of the lower extremity, particularly the first metatarsophalangeal and intertarsal joints, ankles, and knees. The onset and severity of arthritis in acute gout are often dramatic. Pain, tenderness, and swelling occur within several hours and may persist for days to weeks.

Interval Phase of Gout (Intercritical Gout)

An asymptomatic period between gouty attacks may last from months to years. Eventually the recovery between acute attacks becomes incomplete.

Chronic Tophaceous Gout

Chronic gouty arthritis occurs in fewer than one half of patients who experience recurrent acute attacks. Visible tophaceous deposits may be noted within a few years of the initial attack, although the average duration is approximately 12 years. Tophi commonly occur in the synovium and subchondral bone and frequently are noted on the helix of the ear and in the subcutaneous and tendinous tissues of the elbow, hand, foot, knee, and forearm. These deposits may ulcerate with extrusion of chalky masses or urate crystals.

GENERAL PATHOLOGIC FEATURES
Acute Gouty Arthritis

The demonstration of monosodium urate crystals in the synovial fluid is the major criterion for the diagnosis of gouty arthritis. Urate crystals are needle-shaped, with strong negative birefringence when examined under polarized light. During acute attacks of gout, these crystals may be present in large numbers, many within leukocytes in the synovial fluid. Microcrystals of monosodium urate are capable of evoking an acute inflammatory response in the skin, subcutaneous tissues, and joints.

Synovitis in gout is accompanied by a nonspecific inflammatory response in the synovial membrane. Crystals can be identified in detached lining cells and other macrophages and within leukocytes in the synovial fluid.

Chronic Tophaceous Gout

In chronic tophaceous gout, monosodium urate deposition occurs in the articular cartilage, subchondral bone, synovial membrane, and capsular and periarticular tissues. In cartilage, the initial deposits are located within the superficial layers. Nonspecific cartilaginous degenerative changes occur with cartilage fibrillation and erosion. Urates penetrate the entire thickness of cartilage and collect in subchondral osseous areas. Additional foci in the bone result from direct deposition of urates in the bone marrow or from extension from adjacent urate collections within the periosteum, ligaments, tendons, bursae, and soft tissues.

Urate deposits within the thickened synovial villi are surrounded by connective tissue containing giant cells, macrophages, and other inflammatory cells. Inflammatory synovial tissue or pannus grows from the edges of the joint across the irregular cartilaginous surface. Fibrous ankylosis of the joint and secondary osteoarthritic alterations are frequent.

Tophaceous deposits also occur in the joint capsule, tendons, ligaments, and bursae, particularly in the olecranon and prepatellar regions. Extraarticular collections may be noted in the helix or antihelix of the ear, skin of the fingertips, palms, and soles, tarsal plates of the eyelids, nasal cartilage, cornea or sclerotic coats of the eye, aorta, myocardium, aortic and mitral valves, chest wall, tongue, epiglottis, vocal cords, arytenoid cartilage, and penis. As they become larger in size, tophi may calcify or ossify and produce tendon rupture, nerve compressions, and paralysis.

GENERAL RADIOGRAPHIC FEATURES

Although radiographic alterations may accompany initial bouts of acute gouty arthritis, the radiographic evaluation will reveal no abnormalities of articular structures in a great percentage of patients with clinical evidence of gout and symptoms spanning many years. During the acute attack of arthritis, soft tissue prominence or swelling about the involved joint(s) may be evident. As the attack subsides, these radiographic abnormalities will usually disappear. After years of intermittent episodic arthritis, chronic tophaceous gout may lead to permanent radiographic abnormalities.

Soft Tissue Abnormality

Eccentric nodular soft tissue prominence accompanies soft tissue deposition of urates (Fig. 39–1). The lesions are particularly frequent in the feet, hands, ankles, elbows, and knees. Swelling in the olecranon region and the dorsum of the foot is particularly characteristic.

Calcification of a tophus is an unusual finding. The calcific deposits appear as irregular or cloud-like radiodense areas.

Joint Space Abnormality

In gout, the joint space width is remarkably well preserved until late in the course of articular disease (Fig. 39–2). This distinctive radiographic feature relates to the relative integrity of cartilage adjacent to the areas of extensive cartilaginous and osseous destruction. In later stages of the disease, joint space narrowing is frequent, simulating the appearance in rheumatoid arthritis. Bone ankylosis with obliteration of the joint space is extremely rare, except in the interphalangeal joints of the hands and feet and the intercarpal region.

Bone Mineralization Abnormality

Although osteoporosis of subchondral bone can be observed during an acute gouty attack, extensive loss of bone density is not characteristic of this disease. In long-standing gouty arthritis, osteoporosis occurs, probably secondary to disuse atrophy of bone.

Erosions of Bone

Erosions of bone are common in gout. They are produced by tophaceous deposits and may be intraarticular, paraarticular, or located at a considerable distance from the joint (Fig. 39–3). Intraarticular erosions usually commence in the marginal areas of the joint and proceed centrally; paraarticular erosions are eccentric in location, frequently present beneath soft tissue nodules. Gouty erosions may be surrounded by a sclerotic border, producing a "punched out" appearance. As in rheumatoid arthritis, subchondral lytic bone lesions in gout may reveal communication with the joint cavity or appear as discrete cystic radiolucent areas.

In about 40 per cent of patients with gouty erosions of bone, an elevated bone margin or lip extends outward in the

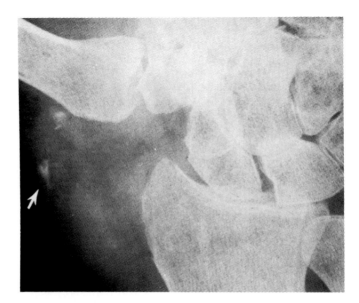

Figure 39–1. Radiographic features of gout: Soft tissue abnormalities. Partial peripheral calcification (arrow) of a tophus is evident on the radial aspect of the wrist.

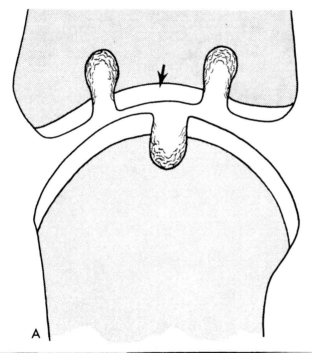

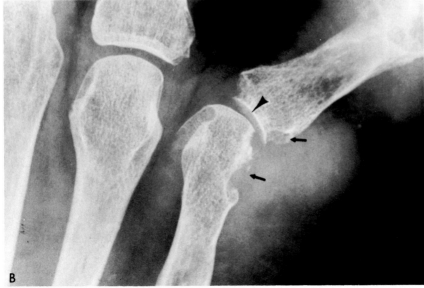

Figure 39–2. Radiographic features of gout: Articular space abnormalities. A Diagram indicating that relatively normal cartilage (arrow) is apparent between areas of cartilaginous and osseous destruction. B Observe that the articular space is only minimally narrowed (arrowhead) despite the presence of nodular soft tissue masses and eccentric osseous erosions (arrows). (From Resnick D: The radiographic manifestations of gouty arthritis. CRC Crit Rev Diagn Imaging 9:265, 1977. Used with permission.)

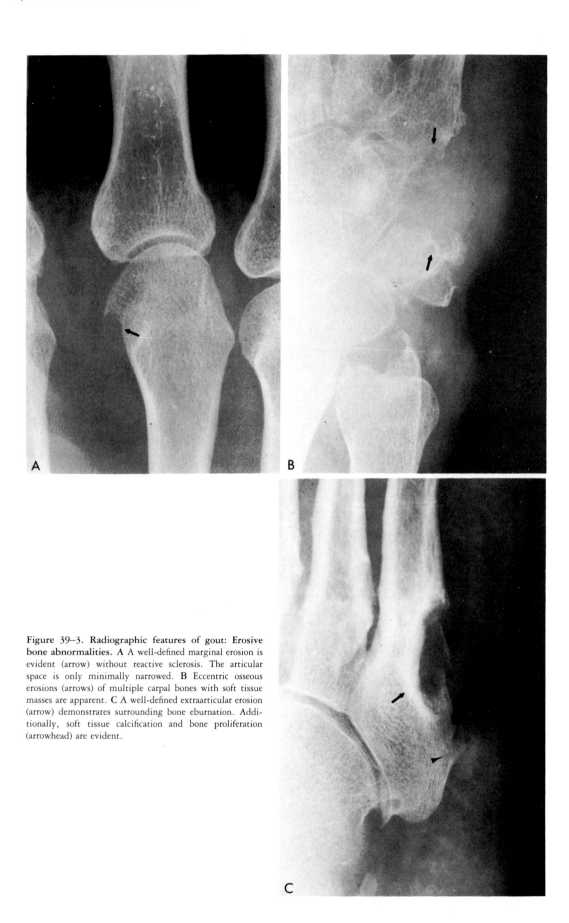

Figure 39–3. Radiographic features of gout: Erosive bone abnormalities. **A** A well-defined marginal erosion is evident (arrow) without reactive sclerosis. The articular space is only minimally narrowed. **B** Eccentric osseous erosions (arrows) of multiple carpal bones with soft tissue masses are apparent. **C** A well-defined extraarticular erosion (arrow) demonstrates surrounding bone eburnation. Additionally, soft tissue calcification and bone proliferation (arrowhead) are evident.

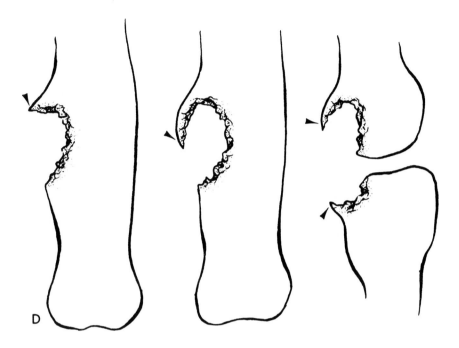

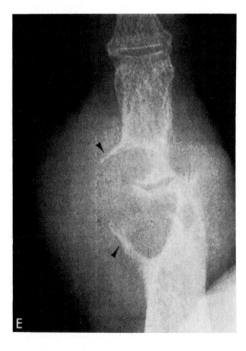

Figure 39–3 *Continued* **D, E** Overhanging margin. This lip of bone (arrowheads) may be evident in intra- or extraarticular locations. (From Resnick D: The radiographic manifestations of gouty arthritis. CRC Crit Rev Diagn Imaging 9:265, 1977. Used with permission.)

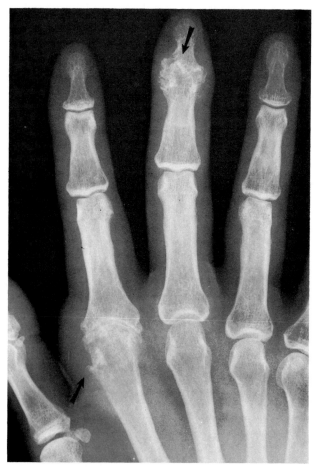

Figure 39–4. Radiographic features of gout: Proliferative bone abnormalities. Considerable productive changes of bone are apparent at the second metacarpophalangeal and third distal interphalangeal joints (arrows).

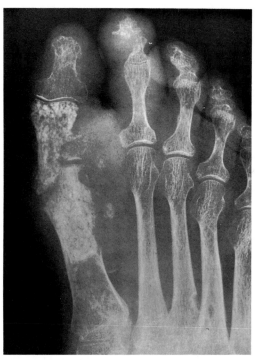

Figure 39–5. Radiographic features of gout: Intraosseous calcification. In this 73 year old woman with gout of 15 years' duration, tophi, and chronic renal disease, observe punctate and circular calcifications in the proximal phalanx and metatarsal bone of the great toe. Extensive soft tissue swelling and calcification about a destroyed first metatarsophalangeal joint are evident.

soft tissues, apparently covering the tophaceous nodule. The overhanging edge may relate to bone resorption beneath the gradually enlarging tophus with periosteal bone apposition at the outer aspect of the involved cortex. Although the appearance is not pathognomonic, it is strongly suggestive of gouty arthritis.

Subperiosteal Apposition of Bone and Proliferative Changes

Bone proliferation is occasionally observed in gout (Fig. 39–4). Club-shaped metacarpal, metatarsal, and phalangeal heads (termed mushrooming), an enlarged ulnar styloid, and thickened diaphyses may be evident. Secondary osteoarthritic alterations in gouty joints are common and may obscure other manifestations of the disease. Associated joint malalignment and subluxation are occasionally noted.

Intraosseous Calcification

Intraosseous calcific deposits occur in approximately 5 per cent of patients with chronic gouty arthritis, tophi, and prominent radiographic abnormalities. Pathologic investigation confirms that the calcification occurs in intraosseous urate deposits, which usually arise from the adjacent articulation.

Intraosseous calcification in gout is seen most frequently in the hands and the feet. Radiographic findings include focal or diffuse calcific collections, usually involving subchondral or subligamentous bone areas, in association with adjacent joint disease, osseous destruction, and involvement of periarticular tissue (Fig. 39–5). The radiographic alterations resemble those of enchondromas or bone infarcts.

DISTRIBUTION OF JOINT INVOLVEMENT

Although the distribution of radiographic abnormalities in gouty arthritis is somewhat variable, some characteristics include asymmetric polyarticular disease, frequent abnormalities in the lower extremities, and common involvement of the feet, hands, wrists, elbows, and knees.

Common Sites of Disease

FOOT ABNORMALITIES (FIGS. 39–6 AND 39–7). The most characteristic site of abnormality in gout is the first metatarsophalangeal joint. Erosions are particularly frequent on the medial and dorsal aspects of the first metatarsal head. Associated soft tissue swelling and hallux valgus deformity frequently are present. Any of the other metatarsophalangeal joints may be involved, particularly the fifth. Involvement of the interphalangeal joint of the great toe and first tarsometatarsal joint occurs, usually in association with changes at the first metatarsophalangeal joint. Interphalangeal joints of other digits may reveal similar abnormalities. Swelling on the dorsum of the foot may be associated with extensive destruction in the tarsometatarsal, intertarsal, and talocalcaneal joints. Calcaneal erosions are not infrequent.

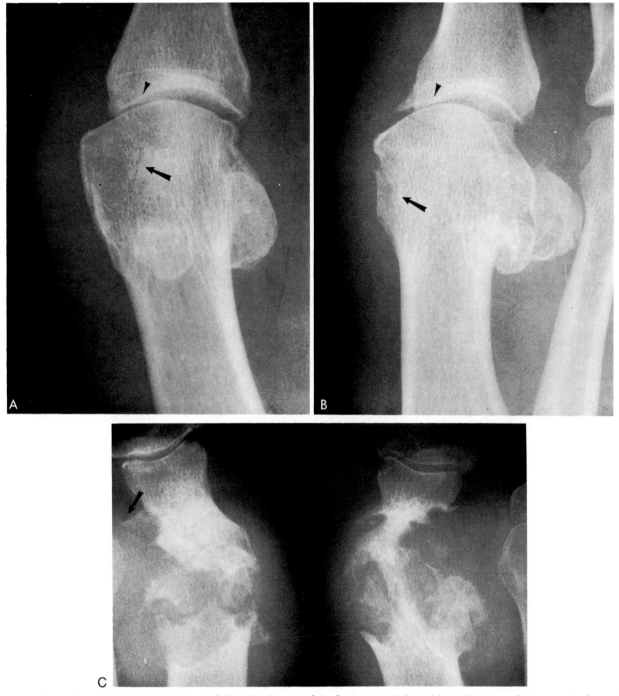

Figure 39–6. Forefoot abnormalities in gout. A, B Early involvement of the first metatarsophalangeal joint. Erosions predominate at the dorsomedial aspect of the metatarsal head (arrows), associated with soft tissue swelling, articular space narrowing (arrowheads), and osteophyte formation. **C** Late findings include extensive bone destruction with overhanging margins and pathologic fractures (arrow). (From Resnick D: The radiographic manifestations of gouty arthritis. CRC Crit Rev Diagn Imaging 9:265, 1977. Used with permission.)

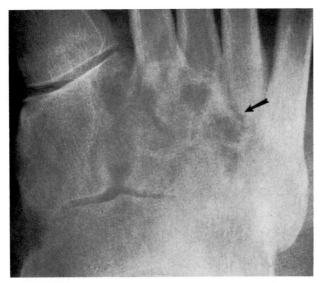

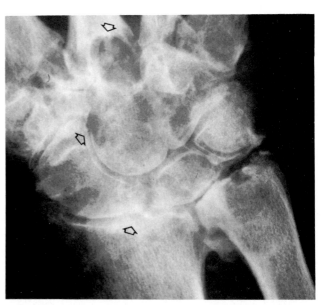

Figure 39–7. Midfoot abnormalities in gout. A typical site of alteration in gout is the tarsometatarsal articulations, where erosions may be extensive (arrow). (From Resnick D: The radiographic manifestations of gouty arthritis. CRC Crit Rev Diagn Imaging 9:265, 1977. Used with permission.)

Figure 39–9. Wrist abnormalities in gout. Diffuse disease of all of the compartments of the wrist is evident. Erosions (arrows) are most prominent at the common carpometacarpal compartment (upper arrow). (From Resnick D: The radiographic manifestations of gouty arthritis. CRC Crit Rev Diagn Imaging 9:265, 1977. Used with permission.)

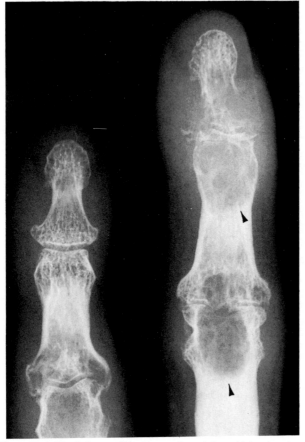

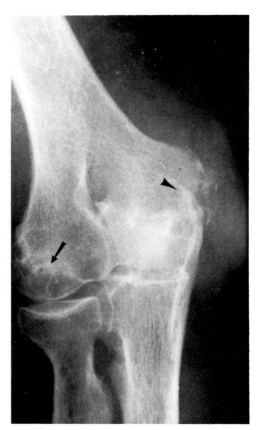

Figure 39–8. Hand abnormalities in gout. Interphalangeal joint alterations include bone erosion and intraosseous defects (arrowheads). (From Resnick D: The radiographic manifestations of gouty arthritis. CRC Crit Rev Diagn Imaging 9:265, 1977. Used with permission.)

Figure 39–10. Elbow abnormalities in gout. Extensive abnormalities consist of multiple subchondral radiolucent areas in the distal part of the humerus (arrow), erosions (arrowhead), and soft tissue swelling.

HAND AND WRIST ABNORMALITIES (FIGS. 39–8 AND 39–9).

Radiographs of the hands and wrists in patients with gout may reveal abnormalities involving distal interphalangeal, proximal interphalangeal, and, to a lesser extent, metacarpophalangeal joints. These hand and wrist alterations lack the symmetry that is characteristic in rheumatoid arthritis. Large erosions of the intercarpal and carpometacarpal articulations occur, and all of the compartments in the wrist may eventually be affected.

ELBOW ABNORMALITIES (FIG. 39–10).

Bursal inflammation commonly produces bilateral soft tissue swelling over the extensor surface of the elbow. Erosive and proliferative changes in the subjacent olecranon process of the ulna are apparent, and the elbow joint itself may be involved.

KNEE ABNORMALITIES (FIG. 39–11).

Marginal erosions in the knee may occur on the medial or lateral aspect of the femur and tibia, or both, in the absence of significant narrowing of the articular space. Cystic lesions of the patella or femur owing to intraosseous tophi may simulate neoplasm. Prepatellar gouty tophi may appear as soft tissue masses with or without calcification.

Uncommon Sites of Disease

SHOULDER ABNORMALITIES. Radiographic changes of the glenohumeral or acromioclavicular joint in gout are not common. Soft tissue swelling, bone erosions and cystic lesions, loss of joint space, and secondary proliferative changes are encountered. Acromioclavicular joint involvement may produce irregular splaying of the distal end of the clavicle.

HIP ABNORMALITIES. Abnormalities of the hip are rare in gout. Previous reports have indicated a high frequency of hyperuricemia or gout in patients with osteonecrosis of the femoral head, but in most of these patients, a definite relationship between the two entities was not established.

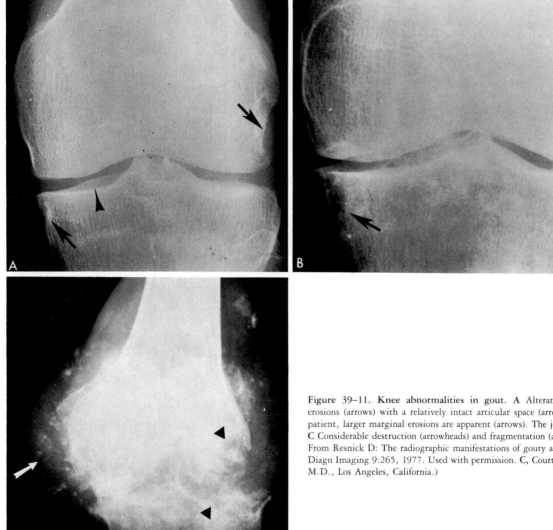

Figure 39–11. Knee abnormalities in gout. **A** Alterations include marginal erosions (arrows) with a relatively intact articular space (arrowhead). **B** In another patient, larger marginal erosions are apparent (arrows). The joint space is narrowed. **C** Considerable destruction (arrowheads) and fragmentation (arrow) are seen. (A, B, From Resnick D: The radiographic manifestations of gouty arthritis. CRC Crit Rev Diagn Imaging 9:265, 1977. Used with permission. C, Courtesy of D. M. Forrester, M.D., Los Angeles, California.)

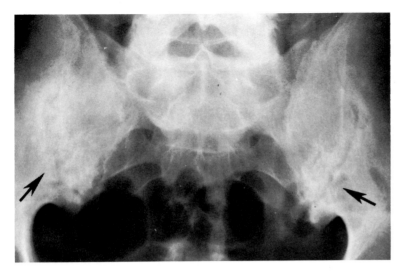

Figure 39–12. Sacroiliac joint abnormalities in gout. Bilateral changes are apparent with erosion and bony eburnation (arrows). (From Resnick D: The radiographic manifestations of gouty arthritis. CRC Crit Rev Diagn Imaging 9:265, 1977. Used with permission.)

Furthermore, monosodium urate deposition in patients with osteonecrosis may be a secondary phenomenon. The presence of necrosis lowers the pH in the neighboring tissues, favoring the local deposition of urates.

SACROILIAC JOINT ABNORMALITIES (FIG. 39–12). The frequency of sacroiliac joint involvement in cases of gout has been reported to be approximately 15 per cent. Irregularity and sclerosis of the articular margins in some patients with gout, however, are falsely interpreted as definite evidence of gouty involvement of the sacroiliac joints; nevertheless these changes are frequent in osteoarthritis alone. Large cystic areas of erosion in the subchondral bone of the ilium and sacrum are more consistent with changes produced by gout. Sacroiliac joint gout has been noted more frequently with early onset disease and demonstrates left-sided predominance.

SPINE ABNORMALITIES (FIG. 39–13). Documented monosodium urate deposition in the spine is exceedingly rare.

Associated radiographic abnormalities in the cervical segment include erosions of the odontoid process or endplates of the vertebral bodies, disc space narrowing, and vertebral subluxation. Spinal cord compression related to urate deposition has been reported as a complication of gout.

COEXISTENT ARTICULAR DISORDERS
Chondrocalcinosis

The reported frequency of chondrocalcinosis in patients with gout is 5 to 33 per cent (Fig. 39–14). These calcific deposits are usually localized in one or two sets of joints, particularly within the menisci of the knee, symphysis pubis, and triangular fibrocartilage of the wrist. Hyaline cartilage calcification or widespread chondrocalcinosis is rare in gouty arthritis. Paraarticular calcification in gouty tophi in the joint capsule, tendons, ligaments, and bursae simulates the soft tissue calcifications that may be observed in calcium pyrophosphate dihydrate crystal deposition disease.

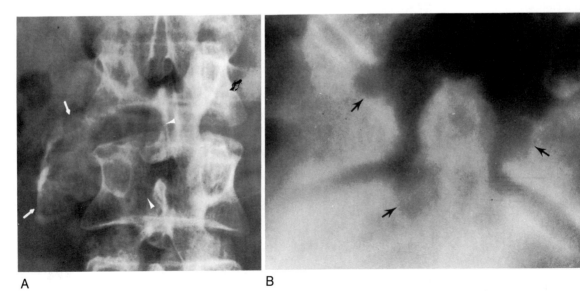

A   B

Figure 39–13. Spinal abnormalities in gout. A A large paraspinal tophus has produced a soft tissue mass (arrows) with erosion of the laminae and articular processes (arrowheads) of two adjacent lumbar vertebrae. (Courtesy of A. Brower, M.D., Washington, D.C.) B On a frontal tomogram, observe erosion of the atlas and axis (arrows) related to gout. Overhanging edges of bone are apparent. (Courtesy of C. Alexander, M.D., Auckland, New Zealand.)

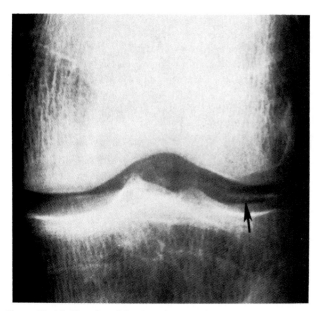

Figure 39–14. Chondrocalcinosis and gout. Fibrocartilaginous deposits of calcium pyrophosphate dihydrate crystals are seen within the menisci of the knee (arrow) in this patient with gout.

Other Coexistent Articular Disorders

Although rheumatoid arthritis and gout are not uncommon diseases, their coexistence is extremely rare. With few exceptions, patients are men in whom gout was the initial disease, followed years later by the development of rheumatoid arthritis. Despite these reports, a negative association between gout and rheumatoid arthritis is well accepted, although its explanation is not clear.

The coexistence of joint infection and gout also is unusual. When septic arthritis and gout coexist, other disorders predisposing to infection, such as renal failure, may also be present.

SPECIAL TYPES OF GOUTY ARTHRITIS
Early Onset Idiopathic Gouty Arthritis

The reported peak age incidence of idiopathic gout has varied from 30 to 50 years. Cases of gout in early life have been reported, but clinical and radiographic abnormalities in idiopathic gout in the first two decades of life are uncommon. In early-onset gouty arthritis, boys and girls are affected with approximately equal frequency. Articular symptoms and signs are similar to those of the adult, as are radiographic abnormalities (Fig. 39–15). The joints most frequently involved are those in the feet and hands.

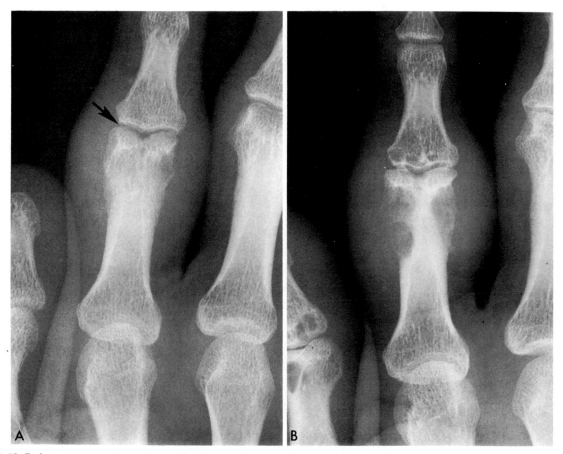

Figure 39–15. Early onset gouty arthritis: Progressive abnormalities over a 2 year period in a 23 year old man with gout. The initial film (**A**) reveals soft tissue swelling and bone destruction of the proximal phalanx (arrow). The subsequent radiograph (**B**) demonstrates the increased severity of the bone and soft tissue changes. (From Resnick D: The radiographic manifestations of gouty arthritis. CRC Crit Rev Diagn Imaging 9:265, 1977. Used with permission.)

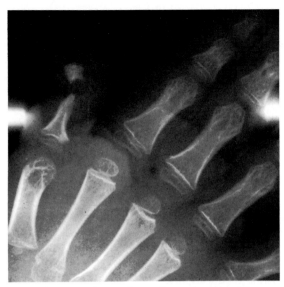

Figure 39–16. Lesch-Nyhan syndrome. Destruction and partial amputation of a phalanx in the hand are seen.

Gout Associated with Hereditary Disease

TYPE I GLYCOGEN STORAGE DISEASE. Patients with type I glycogen storage disease (glucose-6-phosphatase deficiency), a rare hereditary disorder of childhood, may develop gouty arthritis if they live to adulthood. In some of these patients, disabling arthritis may develop in the first decade of life. Gouty nephropathy may also be apparent. Partial deficiency of this enzyme, as opposed to the complete deficiency that characterizes type I glycogen storage disease, has been suggested as an additional factor that may lead to gout or hyperuricemia.

LESCH-NYHAN SYNDROME. The Lesch-Nyhan syndrome consists of spasticity, choreoathetosis, mental retardation, and compulsive self-mutilation manifested as finger- and lip-biting. Boys are affected and the disorder is X-linked (Fig. 39–16). Complete or virtually complete deficiency of hypoxanthine-guanine phosphoribosyltransferase (PRT) activity is associated with the Lesch-Nyhan syndrome. With incomplete deficiency, there may be less extensive purine synthesis, adolescent-onset gouty arthritis, and occasional mild neurologic disease.

Radiographic abnormalities reflect self-mutilation with amputation of soft tissues and osseous structures of the hands. Gouty erosions, retarded skeletal maturation, coxa valga deformities with subluxation of the hips, and soft tissue tophi have been described in this disorder. Additional findings include traumatic changes after seizures, cerebral atrophy, and uric acid calculi in the urinary tract.

Saturnine Gout

The accidental contamination of alcoholic beverages with lead has been recognized for centuries. At times, lead was intentionally added to wines to improve their flavor or prevent spoiling, a practice that was subsequently ruled illegal. Gout occurring as a complication of chronic lead intoxication is designated "saturnine gout." Currently, this form of gout is associated principally with the ingestion of illegally manufactured alcohol (moonshine) and has been observed in many areas of the southeastern portion of the United States. It is caused in large part by decreased urate clearance by the kidneys due to lead nephropathy.

Patients with saturnine gout typically are male, black, aged 45 to 55 years, often azotemic and anemic, but otherwise asymptomatic except for joint disease. Polyarticular involvement, especially in the lower extremities, usually is apparent. Knee abnormalities are characteristic. Radiologic findings resemble those of idiopathic gout.

Gout Associated with Other Clinical Disorders (Secondary Gout)

A number of other disorders may result in hyperuricemia and secondary gout. Myeloproliferative disorders, which are apparent in approximately 5 to 10 per cent of patients with gout, include polycythemia vera, leukemia, lymphoblastoma, myeloid metaplasia, hemolytic anemia, sickle cell anemia, pernicious anemia, thalassemia, multiple myeloma, and Waldenström's hyperproteinemia.

Hyperuricemia may be associated with a variety of endocrine disorders, including hyperparathyroidism, hypoparathyroidism, myxedema, and hypoadrenal states. Additional causes of hyperuricemia and gout are obesity, idiopathic hypercalciuria, psoriasis, myocardial infarction and vascular disease, renal disease, and near-starvation states. Drug-induced gout has been noted in association with diuretic, pyrazinamide, and salicylate therapy.

In many of these disorders, hyperuricemia does not produce joint symptoms. Occasionally clinical and radiographic abnormalities related to gout are present. The radiographic manifestations of secondary and idiopathic gout are, in general, indistinguishable. Secondary gouty arthritis may involve unusual sites and produce radiographic changes in the first two decades of life, however.

DIFFERENTIAL DIAGNOSIS

As radiographic abnormalities in gouty joints appear late in the course of the disease, the diagnosis usually is well established clinically, and the radiologist need only document its extent and severity. Occasionally, the disease is not suspected prior to radiographic examination. The radiographic manifestations frequently are sufficently characteristic to allow a specific diagnosis.

Rheumatoid Arthritis

Rheumatoid arthritis produces radiographic alterations that differ from those of gout, including symmetric joint involvement, fusiform soft tissue swelling, and regional osteoporosis (Table 39–2). Early diffuse joint space loss accompanies marginal erosive changes in the bone. In gout, joint involvement usually is asymmetric in distribution, lobulated eccentric soft tissue masses may be seen, and regional osteoporosis generally is absent. Osseous erosions occur without loss of articular space, and extraarticular defects may be noted. Calcification of rheumatoid nodules has been observed only rarely, whereas calcified tophi are encountered more frequently.

Gout-like radiographic changes characterized by the lack of osteoporosis and the presence of extensive erosions and subchondral cysts without loss of articular space occasionally are reported in men with rheumatoid arthritis.

Table 39–2. RADIOGRAPHIC FEATURES OF GOUT AND RHEUMATOID ARTHRITIS

	Gouty Arthritis	Rheumatoid Arthritis
Distribution	Asymmetric joint involvement	Symmetric joint involvement
Soft tissue swelling	Eccentric	Fusiform
Soft tissue calcification	Occasional	Rare
Osteoporosis	Absent or mild	Moderate or severe
Joint space loss	Frequently absent	Symmetric; occurs early in disease course
Bone erosions	Eccentric	Marginal
	Frequent sclerotic margin	Rare sclerotic margin
	Intra- and extraarticular	Intraarticular
	Overhanging edge	
Malalignment, subluxation	Rare	Common

Psoriatic Arthritis

Psoriatic arthritis may produce radiographic changes that resemble those in gout, and the presence of elevated serum uric acid levels may lead to further diagnostic difficulty. The articular manifestations of psoriasis include progressive destruction of the peripheral joints of the extremities, periosteal proliferation at the margins of the joint, paravertebral ossification, and sacroiliac disease. Osteoporosis generally is not apparent. The metatarsophalangeal joints of the foot (including the first) frequently are abnormal, and a peculiar predilection for the interphalangeal joint of the great toe is well documented. At this latter location, the site and pattern of joint destruction in psoriasis, gout, and rheumatoid arthritis are sufficiently characteristic to allow differentiation among these disorders (Fig. 39–17).

Calcium Pyrophosphate Dihydrate Crystal Deposition Disease

Calcium pyrophosphate dihydrate (CPPD) crystal deposition disease resulting from the presence of intraarticular crystals can produce an acute arthritis with clinical symptoms identical to those of gout, termed the pseudogout syndrome, and radiographic abnormalities consisting of articular and periarticular calcification and a "degenerative" arthropathy. Cartilage calcification, termed chondrocalcinosis, accompanying CPPD crystal deposition disease frequently is widespread and involves hyaline cartilage and fibrocartilage; chondrocalcinosis in gout usually is localized to one or two joints and involves fibrocartilage alone. Structural joint abnormalities of CPPD crystal deposition disease are termed pyrophosphate arthropathy and demonstrate an unusual predilection for the wrist, metacarpophalangeal joints, and knee. They are characterized by joint space narrowing, subchondral sclerosis and cyst formation, bone fragmentation and collapse, and variable osteophyte formation. Pyrophosphate arthropathy may involve the radiocarpal compartment of the wrist and the patellofemoral compartment of the knee selectively. Although the radiographic manifestations of pyrophosphate arthropathy may resemble those of gout, the presence of lobulated soft tissue masses, intact joint spaces, and osseous erosions in gouty arthritis usually permits differentiation of the two disorders (Fig. 39–18). In rare circumstances, tophaceous soft tissue collections are observed in CPPD crystal deposition disease.

Sarcoidosis

Sarcoidosis may produce skeletal abnormalities, particularly in the hand. These alterations include widening of the medullary portion of the bone, a honeycomb configuration, cyst-like lucent osseous defects, and sclerosis. Articular involvement produces either an acute transient type or a persistent chronic type of arthritis. Although granulomatous involvement of the synovium and juxtaarticular bone occurs in the chronic arthritis of sarcoidosis, articular destruction and deformity are unusual.

Amyloidosis

Amyloid infiltration of the articular structures may cause soft tissue masses and cystic and erosive osseous lesions indistinguishable from those of gout. An associated carpal tunnel syndrome is frequent. Marrow infiltration produces diffuse lytic bone defects.

Xanthomatosis

Tendinous xanthomas are particularly frequent on the extensor surface of the hand and foot and in the patellar and Achilles tendon regions. Tuberous xanthomas occur in the subcutaneous tissues of the elbows and knees. Periosteal xanthomas may also appear, particularly in the lower tibia. Clinical findings in these patients are bouts of tendinitis and occasional arthritis. Radiographic changes consist of eccentric soft tissue nodular masses with subjacent bone erosion, findings simulating gouty tophi (Fig. 39–19). Hypercholesterolemia in patients with xanthomatosis is an important laboratory abnormality.

Inflammatory (Erosive) Osteoarthritis and Multicentric Reticulohistiocytosis

Destructive articular abnormalities of the interphalangeal joints, which are noted in both gout and psoriasis, are also apparent in inflammatory (erosive) osteoarthritis and multicentric reticulohistiocytosis. The former disease affects middle-aged and elderly women and produces symmetric joint changes, usually confined to the interphalangeal joints of the fingers, first carpometacarpal joint, and trapezioscaphoid joint. As opposed to the changes in gout, erosions in inflammatory osteoarthritis frequently commence in the central portion of the joint, with subsequent involvement of the marginal bone. The radiographic manifestations in multicen-

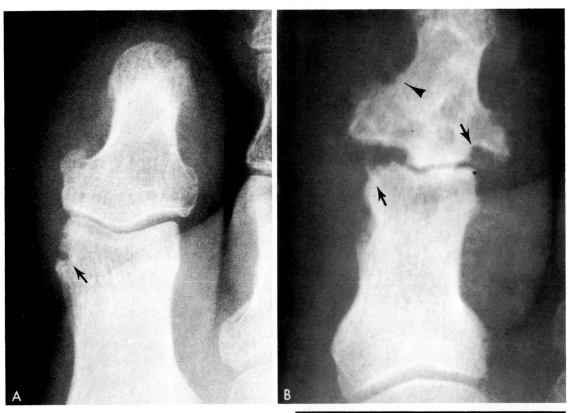

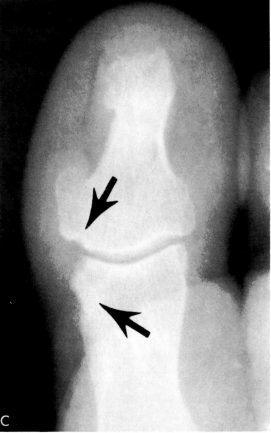

Figure 39–17. Interphalangeal abnormalities in rheumatoid arthritis, psoriasis, and gout. A In rheumatoid arthritis, the most frequent site of bone erosion is on the medial aspect of the distal portion of the proximal phalanx (arrow). B In psoriasis, erosions occur on the medial and lateral aspects of the articulation (arrows) associated with bone proliferation (arrowhead). C In gout, medial (arrows) or lateral erosions may be observed at the interphalangeal joint, but other changes in the foot are generally apparent. (From Resnick D: The radiographic manifestations of gouty arthritis. CRC Crit Rev Diagn Imaging 9:265, 1977. Used with permission.)

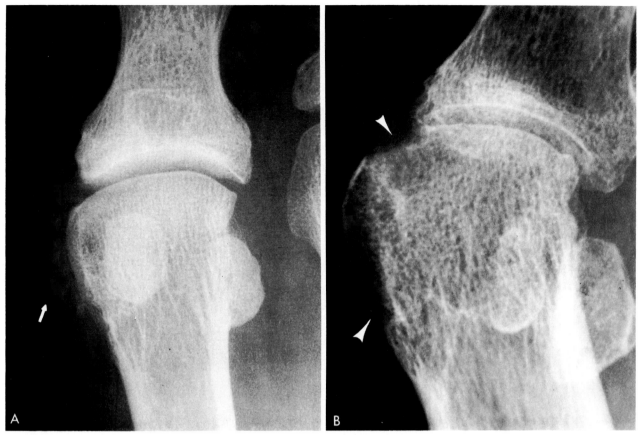

Figure 39–18. Calcium pyrophosphate dihydrate (CPPD) crystal deposition disease versus gout. A In CPPD crystal deposition disease, changes at the first metatarsophalangeal joint may consist of soft tissue calcification (arrow). B In gout, typical marginal and central erosions are observed (arrowheads).

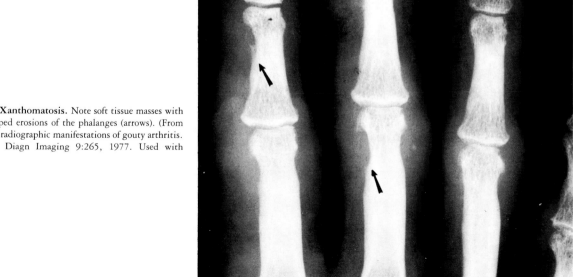

Figure 39–19. Xanthomatosis. Note soft tissue masses with subjacent scalloped erosions of the phalanges (arrows). (From Resnick D: The radiographic manifestations of gouty arthritis. CRC Crit Rev Diagn Imaging 9:265, 1977. Used with permission.)

tric reticulohistiocytosis, a rare systemic disorder primarily affecting skin and synovium, include features similar to those of gout, such as erosions with sharp margins and lack of osteoporosis. Multicentric reticulohistiocytosis produces symmetric joint lesions, and the articular space may be rapidly narrowed. These latter features do not commonly occur in gout.

Degenerative Joint Disease

Gouty arthritis is associated with secondary proliferative alterations of bone, including osteophytosis and subchondral sclerosis. The resulting radiographic appearance is identical to that observed in degenerative joint disease. Abnormalities resembling those of degenerative arthropathy that occur in unusual locations or possess atypical radiographic features may indicate underlying crystal-induced arthropathy.

FURTHER READING

Alarcón-Segovia D, Cetina JA, Diaz-Jouanen E: Sacroiliac joints in primary gout: Clinical and roentgenographic study of 143 patients. AJR *118*:438, 1973.

Barthelemy CR, Nakayama DA, Carrera GF, Lightfoot RW Jr, Wortmann RL: Gouty arthritis: A prospective radiographic evaluation of sixty patients. Skel Radiol *11*:1, 1984.

Bjelle A: Crystals in joints. Clin Rheumatol *2*:103, 1988.

Brailsford JF: The radiology of gout. Br J Radiol *32*:472, 1959.

Forrester DM, Brown JC, Nesson JW: The Radiology of Joint Disease. 2nd Ed. Philadelphia, WB Saunders Co, 1978.

Good AE, Rapp R: Chondrocalcinosis of the knee with gout and rheumatoid arthritis. N Engl J Med *277*:286, 1967.

Halla JT, Ball GV: Saturnine gout: A review of 42 patients. Semin Arthritis Rheum *11*:307, 1982.

Jaffe HL: Metabolic, Degenerative and Inflammatory Disease of Bones and Joints. Philadelphia, Lea & Febiger, 1972.

Lesch M, Nyhan WL: A familial disorder of uric acid metabolism and central nervous system function. Am J Med *36*:561, 1964.

Martel W: The overhanging margin of bone: A roentgenologic manifestation of gout. Radiology *91*:755, 1968.

Resnick D: The radiographic manifestations of gouty arthritis. CRC Crit Rev Diagn Imaging *9*:265, 1977.

Resnick D, Broderick TW: Intraosseous calcifications in tophaceous gout. AJR *137*:1157, 1981.

Resnick D, Reinke RT, Taketa RM: Early-onset gouty arthritis. Radiology *114*:67, 1975.

Seegmiller JE: Human aberrations of purine metabolism and their significance for rheumatology. Ann Rheum Dis *39*:103, 1980.

Watt I, Middlemiss H: The radiology of gout. Clin Radiol *26*:27, 1975.

Calcium Pyrophosphate Dihydrate (CPPD) Crystal Deposition Disease

Donald Resnick, M.D.
Gen Niwayama, M.D.

Until recently, calcium pyrophosphate dihydrate (CPPD) crystal deposition disease has been a commonly overlooked condition. In the last two decades, considerable attention to its various clinical and radiographic manifestations has increased physicians' awareness of this disorder. It is particularly important to realize that chondrocalcinosis can no longer be considered the only significant radiographic feature of CPPD crystal deposition disease. The presence of other intraarticular and periarticular calcifications and structural joint damage must now be regarded as equally characteristic in this disorder. The pattern and distribution of structural joint damage (pyrophosphate arthropathy) are especially distinctive and can be differentiated from the features of degenerative joint disease.

In 1961 and 1962, investigators studying patients with gout-like attacks of arthritis discovered nonurate crystals in the joint fluid. These crystals were subsequently identified as calcium pyrophosphate dihydrate (CPPD) by their x-ray diffraction powder pattern. When the clinical and radiographic findings in these patients were analyzed, it was recognized that the same disease had been previously described as chondrocalcinosis polyarticularis, reflecting the presence of distinctive cartilage calcification on radiographs of affected patients. It thus became clear that patients with a distinctive gout-like pattern of arthritis (pseudogout syndrome) had crystal accumulation within joints (CPPD deposition), which could cause cartilage calcification (chondrocalcinosis). Subsequently, it was learned that other calcium phosphate crystals, including calcium hydroxyapatite, could produce calcific collections in the knee (Table 40–1).

TERMINOLOGY

A variety of names have been used to describe clinical and radiographic manifestations accompanying CPPD crystal deposition. The following terms are most appropriate.

1. *Calcium pyrophosphate dihydrate (CPPD) crystal deposition disease*: a general term for a disorder characterized by the presence of $Ca_2P_2O_7 \cdot 2H_2O$ (calcium pyrophosphate dihydrate or CPPD) crystals in or around joints.

2. *Pseudogout*: a term applied to one of the clinical patterns that may be associated with this crystal deposition. This pattern, characterized by intermittent acute attacks of arthritis, simulates gout.

3. *Chondrocalcinosis*: a term reserved for pathologically or radiologically evident cartilage calcification. In some in-

stances, this calcification may indicate not CPPD crystal deposition but rather deposits of other crystals.

4. *Articular and periarticular calcification*: terms used for pathologically or radiologically evident calcification in and around joints. Chondrocalcinosis is but one of the possible manifestations of such calcification. In some situations, articular and periarticular calcification may not indicate deposits of CPPD crystals but instead reflect accumulations of some other crystal.

5. *Pyrophosphate arthropathy*: a term used to describe a peculiar pattern of structural joint damage occurring in CPPD crystal deposition disease simulating degenerative joint disease but characterized by distinctive features.

CLINICAL SUMMARY

CPPD crystal deposition disease affects both men and women and generally is observed in middle-aged and elderly patients. Varying clinical patterns underscore the ability of this disease to mimic a variety of other conditions, including gout, rheumatoid arthritis, degenerative joint disease, and neuroarthropathy.

TYPE A: PSEUDOGOUT (10 TO 20 PER CENT). The type A pattern of disease is characterized by acute or subacute self-limited attacks of arthritis involving one or several appendicular joints, especially the knee. The attacks, which range in duration from 1 day to several weeks, generally are less painful than attacks of gout and may be provoked by trauma, surgery, or medical illness. This pattern of disease is more frequently apparent in men and may be relieved by colchicine.

Table 40–1. REPORTED FREQUENCY OF CHONDROCALCINOSIS IN THE KNEE*

Author	Number of Cases	Age of Patients	Selection of Material	Method of Study	Frequency of Chondrocalcinosis† (Per Cent)
Tobler (1929)‡	1400	Elderly	Autopsy and surgical specimens	Histologic examination	30
Wolke (1935)	12,268	Wide range	Retrospective	Conventional x-ray	0.42
Bennett et al (1942)	63	Elderly	Cadavers	Histologic study	4.1
McCarty and Haskin (1963)	215	71 years (mean age)	Cadavers	Specimen x-rays, histologic study, and crystal analysis	7 (total) 3.3 (CPPD) 2.3 (DCPD) 1.4 (HA)
Bochner et al (1965)	455	80 years (mean age)	Retrospective and prospective survey	Conventional x-ray	7
Lagier and Baud (1968)	320	Elderly	Cadavers	Histologic study and crystal analysis	6.8 (CPPD)
Schmied et al (1971)	97	64	Prospective control and diabetic survey	Conventional x-ray	4.2
Ellman and Levin (1975)	58	83 years (mean age)	Survey of patients in home for elderly	Industrial film x-ray	28

*After HK Genant: Roentgenographic aspects of calcium pyrophosphate dihydrate crystal deposition disease (pseudogout). Arthritis Rheum 19 (Suppl):324, 1976. Used with permission.
†CPPD, Calcium pyrophosphate dihydrate; DCPD, dicalcium phosphate dihydrate; HA, calcium hydroxyapatite.
‡See original report for complete reference data.

TYPE B: PSEUDO-RHEUMATOID ARTHRITIS (2 TO 6 PER CENT). Characterized by almost continuous acute attacks of arthritis, the type B pattern is associated with symptoms and signs lasting 4 weeks to several months, consisting of morning stiffness, fatigue, synovial thickening, restricted joint motion, and an elevated erythrocyte sedimentation rate.

TYPE C: PSEUDO-OSTEOARTHRITIS (35 TO 60 PER CENT). Chronic progressive arthritis with superimposed acute inflammatory episodes usually is apparent in large articulations, such as the knee and hip. The type C pattern is characterized by bilateral symmetric involvement and flexion contractures, particularly of the knee and elbow.

TYPE D: PSEUDO-OSTEOARTHRITIS (10 TO 35 PER CENT). The type D clinical pattern is characterized by chronic progressive arthritis without acute exacerbations.

TYPE E: ASYMPTOMATIC JOINT DISEASE. Although reports of patients with CPPD crystal deposition disease indicate that symptoms may be absent in 10 to 20 per cent of cases, the frequency of the type E clinical pattern is much higher, as many asymptomatic patients are never seen by a physician. It is probably the most common clinical pattern.

TYPE F: PSEUDONEUROARTHROPATHY (0 TO 2 PER CENT). A less common clinical pattern in CPPD crystal deposition disease, type F, simulates neuroarthropathy.

TYPE G: MISCELLANEOUS PATTERNS (0 TO 1 PER CENT). CPPD crystal deposition disease can produce symptoms that suggest rheumatic fever, psychogenic disease, and trauma. Clinical findings resembling those of ankylosing spondylitis have also been observed.

It is apparent that CPPD crystal deposition disease can appear as an acute or chronic arthritis or as an asymptomatic illness. In the course of the disease, a patient may demonstrate several different clinical patterns.

CLASSIFICATION OF CPPD CRYSTAL DEPOSITION DISEASE

This disease can be conveniently classified into cases that are hereditary, sporadic (idiopathic), or associated with other disorders.

Hereditary cases are not associated with other disease processes. A female predominance is seen in familial cases, with a relatively early age of onset. Many of the sporadic cases have not been examined for possible familial patterns of disease. In this group, the disease usually occurs in middle-aged and elderly patients, and series with both male and female predominance have been recorded.

DISEASES ASSOCIATED WITH CPPD CRYSTAL DEPOSITION DISEASE

Many disorders have been reported in association with CPPD crystal deposition. In most instances, the combination of CPPD crystal deposition disease and another disorder may merely represent the chance occurrence of two diseases.

The following diseases have been reported in association with CPPD crystal deposition disease (Table 40–2).

Diabetes Mellitus

The reported frequency of diabetes mellitus in nonfamilial CPPD crystal deposition disease has varied from below 8 per cent to above 70 per cent. Some investigators, however, have documented the lack of a meaningful association between diabetes mellitus and CPPD crystal deposition.

Table 40–2. SOME CONDITIONS ASSOCIATED WITH CPPD CRYSTAL DEPOSITION

Group A: True association—high probability
1. Primary hyperparathyroidism
2. Familial hypocalciuric hypercalcemia
3. Hemochromatosis
4. Hemosiderosis
5. Hypophosphatasia
6. Hypomagnesemia
7. Bartter's syndrome
8. Hypothyroidism
9. Gout
10. Neuroarthropathy
11. Amyloidosis
12. Localized trauma
    a. Surgery for osteochondritis dissecans
    b. Hypermobility syndrome
13. Corticosteroid therapy (long-term)
14. Aging

Group B: True association—modest probability
1. Hyperthyroidism
2. Nephrolithiasis
3. Diffuse idiopathic skeletal hyperostosis
4. Ochronosis
5. Wilson's disease
6. Hemophilia arthritis

Group C: True association unlikely
1. Diabetes mellitus
2. Hypertension
3. Azotemia
4. Hyperuricemia
5. Gynecomastia
6. Inflammatory bowel disease
7. Rheumatoid arthritis
8. Paget's disease of bone
9. Acromegaly

From McCarty D: Crystals, joints, and consternation. Ann Rheum Dis 42:243, 1983. Used with permission.

Degenerative Joint Disease

The reported frequency of concomitant CPPD crystal deposition and degenerative joint disease has varied from 40 to 70 per cent. The structural joint changes that were described as coexistent degenerative joint disease in some of these patients, however, represented pyrophosphate arthropathy.

Gout and Hyperuricemia

Numerous investigators have described the occurrence of both urate and CPPD crystals in the same joint. The reported frequency of gout in patients with CPPD crystal deposition disease has varied from 0 to 8 per cent. In patients with gout, the reported frequency of chondrocalcinosis has varied from 5 to 32 per cent. Chondrocalcinosis in gouty arthritis usually involves fibrocartilage and is confined to one or several joints. The knee is the most typical site of cartilage calcification.

Hyperparathyroidism

Well-documented descriptions of patients with both primary hyperparathyroidism and chondrocalcinosis have appeared. The reported frequency of hyperparathyroidism in patients with CPPD crystal deposition disease has varied from 0 to 15 per cent. The frequency of chondrocalcinosis in

patients with hyperparathyroidism has been reported as 18 to 40 per cent. A close association of CPPD crystal deposition and hyperparathyroidism is further substantiated by the findings of elevated parathyroid hormone levels in normocalcemic patients with CPPD crystal deposition disease.

CPPD crystal deposition and pseudogout attacks have also been described in patients with chronic renal failure with or without secondary hyperparathyroidism.

Hemochromatosis

Chondrocalcinosis has been observed in about 40 per cent of patients with hemochromatosis, and structural joint changes simulating pyrophosphate arthropathy have frequently been seen in these patients. Chondrocalcinosis has also appeared in patients with secondary hemochromatosis related to hereditary spherocytosis.

Wilson's Disease

An association between CPPD crystal deposition and Wilson's disease has not been well substantiated. Small irregularities of the bone contours and ossicles in Wilson's disease may simulate chondrocalcinosis.

Other Conditions

Tabetic patients with *neuroarthropathy* who reveal CPPD crystal deposition have been identified, and a pathogenic synergism of the two conditions has been suggested.

Several patients with *ochronosis* have revealed synovial deposits of CPPD crystals.

Joint pain and chondrocalcinosis have been described in patients with *hypophosphatasia*.

The simultaneous occurrence of *hypomagnesemia* and CPPD crystal deposition has been reported on numerous occasions.

A large number of disorders have been reported to be associated with CPPD crystal deposition or chondrocalcinosis, or both, including *rheumatoid arthritis, Paget's disease, hemophilia, hypothyroidism, systemic lupus erythematosus, infection, juvenile chronic arthritis, amyloidosis, chronic steroid therapy, familial brachydactyly,* and *osteochondritis dissecans.* In most instances, meaningful associations have not been clearly documented. Evidence would suggest that hypertension, diabetes, azotemia, and gout are not truly associated with CPPD crystal deposits. An association of CPPD crystal deposition disease with "degenerative" joint disease may indicate not the simultaneous occurrence of two processes but rather the appearance of destructive structural articular changes related to CPPD crystal deposition disease itself. The strongest evidence of a significant association of CPPD crystal deposition with another disorder exists for primary *hyperparathyroidism* and *hemochromatosis.*

PATHOGENESIS OF CRYSTAL DEPOSITION AND SYNOVITIS

CPPD crystal deposition generally is first observed in articular cartilage; the earliest site of crystal deposition probably is about the chondrocyte lacunae in the midzonal area. The mechanism by which CPPD crystals are precipitated in cartilage is complex and not fully understood. In the past, it has been popular to suggest that such deposition is an initial step, followed by cartilage degeneration. In recent years, there has been increasing emphasis on local tissue damage as a cause of crystal deposition. The damage to cartilage may be age-related, secondary to trauma, or disease-induced. Cartilage damage may alter proteoglycan concentrations and inhibitory factors, increase inorganic pyrophosphate turnover, or effect some other change that predisposes susceptible individuals to CPPD crystal formation.

Just as the manner in which CPPD crystals are accumulated in cartilage is not clear, the events leading to joint inflammation after such accumulation are not known precisely. The pathogenesis of acute synovitis in this disease may relate to a process of crystal shedding, in which cartilaginous deposits are cast into the articular cavity. Crystal shedding might be exaggerated in conditions associated with significant cartilage destruction, such as infection and neuroarthropathy. The concept of crystal shedding gains additional support from reports documenting the disappearance of radiologically evident chondrocalcinosis during attacks of pseudogout.

GENERAL PATHOLOGIC FEATURES
Crystal Deposition

CPPD crystals may be apparent in cartilage, synovium, capsule, tendons, and ligaments.

CARTILAGE ABNORMALITIES. Crystalline deposits can occur in both fibrocartilage and hyaline cartilage (Fig. 40–1). Fibrocartilaginous collections of CPPD crystals are observed most frequently in the menisci of the knee, triangular fibrocartilage of the wrist, acetabular labra, symphysis pubis, and the anulus fibrosus of the intervertebral disc. Additional sites of fibrocartilaginous deposition include the articular discs of the acromioclavicular and sternoclavicular joints and the glenoid labra.

SYNOVIAL MEMBRANE AND SYNOVIAL FLUID ABNORMALITIES. Both acute and chronic inflammatory changes may be evident in the synovial membrane. Crystals generally are apparent within the inflamed synovial membrane. It is not entirely clear if the crystals within the synovial membrane are deposited there directly or if they migrate from the adjacent cartilage. In the synovial fluid, during acute attacks of inflammation, CPPD crystals are observed within leukocytes.

TENDON AND LIGAMENT ABNORMALITIES. Calcification may occur in tendons and ligaments. These calcifications are most frequently apparent in the Achilles, triceps, quadriceps, and supraspinatus tendons but may also be noted in adjacent bursae, such as the subacromial bursa. Although additional soft tissue calcifications have been noted in patients with this disease, verification that these collections relate to CPPD crystal deposition has not generally been obtained.

Structural Joint Damage

Structural joint damage associated with CPPD crystal deposition disease resembles degenerative joint disease on pathologic as well as radiographic examination (Fig. 40–2). Cartilage fibrillation, erosion, and partial or complete denudation are pathologic findings that correlate with radiographically evident joint space narrowing. The subchondral bone contains thickened trabeculae and multiple cysts. The cysts may or may not communicate with the adjacent articular cavity (Fig. 40–3). Compared with cystic lesions occurring in degenerative joint disease, the cysts of CPPD crystal deposition disease are larger, more numerous, and more widespread.

Bone fragmentation and collapse, which are frequent in this disease, may be related to fracture of these cystic lesions. Intraarticular osseous bodies may be loose within the joint cavity or embedded in the cartilaginous and synovial tissue. The embedded bone is surrounded by synovial proliferation. Although the bone and synovial changes resemble the findings of degenerative joint disease superficially, the extent of osseous fragmentation, embedded cartilage and bone debris, and synovial reaction are more similar to findings observed in neuroarthropathy.

GENERAL RADIOLOGIC FEATURES

The general radiographic features of CPPD crystal deposition disease may be divided into articular and periarticular calcification and pyrophosphate arthropathy (Table 40–3).

Articular and Periarticular Calcification

CPPD crystal deposition disease is associated with calcification of articular and periarticular structures (Fig. 40–4), including cartilage, synovium, capsule, tendons, bursae, ligaments, soft tissues, and vessels. The frequency of radiographically demonstrable articular calcification is greatest in the knees, symphysis pubis, wrists, elbows, and hips. An ideal screening test for articular calcification consists of a postero-anterior radiograph of each wrist, a coned-down anteroposterior radiograph of the symphysis pubis, and anteroposterior radiographs of each knee.

CARTILAGE CALCIFICATION (CHONDROCALCINOSIS). Chondrocalcinosis is most frequent in the knees, wrists, symphysis pubis, elbows, and hips. Chondrocalcinosis may involve fibrocartilage or hyaline cartilage (Fig. 40–5).

Fibrocartilaginous calcification is most common in the menisci of the knee, triangular cartilage of the wrist, symphysis pubis, anulus fibrosus of the intervertebral disc, and acetabular and glenoid labra. Fibrocartilaginous deposits appear as thick, shaggy, irregular radiodense areas, particularly within the central aspect of the joint cavity.

Hyaline cartilage calcification may occur in many locations but is most common in the wrist, knee, elbow, and hip. These deposits are thin and linear and are parallel to and separated from the subjacent subchondral bone.

SYNOVIAL CALCIFICATION. Calcification within the synovial membrane is a common feature of CPPD crystal deposition disease (Fig. 40–6). Synovial deposits are most frequent in the wrist, knee, and metacarpophalangeal and metatarsophalangeal joints. The deposits are cloud-like in appearance, and may simulate idiopathic synovial osteochondromatosis.

CAPSULAR CALCIFICATION. CPPD crystal deposition in joint capsules is observed most commonly in the elbow and metatarsophalangeal joints (Fig. 40–7). These collections appear as fine or irregular linear calcifications that span the joint. They may be associated with joint contractures, particularly in the elbow.

TENDON, BURSA, AND LIGAMENT CALCIFICATION. Tendinous and ligamentous calcification may be observed in the Achilles, triceps, quadriceps, and supra-

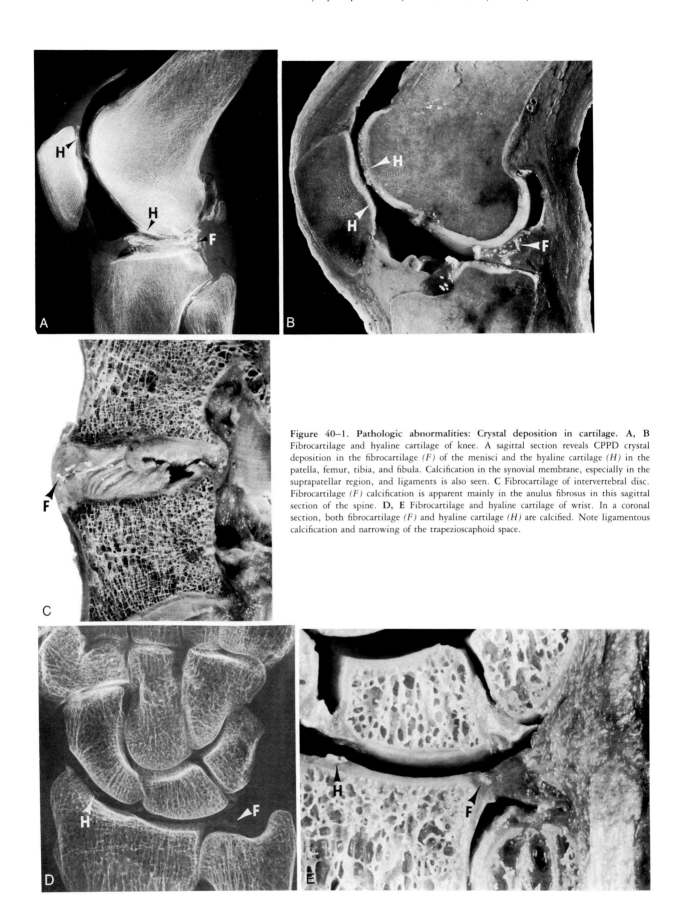

Figure 40–1. Pathologic abnormalities: Crystal deposition in cartilage. A, B Fibrocartilage and hyaline cartilage of knee. A sagittal section reveals CPPD crystal deposition in the fibrocartilage (F) of the menisci and the hyaline cartilage (H) in the patella, femur, tibia, and fibula. Calcification in the synovial membrane, especially in the suprapatellar region, and ligaments is also seen. C Fibrocartilage of intervertebral disc. Fibrocartilage (F) calcification is apparent mainly in the anulus fibrosus in this sagittal section of the spine. D, E Fibrocartilage and hyaline cartilage of wrist. In a coronal section, both fibrocartilage (F) and hyaline cartilage (H) are calcified. Note ligamentous calcification and narrowing of the trapezioscaphoid space.

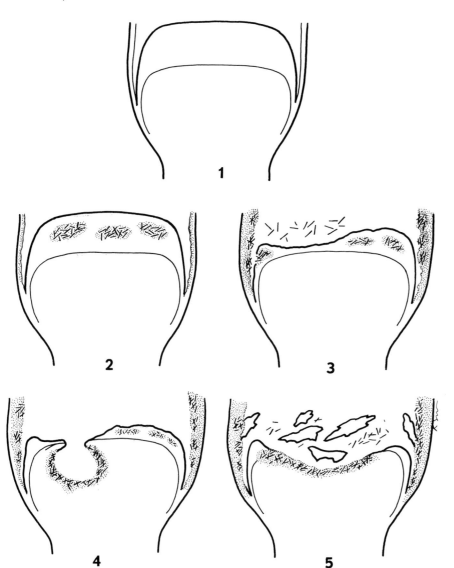

Figure 40–2. **Pathogenesis of pyrophosphate arthropathy.** *1,* The normal situation. *2,* Crystal deposition in hyaline cartilage is apparent. *3,* Cartilage loss, crystal shedding, and synovial deposits are seen with secondary synovial inflammation. *4,* Cystic degeneration and bone sclerosis have occurred. *5,* Fragmentation of bone and cartilage may lead to cartilaginous and osseous debris embedded in the synovial membrane. (Redrawn after McCarty DJ Jr: Calcium pyrophosphate dihydrate crystal deposition disease–1975. Arthritis Rheum *19*[Suppl]:275, 1976. Used with permission.)

Figure 40–3. **Pathologic abnormalities: Cyst formation.** Observe multiple cystic lesions of the femoral head. Cystic communication with the surface of the bone is seen (arrows) on this coronal section.

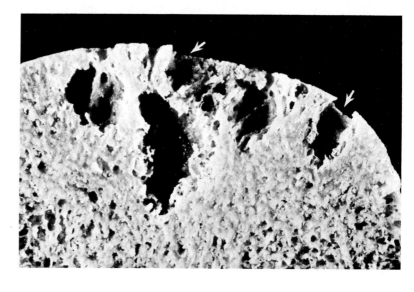

Table 40–3. MOST FREQUENT SITES OF CLINICAL AND RADIOGRAPHIC ABNORMALITIES IN CPPD CRYSTAL DEPOSITION DISEASE

	Clinical Manifestations	Calcification	Arthropathy
Hands	+		+
Wrists	+	+	+
Elbows			+
Shoulders			+
Hips	+	+	
Knees	+	+	+
Ankles	+		
Spine		+	
Pelvis		+	

spinatus tendons as well as the subacromial bursa (Fig. 40–8). In tendons, calcifications appear thin and linear and may extend for considerable distances from the osseous margin. They simulate the findings of idiopathic calcific tendinitis related to calcium hydroxyapatite (HA) crystal deposition but may be more extensive in appearance. In shoulders that demonstrate tendinous and bursal calcification, rotator cuff tears are not infrequent.

It should be emphasized that numerous examples of mixed crystal deposition diseases have been reported (see discussion later in this chapter). CPPD and calcium HA can occur together in one person and, in fact, in a single joint. Therefore, tendon calcification (as well as bursal and synovial calcification) in a patient with CPPD crystal deposition disease can be related to accumulation of HA crystals.

SOFT TISSUE AND VASCULAR CALCIFICATION.

In some patients, poorly defined calcific deposits are seen within the soft tissues and vessels (Figs. 40–7 and 40–9). Tumorous calcific collections, resembling gouty tophi, are observed occasionally.

Pyrophosphate Arthropathy

The structural joint changes associated with CPPD crystal deposition disease are both common and characteristic. These may appear without adjacent or distant articular calcification and, therefore, it is important that these abnormalities be recognized as a manifestation of the disease. Pyrophosphate arthropathy is most common in the knee, wrist, and metacarpophalangeal joints. The distribution is usually bilateral, although symmetric changes may not be present. Pyrophosphate arthropathy simulates, in some ways, degenerative joint disease with articular space narrowing, bone sclerosis, and cyst formation, but it differs from degenerative joint disease in five respects.

1. *Unusual articular distribution.* Although arthropathy is encountered in weight-bearing joints, it is also apparent in sites that are less commonly involved in degenerative joint disease, such as the wrist, elbow, and glenohumeral joint (Fig. 40–10).

2. *Unusual intraarticular distribution.* The distribution of pyrophosphate arthropathy in certain joints is unusual (Fig. 40–11). Thus, isolated or significant involvement of the radiocarpal or trapezioscaphoid joint of the wrist, patellofemoral compartment of the knee, and talocalcaneonavicular articulation of the midfoot may signify CPPD crystal deposition disease.

Text continued on page 488

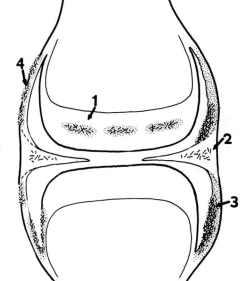

Figure 40–4. Articular and periarticular calcifications. Deposits may be located in hyaline cartilage *(1)*, fibrocartilage *(2)*, synovial membrane *(3)*, and joint capsule *(4)*.

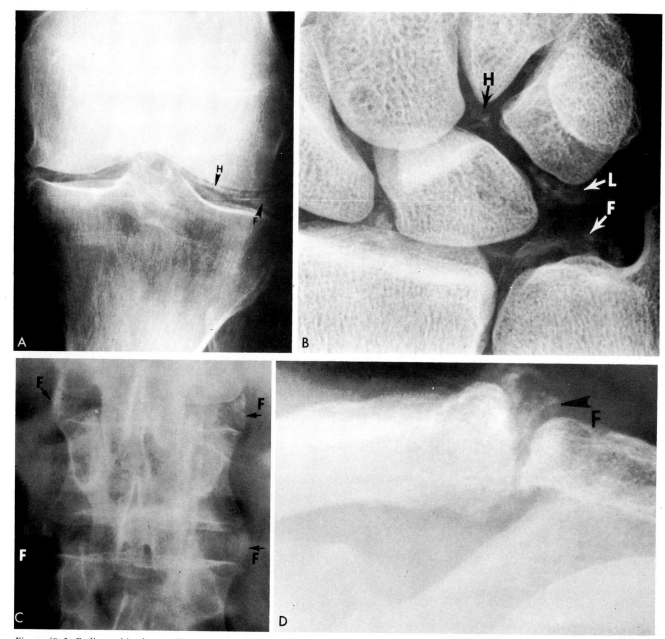

Figure 40–5. Radiographic abnormalities: Chondrocalcinosis. Chondrocalcinosis of fibrocartilage *(F)* is apparent in the menisci of the knee, triangular cartilage of the wrist, anulus fibrosus of the intervertebral discs, and meniscus of the acromioclavicular joint. It is thick and shaggy in character. Hyaline cartilage calcification *(H)*, which is seen in the knee and wrist, is thin and parallels the osseous surface. Possible ligamentous calcification *(L)* is also noted in the wrist. (**A,** From Resnick D, et al: Clinical, radiographic, and pathologic abnormalities in calcium pyrophosphate dihydrate deposition disease (CPPD): Pseudogout. Radiology *122*:1, 1977. Used with permission.)

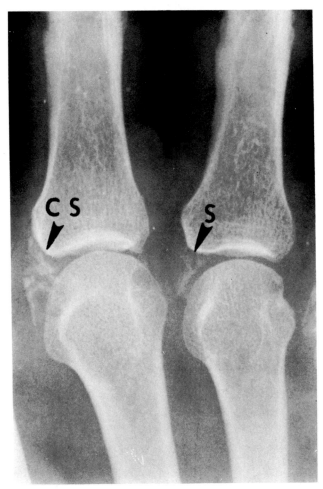

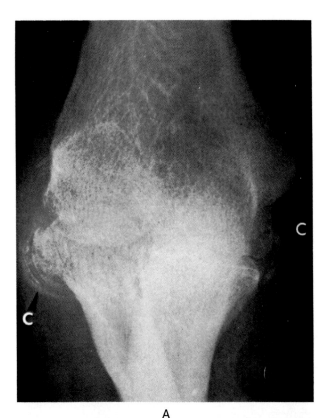

A

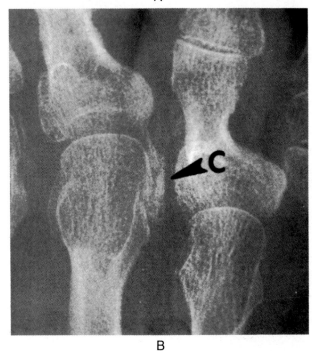

B

Figure 40–6. Radiographic abnormalities: Synovial calcification. Observe synovial (S) and capsular (C) calcification of metacarpophalangeal joints. (From Resnick D, et al: Clinical, radiographic, and pathologic abnormalities in calcium pyrophosphate dihydrate deposition disease (CPPD): Pseudogout. Radiology 122:1, 1977. Used with permission.)

Figure 40–7. Radiographic abnormalities: Capsular calcification. A In the elbow, capsular (C) calcification is associated wtih joint contracture and vascular (V) calcification. B Observe capsular (C) calcification about the metatarsophalangeal joints. (From Resnick D, et al: Clinical, radiographic, and pathologic abnormalities in calcium pyrophosphate dihydrate deposition disease (CPPD): Pseudogout. Radiology 122:1, 1977. Used with permission.)

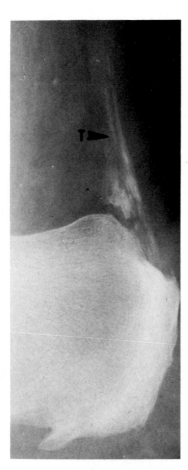

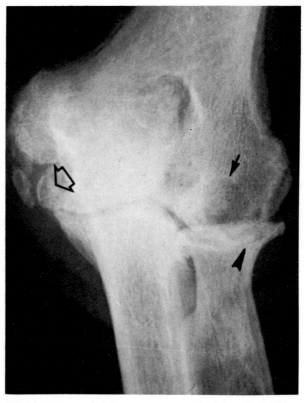

Figure 40–10. Characteristics of pyrophosphate arthropathy: Unusual articular distribution. Changes in the elbow include joint space narrowing, subchondral cysts (solid arrow), deformity of the radial head (arrowhead), and fragmentation (open arrow). (From Resnick D, et al: Clinical, radiographic, and pathologic abnormalities in calcium pyrophosphate dihydrate deposition disease (CPPD): Pseudogout. Radiology, *122*:1, 1977. Used with permission.)

Figure 40–8. Radiographic abnormalities: Tendon, ligament, and soft tissue calcification. Calcification within the Achilles tendon *(T)* is apparent. (From Resnick D, et al: Clinical, radiographic, and pathologic abnormalities in calcium pyrophosphate dihydrate deposition disease (CPPD): Pseudogout. Radiology *122*:1, 1977. Used with permission.)

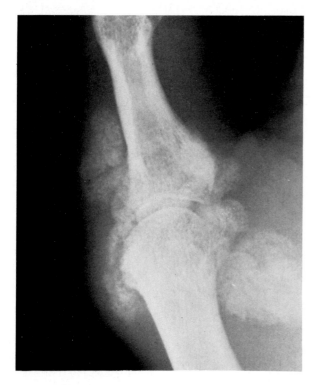

Figure 40–9. Radiographic abnormalities: Tophaceous pseudogout. Intraarticular and periarticular tumoral deposits are evident at the base of the thumb. (Courtesy of G. El Khoury, M.D., Iowa City, Iowa.)

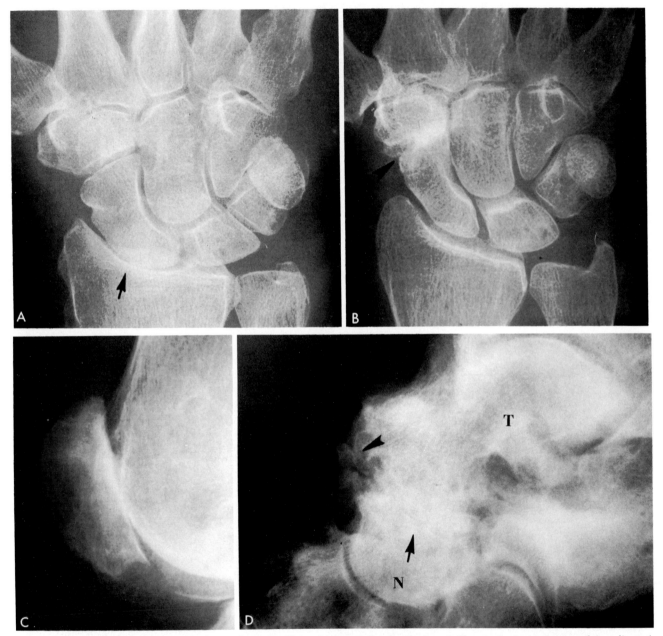

Figure 40–11. Characteristics of pyrophosphate arthropathy: Unusual intraarticular distribution. A Observe selective involvement of the radiocarpal compartment of the wrist (arrow). **B** Considerable abnormality of the trapezioscaphoid space of the midcarpal compartment is seen (arrowhead). **C** Predilection for the patellofemoral compartment of the knee is apparent on this lateral radiograph. **D** Destructive changes (arrowhead) and joint space narrowing (arrow) of the talonavicular area between talus *(T)* and navicular bone *(N)* are characteristic. (**D** From Resnick D, et al: Clinical, radiographic, and pathologic abnormalities in calcium pyrophosphate dihydrate deposition disease (CPPD): Pseudogout. Radiology *122*:1, 1977. Used with permission.)

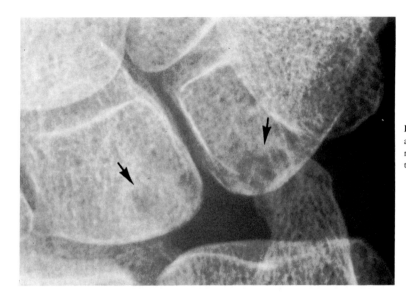

Figure 40–12. Characteristics of pyrophosphate arthropathy: Prominent subchondral cyst formation. Magnification radiography outlines numerous cysts of the lunate and triquetrum (arrows).

3. *Prominent subchondral cyst formation.* The cysts associated with pyrophosphate arthropathy are very numerous and may reach considerable size (Fig. 40–12). Typically they are multiple, subchondral in location, clustered in a group, and surrounded by sclerotic, smudged, and indistinct margins.

4. *Destructive bone changes that are severe and progressive.* Pyrophosphate arthropathy may be associated with extensive and rapid subchondral bone collapse and fragmentation and the appearance of single or multiple intraarticular osseous

bodies (Fig. 40–13). These features resemble those of neuroarthropathy. This destructive arthropathy may be evident in the hips, knees, shoulders, elbows, wrists, symphysis pubis, ankles, and metacarpophalangeal and midtarsal joints.

5. *Variable osteophyte formation.* In some patients, large, irregular bone excrescences are noted about involved joints; in others, joint space narrowing, sclerosis, and fragmentation may be unaccompanied by osteophyte formation, producing a polished, eburnated bone surface (Fig. 40–14).

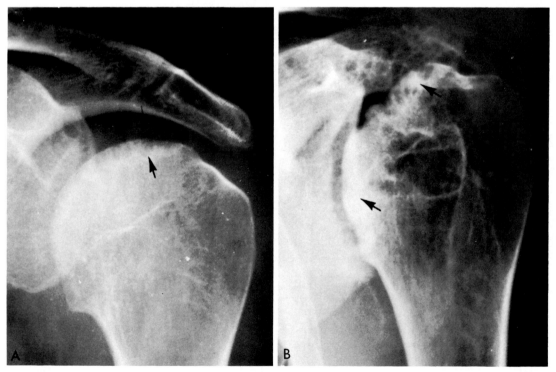

Figure 40–13. Characteristics of pyrophosphate arthropathy: Destructive bone changes that are severe and progressive. Radiographs of the glenohumeral joint obtained 16 months apart outline the rapidity of joint destruction in this disease (arrows). (B From Resnick D, et al: Clinical, radiographic, and pathologic abnormalities in calcium pyrophosphate dihydrate deposition disease (CPPD): Pseudogout. Radiology *122*:1, 1977. Used with permission.)

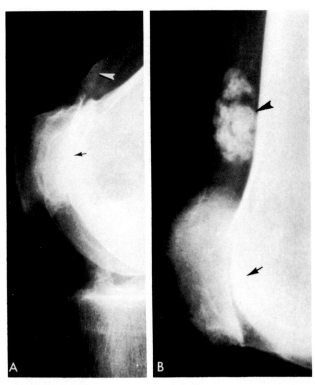

Figure 40–14. Characteristics of pyrophosphate arthropathy: Variable osteophyte formation. A In some persons, large osteophytes (arrowhead) accompany joint space narrowing (arrow). B In other patients, joint space narrowing (arrow) occurs without osteophyte formation. Intraarticular bodies are apparent (arrowhead). (From Resnick D, et al: Clinical, radiographic, and pathologic abnormalities in calcium pyrophosphate dihydrate deposition disease (CPPD): Pseudogout. Radiology 122:1, 1977. Used with permission.)

RADIOLOGIC FEATURES IN SPECIFIC ARTICULATIONS

Knee (Fig. 40–15)

The knee is the joint most commonly involved, both clinically and radiographically. Chondrocalcinosis and synovial calcification may be combined with tendinous and ligamentous deposits in the quadriceps muscle and cruciate ligaments. Intraarticular osseous and calcific bodies are very frequent. Joint effusion, soft tissue swelling, and popliteal cysts may be encountered.

Pyrophosphate arthropathy most commonly involves the medial femorotibial compartment. The patellofemoral compartment is the second most commonly involved area, whereas changes in the lateral femorotibial compartment are less frequent. More importantly, the distribution of knee compartmental alterations in CPPD crystal deposition disease differs from that of degenerative joint disease. Isolated or severe patellofemoral compartmental changes have been stressed as a manifestation of this crystal disease. In this location, extensive compartmental narrowing between the posterior surface of the patella and the anterior surface of the distal end of the femur may be associated with bone eburnation and anterior femoral erosion. These patellofemoral compartmental changes are not specific, because they are observed occasionally in degenerative joint disease, but when they occur as an isolated phenomenon, particularly if severe,

patellofemoral joint alterations should suggest the diagnosis of CPPD crystal deposition disease. Similar manifestations may appear in patients with primary hyperparathyroidism or renal osteodystrophy with or without crystal deposition.

Isolated lateral compartmental alterations, severe flattening of either medial or lateral tibial condyles, and significant varus or valgus angulation are additional characteristics of the knee involvement in this disease.

Wrist (Fig. 40–16)

Calcification in the wrist is observed most commonly in the triangular fibrocartilage, hyaline cartilage of the radiocarpal, midcarpal, and common carpometacarpal joints, synovium, and ligamentous structures, particularly between the scaphoid and lunate and between the lunate and triquetrum. Carpal malalignment with separation of scaphoid and lunate bones may be related to disruption of the intervening interosseous ligament.

The wrist arthropathy of CPPD crystal deposition disease demonstrates unusual predilection for the radiocarpal compartment of the wrist. Joint space narrowing, sclerosis, and discrete subchondral radiolucent lesions are observed between the distal end of the radius and the proximal carpal row. The scaphoid moves proximally and may appear compressed and deformed by the adjacent radius. The lunate may move distally, approaching the capitate and producing a "stepladder" appearance that is very suggestive of this disease. Alterations of the inferior radioulnar compartment are not common. The midcarpal compartment may reveal joint space narrowing; significant abnormalities of the trapezioscaphoid portion of this compartment are observed.

The compartmental distribution of CPPD arthropathy differs considerably from that of degenerative joint disease. The latter disorder affects predominantly the first carpometacarpal and trapezioscaphoid areas, sparing the radiocarpal compartment. Furthermore, the relative paucity of changes at the inferior radioulnar compartment in CPPD crystal deposition disease allows differentiation from rheumatoid arthritis.

Metacarpophalangeal Joints (Fig. 40–17)

Radiographic abnormalities in this location include cartilaginous, capsular, and synovial calcifications and arthropathy. The structural joint changes show predilection for the second and third metacarpophalangeal joints and are characterized by joint space narrowing, sclerosis, cyst formation, and bone collapse, particularly of the metacarpal head. The bone collapse is more prominent in CPPD crystal deposition disease than in degenerative joint disease. Although changes may also be apparent at various interphalangeal joints, they are usually mild. The second and third metacarpophalangeal joints are also involved in hemochromatosis, but changes in the fourth and fifth digits also are not infrequent in this disease. Furthermore, the absence of erosions of the metacarpal heads in CPPD crystal deposition disease differs from the findings of rheumatoid arthritis.

Elbow

Radiographic findings in the elbow include chondrocalcinosis, capsular and synovial calcification, triceps tendon deposits, and arthropathy.

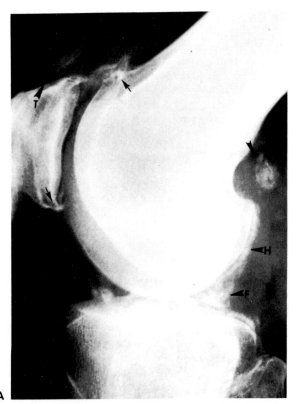
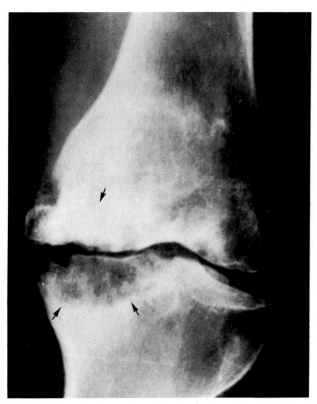

Figure 40–15. Knee abnormalities in CPPD crystal deposition disease. A Findings include hyaline cartilage *(H)*, fibrocartilage *(F)*, and tendon *(T)* calcification, joint space narrowing, osteophyte formation (arrows), and intraarticular osseous bodies (arrowhead). **B** Considerable collapse and fragmentation of the medial femorotibial compartment are visualized (arrows). (B From Resnick D, et al: Clinical, radiographic, and pathologic abnormalities in calcium pyrophosphate dihydrate deposition disease (CPPD): Pseudogout. Radiology *122*:1, 1977. Used with permission.)

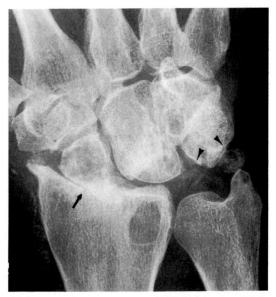

Figure 40–16. Wrist abnormalities in CPPD crystal deposition disease. In addition to chondrocalcinosis and synovial and ligamentous calcification (arrowheads), observe considerable narrowing of the radiocarpal (arrow) and midcarpal compartments, with cyst formation and sclerosis. Note the "stepladder" appearance, with proximal migration of the scaphoid and distal migration of the lunate. (From Resnick D, et al: Clinical, radiographic, and pathological abnormalities in calcium pyrophosphate dihydrate deposition disease (CPPD): Pseudogout. Radiology *122*:1, 1977. Used with permission.)

Hip (Fig. 40–18)

Fibrocartilaginous calcification of the acetabular labra and hyaline cartilage calcification may both be seen. Joint space narrowing may involve the entire joint or be confined to the superolateral aspect. In the latter situation, the changes resemble those of osteoarthritis, whereas with symmetric loss of joint space, the findings are similar to those of rheumatoid arthritis. Additional manifestations of hip involvement in CPPD crystal deposition disease are rapid destruction of the femoral head and acetabulum and protrusio acetabuli deformity.

Glenohumeral Joint

Abnormalities in this location include chondrocalcinosis; capsular, tendinous, and bursal deposits; rotator cuff tears; joint space narrowing; bone eburnation; and cysts.

Ankle, Hindfoot, and Midfoot

Although calcification can be seen about the ankle, arthropathy in this site is unusual. More commonly, the midfoot is altered, particularly the talocalcaneonavicular joint. At this location, the findings resemble those of neuroarthropathy, particularly that associated with diabetes mellitus.

Forefoot

Capsular calcification may be apparent about any metatarsophalangeal joint. In unusual circumstances, cartilage and synovial calcification and soft tissue swelling at the first metatarsophalangeal joint resemble the changes of gout.

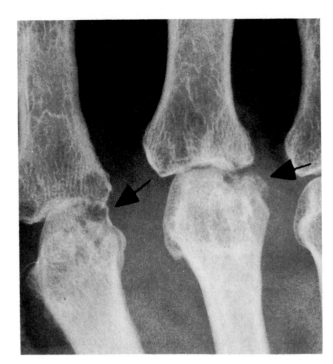

Figure 40–17. Metacarpophalangeal joint abnormalities in CPPD crystal deposition disease. Collapse and fragmentation (arrows) are noted about the second and third metacarpophalangeal joints.

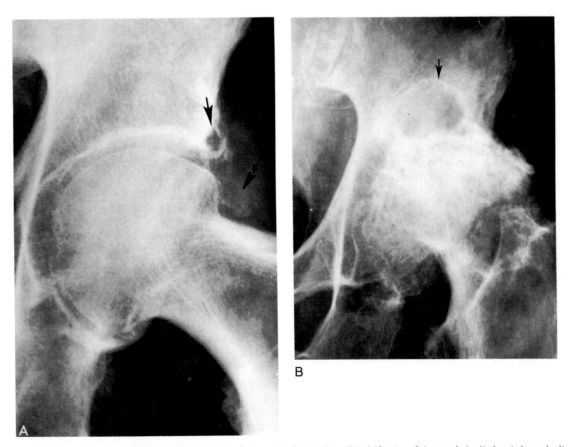

Figure 40–18. Hip abnormalities in CPPD crystal deposition disease. A Fibrocartilage (F) calcification of the acetabular limbus is located adjacent to a small subchondral cystic lesion (arrow). B Considerable flattening and deformity of the femoral head are associated with an elongated lateral acetabular osteophyte and new bone formation on the medial aspect of the femoral neck. The articular space is obliterated and a large subchondral cyst (arrow) is evident. (From Resnick D, et al: Clinical, radiographic, and pathologic abnormalities in calcium pyrophosphate dihydrate deposition disease (CPPD): Pseudogout. Radiology 122:1, 1977. Used with permission.)

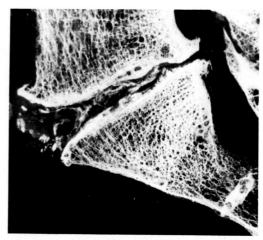

Figure 40–19. Spine abnormalities in CPPD crystal deposition disease. Alterations of the intervertebral disc. In association with widespread discal calcification, disc space loss and bone eburnation are seen in this sagittal section of the lumbosacral junction.

Spine (Figs. 40–19 and 40–20)

Intervertebral discal calcifications are frequent, the deposits initially appearing in the outer fibers of the anulus fibrosus. In this location, calcific collections resemble syndesmophytes of ankylosing spondylitis. CPPD deposits are detected in other spinal tissues as well, including the ligamentum flavum, the posterior longitudinal ligament, the interspinous and supraspinous ligaments, and the interspinous bursae. CPPD crystal accumulation has been documented in the articular cartilage, synovium, and capsule of the apophyseal joints and in the transverse ligament of the atlas.

Disc space narrowing is a common finding in CPPD crystal deposition disease. The narrowing may be extensive, widespread, and associated with considerable vertebral sclerosis; these findings are identical to those occurring in intervertebral osteochondrosis (degenerative disease of the nucleus pulposus). Subluxation of cervical vertebrae may be apparent at any level, including the atlantoaxial junction. Angular deformities relate to collapse and fragmentation of the anterior aspect of the vertebral bodies.

Sacroiliac Joint

Unilateral or bilateral subchondral erosions, sclerosis, and cyst formation may be accompanied by joint space narrowing and bridging osteophytosis. These findings can simulate the appearance of ankylosing spondylitis. Although a vacuum phenomenon has been observed in the sacroiliac joints of patients with CPPD crystal deposition disease, it appears to have little diagnostic significance.

CLINICAL AND RADIOGRAPHIC CORRELATIONS

Investigations correlating the clinical and radiographic findings of CPPD crystal deposition disease have indicated the following:

1. *Clinical pattern of disease and radiographic abnormality.* No definite relationship exists between the clinical pattern of arthritis (e.g., acute, chronic, asymptomatic) and the presence of articular calcification or arthropathy. Even asymptomatic patients may have widespread calcific deposits and severe arthropathy.

2. *Joint symptoms and local (in the same articulation) calcification or arthropathy.* In general, articular calcification is slightly more frequent in symptomatic than in asymptomatic joints. No definite relationship is found between joint symptoms and type of cartilage calcification (fibrocartilage versus hyaline cartilage). In general, the frequency of arthropathy in symptomatic joints is greater than that in asymptomatic joints.

It is apparent that clinical-radiographic dissociation may exist in this disease. Frequently, a patient with significant symptoms in one or more joints reveals no radiographic abnormality in those locations, whereas another individual with absent or mild symptoms will demonstrate both calcification and arthropathy.

3. *Positive crystal aspiration and local calcification or arthropathy.* The frequency and extent of local calcification and arthropathy do not correlate with the success of crystal recovery during joint aspiration. More commonly, the frequency of positive crystal identification from joint aspiration reflects both the presence of acute symptoms with joint effusion and the skill and patience of the microscopist.

4. *Local calcification and local arthropathy.* Arthropathy is consistently more common, although not more severe, in joints with calcification. No relationship is found between the type of chondrocalcinosis (fibrocartilage versus hyaline cartilage) and the presence and severity of arthropathy.

Although calcification and arthropathy frequently coexist in the same joint, either radiographic finding can be identified in the absence of the other. More commonly, calcification precedes arthropathy; instances exist, however, in which arthropathy develops in patients who demonstrate neither local (in the same joint) nor distant (in any joint) calcification on radiographic examination. The absence of radiographically evident calcification in patients with CPPD crystal deposition disease and arthropathy may be related to several factors. Routine radiographic techniques are relatively inadequate in the detection of sparse collections of calcification, such that industrial film may be needed. Additionally, with progressive destruction of joint cartilage, initial calcific deposits may become less evident or disappear.

The absence of cartilage calcification in some patients with arthropathy and intraarticular CPPD crystals may indicate that the primary alteration is one of cartilage degeneration and that secondary calcification occurs. It has been suggested that an "amplification loop" exists in which crystal deposition is favored by age changes in normal cartilage or by tissue deterioration caused by preexisting joint disease. Clinical examples supporting this concept include the detection of CPPD crystals at sites of spinal surgery, the development of chondrocalcinosis subsequent to a scaphoid fracture, and the superimposition of pseudogout on other arthritic processes.

In most patients with CPPD crystal deposition disease who have been followed for several years, the degree of calcification and arthropathy generally remains unchanged. Occasionally patients with moderate or severe structural joint damage and only minimal calcification have developed extensive calcific deposits on subsequent examinations.

DIFFERENTIAL DIAGNOSIS
Intraarticular Calcification

Chondrocalcinosis, particularly of the menisci of the knee, may relate not only to the presence of CPPD crystals but also

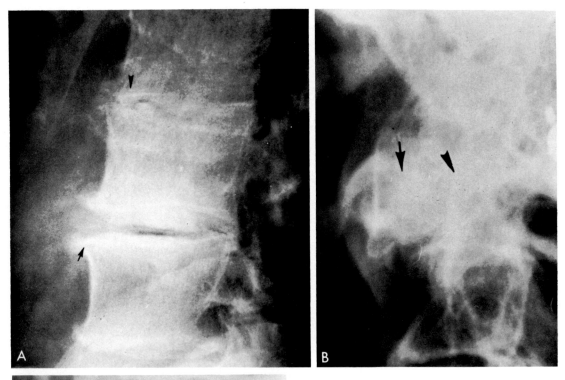

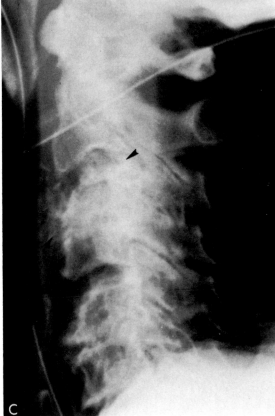

Figure 40–20. Spine abnormalities in CPPD crystal deposition disease. In the lumbar spine, findings are disc space narrowing (arrowhead), vacuum phenomena, sclerosis, and osteophyte formation (arrow). B Atlantoaxial subluxation is indicated by the enlarged space between the anterior arch of the atlas (arrow) and the odontoid process (arrowhead). C Note the obliteration of the disc space between two of the cervical vertebral bodies with anterior osseous fragmentation (arrow). Similar abnormalities can be seen at the level of two lower cervical vertebrae. The third vertebra body (arrowhead) has been extensively resorbed. Joint space narrowing and bone eburnation are present at many apophyseal joints. (From Resnick D, et al: Clinical, radiographic, and pathologic abnormalities in calcium pyrophosphate dihydrate deposition disease (CPPD): Pseudogout. Radiology *122*:1, 1977. Used with permission.)

to the deposition of other crystalline material, such as dicalcium phosphate dihydrate (DCPD) and HA. DCPD deposition produces diffuse, punctate radiodense lesions, whereas HA deposition may produce localized radiodense areas in a single meniscus. Chondrocalcinosis of more than one set of joints usually indicates CPPD crystal deposition. This deposition may be related to familial or sporadic (idiopathic) disease or may occur in association with other disorders, such as primary hyperparathyroidism and hemochromatosis. The diagnosis of hyperparathyroidism is substantiated by the presence of bone resorption elsewhere in the skeleton. The radiographic features of hemochromatosis are closely related to those of idiopathic CPPD crystal deposition disease.

Additional causes of intraarticular radiodense lesions that may simulate CPPD crystal deposition generally produce abnormalities of a single joint. These include meniscal ossicles of the knee; osteochondritis dissecans of the knee, ankle, or elbow; osteonecrosis; and idiopathic synovial osteochondromatosis. Disintegration of articular surfaces with production of single or multiple calcific and ossific dense areas may be seen in a variety of other articular disorders, including neuroarthropathy, steroid-induced arthropathy, infection, gout, and rheumatoid arthritis. In these cases, characteristic signs of the underlying articular disorder usually are apparent. Calcification of intraarticular neoplasms, such as synovial sarcoma and synovial hemangioma, may rarely be encountered.

Intraarticular calcification in one or more locations related to HA crystal deposition has been emphasized in recent years (see Chapter 41). It may occur on an idiopathic basis or secondary to a variety of processes, including osteoarthritis and scleroderma. In general, calcific deposits are tumoral or cloud-like in character, and chondrocalcinosis is unusual. Diagnostic difficulties arise in certain cases of CPPD crystal deposition disease in which homogeneous, tumoral intraarticular calcifications (tophaceous pseudogout) or osteochondral fragments are seen or in those with *both* CPPD and HA crystal accumulation (mixed crystal deposition disease).

Periarticular Calcification

Periarticular radiodense deposits may relate to metastatic calcification, dystrophic calcification, or calcinosis. Such calcification is seen in a variety of disorders, including renal osteodystrophy, idiopathic tumoral calcinosis, collagen diseases, milk-alkali syndrome, and hypervitaminosis D. In these disorders, intraarticular dense lesions generally are not apparent.

Calcific peritendinitis may be associated with deposition of HA crystals in tendons and bursae, particularly about the shoulder. Tendinous calcification in CPPD crystal deposition disease produces similar abnormalities, although the deposits may be more elongated in appearance. Differentiation between these two disorders is aided by the absence of chondrocalcinosis in patients with calcific periarthritis. Deposition of both CPPD and HA crystals can occur in a single joint, however. Chondrocalcinosis related to CPPD crystals can be associated with periarticular calcification related to HA crystals.

Pyrophosphate Arthropathy (Table 40–4)

The arthropathy of CPPD crystal deposition disease closely resembles degenerative joint disease, but, as indicated previously, it involves unusual articulations and compartments and is associated with extensive sclerosis, multiple cysts, bone fragmentation, osseous debris, and variable osteophyte formation.

The degree of bone fragmentation, sclerosis, and collapse encountered in patients with CPPD crystal deposition disease is reminiscent of changes accompanying other disorders, such as neuroarthropathy, steroid-induced arthropathy, osteonecrosis, and infection (Fig. 40–21). The absence of clinical features typical of these other disorders usually ensures accurate diagnosis of CPPD crystal deposition disease in these persons. In addition, joint space narrowing is common in CPPD crystal deposition disease but is not apparent in osteonecrosis until the later stages of the disease. The osseous surfaces in an infected joint are more poorly defined or irregular.

Bone erosion is not a feature of CPPD crystal deposition disease. The absence of erosive change usually aids in distinguishing this condition from rheumatoid arthritis and related synovial disorders, such as psoriatic arthritis and ankylosing spondylitis. The appearance of joint space narrowing, bone eburnation, osteophytosis, and sclerosis in CPPD crystal deposition disease may resemble features of gout. Differentia-

Table 40–4. DIFFERENTIAL DIAGNOSIS OF PYROPHOSPHATE ARTHROPATHY

	Pyrophosphate Arthropathy	Degenerative Joint Disease	Neuroarthropathy	Rheumatoid Arthritis
Common sites	Knee, wrist (radiocarpal), metacarpophalangeal	Hip, knee, interphalangeal of hand, wrist (first carpometacarpal, trapezioscaphoid), first metatarsophalangeal	Tabes: knee, ankle, hip, spine Diabetes: midfoot and forefoot Syringomyelia: upper extremity	Wrist (pancompartmental), metacarpophalangeal, interphalangeal of hand, metatarsophalangeal, knee, shoulder, cervical spine
Articular space narrowing	+	+	±	+
Sclerosis	+	+	+	−
Osteophytosis	±	+	±	−
Erosions	−	−	−	+
Cysts	+	+	±	+
Fragmentation	+	−	+	−

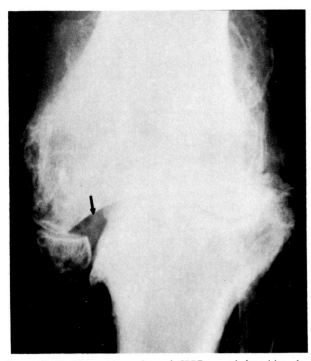

Figure 40–21. Neuroarthropathy and CPPD crystal deposition. In a patient with tabes dorsalis, neuropathic changes of the knee include joint space narrowing, extreme bone eburnation, osteophytosis, fragmentation, and subluxation. Observe chondrocalcinosis in the medial meniscus (arrow). CPPD crystals were obtained on joint aspiration.

tion between gout and CPPD crystal deposition disease is further complicated by the occasional presence of periarticular calcification and chondrocalcinosis in gouty arthritis. In gouty arthritis, however, asymmetric soft tissue swelling and bone erosion, findings not generally seen in CPPD crystal deposition disease, may be noted.

Additional differential diagnostic considerations of pyrophosphate arthropathy depend on the specific articular site of involvement.

KNEE. Although the distribution of compartmental abnormalities in the knee in CPPD crystal deposition disease may be identical to that of degenerative joint disease, isolated patellofemoral compartmental changes are an important diagnostic clue, suggesting the presence of pyrophosphate arthropathy. In degenerative joint disease, patellofemoral changes are frequent, but in most cases they are combined with alterations in the medial femorotibial or, less frequently, the lateral femorotibial compartment. Symmetric loss of joint space in the medial and lateral femorotibial spaces or tricompartmental involvement (medial and lateral femorotibial compartments and patellofemoral compartment) is common in rheumatoid arthritis and infection and is not usually seen in pyrophosphate arthropathy. Patellofemoral compartment erosions may be seen in patients with primary hyperparathyroidism or renal osteodystrophy.

WRIST. Selective involvement of the radiocarpal compartment of the wrist is most characteristic of CPPD crystal deposition disease. Degenerative joint disease in the wrist usually produces changes at the first carpometacarpal and trapezioscaphoid areas rather than at the radiocarpal compartment. After injury, however, osteoarthritis can appear in any

region of the wrist, including the radioscaphoid, radiolunate, and lunate-capitate spaces. Furthermore, radiocarpal compartment changes may occasionally be seen in patients with gout or occupation-related degenerative disease. Rheumatoid arthritis also involves this joint, but additional changes in other compartments of the wrist generally are apparent in this disease. In rheumatoid arthritis, the inferior radioulnar compartment demonstrates extensive abnormalities; this site is not commonly involved in pyrophosphate arthropathy.

METACARPOPHALANGEAL JOINTS. The metacarpophalangeal joints frequently are altered in CPPD crystal deposition disease, and the changes in this location predominate over changes at the interphalangeal articulations. The opposite situation exists in degenerative joint disease; interphalangeal joint abnormalities are extensive, whereas involvement of the metacarpophalangeal joints is less severe. The absence of osseous erosion of the metacarpal heads and proximal phalanges in CPPD crystal deposition disease allows its differentiation from rheumatoid arthritis.

The arthropathies of idiopathic CPPD crystal deposition and of hemochromatosis are very similar, although subtle differences have been defined. Both disorders involve the second and third metacarpophalangeal articulations, but changes in the fourth and fifth digits are more prevalent in hemochromatosis. Peculiar hook-like osteophytes on the radial aspect of the metacarpal heads are also more characteristic of hemochromatosis than of idiopathic CPPD crystal deposition disease. Furthermore, scapholunate separation, or dissociation, is less prevalent in hemochromatosis.

HIP. Asymmetric loss of joint space in the superolateral aspect of this articulation may occur in patients with CPPD crystal deposition disease, mimicking the findings of degenerative joint disease. In other patients with this crystal disorder, symmetric loss of joint space is observed, and the findings are easily differentiated from degenerative disease. In patients with symmetrical disease, the pattern of joint space loss simulates that occurring in various synovial diseases, such as rheumatoid arthritis and ankylosing spondylitis. The degree of bone sclerosis and osteophytosis in CPPD crystal deposition disease allows differentiation of this disorder from rheumatoid arthritis, but the hip involvement of pyrophosphate arthropathy may indeed resemble that of ankylosing spondylitis. The presence of bone fragmentation and collapse and the absence of sacroiliac joint abnormalities in CPPD crystal deposition disease are findings that are not apparent in ankylosing spondylitis.

FOOT. Selective involvement of the talonavicular portion of the talocalcaneonavicular joint is observed in patients with pyrophosphate arthropathy. This distribution of abnormalities is also observed in neuroarthropathy accompanying diabetes mellitus. The absence of significant erosion of the first metatarsophalangeal articulation distinguishes pyrophosphate arthropathy from gouty arthritis.

SPINE. Discal calcification related to CPPD crystal deposition occurs initially in the outer fibers of the anulus fibrosus. With progressive calcification, widespread discal deposits resemble changes of ochronosis. The resemblance between these two disorders is accentuated by the possible occurrence of both peripheral arthropathy and chondrocalcinosis in patients with ochronosis. Widespread discal calcification related to HA crystal deposition is also seen in a variety of disorders, including hyperparathyroidism, and on an idiopathic basis.

Disc space narrowing in the thoracic and lumbar spine in CPPD crystal deposition disease is identical to that seen in intervertebral osteochondrosis (degenerative disease of the nucleus pulposus). Vertebral body sclerosis may be observed in both disorders, but the degree of bone eburnation and the possible occurrence of vertebral body destruction in CPPD crystal deposition disease allow accurate diagnosis.

Cervical spine subluxation, particularly at the atlantoaxial junction, in CPPD crystal deposition disease resembles the findings of rheumatoid arthritis. The absence of discovertebral and apophyseal joint erosions in pyrophosphate arthropathy will distinguish it from rheumatoid arthritis.

Calcification of the posterior longitudinal ligament, ligamenta flava, and interspinous ligaments is related not only to CPPD crystal deposition but also to HA crystal accumulation.

FURTHER READING

Adamson TC III, Resnik CS, Guerra J Jr, Vint VC, Weisman MH, Resnick D: Hand and wrist arthropathies of hemochromatosis and calcium pyrophosphate deposition disease: Distinct radiographic features. Radiology 147:377, 1983.

Dieppe PA, Alexander GJM, Jones HE, Doherty M, Scott DGI, Manhire A, Watt I: Pyrophosphate arthropathy: A clinical and radiological study of 105 cases. Ann Rheum Dis 41:371, 1982.

Leisen J: Calcium pyrophosphate dihydrate deposition disease: Tumorous form. AJR 138:962, 1982.

Ling D, Murphy WA, Kyriakos M: Tophaceous pseudogout. AJR 138:162, 1982.

Martel W, Champion CK, Thompson GR, Carter TL: A roentgenologically distinctive arthropathy in some patients with the pseudogout syndrome. AJR 109:587, 1970.

Martel W, McCarter DK, Solsky MA, Good AE, Hart WR, Braunstein EM, Brady TM: Further observations on the arthropathy of calcium pyrophosphate crystal deposition disease. Radiology 141:1, 1981.

McCarty DJ, Hollander JL: Identification of urate crystals in gouty synovial fluid. Ann Intern Med 54:452, 1961.

McCarty DJ Jr, Kohn NN, Faires JS: The significance of calcium phosphate crystals in the synovial fluid of arthritis patients: The "pseudogout" syndrome. Ann Intern Med 56:711, 1962.

McCarty DJ, Silcox DC, Coe F, Jacobelli S, Reiss E, Genant H, Ellman M: Diseases associated with calcium pyrophosphate dihydrate crystal deposition. Am J Med 56:704, 1974.

Resnick D, Niwayama G, Goergen TG, Utsinger PD, Shapiro RF, Haselwood DH, Wiesner KB: Clinical, radiographic and pathologic abnormalities in calcium pyrophosphate dihydrate deposition disease (CPPD): Pseudogout. Radiology 122:1, 1977.

Resnick D, Pineda C: Vertebral involvement in calcium pyrophosphate dihydrate crystal deposition diesease. Radiographic-pathologic correlation. Radiology 153:55, 1984.

Rynes RI, Merzig EG: Calcium pyrophosphate crystal deposition disease and hyperparathyroidism. A controlled, prospective study. J Rheumatol 5:460, 1978.

Utsinger PD, Zvaifler NJ, Resnick D: Calcium pyrophosphate dihydrate deposition disease without chondrocalcinosis. J Rheumatol 2:258, 1975.

Zitñan D, Sitaj S: Chondrocalcinosis articularis. Section I: Clinical and radiological study. Ann Rheum Dis 22:142, 1963.

Chapter 41

Calcium Hydroxyapatite Crystal Deposition Disease

Donald Resnick, M.D.

Calcium hydroxyapatite (HA) crystal deposition can lead to periarticular accumulations that are associated with typical clinical and radiologic findings. The radiographic manifestations in HA crystal deposition disease are observed most frequently in the shoulder, although similar abnormalities may be apparent at other articular sites. Intraar-ticular alterations have also been documented as a consequence of HA crystal deposition disease, and the combination of both HA and calcium pyrophosphate dihydrate crystal accumulation (mixed calcium phosphate crystal deposition disease) is being identified increasingly frequently.

In the last 20 years, the development of methods such as polarizing microscopy for identifying crystalline deposits in and around joints has led to the elucidation of several disorders that are associated with tissue inflammation: needle-shaped crystals of monosodium urate in patients with gout; calcium pyrophosphate dihydrate (CPPD) crystals in patients who have the pseudogout syndrome; and crystalline depot corticosteroid preparations. Two other crystal types were also identified in human cartilage and extraarticular soft tissues: calcium hydroxyapatite (HA) and calcium orthophosphate dihydrate.

Although the presence of calcification in periarticular soft tissues and tendons, particularly about the shoulder, has been observed for many years, it was not until 1966 that HA was implicated as the material deposited in these calcific collections. HA crystals currently are well recognized as a cause of bursitis and other periarticular inflammatory conditions that may be associated with radiographically demonstrable calcification. In recent years, some investigators have indicated that HA crystals may also be observed in joint fluid and, in this location, can lead to articular manifestations.

The identification of individual HA crystals, or of closely related calcium phosphate crystals, generally is not possible using ordinary or polarized light microscopy owing to their minute size; precise identification requires electron microscopic or radioisotopic techniques or x-ray diffraction analysis. Despite this difficulty, the fact that HA crystals and closely related calcium phosphate compounds are associated with both periarticular and intraarticular abnormalities is now well established.

PERIARTICULAR CRYSTAL DEPOSITION
Clinical Features

Recurrent painful periarticular calcific deposits in tendons and soft tissues have been described by a variety of names, such as peritendinitis calcarea, calcareus tendinitis and bursitis, periarthritis calcarea, calcific tendinitis, peritendinitis and bursitis, and hydroxyapatite rheumatism. These deposits are usually monoarticular in distribution, but they can be polyarticular. The most frequent site of involvement is the shoulder, although involvement of other sites such as the wrist, hand, foot, elbow, hip, neck, and lumbar spine has been described. The disease affects both men and women and is particularly common between 40 and 70 years of age.

Acute symptoms include pain, tenderness on pressure, local edema or swelling, restricted active and passive motion, and mild fever. Chronic symptoms and signs may also be present. In many patients, radiographic deposits are detected when they are entirely asymptomatic. Manual workers are affected more commonly than those who do sedentary work. Laboratory tests generally are unrewarding.

General Pathologic Features

Granular deposits of calcium material (HA) in fibrous connective tissue may be associated with necrosis and loss of fibrous structure and surrounding inflammatory changes. The deposits appear milky or cheesy in consistency and are inspissated or chalk-like in quality.

General Radiologic Features

The radiologic features of periarticular HA crystal deposition depend on the site of involvement. Initially the deposits may appear thin, cloud-like, and poorly defined. With time, they may seem denser, homogeneous, and more sharply delineated. Adjacent osseous tissues may be entirely normal, although osteoporosis, cystic and erosive lesions, reactive sclerosis, and contour irregularities sometimes are apparent.

Sequential radiographic examinations in patients with calcific periarticular deposits reveal varying patterns. In some patients, the deposits remain static for long periods of time, changing little in size or configuration. In other patients, the deposits may enlarge and change shape. Diminution in size and disappearance of deposits likewise are not infrequent, and reappearance of calcification has also been documented. Periarticular amorphous calcific collections in association with

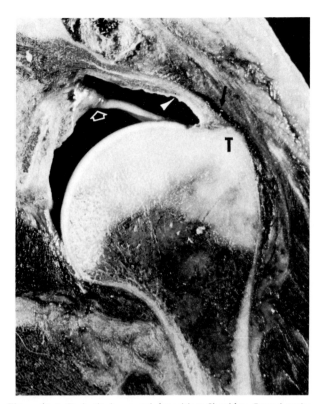

Figure 41–1. Periarticular crystal deposition: Shoulder. Coronal section of the glenohumeral joint showing sites of involvement. Calcific deposits may be located in the tendons of the rotator cuff (arrowhead), particularly near the site of their attachment to the greater tuberosity (*T*), the bicipital tendon at the site of its attachment to the superior rim of the glenoid (open arrow), and the subdeltoid (subacromial) bursa (solid arrow).

some disorders, such as chronic renal disease, may become massive, surrounding the joint.

Cause and Pathogenesis of Crystal Accumulation

The cause and pathogenesis of HA crystal deposition in periarticular tissues are unknown. In the past, it has been attractive to assume that such collections resulted from deposition of calcium in injured and necrotic tissue. More recently, documentation of familial cases, polyarticular distribution, and an increased frequency of certain histocompatibility antigens in these patients suggests that systemic factors may be operational.

Calcific Tendinitis and Bursitis at Specific Sites

SHOULDER. The capsular, tendinous, ligamentous, and bursal tissues about the shoulder are the most common sites of articular and periarticular calcific deposits. These deposits occur in approximately 3 per cent of adults, are bilateral in almost 50 per cent of persons, and are accompanied by clinical manifestation in about 35 per cent of cases.

The radiographic appearance of shoulder calcification will depend on the exact location of the abnormal deposits; commonly they are encountered in the tendons of the rotator cuff, adjacent tendons, and bursae (Fig. 41–1). Several phases or stages of the disease have been recognized (Fig. 41–2). The precise appearance and position of the calcification depend on the phase of the disease process and the specific tendon in which the deposit is located (Fig. 41–3).

Supraspinatus Tendon Calcification. The supraspinatus tendon is the most frequent site of calcification. The deposits are located at the tendinous insertion on the promontory of the greater tuberosity (Fig. 41–4). Radiodense lesions at this site may be seen in profile on external rotation of the shoulder. They may remain in profile on internal rotation, although as

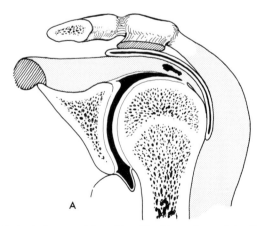
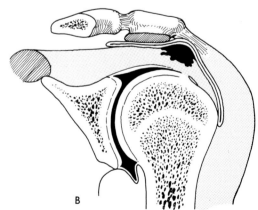

Figure 41–2. Periarticular crystal deposition: Shoulder—phases of the disease. A Silent phase. Subclinical deposition of calcium occurs in the substance of the rotator cuff tendons. **B** Mechanical phase—elevation of bursal floor. As the deposits increase in size, the floor of the subdeltoid (subacromial) bursa is raised.

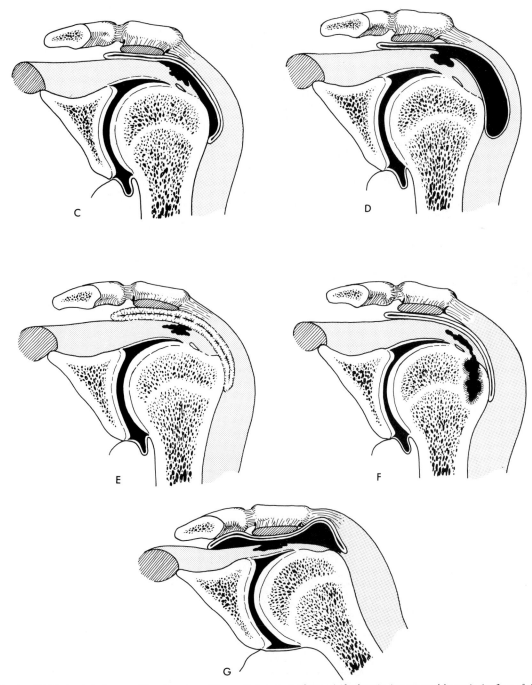

Figure 41–2 *Continued* **C** Mechanical phase—subbursal rupture. Observe that rupture of the calcific deposits has occurred beneath the floor of the bursa. **D** Mechanical phase—intrabursal rupture. The entire deposit is being expelled into the subdeltoid bursa. **E** Adhesive periarthritis stage. Note adduction of the shoulder with adhesive bursitis. **F** Intraosseous loculation. The calcific deposit has extended into the bone. **G** Dumbbell loculation. Rarely, a biloculated deposit may be seen related to pressure from the adjacent coracoacromial ligament. (Redrawn after Moseley HF: Shoulder Lesions. 3rd Ed. Edinburgh, E & S Livingstone, 1969. Used with permission.)

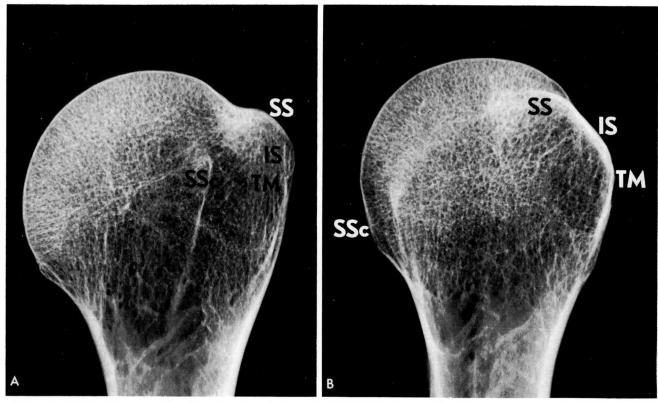

Figure 41–3. **Periarticular crystal deposition: Shoulder—sites of tendon calcification.** A In external rotation, calcification in the supraspinatus *(SS)* tendon is observed adjacent to the greater tuberosity, whereas that in the infraspinatus *(IS)* and teres minor *(TM)* tendons overlies the greater tuberosity. Calcification in the subscapularis *(SSc)* tendon overlies the lesser tuberosity. B In internal rotation, calcification in the infraspinatus *(IS)* and teres minor *(TM)* tendons is seen lateral to the greater tuberosity, that in the supraspinatus *(SS)* tendon is projected over the greater tuberosity, and calcification in the subscapularis *(SSc)* tendon rotates medially, adjacent to the inner margin of the humeral head.

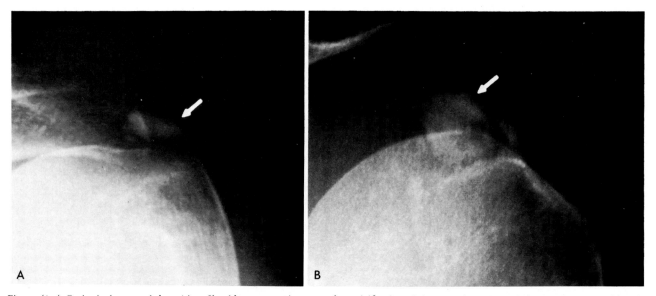

Figure 41–4. **Periarticular crystal deposition: Shoulder—supraspinatus tendon calcification.** A In external rotation, calcification is apparent above the greater tuberosity (arrow). B In internal rotation, calcification moves medially (arrow).

the calcification moves medially in this projection, it may overlie the humeral head.

Infraspinatus Tendon Calcification. Calcification within the substance of the infraspinatus tendon may be projected over the lateral aspect of the humeral head in external rotation because of the attachment of this tendon to the posterior aspect of the greater tuberosity. In internal rotation, the calcification moves laterally and may be seen in profile (Fig. 41–5).

Teres Minor Tendon Calcification. The teres minor tendon attaches to the posterior aspect of the greater tuberosity below the site of attachment of the infraspinatus tendon. Calcification within this tendon is projected over the humeral head in external rotation and moves laterally in internal rotation, where it may be seen in profile (Fig. 41–5).

Subscapularis Tendon Calcification. The subscapularis tendon attaches to the lesser tuberosity of the humerus. Calcification of this tendon is projected over the humeral head in external rotation, related to the anterior position of the lesser tuberosity. This calcification moves medially on internal rotation and can be seen near the inner surface of the humeral head in this position (Fig. 41–5). Calcification is seen tangentially adjacent to the lesser tuberosity in an axillary projection.

Bicipital Tendon Calcification. As the long head of the biceps tendon attaches to the superior aspect of the glenoid fossa after passing through the bicipital groove, calcific tendinitis of this structure appears as a radiodense area in this location, which does not move appreciably on external or internal rotation (Fig. 41–6). The short head of the biceps attaches to the coracoid process. Calcification in this tendon is apparent adjacent to the coracoid tip. Bicipital tendon calcification is also seen along the shaft of the humerus (Fig. 41–6).

Calcification in the subacromial bursa appears as a teardrop-shaped radiodense area adjacent to the superolateral aspect of the joint capsule, which may extend under the greater tuberosity (Fig. 41–7).

ELBOW. Calcification of tendons, ligaments, and bursae about the elbow has been described. These deposits may be observed adjacent to the medial and lateral condyles of the humerus, in the area of the collateral ligaments, at the insertion of the triceps tendon to the ulnar olecranon, and within the olecranon bursa.

HAND AND WRIST. Calcification of tendons and ligaments in periarticular structures of the wrist and, less frequently, the hand has also been encountered. In the vicinity of the wrist, deposits may be noted in or near the tendons of the flexor carpi ulnaris (adjacent to the pisiform) (Fig. 41–8), flexor carpi radialis (on the volar aspect of the radiocarpal joint), common flexors (near the volar aspect of the wrist), and extensor carpi ulnaris (adjacent to the distal ulna and ulnar styloid). In the hand, deposits show predilection for the regions of the metacarpophalangeal joints and fingers.

HIP AND PELVIS. Calcific deposits are frequent in the gluteal insertions into the greater trochanter and in the surrounding bursae (Fig. 41–9). These radiodense regions may also be observed adjacent to the acetabular margin, lesser trochanter, ischial tuberosity, and lateral and medial aspects of the proximal femur.

KNEE. Calcific tendinitis and bursitis may be seen adjacent to the femoral condyles, fibular head, and prepatellar region.

ANKLE, FOOT, AND HEEL. Calcific deposits may occasionally be seen about the ankle, foot, and heel (Fig. 41–10). Involvement may include the tendons of the flexor hallucis brevis, flexor hallucis longus, and peroneus muscles.

NECK. Calcification may appear within the longus colli muscle, the principal flexor of the cervical spine (Fig. 41–11). This muscle originates from the anterior surfaces of the upper three thoracic and the lower three cervical vertebral bodies and inserts on the anterior tubercle of the atlas and the second, third, and fourth cervical vertebrae. Tendinitis in this region may result in acute neck and occipital pain, rigidity, and dysphagia. Radiographic findings include prevertebral soft tissue swelling and amorphous calcification, which is usually seen anterior to the second cervical vertebra, just inferior to the body of the atlas. Resorption of calcification is common and may be complete in 1 to 2 weeks, with disappearance of the soft tissue swelling.

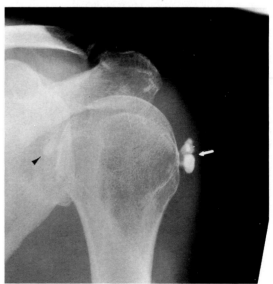

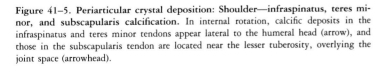

Figure 41–5. Periarticular crystal deposition: Shoulder—infraspinatus, teres minor, and subscapularis calcification. In internal rotation, calcific deposits in the infraspinatus and teres minor tendons appear lateral to the humeral head (arrow), and those in the subscapularis tendon are located near the lesser tuberosity, overlying the joint space (arrowhead).

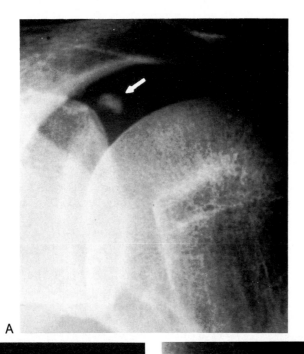

A

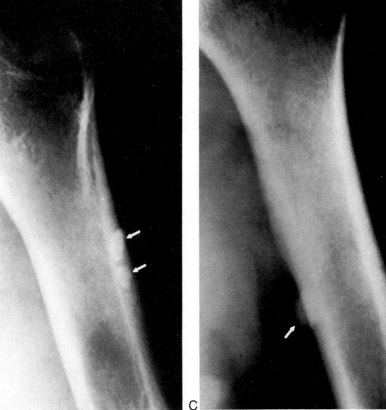

B   C

Figure 41–6. Periarticular crystal deposition: Shoulder—calcification in the biceps. **A** Observe the radiodense shadow (arrow) adjacent to the superior lip of the glenoid, representing calcification in the long head of the biceps. **B, C** In two different patients, calcification in the biceps tendon (arrows) is shown in external rotation (**B**) and internal rotation (**C**) of the humerus. (**B** Courtesy of A. Goldman, M.D., New York, New York; **C** Courtesy of V. Vint, M.D., San Diego, California.)

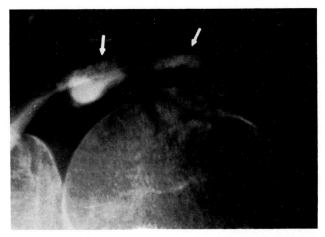

Figure 41–7. **Periarticular crystal deposition: Shoulder—subdeltoid (subacromial) bursal calcification.** Note extensive calcific deposition (arrows) adjacent to the humeral head.

Differential Diagnosis

Tendinitis and bursitis may produce soft tissue swelling without radiographically recognizable calcification. Stenosing tenosynovitis of the abductor pollicis longus and extensor pollicis brevis muscles *(de Quervain's disease)* is well known (Fig. 41–12). An example of noncalcific bursitis is *Haglund's syndrome.* The disorder is characterized clinically by painful soft tissue swelling at the level of the Achilles tendon insertion in the calcaneus, generally in adults and in both men and women. A localized area of soft tissue prominence, termed a "pump bump," may be encountered. The condition appears to be produced by compression of the Achilles tendon and adjacent soft tissues between the os calcis and the shoe.

Calcific tendinitis and bursitis must be distinguished from many disorders that produce periarticular calcification (Table 41–1). Such soft tissue deposits may relate to (1) metastatic calcification, in which a disturbance of calcium and phosphorus metabolism is present; (2) calcinosis, in which calcification

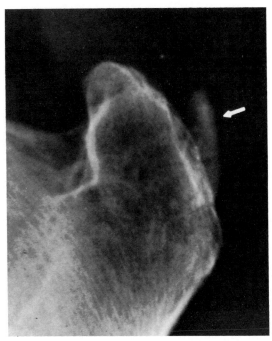

Figure 41–9. **Periarticular crystal deposition: Hip.** Note calcification (arrow) in the gluteal insertion.

of skin and of subcutaneous and connective tissue occurs in the presence of normal calcium metabolism; and (3) dystrophic calcification, in which calcium deposition occurs in devitalized tissues. Metastatic calcification is common in renal osteodystrophy, and periarticular deposits in this condition represent HA crystal accumulation (Fig. 41–13). Periarticular metastatic calcification may also be observed in hypoparathyroidism, sarcoidosis, hypervitaminosis D, milk-alkali syndrome, and numerous other conditions. These deposits appear as radiodense areas of variable size, which may be observed in

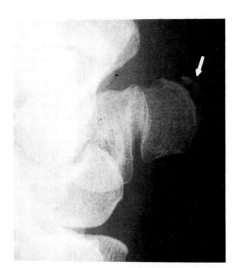

Figure 41–8. **Periarticular crystal deposition: Wrist.** Calcification (arrow) is apparent on the undersurface of the pisiform within the tendon of the flexor carpi ulnaris muscle.

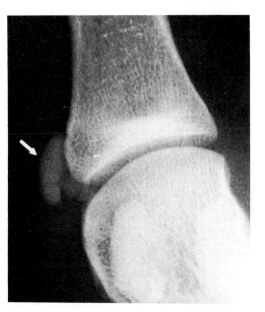

Figure 41–10. **Periarticular crystal deposition: Foot.** Observe homogeneous calcification (arrow) adjacent to the first metatarsophalangeal joint.

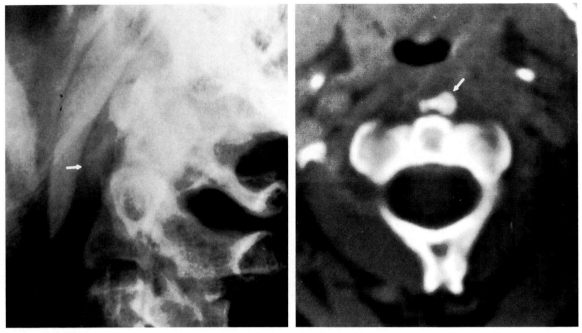

Figure 41–11. Periarticular crystal deposition: Neck. A lateral radiograph **(A)** and transaxial computed tomographic image **(B)** at the level of the base of the odontoid process document calcification (arrows) within the longus colli muscle. Symptoms and imaging abnormalities disappeared over a period of weeks. (Courtesy of G. Greenway, M.D., Dallas, Texas.)

multiple (and often symmetric) locations in periarticular and other soft tissue sites. Generalized calcinosis may be seen in (idiopathic) calcinosis interstitialis universalis (Fig. 41–14), collagen diseases such as scleroderma and dermatomyositis, and (idiopathic) tumoral calcinosis (Fig. 41–15). Localized or

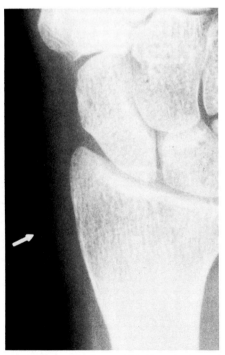

Figure 41–12. De Quervain's disease. This disease is characterized by soft tissue swelling (arrow) on the radial aspect of the wrist related to inflammation of the tendons of the abductor pollicis longus and extensor pollicis brevis muscles.

widespread dystrophic calcification may appear in degenerative, necrotic, neoplastic, and inflammatory foci.

Calcific tendinitis and bursitis should be differentiated from causes of soft tissue ossification (Table 41–2). Frequently this is possible because ossified masses reveal trabecular patterns. Soft tissue ossification is frequent after trauma (myositis ossificans), neurologic injury (Fig. 41–16), and burns and may also accompany fibrodysplasia (myositis) ossificans progressiva, soft tissue sarcomas, pseudomalignant osseous tumor of soft tissue, postsurgical scars, and varicose veins.

Bone excrescences at sites of tendon and ligament attachment to bone may be seen as an isolated phenomenon or as part of the ossifying diathesis of diffuse idiopathic skeletal hyperostosis. In these instances, trabeculae can be identified extending from the parent bone into the tendon.

Calcific tendinitis may appear in CPPD crystal deposition disease, owing to CPPD crystal accumulation within the tendinous structures. Other findings, such as chondrocalcinosis and pyrophosphate arthropathy, also are observed.

Clinical and radiologic similarity may exist between calcific tendinitis and gouty arthritis. Articular and periarticular

Table 41–1. SOME CONDITIONS ASSOCIATED WITH PERIARTICULAR CALCIFICATION

Calcific tendinitis and bursitis
Collagen disease
Hyperparathyroidism and renal osteodystrophy
Hypoparathyroidism
Hypervitaminosis D
Milk-alkali syndrome
Idiopathic tumoral calcinosis
Articular disorders: CPPD crystal deposition
    disease, gout, infection
Sarcoidosis

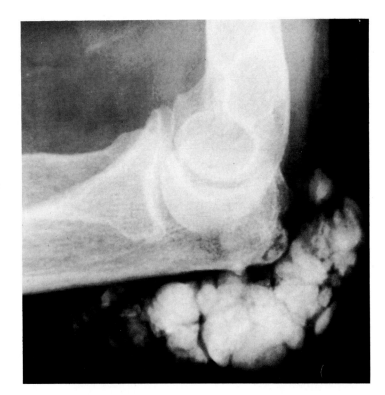

Figure 41–13. **Renal osteodystrophy.** Large radiodense collections about the elbow are typical of calcifications in this disorder.

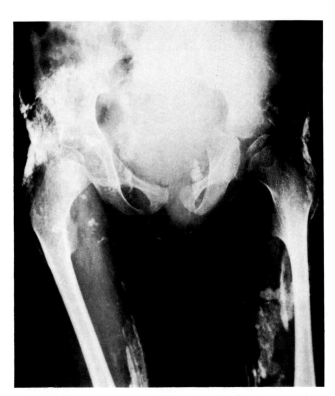

Figure 41–14. **Calcinosis interstitialis universalis.** Plaque-like soft tissue calcification is apparent in this child.

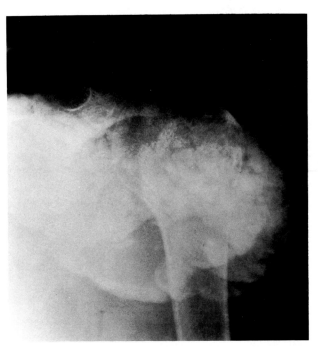

Figure 41–15. **Idiopathic tumoral calcinosis.** Observe large sac-like collections of calcification about the shoulder.

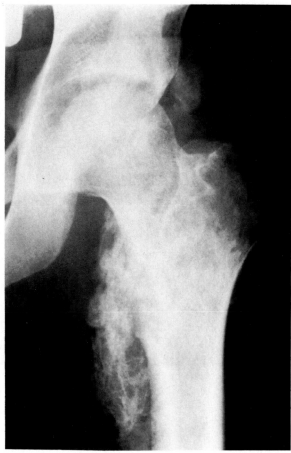

Figure 41–16. Heterotopic ossification after neurologic injury. In a paralyzed patient, ossification about the acetabulum and proximal femur can be seen.

inflammation with erythema, increased heat, swelling, and tenderness is seen in both conditions. Patients with both disorders may reveal soft tissue swelling and calcific accumulation. In gout, additional radiographic findings, such as osseous erosion, are usually apparent.

INTRAARTICULAR CRYSTAL DEPOSITION

The concept of intraarticular HA crystal deposition has been studied extensively in recent years. Investigations of elderly women who had painful shoulders with decreased mobility or stability have revealed radiographic evidence of disruption of the rotator cuff and microspheroids containing HA crystals in synovial fluid. The fluid also revealed activated collagenase and neutral protease activity. A pathogenetic scheme for the disorder, termed *"Milwaukee shoulder"* syndrome, has been developed: The HA mineral phase develops in altered

---

Table 41–2. SOME CONDITIONS ASSOCIATED WITH SOFT TISSUE OSSIFICATION

Myositis ossificans traumatica
Fibrodysplasia (myositis) ossificans progressiva
Neurologic injury
Burn
Pseudomalignant osseous tumor of soft tissue

---

capsular or synovial tissue or in degenerative articular cartilage; crystals are released into the synovial fluid together with their tissue matrix to form the observed microspheroids; these particles are then engulfed by the fixed macrophage–like synovial cells, inducing the release of collagenase and neutral protease; the released enzymes attack the periarticular tissues, including the rotator cuff, resulting in additional release of crystals into the synovial fluid; rotator cuff disruption ensues; and progressive deterioration results from joint instability, with recurrent cycles of mineral phase formation.

On the basis of evidence contained in these investigations as well as others, HA crystal deposition appears to play an important role in the degeneration of cartilaginous, osseous, and soft tissue structures in and about joints. Although the initial observations were related to disintegration of the glenohumeral articulation, the concept has been applied to other sites, including the knee, elbow, hip, and midtarsal articulations.

Radiographic and Pathologic Features

CALCIFICATION. HA crystal accumulation in joints can lead to intraarticular calcification. Although cartilage calcification, or chondrocalcinosis, has occasionally been noted, other patterns of calcification are more typical. Crystal deposition can involve the synovial membrane or capsule and usually leads to amorphous or cloud-like radiodense areas within the joint (Fig. 41–17).

Calcification related to HA crystal deposition can occur in an articulation that is otherwise normal, in which site it may lead to subsequent deterioration of the joint, or it can develop in an articulation with preexisting abnormalities. In this regard, visible radiodense lesions related to HA crystal deposition may occur within the joints of patients with scleroderma as well as osteoarthritis. Although usually evident in the small articulations of the hand and wrist, HA crystal accumulation leading to calcification in large joints is reported. Women are affected more frequently than men, and adults are affected much more commonly than children.

ARTHROPATHY. Structural joint damage is observed in some patients with intraarticular HA crystal accumulation. This has been investigated most extensively in the shoulder (Milwaukee shoulder syndrome). At this site, radiographic findings include loss of joint space, destruction of bone, subchondral sclerosis, intraarticular osseous debris, and joint disorganization and deformity (Fig. 41–18). Associated disruption of the rotator cuff allows the humeral head to become displaced in a superior direction and leads to narrowing of the acromiohumeral space. In the presence of a massive tear of the rotator cuff, the displaced humeral head can severely erode the anterior portion of the acromion, distal portion of the clavicle, glenoid cavity, and coracoid process. The resulting articular disease is termed *cuff tear arthropathy* by some investigators, who believe that the initial alteration is not HA crystal accumulation but rather disruption of the rotator cuff, which is followed by leakage of synovial fluid, deterioration of cartilage nutrition, and mechanical derangement of the joint.

An association of arthropathy in the shoulder and arthropathy in other joints, especially the knee, is reported. Typically, unicompartmental alterations in the lateral femorotibial space are seen, leading to joint space narrowing, collapse of the articular surfaces of the tibia and femur, bone sclerosis

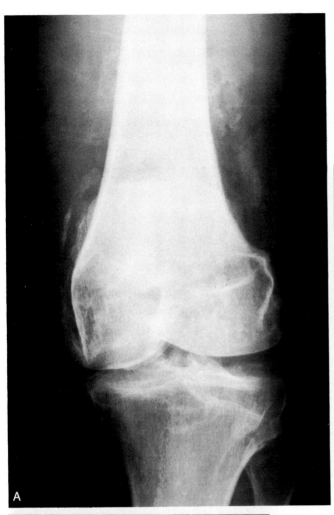

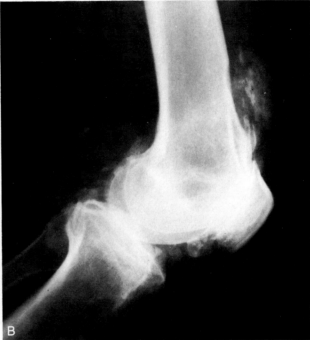

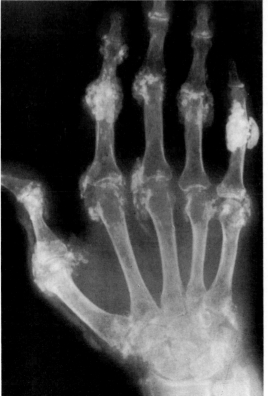

Figure 41–17. Intraarticular crystal deposition: Calcification. A, B Observe extensive amorphous intraarticular calcifications, especially within the suprapatellar pouch. Aspiration revealed HA crystals without CPPD crystal deposition. **C** The radiograph reveals periarticular and intraarticular calcification involving the hand and the wrist. The opposite side was affected similarly. A synovial biopsy of a proximal interphalangeal joint documented presence of HA crystal deposition. (**A,** From Bonavita JA, et al: Hydroxyapatite deposition disease. Radiology *134*:621, 1980. Used with permission.)

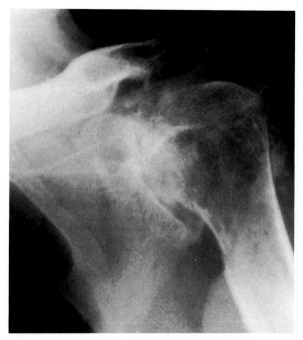

Figure 41–18. Intraarticular crystal deposition: Arthropathy—Milwaukee shoulder syndrome. The radiographic characteristics of this syndrome include joint space narrowing, subchondral sclerosis, and erosion of the undersurface of the clavicle and acromion.

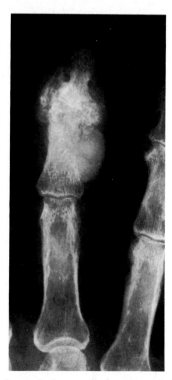

Figure 41–19. Intraarticular crystal deposition: Arthropathy. Note calcification within and around a distal interphalangeal joint associated with interosseous space narrowing and osteophytosis. (Courtesy of V. Vint, M.D., San Diego, California.)

Table 41–3. SOME CAUSES OF SEVERE DESTRUCTION OF GLENOHUMERAL JOINT

Milwaukee shoulder syndrome*
Cuff-tear arthropathy*
CPPD crystal deposition disease
Neuroarthropathy
Alkaptonuria
Infection
Idiopathic chondrolysis*
Senile hemorrhagic shoulder syndrome*
Ischemic necrosis
Rheumatoid arthritis

*These may represent four names for a single disease.

and fragmentation, and valgus angulation. The patellofemoral compartment may also be affected, and chondrocalcinosis occasionally is evident. Analysis of the synovial fluid in the knee commonly indicates CPPD crystal deposition, evidence that supports the existence of diseases related to a mixture of calcium phosphate crystals (see later discussion). Additional joints, such as the hip and small joints of the hand and feet, may be involved.

HA crystal deposition may be associated with arthropathy of the interphalangeal and metacarpophalangeal joints of the hand (Fig. 41–19). Changes resemble those of osteoarthritis, with narrowing of the interosseous space and osteophytes.

Differential Diagnosis

The radiographic manifestations of intraarticular HA crystal deposition disease are similar to those of osteoarthritis and CPPD crystal deposition disease. In the knee, the arthropathy associated with HA crystal accumulation is more aggressive than osteoarthritis and involves the lateral femorotibial or patellofemoral space, or both; in osteoarthritis, changes predominate in both the medial femorotibial and the patellofemoral compartments. Osteoarthritis of the glenohumeral joint is accompanied by minor radiographic alterations unlike the severe abnormalities of apatite arthropathy. Other disorders of the shoulder, such as alkaptonuria, infection, neuroarthropathy, and idiopathic chondrolysis, resemble the arthropathy of HA crystal deposition disease (Table 41–3).

Apatite arthropathy most simulates pyrophosphate arthropathy and, as indicated later, the two may coexist in the same person or in the same joint. In general, HA crystal accumulation does not produce chondrocalcinosis but leads to homogeneous, cloud-like intraarticular radiodense shadows with or without capsular calcification. Both disorders apparently can produce severe and progressive degenerative-like abnormalities of joints.

MIXED CALCIUM PHOSPHATE CRYSTAL DEPOSITION

Inspection of synovial fluid or cartilage in patients has documented on numerous occasions the coexistence of HA and CPPD crystals. Both crystals can cause an inflammatory response, and both are associated with cartilage degeneration and a degenerative-like arthropathy. When the crystals occur together, it is difficult to identify precisely their relative roles in the production of joint damage. The diagnosis of such mixed crystal deposition disease may be elusive to the clinician, who generally attempts to determine a single cause for articular symptoms and signs, and to the crystallographer, who might easily overlook the presence of a second type of crystal in the excitement after identification of the first.

The radiologist is also faced with a diagnostic challenge in cases of mixed calcium phosphate crystal deposition disease. Calcification within or outside a joint is a manifestation of both HA and CPPD crystal accumulation. Although subtle differences exist in the pattern of calcification in these two disorders, calcific deposits in synovium, capsule, and tendon are common to both. A diagnostic clue is provided by cartilage calcification (chondrocalcinosis), which, when widespread, is much more characteristic of CPPD crystal deposition than of HA crystal accumulation. Conversely, diffuse amorphous calcification within the joint is more typical in HA crystal deposition. Problems in diagnosis arise in cases of (1) CPPD crystal deposition disease associated with tumoral calcific collections ("tophaceous pseudogout"), which may occur in the absence of chondrocalcinosis; (2) CPPD crystal deposition disease associated with widespread synovial osteochondromatosis, in which the osteochondromas themselves are composed mainly of apatite crystals; and (3) HA crystal deposition disease accompanied by calcific foci in the hyaline cartilage or fibrocartilage.

Certain radiographic signs should raise the possibility of mixed calcium phosphate crystal deposition disease. There appears to be an association of intraarticular accumulation of CPPD crystals (in the form of chondrocalcinosis) and periarticular accumulation of HA crystals (in the form of capsular and tendinous calcification). The presence of both disorders should be suspected if radiographs reveal extensive cartilage calcification (indicative of CPPD crystal deposition) *and* diffuse capsular calcification or dense homogeneous calcific collections at tendinous insertions (indicative of HA crystal deposition).

It is the Milwaukee shoulder syndrome and its manifestations in additional joints that appear to represent the most extensive example of mixed calcium phosphate crystal deposition disease. Although analysis of fluid in the glenohumeral joint documents the accumulation of apatite crystals, widespread chondrocalcinosis in other joints and the recovery of CPPD crystals from the shoulder or elsewhere confirm that a second crystalline disorder is also present. Furthermore, structural joint damage in the knees, with predilection for the lateral femorotibial or patellofemoral compartment, is consistent with the arthropathy of CPPD crystal deposition disease. It is not clear in these cases whether the occurrence of two crystals (HA and CPPD crystals) leads to a unique arthrosis dissimilar from that accompanying the presence of either crystal alone; it is certain, however, that the resulting joint damage differs considerably from osteoarthritis.

FURTHER READING

Bonavita JA, Dalinka MK, Schumacher HR Jr: Hydroxyapatite deposition disease. Radiology *134*:621, 1980.

Codman EA: The Shoulder, Boston, Thomas-Todd Co, 1934.

Dieppe PA, Doherty M, MacFarlane DG, Hutton CW, Bradfield JW, Watt I: Apatite associated destructive arthritis. Br J Rheumatol *23*:84, 1984.

Halverson PB, McCarty DJ: Clinical aspects of basic calcium phosphate crystal deposition. Rheum Dis Clinics North Am *14*:427, 1988.

Halverson PB, McCarty DJ: Patterns of radiographic abnormalities associated with basic calcium phosphate and calcium pyrophosphate dihydrate crystal deposition in the knee. Ann Rheum Dis *45*:603, 1986.

Halverson PB, McCarty DJ, Cheung HS, Ryan LM: Milwaukee shoulder syndrome: Eleven additional cases with involvement of the knee in seven (basic calcium phosphate crystal deposition disease). Semin Arthritis Rheum *14*:36, 1984.

Martin JF, Brogdon BG: Peritendinitis calcarea of the hand and wrist. AJR *78*:74, 1957.

McCarty DJ, Gatter RA: Recurrent acute inflammation associated with focal apatite crystal deposition. Arthritis Rheum *9*:804, 1966.

McCarty DJ, Halverson PB, Carrera GF, Brewer BJ, Kozin F: "Milwaukee shoulder"—association of microspheroids containing hydroxyapatite crystals, active collagenase, and neutral protease with rotator cuff defects. I. Clinical aspects. Arthritis Rheum *24*:464, 1981.

Neer CS II, Craig EV, Fukuda H: Cuff-tear arthropathy. J Bone Joint Surg [Am] *65*:1232, 1983.

Newmark H III, Forrester DM, Brown JC, Robinson A, Olken SM, Bledsoe R: Calcific tendinitis of the neck. Radiology *128*:355, 1978.

Pavlov H, Heneghan MA, Hersh A, Goldman AB, Vigorita V: The Haglund syndrome: Initial and differential diagnosis. Radiology *144*:83, 1982.

Schumacher HR, Somlyo AP, Tse RL, Maurer K: Arthritis associated with apatite crystals. Ann Intern Med *87*:411, 1977.

Uhthoff HK, Sarkar K, Maynard JA: Calcifying tendinitis. A new concept of its pathogenesis. Clin Orthop *118*:164, 1976.

ViGario DG, Keats TE: Localization of calcific deposits in the shoulder. AJR *108*:806, 1970.

Chapter 42

Hemochromatosis and Wilson's Disease

Donald Resnick, M.D.

The skeletal manifestations of hemochromatosis include osteoporosis, chondrocalcinosis, and a distinctive arthropathy characterized by joint space narrowing, subchondral cyst formation, and osteophytes, which has predilection for the metacarpophalangeal joints and wrists. These abnormalities resemble the findings of calcium pyrophosphate dihydrate (CPPD) crystal deposition disease but are associated with more uniform loss of joint space and a less progressive course.

Wilson's disease is associated with distinctive skeletal abnormalities, which include osteopenia, bone fragmentation and cyst formation, ossicles, poorly defined subchondral bone, and osteochondritis dissecans. These findings superficially resemble the changes in hemochromatosis and idiopathic CPPD crystal deposition disease.

HEMOCHROMATOSIS

Hemochromatosis is recognized as a rare disorder characterized pathologically by tissue damage produced by iron deposition. Specific clinical manifestations relate to the site of abnormal iron accumulation: Iron within the parenchymal cells of the liver is associated with hypertrophy and cirrhosis; iron deposits in the pancreas result in diabetes; iron and melanin accumulations in the skin produce abnormal pigmentation; and cardiac deposition of iron results in heart failure. The disease can be further classified into primary (endogenous or idiopathic) and secondary hemochromatosis. Primary hemochromatosis is believed to be a consequence of a genetically determined error of metabolism in which an unexplained increased absorption of iron occurs from the gastrointestinal tract. Secondary hemochromatosis is associated with an increased intake and accumulation of iron of known cause, such as alcoholic cirrhosis, multiple blood transfusions, refractory anemia, and chronic excess oral iron ingestion. The disease is diagnosed by detection of elevated serum iron concentration and increased saturation of the plasma iron binding protein transferrin combined with a typical histologic appearance on liver biopsy.

Clinical Features

Most patients with primary hemochromatosis become symptomatic between the ages of 40 and 60 years. The disorder is 10 to 20 times more frequent in men than in women, and women with this disorder frequently report absent or scanty menses. Initial clinical manifestations relate to the classic triad of the disease: cirrhosis, skin pigmentation, and diabetes. Subsequent complaints relate to ascites and cardiac failure.

The arthropathy associated with hemochromatosis is manifested as a noninflammatory condition involving initially the small joints of the hands and eventually large joints. Joint symptoms generally occur late in the disease and include pain, swelling, and stiffness. Involvement usually is symmetric, and the arthropathy generally is progressive in nature. Attacks of acute arthritis, presumably related to the presence of calcium pyrophosphate dihydrate (CPPD) crystals, may be superimposed on the chronic progressive "degenerative-like" joint disease.

Laboratory analysis reveals nonreactive serum rheumatoid factor, normal or slightly elevated erythrocyte sedimentation rate, and normal or depressed levels of serum uric acid. Joint aspiration demonstrates noninflammatory synovial fluid.

Pathologic Features

Articular abnormalities consist of two major features: (1) abnormal amounts of hemosiderin granules, and (2) CPPD crystal deposition. Accumulation of both iron and CPPD crystals may occur in the same joint.

SYNOVIAL MEMBRANE ABNORMALITIES. Hemosiderin granules are seen either in the synovioblasts or in the perivascular histiocytes. The extent of synovial iron deposition may relate to the degree of total body iron overload and may decrease after phlebotomy therapy. Increased synovial tissue deposition of iron is not limited to hemochromatosis but may also be observed in rheumatoid arthritis, degenerative disease, pigmented villonodular synovitis, hemophilia, and hemarthrosis.

Synovial inflammation is not a major histologic feature of hemochromatosis. In contrast to the situation in rheumatoid arthritis, synovial villus formation is not a prominent macroscopic feature in hemochromatosis.

CPPD crystals may be seen in the synovium, particularly in the superficial layers of the membrane.

CARTILAGE ABNORMALITIES. Chondrocalcinosis occurs in as many as 30 per cent of patients with hemochromatosis as an isolated phenomenon or in association with structural joint damage. Calcification, which relates to CPPD crystal deposition, involves predominantly the fibrocartilage and hyaline cartilage of the knee but also is frequent in the symphysis pubis, wrist, and intervertebral disc. Cartilaginous fibrillation and erosion with partial or complete denudation may be observed. Most investigators have failed to detect hemosiderin within fibrocartilage or hyaline cartilage, although fine hemosiderin granules may be seen in superficial chondrocytes.

BONE ABNORMALITIES. The osseous abnormalities in hemochromatosis are similar to those noted in idiopathic CPPD crystal deposition disease. Specifically, the presence of bone eburnation and cysts and the absence of significant osteophyte formation are findings of hemochromatosis. As CPPD crystal deposition is a documented feature of hemochromatosis, the bone changes in this disease, at least in part, may indeed be related to the occurrence of these crystals.

Radiographic Features

OSTEOPOROSIS. The reported frequency of osteoporosis in patients with hemochromatosis has varied from 25 to 58 per cent. Osteoporosis may involve either the axial or the appendicular skeleton. Osteoporosis of vertebral bodies produces biconcave deformities or "fish vertebrae," which are identical to those occurring in other forms of osteoporosis.

ARTICULAR CALCIFICATION. The reported frequency of chondrocalcinosis related to CPPD crystal deposi-

tion in patients with hemochromatosis has varied from approximately 20 to 60 per cent. It is most frequently observed in the wrists, knees, symphysis pubis, intervertebral discs, shoulders, and hips, and it may involve fibrocartilage or hyaline cartilage (Fig. 42–1). The distribution of chondrocalcinosis is similar or identical to that associated with idiopathic CPPD crystal deposition disease. Fibrocartilage calcification, which is frequent in the triangular fibrocartilage of the wrist, menisci of the knee, symphysis pubis, and intervertebral disc, appears as thick, shaggy radiodense lesions, commonly within the central portion of the joint; hyaline cartilage calcification appears as linear or curvilinear radiodense areas paralleling the subchondral osseous surface. In the intervertebral disc, CPPD crystal deposition occurs in the outer fibers of the anulus fibrosus.

Additional articular and periarticular calcification is rarely recorded in patients with hemochromatosis.

STRUCTURAL JOINT DAMAGE OR ARTHROPATHY. The reported frequency of structural joint damage in hemochromatosis has ranged from 24 per cent to 50 per cent. The arthropathy superficially resembles degenerative joint disease, with joint space narrowing, sclerosis, and osteophytosis, but in hemochromatosis it demonstrates definite characteristics in its distribution and appearance that enable it to be recognized on radiographic examination. Arthropathy in hemochromatosis is almost identical to arthropathy in idiopathic CPPD crystal deposition disease, sharing the following features:

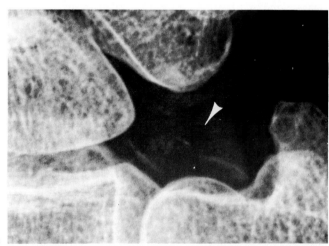

A

Figure 42–1. Radiographic findings in hemochromatosis: Chondrocalcinosis. A Magnification radiography outlines calcium deposits (arrowhead) of cartilage in the wrist. B Diffuse chondrocalcinosis of both fibrocartilage and hyaline cartilage is present in the knee. C In the symphysis pubis, chondrocalcinosis (arrowhead) of fibrocartilage is apparent.

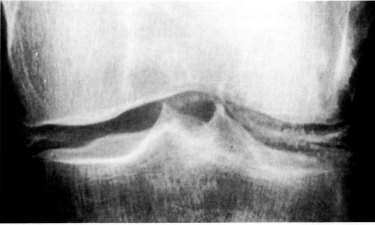

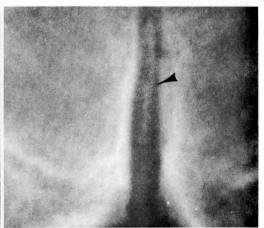

B   C

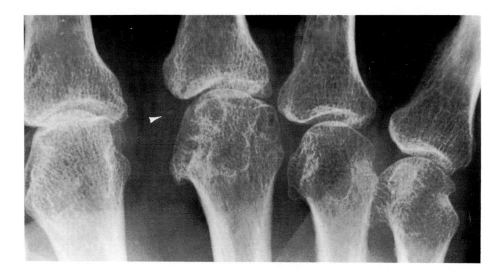

Figure 42–2. Radiographic findings in hemochromatosis: Metacarpophalangeal joint arthropathy. Involvement of all of the metacarpophalangeal joints is characterized by articular space narrowing, surface irregularity, small cystic lesions, beak-like osteophytes, focal calcifications (arrowhead), and mild osteoporosis.

1. *Involvement of unusual articular sites*. Arthropathy may produce abnormalities at joints that are not commonly involved in degenerative joint disease, such as the metacarpophalangeal joints, midcarpal and radiocarpal compartments of the wrists, elbows, and glenohumeral joints.

2. *Formation of large subchondral cystic lesions*. Arthropathy may be associated with multiple cysts in the subchondral bone, which can, on occasion, reach large size.

3. *Uniform loss of articular space*. Arthropathy may be characterized by symmetric loss of articular space, an unusual finding in degenerative joint disease. The joint space loss is associated with subchondral bone eburnation and cyst formation.

Although it is difficult to differentiate the arthropathy of hemochromatosis and that of idiopathic CPPD crystal deposition disease, several subtle findings appear more typical of hemochromatosis:

1. *Predilection for the metacarpophalangeal joints*. These joints are the most characteristic sites of involvement in hemochromatosis (Fig. 42–2). Abnormalities are particularly frequent in the second and third metacarpophalangeal joints. The first,

fourth, and fifth metacarpophalangeal joints and the interphalangeal joints are less commonly abnormal.

Involvement of the metacarpophalangeal joints is associated with symmetric or asymmetric loss of articular space, well-defined subchondral bone eburnation, sharply marginated 1 to 3 mm cysts, osteophytes on the medial aspect of the metacarpal head, and flattening or mild collapse of the osseous surface. Findings in the metacarpophalangeal joints that are more characteristic of hemochromatosis than of idiopathic CPPD crystal deposition disease include more prevalent joint space narrowing in these joints, including those in the fourth and fifth digits, and peculiar hook-like osteophytes on the radial aspect of the metacarpal heads.

2. *Widespread abnormalities of the wrist*. Involvement of the carpal bones may be noted in 30 to 50 per cent of patients (Fig. 42–3). Findings include joint space narrowing, sclerosis, and cyst formation. Although the radiocarpal compartment may be affected as in idiopathic CPPD crystal deposition disease, this compartment occasionally is unaffected in the arthropathy of hemochromatosis. In these cases, diffuse involvement of the midcarpal, common carpometacarpal, and first carpometacarpal compartments may be observed. Furthermore, the prevalence of scapholunate separation (or dis-

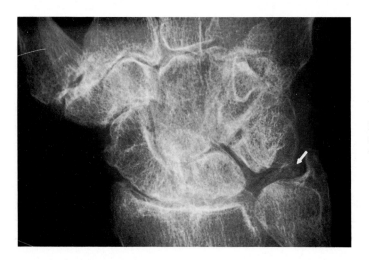

Figure 42–3. Radiographic findings in hemochromatosis: Wrist arthropathy. Observe chondrocalcinosis (arrow) and diffuse narrowing of the radiocarpal, midcarpal, and first carpometacarpal joints.

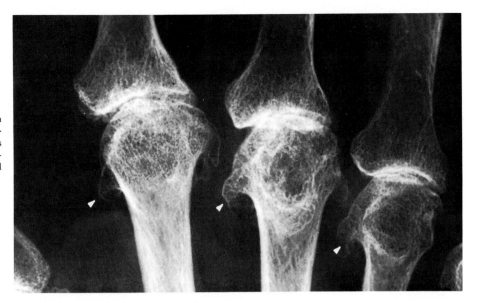

Figure 42–4. Radiographic findings in hemochromatosis: Unusual pattern of osteophytosis. Note beak-like excrescences (arrowheads), particularly on the radial aspect of the flattened and sclerotic metacarpal heads.

sociation) is lower, and the combination of metacarpophalangeal joint space narrowing without radiocarpal joint space narrowing is higher in patients with hemochromatosis than in those with idiopathic CPPD crystal deposition disease.

3. *Slowly progressive alterations*. The arthropathy of hemochromatosis may be slowly progressive. Rapidly developing changes are more characteristic of idiopathic CPPD crystal deposition disease.

4. *Unusual pattern of osteophytosis*. Beak-like osteophytes of the metacarpal heads are particularly characteristic (Fig. 42–

4). Similarly, osteophytes may be apparent about other involved sites, such as the hip and glenohumeral joint.

The arthropathy of hemochromatosis may be widespread throughout the skeleton (Fig. 42–5). Reports of involvement of the hand and wrist, elbow, glenohumeral joint, hip, knee, ankle, foot, and spine have appeared. At most of these skeletal sites, radiographic abnormalities include joint space narrowing, bone eburnation, subchondral cyst formation, and osteophytosis. Chondrocalcinosis may or may not be apparent in the involved joint.

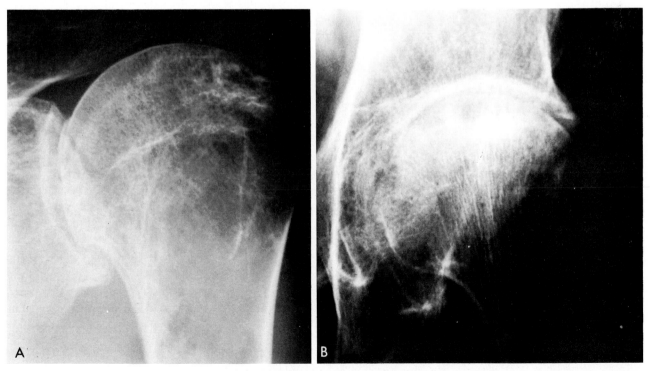

Figure 42–5. Radiographic findings in hemochromatosis: Arthropathy at multiple articular sites. **A** In the glenohumeral joint, findings are joint space narrowing and contour irregularities. **B** In the hip, abnormalities include symmetric loss of joint space, sclerosis, and cysts.

Pathogenesis of Chondrocalcinosis and Arthropathy

The mechanism leading to cartilage calcification and arthropathy in hemochromatosis is not known. Some investigators believe that cartilaginous changes constitute the initial abnormality, which is followed by calcification. It may be speculated that iron deposition itself may lead to abnormality of cartilage. Arthropathy has been described in association with the iron overload of repeated blood transfusions and in additional cases of spherocytosis and sideroblastic anemia. In addition, *Kashin-Beck disease,* a degenerative arthropathy occurring in certain parts of the Soviet Union and Manchuria, has been attributed by some observers to chronic ingestion of drinking water with elevated levels of iron.

Iron inhibits pyrophosphatase activity in cartilage in vitro and thereby can lead to precipitation of CPPD crystals. After such precipitation, sequential abnormalities might lead to the arthropathy of hemochromatosis, much as they might contribute to the arthropathy of idiopathic CPPD crystal deposition disease.

Differential Diagnosis

In most patients with hemochromatosis, clinical manifestations of the disease allow accurate diagnosis. In some patients, articular changes may represent the presenting or predominant manifestation of the disorder. In such cases it is imperative to differentiate the radiographic manifestations of hemochromatosis from those associated with other disorders.

ARTICULAR CALCIFICATION. Chondrocalcinosis associated with hemochromatosis is almost identical to that associated with idiopathic CPPD crystal deposition disease and primary hyperparathyroidism. Chondrocalcinosis in hemochromatosis is readily differentiated from other intraarticular and periarticular calcifications that can be observed in a variety of disorders.

ARTHROPATHY. The arthropathy of hemochromatosis can easily be differentiated from that of rheumatoid arthritis, seronegative spondyloarthropathies, and gout. It differs from degenerative joint diseases in its distribution and appearance;

involvement of unusual joints and the presence of uniform loss of articular space, multiple cystic lesions, distinctive osteophytes, and mild collapse and flattening of bone allow differentiation of this disease from degenerative joint disease in most persons.

The arthropathy of hemochromatosis is almost identical to that of idiopathic CPPD crystal deposition disease (Table 42–1). Subtle differences in hemochromatosis may include involvement of all of the metacarpophalangeal joints, including the fourth and fifth, as well as the midcarpal and common carpometacarpal joints, the presence of osteoporosis and distinctive beak-like osteophytes, and the absence of rapidly progressive neuropathic-like joint damage (Fig. 42–6).

WILSON'S DISEASE

Wilson's disease (hepatolenticular degeneration) is a rare autosomal, recessively inherited disorder characterized by degenerative changes in the brain, particularly the basal ganglia, cirrhosis of the liver, and diagnostic Kayser-Fleischer rings of greenish-brown pigment at the limbus of the cornea.

The primary abnormality in Wilson's disease is not known. It is certain, however, that the clinical symptoms and signs of Wilson's disease result from relentless accumulation of copper in the body. Currently, it has been confirmed that there is both increased tissue copper and elevated urinary copper excretion in this disease. Copper concentration is increased in the liver, the brain, and other tissues; levels of serum copper and copper-binding protein (ceruloplasmin) generally are decreased. Mobilization of copper from the body may produce clinical improvement in patients with Wilson's disease.

Clinical Features

The disease may be slightly more common in men than in women. The age of onset is variable. Symptoms and signs usually become apparent between the ages of 5 and 40 years.

Lenticular degeneration leads to neurologic symptoms, which include tremor, rigidity, dysarthria, incoordination, and personality change. Clinical evidence of hepatic disease is minimal, although pathologic evidence of cirrhosis generally is obtained at autopsy examination. Diagnostic eye changes are greenish-brown rings, which are most marked at the superior and inferior aspects of the cornea. Renal tubular disease in many patients becomes manifest as aminoaciduria, proteinuria, phosphaturia, glucosuria, and uricosuria.

Articular alterations are unusual in children but may be observed in as many as 50 per cent of adults. They frequently are asymptomatic, although pain and swelling may occasionally be observed. Many joints are involved, including those in the hand, wrist, elbow, shoulder, hip, and knee.

Osteopenia has been described in 25 to 50 per cent of patients with Wilson's disease. It may lead to fractures.

Pathologic Features

Synovial biopsy findings have included microvillus formation, with inflammatory changes and vasculitis. The osteopenia of Wilson's disease has been attributed to osteoporosis and osteomalacia.

Radiographic Features

OSTEOPENIA. Osteopenia is most apparent in the hands, feet, and spine and may be associated with a high frequency

Table 42–1. HEMOCHROMATOSIS, WILSON'S DISEASE, AND IDIOPATHIC CPPD CRYSTAL DEPOSITION DISEASE

	Hemochromatosis	Wilson's Disease	Idiopathic CPPD Crystal Deposition Disease
Osteopenia	+	+	–
Chondrocalcinosis	+*	?‡	+
Additional calcification	±	?‡	+
Joint space narrowing	+	+	+
Subchondral cysts	+	+	+
Rapid progression	±	–	+
Involvement of unusual articular sites	+†	+	+

*Hemochromatosis may reveal more prominent hyaline cartilage calcification than idiopathic CPPD crystal deposition disease.

†Wrist involvement in hemochromatosis may be more diffuse and metacarpophalangeal joint involvement may be more widespread than in idiopathic CPPD crystal deposition disease.

‡Bone fragmentation in Wilson's disease may resemble intraarticular and periarticular calcification.

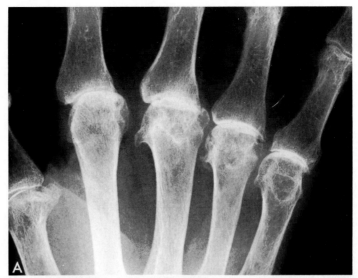

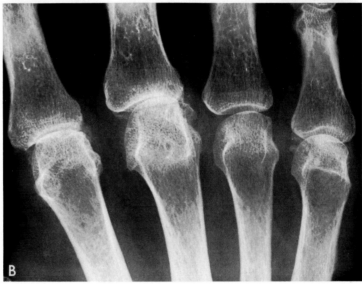

Figure 42–6. Hemochromatosis versus idiopathic CPPD crystal deposition disease. A Hemochromatosis. Note uniform loss of joint space at all metacarpophalangeal joints, including the fourth and fifth. Significant "crumbling" of the metacarpal heads is evident, especially in the third digit. Beak-like osseous excrescences are arising from the radial aspect of the metacarpal heads, particularly the third and fourth. Abnormal calcification is not apparent. **B** Idiopathic CPPD crystal deposition disease. Loss of joint space is evident in the second and third metacarpophalangeal joints, with relative sparing of those in the fourth and fifth digits. Slight flattening of the metacarpal heads and abnormal calcification about the metacarpophalangeal joints are seen. Small osteophytes are arising from the radial aspect of the second and third metacarpal heads, but they are not nearly so apparent as in **A**.

of fractures. Rickets and osteomalacia as well as Fanconi's syndrome have been reported in patients with Wilson's disease.

CHONDROCALCINOSIS. Cartilage calcification in Wilson's disease is rare. The nature of the calcific deposits has not been studied, although it has been attractive to relate them to CPPD crystal accumulation. Considering the frequency of idiopathic CPPD crystal deposition disease and the presence of bone fragmentation in Wilson's disease, which might be confused with chondrocalcinosis, caution must be exerted in reporting a true association of Wilson's disease and CPPD crystal deposition.

ARTHROPATHY. Reports of articular manifestations in Wilson's disease have described subchondral bone fragmentation, cyst formation, cortical irregularities, and sclerosis in the wrist, hand, foot, hip, shoulder, elbow, and knee (Fig. 42–7). These abnormalities may be apparent in half of persons affected with the disease.

Radiodense lesions occur centrally and at the joint margins and may be associated with joint space narrowing. Distinct ossicles may appear, which possess complete cortices (Fig.

42–8). The subchondral bone is irregular and indistinct, and subchondral cystic lesions are also seen. Focal areas of fragmentation of the articular surface can be observed in the metacarpophalangeal, interphalangeal, and wrist joints; in the knee, the findings resemble those of osteochondritis dissecans.

The cause of bone fragmentation in Wilson's disease is obscure. Because of their spasticity and tremors, patients with Wilson's disease may be prone to suffer minor injuries, producing cartilaginous and osseous damage. Joint hypermobility has also been recorded in patients with Wilson's disease, and it could also lead to repetitive trauma and bone fragmentation.

Joint space loss confined to the patellofemoral space has been observed in Wilson's disease (Fig. 42–9). This change resembles the patellofemoral arthropathy of CPPD crystal deposition disease.

Additional radiographic characteristics of arthropathy in Wilson's disease are small or absent joint effusions, peculiar tongue-like osteophytes at bone prominences such as those about the elbows and ankles, and fluffy periostitis of the trochanters and inferior surface of the calcaneus (Fig. 42–10).

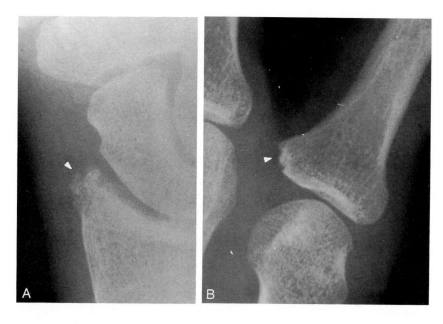

Figure 42–7. Radiographic findings in Wilson's disease: Bone irregularity. Observe osseous irregularity in the radial styloid process and base of a proximal phalanx (arrowheads). (Courtesy of C. Alexander, M.D., Auckland, New Zealand.)

Irregularity of vertebral body contour may resemble the changes of Scheuermann's disease.

Pathogenesis of Arthropathy

The pathogenesis of articular abnormalities in Wilson's disease remains unknown. Tremor and spasticity as well as joint hypermobility could lead to recurrent trauma, with bone irregularity, fragmentation, and fracture. The possible association of Wilson's disease and CPPD crystal deposition may relate to pyrophosphatase inhibition by heavy metal ions, such as copper.

Renal tubular dysfunction in some patients with Wilson's disease may contribute to rickets or osteomalacia. Furthermore, hepatic dysfunction associated with cirrhosis may produce osteoporosis.

Differential Diagnosis

Although reports emphasize that articular abnormalities in Wilson's disease may be confused with degenerative joint disease, these two disorders can be distinguished by close inspection of the radiographs. The distribution of articular abnormality in Wilson's disease includes predilection for the small joints of the hands and wrists, particularly the meta-

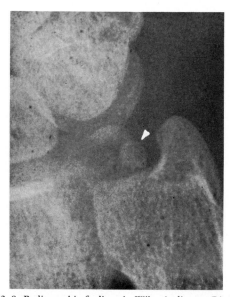

Figure 42–8. Radiographic findings in Wilson's disease: Distinct ossicles. One or more ossicles (arrowhead) are present about the distal end of the ulna, resembling chondrocalcinosis. (Courtesy of M. Dalinka, M.D., Philadelphia, Pennsylvania.)

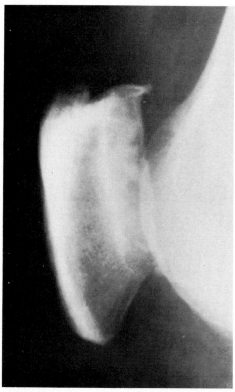

Figure 42–9. Radiographic findings in Wilson's disease: Patellar and patellofemoral abnormalities. Observe cystic lesions and osteophytes in the posterior surface of the patella and bone proliferation at the site of attachment of the quadriceps tendon. (Courtesy of C. Alexander, M.D., Auckland, New Zealand.)

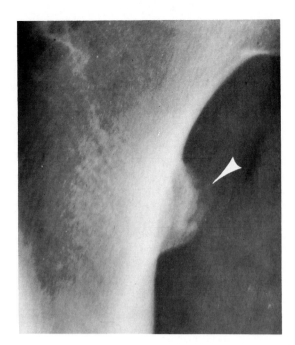

Figure 42–10. Radiographic findings in Wilson's disease: Bone proliferation. Observe fluffy bone production on the lesser trochanter (arrowhead). (From Golding D, Walshe JM: Arthropathy of Wilson's disease. Study of clinical and radiological features in 32 patients. Ann Rheum Dis 36:99, 1977. Used with permission.)

carpophalangeal joints; this distribution is not observed in osteoarthritis. Bone fragmentation and irregular osseous surfaces in Wilson's disease differ from findings in degenerative joint disease. Some articular manifestations of Wilson's disease are identical to those of osteochondritis dissecans, whereas others simulate hypophosphatasia or Scheuermann's disease.

The arthropathy of Wilson's disease most resembles idiopathic CPPD crystal deposition disease and hemochromatosis (Table 42–1). Both of these latter disorders are associated with CPPD crystal deposition; a definite association of Wilson's disease and CPPD crystal deposition is not proved. The distribution of joint alterations is similar in Wilson's disease, hemochromatosis, and idiopathic CPPD crystal deposition disease. In Wilson's disease, distinctive findings are multiple small ossicles and poor definition of the subarticular bone.

FURTHER READING

Adamson TC III, Resnik CS, Guerra J Jr, Vint VC, Weisman MH, Resnick D: Hand and wrist arthropathies of hemochromatosis and calcium pyrophosphate deposition disease: Distinct radiographic features. Radiology 147:377, 1983.

Finby N, Bearn AG: Roentgenographic abnormalities of the skeletal system in Wilson's disease (hepatolenticular degeneration). AJR 79:603, 1958.

Hamilton E, Williams R, Barlow KA, Smith PM: The arthropathy of idiopathic haemochromatosis. Q J Med 37:171, 1968.

Hirsch JH, Killien C, Troupin RH: The arthropathy of hemochromatosis. Radiology 118:591, 1976.

Mindelzun R, Elkin M, Scheinberg IH, Sternlieb I: Skeletal changes in Wilson's disease. A radiological study. Radiology 94:127, 1970.

Schumacher HR Jr: Hemochromatosis and arthritis. Arthritis Rheum 7:41, 1964.

Yu-zhang X, Xue-zhe Z, Xian-hao X, Zhen-xin Z, Ying-kun F: Radiologic study of 42 cases of Wilson's disease. Skel Radiol 13:114, 1985.

Chapter 43

Alkaptonuria

Donald Resnick, M.D.

Alkaptonuria is a rare hereditary disorder resulting from an inability to metabolize homogentisic acid. Clinical and radiographic findings relate to homogentisic aciduria and ochronosis. The latter feature is accompanied by typical radiographic and pathologic findings in both spinal and extraspinal sites. The most characteristic manifestations of ochronosis are widespread discal calcification, with loss of height of the intervertebral disc, and a distinctive arthropathy of axial and extraaxial joints. Careful evaluation of the radiographs will usually allow accurate diagnosis, differentiating this condition from degenerative joint disease and ankylosing spondylitis, the two most likely disorders with which it may be confused.

Alkaptonuria is a rare hereditary metabolic disorder characterized by absence of the enzyme homogentisic acid oxidase. This defect leads to the accumulation of homogentisic acid, which is produced during the metabolism of phenylalanine and tyrosine. When urine is allowed to stand, the homogentisic acid is oxidized to a melanin-like product, which explains why the urine will gradually turn dark. The term alkaptonuria is derived from an Arabic word meaning "alkali" and a Greek word meaning "to suck up avidly," and it has been used to explain the change in color that is observed when urine is alkalinized. Alkaptonuria also is applied as a general designation of the disease. Ochronosis describes the abnormal brown-black pigmentation that may be observed in various connective tissues. Ochronotic arthropathy results from the pigmented deposits in the joints of the appendicular and axial skeleton.

PATHOGENESIS

In the normal situation, the enzyme homogentisic acid oxidase is active in the metabolism of homogentisic acid, so that the latter substance is not detected in either the urine or the plasma. In alkaptonuria, absence of activity of the enzyme is documented in biopsy material from the kidney or liver, and homogentisic acid is found in the plasma and urine. Homogentisic acid can be oxidized to an ochronotic pigment either by enzymatic action or by the presence of oxygen and alkali, the latter situation applying to the urine. The pigment has high affinity for cartilage and connective tissue macromolecules.

GENERAL CLINICAL FEATURES

Alkaptonuria has a worldwide distribution. The disorder affects both men and women. The majority of familial cases reveal a single autosomal recessive type of inheritance, whereas a minority show a dominant pattern of inheritance.

In general, alkaptonuria is asymptomatic until adult life, although it will almost inevitably progress to ochronosis and arthropathy. Ochronotic pigmentation is rarely observed before the age of 20 or 30 years. It first appears as mild pigmentation of the ears or the sclerae. Perspiration in the axillary and genital areas may cause discoloration of the skin, leading to staining of clothing.

Ochronotic arthropathy is a manifestation of long-standing alkaptonuria. Symptoms and signs usually appear in the fourth decade of life. Initial clinical manifestations may be seen in the hips, knees, and shoulders, with pain and limitation of motion. Joint effusions result from fragmentation of friable cartilage. Stiffness and low back pain, obliteration of the normal lumbar curve, thoracic kyphosis, and restriction of motion are spinal manifestations of the disease. The elderly patient with alkaptonuria may be completely disabled.

Symptoms and signs of alkaptonuria may relate to ochronotic deposition in other organs, including the cardiovascular and genitourinary systems and upper respiratory tract.

GENERAL PATHOLOGIC FEATURES

Abnormal pigmentation of the connective tissue may be observed in the sclera; cornea; laryngeal, tracheal, bronchial, and costal cartilages; tympanic membrane; aortic intima; heart valves; kidney; and prostate. Pigment may also be deposited in articular cartilage, tendons, and ligaments. The chemical characteristics of the pigment resemble those of melanin. It is presumed to be a polymer derived from homogentisic acid.

In the large diarthrodial joints, pigmentation of fibrocartilage and hyaline cartilage is seen. Segmental fragmentation of superficial cartilage leads to a shaggy, irregular cartilaginous surface with exposure of severely pigmented deeper layers. With further denudation of cartilage, the sclerotic subchondral bone is exposed. Displaced pieces of cartilage and bone may locate in the synovial membrane. Foreign body reaction, synovial polyp formation, and osteochondral bodies are observed.

In the vertebral column, the earliest findings are seen in the lumbar spine. The pigmented discs become hard and brittle. Bone proliferation, originating from the vertebral body, may isolate disc fragments and lead to ankylosis between vertebral bodies. Calcification of the intervertebral disc may

518

become extreme; the calcareous deposits are composed of calcium hydroxyapatite. Pigment may be identified in various vertebral ligaments.

GENERAL RADIOLOGIC FEATURES (TABLE 43–1)
Spinal Abnormalities

Discal calcification is the most characteristic abnormality of the spine (Fig. 43–1). The calcium deposits are found predominantly in the inner fibers of the anulus fibrosus. They consist of apatite crystals and are considered dystrophic in nature. Calcification may appear in any segment of the vertebral column but has predilection for the intervertebral discs of the lumbar spine. The calcific collections are accentuated by the presence of osteoporosis of the neighboring vertebral bodies.

Narrowing of the intervertebral disc space is also a characteristic manifestation of alkaptonuria (Fig. 43–1). Vacuum phenomena, with linear or circular radiolucent collections of gas overlying the intervertebral disc at multiple levels, are also suggestive of this diagnosis (Fig. 43–2). With further loss of disc space, the calcific deposits may become obscured. Progressive ossification of the discs may be seen, with formation of marginal intervertebral bridges and obliteration of

Table 43–1. DIAGNOSTIC FEATURES OF OCHRONOTIC ARTHROPATHY

Spinal Abnormalities
   Osteoporosis of vertebral bodies
   Calcification and ossification of intervertebral discs
   Disc space narrowing with vacuum phenomena
   Small or absent osteophytes
   Loss of lumbar lordosis

Extraspinal Abnormalities
   Involvement of sacroiliac joints, symphysis pubis, and large
      peripheral joints
   Joint space narrowing
   Bone sclerosis
   Collapse and fragmentation with intra-articular osseous bodies
   Small or absent osteophytes
   Tendinous calcification, ossification, and rupture
   Unusual involvement of hands, wrists, feet, elbows, and ankles

the intervertebral space (Fig. 43–3). These bridges resemble the syndesmophytes of ankylosing spondylitis.

Severe changes may be apparent in long-standing disease, with progressive kyphosis, osteoporosis, obliteration of intervertebral disc spaces, and bone bridging, with a bamboo spine. The appearance of a bamboo spine may lead to an erroneous diagnosis of ankylosing spondylitis.

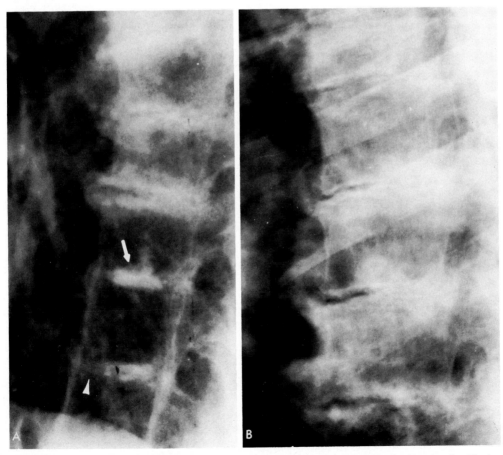

Figure 43–1. Radiographic features of alkaptonuria: Thoracic spine. A Alterations include discal calcification (arrow) and ossification (arrowhead), disc space loss, vertebral body osteoporosis with marginal sclerosis, and mild osteophytosis. **B** In another patient, the most obvious abnormalities are disc space loss, vertebral body marginal sclerosis, and anterior osteophytes.

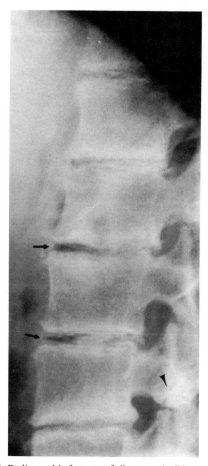

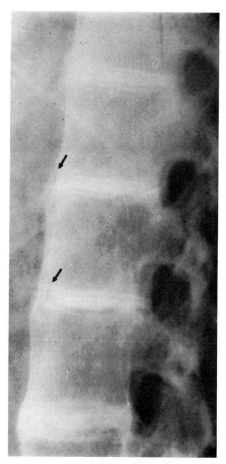

Figure 43–2. Radiographic features of alkaptonuria: Disc space narrowing and vacuum phenomena. Observe linear radiolucent areas (arrows) superimposed on multiple narrowed intervertebral discs. Discal calcification is not prominent. Apophyseal joint space narrowing is seen. Note spondylolysis of a lower lumbar vertebra (arrowhead).

Figure 43–3. Radiographic features of alkaptonuria: Spinal ossification. Diffuse extensive discal calcification is seen. Observe marginal discal ossification (arrows) simulating the findings of ankylosing spondylitis. The apophyseal joints are narrowed or fused.

Extraspinal Abnormalities

At the symphysis pubis, joint space narrowing, calcification, bone eburnation, and fragmentation may be seen. Similarly, at the sacroiliac articulations, joint space narrowing, sclerosis, and osteophytosis can be apparent (Fig. 43–4).

The knee is the most common site of peripheral abnormality (Fig. 43–5). Findings in this location simulate those of uncomplicated degenerative joint disease, with effusion, joint space narrowing, and bone sclerosis. Differences between these two diseases may include isolated involvement of the lateral femorotibial compartment, relatively symmetric involvement of both medial and lateral femorotibial compartments, bone collapse and fragmentation with multiple radiopaque intraarticular bodies, meager osteophytosis, and tendinous calcification in alkaptonuria.

Radiographic findings in the hip may be identical to changes of degenerative joint disease with joint space narrowing and sclerosis. In some patients with this disease, symmetric loss of joint space, severe destruction with fragmentation and formation of intraarticular cartilaginous and osseous bodies, and tendinous calcification and ossification permit differentiation from typical degenerative alterations (Fig. 43–6).

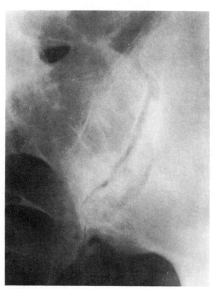

Figure 43–4. Radiographic features of alkaptonuria: Sacroiliac joint. Diffuse narrowing of the articular space is associated with irregularity of subchondral bone and sclerosis. The articular margins are more sharply defined than would be expected in anklyosing spondylitis.

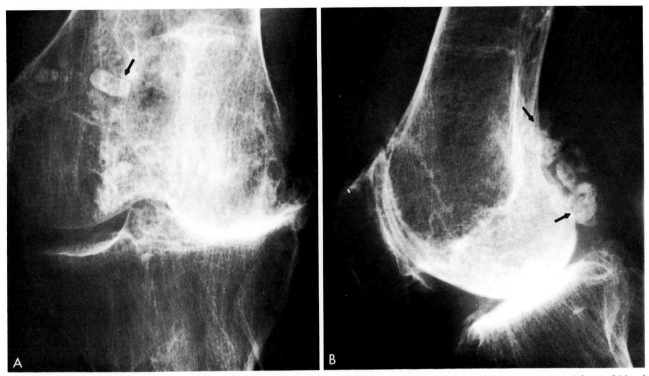

Figure 43–5. Radiographic features of alkaptonuria: Knee. In this patient, abnormalities include joint space narrowing in the lateral femorotibial and patellofemoral compartments associated with bone sclerosis, small osteophytes, and multiple intraarticular osseous bodies (arrows).

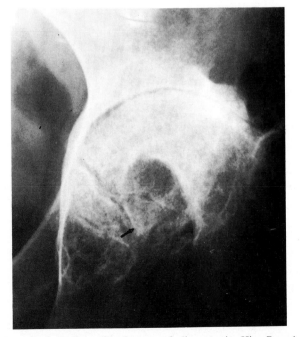

Figure 43–6. Radiographic features of alkaptonuria: Hip. Extensive resorption and flattening of the femoral head is associated with a bizarre radiographic appearance. Findings include joint space narrowing, mild acetabular protrusion, and bone fragmentation (arrow).

Involvement of the small joints of the hands and feet, the elbow, the glenohumeral joint, and the ankle is not common.

DIFFERENTIAL DIAGNOSIS
Spinal Manifestations

Discal calcification in this disease may be confused with that accompanying other disorders (Table 43–2). Dystrophic calcification of the nucleus pulposus is not infrequent. In these instances, the radiodense collections generally are globular in appearance and confined to the central portion of the

Table 43–2. DISCAL CALCIFICATION*

Diagnosis	Site of Calcification†	Nature of Calcification‡
Ochronosis	AF; NP	HA
CPPD crystal deposition disease		
Sporadic	AF	CPPD
Familial	AF; NP	?
Hemochromatosis	AF; NP	CPPD
Hyperparathyroidism	AF; NP	CPPD
Acromegaly	AF; NP	HA
Poliomyelitis	AF; NP	?
Amyloidosis	AF; NP	?
Spinal fusion	NP	?

*Reprinted by permission from Weinberger A, Myers AR: Intervertebral disc calcification in adults: A review. Semin Arthritis Rheum 18:69–75, 1978.

†AF, Anulus fibrosus; NP, nucleus pulposus.

‡HA, Calcium hydroxyapatite; CPPD, calcium pyrophosphate dihydrate.

intervertebral disc. This pattern of calcification usually is not widespread and can be differentiated readily from diffuse discal calcification at multiple levels in the spines of patients with alkaptonuria.

Calcification of the intervertebral disc may be seen as a secondary phenomenon in patients with primary disorders that lead to spinal ankylosis. This calcification may result from abnormal nutrition of the intervertebral disc associated with lack of mobility. Thus, discal calcification can be noted in patients with ankylosing spondylitis, diffuse idiopathic skeletal hyperostosis (DISH), juvenile-onset rheumatoid arthritis, Klippel-Feil deformities, and surgical fusions of the spine.

Discal calcification is also observed in CPPD crystal deposition disease. In this disorder, the deposits predominate in the outer fibers of the anulus fibrosus.

Disc space loss, vacuum phenomena, and vertebral body marginal sclerosis accompany intervertebral osteochondrosis. The findings generally are not so pronounced or widespread as in alkaptonuria. Nonetheless, the possibility of alkaptonuria must be considered in any patient whose radiographs reveal loss of height of multiple intervertebral discs, particularly if the changes occur in a middle-aged patient and are accompanied by multiple vacuum phenomena, discal calcification, vertebral fusion, and kyphosis.

Discal ossification with fusion of vertebral bodies, a finding in alkaptonuria, may resemble abnormalities in ankylosing spondylitis. In long-standing alkaptonuria, a bamboo spine may again simulate that in ankylosing spondylitis, although additional skeletal manifestations allow differentiation of these two disorders.

Extraspinal Manifestations

Involvement of extraspinal sites in patients with alkaptonuria may lead to a radiographic appearance that is reminiscent of degenerative joint disease. Certain features of ochronotic arthropathy usually permit its identification in these individuals (Table 43–3):

1. *Involvement of unusual articular sites.* An arthropathy of the glenohumeral joint resembling that of severe degenerative articular disease should suggest the diagnosis of alkaptonuria, as it is unusual to observe considerable findings of degenerative joint disease in this location without a history of significant trauma. Similarly, severe changes in the sacroiliac or symphyseal joints may be a clue to the presence of ochronotic arthropathy.

2. *Unusual patterns of joint space loss.* Ochronotic arthropathy of the knee may lead to isolated lateral femorotibial compartment changes or to symmetric loss of articular space in both the medial and lateral femorotibial compartments. These patterns are unusual in degenerative joint disease. Furthermore, symmetric loss of joint space in the hip and shoulder is seen in alkaptonuria.

Table 43–3. OCHRONOTIC ARTHROPATHY VERSUS DEGENERATIVE JOINT DISEASE

Ochronotic Arthropathy	Degenerative Joint Disease
Involvement of hips, shoulders, knees, sacroiliac joints, and symphysis pubis	Involvement of hips, knees, and hands
Asymmetric or symmetric joint space loss	Asymmetric joint space loss
Absent or meager osteophytosis	Prominent osteophytosis
Small cystic lesions	Small or large cystic lesions
Collapse, fragmentation, and intraarticular osseous bodies	No collapse or fragmentation
Tendon abnormalities	No tendon abnormalities

3. *Severe abnormalities with extreme sclerosis, fragmentation, and intraarticular cartilaginous and osseous bodies.* The severity of the changes accompanying ochronotic arthropathy may be greater than is usually seen in degenerative joint disease. The production of multiple intraarticular bodies is particularly characteristic.

The peculiar pattern of "degenerative" arthropathy that is characteristic of alkaptonuria may be simulated by other disorders, such as CPPD crystal deposition disease, calcium hydroxyapatite (HA) crystal deposition disease, acromegaly, and epiphyseal and spondyloepiphyseal dysplasias. In CPPD crystal deposition disease, the presence of chondrocalcinosis and capsular and synovial calcification and the absence of diffuse discal calcification are helpful diagnostic clues. Tendinous calcification may be observed in both diseases. The arthropathy of calcium HA crystal deposition disease includes bone fragmentation and sclerosis, findings seen in alkaptonuria, although cloud-like intraarticular and periarticular calcification in the former disorder is an important diagnostic feature. Arthropathy accompanying acromegaly and epiphyseal and spondyloepiphyseal dysplasias may be confused with ochronotic arthropathy, particularly in the hip, knee, and glenohumeral joints. Additional skeletal manifestations in these disorders ensure proper diagnosis. Destructive arthropathy in alkaptonuria may occasionally simulate neuroarthropathy.

FURTHER READING

Justesen P, Andersen PE Jr: Radiologic manifestations in alcaptonuria. Skel Radiol *11*:204, 1984.

Lagier R, Sitaj S: Vertebral changes in ochronois. Anatomical and radiological study of one case. Ann Rheum Dis *33*:86, 1974.

Laskar RH, Sargison KD: Ochronotic arthropathy. A review with four case reports. J Bone Joint Surg [Br] *52*:653, 1970.

Pomeranx MM, Friedman LJ, Tunick IS: Roentgen findings in alkaptonuric ochronosis. Radiology *37*:295, 1941.

Thompson MM Jr: Ochronosis. AJR *78*:46, 1957.

Chapter 44

Other Crystal-Induced Diseases

Donald Resnick, M.D.

Other crystals besides monosodium urate, calcium pyrophosphate dihydrate, and calcium hydroxyapatite crystals can lead to articular and osseous abnormalities. Cholesterol crystals are identified in patients with rheumatoid arthritis as well as osteoarthritis, appear to reflect local rather than systemic alterations, and may be responsible for low grade synovial inflammation. Corticosteroid preparations, when injected into joints, are accompanied by a mild synovial inflammatory response. Accumulation of calcium oxalate crystals is seen in both primary and secondary oxalosis, the latter most typically occurring as a complication of chronic renal disease. Destructive lesions of the metaphyseal regions of tubular bones, discovertebral regions and, perhaps, joints become apparent.

When synovial fluid is examined with polarizing light microscopy, a variety of crystals can be identified, which may provide an immediate clue to the precise cause of articular symptoms and signs. Previous chapters have discussed three basic crystal-induced arthropathies: monosodium urate crystal deposition disease (gout); calcium pyrophosphate dihydrate (CPPD) crystal deposition disease (pseudogout and other clinical presentations); and calcium hydroxyapatite (HA) crystal deposition disease. Additional types of crystals are encountered occasionally. In some cases, they represent no more than artifacts, unrelated to articular pathology; in other instances, they may cause or accompany significant joint abnormalities.

CHOLESTEROL CRYSTALS

Crystals of cholesterol have been recognized in synovial fluid on numerous occasions, especially in patients with rheumatoid arthritis. The exact origin of cholesterol crystals within the joint is unknown, although local rather than systemic factors appear more important. The known relationship of cholesterol crystal deposition and an underlying disorder such as rheumatoid arthritis or osteoarthritis lends support to the concept that these crystals are responsible for low grade synovial inflammation and, perhaps, cartilage damage. Less clear is the existence of a specific cholesterol-induced crystal arthropathy.

CORTICOSTEROIDS

Corticosteroid preparations for intraarticular injections are suspensions of microcrystals that may persist for some time and be misinterpreted as monosodium urate or CPPD during polarizing microscopy. The use of intrasynovial corticosteroid therapy has been followed inconstantly by local exacerbations of symptoms in the treated joints. This phenomenon usually commences within 1 to 3 days after the injection and persists for several days.

Structural joint damage may be observed in some patients after intraarticular corticosteroid injection (see Chapter 65).

CALCIUM OXALATE (OXALOSIS)

Deposition of calcium oxalate crystals in tissue occurs in two main situations: as a rare primary hereditary process, or, more commonly, as a secondary or acquired process, usually in association with chronic renal disease.

Primary Oxalosis

This disorder, which is inherited as an autosomal recessive trait, is divided into two forms: type 1, glycolic aciduria due to the absence of alpha-ketoglutarate-glyoxylate carboxylase activity; and type 2, 1-glyceric aciduria due to a defect of D-glycerate-dehydrogenase. Overproduction of oxalate related to these enzyme defects is accompanied by its accumulation in various tissues. Damage to the kidneys in the form of calcium oxalate nephrolithiasis and nephrocalcinosis produces progressive renal failure and uremia. Extrarenal accumulation of calcium oxalate occurs in the small arteries, eyes, soft tissues, and bone.

Both boys and girls are affected. Clinical manifestations generally become apparent before the age of 5 years and are mainly the result of renal accumulation of calcium oxalate crystals. Calculi and pyelonephritis are observed. Radiographic examination of the genitourinary system may reveal small, contracted kidneys with parenchymal calcification (Fig. 44–1).

Irregular transverse sclerotic bands in the metaphyseal segments of tubular bones, including the femur, humerus, tibia, fibula, metacarpal and metatarsal bones, and phalanges, are observed. These bands extend into the epiphyses, and narrow translucent zones are seen at the level of the physis between the epiphyseal and metaphyseal components. Similar radiodense regions can appear in subchondral areas in the humeri and femora, resembling the findings of ischemic

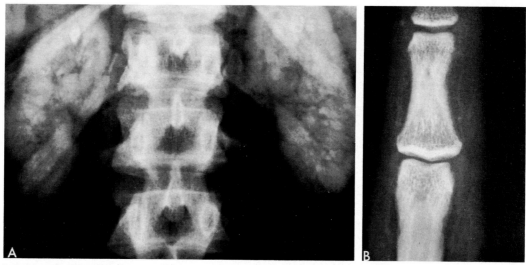

Figure 44–1. Primary oxalosis: Radiographic abnormalities. A A preliminary film from an intravenous pyelogram, before the injection of contrast material, reveals bilateral diffuse calcification within contracted kidneys. **B** Findings include vascular calcification and subperiosteal bone resorption in a finger.

necrosis, whereas in the spine, sclerotic zones at the top and bottom of the vertebral bodies simulate the rugger-jersey appearance of renal osteodystrophy. Eventually, chronic renal failure can lead to widespread skeletal abnormalities of renal osteodystrophy, such as subperiosteal bone resorption and diffuse osteosclerosis (Fig. 44–1). Multiple pathologic fractures and vascular and soft tissue calcification have been seen.

Histologic investigation indicates that the sclerotic regions in the tubular bones represent, in large part, deposition in the marrow of calcium oxalate crystals. A foreign body giant cell reaction results, which stimulates new bone formation. Massive deposits of calcium oxalate are associated with resorption and disappearance of trabeculae, cystic lesions, fracture, and deformities such as acetabular protrusion.

Secondary Oxalosis

Oxalosis is a recognized complication of other diseases, especially renal disorders; secondary forms of oxalosis are also related to ingestion of substances that either contain the oxalate ion or are metabolized to oxalate (rhubarb, ethylene glycol) and to bowel disorders that cause malabsorption and steatorrhea. Calcium oxalate is deposited in the body's tissues. The deposits occur primarily in the kidney itself. Other organs that are involved include the myocardium, thyroid gland, spleen, liver, lymph nodes, brain, salivary glands, dentin, dental pulp, arteries and veins, and musculoskeletal tissues.

Sites of crystal deposition in osseous tissue in secondary oxalosis are the hypertrophic zone of the physes, the bone marrow in the metaphyses, and areas of tissue necrosis associated with former fracture. Trabecular condensation accounts for the resulting radiodensity and cystic appearance evident on the radiographs. Articular manifestations have been reported in multiple locations, including the knees, wrists, and metacarpophalangeal and interphalangeal joints. In addition to juxtaarticular osteoporosis, radiographs may reveal capsular and cartilage calcification (chondrocalcinosis), the latter unrelated to CPPD crystal deposition (Fig. 44–2).

The radiographic characteristics of musculoskeletal involve-

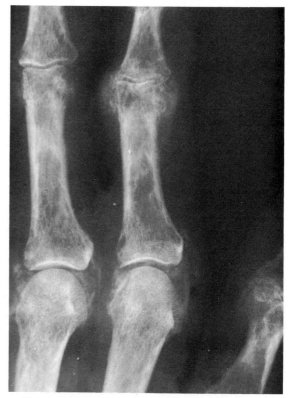

Figure 44–2. Secondary oxalosis. Radiologic abnormalities. A radiograph reveals periarticular and intraarticular calcification. The latter is within the capsule, synovium, and, possibly, the cartilage. Minimal subperiosteal bone resorption is suggested. Similar findings were apparent on the opposite side, and chondrocalcinosis in the knees was seen. Synovial fluid from the knees revealed positively birefringent chunks and rod-shaped crystals, which proved to be calcium oxalate. (Courtesy of R. Schumacher, M.D., Philadelphia, Pennsylvania.)

ment in secondary oxalosis present diagnostic difficulties. Chondrocalcinosis, as well as calcification in the joint capsule and tendons, can relate to CPPD, calcium HA, or calcium oxalate crystal deposition (or any combination of the three) in patients with chronic renal disease. Bone erosions can potentially relate to any of these crystals or to secondary hyperparathyroidism. Discovertebral destruction, a recently recognized complication of renal dialysis, may represent an additional manifestation of calcium oxalate crystal accumulation, although subchondral resorption due to secondary hyperparathyroidism, amyloidosis, or HA or CPPD crystal deposition can lead to a similar aberration. Sclerosis in metaphyseal segments of tubular bones is a finding of secondary (as well as primary) oxalosis, although apparently it can be seen in chronic renal disease without oxalate deposition.

FURTHER READING

Brancaccio D, Poggi A, Ciccarelli C, Bellini F, Galmozzi C, Poletti I, Maggiore Q: Bone changes in end-stage oxalosis. AJR *136*:935, 1981.

Day DL, Scheinman JI, Mahan J: Radiological aspects of primary hyperoxaluria. AJR *146*:395, 1986.

Fam AG, Sugai M, Gertner E, Lewis A: Cholesterol "tophus." Arthritis Rheum *26*:1525, 1983.

Martijn A, Thijn CJP: Radiologic findings in primary hyperoxaluria. Skel Radiol 8:21, 1982.

McCarty DJ Jr, Hogan JM: Inflammatory reaction after intrasynovial injection of microcrystalline adrenocorticosteroid esters. Arthritis Rheum 7:359, 1964.

Milgram JW, Salyer WR: Secondary oxalosis of bone in chronic renal failure. A histopathological study of three cases. J Bone Joint Surg [Am] *56*:387, 1974.

Zuckner J, Uddin J, Gantner GE Jr, Dorner RW: Cholesterol crystals in synovial fluid. Ann Intern Med *60*:436, 1964.

SECTION VII

SPECIFIC TARGET AREAS OF ARTICULAR DISEASES

CASE VII

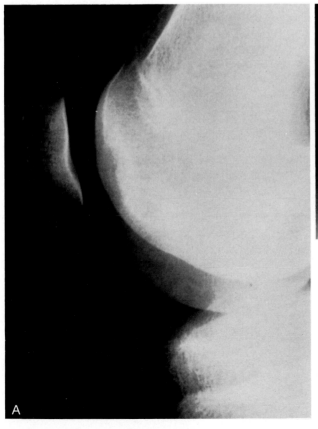

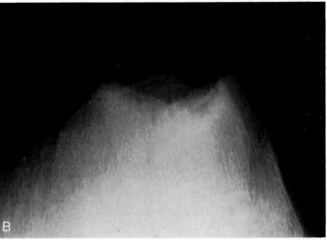

A 15 year old boy developed pain in the anterior aspect of the knee. He had no history of acute injury.

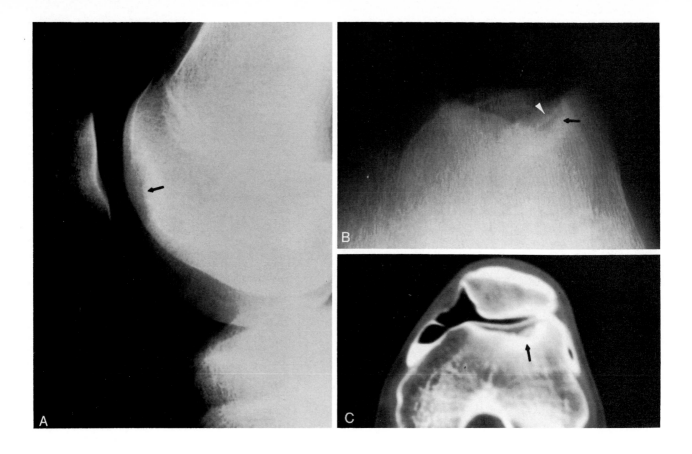

Lateral (*A*) and axial (*B*) radiographs of the knee reveal an ovoid area of irregularity or erosion involving the anterior aspect of the lateral condyle (arrows). On the latter radiograph, an ossific radiodense region (arrowhead) is evident in the area of abnormality. A transaxial computed tomographic scan (*C*) that was obtained after the introduction of positive contrast material and air into the knee shows the lesion and a radiodense spicule (arrow). The subjacent bone in the femur is sclerotic, and the overlying articular cartilage appears intact.

Although initial diagnostic considerations might include a variety of neoplasms, particularly chondroblastoma, and subchondral cystic lesions, the imaging abnormalities are pathognomonic of an osteochondral fracture, or osteochondritis dissecans. Osteochondritis dissecans is most frequently observed in the knee, especially on the lateral aspect of the medial femoral condyle. Involvement of the anterior portion of the lateral femoral condyle, however, is also well recognized, particularly in physically active adolescent individuals. The precise radiographic appearance of osteochondritis dissecans depends on the extent of osseous abnormality, although a saucer-like area of osseous irregularity, as in the test case, is most typical. On the lateral radiograph, the osteochondral defect in the lateral condyle generally is seen in the distal portion of the femur at the level of the superior or middle region of the patella; it is not apparent on the frontal and "tunnel" radiographic projections. Axial radiographs of the patella, particularly the Merchant projection, will show that the defect resides in the anterior aspect of the lateral condyle. Arthrography alone, arthrography combined with conven-

tional or computed tomography, or magnetic resononance imaging may be useful in defining the status of the overlying articular cartilage.

Osteochondritis dissecans involving the distal portion of the femur must be differentiated from ischemic necrosis of bone, which also commonly affects the femur. Osteonecrosis may relate to a variety of causative factors, including corticosteroid medication, or have an idiopathic basis. Features that generally allow differentiation of ischemic necrosis from osteochondritis dissecans are an appropriate history and involvement of the weight-bearing surface of the femur as well as other sites. Neuropathic disease, particularly that related to congenital insensitivity to pain, occasionally may lead to radiographic abnormalities of the femur that simulate those of osteochondritis dissecans or ischemic necrosis.

FINAL DIAGNOSIS: Osteochondral fracture (osteochondritis dissecans) of the lateral femoral condyle.

FURTHER READING

Pages 817–821 and the following:

1. Cayea PD, Pavlov H, Sherman MF, Goldman AB: Lucent articular lesion in the lateral femoral condyle: Source of patellar femoral pain in the athletic adolescent. AJR *137*:1145, 1981.
2. Mesgarzadeh M, Sapega AA, Bonakdarpour A, Revesz G, Moyer RA, Maurer A, Alburger PD: Osteochondritis dissecans: Analysis of mechanical stability with radiography, scintigraphy, and MR imaging. Radiology *165*:775, 1987.

(Case VII, courtesy of Kenneth A. Jurist, M.D., Warren, Michigan.)

528

Chapter 45

Temporomandibular Joint

William A. Murphy, M.D.

Temporomandibular joint (TMJ) pain and dysfunction are important clinical problems. In the last 10 years, radiologists have had a major impact on TMJ diagnosis because of a technologic explosion of imaging methods. Foremost among these have been arthrography, computed tomography, and, more recently, magnetic resonance imaging. Although many controversies continue, the recent impact of newer imaging techniques on the diagnosis of TMJ disorders is undeniable.

The temporomandibular joint (TMJ) is afflicted by many osseous and soft tissue conditions, and because of its particular anatomic structure and location, it is subject to a unique biomechanical environment and set of pathologic conditions.

ANATOMY

The temporomandibular joint is an articulation between the condyle of the mandible and the mandibular fossa and articular eminence of the temporal bone. The condylar and temporal bone components of the TMJ are maintained in apposition by muscles, ligaments, and joint capsule. The capsule attaches about the joint margins and is reinforced laterally by a strong temporomandibular ligament and medially by two weaker ligaments. Branches of the mandibular division of the trigeminal nerve innervate the joint. Similarly, branches of the superficial temporal and maxillary arteries provide the blood supply.

Osseous Anatomy

Important osseous landmarks in the lateral projection are the cortical and trabecular elements of the condyle, mandibular fossa, temporal eminence, and auditory canal (Fig. 45–1). The long axis of the mandibular condyle, the articulating surface of the bone, lies perpendicular to the mandibular ramus. The articulating surface of the temporal bone is composed of the mandibular fossa and the articular eminence. The plate of bone between the mandibular fossa and the middle cranial fossa is quite thin.

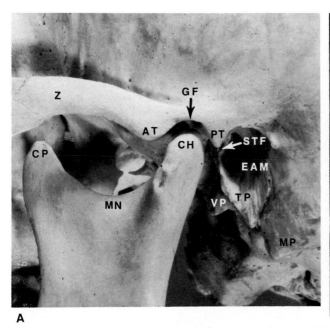
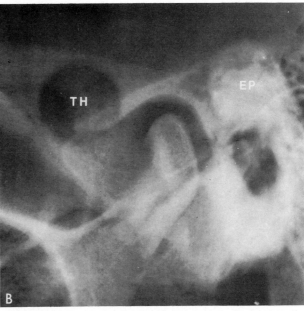

Figure 45–1. Lateral perspective of normal adult osseous anatomy. A Surface photograph of the skull. **B** Magnified lateral projection (closed mouth position). The following anatomic landmarks can be identified: Z, zygoma; GF, glenoid (mandibular) fossa; AT, anterior glenoid tubercle (articular eminence); PT, posterior glenoid tubercle; CH, condylar head; CP, coronoid process; STF, squamotympanic fissure; EAM, external auditory meatus; VP, vaginal process; TP, tympanic process; MP, mastoid process; TH, threaded hole in radiographic positioning device; EP, ear plug.

529

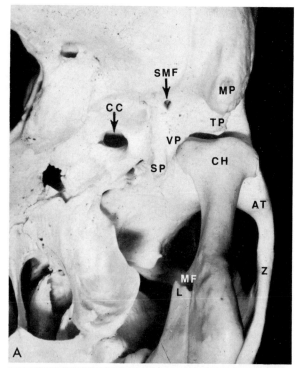

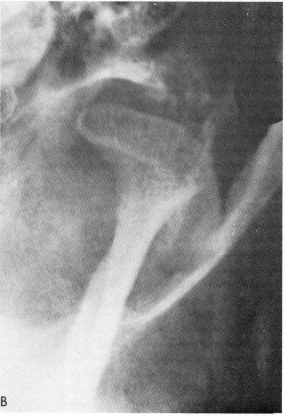

Figure 45–2. Frontal (Towne) perspective of the normal adult osseous anatomy. A Surface photograph of the skull. B Magnified Towne projection (closed mouth position). The following anatomic landmarks can be identified: CC, Carotid canal; SMF, stylomastoid foramen; SP, styloid process; VP, vaginal process; MP, mastoid process; TP, tympanic process; CH, condylar head; AT, anterior glenoid tubercle; MF, mandibular foramen; L, lingula; Z, zygoma.

Major osseous landmarks in the frontal (Towne) projection are portions of the condyle, including its neck and medial and lateral poles (Fig. 45–2). Medially, the mandibular fossa is limited by an osseous ridge that is a barrier to medial dislocation of the condyle.

In both lateral (sagittal) and frontal (coronal or Towne) perspectives, the joint surfaces are smooth, and the joint space is of nearly uniform thickness along the articulating surfaces. The condyle rests symmetrically within the fossa. The joint surfaces are covered by fibrocartilage rather than hyaline cartilage. A synovial membrane lines those parts of the joint that are not covered by fibrocartilage.

Soft Tissue Anatomy

The major soft tissue structure of the TMJ is an articular disc (meniscus) that is interposed between the adjacent osseous elements (Fig. 45–3). The disc separates the joint into two synovial articulations, one superior, between the temporal bone and the disc, and the other inferior, between the disc and the condylar head. The disc is thin centrally and ridged or thickened peripherally. It is attached to capsular, ligamentous, and other soft tissue structures about its entire periphery.

The disc is a biconcave fibrocartilaginous structure. In the sagittal perspective, the anterior and posterior ridges of the disc are prominent and are termed (anterior and posterior) bands. The anterior band of the disc is smaller than the posterior band and attaches to the anterior margin of the articular eminence and to the anteroinferior aspect of the articular margin of the condyle. The posterior band of the disc blends with a highly vascular and innervated areolar tissue termed the bilaminar zone.

With the jaw closed, the disc is positioned between the condyle and the fossa such that the posterior band is located between the apex of the condyle and the depth of the fossa. As the jaw opens, the disc and condyle move forward in a complex coordinated fashion. The result is that the thin central portion of the disc maintains a position between the juxtaposed articular surfaces of the condyle and eminence.

IMAGING METHODS
Radiography

Conventional radiography has been considered best suited for display of osseous anatomy and the general positional relationship of the condyle with respect to the mandibular fossa; however, obtaining optimal images has been technically demanding and not always successful.

TRANSCRANIAL RADIOGRAPHY. When patient positioning and beam centering are optimal, conventional transcranial lateral films provide an acceptable profiled image for study of TMJ anatomy and range of motion (Fig. 45–4). A logical method to improve lateral transcranial radiography is to standardize head positioning, and several devices have been developed to accomplish this. A more recent advancement in TMJ imaging was the marriage of a positioning device to an x-ray unit capable of direct geometric magnification. This method provides both minute radiologic detail and dependable positioning of a small, inaccessible anatomic structure (Fig. 45–5).

Conventional tomography (laminagraphy) for the radiologic diagnosis of TMJ problems generally reveals a greater number of osseous changes than do conventional radiographs (Fig. 45–6). The method has several disadvantages, however, in-

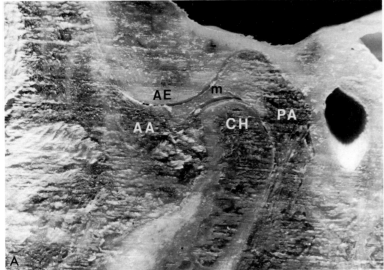

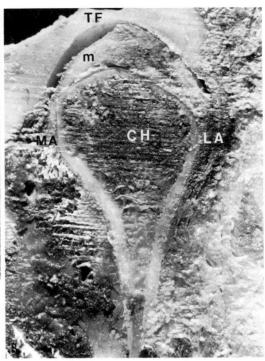

Figure 45–3. Normal soft tissue anatomy of the temporomandibular joint. A Sagittal section shows disc or meniscus (m) separating the articular eminence (AE) from the condylar head (CH). Anterior (AA) and posterior (PA) meniscal attachments are broadly based in the adjacent soft tissues. **B** Coronal section shows the meniscus (m) separating the temporal fossa (TF) from the condylar head (CH). Meniscal attachments to the condylar head are thin medially (MA) and thick laterally (LA).

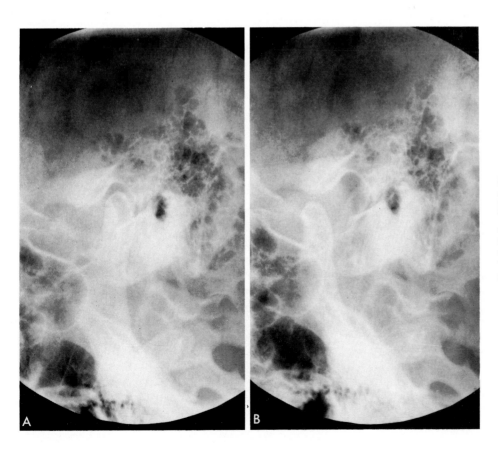

Figure 45–4. Contact transcranial lateral view. A The closed TMJ is projected free of other cranial structures. The condylar head and mandibular fossa are profiled. **B** The open mouth view shows the normal range of motion, and the bone structures remain profiled. The TMJ makes up less than 10 per cent of this image.

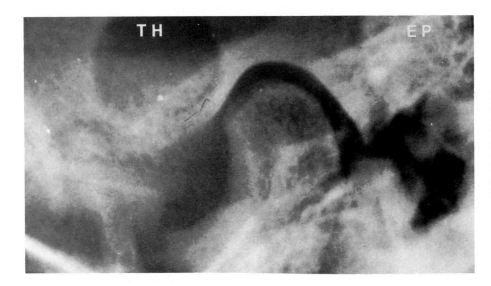

Figure 45–5. Magnification lateral image of a normal TMJ in closed mouth position. Bone detail is exquisite, and the TMJ constitutes about 50 per cent of the overall image. Side-by-side round artifacts result from the positioning device; the lucent area is the threaded ear plug hole (TH) and the dense area is the ear plug (EP) itself.

cluding being relatively time consuming, requiring the attention of a physician, and involving a relatively high radiation exposure. Since the introduction of newer imaging methods, conventional tomography has diminished in importance as a technique for evaluating the TMJ.

OTHER RADIOGRAPHIC PROJECTIONS. The *Towne projection* provides a frontal or coronal image of the condylar head and mandibular fossa of the temporal bone (Fig. 45–2). It reveals detailed osseous features of the medial and lateral poles of the condylar head, the posterosuperior cortical surface, and the condylar neck. An angle of approximately 30 degrees is optimal, because at this angle the TMJ is projected free of the mastoid air cells.

The *submentovertical (base) projection* also images the medial and lateral condylar poles. Anterior and posterior cortical surfaces are profiled, and information is provided about adjacent bone structures at the base of the skull (Fig. 45–7).

The *panoramic radiographic projection* provides an excellent survey of the mandible and dentition. It images both TMJs simultaneously and may reveal disease processes of these joints, the mandible, or the teeth (Fig. 45–8).

CLINICAL ASPECTS OF RADIOGRAPHY. The size and shape of the left and right condyles and mandibular fossae are symmetric in normal persons. The cortices are thin and smooth and encase finely trabeculated bone. The earliest osseous abnormalities appear in the condyle and may consist of erosions, spurs, and sclerosis. Changes in the eminence generally follow condylar changes and consist of sclerosis and remodeling.

The condyle generally is positioned centrally with respect to the mandibular fossa in normal, asymptomatic individuals. Likewise, many patients with symptoms will have a condyle that is positioned posteriorly with respect to the fossa (retropositioned). Normal persons show variation in condyle position, however, and symptomatic people may have an isocentric condylar position.

Normal, asymptomatic persons are capable of a range of joint motion such that with full jaw opening the condyle reaches the apex of the eminence and usually passes beyond it (Fig. 45–4).

Sectional Imaging

COMPUTED TOMOGRAPHY. Depending on the individual computed tomographic (CT) unit being operated, one or more methods of TMJ imaging are available. In general, transaxial scans of the TMJ have not been useful. Instead, sagittal scans have been adopted, obtained either by reformatting data from a stack of transaxial images or by positioning the patient so that direct sagittal images are possible.

CT is very useful for evaluation of osseous anatomy. The greater emphasis, however, has been on the detection of internal derangement of the disc (Fig. 45–9). Displaced discs are detected by CT with high sensitivity, accuracy, and positive predictive value (greater than 90 per cent) by whatever method is employed so long as it is technically well performed.

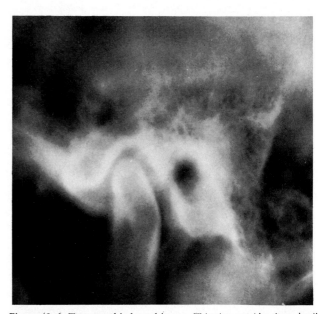

Figure 45–6. **Tomographic lateral image.** This view provides sharp detail of a 5 mm section of a normal TMJ in closed mouth position.

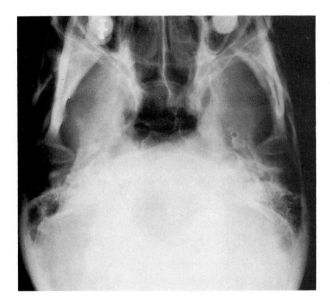

Figure 45–7. Contact submentovertical (base) projection. This view also surveys cranial anatomy surrounding the TMJ. Medial and lateral poles and anterior and posterior cortices of the condylar heads are well shown.

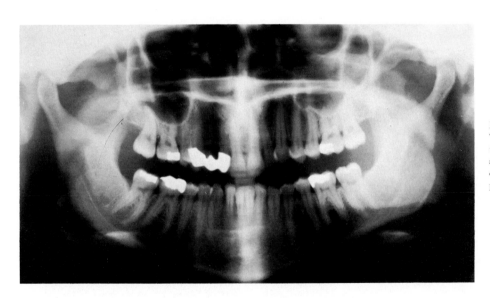

Figure 45–8. Panoramic radiograph. The panoramic view shows mandible, dental structures, and TMJs in a single image, a useful survey for dental or periarticular disease that might be manifested as TMJ pain.

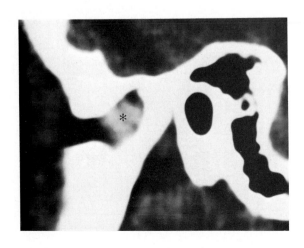

Figure 45–9. Computed tomography of TMJ. CT direct sagittal section at a soft tissue window setting showing a soft tissue mass (asterisk) anterior to condyle, diagnostic of a dislocated disc. (Courtesy of K. Bell, M.D., New Orleans, Louisiana.)

The advantages of CT are its sectional display of osseous and soft tissue anatomy and its noninvasive nature. Its disadvantages are that the method is technically demanding and difficult to perform well, it fails to delineate the condition of the disc, and it provides no dynamic functional information.

MAGNETIC RESONANCE IMAGING. Magnetic resonance (MR) imaging provides greater inherent soft tissue contrast than any other imaging method. For TMJ imaging, the sagittal plane has been emphasized. Surface coils have been employed to improve the signal-to-noise ratio, increase the spatial resolution, and decrease the section thickness. Spin density (long TR, short TE) or T1 weighted (short TR, short TE) spin echo sequences provide better contrast than do T2 weighted (long TR, long TE) sequences for TMJ imaging.

Like CT, MR imaging is an excellent method for demonstration of disc position (Fig. 45–10). It performs as well as arthrography in the demonstration of disc position but less well in the demonstration of disc condition or dynamic function.

Arthrography

Arthrography should be considered the primary method for complete analysis of internal derangement and the method of examining the disc against which all other techniques are measured.

In general, after cleansing of the preauricular skin, a disposable needle (scalp needle) is inserted through the skin anterior to the tragus and into a joint space. Either the lower joint space is examined alone or both lower and upper joint spaces are studied. Under most circumstances, the position of the disc and its functional relationship to the condyle are revealed by opacification of the lower space. When imaging

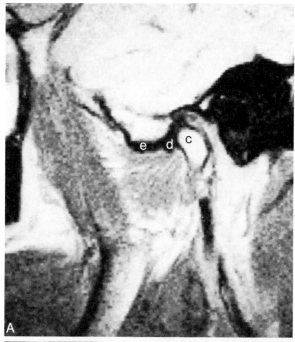

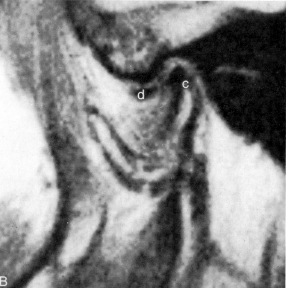

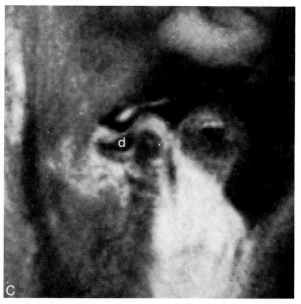

Figure 45–10. Magnetic resonance imaging of TMJ. A Direct sagittal section of normal volunteer shows bright signal from condylar marrow (c) and low signal from eminence of temporal bone (e). Low signal disc (d) is interposed between condyle and fossa. **B** Direct sagittal section of patient with clinical evidence of a dislocated disc that does not reduce shows low signal disc (d) located anterior to the condyle (c). **C** Similar section of same patient with jaw opened to point of lock shows persistent anterior position of dislocated disc (d). (Courtesy of W. G. Totty, M.D., St. Louis, Missouri.)

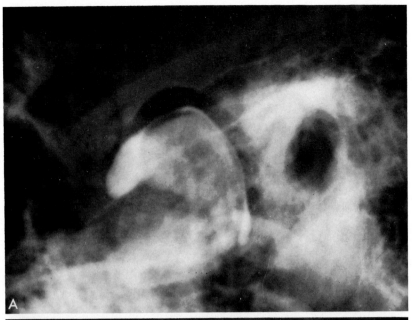

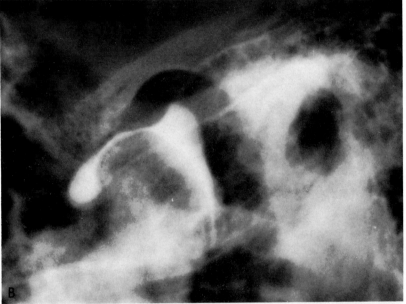

Figure 45-11. Arthrography of normal TMJ. A
Mouth closed. Contrast agent fills the inferior joint
space and outlines the undersurface of the disc. In
this closed position, the anterior recess is full and
has a biconvex contour and a vertical teardrop
orientation and configuration. The posterior recess
is collapsed against the condyle. B Mouth half
opened: Contrast agent has redistributed as the
anterior recess begins to close and the posterior
recess begins to open. The posterior band of disc is
clearly seen at the 12 o'clock position above the
condyle as it indents the contrast material that fills
the posterior recess. C Mouth fully opened: Contrast
agent is now squeezed out of the anterior recess,
which is collapsed against the condyle. The posterior
recess is full and the posterior band of disc is behind
the condyle.

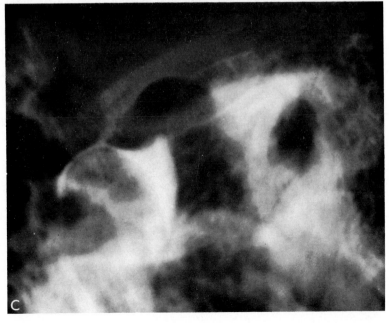

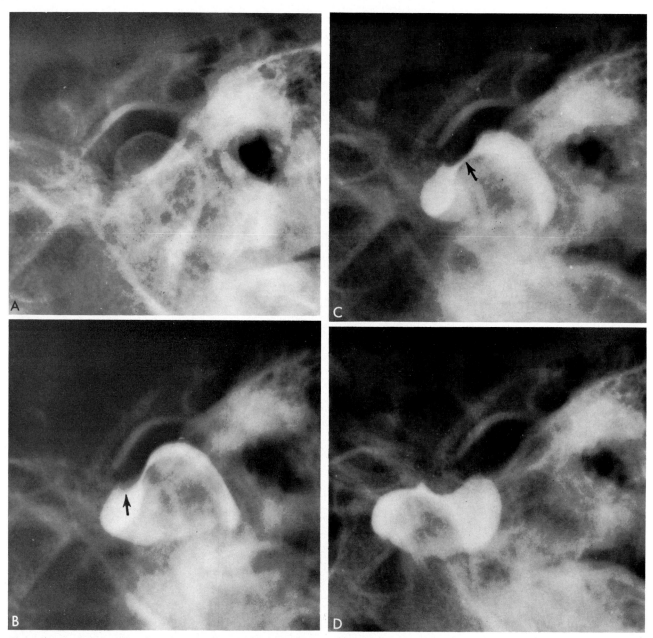

Figure 45–12. Arthrography of an abnormal TMJ showing disc dislocation with reduction. A Mouth closed: Magnification transcranial radiograph shows normal osseous anatomy and isocentric condyle position in the mandibular fossa. **B** Mouth closed: Contrast agent fills the inferior joint space and outlines the undersurface of the disc. Note that the posterior band of the disc is located anterior to the condyle (arrow) and bulges prominently in the anterior recess (compare with Fig. 45–11A). This is diagnostic of an anterior dislocation of the disc. **C** Mouth half opened: Contrast agent has redistributed, and the condyle has moved onto the posterior band (arrow), which is now compressed between the condyle and the eminence (compare with Fig. 45–11B). **D** Mouth fully opened: Condyle has now translated anterior to the eminence and, in doing so, has crossed the prominent thick posterior band, causing a click. The posterior band is now in a normal position posterior to the condyle.

Table 45–1. ALDERMAN'S CLASSIFICATION OF TMJ DISORDERS

EXTRACAPSULAR DISORDERS

Psychophysiologic: Tension, anxiety, oral habits
Iatrogenic: Misdirected mandibular nerve block, excessive depression of the mandible during anesthesia or oral procedures
Traumatic: Blow to the face not involving fractures
Dental: Occlusal abnormalities; periapical or periodontal lesions; mobile, sensitive or damaged teeth; ulcerations
Infectious: Secondary, outside the joint
Otologic: Otitis media or external ear infection
Neoplastic: Parotid gland, nasopharyngeal tumor

INTRACAPSULAR DISORDERS

Congenital: Agenesis, hyperplastic or hypoplastic condyle
Infectious: Primary bacterial infection within the joint
Arthritic: Rheumatoid arthritis, osteoarthritis, psoriatic arthritis, juvenile chronic arthritis
Traumatic: Fractures, disc tears
Functional: Subluxation, dislocation, disc derangement, hypermobility, ankylosis
Neoplastic: Benign or malignant tumors

the joint after instillation of the contrast agent, it is important to videotape the functional anatomy to display and record the dynamic aspects of disc dysfunction.

TMJ arthrography provides a demonstration of both osseous and soft tissue anatomy augmented by dynamic information (Fig. 45–11). It indicates the presence of disc perforation, gives an estimate of its size, and documents the presence of a dislocation of the disc and whether or not the disc reduces. The dynamic evaluation correlates the occurrence of clicks with protrusive or retrusive condylar translation and allows estimation of the magnitude of the effort necessary to recapture the disc. The degree of disc deformation is also documented (Fig. 45–12). If disc reduction does not occur, and clicks are still present, this information is provided. Likewise, the degree of limitation of joint motion is shown. Arthrography also is a useful adjunct to management of patients undergoing

conservative or surgical therapy and for those with persistent pain or dysfunction after therapeutic intervention.

DISORDERS

Disorders of the TMJ region can be divided into two general categories, extracapsular and intracapsular (Table 45–1). Extracapsular disorders are seen frequently by clinicians and often are classified as a myofascial pain–dysfunction syndrome. Many of the extracapsular disorders have a known cause, such as a form of trauma or local inflammation. Many others have no obvious cause, however. In these extracapsular conditions, results of radiography, arthrography, and sectional imaging are normal. Conversely, imaging studies in patients with intracapsular disorders usually reveal a structural or functional abnormality.

Congenital or Developmental Disorders

Congenital TMJ disturbances generally relate to abnormalities of development in the first branchial arch, resulting in agenesis, hypoplasia, or hyperplasia of the mandible. The defects may be focal, diffuse, unilateral, or bilateral.

Many other congenital or developmental diseases may affect the mandible and temporomandibular joints (Fig. 45–13). They may cause functional or arthritic disturbances.

Tumors and Tumor-like Disorders

Tumors of the temporomandibular joint are rare. Most often the joint is affected secondarily by extension of a mandibular neoplasm, such as an osteosarcoma or a metastasis (Fig. 45–14). Intraarticular tumor-like processes include osteocartilaginous loose bodies, synovial (osteo)chondromatosis, and pigmented villonodular synovitis.

Traumatic Disorders

Injury to the mandible or a direct blow to the temporomandibular joint is a common cause of TMJ pain and dysfunction. The trauma may result in soft tissue or osseous injury, or a combination of the two. Evaluation of the effect

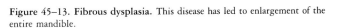

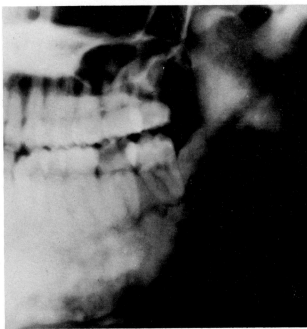

Figure 45–13. Fibrous dysplasia. This disease has led to enlargement of the entire mandible.

of trauma to this region must include an analysis of the mandible, the dental occlusion, and the temporomandibular joint. A particularly useful view is the panoramic radiograph, providing the best available method to survey the entire mandible and dentition. CT also is an important diagnostic method, allowing analysis of complicated fractures.

Mandibular fractures commonly relate to a direct force applied to the face. The mandible is a ring-like structure; therefore, when one fracture is discovered, another mandibular fracture should be sought. The second fracture may be ipsilateral or contralateral to the first. When forces are applied directly to the chin and the mandible does not fracture, the energy may be dissipated into the temporomandibular joint. Usually, the TMJ disc will cushion the impact or be injured. Sometimes, however, the temporal bone will fracture.

Fractures of the mandible are classified according to their anatomic location, which includes the condylar head, condylar neck, and coronoid process as well as the mandibular ramus, angle, body, and symphysis (Fig. 45–15). Condylar fractures are subdivided according to an intracapsular or extracapsular location, displacement at the fracture site, and position of the condylar head with respect to the mandibular fossa of the temporal bone (Table 45–2).

Intracapsular fractures of the condylar head occur infrequently. The fracture fragments usually are impacted (Fig. 45–16), although they may be rotated or even comminuted. Extracapsular condylar neck fractures may be nondisplaced or displaced, and the condylar head may remain in the mandibular fossa (Fig. 45–17) or be dislocated.

Although methods of treatment of mandibular fractures are varied, certain general therapeutic goals can be identified: (1) achieve fracture union with the most anatomically correct reduction possible, (2) preserve normal dental occlusion, (3)

Table 45–2. FRACTURES OF THE MANDIBULAR CONDYLE

   I. Intracapsular head fracture
      A. Nondisplaced
      B. Displaced
  II. Extracapsular neck fracture
      A. Nondisplaced
      B. Displaced—head located
      C. Displaced—head dislocated
 III. Extracapsular subcondylar fracture
      A. Nondisplaced
      B. Displaced

maintain a full range of pain-free TMJ mobility, and (4) ensure the best possible cosmetic appearance.

Complications of mandibular fractures are numerous. Direct complications of the fracture include loss of teeth, malunion or nonunion, displacement with deformity, and infection. Secondary complications of trauma often are more severe and include malocclusion and TMJ internal derangement, both of which result in pain and malfunction. Furthermore, TMJ ankylosis may follow a condylar fracture. It may result from hemarthrosis or fracture healing if the disc becomes adherent to the condylar head, mandibular fossa, or both. Ankylosis may also develop owing to immobility during interdental fixation.

A prosthetic replacement of the condylar head and neck may be implanted in selected cases after fracture or in advanced arthritis with ankylosis. Many types of prostheses and surgical methods have been used in the replacement of the articular surface of the condyle and eminence. Among these are a variety of metal and plastic components, substances that are interposed between the articulating surfaces, and various

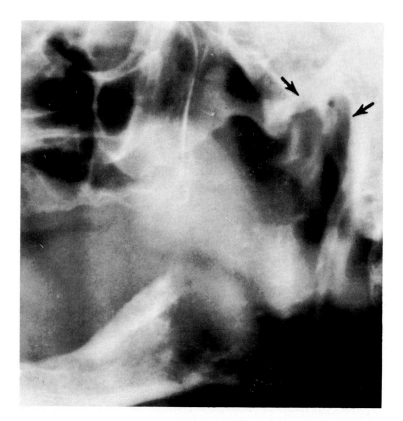

Figure 45–14. Metastatic lung carcinoma in the ascending ramus of the mandible. The condylar head is floating freely (arrows) in the mandibular fossa.

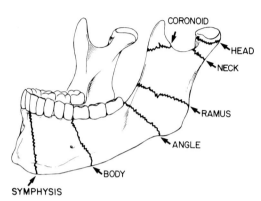

Figure 45–15. Locations of various mandibular fractures.

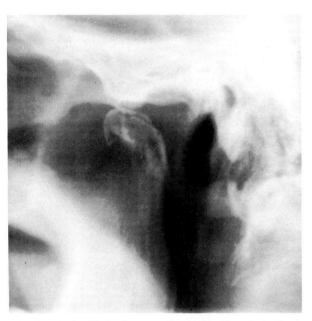

Figure 45–16. Mandibular fractures. Panoramic radiograph showing intracapsular condylar head fracture with impaction of fracture fragments.

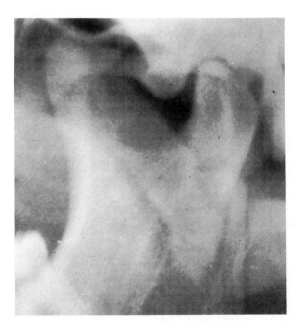

Figure 45–17. Mandibular fracture. Low condylar neck fracture with the condyle still seated in the mandibular fossa.

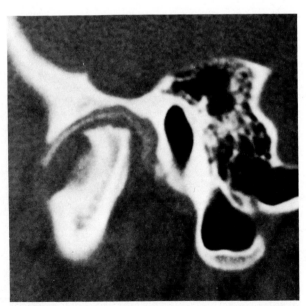

Figure 45–18. Treatment of mandibular fracture. Computed tomography in the sagittal plane shows a Teflon sheet interposed between the deformed surfaces of the condyle and mandibular fossa. (Courtesy of K. Bell, M.D., New Orleans, Louisiana.)

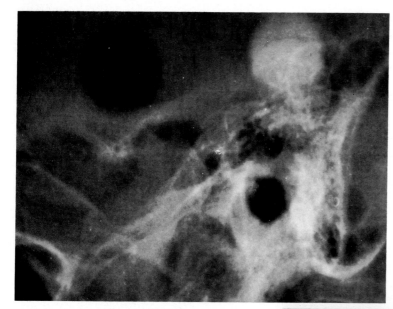

Figure 45–19. Seropositive rheumatoid arthritis. The joint space is very narrow, periarticular osteopenia is advanced, and bone erosions are large and diffuse.

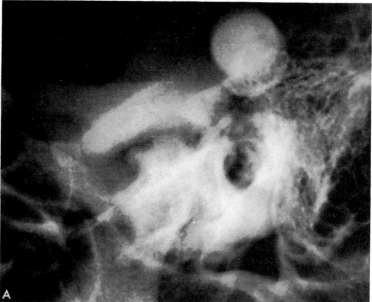

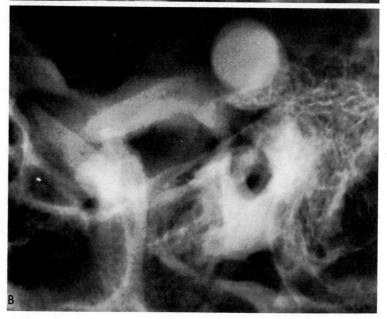

Figure 45–20. Osteoarthritis in both closed (A) and open (B) mouth positions. Despite advanced joint space loss, large osteophytes, remarkable reformation of the mandibular fossa, and dense osteosclerosis, functional motion is relatively maintained.

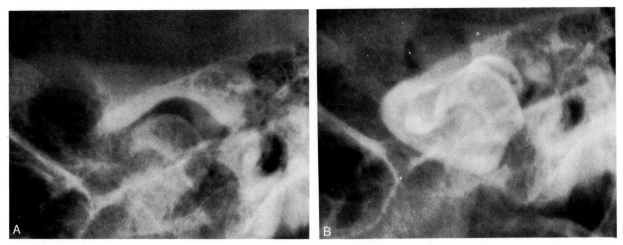

Figure 45–21. **Moderately advanced osteoarthritis associated with a perforated and dislocated disc. A** Magnification transcranial radiograph shows focal narrowing of the joint space, condylar spur formation, flattening of the eminence, and sclerosis of the apposing articular bone. **B** Inferior space arthrogram shows perforation with anterior dislocation of the disc.

autografts (such as muscle). A more recent approach has been to implant a thin sheet of Teflon (Fig. 45–18). Additional methods include condylar shaving, condylectomy, and eminectomy.

Infectious Disorders

Pyogenic or granulomatous infections of the TMJ are uncommon. They may occur as a result of hematogenous seeding from a distant infection, but more commonly they develop as a direct extension of oral infections or after TMJ surgery. The radiologic findings are similar to those of rheumatoid arthritis.

Articular Disorders

TMJ arthritis is a common problem. Many patients have osteoarthritis, usually secondary to internal derangement of the disc. Gout and pseudogout, as well as rheumatoid arthritis, juvenile chronic arthritis, psoriatic arthritis, ankylosing spondylitis, and systemic lupus erythematosus, may all affect the TMJ. Many of these diseases may be indistinguishable both clinically and radiologically. In rheumatoid arthritis and related disorders, osteopenia, joint space narrowing, and bone erosion or production may be evident (Fig. 45–19).

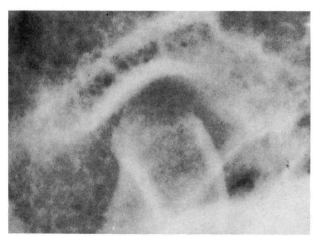

Figure 45–22. **Erosive phase of osteoarthritis.** Magnification transcranial radiograph shows a moderately advanced erosion of the condyle with resorption of the cortex and exposure of a roughened surface.

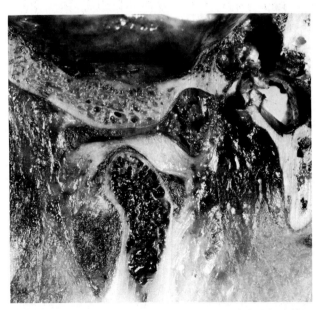

Figure 45–23. **TMJ compartments.** Sagittal section with the joint halfway through translation shows a biconcave disc interposed between the condyle and the eminence dividing the TMJ into superior and inferior compartments. These compartments are distended with latex. Note how much larger the superior compartment is compared with the inferior compartment.

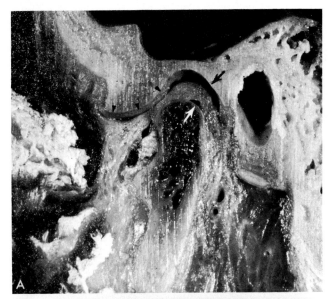

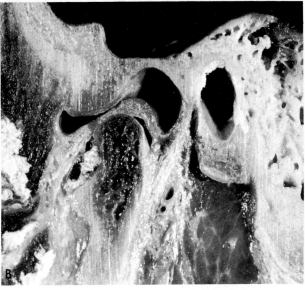

Figure 45–24. Functional anatomy of the temporomandibular joint. **A** Sagittal section of a fresh specimen in a slightly open mouth position shows posterior sulci (arrows) beginning to open. Articular cartilage (arrowheads) covers the articular eminence. Note that the posterior band of the disc is at the 12 o'clock position. **B** In the intermediate open mouth position, the posterior and anterior superior sulci are open. Note that the thin region of the disc stays between the articular surfaces and that changes in the joint shape are primarily a result of changes in the soft tissues about the sulci. Note also that translation is due primarily to motion of the disc with respect to the eminence.

Osteoarthritis of the TMJ generally is similar in radiologic appearance to osteoarthritis of other joints. Joint space narrowing, bone erosion, osteosclerosis, osteophytosis, and remodeling are seen (Fig. 45–20). Cartilage loss may be the predominant feature. Osteophytes may vary in size from small to large, and typically they develop at the margins of the articular surface. The degree of bone sclerosis and remodeling can be quite pronounced. Even with advanced osteoarthritis, a remarkable range of joint mobility may be retained. Fibrous or bone ankylosis rarely occurs in osteoarthritic joints.

It is now well recognized that a major fraction of TMJ osteoarthritis follows the development of an internal derangement, the frequency increasing with increasing duration of internal derangement. Osteoarthritis is closely associated with disc dislocation, joint locking, disc perforation, and disc fragmentation (Fig. 45–21). It is less well recognized that osteoarthritis of the TMJ commonly is erosive in the early or acute stages (Fig. 45–22).

Internal Derangement

Internal derangement is the most frequent disorder of the TMJ. Although estimates of prevalence vary, most investigators agree that between 20 and 30 per cent of the adult population have signs and symptoms of TMJ internal derangement. Women are affected clinically 3 to 5 times more frequently than are men. The average age at diagnosis in both men and women is in the fourth decade of life. Although most internal derangement has an insidious onset, with no obvious etiologic factors, trauma is considered to be a major cause.

An understanding of internal derangement of the TMJ requires knowledge of normal functional anatomy. The disc separates the TMJ into superior and inferior compartments (Fig. 45–23). A complex, dynamic relationship exists among the condyle, disc, and temporal eminence. Although the disc is restrained by its attachments, specific movements are permitted. Throughout all phases of normal joint mobility,

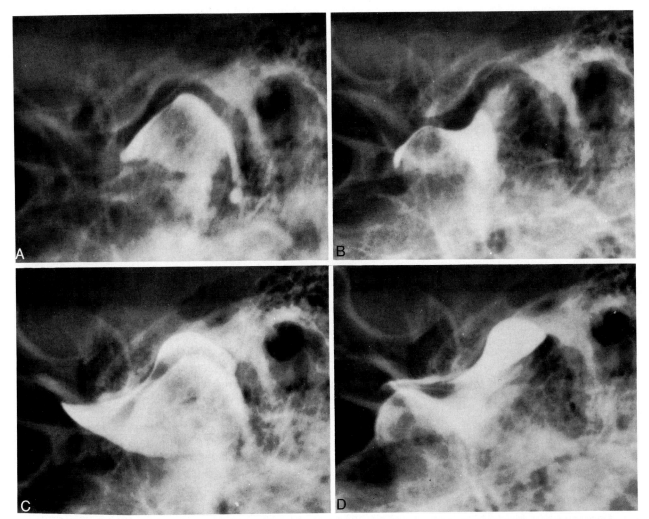

Figure 45–25. Arthrography of normal functional anatomy. A, B Inferior compartment arthrogram. Mouth closed (**A**): Posterior band of disc is at the 12 o'clock position with respect to condyle. The anterior recess (sulcus) is smooth. Mouth opened (**B**): Note that the posterior band is now dorsal to the condyle, indicating posterior rotation of the disc with respect to the condyle. Note also that the disc-condyle complex has moved to the apex of the eminence. **C, D** Bicompartment arthrogram in the same joint as in **A** and **B**. Mouth closed (**C**): Contrast in both the superior and the inferior compartments outlines both surfaces of the disc and shows similar features as in **A**. Mouth opened (**D**): Note similar features to those in **B**. Note also how retrodiscal soft tissues are drawn forward and how posterior recesses change shape.

meniscal motion is closely coordinated with condylar motion, and the left and right TMJs act synchronously. The meniscus itself is somewhat pliable, but most of the necessary soft tissue deformation occurs in the periarticular structures and through alterations in the configuration of the joint recesses.

With the mouth closed, the disc is situated deep in the mandibular fossa with the posterior band at the 12 o'clock position between the condyle and temporal bone. The posterior sulci of both joint compartments are collapsed (Fig. 45–24). Initial opening of the mouth is accompanied by a hinge action that takes place in the inferior compartment as the condyle rotates on the disc. The disc-condyle complex translates forward as it glides along the eminence. Simultaneously, the disc rotates with respect to the condyle. During mouth opening, the disc rotates posteriorly such that the posterior band comes to rest dorsal to the condyle when the mouth is fully open (Fig. 45–25). As the mouth closes, the relation-

ships reverse, and the disc rotates anteriorly with respect to the condyle as the disc-condyle complex glides into the fossa. This entire process is smooth, continuous, and synchronous.

Internal derangement is characterized by anterior subluxation or dislocation of the disc with respect to both the condyle and the fossa, owing primarily to ligamentous laxity. The displaced disc is an anatomic impediment to normal function. It results in irregular or limited joint movements that are characterized clinically as clicks or locks.

A click is a friction event that occurs when the disc and the condyle move in opposite directions momentarily as the disc is pinched between the condyle and eminence. Clicks are a result of disc malposition that places the thick posterior band anterior to the condyle (Fig. 45–26). During mouth opening, the posterior band moves posteriorly instantaneously, producing an opening click and reducing the dislocation. During closure, the posterior band moves anteriorly,

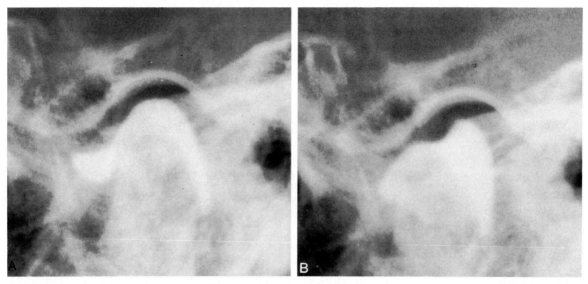

Figure 45–26. Mid-opening click. A Anterior dislocation of disc with the mouth about one-third opened. The posterior band is squeezed between the condyle and the eminence. **B** With mouth half opened, the disc has been recaptured (resulting in a click) as the posterior band crossed between the condyle and eminence, returning the disc to its normal position.

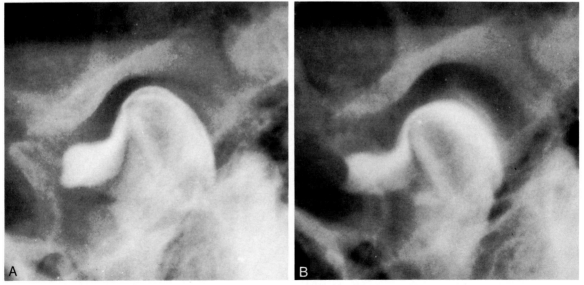

Figure 45–27. Acute TMJ lock. A Closed mouth position shows an anterior dislocation of the disc with deformation of the shape of the anterior recess. **B** Maximum opening of the mouth results in severe restriction of joint motion. Note the greater deformity of the anterior recess as the disc folds forward.

instantaneously producing a closing click and resulting in a redislocation of the disc. The phenomenon of combined opening and closing clicks is termed reciprocal clicking.

Locking is the result of a dislocated disc that will not reduce. An acute lock generally is painful and associated with very limited function (Fig. 45–27). With time, the bilaminar zone (retrodiscal tissue) usually stretches such that pain diminishes and considerable range of motion is regained.

Perforations may be associated with communication of the inferior and superior joint compartments (Fig. 45–21). These perforations may develop in the disc tissue but are more common in the retrodiscal tissues. Most perforations are associated with dislocated discs.

Pain and dysfunction may also result from adhesions in and around the joint. These may follow infection, hemarthrosis, fracture, radiotherapy, or surgery. The result is diminished volume of the joint compartments and a clinically frozen joint.

FURTHER READING

Helms CA, Morrish RB Jr, Kircos LT, Katzberg RW, Dolwick MF: Computed tomography of the meniscus of the temporomandibular joint: Preliminary observations. Radiology 145:719, 1982.

Helms CA, Vogler JB III, Morrish RB Jr, Goldman SM, Capra RE, Proctor E: Temporomandibular joint internal derangements: CT diagnosis. Radiology 152:459, 1984.

Kaplan PA, Tu HK, Sleder PR, Lydiatt DD, Lancy TJ: Inferior joint space arthrography of normal temporomandibular joints: Reassessment of diagnostic criteria. Radiology 159:585, 1986.

Katzberg RW, Bessette RW, Tallents RH, Plewes DB, Manzione JV, Schenck JF, Foster TH, Hart HR: Normal and abnormal temporomandibular joint: MR imaging with surface coil. Radiology 158:183, 1986.

Katzberg RW, Keith DA, Guralnick WC, Manzione JV Jr, Ten Eick WR: Internal derangements and arthritis of the temporomandibular joint. Radiology 146:107, 1983.

Manco LG, Messing SG, Busino LJ, Fasulo CP, Sordill WC: Internal derangements of the temporomandibular joint evaluated with direct sagittal CT: A prospective study. Radiology 157:407, 1985.

Murphy WA: Arthrography of the temporomandibular joint. Radiol Clin North Am 19:365, 1981.

Murphy WA, Adams RJ, Gilula LA, Barbier JY: Magnification radiography of the temporomandibular joint: Technical considerations. Radiology 133:524, 1979.

Thompson JR, Christiansen E, Sauser D, Hasso AN, Hinshaw DB Jr: Dislocation of the temporomandibular joint meniscus: Contrast arthrography vs. computed tomography. AJR 144:171, 1985.

Updegrave WJ: Radiography of the temporomandibular joints. Semin Roentgenol 6:381, 1971.

Yune HY, Hall JR, Hutton CE, Klatte EC: Roentgenologic diagnosis in chronic temporomandibular joint dysfunction syndrome. AJR 118:401, 1973.

Chapter 46

Target Area Approach to Articular Diseases

Donald Resnick, M.D.

The target area approach is a useful concept in the radiographic evaluation of articular diseases. The pattern of distribution of the lesions in each of the diseases is remark- *ably constant. Furthermore, because this pattern varies from one disorder to the next, it may be used for accurate differential diagnosis in many cases.*

An accurate radiologic diagnosis of joint disease is based on evaluation of two fundamental parameters: the morphology of the articular lesions and their distribution in the body. Morphologic characteristics vary among the disorders in response to the underlying pathologic aberrations; these characteristics provide essential diagnostic clues. Equally important in the interpretation of the radiographs is the evaluation of the distribution of articular lesions. There is a remarkable proclivity of certain disorders to affect specific joints (and regions of those joints), which is largely unexplained. Radiographic analysis of the distribution of articular lesions is termed the "target area" approach. The basic rules for this analysis in extraspinal locations are summarized in this chapter, but they must be interpreted cautiously. Although a specific disorder may characteristically appear in one or two

sites with relative sparing of other locations, it should *never* be said that the condition *never* affects these other sites because, almost invariably, such a statement will lead to error. The target area approach dictates locations that are involved predominantly in a disease process, not those that are involved exclusively.

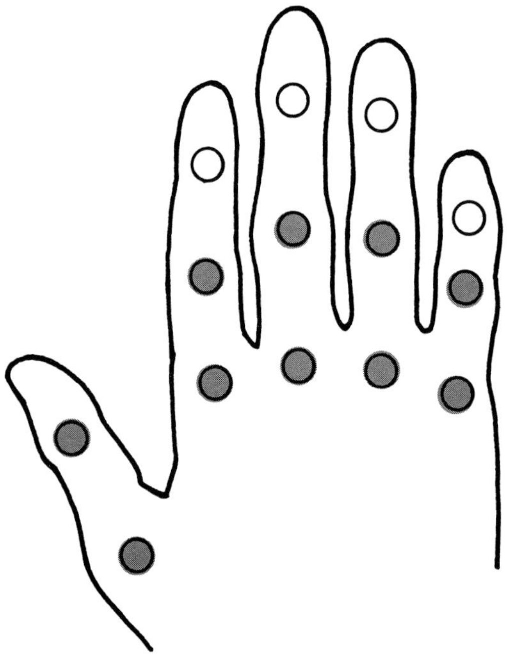

HAND

The joints of the hand consist of the distal interphalangeal, proximal interphalangeal, and metacarpophalangeal joints of the second to fifth digits and the metacarpophalangeal and interphalangeal joints of the thumb.

Rheumatoid Arthritis (Fig. 46–1)

Both hands are affected in a relatively symmetric fashion. Major alterations appear in all five metacarpophalangeal joints, the proximal interphalangeal articulations, and the interphalangeal joint of the thumb. Abnormalities in the distal interphalangeal articulations are less frequent, are mild, and rarely occur in the absence of changes in more proximal locations. When severe, they may indicate a second process (e.g., degenerative joint disease). The earliest changes are most frequently apparent in the second and third metacarpophalangeal joints and the third proximal interphalangeal joint. Fusiform soft tissue swelling, regional osteoporosis, diffuse loss of interosseous space, and marginal and central bone erosions are the observed findings.

Juvenile Chronic Arthritis (Fig. 46–2)

A symmetric or asymmetric distribution can be evident. Juvenile chronic arthritis can affect any joint of the hand, including the distal interphalangeal joints, and its exact pattern is influenced by the specific type of disease that is present (juvenile-onset adult type rheumatoid arthritis, Still's disease, and so forth). The degree of osteoporosis, joint space narrowing, and osseous erosion is variable, and bone proliferation (periostitis and intraarticular fusion) may be a prominent finding.

Figure 46–1. Rheumatoid arthritis.

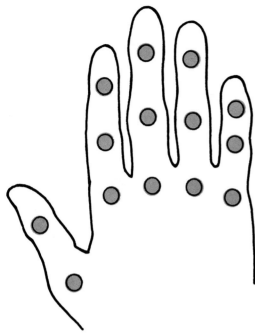

Figure 46–2. Juvenile chronic arthritis.

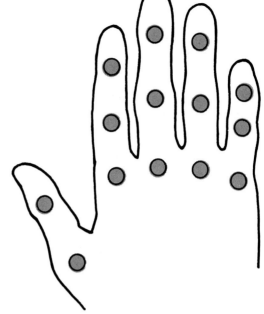

Figure 46–3. Ankylosing spondylitis, psoriatic arthritis, and Reiter's syndrome.

Ankylosing Spondylitis (Fig. 46–3)

Bilateral and asymmetric findings predominate. Distal interphalangeal, proximal interphalangeal, and metacarpophalangeal joints as well as the interphalangeal joint of the thumb can be affected, although the findings in the distal interphalangeal joints generally are less marked than in more proximal locations. Osteoporosis, joint space diminution, osseous erosions, and deformities are less striking in this disease than in rheumatoid arthritis. Osseous proliferation can be exuberant.

Psoriatic Arthritis (Fig. 46–3)

The distribution of this disease is widely variable. Bilateral asymmetric polyarticular changes are most characteristic, with predilection for the interphalangeal joints. In many patients, the extent of distal interphalangeal joint abnormalities is striking. Osteoporosis may be absent and intraarticular osseous fusion and periarticular osseous excrescences can be evident, allowing differentiation from rheumatoid arthritis. Psoriatic arthritis may be accompanied by a ray-like distribution in which one or two digits are involved extensively and others are unaffected. In other psoriatic patients, however, a symmetric polyarthritis can be identical to rheumatoid arthritis in its distribution.

Reiter's Syndrome (Fig. 46–3)

Asymmetric changes are most typical. Monoarticular or pauciarticular disease can affect any joint of the hand, including the distal interphalangeal joints. Its features are virtually identical to those of psoriatic arthritis or ankylosing spondylitis, with lack of osteoporosis and presence of exuberant periostitis. Intraarticular osseous fusion and prominent soft tissue swelling (sausage digit) also can be noted.

Degenerative Joint Disease (Osteoarthritis) (Fig. 46–4)

Bilateral, symmetric, or asymmetric findings can be observed. Distal interphalangeal and proximal interphalangeal joints generally are affected to a greater degree than metacarpophalangeal joints, although joint space narrowing is not infrequent at the last location. Isolated abnormalities may appear at the distal interphalangeal or proximal interphalangeal joints, but changes are rarely isolated to the metacarpo-

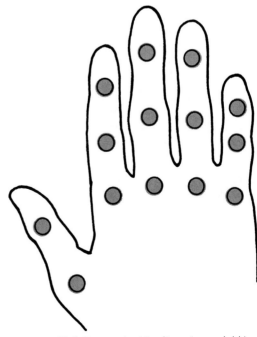

Figure 46–4. Degenerative joint disease (osteoarthritis).

phalangeal joints. In interphalangeal articulations, loss of interosseous space, subchondral eburnation, marginal osteophytes, and small ossicles appear. Findings suggesting a disease other than osteoarthritis are marginal erosions in distal or proximal interphalangeal joints, or both, and prominent osteophytes or erosions in metacarpophalangeal articulations.

Inflammatory (Erosive) Osteoarthritis (Fig. 46–5)

A bilateral, symmetric, or asymmetric distribution is encountered. The distribution of this disorder is similar to that in nonerosive osteoarthritis, with distal interphalangeal and proximal interphalangeal joint abnormalities predominating over those in the metacarpophalangeal joints. The morphologic aspects of the alterations can be indistinguishable from those of noninflammatory osteoarthritis, although the presence of centrally located osseous defects in combination with osteophytosis allows this specific diagnosis to be made. Erosions at metacarpophalangeal joints are extremely rare in inflammatory osteoarthritis.

Systemic Lupus Erythematosus (Fig. 46–6)

A deforming, nonerosive arthropathy with a bilateral and symmetric distribution affecting metacarpophalangeal and interphalangeal joints of all of the digits, including the thumb, characterizes one type of joint abnormality in this disease. Osteonecrosis at one or more metacarpophalangeal joints is a second pattern of articular disease in systemic lupus erythematosus. Finally, some patients reveal a rheumatoid arthritis–like condition and may, in fact, have coexistent rheumatoid arthritis, mixed connective tissue disease, or an overlap syndrome.

Scleroderma and Polymyositis (Fig. 46–7)

A bilateral erosive arthritis showing predilection for the distal interphalangeal and, to a lesser extent, the proximal interphalangeal joints has been observed in some patients

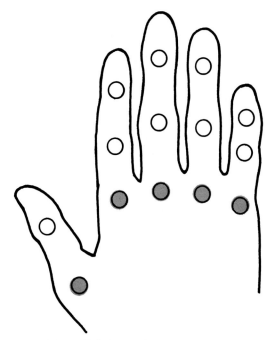

Figure 46–6. Systemic lupus erythematosus.

with scleroderma. Features may resemble psoriatic arthritis or inflammatory (erosive) osteoarthritis. A similar pattern of joint disease is rarely encountered in patients with polymyositis. In both of these diseases, more characteristic findings, such as soft tissue calcification and tuftal resorption, are usually evident.

Gouty Arthritis (Fig. 46–8)

A bilateral and asymmetric process predominates. Changes may appear in distal interphalangeal, proximal interphalangeal, or metacarpophalangeal joints, consisting of lobulated soft tissue masses, eccentric intra- and extraarticular osseous

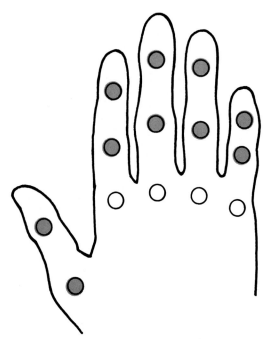

Figure 46–5. Inflammatory (erosive) osteoarthritis.

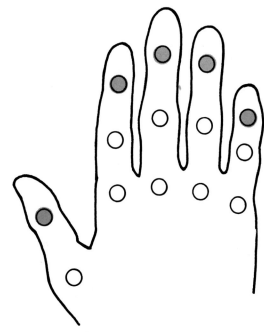

Figure 46–7. Scleroderma and polymyositis.

erosions, preservation of joint space, proliferation of bone (mushrooming or overhanging edges), and lack of osteoporosis.

Calcium Pyrophosphate Dihydrate (CPPD) Crystal Deposition Disease (Fig. 46–9)

Idiopathic CPPD crystal deposition disease or that associated with hemochromatosis produces bilateral, relatively symmetric changes that predominate at the metacarpophalangeal joints. In both disorders, changes are most frequent in the second and third metacarpophalangeal joints; in hemochromatosis, the fourth and fifth digits are more commonly involved than in idiopathic CPPD crystal deposition disease. Furthermore, in hemochromatosis, beak-like osseous excrescences arising from the radial aspect of the metacarpal heads are distinctive. In both disorders, findings may also be evident at distal interphalangeal and proximal interphalangeal joints, although generally they are mild in comparison with those of the metacarpophalangeal joints. The latter findings may resemble degenerative joint disease, but their isolation to the metacarpophalangeal articulations and the possible presence of intraarticular or periarticular calcification allow an accurate diagnosis.

Other Diseases

Multicentric reticulohistiocytosis can lead to significant abnormalities of both hands that usually are most striking in the distal interphalangeal and, to a lesser extent, the proximal interphalangeal joints. *Thermal injuries*, including frostbite and burns, may produce alterations that also predominate in distal locations. In some cases, the joints of the thumb are spared in frostbite. *Hyperparathyroidism* (and renal osteodystrophy) can lead to a peculiar "erosive" arthritis of the digits that affects distal interphalangeal, proximal interphalangeal, or metacarpophalangeal joints of both hands. In most cases, the changes are combined with subperiosteal resorption along the radial aspect of the proximal and middle phalanges and in the terminal tufts. In *rheumatic fever*, a deforming, nonerosive arthropathy (Jaccoud's arthropathy) predominates in the fourth and fifth digits. At this site, ulnar deviation of the metacarpophalangeal joints may be associated with deformity of the proximal interphalangeal or distal interphalangeal joints. *Septic arthritis* of the metacarpophalangeal joints may follow a fist fight in which the fist is cut when striking the opponent's teeth, allowing direct access of organisms into the joint cavity. *Calcium hydroxyapatite crystal deposition disease* leads to intraarticular and periarticular calcification in interphalangeal locations and may be combined with a "degenerative"-like arthropathy. *Wilson's disease* produces indistinct and irregular subchondral bone in the metacarpophalangeal and interphalangeal joints.

WRIST

The major compartments of the wrist are summarized in Table 46–1 and Figure 46–10.

Rheumatoid Arthritis (Fig. 46–11)

A bilateral and symmetric process is usually evident. Initial abnormalities predominate in the radiocarpal, inferior radioulnar, and pisiform-triquetral compartments and are associated with tenosynovitis, especially in the sheath of the extensor carpi ulnaris tendon. There is often simultaneous involvement

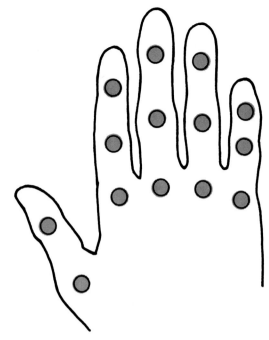

Figure 46–8. Gouty arthritis.

of the midcarpal and common carpometacarpal compartments. It is unusual to note extensive changes in the radiocarpal, inferior radioulnar, and pisiform-triquetral compartments without the others being affected to some degree. Thus, early in the course of the disease, all of the compartments of the wrist are affected.

Juvenile Chronic Arthritis (Fig. 46–12)

The pattern of wrist involvement is variable. In some forms of juvenile chronic arthritis, all of the carpal bones migrate toward the bases of the metacarpals, reflecting joint space loss

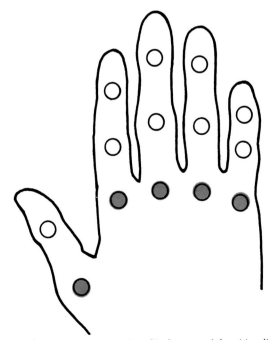

Figure 46–9. Calcium pyrophosphate dihydrate crystal deposition disease.

Table 46–1. MAJOR COMPARTMENTS OF THE WRIST

Compartment	Location
Radiocarpal	Between the distal end of the radius and the proximal carpal row
Midcarpal	Between the distal and the proximal carpal rows
Common carpometacarpal	Between the distal carpal row and the bases of the four ulnar metacarpals
First carpometacarpal	Between the trapezium and the base of the first metacarpal
Inferior radioulnar	Between the distal ends of the radius and ulna, separated from the radiocarpal compartment by the triangular fibrocartilage of the wrist
Pisiform-triquetral	Between the pisiform and triquetrum

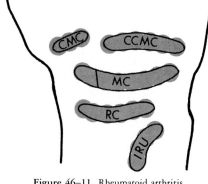

Figure 46–11. Rheumatoid arthritis.

in the midcarpal and common carpometacarpal compartments. In fact, eventual osseous fusion of the proximal and distal carpal rows and bases of the four ulnar metacarpals may be seen, with relative sparing of the first carpometacarpal and radiocarpal compartments. A similar pattern of disease may be apparent in some patients with adult-onset Still's disease.

Ankylosing Spondylitis, Psoriatic Arthritis, and Reiter's Syndrome (Fig. 46–13)

Asymmetric findings in the wrist can appear during the course of any of these three disorders. Pancompartmental changes, especially in psoriatic arthritis and ankylosing spondylitis, can be seen. Although similar to rheumatoid arthritis, these disorders are associated with less frequent and extensive wrist disease, the absence of osteoporosis, and the presence of poorly defined osseous excrescences or "whiskers."

Degenerative Joint Disease (Osteoarthritis) (Fig. 46–14)

In the absence of significant accidental or occupational trauma, degenerative joint disease of the wrist is virtually limited to the first carpometacarpal and trapezioscaphoid areas. One or both wrists may be involved, and findings can be isolated to or predominate in either one of these two sites.

At the first carpometacarpal joint, radial subluxation of the metacarpal base can be evident, whereas at the trapezioscaphoid area of the midcarpal compartment, joint space narrowing and eburnation may be the only findings.

In the presence of occupational or accidental trauma, more widespread alterations of the wrist may be detected. Thus, abnormalities of the radiocarpal and midcarpal compartments can follow a scaphoid fracture of Kienböck's disease, changes at the inferior radioulnar compartment can appear after a subluxation or dislocation about the distal ulna, and abnormalities of the radiocarpal and midcarpal areas can be observed in pneumatic tool operators or professional athletes. Posttraumatic abnormalities may eventually become severe and widespread, leading to a pattern that is designated scapholunate advanced collapse.

Inflammatory (Erosive) Osteoarthritis (Fig. 46–14)

A bilateral symmetric or asymmetric appearance can be noted. Changes predominate along the radial aspect of the wrist at the first carpometacarpal and trapezioscaphoid areas, a distribution identical to that in noninflammatory osteoarthritis. At these sites, joint space narrowing and eburnation predominate, although, rarely, erosive abnormalities may be detected. More widespread involvement of the wrist in this

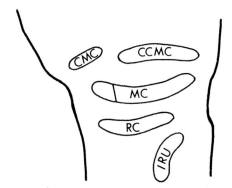

Figure 46–10. Articulations of the wrist. *RC,* Radiocarpal compartment; *IRU,* inferior radioulnar compartment; *MC,* midcarpal compartment; *CCMC,* common carpometacarpal compartment; *CMC,* first carpometacarpal compartment. The pisiform-triquetral compartment is not shown. The trapezioscaphoid region of the midcarpal joint is separated by a vertical line from the remainder of this joint.

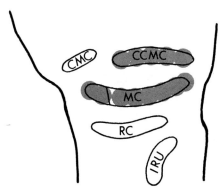

Figure 46–12. Juvenile chronic arthritis and adult-onset Still's disease.

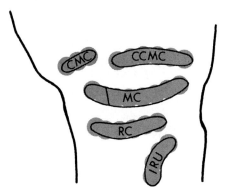

Figure 46–13. Ankylosing spondylitis, psoriatic arthritis, and Reiter's syndrome.

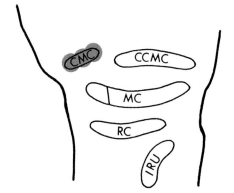

Figure 46–15. Scleroderma.

condition, particularly when the radiocarpal or inferior radioulnar compartment or both are altered, may indicate the superimposition of rheumatoid arthritis or a crystal-induced arthropathy.

Scleroderma (Fig. 46–15)

Selective involvement of one or both first carpometacarpal and inferior radioulnar compartments has been noted in some patients with scleroderma. The changes at the first carpometacarpal joints consist of scalloped erosions of the base of the metacarpal and adjacent trapezium and may relate to mechanical attrition caused by radial and proximal subluxation of the metacarpal. In fact, similar alterations of the first carpometacarpal joint can be encountered in other diseases in which tendinous and muscular imbalances are apparent, such as systemic lupus erythematosus, polymyositis, and Ehlers-Danlos syndrome. In scleroderma, intraarticular and periarticular calcification can frequently be observed about the altered joint.

The involvement of the inferior radioulnar compartment in scleroderma consists of soft tissue swelling and erosion of the distal portion of the ulna.

Gouty Arthritis (Fig. 46–16)

In long-standing gouty arthritis, bilateral symmetric or asymmetric changes can be observed in the wrist. A pancompartmental distribution, similar to that in rheumatoid arthritis, may be apparent. Of diagnostic significance, the common

carpometacarpal compartment may be the site of the most extensive abnormality in this disease. At this site, scalloped erosions of the bases of one or more of the four ulnar metacarpals are seen. Additional findings, such as the absence of osteoporosis and the presence of eccentric erosions with sclerotic margins, lobulated soft tissue masses, and preservation of joint space, also aid in the differentiation of gouty arthritis from rheumatoid arthritis.

Calcium Pyrophosphate Dihydrate Crystal Deposition Disease (Fig. 46–17)

This disorder leads to bilateral symmetric or asymmetric changes that reveal a distinct predilection for the radiocarpal compartment of the wrist. At this site, extensive narrowing or obliteration of the space between the distal portion of the radius and scaphoid may be combined with sclerosis and fragmentation of apposing osseous surfaces, "incorporation" of the scaphoid into the articular surface of the distal end of the radius, prominent cysts, and calcifications, especially of the triangular fibrocartilage. Elsewhere in the wrist, severe involvement of the trapezioscaphoid area of the midcarpal compartment and the first carpometacarpal compartment may be apparent. The inferior radioulnar compartment is relatively spared. Changes in the wrist in hemochromatosis resemble those of idiopathic calcium pyrophosphate dihydrate crystal deposition disease, with a greater tendency for diffuse involvement and a lesser frequency of separation, or dissociation, of the scaphoid and lunate.

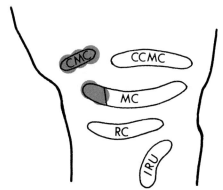

Figure 46–14. Degenerative joint disease (osteoarthritis) and inflammatory (erosive) osteoarthritis.

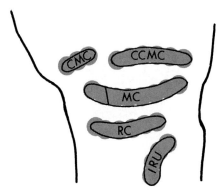

Figure 46–16. Gouty arthritis.

Other Diseases

Septic arthritis of the wrist, owing to bacterial, mycobacterial, or fungal agents, leads to monoarticular disease. Although initially one compartment may be involved, pancompartmental disease is the rule in neglected infection. *Amyloidosis* can also affect one or both wrists. In this disease, localization to the inferior radioulnar compartment is not unusual. A peculiar variety of *osteolysis*, appearing in young individuals, can lead to progressive involvement of the carpus and tarsus. The resulting radiographic abnormalities may resemble those in juvenile chronic arthritis. *Wilson's disease* is associated with indistinct subchondral bone in the distal portion of the radius and peculiar ossicles in the wrist. *Calcium hydroxyapatite crystal deposition disease* is associated with curvilinear calcification in the flexor carpi ulnaris tendon, adjacent to the pisiform.

FOREFOOT

The joints of the forefoot include the distal interphalangeal, proximal interphalangeal, and metatarsophalangeal articulations of the second to fifth digits and the interphalangeal and metatarsophalangeal articulations of the great toe.

Rheumatoid Arthritis (Fig. 46–18)

A bilateral and symmetric process of the forefoot represents one of the earliest and most frequent radiographic findings in rheumatoid arthritis. Typically, the predominant changes occur at one or more metatarsophalangeal joints and the interphalangeal joint of the great toe. Significant involvement of the proximal interphalangeal and distal interphalangeal articulations of the second to fifth toes is infrequent. At the metatarsophalangeal joints, abnormalities are encountered most commonly on the medial aspect of the metatarsal heads of the second to fourth digits and on the medial and lateral aspects of the metatarsal head of the fifth digit. At the interphalangeal joint of the great toe, a typical erosion appears on the medial aspect of the distal portion of the proximal phalanx. Changes on the lateral aspect of this joint are less frequent and less extensive; furthermore, widespread intraarticular destruction at this location is less common in rheumatoid arthritis than in psoriatic arthritis, Reiter's syndrome, or gouty arthritis.

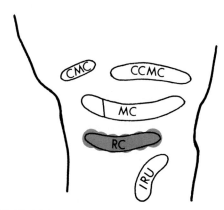

Figure 46–17. Calcium pyrophosphate dihydrate crystal deposition disease.

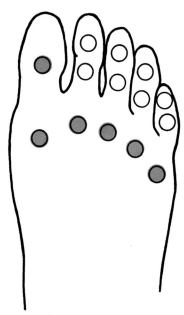

Figure 46–18. Rheumatoid arthritis.

Ankylosing Spondylitis, Psoriatic Arthritis, and Reiter's Syndrome (Figs. 46–19 and 46–20)

In ankylosing spondylitis, symmetric or asymmetric abnormalities may appear at the metatarsophalangeal joints and the interphalangeal joint of the great toe. Findings in the proximal interphalangeal and distal interphalangeal joints of the second to fifth toes are infrequent and mild.

Psoriatic arthritis can be associated with a bilateral symmetric or asymmetric or unilateral process, with or without a ray-like pattern, leading to considerable abnormalities of the forefoot. The most severe changes are commonly seen at the metatarsophalangeal joints and the interphalangeal joint of the great toe. At the latter site, the degree of osseous destruction is greater in this disease than in any other articular disorder. Prominent erosions and intraarticular osseous fusion can be evident at other interphalangeal joints as well. In this fashion, the distribution of changes in psoriatic arthritis differs from that in rheumatoid arthritis.

Asymmetric or unilateral abnormalities of the forefoot are frequent in Reiter's syndrome. Fewer joints are affected in this disorder than in rheumatoid arthritis or psoriatic arthritis. Any joint of the forefoot is a potential site of abnormality, however. Selective involvement of the interphalangeal joint of the great toe can be encountered, similar to that seen in psoriatic arthritis.

Degenerative Joint Disease (Osteoarthritis) (Fig. 46–21)

The first metatarsophalangeal joint is affected most frequently in degenerative joint disease. A unilateral or bilateral distribution can be evident, and changes include loss of interosseous space, eburnation, osteophytosis, and even hallux valgus deformity.

Gouty Arthritis (Fig. 46–22)

Bilateral symmetric or asymmetric changes in gouty arthritis can appear in any joint of the forefoot. The characteristic distribution includes the first metatarsophalangeal joint

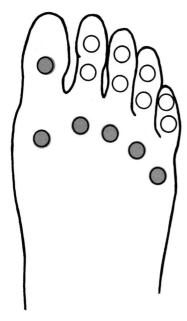

Figure 46–19. Ankylosing spondylitis.

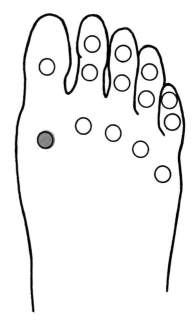

Figure 46–21. Degenerative joint disease (osteoarthritis).

and, to a lesser degree, the interphalangeal joint of the great toe. Prominent changes about other metatarsophalangeal and interphalangeal joints are not infrequent, however. At any involved site, a large soft tissue mass commonly indicates the presence of a tophus.

Neuroarthropathy (Fig. 46–23)

Neuropathic joint disease, particularly in diabetic patients, frequently affects the forefoot in a bilateral distribution. Metatarsophalangeal joint abnormalities predominate, although with progressive disease a great degree of phalangeal resorption can be evident. Other causes of neuroarthropathy, such as leprosy and alcoholism, can occasionally produce a similar pattern of disease.

Other Diseases

Infrequently, metatarsophalangeal joint abnormalities may be seen in *calcium pyrophosphate dihydrate crystal deposition disease, scleroderma, systemic lupus erythematosus,* and *Jaccoud's arthropathy. Infectious processes* of the foot not infrequently follow diabetes mellitus and local puncture wounds.

MIDFOOT AND HINDFOOT

The major joints of the midfoot and hindfoot are the "posterior" subtalar, talocalcaneonavicular, calcaneocuboid, cuneonavicular, cuneocuboid, and medial, intermediate, and lateral tarsometatarsal joints (Fig. 46–24). They are best observed on the oblique rather than the anteroposterior radiograph of the foot.

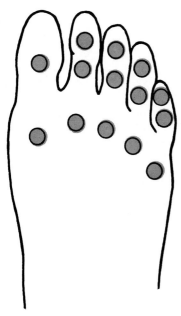

Figure 46–20. Psoriatic arthritis and Reiter's syndrome.

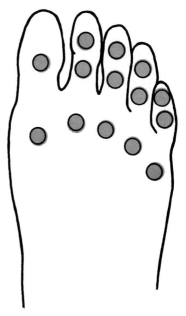

Figure 46–22. Gouty arthritis.

Rheumatoid Arthritis (Fig. 46–25)

As in the wrist, rheumatoid arthritis frequently affects all of the joints of the midfoot, commonly in association with changes at the metatarsophalangeal joints. Bilateral and symmetric abnormalities predominate. The most typical sites of involvement are the talonavicular portion of the talocalcaneonavicular joint, the tarsometatarsal joints, and the "posterior" subtalar joint. Initial abnormalities consist of superficial osseous erosions and diffuse joint space narrowing. These may eventually progress to the extent that the tarsus becomes a single ossified mass.

Juvenile Chronic Arthritis (Fig. 46–25)

Any of the joints of the midfoot can be affected in juvenile chronic arthritis. Bone ankylosis of the tarsal bones and bases of the metatarsal bones of both feet may eventually be encountered.

Degenerative Joint Disease (Osteoarthritis) (Fig. 46–26)

Abnormalities of the first tarsometatarsal joint in one or both feet represent the most typical pattern of degenerative joint disease in the midfoot. The findings, consisting of joint space narrowing, sclerosis, and osteophytosis, can simulate those of gout. After injury, alterations at other tarsometatarsal or intertarsal joints may be apparent.

Gouty Arthritis (Fig. 46–27)

Although any of the joints of the midfoot can be affected, predilection for the tarsometatarsal articulations exists. A bilateral symmetric or asymmetric process is most frequent. Prominent osseous erosions of the bases of one or more metatarsal bones are especially characteristic, usually combined with findings in more distal locations. Many of the changes predominate on the dorsal aspect of the foot.

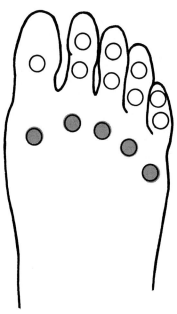

Figure 46–23. Neuroarthropathy.

Calcium Pyrophosphate Dihydrate Crystal Deposition Disease (Fig. 46–28)

Considerable osseous destruction and fragmentation in a bilateral distribution about the talonavicular aspect of the talocalcaneonavicular joint represent an infrequent but distinctive pattern in this disorder. The apposing surfaces of the talus and the navicular are progressively destroyed, and the appearance and distribution are difficult to distinguish from those accompanying the neuroarthropathy of diabetes mellitus.

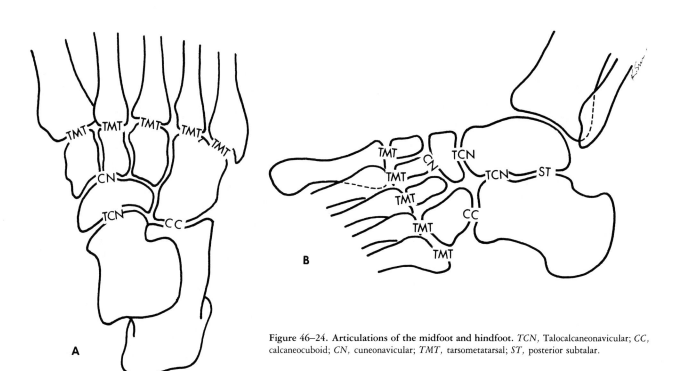

Figure 46–24. Articulations of the midfoot and hindfoot. *TCN*, Talocalcaneonavicular; *CC*, calcaneocuboid; *CN*, cuneonavicular; *TMT*, tarsometatarsal; *ST*, posterior subtalar.

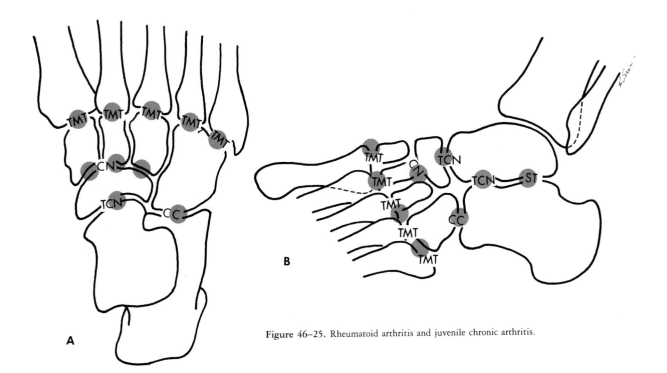

Figure 46–25. Rheumatoid arthritis and juvenile chronic arthritis.

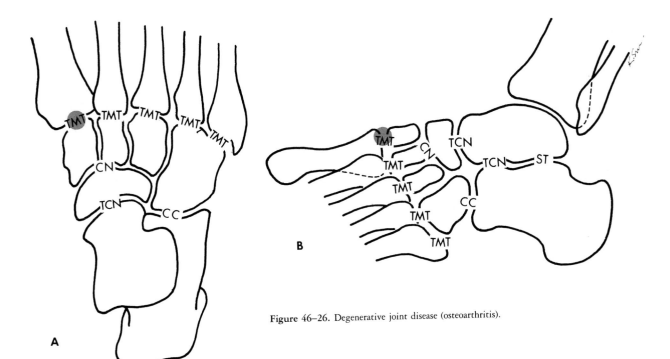

Figure 46–26. Degenerative joint disease (osteoarthritis).

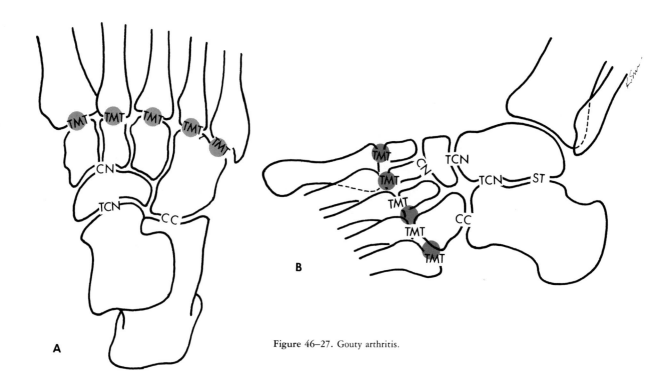

Figure 46–27. Gouty arthritis.

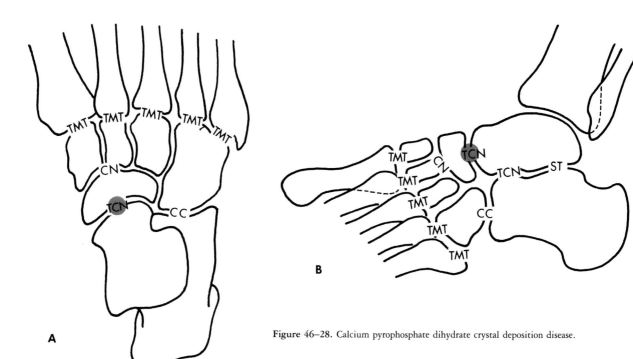

Figure 46–28. Calcium pyrophosphate dihydrate crystal deposition disease.

Neuroarthropathy

The midfoot or hindfoot is not an infrequent site of involvement in certain disorders that lead to neuroarthropathy, such as diabetes mellitus and leprosy. Tarsal disintegration with extension to the bases of the metatarsal bones may be combined with changes at one or more metatarsophalangeal joints. In some cases, fragmentation and subluxation at the tarsometatarsal joints simulate the appearance of a Lisfranc's fracture-dislocation.

CALCANEUS

Five potential target areas exist on the calcaneus: (1) the superior surface; (2) the posterior surface above the attachment of the Achilles tendon; (3) the posterior surface at the site of attachment of the Achilles tendon; (4) the plantar surface at the site of attachment of the plantar aponeurosis; and (5) the plantar surface anterior to the attachment of the aponeurosis (Fig. 46–29). Of fundamental importance is the intimate relationship of a synovium lined sac, the retrocalcaneal bursa, to the posterosuperior aspect of the calcaneus as it lies between the Achilles tendon and the osseous surface.

Rheumatoid Arthritis (Fig. 46–30)

Retrocalcaneal bursitis leads to unilateral or bilateral calcaneal erosions in both site 1 and site 2. An adjacent soft tissue mass projecting into the preachilles fat pad frequently is evident. Well-defined posterior (site 3) and plantar (site 4) calcaneal spurs are also typical. They are not specific, as identical abnormalities can be evident in "normal" individuals. Plantar osseous erosions of considerable size are distinctly unusual. Achilles tendinitis producing an enlarged or poorly defined tendinous outline can be seen.

Ankylosing Spondylitis and Psoriatic Arthritis (Fig. 46–31)

Similar abnormalities occur in both ankylosing spondylitis and psoriatic arthritis, frequently in a bilateral distribution. Retrocalcaneal bursitis leads to osseous erosions that predominate at site 2. The changes, which may occasionally be combined with alterations at site 1, resemble the findings in rheumatoid arthritis, although reactive bone formation may be more prominent. Well-defined calcaneal spurs at the site of attachment of the Achilles tendon (site 3) can also be observed, a nonspecific finding. On the plantar aspect of the bone, at sites 4 and 5, poorly marginated erosions, reactive sclerosis, and ill-defined spurs may be detected. The out-

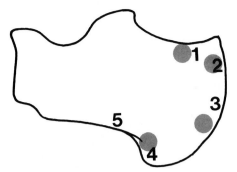

Figure 46–30. Rheumatoid arthritis.

growths are more irregular and the degree of sclerosis is more prominent in these disorders than in rheumatoid arthritis. Achilles tendon thickening can be seen.

Reiter's Syndrome (Fig. 46–32)

In Reiter's syndrome, unilateral or bilateral alterations can be encountered. Retrocalcaneal bursitis produces erosions at sites 1 and 2 that resemble the findings in rheumatoid arthritis. Abnormalities at site 3, including well-defined calcaneal excrescences, are less frequent than in psoriatic arthritis, ankylosing spondylitis, and rheumatoid arthritis, probably reflecting the younger age of the patients. On the plantar aspect of the bone, osseous erosions and poorly defined bone formation predominate at site 4. The irregular spurs that develop may become better defined over an extended period of time.

Gouty Arthritis (Fig. 46–33)

Tophaceous nodules in and about the Achilles tendon can lead to erosions at sites 2 and 3. The findings are combined with other, more typical changes at the metatarsophalangeal and interphalangeal joints.

Calcium Pyrophosphate Dihydrate Crystal Deposition Disease (Fig. 46–34)

Calcific collections consisting of calcium pyrophosphate dihydrate crystals can be deposited in the Achilles tendon and plantar aponeurosis of one or both feet. The deposits are linear in configuration and may be of considerable length. Similar abnormalities may be seen in calcium hydroxyapatite crystal deposition disease.

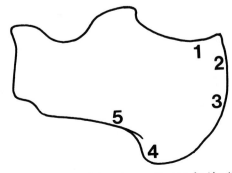

Figure 46–29. Target areas of the calcaneus (see text for identification of numbered areas)

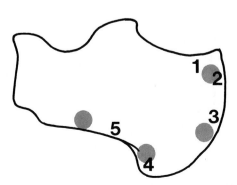

Figure 46–31. Ankylosing spondylitis and psoriatic arthritis.

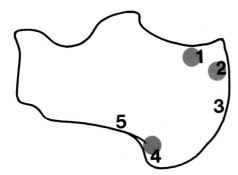

Figure 46–32. Reiter's syndrome.

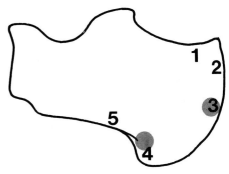

Figure 46–34. Calcium pyrophosphate dihydrate crystal deposition disease, xanthomatosis, and diffuse idiopathic skeletal hyperostosis.

Xanthomatosis (Fig. 46–34)

Tendinous xanthomas can appear in the Achilles tendon and the plantar aponeurosis in a unilateral or bilateral distribution. They produce eccentric soft tissue masses that do not calcify. On rare occasions, they may erode subjacent bone.

Diffuse Idiopathic Skeletal Hyperostosis (Fig. 46–34)

Well-defined outgrowths of variable size occur at the sites of bone attachment of the Achilles tendon and plantar aponeurosis (sites 3 and 4). Generally, both sides are affected in a relatively symmetric fashion, and the excrescences may reach considerable size. Rarely, bone protuberances may appear on the anterior plantar aspect of the calcaneus (site 5).

Other Diseases

Hyperparathyroidism can lead to subligamentous erosion at site 4, as well as subtle defects elsewhere in the calcaneus, including site 1 (Fig. 46–35). Both feet usually are affected, and, in general, other findings are present elsewhere in the skeleton. *Haglund's syndrome* is characterized by retrocalcaneal bursitis with a soft tissue mass at sites 1 and 2.

KNEE

It is useful to analyze separately three major areas or spaces of the knee: the medial femorotibial space, the lateral femorotibial space, and the patellofemoral space. Anteroposterior radiographs allow analysis of the medial and lateral femorotibial compartments, an analysis that can be improved by obtaining radiographs with the patient standing. Lateral and axial radiographs allow evaluation of the patellofemoral compartment.

Rheumatoid Arthritis (Fig. 46–36)

Rheumatoid arthritis usually leads to alterations that are bilateral and symmetric in distribution and affect both medial and lateral femorotibial compartments to an equal degree. The findings consist of diffuse joint space narrowing that may be combined with osteoporosis, superficial and deep marginal or central osseous erosions, and subchondral sclerosis, especially in the tibia. Crumbling of the osteoporotic bone of the tibia in combination with ligamentous abnormalities may create varus or valgus angulation of the knee.

Involvement of the patellofemoral space often is combined with involvement of the other two compartments in the rheumatoid knee. Although not invariably present, tricompartmental abnormalities that are of equal severity are most suggestive of rheumatoid arthritis.

Ankylosing Spondylitis, Psoriatic Arthritis, and Reiter's Syndrome (Fig. 46–37)

Any of these three disorders can affect one or both knees. A tricompartmental distribution may be encountered, although the degree of joint space narrowing, osteoporosis, and osseous erosion is less than in rheumatoid arthritis, and the extent of periosteal proliferation or "whiskering" may be pronounced.

Degenerative Joint Disease (Osteoarthritis) (Fig. 46–38)

A unilateral or bilateral distribution can be seen. Asymmetric involvement of the medial and lateral femorotibial compartments predominates, frequently in combination with

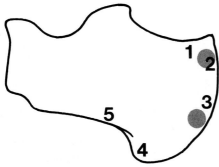

Figure 46–33. Gouty arthritis.

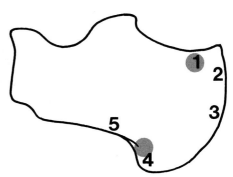

Figure 46–35. Hyperparathyroidism.

significant patellofemoral compartmental disease. Thus, bi-compartmental rather than tricompartmental findings are evident radiographically. In most instances, it is the medial femorotibial compartment that is affected more severely, and the asymmetric nature of the process may lead to moderate or severe varus deformity. Severe alterations in the lateral femorotibial compartment and valgus deformity are far less common on radiographs of the osteoarthritic knee.

Isolated abnormalities of the patellofemoral compartment are relatively unusual in degenerative joint disease of the knee. The detection of joint space narrowing, sclerosis, and osteophytosis in this location in the absence of similar changes in either the medial or lateral femorotibial space should initiate a search for other disease processes, such as calcium pyrophosphate dihydrate crystal deposition disease. Rarely, findings are restricted to the patellofemoral space in degenerative joint disease, perhaps representing a sequela of chondromalacia.

Calcium Pyrophosphate Dihydrate Crystal Deposition Disease (Fig. 46–39)

The distribution of abnormalities of the knee in patients with calcium pyrophosphate dihydrate crystal deposition disease is somewhat variable. Usually both knees are affected, although the changes may be asymmetric in extent and severity. The medial femorotibial and patellofemoral compartments commonly are affected simultaneously, a distribution that is identical to that in osteoarthritis. In these cases, the greater extent of osseous destruction and fragmentation may allow accurate differentiation of calcium pyrophosphate dihydrate crystal deposition disease from osteoarthritis. Lateral femorotibial compartmental changes with or without medial femorotibial compartmental abnormalities can also be encountered in this disease and, in some instances, may lead to impressive valgus deformity of the knee. Furthermore, findings isolated to the patellofemoral compartment are also observed in some patients. In fact, a "degenerative"-like arthropathy of the patellofemoral compartment appearing in the absence of significant medial or lateral femorotibial space alterations raises the possibility that this disease is present.

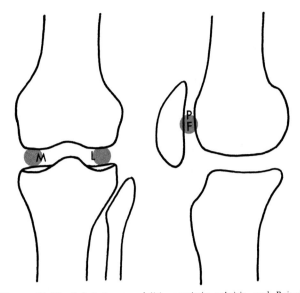

Figure 46–37. Ankylosing spondylitis, psoriatic arthritis, and Reiter's syndrome.

Other Diseases

In addition to subperiosteal resorption of bone along the medial aspect of the tibia, *hyperparathyroidism* can produce distinctive types of articular abnormality on radiographs of the knee. Subchondral resorption of bone may be evident in any compartment, usually in a bilateral but not necessarily symmetric distribution. The changes, consisting of poorly defined "erosion" and sclerosis, may be especially marked in the patellofemoral areas, and a concave posterior patellar surface may appear to wrap itself about the anterior portion of the femur (Fig. 46–40).

Septic arthritis affecting the knee can become evident initially in any compartment. As in rheumatoid arthritis, the alterations then can spread to all areas of the joint (including the proximal tibiofibular space), producing tricompartmental disease. A unilateral distribution is most frequent.

Neuroarthropathy accompanying tabes dorsalis or, more rarely, other diseases with neurologic deficit can lead to

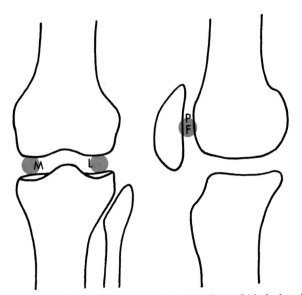

Figure 46–36. Rheumatoid arthritis. *M*, Medial femorotibial; *L*, lateral femorotibial; *PF*, patellofemoral.

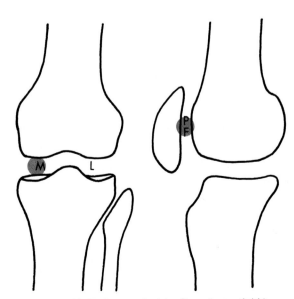

Figure 46–38. Degenerative joint disease (osteoarthritis).

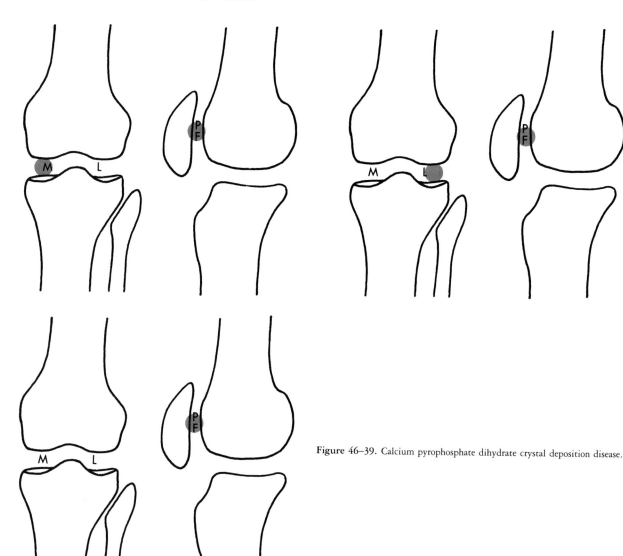

Figure 46–39. Calcium pyrophosphate dihydrate crystal deposition disease.

involvement of one or both knees with sclerosis, fragmentation, subluxation, and disorganization of the joint.

Calcium hydroxyapatite crystal deposition disease or *mixed calcium phosphate crystal deposition disease* has a distinctive appearance in the knee. Involvement predominates in the lateral femorotibial compartment, leading to osseous collapse and fragmentation, and may be combined with changes in the shoulder.

Ischemic necrosis commonly involves the distal portion of the femur or, to a lesser extent, the proximal part of the tibia. It may relate to an underlying condition, such as corticosteroid medication, or occur on an idiopathic basis. The medial side of the knee typically is affected.

Wilson's disease is associated with abnormality of the patellofemoral compartment (Fig. 46–40). In *alkaptonuria*, changes resemble those of osteoarthritis, although isolated involvement of the lateral femorotibial compartment and considerable bone collapse and fragmentation are encountered.

HIP

In evaluating articular disorders that affect the hip, it is useful to define the nature or location of any accompanying joint space loss. With diminution of the articular space, the femoral head migrates in one of three basic directions with respect to the adjacent acetabulum. If the loss is confined to the superior aspect of the joint, the femoral head moves in an upward or superior direction; if the loss is confined to the inner third of the articulation, the femoral head migrates in a medial direction; and if the joint space loss involves the entire articulation, the femoral head migrates in an axial direction along the axis of the femoral neck (Fig. 46–41). Certain disorders are associated with characteristic patterns of femoral head migration.

Rheumatoid Arthritis (Fig. 46–42)

In rheumatoid arthritis, the entire articular cartilaginous coat of the femoral head and acetabulum typically is affected

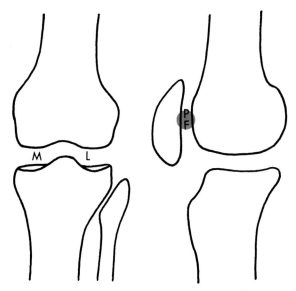

Figure 46–40. Hyperparathyroidism and Wilson's disease.

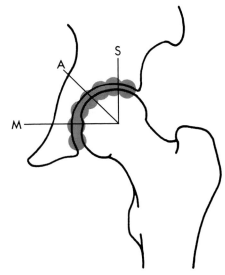

Figure 46–42. Rheumatoid arthritis and ankylosing spondylitis.

in a bilateral and symmetric fashion. Thus, with progressive chondral destruction, diffuse loss of the interosseous space occurs with axial migration of the femoral head with respect to the acetabulum. This finding usually is accompanied by marginal and central osseous erosions and cysts and even localized sclerosis. Osteophytosis is not a prominent feature.

Juvenile Chronic Arthritis

The frequency and type of hip involvement in juvenile chronic arthritis are influenced by the specific variety of disease that is present (e.g., juvenile-onset adult type seropositive rheumatoid arthritis, Still's disease, juvenile-onset ankylosing spondylitis). In some patients, diffuse loss of joint space with concentric narrowing of the joint results in axial migration of the femoral head and a radiographic picture that resembles that in adult-onset rheumatoid arthritis. In others, osseous erosions may be unaccompanied by loss of interosseous space. In patients with juvenile-onset ankylosing spondylitis,

the radiographic findings are similar to those in adult-onset ankylosing spondylitis and may eventually be characterized by bone ankylosis of the joint.

Ankylosing Spondylitis (Fig. 46–42)

A bilateral and symmetric pattern consisting of axial migration of the femoral head due to diffuse loss of joint space is seen. Although this pattern is identical to that seen in rheumatoid arthritis, the presence of osteophytosis, commencing on the superolateral aspect of the femoral head and progressing as a collar about the femoral head-neck junction, is distinctive of ankylosing spondylitis. Indeed, the combination of axial migration of the femoral head and osteophyte formation is most characteristic of ankylosing spondylitis and calcium pyrophosphate dihydrate crystal deposition disease. Rarely, patients with degenerative joint disease may reveal symmetric loss of interosseous space, but the usual pattern in this disease is dominated by superior or medial loss of joint space. In ankylosing spondylitis, acetabular and femoral cysts, mild acetabular protrusion, and partial or complete intraarticular bone ankylosis can be observed.

Psoriatic Arthritis and Reiter's Syndrome

Hip involvement is unusual in both psoriatic arthritis and Reiter's syndrome. Occasionally a patient with either disease may reveal concentric loss of joint space resembling that in rheumatoid arthritis, and, rarely, patients with psoriatic arthritis will have more extensive osseous destruction leading to a blunted and eroded femoral head.

Degenerative Joint Disease (Osteoarthritis) (Fig. 46–43)

Unilateral or bilateral alterations can be delineated. Most commonly, loss of interosseous space is maximal on the upper aspect of the articulation, resulting in superior migration of the femoral head with respect to the acetabulum. Less frequently, medial loss of joint space is seen, which may be associated with mild protrusio acetabuli deformity. Rarely, axial migration of the femoral head indicates diffuse loss of the cartilaginous surfaces of the femur and acetabulum. In all

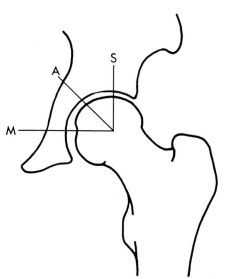

Figure 46–41. Patterns of migration of the femoral head. S, Superior migration; A, axial migration; M, medial migration.

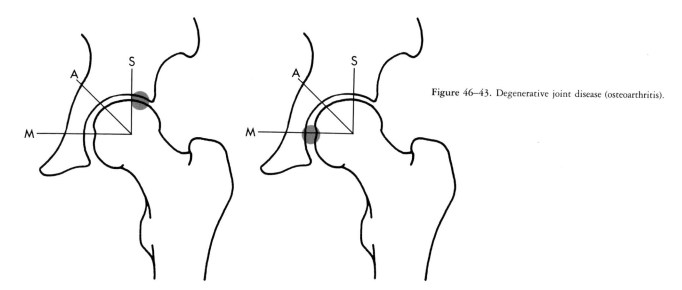

Figure 46–43. Degenerative joint disease (osteoarthritis).

cases of degenerative joint disease, femoral and acetabular osteophytes, sclerosis, and cyst formation are common, and thickening or buttressing of the medial femoral cortex is apparent.

Gouty Arthritis

Hip involvement is unusual in gouty arthritis. Rarely, osseous erosion or osteonecrosis can be seen.

Calcium Pyrophosphate Dihydrate Crystal Deposition Disease (Fig. 46–44)

The arthropathy of calcium pyrophosphate dihydrate crystal deposition disease may involve one or both hips. It is characterized by symmetric loss of joint space with axial migration, sclerosis, cyst formation, and osteophytosis. The degree of osseous collapse and fragmentation may be extreme, and the resulting radiographic features may be misinterpreted as neuroarthropathy or osteonecrosis. Additional findings, such as chondrocalcinosis of the acetabular labrum and symphysis pubis, aid in correct diagnosis.

Osteonecrosis

Although osteonecrosis of one or both femoral heads can accompany a vast number of diseases, the joint space is remarkably preserved in most cases, even in the presence of significant bone collapse and fragmentation. In long-standing cases, secondary degenerative joint disease can result, owing to the incongruity of the apposing articular surfaces. In these instances, loss of joint space usually predominates in the superior aspect of the joint, leading to superior migration of the femoral head with respect to the acetabulum. Occasionally, loss of joint space is more diffuse, involving the entire articulation.

Neuroarthropathy

Disintegration of osseous and cartilaginous tissue in one or both hips can be a manifestation of neuroarthropathy. In these cases, tabes is the most typical underlying disorder.

Other Diseases

In *Paget's disease*, involvement of paraarticular osseous tissue can lead to secondary degenerative joint disease. The radio-

graphic findings are influenced by the distribution of pagetic changes; the pattern of joint space loss may differ in cases in which the acetabulum is affected alone, in those in which both the acetabulum and femur are affected, and in those in which the femur is the only site of involvement. Because of these variations, any pattern of femoral head migration can appear in Paget's disease; instances of medial, axial, or superior migration are recognized. The diagnosis is facilitated by the recognition of Paget's disease in the adjacent bone.

Idiopathic chondrolysis of the hip is rare, but it is associated with diffuse loss of joint space and axial migration of the femoral head with respect to the acetabulum. The appearance may closely resemble that of infection.

Regional migratory osteoporosis and *transient osteoporosis of the hip* are self-limited conditions that can produce periarticular osteoporosis that improves spontaneously over several months. A unilateral distribution is typical, and, when transient osteoporosis affects a woman in the third trimester of pregnancy, the left hip is involved almost invariably. Preservation of joint space and the absence of significant defects in the

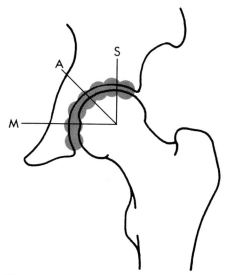

Figure 46–44. Calcium pyrophosphate dihydrate crystal deposition disease.

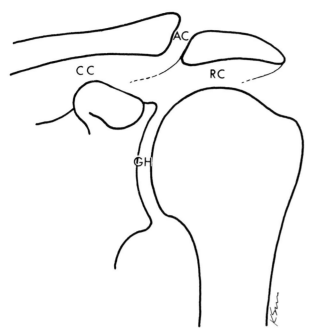

Figure 46–45. Target areas of the shoulders. *GH*, Glenohumeral joint; *AC*, acromioclavicular joint; *CC*, coracoclavicular ligament; *RC*, rotator cuff.

subchondral bone plate are features of regional osteoporosis that allow its differentiation from infection.

Infections of the hip can have a bacterial, mycobacterial, or fungal cause. Joint space loss, which generally is diffuse in nature, is a fundamental finding in all infectious disorders, although the rapidity of the loss is influenced by the nature of the causative organism; rapid loss of interosseous space is characteristic of pyogenic (bacterial) infection, whereas slow loss is typical of tuberculosis and fungal disorders. Other findings, such as osteoporosis and marginal and central osseous erosions, are also influenced by the specific cause of the infection.

Pigmented villonodular synovitis and *idiopathic synovial osteochondromatosis* are two disorders that can produce monoarticular disease of the hip. In both conditions, soft tissue swelling and osseous erosions may appear in the absence of joint space narrowing and osteoporosis, although the last two findings are also evident in some cases. The presence of cystic erosions of the femoral neck on plain films and of intraarticular masses on arthrograms in both conditions and the detection of calcific or ossific foci in idiopathic synovial osteochondromatosis are important diagnostic clues.

Familial acetabular protrusion (Otto pelvis) leads to bilateral abnormalities, especially in women, characterized by protrusio acetabuli deformity and, eventually, joint space loss.

Cartilage atrophy, secondary to disuse, immobilization, or paralysis, produces diffuse loss of joint space and axial migration of the femoral head. Osteoporosis is evident.

Alkaptonuria has variable manifestations in the hip, although joint space loss is frequent.

Irradiation can lead to collapse of the femoral head, fragmentation of the acetabulum, acetabular protrusion, and concentric joint space loss.

SHOULDER

In the shoulder region, there are three potential target areas that can be affected in various articular disorders: the glenohumeral joint, the acromioclavicular joint, and the undersurface of the distal clavicle at the site of attachment of the coracoclavicular ligament (Fig. 46–45).

Rheumatoid Arthritis (Fig. 46–46)

All three target areas on both sides of the body can be involved in rheumatoid arthritis. Glenohumeral joint alterations consist of osteoporosis, symmetric loss of joint space, and marginal osseous erosions, predominantly on the superolateral aspect of the humeral head. Associated atrophy or tear of the rotator cuff may lead to slow or rapid elevation of the humeral head with respect to the glenoid cavity and narrowing of the acromiohumeral head distance.

Acromioclavicular joint erosion with widening of the articular space is a recognized manifestation of this disease. Bone defects appear on both the acromial and the clavicular aspects of the joint, and the margins of the distal end of the clavicle may assume a tapered appearance. Similarly, scalloped erosion on the undersurface of the distal end of the clavicle opposite the coracoid process is an additional manifestation of rheumatoid arthritis, although almost invariably it is recognized in the later stages of the disease, at a time when other manifestations are evident.

Ankylosing Spondylitis (Fig. 46–46)

The changes about the shoulder in ankylosing spondylitis resemble those in rheumatoid arthritis. Glenohumeral joint involvement leads to joint space narrowing and osseous erosion. A large bone defect, the "hatchet" deformity, can appear on the superolateral aspect of the humeral head, which is distinctive. The absence of osteoporosis and the presence of bone proliferation about the osseous erosions are also helpful in diagnosis.

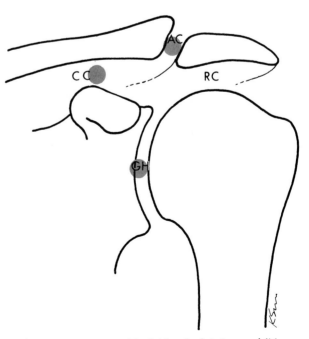

Figure 46–46. Rheumatoid arthritis and ankylosing spondylitis.

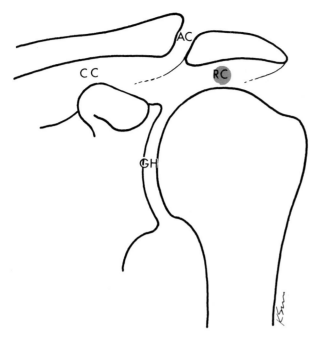

Figure 46–47. Rotator cuff degeneration.

Osseous erosions about the acromioclavicular joint and along the undersurface of the distal end of the clavicle can also be noted in ankylosing spondylitis. Adjacent bone proliferation along the inferior portion of the clavicle is more common and exuberant in this disease than in rheumatoid arthritis.

Degenerative Joint Disease (Fig. 46–47)

Although severe abnormalities in the glenohumeral joint are not typical of uncomplicated osteoarthritis unless significant accidental or occupational trauma has occurred, mild alterations consisting of joint space narrowing, sclerosis, and osteophytosis can be seen even in the absence of such trauma. Degeneration and disruption of the rotator cuff are frequent in elderly persons, producing elevation of the humeral head. Although the appearance may simulate that of rotator cuff injury in rheumatoid arthritis, the initial absence of significant glenohumeral joint involvement in association with degeneration of the cuff is noteworthy. Furthermore, the appearance of an osseous excrescence on the anteroinferior surface of the acromion is a degenerative alteration responsible for or accompanying the shoulder impingement syndrome.

Acromioclavicular joint degeneration is frequent in middle-aged and elderly persons. Changes are usually mild in nature, consisting of articular space narrowing and eburnation. Proliferative degenerative abnormalities along the inferior surface of the distal end of the clavicle are not conspicuous in the absence of significant injury, especially subluxation or dislocation of the acromioclavicular joint.

Calcium Pyrophosphate Dihydrate Crystal Deposition Disease (Fig. 46–48)

Both the glenohumeral and acromioclavicular joints can be affected in this disease, although the abnormalities are less extensive than changes in other joints, such as the wrist, the metacarpophalangeal joints, and the knee. Fibrocartilage or hyaline cartilage calcification, articular space narrowing, sclerosis, and osteophytosis can appear at either shoulder location.

Although the findings may be reminiscent of those in degenerative joint disease, the absence of a history of trauma and the presence of calcific deposits and extensive osseous alterations are features that suggest calcium pyrophosphate dihydrate crystal deposition disease.

Calcium Hydroxyapatite Crystal Deposition Disease

The deposition of calcium hydroxyapatite crystals in the shoulder is responsible for periarticular cloud-like calcification in the rotator cuff or subacromial (subdeltoid) bursa. The presence of crystals may also be instrumental in causing a distinctive arthropathy, the Milwaukee shoulder syndrome, that is characterized by destruction of bone and cartilage and deterioration of the rotator cuff.

Other Diseases

Alkaptonuria (ochronosis) can lead to an arthropathy resembling degenerative joint disease of the glenohumeral joint in one or both shoulders. Similarly, in *acromegaly*, osteophytosis can be evident in this site, especially on the inferior aspect of the humeral head. *Hyperparathyroidism* leads to osseous resorption of the distal end of the clavicle and adjacent acromion as well as of the inferior aspect of the clavicle at the site of attachment of the coracoclavicular ligament. Erosions in the humeral head are also identified. *Posttraumatic changes* include osteolysis of the distal end of the clavicle, and degenerative joint disease may be seen in association with recurrent posterior dislocation of the glenohumeral joint.

SACROILIAC JOINT

The most important aspect in the differential diagnosis of diseases that affect the sacroiliac joint is the distribution of the abnormalities. Findings can be bilateral and symmetric, bilateral and asymmetric, or unilateral (Fig. 46–49). In nearly every instance, the synovial portion of the joint (the lower one half or two thirds of the interosseous space between

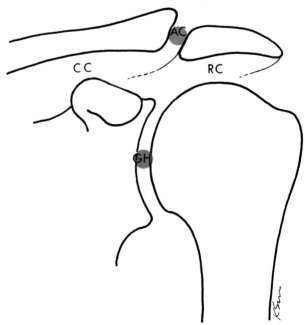

Figure 46–48. Calcium pyrophosphate dihydrate crystal deposition disease.

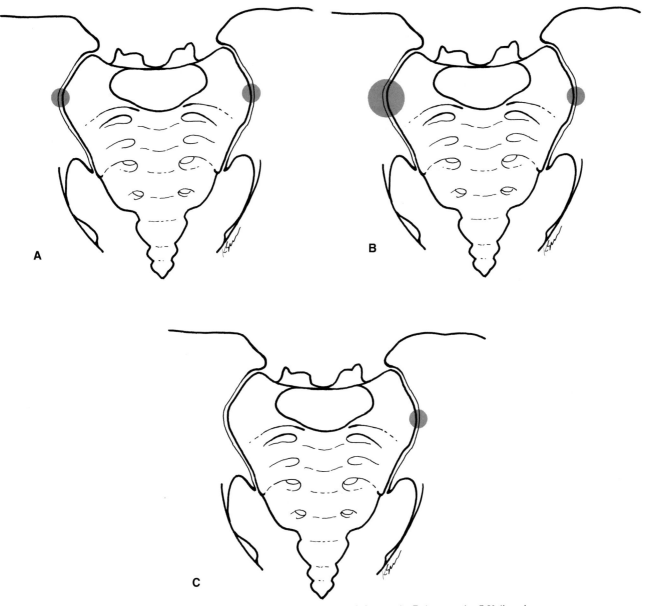

Figure 46–49. Distribution of sacroiliac joint changes. **A** Symmetric. **B** Asymmetric. **C** Unilateral.

sacrum and ilium) is affected to a greater degree than the ligamentous portion (that area above the synovium-lined space).

Rheumatoid Arthritis (Fig. 46–49*B,C*)

Abnormalities of the sacroiliac joint in rheumatoid arthritis generally are a minor feature of the disease. Bilateral asymmetric or unilateral changes predominate, consisting of joint space narrowing, superficial osseous erosions, minor sclerosis, and absence of widespread bone ankylosis.

Juvenile Chronic Arthritis

The frequency and appearance of sacroiliac joint changes in juvenile chronic arthritis depend on the subgroup of disease that is present. Changes usually are not prominent unless

juvenile-onset ankylosing spondylitis is evident. In this case, a bilateral and symmetric distribution is encountered.

Ankylosing Spondylitis (Fig. 46–49*A*)

The classic findings in this disease are bilateral and symmetric in distribution. Erosions, sclerosis, and bone ankylosis of the synovial joint frequently are combined with poorly defined osseous margins in the ligamentous aspect of the joint. Occasionally, initial radiographs will reveal asymmetric abnormalities. In all cases, iliac abnormalities predominate.

Psoriatic Arthritis and Reiter's Syndrome (Fig. 46–49*A–C*)

The distribution of abnormalities is variable in psoriatic arthritis and Reiter's syndrome. Changes may be bilateral and symmetric, bilateral and asymmetric, or unilateral. Osseous erosion and sclerosis are similar to the findings in ankylosing spondylitis, although joint space narrowing and bone ankylosis occur with decreased frequency. Proliferation of bone in the ilium and sacrum above the synovial aspect of the joint may be prominent, particularly in Reiter's syndrome.

Degenerative Joint Disease (Osteoarthritis) (Fig. 46–49A–C)

Osteoarthritis of the sacroiliac joint can be unilateral or bilateral in distribution. Unilateral abnormalities in conjunction with osteoarthritis of the contralateral hip may be encountered. Findings include joint space narrowing, sclerosis, and osteophytosis. The bone excrescences predominate on the anterosuperior and anteroinferior aspects of the joint. Erosions are not prominent, and paraarticular rather than intraarticular ankylosis predominates.

Gouty Arthritis (Fig. 46–49A–C)

Abnormalities of the sacroiliac joint can be seen in patients with long-standing tophaceous gout. Bilateral symmetric, bilateral asymmetric, or unilateral alterations consisting of large erosions and reactive sclerosis are found.

Other Diseases

Sacroiliitis accompanying *inflammatory bowel diseases* is bilateral and symmetric in distribution and cannot be differentiated from that seen in ankylosing spondylitis (Fig. 46–49A). In *hyperparathyroidism*, subchondral resorption of bone, especially in the ilium, produces bilateral and symmetric changes consisting of joint space widening and reactive sclerosis (Fig. 46–49A). Unilateral abnormalities are typical of sacroiliac joint *infection* (Fig. 46–49C). Such infection can be related to bacterial, mycobacterial, or fungal agents and is not infrequent in the drug abuser. *Osteitis condensans ilii* produces bilateral and symmetric alterations in young women consisting of well-defined triangular sclerosis of the inferior aspect of the ilium (Fig. 46–49A). Sacroiliac joint involvement may also accompany *familial Mediterranean fever, relapsing polychondritis, Behçet's syndrome, alkaptonuria, immobilization,* and *disuse.*

SECTION VIII

METABOLIC AND ENDOCRINE DISEASES

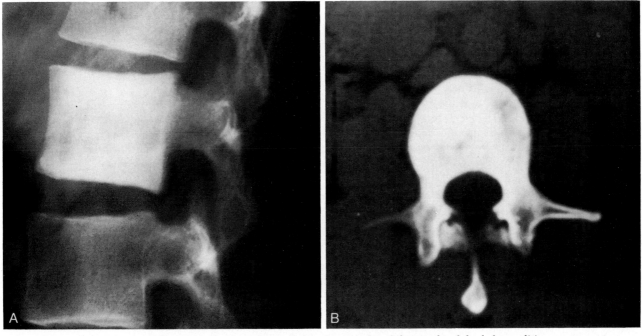

This 37 year old man complained of back pain. A bone scan (not shown) confirmed that no other skeletal abnormalities were present.

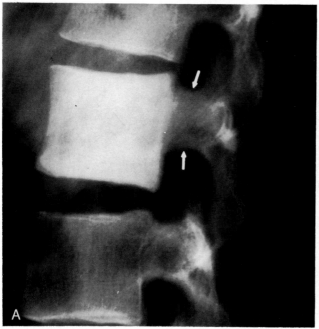 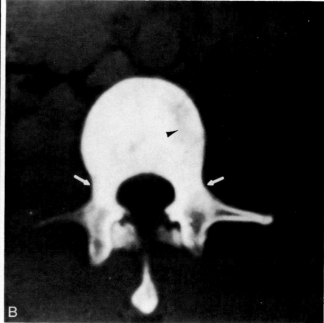

A lateral radiograph (A) reveals osteosclerosis involving the second lumbar vertebra. The vertebral body is of increased radiodensity, especially in its superior and inferior portions, with patchy radiolucent areas centrally. The size of the vertebral body appears normal, and there is mild narrowing of the intervertebral disc space between the first and second lumbar vertebrae. One or both pedicles of the second lumbar vertebra also are sclerotic with thickened cortices (arrows). Transaxial computed tomography (B) confirms the existence of osteosclerosis affecting both the vertebral body and the pedicles (arrows). Some radiolucent areas within the vertebral body (arrowhead) are observed. The spinal canal is of normal size and configuration.

The radiographic appearance is that of an ivory vertebra. Possible causes of this appearance include skeletal metastasis, lymphoma, plasmacytoma, chordoma, Paget's disease, chronic osteomyelitis, and discogenic sclerosis. Some of these diagnoses, however, can be eliminated immediately as unlikely possibilities. Bone sclerosis related to discogenic disease (intervertebral osteochondrosis) would be expected to be associated with considerable disc space loss and vacuum phenomena, would not generally be confined to a single vertebra, and would not explain osteosclerosis affecting the pedicles. Although chronic osteomyelitis can lead to osteosclerosis of a vertebral body, the diffuse sclerotic pattern illustrated in Case VIII would be an unusual finding of infection. Furthermore, involvement of adjacent intervertebral disc spaces and vertebrae is typical of infectious spondylitis, and alterations of the pedicles would be unexpected in this condition. Skeletal metastasis is a well known cause of an ivory vertebra, but involvement of other vertebrae and extravertebral abnormalities generally are observed. Plasmacytoma and chordoma are unusual causes of an ivory vertebra, and the pattern of pedicle involvement evident in the test case is not typical of either of these tumors.

Of the diagnostic choices, lymphoma and Paget's disease are most likely. Of the various types of lymphoma, Hodgkin's disease is the one that most typically produces osteosclerosis, a finding that is observed in 15 to 45 per cent of cases. The spine is a frequent site of osseous involvement in Hodgkin's disease, and an ivory vertebra may be seen. Multiple skeletal lesions occur with a greater frequency than solitary lesions, however, so that the occurrence of a single ivory vertebra, as in this test case, would not be common in Hodgkin's disease. Still, the diagnosis of Hodgkin's disease must be given careful consideration.

Paget's disease represents the best diagnostic possibility for the radiographic abnormalities illustrated in Case VIII. Approximately 3 to 5 per cent of patients with Paget's disease are younger than 40 years, and the spine is affected in 30 to 75 per cent of patients with this disorder. Monostotic involvement occurs in 10 to 35 per cent of cases of Paget's disease, and the axial skeleton commonly is affected in such cases. Therefore, Paget's disease involving one skeletal site, a lumbar vertebra, is a reasonable diagnostic possibility. This disorder is more certain if radiographs of the involved lumbar vertebra reveal a picture-frame appearance in which condensation of bone is seen along the peripheral margins of the vertebral body. More homogeneous vertebral osteosclerosis, as in this test case, is a recognized manifestation of Paget's disease, however. Furthermore, involvement of the pedicles may be evident in this disorder. Indeed, it is such involvement that provides an important diagnostic clue in the present case. On the lateral radiograph (A), cortical thickening and an increase in the vertical dimensions of the pedicles can be observed, findings characteristic of Paget's disease.

A biopsy of the affected lumbar vertebra in the test case confirmed the diagnosis of Paget's disease.

FINAL DIAGNOSIS: Paget's disease.

FURTHER READING

Pages 606 and 607 and the following:

1. Groh JA: Mono-osteitic Paget's disease as a clinical entity. Roentgenologic observations in nine cases. AJR 50:230, 1943.
2. Resnick D: Paget disease of bone: Current status and a look back to 1943 and earlier. AJR 150:249, 1988.
3. Schreiber MH, Richardson GA: Paget's disease confined to one lumbar vertebra. AJR 90:271, 1963.

(Case VIII, courtesy of R. Kerr, M.D., Los Angeles, California.)

Chapter 47

Osteoporosis

Donald Resnick, M.D.
Gen Niwayama, M.D.

Osteoporosis is an extremely common metabolic disorder that can accompany a variety of disease processes. It can conveniently be divided into generalized, regional, and localized types.

Localized osteoporosis commonly is associated with focal skeletal lesions, such as neoplasm and infection.

Generalized osteoporosis accompanies certain age-related conditions (senile and postmenopausal state); endocrine disorders such as acromegaly, hyperthyroidism, hyperparathyroidism, and Cushing's disease; pregnancy; heparin administration; and alcoholism. This type of osteoporosis, which must be distinguished from that accompanying other metabolic disorders, such as osteomalacia and hyperparathyroidism (osteitis fibrosa cystica), predominates in the axial skeleton, with major effect on the vertebrae. Abnor-

malities of the appendicular skeleton are mild, consisting of uniform loss of osseous density (osteopenia). In the vertebral bodies, characteristic changes in radiolucency, trabecular pattern, and osseous contour are encountered.

Regional osteoporosis accompanies disuse or immobilization, the reflex sympathetic dystrophy syndrome, and transient regional osteoporosis. Changes predominate in the appendicular skeleton. A more aggressive type of bone resorption in these conditions can lead to cortical bone changes at endosteal, intracortical, and subperiosteal bone envelopes and to spongy bone changes at subchondral and metaphyseal locations.

Additional manifestations of osteoporosis include acute and insufficiency stress fractures and bone bars (reinforcement lines).

Osteoporosis is the most frequent metabolic bone disease. In this disorder, there is a generalized decrease in bone mass, although the remaining bone is structurally normal as determined by histologic and chemical analysis. Routine radiographic procedures are not helpful in the early detection of this metabolic condition, as it has been estimated that 30 to 50 per cent of skeletal calcium must be lost before a change appears on the radiographs. Because of this inadequacy, newer diagnostic techniques have been used for the earlier detection and the quantitation of osteoporosis (see Chapter 18). When severe or of long duration, osteoporosis produces characteristic radiographic abnormalities.

Osteoporosis is characterized by qualitatively normal but quantitatively deficient bone. Radiographs in patients with osteoporosis reveal increased radiolucency of bone, a finding that is best termed osteopenia, meaning "poverty of bone." The discovery of osteopenia on a radiograph does not allow a precise diagnosis of osteoporosis, however, as this finding is present in a variety of conditions that lead to rarefied or radiolucent bone. Osteopenia occurs when bone resorption exceeds bone formation no matter what the specific pathogenesis (Table 47–1). Diffuse osteopenia is found in osteoporosis, osteomalacia, hyperparathyroidism, neoplasm, and a variety of other conditions. Once osteopenia is discovered, radiographs must be searched carefully for additional and more specific abnormalities; for example, osteomalacia can lead to characteristic linear radiolucent areas termed Looser's zones; hyperparathyroidism can produce aggressive subperiosteal and subchondral resorption of bone; and neoplasms, such as plasma cell myeloma, can be associated with focal skeletal radiolucent

Table 47–1. MAJOR CAUSES OF DIFFUSE OSTEOPENIA

Osteoporosis
Osteomalacia
Hyperparathyroidism
Neoplasm

lesions. Osteoporosis, too, can lead to additional radiographic findings, but, in general, these findings are not specific. Thus, the accurate diagnosis of osteoporosis rests on the radiologic findings of osteopenia coupled with typical clinical and histologic features. The inclusion of the clinical and histologic features in the definition of osteoporosis is required owing to the loss of bone that occurs normally in all persons as they age, a process that is more prominent in women than in men. Osteoporosis is established when the decrease in bone mass is greater than that expected for a person of a given age, sex, and race, and when it results in structural bone failure manifested by fractures. These fractures are most typical in the spine, proximal portion of the femur, and distal portion of the radius; they are produced by trabecular or cortical bone loss, or both, depending on the site of involvement.

ETIOLOGY

Osteoporosis can be classified as generalized (involving the major portion of the skeleton, particularly its axial component), regional (involving one segment of the skeleton), or localized (single or multiple focal areas of osteoporosis). There are many causes of generalized, regional, and localized osteoporosis. Localized osteoporosis may accompany focal skeletal

Table 47–2. MAJOR CAUSES OF GENERALIZED OSTEOPOROSIS

Age-related conditions (senile and postmenopausal states)

Medications
  Steroids
  Heparin

Endocrine states
  Hyperthyroidism
  Hyperparathyroidism
  Cushing's disease
  Acromegaly
  Pregnancy
  Diabetes mellitus
  Hypogonadism

Deficiency states
  Scurvy
  Malnutrition
  Calcium deficiency

Alcoholism

Chronic liver disease

Anemic states

Osteogenesis imperfecta

Idiopathic condition

---

lesions such as arthritis, infection, and neoplasm, and it is often overshadowed by the radiographic features of the primary process itself.

Generalized Osteoporosis

The osseous manifestations of conditions leading to generalized osteoporosis predominate in the axial skeleton and proximal long bones of the appendicular skeleton. Abnormalities of the spine are particularly prominent, leading not only to osteopenia but also to changes in vertebral contour characterized by biconcave vertebral bodies ("fish vertebrae") and collapse. In both the axial and the appendicular skeleton, the decrease in radiodensity usually is uniform in nature, although some differences are apparent in the distribution and appearance of osteopenia among the various diseases that produce generalized osteoporosis (Table 47–2).

AGE-RELATED OSTEOPOROSIS (FIG. 47–1). Senescent osteoporosis and postmenopausal osteoporosis constitute the most common causes of generalized osteoporosis. The reported frequency of osteoporosis in older persons has varied, influenced considerably by a number of factors, including the diagnostic method used to detect osteoporosis and the person's sex, hormone balance, skeletal size, level of exercise or activity, and nutritional status. In general, there is a gradual loss of skeletal mass beginning in the fifth or sixth decade of life in men and in the fourth decade in women. After the age of about 50 years, bone loss occurs at a rate of 0.4 per cent each year in men; after the age of approximately 35 years, women lose bone at a yearly rate of 0.75 to 1 per cent, which increases to a rate of 2 to 3 per cent after the menopause. Although loss of both compact and trabecular bone occurs in older men and women, the magnitude of the loss of compact bone in women after the menopause is much greater than that in men.

Patients with age-related osteoporosis may be entirely asymptomatic, although significant loss of bone mass may be accompanied by various clinical findings. Bone pain, particularly in the back, may be associated with loss of height due to vertebral compression. Increased thoracic kyphosis is apparent. Neurologic complications are unusual. Fractures of the femoral neck occur spontaneously or after minor trauma and may be accompanied by fractures of the ribs, humerus, or radius. Laboratory analysis generally yields unremarkable results (Table 47–3).

The pathogenesis of age-related osteoporosis is not clear, although the importance of loss of ovarian function with resultant estrogen deficiency in the evolution of postmenopausal osteoporosis has been emphasized for more than 45 years. The mechanism that accounts for bone loss is not clear, however. Whatever the precise mechanism, the apparent

---

Table 47–3. LABORATORY DIAGNOSIS OF METABOLIC BONE DISEASE*†

	Serum Levels					Urine Levels		
	Ca	P	AP	Urea or Creatinine	PTH	Ca	Tubular Resorption of Phosphate	Hydroxy-proline
Age-related osteoporosis	N	N	N	N	N	N	N	N; I
Osteogenesis imperfecta	N	N	N	N	N	N	N	N
Hyperthyroidism	N; I	N	N	N	N; D	I	N	I
Hyperparathyroidism								
Primary	I	D	N; I	N; I	I	N; I	D	I
Secondary	N; D	I	I	I	I	D	D	I
"Tertiary"	I	N; D	N; I	N; I	I	N; I	D	I
Hypoparathyroidism	D	I	N	N	D	D	I	N
Pseudohypoparathyroidism	D	I	N	N	N; I	D	I	N
Pseudopseudohypoparathyroidism	N	N	N	N	N	N	N	N
Paget's disease	N	N	I	N	N	N	N	I
Rickets or osteomalacia								
Vitamin D deficiency	D	D	I	N	I	D	D	N
Vitamin D refractory	N	D	I	N; I	N; I	D	D	N
Hypophosphatasia	N; I	N	D	N	?	N; I	N	D

*After Goldsmith RS: Laboratory aids in the diagnosis of metabolic bone disease. Orthop Clin North Am 3:545, 1972. Used with permission.
†N, normal; I, increased; D, decreased; Ca, calcium; P, phosphorus; AP, alkaline phosphatase; PTH, parathyroid hormone.

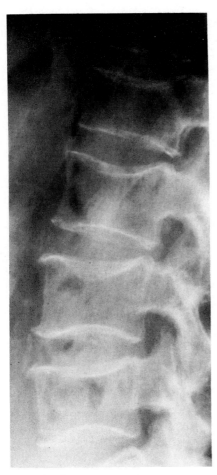

Figure 47–1. Age-related (postmenopausal) osteoporosis. In this elderly woman, a lateral radiograph of the lumbar spine outlines increased lucency and biconcave deformity ("fish vertebra") of multiple vertebral bodies.

relationship between loss of ovarian function and osteoporosis after the menopause—a relationship that is supported by the occurrence of osteoporosis in young oophorectomized women, in female athletes with secondary amenorrhea, in women with hyperprolactinemia, and in patients with Turner's syndrome—has led to preventive and therapeutic use of estrogen.

HYPERPARATHYROIDISM. Osteoporosis may occur during the course of hyperparathyroidism. The characteristic skeletal changes in this disease relate to increased rates of both bone resorption and bone formation. Superimposed on osteoporosis are the typical findings of osteitis fibrosa cystica (see Chapter 52).

STEROID-INDUCED OSTEOPOROSIS (FIG. 47–2). Osteoporosis occurring during the course of either Cushing's syndrome or exogenous (iatrogenic) hypercortisolism is well known (see Chapters 53 and 65). Histologic studies have revealed decreased bone formation and increased bone resorption. Laboratory analysis reveals negative calcium balance and hypercalciuria. Radiographic evaluation indicates the usual findings of osteoporosis, although peculiar condensation of bone at the margins of the vertebral bodies and involvement of extraspinal sites may be encountered. Furthermore, insufficiency fractures in the axial (pelvis) and appendicular skeleton are characteristic and easily overlooked.

HYPERTHYROIDISM. Osteoporosis in hyperthyroidism is associated with an increase in both bone resorption and bone formation. Hypercalcemia, hypercalciuria, hyperphos-

phatemia, and elevation of serum levels of alkaline phosphatase can occur. Radiologic findings are typical of osteoporosis, although rapid progression prior to treatment and rapid improvement after therapy can be evident (see Chapter 51).

ACROMEGALY. Osteoporosis can occur in acromegaly, in which disorder there is a negative calcium, phosphorus, and nitrogen balance (see Chapter 50).

PREGNANCY AND RELATED CONDITIONS. Although uncommon, osteoporosis may be observed in childbearing women. Its cause in this clinical setting has not been determined. Osteoporosis appearing in association with pregnancy or lactation is accompanied by normal results on histologic and serum and urinary laboratory analysis.

HEPARIN-INDUCED OSTEOPOROSIS. The development of osteoporosis has been documented in patients who are receiving large doses of heparin (greater than 15,000 units per day). The changes may be reversible with cessation of therapy. The mechanism of osteoporosis in these patients is not known. The activity of mast cells (which store heparin) may be an important factor in heparin-induced osteoporosis. Typical radiographic findings in the spine include osteopenia and vertebral compression.

ALCOHOLISM. Alcoholic patients reveal a reduced bone mass compared with controls and increased bone fragility, manifested as a high rate of occurrence of fractures. The cause of this loss in bone mineral is not known.

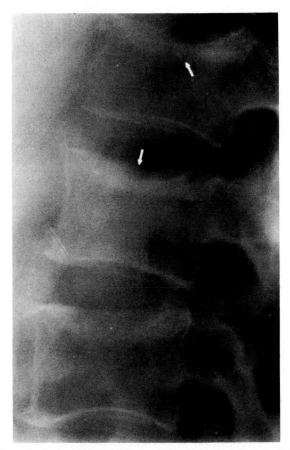

Figure 47–2. Steroid-induced osteoporosis. A lateral radiograph of the lumbar spine outlines osteoporosis and compressed vertebral bodies with peripheral condensation of bone (arrows). This latter feature, which leads to radiodense superior and inferior vertebral margins, is characteristic of exogenous or endogenous hypercortisolism.

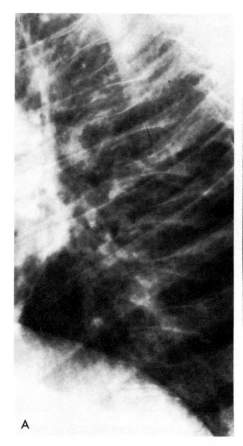

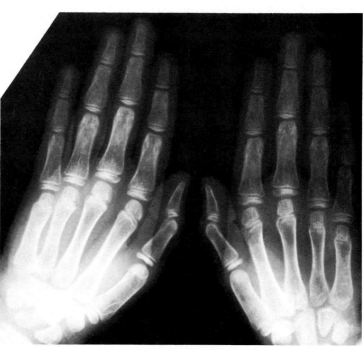

B

Figure 47–3. Idiopathic juvenile osteoporosis. This 11 year old girl developed progressive osteoporosis of bones in the appendicular and axial skeleton. There was no clinical evidence of blue sclerae or deafness. Laboratory evaluation was unremarkable. Family history was noncontributory. **A** A lateral radiograph of the thoracic spine reveals severe compression and collapse of multiple radiolucent vertebral bodies. The disc spaces appear ballooned. **B** A radiograph of the hands outlines osteopenic bones with thinned cortices.

A

IDIOPATHIC JUVENILE OSTEOPOROSIS (FIG. 47–3). Idiopathic juvenile osteoporosis is an uncommon, self-limited disease of childhood. Clinically affected children come to medical attention about 2 years before puberty with spinal and extraspinal symptoms. On radiographic examination, osteoporosis of the spine may be combined with vertebral collapse. Kyphosis represents the characteristic spinal complication. Although transverse and oblique fractures may occur in the bones of the peripheral skeleton a more typical feature appears to be metaphyseal injury, especially about the knees and ankles, a finding that is less common in osteogenesis imperfecta, the disease that is most likely to be confused with idiopathic juvenile osteoporosis. The pathologic aberrations in idiopathic juvenile osteoporosis include a quantitative rather than a qualitative change in bone characterized by an increase in bone resorption surface. Despite an increase in osteoclastosis, most laboratory parameters yield normal results.

The major problem in differential diagnosis is distinguishing idiopathic juvenile osteoporosis from osteogenesis imperfecta (Fig. 47–4). Osteogenesis imperfecta congenita appears in early infancy with distinctive features. Osteogenesis imperfecta tarda forms may not produce abnormalities until later childhood or adolescence. Osteogenesis imperfecta (see Chapter 73) may be associated with blue sclerae; progressive cranial, facial, and pelvic deformities; and a qualitative abnormality of bone on histologic examination, findings not evident in idiopathic juvenile osteoporosis. In osteogenesis imperfecta, thin cortices of the diaphyses lead to characteristic fractures

of the shaft. Other childhood disorders, such as leukemia, homocystinuria, Cushing's disease, and juvenile chronic arthritis, usually are easily differentiated from idiopathic juvenile osteoporosis.

OTHER DISORDERS. Generalized osteoporosis may accompany plasma cell myeloma, Gaucher's disease and glycogen storage disease, anemias, nutritional deficiencies, diabetes mellitus, immunodeficiency states, and chronic liver disease.

DIFFERENTIAL DIAGNOSIS. The differentiation between generalized osteoporosis and osteomalacia, especially in adults, may be extremely difficult on the basis of radiographic abnormalities and ultimately may require histologic evaluation of skeletal tissue. In infants and children, the presence of rickets with its characteristic metaphyseal changes represents a valuable diagnostic clue. Accurate diagnosis becomes important in infants, particularly those receiving long-term intravenous hyperalimentation, in whom the development of rickets may lead to multiple fractures that contribute to an erroneous diagnosis of osteogenesis imperfecta, the child abuse syndrome, or copper deficiency (Fig. 47–5).

In adults with osteomalacia, diffuse osteopenia simulates generalized osteoporosis. In osteomalacia, however, trabeculae may appear indistinct and the interface of cortical and medullary bone may be obscured. More helpful is the identification of osseous deformity (such as acetabular protrusion and a bell-shaped thorax) and insufficiency fractures (pseudo-fractures), which are most frequent in the pubic rami, medial portion of the femoral neck, axillary margins of the ribs, scapula, and, occasionally, the tubular bones (Fig. 47–6). In

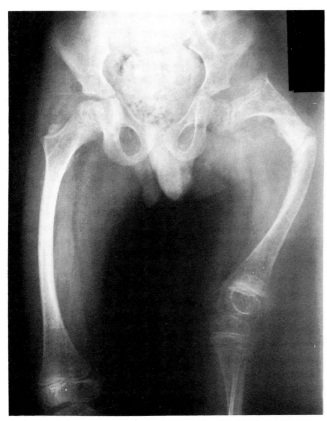

Figure 47–4. Osteogenesis imperfecta. In a child, observe the generalized osteoporosis, cortical diminution, and osseous deformity and fracture.

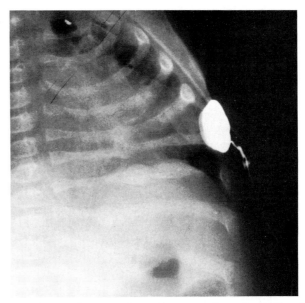

Figure 47–5. Rickets secondary to intravenous hyperalimentation. In this infant multiple fractures of the ribs simulate those seen in the child abuse syndrome. (Courtesy of M. Dalinka, M.D., Philadelphia, Pennsylvania.)

some forms of osteomalacia, additional distinctive alterations are apparent (see Chapter 48). X-linked hypophosphatemic osteomalacia (or rickets) is associated with a generalized enthesopathy in which bone proliferation at sites of tendon and ligament attachment and tendinous, ligamentous, and capsular calcification become evident; calcification of cartilage and small ossicles may also be noted. Atypical axial osteomalacia is characterized by involvement of the spine and pelvis, a coarsened trabecular pattern (particularly in the cervical region), normal or near-normal laboratory values, and osteomalacia on histologic analysis. Adult men and women are affected, and a family history of the disease is sometimes encountered.

Primary or secondary hyperparathyroidism generally leads to diagnostic abnormalities in addition to osteopenia; aggressive bone resorption occurs in subperiosteal, intracortical, endosteal, subligamentous, and subchondral locations. In patients with renal osteodystrophy, these changes are accompanied by osteosclerosis, osteomalacia, and vascular, soft tissue, and periarticular calcification (see Chapter 52).

Fibrogenesis imperfecta ossium is a rare disorder of bone characterized by the formation of abnormal collagen fibers in osteoid that are not birefringent when examined under polarized light (see Chapter 73). The age of onset of disease is variable. The disorder leads to crippling deformity and death. A consistent biochemical abnormality is elevation of serum levels of alkaline phosphatase. Radiographic alterations include amorphous sclerosis of the medullary cavity, or a fishnet or basket-weave trabecular appearance (Fig. 47–7). Os-

seous protuberances, especially in the pelvis, scapula, and proximal portion of the femur, are characteristic. Pathologic fractures in the axial and appendicular bones are frequent.

Regional Osteoporosis

Osteoporosis confined to a segment of the body is associated with disorders of the appendicular skeleton. The classic

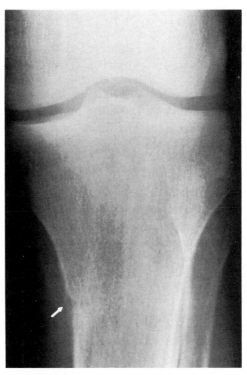

Figure 47–6. Osteomalacia. Observe an insufficiency fracture in the medial aspect of the left tibial metaphysis (arrow). (Courtesy of G. Greenway, M.D., Dallas, Texas.)

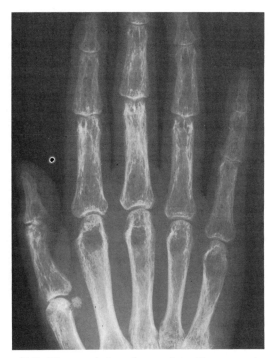

Figure 47–7. Fibrogenesis imperfecta ossium. Note osteopenia and a coarsened trabecular pattern in the metacarpal bones and phalanges. The interface between the cortex and the medullary canal is obliterated, and there is no evidence of subperiosteal resorption. (Courtesy of P. Kline, M.D., San Antonio, Texas.)

Table 47–4. MAJOR CAUSES OF REGIONAL OSTEOPOROSIS

Immobilization and disuse
Reflex sympathetic dystrophy syndrome
Transient regional osteoporosis
   Transient osteoporosis of the hip
   Regional migratory osteoporosis

months; the findings appear initially in the appendicular skeleton. Spinal abnormalities are not prominent. The radiographic patterns are uniform osteoporosis (most common type), speckled or spotty osteoporosis (characterized by small, spheroid lucent areas most frequently in periarticular regions and in the carpal and tarsal areas), band-like osteoporosis (in the subchondral or metaphyseal regions), and cortical lamellation or scalloping (translucency of the outer or inner aspects of the cortex). These radiographic appearances may simulate those of malignancy.

In association with osteoporosis of disuse, patients may reveal hypercalcemia and hypercalciuria. Serum phosphorus levels may also be elevated during disuse. The pathogenesis of disuse osteoporosis is debated.

Although a regional distribution is the hallmark of disuse osteoporosis, generalized or scattered patterns may be observed

example of such a disorder is osteoporosis accompanying disuse or immobilization of a limb or portion of a limb. Other examples include the reflex sympathetic dystrophy syndrome and transient regional osteoporosis (Table 47–4).

The radiographic patterns of regional osteoporosis are variable. Uniform osteopenia may accompany regional osteoporosis of long duration, such as that associated with chronic disuse in patients who are paralyzed or who have undergone amputation. Band-like osteopenia (in the subchondral or metaphyseal regions) and patchy osteopenia (particularly in the epiphyses) may indicate a more acutely developing osteoporosis, such as that occurring in the reflex sympathetic dystrophy syndrome. In acute osteoporosis, both cortical and spongy bone can show dramatic alterations. The cortical abnormalities, which include subperiosteal, intracortical, and endosteal erosion, may require high quality radiography for their detection.

OSTEOPOROSIS OF IMMOBILIZATION AND DISUSE (FIG. 47–8). This type of osteoporosis occurs most characteristically in the immobilized regions of patients with fractures, motor paralysis due to central nervous system disease or trauma, and bone and joint inflammation.

In humans, disuse osteoporosis is associated with a negative calcium balance, the source of which is the skeleton. The radiographic appearance of osteoporosis depends on many factors, including the age of the patient (osteoporosis appears sooner in younger individuals) and the extent and duration of the negative calcium balance (osteoporosis is more severe when calcium loss is more prominent). After paralysis or immobilization, osteoporosis generally appears within 2 or 3

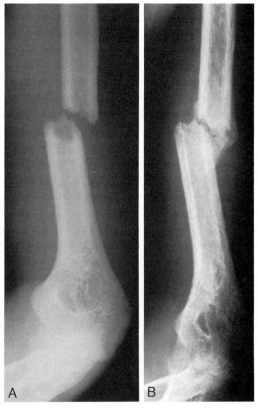

Figure 47–8. Osteoporosis of immobilization and disuse: Fracture. Radiographs obtained immediately after a fracture of the humeral shaft (**A**) and two months later (**B**) are shown. Observe in **B** the extent of the osteopenia both above and below the healing fracture. Note intracortical radiolucent lines.

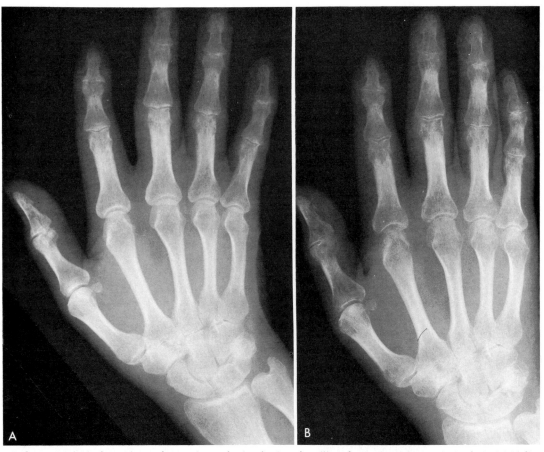

Figure 47–9. Reflex sympathetic dystrophy syndrome. A man developed pain and swelling after a minor injury to the hand. An initial film (**A**) outlines mild periarticular osteoporosis and soft tissue swelling. Six weeks later (**B**), osteoporosis is much more exaggerated. The periarticular osteoporosis simulates the appearance of rheumatoid arthritis.

in unusual circumstances. This phenomenon has been noted in quadriplegic persons and may be observed in astronauts as a result of weightlessness owing to lack of gravitational force.

REFLEX SYMPATHETIC DYSTROPHY SYNDROME (FIG. 47–9). The reflex sympathetic dystrophy syndrome (RSDS) is a distinct entity that is produced in a variety of clinical situations. Some of the many terms applied to RSDS are causalgia, Sudeck's atrophy, algodystrophy, shoulder-hand syndrome, and reflex sympathetic dystrophy. Any neurally related visceral, musculoskeletal, neurologic, or vascular condition is a potential source for RSDS. Reported associated conditions have included myocardial infarction; cerebrovascular disorders; degenerative disease of the cervical spine; discal herniation; polymyalgia rheumatica; posttraumatic, postsurgical, and postinfectious states; calcific tendinitis; vasculitis; and neoplasm. The RSDS is less frequent in children than in adults.

The pathogenesis of RSDS is not entirely clear. The most widely held theory is that of the "internuncial pool" in which it is assumed that an injury or lesion produces painful impulses that travel via afferent pathways to the spinal cord, where a series of reflexes are initiated that spread via the interconnecting pool of neurons. These latter reflexes stimulate the lateral and anterior tracts, provoking efferent pathways that travel to the peripheral nerves, producing the local findings of the RSDS.

Clinical symptoms and signs are variable. They may be evident in any involved site, although the characteristic distribution is the shoulder and hand. Initially (at any site), stiffness, pain, tenderness, and weakness may be associated with swelling, vasomotor changes, hyperesthesia, and disability. The duration of the RSDS varies, and, in some cases, findings may persist for years, becoming irreversible.

Soft tissue swelling and regional osteoporosis are the most important radiographic findings. Fine-detail radiography has revealed five types of bone resorption: (1) Resorption of cancellous bone in the metaphyseal region leads to band-like, patchy, or periarticular osteoporosis; (2) subperiosteal bone resorption is similar to that occurring in cases of hyperparathyroidism; (3) intracortical bone resorption produces excessive striation or tunneling in cortices; (4) endosteal bone resorption, which is the region of greatest bone mineral loss in this condition, causes initial excavation and scalloping of the endosteal surface, with subsequent uniform remodeling of the endosteum and widening of the medullary canal; and (5) subchondral and juxtaarticular erosion may lead to small periarticular erosions and intraarticular gaps in the subchondral bone. Because of the widespread nature and severity of bone resorption in RSDS, the radiographs may reveal rapid and severe osteopenia, particularly in periarticular regions, which simulates the appearance of primary articular disorders. The absence of significant intraarticular erosions and joint space loss usually allows accurate differentiation of RSDS from these various arthritides. The preservation of joint space cannot be overemphasized as a characteristic finding in this syndrome.

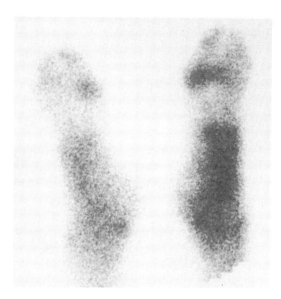

Figure 47–10. Reflex sympathetic dystrophy syndrome: Scintigraphic abnormalities. A delayed image during a bone scan shows abnormal uptake of the radionuclide in the midfoot and forefoot on the left side with similar but mild changes in the opposite foot.

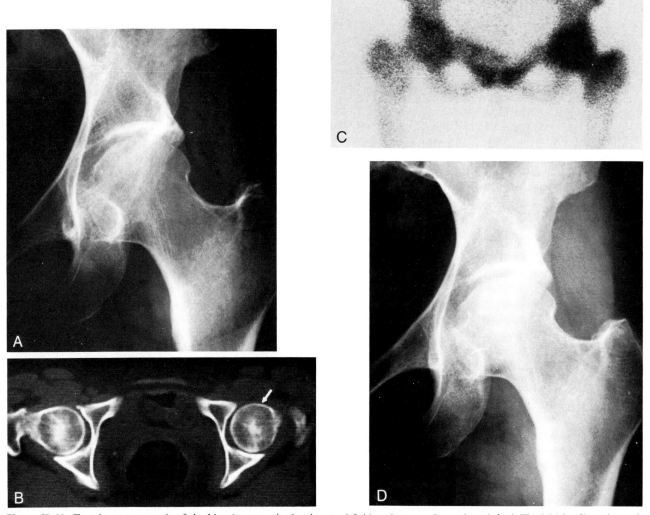

Figure 47–11. Transient osteoporosis of the hip. A woman developed severe left hip pain over a 3 month period. **A** The initial radiograph reveals osteopenia of the left femoral head and neck. The joint space is normal. **B** Computed tomography demonstrates that the cortex of the involved femoral head is diffusely thinned (arrow). There is little difference in the radiodensity of the spongiosa in the affected femoral head when compared with that on the opposite side. **C** Intense accumulation of the bone-seeking radionuclide in the left femoral head and neck is evident. **D** Five months later, the left hip appears normal. (Courtesy of G. Greenway, M.D., Dallas, Texas.)

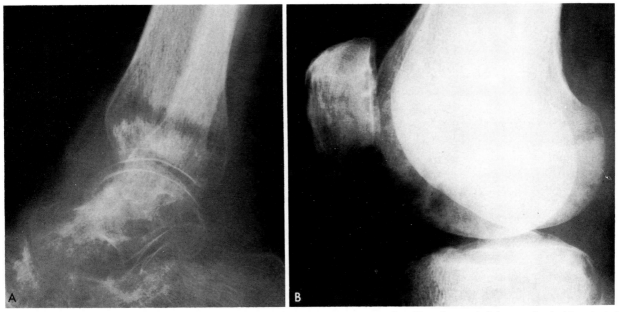

Figure 47–12. Regional migratory osteoporosis. Typical in this condition are transient pain and swelling of one articulation associated with periarticular osteoporosis, followed by spontaneous improvement and involvement of an adjacent articulation. Observe the soft tissue swelling and band-like osteopenia of the tibia and talus (**A**) and the spotty osteoporosis of the distal part of the femur and patella (**B**).

Bone and joint scintigraphy also demonstrates typical abnormalities in RSDS, which may antedate clinical and radiographic changes. Joint imaging with ^{99m}Tc-pertechnetate reveals increased radionuclide accumulation in articular regions. Bone-seeking agents reveal a similar increased accumulation in involved bones in RSDS (Fig. 47–10). This appears to be related to increased blood flow.

Radiographic and scintigraphic analyses reveal that RSDS is a bilateral process; the abnormalities are much more marked on one side compared with the other. Almost universally, an entire extremity distal to an affected site is altered, although the changes on the less involved extremity may appear patchy in distribution. Rarely, a segmental pattern affecting only a portion of an extremity may be encountered. This localized form of RSDS may lead to involvement of one or several digits of the hand or foot or a portion of an articular surface.

Synovial biopsies in symptomatic articulations demonstrate edema, proliferation of synovial lining cells and capillaries, fibrosis of the subsynovium, and perivascular infiltration with chronic inflammatory cells. In affected bone, increased vascularity, osteocytic degeneration, and prominent osteoclastic activity are observed.

TRANSIENT REGIONAL OSTEOPOROSIS. Transient regional osteoporosis is an appropriate term for conditions that share certain features: rapidly developing osteoporosis affecting periarticular bone; self-limited and reversible nature; and the absence of clear-cut evidence of inciting events, such as trauma and immobilization. There are two important diseases that fall into this category: transient osteoporosis of the hip and regional migratory osteoporosis.

Transient Osteoporosis of the Hip (Fig. 47–11). This condition typically is seen in young and middle-aged adults, particularly men. In male patients, either hip may be involved; in female patients, the left hip is affected almost exclusively, and the disease frequently occurs in the third trimester of pregnancy. Hip pain begins spontaneously, without an antecedent history of trauma or infection, is aggravated by weight-bearing, and usually progresses within a few weeks, becoming severe enough to produce a limp. The clinical findings regress in 2 to 6 months without permanent sequelae.

Joint fluid may be increased in quantity, and synovial biopsy either yields normal results or shows mild chronic inflammatory changes.

Radiographic findings are characteristic. Progressive and marked osteoporosis of the femoral head, which begins several weeks after the onset of clinical abnormalities, is associated with less extensive involvement of the femoral neck and acetabulum. The femoral subchondral bone plate is thin but otherwise intact. The joint space is normal. Restoration of normal radiographic density of the bone takes place rapidly. Radionuclide studies using bone-seeking agents reveal abnormal accumulation of isotope prior to radiographically demonstrable osteoporosis. Computed tomography shows osteopenia with cortical thinning. Magnetic resonance imaging may show decreased signal intensity in affected sites.

The cause of this condition is unknown. Its similarity to RSDS suggests a related neurogenic pathogenesis. Of particular interest was the observation that transient osteoporosis of the hip could occasionally be bilateral in distribution or involve other joints, suggesting a relationship with regional migratory osteoporosis.

Regional Migratory Osteoporosis (Fig. 47–12). The second form of transient osteoporosis is migratory in nature. Abnormalities of the hip are less frequent than abnormalities in other areas, particularly the knee, the ankle, and the foot. The disorder occurs more frequently in men than in women and usually becomes evident in the fourth or fifth decade of life. It is characterized by local pain and swelling, which develop rapidly, last up to 9 months, and then diminish and disappear. Subsequent involvement occurs in other regions of the same or opposite extremity. Several recurrences can occur successively within 2 years or be separated by 2 years or a

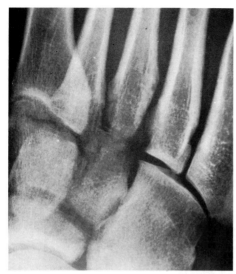

Figure 47–13. Partial transient osteoporosis: Radial type. Note osteopenia involving principally the second and third metatarsal bases, adjacent cuneiforms, and a portion of the tarsal navicular. (Courtesy of M. Dalinka, M.D., Philadelphia, Pennsylvania.)

longer period of time. Radiographic evidence of osteoporosis becomes apparent within weeks or months of the onset of clinical findings. It too progresses rapidly, diminishes subsequently, and appears at other sites. The joint space is not narrowed, nor is there evidence of intraarticular erosion. Bone scanning reveals increased activity in involved areas. Laboratory analysis may document an increase in the urinary excretion of calcium, hydroxyproline, and fluoride.

The migratory nature of the syndrome is the major feature that differentiates this condition from transient osteoporosis of the hip. Usually the joint nearest to the diseased one is the next to be involved. There may be overlap of clinical features so that more than one joint can be symptomatic at any given time. Rarely, cases demonstrating similar clinical and radiographic features remain isolated in a single joint.

A variant of this syndrome, termed partial transient osteoporosis, leads to osteopenia of a portion of an articulation. In the radial type of partial transient osteoporosis (Fig. 47–13), one or two rays of a hand or foot are affected. Changes may extend from the carpus through the metacarpus to the phalanges of the hand, or from the tarsus through the metatarsus to the phalanges of the foot. In the zonal type of partial transient osteoporosis, involvement of the knee is characterized by abnormality of the medial or lateral condyle of the femur, and involvement of the hip is characterized by abnormality of a single quadrant of the femoral head. Spontaneous recovery occurs in both the radial and the zonal forms of the disease.

Histologic evaluation of synovium in regional migratory osteoporosis delineates thickened tissue with chronic inflammatory cellular reaction. The bone itself is osteoporotic.

The pathogenesis of this condition is not known, although it has been linked to the reflex sympathetic dystrophy syndrome and transient osteoporosis of the hip.

DIFFERENTIAL DIAGNOSIS. The accurate diagnosis of regional osteoporosis associated with disuse is not difficult. That associated with the reflex sympathetic dystrophy syndrome, transient osteoporosis of the hip, and regional migra-

tory osteoporosis may simulate other conditions. Septic arthritis can lead to regional osteoporosis; however, joint space narrowing and osseous erosion eventually are observed in infection, whereas in regional osteoporosis, these findings are not apparent. Similarly, in rheumatoid arthritis, intense synovial inflammation can produce significant cartilaginous and osseous destruction. In addition, symmetric involvement of multiple joints is characteristic of rheumatoid arthritis. Monarticular processes such as pigmented villonodular synovitis and idiopathic synovial osteochondromatosis may lead to clinical and radiographic findings that simulate those of regional osteoporosis. Monarticular involvement of the hip or other joints also is not infrequent in osteonecrosis (Fig. 47–14). In osteonecrosis, the presence of osteoporosis on radiographic examination, increased radionuclide accumulation on scintigraphic examination, and the absence of articular space narrowing are findings that are identical to those in regional osteoporosis. Patchy osteosclerosis and osseous collapse are additional manifestations of osteonecrosis.

RADIOGRAPHIC-PATHOLOGIC CORRELATION
General Distribution of Abnormalities

Generalized osteoporosis is most prominent in the axial skeleton, particularly the vertebral column, the pelvis, the ribs, and the sternum (Fig. 47–15). Eventually, less extensive changes may become evident in the long and short tubular bones of the appendicular skeleton. Cranial vault alterations

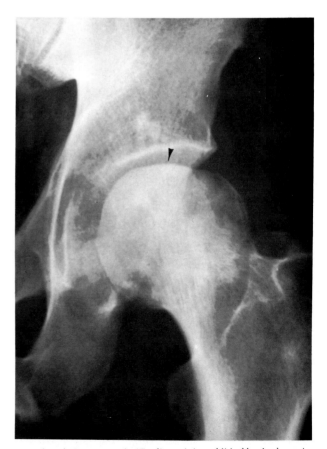

Figure 47–14. Osteonecrosis. The diagnosis is established by the depression of the articular surface of the femoral head (arrowhead), which is associated with patchy lucency and sclerosis.

usually are mild. In regional osteoporosis, alterations in the appendicular skeleton predominate over those in the axial skeleton.

Spine

The diagnosis of osteoporosis of the spine is made on the basis of changes in radiolucency of the bone, in trabecular pattern, and in shape of the vertebral bodies.

CHANGE IN RADIOLUCENCY (FIG. 47–16). Osteoporosis produces increased radiolucency of vertebral bone. Associated vertebral compression, however, can lead to increase in bone density due to compaction of trabeculae and callus formation.

CHANGE IN TRABECULAR PATTERN (FIG. 47–16). In osteoporosis, individual trabeculae are thinned, and some are lost. The changes are more prominent in the horizontal trabeculae than in the vertical trabeculae. In fact, relative accentuation of the vertical trabeculae leads to vertical radiodense striations (bars), which simulate the appearance of a hemangioma (Fig. 47–17). Furthermore, in osteoporosis, a distinct but thinned subchondral bone plate becomes evident in the superior and inferior portions of the vertebral body.

CHANGE IN SHAPE OF THE VERTEBRAL BODIES (TABLE 47–5). Characteristic abnormalities of vertebral shape are observed in osteoporosis, which must be distinguished from normal variations of vertebral contour as well as from artifacts produced by improper radiographic examination (Fig. 47–18). Several alterations of vertebral shape can be identified: *wedge-shaped* vertebrae, with a reduced anterior border but normal posterior border; *biconcavity* or "fish vertebrae," in which the central portion of the vertebral body is not as high as the anterior or posterior border; and *compression*, in which both the anterior and the posterior vertebral heights

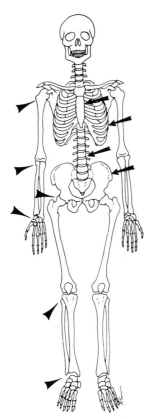

Figure 47–15. Osteoporosis: Distribution of abnormalities. Generalized versus regional osteoporosis. In generalized osteoporosis (arrows, on right half of diagram), the spine, the pelvis, the ribs, and the sternum are affected most commonly. In regional osteoporosis (arrowheads, on left half), the appendicular skeleton is the predominant site of alterations, particularly in periarticular regions.

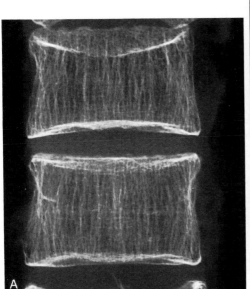
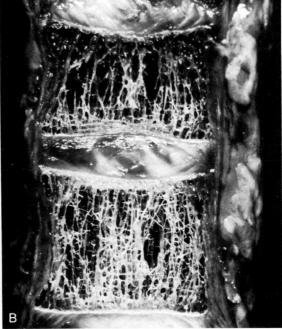

Figure 47–16. Osteoporosis: Spine—changes in radiolucency and trabecular pattern. In two different cadaveric spines, observe accentuation of the vertical trabeculae with preferential resorption of horizontal trabeculae. Additional findings characteristic of osteoporosis are the depression of the superior margin of the vertebral body and a distinct but thinned bone plate at the superior and inferior surfaces of the vertebral bodies.

Table 47–5. ABNORMALITIES OF VERTEBRAL BODY SHAPE

Abnormality	Common Causes	Characteristics
Biconcave ("fish") vertebrae	Osteoporosis Osteomalacia Paget's disease Hyperparathyroidism	Arch-like contour defects of superior and inferior vertebral surfaces, particularly in the lower thoracic and lumbar areas
Cupid's bow vertebrae	Normal	Parasagittal concavities on the inferior surface of the lower lumbar vertebrae
Butterfly vertebrae	Congenital	Funnel-like defect through vertebra dividing it into right and left halves
Cartilaginous nodes	Scheuermann's disease Trauma Hyperparathyroidism Intervertebral osteochondrosis	Depression and discontinuity of the vertebral endplate with intraosseous lucency and surrounding sclerosis
"H" vertebrae	Sickle cell anemia Gaucher's disease	Step-like central depression of the vertebral endplates

are decreased. In osteoporosis, wedging, biconcavity, and compression may all be apparent. Wedge-shaped vertebral bodies are common (particularly in the thoracic region, owing to the normal thoracic kyphosis), as the vertebra is strengthened posteriorly by the neural arch and paravertebral muscles. Vertebral compression is frequently combined with wedging. Both wedging and compression in osteoporosis indicate a fracture of the vertebral body (Fig. 47–19).

"Fish Vertebrae." Increased concavity of the vertebral bodies in osteoporosis produces typical "fish vertebrae," so called because radiographs of the spine of normal fish show a series of biconcave vertebral bodies. Biconcave deformities of the vertebral bodies are characteristic of disorders in which there is diffuse weakening of the bone (Fig. 47–20). One such disorder is osteoporosis, although similar abnormalities may be seen in osteomalacia, Paget's disease, hyperparathyroidism, and neoplasm. In all of these diseases, osseous deformity results from the expansile pressure of the adjacent intervertebral discs, which leads to thinning and stretching of the cartilaginous endplates without disruption.

"Fish vertebrae" are particularly common in the lower thoracic and upper lumbar spine. In the middle and upper thoracic spine, a normal dorsal kyphosis exists, with maximum pressure on the anterior surface of the vertebra. In this region, osseous weakening leads to anterior wedging of the vertebral body, with increasing kyphosis. At any spinal level, if the nucleus pulposus is abnormal, "fish vertebrae" do not develop, but diffuse flattening of the vertebral body is noted.

"Fish vertebrae" complicating osteoporosis must be differentiated from "fish vertebrae" in other metabolic disorders as well as from certain normal and abnormal changes in vertebral shape. In osteomalacia, biconcave vertebral deformities are smoother than those in osteoporosis and involve superior and inferior margins of the vertebral body with equal severity (Fig. 47–21). In addition, wedging and compression of vertebrae are unusual. In osteoporosis, the weakened and

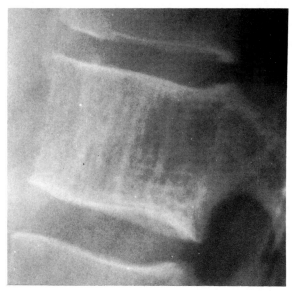

Figure 47–17. **Hemangioma.** Note the typical characteristics of a hemangioma of a vertebral body: increased radiolucency and coarse vertical trabeculae producing a spongy appearance.

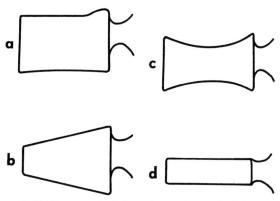

Figure 47–18. **Osteoporosis: Spine—changes in vertebral shape.** *a*, In the normal situation, the superior and inferior vertebral outlines are relatively parallel, although a slight elevation or protuberance can be seen at the posterosuperior aspect of the vertebral bodies. *b*, Wedge-shaped vertebrae relate to collapse of the anterior aspect of the vertebral body. *c*, Biconcave or "fish vertebrae" are characterized by biconcave deformity of the superior and inferior surfaces of the vetebral body. *d*, Flattened or "pancake" vertebrae are associated with compression of the entire vertebral surface.

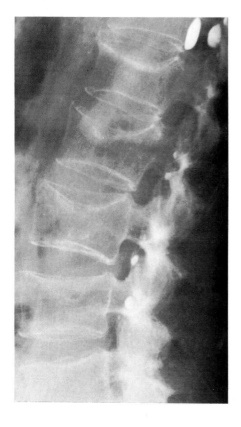

Figure 47–19. Osteoporosis: Vertebral compression. Multiple compression fractures of the vertebral bodies are seen. Note that the osseous depressions involve mainly the central portion of the superior bone plate and are accompanied by an increase in radiodensity at the fracture site in the first and second lumbar vertebral bodies. Acutely, such radiodense areas may represent compression of trabeculae; subacutely or chronically, they may indicate new bone formation at the site of fracture.

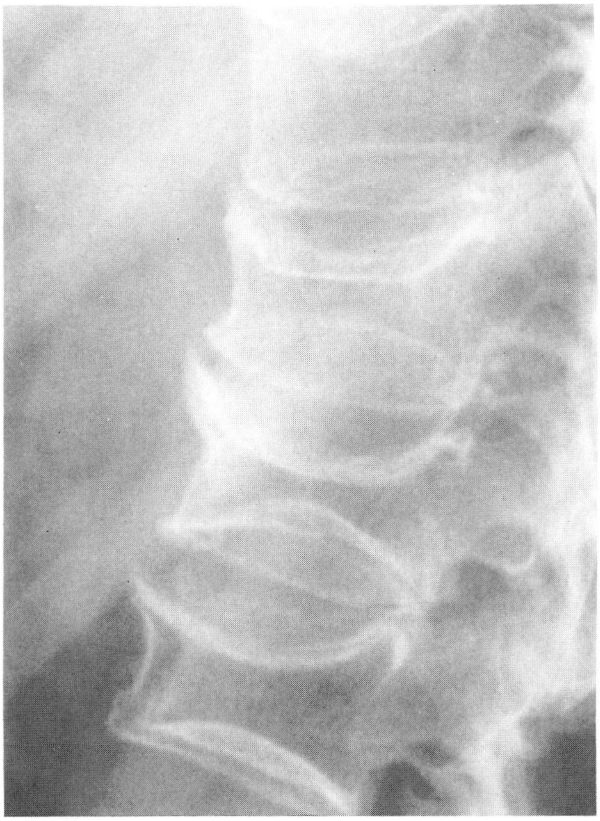

Figure 47–20. Osteoporosis: "Fish vertebrae." A lateral radiograph of the lumbar spine reveals severe osteoporosis with multiple "fish vertebrae." Note that the superior and inferior surfaces of the vertebral bodies are not involved to the same extent. Note also that the subchondral bone plates appear dense compared with the lucent central portion of the vertebral bodies.

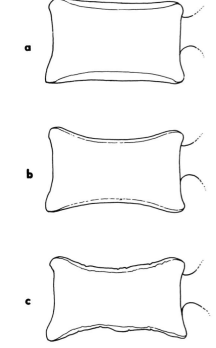

Figure 47–21. "Fish vertebrae": Differential diagnosis of osteoporosis and osteomalacia. The normal vertebra *(a)* becomes biconcave in outline in both osteomalacia *(b)* and osteoporosis *(c)*. In osteomalacia, however, the indentation of the osseous surface is smooth, and both superior and inferior borders are involved to approximately the same degree. In osteoporosis, the depression is more angular or irregular, and superior and inferior surfaces of the vertebral body are frequently involved to different degrees.

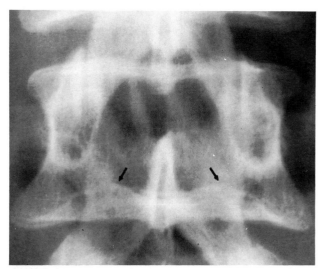

Figure 47–22. Cupid's bow contour. A frontal radiograph of a lower lumbar vertebral body reveals a normal variation of vertebral outline, the Cupid's bow contour. Observe smooth parasagittal concavities on the inferior surface of the vertebral body (arrows).

brittle bone leads to more irregular collapse, and the upper and lower margins of the vertebrae are not involved to similar degrees. In osteomalacia, adjacent vertebrae are affected to the same extent, although the lumbar spine may be involved more severely than the thoracic spine; in osteoporosis, abnormalities of vertebral shape may be distributed unevenly throughout the spine, and several affected vertebrae may be separated by relatively normal vertebrae.

Cupid's-bow contour is a name applied to a normal concavity on the inferior aspect of the third, fourth, and fifth lumbar vertebral bodies, which may resemble the biconcave changes of "fish vertebrae" (Fig. 47–22). When viewed from the front, parasagittal concavities on the undersurface of the vertebrae resemble a bow, pointing cephalad. On lateral views, these vertebral depressions are located posteriorly.

Abnormalities of vertebral shape other than "fish vertebrae" can accompany many diseases. Incomplete embryologic regression of the chorda dorsalis alters vertebral contour and can lead to sagittal clefts in the vertebral body, producing a distinctive butterfly configuration (Fig. 47–23). The superior and inferior surfaces of the divided vertebral body are depressed and assume a funnel-shaped defect through which two adjacent discs are connected; the lateral aspects of the vertebral bodies appear broadened. Extensive osseous destruction in neoplasm and infection can lead to irregular vertebral collapse. In infection, discal destruction with disc space narrowing is characteristic.

Cartilaginous (Schmorl's) Nodes. In addition to "fish vertebrae," a second contour defect can be apparent in many metabolic disorders, including osteoporosis, which can be attributed to displacement of a portion of the intervertebral disc into the vertebral body (Fig. 47–24). These discal protrusions are called cartilaginous or Schmorl's nodes. They occur when the cartilaginous plate of the vertebral body has been disrupted. Such disruption can be produced by an intrinsic abnormality of the plate itself or by alterations in the subchondral bone of the vertebral body. Whatever the cause of the damage to the cartilaginous endplate or to the

subchondral bone of the vertebral body, a weakened area is created that no longer can resist the expansive pressure of the adjacent nucleus pulposus. This pathogenetic scheme explains the appearance of cartilaginous nodes in such diverse osseous processes as osteoporosis, osteomalacia, Paget's disease, hyperparathyroidism, infection, and neoplasm, and such cartilaginous processes as degenerative disc disease (intervertebral [osteo]chondrosis), infection, and juvenile kyphosis (Scheuermann's disease).

The radiographic evidence of cartilaginous node formation is based on the presence of a break in the subchondral bone plate (corresponding to the site of discal displacement), a lucent area of varying size bordering on the intervertebral disc (corresponding to the amount of protruded disc material), and a small degree of surrounding bone sclerosis (corresponding to trabecular condensation and thickening).

Proximal Portion of the Femur

The analysis of the trabecular pattern of the upper end of the femur has been emphasized as an index of osteoporosis (Fig. 47–25). In this region, five anatomic groups of trabeculae can be identified:

1. *Principal compressive group.* This group comprises the uppermost compression trabeculae, which extend from the medial cortex of the femoral neck to the upper portion of the femoral head in slightly curved radial lines. It contains the thickest and most densely packed trabeculae in the region.

2. *Secondary compressive group.* Those trabeculae that arise from the medial cortex of the shaft below the principal compressive group form this group. They curve upward and slightly laterally toward the greater trochanter and the upper portion of the femoral neck. These trabeculae are thin and widely spaced.

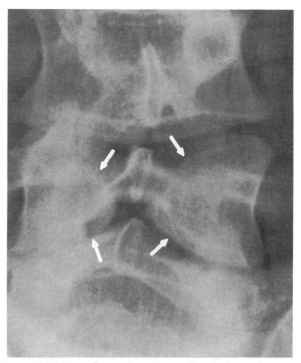

Figure 47–23. Butterfly vertebrae. Among the spinal anomalies present in this patient, observe a typical butterfly vertebra (arrows).

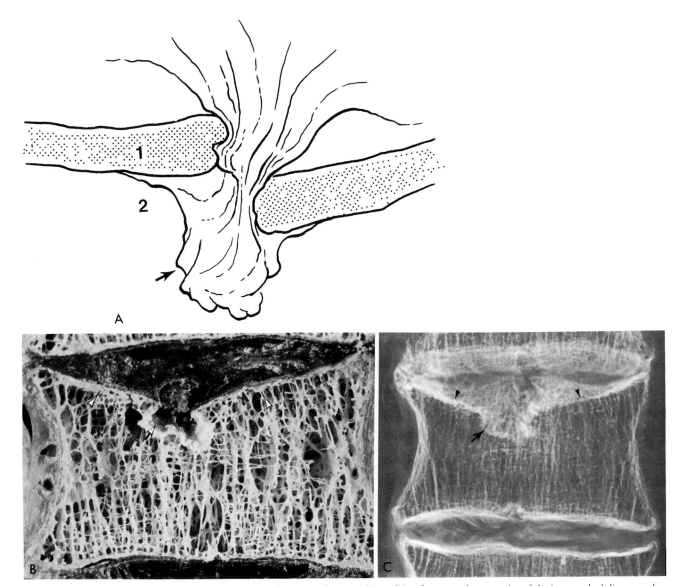

Figure 47–24. Osteoporosis: Cartilaginous (Schmorl's) nodes. A Cartilaginous (Schmorl's) nodes occur when a portion of the intervertebral disc protrudes into the vertebral body (arrow) through a gap in the cartilaginous endplate (1) and subchondral bone plate (2). **B, C** A photograph and radiograph of a coronal section reveal depression of the subchondral bone (arrowheads). A cartilaginous node (arrows) has resulted from disruption of the cartilage and bone plates. It has created a radiolucent defect within the bone with a small rim of sclerosis. A small cartilaginous node is noted on the opposite side of the vertebral body (**B, C,** From Resnick D, Niwayama G: Intravertebral disk herniations: Cartilaginous (Schmorl's) nodes. Radiology 126:57, 1978. Used with permission.)

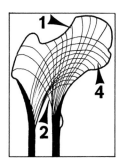

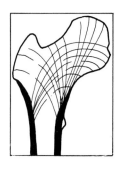
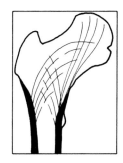
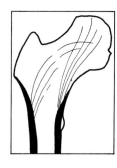

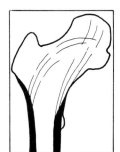
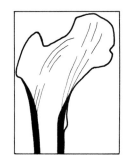
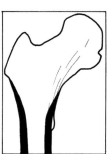

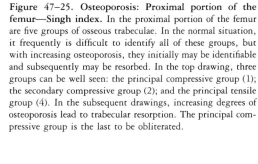

Figure 47–25. Osteoporosis: Proximal portion of the femur—Singh index. In the proximal portion of the femur are five groups of osseous trabeculae. In the normal situation, it frequently is difficult to identify all of these groups, but with increasing osteoporosis, they initially may be identifiable and subsequently may be resorbed. In the top drawing, three groups can be well seen: the principal compressive group (1); the secondary compressive group (2); and the principal tensile group (4). In the subsequent drawings, increasing degrees of osteoporosis lead to trabecular resorption. The principal compressive group is the last to be obliterated.

3. *Greater trochanter group.* This group is composed of slender and poorly defined tensile trabeculae, which arise laterally below the greater trochanter and extend upward to terminate near its superior surface.

4. *Principal tensile group.* The trabeculae that arise from the lateral cortex below the greater trochanter and extend in a curvilinear fashion superiorly and medially across the femoral neck, ending in the inferior portion of the femoral head, form the thickest tensile trabeculae.

5. *Secondary tensile group.* These trabeculae arise from the lateral cortex below the principal tensile group. They extend superiorly and medially to terminate after crossing the middle of the femoral neck.

In the femoral neck, a triangular area, Ward's triangle, contains thin and loosely arranged trabeculae. This area is enclosed by trabeculae from the principal compressive, secondary compressive, and tensile groups.

Patterns of trabecular loss may correlate with increasing severity of osteoporosis (Fig. 47–25). With early trabecular resorption, the structure of the principal compressive and principal tensile trabecular groups is accentuated. Ward's triangle may become more prominent. With an increased degree of trabecular resorption, tensile trabeculae are reduced in number. With further increase in trabecular resorption, the outer portion of the principal tensile trabeculae opposite the greater trochanter disappears. As osteoporosis increases in severity, resorption of all trabecular groups occurs, with the exception of bone trabeculae in the principal compressive group. With severe osteoporosis, even these latter trabeculae are partially or completely obliterated.

The value of this trabecular pattern (termed the Singh index) as a gauge to the severity of osteoporosis is debated. Furthermore, attempts to use trabecular patterns at other sites, such as the calcaneus, as an indicator of the presence and severity of osteoporosis have met with mixed success.

Cortex of the Tubular Bones

There are three specific sites at which osseous resorption of bone cortices may become apparent (Table 47–6) (Fig. 47–26). A cellular, vascularized membrane covering the endosteal surface of the cortex may be called the endosteal envelope; an intracortical (haversian) envelope constitutes the surfaces within the cortical bone (haversian and Volkmann's canals); and a periosteal envelope covers the surface of the cortex. The response to stimuli induced by various endocrine and metabolic disorders is not always identical in these three bone envelopes. It is for this reason that careful investigation of cortical bone in the hand may provide important differential diagnostic clues.

Endosteal resorption produces scalloped concavities on the inner margin of the cortex, enlarging the marrow cavity. Intracortical resorption is characterized by the appearance of

Table 47–6. PATTERNS OF OSSEOUS RESORPTION IN TUBULAR BONES

Site	Pattern
Cortex	
Endosteal	Diffuse cortical thinning or scalloped erosions
Intracortical	Cortical radiolucent areas or striations
Periosteal	Subperiosteal erosions
Spongiosa	
Subchondral	Linear, band-like, or spotty radiolucent areas
Metaphyseal	Band-like radiolucent areas
Diffuse	Homogeneous or spotty radiolucent areas

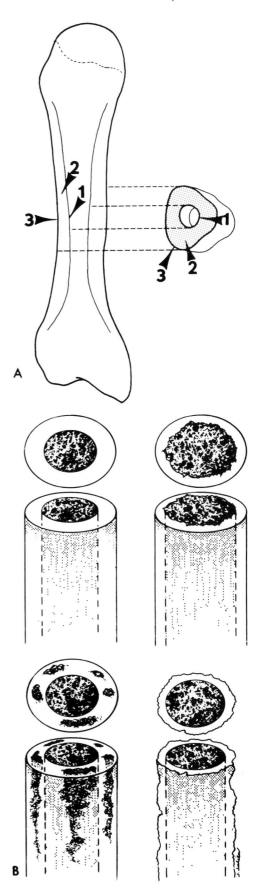

prominent longitudinal striations within the cortex. The detection of several radiolucent striae deep within a localized portion of the cortex can be a normal finding. An increased number of striae with wider distribution is indicative of an abnormal situation. In some instances, abnormal linear resorption may localize to the outer cortical area, simulating subperiosteal bone resorption or even periosteal bone formation—pseudoperiostitis. Abnormal linear radiolucent areas within the cortex can be detected in such disorders as hyperparathyroidism, hyperthyroidism, acromegaly, osteomalacia, renal osteodystrophy, disuse osteoporosis, and the reflex sympathetic dystrophy syndrome. Cortical lucent lesions are generally not apparent in low bone turnover states, such as senile or postmenopausal osteoporosis and Cushing's disease.

Subperiosteal resorption produces irregularity and poor definition of the outer surface of the cortex. It becomes prominent in diseases of rapid bone turnover, particularly hyperparathyroidism. Moderate to severe subperiosteal resorption is virtually specific for this condition.

Cortical resorption, which can be detected using magnification radiography, can be quantitated with radiographic morphometry. This procedure consists of measuring cortical dimensions on a radiographic film with a suitable caliper. Although it is applicable to various sites, radiographic morphometry is usually performed on the hands using the shaft of a metacarpal bone, particularly the second (Fig. 47–27).

Spongiosa in the Appendicular Skeleton

The spongy bone undergoes early and significant changes in osteoporosis and related metabolic conditions (Table 47–6). Several radiographic patterns can be distinguished in the tubular bones and the carpal and tarsal areas: diffuse or homogeneous osteoporosis; speckled or spotty osteoporosis, which is particularly prominent in periarticular areas; and

Figure 47–26. Cortex of tubular bones: Sites of osseous resorption. A Three envelopes exist at which cortical resorption may occur. These are the endosteal envelope (1), intracortical (haversian) envelope (2), and periosteal envelope (3). B Diagram indicates the normal situation (top left), endosteal resorption (top right), intracortical resorption (bottom left), and subperiosteal resorption (bottom right).

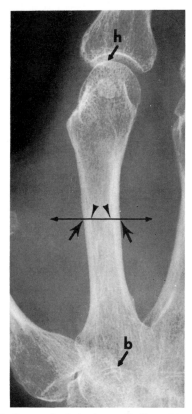

Figure 47–27. Cortex of tubular bones: Radiographic morphometry.
Normal measurements. The length of the metacarpal is measured from the
most distal point of its base (b) to the most distal point of its head (h). The
midpoint is found and a line can be drawn across the shaft. Measurements
are then made of the outer diameter or width (W—between arrows), the
marrow cavity width (m—between arrowheads), and the combined cortical
thickness (CCT = W − m). (From Garn SM, et al: Bone measurement in
the differential diagnosis of osteopenia and osteoporosis. Radiology *100*:509,
1971. Used with permission.)

linear and band-like osteoporosis in subchondral and metaphyseal areas (Figs. 47–28 and 47–29). In postmenopausal
or senile osteoporosis, diffuse osteoporosis is most characteristic; in the reflex sympathetic dystrophy syndrome and
immobilization states, speckled, linear, or band-like patterns
may become prominent. In children, extensive metaphyseal
osteopenia can simulate the appearance of an infection.

In subchondral locations, linear radiolucent bands in osteoporosis produce thinning of the overlying bone plate and
small areas of osseous disruption. The absence of large gaps
in the subchondral bone plate and of joint space narrowing
allows differentiation of osteoporosis from rheumatoid arthritis; the absence of significant bone collapse facilitates its
differentiation from osteonecrosis. The degree of periarticular
bone resorption in osteoporosis, however, can become striking, leading to an erroneous diagnosis of arthritis, infection,
or even neoplastic disease.

Additional Skeletal Manifestations of Osteoporosis

FRACTURES. Acute fractures are an important complication of osteoporosis. The most common sites of fractures
are the vertebral bodies, the neck and intertrochanteric region
of the femur, the distal portion of the radius, and the humeral
neck. Although attempts have been made to define the
importance of trabecular bone loss or cortical bone loss, or
both, as factors contributing to such fractures, there is no
uniform agreement on the subject. In general, it appears that
trabecular bone loss is more significant than cortical bone loss
in the pathogenesis of fractures in the spine and distal portion
of the radius. Certainly loss of cortical bone must be considered important in the pathogenesis of femoral fractures,
although other factors, such as a tendency to fall, are
important determinants of which elderly persons will have
fractures.

The insufficiency type of stress fracture may appear in
patients with osteoporosis. The typical sites of involvement
are the symphysis pubis (Fig. 47–30) and pubic rami, sacrum
(Fig. 47–31), supraacetabular area, other regions of the bony
pelvis, femoral neck, proximal and distal portions of the

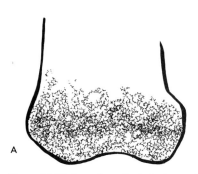
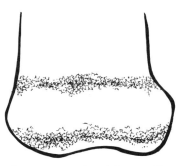
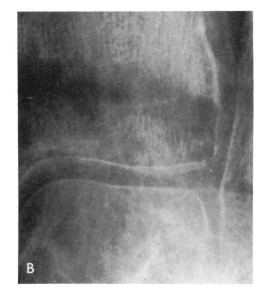

Figure 47–28. Spongiosa of tubular bones: Sites of osseous resorption. A Patterns of bone
loss include band-like radiolucent areas in the metaphysis or subchondral bone (drawing on
right) and homogeneous periarticular radiolucent areas (drawing on left). **B** Band-like resorption:
Metaphyseal and subchondral linear radiolucent areas are evident.

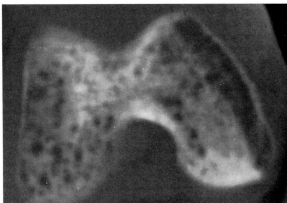

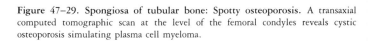

Figure 47–29. Spongiosa of tubular bone: Spotty osteoporosis. A transaxial computed tomographic scan at the level of the femoral condyles reveals cystic osteoporosis simulating plasma cell myeloma.

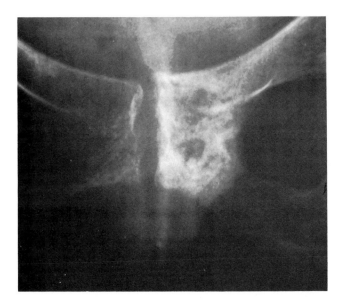

Figure 47–30. Osteoporosis: Insufficiency fracture—symphysis pubis. The radiographic appearance of such fractures includes irregular osteolysis and osteosclerosis simulating a malignant neoplasm. (Courtesy of V. Vint, M.D., San Diego, California.)

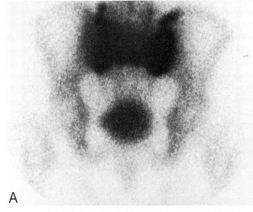

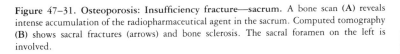

Figure 47–31. Osteoporosis: Insufficiency fracture—sacrum. A bone scan **(A)** reveals intense accumulation of the radiopharmaceutical agent in the sacrum. Computed tomography **(B)** shows sacral fractures (arrows) and bone sclerosis. The sacral foramen on the left is involved.

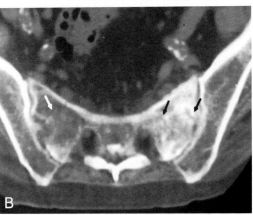

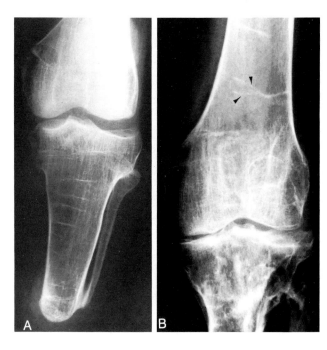

Figure 47–32. Reinforcement lines (bone bars): Radiographic abnormalities—association with chronic osteoporosis. A Observe numerous thick bone bars in the metaphysis and diaphysis of the tibia in association with diffuse osteopenia in a patient who had had his leg amputated many years previously. In large part, the bars extend completely across the medullary canal. (Courtesy of P. Kaplan, M.D., Omaha, Nebraska.) B In a different patient with a remote history of a tibial and fibular fracture, diffuse osteopenia is accompanied by horizontally and obliquely oriented bone bars in the femoral metaphysis and diaphysis. One of these is branching (arrowheads).

tibia, and sternum. Potential contributing factors include rheumatoid arthritis and corticosteroid or radiation therapy.

Insufficiency fractures of the pubic rami may be accompanied by considerable osteolysis and fragmentation of bone, findings that simulate a malignant tumor. Those of the sacrum are associated with a characteristic scintigraphic pattern in which vertical and horizontal regions of increased accumulation of the bone-seeking radiopharmaceutical agent produce a configuration that is referred to as the "H" pattern. Insufficiency fractures of the supraacetabular bone produce poorly defined zones of increased radiodensity of variable size. All of these pelvic fractures may occur in isolation but are often observed in various combinations. Similar fractures of the tibial plateau resemble osteoarthritis or spontaneous osteonecrosis, whereas those of the sternum are secondary to progressive kyphosis in the osteoporotic thoracic spine.

REINFORCEMENT LINES (BONE BARS). In patients with chronic osteopenia, usually related to osteoporosis associated with disuse mandated by neurologic injury, physical trauma, surgical amputation, or debilitating illness, radiographs of the tubular bones, particularly the femur and tibia, commonly reveal strands of trabeculae of variable thickness, extending partially or completely across the marrow cavity (Fig. 47–32). They frequently branch and are oriented at right angles to the cortex in the diaphysis or in an oblique fashion in the metaphysis. These strands, which are referred to as reinforcement lines or bone bars, are evident in both adults and children. Their linear nature is readily apparent when they are viewed en face; punctate or short linear dense foci, simulating bone infarction or a cartilaginous tumor, are evident when they are seen in profile.

Biomechanical principles are important in the formation of bone bars. Many of the bone bars correspond in position and in curvature to the lines of maximum compressive stress. It appears likely that some of the bars of bone in the osteopenic skeleton are the body's attempt at reinforcement as a response to normal stresses. Bone bars are not a prominent feature in diseases associated with rapid osteopenia, such as the reflex sympathetic dystrophy syndrome and acute neurologic injury. They appear to represent a response to prolonged stress in which existing normal trabeculae within the medullary canal are reinforced by the slow deposition of new bone.

FURTHER READING

Arnstein AR: Regional osteoporosis. Orthop Clin North Am 3:585, 1972.

Cooper KL: Insufficiency fractures of the sternum: A consequence of thoracic kyphosis? Radiology 167:471, 1988.

Cooper KL, Beabout JW, Swee RG: Insufficiency fractures of the sacrum. Radiology 156:15, 1985.

Cummings SR: Are patients with hip fractures more osteoporotic? Review of the evidence. Am J Med 78:487, 1985.

De Smet AA, Neff JR: Pubic and sacral insufficiency fractures: Clinical course and radiologic findings. AJR 145:601, 1985.

Dietz GW, Christensen EE: Normal "cupid's bow" contour of the lower lumbar vertebrae. Radiology 121:577, 1976.

Genant HK, Kozin F, Bekerman C, McCarty DJ, Sims J: The reflex sympathetic dystrophy syndrome. A comprehensive analysis using fine-detail radiography, photon absorptiometry and bone and joint scintigraphy. Radiology 117:21, 1975.

Houang MTW, Brenton DP, Renton P, Shaw DG: Idiopathic juvenile osteoporosis. Skel Radiol 3:17, 1978.

Kozin F, McCarty DJ, Simms J, Genant H: The reflex sympathetic dystrophy syndrome. I. Clinical and histologic studies: Evidence for bilaterality, response to corticosteroids and articular involvement. Am J Med 60:321, 1976.

Lequesne M, Kerboull M, Bensasson M, Perez C, Dreiser R, Forest A: Partial transient osteoporosis. Skel Radiol 2:1, 1977.

McCord WC, Nies KM, Campion DS, Louie JS: Regional migratory osteoporosis. A denervation disease. Arthritis Rheum 21:834, 1978.

Naides S, Resnick D, Zvaifler N: Idiopathic regional osteoporosis. J Rheumatol 12:763, 1985.

Resnick D, Niwayama G: Intravertebral disk herniations: Cartilaginous (Schmorl's) nodes. Radiology 126:57, 1978.

Rosen RA: Transitory demineralization of the femoral head. Radiology 94:509, 1970.

Singh M, Nagrath AR, Maini PS: Changes in trabecular pattern of the upper end of the femur as an index of osteoporosis. J Bone Joint Surg [Am] 52:457, 1970.

Chapter 48

Rickets and Osteomalacia

Michael J. Pitt, M.D.

The terms rickets and osteomalacia encompass a group of disorders with similar gross pathologic, histologic, and radiologic findings. Etiologic factors include abnormalities of vitamin D metabolism and syndromes resulting primar-ily from renal tubular phosphate loss. Significant advances in the understanding of vitamin D metabolism over the past decade have yielded new insights into these syndromes.

The terms rickets and osteomalacia describe a group of diseases demonstrating similar gross pathologic, radiologic, and histologic abnormalities. The pathologic changes result from an interruption in orderly development and mineralization of the growth plate (rickets) or from inadequate or delayed mineralization of osteoid in mature cortical and spongy bone (osteomalacia). Therefore, prior to growth plate fusion, rickets and osteomalacia coexist.

The radiologic findings in affected bones and cartilage reflect the gross pathologic and histologic abnormalities. Although the general radiographic findings in all of the rachitic and osteomalacic syndromes are similar, some distinctive features may be of help in sorting out the various disease entities.

BIOCHEMISTRY OF VITAMIN D

Progress in the understanding of vitamin D metabolism has occurred at an exponentially rapid pace in the past 25 years, resulting in basic modifications of long-standing views. Until recently it was generally assumed that vitamin D was a vitamin and was metabolically unaltered prior to discharging its physiologic function. It has now been established that "vitamin D" (Fig. 48–1) is a prohormone that requires two sequential hydroxylations before the active hormonal form, 1,25-dihydroxyvitamin D_3 (1,25[OH]$_2$D$_3$), is produced. Two prohormonal forms of 1,25(OH)$_2$D are found in humans: vitamin D_3 and vitamin D_2. Vitamin D_3 is the natural, endogenously produced compound resulting from interaction of ultraviolet light with a cholesterol derivative, 7-dehydrocholesterol, in the deeper layers of the skin. The mechanism of this reaction is incompletely understood. Small amounts of exogenous vitamin D_3 may be derived from dietary sources, such as dairy products and fish liver oils. Vitamin D_2 is artificially prepared by irradiation of ergosterol obtained from yeast or fungi and is the compound used for food supplementation and pharmaceutical preparations.

Both vitamin D_3 and vitamin D_2 are hydroxylated at the carbon 25 position to form 25-OH-D$_3$ and 25-OH-D$_2$, respectively. This occurs predominantly in the liver but has also been noted in extrahepatic sites, such as the intestine and kidney. When both vitamin D_3 and vitamin D_2 are available in adequate amounts, the major portion of the circulating 25-hydroxylated form is 25-OH-D$_3$, which circulates bound to a specific binding protein.

Under physiologic conditions, 25-OH-D is further hydroxylated at the carbon 1 position, producing the physiologically active form of the hormone, 1,25(OH)$_2$D$_3$. The 1α hydroxylating enzyme (25-OH-D-1α hydroxylase) is found exclusively in renal tissue. The production of 1,25(OH)$_2$D is directly related to body needs and is closely regulated by multiple factors, which may be integrated into classic hormonal feedback loops. In comparison to 25-OH-D, the serum levels of 1,25(OH)$_2$D$_3$ are relatively low. 1,25(OH)$_2$D$_3$ is produced and metabolized rapidly, and, unlike 25-OH-D, has no significant tissue stores.

Although the kidney is the major site of formation and

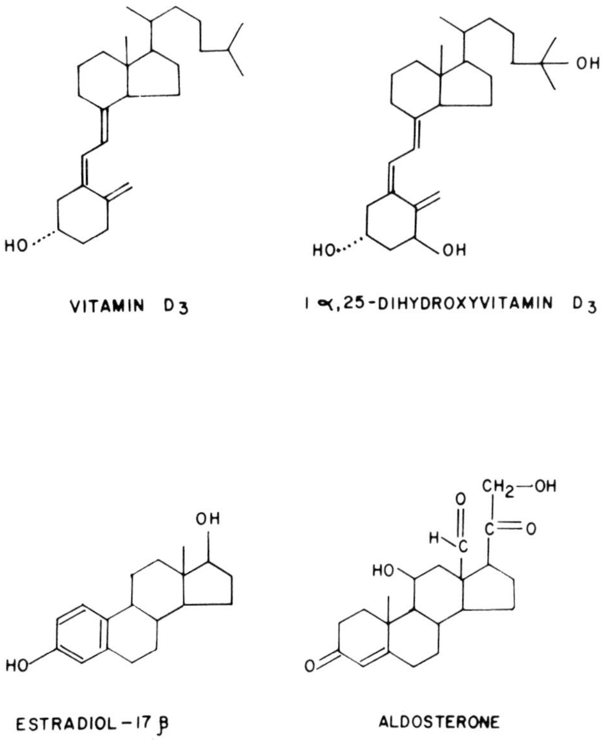

Figure 48–1. Chemical structures of vitamin D_3 and the active hormonal form, 1,25(OH)$_2$D$_3$. Note the structural similarities to other steroid hormones. (From Pitt MJ, Haussler MR: Vitamin D: Biochemistry and clinical applications. Skel Radiol 1:191, 1977. Used with permission.)

regulation of 1,25-(OH)$_2$D under *physiologic* conditions, extrarenal formation also occurs. Production of 1,25(OH)$_2$D by the placenta (which also produces other hormones) probably plays a direct role in fetal bone and mineral metabolism. In vitro formation of 1,25(OH)$_2$D in bone has also been demonstrated, suggesting that 1,25(OH)$_2$D may be produced at its major target site as well. Extrarenal production of 1,25(OH)$_2$D also has been reported in association with abnormal states including sarcoidosis and lymphoma.

Action of Vitamin D

The long-recognized functions of vitamin D are the homeostatic maintenance of serum calcium and phosphorus levels and the mineralization of bone. The physiologic form of the vitamin, 1,25(OH)$_2$D$_3$, acts on two main target organs—the intestine and bone. The kidney and the parathyroid glands are also sites of action.

INTESTINES. 1,25(OH)$_2$D acts on the intestine to increase the absorption of calcium and phosphorus. Although it has been well established that 1,25(OH)$_2$D increases intestinal calcium transport, its influence on phosphate absorption from the intestine has only recently been defined. In addition to passive absorption of phosphorus in conjunction with the active intestinal transport of calcium, active phosphate transporting mechanisms in response to vitamin D have also been demonstrated.

BONE. In the skeleton, 1,25(OH)$_2$D has two actions, which initially appear to be diametrically opposed: mobilization of calcium and phosphorus from previously formed bone and promotion of maturation and mineralization of organic matrix.

1,25(OH)$_2$D mobilizes calcium and phosphorus from previously formed bone by stimulating osteocytic osteolysis and in this way participates in the breakdown process occurring as part of skeletal homeostasis. The process requires the presence of both 1,25(OH)$_2$D and parathyroid hormone.

The presence of vitamin D clearly is essential for adequate deposition of bone mineral. Two hormonal roles are possible: the maintenance of adequate serum calcium and phosphorus levels or a direct effect on skeletal tissue (or both). Vitamin D's role in the preservation of normal serum levels of calcium and phosphorus has likewise been firmly established. Low levels of serum calcium or phosphorus, or both, regardless of cause (e.g., deficiency of 1,25[OH]$_2$D, diet, renal loss) are important factors in the development of rickets and osteomalacia. Clinical experience shows a poor correlation between the serum calcium and phosphorus concentrations and the severity of rachitic and osteomalacic states, however. Administration of vitamin D in these conditions can result in a positive bone mineralization response, which precedes correction of the serum calcium and phosphorus levels. Therefore, there is a distinct possibility that vitamin D metabolites have a direct effect on bone cells and matrix during the process of mineralization.

KIDNEY AND PARATHYROID GLANDS. Although the intestine and skeleton are the major targets of 1,25(OH)$_2$D$_3$ action, the kidney and parathyroid glands are also target organs affected by vitamin D. It appears that vitamin D has a direct effect on proximal renal tubular function. Furthermore, direct action of 1,25(OH)$_2$D$_3$ on the parathyroid glands has been demonstrated, with resulting suppression of parathyroid hormone secretion.

Regulators of 1,25(OH)$_2$D$_3$ Production

Considerable evidence exists to justify classifying vitamin D as a hormone. As with other hormones, only one specific organ, the kidney, produces the substance using the substrates formed in extrarenal sites. 1,25(OH)$_2$D$_3$ is secreted and transported to target organs, where it has an intranuclear mechanism of action resembling that of other steroid hormones. The renal production of 1,25(OH)$_2$D$_3$ is closely supervised by several factors that may be integrated into classic endocrine loops with typical feedback features. The established regulators are the levels of serum calcium, parathyroid hormone, and serum phosphate. Less certain are the roles of 1,25(OH)$_2$D itself, calcitonin, corticosteroids, sex hormones, thyroid hormone, and growth hormones.

CALCIUM AND PARATHYROID HORMONE. Although calcium and parathyroid hormone exert a significant regulatory influence on 1,25(OH)$_2$D formation, the issue of how this is accomplished remains to be more completely defined. Available data suggest that the increase in 1,25(OH)$_2$D$_3$ that is elicited by low serum calcium levels is mediated primarily by the parathyroid hormone, although the need for and importance of parathyroid hormone in this loop have been questioned. It is generally agreed that under acute conditions stimulation of 1,25(OH)$_2$D production by signals stemming from low calcium levels is mediated primarily by parathyroid hormone. Physiologically, in the absence of parathyroid hormone deficient or resistant states, this is most likely the important operative mechanism. In situations in which chronic parathyroid hormone deficiency or resistance exists, the body apparently has the adaptive capacity to produce 1,25(OH)$_2$D$_3$ in response to low serum calcium levels.

PHOSPHATE. Dietary and serum inorganic phosphorus levels significantly influence and regulate 1,25(OH)$_2$D$_3$ formation. Hypophosphatemia is frequently noted in the deficiency rachitic states, however, and is probably the primary factor in the development of rickets and osteomalacia in the syndromes associated with renal tubular phosphate loss (e.g., X-linked hypophosphatemia and Fanconi syndromes). Indeed, depression of serum phosphate may be of more importance than low calcium levels in the development of rickets and osteomalacia. Low dietary phosphate levels are associated with increased levels of 25-OH-D-1α hydroxylase activity and increased serum levels of 1,25(OH)$_2$D$_3$. Hypophosphatemia directly stimulates 1,25(OH)$_2$D$_3$ production; in contrast to the acute hypocalcemic signal, this effect is independent of parathyroid hormone.

1,25(OH)$_2$D$_3$ (A SELF-REGULATOR). 1,25(OH)$_2$D$_3$ affects its own production by both direct and indirect means. The indirect influence occurs through suppression of parathyroid hormone secretion. A direct negative feedback effect of 1,25(OH)$_2$D$_3$ on its own production has been demonstrated. Suppression of enzymatic conversion of 25-OH-D$_3$ to 1,25(OH)$_2$D$_3$ in isolated renal tubules occurs in the presence of 1,25(OH)$_2$D$_3$.

SUMMARY OF REGULATORY CONTROLS. Two main regulatory loops initiated by low serum calcium and low serum phosphate levels, respectively, may be postulated (Fig. 48–2). Acute depressions of serum calcium concentration signal the production of parathyroid hormone, which in turn stimulates 1,25(OH)$_2$D$_3$ production. Serum calcium and phosphate levels rise owing to the subsequent action of

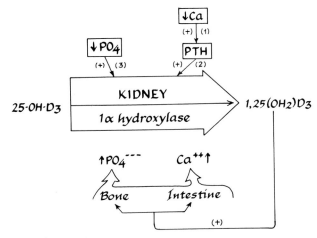

Figure 48–2. Regulatory loops initiated by low serum calcium and low serum phosphate levels. 25-OH-D is converted in the kidney to 1,25(OH)₂D by the action of the renal enzyme 1α-hydroxylase. This reaction is regulated by serum phosphate (3) and parathyroid hormone (2). Serum calcium (1) indirectly influences the reaction through its effect on the parathyroid glands. The two main target organs of 1,25(OH)₂D action, bone and intestine, are depicted. A plus (+) indicates a stimulatory effect. (From Pitt MJ, et al: Current concepts of vitamin D metabolism: Correlation with clinical syndromes. Crit Rev Radiol Sci 10:135, 1977. Used with permission.)

tive of both lesions are present in individuals affected prior to growth plate fusion. Although rickets and osteomalacia may coexist, it is convenient and classic to describe each separately.

The structure of the normal growth plate must be understood before the changes of rickets may be appreciated. The typical growth plate, a complex structure composed of fibrous, cartilaginous, and osseous tissues, is located at the ends of long bones and situated between the epiphysis and the metaphysis. Although the growth plate is in apposition to the epiphysis, it is functionally part of the shaft. Therefore, the commonly used term "epiphyseal plate" is inaccurate. The usual growth plate is discoid in configuration, but variations are present depending on the specific anatomic location.

Histologically, the cellular arrangement of the normal growth plate is characterized by *order* (Fig. 48–3). From epiphyseal to metaphyseal side, there is a progressive increase in the number and size of cartilage cells and a development of cell columns aligned with the long axis of the shaft. Zones of development may be identified:

1. *The reserve zone* (also termed resting or germinal zone) is subjacent to the epiphysis. The cartilage cells are few in number, are randomly situated either singly or in pairs, and are spherical in shape. They are not resting, are not germinal

1,25(OH₂)D₃ on the intestine and to the combined effects of parathyroid hormone and 1,25(OH)₂D₃ on bone, causing calcium and phosphate mobilization. The elevation of serum phosphate level is negated by increased renal excretion of phosphate as a result of parathyroid action on the renal tubules. The net result is an increase in serum calcium levels.

The hypophosphatemic signal directly stimulates 1,25(OH)₂D production. Elevation of serum phosphate and calcium levels results from 1,25(OH)₂D action on the intestine, bone, and kidney. Subsequent suppression of parathyroid hormone secretion, resulting from the 1,25(OH)₂D-induced elevation of serum calcium concentration and the direct suppressive effect of 1,25(OH)₂D on the parathyroid glands, together with the hypercalcemia, leads to an increase in urinary calcium excretion but a decrease in urinary phosphate excretion. 1,25(OH)₂D may also increase serum phosphate concentration by mobilization of phosphate from soft tissue stores. The total sequence accounts for a net increase in serum phosphate concentration.

1,25(OH)₂D acts to close each of these controlling loops by (directly and indirectly) depressing its own formation. The role of calcitonin and other hormones awaits further investigation.

STRUCTURAL PATHOANATOMY OF RICKETS AND OSTEOMALACIA
Gross Pathology and Histology

Regardless of their causes, the rachitic and osteomalacic syndromes display remarkably similar histologic and radiographic features. The characteristic changes of rickets are identified in the growth plates prior to closure; abnormalities of osteomalacia are seen in mature areas of trabecular and cortical bone. Because rickets and osteomalacia result from the same pathophysiologic mechanisms, findings representa-

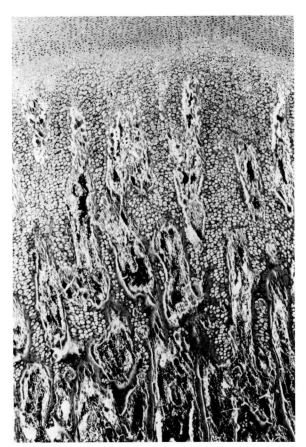

Figure 48–3. Normal chick growth plate with zone of proliferation at top. Observe orderly cartilaginous cell columns with zone of primary spongiosa at bottom. (Hematoxylin and eosin stain, 200×.) (From Pitt MJ, et al: Current concepts of vitamin D metabolism: Correlation with clinical syndromes. Crit Rev Radiol Sci 10:140, 1977. Used with permission.)

cells, and are not small in comparison with cells in the proliferative zone. Their function may be nutritional as they store various materials, particularly lipids.

2. *The proliferating zone* is where the chondrocytes become flattened and arranged into longitudinal, parallel columns. These are the only cells in the cartilaginous portion of the growth plate that actively divide. The function of this zone is matrix production and cellular proliferation.

3. *The hypertrophic zone* is a region that may be further subdivided into zones of *maturation, degeneration,* and *provisional calcification.* The change in cell morphology from the proliferative to the hypertrophic zones is usually abrupt and marked by sphericity and progressive enlargement. Cells nearing the metaphyseal side of the growth plate become quite large and vacuolated, with the last cells in the column becoming nonviable. The upper portions of this zone are active metabolically, and calcification of intervening cartilage matrix occurs.

4. *The zones of primary and secondary spongiosa* are located in the metaphysis immediately subjacent to the growth plate. Cartilage bars are partially or completely calcified and become ensheathed with osteoblasts, which produce layers of osteoid. Bone is produced by endochondral ossification.

The rachitic lesion displays disorganization in the growth plate and subjacent metaphysis (Fig. 48–4). The resting and

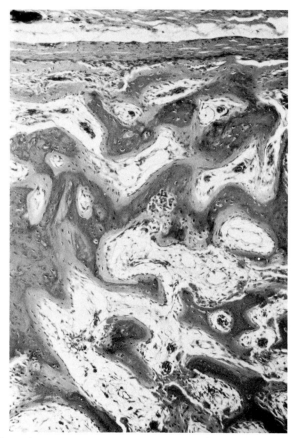

Figure 48–5. Osteomalacic cortex and subcortical spongy bone from metaphyseal region of a vitamin D–deficient chick. Trabeculae are thinned and irregular in shape and distribution. Sheaths of lightly stained osteoid almost equal the girth of bone in the trabeculae. Interspicular tissue is loosely fibrocartilaginous. (Hematoxylin and eosin stain, 500×.) (From Pitt MJ, et al: Current concepts of vitamin D metabolism: Correlation with clinical syndromes. Crit Rev Radiol Sci 10:141, 1977. Used with permission.)

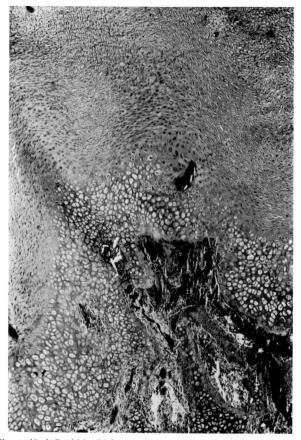

Figure 48–4. Rachitic chick growth plate with thick disordered hypertrophic zone virtually filling the field. Epiphyseal side appears at top. (Hematoxylin and eosin stain, 200×.) (From Pitt MJ, et al: Current concepts of vitamin D metabolism: Correlation with clinical syndromes. Crit Rev Radiol Sci 10:140, 1977. Used with permission.)

proliferative zones of the cartilaginous growth plate are not altered significantly from the normal pattern. The zone of maturation is grossly abnormal, however, with a disorganized increase in the number of cells and a loss of normal columnar pattern. This cell mass results in an increase in length and width of the growth plate. Concomitantly, vascular intrusion from the metaphysis and subsequent calcification of the intervening cartilaginous bars are decreased and grossly disordered. Defective mineralization in the zone of primary spongiosa and a lack of proper formation of bone lamellae and haversian systems occur.

Osteomalacia (Fig. 48–5) is characterized by abnormal quantities of osteoid (inadequately mineralized bone matrix) coating the surfaces of trabeculae and lining the haversian canals in the cortex ("osteoid seams"). Trabeculae become thin and decrease in number. In the cortex, the haversian systems become irregular and large channels develop. Osteoid seams are not pathognomonic for osteomalacia and may be found in other states of high bone turnover. In osteomalacia, however, there is an increase in both the number and width of these osteoid seams. Looser's lines or Milkman's pseudofractures, which are radiographically diagnostic of osteomalacia, are composed of focal accumulations of osteoid. Osteitis fibrosa cystica frequently is superimposed on the lesions of rickets and osteomalacia, reflecting hyperparathyroidism (secondary to the low serum calcium level). This feature is particularly prominent in renal osteodystrophy.

Radiologic Diagnosis of Rickets and Osteomalacia

RICKETS. Rachitic changes are more obvious in regions of the most active growth. Therefore, in order of decreasing sensitivity, the sites of highest radiographic yield would be the costochondral junctions of middle ribs, the distal part of the femur, the proximal part of the humerus, both ends of the tibia, and the distal ends of the ulna and radius.

Nonspecific radiographic features of rickets include a general retardation in body growth and osteopenia. Characteristic changes at the growth plate reflect the disordered increase in cell growth in the zone of hypertrophy, coupled with the deficient mineralization of the zone of provisional calcification (Fig. 48–6). Slight axial widening at the growth plate represents the earliest specific radiographic change. This is followed by a decrease in density at the zone of provisional calcification (on the metaphyseal side of the growth plate). As the disease progresses, further widening of the growth plate occurs, and the zone of provisional calcification becomes

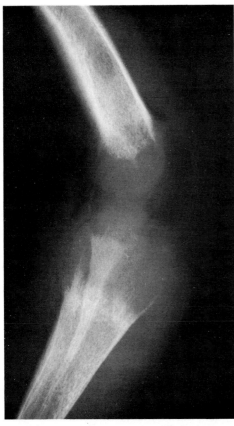

Figure 48–6. Knee radiograph of 6 week old chick showing advanced dietary deficiency rickets. Observe the advanced demineralization and disorganization in the metaphysis subjacent to the enlarged (unmineralized) growth plates. A thin rim of circumferential new bone is seen surrounding the rachitic growth plate in the tibia. Also note the thickened, blunted posterior femoral cortex representing an increase in inadequately mineralized osteoid. (From Pitt MJ, et al: Current concepts of vitamin D metabolism: Correlation with clinical syndromes. Crit Rev Radiol Sci 10:144, 1977. Used with permission.)

irregular. Disorganization and "fraying" of the spongy bone occur in the metaphyseal region. Widening and cupping of the metaphysis can be explained by the chaotic cartilage cell growth in the zone of maturation, which deposits an increased cell mass in both the longitudinal and the latitudinal axes; this bulky mass places abnormal stress on the growth plate with inward protrusion on the more central areas of the metaphysis. On occasion, a thin bony margin is seen extending from the peripheral portions of the metaphysis surrounding the uncalcified cartilage mass (Fig. 48–6).

Conceptually, the ossified center of the epiphysis is surrounded by cartilage cells, which are organized in a similar fashion to the growth plate. The peripheral rim of the ossified epiphyseal nucleus is analogous to the zone of provisional calcification. Changes similar to those seen in the growth plate are present, consisting of deossification and unsharpness of the ossified periphery.

The bulky growth plates at the shaft bone-cartilage junctions of long bones and ribs explain some of the characteristic physical findings of rickets. Swelling about joints is typical and a "rachitic rosary" develops at the costochondral junctions of the middle ribs. These latter areas are weakened, and frequently they are depressed. An additional semicoronal impression may be found at the costal attachment of the diaphragm (Harrison's groove).

The deformities caused by rickets exhibit different patterns, depending on the child's age when the disease develops. The head is particularly affected during the first months of life. During this period, the skull must accommodate to the most rapidly growing organ, the brain. The rapid accommodation by the skull is associated with excess osteoid formation, particularly at the central margins and outer table. Resorption at the inner table continues. The thin calvarium is subject to supine postural influences, resulting in posterior flattening. Continued accumulation of osteoid in the frontal and parietal regions results in the squared configuration known as craniotabes.

During infancy and early childhood, the long bones show the greatest deformity, both at the cartilage-shaft junctions and in the diaphyses. The characteristic bowing deformities of the arms and legs can be related to the sitting position assumed by the infant and child. Bowing is also a result of displacement of the growth centers owing to asymmetric musculotendinous pulls on the weakened growth plate. For example, the saber shin deformity of the tibia results from the strong posterior pull of the Achilles tendon on the calcaneus.

With increasing age the effects of weight-bearing become prominent. Scoliosis frequently develops and, coupled with bending deformities of long bones, results in an overall decrease in height. The intervertebral discs expand, producing concave impressions on the vertebral endplates. The skull shows basilar invagination, and intrusion of the hip and spine into the soft pelvis produces a triradiate configuration. The sacral orientation becomes more horizontal.

OSTEOMALACIA. The radiographic confirmation of osteomalacia is difficult. Many changes, such as osteopenia, are nonspecific. Areas of spongy bone show a decrease in the total number of trabeculae, owing to a loss of secondary trabeculae. The remaining trabeculae appear prominent and project a "coarsened" pattern; careful attention to their margins reveals an unsharpness reflecting the inadequately mineralized coats

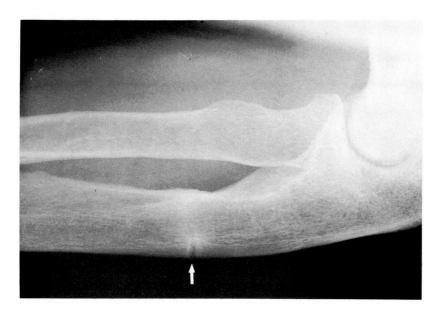

Figure 48–7. Pseudofracture (arrow) in adult patient with X-linked hypophosphatemic osteomalacia occurring in characteristic location in proximal ulna. Note bowing of ulna. (From Pitt MJ, et al: Current concepts of vitamin D metabolism: Correlation with clinical syndromes. Crit Rev Radiol Sci 10:145, 1977. Used with permission.)

of osteoid. Lucent sites in the cortex reflect accumulations of osteoid and widened, irregular haversian canals.

Pseudofractures or Looser's zones may precede other radiographic changes. These lucent areas are oriented at right angles to the cortex and incompletely span the diameter of the bone. They tend to occur in characteristic sites, such as the axillary margins of the scapula, ribs, superior and inferior pubic rami, inner margins of the proximal femora, and posterior margins of the proximal ulnae (Fig. 48–7). Pseudofractures typically are bilateral and symmetric. Sclerosis often demarcates the intraosseous margins; new bone on the periosteal aspect suggests callus. Radiolucent areas similar to pseudofractures may be found in bones affected by Paget's disease and fibrous dysplasia. The radiolucent zones in these diseases, however, are confined to the affected bone and, unlike pseudofractures, are not generalized.

The mechanism of formation of Looser's zones is not clearly defined. They have been attributed to a mechanical erosive process on the softened cortex from adjacent blood vessels and to accelerated bone turnover at sites of stress.

CLINICAL SYNDROMES

The terms rickets and osteomalacia encompass a group of disorders with similar gross pathologic, histologic, radiologic, and biochemical findings but diverse causes. An etiologic approach to the rachitic and osteomalacic disorders, as shown in Figure 48–8, includes the following:

1. Abnormalities of vitamin D metabolism:
   Abnormalities in prohormone vitamin D
   Abnormalities in 25-OH-D
   Abnormalities in 1,25(OH)$_2$D

2. Rachitic and osteomalacic syndromes resulting primarily from renal tubular *phosphate loss*.

3. Rachitic and osteomalacic syndromes that do not show abnormalities of vitamin D metabolism or aberrations of calcium or phosphorus metabolism.

Table 4–1 lists useful points in diagnosing specific syndromes.

Vitamin D Deficiency

Classic vitamin D deficiency rickets is uncommonly encountered in the United States today owing to the widespread addition of synthetic vitamin D$_2$ to foods, notably dairy products and bread. The natural source of vitamin D for humans, however, is not dietary. Rather, humans depend mainly on the ultraviolet rays of the sun for endogenous conversion of 7-dehydrocholesterol in the skin to the prohormone vitamin D$_3$ (cholecalciferol). Therefore, a reasonable degree of exposure to the sun should prevent the development of rickets and osteomalacia in the normal person whose diet contains adequate amounts of calcium and phosphorus.

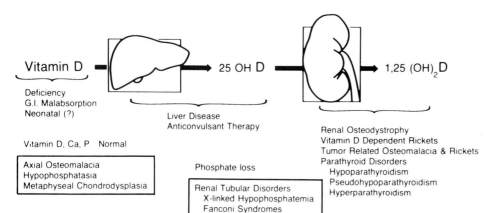

Figure 48–8. Etiologic approach to the rachitic and osteomalacic syndromes. This approach is organized in a framework of (1) abnormalities of vitamin D; (2) syndromes secondary to renal tubular loss of phosphate; and (3) syndromes in which there is known abnormality of vitamin D metabolism or calcium-phosphorus homeostasis.

Table 48–1. RADIOGRAPHIC FEATURES OF SPECIFIC RACHITIC AND OSTEOMALACIC STATES

1. Nonspecific radiographic changes of rickets and osteomalacia
   a. Patients less than 6 months of age: Consider biliary atresia, vitamin D–dependent rickets, hypophosphatasia, and rickets associated with prematurity.
   b. If there is resistance to usual doses of vitamin D (in the absence of chronic glomerular renal disease): Consider a renal tubular disorder, tumor association, hypophosphatasia, or metaphyseal chondrodysplasia, type Schmid. Note: *Mild* changes of secondary hyperparathyroidism may be present.
2. Renal osteodystrophy (uremic osteopathy): Radiographic changes of secondary hyperparathyroidism are usually present and predominate over the pattern of deossification. Osteosclerotic foci, particularly in the spine adjacent to the cartilaginous endplates (rugger-jersey spine), are characteristic. Vascular calcification of the Mönckeberg type and, less commonly, large "tumoral" deposits of amorphous calcification may be identified, particularly around joints.
3. X-linked hypophosphatemia
   a. Children: Rachitic changes at the growth plates are usually only mild to moderate in degree. General osteoporosis is uncommon and the bones, although bowed, are "strong" in appearance.
   b. Adults: Generalized increase in bone density may be present, particularly in the axial skeleton. Changes may suggest ankylosing spondylitis. Characteristic is paravertebral calcification, multiple small ossified dense areas near joints, and new bone formation at ligamentous and tendinous attachments in the extremities. Biochemical tests reveal hyperphosphaturia with low serum phosphate concentration.
4. Axial osteomalacia: Radiographic abnormalities are confined to axial skeleton. Dense, coarse trabecular pattern is most marked in the cervical region. Lumbar spine, pelvis, and ribs are also involved. The skull is normal. This disorder affects men, symptoms are minimal, and biochemical values are within normal limits.
5. Primary biliary cirrhosis: Mild to moderate generalized deossification. Hands show small, asymmetric, intracapsular marginal erosions. Symptoms are mild; the arthritis is nondeforming.
6. Hypophosphatasia: Varies in severity. Newborn infants may show advanced demineralization. Rachitic growth plates show characteristic multiple lucent extensions into the metaphyses. Wormian bones and craniosynostosis may be present.
7. Metaphyseal chondrodysplasia, type Schmid: Multiple small bone projections extend from metaphyses into rachitic growth plates. Long bones maintain normal density. Skull is within normal limits. Spontaneous healing occurs.

In worldwide perspective, deficiency rickets and osteomalacia still represent a health problem. In the United Kingdom, the occurrence of rickets and osteomalacia among the immigrant Indian and Pakistani population is significant. The factors contributing to the development of rickets and osteomalacia in the British Asian population are multiple; however, ethnic traditions and dietary patterns are most contributory. The custom of Asian girls and women to remain indoors and wear traditional dress decreases their exposure to the sun, thus limiting endogenous production of vitamin D. Chupatti flour, a dietary staple in this group, is also an important factor. The high phytate content in the wheat fiber binds to calcium and zinc and results in increased fecal loss. In addition, lignin, a component of the wheat fiber, binds to bile acids and increases their fecal excretion. Vitamin D may combine with this fiber-bile acid complex and be unavailable for absorption.

Deficiency rickets and osteomalacia have been reported even in sun-rich areas. Again, custom and diet are major factors. In Nigeria, deficiency rickets may relate to the custom of purdah, in which mothers and their children are inadequately exposed to the sun. In the United States, among followers of food cults and food fads, reports of rickets in children on vegetarian diets have appeared.

In developed countries, it is important to appreciate the occurrence of osteomalacia in the elderly, particularly those patients who are house-bound or institutionalized for long periods. Although decreased exposure to the sun is a prime cause, other postulated factors include deficient intake of oral vitamin D_2, intestinal malabsorption of the elderly, and lower vitamin D hydroxylase activity in the liver and kidney.

Although "deficiency" rickets (and osteomalacia) usually connotes a lack of vitamin D, insufficiencies of calcium or phosphorus, or both, should also be considered. Rickets secondary to phosphorus deficiency usually is a result of congenital or acquired renal disease. Proximal renal tubular dysfunction with defective absorption of phosphorus is seen in X-linked hypophosphatemia and Fanconi syndromes. Phosphate loss may also complicate hemodialysis, cadaveric renal transplantation, or excessive ingestion of aluminum hydroxide, which binds phosphate in the gut. Rickets secondary to insufficient calcium in the diet is rare.

Gastrointestinal Malabsorption

Disorders of the small bowel, hepatobiliary system, and pancreas associated with intestinal malabsorption are the most common causes of vitamin D deficiency in the United States. Rickets and osteomalacia may develop in many small bowel malabsorptive states, including sprue, gluten-sensitive enteropathy (celiac disease) (Fig. 48–9), regional enteritis, sclero-

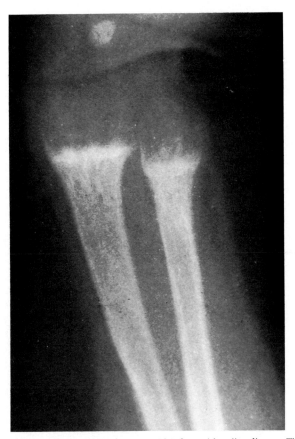

Figure 48–9. Rickets in a 4 month old infant with celiac disease. The metaphysis is demineralized and disorganized. Metaphyseal widening reflects the enlarged growth plate.

derma, and even unusual conditions such as multiple jejunal diverticula or stagnant (blind) loop syndromes. Decreased absorption and excessive fecal loss of both vitamin D and (probably) calcium are contributory. Rickets and osteomalacia have also been reported after small bowel or gastric resection.

Malabsorption associated with pancreatic insufficiency, even when pronounced, is infrequently associated with osteomalacia. Children with cystic fibrosis, in contrast to other malabsorptive diseases, seldom develop rickets.

Rickets Associated with Prematurity (Neonatal Rickets)

Abnormal mineral homeostasis with low serum levels of calcium and phosphorus is a well recognized complication in low birth weight premature infants. Although uncommon, radiographic evidence of metabolic bone disease, predominantly rickets and osteomalacia, is being recognized and reported. Affected infants are usually below 1000 gm birth weight or of less than 28 weeks' gestation. Although bone disease usually appears at about 12 weeks of age, it may develop later, particularly in situations in which prolonged parenteral nutrition is required (Fig. 48–10).

The pathogenesis of the bone disease can be related to a combination of nutritional, metabolic, and sometimes iatrogenic factors. Skeletal development is occurring at a very rapid rate during the last trimester of pregnancy. Therefore, the requirements for calcium, phosphorus, and vitamin D of the premature infant are greater than those of the infant born at term. This increased need usually is not provided for in the diet. Human milk and standard infant formulas, which are adequate for the term baby, have insufficient amounts of

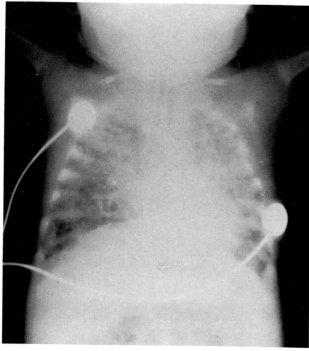

Figure 48–10. Four month old infant with generalized rachitic changes. Observe demineralization and disorganization of proximal humeral metaphyses. Respiratory distress syndrome developed after premature birth, with subsequent development of bronchopulmonary dysplasia. Parenteral nutrition provided inadequate amounts of vitamin D and calcium.

vitamin D, phosphorus, and probably calcium for the premature infant. It also is possible that the rickets of prematurity is related to abnormal vitamin D metabolism, perhaps to immaturity of $1,25(OH)_2D$ receptors in the intestine, bone, and other tissues rather than to a deficiency in $1,25(OH)_2D$ itself.

Liver Disease

Metabolic bone disease, termed hepatic osteodystrophy, is a well-recognized complication of chronic biliary ductal and hepatocellular disorders. Both osteoporosis and osteomalacia are found histologically. Although many patients are asymptomatic, morbidity relating to bone pain, tenderness, and fractures may be significant, particularly in patients with primary biliary cirrhosis and other chronic cholestatic diseases.

When present, radiologic changes are usually those of nonspecific osteopenia. Pseudofractures indicate the presence of osteomalacia. Hypertrophic osteoarthropathy and articular abnormalities have been reported but are not common (see Chapter 27).

Like renal osteodystrophy, the cause of hepatic osteodystrophy is multifactorial. Because the liver is the major site for the initial hydroxylation of vitamin D, abnormalities in vitamin D metabolism might be expected. 25-Hydroxylation activity of the liver appears to be almost normal, however. The low serum levels of 25-OH-D are more likely a reflection of inadequate amounts of prohormone resulting from decreased exposure to ultraviolet light, decreased vitamin D supplementation, and, particularly if steatorrhea is present, malabsorption of vitamin D.

Rickets developing in patients with neonatal hepatitis may be more common than is generally appreciated. Furthermore, because bile salts are necessary for the absorption of vitamin D, biliary duct obstruction, such as that which occurs in congenital biliary atresia (usually extrahepatic duct involvement), may be associated with typical rachitic changes, which may appear before 6 months of age.

Anticonvulsant Drug-Related Rickets and Osteomalacia

Rickets and osteomalacia may be seen both histologically and radiographically in patients receiving anticonvulsant drug therapy, particularly phenobarbital and phenytoin (Dilantin). The frequency of clinical bone disease and abnormal radiographic changes in these patients is probably low. Although the mechanisms responsible for the production of rickets and osteomalacia are incompletely understood, decreased exposure to sunlight in institutionalized patients and interference with vitamin D metabolism by the anticonvulsant drugs themselves may be involved. The mechanism of action of the various anticonvulsant drugs differs with regard to the development of bone disease. Although both phenytoin and phenobarbital induce hepatic hydroxylase activity, phenytoin, but not phenobarbital, also decreases intestinal absorption of calcium, apparently by decreasing the activity of vitamin D–dependent calcium binding protein. These findings may implicate phenytoin as the most important anticonvulsant drug in the development of osteomalacia.

The reported frequency of radiographic changes of rickets and osteomalacia in association with anticonvulsant drug therapy has varied. When present, the radiographic changes are nonspecific and cannot be differentiated from rickets or osteomalacia resulting from other causes. Changes of osteomalacia may be quite severe, particularly in nonambulatory, long-term institutionalized patients. Long-term phenytoin therapy, in addition to producing radiographic evidence of rickets, may also be associated with diffuse calvarial thickening, dental root abnormalities varying from widespread resorption to stumpy shortening, cleft palate, and occasional syndactyly.

Renal Osteodystrophy (Uremic Osteopathy)

The bone disease associated with chronic renal failure results from multiple complex factors. Although the pathogenesis remains incompletely explained, two main mechanisms (probably acting in concert) are responsible: secondary hyperparathyroidism and abnormal vitamin D metabolism.

SECONDARY HYPERPARATHYROIDISM. Secondary hyperparathyroidism is consistently noted in untreated uremia occurring early in the course of the disease. Parathyroid hormone levels may be significantly increased and frequently are higher than the levels reached in primary hyperparathyroidism. The secondary hyperparathyroidism is provoked by hypocalcemia, which results from several different mechanisms; phosphate retention is the major factor. Phosphate retention becomes more constant with moderate to advanced renal failure, and the elevated serum phosphate concentration reciprocally depresses serum calcium level (calcium × phosphorus ion product).

ABNORMAL VITAMIN D METABOLISM. The singular importance of the kidney as the only organ capable of producing the physiologically active form of vitamin D, $1,25(OH)_2D$, has been emphasized earlier in this chapter. It would therefore be anticipated that loss of renal tissue in acquired renal disease would be associated with low levels of $1,25(OH)_2D$. The hyperphosphatemia of renal failure also inhibits $1,25(OH)_2D$ production.

HISTOLOGY AND RADIOLOGY. The histologic and radiographic findings in chronic renal failure reflect hyperparathyroidism and deficiency of $1,25(OH)_2D$: The major abnormalities are osteitis fibrosa cystica, osteomalacia or rickets (or both), osteosclerosis (representing areas of increased bone volume), and osteoporosis (see also Chapter 52). The reported predominance of these features varies and does not correlate well with clinical or laboratory signs.

Histologic evidence of secondary hyperparathyroidism is invariably present and is usually the dominant finding. The extent of bone resorption depends on the duration and degree of elevation of parathyroid hormone concentration. Osteomalacia or rickets, or both, is present in variable degrees and in several patterns. An increase in the number of osteoid borders or seams surrounding trabecular bone frequently is present but may result from either parathyroid hormone excess or vitamin D deficiency. Osteomalacia is a comparatively infrequent finding.

Radiographic abnormalities in chronic renal disease are found in both the bones and the soft tissues. Bone changes reflect the abnormal histology and display secondary hyperparathyroidism, rickets or osteomalacia, or both, and osteosclerosis (Fig. 48–11). A combination of these abnormalities frequently is present.

Rickets may be the presenting feature and the first indication of chronic renal disease in children. Osteitis fibrosa cystica may also be quite conspicuous. General retardation of

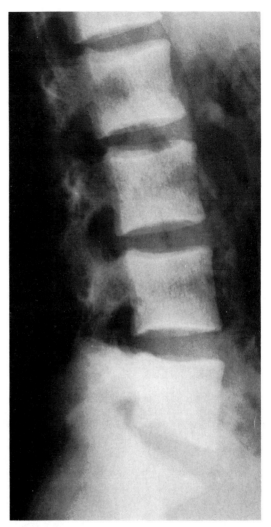

Figure 48–11. Chronic renal disease. Areas of increased sclerosis subjacent to the cartilaginous plates (rugger-jersey spine) are demonstrated in a patient with chronic renal failure.

growth is noted as the disease progresses. In adults, the earliest radiographic changes are usually found in the hands. Subperiosteal resorption of bone on the radial aspects of the middle phalanges of the index and long fingers is identified. A similar lack of definition may be seen in the cortex of the phalangeal tufts. With more advanced disease, other bones show evidence of subperiosteal resorption in concave areas ("cutback zones"), such as the medial margins of the femoral necks and inner aspects of the proximal tibiae. Widening of various joints, such as the acromioclavicular and sacroiliac joints and symphysis pubis, may occur secondary to subchondral resorption of bone and replacement fibrosis. Brown tumors, previously thought to be unusual in uremic osteopathy, are being seen and reported with increasing frequency.

Areas of increased density (osteosclerosis) frequently are seen in uremic osteopathy and histologically represent accumulations of excessive osteoid. These areas are characteristic in the spine, subjacent to the cartilaginous plates, and account for the characteristic rugger-jersey appearance (Fig. 48–11). Areas of increased sclerosis are also noted in the pelvis and metaphyses of long bones.

Soft tissue calcifications in uremia may be visceral or

nonvisceral. Visceral calcification occurs in the heart, lungs, skeletal muscle, stomach, and kidneys. With the exception of the kidneys and lungs, these changes are rarely detected radiographically. Nonvisceral calcification occurs in the eyes, skin, periarticular areas, and arteries. The calcium deposition in visceral areas is amorphous; nonvisceral calcified areas demonstrate a hydroxyapatite composition almost identical to that of uremic bone. Vascular calcification is of the Mönckeberg type and probably is a reflection of hyperphosphatemia. Accumulations of amorphous calcium in periarticular regions are also a reflection of increased serum phosphate levels. These deposits can become quite large; they may be single or multiple and appear multiloculated (Fig. 48–12). These masses may be painful, and they often drain spontaneously through the skin. Periarticular calcification in the capsule and tendons of both large and small joints is not uncommon. Chondrocalcinosis, a feature of primary hyperparathyroidism, is less common in advanced renal failure.

Hereditary Vitamin D–Dependent Rickets

Hereditary vitamin D–dependent rickets, also termed pseudovitamin D–dependent rickets, is a rare disorder characterized by the clinical, radiographic, and biochemical features

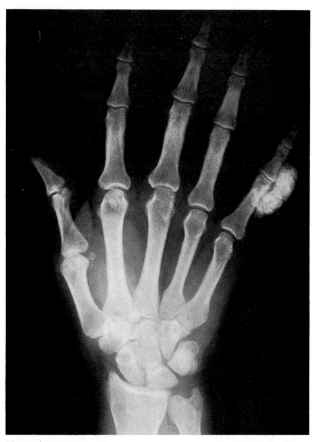

Figure 48–12. Tumoral calcinosis adjacent to the proximal interphalangeal joint of the little finger in a patient with chronic renal failure. Note the septated appearance of the calcium deposits. This patient had received large doses of vitamin D. Secondary hyperparathyroidism is reflected by the unsharpness of the phalangeal tufts and the subperiosteal bone resorption on the radial aspects of the middle phalanges of the index and long fingers.

of vitamin D deficiency. Vitamin D intake is normal, however, and there is no evidence of other disease states, such as intestinal malabsorption and liver or kidney disorders, which would account for derangement in vitamin D metabolism. Symptoms may be present as early as 3 months of age (in contrast to the later onset of nutritional rickets), with most patients being symptomatic by 1 year of age. Rachitic bone changes may be severe and rapidly progressive, with pathologic fractures. Although hypophosphatemia is present, the primary rachitogenic factor is hypocalcemia, which results from a decrease in intestinal calcium absorption; secondary hyperparathyroidism follows. The effect of elevated parathyroid hormone levels on the kidney is responsible for the hyperphosphaturia, aminoaciduria, and hypophosphatemia.

Tumor-Associated Rickets and Osteomalacia

Hypophosphatemic vitamin D–refractory rickets and osteomalacia in association with various neoplasms have been recognized with increasing frequency. The associated neoplasms have occurred in children and adults, are located in soft tissues or bone, and vary in size. The lesions typically are vascular and often show foci of new bone formation; the most frequent histologic diagnosis has been hemangiopericytoma. Although most of the neoplasms have been of mesenchymal origin, the syndrome has been reported in association with prostatic carcinoma and with oat cell carcinoma of the lung. Bone lesions have included nonossifying fibroma, giant cell tumor, osteoblastoma, and a non-neoplastic disease—fibrous dysplasia. Although the tumors usually are histologically benign, some may be malignant. Patients frequently have generalized muscle weakness. Radiographic changes of rickets and osteomalacia may be advanced. Hypophosphatemia is the predominant biochemical feature and is secondary to failure of renal tubular reabsorption of phosphate. Serum calcium level is within normal limits. Serum alkaline phosphatase concentration usually is elevated. Parathyroid hormone levels generally are within normal limits.

The cause of the decreased renal tubular absorption of phosphate remains unidentified. Circumstantial evidence suggests the presence of a tumor-elaborated humoral substance that directly affects renal phosphate absorption in the proximal tubule.

Rickets and Osteomalacia Secondary to Phosphate Loss

A number of rachitic and osteomalacic syndromes have been identified, which, although differing in genetic and clinical features, share one or several renal tubular abnormalities: renal phosphate loss with secondary hypophosphatemia, glycosuria, aminoaciduria, renal tubular acidosis, hypokalemia, and vasopressin-resistant polyuria. These diseases are collectively designated Fanconi syndromes. The most common is cystinosis; tyrosinemia and the oculocerebrorenal syndrome (Lowe's syndrome) are other, less common examples. In addition to congenital diseases, similar acquired renal tubular disorders may be secondary to drug toxicity, heavy metal intoxication, paraproteinemias, and tumors.

X-LINKED HYPOPHOSPHATEMIA. X-linked hypophosphatemia (also known as familial vitamin D–resistant rickets) is the most common form of renal tubular rickets and osteomalacia. The classic syndrome is genetically transmitted as an X-linked dominant trait, with men being affected to a

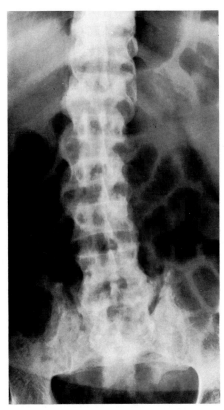

Figure 48–13. X-linked hypophosphatemia. Multifocal areas of paravertebral ossification are similar to those in diffuse idiopathic skeletal hyperostosis or ankylosing spondylitis. Abnormalities of both sacroiliac joints result from ossification of the anterior sacroiliac ligaments.

linked hypophosphatemia and may lead to symptoms. In the pelvis, multiple sites of calcification may involve the acetabulum, iliolumbar ligaments, and sacroiliac ligaments. The appendicular skeleton shows multiple sites of new bone formation at various muscle and ligament attachments. Separate small ossicles may develop around various joints, particularly those in the carpus (Fig. 48–14).

X-linked hypophosphatemia and the various Fanconi syndromes produce rickets and osteomalacia principally by renal tubular phosphate loss. It has been suggested that there are two separate renal tubular mechanisms for phosphate resorption: a parathyroid hormone–sensitive component, which is responsible for about two thirds of the total net resorption, and an additional system, which is responsive to the serum calcium level. The parathyroid hormone–sensitive component is completely absent in male patients with X-linked hypophosphatemia and is partially absent in female patients, perhaps explaining the phosphaturia that is characteristic of this condition. Abnormalities in vitamin D metabolism also have been demonstrated in both X-linked hypophosphatemia and the Fanconi syndromes. The relative importance of these abnormalities is uncertain but they may contribute to the pathogenesis of the bone disease.

Atypical Axial Osteomalacia

Atypical axial osteomalacia is a rare condition in which radiographic changes are characteristic. Skeletal involvement is axial, with sparing of appendicular sites (Fig. 48–15). A dense, coarse trabecular pattern involves primarily the cervical

greater degree than women. The syndrome is characterized by lifelong hypophosphatemia that is secondary to renal tubular phosphate loss, decreased intestinal absorption of calcium, and normal serum levels of calcium. Rickets generally appears between 12 and 18 months of age. Remission usually follows growth plate closure, but recurrence of symptoms is common later in life. Patients typically are short, bowlegged, and stocky. Systemic signs such as muscle weakness and hypotonia are absent. The development and severity of rickets may differ among patients with the classic syndrome.

Radiographic features may allow the specific diagnosis of this syndrome. Rachitic changes at the growth plates, in themselves nonspecific, usually are of only mild degree. Osteopenia is not prominent. Bowing of long bones, particularly of the lower extremities, may occur, but deformity frequently is minimal. With increasing age, the trabecular pattern becomes coarsened. Looser's zones may be present and can be complicated by complete fractures. By adulthood, a generalized increase in bone density, especially in the axial skeleton, is characteristic. Enthesopathic calcification and ossification may develop in the paravertebral ligaments, anulus fibrosus, and capsules of apophyseal and appendicular joints (Figs. 48–13 and 48–14). The spinal changes may resemble those of ankylosing spondylitis or diffuse idiopathic skeletal hyperostosis. In contrast to ankylosing spondylitis, however, the sacroiliac joints in X-linked hypophosphatemia show no bone erosions. Narrowing of the lumbar canal secondary to decreased growth of the pedicles is a frequent finding in X-

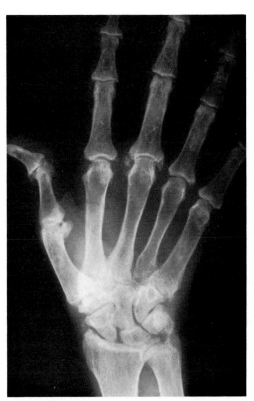

Figure 48–14. X-linked hypophosphatemia. Small ossicles are noted at the radial aspect of the wrist, and ossification of triangular fibrocartilage is present. Capsular ossification is noted at multiple interphalangeal and metacarpophalangeal joints.

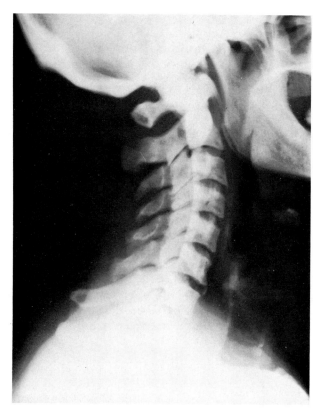

Figure 48–15. Atypical axial osteomalacia. A dense, coarse trabecular pattern involves the cervical spine. The appendicular skeleton was normal. (Courtesy of D. Resnick, M.D., San Diego, California.)

spine but is also present in the lumbar spine, pelvis, and ribs. Looser's zones have not been identified.

All reported patients have been men. Their general health is good, symptoms are minimal, and the biochemical findings are within normal limits. Biopsy of the involved areas demonstrates typical osteomalacia. There is no response to vitamin D therapy.

Hypophosphatasia

Hypophosphatasia is a rare disorder, genetically transmitted in an autosomal recessive pattern and characterized by defective skeletal mineralization resembling that of rickets and osteomalacia, low serum alkaline phosphatase levels, and abnormal amounts of phosphoethanolamine in the urine and blood. Although most patients are diagnosed during infancy or childhood, in some patients the condition may not be recognized until adult life. The most severely affected infants usually die soon after birth. Generalized deficient or absent mineralization is noted radiologically. Fractures with deformity and shortening of the extremities occur.

Patients surviving infancy display varying degrees of skeletal involvement. The growth plates demonstrate irregular, often prominent, lucent extensions into the metaphysis representing uncalcified bone matrix (Fig. 48–16). A coarse trabecular pattern, bowing deformities with or without healing fractures, and subperiosteal new bone accumulation may be present. Craniosynostosis involving all sutures is common, and wormian (intersutural) bones may be identified.

Uncommonly, the disease may be manifested first in

adulthood, with fractures that occur after minor injury and that heal slowly. Radiography suggests osteomalacia with a coarse trabecular pattern, bowing deformities, Looser's zones, and subperiosteal bone formation. A small skull may be present as a result of craniosynostosis. Calcification of ligamentous and tendinous attachments to bone and in paravertebral areas has been described.

Metaphyseal Chondrodysplasia (Type Schmid)

Metaphyseal chondrodysplasias encompass a variety of disorders that have in common generalized symmetric disturbance of endochondral bone formation, primarily at the metaphyses. The type described by Schmid is the most common and has radiologic features very similar to those of X-linked hypophosphatemic rickets (vitamin D–resistant rickets). Normal levels of serum phosphorus, alkaline phosphatase, and calcium differentiate these disorders from other rachitic syndromes.

The disease becomes manifested in childhood with short stature, bowing of long bones, and an accentuated lumbar lordosis with a waddling gait. The clinical course is benign. The disease is transmitted in an autosomal dominant pattern, but spontaneous mutations occur.

In the child, radiographs show widening of the growth plates, particularly in the more rapidly growing areas. In contrast to usual rickets, the metaphysis is well mineralized and may actually show increased density. Fine, spur-like

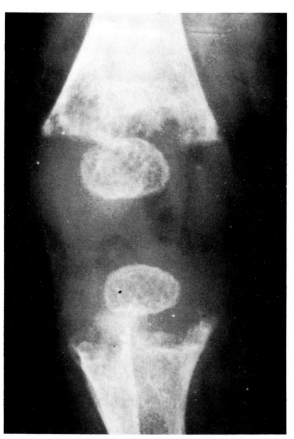

Figure 48–16. Hypophosphatasia. Deossification is present adjacent to the growth plates. Characteristic radiolucent areas extend from the growth plates into the metaphysis.

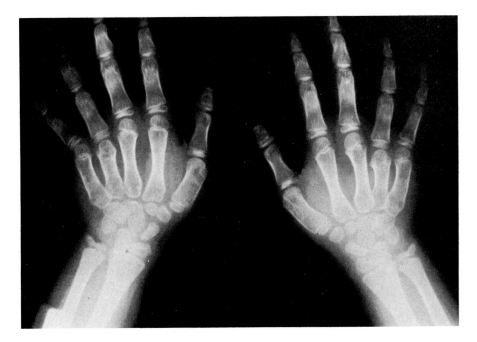

Figure 48–17. Pseudohypoparathyroidism (Albright's hereditary osteodystrophy). In a 9 year old boy, note shortening of all metacarpals, particularly the fourth.

projections of organized bone may extend into the growth plate from the metaphysis. The long bones are bowed. There is a notable absence of Looser's zones or signs of secondary hyperparathyroidism. The lesions tend to heal spontaneously.

Pseudohypoparathyroidism and Pseudopseudohypoparathyroidism

The term pseudohypoparathyroidism was introduced by Albright and associates to describe patients who presented a characteristic phenotype consisting of short stature, round face, short neck, and shortening of metacarpals, particularly the first, fifth, and fourth (Fig. 48–17) that was accompanied by low serum calcium and high serum phosphorus levels consistent with hypoparathyroidism. Administration of parathyroid hormone in these patients did not result in the normally expected increase in urinary phosphate levels, leading investigators to postulate the existence of an end-organ (kidney) unresponsiveness to parathyroid hormone. Patients were subsequently described who had the characteristic phenotype of pseudohypoparathyroidism with normal blood chemistry values, and the term pseudopseudohypoparathyroidism was applied to this condition. The renal response to parathyroid hormone in this latter group of patients is normal.

Both pseudohypoparathyroidism and pseudopseudohypoparathyroidism have the same phenotype. The parathyroid glands are intrinsically normal. Parathyroid hormone levels are normal in pseudopseudohypoparathyroidism and elevated in pseudohypoparathyroidism, the latter a consequence of the ineffective hormone action at the kidney with secondary hyperphosphatemia and hypocalcemia. Patients have been described who exhibit this same phenotype but who have true hypoparathyroidism. Parathyroid hormone levels are low, and there is a proper target-organ response to the administration of parathyroid hormone. These patients would be classified as having pseudopseudohypoparathyroidism. To clarify the distinctions between these disorders, it has been proposed that the condition with the phenotypic changes originally described by Albright be termed Albright's hereditary osteodystrophy (distinct from Albright's syndrome, which consists

of fibrous dysplasia, precocious puberty, and café-au-lait spots). Hypoparathyroid states should be classified as either true hormone-deficient or hormone-resistant forms. Patients with Albright's hereditary osteodystrophy may exhibit target-organ (kidney and bone) unresponsiveness to parathyroid hormone (pseudohypoparathyroidism) or may exhibit a normal target-organ responsiveness (pseudopseudohypoparathyroidism with normal parathyroid hormone levels or pseudopseudohypoparathyroidism with true deficiency of parathyroid hormone) (see Chapter 52).

FURTHER READING

Albright F, Burnett CH, Smith PH, Parson W: Pseudohypoparathyroidism—an example of Seabright-Bantam syndrome (report of 3 cases). Endocrinology 30:922, 1942.

Burnstein MI, Kottamasu SR, Petitifor JM, Sochett E, Ellis BI, Frame B: Metabolic bone disease in pseudohypoparathyroidism: Radiologic features. Radiology 155:351, 1985.

Brighton CT: Structure and function of the growth plate. Clin Orthop 136:22, 1978.

Dent CE: Rickets (and osteomalacia), nutritional and metabolic (1919–1969). Proc R Soc Med 63:401, 1970.

Dent CE, Normand ECS: Metaphysial dysostosis, type Schmid. Arch Dis Child 39:444, 1964.

Frame B, Frost HM, Ormond RS, Hunter RB: Atypical osteomalacia involving the axial skeleton. Ann Intern Med 55:632, 1961.

Frymoyer JW, Hodgkin W: Adult-onset vitamin D–resistant hypophosphatemic osteomalacia. J Bone Joint Surg [Am] 59:101, 1977.

Kidd GS, Schaaf M, Adler RA, Lassman MN, Wray HL: Skeletal responsiveness in pseudohypoparathyroidism: A spectrum of clinical disease. Am J Med 68:772, 1980.

Kolb FO, Steinbach HL: Pseudohypoparathyroidism with secondary hyperparathyroidism and osteitis fibrosa. J Clin Endocrinol Metab 22:59, 1962.

Linovitz RJ, Resnick D, Keissling P, Kondon JJ, Schler B, Nejdl RJ, Rowe JH, Deftos LJ: Tumor-induced osteomalacia and rickets: A surgically curable syndrome, report of two cases. J Bone Joint Surg [Am] 58:419, 1976.

Lyles KW, Berry WR, Haussler M, Harrelson JM, Drezner MK: Hypophosphatemic osteomalacia: Association with prostatic carcinoma. Ann Intern Med 93:275, 1980.

Mankin HJ: Rickets, osteomalacia, and renal osteodystrophy—Part I. J Bone Joint Surg [Am] 56:101, 1974.

Mankin HJ: Rickets, osteomalacia, and renal osteodystrophy—Part II. J Bone Joint Surg [Am] 56:352, 1974.

Nelson AM, Riggs BL, Jowsey JO: Atypical axial osteomalacia, report of four cases with two having features of ankylosing spondylitis. Arthritis Rheum 21:715, 1978.

Polisson RP, Martinez S, Khoury M, Harrell RM, Lyles KW, Friedman N, Harrelson JM, Reisner E, Drezner MK: Calcification of entheses associated with X-linked hypophosphatemic osteomalacia. N Engl J Med 313:1, 1985.

Renton P, Shaw DG: Hypophosphatemic osteomalacia secondary to vascular tumors of bone and soft tissue. Skel Radiol 1:21, 1976.

Reynolds WA, Karo JJ: Radiologic diagnosis of metabolic bone disease. Orthop Clin North Am 3:521, 1972.

Shapiro R: Radiologic aspects of renal osteodystrophy. Radiol Clin North Am 10:557, 1972.

Spiegel AM, Levine MA, Marx SJ, Aurbach GD: Pseudohypoparathyroidism: The molecular basis for hormone resistance—a retrospective. N Engl J Med 307:679, 1982.

Steinbach HL, Noetzli M: Roentgen appearance of the skeleton in osteomalacia and rickets. AJR 91:955, 1964.

Steinbach HL, Kolb FO, Gilfillan R: A mechanism of the production of pseudofractures in osteomalacia (Milkman's syndrome). Radiology 62:388, 1954.

Turner ML, Dalinka MK: Osteomalacia: Uncommon causes. AJR 133:539, 1979.

Chapter 49

Paget's Disease

Donald Resnick, M.D.
Gen Niwayama, M.D.

Paget's disease is a common disorder of middle-aged and elderly patients, characterized by excessive and abnormal remodeling of bone. Its radiographic features are virtually diagnostic, including an initial osteolytic phase, most common in the skull and tubular bones, and a subsequent osteosclerotic phase, particularly in the axial skeleton. An enlarged bone with increased radiodensity and accentuated trabecular pattern is typical. Involvement of specific sites leads to characteristic radiographic signs, including the cotton-wool cranial vault and the picture frame vertebral body. Complications associated with Paget's disease are insufficiency fractures, neurologic symptoms and signs, skeletal deformities, neoplasms, and articular alterations.

Paget's disease (osteitis deformans) is a condition of unknown cause affecting approximately 3 per cent of the population over the age of 40 years. The disease varies considerably in severity: Commonly it is a process localized to one or several regions of the skeleton without significant clinical findings; occasionally it is widespread and severe, producing extensive osseous abnormality and deformity. Paget's disease demonstrates certain geographic and racial characteristics: It appears to be particularly common in inhabitants of Australia, Great Britain, and certain areas of continental Europe; it is not uncommon in the United States; and it is extremely rare among the Chinese. The disease is characterized by excessive and abnormal remodeling of bone. Its active phase is associated with aggressive bone resorption and formation, whereas its quiescent phase is associated with a diminished rate of bone turnover. The combination of osseous resorption and apposition produces a diagnostic pathologic and radiographic appearance in which irregular bone fragments with a thickened and disorganized trabecular (mosaic) pattern are visualized as coarsened and enlarged osseous trabeculae on radiographic evaluation.

CLINICAL FEATURES

Paget's disease is common, particularly in middle-aged and elderly persons. Indeed, the disease is present in approximately 10 to 11 per cent of patients over the age of 80 years. Rarely, Paget's disease is documented in patients under 40 years old. It is more common in men than in women.

In many patients, the disorder is first diagnosed as an incidental finding on radiographs obtained for unrelated purposes. In patients with symptoms, clinical findings vary with the distribution of the disease. Local pain and tenderness frequently are present at an affected skeletal site. Increasing size of a bone may produce clinical findings, such as enlarging head size or progressing prominence of the shins. Skeletal deformities include kyphosis and bowing of the long bones of the extremities. Osseous involvement may lead to pathologic fracture, with resulting pain and angulation, or to

stiffness and reduced mobility of joints. Neurologic deficits, such as muscle weakness, paralysis, and rectal and vesical incontinence, result from impingement on the spinal cord. Similar deficits may accompany platybasia owing to involvement of the base of the skull, although compression of cranial nerves in their foramina is not very common.

Congestive heart failure has been noted in patients with Paget's disease. Initially, investigators thought that this complication was due to the presence of arteriovenous shunts in the involved bone, but these observations have not been confirmed. It now seems probable that high output congestive failure is related to hyperemia and increased blood flow in pagetic bone.

Laboratory analysis in Paget's disease generally reveals elevated serum levels of alkaline phosphatase and hydroxyproline and urinary levels of hydroxyproline. These biochemical abnormalities vary with the distribution and activity of disease; in patients with limited skeletal involvement or inactive disease, aberrations in laboratory values may be absent or not pronounced. Usually serum levels of calcium, phosphorus, and acid phosphatase are normal in patients with Paget's disease.

ETIOLOGY

Although the etiologic factors responsible for Paget's disease are not entirely clear, it is a viral cause of the disease that has gained support in recent years. Active pagetic bone is characterized by the presence of giant osteoclasts containing large numbers of nuclei. Intranuclear inclusion bodies have been identified in these cells, which are not observed in osteoblasts or osteocytes of pagetic bone or in osseous tissue derived from patients with a variety of other skeletal disorders. Ultrastructural characteristics of the pagetic osteoclasts are similar to those that are observed in disorders produced by certain viruses, specifically subacute sclerosing panencephalitis related to a paramyxovirus of the measles group. Additional morphologic evidence for a viral cause includes the following: The dense fibrillar material associated with some of the inclusions is similar to that found in the nuclei of virus-infected cells; filament bundles and spindle-shaped structures enclosed in double membranes observed in the cytoplasm of some osteoclasts are considered an indirect cellular response to viral attack; and the very presence of enormous osteoclasts in pagetic bone is compatible with abnormalities noted with in vitro measles virus infection. The identification of similar intranuclear inclusions within giant cell tumors in patients with Paget's disease is further evidence supporting a viral cause of the disorder. In addition, significant and sustained viral antibody titers against the measles virus have been detected in a few patients with Paget's disease. The minimal degree of inflammation and the absence of considerable inflammatory cells in bone and peripheral blood in Paget's disease are compatible with a response to a chronic infection. Viral infections may require several years for clinical expression, consistent with the advanced age of most patients with Paget's disease. Furthermore, geographic and familial clustering is typical of an infectious process, and viruses may selectively affect a single organ system, such as the skeletal tissue, of patients with Paget's disease.

PATHOPHYSIOLOGY

Paget's disease evolves through various stages or phases of activity, followed by an inactive or quiescent stage. Its initial characteristic is an intense wave of osteoclastic activity with resorption of normal bone by giant multinucleated cells. Subsequently, excessive and disorganized new bone formation owing to a vigorous osteoblastic response leads to the appearance of osseous tissue that is architecturally abnormal, consisting of primitive or woven bone with increased vascularity and a pronounced connective tissue reaction. After a variable period of time, osteoclastic activity may decrease, although deposition of abnormal bone continues. Some of the immature woven bone may be replaced by normal-appearing lamellar bone. Microscopic evaluation reveals distortion of the normal trabecular appearance with a mosaic pattern of irregular cement lines joining areas of lamellar bone. Eventually, osteoblastic activity also declines, and the condition becomes quiescent or inactive. In this stage, sclerotic bone is observed, and evidence of continued resorption and increased cellular activity is minimal or absent.

As Paget's disease commonly is accompanied by widespread involvement of the skeleton, each lesion demonstrates its own pathophysiology with a unique rate of progression. At any one time, multiple stages or phases of the disease process can be identified in different skeletal regions.

RADIOGRAPHIC-PATHOLOGIC CORRELATION
General Stages of the Disease Process (Table 49–1)

An initial phase of intense osteoclastic activity with resorption of bone trabeculae may be detected on radiographs as an "osteolytic" form of the disease (Fig. 49–1). This radiographic appearance is particularly common in the skull, at which site it is termed osteoporosis circumscripta. Osteolysis in the cranial vault is observed most frequently in the frontal or occipital region and may progress to involve the entire skull. The advancing radiolucent lesion may be sharply delineated from the adjacent normal bone. This osteolytic phase may be followed by bone sclerosis and condensation.

The osteolytic phase of Paget's disease may be apparent

Table 49–1. STAGES OF PAGET'S DISEASE

Stage	Most Common Sites	Appearance
Active		
Osteolytic	Cranial vault	Osteoporosis circumscripta
	Long tubular bones	Subchondral location; advancing wedge of radiolucency
Osteolytic or osteosclerotic, or both	Cranial vault	Osteoporosis circumscripta; focal radiodense lesions
	Pelvis	Patchy radiolucency and radiodensity
	Long tubular bones	Diaphyseal radiolucent lesion; epiphyseal and metaphyseal radiodense region
Inactive		
Osteosclerotic	Cranial vault	"Cotton-wool" appearance; thickened cranial vault; basilar invagination
	Spine	"Picture frame" vertebral body; ivory vertebral body
	Pelvis	Thickening of pelvic ring; focal or diffuse radiodense lesions
	Long tubular bones	Epiphyseal predilection; coarse trabeculae; widened and deformed bone

elsewhere in the skeleton, particularly in the long bones. In tubular bones, osteolysis almost invariably begins in the subchondral regions of the epiphysis and subsequently extends into the metaphysis and diaphysis; occasionally, the disease may appear at both ends of an involved bone, but only exceptionally is Paget's disease apparent in the diaphysis without involvement of the epiphysis. When present, this latter feature typically occurs in the tibia. As the disease progresses, osteolysis may advance into the diaphysis as a V- or wedge-shaped radiolucent area, clearly demarcated from the adjacent bone. This appearance has been likened to a blade of grass or flame. Within the area of radiolucency, remaining trabeculae may appear thickened, although frequently they are obliterated and a hazy "ground glass" or "washed-out" pattern is observed. The involved bone commonly is enlarged or widened, and pathologic fractures may be evident.

Radiographic evidence of increased density or sclerosis of bone may be seen in both the active and inactive stages of the disease (Figs. 49–2 and 49–3). Coarsened trabeculae produce focal or widespread areas of radiodensity, which may be superimposed on lytic foci. Cortical thickening, enlargement of bone, and coarsened trabeculae are prominent. Eventually, radiographic evidence of osteolysis may be absent, and the radiographic picture is entirely that of osteosclerosis.

General Distribution of the Disease (Fig. 49–4)

Paget's disease predominates in the axial skeleton. Particularly characteristic is involvement of the pelvis (30 to 75 per cent); sacrum (30 to 60 per cent); spine (30 to 75 per cent), especially the lumbar segment; and skull (25 to 65 per cent). Additionally, the proximal long bones, particularly the femur (25 to 35 per cent), commonly are affected. Abnormalities of the axial skeleton or proximal part of the femur are present in approximately 75 to 80 per cent of cases. Furthermore, the shoulder girdle is not infrequently altered. In fact, no bone is exempt, although changes in the ribs, fibula, and

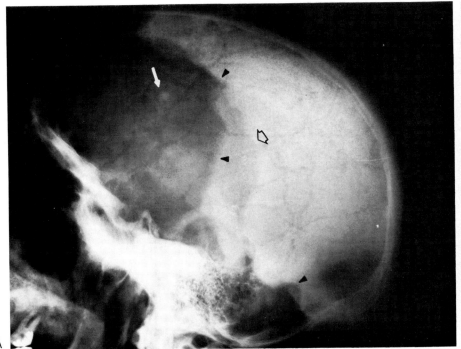

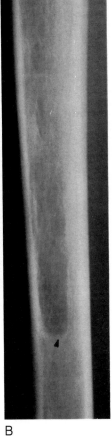

Figure 49–1. **General stages of Paget's disease: Osteolytic stage.** **A** Cranial vault. An example of osteoporosis circumscripta. The osteolytic bone usually commences in the frontal or occipital area of the skull. Its advancing edge (arrowheads) is well demarcated from adjacent normal bone. Focal radiodense areas (arrow) within the areas of osteolysis are apparent. In some locations, involvement of a portion of the cranial vault has created beveled margins (open arrow). **B** Tubular bones. An advancing wedge-shaped radiolucent edge (arrowhead) is observed in the femur.

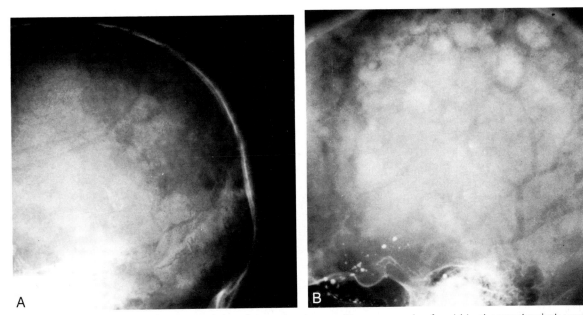

Figure 49–2. **General stages of Paget's disease: Osteolytic and osteosclerotic stage.** These two examples of cranial involvement show both osteolysis and osteosclerosis. Radiodense foci in **A** are occurring in an area of osteoporosis circumscripta. In **B**, more extensive osteosclerosis, producing the "cotton-wool" appearance, is seen.

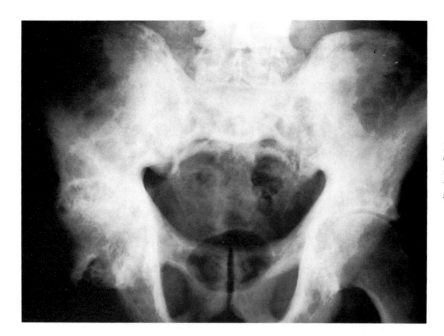

Figure 49–3. General stages of Paget's disease: Osteosclerotic stage. In this example of long-standing disease, diffuse osteosclerosis throughout the pelvis, including the sacrum, is evident. Note degenerative joint disease in the right hip.

small bones in the hand and foot are infrequent. In some patients, the disease is initially or totally monostotic, a pattern that is evident in 10 to 35 per cent of cases.

Involvement of Specific Sites

CRANIUM (FIGS. 49–1 AND 49–2). Pagetic alterations of the skull vary from typical osteoporosis circumscripta to widespread sclerosis. Focal radiodense areas may be observed, termed the "cotton-wool" appearance. Cranial thickening occasionally is extensive, particularly in frontal regions, and both bone sclerosis and thickening may be asymmetrically distributed. As opposed to exuberant facial changes that may be seen in fibrous dysplasia, extensive alterations of the facial bones in Paget's disease are infrequent, although maxillary and mandibular changes may be observed, including radiodense lesions termed cementomas, which can displace teeth and result in malocclusion.

Basilar invagination is seen in about one third of patients with Paget's disease of the skull. This complication is more frequent in women than in men and increases in frequency with progressive severity of the disease. Basilar invagination is characterized by upward protrusion of the foramen magnum and surrounding bone owing to the effect of gravity and muscle pull. It may be associated with neurologic symptoms and signs caused by compression of the contents of the upper cervical canal and posterior fossa. Additional clinical findings relate to impingement on other cranial nerves by the enlarging pagetic bone.

VERTEBRAL COLUMN (FIGS. 49–5 AND 49–6). Paget's disease frequently involves the vertebral column, particularly the lumbar spine and the sacrum. Thoracic and cervical involvement and monostotic disease of the spine can be observed. Five mechanisms have been emphasized in the pathogenesis of neurologic complications of such involvement: collapse of affected vertebral bodies; increased vascularity of pagetic bone, which "steals" blood from the spinal cord; mechanical interference with the spinal cord blood supply; narrowing of the spinal canal owing to new bone formation; and stenosis of neural foramina resulting from involvement of

vertebral posterior elements. In the lumbar spine, Paget's disease can lead to compression of the cauda equina and encroachment on the foramina. In the thoracic spine, cord compression and intervertebral foraminal impingement may be seen. With cervical involvement, Paget's disease can lead to cord compression. Pagetic abnormalities of the vertebral

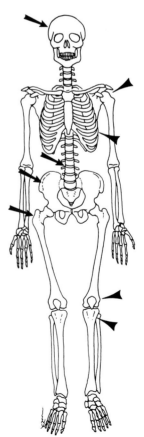

Figure 49–4. General distribution of Paget's disease. Very common (arrows) and common (arrowheads) sites are indicated.

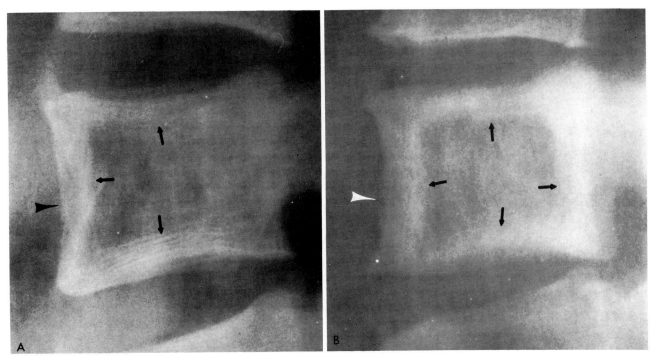

Figure 49–5. Radiographic abnormalities in Paget's disease: Spine. "Picture-frame" vertebral bodies. Condensation of bone can be seen along the peripheral margins (arrows) on lateral radiographs of the spine in two patients with Paget's disease. Observe straightening or convexity of the anterior surface of the bone (arrowheads), and involvement of the pedicles.

body at any level can lead to collapse, a complication that may induce acute compression of the spinal cord.

The vertebral bodies and posterior elements may be altered. Enlarged, coarsened trabeculae are observed, and condensation of bone may be especially prominent along the contours of the vertebral body. In this situation, the highlighted contour of the involved vertebra resembles a picture frame, an appearance that is diagnostic of this condition. In some patients, uniform increase in osseous density is seen, producing an ivory vertebra, and differentiation of Paget's disease from other causes of ivory vertebrae, such as metastasis and lymphoma, may be difficult. In this situation, if the vertebra is enlarged, the diagnosis of Paget's disease is usually assured. It must be stressed, however, that such enlargement may not be apparent.

Alterations in shape of involved vertebral bodies in Paget's disease are common, reflecting the structural weakness of the altered bone. Biconcave deformities termed "fish vertebrae" are identical to those occurring in metabolic disorders such as osteoporosis, osteomalacia, and hyperparathyroidism. Infrequently, complete collapse of the vertebral bodies is observed in Paget's disease, and an adjacent soft tissue mass can be seen.

Pagetic changes in the posterior elements may occur in conjunction with vertebral body abnormalities or as an isolated spinal manifestation of the disease. With pediculate involvement, increased radiodensity may simulate osteoblastic metastasis. Osteolytic features commonly predominate in the sacrum.

PELVIS (FIG. 49–3). Manifestations of Paget's disease in the pelvis usually include both bone resorption and bone formation. Initial trabecular thickening may be evident along the inner contour of the pelvis. The iliopubic and ilioischial

lines may be prominent, with little other osseous abnormality of the pelvis. Thickening in these areas must be distinguished from irregularity of the iliopubic contour, which is frequent in normal elderly persons, and from calcification of Cooper's ligament. The periphery of the iliac bone may appear radiodense, with a relatively lucent central portion. Iliac sclerosis

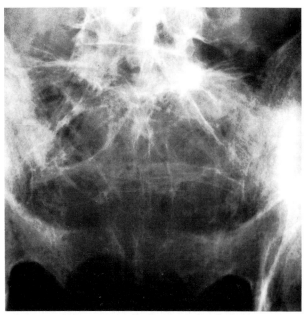

Figure 49–6. Radiographic abnormalities in Paget's disease: Sacrum. Although the sacrum reveals few trabeculae and the entire bone is osteopenic, the remaining trabecular pattern is coarsened, diagnostic of Paget's disease.

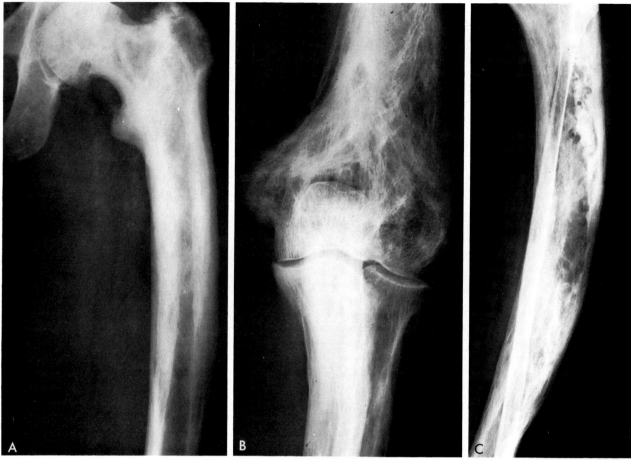

Figure 49–7. Radiographic abnormalities in Paget's disease: Additional sites. A Femur. Alterations extend from the femoral head to the middiaphyseal region. The cortex is thickened and there is cortical encroachment on the medullary canal. Observe the coarse trabecular pattern. **B** Humerus, radius, and ulna. Coarsely trabeculated bone is associated with radiolucent regions of varying size. The osseous outlines are enlarged. **C** Tibia. On a lateral radiograph, typical Paget's disease of the tibia is associated with exaggerated anterior curvature. Note the lack of fibular involvement. **D** The characteristic findings of Paget's disease are observed throughout an entire metacarpal.

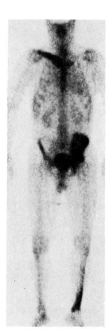

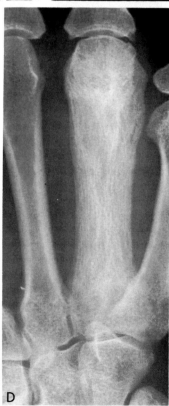

Figure 49–8. Scintigraphic abnormalities in Paget's disease: Bone-seeking agents (technetium polyphosphate), osteosclerotic phase. Observe the accentuated uptake of radionuclide in the left hemipelvis, distal portion of the left tibia, and right clavicle. The scintigraphic pattern is virtually diagnostic of Paget's disease.

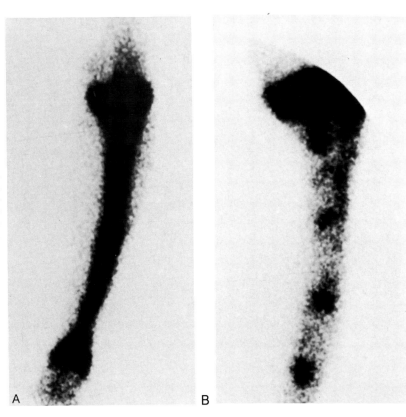

Figure 49–15. Treatment of Paget's disease: Thyrocalcitonin—scintigraphic improvement. Bone scans show initially, intense accumulation of the radionuclide in the tibia (A) with partial resolution over a 2 year period during treatment with thyrocalcitonin (B). The residual activity on the second scan corresponded in position to sites of insufficiency fractures.

A   B

Scintigraphy, in comparison to radiography, possesses advantages in monitoring the response of pagetic bone to any of these therapeutic agents. A distinct decrease in radionuclide accumulation in diseased areas is characteristic of the pagetic response to treatment (Fig. 49–15). In general, there is good correlation of scintigraphic and biochemical parameters of disease activity. Recurrence of the disorder typically is accompanied scintigraphically by a rise in activity in one or more bones in a diffuse or circumscribed pattern, or by spread of disease into an adjacent normal bone.

DIFFERENTIAL DIAGNOSIS

General Features

Although the initial lytic phase of Paget's disease may present some difficulties for the inexperienced observer, its radiographic features are diagnostic. Epiphyseal involvement, sharply demarcated bone lysis, and an advancing wedge of radiolucency allow accurate diagnosis. Widespread sclerosis, which can be apparent in Paget's disease of long duration, also has specific characteristics, such as bone enlargement and

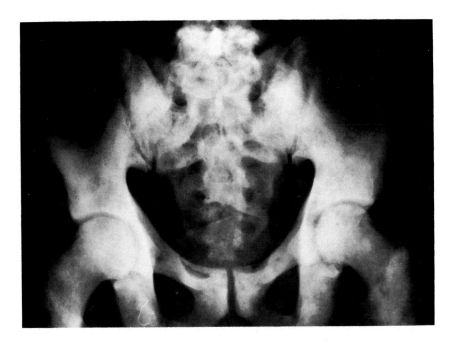

Figure 49–16. Skeletal metastasis from carcinoma of the prostate. Patchy osteosclerosis is observed in the pelvis, spine, sacrum, and proximal portions of the femora. A coarsened trabecular pattern, which is evident in Paget's disease, is not seen in skeletal metastases.

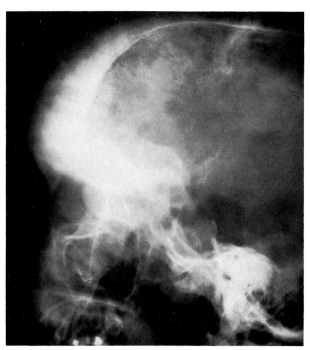

Figure 49–17. Fibrous dysplasia. Characteristic hyperostosis and calvarial thickening can be seen in the frontal regions. The facial bones are also affected.

a coarsened trabecular pattern, which can be distinguished from findings associated with other diseases. Diffuse increased skeletal radiodensity may be observed in bone metastasis (particularly from prostatic carcinoma) (Fig. 49–16), myelofibrosis, fluorosis, mastocytosis (urticaria pigmentosa), renal osteodystrophy, fibrous dysplasia, and tuberous sclerosis. Additional findings in these other disorders ensure their recognition. For example, hepatosplenomegaly (myelofibrosis, mastocytosis), ligamentous ossification (fluorosis), focal radiodensity (mastocytosis and tuberous sclerosis), characteristic bowing deformities and "ground glass" appearance (fibrous dysplasia), and subperiosteal and subchondral bone resorption (renal osteodystrophy) are abnormalities associated with these other diseases.

Axial osteomalacia is a rare disorder, confined to the axial skeleton (see Chapter 48). The radiographic findings may simulate those of Paget's disease. Fibrogenesis imperfecta ossium is another rare disease observed in elderly patients, associated with coarse trabeculation, spontaneous fractures, and deformity (see Chapter 73).

Familial idiopathic hyperphosphatasia (osteitis deformans in children, "juvenile" Paget's disease, hyperostosis corticalis) is a rare disorder of bone occurring in children, associated with progressive skeletal deformities, coarsely trabeculated and widened bone, and elevated serum alkaline phosphatase and urinary hydroxyproline levels. Although some characteristics of this disorder resemble those of Paget's disease, familial idiopathic hyperphosphatasia occurs in younger patients, and epiphyses may not be involved.

Calvarial Hyperostosis

Paget's disease of the skull can be confused with other disorders associated with calvarial hyperostosis. These include hyperostosis frontalis interna, fibrous dysplasia, anemias, and skeletal metastasis. Hyperostosis frontalis interna predominates in women and produces thickening of the inner table of the frontal squama. Fibrous dysplasia may cause gross enlargement of the skull, although facial involvement is particularly characteristic (Fig. 49–17). Certain anemias, such as sickle cell anemia and thalassemia, produce thickening of the cranial vault and a radiating trabecular pattern (hair-on-end appearance). The base of the skull is generally spared. Osteoblastic metastasis can simulate the "cotton-wool" radiodense lesions of Paget's disease.

Vertebral Sclerosis

Condensation of the periphery of a vertebral body, the picture frame vertebra, is diagnostic of Paget's disease. It differs from the accentuated vertical trabeculae of hemangiomas and the rugger-jersey spine of renal osteodystrophy. Some patients with Paget's disease reveal diffuse sclerosis of an entire vertebral body, the ivory vertebra, which can simulate skeletal metastasis and lymphoma.

Pelvic Abnormalities

Although pelvic sclerosis in Paget's disease can mimic the findings of osteoblastic metastasis, asymmetric or unilateral distribution, accentuated trabecular pattern, and enlargement of the involved bone are typical of Paget's disease.

FURTHER READING

Altman RD, Collins B: Musculoskeletal manifestations of Paget's disease of bone. Arthritis Rheum 23:1121, 1980.

Barry HC: Paget's Disease of Bone. Edinburgh, E&S Livingstone, 1969.

Bowerman JW, Altman J, Hughes JL, Zadek RE: Pseudo-malignant lesions in Paget's disease of bone. AJR 124:57, 1975.

Goldman AB, Bullough P, Kammermans S, Ambos M: Osteitis deformans of the hip joint. AJR 128:601, 1977.

Greditzer HG III, McLeod RA, Unni KK, Beabout JW: Bone sarcomas in Paget disease. Radiology 146:327, 1983.

Hamdy RC: Paget's Disease of Bone. Assessment and Management. New York, Praeger Publishers, 1981.

Jacobs P: Osteolytic Paget's disease. Clin Radiol 25:137, 1974.

Mills BG, Singer FR: Nuclear inclusions in Paget's disease of bone. Science 194:201, 1976.

Murphy WA, Whyte MP, Haddad JG Jr: Paget bone disease: Radiologic documentation of healing with human calcitonin therapy. Radiology 136:1, 1980.

Paget J: On a form of chronic inflammation of bones (osteitis deformans). Med Chir Tr 60:37, 1877.

Resnick D: Paget disease of bone: Current status and a look back to 1943 and earlier. AJR 150:249, 1988.

Singer FR, Mills BG: Evidence for a viral etiology of Paget's disease of bone. Clin Orthop 178:245, 1983.

Smith J, Botet JF, Yeh SDJ: Bone sarcomas in Paget's disease: A study of 85 patients. Radiology 152:583, 1984.

Steinbach HL: Some roentgen features of Paget's disease. AJR 86:950, 1961.

Wick MR, McLeod RA, Siegal GP, Greditzer HG III, Unni KK: Sarcomas of bone complicating osteitis deformans (Paget's disease). Fifty years' experience. Am J Surg Pathol 5:47, 1981.

Wilner D, Sherman RS: Roentgen diagnosis of Paget's disease (osteitis deformans). Med Radiogr Photogr 42:35, 1966.

Zlatkin MB, Lander PH, Hadjipavlou AG, Levine JS: Paget's disease of the spine: CT with clinical correlation. Radiology 160:155, 1986.

Chapter 50

Pituitary Disorders

Donald Resnick, M.D.

In acromegaly, bone alterations result from the effects of elevated levels of serum growth hormone on the adult skeleton. Endochondral bone formation is reactivated and periosteal bone formation is stimulated in association with connective tissue proliferation. These changes lead to characteristic radiographic findings, including increased soft tissue thickness and bone overgrowth. Joint abnormalities result from chondrocyte proliferation in articular cartilage. Radiographically, joint space narrowing, bone sclerosis,

cyst formation, and osteophytosis are seen, which simulate the changes of primary degenerative joint disease.

In hypopituitarism, abnormalities of bone development result from damage to the anterior lobe of the pituitary gland. Delays occur in appearance, growth, fusion, and disappearance of ossification centers. Absence of closure of the physes is seen radiographically. Clinical findings include immature body proportions and facial features and a delay in the eruption of secondary teeth.

ACROMEGALY AND GIGANTISM

Growth hormone (somatotropin) hypersecretion can be associated with acidophilic or chromophobic adenomas of the anterior lobe of the pituitary gland. Less frequently, such hypersecretion is associated with diffuse hyperplasia of the acidophil cells or no histologic abnormality at all. In the immature skeleton, in which the growth plates are still open, growth hormone hypersecretion leads to excessive proportional growth of bone (e.g., in both length and width) owing to direct hormonal stimulation of endochondral bone formation at the physeal growth plates. The resulting syndrome is termed hyperpituitary gigantism. In the mature skeleton, growth hormone hypersecretion may reactivate endochondral bone formation at various existing cartilage-bone junctions (such as the costochondral junctions) and induce periosteal bone formation, leading to widening of osseous structures. The term acromegaly reflects this overgrowth of bone in association with enlargement of soft tissue, which is particularly prominent in the acral parts (hands, feet, lower jaw) of the skeleton.

General Clinical Features

Typically the onset of symptoms and signs of acromegaly is in the third or fourth decade of life. The physical appearance of a patient with hyperpituitary gigantism is essentially that of a tall, normally proportioned individual, whereas a patient with acromegaly may reveal a large mandible, producing a "lantern jaw" appearance, poor dental occlusion, coarsening of facial features, prominence of the forehead, deepening of the voice, and prominence of the tongue. The hands appear broad and spade-like, and the fingers are separated and blunted. Hypersecretion of growth hormone also affects other organ systems, producing thickening of the skin, enlargement of abdominal viscera, thyroid gland hypertrophy, and cardiomegaly. Associated endocrine alterations may be observed, including diabetes mellitus (12 to 25 per cent), persistent lactation (4 per cent), increased secretion of cortisol by the

adrenal cortex, and increased frequency of parathyroid and pancreatic islet cell adenomas.

Owing to the insidious nature of the disease, there may be a considerable delay before the acromegalic patient seeks medical attention. Headaches and visual disturbances are common presenting features, as are loss of libido in men and cessation of menstruation in women.

Rheumatic complaints are common in patients with acromegaly. Articular symptoms and signs appear to relate to overstimulation of cartilaginous tissue. Rheumatic manifestations generally begin after 20 years of age and are equally frequent in men and women. Five types of rheumatic complaints may be encountered (Table 50–1).

BACKACHE. Approximately 50 per cent of acromegalic patients have backache, particularly of the lower spine. Painful kyphosis of the thoracic spine also may be observed.

LIMB ARTHROPATHY. Arthropathy is most common in the large joints, such as the knees, shoulders, and hips. Symptoms and signs include soft tissue swelling, crepitus, and minimal pain and tenderness. Synovial effusions are uncommon. In later stages of the articular disease, secondary degenerative changes, particularly in the hip and knee, may produce pain, limitation of motion, deformity, and angulation.

COMPRESSION NEUROPATHY. Compression neuropathies are due to connective tissue and bone overgrowth. The carpal tunnel syndrome is particularly characteristic. Spinal cord compression with long tract signs also has been noted. This may relate to narrowing of the spinal canal from soft tissue overgrowth and hypertrophy of the vertebrae.

Table 50–1. RHEUMATIC COMPLAINTS IN ACROMEGALY

Backache
Limb arthropathy
Compression neuropathy
Neuromuscular symptoms
Raynaud's phenomenon

615

NEUROMUSCULAR SYMPTOMS. Fatigue and lethargy are two common clinical findings in acromegaly. Muscle wasting generally is not a prominent feature. Neurologic changes, including peripheral neuropathy, are also encountered.

RAYNAUD'S PHENOMENON. This is a relatively uncommon manifestation of the disease.

Pathologic Features of Skeletal Involvement (Table 50–2)

STIMULATION OF ENDOCHONDRAL OSSIFICATION. In patients whose growth plates are not yet closed, excessive growth hormone results in exaggerated longitudinal growth of the skeleton. In the young, true gigantism may result, whereas in persons in whom the cartilaginous growth plates are near fusion, some increase in longitudinal growth is observed, but gigantism is relatively mild. After closure of the growth plates, excessive secretion of growth hormone can result in reactivation of endochondral bone formation at certain chondroosseous junctions, such as the costochondral area of the rib. Resultant enlargement of the costochondral junctions is termed the acromegalic rosary.

STIMULATION OF PERIOSTEAL BONE FORMATION. In acromegaly, subperiosteal bone formation is observed at specific sites. In the skull, this form of bony proliferation is apparent on the alveolar margins of the maxilla and mandible, with resultant deepening of the alveolar sockets and separation of the teeth. Subperiosteal new bone formation and articular cartilage stimulation produce distinctive changes along the mental eminence of the mandible and mandibular rami, with enlargement and forward protrusion of the entire mandible. Bone deposition is also characteristic in the supraorbital ridges, facial bones, and calvarial vault.

Subperiosteal and subligamentous bone formation may result in thickening and irregularity of the cortices of the shafts of the tubular bones, prominence of various tuberosities, and osteophytosis. These alterations account for the enlargement of the phalanges, metacarpals, and metatarsals.

Both the transverse and the sagittal diameters of the vertebral bodies increase owing to prominent subperiosteal bone deposition. The vertebral bodies appear short in height and elongated in sagittal and transverse planes. These abnormalities are associated with an increase in size of the intervertebral disc, which is produced by marginal subperichondrial formation of cartilage. Osteophytes of the vertebral column may be a prominent feature.

BONE FORMATION AND BONE RESORPTION. It appears that subperiosteal and endosteal bone proliferation in acromegaly occurs simultaneously with increased bone resorption. In most sites, bone apposition exceeds bone resorption; occasionally however, the opposite may be true, in which case decreased bone thickness is observed.

ARTICULAR CARTILAGE ALTERATIONS. Increased growth hormone secretion can lead to proliferation of articular cartilage. Ulceration and fissuring of superficial cartilage may progress to involve deeper layers. A continuous cycle apparently occurs, with progressive cartilaginous fragmentation and denudation, disordered joint mechanics, and tissue repair with remodeling (Fig. 50–1). The regeneration process is associated with fibrocartilaginous plugs within cartilage and articular margins and capsule that become hypertrophied, calcified, and ossified. Widespread osteophytic outgrowths are seen in association with subchondral cyst formation. The

Table 50–2. RADIOGRAPHIC-PATHOLOGIC CORRELATION IN ACROMEGALY

Pathologic Features	Radiographic Features
Stimulation of endochondral bone formation	Enlargement of costochondral junctions Thickening of intervertebral discs
Stimulation of periosteal bone formation	Mandibular enlargement Thickening of the cranial vault Prominence of the supraorbital ridges and facial structures Cortical thickening of tubular bones Enlargement of phalangeal tufts Increase in anteroposterior and transverse diameters of vertebral bodies
Stimulation of subligamentous bone formation	Calcaneal spurs Excrescences on patella, tuberosities, trochanters
Stimulation of bone resorption	Overtubulation of phalanges, metacarpals, metatarsals Intracortical striations Medullary widening Vertebral scalloping
Proliferation of articular cartilage	Widening of articular spaces
Cartilaginous degeneration and regeneration	Narrowing of articular spaces Periarticular calcifications and ossifications Osteophytosis
Connective tissue hyperplasia	Increased thickness of skin (e.g., heel-pad)
Pituitary neoplasm	Sella turcica abnormalities

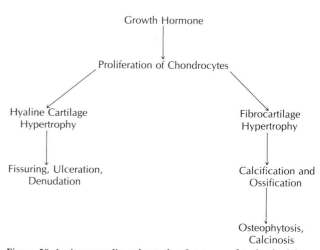

Figure 50–1. Acromegalic arthropathy: Summary of pathophysiology. Excess circulating growth hormone stimulates chondrocyte proliferation. Hypertrophy of both hyaline cartilage and fibrocartilage occurs. Fissuring, ulceration, and denudation of the hyaline cartilage lead to degeneration of the articular surface. Calcification and ossification of fibrocartilage are associated with formation of osteophytes and calcinosis. Brisk fibrocartilaginous regeneration is characteristic, producing thickened cartilage, enlarged bones, and hypertrophy of periarticular soft tissues.

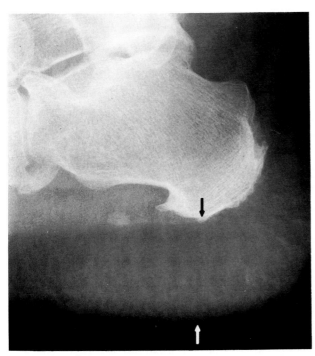

Figure 50-2. Acromegaly: Radiographic features—increase in skin thickness. Observe prominence of the soft tissues of the heel with associated hyperostosis and osteophytosis of the calcaneus. One technique of measurement of these soft tissues evaluates the shortest distance between the calcaneus and plantar skin surface (between arrows).

eventual features of the exuberant regenerative process of acromegaly are an enlarged articulation with thickened ulcerative cartilage, hypertrophied periarticular tissue, calcinosis, osteophytosis, and periosteal bone formation at insertion sites of tendons, ligaments, and capsule.

The synovial membrane may show a mild, nonspecific, villous synovitis with a fatty tissue core and increased vascularity. Skin hypertrophy is also apparent.

Radiologic Features of Skeletal Involvement

CHANGES IN SKIN THICKNESS (FIG. 50-2). Numerous articles have reported the potential use of radiographic measurements of skin thickness, particularly heel-pad thickness, in the diagnosis of acromegaly. Despite some inconsistencies in the value of heel-pad thickness measurements because of its variation with body weight, values greater than 23 mm in men and 21.5 mm in women are suggestive of acromegaly, and values greater than 25 mm in men and 23 mm in women are even more diagnostic of this disease if local causes of skin thickening are excluded.

ABNORMALITIES OF THE SKULL (FIG. 50-3). Radiographic manifestations of the skull in patients with acromegaly include sella turcica alterations (such as enlargement, rarefaction, and destruction of the dorsum of the sella and osteopenia of the anterior and posterior clinoid processes), prominence and enlargement of the frontal and maxillary sinuses, excessive pneumatization of the mastoids, prominence of the occipital protuberance (particularly in men), thickening or, less commonly, thinning of the cranial vault, prominence of the supraorbital ridges and zygomatic arches, enlargement and elongation of the mandible, widening of the mandibular angle, and anterior tilting, separation, and hypercementosis of the teeth.

ABNORMALITIES OF THE HAND AND WRIST (FIG. 50-4). Radiographic findings of acromegaly in the hand include soft tissue thickening of the fingers, thickening and squaring of the phalanges and metacarpals, overtubulation or overconstriction of the shafts of the phalanges, abnormally wide articular spaces, bone excrescences at sites of tendon and ligament attachment to bone, and prominence of the ungual tufts. Bone enlargement can be observed about the wrist as well.

The sesamoid index, which consists of measurements of the size of the medial sesamoid at the first metacarpophalangeal joint, has been used in the early diagnosis of acromegaly. On a nonmagnified radiograph of the hand exposed at a 36 inch focus-film distance, the greatest diameter of this bone is multiplied by the greatest diameter of the same sesamoid image that is perpendicular to the first measurement. Although the reliability of the sesamoid index in diagnosing acromegaly has been questioned, a sesamoid index of greater than 40 in men and greater than 32 in women is suggestive of acromegaly, and a sesamoid index below 30 militates against but does not exclude the diagnosis of acromegaly.

Other measurements of the hand that have been used to diagnose acromegaly are given in Table 50-3.

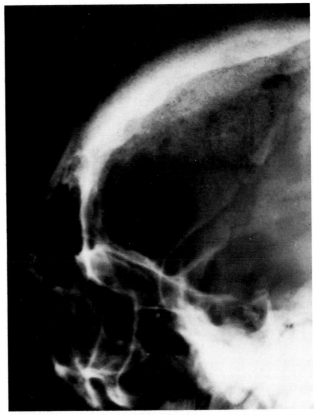

Figure 50-3. Acromegaly: Radiographic features—skull abnormalities. Findings include increased thickness of the cranial vault, prominent sinuses and supraorbital ridges, and enlarged sella turcica.

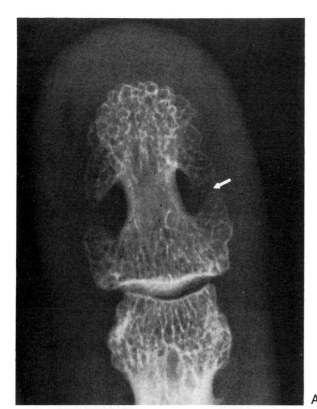

A

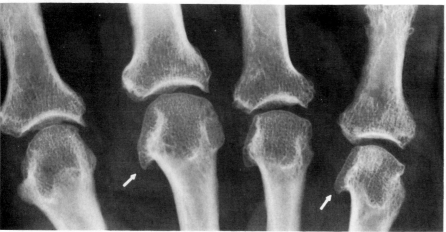

B

Figure 50–4. Acromegaly: Radiographic features—abnormalities of the hand. **A** Terminal phalanges: Typical findings include soft tissue prominence and enlargement of the tuft and base of the terminal phalanges. Note the formation of pseudoforamina (arrow). **B** Metacarpophalangeal joints. Observe widening of some articular spaces and narrowing of others and beak-like osteophytes on the medial aspect of the metacarpal heads (arrows).

Table 50–3. BONE AND SOFT TISSUE MEASUREMENTS SUGGESTIVE OF ACROMEGALY

Heel-pad thickness	>23 mm (men)
	>21.5 mm (women)
Sesamoid index (first MCP* joint)	>40 (men)
	>32 (women)
Tuftal width (third finger)	≥12 mm (men)
	≥10 mm (women)
Joint space thickness (second MCP joint)	>2.5 mm (men and women)
Phalangeal soft tissue thickness (proximal midphalanges)	≥27 mm (men)
	≥26 mm (women)

*MCP, Metacarpophalangeal.

ABNORMALITIES OF THE FOOT (FIG. 50–5). Radiographic changes in the foot resemble those in the hand. Thickening of the soft tissues of the toes, enlargement of the sesamoid bones and articular spaces (particularly at the metatarsophalangeal joints), and prominence of the metatarsal heads are seen. The terminal tufts become prominent, and exostoses arise from the terminal phalangeal base, extending distally. Proliferation at sites of tendon and ligament attachments such as the calcaneus, thickening of the metatarsal shafts, and constriction of the shafts of the proximal phalanges may be observed.

ABNORMALITIES OF THE VERTEBRAL COLUMN (FIG. 50–6). Elongation and widening of the vertebral bodies are noted in some patients with acromegaly. These findings

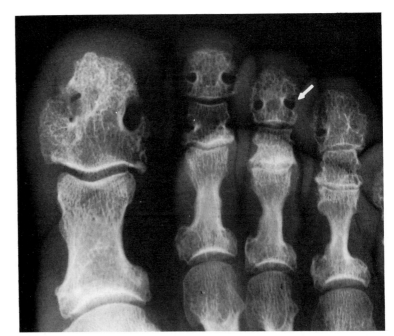

Figure 50–5. Acromegaly: Radiographic features—abnormalities of the foot. Findings are soft tissue enlargement, prominence of the tufts and bases of the terminal phalanges, and pseudoforamina (arrow).

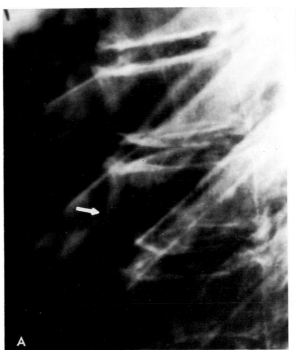

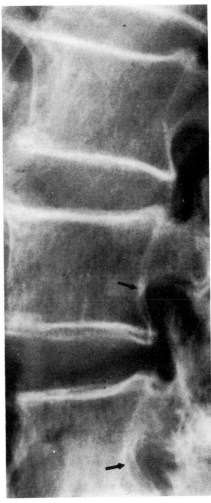

Figure 50–6. Acromegaly: Radiographic features—abnormalities of the spine. A In the thoracic spine, note bone formation on the anterior aspect of the vertebrae (arrow) producing an increase in the anteroposterior diameter of the vertebral bodies. **B** In another patient, observe exaggerated concavity on the posterior aspect of multiple lumbar vertebral bodies (arrows).

are most frequent in the thoracic and lumbar spinal regions. Anterior and lateral osteophytes of the thoracic and lumbar vertebrae may be extensive, but posterior deposition of bone is less frequent. Increased height of the intervertebral disc space, particularly in the lumbar region, hypertrophic changes about apophyseal joints, increased thoracic kyphosis, and increased lumbar lordosis are additional manifestations of acromegaly.

Exaggeration of the normal concavity on the posterior aspect of the vertebral bodies is a recognized abnormality in this disease. This finding, related to excessive resorption of bone, frequently is associated with apposition of bone on the anterior margin of the vertebrae. The cause of scalloping of the posterior margins of the vertebral bodies in acromegaly is not clear. Although it is reasonable to attribute scalloping to the well-documented hyperplasia of soft tissue that occurs in acromegaly, this theory does not adequately explain the predilection of the changes for the lumbar region and the absence of more widespread canal enlargement. It should also be recognized that scalloping of vertebral bodies is not diagnostic of this condition, being found in a variety of disease processes.

Cauda equina compression may be apparent in patients with acromegaly. Back pain can simulate the findings of a herniated intervertebral disc. The changes may be due to soft tissue and bone overgrowth superimposed on a narrow lumbar spinal canal.

ABNORMALITIES OF THE THORACIC CAGE. The thorax may appear enlarged owing to elongation of the ribs. Elevation of the lower portion of the sternum and an increased angulation of the sternal angle have been observed.

MISCELLANEOUS ABNORMALITIES. Bone proliferation occurs at sites of tendon and ligament attachment to bone (Fig. 50–7). Particularly characteristic are excrescences on the undersurface of the calcaneus, the anterior margin of the patella, the trochanters of the femur, the tuberosities of the humerus, and the undersurface of the distal clavicle.

ARTICULAR ABNORMALITIES. Radiologic abnormalities of the peripheral joints in acromegaly are seen most

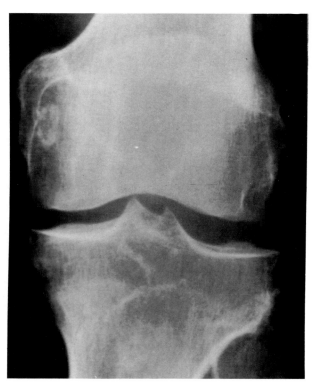

Figure 50–8. Acromegaly: Radiographic features—cartilage hypertrophy. Joint space widening is apparent in the knee.

frequently in the knees, hips, and shoulders. These abnormalities can be divided into two types: cartilage hypertrophy and cartilaginous and osseous degeneration.

Cartilage Hypertrophy (Fig. 50–8). Gross thickening of the cartilage is associated with radiographically evident widening of the articular space. Widening of the joint space may be apparent in any joint, although it is observed most frequently in the metacarpophalangeal, metatarsophalangeal, and interphalangeal joints. Softening and thickening of the capsular and ligamentous structures produce joint laxity.

Cartilaginous and Osseous Degeneration (Fig. 50–9). In later stages of the disease, cartilage fibrillation and erosion lead to secondary degenerative alterations. Initially, osteophytes are seen, and the combination of osteophyte formation and a normal or widened joint space is suggestive of acromegaly. Joint space narrowing, cyst formation, sclerosis, and progressive osteophytosis are seen subsequently. The eventual appearance resembles that of primary degenerative disease; however, involvement of articular sites such as the shoulder and elbow, which are not commonly affected in degenerative joint disease, the presence of prominent osteophytes and bone excrescences, and the documentation of typical findings of acromegaly elsewhere in the skeleton usually allow accurate diagnosis of this disease. Beak-like osteophytes on the inferior aspect of the humeral head, lateral aspect of the acetabulum, medial portion of the femoral head, superior margin of the symphysis pubis, and radial aspect of the metacarpals or tibial aspect of the metatarsals are characteristic of acromegaly. Small collections of calcification or ossification within or around the articular space have been described in patients with acromegaly, and chondrocalcinosis attributable to CPPD crystal deposition, particularly in the knee, is occasionally encountered in these individuals.

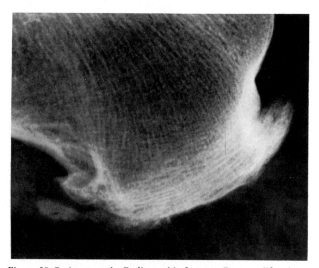

Figure 50–7. Acromegaly: Radiographic features. Bone proliferation at sites of tendon and ligament attachment. Note proliferation along the posterior and inferior aspects of the calcaneus.

Differential Diagnosis

The combination of radiographic findings in acromegaly is sufficiently characteristic that accurate diagnosis is not difficult, particularly in advanced cases, although individual radiographic signs, such as increased soft tissue width, tuftal prominence, and vertebral scalloping, which are apparent in this disease, may be noted in other disorders. The early radiographic diagnosis of acromegaly relies on a variety of measurements, especially in the hands and feet, which discriminate patients with this disease from normal persons (Table 50–3).

GENERAL RADIOGRAPHIC FEATURES. An acromegaly-like syndrome has been associated with pachydermoperiostosis. The characteristic features of this familial syndrome are digital clubbing, coarsening of facial features, furrowing and oiliness of the skin, and periosteal new bone formation (Fig. 50–10). Some radiographic findings are similar to those of acromegaly, with enlarged sinuses, prominent supraorbital ridges, and thickening of the phalanges. The sella turcica is not enlarged, however.

THICKENING OF SOFT TISSUES. Although soft tissue thickening at certain sites, such as the phalanges and heel, can be reliable indicators of acromegaly, similar thickening can be seen in other diseases, related to edema, hemorrhage, exudation, or fatty tissue infiltration. Long-term phenytoin therapy has been accompanied by thickening of the heel-pad.

SCALLOPED VERTEBRAE. Exaggerated concavity of the posterior surface of the vertebral bodies is recognized in acromegaly. It is also seen in a variety of other disease processes (Table 50–4).

ARTICULAR ABNORMALITIES. The initial phase of acromegalic joint disease is manifested as increased articular space and enlargement of the osseous surfaces. These radiographic findings are easily differentiated from those accompanying other disease processes. The later stages of acromegalic joint disease include findings such as joint space narrowing, cyst formation, sclerosis, and osteophytosis, which are similar to the abnormalities of primary degenerative joint disease. In some patients with acromegaly, involvement of weight-bearing joints such as the hip and knee simulates the distribution of primary degenerative joint disease, although in other patients, non–weight-bearing joints such as the shoulder and elbow are involved, a distribution that is unusual in primary degenerative joint disease. Furthermore, prominent osteophytes and beak-like excrescences of articular bone surfaces are characteristic in acromegaly. In fact, these outgrowths may be apparent before joint space loss becomes evident.

HYPOPITUITARISM

Damage to the anterior lobe of the pituitary gland during the period of skeletal growth leads to abnormality of osseous

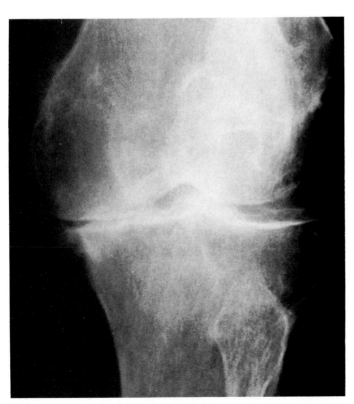

Figure 50–9. Acromegaly: Radiographic features—cartilaginous and osseous degeneration. In the knee, narrowing of both the medial and lateral femorotibial compartments is seen with sclerosis and osteophytosis.

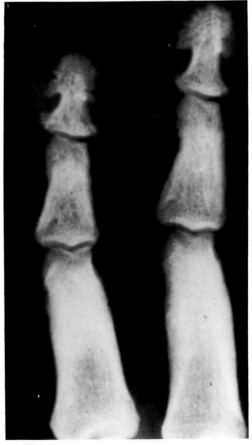

Figure 50–10. Pachydermoperiostosis. Findings include soft tissue prominence, thickening of all the phalanges, and enlargement of phalangeal tufts.

Table 50–4. SOME CAUSES OF SCALLOPED VERTEBRAL BODIES*

1. Increased intraspinal pressure
   a. Intradural neoplasms
   b. Intraspinal cysts
   c. Syringomyelia and hydromyelia
   d. Communicating hydrocephalus

2. Dural "ectasia"
   a. Marfan's syndrome
   b. Ehlers-Danlos syndrome
   c. Neurofibromatosis

3. Bone resorption
   a. Acromegaly

4. Congenital disorders
   a. Achondroplasia
   b. Morquio's disease
   c. Hurler's syndrome

5. Physiologic scalloping

*From Mitchell GE, et al: The various causes of scalloped vertebrae with notes on their pathogenesis. Radiology 89:67, 1967. Used with permission.

development. The cause of damage is variable and includes neoplasms (adenomas, craniopharyngioma, pituitary carcinoma, metastasis), infection (pyogenic, tuberculous, fungal), granulomas (histiocytosis, sarcoidosis), injury, and vascular insult. In approximately 10 per cent of cases, hypopituitarism is familial, probably related to transmission of a recessive gene or, less commonly, a dominant gene. The effect on the skeleton is a delay in appearance and growth of ossification

centers and a similar delay in their fusion and disappearance (Fig. 50–11). On histologic examination, the growth plate is observed to remain open and its metaphyseal side is "closed off" as osseous tissue abuts on the cartilaginous tissue. Eventually the growth plate may disappear, although osseous fusion occurs at an advanced age.

Clinically, growth failure usually is recognized when the child is 1 to 3 years of age and, if the condition is untreated, continued slow growth at the rate of 50 to 60 per cent of normal occurs throughout childhood. Findings include immature body proportions and facial features, abnormal distribution of fat, and delay in eruption of secondary teeth. Mental development generally correlates with the chronologic age.

In patients with hypopituitarism, treatment with human growth hormone results in an increase in skeletal maturation paralleling the increase in chronologic age and an increase in cortical thickness. The growth plates may widen. In rare instances, slipping of the femoral capital epiphysis may occur before or during growth hormone therapy in patients with pituitary dysfunction. The exact mechanism for epiphyseal displacement in these persons is not known.

The differential diagnosis of pituitary dwarfism includes psychosocial dwarfism, hypothyroidism, gonadal dysgenesis (Turner's syndrome), malnutrition, diabetes mellitus, occult systemic inflammatory diseases, chronic renal disease, and a variety of skeletal disorders, including achondroplasia, forms of rickets, pseudohypoparathyroidism, and neurofibromatosis (Table 50–5). Most of these conditions are easily differentiated from pituitary dwarfism, which is important, as the latter disease probably accounts for fewer than 10 per cent of cases of short stature in children.

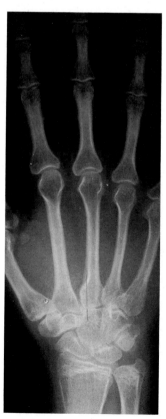

Figure 50–11. Hypopituitarism: Delayed skeletal maturation. In this 23 year old woman, a marked reduction in the rate of skeletal maturation is confirmed by the absence of closure of the physes of the distal portions of the radius and ulna. Osteopenia is evident.

Table 50–5. SOME CAUSES OF SHORT STATURE

Endocrine Disorders
   Hypopituitarism
   Hypothyroidism
   Diabetes mellitus
   Hypercortisolism
   Congenital adrenal hyperplasia
   Deficient somatomedin production (Laron dwarfism)

Chronic Disorders of Major Organ Systems
   Chronic renal disease
   Congenital heart disease
   Juvenile chronic arthritis
   Sickle cell anemia
   Malabsorption syndromes

Skeletal Disorders
   Achondroplasia
   Osteochondrodysplasias
   Pseudohypoparathyroidism and pseudopseudo-
      hypoparathyroidism
   Rickets

Chromosomal Aberrations
   Gonadal dysgenesis
   Trisomy conditions

Miscellaneous Disorders
   Malnutrition
   Familial short stature
   Inborn errors of metabolism
   Intrauterine infections
   Systemic inflammatory diseases
   Renal tubular disorders
   Psychosocial dwarfism
   Neurologic disorders

FURTHER READING

Anton HC: Hand measurements in acromegaly. Clin Radiol 23:445, 1972.

Bluestone R, Bywaters EGL, Hartog M, Holt PJL, Hyde S: Acromegalic arthropathy. Ann Rheum Dis 30:243, 1971.

Hernandez RJ, Poznanski AW, Hopwood NJ: Size and skeletal maturation of the hand in children with hypothyroidism and hypopituitarism. AJR 133:405, 1979.

Jaffe HL: Metabolic, Degenerative and Inflammatory Diseases of Bones and Joints. Philadelphia, Lea & Febiger, 1972.

Lang EK, Bessler WT: The roentgenologic features of acromegaly. AJR 86:321, 1961.

Layton MW, Fudman EJ, Barkan A, Braunstein EM, Fox IH: Acromegalic arthropathy. Characteristics and response to therapy. Arthritis Rheum 31:1022, 1988.

Lin SR, Lee KF: Relative value of some radiographic measurements of the hand in the diagnosis of acromegaly. Invest Radiol 6:426, 1971.

Mitchell GE, Lourie H, Berne AS: The various causes of scalloped vertebrae with notes on their pathogenesis. Radiology 89:67, 1967.

Steinbach HL, Feldman R, Goldberg MB: Acromegaly. Radiology 72:535, 1959.

Chapter 51

Thyroid Disorders

Donald Resnick, M.D.

Distinctive osseous, articular, and soft tissue alterations may accompany hyperthyroid and hypothyroid states. These alterations underscore the importance of thyroid hormone in regulating normal growth, development, and maturation of tissue.

Thyroxine and triiodothyronine are active thyroid hormones that increase the turnover of protein, carbohydrate, fat, and mineral. They circulate in the blood, largely bound to serum proteins, although small quantities are in an active free form. Excessive thyroid hormone produces catabolism of protein and loss of connective tissue; a deficiency causes defects in bone growth and development.

HYPERTHYROIDISM

Thyrotoxicosis is a general term indicating biochemical and physiologic abnormalities that result from excessive quantities of the thyroid hormones; the term hyperthyroidism is used to describe this syndrome when it is the result of overproduction of these hormones by the thyroid gland itself rather than of abnormalities that have not originated in this gland. Of the many forms of thyrotoxicosis, toxic diffuse goiter (Graves' disease or Basedow's disease) and toxic nodular goiter produced by single or multiple adenomas are most common. Clinical manifestations of thyrotoxicosis include symptoms such as fatigue, weakness, nervousness, hypersensitivity to heat, hyperhidrosis, weight loss, tachycardia, palpitation, eye complaints, and diarrhea; physical signs may include enlargement of the neck, rapid heart beat, tremor, thyroid bruit, and abnormalities of the eye. Musculoskeletal abnormalities also are well known (Table 51–1).

Bone Resorption

In patients with endogenous or exogenous hyperthyroidism, elevation of serum calcium concentration is apparent. Additional laboratory findings are elevated levels of serum phosphorus and alkaline phosphatase and hypercalciuria. These features underscore the presence of excessive bone turnover with a negative calcium balance, although the mechanism by which this occurs is not known.

The reported frequency of radiographically detectable bone disease in patients with hyperthyroidism has varied from 3.5 to 50 per cent. The changes are more common in men than in women, and, in women, predominate after the menopause. Most individuals with bone abnormalities have had hyperthyroidism for longer than 5 years. Such abnormalities may be associated with pain, fracture, and deformities, which include reduction in height and exaggerated dorsal kyphosis. Spontaneous fractures in hyperthyroidism are frequent and, in

Table 51–1. MUSCULOSKELETAL ABNORMALITIES OF HYPERTHYROIDISM

> Hyperthyroid osteopathy
> Accelerated skeletal maturation
> Myopathy

addition to vertebral body collapse, may be seen in the femoral neck and other tubular bones. Clinical as well as radiographic findings may appear quickly, progress rapidly, and stabilize or improve with appropriate treatment of thyrotoxicosis.

The radiographic features of bone loss in hyperthyroidism simulate those associated with other varieties of osteoporosis, although hyperthyroid osteopathy may lead to bone loss not only in the vertebral column but also in the pelvis, cranium, hands, and feet. Osteoporosis, vertebral compression, and kyphosis (or kyphoscoliosis) are seen (Fig. 51–1). Osteoporosis produces typical rarefaction of the midportion of the vertebral body and "fish vertebrae" with exaggerated biconcave deformity of the vertebral body. These changes are more pronounced in the thoracic and lumbar spine. In the skull, focal rarefaction of bone, particularly in the frontal region, may produce a radiographic picture reminiscent of that in multiple myeloma. Osteoporosis is also observed in the hands and feet of patients with hyperthyroidism.

The qualitative and quantitative histologic findings in hyperthyroid osteopathy suggest the presence of both hyperosteoclastosis and hyperosteoblastosis, which are more prominent in cortical bone than in trabecular bone. Both bone resorption and bone formation are increased, but resorption is the more dominant abnormality. Osteopenia, deformity, and even pathologic fracture are the observed radiologic alterations.

Additional Musculoskeletal Abnormalities

Hyperthyroidism in children is associated with acceleration of skeletal maturation. Premature craniosynostosis can be evident.

Myopathy is frequent in hyperthyroidism, especially in men, and its symptoms and signs may simulate arthritis. Weakness, cramps, and muscular tenderness are observed. Neurologic manifestations of hyperthyroidism include pe-

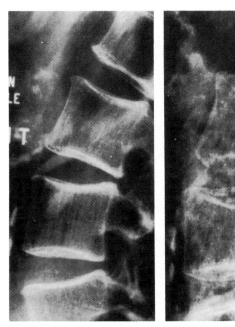

Figure 51–1. Hyperthyroidism: Spinal abnormalities. Radiographs obtained five months apart reveal the rapid course of vertebral osteoporosis that may accompany thyrotoxicosis. On the later film (right), increased radiolucency of the vertebral bodies and biconcave deformities are apparent. (From Meunier PJ, et al: Bony manifestations of thyrotoxicosis. Orthop Clin North Am 3:745, 1972. Used with permission.)

Table 51–2. CLINICAL AND RADIOGRAPHIC FEATURES OF THYROID ACROPACHY

Exophthalmos
Soft tissue swelling
Pretibial myxedema
Clubbing
Periositis

ripheral neuropathy, corticospinal tract disease, chorea, seizures, and psychiatric disorders.

THYROID ACROPACHY

Thyroid acropachy is an unusual manifestation of thyroid disease that may be seen in approximately 0.5 to 1 per cent of patients with thyrotoxicosis. This condition usually is observed after treatment of hyperthyroidism, at which time the patient may be euthyroid or hypothyroid. It can occur at any age, and men and women are affected equally.

Clinical findings in thyroid acropachy include exophthalmos, painless soft tissue swelling of the fingers and toes, pretibial myxedema, and clubbing of the fingers (Table 51–2).

Radiographic and Pathologic Findings

Radiographic abnormalities are virtually diagnostic (Fig. 51–2). Periosteal bone formation is seen in the diaphyses of the metacarpals, metatarsals, and proximal and middle phalanges, although this change may be visualized occasionally at other sites, including the long bones. Periostitis is more prominent on the radial aspect of the bone, and it tends to

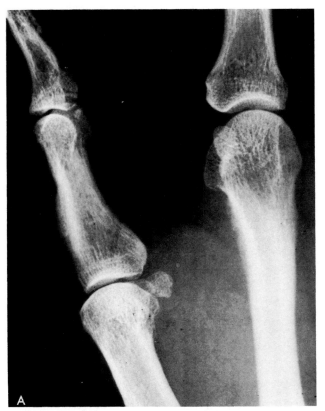

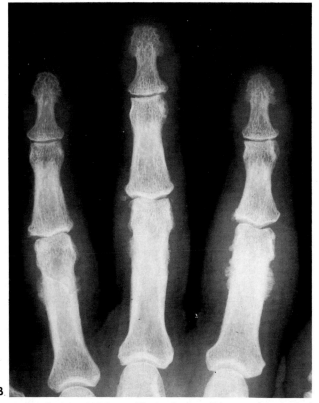

Figure 51–2. Thyroid acropachy. A Observe thick shaggy periostitis, asymmetric in distribution, which has predilection for the radial aspect of the proximal phalanx of the first digit and the second metacarpal. (Courtesy of V. Schiappacasse, M.D., Santiago, Chile.) B In a different patient, observe soft tissue swelling, clubbing, and spiculated or feathery periostitis in the proximal phalanges. Less extensive changes are seen in middle phalanges and terminal tufts. (Courtesy of L. Santini, M.D., Danville, Pennsylvania.)

be dense and solid in appearance, with a feathery contour. Soft tissue swelling in the hands and feet, phalangeal tufts, and anterior tibial region is observed. The osseous abnormalities generally are not progressive; correcting the thyroid function has little or no effect on the acropachy.

The cause of thyroid acropachy is not known.

Differential Diagnosis

Thyroid acropachy must be differentiated from other disorders associated with periosteal bone formation (Table 51–3). In hypertrophic osteoarthropathy, periosteal bone formation is observed most commonly in the tibia, fibula, radius, and ulna. Changes limited to the hands and feet are unusual in this condition. Furthermore, the feathery pattern of bone proliferation that is seen in thyroid acropachy is not typical of hypertrophic osteoarthropathy.

Pachydermoperiostosis is associated with typical facies, soft tissue prominence of the hands, and periostitis. Periosteal bone formation occurs generally in a symmetric pattern in the tibia, fibula, radius, and ulna, although the hands may also be affected. Periostitis in this disorder is not limited to the diaphysis but may be exuberant at the metaphyseal and epiphyseal areas.

Hypervitaminosis A and venous stasis may produce periosteal bone proliferation, but clinical and radiographic features allow accurate diagnosis of these conditions. Fluorosis is associated with more extensive abnormality of the axial skeleton and long bones. Periosteal bone formation in acromegaly and vasculitides such as periarteritis nodosa is readily distinguished from changes of thyroid acropachy. Infectious and traumatic disorders reveal alterations in addition to periostitis.

HYPOTHYROIDISM

Hypothyroidism and myxedema are terms describing a clinical state of thyroxine and triiodothyronine deficiency. The deficiency may be divided into a primary form, in which the thyroid gland itself is involved, and a secondary form, which involves a deficiency in thyroid stimulating hormone. There are many causes of hypothyroidism, including atrophy; thyroid gland destruction after radioactive iodine therapy or surgery; thyroiditis, which may be acute or chronic (Hashimoto's disease); infiltrative disorders, such as lymphoma, cystinosis, amyloidosis, and metastasis; deficiency in iodine or iodine metabolism; use of certain medications; and a variety of pituitary disorders.

In infants, thyroid deficiency results in cretinism, and in children it produces juvenile myxedema, with mental retardation and developmental abnormalities. Symptoms and signs include lethargy, constipation, enlarged tongue, abdominal distention, hypotonia, dry hair and skin, and delayed dentition. In adults, the disease is more frequent in women than in men and can be associated with dry, coarse skin and hair, fatigue, lethargy, edema, hoarseness, constipation, paresthesias, and bradycardia as well as other symptoms and signs (Table 51–4).

In adult-onset hypothyroidism, bone abnormalities are mild. In cretinism and juvenile myxedema, however, skeletal manifestations are marked. Delayed bone maturation is most characteristic, and in the infant, absence of the epiphyses in the distal portion of the femur and proximal portion of the

Table 51–3. SOME CONDITIONS ASSOCIATED WITH PERIOSTITIS OF MULTIPLE BONES

Hypertrophic osteoarthropathy
Pachydermoperiostosis
Thyroid acropachy
Hypervitaminosis A
Venous stasis
Fluorosis
Leukemia
Vascular insufficiency
Infection
Trauma

tibia is an important radiographic clue. In older children, abnormal epiphyseal maturation leads to distinctive radiographic findings, with fragmented irregular epiphyseal contours, termed epiphyseal dysgenesis. Delayed dental development is a concomitant feature of the disease. Retardation in growth in these patients may simulate that associated with growth hormone deficiency.

Altered Development of Bone

Although skeletal retardation may be seen in other disorders, usually it is more severe in hypothyroidism than in these other conditions (Fig. 51–3), and the diagnosis of hypothyroidism is suspect if a child has normal maturation. The radiographic confirmation of delayed skeletal maturation relies on a delay in appearance and growth of epiphyseal ossification centers and is most facilitated in the infant by examination of the knees (or feet). Evaluation of the bones of the hand is less helpful as in normal situations the carpal bones are not ossified at birth. This abnormality of epiphyseal development is accompanied by alterations in development of synchondroses (e.g., between segments of sternum and sacrum) and sutures; physeal growth plates and sutures may persist well beyond the age at which they should normally have disappeared.

On histologic examination, the persisting physeal growth plate reveals little evidence of cartilage cellular proliferation. The plate is "closed off" by osseous tissue of the metaphysis.

In the skull, growth retardation is particularly striking at the base of the cranium. Decreased growth of the sphenooccipital synchondrosis produces brachycephaly. Enlargement of

Table 51–4. REPORTED MUSCULOSKELETAL ABNORMALITIES OF HYPOTHYROIDISM

Retarded skeletal maturation
Accessory sutural bones
Epiphyseal dysgenesis
Epiphyseal deformity with secondary
  degenerative joint disease
Gibbus deformity
Dystrophic calcification
Carpal tunnel syndrome
Synovial effusion; tenosynovitis
Myopathy
Neuropathy
Soft tissue edema
Osteoporosis
Slipped capital femoral epiphysis
Ligamentous laxity
Calcium pyrophosphate dihydrate crystal deposition

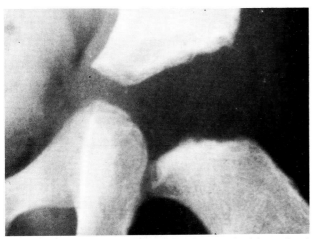

Figure 51–3. Hypothyroidism: Delayed ossification of epiphyses. In a 3 year old child with hypothyroidism, the capital femoral epiphysis has not yet ossified.

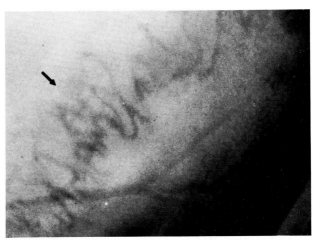

Figure 51–5. Hypothyroidism: Prominent sutures with accessory (wormian) bones (arrow).

the sella turcica is observed (Fig. 51–4). Additional cranial findings in hypothyroidism include prominent sutures with accessory (wormian) bones (which can also be seen in osteogenesis imperfecta, cleidocranial dysostosis, and other conditions), underdevelopment of the paranasal sinuses and mastoid air cells, and a prognathous lower jaw (Fig. 51–5).

In addition to delay in the appearance of epiphyseal centers, the pattern of ossification within these centers may be altered in hypothyroidism. Ossification proceeds from multiple centers rather than from a single site, and the resulting irregular appearance is termed epiphyseal dysgenesis (Fig. 51–6).

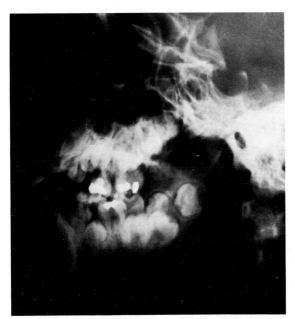

Figure 51–4. Hypothyroidism: Cranial and facial abnormalities. In a 21 year old man with cretinism, findings include an enlarged sella turcica, prominent lower jaw and delayed dental development. (Courtesy of S. Hilton, M.D., San Diego, California.)

Epiphyseal dysgenesis is particularly frequent in the femoral and humeral heads and tarsal navicular bone. The fragmented epiphysis can simulate the appearance of osteonecrosis and lead to a mistaken diagnosis of Legg-Calvé-Perthes disease. It is important to realize that epiphyseal dysgenesis is not the result of vascular insufficiency. It relates to an aberration of the ossification pattern in the involved epiphysis, in which islands of endochondral ossification are observed. When the patient is treated, coalescence of the fragments may lead to disappearance of epiphyseal dysgenesis within a year or two. With delayed or inadequate therapy, epiphyseal abnormalities may result in secondary articular degeneration.

Increased radiopacity of epiphyses as well as metaphyses also has been noted in patients with hypothyroidism. Unfused apophyses may be seen.

Spinal findings in hypothyroidism are particularly prominent at the thoracolumbar junction, at which site short and bullet-shaped twelfth thoracic and first lumbar vertebral bodies may be visualized (Fig. 51–7). A gibbus deformity may result. Additional vertebral alterations that have been noted in hypothyroidism are relatively widened intervertebral disc spaces and increased distance between the anterior arch of the atlas and the odontoid process of the axis. Thoracic cage deformities may be apparent. Also, a distinctive osseous projection in the midportion of the metaphyses of the distal phalanges has been described.

Additional Rheumatologic Manifestations

An entrapment neuropathy, including the carpal tunnel syndrome caused by median nerve compression at the wrist, is seen in approximately 7 per cent of patients with hypothyroidism.

Muscular cramps and stiffness also are common in hypothyroidism, with predilection for the calves, thighs, and shoulders. Myxomatous infiltration of soft tissues causes prominence of these tissues.

Articular findings are less prominent than those related to neuropathy and myopathy. Thickening of periarticular soft tissues and effusions are rarely encountered.

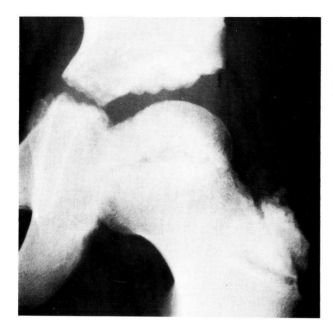

Figure 51–6. Hypothyroidism: Epiphyseal dysgenesis. Irregularity of the apophysis of the greater trochanter and acetabular margin is associated with flattening and deformity of the proximal capital femoral epiphysis.

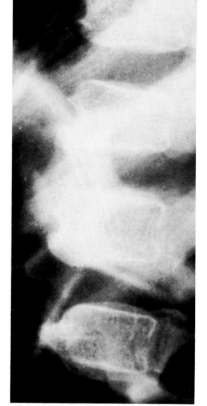

Figure 51–7. Hypothyroidism: Spinal abnormalities. Note bullet-shaped vertebrae and beak-like anterior surfaces of the vertebral bodies.

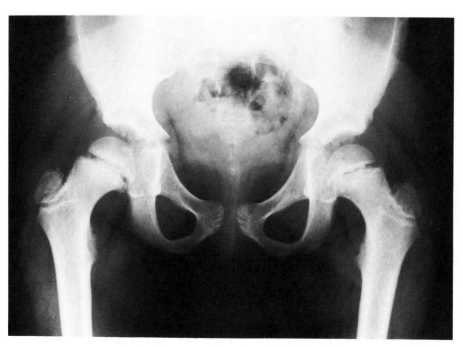

Figure 51–8. Hypothyroidism: Slipped capital femoral epiphyses. A frontal radiograph of the pelvis shows bilateral slipped capital femoral epiphyses with widened and irregular physes. Evaluation revealed decreased bone age and, subsequently, the diagnosis of hypothyroidism was verified. (Courtesy of G. Greenway, M.D., Dallas, Texas.)

Slipped Capital Femoral Epiphysis

Slipped capital femoral epiphyses may occur in patients with hypothyroidism who may or may not have been started on treatment. Although usually seen in prepubescent subjects, the complication occasionally is apparent in the more sexually mature man or woman. A bilateral or unilateral distribution is evident. Typical radiographic features are encountered (Fig. 51–8). The cause of this complication in treated or untreated hypothyroidism is not known.

FURTHER READING

Bonakdarpour A, Kirkpatric JA, Renzi A, Kendall N: Skeletal changes in neonatal thyrotoxicosis. Radiology 102:149, 1972.

Borg SA, Fitzer PM, Young LW: Roentgenologic aspects of adult cretinism. Two case reports and review of the literature. AJR 123:820, 1975.

Hernandez RJ, Poznanski AK: Distinctive appearance of the distal phalanges in children with primary hypothyroidism. Radiology 132:83, 1979.

Hernandez RJ, Poznanski AW, Hopwood NJ: Size and skeletal maturation of the hand in children with hypothyroidism and hypopituitarism. AJR 133:405, 1979.

Jaffe HL: Metabolic, Degenerative and Inflammatory Diseases of Bones and Joints. Philadelphia, Lea & Febiger, 1972.

Lintermans JP, Seyhnaeve V: Hypothyroidism and vertebral anomalies. A new syndrome? AJR 109:294, 1970.

Meunier PJ, S-Bianchi GG, Edouard CM, Bernard JC, Courpron P, Vignon GE: Bony manifestations of thyrotoxicosis. Orthop Clin North Am 3:745, 1972.

Moorefield WG, Urbaniak JR, Ogden WS, Frank JL: Acquired hypothyroidism and slipped capital femoral epiphysis. Report of three cases. J Bone Joint Surg [Am] 58:705, 1976.

Scanlon GT, Clemett AR: Thyroid acropachy. Radiology 83:1039, 1964.

Wietersen FK, Balow RM: The radiologic aspects of thyroid disease. Radiol Clin North Am 5:255, 1967.

Chapter 52

Parathyroid Disorders and Renal Osteodystrophy

Donald Resnick, M.D.
Gen Niwayama, M.D.

Elevated levels of parathyroid hormone occurring in primary and secondary hyperparathyroidism produce considerable osseous erosion involving subperiosteal, intracortical, endosteal, trabecular, subchondral, and subligamentous foci. In renal osteodystrophy, the changes of secondary hyperparathyroidism are combined with additional features, including osteomalacia, osteoporosis, and soft tissue and vascular calcification, findings that may become exaggerated or arrested after hemodialysis and renal transplantation.

Depressed levels of parathyroid hormone may be associated with osteosclerosis, subcutaneous and basal ganglion calcification, and spinal abnormalities simulating diffuse idiopathic skeletal hyperostosis. Pseudohypoparathyroidism and pseudopseudohypoparathyroidism may be associated with abnormalities in skeletal maturation and development, peculiar exostoses, and soft tissue calcification and ossification.

Parathyroid hormone is essential for the proper transport of calcium and other ions in bone, intestine, and kidney. Its initial effect on bone is to promote release of calcium into the blood, and a second action is to stimulate extensive bone remodeling. Alterations of parathyroid function cause breakdown in calcium homeostasis, leading to characteristic pathologic and radiographic abnormalities.

HYPERPARATHYROIDISM
General Features

Hyperparathyroidism is a general term indicating an increased level of parathyroid hormone in the blood. The condition generally is divided into three types: primary, secondary, and tertiary.

In *primary hyperparathyroidism* increased parathyroid hormone secretion occurs as a result of abnormality in one or more of the parathyroid glands. Autonomous hyperfunction of these glands results from a variety of causes, including diffuse hyperplasia (10 to 40 per cent of cases), single (50 to 80 per cent) or multiple (10 per cent) adenomas, and, rarely, carcinoma. The fundamental biochemical parameter of the disease is persistent hypercalcemia, although some patients with primary hyperparathyroidism demonstrate intermittent hypercalcemia or normal total serum calcium concentrations.

Secondary hyperparathyroidism is associated with abnormalities in function of the parathyroid glands induced by a sustained hypocalcemic stimulus, usually resulting from chronic renal failure or, occasionally, from malabsorption states. Pathologic examination generally reveals hyperplasia of all four parathyroid glands, plasma calcium levels are normal or low, and serum inorganic phosphate levels are high (chronic renal disease) or low (intestinal malabsorption). Renal abnormality is associated with soft tissue and skeletal changes, termed *renal osteodystrophy*.

Tertiary hyperparathyroidism occurs in patients with chronic renal failure or malabsorption and long-standing secondary hyperparathyroidism who develop relatively autonomous parathyroid function and hypercalcemia.

It is the elevation of serum levels of parathyroid hormone with subsequent hypercalcemia that provides the most important clue in diagnosing hyperparathyroidism; it should be emphasized, however, hypercalcemia is a known complication of other disease states (Table 52–1). Indeed, hypercalcemia develops in 10 to 20 per cent of patients with malignancy. The syndrome consisting of hypercalcemia of malignancy in the absence of demonstrable skeletal metastasis or primary hyperparathyroidism is termed *pseudohyperparathyroidism*. Serum biochemical parameters in this syndrome are consistent with a status of suppressed parathyroid function and support the concept of a humoral substance, distinct from parathyroid hormone, that is elaborated by the tumors.

In addition to hypercalcemia, laboratory abnormalities in hyperparathyroidism include hypophosphatemia, hyperphosphatasia, hypercalciuria, and, less constantly, a tendency toward hyperchloremic acidosis, hydroxyprolinuria, hyperglycemia, hyperuricemia, and hypomagnesemia.

In general, clinical findings in hyperparathyroidism are most commonly attributable to renal, skeletal, and gastrointestinal changes. The patient's initial complaints frequently are attributable to the presence of urinary tract calculi and nephrolithiasis, peptic ulcer disease, or pancreatitis. Symptomatic bone disease may be observed in 10 to 25 per cent of patients and may consist of tenderness, pain, swelling, and deformity. Alterations in the central nervous system, skin,

Table 52–1. DIFFERENTIAL DIAGNOSIS OF HYPERCALCEMIA

Artifactual Disorders
  Hyperproteinemia
    Venous stasis during blood collection
    Hyperalbuminemia (e.g., hyperalimentation)
    Hypergammaglobulinemia (e.g., myeloma, sarcoidosis)
Malignancy
  Solid tumors (primarily breast cancer)
  Hematologic disorders
    Myeloma
    Lymphoma
    Leukemia
Endocrinologic Disorders
  Primary hyperparathyroidism
  Multiple endocrine adenomatoses, types I and II
  Ectopic hyperparathyroidism (malignancy, predominantly lung cancer)
  Secondary hyperparathyroidism (e.g., renal failure)
  Hyperthyroidism
  Hypoadrenalism (usually after acute steroid withdrawal)
Drugs
  Vitamin A intoxication
  Vitamin D intoxication
  Thiazides
  Calcium
    Milk-alkali syndrome (ingestion of absorbable antacid calcium-containing preparations—e.g., calcium carbonate)
    Dialysis (with dialysate calcium concentration >7.0 mg/dl)
Granulomatous Disorders
  Sarcoidosis
  Tuberculosis
  Histoplasmosis
  Berylliosis
  Rheumatoid arthritis (primarily during immobilization)
Pediatric Disorders
  Infantile hypercalcemia
  Hypophosphatasia
Immobilization
  Paget's disease
  Growth
Miscellaneous Disorders
  Pheochromocytoma
  Idiopathic periostitis
  Post–renal transplant surgery
  Benign familial hypercalcemia
  Diuretic phase of acute renal failure

(From Aviolo LV, Raisz LG: Bone metabolism and disease. In Bondy PK, Rosenberg LE (Eds): Metabolic Control and Disease. 8th Ed. Philadelphia, WB Saunders, 1980, p 1734. Used with permission.)

and cardiovascular system may also contribute to the clinical picture.

Fundamental Characteristics of Bone Involvement

Although hyperparathyroidism is accompanied by an increase in the ratio of osteoclasts to osteoblasts, parathyroid hormone influences all three types of bone cells—osteoclasts, osteoblasts, and osteocytes. Histologic examination of osseous tissue demonstrates osteitis fibrosa cystica, with replacement of marrow elements by highly vascular fibrous tissue, as well as the changes of osteoporosis and osteomalacia. Initially, exaggerated osteoclastic activity is evident on the surface of trabeculae within the cancellous bone and on the walls of the haversian canals within the cortical bone. Subsequently, osteofibrosis is associated with localized cysts or brown tumors, rarefied and thinned cortices, distorted and blurred cancellous trabeculae, infractions, fractures, and deformities.

Bone Resorption

Resorption of osseous tissue is evident on histologic and radiologic examination in patients with primary (or secondary) hyperparathyroidism. Although many skeletal sites are affected, the sensitivity of bone resorption in the hands in the early stages of the disease has been documented repeatedly, indicating that high quality radiography of this region is adequate in detecting and monitoring the course of skeletal changes in primary and secondary hyperparathyroidism.

It is convenient to categorize bone resorption as subperiosteal, intracortical, endosteal, subchondral, trabecular, and subligamentous in type. Localized lesions or brown tumors may also be seen.

SUBPERIOSTEAL BONE RESORPTION (FIG. 52–1). Subperiosteal resorption of cortical bone is virtually diagnostic of hyperparathyroid bone disease. Although this change may be visualized in various skeletal locations, it is most frequent along the radial aspect of the phalanges of the hand, particularly in the middle phalanges of the index and middle fingers. A lace-like appearance of the phalangeal bone may progress to a spiculated contour and, eventually, to complete resorption of the entire cortex. Additional sites of subperiosteal resorption include the phalangeal tufts; medial aspect of the proximal portion of the tibia, humerus, and femur; superior and inferior margins of the ribs; and lamina dura.

Subperiosteal resorption of bone may also be apparent at the *margins* of certain joints, accounting for one "articular" manifestation of hyperparathyroidism (Table 52–2) (Fig. 52–2). Although this may be noted about the acromioclavicular, sternoclavicular, and sacroiliac joints and symphysis pubis, periarticular subperiosteal resorption may be especially prominent in the hand, wrist, and foot. The erosions that are created can simulate the appearance of rheumatoid arthritis, although they may be located slightly farther from the joint margin and are almost always associated with typical subperiosteal resorption of the adjacent phalangeal shafts. Furthermore, they predominate on the ulnar aspect of the metacarpal heads (compared with a radial predilection in rheumatoid arthritis), involve the distal interphalangeal joints with relative sparing of the proximal interphalangeal joints (compared with the opposite situation in rheumatoid arthritis), are associated with a normal-appearing joint space (whereas early joint space narrowing is typical of rheumatoid arthritis), and are characterized by a shaggy, irregular osseous contour with bone "whiskering" (in comparison to rheumatoid arthritis, in which bone proliferation is mild or absent).

It should be stressed that although other forms of bone resorption are frequent in hyperparathyroidism, subperiosteal resorption is the most useful diagnostic sign, and changes in the phalanges are among the initial osseous manifestations of the disease. Other disorders can occasionally be associated with subperiosteal resorption of bone, particularly as a localized phenomenon.

INTRACORTICAL BONE RESORPTION (FIG. 52–3). Osteoclastic resorption of bone within cortical haversian canals can produce radiographically detectable intracortical linear striations. These are best observed in the cortex of the second metacarpal. The findings are not specific, being seen in other disorders with rapid bone turnover, such as acromegaly and hyperthyroidism. In hyperparathyroidism, intracortical resorption of bone is almost always associated with subperiosteal resorption.

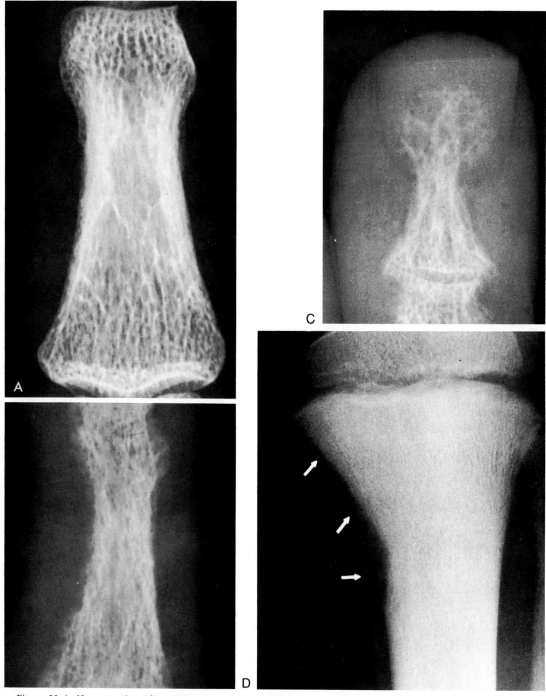

Figure 52–1. Hyperparathyroidism: Subperiosteal bone resorption. A, B Phalanges. Examples of mild (**A**) and severe (**B**) subperiosteal resorption. Early findings include lace-like bone resorption, particularly on the radial aspect of the middle phalanges. This pattern may progress to severe cortical destruction with loss of definition between cortex and spongiosa. **C** Phalangeal tuft. An example of tuftal resorption. **D** Proximal tibia. Subperiosteal resorption is particularly prominent on the medial aspect of this bone (arrows).

Table 52–2. ARTICULAR MANIFESTATIONS OF HYPERPARATHYROIDISM

Mechanism	Characteristic Sites	Characteristic Appearance
Subperiosteal bone resorption	Hands, wrists, feet	Marginal erosions with adjacent bone resorption and proliferation
Subchondral bone resorption	Sacroiliac, sternoclavicular, and acromioclavicular joints; symphysis pubis; discovertebral junction; large and small joints of the appendicular skeleton	Subchondral erosions, weakening, and collapse
Subligamentous bone resorption	Trochanters, ischial tuberosities, humeral tuberosities, calcanei, distal clavicles	Osseous erosion with reactive bone formation
CPPD crystal deposition	Knees, wrists, and symphysis pubis	Chondrocalcinosis; pyrophosphate arthropathy (rare)
Urate crystal deposition	Various sites	Soft tissue swelling, osseous erosions
Tendon and ligament laxity	Sacroiliac and acromioclavicular joints; spine	Joint instability, soft tissue swelling, osseous erosion, dislocation, and subluxation
Tendon avulsion and rupture	Quadriceps, infrapatellar, triceps, flexor and extensor finger tendons	Subluxation and dislocation

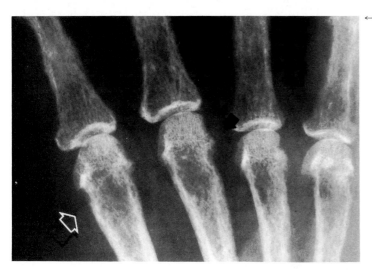

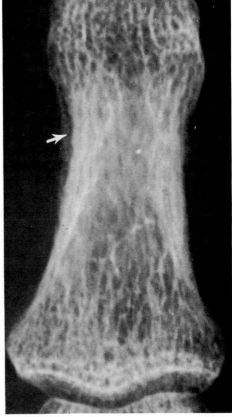

Figure 52–2. **Hyperparathyroidism: Subperiosteal bone resorption—juxtaarticular erosions.** Metacarpophalangeal joint abnormalities. Erosions occur on the radial (open arrow) and ulnar (solid arrow) aspects of the metacarpal heads and proximal phalanges. Although in some places the erosions are intraarticular, they extend outside the joint. Observe the shaggy irregular osseous contour. The articular spaces are relatively normal. Subperiosteal bone resorption is also evident. (From Resnick D: Erosive arthritis of the hand and wrist in hyperparathyroidism. Radiology *110:*263, 1974. Used with permission.)

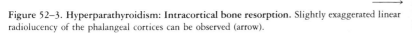

Figure 52–3. **Hyperparathyroidism: Intracortical bone resorption.** Slightly exaggerated linear radiolucency of the phalangeal cortices can be observed (arrow).

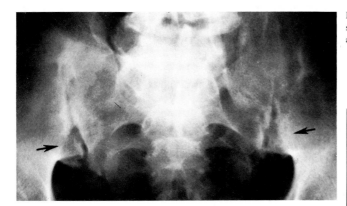

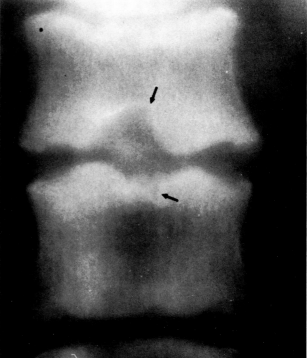

Figure 52–4. Hyperparathyroidism: Subchondral bone resorption—sacroiliac joint. Observe the irregular osseous surface on the ilium and adjacent reactive sclerosis (arrows). A paraarticular osteophyte is also apparent.

Figure 52–5. Hyperparathyroidism: Subchondral bone resorption—discovertebral junction. Frontal tomography in a patient with renal osteodystrophy reveals extensive subchondral resorption of bone at the discovertebral junction. Note cartilaginous (Schmorl's) nodes (arrows) producing irregular depressions in the osseous surface, reactive sclerosis, and narrowing of the disc space. (Courtesy of J. Mink, M.D., Los Angeles, California.)

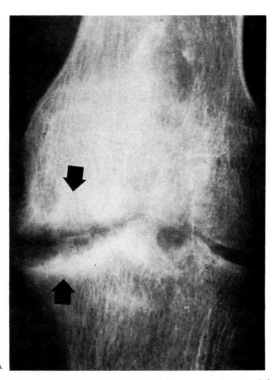

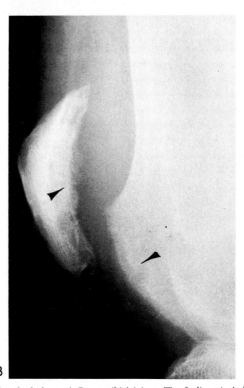

A   B

Figure 52–6. Hyperparathyroidism: Subchondral bone resorption—peripheral articulations. A Femorotibial joints. The findings include irregularity and depression of the articular surface simulating infection (arrows). (From Resnick D, Niwayama G: Subchondral resorption of bone in renal osteodystrophy. Radiology *118*:315, 1976. Used with permission.) **B** Patellofemoral joint. Observe considerable erosion with deformity of the posterior surface of the patella and resorption on the anterior surface of the femur (arrowheads). (Courtesy of R. Shapiro, M.D., and K. Weisner, M.D., Sacramento, California.)

ENDOSTEAL BONE RESORPTION. Osteoclastic resorption occurs along the endosteal surface of bone, particularly in the hands. Radiographic features include localized pocket-like or scalloped defects along the inner margin of the cortex, which are reminiscent of abnormalities occurring in multiple myeloma, and more generalized thinning of the cortex, which can simulate the appearance of osteoporosis. Endosteal bone resorption is rarely an isolated or predominant feature of hyperparathyroidism.

SUBCHONDRAL BONE RESORPTION (FIGS. 52–4 TO 52–6). Subchondral resorption of bone is a common manifestation of hyperparathyroidism, accounting for a second "articular" finding in this disease. This type of resorption is most frequent in the sacroiliac, sternoclavicular, and acromioclavicular joints, symphysis pubis, and discovertebral junctions, although it is also observed in large and small joints of the appendicular skeleton. Weakening and collapse of the osseous surface are accompanied by depression of the overlying cartilage. Juxtaarticular bone surfaces may demonstrate concomitant subperiosteal resorption.

Subchondral resorption in the sacroiliac joints may lead to radiographic findings simulating those of ankylosing spondylitis. Osseous erosion and reactive new bone formation produce a poorly defined and sclerotic articular margin and "pseudo-widening" of the joint space (Fig. 52–7). As in ankylosing spondylitis, the classic sacroiliac joint changes in hyperparathyroidism are usually bilateral and symmetric in distribution.

Subchondral resorption is also common at the acromioclavicular and sternoclavicular joints. The changes are usually symmetric in distribution. They are equally severe on the sternum and clavicle at the sternoclavicular joint and more severe on the clavicle than on the acromion at the acromioclavicular joint. Although resorption of the distal end of the clavicle is not a specific sign of hyperparathyroidism, it is helpful in diagnosis. Subchondral resorption is also evident

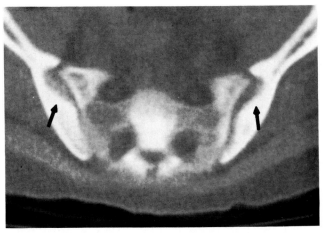

Figure 52–7. Hyperparathyroidism: Subchondral bone resorption—sacroiliac joints. A transaxial computed tomographic image reveals bilateral and symmetric abnormalities (arrows).

at the discovertebral junctions. Changes in the vertebral bodies beneath the cartilaginous endplates produce areas of structural weakening, allowing displacement of disc material or formation of cartilaginous (Schmorl's) nodes.

Subchondral bone collapse in the peripheral skeleton also has been described. This finding is particularly frequent in the knee but may also be observed in other large and small appendicular joints.

TRABECULAR BONE RESORPTION (FIG. 52–8). Trabecular resorption occurs throughout the skeleton in hyperparathyroidism, particularly in the advanced stages of the disease. Such resorption within the cranium is especially striking. The diploë is replaced by connective tissue containing newly formed trabeculae, and definition between the diploic portion of the skull and the inner and outer tables is

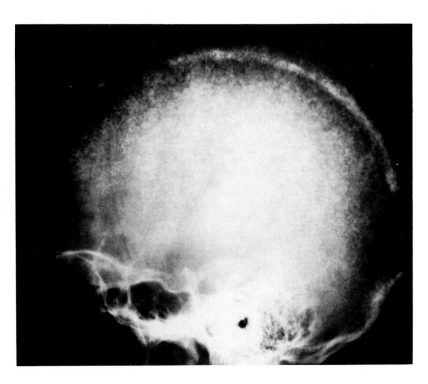

Figure 52–8. Hyperparathyroidism: Trabecular bone resorption—cranial vault. The lateral radiograph outlines the characteristic mottling of the vault. Alternating areas of lucency and sclerosis produce the "salt and pepper" appearance.

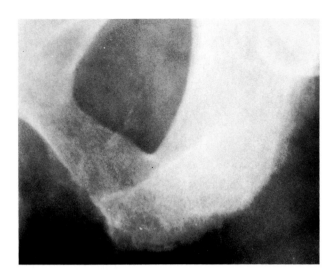

Figure 52–9. Hyperparathyroidism: Subligamentous bone resorption—ischial tuberosity. Erosion of bone has produced a poorly defined, irregular osseous surface.

lost. On radiographs, an osteopenic (decreased radiodensity) and speckled appearance is termed the "salt and pepper" skull.

SUBLIGAMENTOUS BONE RESORPTION (FIG. 52–9). Osseous resorption occurs at sites of tendon and ligament attachment to bone. This is particularly frequent at the trochanters, ischial and humeral tuberosities, elbow, inferior surface of the calcaneus, and inferior aspect of the distal end of the clavicle.

BROWN TUMORS (FIG. 52–10). Brown tumors or osteoclastomas are characteristic of primary hyperparathyroidism, although they are noted in secondary hyperparathyroidism as well. Brown tumors represent localized accumulations of fibrous tissue and giant cells, which can replace bone and may even produce osseous expansion. They may subsequently undergo necrosis and liquefaction, producing cysts. Brown tumors appear as single or multiple well-defined lesions of the axial or appendicular skeleton. Common sites of involvement are the facial bones, pelvis, ribs, and femora. With removal of the parathyroid adenoma, brown tumors may demonstrate healing with increased radiodensity.

Bone Sclerosis

Increased amounts of trabecular bone can occur in patients with hyperparathyroidism and create abnormal radiodensity on skeletal radiographs. This is observed far more frequently

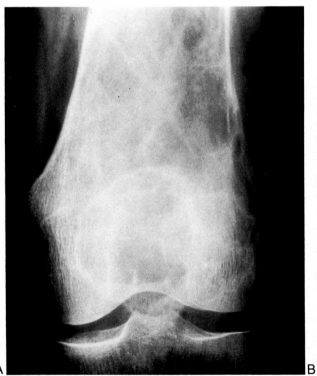
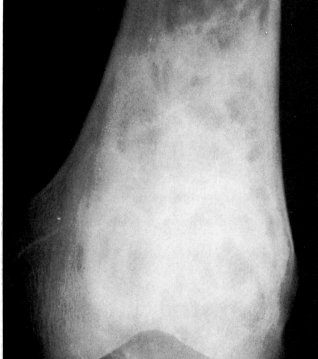

A   **B**

Figure 52–10. Hyperparathyroidism: Brown tumors. Brown tumor of the distal part of the femur before (A) and after (B) removal of parathyroid adenoma. Increased radiodensity of the lesion after surgery is evident.

in patients with renal osteodystrophy and secondary hyperparathyroidism, although it may be apparent in primary hyperparathyroidism as well. In patients with secondary hyperparathyroidism diffuse increase in bone density may be seen. In patients with primary hyperparathyroidism, bone sclerosis may be localized or patchy in distribution, apparent in the metaphyseal regions of the long bones, the skull, or the vertebral endplates.

The mechanism of bone sclerosis in hyperparathyroidism is not clearly defined.

Chondrocalcinosis (Calcium Pyrophosphate Dihydrate Crystal Deposition)

The association of primary hyperparathyroidism and calcium pyrophosphate dihydrate (CPPD) crystal deposition is well known. CPPD crystal deposition may also occur in chronic renal disease, although its frequency is much lower than in primary hyperparathyroidism. Radiographic evidence of such crystal deposition has been reported in 18 to 40 per cent of patients with hyperparathyroidism.

Additional Rheumatic Manifestations

In addition to subchondral osseous resorption leading to collapse and fragmentation of bone, subperiosteal bone resorption leading to periarticular erosions, subligamentous osseous resorption with erosion at ligamentous attachments to bone, and CPPD crystal deposition that may lead to the pseudogout syndrome, other rheumatic manifestations of hyperparathyroidism may be encountered (Fig. 52–11).

Parathyroid hormone may affect ligaments and tendons themselves. The resultant capsular and ligamentous laxity may contribute to joint instability, traumatic synovitis, and cartilaginous and osseous destruction. Furthermore, the occurrence of spontaneous tendon avulsion in patients with hyperparathyroidism has been attributed to the direct effect of parathyroid hormone on connective tissue. Similar reports of tendinous ruptures have been seen in patients on chronic hemodialysis with secondary hyperparathyroidism. Tendon rupture in either primary or secondary hyperparathyroidism can involve one or multiple sites, including the quadriceps, infrapatellar, and triceps tendons, as well as the flexor and extensor tendons of the fingers.

Monosodium urate crystals and clinical gout have been described in patients with hyperparathyroidism.

Hyperparathyroidism in Infants and Children

Congenital primary hyperparathyroidism is a rare disorder occurring in infants, demonstrating autosomal recessive inheritance. Symptoms and signs include hypotonicity, respiratory distress, fever, dehydration, constipation, anorexia, lethargy, vomiting, dysphagia, craniotabes, and hepatosplenomegaly. Hypercalcemia generally is present. Radiographs may reveal severe bone disease with subperiosteal resorption, periosteal bone formation, trabecular reduction, extensive erosions of tubular bones, and pathologic fractures. Rib fractures with callus formation resemble pulmonary infiltrates.

A second disorder, *transient hyperparathyroidism of the neonate,* is secondary to hypoparathyroidism in the mother. The radiographic changes are similar to congenital primary hyperparathyroidism, although they resolve rapidly.

In older children, skeletal involvement in hyperparathy-roidism is characterized by osteopenia, genu valgum, fractures, cystic lesions of bone, and clubbing of the fingers. Renal involvement and rickets-like changes with metaphyseal irregularity may be observed.

Familial Hypercalcemia

Specific and distinct syndromes of familial hypercalcemia have been identified including several types of disorders accompanied by tumors of multiple endocrine glands and familial hypocalciuric hypercalcemia (Table 52–3).

Familial multiple endocrine neoplasia (MEN), type I, which is also referred to as multiple endocrine adenomatosis (MEA) and Wermer's syndrome, is an autosomal dominant disease associated with primary hyperparathyroidism (95 per cent of cases) and, less frequently, excessive secretion of gastrin (20 to 40 per cent of cases), insulin (2 to 10 per cent of cases), other pancreatic islet peptides (rare), and anterior pituitary peptides (rare). Nonsecretory neoplastic masses, including lipomas, pituitary chromophobe adenomas, carcinoid tumors, and adrenal and thyroid adenomas, also occur. Familial

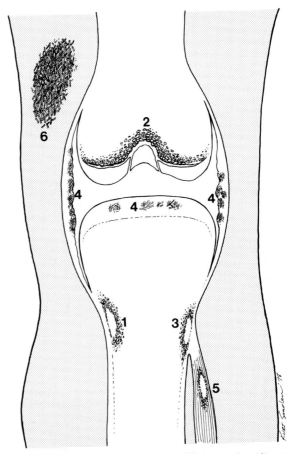

Figure 52–11. Rheumatic manifestations of hyperparathyroidism (and renal osteodystrophy). Findings may relate to subperiosteal resorption at the margins of the joint (1), subchondral resorption leading to cartilage and bone disintegration and fragmentation (2), subligamentous resorption (3), intraarticular crystal deposition (CPPD, monosodium urate) in cartilage, synovium, and capsule (4), tendinous and ligamentous injury and rupture (5), and periarticular crystal deposition (monosodium urate, calcium hydroxyapatite) in soft tissues (6). Amyloidosis may also be evident.

Table 52–3. MAJOR FEATURES IN SYNDROMES OF FAMILIAL HYPERCALCEMIA

	Multiple Endocrine Neoplasia, Type I	Multiple Endocrine Neoplasia, Type II*	Hypocalciuric Hypercalcemia
Inheritance	Autosomal dominant	Autosomal dominant	Autosomal dominant
Penetrance of hypercalcemia, first decade	Low	Low	High
Associated endocrinopathy	Islet cell; anterior pituitary	Medullary thyroid cancer; pheochromocytoma	None
Unique biochemical features	Hypergastrinemia	Hypercalcitoninemia	Relative hypocalciuria
Subtotal parathyroidectomy	Useful	Useful	Usually no benefit

*Multiple endocrine neoplasia, type IIB, rarely has hypercalcemia or hyperparathyroidism.
(From Aurbach GD, Marx SJ, Spiegel AM: Parathyroid hormone, calcitonin, and the calciferols. *In* Williams RH [Ed]: Textbook of Endocrinology. 7th Ed. Philadelphia, WB Saunders Co, 1985, p 1176. Used with permission.)

multiple endocrine neoplasia, type IIA, also called Sipple's syndrome, is inherited as an autosomal dominant trait with very high penetrance for medullary thyroid carcinoma in adults. Abnormalities of other endocrine glands, particularly primary parathyroid hyperplasia and pheochromocytoma, occur in approximately one third of cases, but malignant change related to these other endocrine aberrations is rare. A variant of this type of familial multiple endocrine neoplasia, type IIB or III, is characterized by overgrowth of neural elements and the development of mucosal neuromas, thickened corneal nerves, and intestinal ganglioneuromatosis. Additional features include joint laxity, slender body habitus, pes cavus, talipes equinovarus, abnormal spinal curvature, muscle weakness, and pectus excavatum or carinatum. MEN type IIB is a serious disorder with a high mortality rate, owing mainly to metastasis from the medullary thyroid carcinoma.

Familial hypocalciuric hypercalcemia, also called familial benign hypercalcemia, is a rare disorder of unknown cause characterized by autosomal dominant inheritance with high penetration for expression of hypercalcemia at all ages. The syndrome is associated with lifelong hypercalcemia, low urinary calcium excretion, the absence of prominent symptoms and signs, and the failure of subtotal parathyroidectomy to decrease plasma calcium levels. Superficially, familial hypocalciuric hypercalcemia resembles asymptomatic primary hyperparathyroidism; in the former condition, however, there is no significant reduction of bone mass in the axial or appendicular skeleton, and the prevalence of fractures is not increased.

Differential Diagnosis

Subperiosteal bone resorption in hyperparathyroidism is the most helpful diagnostic clue on the radiographs. Widespread subperiosteal resorption is confined to hyperparathyroid bone disease; focal areas of subperiosteal bone resorption may be seen adjacent to a variety of soft tissue processes. Intracortical bone resorption may be noted in disease states characterized by rapid bone turnover, such as hyperthyroidism and acromegaly, whereas endosteal bone resorption can be produced by osteoporosis or marrow-containing disorders, such as multiple myeloma. Some degree of subchondral bone resorption may accompany osteoporosis, but extensive resorption and collapse of articular surfaces are not common features of this condition. The severely fragmented subchondral bone surface that may accompany hyperparathyroidism may simulate the findings of septic arthritis, osteonecrosis, or crystal-induced arthropathy. In addition, the presence of these changes in certain joints necessitates inclusion of other differential diagnostic possibilities: In the interphalangeal joints of the hand, the findings may resemble inflammatory osteoarthritis, psoriasis, or even rheumatoid arthritis; in the sacroiliac joints and symphysis pubis, the differential diagnosis includes ankylosing spondylitis and its variants; in the acromioclavicular and sternoclavicular joints, hyperparathyroid subchondral bone resorption may simulate the changes of rheumatoid arthritis or ankylosing spondylitis; in the patellofemoral joints, the appearance is almost identical to that in Wilson's disease and CPPD crystal deposition disease; and at the discovertebral junction, hyperparathyroidism with subchondral resorption resembles infection, neuroarthropathy, or degenerative disc disease. Subligamentous bone resorption in hyperparathyroidism may simulate the changes that can be seen in ankylosing spondylitis and related disorders. Localized areas of osseous resorption (brown tumors) in hyperparathyroidism resemble a variety of neoplastic or neoplastic-like diseases, particularly giant cell tumor and fibrous dysplasia.

Bone sclerosis is a radiographic finding of hyperparathyroidism that can also be confused with changes in other diseases. The rugger-jersey spine is a relatively specific finding of the disease, although a somewhat similar vertebral sclerosis may occur in Paget's disease (leading to the "picture frame" vertebral body) and osteoporosis (particularly that associated with excess endogenous or exogenous steroid hormones). Diffuse bone sclerosis, which is more frequent in secondary hyperparathyroidism, also is seen in many other diseases, such as myelofibrosis, fluorosis, mastocytosis (urticaria pigmentosa), anemia (particularly sickle cell anemia), neoplasm (especially metastasis), irradiation, hypoparathyroidism, sarcoidosis, and Paget's disease.

CPPD crystal deposition in primary and (less commonly) secondary hyperparathyroidism is identical to that occurring in idiopathic CPPD crystal deposition disease and hemochromatosis. Any patient with chondrocalcinosis should be evaluated for the presence of hyperparathyroidism. Monosodium urate crystal deposition in hyperparathyroidism leads to secondary gout, which resembles primary gout.

In infants and children, periostitis and extensive bone resorption in hyperparathyroidism may simulate the findings of syphilis or leukemia, whereas metaphyseal destruction in the long bones in hyperparathyroidism produces a radiographic picture identical to that of rickets.

RENAL OSTEODYSTROPHY
General Features

In the presence of chronic renal insufficiency, the parathyroid glands undergo hyperplasia of the chief cells, the effect being generally attributable to phosphate retention and consequent lowering of serum calcium level. Secondary hyperparathyroidism also is seen in other conditions, such as malabsorption states, osteomalacia, and pseudohypoparathyroidism. It is but one of the skeletal changes that occur in patients with chronic renal disease. As normal function of the kidney is fundamental to the proper metabolism of vitamin D, renal diseases can lead to rickets and osteomalacia.

Renal osteodystrophy is a term applied to the bone disease that is apparent in patients with chronic renal failure. The pathologic and radiologic findings can be divided into hyperparathyroidism, rickets and osteomalacia, osteoporosis, soft tissue and vascular calcification, and miscellaneous alterations.

Hyperparathyroidism

The abnormalities associated with hyperparathyroidism may become manifest in renal osteodystrophy, including subperiosteal, intracortical, endosteal, trabecular, subchondral, and subligamentous bone resorption, brown tumors, bone sclerosis, and chondrocalcinosis. The frequency of some of these findings is different in renal osteodystrophy with secondary

Table 52–4. PRIMARY VERSUS SECONDARY HYPERPARATHYROIDISM

Finding	Primary Hyperparathyroidism	Secondary Hyperparathyroidism*
Brown tumors	Common	Less common
Osteosclerosis	Rare	Common
Chondrocalcinosis	Not infrequent	Rare
Periostitis	Rare	Not infrequent

*Additional findings of renal osteodystrophy are observed in association with secondary hyperparathyroidism, including rickets, osteomalacia, and soft tissue and vascular calcification.

hyperparathyroidism compared with primary hyperparathyroidism (Table 52–4). It should be noted, however, that modern techniques allow the diagnosis of primary hyperparathyroidism to be made at an early stage, when bone abnormalities are not extensive; therefore, many of the osseous changes originally believed to be more frequent in primary than in secondary hyperparathyroidism currently are found to be more typical of the latter.

Osteosclerosis is a well-known feature of renal osteodystrophy (Fig. 52–12). It predominates in the axial skeleton with involvement of the pelvis, ribs, and superior and inferior portions of the vertebral bodies (rugger-jersey spine), although

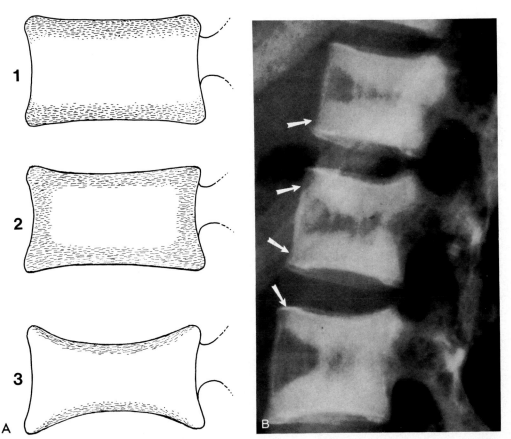

Figure 52–12. Renal osteodystrophy: Osteosclerosis—vertebral bodies. A Vertebral osteosclerosis in renal osteodystrophy is characterized by band-like sclerosis on the superior and inferior surfaces of the vertebral body (1), an appearance that is termed the rugger-jersey spine. In Paget's disease (2), sclerosis around the entire vertebral body resembles a picture frame. In osteoporosis (3), particularly that associated with steroid excess, biconcave vertebral bodies ("fish vertebrae") may be associated with condensation of bone. **B** An example of a rugger-jersey spine. Condensation of bone in the superior and inferior margins of the vertebral bodies (arrows) is not associated with osseous collapse.

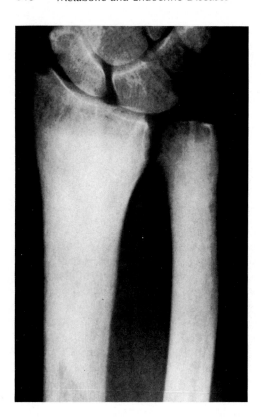

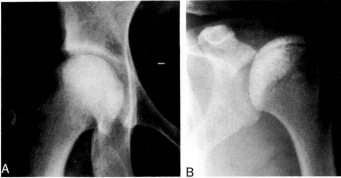

Figure 52–13. Renal osteodystrophy: Osteosclerosis—appendicular skeleton. Findings include osteosclerosis of the diaphyses and metaphyses of the radius and ulna. (Courtesy of L. Cooperstein, M.D., Pittsburgh, Pennsylvania.)

Figure 52–14. Renal osteodystrophy: Osteosclerosis—appendicular skeleton. Multiple small, punctate, mottled radiodense lesions, resembling the findings of ischemic necrosis, are evident in the epiphyseal regions of the tubular bones. (From Garver P, et al: Epiphyseal sclerosis in renal osteodystrophy simulating osteonecrosis. AJR *136*:1239, 1981. Copyright 1981, American Roentgen Ray Society. Used with permission.)

the appendicular skeleton (Fig. 52–13) may also be involved, particularly the metaphyseal regions of long bones. Less commonly, epiphyseal sclerosis resembling ischemic necrosis is seen (Fig. 52–14). It is popular to ascribe osteosclerosis in renal osteodystrophy to hyperparathyroidism, as increased bone radiodensity is also seen in primary hyperparathyroidism (see previous discussion), although other theories for increased bone density have been suggested.

Chondrocalcinosis attributable to CPPD crystal deposition is much more frequent in primary hyperparathyroidism than in renal osteodystrophy. Indeed, widespread chondrocalcinosis and pyrophosphate arthropathy are unusual manifestations of the latter disorder.

Periosteal neostosis is a term applied to periosteal bone formation in patients with renal osteodystrophy (Fig. 52–15). Its frequency is estimated to be 8 to 25 per cent in such patients, and periostitis is more frequent in those with severe skeletal abnormalities. Periosteal neostosis is observed most commonly in the metatarsals, femur, and pelvis, although it may occur elsewhere, including the humerus, radius, ulna, tibia, metacarpals, and phalanges. With regard to pathogenesis, periosteal neostosis has generally been considered to be a manifestation of hyperparathyroidism, although alternative explanations exist.

Rickets and Osteomalacia

The cause of osteomalacia in chronic renal disease prior to dialysis treatment is not clear; however, as the kidney is essential in the further hydroxylation of 25-hydroxycholecalciferol to 1,25-dihydroxycholecalciferol, the active form of vitamin D, absence of this metabolite in patients with chronic renal disease could theoretically lead to abnormality of bone. Furthermore, patients with renal failure have malabsorption

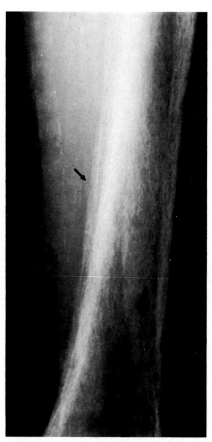

Figure 52–15. Renal osteodystrophy: Periosteal neostosis. Frontal radiograph of the femur in a patient with renal osteodystrophy outlines laminated periosteal new bone formation (arrow). Vascular calcification and bone abnormalities are present.

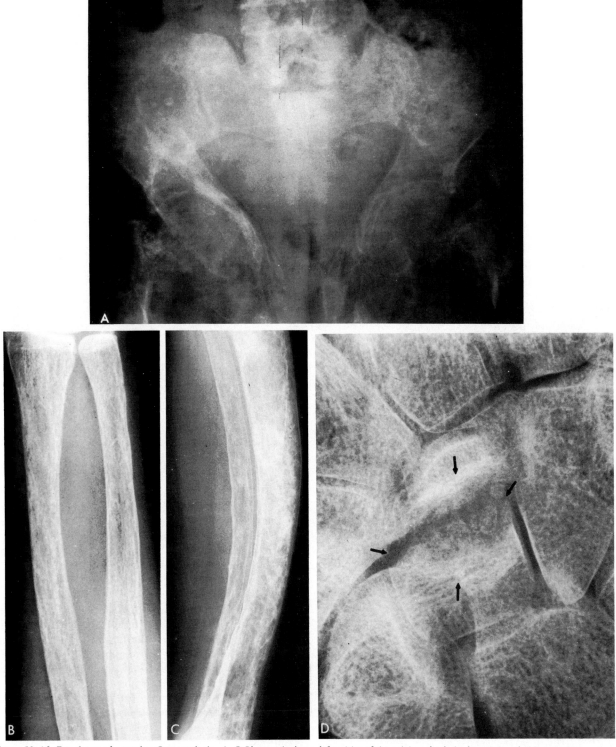

Figure 52–16. Renal osteodystrophy: Osteomalacia. A–C Observe the bone deformities of the pelvis and tubular bones. Acetabular protrusion, coxa vara, and bowing of the radius, ulna, tibia, and fibula are seen. Trabecular detail is virtually absent. **D** Pseudofracture of the capitate. A spontaneously occurring complete fracture (arrows) has resulted in separation of bone fragments and reactive sclerosis.

of calcium from the gut, which can also contribute to bone disease. Osteomalacia may also relate to vitamin D deficiency as well as resistance, the deficiency occurring as a result of anorexia and inadequate diet, increased requirement of hyperparathyroid bone, and abnormality of a hepatic enzyme system.

The radiographic features of osteomalacia in chronic renal disease are not prominent or easily separated from those related to other forms of bone disease in renal osteodystrophy. When present, such features include osteopenia (decrease in radiodensity of bone), which is also a sign of osteitis fibrosa cystica itself, and Looser's zones (Fig. 52–16). These latter abnormalities are narrow radiolucent bands, frequently symmetric in distribution and perpendicular to the osseous

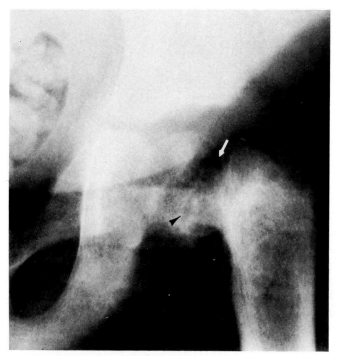

Figure 52–17. Renal osteodystrophy: Rickets. Note metaphyseal irregularity and resorption (arrow), with surrounding sclerosis, and severe coxa vara. The growth plate (arrowhead) is oriented in a vertical position, which may predispose to epiphyseal slipping.

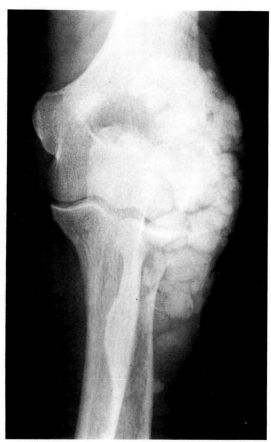

Figure 52–18. Renal osteodystrophy: Soft tissue calcification. Extensive "tumoral" calcification is apparent in the periarticular regions of the elbow.

surface. Looser's zones are most common in the pubic rami, ilii, ribs, femoral necks, scapulae, and long bones. Radiographic features consistent with rickets include osteopenia, irregularity and widening of the growth plate, and poor definition of the epiphysis (Fig. 52–17).

Slipped epiphyses have been described in chronic renal disease in children. The capital femoral epiphysis is by far the most common site of involvement. Bilateral involvement is frequent. Three radiographic signs may precede slipping of the capital femoral epiphysis in renal osteodystrophy: bilateral subperiosteal erosion on the medial aspect of the femoral neck; increase in width of the cartilaginous growth plate; and bilateral coxa vara. Histologic evidence suggests that epiphyseal slipping in chronic renal disease is related to hyperparathyroidism itself.

Osteoporosis

A diminution of bone volume occurs in renal osteodystrophy, which may be characterized as osteoporosis. On radiographs, decreased bone density or osteopenia is evident, although the diminished radiodensity is attributable not only to osteoporosis but also to osteitis fibrosa cystica and osteomalacia. Pathologic fractures may become evident.

Soft Tissue and Vascular Calcification

Although calcification may be observed in the soft tissues and vessels of patients with primary hyperparathyroidism, it is much more frequent in patients with renal osteodystrophy.

Soft tissue calcification in patients with chronic renal failure occurs when multiplication of the respective concentrations (in mg/dl) of plasma calcium and plasma phosphorus produces a value greater than 70.

Soft tissue deposits can occur in multiple sites, including corneal and conjunctival tissue, viscera, vasculature, and subcutaneous and periarticular tissue (Fig. 52–18). Accumulated evidence has suggested that the chemical nature of the deposited crystal varies according to the anatomic site that is involved: In subcutaneous tissues, vessels, and periarticular regions, calcium hydroxyapatite material is observed; in viscera such as the heart, lung, and muscle, magnesium whitlockite–like material is found.

Periarticular deposits may reach considerable size and produce striking tumoral radiodense areas, particularly in the hips, knees, shoulders, and wrists. Bilateral symmetric deposits about multiple joints are not uncommon. Osseous erosions beneath periarticular calcific collections and associated intraarticular calcium hydroxyapatite crystal deposition have been described.

Miscellaneous Abnormalities

Patients with chronic renal insufficiency have hyperuricemia and may develop secondary gouty arthritis. Radiographic features resemble those of primary gout, although in secondary gout, atypical articular sites may be affected. Oxalosis of bone may develop as a rare secondary manifestation of chronic renal failure (see Chapter 44).

Table 52–5. MUSCULOSKELETAL ABNORMALITIES FOLLOWING DIALYSIS AND RENAL TRANSPLANTATION

Hyperparathyroidism
Osteomalacia and rickets
Osteosclerosis
Fractures
Soft tissue and vascular calcification
Osteomyelitis and septic arthritis
Osteonecrosis
Crystal deposition
Amyloidosis
Digital clubbing
Aluminum toxicity
Dialysis cysts
Olecranon bursitis

Musculoskeletal Abnormalities Following Dialysis (Table 52–5)

In the vast majority of patients with chronic renal failure who are placed on maintenance hemodialysis, many of the bone changes of renal osteodystrophy resolve provided that the hemodialysis is of adequate quality and duration (Fig. 52–19). It should be emphasized, however, that a general statement regarding the osseous response to hemodialysis is difficult owing to the complex histologic aberrations in renal osteodystrophy. In poorly managed patients on dialysis, increasing osteopenia may be observed in association with spontaneous fractures. These fractures are most frequent in the ribs, although they are seen at other skeletal sites, including the femoral necks, vertebrae, pubic rami, tibiae, and metatarsals.

It is now generally believed that the primary cause of the progression of skeletal abnormalities in patients on chronic regular hemodialysis is osteomalacia attributable to aluminum intoxication (Fig. 52–20). Clinical characteristics of this syndrome include bone pain, myopathy, fracture, and dialysis encephalopathy. High aluminum levels in tissues, including the brain and bone as well as various articular structures, support the speculation that aluminum toxicity is involved in this syndrome. The source of the aluminum can be related to the contents of phosphate binding gels or the ambient water or dialysate. Reversal of the findings may follow the removal of sources of aluminum contamination.

Soft tissue and vascular calcification is frequent in patients undergoing hemodialysis. When compared to similar calcification present prior to the onset of dialysis, reversal of periarticular and, less commonly, vascular calcification may be seen during dialysis. Progression of such calcification, however, is a more typical finding.

Septicemia, osteomyelitis, and septic arthritis are well-recognized complications of hemodialysis (as well as of renal transplantation). Osteomyelitis and septic arthritis may occur at any site, and any type of organism may be implicated. Typical radiologic signs of infection will become apparent, although radionuclide examination will usually allow earlier diagnosis of infection in these patients.

Ischemic necrosis of bone may complicate the administration of steroids in patients with chronic renal disease undergoing dialysis. (This same complication is well recognized after renal transplantation and is discussed later in this chapter.)

A peculiar pattern of spondyloarthropathy has been identified in a few patients with chronic renal disease who have been undergoing hemodialysis. Middle-aged or elderly men or women who have been hemodialyzed for a period of years are affected. Mild to moderate back or neck pain is seen. Single or multiple spinal levels, especially in the cervical or lumbar segment, reveal progressive radiographic abnormalities characterized by loss of intervertebral disc space, erosion of subchondral bone in the neighboring vertebral bodies, and new bone formation (Fig. 52–21). The findings resemble infection, neuroarthropathy, severe intervertebral (osteo)chondrosis, or CPPD crystal deposition disease. Histologic analysis indicates the absence of infection, although the precise

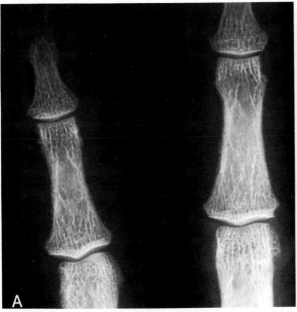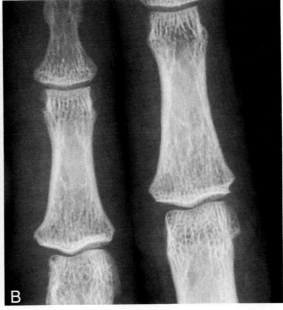

Figure 52–19. Renal osteodystrophy: Resolution of skeletal abnormalities during hemodialysis. Radiographs obtained 4 years apart reveal significant improvement in the osseous abnormalities.

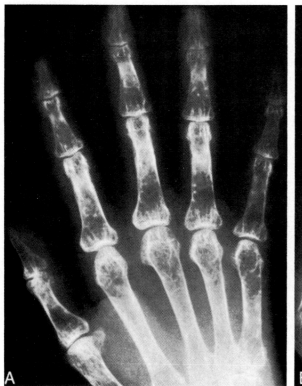
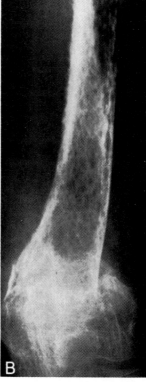

Figure 52–20. Renal osteodystrophy: Aluminum intoxication during hemodialysis. **A** A radiograph of the hand reveals marked osteopenia with indistinctness of the cortical margins and trabeculae. **B** The radiograph of the lower femur shows osteopenia, cortical tunneling, and a supracondylar fracture with insignificant callus formation 1 year after the injury. (From Llewellyn CH, et al: Case report 288. Skel Radiol *12*:233, 1984. Used with permission.)

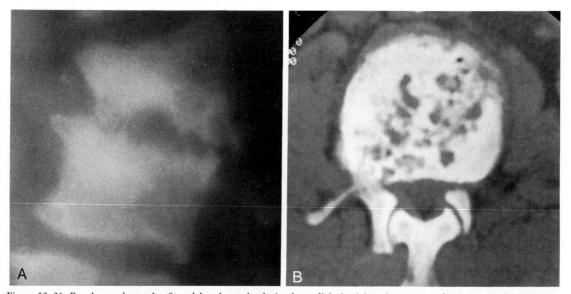

Figure 52–21. Renal osteodystrophy: Spondyloarthropathy during hemodialysis. A lateral tomogram of the spine (**A**) delineates loss of height of the intervertebral disc, erosion of the subchondral bone of two adjacent vertebral bodies, extreme bone sclerosis, and subluxation. The findings resemble those of infection, CPPD crystal deposition disease, cartilaginous node formation, or neuroarthropathy. A transaxial computed tomographic image (**B**) shows multiple radiolucent foci within a sclerotic vertebral body. (Courtesy of P. Kaplan, M.D., Omaha, Nebraska.)

cause of the abnormalities is not clear. The lack of biochemical evidence of hyperparathyroidism makes subchondral resorption of bone an unlikely factor. Hydroxyapatite or oxalate crystal deposition in the vertebral lesions in some cases suggests the importance of crystalline accumulation in the pathogenesis of the spondyloarthropathy of hemodialysis. Amyloidosis may also be involved.

The carpal tunnel syndrome occurring in uremic patients receiving hemodialysis is well recognized and usually is attributed to alterations in vascular hemodynamics at the access site, resulting in edema, venous distention, and secondary compression of the median nerve within the carpal canal. Histologic features indicate amyloid deposition in the synovium and adjacent tendons in some patients, however. Amyloid accumulation also occurs in accompanying small cystic lesions in the carpal bones (Fig. 52–22).

Several additional musculoskeletal manifestations of hemodialysis are worthy of note. Olecranon bursitis, called dialysis elbow, may be seen in patients on long-term hemodialysis as a consequence of the sustained pressure on the elbow related to the position of the arm during treatment. Digital clubbing confined to one or more fingers may be induced by anoxia distal to the fistulae, and aneurysms with or without calcification may appear at the site of shunt. Hemarthrosis has also been reported in hemodialyzed patients, perhaps related to heparin administration or abnormal platelet function.

Bone disease and soft tissue calcification have also been observed in uremic patients undergoing peritoneal dialysis. Some investigators suggest that the frequency and severity of the osseous and soft tissue changes are less with this therapeutic technique than with hemodialysis.

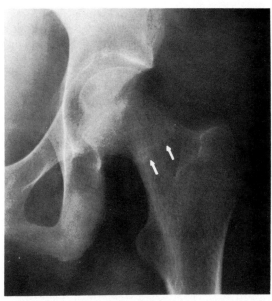

Figure 52–23. Renal osteodystrophy: Insufficiency fracture after renal transplantation. The classic radiographic features of such a fracture in the femoral neck are evident. Observe linear condensation of bone (arrows). (Courtesy of M. Dalinka, M.D., Philadelphia, Pennsylvania.)

Musculoskeletal Abnormalities After Renal Transplantation

The occurrence of osteonecrosis after renal transplantation is well known. Osteonecrosis usually becomes evident from 4 to 36 months after the surgery. It generally is assumed that osteonecrosis in the posttransplant period is attributable to steroid medications, although patients with severe secondary hyperparathyroidism being treated with chronic hemodialysis who have not received steroids or undergone renal transplantation may develop osteonecrosis. The reported frequency of osteonecrosis after renal transplantation has varied from 1.4 to 40 per cent. The most common site of osteonecrosis after renal transplantation is the femoral head; additional sites are the distal part of the femur, humeral head, talus, humeral condyles, cuboid, and carpal bones. Typical radiographic and pathologic features of osteonecrosis are encountered (see Chapter 70).

Spontaneous fractures are not infrequent after renal transplantation. This complication occurs within 1 month or as long as 5 years after the surgery. Multiple fractures, particularly in the axial skeleton, are typical. The ribs, pubic rami, and vertebrae are favored fracture locations, although short and long tubular bones may also be affected (Fig. 52–23). Fracture healing generally is normal.

As in the case of hemodialysis, bone and joint infection may be noted after renal transplantation. The predisposing factors include decreased host resistance owing to the presence of a chronic debilitating disease and the administration of steroids and immunosuppressive agents.

Differential Diagnosis

In renal osteodystrophy, the radiographic features of hyperparathyroidism must be distinguished from those accompanying primary hyperparathyroidism. In secondary hyperparathyroidism, diagnostic features include an increased frequency of vascular and soft tissue calcification, more com-

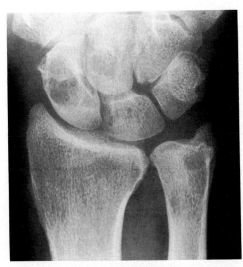

Figure 52–22. Renal osteodystrophy: Carpal tunnel syndrome and amyloid deposition during hemodialysis. Observe soft tissue swelling and cystic lesions in the scaphoid, lunate, capitate, and ulna. During a carpal tunnel release, a biopsy of the synovium and distal portion of the ulna revealed tissue that demonstrated chronic synovitis with amyloid deposition in both the synovium and the bone.

mon and widespread bone sclerosis, and a decreased frequency of chondrocalcinosis. Diffuse osteosclerosis in renal osteodystrophy may be prominent and, although usually accompanied by other radiographic changes of renal osteodystrophy, must be differentiated from the increased radiodensity associated with various other endocrine, metabolic, and neoplastic diseases. Periosteal neostosis in renal osteodystrophy produces diffuse periosteal bone formation, a finding that can also occur with hypertrophic osteoarthropathy, neoplasm, and infection.

Osteomalacia in chronic renal disease produces decreased radiodensity of bone, a finding that lacks specificity. Occasionally, Looser's zones appear identical to those accompanying other types of osteomalacia. Rachitic changes of renal osteodystrophy are almost identical to those accompanying rickets related to dietary deficiencies and chronic renal tubular disorders. Slipped epiphyses and genu valgum deformities are features that may be more common in the rickets of renal osteodystrophy.

Periarticular calcification is found not only in renal osteodystrophy but also in various collagen diseases, hypervitaminosis D, milk-alkali syndrome, idiopathic tumoral calcinosis, and calcium hydroxyapatite crystal deposition disease. The periarticular, soft tissue, and vascular calcifications of renal osteodystrophy usually are accompanied by other radiographic changes of the disorder.

HYPOPARATHYROIDISM
General Features

Hypoparathyroidism is characterized by hypocalcemia and its neuromuscular symptoms and signs. The disease may result from a deficiency in parathyroid hormone production or an end-organ resistance to the action of the hormone. Deficiency of parathyroid hormone most commonly occurs as a result of excision or trauma to the parathyroid glands during thyroid surgery, although it can also occur as idiopathic hypoparathyroidism in which the parathyroid glands are usually absent or atrophied. End-organ unresponsiveness to parathyroid hormone is seen in pseudohypoparathyroidism and pseudopseudohypoparathyroidism. Rare forms of hypoparathyroidism are seen after radiation damage to the gland and as a response of an infant to hyperparathyroidism in the mother.

Postsurgical hypoparathyroidism occurs in fewer than 13 per cent of thyroidectomies, may be unrecognized for years, and becomes evident clinically during pregnancy and lactation. Idiopathic hypoparathyroidism usually occurs in childhood, girls being more commonly affected than boys. The disease is rare in blacks. A familial occurrence is noted occasionally. The disorder may be characterized by the presence of circulating antibodies to the parathyroid, adrenal, and thyroid glands, supporting the concept that idiopathic hypoparathyroidism may be a part of a generalized autoimmune disease.

General radiographic abnormalities of hypoparathyroidism include thickening of the cranial vault and facial bones; increased intracranial pressure with sutural diastasis; calcification of the basal ganglia and rarely the choroid plexus and the cerebellum; ventricular dilatation; dental abnormalities such as hypoplasia of enamel and dentin, delay or failure of eruption, blunting of the roots, and thickening of the lamina dura; and gastrointestinal hypersecretion and spasm.

Table 52–6. RADIOGRAPHIC FEATURES OF THE SKELETON IN HYPOPARATHYROIDISM
Osteosclerosis
Calvarial thickening
Hypoplastic dentition
Subcutaneous calcification
Basal ganglion calcification
Premature physeal fusion
Spinal ossification

Skeletal Abnormalities (Table 52–6)

Osteosclerosis, which may be generalized or localized, is the most common skeletal abnormality of hypoparathyroidism. Typically radiographic findings of hypoparathyroidism (and pseudohypoparathyroidism) include increased radiodensity of the skeleton, calvarial thickening, and hypoplastic dentition (Fig. 52–24). Also noteworthy are peculiar bandlike areas of increased radiodensity in the metaphyses of long bones associated with increased density of the iliac crest and marginal sclerosis of the vertebral bodies.

Subcutaneous calcification may be seen, especially about the hips and shoulders. The deposits generally are asymptomatic, although painful calcific periarthritis is reported in this condition.

In rare situations, distinctive abnormalities of the spine have been reported in patients with hypoparathyroidism. These patients reveal pain, stiffness, and limitation of spinal motion. Radiographic evaluation outlines calcification of the

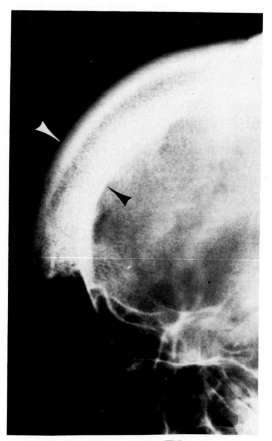

Figure 52–24. Hypoparathyroidism: Calvarial thickening. In a lateral radiograph of the anterior aspect of the skull, observe thickening of the cranial vault (arrowheads) with narrowing of the diploic space.

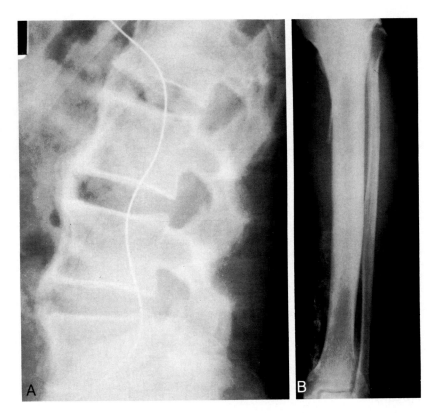

Figure 52–25. Hypoparathyroidism: Enthesopathy and soft tissue calcification. A Changes resemble those of diffuse idiopathic skeletal hyperostosis, including flowing anterior vertebral ossification. **B** Soft tissue calcification in the calf and bone excrescences arising from the proximal portion of the tibia are evident. (Courtesy of P. Cockshott, M.D., Hamilton, Ontario, Canada.)

anterior longitudinal ligament and posterior paraspinal ligaments with spinal osteophytes (Fig. 52–25). In some cases, these spinal changes are associated with bone proliferation about the pelvis, hip, and long bones in addition to soft tissue and tendon calcification. These changes resemble or are identical to those of diffuse idiopathic skeletal hyperostosis.

Differential Diagnosis

Widespread osteosclerosis, which may be identified in hypoparathyroidism, is also seen in certain other disorders, including osteoblastic metastasis, myelofibrosis, Paget's disease, fluorosis, renal osteodystrophy, sickle cell anemia, and mastocytosis. In hypoparathyroidism (and pseudohypoparathyroidism), additional findings such as calvarial thickening and hypoplastic dentition are helpful clues. Hypoplastic dentition is also seen in a variety of congenital syndromes, including cleidocranial dysostosis and pyknodysostosis, and a number of other endocrine disorders, such as hypopituitarism and hypothyroidism. Sclerosis of the metaphyseal region of the long bones, which is seen in some patients with hypoparathyroidism, is not specific. A similar finding may be noted in systemic illnesses in infancy and childhood, leukemia during treatment, heavy metal poisoning, hypothyroidism, healing scurvy, and hypervitaminoses.

Basal ganglion calcification is particularly characteristic of hypoparathyroidism and pseudohypoparathyroidism. It is also seen without known cause in infectious disorders such as toxoplasmosis and cytomegalic inclusion disease, in Fahr's syndrome (ferrocalcinosis), and after radiation therapy or exposure to toxic substances such as carbon monoxide. Also, subcutaneous calcification, seen in hypoparathyroidism and pseudohypoparathyroidism, also is observed in collagen diseases, hypervitaminosis D, milk-alkali syndrome, and renal osteodystrophy.

PSEUDOHYPOPARATHYROIDISM AND PSEUDOPSEUDOHYPOPARATHYROIDISM
General Features

Pseudohypoparathyroidism (PHP) is a heritable disorder that shares many features with idiopathic hypoparathyroidism, including hypocalcemia, hyperphosphatemia, and basal ganglion and soft tissue calcification. PHP differs from idiopathic hypoparathyroidism in several respects; it involves an end-organ resistance to the action of parathyroid hormone, and it is associated with a characteristic somatotype, which includes short stature, obesity, round face, and brachydactyly. Additional clinical findings of this disease are abnormal dentition, mental retardation, strabismus, dermatoglyphic abnormalities, and impaired taste and olfaction. Typical radiographic features of PHP are short metacarpals, metatarsals, and phalanges, exostoses, cone epiphyses, and wide bones. In some cases, changes of secondary hyperparathyroidism are seen (see later discussion).

PHP is more frequent in women than in men and appears to be transmitted as an X-linked dominant trait. It usually is diagnosed in the second decade of life. Affected individuals reveal increased levels of serum phosphorus, decreased concentrations of serum calcium, and diminished phosphaturia.

Excessive secretion of parathyroid hormone has been demonstrated in some patients with PHP. In fact, an apparently rare variation of PHP is characterized by renal unresponsiveness to parathyroid hormone but with a normal osseous response to the hormone. The condition, termed pseudohypoperparathyroidism, is associated with histologic and radiographic findings similar to those of renal osteodystrophy.

Pseudopseudohypoparathyroidism (PPHP) is the normocalcemic form of PHP. Patients with PPHP possess the same somatic abnormalities as those with PHP. The two diseases, PHP and PPHP, may occur in the same family, suggesting

Table 52–7. RADIOGRAPHIC FEATURES OF THE SKELETON IN PHP AND PPHP*

Soft tissue calcification and ossification
Basal ganglion calcification
Premature physeal fusion
Metacarpal and metatarsal shortening
Calvarial thickening
Exostoses
Abnormalities of bone density
Bowing deformities

*PHP, Pseudohypoparathyroidism; PPHP, pseudopseudohypoparathyroidism.

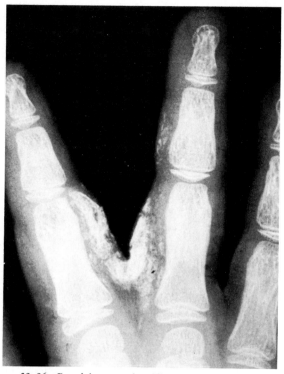

Figure 52–26. Pseudohypoparathyroidism: Soft tissue calcification. Plaque-like calcification of the subcutaneous tissue of the second and third digits is observed.

that they are closely associated. Both conditions have been grouped together under the term Albright's hereditary osteodystrophy (see Chapter 48).

Skeletal Abnormalities (Table 52–7)

Skeletal abnormalities in PHP and PPHP include shortening of all of the metacarpals with premature fusion of the growth plates, broad and short phalanges with pseudoepiphyses, and soft tissue calcification or ossification (Fig. 52–26).

In most reports of PHP and PPHP, metacarpal shortening is frequently observed in the first, fourth, and fifth digits; metatarsal shortening shows predilection for the first and fourth digits (Fig. 52–27). Additional findings have included

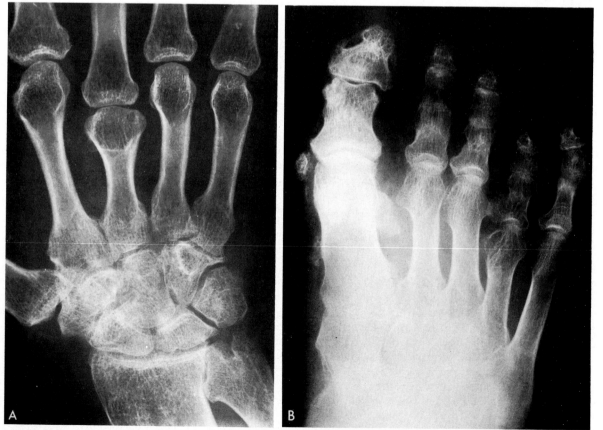

Figure 52–27. Pseudohypoparathyroidism: Metacarpal and metatarsal shortening. A Shortening of all of the metacarpal bones is evident, although the most severe abnormality is present in the third digit. Note irregularity of the distal part of the ulna and carpal bones, with joint space narrowing and sclerosis. **B** Shortening of all of the metatarsal bones, particularly the fourth, is associated with soft tissue ossification on the medial aspect of the first digit.

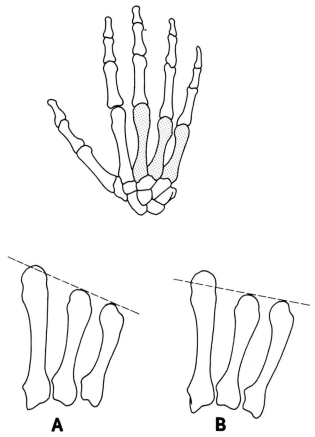

Figure 52–28. Pseudohypoparathyroidism and pseudopseudohypoparathyroidism: Positive metacarpal sign. Normally, a line drawn tangential to the heads of the fourth and fifth metacarpal bones will not intersect the end of the third metacarpal bone or will just contact its articular surface (**A**). A positive metacarpal sign is present when such a line intersects the third metacarpal bone (**B**).

basal ganglion calcification, calvarial thickening, bowing of the extremities, and exostoses. The exostoses frequently project at right angles to the bone, differing from the appearance of multiple hereditary exostoses, in which outgrowths usually are directed away from joints.

The shortening of the metacarpals may lead to a positive metacarpal sign (Fig. 52–28). This sign is not specific for PHP and PPHP, being positive in other congenital conditions, such as the basal cell nevus syndrome, multiple epiphyseal dysplasia, and Beckwith-Wiedemann syndrome, as well as in acquired conditions, such as juvenile chronic arthritis, sickle cell anemia with infarction, trauma, and neonatal hyperthyroidism.

Differential Diagnosis

Radiographic abnormalities of the hand in PHP and PPHP are almost identical. Additionally, these hand abnormalities resemble findings in acrodysostosis, Turner's syndrome, and brachydactyly E and D. Some radiographic features of PHP and PPHP resemble findings of myositis (fibrodysplasia) ossificans progressiva and multiple hereditary exostoses.

FURTHER READING

Bywaters EGL, Dixon ASJ, Scott JT: Joint lesions of hyperparathyroidism. Ann Rheum Dis 22:171, 1963.

Dodds WJ, Steinbach HL: Primary hyperparathyroidism and articular cartilage calcification. AJR 104:884, 1968.

Doppman JL: Multiple endocrine syndromes—a nightmare for the endocrinologic radiologist. Semin Roentgenol 20:7, 1985.

Elmstedt E: Avascular bone necrosis in the renal transplant patient: A discriminant analysis of 144 cases. Clin Orthop 158:149, 1981.

Fenves AZ, Emmett M, White MG, Greenway G, Michaels DB: Carpal tunnel syndrome with cystic bone lesions secondary to amyloidosis in chronic hemodialysis patients. Am J Kid Dis 7:130, 1986.

Garrett P, McWade M, O'Callaghan J: Radiological assessment of aluminum-related bone disease. Clin Radiol 37:63, 1986.

Genant HK, Baron JM, Strauss FH II, Paloyan E, Jowsey J: Osteosclerosis in primary hyperparathyroidism. Am J Med 59:104, 1975.

Genant HK, Heck LL, Lanzl LH, Rossmann K, Horst JV, Paloyan JE: Primary hyperparathyroidism. A comprehensive study of clinical, biochemical, and radiographic manifestations. Radiology 109:513, 1973.

Goldman AB, Lane JM, Salvati E: Slipped capital femoral epiphyses complicating renal osteodystrophy: A report of three cases. Radiology 126:333, 1978.

Greenfield GB: Roentgen appearance of bone and soft tissue changes in chronic renal disease. AJR 116:749, 1972.

Griffiths HJ, Ennis JT, Bailey G: Skeletal changes following renal transplantation. Radiology 113:621, 1974.

Kaplan P, Resnick D, Murphey M, Heck L, Phalen J, Egan D, Rutsky E: Destructive noninfectious spondyloarthropathy in hemodialysis patients: A report of four cases. Radiology 162:241, 1986.

Kriegshauser JS, Swee RG, McCarthy JT, Hauser MF: Aluminum toxicity in patients undergoing dialysis: Radiographic findings and prediction of bone biopsy results. Radiology 164:399, 1987.

Kuntz D, Naveau B, Bardin T, Drueke T, Treves R, Dryll A: Destructive spondyloarthropathy in hemodialyzed patients. A new syndrome. Arthritis Rheum 27:369, 1984.

Meema HE, Oreopoulos DG, Rabinovich S, Husdan H, Rapoport A: Periosteal new bone formation (periosteal neostosis) in renal osteodystrophy. Relationship to osteosclerosis, osteitis fibrosa, and osteoid excess. Radiology 110:513, 1974.

Milgram JW, Salyer WR: Secondary oxalosis of bone in chronic renal failure. J Bone Joint Surg [Am] 56:387, 1974.

Poznanski AK, Werder EA, Giedion A, Martin A, Shaw H: The pattern of shortening of the bones of the hand in PHP and PPHP—a comparison with brachydactyly E, Turner syndrome, and acrodysostosis. Radiology 123:707, 1977.

Pugh DG: Subperiosteal resorption of bone. A roentgenologic manifestation of primary hyperparathyroidism and renal osteodystrophy. AJR 66:577, 1951.

Resnick D: Abnormalities of bone and soft tissue following renal transplantation. Semin Roentgenol 13:329, 1978.

Resnick D, Niwayama G: Subchondral resorption of bone in renal osteodystrophy. Radiology 118:315, 1976.

Steinbach HL, Young DA: The roentgen appearance of pseudohypoparathyroidism (PH) and pseudo-pseudohypoparathyroidism (PPH). Differentiation from other syndromes associated with short metacarpals, metatarsals and phalanges. AJR 97:49, 1966.

Steinbach HL, Gordan GS, Eisenberg E, Crane JT, Silverman S, Goldman L: Primary hyperparathyroidism: A correlation of roentgen, clinical and pathologic features. AJR 86:329, 1961.

Steinbach HL, Rudhe U, Jonsson M, Young DA: Evolution of skeletal lesions in pseudohypoparathyroidism. Radiology 85:670, 1965.

Steinberg H, Waldron BR: Idiopathic hypoparathyroidism: Analysis of 52 cases, including report of new case. Medicine 31:133, 1952.

Sundaram M, Phillipp SR, Wolverson MK, Riaz MA, Rao BJ: Ungual tufts in the follow-up of patients on maintenance dialysis. Skel Radiol 5:247, 1980.

Weller M, Edeiken J, Hodes PJ: Renal osteodystrophy. AJR 104:354, 1968.

Chapter 53

Disorders of Other Endocrine Glands and of Pregnancy

Donald Resnick, M.D.

Various musculoskeletal manifestations may accompany endocrine disorders such as Cushing's syndrome, congenital adrenal hyperplasia, Addison's disease, pheochromocytoma, neuroblastoma, and diabetes mellitus. Furthermore, certain complications are apparent in women after pregnancy. In Cushing's disease, osteoporosis is most typical and, although osteonecrosis is seen occasionally, it is not as frequent as in cases of exogenous hypercortisolism. The list of disorders that may be associated with diabetes includes crystal-induced arthropathy (gout and calcium pyrophos-phate dihydrate crystal deposition disease), soft tissue contractures, osteomyelitis, septic arthritis, and neuroarthropathy. Musculoskeletal anomalies, including the caudal regression syndrome and the combination of unusual facies and femoral hypoplasia, are identified in some infants born of diabetic mothers. After normal pregnancy, osteitis condensans ilii and osteitis pubis may be apparent, and a similar-appearing abnormality of the clavicle has been described.

Several additional endocrine disorders may be associated with significant abnormalities of the skeleton. In addition, musculoskeletal manifestations accompanying or following pregnancy are well recognized.

CUSHING'S DISEASE
General Features

Cushing's syndrome is caused by the presence of excessive amounts of adrenocortical glucocorticoid steroids in the body. This excess may be induced by hyperplasia or hyperfunctioning tumors of the adrenal cortex (endogenous Cushing's disease) or by excessive administration of corticosteroid medication (exogenous Cushing's disease). Endogenous Cushing's disease usually results from adrenal hyperplasia, less commonly from adenoma or carcinoma of the adrenal gland, and rarely from neuroblastoma, anterior pituitary neoplasm, ectopic adrenal tissue, and ectopic adrenocorticotropic hormone (ACTH)–producing tumors. The disease can occur at any age but is most frequent in women between the ages of 20 and 60 years. Easy bruisability and the development of purpura may be early manifestations. In women, menstrual abnormalities may herald the onset of the disease. Generalized obesity, muscle weakness, emotional disturbance, and backache are additional common symptoms. On physical examination, patients may demonstrate moon face (increased fullness of the face and cheeks), buffalo hump (fatty deposition over the dorsal spine), increased transparency of the skin, purple striae, abnormal distribution of hair with hirsutism, hypertension, and bone tenderness. In children, short stature is observed. Laboratory tests reveal leukocytosis and a glucose tolerance test with results characteristic of diabetes mellitus.

Osteoporosis

Osteopenia in Cushing's syndrome is most pronounced in the vertebral column, pelvis, ribs, and cranial vault. Radiographic examination reveals typical findings of osteoporosis. In the spine, diminished bone density, biconcave deformities of vertebral bodies ("fish vertebrae"), compression fractures, and exaggerated kyphosis are apparent (Fig. 53–1). The

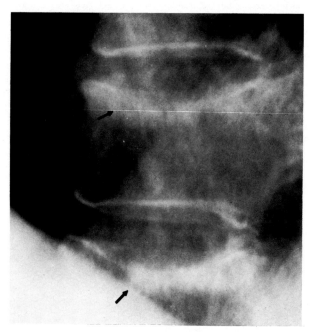

Figure 53–1. Endogenous and exogenous Cushing's disease: Vertebral osteoporosis. A lateral radiograph outlines osteoporosis of the vertebrae, collapse of vertebral bodies, and condensation of bone (arrows) at the vertebral margins.

appearance is not unlike that in other disorders associated with osteoporosis, although increased radiodensity of the superior and inferior margins of compressed or collapsed vertebral bodies, related to the presence of exuberant callus, allows specific diagnosis in some patients with Cushing's disease. Furthermore, in Cushing's syndrome, peculiar patchy radiolucent areas in the cranial vault are evident. The ribs are also involved, and rib fractures, which are frequent in Cushing's syndrome, may heal with abundant callus formation. Osteoporosis of the pelvis may be associated with protrusio acetabuli.

Osteoporosis, vertebral compression, and kyphosis may also occur with exogenous corticosteroid therapy. The degree of osteoporosis may be influenced by the type and dose schedule of administered steroids.

Osteonecrosis

Osteonecrosis is a well-recognized complication of exogenous hypercortisolism but is not commonly recorded in endogenous hypercortisolism. Osteonecrosis in this latter situation most frequently involves the femoral head, although changes in the humeral head have also been noted. When osteonecrosis occurs in Cushing's syndrome, typical radiographic features are evident, with subchondral curvilinear radiolucent shadows, osteoporosis, osteosclerosis, bone collapse and fragmentation, and a relatively normal articular space.

Other Musculoskeletal Abnormalities

Delayed skeletal maturation, growth recovery lines, decreased osteophyte formation about abnormal joints, and loss of the lamina dura can rarely be observed in Cushing's disease. Soft tissue changes relate to redistribution of fat, leading to accumulation of fatty tissue in the trunks of adults and in the trunks and extremities of children. Muscle atrophy and mediastinal and retroperitoneal fat deposition may be noted.

CONGENITAL ADRENAL HYPERPLASIA

This condition, originally called the adrenogenital syndrome, is related to a relative or absolute loss of one of the various enzymes that are involved in the conversion of cholesterol to normal hormonal steroids. This defect leads to the secretion of excessive amounts of ACTH, with resultant adrenal hyperplasia. The clinical picture varies, but the most frequent type of intersex problem is female pseudohermaphroditism. Virilization of the female infant usually is present at birth or, less frequently, appears in the first few months of life. Accelerated growth is seen initially but premature physeal closure may eventually lead to short stature. Additional musculoskeletal manifestations include accelerated dental maturation, prominent musculature, and premature calcification of the costal cartilages.

ADDISON'S DISEASE

Destruction of the adrenal cortex leading to Addison's disease can be attributed to a variety of processes, including infections and infiltrating neoplasms, although most commonly idiopathic atrophy of the adrenal glands is observed. The clinical manifestations usually are insidious and related to deficiencies of aldosterone and cortisol. Musculoskeletal manifestations are not frequent or prominent. Radiographs may reveal calcification in the adrenal glands, external ear, periarticular areas, and costal cartilages, and skeletal maturation may be delayed.

PHEOCHROMOCYTOMA

A pheochromocytoma arises from chromaffin elements, typically in the adrenal medulla but also in the paraaortic and thoracic sympathetic chains, the organs of Zuckerkandl, the carotid body, and the urinary bladder. Adults between the ages of 30 and 50 years are usually affected. Clinical abnormalities frequently are related to the increased production of catecholamines, leading to hypertension, flushing or blanching, palpitations, excessive sweating, headache, anorexia, weight loss, decreased gastrointestinal motility, and psychosis. Osteolytic and osteosclerotic regions in the metaphyses of the tubular bones of children, presumably related to ischemia and infarction, have been reported. A second osseous abnormality relates to sites of metastasis, which predominate in the axial skeleton. Single or multiple osteolytic lesions occur and may lead to bone expansion and fracture.

NEUROBLASTOMA

Tumors of the sympathetic nervous system generally are classified as neuroblastoma, ganglioneuroblastoma, and ganglioneuroma. Of these, neuroblastoma is most frequent and usually arises in the adrenal medulla. Neuroblastoma is characterized by rapid growth and widespread metastases. Approximately 80 per cent of patients are children less than 5 years of age. At the time that the neuroblastoma is discovered, skeletal metastases are frequent (see Chapter 80). Bilateral osseous lesions, especially in the metaphyseal segments, are typical (Fig. 53–2). Osteolytic lesions with per-

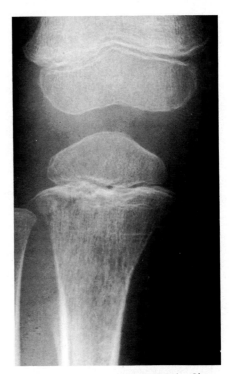

Figure 53–2. Neuroblastoma: Skeletal metastasis. Observe permeative bone destruction and periostitis in the metaphysis of the tibia. Growth recovery lines are also evident.

meative bone destruction predominate. In the skull, increased intracranial pressure, owing to leptomeningeal involvement and leading to sutural diastasis, vertical osseous striations extending from the outer table, and soft tissue swelling are seen. Additional manifestations of the skeletal metastases include "floating" teeth related to mandibular involvement, vertebral collapse, rib alterations with extrapleural extension, and pelvic bone destruction. The differential diagnosis includes Ewing's sarcoma, lymphomas, leukemias, and metastases from other tumors, such as rhabdomyosarcoma, medulloblastoma, retinoblastoma, and Wilms' tumor.

DIABETES MELLITUS

General Features

Numerous musculoskeletal disorders have been described in conjunction with diabetes mellitus (Table 53–1).

Gouty Arthritis

The relationship between diabetes mellitus and gouty arthritis is not well defined. The evidence suggests that the prevalence of diabetes in patients with gout is related to the high frequency of obesity in hyperuricemic subjects.

Calcium Pyrophosphate Dihydrate (CPPD) Crystal Deposition Disease

The frequency of diabetes mellitus in patients with CPPD crystal deposition disease may be quite high, as may be the frequency of CPPD crystal accumulation in persons with diabetes mellitus (see Chapter 40). A true association of diabetes mellitus and CPPD crystal deposition disease is not clear at this time, however.

Soft Tissue Syndromes

PERIARTHRITIS. Periarthritis produces a painful stiff shoulder characterized by loss of joint motion, without evidence of intraarticular disease. Periarthritis of the shoulder may be four or five times more common in diabetic patients than in nondiabetic patients. On radiographic examination, patients with periarthritis may reveal no abnormality, although calcific bursitis or tendinitis may be apparent. Capsular fibrosis and thickening are pathologic findings in this condition.

Glenohumeral joint periarthritis can be accompanied by the shoulder-hand syndrome. Clinical findings include stiffness and pain of one or both hands, followed by diffuse swelling, warmth, erythema, tenderness, and hyperhidrosis of the hands. Subsequently, swelling decreases and atrophy of the skin and muscle, osteopenia, and thickening and contracture of the palmar fascia are noted. The syndrome may resolve spontaneously or be followed by permanent limb disability.

DIABETIC CHEIROARTHROPATHY. A condition sharing some clinical features with the shoulder-hand syndrome has been described in as many as 40 per cent of patients with insulin-requiring juvenile diabetes. Characteristic findings of this syndrome, which is variously termed diabetic cheiroarthropathy and diabetic hand syndrome, are mild to moderately severe joint contractures of the fingers, thickening of the skin on the dorsum of the hand, and short stature. Occasionally other joints may be involved. On rare occasions, cases of this syndrome have been identified in adults with insulin-dependent or non-insulin–dependent diabetes.

DUPUYTREN'S CONTRACTURE. A high frequency of Dupuytren's contracture has been recognized in patients with diabetes. Similarly, diabetes mellitus is not infrequent in patients who reveal Dupuytren's contracture. This condition develops insidiously as nodular or plaque-like thickening of the palmar fascia. Extension of the fibrous process to the metacarpophalangeal and proximal interphalangeal joints may result in finger contracture (Fig. 53–3).

FLEXOR TENOSYNOVITIS. Flexor tenosynovitis (trigger finger, stenosing tenovaginitis) refers to a condition of one or more fingers associated with snapping, pain, locking, and limitation of motion of the interphalangeal joint owing to obstruction of the flexor tendon in a constricted tendon sheath. The sheath is thickened, with local inflammatory changes and fibrosis. Some reports suggest that diabetes mellitus may be apparent in 10 to 30 per cent of patients with flexor tenosynovitis.

Table 53–1. MUSCULOSKELETAL MANIFESTATIONS OF DIABETES MELLITUS

Gout*
CPPD crystal deposition disease*
Degenerative joint disease*
DISH
Soft tissue syndromes
  Periarthritis
  Diabetic cheiroarthropathy
  Dupuytren's contracture
  Flexor tenosynovitis
  Carpal tunnel syndrome
Osteomyelitis
Septic arthritis
Neuroarthropathy
Forefoot osteolysis

*Possible association.

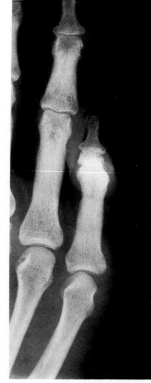

Figure 53–3. Diabetes mellitus and Dupuytren's contracture. Observe flexion contracture at the fifth proximal interphalangeal joint in this diabetic patient.

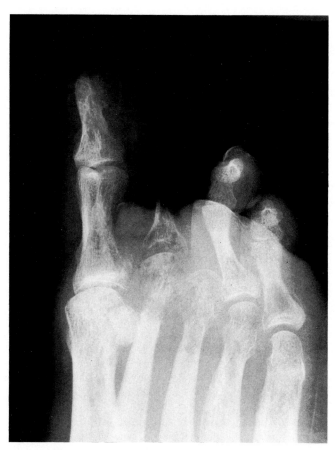

Figure 53–4. Diabetes mellitus: Association of osteomyelitis and septic arthritis. A radiograph illustrates soft tissue and osseous infection in a foot of a patient with diabetes, with associated skin ulceration. A previous resection of the second and third toes had been accomplished. The radiograph outlines soft tissue swelling, radiolucency of the soft tissues, and osseous destruction of the second and third metatarsal heads.

CARPAL TUNNEL SYNDROME. The carpal tunnel syndrome results from entrapment of the median nerve within the carpal tunnel on the volar aspect of the wrist. Although 40 to 50 per cent of cases of carpal tunnel syndrome have no apparent cause, any process associated with a mass in and around the carpal tunnel can produce this syndrome. Tissue infiltration in leukemia, sarcoidosis, amyloidosis, and neoplasm; tissue edema in acromegaly and hypothyroidism; tissue hemorrhage following trauma; and tissue inflammation in rheumatoid arthritis, systemic lupus erythematosus, dermatomyositis, gout, and CPPD crystal deposition disease are potential causes. The frequency of diabetes mellitus in patients with the carpal tunnel syndrome has been reported as 5 to 17 per cent. An increased occurrence of this syndrome in diabetes may be due to ischemic changes related to microvascular disease.

Osteomyelitis and Septic Arthritis

Soft tissue ulceration and infection, which are frequent in diabetes, may lead to contamination of contiguous bones and joints (see Chapter 59). This sequence is particularly frequent in the diabetic foot (Fig. 53–4). Initial soft tissue lesions in the foot in diabetes are particularly frequent beneath the first and fifth metatarsophalangeal joints and the calcaneus at pressure points. The radiographic findings include defects in

soft tissue contour, loss of tissue planes, and swelling. As the infection reaches the bone, the radiographic findings of osteomyelitis and septic arthritis become evident.

Neuroarthropathy

In recent years, diabetes has surpassed syphilis as the leading cause of neuroarthropathy (see Chapter 69). The arthropathy appears to be a direct sequela of diabetic peripheral neuropathy, with loss of pain and proprioceptive sensations. Aggravating factors in the diabetic patient are vascular changes, trauma, and infection.

Diabetic neuroarthropathy frequently involves the tarsometatarsal, intertarsal, and metatarsophalangeal joints (Fig. 53–5). Abnormalities of the ankle and interphalangeal joints are less frequent. Occasionally changes occur at other sites, including the knee, spine, and joints of the upper extremity. The radiographic and pathologic picture may be a composite of both neuropathic disease and infection. Osteolysis and resorptive changes may predominate over fragmentation and productive abnormalities. Spontaneous fractures and dislocations are not infrequent. In this regard, diabetic neuroarthropathy with findings resembling a Lisfranc fracture-dislocation at the tarsometatarsal joints is well recognized.

Forefoot Osteolysis

A distinct osteolysis of the forefoot in patients with diabetes mellitus is characterized by osteoporosis of the distal meta-

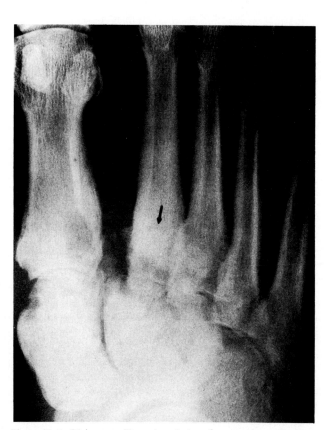

Figure 53–5. Diabetes mellitus: Association of neuroarthropathy. Note the degree of sclerosis, fragmentation, and subluxation of the tarsometatarsal joints (arrow). This radiograph illustrates a common site of occurrence and appearance of neuroarthropathy in diabetic patients.

tarsals and proximal phalanges. Progressive osteolysis some-times becomes apparent. The process may terminate at any stage, and resolution may commence with restoration of bone architecture. The cause of this condition is not clear, although it is possible that sympathetic nerve dysfunction is an impor-tant factor.

Osteopenia

Osteopenia is a well-recognized manifestation of insulin-treated diabetes mellitus in patients of all ages. Although correlation of bone loss with the severity of the disorder is poor, bone loss is particularly marked initially and in the younger age groups. The pathogenesis of diabetic osteopenia is not clear. Potential factors present in uncontrolled diabetes include glycosuria, calciuria, phosphaturia, systemic acidosis, and other hormonal aberrations.

Vascular Calcification

Arterial calcifications commonly are observed during ra-diography in patients with diabetes mellitus. Arterial calci-fications of the media, rather than intimal calcifications, are the typical lesion of diabetes mellitus and lead to regular, diffuse, and fine-grained collections generally affecting the whole circumference of the vessel and accumulating in rings. Calcification in the interdigital arteries of the feet can aid in the diagnosis of clinically unsuspected diabetes as these vessels rarely exhibit calcification in nondiabetic persons.

LIPOATROPHIC DIABETES
General Features

Features of lipoatrophic diabetes include insulin-resistant diabetes, hepatosplenomegaly, hyperlipidemia, hypermeta-bolism, accelerated growth and maturation, muscular over-development, hirsutism, hyperpigmentation, and progressive loss of adipose tissue without ketosis. Additional clinical features are cutaneous xanthomas, protuberant abdomen, corneal opacities, and mental retardation.

Lipoatrophic diabetes may be congenital or acquired. In the congenital form, there is paucity of fat at the time of birth, and diabetes commonly appears in the second decade of life. In acquired lipodystrophy, a relationship may exist with previous infections, such as pertussis and mumps. This form of the disease is more common in women than in men and may have its onset after difficult labor and delivery. The cause of either form of this disorder is unknown.

Radiographic Findings

The most striking radiographic finding is decrease or absence of body fat. A markedly advanced bone age may be seen in children with this syndrome. Thickening of the diaphyseal cortices, metaphyseal sclerosis, and hypertrophy of the epiphyses have been described in the long bones. Small cystic lesions may appear in the metaphysis. Changes in the skull may include dolichocephaly, brachycephaly, calcification of the falx cerebri, thickening of the calvarium, and advanced dentition. Evidence of organomegaly may be seen in the chest and abdomen.

Cystic and sclerotic foci are particularly common in peri-articular regions, and the findings may resemble those of osteonecrosis or osteopoikilosis (Fig. 53–6). The regions of increased density may extend into the metaphysis and involve the margins of the vertebral bodies. It has been suggested that the radiodense foci represent osteoblastic reaction to loss of fat in the bone marrow.

This condition should be differentiated from partial lipo-dystrophy, in which loss of facial, trunk, and upper extremity fat is apparent in children between the ages of 5 and 15 years. Decrease in subcutaneous fat may be seen in hyperthy-roidism, anorexia nervosa, progeria, and various other con-genital and acquired disorders. The gigantism of lipoatrophic diabetes must be distinguished from pituitary and cerebral gigantism. In pituitary gigantism, increased subcutaneous fat and typical osseous changes are apparent, whereas in cerebral gigantism, there is excessive body fat and absence of hepato-splenomegaly.

ANOMALIES IN INFANTS OF DIABETIC MOTHERS

Hyperinsulinemia in the fetus of a diabetic mother is presumed to be the result of maternal hyperglycemia, as insulin itself does not traverse the placental barrier. The elevated levels of insulin can promote abnormal growth, which is manifested in the newborn infant as visceromegaly and increased body fat. The frequency of more serious anom-alies and even death in the infants of women with diabetes mellitus is difficult to define owing to wide variations in the criteria used to diagnose maternal diabetes and in the severity of the disease. It is generally believed, however, that the frequency of congenital anomalies in the offspring of diabetic mothers may be as high as 20 per cent.

A wide variety of congenital abnormalities is observed in such infants. These include respiratory anomalies; cardiomy-opathy and congenital heart disease; hyperviscosity, throm-bosis, and hemorrhage; renal anomalies; the small left colon syndrome; and alterations in the musculoskeletal system.

Sacrococcygeal agenesis, or the caudal regression syndrome, is one of the most specific anomalies in these infants. Approximately 20 per cent of individuals with this syndrome are the children of diabetic mothers and approximately 16 per cent of children born to diabetic mothers have sacral anomalies. Agenesis varies in severity (Fig. 53–7). Associated abnormalities include meningocele, arthrogryposis, hip dis-locations, flexion contractures of the knees and hips, foot deformities, and urinary tract anomalies.

An additional skeletal malformation syndrome, consisting of unusual facies and femoral hypoplasia, has been identified in the infants of diabetic mothers. Additional, less constant findings are Sprengel's deformity, radiohumeral or radioulnar synostosis, abnormal ribs, vertebral anomalies, and foot de-formities.

DISORDERS AND COMPLICATIONS OF PREGNANCY

The major radiographic findings associated with physiologic and pathologic changes during pregnancy occur at the sacro-iliac joints and symphysis pubis. Bone eburnation about the sacroiliac joint is termed osteitis condensans ilii, whereas that at the symphysis pubis is termed osteitis pubis. Although either of the two conditions may be apparent in nulliparous women or even men, both are observed most frequently in multiparous women.

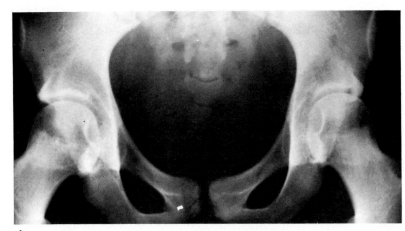

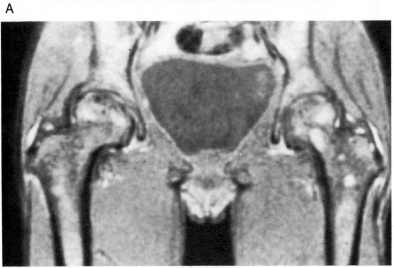

Figure 53–6. Lipoatrophic diabetes. A Note increased radiodensity in the femoral necks. **B** In a different patient, a coronal magnetic resonance image shows patchy areas of decreased signal intensity in the marrow of the proximal portion of the femora. (**A** From Gold RH, Steinbach HL: Lipoatrophic diabetes mellitus (generalized lipodystrophy): Roentgen findings in two brothers with congenital disease. AJR *101*:884, 1967. Copyright 1967, American Roentgen Ray Society. Used with permission.)

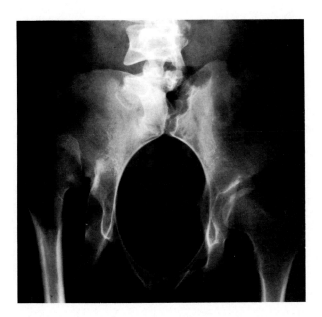

Figure 53–7. Anomalies in children of diabetic mothers: Caudal regression syndrome. Aplasia of the lower lumbar spine and sacrum is associated with pelvic and acetabular deformity and dislocation of the right hip. (Courtesy of S. Hilton, M.D., San Diego, California.)

Osteitis Condensans Ilii

This is a condition of the pelvis that involves predominantly the ilium adjacent to the sacroiliac joint. It is usually a bilateral and relatively symmetric process of women; rarely, men may be affected, and asymmetric or unilateral changes may be observed. Osteitis condensans ilii is associated with well-defined triangular sclerosis on the iliac aspect of the sacroiliac joint (Fig. 53–8). The bone eburnation involves the inferior portion of the bone, and the apex of the sclerosis extends into the auricular portion of the ilium. The subchondral bone generally is well defined. Significant narrowing of the sacroiliac joint and extensive involvement of the sacrum are distinctly unusual. The condition may resolve with time.

The cause of osteitis condensans ilii is not clear. The predominant theory suggests that the condition is secondary to mechanical stress across the sacroiliac joint coupled with increased vascularity during pregnancy. Additional radiographic manifestations of articular degeneration, such as osteophytosis and cyst formation, can be observed.

Although some authors have difficulty distinguishing between the sacroiliac joint changes of osteitis condensans ilii and ankylosing spondylitis (Table 53–2), it generally is easy to differentiate the two conditions. Both conditions are characterized by bilateral, symmetric sacroiliac joint abnormalities; however, osseous erosion, indistinctness of subchondral bone, joint space narrowing, sacral involvement, and

Table 53–2. OSTEITIS CONDENSANS ILII (OCI) VERSUS ANKYLOSING SPONDYLITIS (AS)

	OCI	AS
Age	Young adults	Young adults
Sex	Women > men	Men > women
Clinical symptoms, signs	Absent or mild	Mild to severe
HLA-B27	Present in 8% (same as controls)	Present in 90%
Sacroiliac joint abnormalities		
Distribution	Bilateral, symmetric; iliac	Bilateral, symmetric; iliac > sacral
Sclerosis	Well defined	Ill defined
Joint space	Normal	Narrowed
Erosion	Absent	Common
Bone ankylosis	Absent	Common
Spinal abnormalities	Absent	Common
Symphysis pubis abnormalities	Less common	More common

ligamentous ossification are features that are usually prominent in ankylosing spondylitis and absent in osteitis condensans ilii.

Osteitis Pubis

Osteitis pubis is a painful condition of the symphysis pubis that may become apparent within one or more months after delivery or other pelvic operations. In men, it is particularly frequent after prostatic (or bladder) surgery. Clinical findings are characterized by local pain and tenderness, muscle spasm, and unstable gait.

The radiographic appearance of osteitis pubis includes mild to severe subchondral bone irregularity of the symphysis pubis with resorption (Fig. 53–9). The condition usually involves both pubic bones in a symmetric fashion, although asymmetric or unilateral findings occasionally are encountered. Restoration of the osseous surface with disappearance of the sclerosis may be associated with bone ankylosis of the articulation.

Local aspiration has occasionally revealed an abscess cavity, and antibiotics can produce some relief of symptoms, observations that have led some investigators to speculate that the condition represents a low-grade infection. A more aggressive and progressive course is characteristic of infective osteitis pubis, however, although sterile and infective inflammatory changes of the symphysis pubis are similar.

The differential diagnosis of osteitis pubis includes not only trauma (tendon avulsion) and infection but also inflammatory articular disorders. Ankylosing spondylitis and psoriatic arthritis can produce erosion, sclerosis, and resorption of the pubis, combined with more typical abnormalities at other sites. Subchondral resorption of bone in primary and secondary hyperparathyroidism and stress or insufficiency fractures in this condition as well as osteomalacia and osteoporosis can produce abnormalities that simulate osteitis pubis.

Ischemic Necrosis of Bone

Disseminated intravascular coagulation is a recognized complication of pregnancy, which may be related, in part, to

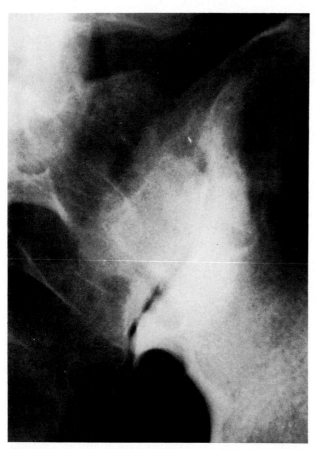

Figure 53–8. Osteitis condensans ilii. Typical radiographic features are well-defined sclerosis on the iliac aspect of the joint, triangular in shape. The joint space is relatively well defined.

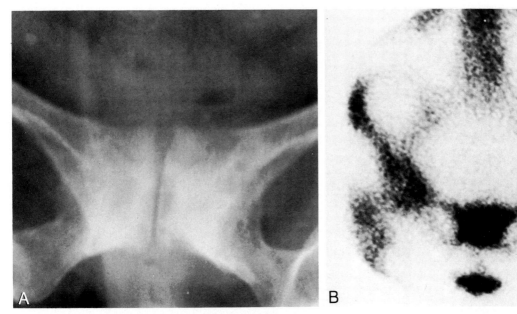

Figure 53–9. Osteitis pubis. A The radiograph reveals considerable bone sclerosis on both sides of the symphysis with narrowing of the joint space. **B** Marked increased accumulation of the bone-seeking radiopharmaceutical agent is observed. (Courtesy of M. Austin, M.D., Newport Beach, California.)

amnionic fluid embolization. In rare instances, ischemic necrosis of bone marrow may be associated with disseminated intravascular coagulation. Although such necrosis generally is patchy in distribution, it may become widespread. Radiographic findings typically are unremarkable.

Well-documented instances of ischemic necrosis of bone related to pregnancy also have been reported. Ischemic necrosis usually is identified in close association with childbirth, and the femoral head or, less commonly, the humeral head is the principal target area.

Transient Osteoporosis of the Hip

As is discussed in Chapter 47, periarticular osteoporosis of the hip has been identified in women during the third trimester of pregnancy and, occasionally, it has been described inappropriately as ischemic necrosis. Affected persons reveal joint pain, an antalgic limp, and restricted hip motion. The left side is involved almost exclusively. The cause of the condition is unknown.

MISCELLANEOUS DISORDERS
Osteitis Condensans (Condensing Osteitis) of the Clavicle

Although this relatively newly described condition is not a complication of pregnancy, it does share morphologic and radiologic features with osteitis condensans ilii and osteitis pubis. Patients with osteitis condensans of the clavicle are women averaging 40 years of age and with a history of stress to the region of the sternoclavicular joint, usually associated with heavy lifting or sports activity. Radiographs reveal bone sclerosis and mild enlargement of the inferomedial aspect of the clavicle, as well as osteophytes in the inferior margin of the clavicular head (Fig. 53–10). The sternoclavicular joint space is not narrowed, and adjacent soft tissue and osseous structures are not affected. In addition to scintigraphy, which demonstrates increased accumulation of bone-seeking radio-

pharmaceutical agents, computed tomography can be used to document the extent of bone involvement. Rarely, similar lesions are identified in the sternum, symphysis pubis, or spine.

The cause of condensing osteitis of the clavicle is unknown. Its occurrence in women of childbearing age suggests a common etiologic agent with osteitis condensans ilii, and stress-induced changes are most likely.

The differential diagnosis of this clavicular lesion is limited. The most difficult entity to exclude is ischemic necrosis of the medial clavicular epiphysis (Friedrich's disease), a rare disorder that typically occurs in children and adolescents and is believed to be attributable to direct trauma or to an embolic event that results in obliteration of the vascular supply to the medial clavicular epiphysis. Radiographs reveal osteosclerosis of the entire clavicular head, and necrotic bone may be recognized on biopsy. The disease appears to be a benign, self-limited process.

Sternocostoclavicular hyperostosis is a second disease that affects the medial end of the clavicle. Hyperostosis of the clavicle, sternum, and upper anterior ribs with ossification of intervening soft tissues is observed. This condition is more common in older patients and in men, usually is bilateral, and often is accompanied by pustular lesions of the palms and soles (pustulosis palmaris et plantaris).

Pyarthrosis of the sternoclavicular joint, especially the type seen in intravenous drug abusers, may mimic condensing osteitis of the clavicle, as may osteoarthritis of the sternoclavicular joint.

Cleidometaphyseal (recurrent multifocal or plasma cell) osteomyelitis is an unusual syndrome, seen in children and adolescents, leading to symmetric lesions of tubular bones and clavicles. Hyperostosis is a prominent feature of clavicular involvement, producing enlargement of the bone that resembles the findings in sternocostoclavicular hyperostosis.

Other causes of clavicular sclerosis and enlargement, such

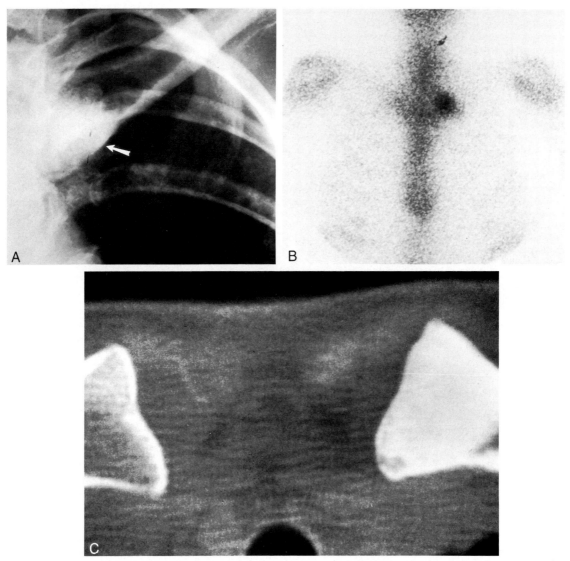

Figure 53–10. Condensing osteitis of the clavicle. A The radiograph reveals increased density and enlargement of the inferomedial aspect of the left clavicle (arrow). **B** Increased accumulation of the bone-seeking radiopharmaceutical agent is evident. **C** A transaxial computed tomographic image documents the increased radiodensity of the medial end of the left clavicle. (Courtesy of W. Murray, M.D., Boise, Idaho.)

as Paget's disease, fibrous dysplasia, syphilis, and osteoid osteoma, do not realistically enter into the differential diagnosis of condensing osteitis.

FURTHER READING

Barnes WC, Malament M: Osteitis pubis. Surg Gynaecol Obstet *117*:277, 1963.

Brower AC, Sweet DE, Keats TE: Condensing osteitis of the clavicle: A new entity. AJR *121*:17, 1974.

Cone RO, Resnick D, Goergen TG, Robinson C, Vint V, Haghighi P: Condensing osteitis of the clavicle. AJR *141*:387, 1983.

Dunn V, Nixon GW, Jaffe RB, Condon VR: Infants of diabetic mothers: Radiographic manifestations. AJR *137*:123, 1981.

Gold RH, Steinbach HL: Lipoatrophic diabetes mellitus (generalized lipodystrophy): Roentgen findings in two brothers with congenital disease. AJR *101*:884, 1967.

Gray RG, Gottlieb NL: Rheumatic disorders associated with diabetes mellitus: Literature review. Semin Arthritis Rheum 6:19, 1976.

James RE, Baker HL, Scanlon PW: The roentgenologic aspects of metastatic pheochromocytoma. AJR *115*:783, 1972.

Johnson JP, Carey JC, Gooch WM III, Petersen J, Beattie JF: Femoral hypoplasia—unusual facies syndrome in infants of diabetic mothers. J Pediatr *102*:866, 1983.

Kincaid OW, Hodgson JR, Dockerty MB: Neuroblastoma: A roentgenographic and pathologic study. AJR 78:420, 1957.

Madell SH, Freeman LM: Avascular necrosis of bone in Cushing's syndrome. Radiology *83*:1068, 1969.

Mendelson EB, Fisher MR, Deschler TW, Rogers LF, Hendrix RW, Spies S: Osteomyelitis in the diabetic foot: A difficult diagnostic challenge. RadioGraphics 3:248, 1983.

Numaguchi Y: Osteitis condensans ilii, including its resolution. Radiology 98:1, 1971.

Pognowska MJ, Collins LC, Dobson HL: Diabetic osteopathy. Radiology 89:265, 1967.

Segal G, Kellogg DS: Osteitis condensans ilii. AJR *71*:643, 1954.

Sinha S, Munichoodappa CS, Kozak GP: Neuro-arthropathy (Charcot joints) in diabetes mellitus (clinical study of 101 cases). Medicine *51*:191, 1972.

DISEASES OF THE HEMATOLOGIC AND HEMATOPOIETIC SYSTEMS

CASE IX

LEVEL OF DIFFICULTY: 1

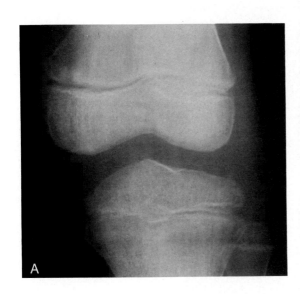

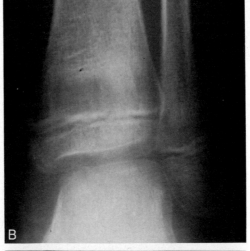

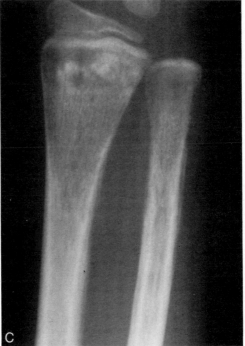

An 8 year old boy had weight loss, fatigue, bone pain, and neutropenia.

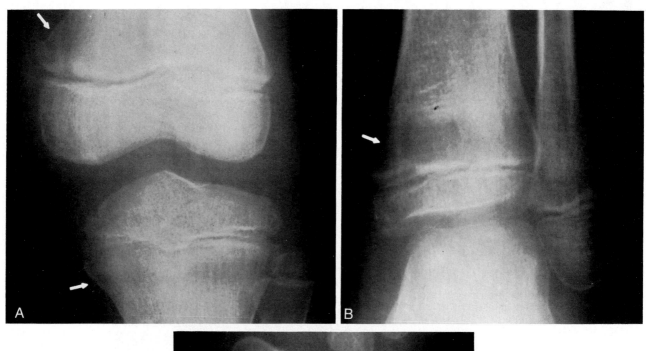

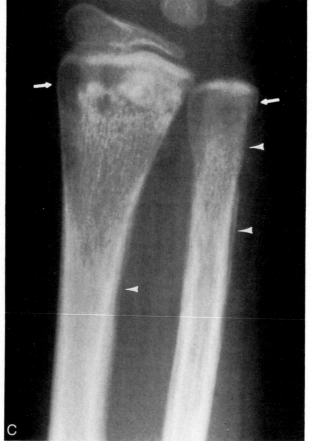

Radiographs of the knee (A), ankle (B), and forearm (C) reveal osteopenia. In addition, radiolucent bands can be seen in the metaphyseal region of the proximal portion of the tibia and distal portions of the femur, tibia, radius, and ulna (arrows). Areas of osteolysis and periostitis are also noted (arrowheads), and patchy osteosclerosis is seen in the radius.

The radiographic findings are virtually diagnostic of acute leukemia. Acute leukemia in children dominates in the first few years of life, particularly between the ages of 2 and 5 years. The vast majority of such cases are lymphoblastic in origin. Although some children with acute leukemia are asymptomatic, bone and joint pain, lymphadenopathy, and splenomegaly may be observed.

Radiographic features are evident in over 50 per cent of children with acute leukemia. The findings include diffuse osteopenia, radiolucent and radiodense metaphyseal bands, osteolytic lesions, periostitis and, less commonly, osteosclerosis. The metaphyseal radiolucent bands represent a nonspecific radiographic abnormality that probably indicates disruption of normal osteogenesis. The bands are observed most commonly in areas of rapid bone growth, such as about the knee and wrist. Their presence in an older child is most suggestive of the diagnosis of leukemia.

Osteolytic lesions and periostitis, which are evident in more than 30 per cent of children with acute leukemia, are indicative of abnormal cellular proliferation. These changes predominate in the long tubular bones, although other osseous sites may be affected. During treatment of the disease, lytic lesions may resolve, although they may reappear during relapse.

Although additional diagnoses, such as syphilis, juvenile chronic arthritis, hyperparathyroidism, sickle cell anemia, and neuroblastoma, may be considered on the basis of clinical and radiographic abnormalities, the diagnosis of acute leukemia is most likely in a child who has a combination of metaphyseal radiolucent bands, periostitis, and osteolysis that are symmetrically distributed and predominate in the tubular bones.

A biopsy of the bone marrow in this 8 year old boy confirmed the diagnosis of acute lymphoblastic leukemia.

FINAL DIAGNOSIS: Acute lymphoblastic leukemia.

FURTHER READING
Pages 703 to 705 and the following:

1. Benz G, Brandeis WE, Willich E: Radiological aspects of leukemia in childhood. An analysis of eighty-nine children. Pediatr Radiol 4:201, 1976.
2. Simmons CR, Harle TS, Singleton EB: The osseous manifestations of leukemia in children. Radiol Clin North Am 6:115, 1968.

(Case IX, courtesy of Naval Hospital, San Diego, California.)

Chapter 54

Hemoglobinopathies and Other Anemias

Donald Resnick, M.D.

The hemoglobinopathies are associated with characteristic abnormalities of the skeleton. In general, these changes are related to marrow hyperplasia, vascular occlusion, and several additional problems, including fracture and infection. Although these features are apparent in almost all of the hemoglobin disorders, their severity varies from one to another, permitting, in some instances, differentiation among these disorders. Articular manifestations in hemoglobinopathies can be attributed to epiphyseal osteonecrosis, growth disturbances, osseous weakening, infection, crystal deposition, hemarthrosis, and synovial membrane microvascular obstruction.

Anemia should be regarded as a clinical finding rather than as a specific disease. It is characterized by a reduction in the blood's capacity to transport oxygen. Oxygen combined with hemoglobin is transported by the red cell; therefore, anemia occurs when the circulating red cell mass is abnormally low. As the red cell mass generally is correlated with the concentration of hemoglobin or the hematocrit, anemia is usually accompanied by a decrease in hemoglobin concentration (below 13.5 gm/dl in men and 12.0 gm/dl in women) and a fall in hematocrit.

Hemoglobin represents approximately one third of the wet weight of the red blood cell and 95 per cent of its dry weight. Ninety-seven per cent of the molecule consists of the polypeptide chains of globin and 3 per cent of the heme groups. The structure of 97 per cent of the hemoglobin in the normal adult, consisting of two pairs of coiled polypeptide chains, two alpha chains composed of 141 amino acids and two beta chains composed of 146 amino acids, is termed Hb A. A smaller fraction of hemoglobin (approximately 2 per cent) termed Hb A2 may also be found; this fraction contains a different second set of polypeptide chains. In the fetus, another type of hemoglobin is found, termed Hb F. This hemoglobin is present in infants at birth, varying in concentrations from 60 per cent to 90 per cent. It generally decreases in concentration during the neonatal period and, in most infants, it has almost disappeared by 4 months of age, by which time Hb A becomes predominant. In the adult, Hb F makes up the remaining 1 per cent of the hemoglobin.

The clinical manifestations of anemia are variable, being influenced by its rate of development and the status or function of the cardiovascular, cerebrovascular, and renal systems. Characteristic abnormalities include exertional dyspnea, tachycardia, claudication, vertigo, and angina. Specific types of anemia are sometimes associated with typical clinical clues, including the cholelithiasis seen in chronic hemolytic states and the bone pain and tenderness accompanying osseous metastasis with compromise of the bone marrow.

The hypoxia of anemia represents a stimulus for increased erythropoiesis through the action of the hormone erythropoietin, formed principally in the kidneys. In the presence of bone marrow compromise, extramedullary sites, such as the liver and the spleen, become actively involved in hematopoiesis.

SICKLE CELL ANEMIA
General Features

Sickle cell disease is a term that describes all conditions characterized by the presence of Hb S. These conditions include sickle cell anemia (Hb S-S), sickle cell trait (Hb A-S), and diseases in which Hb S is combined with another abnormal hemoglobin. Hb S is characterized by a normal alpha chain and an abnormal beta chain, in which valine has replaced glutamic acid. It has been estimated that the sickle cell trait exists in approximately 7 per cent and sickle cell anemia occurs in approximately 0.3 to 1.3 per cent of North American blacks.

Clinical Features

Symptomatic, painful crises (pain, fever, icterus, nausea) usually commence during the second or third year of life. The basic pathogenesis of the sickle crisis appears to be deformation of red blood cells, which produces vasoocclusion and tissue death. Sickle cells are rigid, are the ones that accumulate at the entrance of narrow capillaries, and have the greatest effect on resistance to blood flow through the microcirculation. Ischemia is the clinical (as well as radiologic and pathologic) consequence of these cellular characteristics. Pain and tenderness frequently are related to infarction of bone marrow. The sickle cell crisis can resolve, and the patient may be free of clinical manifestations for a long period of time prior to the onset of a second crisis. In patients with sickle cell trait, painful crises usually are not apparent unless the patient is exposed to an atmosphere low in oxygen.

Although sickle cell anemia rarely has its clinical onset in infants prior to the age of 6 months because of the persistence of Hb F, fever, pallor, and swelling of the hands are observed in children with this disease, apparently related to infarction of the small tubular bones. This "hand-foot" syndrome or dactylitis is most frequent between the ages of 6 months and 2 years.

Other clinical manifestations that may be apparent in sickle cell anemia are hepatosplenomegaly, cardiac enlargement, chronic leg ulcers, osteomyelitis, septic arthritis, pulmonary abnormalities, abdominal pain, cholelithiasis, jaundice, peptic ulcer disease, hematuria, priapism, neurologic findings, and lymphadenopathy. Death may result from infection, cardiac decompensation, or thrombosis of various organs.

Radiographic and Pathologic Features

MARROW HYPERPLASIA (FIG. 54–1). Hypercellularity of the bone marrow in this disease is a response to anemia of long duration. Marrow hyperplasia produces widening of the medullary cavities and rarefaction of remaining trabeculae in the spongiosa and cortex. Associated radiographic abnormalities, which are most prominent in the axial skeleton, include increased radiolucency of osseous tissue, fewer and more accentuated bone trabeculae, and cortical thinning.

In the skull, diffuse widening of the diploic space is associated with thinning of both the outer and inner tables of the skull. The entire cranial vault except for the base of the occiput is involved. Focal radiolucent areas simulate metastasis or myeloma. In rare instances, osteosclerosis of the cranium is observed, perhaps related to myelofibrosis. The facial bones, with the exception of the mandible, generally are not involved in sickle cell anemia. Mandibular involvement, however, is common. Increased radiolucency and a coarsened trabecular pattern are characteristic. Prominence of the lamina dura may be observed.

In sickle cell anemia, increased radiolucency of the vertebral bodies, prominence of vertical trabeculae, and smooth deformity of the contour of the vertebral bodies ("fish vertebrae") owing to compression by the adjacent intervertebral discs are common. These changes are not specific, although squared-off indentations of the vertebral bodies are virtually diagnostic of sickle cell anemia or related disorders. This abnormality of vertebral contour apparently relates to bone infarction and arrested growth (see later discussion).

Marrow hyperplasia in bones of the thorax and extremities may also lead to osteoporosis and cortical thinning. The findings in the appendicular skeleton are not so prominent in the adult as in the child because of the normal fatty infiltration of the marrow of the extremities that occurs with advancing age.

VASCULAR OCCLUSION. Osteonecrosis is the sequela of the sickling phenomenon in which sequestration of cells occurs. Patients with osteonecrosis reveal fever, soft tissue swelling, bone pain and tenderness, and leukocytosis.

Sickle Cell Dactylitis (Fig. 54–2). In children between the ages of 6 months and 2 years, osteonecrosis may involve the small tubular bones of the hands and feet, leading to the "hand-foot" syndrome or dactylitis. The syndrome may be present in as many as 20 to 50 per cent of children with sickle cell anemia. Clinical manifestations include soft tissue swelling, pain, tenderness, elevated temperature, and limitation of motion.

In the early stages of sickle cell dactylitis, soft tissue swelling frequently is seen. Within 1 to 2 weeks, symmetrically distributed patchy radiolucency of the shaft with surrounding periostitis is observed, especially in the metacarpals, metatarsals, and phalanges. Focal osteosclerosis is also seen. The findings resemble those of osteomyelitis. Eventually, during a period of several months, bone reconstitution may lead to a completely normal osseous shadow.

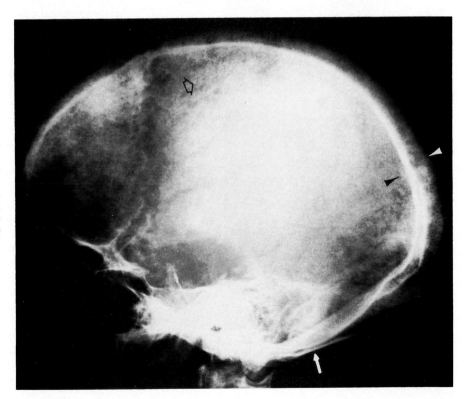

Figure 54–1. Sickle cell anemia: Marrow hyperplasia. A lateral view of the skull demonstrates widening of the diploic space (arrowheads). The base of the occiput is spared (arrow). Focal areas of increased radiodensity (open arrow) may represent myelofibrosis or healing infarcts.

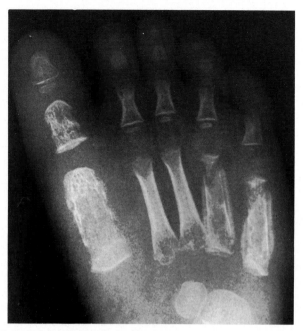

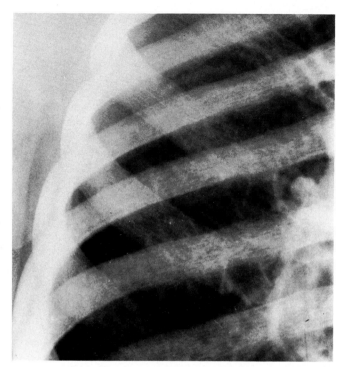

Figure 54–2. Sickle cell anemia: Vascular occlusion—sickle cell dactylitis. Observe soft tissue swelling, small osteolytic lesions (especially in the proximal phalanx of the great toe and the first, fourth, and fifth metatarsal bones), areas of more prominent osteolysis (including the distal portions of the fourth and fifth metatarsals), focal osteosclerosis, and periostitis. (Courtesy of P. Kaplan, M.D., Omaha, Nebraska.)

Figure 54–4. Sickle cell anemia: Vascular occlusion—infarction of ribs. Diffuse sclerosis has resulted in a coarsened trabecular pattern.

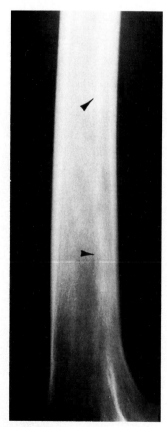

Figure 54–3. Sickle cell anemia: Vascular occlusion—diaphyseal infarction of larger tubular bones. A typical example of a bone-within-bone appearance owing to diaphyseal infarction. Observe linear sclerosis beneath the cortex (arrowheads) on this lateral view of the femur.

Diaphyseal Infarction of Larger Tubular Bones (Fig. 54–3). The diaphyses and epiphyses of long tubular bones are common sites of infarction in sickle cell anemia. The most frequent site of infarction is the proximal aspect of the femur, although the proximal part of the humerus, distal end of the femur, proximal part of the tibia, and other locations may be affected.

Extensive infarction of the shaft is associated with patchy lucency and sclerosis of the medullary bone. In addition, the diaphysis may be broadened or enlarged by the appearance and incorporation of subperiosteal new bone. On radiographic examination, such bone appears initially as a linear radiodense area adjacent to the cortex, which may extend along the entire shaft. Along the inner surface of the cortex, laminated new bone formation in response to infarction can produce concentric cylinders of bone paralleling the cortical surface. On radiographs, discrete linear bands beneath the cortical bone produce a bone-within-bone appearance, which is diagnostic of osteonecrosis.

Infarction of Other Bones (Fig. 54–4). Osteosclerosis in association with medullary infarction of bone is particularly common in the pelvis, spine, thorax, tibia, and fibula, producing increased radiodensity of bone and a coarsened trabecular pattern. Sclerosis in the terminal phalanges of the hand also has been observed (Fig. 54–5). Furthermore, sternal abnormalities, presumably related to infarction, have also been noted in patients with sickle cell anemia.

Epiphyseal Infarction (Fig. 54–6). Epiphyseal infarcts in sickle cell anemia are frequent and are more prevalent in adults than in children. Occasionally in older children, infarction of the capital femoral epiphysis leads to an appearance simulating that of Legg-Calvé-Perthes disease. Epiphyseal infarction commonly is bilateral in distribution, with predilection for the capital femoral and proximal humeral epiphyses. Occasionally, other sites are affected, including the distal end of the femur, proximal part of the tibia, and distal end of the humerus.

Osteonecrosis of the epiphysis in the adult with sickle cell anemia mimics the necrosis and collapse of epiphyses that accompany other processes, including steroid-induced and fracture-related conditions. Focal lucency and sclerosis, subchondral linear or curvilinear radiolucent shadows, collapse, and fragmentation are evident in involved epiphyses. Although collapse and disintegration of epiphyses, followed by the development of osteoarthritis, may be observed in weight-bearing areas such as the hip, epiphyseal necrosis in non–weight-bearing sites may lead to osteosclerosis without significant loss of epiphyseal contour. This is frequent in the proximal portion of the humerus, where alternating areas of lucency and sclerosis produce a "snow-capped" appearance.

Growth Disturbances (Fig. 54–7). Damage to epiphyseal circulation may produce arrested or decreased cartilage proliferation in the growth plate, leading to shortening of the bone. Ingrowth of blood vessels from the metaphysis may cause osseous fusion, particularly in the central portion of the growth plate. Cone-shaped epiphyses and inverted V, "cup," or "channel" deformities of the adjacent metaphyses are observed in sickle cell anemia, although similar changes occur in many other disorders, including congenital diseases, infection, trauma, and radiation injury.

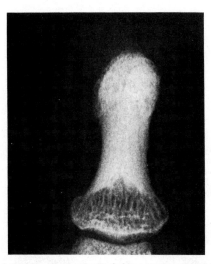

Figure 54–5. Sickle cell anemia: Probable vascular occlusion—phalangeal sclerosis. (From Sebes JI, Brown DL: Terminal phalangeal sclerosis in sickle cell disease. AJR *140*:763, 1983. Copyright 1983, American Roentgen Ray Society. Used with permission.)

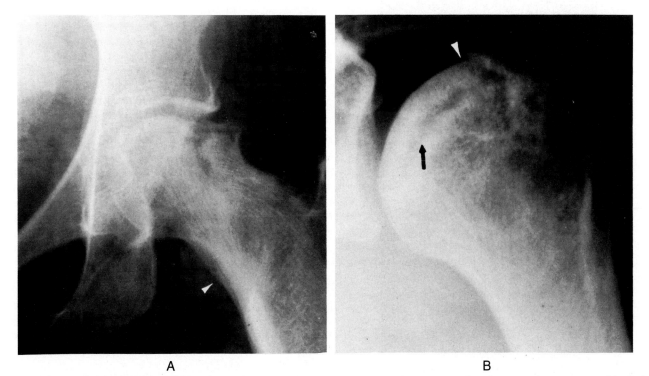

A   B

Figure 54–6. Sickle cell anemia: Vascular occlusion—epiphyseal infarction. A Changes of osteonecrosis of the femoral head are characterized by focal areas of sclerosis and collapse, with irregularity of the articular surface. Observe lateral femoral osteophytes and buttressing (arrowhead) of the femoral neck. B A "snow-capped" appearance of the humeral head is due to patchy sclerosis. Collapse of the articular surface (arrowhead) and subchondral fractures (arrow) are evident.

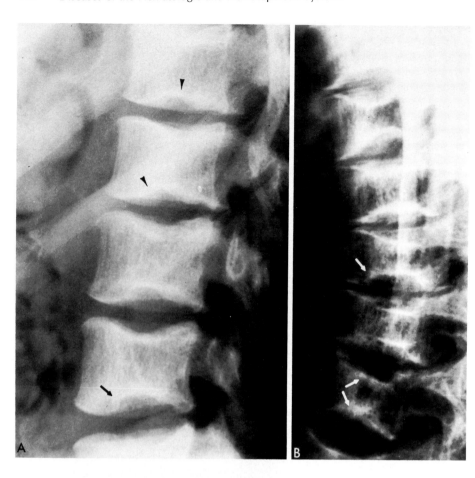

Figure 54–7. Sickle cell anemia: Growth disturbance—H vertebrae. A, B Two examples of H vertebrae characterized by central indentations of the vertebral bodies. Initially the abnormalities may simulate cartilaginous nodes or "fish vertebrae" (arrowheads), although eventually typical squared-off indentations are observed (arrows).

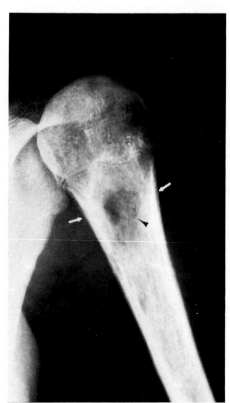

Figure 54–8. Sickle cell anemia: Osteomyelitis. Salmonella infection of the humerus has led to lytic lesions (arrowhead) with surrounding periostitis (arrows). This organism may produce symmetric diaphyseal osteomyelitis of long tubular bones in patients with sickle cell anemia.

Tibiotalar deformity has been mentioned as a radiographic finding in sickle cell anemia. This deformity, which consists of slanting of the articular surfaces of the distal part of the tibia and the talus, had previously been emphasized as a characteristic abnormality of hemophilia, juvenile-onset rheumatoid arthritis, and multiple epiphyseal dysplasia.

Central depression of the vertebral bodies may represent an additional growth disturbance of sickle cell anemia. The resulting deformity of the vertebra consists of squared-off endplate depressions, the "H" vertebra. It has been postulated that this deformity results from ischemia of the central portion of the vertebral growth plate. The radiographic picture is easily distinguished from the smooth biconcave contour defects of vertebral bodies that characterize many metabolic disorders. Although H vertebrae occasionally are described in other conditions, including thalassemia, Gaucher's disease, congenital hereditary spherocytosis, and osteoporosis, their appearance is very suggestive of the diagnosis of sickle cell anemia. In addition, exaggerated anterior vertebral notching, perhaps related to venous stasis, has been described in sickle cell disease.

MISCELLANEOUS FINDINGS

Fractures. Fractures in the appendicular and axial skeleton in patients with sickle cell anemia can occur spontaneously or after minor trauma. In the long tubular bones, marrow hyperplasia produces cortical thinning, which predisposes to this complication.

Osteomyelitis and Septic Arthritis (Fig. 54–8). Patients with sickle cell anemia are susceptible to bacterial infection. This susceptibility relates to a variety of causes: tissue injury from vascular insult with infarction; increased exposure to infection because of multiple hospitalizations; impaired phagocytosis at low oxygen tensions; and decreased splenic function attributable to fibrosis. Bone and joint infections in sickle cell anemia are caused by salmonellae in over 50 per cent of cases. It is suggested that these organisms gain entry to the bloodstream as a result of intestinal infarction produced by sickling within mesenteric vessels. Staphylococci represent a second common cause of osteomyelitis in sickle cell anemia. Additional organisms that may be implicated in these infections are pneumococci, Serratia, Haemophilus, and *Escherichia coli*.

Osteomyelitis is most frequent in the long tubular bones. Infection, particularly that associated with salmonellae, may produce symmetric involvement with diaphyseal localization. The findings of osteomyelitis in patients with sickle cell anemia may simulate those of osteonecrosis, with fever, bone pain, and leukocytosis on clinical evaluation, and with osteolysis and periostitis on radiographic evaluation. Involucrum formation, cortical sequestration, fracture, soft tissue abscesses, and sinus tracts are later manifestations of infection.

Septic arthritis complicating sickle cell anemia is less frequent than osteomyelitis. Implicated organisms have included staphylococci, *E. coli*, Enterobacter, salmonellae, and, rarely, anaerobic species.

Crystal Deposition. Hyperuricemia occurs in some patients with sickle cell anemia. The frequency of clinical attacks of gout is low, however.

Hemarthrosis. Although hemarthrosis may accompany osteonecrosis with epiphyseal collapse in patients with sickle cell anemia, this is not a common complication of the disease.

Joint Effusions. Joint effusions in sickle cell anemia that are not associated with infection, crystal deposition, or hemarthrosis are relatively common. These effusions, which most frequently involve the knee and elbow, are associated with clinical manifestations of crises and presumably relate to synovial ischemia.

Radionuclide Features

Bone marrow in normal adults is located predominantly in the axial skeleton and proximal portions of femora and humeri; in patients with various anemias, the marrow expands symmetrically to occupy long bones and skull. During asymptomatic periods, patients with sickle cell anemia may reveal focal areas of decreased uptake on bone marrow scanning, which can probably be attributed to sites of previous infarction. During a crisis, additional areas without radionuclide activity are found, surrounded by active marrow.

Bone scanning agents such as ^{99m}Tc-polyphosphate demonstrate uptake related to the integrity of blood flow and the presence of new bone formation. In patients with sickle cell anemia, marrow expansion is associated with increased blood flow and an increased accumulation of radionuclide in the skeleton. Immediately after a crisis, an area of infarction may demonstrate decreased or absent radionuclide activity (Fig. 54–9). One to 2 weeks after the crisis, increased activity by bone scanning occurs owing to reactive bone formation about the area of infarction. This abnormal activity may persist for several months.

It has been suggested that scanning with both bone- and bone-marrow–seeking radionuclides allows differentiation of

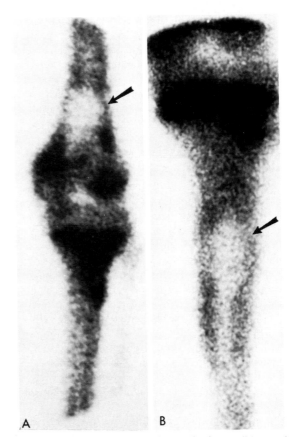

Figure 54–9. Sickle cell anemia: Radionuclide abnormalities—technetium polyphosphate bone scanning. Examples of diaphyseal infarctions of the distal part of the femur (A) and proximal part of the tibia (B) associated with focal decreased accumulation of radionuclide are seen (arrows). Increased metaphyseal activity is apparent.

osteomyelitis and osteonecrosis in patients with sickle cell anemia. The combination of a large defect on the bone marrow scan and a smaller defect on the bone scan is typical of osteonecrosis.

Marrow scans with ^{99m}Tc-sulfur colloid may also outline sites of extramedullary hematopoiesis in sickle cell anemia or related disorders.

SICKLE CELL TRAIT

Sickle cell trait is characterized by the presence of Hb A-S. It can be associated with sickling if the blood is exposed to low oxygen tension. Patients with sickle cell trait are not jaundiced or anemic, and hyperplasia of bone marrow is not present. Musculoskeletal findings related to sickle cell trait are of low frequency, although osteonecrosis of the femoral head has been reported in some patients.

SICKLE CELL–HEMOGLOBIN C DISEASE

The observation that parents of atypical patients with sickle cell disease might not demonstrate sickling led to the discovery of hemoglobin C and of the hemoglobinopathy termed sickle cell–hemoglobin C disease. The clinical disability is less severe than homozygous sickle cell disease (sickle cell anemia), and the diagnosis often is not established until adulthood.

Marrow hyperplasia in sickle cell–hemoglobin C disease may result in calvarial alterations in 25 per cent of patients. The reported changes in the skull include granular osteoporosis, diploic widening, and thinning of the outer table. Spinal abnormality may be seen with biconcavity of the vertebral bodies and narrowing of the intervertebral discs. Osteonecrosis of the femoral and humeral heads also may be apparent (Fig. 54–10).

SICKLE CELL–THALASSEMIA DISEASE

Sickle cell–thalassemia disease is caused by the inheritance of one gene for hemoglobin S and one gene for thalassemia. Some patients with this disease have manifestations that are almost identical to those associated with sickle cell anemia; other patients are entirely asymptomatic. Ischemic changes in the skeleton in sickle cell–thalassemia disease are common, leading to patchy sclerosis and lucency and a bone-within-bone appearance, and diaphyseal and epiphyseal infarcts are most common in the proximal epiphyses of femora and humeri, causing lucency, sclerosis, collapse, and fragmentation. H vertebrae also are encountered in sickle cell–thalassemia disease.

Signs of marrow hyperplasia consist of cortical thinning and osteoporosis of the long tubular bones, biconcave deformities of the spine, thickening of the cranial vault with a mild hair-on-end appearance, and thinning of the outer table in the skull.

Osteomyelitis and septic arthritis also may occur in sickle cell–thalassemia disease.

THALASSEMIA
General Features

In 1925, a form of severe anemia associated with splenomegaly and bone abnormalities was described, which was designated thalassemia, from the Greek word for "the sea," because affected patients were of Mediterranean origin. It is now known that thalassemia is not a single disease but a group of disorders related to an inherited abnormality of globin production. There are two main groups of thalassemia: Alpha-thalassemia is characterized by a deficiency of alpha globin chain synthesis; beta-thalassemia is characterized by a deficiency of beta globin chain synthesis. As hemoglobin F contains alpha chains, the fetus is affected by alpha-thalassemia; beta-thalassemia becomes apparent after the newborn period as hemoglobin A replaces hemoglobin F. Several distinct disorders exist within these groups. Furthermore, thalassemia may exist in a homozygous form, called thalassemia major, or a heterozygous form, termed thalassemia minor or minima. Thalassemia intermedia represents a poorly defined intermediate variety of the disease. Although thalassemia has been denoted as "Mediterranean anemia" because of its peculiar geographic distribution with involvement of persons of Italian or Greek descent, this hemolytic anemia can be seen in people from other areas as well.

Clinical Features

Homozygous beta-thalassemia (thalassemia major) is characterized by severe anemia, prominent hepatosplenomegaly, and early death, often in childhood. Heterozygous beta-thalassemia (thalassemia minor) generally is associated with mild clinical findings, including slight to moderate anemia, splenomegaly, and jaundice.

With respect to alpha-thalassemia, the most severe form is hydrops fetalis with Bart's hemoglobin, in which there is a complete absence of alpha chain production. The disease, which is almost exclusively seen in Southeast Asia, leads to death in utero or at birth.

Radiographic and Pathologic Features
MARROW HYPERPLASIA (FIGS. 54–11 TO 54–14). The radiographic and pathologic features of beta-thalassemia are due in large part to marrow hyperplasia. Initially, both the axial and the appendicular skeleton is altered, but as the patient reaches puberty, the appendicular skeletal changes diminish, owing to normal regression of the marrow from the

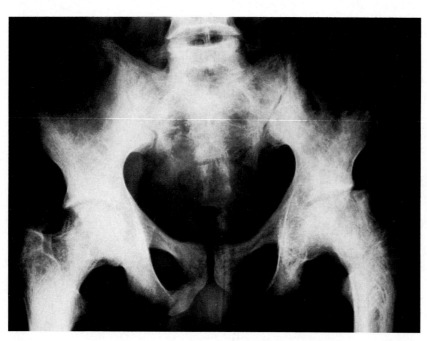

Figure 54–10. Sickle cell–hemoglobin C disease: Vascular occlusion. Diffuse osteosclerosis of the pelvis and proximal portions of the long bones is associated with osteonecrosis of the femoral heads. Significant collapse of the left femoral head is apparent.

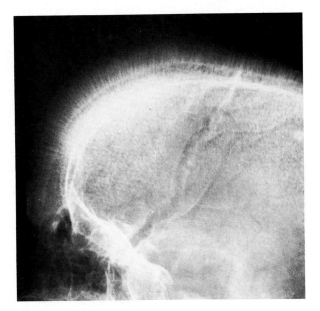

Figure 54–11. Thalassemia major: Marrow hyperplasia—skull. A lateral radiograph of the skull delineates striking abnormalities. Bone proliferation on the outer table of the vault has created a hair-on-end appearance, with dense radial striations traversing the thickened calvarium. Bone overgrowth in the face with decreased sinus aeration is also evident.

peripheral skeleton. The changes in thalassemia major are much more severe than those in thalassemia minor.

In the skull, the frontal bones reveal the earliest and most severe changes, and the inferior aspect of the occiput is usually unaltered. Findings include granular osteoporosis, widening of the diploic space, and thinning of the outer table. Bone proliferation on the outer table of the vault leads to a hair-on-end appearance (Fig. 54–11). This appearance, is characterized by dense radial striations traversing the thickened calvarium, which appear to extend beyond the outer table.

In thalassemia, marrow hyperplasia involves the facial bones as well. In infancy and early childhood, osseous expansion of the nasal and temporal bones leads to obliteration of the air spaces of the paranasal sinuses. Maxillary alterations can produce lateral displacement of the orbits, leading to hypertelorism, malocclusion of the jaws, and displacement of dental structures, resulting in "rodent" facies (Fig. 54–12). The striking facial abnormalities accompanying this disease are rarely seen in other anemias. Furthermore, the extent and severity of cranial vault changes, including the hair-on-end appearance, are much greater in thalassemia than in other anemic disorders.

Osteoporosis is evident in the vertebral bodies. Reduction in the number of trabeculae, thinning of the subchondral bone plates, accentuation of vertical trabeculation, and biconcave deformities ("fish vertebrae") are observed. Rarely, central squared-off vertebral depressions or H vertebrae, characteristic of sickle cell anemia, are noted in thalassemia major.

Medullary hyperplasia is also evident in the ribs, pelvis, and clavicles, as well as the bones of the appendicular skeleton (Fig. 54–13). The posterior aspects of multiple ribs frequently reveal significant expansion, cortical thinning, and osteoporosis (Fig. 54–14). Similarly, the tubular bones reveal a widened marrow cavity, cortical thinning, and a coarse, trabeculated appearance. The contour of some of the long bones is altered; normal concavity is lost, and the bones may have a straight or convex appearance. Widening of the metaphyses and epiphyses resembles an Erlenmeyer flask.

GROWTH DISTURBANCES. Modeling deformity with an Erlenmeyer flask tubular bone is only one of the growth disturbances that may be encountered in patients with thalassemia. Near the ends of long bones, it is common to detect irregular transverse radiodense (growth recovery) lines in patients with this disorder.

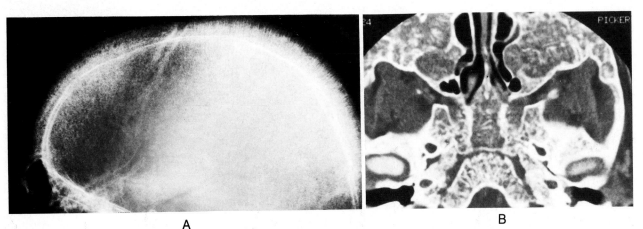

A   B

Figure 54–12. Thalassemia major: Marrow hyperplasia—skull and face. A hair-on-end appearance is well shown on the routine radiograph (A), and the overgrowth of the facial bones is delineated with transaxial computed tomography (B). (Courtesy of S. Kursunoglu, M.D., San Diego, California.)

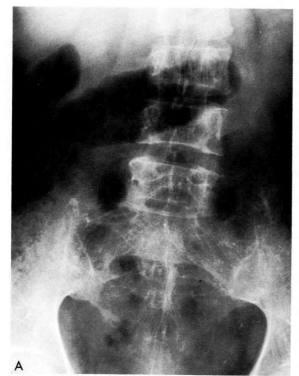

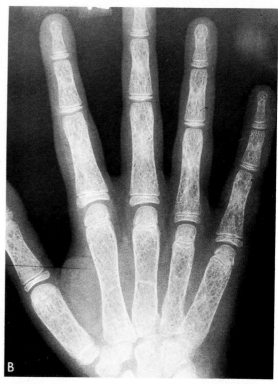

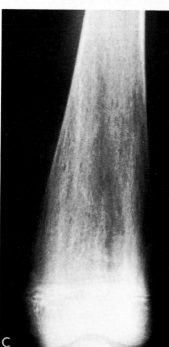

Figure 54–13. Thalassemia major: Marrow hyperplasia—axial and appendicular skeleton. A Pelvis and spine. Osteoporosis of the pelvis and vertebrae is evident. Mild biconcave deformities of the vertebral bodies can be seen. The sacroiliac joints are poorly defined. **B** Hands. Note osteoporosis, a reticulated trabecular pattern, widening of the medullary cavity, thinned cortices, and mild osseous expansion. **C** Femur. Erlenmeyer flask deformity is apparent, with loss of normal concavity and straightening or convexity of the osseous contour, particularly along the medial aspect of the bone.

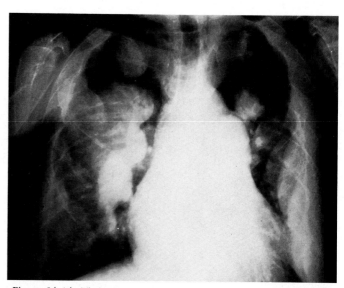

Figure 54–14. Thalassemia major: Marrow hyperplasia—axial skeleton. Widespread and marked involvement of the ribs is associated with osteopenia, cortical thinning, and bone expansion. The entire thorax and the humeri are affected.

670

Premature fusion of the physes (growth plates) in the tubular bones of the extremities, which has been noted in 10 to 15 per cent of patients with thalassemia major, generally occurs after the age of 10 years and is most frequent in the proximal part of the humerus and distal part of the femur. Shortening and deformity of the extremity may be apparent. In the humerus, varus deformity is characteristic.

FRACTURES (FIG. 54–15). Spontaneous fractures are not uncommon in patients with thalassemia. They are most frequent in the bones of the lower extremity, particularly the femur, in the bones of the forearm, and in the vertebrae. Fractures are not unexpected in view of the severe osteopenia that is common in this condition and the increased life expectancy of patients related to more adequate transfusion therapy.

CRYSTAL DEPOSITION. Secondary hemochromatosis resulting from repeated transfusions can be seen in patients with thalassemia. Arthropathy in these patients resembles that of primary hemochromatosis. Calcium pyrophosphate dihydrate (CPPD) crystal deposition may lead to chondrocalcinosis.

Hyperuricemia and acute gouty arthritis may appear during the clinical course of thalassemia.

EXTRAMEDULLARY HEMATOPOIESIS. Extramedullary hematopoiesis represents the body's attempt to maintain erythrogenesis when there is an important alteration in blood cell population. It is observed in a variety of processes that have in common a change in bone marrow content. These processes include destruction of marrow by neoplasm or toxin, myeloproliferative disorders, and hemolytic anemias; extramedullary hematopoiesis is a well-recognized phenomenon in thalassemia. Its mechanism, appearance, and location vary somewhat among these disorders: in those instances in which the marrow is destroyed or is inefficient, focal areas of hematopoiesis appear in the liver, spleen, and lymph nodes, probably arising from multipotential stem cells; in hemolytic disorders, such as thalassemia, in which the marrow has accelerated activity, extraosseous herniation of medullary tissue is observed.

In thalassemia, posterior paravertebral mediastinal masses (Fig. 54–16), representing sites of extramedullary hematopoiesis, result from extraosseous extensions of medullary tissue derived from vertebral bodies and ribs. Radiographs of the ribs in such cases document expanded and thinned cortices and cortical perforations with lobulated soft tissue masses. Spinal cord compression owing to extradural hematopoietic tissue may occur. Extramedullary hematopoiesis in thalassemia as well as in other anemias also can involve additional sites, including the retroperitoneal space and pelvis.

MISCELLANEOUS ABNORMALITIES. Enlargement of nutrient foramina in the phalanges of the hand has been identified in beta-thalassemia. The finding, which is also observed in Gaucher's disease, presumably is related to either an increased arterial supply, an increased venous return, or both, to or from the hyperactive and hyperemic bone marrow. Tortuous and widened vascular channels in the skull have also been seen in this disease.

Other Diagnostic Techniques

Iron overload resulting from repeated blood transfusions in thalassemia is associated with a reduction in skeletal uptake of phosphorus-containing bone-seeking radiopharmaceutical

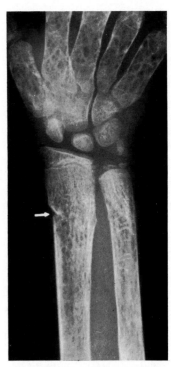

Figure 54–15. Thalassemia major: Fractures. An example of extreme osteoporosis in the upper extremity. The cortices are extensively thinned or absent. A fracture can be observed (arrow).

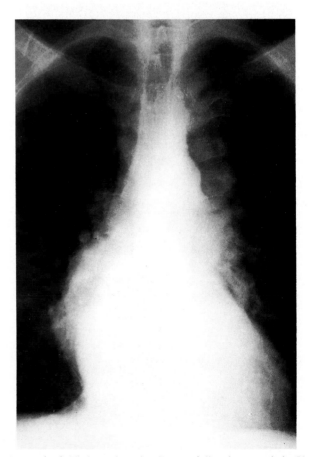

Figure 54–16. Thalassemia major: Extramedullary hematopoiesis. Bilateral lobulated posterior mediastinal masses can be seen. The heart is enlarged.

agents and an increase in renal and soft tissue radioactivity. Similarly, sites of extramedullary hematopoiesis can be analyzed using radionuclide techniques.

Computed tomography can document the abnormal deposition of iron that follows multiple blood transfusions in patients with thalassemia (or other anemias). This can be evident in the liver, spleen, bowel, pancreas, lymph nodes, and additional organs. This technique can also be used to document sites of extramedullary hematopoiesis, particularly in the posterior mediastinum, spinal canal, and pelvis.

Magnetic resonance imaging is an additional diagnostic method that has been used in some patients with thalassemia. The intensity of the image obtained with magnetic resonance provides an assessment of the amount of iron that is deposited in the tissues of the body (Fig. 54–17).

IRON DEFICIENCY ANEMIA

In children, iron deficiency anemia results from insufficient intake or excessive loss of iron during the first 6 months of life, which depletes the iron that was stored during late prenatal life. This type of anemia is most frequent between 9 months and 2 years of age.

Skeletal abnormalities generally are mild. Marrow hyperplasia may result in changes of the cranial vault. Thinning of the outer table and diploic widening are observed in the

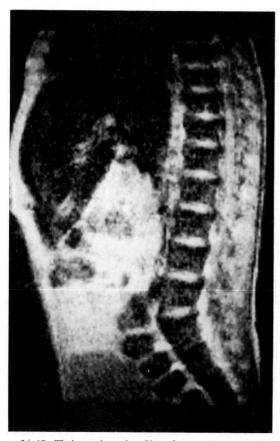

Figure 54–17. Thalassemia major: Use of magnetic resonance imaging—assessment of iron deposition. In this midsagittal image of a 14 year old child, there is depression of the spin echo signal intensity in the liver and bone marrow. Increased signal intensity was present in the muscles and kidneys. (Courtesy of R. Brasch, M.D., San Francisco, California.)

frontal, parietal, or occipital bone. As in cases of hemolytic anemia, the occipital squamosa inferior to the internal occipital protuberance is unaffected in this disease. Radial striations extending from the outer table are rare and usually are mild in iron deficiency anemia. Furthermore, facial involvement is not apparent. Osteoporosis of other sites has been noted, including the long and short tubular bones.

HEREDITARY SPHEROCYTOSIS

This hemolytic anemia, which is inherited as an autosomal dominant disorder, is worldwide in distribution but most common in northern Europeans. It is characterized by abnormally shaped red blood cells or spherocytes in the peripheral blood, which are hemolyzed in the spleen. The onset of disease varies from early infancy to adulthood, although the majority of cases become evident in late childhood and early adolescence. Clinical features include anemia, jaundice, and splenomegaly. Gallstones and chronic leg ulcerations are two other potential manifestations of this disorder.

Compensatory hyperplasia of the bone marrow occurs with extension of red marrow into the diaphyses of long bones. In the cranial vault, diploic widening and thinning of the outer table are evident. Rarely, hair-on-end striations and medullary widening with osteoporosis in long bones are seen. Significant long bone changes are indeed unusual, however. Occasionally, extramedullary hematopoiesis results in paravertebral masses simulating infection or tumor.

HEREDITARY ELLIPTOCYTOSIS

In hereditary elliptocytosis, red cells are oval or elliptical in shape. The disorder is closely linked to hereditary spherocytosis, as some families contain members with elliptocytosis and other members with spherocytosis. Hemolysis occurs in the spleen. The bone abnormalities are largely undescribed.

NONSPHEROCYTIC HEMOLYTIC ANEMIA

Nonspherocytic hemolytic anemia is a designation that can be used for hereditary hemolytic processes not attributable to thalassemia, spherocytosis, elliptocytosis, or one of the hemoglobinopathies. The two most important disorders in this category are pyruvate kinase deficiency and glucose-6-phosphate dehydrogenase deficiency anemias. Radiographic changes have been documented in association with deficiency of pyruvate kinase. Marrow hyperplasia producing osteoporosis, diploic widening, and thinning of the outer table in the cranial vault is a finding identical to that in other anemias. Unlike the case with thalassemia, the facial bones and sinuses are unaffected. Splenectomy may result in improvement of the anemia and in partial resolution of the skull changes.

MISCELLANEOUS ANEMIAS

Hemolytic disease of the newborn (erythroblastosis fetalis) is associated with excessive destruction of the erythrocytes beginning in fetal life, usually owing to Rh incompatibility between the blood of the fetus and that of the mother. Clinical and radiographic findings include soft tissue edema ("halo sign"), loss of muscle and fat planes in the soft tissues, and metaphyseal lucency and sclerosis.

Fanconi's anemia consists of severe refractory hypoplastic anemia with pancytopenia, brown pigmentation of the skin, and multiple congenital anomalies. The onset of this anemia frequently is delayed until the end of the first decade of life. Radiographic findings include anomalies of the radius and radial side of the hand, ranging from hypoplasia to aplasia of osseous structures, short stature, microcephaly, delayed ossification, congenital dislocation or subluxation of the hip, and renal anomalies.

The syndrome of thrombocytopenia and absent radius (TAR syndrome) resembles Fanconi's anemia. It consists of congenital hypomegakaryocytic thrombocytopenia, severe hemorrhages, and skeletal anomalies. The last-mentioned include bilateral absence of the radius, shortening of the ulna, dysplasia of the knee, and osseous deformity. The presence of five digits in the hand in the TAR syndrome differs from the absence of the thumb that is seen in Fanconi's anemia. Furthermore, the TAR syndrome generally is evident in the first few years of life, whereas Fanconi's anemia has a later onset.

DIFFERENTIAL DIAGNOSIS
Differentiation Among the Anemias (Table 54–1)

Extensive thickening of the cranial vault associated with marked diploic expansion and a hair-on-end appearance is most characteristic of thalassemia. Its occurrence in patients with sickle cell anemia has been overemphasized. Some thickening of the cranial vault can be apparent in sickle cell–hemoglobin C disease, sickle cell–thalassemia disease, iron deficiency anemia, hereditary spherocytosis, and pyruvate kinase deficiency, but widespread and severe skull alterations are rare in these disorders. Severe facial changes are limited to thalassemia.

Changes of marrow hyperplasia in the peripheral skeleton are most common and marked in thalassemia. In this disease, abnormality can occur in long and short tubular bones, although the changes may regress and disappear with advancing age. In children with sickle cell anemia, osteoporosis and cortical thinning in the small tubular bones of the hands and feet can be seen, although the findings generally are mild. In the adult with sickle cell anemia, the findings of marrow hyperplasia in the peripheral skeleton are overshadowed by findings of multiple bone infarcts. In iron deficiency anemia and sickle cell–thalassemia disease, changes of marrow hyperplasia in the tubular bones are absent or mild.

Bone infarction is particularly common in sickle cell anemia and sickle cell–hemoglobin C disease. Ischemic skeletal changes are less frequent in sickle cell–thalassemia disease and sickle cell trait and are not characteristic of thalassemia or iron deficiency anemia. Diaphyseal infarction with surrounding sclerosis producing a bone-within-bone appearance is suggestive of sickle cell anemia or sickle cell–hemoglobin C disease, being rare in other anemias. Infarction of the small bones of the hands and feet in children producing dactylitis and the hand-foot syndrome is almost diagnostic of sickle cell anemia.

Abnormalities of vertebral body contour with squared-off compressions of the vertebrae (H vertebrae) occur in sickle cell anemia, sickle cell–hemoglobin C disease, and sickle cell–thalassemia disease, although such abnormalities may be seen in thalassemia and in other conditions, such as Gaucher's disease. Flaring of the ends of the tubular bones, the Erlenmeyer flask appearance, is most suggestive of thalassemia. This finding, too, can be seen in disorders other than anemias. Premature fusion of the growth plate has been described in both sickle cell anemia and thalassemia.

Osteopenia, which may be found in many of the anemic disorders, leads to osseous weakening, predisposing to skeletal fractures. Pathologic fractures have been noted in sickle cell anemia and thalassemia.

Osteomyelitis, particularly that associated with Salmonella infection, is a known complication of sickle cell anemia, although infections of bones and joints can be observed in thalassemia and other hemoglobinopathies.

Secondary hemochromatosis with or without CPPD crystal

Table 54–1. CHARACTERISTIC SKELETAL FINDINGS IN THE ANEMIAS

Disease	Marrow Hyperplasia			Bone infarction		Growth Disturbances		Fractures	Osteomyelitis and Septic Arthritis	Crystal Deposition	
	Cranial Vault	Facial Bones	Tubular Bones	Long Tubular Bones	Hands, Feet	H Vertebrae	Flaring of Tubular Bones			Calcium Pyrophosphate Dihydrate	Monosodium Urate
Sickle cell anemia	+		+	+	+	+		+	+		+
Sickle cell trait				+					+		
Sickle cell–hemoglobin C disease	+			+		+					
Sickle cell–thalassemia disease	+		+	+		+			+		
Thalassemia	+	+	+			+	+	+	+	+	+
Iron deficiency anemia	+		+								
Spherocytosis	+									+	
Nonspherocytic hemolytic anemia	+										

deposition may complicate repeated blood transfusions in thalassemia, spherocytosis, and hypoplastic and sideroblastic anemias. Hyperuricemia and gouty arthritis occur with sickle cell anemia and thalassemia and, occasionally, in other anemias as well.

Differentiation of Anemia from Other Conditions

In anemic disorders, diffuse skeletal abnormality characterized by decreased radiographic density (osteopenia) indicates marrow hyperplasia. Other primary marrow diseases, such as Gaucher's disease and Niemann-Pick disease, are associated with similar findings. Osteopenia may also accompany osteogenesis imperfecta, idiopathic juvenile osteoporosis, hyperparathyroidism, and leukemia as well as other diseases. In sickle cell anemia, infarction in the long tubular bones of the appendicular skeleton and in portions of the axial skeleton may lead to increased radiodensity with a coarsened trabecular pattern simulating the changes of renal osteodystrophy, myelofibrosis, and osteomalacia.

Thickening of the cranial vault is a radiographic finding that is apparent in many disorders. In anemias, this thickening frequently involves the entire cranium with the exception of the inferior aspect of the occipital bone and base of the skull. Fibrous dysplasia and leontiasis ossea can lead to excessive hyperostosis of the skull, but changes usually predominate in the frontal regions and face. Hyperostosis frontalis interna generally is confined to the anterior aspect of the cranial vault, whereas acromegaly, Paget's disease, and hypoparathyroidism may produce diffuse thickening of the cranium.

Epiphyseal and diaphyseal bone infarction occurs not only in anemia but also in other diseases. Epiphyseal ischemia, particularly of the femoral head, is noted in endogenous and exogenous corticosteroid excess, caisson disease, Gaucher's disease, collagen disorders, alcoholism with pancreatitis, and radiation therapy, as well as after trauma and in many other processes. Diametaphyseal ischemia is seen in association with steroid administration, caisson disease, pancreatitis, and Gaucher's disease.

Abnormality of vertebral body contour characterized by step-like depressions of the osseous surface, the H vertebra, is a relatively specific radiographic sign of anemia. It has been noted rarely in other conditions, including Gaucher's disease. The H vertebra with its abrupt endplate indentations can be distinguished from the "fish vertebra," which has a smooth biconcave appearance. "Fish vertebrae" may be observed in anemias, but the changes are not specific, as they appear in all forms of osteoporosis and in osteomalacia, hyperparathyroidism, Paget's disease, and neoplasm.

The findings of sickle cell dactylitis may simulate the changes of other disorders associated with destruction and periostitis of small tubular bones in the hands and feet. Dactylitis may be apparent in tuberculosis, syphilis, leprosy, and fungal and pyogenic disorders. Furthermore, periostitis of small tubular bones with or without bone destruction can accompany leukemia, scurvy, hypervitaminosis A, trauma, and infantile cortical hyperostosis.

Extramedullary hematopoiesis accompanying thalassemia and, less commonly, other anemias leads to enlargement of the posterior portions of the ribs, simulating the findings in fibrous dysplasia, and lobulated posterior mediastinal masses resembling neoplasm. With regard to the rib lesions, multiplicity, bilaterality, and the known presence of an anemia generally allow differentiation of sites of extramedullary hematopoiesis from the other causes of rib expansion.

FURTHER READING

Agarwal KN, Dhar N, Shah MM, Bhardwaj OP: Roentgenologic changes in iron deficiency anemia. AJR 110:635, 1970.

Barton CJ, Cockshott WP: Bone changes in hemoglobin SC disease. AJR 88:523, 1962.

Bohrer SP: Growth disturbances of the distal femur following sickle cell bone infarcts and/or osteomyelitis. Clin Radiol 25:221, 1974.

Brasch RC, Wesbey GE, Gooding CA, Koerper MA: Magnetic resonance imaging of transfusional hemosiderosis complicating thalassemia major. Radiology 150:767, 1984.

Caffey J: Cooley's anemia: A review of the roentgenographic findings in the skeleton. AJR 78:381, 1957.

Cooley TB, Lee P: A series of cases of splenomegaly in children with anemia and peculiar bone changes. Trans Am Pediatr Soc 37:29, 1925.

Currarino G, Erlandson ME: Premature fusion of epiphyses in Cooley's anemia. Radiology 83:656, 1964.

Fink IJ, Pastakia B, Barranger JA: Enlarged phalangeal foramina in Gaucher disease and B-thalassemia major. AJR 143:647, 1984.

Janus WL, Dietz MW: Osseous changes in erythroblastosis fetalis (21 cases). Radiology 53:59, 1949.

Juhl JH, Wesenberg RL, Gwinn JL: Roentgenographic findings in Fanconi's anemia. Radiology 89:646, 1967.

Kaplan PA, Asleson RJ, Klassen LW, Duggan MJ: Bone marrow patterns in aplastic anemia: 1.5-T MR imaging. Radiology 164:441, 1987.

Lawson JP, Ablow RC, Pearson HA: The ribs in thalassemia. I. The relationship to therapy. Radiology 140:663, 1981.

Lawson JP, Ablow RC, Pearson HA: The ribs in thalassemia. II. The pathogenesis of the changes. Radiology 140:673, 1981.

Lutzker LG, Alavi A: Bone and marrow imaging in sickle cell disease: Diagnosis of infarction. Semin Nucl Med 6:83, 1976.

O'Hara AE: Roentgenographic osseous manifestations of the anemias and the leukemias. Clin Orthop 52:63, 1967.

Pauling L, Itano HA, Singer SJ, Wells IC: Sickle cell anemia, a molecular disease. Science 110:543, 1949.

Reynolds J: The Roentgenological Features of Sickle Cell Disease and Related Hemoglobinopathies. Springfield, Ill, Charles C Thomas, 1965.

Reynolds J: A re-evaluation of the "fish vertebra" sign in sickle cell hemoglobinopathy. AJR 97:693, 1966.

Sebes JI, Brown DL: Terminal phalangeal sclerosis in sickle cell disease. AJR 140:763, 1983.

Chapter 55

Plasma Cell Dyscrasias and Dysgammaglobulinemias

Donald Resnick, M.D.

Musculoskeletal findings occur in various plasma cell dyscrasias and dysgammaglobulinemias. In plasma cell myeloma, widespread or localized osteolysis can be attributed, in large part, to plasma cell infiltration in the bone marrow. Accompanying amyloid deposition in some patients may become manifest as articular and periarticular alterations. Additional joint findings in plasma cell myeloma may be related to secondary gout, infection, and hemarthrosis. Skeletal and articular manifestations of Waldenström's macroglobulinemia resemble those of plasma cell myeloma. Amyloidosis, which can occur in both plasma cell myeloma and Waldenström's macroglobulinemia, can also be apparent in a primary form without antecedent cause or in a secondary form in various other conditions. In both primary and secondary types, amyloid deposition can lead to significant bone and joint changes, including osteoporosis, osseous lytic lesions, and tumorous foci in both articular and extraarticular locations. Finally, syndromes related to antibody deficiency (agammaglobulinemia, hypogammaglobulinemia) are associated with recurrent and severe infections that may involve bones and joints and a rheumatoid arthritis–like chronic asymmetric polyarthritis.

Plasma cells are the functional unit of the immune defense system. They are found in various areas of the human body, particularly in the lymph nodes, the bone marrow, and the submucosa of the gastrointestinal tract, and they are responsible for antibody synthesis. Plasma cells are the principal source of immunoglobulins, proteins of high molecular weight, which function as antibodies as they circulate throughout the tissues. In the presence of infectious disease (as well as other disorders), the number of plasma cells within the bone marrow increases, resulting in a similar increase in the production of immunoglobulins. This response is termed plasmacytosis and is a normal consequence of infection. When plasma cell proliferation appears as an inappropriate or uncontrolled event, a disease state exists. Several diseases can be manifested in this fashion and are grouped together as plasma cell dyscrasias. Related conditions such as agammaglobulinemia and hypogammaglobulinemia are associated with a decrease in concentration of plasma gamma globulins and a concomitant impairment of antibody formation.

Plasma cell dyscrasias are characterized by (1) the uncontrolled proliferation of plasma cells in the absence of an identifiable antigenic stimulus; (2) the elaboration of electrophoretically and structurally homogeneous monoclonal, M type (plasma cell myeloma, macroglobulinemia) gamma globulins or excessive quantities of homogeneous polypeptide subunits of these proteins (Bence Jones proteins, H chains), or both; and (3) a commonly associated deficiency in the synthesis of normal immunoglobulins. Some of these dyscrasias, such as plasma cell myeloma, macroglobulinemia, amyloidosis, and heavy chain diseases, have a typical constellation of clinical manifestations that permits specific diagnosis, whereas others initially or ultimately defy precise classification. Disease states in the latter category include premyeloma, essential hypergammaglobulinemia, essential cryoglobulinemia, dysgammaglobulinemia, and idiopathic monoclonal gammopathy.

Plasma cell dyscrasias result in the synthesis of large quantities of a single protein related to one of the major classes of immunoglobulins. There are five major classes of antigenetically distinct immunoglobulins: IgG, IgM, IgA, IgD, IgE. All of these consist of two identical heavy (H) chains linked to two identical light (L) chains. The type of immunoglobulin that is being elaborated abnormally can be identified by its electrophoretic pattern and varies among the plasma cell dyscrasias. For example, in patients with multiple myeloma, IgG predominates, followed, in order of decreasing frequency, by IgA, IgD, IgM, and IgE. In Waldenström's macroglobulinemia, the elaboration of large amounts of IgM globulins is apparent. Furthermore, a subunit of one of these proteins may be identified in some of these dyscrasias; in multiple myeloma, large quantities of Bence Jones proteins (representing free light chains) are common.

PLASMA CELL MYELOMA

Plasma cell myeloma (myelomatosis, Kahler's disease, plasmacytic myeloma, multiple myeloma, plasmacytoma) is a malignant disease of plasma cells that usually originates in the bone marrow but may involve other tissues as well.

Clinical Features

Plasma cell myeloma represents approximately 1 per cent of all malignancies and 10 to 15 per cent of malignancies of the hematologic system. The disease usually occurs between the ages of 40 and 80 years, predominantly in older patients.

It appears to be slightly more common in men than in women. Myeloma is particularly common in blacks.

In large part, clinical findings in this disease are a consequence of excessive proliferation of abnormal plasma cells, creating a mechanical burden that compromises the skeleton by displacing and eroding bone trabeculae. Symptoms include bone pain, weakness, fatigue, and the presence of deformities such as exaggerated kyphosis and loss of height. Additionally, fever, weight loss, bleeding, and neurologic signs may be seen. Physical signs include fever, pallor, purpura, hepatosplenomegaly, bone tenderness, and extramedullary tumefaction. The major causes of death in patients with myeloma are infection and renal failure.

Laboratory investigation outlines moderate or severe anemia, elevated erythrocyte sedimentation rate, a normal or slightly elevated leukocyte count, a positive Coombs' test (10 per cent), thrombocytopenia (13 per cent), and a positive serologic test for rheumatoid factor (8 per cent). Hypercalcemia (25 to 50 per cent) and hyperuricemia may be observed.

Most patients with plasma cell myeloma demonstrate an increase in the total serum protein concentration, usually owing to an increase in the globulin fraction. When patients with plasma cell myeloma are grouped according to the type of protein produced by the tumor, approximately 55 to 60 per cent have IgG myeloma, 20 per cent have IgA myeloma, and 1 to 2 per cent have IgD myeloma; IgE and IgM

myelomas are rare. Accumulation of a light chain protein may be observed in 20 to 25 per cent of patients. On rare occasions, no abnormal protein is observed, a phenomenon called nonsecretory myeloma.

Urinary electrophoresis in patients with myeloma may demonstrate abnormalities when the serum electrophoretic pattern is entirely normal. Bence Jones proteinuria is apparent in 40 to 60 per cent of patients with this disease. Increased serum viscosity also is a common feature in plasma cell myeloma. Associated clinical manifestations include bleeding, decrease of visual acuity, retinopathy, dizziness, confusion, neurologic symptoms, and congestive heart failure. Hyperviscosity can lead to bone infarction in patients with myeloma (as well as macroglobulinemia).

Additional laboratory studies that are important in establishing a diagnosis of plasma cell myeloma are bone biopsy and bone marrow aspiration. Plasmacytosis of the marrow usually is evident, which is associated with cellular immaturity, increased pleomorphism, and frequent mitoses. Marrow involvement in myeloma is most frequent in the vertebrae, pelvis, ribs, and skull.

Although the cause of plasma cell proliferation in myeloma is not clear, the detrimental effect of such proliferation on the skeleton is well known. Focal intraosseous collections of plasma cells are surrounded by areas of increased osteoclastic activity. Initially, this osteoclastosis was attributed to differentiation of plasma cells into osteoclasts, although it is now known that plasma cells can produce an osteoclastic stimulating factor that may be responsible for the osteolytic lesions that are characteristic of myeloma.

Radiologic Features

GENERAL ABNORMALITIES. In almost all patients, the predominant pattern of plasma cell myeloma is osteolysis. Rarely, focal or diffuse sclerotic lesions are seen. Although multiple sites of involvement are characteristic, solitary lesions, or plasmacytomas, may exist for prolonged periods of time.

Typically, the axial skeleton is the predominant site of abnormality (Fig. 55–1). Multiple lesions are most common in the vertebral column, ribs, skull, pelvis, and femur, in descending order of frequency. Solitary plasmacytomas reveal a similar distribution, although well over 50 per cent of these lesions are located in the vertebrae. Diffuse lesions of the appendicular skeleton have been described in plasma cell myeloma, usually accompanying extensive involvement of the axial skeleton. Mandibular abnormalities are observed in approximately one third of patients with myeloma.

Classically, multiple myeloma is first manifested as widespread osteolytic lesions with discrete margins, which appear uniform in size (Fig. 55–2). These characteristic morphologic features are seen much less frequently in bone metastasis. Although smaller areas may coalesce into larger segments of destruction in myeloma, such large foci are seen more commonly in skeletal metastasis. Particularly distinctive in plasma cell myeloma is a subcortical elliptical radiolucent shadow, which is observed most often in the long tubular bones. The subcortical defects cause erosion of the inner margins of the cortex and create a scalloped contour throughout the endosteal bone. This appearance is highly suggestive of plasma cell myeloma, is occasionally seen in cases of rapid and aggressive osteoporosis, and is unusual in skeletal metastasis, in which

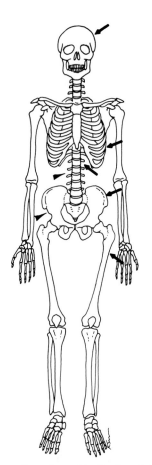

Figure 55–1. Plasma cell myeloma: Distribution of abnormalities. The most common sites of multiple lesions of myeloma are indicated on the right half of the diagram (arrows). These include the spine, the pelvis, the ribs, and the skull. The most common sites of solitary plasmacytoma are indicated on the left (arrowheads). These include the spine and the pelvis.

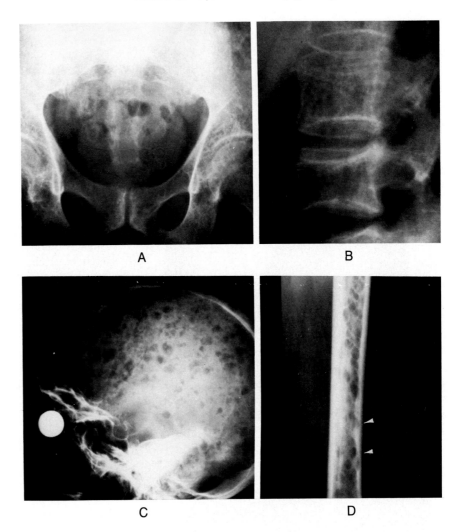

Figure 55–2. Plasma cell myeloma: Multiple lytic lesions. A Pelvis. Although the major radiographic pattern is one of diffuse osteopenia, some lytic lesions can be identified, particularly in the ilium, the ischium, and the pubis. **B** Spine. On a lateral radiograph of the lumbar spine, observe lytic lesions of multiple vertebral bodies with evidence of vertebral compression. Pediculate involvement is mild. **C** Skull. Well-circumscribed radiolucent lesions without surrounding sclerosis are obvious. They are relatively uniform in size, a feature that is more suggestive of myeloma than skeletal metastasis. The radiodense area overlying the orbit represents an eye prosthesis. **D** Femur. On this frontal radiograph, striking radiolucent lesions are seen throughout the diaphysis, producing scalloping of the endosteal margin of the cortex (arrowheads). This latter feature is particularly characteristic of plasma cell myeloma.

rapid cortical expansion and disruption are more characteristic. Expansile bone lesions of considerable size can be seen in both plasma cell myeloma and skeletal metastasis.

Diffuse skeletal osteopenia without well-defined areas of lysis can also be observed in plasma cell myeloma, simulating the appearance of osteoporosis.

Sclerosis in plasma cell myeloma generally is seen after pathologic fracture, irradiation, or chemotherapy, although it can occasionally be noted in conjunction with untreated lesions. Solitary sclerotic lesions are more common in the ribs, sternum, and ilium. Diffuse sclerosis is apparent in fewer than 3 per cent of patients with plasma cell myeloma (Fig. 55–3). It can simulate the appearance of osteoblastic metastasis, lymphoma, mastocytosis, renal osteodystrophy, and myelofibrosis. The cause of osteosclerosis in plasma cell myeloma is unknown.

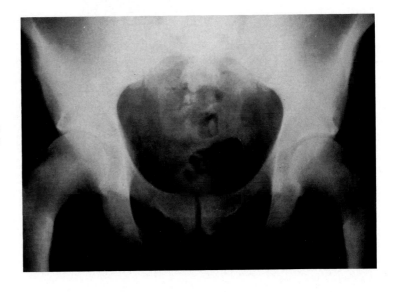

Figure 55–3. Plasma cell myeloma: Osteosclerosis. Diffuse osteosclerosis is seen in the pelvis and proximal portions of the femora.

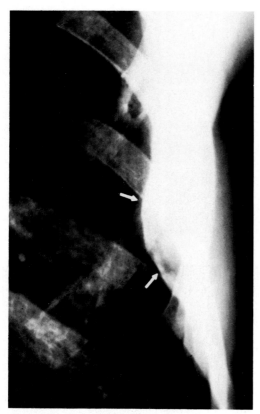

Figure 55–4. Plasma cell myeloma: Soft tissue mass. Extrapleural masses (arrows) frequently accompany rib involvement in this disease.

Plasma cell myeloma involving bone, particularly the ribs or vertebral column, often initiates an adjacent soft tissue mass (Fig. 55–4). Extensive paraspinal or extrapleural masses are observed, which may seem out of proportion to the degree of bone disease.

SPECIFIC SITES OF INVOLVEMENT. In the skull, numerous discrete lytic areas of uniform size are more common in plasma cell myeloma than in skeletal metastasis. Myeloma may demonstrate a predilection for mandibular involvement, an uncommon site for skeletal metastasis. Sternal involvement in myeloma may lead to pathologic fracture.

In the spine, preferential destruction of the vertebral bodies with sparing of the posterior elements has been emphasized as a differential point favoring the diagnosis of myeloma rather than osteolytic metastasis. Paraspinal extension of tumor is quite characteristic of myeloma. Scalloping of the anterior margins of the vertebral bodies is noted in both plasma cell myeloma and metastasis.

Preferential involvement of the distal end of the clavicle, acromion, glenoid, and ulnar olecranon is seen in myeloma (Fig. 55–5), whereas this distribution is less common in metastatic disease involving the skeleton.

Radionuclide Examination

Although radionuclide examination using various technetium bone-seeking pharmaceutical agents is valuable in the early detection of most neoplastic processes of the skeleton, the results of this examination are less predictable in patients with myeloma (Fig. 55–6). False-negative scans are not uncommon in this disease, as the small, osteolytic lesions of myeloma may not concentrate the radionuclide. The current belief is that the radionuclide examination in patients with

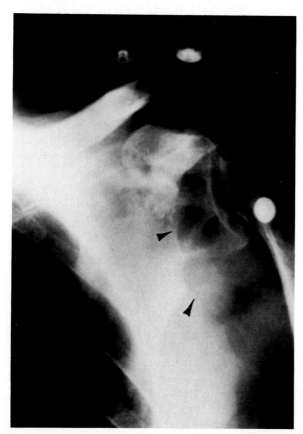

Figure 55–5. Plasma cell myeloma: Shoulder involvement. Observe extensive destruction of the glenoid and adjacent scapula (arrowheads).

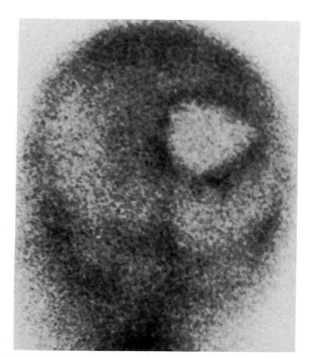

Figure 55–6. Plasma cell myeloma: Scintigraphic abnormalities. Observe a large lesion of the cranial vault whose center shows a relative lack of accumulation of the bone-seeking radiopharmaceutical agent ("cold" lesion) with a peripheral rim of augmented radionuclide activity. This appearance is termed the doughnut sign.

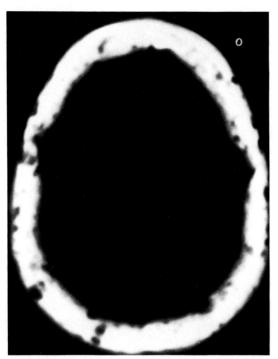

Figure 55–7. Plasma cell myeloma: Computed tomographic abnormalities—skull. Note osteolytic lesions throughout the cranium.

myeloma does not reveal all lesions and that radiography is a more valuable technique in the assessment of the distribution of the lesions, with the possible exception of rib abnormalities, which may be seen more easily with scintigraphy. In fact, fractures account for augmented radionuclide uptake in a large percentage of patients with myeloma. Rarely, soft tissue accumulation of radionuclides in patients with myeloma may correspond to sites of calcification or of nodules containing amyloid.

Although the radiographic examination appears to be more sensitive than scintigraphy in detecting the osseous alterations of plasma cell myeloma, it is far from ideal as an imaging method in monitoring the course of the disease. Reports indicate that scintigraphy is a potential aid in following patients with myeloma who are receiving chemotherapy; remission is characterized by significant regression or disappearance of scintigraphic abnormalities in many of these patients.

Computed Tomography and Magnetic Resonance Imaging

Computed tomography is valuable in delineating lesions within the medullary canal, whether they be sites of metastasis, infection, or myeloma (Figs. 55–7 and 55–8). The technique is well suited for the evaluation of patients in whom myeloma is suspected on the basis of clinical and laboratory parameters and in whom radiographs are normal. In such persons, computed tomography may outline typical spinal lesions of the disease. Furthermore, this technique can be used to detect the extent of osseous and soft tissue involvement in patients with well-documented myeloma.

Magnetic resonance imaging is capable of delineating the degree of marrow involvement in many disorders, including lymphoma, leukemia, Gaucher's disease, and plasma cell myeloma. The normally intense signal derived from marrow fat is diminished as a result of tumor or cellular infiltration.

Plasmacytoma

Myeloma can occur as a solitary lesion of bone. Laboratory analysis may reveal the same abnormalities as occur in disseminated myelomatosis, although in some patients with solitary plasmacytoma, serologic tests are negative or abnormal patterns of serum electrophoresis disappear after excision of the tumor.

Many cases of apparently solitary plasmacytoma reveal multiple lesions if followed for a long period of time. In other patients, solitary lesions may never demonstrate evidence of dissemination even when persons are followed for 20 to 30 years. These varying results have led to a controversy regarding the very existence of solitary plasmacytoma. Two strict criteria have been suggested as prerequisites for the diagnosis of such a lesion: survival for longer than 12 years without evidence of dissemination and negative histologic examination of all bones at necropsy.

Solitary plasmacytoma, as compared with multiple myeloma, is rare, affects younger patients, commonly is accompanied by neurologic manifestations, and can simulate giant cell tumor on radiologic examination. It is most frequent in the spine and pelvis although it may occur at other skeletal sites or in extraskeletal locations, particularly the nasal cavities, paranasal sinuses, or upper airways (Figs. 55–9 and 55–10). A multicystic expansile lesion with thickened trabeculae or a purely osteolytic focus without expansion may be observed. Sclerotic lesions have also been identified and, in fact, solitary plasmacytoma may appear as a radiodense vertebral body, the ivory vertebra.

Solitary plasmacytoma of the spine deserves special emphasis. This diagnosis must be considered in any middle-aged or

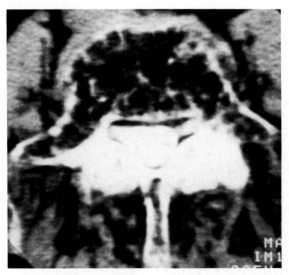

Figure 55–8. Plasma cell myeloma: Computed tomographic abnormalities—spine. Osteolytic foci are apparent in the vertebral body, pedicles, and transverse and spinous processes.

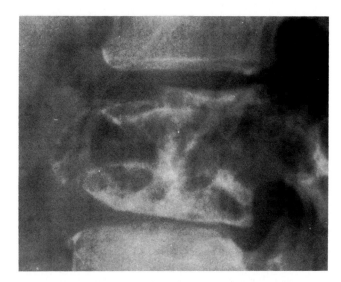

Figure 55–9. Plasmacytoma: Spine. Observe a radiolucent lesion involving the third lumbar vertebal body, with osseous collapse and extension into the pedicles.

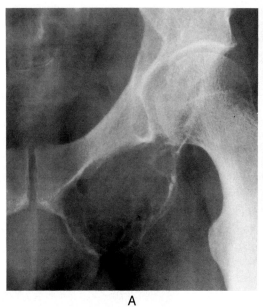

A

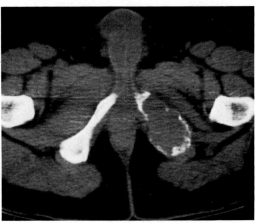

B

Figure 55–10. Plasmacytoma: Pelvis. A radiograph (**A**) reveals an expansile trabeculated lesion of the ischium. A transaxial computed tomogram (**B**) reveals the expansile lesion, cortical thinning and perforation, and the absence of a soft tissue mass. (Courtesy of G. Greenway, M.D., Dallas, Texas.)

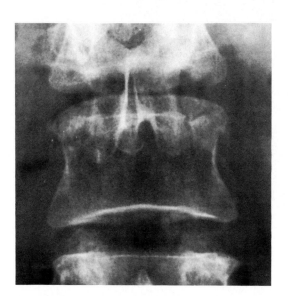

Figure 55–11. Plasmacytoma: Vertebral arch. In this patient, the spinous process, laminae, articular processes, and pedicles are destroyed. (Courtesy of J. Slivka, M.D., San Diego, California.)

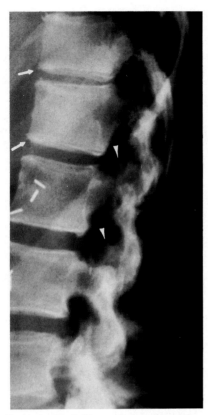

Figure 55–12. Syndrome of plasma cell dyscrasia, polyneuropathy, and endocrine disturbances (POEMS syndrome). On a lateral radiograph of the lumbar spine, observe peculiar proliferative changes about the apophyseal joints (arrowheads) and, to a lesser extent, the discovertebral junctions (arrows). The bones appear radiodense.

elderly patient with a single osteolytic lesion of a vertebral body or, less commonly, a vertebral arch (Fig. 55–11). An involved vertebral body may collapse, or the lesion may extend across the intervertebral disc to invade the adjacent vertebral body.

Rheumatologic Manifestations

NEUROLOGIC FINDINGS. Sciatica and brachial neuralgia are encountered in patients with spinal disease, related to nerve root pressure. In addition, patients with sclerotic plasma cell myeloma (or rarely osteolytic myeloma) may reveal an associated peripheral neuropathy.

POEMS SYNDROME. A syndrome of plasma cell dyscrasia, chronic progressive polyneuropathy, and endocrine disturbances, including diabetes mellitus, has been recognized (Figs. 55–12 and 55–13). Additional characteristics of this syndrome are thickening and pigmentation of the skin, edema, excess perspiration, hirsutism, impotence, gynecomastia or amenorrhea, and hepatosplenomegaly. The syndrome is more frequent in men and has its onset at a young age. Sclerotic plasmacytomas are evident in most cases, particularly in the spine and pelvis. Bone proliferation also is apparent at sites of tendon and ligament attachment to bone. Particularly characteristic are irregular bone excrescences involving the posterior elements of the spine, including the articular, transverse, and spinous processes. Similar findings

are observed about the sacroiliac and costovertebral joints. The cause of this syndrome is not known.

The acronym POEMS has been used to facilitate recognition of the most constant features of this syndrome—polyneuropathy (P), organomegaly (O), endocrinopathy (E), M proteins (M), and skin changes (S).

POLYARTHRITIS AND AMYLOID DEPOSITION. Plasma cell myeloma may be manifested as a polyarthritis that superficially resembles rheumatoid arthritis. Soft tissue nodules in periarticular locations, carpal tunnel syndrome, and macroglossia may also be apparent. Radiographs can demonstrate soft tissue masses, periarticular swelling, and osseous erosion. Synovial biopsy or autopsy examination outlines amyloid deposition within the synovium, the para-articular tissues including muscle, and the carpal tunnel.

Amyloidosis occurs in approximately 15 per cent of patients with plasma cell myeloma. The distribution of amyloid in these patients resembles that in primary amyloidosis. Rarely, a circumscribed mass of amyloid may be identified within a plasmacytoma in the skeleton. Its presence can be suspected when areas of calcification are evident in the lesion. The resulting radiographic abnormalities resemble those of chondrosarcoma (Fig. 55–14).

GOUTY ARTHRITIS. There are several reports of an association of plasma cell myeloma and gout.

INFECTION. Hypogammaglobulinemia in myeloma re-

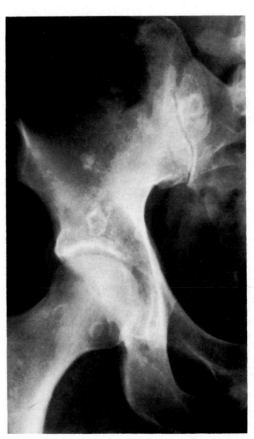

Figure 55–13. Syndrome of plasma cell dyscrasia, polyneuropathy, and endocrine disturbances (POEMS syndrome). The radiograph outlines many sclerotic lesions of the ilium, sacrum, and femur.

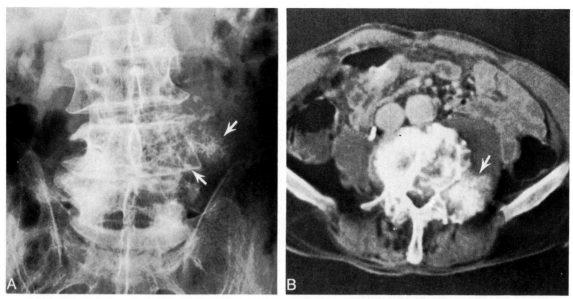

Figure 55–14. Plasmacytoma with amyloid deposition. A Observe an osteolytic lesion with calcification (arrows) in the fourth lumbar vertebra. **B** A transaxial computed tomographic image shows the extent of bone destruction and the presence of calcification (arrow). (Courtesy of J. Castello, M.D., Madrid, Spain.)

sults in impairment in humoral immunity and an increased susceptibility to infection. The most frequent sites of infection are the lung and the urinary tract, although soft tissue involvement is also common. Osteomyelitis and septic arthritis may be seen.

Differential Diagnosis

Widespread osteolytic lesions in a middle-aged or elderly patient should arouse suspicion of myeloma or skeletal metastasis (Table 55–1). Certain features favor the diagnosis of myeloma, including symmetrically distributed lesions of equal size without adjacent sclerosis; subcortical lucent areas with endosteal scalloping; involvement of the mandible, shoulder girdle, and elbow region; and spinal lesions with preservation of the pediculate shadow. None of these characteristics is pathognomonic of myeloma, however. Additional disorders may also be associated with widespread osteolysis, including macroglobulinemia, leukemia, histiocytosis, vascular tumors, infections such as tuberculosis and fungal disease, fibrous dysplasia, hyperparathyroidism, pancreatitis with fat necrosis, and Weber-Christian disease.

Diffuse osteosclerosis is unusual in plasma cell myeloma. When present, the pattern simulates that associated with myelofibrosis, osteoblastic metastasis, sickle cell anemia, Paget's disease, fibrous dysplasia, lymphoma, mastocytosis, tuberous sclerosis, renal osteodystrophy, and sarcoidosis.

Single (or several) lytic foci in myeloma are difficult to distinguish from many other primary and secondary skeletal neoplasms and infections. Expansile myelomatous lesions can simulate skeletal metastasis (particularly from thyroid and renal carcinoma), brown tumors of hyperparathyroidism, fibrous dysplasia, angiomatous lesions, hemophilic pseudotumors, and several primary bone tumors. In addition, single (or several) sclerotic foci in myeloma are not diagnostic. Osteoblastic metastasis, bone sarcomas, lymphoma, fibrous dysplasia, and infection can produce similar radiodense shadows.

WALDENSTRÖM'S MACROGLOBULINEMIA
Clinical Features

Macroglobulinemia is a disorder of middle-aged and elderly persons. Its symptoms include weakness, weight loss, a

Table 55–1. PLASMA CELL MYELOMA VERSUS SKELETAL METASTASIS

	Plasma Cell Myeloma	Skeletal Metastasis
Distribution and common sites	Symmetric Axial skeleton; proximal long bones; shoulder and elbow region	Asymmetric Axial skeleton; proximal long bones
Predominant pattern	Osteolytic lesions > osteosclerotic lesions Diffuse osteopenia (common) Diffuse osteosclerosis (rare)	Osteolytic or osteosclerotic lesions Diffuse osteopenia (rare) Diffuse osteosclerosis (common with prostatic carcinoma)
Morphology of lesions	Well-circumscribed lesions of uniform size Medullary or subcortical lucent lesions with cortical scalloping Expansile lesions or soft tissue mass or both (common in ribs, spine)	Poorly circumscribed lesions of varying size Medullary, subcortical, or cortical lucent lesions with cortical destruction Expansile lesions or soft tissue mass or both (common with thyroid and renal carcinoma)

bleeding diathesis, dyspnea, and personality changes; physical findings include retinal hemorrhages, hepatosplenomegaly, and lymphadenopathy. Laboratory analysis outlines anemia, elevated erythrocyte sedimentation rate, increased serum viscosity, hyperglobulinemia, and increased cerebrospinal fluid protein. Immunoelectrophoresis demonstrates globulins (IgM) with a large effective weight and size. Amyloidosis may be a complicating condition in approximately 10 per cent of cases.

Cellular infiltration (lymphocytes, plasma cells, histiocytes, and mast cells) into various organs accounts for the clinical and radiologic manifestations of this disease. Involvement of the lung and gastrointestinal tract is well documented. Histologic abnormalities in osseous and synovial tissue are also described.

Skeletal Manifestations

Skeletal findings in Waldenström's macroglobulinemia are similar to those of multiple myeloma. Osteopenia, widening of the marrow spaces, and endosteal erosion are evident. Vertebral collapse is encountered. Osteolytic lesions can also be observed; these lesions can be solitary or multiple, and they may be small or large. Involvement of the pelvis, perhaps with predilection for the paraacetabular regions, is not uncommon. As is true in myeloma, the role of scintigraphy in the evaluation of bone lesions in Waldenström's macroglobulinemia is not clear.

Ischemic necrosis of the femoral or humeral head(s), which could be related to hyperviscosity of the blood, may be an additional manifestation of Waldenström's macroglobulinemia.

Rheumatologic Manifestations

Amyloid deposition in peri- and intraarticular locations in patients with macroglobulinemia has been described. The resulting arthropathy may simulate rheumatoid arthritis because of the presence of subcutaneous nodules, symmetric synovial thickening, and osseous erosions. Secondary gouty arthritis also can be observed in patients with Waldenström's macroglobulinemia.

AMYLOIDOSIS

Amyloidosis is not a rare phenomenon. Several different types are recognized:

PRIMARY AMYLOIDOSIS. The primary form of amyloidosis occurs without coexistent or antecedent disease. It most frequently involves certain mesenchymal structures, such as the heart, muscle, tongue, synovial membrane, and perivascular connective tissue. In many patients, primary amyloidosis is associated with multiple myeloma.

SECONDARY AMYLOIDOSIS. The secondary form is associated with various chronic diseases, including rheumatoid arthritis, sepsis, neoplasm, inflammatory disorders, and familial Mediterranean fever. Amyloid deposition in the secondary type shows predilection for the liver, spleen, kidneys, and adrenals.

HEREDOFAMILIAL AMYLOIDOSIS. An increasing number of heredofamilial amyloid syndromes have been described. These can be classified by the site of predominant organ involvement. Thus, heredofamilial amyloidoses include neuropathies, nephropathies, cardiomyopathies, and miscellaneous types.

SENILE AMYLOIDOSIS. Senile amyloidosis refers to a type that increases with age.

LOCALIZED AMYLOID TUMORS. In this type of amyloidosis, focal growths occur in the larynx, trachea, bronchi, and rarely skin (lichen amyloidosus).

Clinical Features

Primary amyloidosis is more frequent in men than in women and its onset generally is between the ages of 40 and 80 years. Clinical manifestations include heart failure, macroglossia, hypertension, lymphadenopathy, weight loss, purpura, scleroderma-like skin changes, and joint pain. Hepatosplenomegaly and renal abnormality may become evident, although the liver, spleen, and kidney are involved more frequently in secondary amyloidosis.

Secondary amyloidosis can develop at any age, depending on the underlying disease process. Amyloid deposition in the kidneys leads to the nephrotic syndrome. Hepatosplenomegaly and adrenal insufficiency may become apparent. Amyloidosis of the gastrointestinal tract may be manifested as obstruction, malabsorption, hemorrhage, protein loss, and diarrhea.

Amyloidosis occurring in association with plasma cell myeloma may be difficult to detect because of the presence of significant clinical findings related to this latter disease. Renal involvement and hepatosplenomegaly can be apparent.

Localized amyloid tumors of the respiratory tract may cause hoarseness, dyspnea, epistaxis, dysphagia, and hemoptysis.

Heredofamilial amyloidoses are associated with neurologic, cardiac, and renal abnormalities.

Although no laboratory examination is pathognomonic of amyloidosis, the diagnosis can be substantiated by performance of the Congo red test. This test depends on the removal from the blood of injected dye by selective absorption by amyloid deposits. Tissue biopsy (gingiva, rectum, liver, spleen, kidney) may be required.

Musculoskeletal Features

Osseous and articular abnormalities in amyloidosis are the result of amyloid deposition in bone, synovium, and soft tissue. Additionally, musculoskeletal features may be indicative of an underlying disease process, such as myeloma, macroglobulinemia, or chronic osteomyelitis.

AMYLOIDOSIS COMPLICATING RHEUMATOLOGIC DISORDERS. The reported frequency of amyloidosis in rheumatoid arthritis has varied from 5 to 25 per cent. Amyloidosis rarely develops in patients with rheumatoid arthritis who have had their disease for less than 2 years. Amyloidosis developing in children is most frequently secondary to juvenile-onset rheumatoid arthritis, although it sometimes also complicates chronic suppurative diseases and familial Mediterranean fever in this age group. Amyloidosis may occur during the course of ankylosing spondylitis, Reiter's disease, psoriatic arthritis, and intestinal arthropathies.

Amyloid deposition may be apparent in collagen disorders such as systemic lupus erythematosus, dermatomyositis, polyarteritis nodosa, and Gaucher's disease. The deposits can be recognized as an incidental finding in the articular capsule, cartilage, and synovial membrane of patients with osteoarthritis, and within joints of elderly asymptomatic individuals.

Amyloidosis complicating familial Mediterranean fever deserves special emphasis. As many as 30 per cent of patients with this disorder may develop secondary amyloidosis, and this complication can ultimately lead to the patient's death from renal failure.

BONE LESIONS (TABLE 55-2). Osteoporosis, lytic lesions of bone, and pathologic fractures may be observed (Fig. 55–15). Radiolucent areas of variable size are detected within medullary and cortical bone, particularly in the proximal portions of the femur and humerus. These lesions produce scalloping along the endosteal margin of the cortex, simulating the appearance of plasma cell myeloma. They are produced by focal deposits of amyloid. Secondary occlusion of blood vessels related to perivascular amyloidosis can lead to osteonecrosis of epiphyses with collapse. Amyloidosis also can produce vertebral osteoporosis and collapse.

There are occasional reports of tumorous lesions of bone containing amyloid. These lesions predominate in patients with plasma cell myeloma and coexistent amyloidosis. Pathologic fractures, especially in the spine and proximal portion of the femur, complicate localized "amyloidomas." Calcification within these lesions may be evident.

ARTICULAR AND PERIARTICULAR LESIONS. The articular manifestations of amyloidosis are characterized by the accumulation of this substance in synovial tissue, other intraarticular structures, peritendinous areas, and surrounding soft tissue (Figs. 55–16 and 55–17). Soft tissue amyloid deposition produces nodules resembling those of rheumatoid arthritis. Amyloid nodules are particularly prominent in the olecranon region, hand, and wrist. Extensive infiltration about the shoulders produces rubbery masses that are accentuated by surrounding muscle atrophy, resembling the shoulder pads

worn by football players. Similar deposits in the carpal canal lead to the carpal tunnel syndrome.

The clinical findings of amyloid joint disease resemble the manifestations of rheumatoid arthritis. Bilateral symmetric arthritis of large and small joints is seen in both disorders. This clinical difficulty in distinguishing patients with amyloidosis from those with rheumatoid arthritis is accentuated by the pathologic observation that rheumatoid arthritis is frequently associated with articular deposits of amyloid.

Amyloidosis may lead to joint contractures; such contractures can appear in any joint, including those of the fingers.

The radiographic findings of joint involvement in amyloidosis reflect this intraarticular and periarticular distribution of amyloid (Table 55–2). Asymmetric soft tissue masses, periarticular osteoporosis, widening of the articular space, subchondral cysts, and erosions are seen. Subluxation, lytic lesions of bone, and pathologic fractures are additional manifestations. Involvement frequently is bilateral in distribution. Although the radiographic appearance is reminiscent of that in rheumatoid arthritis, extensive soft tissue nodular masses, well-defined cystic lesions with or without surrounding sclerosis, and preservation of joint space are more characteristic of amyloid joint disease.

Extensive joint destruction occasionally is encountered in amyloidosis. This may result from osteonecrosis of epiphyseal surfaces or neuroarthropathy. Rarely, erosive arthritis of the hands and wrists has been noted in patients with heredofamilial amyloidosis.

Differential Diagnosis

BONE LESIONS. Diffuse lytic lesions in amyloidosis are indistinguishable from those accompanying skeletal metastasis and plasma cell myeloma. Bone lysis in Waldenström's macroglobulinemia also is virtually identical to that accompanying amyloidosis.

Localized destructive lesions of the skeleton in amyloidosis resemble sites of metastasis or a primary bone neoplasm. They generally are well marginated and located in the spine or the metaphyseal and diaphyseal regions of tubular bones, especially the femur. A soft tissue mass is common, but periostitis is rare.

ARTICULAR LESIONS. Articular lesions in amyloidosis are characterized by bulky soft tissue masses, well-defined erosions and cysts, and preservation of joint space. These features can usually be distinguished from those of rheumatoid arthritis, which is associated with symmetric soft tissue swelling, early joint space loss, and marginal erosions of bone. Amyloid joint disease shares many radiographic characteristics with gouty arthritis and xanthomatosis, although clinical and laboratory manifestations of these latter disorders

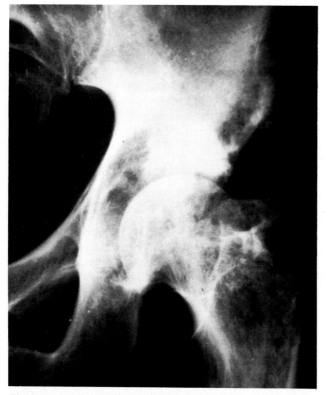

Figure 55–15. Amyloidosis: Lytic lesions and osteoporosis. Osteolytic lesions with reactive sclerosis can be seen in the ilium and proximal femur.

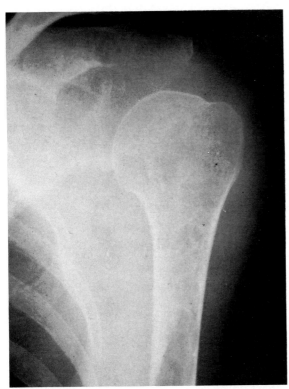

Figure 55–16. Amyloidosis: Soft tissue abnormalities. Patients with amyloidosis may have hard, rubbery masses about the shoulders resembling in appearance the shoulder pads worn by football players. Radiographs in such patients may indicate the degree of soft tissue swelling and associated osteoporosis of underlying bones.

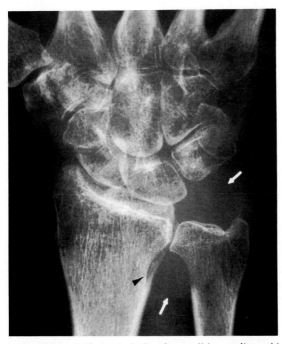

Figure 55–17. Amyloidosis: Articular abnormalities—radiographic alterations. Complete workup in this patient revealed the presence of amyloidosis complicating plasma cell myeloma. Observe soft tissue swelling and osteoporosis. A distended inferior radioulnar joint can be seen (arrows) with associated osseous erosion (arrowhead).

usually ensure their accurate diagnosis. The arthropathy of amyloidosis also resembles pigmented villonodular synovitis; distinguishing features of the former include multiple sites of involvement, juxtaarticular osteoporosis, and the older age of the patients.

AGAMMAGLOBULINEMIA AND HYPOGAMMAGLOBULINEMIA

General Features

Agammaglobulinemia and hypogammaglobulinemia are syndromes associated with considerable impairment of antibody formation and, in most instances, depressed levels of plasma gamma globulins. These disorders may arise from either a diminished rate of synthesis of gamma globulins (primary form) or an increased rate of catabolism or loss of gamma globulins (secondary form). The primary form of agammaglobulinemia may be congenital or acquired. The secondary form of hypogammaglobulinemia results from gamma globulin loss in the intestine, urine, or skin.

The clinical manifestations of agammaglobulinemia and hypogammaglobulinemia are characterized by recurrent and severe infections, most commonly related to bacterial organisms. The types of infection encountered include sinusitis, otitis media, conjunctivitis, pneumonia, meningitis, septic arthritis, and furunculosis. Tuberculosis and fungal disorders can also be apparent.

Musculoskeletal Abnormalities

A chronic inflammatory polyarthritis that resembles rheumatoid arthritis is seen in 10 to 30 per cent of patients with agammaglobulinemia and hypogammaglobulinemia. It is more frequent in men than in women and in children than in adults. Asymmetric involvement is more characteristic of agammaglobulinemia than of rheumatoid arthritis. Symptoms and signs may be transient or persistent, although permanent joint damage is uncommon. Subcutaneous nodules may appear in the elbows and elsewhere. Radiographs reveal soft tissue swelling, periarticular osteoporosis, joint space narrowing, and deformities without osseous erosions. The radiographic appearance is reminiscent of Jaccoud's arthropathy and that accompanying systemic lupus erythematosus.

FURTHER READING

Bardwick PA, Zvaifler NJ, Gill GN, Newman D, Greenway GD, Resnick DL: Plasma cell dyscrasia with polyneuropathy, organomegaly, endocrinopathy, M protein, and skin changes: The POEMS syndrome. Medicine 59:311, 1980.

Barnett EV, Winkelstein A, Weinberger HJ: Agammaglobulinemia with polyarthritis and subcutaneous nodules. Am J Med 48:40, 1970.

Bataille R, Chevalier J, Rossi M, Sany J: Bone scintigraphy in plasma-cell myeloma. A prospective study of 70 patients. Radiology 145:801, 1982.

Clarisse PDT, Staple TW: Diffuse bone sclerosis in multiple myeloma. Radiology 99:327, 1971.

Grayzel AI, Marcus R, Stern R, Winchester RJ: Chronic polyarthritis associated with hypogammaglobulinemia. A study of two patients. Arthritis Rheum 20:887, 1977.

Gootnick LT: Solitary myeloma: Review of sixty-one cases. Radiology 45:385, 1945.

Grossman RE, Hensley GT: Bone lesions in primary amyloidosis. AJR 101:872, 1967.

Heiser S, Schwartzman JJ: Variation in the roentgen appearance of the skeletal system in myeloma. Radiology 58:178, 1952.

Jacobson HG, Poppel MH, Shapiro JH, Grossberger S: The vertebral pedicle sign: A roentgen finding to differentiate metastatic carcinoma from multiple myeloma. AJR 80:817, 1958.

Katz GA, Peter JB, Pearson CM, Adams WS: The shoulder-pad sign—a diagnostic feature of amyloid arthropathy. N Engl J Med *288*:354, 1973.

Meszaros WT: The many facets of multiple myeloma. Semin Roentgenol 9:219, 1974.

Mundy GR, Raisz LG, Cooper RA, Schechter GP, Salmon SE: Evidence for the secretion of an osteoclast stimulating factor in myeloma. N Engl J Med *291*:1041, 1974.

Renner RR, Smith JR: Plasma cell dyscrasias (except myeloma). Semin Roentgenol 9:209, 1974.

Renner RR, Nelson DA, Lozner EL: Roentgenologic manifestations of primary macroglobulinemia (Waldenström). AJR *113*:499, 1971.

Resnick D, Greenway GD, Bardwick PA, Zvaifler NJ, Gill GN, Newman DR: Plasma-cell dyscrasia with polyneuropathy, organomegaly, endocrinopathy, M-protein, and skin changes: The POEMS syndrome. Radiology *140*:17, 1981.

Subbarao K, Jacobson HG: Amyloidosis and plasma cell dyscrasias of the musculoskeletal system. Semin Roentgenol *21*:139, 1986.

Tong D, Griffin TW, Laramore GE, Kurtz JM, Russell AH, Groudine MT, Herron T, Blasko JC, Tesh DW: Solitary plasmacytoma of bone and soft tissues. Radiology *135*:195, 1980.

Vermess M, Pearson KD, Einstein AB, Fahey JL: Osseous manifestations of Waldenström's macroglobulinemia. Radiology *102*:497, 1972.

Weinfeld A, Stern MH, Marx LH: Amyloid lesions of bone. AJR *108*:799, 1970.

Chapter 56

Lipidoses, Histiocytoses, and Hyperlipoproteinemias

Donald Resnick, M.D.

Musculoskeletal findings are a significant part of the lipidoses, histiocytoses, and hyperlipoproteinemias. In Gaucher's disease, osteonecrosis and modeling deformities of long bones are characteristic. The findings in Niemann-Pick disease may resemble those of Gaucher's disease, although osteonecrosis is not encountered. This latter abnormality is detected in Fabry's disease.

In multicentric reticulohistiocytosis skeletal involvement can lead to a symmetric destructive polyarthritis with predilection for the interphalangeal joints of the hands and feet.

The histiocytoses consist of three disorders—eosinophilic granuloma, Hand-Schüller-Christian disease, and Letterer-Siwe disease—that share numerous radiologic and pathologic features. Single or multiple osteolytic lesions may be apparent in any of these three disorders.

Erdheim-Chester disease is an unusual lipidosis leading to characteristic skeletal abnormalities. Sinus histiocytosis with massive lymphadenopathy is a self-limited disease associated with osteolytic lesions. Malignant histiocytosis, on the other hand, produces similar bone abnormalities but has a poor prognosis.

The hyperlipoproteinemias are divided into five types according to the predominant lipoprotein pattern. Manifestations of these disorders include xanthomatous collections in soft tissue, tendon, subperiosteal and intraosseous locations, gout, arthralgias, and arthritis.

Membranous lipodystrophy is a rare disorder characterized by neuropsychiatric manifestations and symmetrically distributed osteolytic areas in the appendicular skeleton.

There is no uniform agreement regarding the classification of lipid storage and histiocytic disorders partly because of a lack of clear understanding of the cause and pathogenesis of many of these processes. A classification system of these diseases, based on a composite of reported systems, is given in Table 56–1. Some of the disorders produce prominent musculoskeletal abnormalities.

GAUCHER'S DISEASE

General Features

Gaucher's disease is a rare familial disorder of cerebroside metabolism in which abnormal accumulation of lipid material occurs in the reticuloendothelial cells of the body. The disease affects both men and women and may develop at any age, although it is particularly frequent in childhood and early adult life. Many patients are Ashkenazic Jews.

The manifestations of Gaucher's disease can be attributed to accumulation of Gaucher cells (a reticulum cell) in various tissues of the body. Proliferation of Gaucher cells in the liver and spleen leads to hepatosplenomegaly. Similarly, accumulation of these cells in the lymph nodes produces lymphadenopathy, and in the brain, it leads to cellular proliferation and degeneration in the cerebral cortex. Cellular infiltration also occurs in the lungs, kidneys, tonsils, thyroid, thymus, intestines, and adrenals. Accumulation of Gaucher cells in the bone marrow may cause osseous destruction, hematologic abnormalities, and articular manifestations.

Table 56–1. LIPID STORAGE AND HISTIOCYTIC DISORDERS

Lipid Storage Diseases
    Gaucher's disease (glucosylceramide lipidosis)
    Niemann-Pick disease (sphingomyelin lipidosis)
    Fabry's disease (glycolipidosis)
    Refsum's disease (phytanic acid storage disease)
    Krabbe's disease (galactosylceramide lipidosis)
    Metachromatic leukodystrophy (sulfatide lipidosis)
    Farber's lipogranulomatosis (ceramidase deficiency)
    Gangliosidoses
    Sea-blue histiocytosis
    Tay-Sachs disease
    Fucosidosis

Reactive Histiocytoses
    Multicentric reticulohistiocytosis
    Histiocytosis X
    Lipid granulomatosis (Erdheim-Chester disease)
    Sinus histiocytosis with lymphadenopathy
    Erythrophagocytic lymphohistiocytosis

Neoplastic Histiocytoses
    Acute monocytic leukemia
    Chronic myelomonocytic leukemia
    Histiocytic lymphoma
    Malignant histiocytosis (histiocytic medullary reticulosis)

Disorders of Lipoprotein Metabolism
    Hyperlipoproteinemias
    Hypolipoproteinemias

Miscellaneous Disorders
    Membranous lipodystrophy

Clinical Features

Gaucher's disease has been divided into three clinical forms; common to all three types are recessive inheritance, hepatosplenomegaly, deficient acid β-glucosidase activity, elevated nontartrate-inhibitable acid phosphatase activity, and characteristic Gaucher cells in the bone marrow. Type 1 disease, termed chronic non-neuronopathic or "adult" Gaucher's disease, is the most frequent, occurring in Ashkenazic Jews and leading to clinical manifestations that may initially appear in childhood but worsen as the patient enters the second and third decades of life. Such manifestations include pain, a protuberant abdomen, fever, growth disturbance, respiratory distress, pneumonia, and diffuse yellow-brown skin pigmentation. Laboratory findings include microcytic anemia, leukopenia, and a decreased number of platelets in association with easy bruisability and a bleeding diathesis. Bone involvement is common.

Type 2, acute neuronopathic Gaucher's disease, is a rare, fatal neurodegenerative disorder, with no particular ethnic predilection, which becomes manifest clinically shortly after birth or in the first few months of life. Neurologic manifestations include head retraction, spasticity, strabismus, mental retardation, loss of sensation, and seizures. Bone abnormalities are limited. The average time of survival is approximately 1 year.

Type 3 subacute neuronopathic (juvenile) Gaucher's disease is uncommon and is characterized by hepatosplenomegaly. Neurologic and skeletal manifestations appear during childhood or adolescence, and the majority of the affected children have convulsions. Additional manifestations are hypertonicity, lack of coordination and strabismus.

The presence of enlarged lipid-laden histiocytes, the Gaucher cells, represents the hallmark of all types of the disease. Gaucher cells are particularly prominent in the spleen, the bone marrow, and the lymph nodes.

Musculoskeletal Abnormalities

Osteoarticular findings may be minimal in young infants with the acute, fulminant variety of disease. They are more pronounced in older infants, children, and adults who suffer from the more chronic form of Gaucher's disease. In some patients, evidence of skeletal disease can be the earliest and most prominent feature.

MARROW INFILTRATION (FIG. 56-1). Accumulation of Gaucher cells within the bone marrow is associated with cellular necrosis, fibrous proliferation, and resorption of trabeculae. These pathologic skeletal changes become manifest on radiographs as increased radiolucency of bone and cortical scalloping and thinning. They predominate in the axial skeleton and proximal long bones, especially the femur, and they are usually bilateral in distribution. Even the small tubular bones of the hands and feet may reveal osteopenia and a coarsened trabecular pattern. Isolated focal destructive areas can create radiolucent shadows with geographic or motheaten patterns of destruction.

In the spine, cellular infiltration results in loss of trabeculae with increased radiolucency of the vertebral bodies and multiple compression fractures. Kyphosis, gibbus deformity, and bone ankylosis across the intervertebral disc may eventually become apparent. In the calvarium, trabecular destruction and thinning of both the outer and inner tables can be seen.

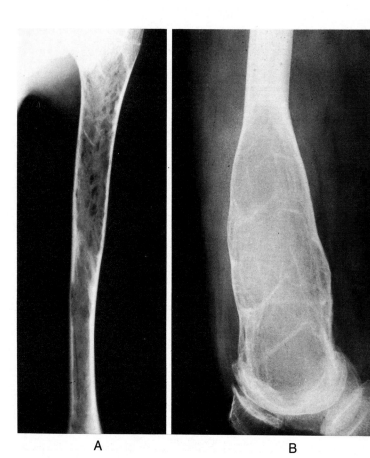

Figure 56-1. Gaucher's disease: Marrow infiltration. A The radiographic abnormalities of the humerus include osteopenia, osteolytic lesions, medullary widening, and cortical diminution. The resemblance to features of plasma cell myeloma is obvious. B Observe the long expansile lesion of the distal femur with a ground-glass appearance, crossing trabeculae, and cortical diminution.

A   B

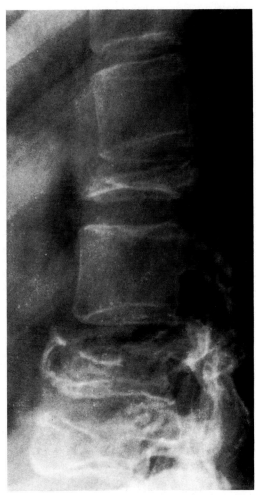

Figure 56–2. Gaucher's disease: Fractures. Vertebral fracture and collapse in this disease are particularly frequent. In this case, marrow replacement has led to dramatic collapse of multiple vertebral bodies, some of which have been reduced to a flattened structure (vertebra plana).

FRACTURES (FIG. 56–2). Infiltration of the marrow spaces with Gaucher cells and trabecular resorption may result in pathologic fractures, especially in the vertebral column. The involved vertebral body may become completely flattened (vertebra plana). This appearance, which is identical to that accompanying the histiocytoses, can be evident at multiple levels, associated with paravertebral soft tissue swelling.

Fractures are also observed in the ribs and in the long bones of the appendicular skeleton, particularly the femur, the tibia, and the humerus. Fracture of the femoral neck is associated with coxa vara deformity.

MODELING DEFORMITIES (FIG. 56–3). One of the most characteristic osseous manifestations of chronic Gaucher's disease is modeling deformities, particularly in the appendicular skeleton. Expansion of the contour of the long tubular bones is most frequent in the lower ends of both femoral shafts. It results in loss of the normal concavity of the bone outline. The appearance of a straightened or convex osseous margin, which has been termed an Erlenmeyer flask deformity, is very suggestive of the diagnosis of Gaucher's disease, particularly if it is associated with epiphyseal osteonecrosis.

Peculiar step-like depressions of the superior and inferior margins of the vertebral bodies (Fig. 56–4) have been described in Gaucher's disease, identical to those that are typical of sickle cell anemia and other hemoglobinopathies. This deformity has been termed the "H" vertebra because of its resemblance to this capital letter. H vertebrae in Gaucher's disease could possibly relate to ischemia resulting from both extrinsic compression and intrinsic abnormality of vessels. An alternative theory suggests that the "stepped" vertebral body in Gaucher's disease is caused by initial collapse of the vertebral body, with subsequent growth recovery peripherally.

OSTEONECROSIS (FIG. 56–5). Osteonecrosis of epiphyses and diaphyses is well recognized in Gaucher's disease. In the shafts of long bones, alternating radiolucency and sclerosis appear with associated periostitis. In the cortex, an inner layer of new bone formation, which does not merge with the overlying cortical bone, produces a bone-within-bone appearance identical to that seen in sickle cell anemia.

Radiologic and pathologic evidence of epiphyseal bone necrosis can be visualized in one or both femoral heads, humeral heads, and tibial plateaus. Other skeletal sites may also be involved. The pathogenesis of epiphyseal necrosis in Gaucher's disease apparently is related to compression of intraosseous sinusoids and lumina by masses of Gaucher cells and macrophages. The resulting radiographic picture of osteonecrosis is identical to that accompanying many other diseases. Secondary degenerative joint disease may appear.

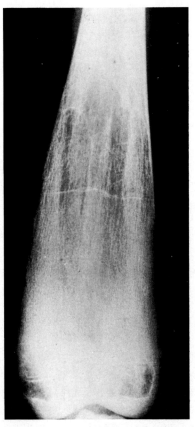

Figure 56–3. Gaucher's disease: Modeling deformities. An example of Erlenmeyer flask deformities of the distal femur. Note the expansion of the contour of the bone, with straightening and convexity of the osseous margin, particularly along the medial aspect of the metaphysis.

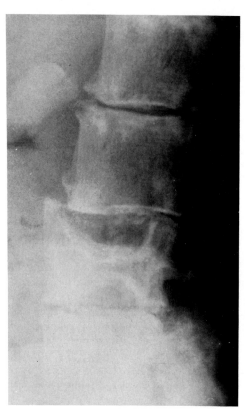

Figure 56–4. Gaucher's disease: Modeling deformities. Step-like deformity of a lumbar vertebral body and severe loss of height of multiple intervertebral discs are seen. The precise cause of these changes is not clear. (Courtesy of V. Vint, M.D., San Diego, California.)

INFECTION (FIG. 56–6). Patients with Gaucher's disease have an increased susceptibility to development of bone infection. The pathogenesis of infection in these patients may be identical to that observed in sickle cell anemia and related disorders. Bone necrosis, hemorrhage, and lipid-containing marrow tissue produce an ideal environment for bacterial proliferation. Infection may involve any skeletal site and may be caused by various organisms, including salmonellae.

Differential Diagnosis

Generalized osteopenia is not a specific sign of Gaucher's disease. This finding also is apparent in a variety of metabolic (osteoporosis, osteomalacia, and hyperparathyroidism), hematologic (sickle cell anemia and thalassemia), and neoplastic disorders (plasma cell myeloma and leukemia). In Gaucher's disease, localized lucent areas and cystic lesions producing a honeycomb appearance may simulate findings of plasma cell myeloma, amyloidosis, and skeletal metastasis.

Generalized or localized osteosclerosis likewise is not specific for Gaucher's disease, occurring also in skeletal metastasis, tuberous sclerosis, mastocytosis, myelofibrosis, and Hodgkin's disease. In Gaucher's disease, the sclerosis includes a coarsened trabecular pattern and a bone-within-bone appearance, a finding that is not apparent in these other disorders. Similar changes can be seen in sickle cell anemia

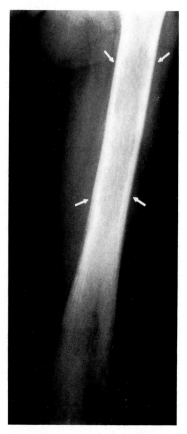

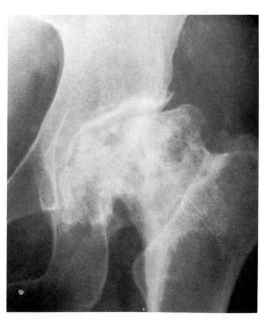

Figure 56–5. Gaucher's disease: Osteonecrosis. The radiograph delineates ischemic necrosis of the femoral head with collapse of bone and secondary osteoarthritis. (Courtesy of G. Greenway, M.D., Dallas, Texas.)

Figure 56–6. Gaucher's disease: Osteomyelitis. Poorly defined radiolucency of the upper femoral shaft is associated with periosteal bone formation (arrows) in a patient with Gaucher's disease and documented Salmonella osteomyelitis. Observe the Erlenmeyer flask deformity of the distal part of the femur.

**Table 56–2. CONDITIONS CHARACTERIZED
BY ERLENMEYER FLASK DEFORMITY**

Gaucher's disease
Niemann-Pick disease
Anemias
Fibrous dysplasia
Metaphyseal dysplasia (Pyle's disease)
Osteopetrosis
Heavy metal poisoning

and its variants, however, the similarity being related to the occurrence of bone infarction and necrosis in these anemias and Gaucher's disease. Furthermore, epiphyseal osteonecrosis also is observed in both Gaucher's disease and hemoglobinopathies. Epiphyseal osteonecrosis is apparent in Cushing's syndrome and exogenous hypercortisolism, pancreatitis, caisson disease, collagen disorders, and numerous other diseases as well. Diametaphyseal osteonecrosis is a manifestation of Gaucher's disease, hemoglobinopathies, pancreatitis, hypercortisolism, and caisson disease.

An Erlenmeyer flask appearance is seen in Gaucher's disease and other disorders (Table 56–2). The diagnosis of Gaucher's disease should be considered in a patient with hepatosplenomegaly who demonstrates widespread osteopenia with a coarsened trabecular pattern, focal osteosclerosis, ischemic necrosis of the proximal capital femoral epiphyses, and flaring or Erlenmeyer flask deformities of the distal portions of the femurs.

NIEMANN-PICK DISEASE

General Features

Niemann-Pick disease is a rare, genetically determined disorder characterized by the widespread accumulation of lipid, particularly sphingomyelin, in the body. Currently it is recognized that Niemann-Pick disease is not a single entity. Five types of sphingomyelin lipidoses are recognized:

TYPE A. Acute neuronopathic form characterized by rapidly fatal disease of infancy with involvement of both viscera and nervous system and with a severe deficiency of sphingomyelinase.

TYPE B. Chronic form without nervous system involvement, characterized by visceral involvement in infants and a moderate to severe deficiency of sphingomyelinase.

TYPE C. Subacute (juvenile) form with neurologic abnormalities in childhood, usually leading to death by adolescence and with questionable sphingomyelinase deficiency.

TYPE D. Nova Scotia form, in which patients, other than having an ancestry in Nova Scotia, resemble those in Type C.

TYPE E. Indeterminate form, occurring in adults with visceral involvement and with questionable sphingomyelinase deficiency.

Clinical Features

The clinical manifestations vary with the specific type of the disease. The sex distribution is approximately equal, and many of the patients are of Jewish background. In general, symptoms and signs become apparent during infancy and progress rapidly, leading to the patient's demise. Findings in these infants may include jaundice, hepatosplenomegaly,

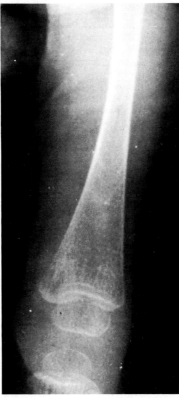

Figure 56–7. Niemann-Pick disease: Marrow infiltration. The distal femoral shaft is both osteopenic and expanded.

abdominal enlargement, lymphadenopathy, emaciation, blindness, anemia, and thrombocytopenia. Some affected individuals may live into adolescence.

The diagnosis is suggested by identification of foam cells in marrow aspirates or tissue biopsy specimens and confirmed by the chemical determination of a predominant increase in sphingomyelin in abnormal tissue.

Musculoskeletal Abnormalities

Accumulation of lipid-containing foam cells occurs in the bone marrow, particularly in children who have a type of Niemann-Pick disease that is compatible with longer life (type B). Resultant radiographic findings are osteopenia, medullary widening, and cortical diminution (Fig. 56–7), findings that are similar to those of Gaucher's disease and thalassemia. Modeling deformities in Niemann-Pick disease also are similar to those of Gaucher's disease, with straightening and convexity of the distal femoral contour. Additional features are coxa valga deformity, notched upper lumbar vertebrae, osseous defects of the proximal medial humerus, epiphyseal stippling, and delayed ossification of various secondary centers.

Differential Diagnosis

The skeletal manifestations of Niemann-Pick disease are similar to those of Gaucher's disease (Table 56–3). Unlike Gaucher's disease, however, Niemann-Pick disease has not been associated with epiphyseal osteonecrosis or with a high frequency of well-circumscribed radiolucent lesions.

Table 56–3. MUSCULOSKELETAL MANIFESTATIONS OF GAUCHER'S DISEASE AND NIEMANN-PICK DISEASE

	Gaucher's Disease	Niemann-Pick Disease
Osteopenia	+	+
Cortical thinning or erosion	+	+
Coarsened trabecular pattern	+	+
Lytic lesions	+	−
Modeling deformity	+	+
Osteonecrosis	+	−

FABRY'S DISEASE
General Features

Fabry's disease or glycosphingolipidosis is a hereditary, X-linked systemic disorder characterized by accumulation in various tissues of ceramide trihexoside. This accumulation of lipid may lead to the patient's death by the fifth or sixth decade of life because of renal failure and hypertension with cardiac and neurologic complications.

Clinical manifestations include skin lesions, fever, pain, paresthesias, azotemia, hypertension, cardiomegaly, myocardial infarction, seizures, sensory deficits, dizziness, aphasia, and cerebral hemorrhage. The diagnosis is established by the detection of the characteristic skin lesion, corneal epithelial dystrophy, and abnormal levels of birefringent lipid material in the skin or kidney.

Musculoskeletal Abnormalities

Periarticular swelling in the knees, elbows, and small joints of the fingers may appear in Fabry's disease. Osteonecrosis, related to lipid infiltration in marrow and vessel walls, is observed at many sites, including the femoral head and talus.

FARBER'S LIPOGRANULOMATOSIS

Farber's disease is a rare and progressive disorder of infancy and early childhood, transmitted as an autosomal recessive characteristic, which is accompanied by hoarseness, aphonia, painful and swollen joints, brownish desquamating dermatitis, subcutaneous and periarticular nodules, and pulmonary abnormalities. The basic defect in this disease is a deficiency of acid ceramidase activity, leading to accumulation of ceramide in the kidneys, liver, lungs, lymph nodes, and subcutaneous tissue.

Affected persons appear normal at birth, but, in the first weeks or months of life, soft tissue swelling in the limbs becomes evident, leading to nodular thickening about joints and tendon sheaths. These nodules are seen in the hands, wrists, elbows, and ankles, as well as the conjunctivae, nostrils, ears, skull, and spine. The bones, cartilage, and soft tissues are infiltrated with macrophages, histiocytes, and foam cells containing lipid material. Radiographic findings include soft tissue swelling, periarticular masses, and juxtaarticular bone erosions.

No specific therapy has proved effective, so that rapid progression leading to the patient's demise in 1 or a few years is typical.

GENERALIZED (G_{M1}) GANGLIOSIDOSIS

Generalized gangliosidosis is an inherited liposomal storage disease caused by a deficiency of G_{M1}-ganglioside-β-galactosidase, leading to accumulation of ganglioside G_{M1} in various tissues, including the nervous system. Several clinical varieties have been described, which differ principally in the time of onset of disease, the pattern of specific organic dysfunction, and the degree of neurologic deterioration. Common clinical manifestations of generalized (G_{M1}) gangliosidosis, which appear in the first few months of life, are mental retardation, a cherry-red spot in the macula, hepatomegaly, and osseous deformities. Early death is the rule.

Radiographic abnormalities related to the musculoskeletal system include diffuse osteopenia, a delay in bone maturation, thickening of the calvarium, horizontally oriented ribs, flattening and beaking of the vertebral bodies, flared iliac wings, acetabular dysplasia, epiphyseal fragmentation, and slender tubular bones. Foam cells are present in the bone marrow.

MULTICENTRIC RETICULOHISTIOCYTOSIS
General Features

Multicentric reticulohistiocytosis is an uncommon systemic disease of unknown cause that becomes apparent in adult life and that is characterized by the proliferation of histiocytes in the skin, the mucosa, the subcutaneous tissues, the synovia, and, on occasion, the bone and periosteum. Other names for the disorder include lipoid dermatoarthritis, and giant cell reticulohistiocytosis.

Clinical Features

The clinical onset of multicentric reticulohistiocytosis is most frequent in middle age, although cases occurring in adolescence and senescence are known. Women are more frequently affected than men. In most patients, polyarthritis is the first manifestation of the disease, followed after months to years by a nodular eruption of the skin. These nodules are common in the ears, nose, scalp, face, dorsum of the hands, forearms, and elbows. Small tumefactions are characteristic about the nail folds. Mucosal papules occur in 50 per cent of patients.

Polyarticular manifestations are symmetric in distribution and involve, in descending order of frequency, the interphalangeal joints of the fingers, knees, shoulders, wrists, hips, ankles, feet, elbows, spine, and temporomandibular joints. Clinical findings resemble those of rheumatoid arthritis. One difference from this latter disease, however, is the increased frequency of distal interphalangeal changes. Almost 50 per cent of patients with multicentric reticulohistiocytosis develop arthritis mutilans.

Patients also may reveal xanthelasmas. Xanthomas involve predominantly the eyelids. Tendon sheath swelling, hypertension, lymphadenopathy, ganglia, erythema, joint hypermobility, and pathologic fractures are other clinical manifestations. A variety of tumors have also been described in association with multicentric reticulohistiocytosis, including carcinomas in many different sites, such as the colon, bronchus, breast, and cervix.

Some characteristics of laboratory examination in this disease are anemia, hypercholesterolemia, and elevated erythrocyte sedimentation rate.

Table 56–4. RADIOGRAPHIC CHARACTERISTICS OF MULTICENTRIC RETICULOHISTIOCYTOSIS

Bilateral symmetric involvement
Predilection for the interphalangeal joints of hand, foot
Atlantoaxial subluxation
Marginal erosions
Absence of osteoporosis
Soft tissue nodules

Radiologic Abnormalities (Table 56–4)

The radiologic features of musculoskeletal involvement in multicentric reticulohistiocytosis include bilateral symmetric involvement; predilection for the interphalangeal joints of the hand and foot; early and severe involvement of the atlantoaxial joint; erosive arthritis beginning at the margins of the joint and spreading centrally, producing separation of osseous surfaces; lack of significant periarticular osteoporosis or periosteal bone formation; and uncalcified nodules of skin, subcutaneous tissues, and tendon sheaths. These radiographic features may become severe and destructive.

The most characteristic and common site of involvement is the interphalangeal joints of the hands (Fig. 56–8). The metacarpophalangeal and carpal joints are also affected. Typical findings include soft tissue swelling and marginal erosions, with a symmetric distribution. The erosions are well circumscribed, resembling the defects of gouty arthritis. The articular space may be widened or narrowed. Progression of disease leads to dramatic resorption of the phalanges, foreshortening of the fingers, and an end-stage arthritis mutilans. Abnormalities of the feet resemble those of the hands (Fig. 56–9).

Changes may be evident in the glenohumeral and acromioclavicular joints, hip, knee, elbow, and ankle (Fig. 56–10). Bilateral and symmetric involvement usually is apparent. Abnormalities in the sacroiliac joint include erosion and obliteration, with bone ankylosis of the articular space. Although this process may be bilateral and symmetric, the absence of adjacent sclerosis aids in distinguishing multicentric reticulohistiocytosis from ankylosing spondylitis.

Severe destructive abnormalities in the cervical spine have been emphasized in multicentric reticulohistiocytosis. Subluxation at the atlantoaxial joint can be an early manifestation of the disease. Eventual findings resemble those of rheumatoid arthritis, although they may be even more severe.

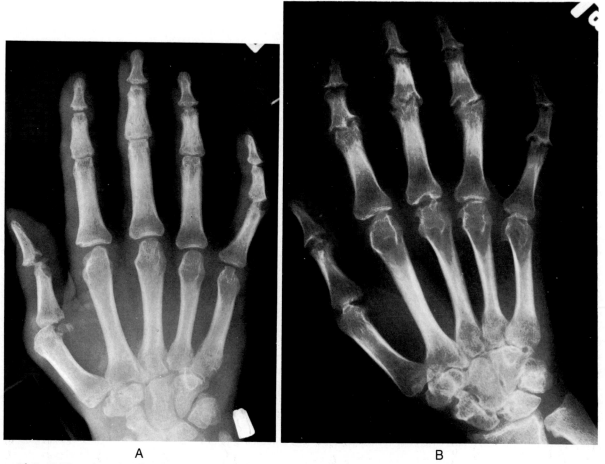

Figure 56–8. Multicentric reticulohistiocytosis: Hand and wrist involvement. A Radiograph demonstrates well-circumscribed marginal erosions accompanied by nodular soft tissue swelling affecting all metacarpophalangeal and interphalangeal joints. In addition, erosions can be observed in several of the carpal bones, including the scaphoid and trapezium. (From Gold RH, et al: Multicentric reticulohistiocytosis (lipoid dermatoarthritis). AJR *124*:610, 1975. Copyright 1975, American Roentgen Ray Society. Used with permission.) **B** In a differnt patient, radiograph reveals well-defined erosions of interphalangeal and metacarpophalangeal joints as well as throughout the wrist. (Courtesy of A. Brower, M.D., Washington, D.C.)

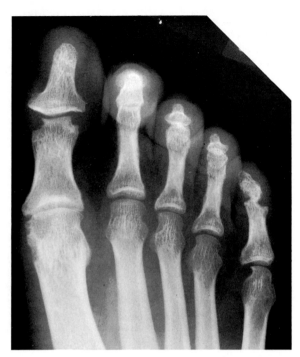

Figure 56–9. Multicentric reticulohistiocytosis: Foot involvement.
Nearly all joints manifest well-circumscribed marginal erosions. Osteoporosis and periostitis are not evident. Soft tissue swelling is apparent. (From Gold RH, et al: Multicentric reticulohistiocytosis (lipoid dermatoarthritis). AJR *124*:610, 1975. Copyright 1975, American Roentgen Ray Society. Used with permission.)

Pathologic Abnormalities

The skin lesions consist of a granulomatous infiltration of histiocytic multinucleated giant cells, which contain large amounts of periodic acid–Schiff (PAS)-positive material. Similar lesions may be seen in the mucous membranes, liver, kidney, lymph nodes, muscle, subcutaneous tissue, bone, nail bed, and endocardium. Although the pathologic aberrations in the synovial tissues in multicentric reticulohistiocytosis resemble those of rheumatoid arthritis, in rheumatoid disease there is more severe inflammation, more extensive villous hypertrophy, and many giant cells that do not contain foamy or granular cytoplasm.

Differential Diagnosis (Table 56–5)

The early erosive changes at the margins of joints in multicentric reticulohistiocytosis resemble the erosions in rheumatoid arthritis, psoriasis, ankylosing spondylitis, and Reiter's syndrome. Although symmetry of involvement and absence of new bone formation are seen in both multicentric reticulohistiocytosis and rheumatoid arthritis, periarticular osteoporosis and early joint space loss are more characteristic of rheumatoid arthritis. In addition, significant destructive changes of distal interphalangeal joints are not common in rheumatoid arthritis but represent an important finding in multicentric reticulohistiocytosis. Atlantoaxial subluxation may be seen in both conditions. Distinguishing features in psoriasis are asymmetric involvement, new bone formation and proliferation with poorly defined erosive alterations, and intraarticular bone ankylosis. The character of erosions in

Reiter's syndrome and ankylosing spondylitis resembles that of psoriasis (poorly defined erosive change with proliferation), differing from the erosions in multicentric reticulohistiocytosis. In addition, the distribution of articular involvement in both Reiter's syndrome and ankylosing spondylitis is characteristic.

Inflammatory (erosive) osteoarthritis and scleroderma are two other diseases that may be associated with osseous erosion of interphalangeal joints. In the former disease, erosive changes may predominate in the central portion of the joint and may be associated with osteophytosis and intraarticular bone ankylosis. These features are not part of the radiographic picture of multicentric reticulohistiocytosis. Distal interphalangeal joint erosions in scleroderma are unusual, and, when present, are associated with more typical findings, such as tuftal resorption and soft tissue calcification.

Gouty arthritis is characterized by soft tissue nodular masses, sharply marginated erosions, preservation of joint space, and lack of osteoporosis, radiographic findings that are identical to those of multicentric reticulohistiocytosis. An asymmetric distribution, partially calcified soft tissue masses, and bone production with overhanging edges are findings of gout that are not apparent in multicentric reticulohistiocytosis.

HISTIOCYTOSIS X
General Features

The three major conditions in the category of histiocytosis X are eosinophilic granuloma, Hand-Schüller-Christian disease, and Letterer-Siwe disease. Although the term histiocytosis X has been used as a comprehensive designation for these three conditions, some authors regard these disorders as unrelated. The three forms are divided according to the following scheme: eosinophilic granuloma is the mildest form, which may present as single or multiple lesions of bone;

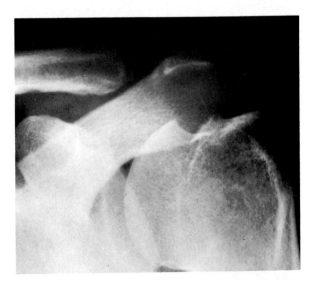

Figure 56–10. Multicentric reticulohistiocytosis: Involvement of the shoulder. Extensive osseous erosions on the lateral aspect of the humeral head and distal end of the clavicle can be seen. The erosions are well defined. The joint space is not narrowed. (From Gold RH, et al: Multicentric reticulohistiocytosis (lipoid dermatoarthritis). AJR *124*:610, 1975. Copyright 1975, American Roentgen Ray Society. Used with permission.)

Table 56–5. DIFFERENTIAL DIAGNOSIS OF MULTICENTRIC RETICULOHISTIOCYTOSIS

	Symmetric Involvement	Involvement of DIP Joints*	Marginal Erosions	Osteoporosis	Intra-articular Bone Ankylosis	Atlantoaxial Subluxation	Soft Tissue Nodules
Multicentric reticulohistiocytosis	+	+	+	−	−	+	+
Rheumatoid arthritis	+	−	+	+	−	+	+
Psoriatic arthritis	±	+	+	−	+	+	−
Inflammatory (erosive) osteoarthritis	+	+	±	−	+	−	−
Gouty arthritis	±	+	+	−	−	−	+

*DIP, Distal interphalangeal.

Hand-Schüller-Christian disease is the most varied form, with chronic dissemination of osseous lesions; and Letterer-Siwe disease is the acute form, with rapid dissemination and poor clinical prognosis.

Although clear distinction among these three forms of histiocytoses frequently is difficult on the basis of clinical and radiologic manifestations, evidence supporting the intimate relationship of eosinophilic granuloma, Hand-Schüller-Christian disease, and Letterer-Siwe disease is the identification in all three entities of specific histiocytic cells (Langerhans cells) containing cytoplasmic inclusion bodies (Langerhans granules or X bodies). Although similar granules have been found in normal persons and in patients with unrelated disorders, the Langerhans cells are believed by many investigators to be of histiocytic origin and virtually diagnostic of the histiocytoses. Furthermore, such cells reveal intense phagocytic activity and mobility, features that may account for the proclivity of the histiocytoses to disseminate widely in the body's tissues. Despite such histologic evidence, many other observers maintain that the three disorders are unrelated, emphasizing the differing clinical manifestations of the processes. Early and diffuse organ involvement and rapid patient demise, characteristics of Letterer-Siwe disease, support its classification as a malignant lymphoma. At the other end of the spectrum, eosinophilic granuloma certainly is benign in its clinical characteristics, resembling more an inflammatory process than a neoplasm. Hand-Schüller-Christian disease is believed by some to be a multifocal variety of eosinophilic granuloma.

The precise cause of the histiocytoses is no clearer than the relationship among its various component diseases.

Eosinophilic Granuloma

Eosinophilic granuloma is characterized by single or multiple skeletal lesions occurring predominantly in children, adolescents, or young adults. It represents approximately 70 per cent of the total number of cases of histiocytosis X, and it is more common in men than in women and in whites than in blacks. Clinical manifestations include local pain, tenderness, and swelling or a soft tissue mass related to adjacent skeletal lesions. Fever and leukocytosis may also be apparent.

Solitary lesions predominate over multiple lesions. The most common sites of involvement are the skull, mandible, spine, ribs, and long bones. When tubular bones are affected, diaphyseal and metaphyseal localization is more frequent than

epiphyseal localization. Epiphyseal lesions may cross an open physeal plate.

In long bones, the lesions appear radiographically as radiolucent areas, particularly in the medullary cavity (Fig. 56–11). With further growth of the lesion, endosteal erosion of the cortex and periosteal new bone formation are seen. The appearance can simulate that of osteomyelitis or malignant neoplasm, such as Ewing's sarcoma and lymphoma. In ribs, single or multiple lesions can lead to pathologic fractures (Fig. 56–12). In the skull and pelvis, the lytic areas may be particularly well defined with or without surrounding sclerosis (Fig. 56–13). A radiodense focus within a lytic cranial lesion has been termed a "button" sequestrum (Fig. 56–14). Nonuniform growth of the lesion leads to beveled bone margins

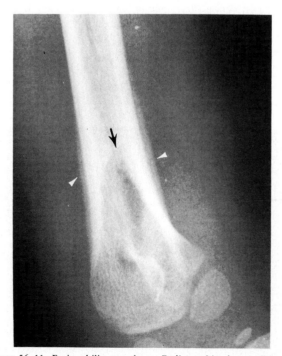

Figure 56–11. Eosinophilic granuloma: Radiographic abnormalities—tubular bones of appendicular skeleton. A typical lesion of the distal part of the humerus in this child consists of an area of osteolysis (arrow) and thick, linear periosteal bone formation (arrowheads).

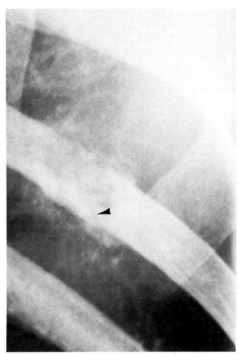

Figure 56–12. **Eosinophilic granuloma: Radiographic abnormalities—ribs.** A poorly defined osteolytic lesion is evident. A pathologic fracture (arrowhead) extends across the lesion. (Courtesy of G. Greenway, M.D., Dallas, Texas.)

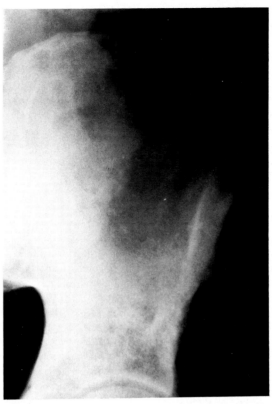

Figure 56–13. **Eosinophilic granuloma: Radiographic abnormalities—axial skeleton.** Extensive osteolytic lesions of the ilium are associated wtih surrounding sclerosis. The degree of increased radiodensity in this case is somewhat unusual.

and unequal destruction of the inner and outer tables of the vault. In the mandible, radiolucent lesions about the teeth may lead to loss of supporting bone and a "floating teeth" appearance.

Vertebral destruction can lead to a flattened vertebral body, termed vertebra plana, a finding that is much more frequent in children than in adults (Fig. 56–15). Eosinophilic granuloma, however, also can produce bubbly, lytic, expansile lesions of both the vertebral bodies and posterior osseous elements without significant collapse. Thoracic and lumbar

spine involvement predominates, and involvement of adjacent vertebrae is sometimes seen. A paraspinal mass can be evident.

The gross pathologic abnormalities of eosinophilic granuloma include a soft hemorrhagic lesion consisting of reticulum cells, multinucleated giant cells, eosinophils, lymphocytes, and plasma cells.

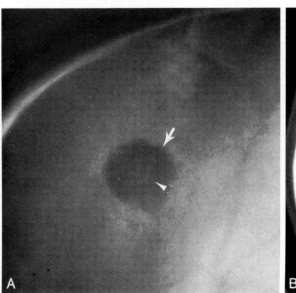

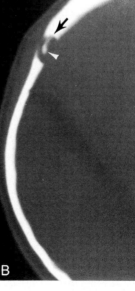

Figure 56–14. **Eosinophilic granuloma: Radiographic abnormalities—"button" sequestrum.** A plain film (**A**) and computed tomographic image (**B**) show an osteolytic lesion (arrows) with a radiodense sequestrum (arrowheads).

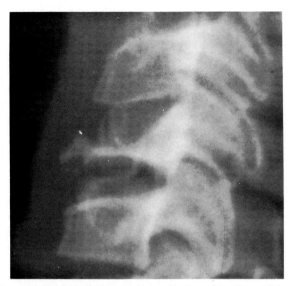

Figure 56–15. Eosinophilic granuloma: Radiographic abnormalities—vertebra plana. Observe the flattened fourth cervical vertebral body. (Courtesy of T. Yochum, D.C., Denver, Colorado.)

Hand-Schüller-Christian Disease

The classic triad of Hand-Schüller-Christian disease consists of diabetes insipidus, unilateral or bilateral exophthalmos, and single or multiple areas of bone destruction. This triad, however, may be apparent in fewer than 10 per cent of patients. Hand-Schüller-Christian disease predominates in children. The fundamental pathologic lesion is a histiocytic granuloma in which the histiocytes are filled with cholesterol.

Clinical characteristics are otitis media; cutaneous involvement with eczema, xanthomatosis, and soft tissue nodules; ulceration of the gums; lymphadenopathy; and hepatosplenomegaly. Visceral involvement of the lungs, kidneys, brain, liver, and spleen is observed. Anemia is a grave prognostic sign. In general, the disease runs a protracted course.

The skeletal lesions of Hand-Schüller-Christian disease may be widely disseminated (Fig. 56–16). The radiographic manifestations of individual lesions are similar to those of eosinophilic granuloma. In the skull, confluent areas of destruction may isolate islands of bone, creating the geographic skull. Similar findings in the mandible with isolation of teeth is termed the "floating teeth" appearance. The diagnosis of Hand-Schüller-Christian disease or a related histiocytosis should be considered in any infant or child with osteolytic lesions of the pelvis or skull.

Initially, the histologic picture of Hand-Schüller-Christian disease may closely resemble that of eosinophilic granuloma. With time, the lesions undergo necrosis and contain some mature histiocytes with decrease in the number of inflammatory cells. Eventually the lipogranulomatous stage occurs, marked by histiocytic multinucleated giant cells, hemosiderin, necrosis, and cholesterol crystals.

The outcome in Hand-Schüller-Christian disease is variable. In some instances, bone lesions resolve gradually; in other instances, the lesions progress. The prognosis worsens with involvement of multiple organ systems, and the disease is fatal in 10 to 30 per cent of cases.

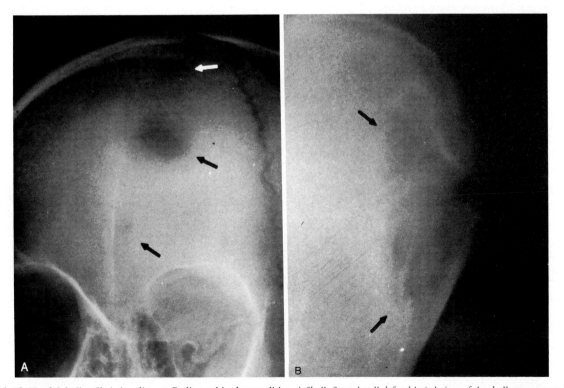

Figure 56–16. Hand-Schüller-Christian disease: Radiographic abnormalities. A Skull. Several well-defined lytic lesions of the skull are apparent (arrows). Some of these have beveled margins. B Pelvis. A large lytic lesion of the lateral aspect of the ilium is surrounded by a thin rim of sclerosis (arrows).

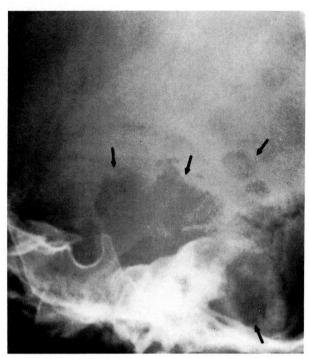

Figure 56–17. Letterer-Siwe disease: Radiographic abnormalities. Note the confluent areas of bone destruction (arrows) at the base of the skull.

Letterer-Siwe Disease

Letterer-Siwe disease is a relatively acute syndrome that is most frequent in children below the age of 3 years. It is characterized by histiocytic proliferation in multiple visceral organs. The frequency of this form is lower than that of eosinophilic granuloma and Hand-Schüller-Christian disease, composing approximately 10 per cent of all the histiocytoses.

Clinical manifestations include febrile episodes, cachexia, hepatosplenomegaly, lymphadenopathy, purpuric skin eruption, hyperplasia of the gums, and progressive anemia. The course generally is rapidly progressive, most patients dying within 1 or 2 years. Diagnosis is established by biopsy of bone marrow or lymph nodes.

Single or multiple areas of bone destruction are observed, particularly in the calvarium, base of the skull, and mandible (Fig. 56–17). Histologically and radiologically, the bone lesions simulate those in eosinophilic granuloma.

Disease Prognosis and Evolution of Osseous Abnormalities

Involvement of tissues other than those of the musculoskeletal system is most typical of Hand-Schüller-Christian disease and Letterer-Siwe disease although each of the histiocytoses can affect other systems. Pulmonary involvement in eosinophilic granuloma may lead to a honeycomb appearance. In general, the prognosis of any of the types of histiocytosis X is related to the location and the extent of organ involvement. The greater the number of tissues that are affected, the poorer is the prognosis. The prognosis of the histiocytoses is also related to the age of the patient at the time of onset of clinical abnormalities; generally, the younger the individual, the poorer the prognosis.

Complicating any analysis of disease prognosis of the histiocytoses and the choice of appropriate therapeutic agents is the documentation that osseous as well as extraosseous lesions may resolve spontaneously. During healing, osteolytic lesions in extraspinal locations typically develop bone sclerosis, periosteal reaction, and cortical thickening. Alternatively, enlargement of foci of osseous destruction or the appearance of new areas of lysis is a finding indicative of an unfavorable prognosis. The typical healing response of those spinal lesions that have produced vertebra plana is partial reconstitution of vertebral height.

Intralesional injection of corticosteroid preparations has become a popular method of treatment of the histiocytoses in recent years. Progressive healing of the osseous lesions generally becomes detectable radiographically after 2 to 4 months. Clinical improvement accompanies the radiographic changes. The mechanism of action of the corticosteroid preparation after intralesional administration is not clear.

Scintigraphy

In general, bone scintigraphy has proved to be less sensitive than radiography in detecting osseous lesions in the histiocytoses. Use of ^{67}Ga-citrate and ^{99m}Tc-sulfur colloid bone marrow scanning offers no additional advantages. When bone scan findings are present, osseous lesions in histiocytosis X demonstrate a spectrum of radionuclide abnormalities ranging from "cold" areas with decreased or absent accumulation of the radionuclide to areas of augmented activity (Fig. 56–18).

Differential Diagnosis

The predominant pattern of the histiocytoses is osteolysis. Osteolytic lesions may be single or multiple. Single lytic defects must be differentiated from neoplastic and inflammatory lesions as well as fibrous dysplasia. Multiple lytic lesions may simulate infection, skeletal metastasis, leukemia, lymphoma, hyperparathyroidism with brown tumors, and Gaucher's disease.

LIPID GRANULOMATOSIS (ERDHEIM-CHESTER DISEASE)

Lipid granulomatosis is an unusual lipidosis that differs from other lipidoses. The clinical manifestations are not well

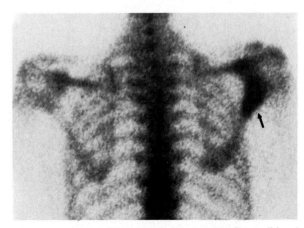

Figure 56–18. Eosinophilic granuloma: Scintigraphic abnormalities. An area of increased uptake (arrow) of a bone-seeking radiopharmaceutical agent is indicative of a lesion in the scapula.

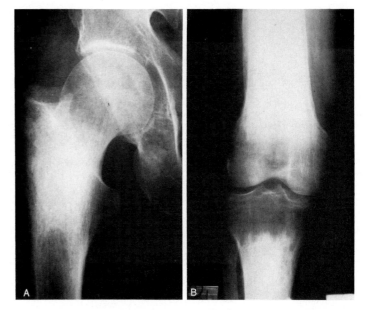

Figure 56–19. Erdheim-Chester disease. Observe the sclerotic lesion of the proximal portion of the right femur (**A**) and distal part of the femur and tibia (**B**). The epiphyses are spared, and the opposite side was similarly involved. (Courtesy of G. Greenway, M.D., Dallas, Texas.)

defined, although men and women in the fifth through seventh decades appear to be affected. Cardiac and pulmonary manifestations owing to liberation of cholesterol from foam cells and xanthomatous patches in the eyelids may be seen. Chronic lipogranulomatous pyelonephritis also has been reported. Patients may be entirely asymptomatic, however.

The major long bones of the limbs are invariably affected, whereas axial skeletal involvement is unusual. A patchy or diffuse increase in density, coarsened trabecular pattern, medullary sclerosis, and cortical thickening appear in the diaphysis and metaphysis, with minor changes or sparing of the epiphysis (Fig. 56–19). Symmetry is the rule. Bone scans demonstrate increased accumulation of isotope in areas of radiographic abnormality. Gallium imaging may reveal a similar distribution.

Pathologic findings in the skeleton resemble those in extraskeletal sites, where extensive lipogranulomatous changes in internal organs and even retroperitoneal xanthogranulomas may be observed. The pathologic aberrations most resemble those of Hand-Schüller-Christian disease. The relationship of Erdheim-Chester disease to the histiocytoses is not known, however.

SINUS HISTIOCYTOSIS WITH LYMPHADENOPATHY

Sinus histiocytosis with massive lymphadenopathy, or Rosai-Dorfman disease, is a non-neoplastic, self-limited disease of unknown cause occurring predominantly in the first two decades of life, especially in black patients. The disease is characterized by painless bilateral cervical adenopathy, adenopathy in other lymph node chains, fever, elevated erythrocyte sedimentation rate, neutrophilic leukocytosis, occasional eosinophilia, and hypergammaglobulinemia. Extranodal sites of involvement include the upper respiratory tract, salivary glands, orbits, eyelids, testes, and bone.

Osseous manifestations of this disease are generally restricted to multiple or, less frequently, solitary osteolytic lesions (Fig. 56–20) involving principally the long tubular bones but also the skull, pelvis, vertebral bodies, phalanges, metacarpals, and ribs. The lesions usually are asymptomatic. Intralesional calcification and periostitis are absent. Surrounding sclerosis is sometimes apparent. Serial radiographs may reveal a continuous decrease in the size of the lytic defects with eventually their complete disappearance.

MALIGNANT HISTIOCYTOSIS

The major features of malignant histiocytosis (histiocytic medullary reticulosis) are a variable age of onset, fever, weight

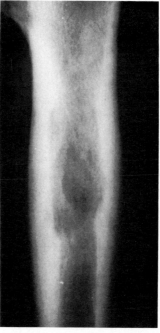

Figure 56–20. Sinus histiocytosis with lymphadenopathy. An osteolytic lesion is apparent in the femur. (Courtesy of D. Sartoris, M.D., San Diego, California.)

Table 56–6. HYPERLIPOPROTEINEMIAS

Type	Lipoprotein Abnormality	Primary Form	Secondary Forms	Xanthomas	Arthralgia or Arthritis	Hyper-uricemia
I	Chylomicrons	Autosomal recessive	Diabetes mellitus Pancreatitis Alcoholism	Skin		
II	Beta-lipoprotein	Autosomal dominant	Hypothyroidism Myeloma Macroglobulinemia Obstructive hepatic disease	Skin Tendinous Tuberous Subperiosteal	+	
III	Beta- or prebeta-lipoprotein	Autosomal recessive (?)	Diabetes mellitus Hypothyroidism	Skin Tendinous Tuberous Subperiosteal		+
IV	Prebeta-lipoprotein	Autosomal recessive	Diabetes mellitus Pancreatitis Alcoholism Hypothyroidism Glycogen storage disease Gaucher's disease Gout Hypercalcemia	Skin Tuberous Intraosseous	+	+
V	Prebeta-lipoprotein, chylomicrons	Autosomal dominant (?)		Skin		+

loss, hepatosplenomegaly, jaundice, and progressive pancytopenia. Histiocytic infiltration in lymph nodes, liver, spleen, and bone marrow is observed. Radiographically evident bone lesions, although uncommon, appear as osteolytic foci with sclerotic margins or, less commonly, areas of osteosclerosis. The pelvis, spine, and tubular bones are involved. These lesions may disappear during treatment. The prognosis of the disease is poor, as most patients die within 6 months of the onset of symptoms and signs. Rarely, partial or complete remissions are seen.

HYPERLIPOPROTEINEMIAS
General Features

Primary familial hyperlipoproteinemias comprise a group of heritable diseases associated with an increase in plasma concentrations of cholesterol or triglycerides. Currently, these diseases are subdivided into five major types according to the plasma lipoprotein pattern (Table 56–6).

TYPE I HYPERLIPOPROTEINEMIA. Primary type I hyperlipoproteinemia is related to a hereditary abnormality in chylomicron removal in which there is a deficiency in plasma postheparin lipoprotein lipase activity. The plasma appears milky, plasma cholesterol levels are normal or slightly increased, and plasma triglyceride levels are elevated. Type I hyperlipoproteinemia may occur in a secondary form in diabetes mellitus, pancreatitis, and alcoholism. Most patients with primary type I hyperlipoproteinemia are diagnosed in the first or second decade of life. Clinical findings include lipemia retinalis, hepatosplenomegaly, abdominal pain, and pancreatitis.

TYPE II HYPERLIPOPROTEINEMIA (FAMILIAL HYPERCHOLESTEROLEMIA). Type II, the most common type, is related to an increase in the plasma concentration of low density lipoproteins or beta-lipoproteins. Type II is further divided into two subgroups, types IIA and IIB; the former is characterized by an excess of beta-lipoproteins and

the latter by an excess of both beta- and prebeta-lipoproteins. In its primary form, type II hyperlipoproteinemia is an autosomal dominant hereditary abnormality. It may also occur secondarily to hypothyroidism, plasma cell myeloma, mac-

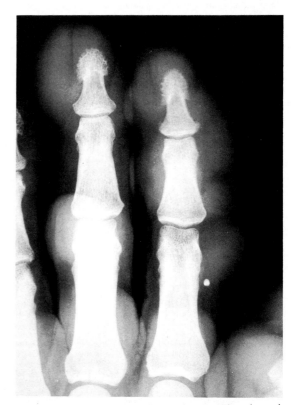

Figure 56–21. Hyperlipoproteinemia: Xanthomas without bone abnormalities. A radiograph reveals asymmetric soft tissue masses in periarticular and periosseous locations. Neither soft tissue calcification nor significant osseous erosions are evident.

roglobulinemia, and obstructive liver disease. The diagnosis of primary type II hyperlipoproteinemia usually is established in early childhood. The findings include xanthomas and premature coronary, cerebral, and peripheral vascular disease.

TYPE III HYPERLIPOPROTEINEMIA ("BROAD-BETA" DISEASE). Type III, an uncommon type, is associated with beta- or prebeta-lipoprotein abnormality. In its primary form, type III hyperlipoproteinemia may be an autosomal recessive disorder. Rarely it occurs secondarily to severe insulinopenic diabetes and hypothyroidism. Primary type III hyperlipoproteinemia may not be detected until the third, fourth, or fifth decade of life. Xanthomas and premature peripheral vascular disease are apparent.

TYPE IV HYPERLIPOPROTEINEMIA. Type IV is characterized by the presence of increased low density lipoproteins or prebeta-lipoproteins without chylomicronemia. In its primary form, the disease appears to be an autosomal recessive disorder. Type IV hyperlipoproteinemia may be secondary to diabetes mellitus, pancreatitis, alcoholism, hypothyroidism, glycogen storage disease, Gaucher's disease, gout, and hypercalcemia. In its primary form, the disease rarely is detected below the age of 20 years. Xanthomas, hyperuricemia, and coronary vascular disease may be evident.

TYPE V HYPERLIPOPROTEINEMIA. Type V is similar to type IV, with an increase in low density lipoproteins and chylomicrons. In its primary form, it is probably an autosomal dominant hereditary disease that rarely is manifested clinically in childhood. Xanthomas, hyperuricemia, abdominal pain, hepatosplenomegaly, paresthesias, and lipemia retinalis can be detected.

Musculoskeletal Abnormalities

XANTHOMA. Xanthomas may be apparent in all five types of hyperlipoproteinemia and in primary and secondary forms of the disease. Xanthomas can be classified as follows:

1. Eruptive xanthomas: Papules containing triglycerides on the knees, buttocks, back, and shoulders.

2. Tendinous xanthomas: Localized deposits in the tendons of the hand, the patellar tendon, the Achilles tendon, the plantar aponeurosis, and the peroneal tendons, and around the elbow and lower tibia.

3. Tuberous xanthomas: Soft subcutaneous masses, which occur over extensor surfaces.

4. Subperiosteal and osseous xanthomas: Lipid deposits, which occur beneath the periosteum or within the spongiosa, leading to osteolytic defects, periosteal or endosteal erosion of the cortex, and even osteonecrosis.

Tuberous and tendinous xanthomas produce nodular masses in soft tissue and tendons (Fig. 56–21). These rarely calcify. Subperiosteal xanthomas are associated with scalloping of the external cortical surface (Fig. 56–22). Intramedullary lipid deposition leads to lytic defects, endosteal erosion, subchondral collapse, juxtaarticular erosive changes, and pathologic fractures. In general, the bone defects are well defined.

GOUT. Hyperuricemia and clinical gout have been reported in association with types III, IV, and V hyperlipoproteinemias. Typical radiographic findings of gout may be encountered in patients with hyperuricemia.

ARTHRALGIAS AND ARTHRITIS. In type II hyperlipoproteinemia, a migratory polyarthritis may be detected affecting large and small peripheral articulations. Symptoms

and signs may simulate the findings of rheumatic fever. Soft tissue swelling may be observed on radiographs.

Arthralgias may occur in patients with type IV hyperlipoproteinemia. Joint pain, tenderness, and stiffness may be evident, but synovitis is not detectable.

Cerebrotendinous Xanthomatosis

Cerebrotendinous xanthomatosis is a rare disease characterized by xanthomas, cataracts, progressive cerebellar ataxia, and dementia. Accumulation of cholesterol and cholesterol-like crystals occurs in the white matter of the brain and in xanthomas. Serum cholesterol levels are normal or low and cholestanol levels are markedly elevated. Cerebrotendinous xanthomatosis is probably an autosomal recessive disorder, whose biochemical basis is not known.

Differential Diagnosis

One radiographic characteristic of the hyperlipoproteinemias—eccentric masses without calcification—can be simulated by changes in gouty arthritis. This similarity is accentuated by the localization of masses to periarticular soft tissues, tendons, and subperiosteal and osseous areas, by the adjacent bone lysis, and by the simultaneous occurrence of both hyperlipidemia and hyperuricemia. The osseous erosions in both disorders share common features, including well-defined margins, eccentricity, and intra- and extraarticular distribution. The soft tissue swelling of gout may contain radiographically evident calcification, a finding that is not characteristic of xanthoma.

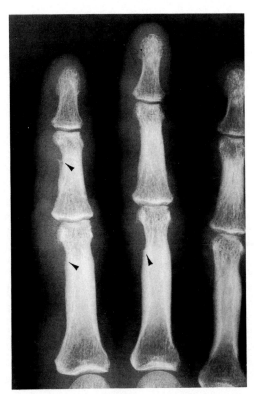

Figure 56–22. Hyperlipoproteinemia: Xanthomas with bony abnormalities. Observe nodular soft tissue masses with subjacent osseous erosion (arrowheads). The osseous defects are eccentric and well defined. Osteoporosis and joint space narrowing are not apparent.

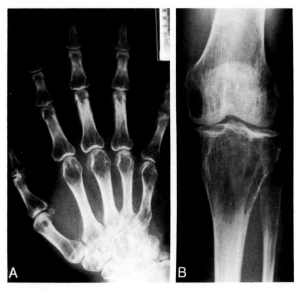

Figure 56–23. Membranous lipodystrophy: Radiographic abnormalities. A Observe symmetric radiolucent lesions involving virtually all of the bones of the hand and wrist. The opposite side was similarly affected. B Poorly defined osteolytic areas in the metaphyseal and epiphyseal regions of the femur, tibia, and fibula are associated with mild expansion of the bone. Similar lesions were present on the opposite side. (Courtesy of I. Sugiura, M.D., Nagoya, Japan.)

Subperiosteal xanthomas in hyperlipoproteinemias produce subjacent bone erosion. This appearance resembles subperiosteal erosion of hyperparathyroidism.

MEMBRANOUS LIPODYSTROPHY

Membranous lipodystrophy, also termed polycystic lipomembranous osteodysplasia, is a rare hereditary disorder of adipose tissue affecting several organ systems but especially the bones and brain. Prominent neuropsychiatric manifestations relating to sclerosing leukoencephalopathy account for the frequent discovery of membranous lipodystrophy in patients in mental hospitals. There is strong evidence that the disease is of autosomal recessive inheritance.

Clinical characteristics include the appearance of painful bones and joints in the second or third decade of life. Subsequently, neuropsychiatric symptoms and signs resembling those of Alzheimer's disease appear and progress rapidly, often culminating in death by the fourth or fifth decade of life. Histologic abnormalities are observed in the fat cells throughout the body.

Osseous alterations dominate the early phases of the disease. The osseous lesions occur as early as infancy, although they are more typically seen in childhood. Symmetric radiolucent lesions appear in the tubular bones of the extremities, carpus, tarsus, metacarpals, metatarsals, and phalanges (Fig. 56–23). The axial skeleton is spared. The cystic areas have poorly defined margins and are unassociated with sclerotic reaction. Bone deformities result from pathologic fractures. Serial radiographic examinations document either little change in

the size of the lesions or slow progression. Pathologically, cystic areas in the bone contain jellylike material that is PAS-positive, suggesting a glycoprotein structure.

The cause of membranous lipodystrophy is unknown. The differential diagnosis of the radiographic changes in the bones includes fibrous dysplasia, hyperparathyroidism, neurofibromatosis, sarcoidosis, lymphangiomatosis, and hemangiomatosis. Knowledge of accompanying neuropsychiatric symptoms and signs combined with radiographic features consisting of symmetric osseous lesions confined to the appendicular skeleton aids in correct diagnosis of this unusual disease.

FURTHER READING

Barrow MV, Holubar K: Multicentric reticulohistiocytosis. A review of 33 patients. Medicine 48:287, 1969.

Cohen M, Zornoza J, Cangir A, Murray JA, Wallace S: Direct injection of methylprednisolone sodium succinate in the treatment of solitary eosinophilic granuloma of bone. A report of 9 cases. Radiology 136:289, 1980.

Dee P, Westgaard T, Langholm R: Erdheim-Chester disease: Case with chronic discharging sinus from bone. AJR 134:837, 1980.

Dunnick NR, Parker BR, Warnke RA, Castellino RA: Radiographic manifestations of malignant histiocytosis. AJR 127:611, 1976.

Gold RH, Metzger AL, Mirra JM, Weinberger HJ, Killebrew K: Multicentric reticulohistiocytosis (lipoid dermatoarthritis). An erosive polyarthritis with distinctive clinical, roentgenographic, and pathologic features. AJR 124:610, 1975.

Greenfield GB: Bone changes in chronic adult Gaucher's disease. AJR 110:800, 1970.

Hasegawa Y, Inagaki Y: Membranous lipodystrophy (lipomembranous polycystic osteodysplasia). Two case reports. Clin Orthop 181:229, 1983.

Jaffe HL: Metabolic, Degenerative and Inflammatory Diseases of Bones and Joints. Philadelphia, Lea & Febiger, 1972.

Jaffe HL, Lichtenstein L: Eosinophilic granuloma of bone. A condition affecting one, several or many bones, but apparently limited to the skeleton and representing the mildest clinical expression of the peculiar inflammatory histiocytosis also underlying Letterer-Siwe Disease and Schüller-Christian disease. Arch Pathol 37:99, 1944.

Kaye JJ, Freiberger RH: Eosinophilic granuloma of the spine without vertebra plana. A report of two unusual cases. Radiology 92:1188, 1969.

Lachman R, Crocker A, Schulman J, Strand R: Radiological findings in Niemann-Pick disease. Radiology 108:659, 1973.

Levin B: Gaucher's disease. Clinical and roentgenologic manifestations. AJR 85:685, 1961.

Lichtenstein L: Histiocytosis X. Integration of eosinophilic granuloma of bone, "Letterer-Siwe Disease" and "Schüller-Christian" disease as related manifestations of a single nosologic entity. Arch Pathol 56:84, 1953.

Owman T, Sjoblad ST, Gothlin J: Radiographic skeletal changes in juvenile GM₁-gangliosidosis. ROFO 132:682, 1980.

Pastershank SP, Yip S, Sodhi HS: Cerebrotendinous xanthomatosis. J Can Assoc Radiol 25:282, 1974.

Ponseti I: Bone lesions in eosinophilic granuloma, Hand-Schüller-Christian disease, and Letterer-Siwe disease. J Bone Joint Surg [Am] 30:811, 1948.

Puczynski MS, Demos TC, Suarez CR: Sinus histiocytosis with massive lymphadenopathy: Skeletal involvement. Pediatr Radiol 15:259, 1985.

Resnick D, Greenway G, Genant H, Brower A, Haghighi P, Emmett M: Erdheim-Chester disease. Radiology 142:289, 1982.

Rosai J, Dorfman RF: Sinus histiocytosis with massive lymphadenopathy. A newly recognized benign clinicopathologic entity. Arch Pathol 87:63, 1969.

Siegelman SS, Schlossberg I, Becker NH, Sachs BA: Hyperlipoproteinemia with skeletal lesions. Clin Orthop 87:228, 1972.

Waite RJ, Doherty PW, Liepman M, Woda B: Langerhans cell histiocytosis with the radiographic findings of Erdheim-Chester disease. AJR 150:869, 1988.

Warnke RA, Kim H, Dorfman RF: Malignant histiocytosis (histiocytic medullary reticulosis). I. Clinicopathologic study of 29 cases. Cancer 35:215, 1975.

Chapter 57

Myeloproliferative Disorders

Donald Resnick, M.D.
Parviz Haghighi, M.D.

Musculoskeletal abnormalities accompany a variety of myeloproliferative disorders. In leukemias, such abnormalities are particularly frequent in children. Osseous involvement from the primary disease leads to local symptoms and signs. Synovial involvement owing to leukemic infiltration and hemorrhage can result in articular findings. Hyperuricemia and secondary gout can complicate this disease. Bone destruction and secondary gout also may be observed in the lymphomas. Sjögren's syndrome is associated with an arthritis that usually appears identical to rheumatoid arthritis. In systemic mastocytosis, characteristic skeletal abnormalities include focal or diffuse lytic or sclerotic lesions. Polycythemia vera may be characterized by osteonecrosis, osteopenia, and hyperuricemia. Myelofibrosis can be accompanied by osteosclerosis, particularly in the axial skeleton. In addition, hyperuricemia and secondary gout are relatively common in this disorder.

Certain myeloproliferative disorders are associated with skeletal manifestations that can constitute an initial or dominant part of the entire clinical picture. Included in these are leukemias, lymphomas, Sjögren's syndrome, systemic mastocytosis (urticaria pigmentosa), polycythemia vera, and myelofibrosis.

LEUKEMIAS
General Features

It is convenient to divide the leukemias into acute and chronic forms (Table 57–1). Acute leukemia can affect both children and adults. In children, acute leukemia almost always is lymphoblastic in cell origin, and the survival time is limited to approximately 1 year; in adults, acute leukemia frequently is myeloid in cell origin. Chronic leukemia may be granulocytic or lymphocytic; chronic lymphocytic leukemia is closely related to lymphosarcoma. The chronic types of leukemia have a peak age of onset of 35 to 55 years and an average survival time of approximately 3 years.

Acute Childhood Leukemia

Acute leukemia in children is a disease of the first few years of life, the peak frequency occurring between 2 and 5 years of age. Approximately 80 per cent of cases are lymphoblastic in origin, 10 per cent are myeloblastic, and 10 per cent are of other cellular origin. Acute myeloblastic leukemia may have a paucity of clinical signs. In acute lymphoblastic leukemia, however, lymphadenopathy and splenomegaly may be seen. Other findings in children with leukemia may cause confusion with rheumatic fever, juvenile chronic polyarthritis, or osteomyelitis. Arthralgias and arthritis have been reported in 12 to 65 per cent of patients. These joint manifestations are attributable to hemorrhage or to leukemic masses in metaphyseal periosteum, subarticular bone, and synovium.

SKELETAL ABNORMALITIES. Radiographic changes in the skeleton in acute leukemia are reported in 50 to 70 per cent of cases. They include the following:

Diffuse Osteopenia (15 to 100 Per Cent). Osteopenia with medullary widening and cortical thinning in tubular bones and vertebral compression is encountered. Osteopenia may progress slowly without treatment or improve with therapy.

Radiolucent and Radiodense Metaphyseal Bands (10 to 55 Per Cent) (Fig. 57–1). Symmetric metaphyseal band-like radiolucent areas are observed in leukemia and other chronic childhood illnesses. This nonspecific finding probably reflects an interference with proper osteogenesis. As a consequence, it is most commonly seen at sites of rapid bone growth, including the distal parts of the femur and radius and the proximal portions of the tibia and humerus. After the age of 2 years, radiolucent metaphyseal bands are more characteristic of leukemia than of any other condition. Histologically, the radiolucent lesions of the metaphysis are not associated with leukemic cell infiltration. Osseous weakening at radiolucent

Table 57–1. SKELETAL ALTERATIONS IN THE LEUKEMIAS*

	Acute Childhood Leukemia	Acute Adult Leukemia	Chronic Leukemia
Osteopenia	+ +	+ +	+
Metaphyseal abnormalities	+ +	+	−
Osteolysis	+ +	+ +	+
Periostitis	+ +	+	+
Osteosclerosis	+	+	+
Articular abnormalities	+ +	+	+

*+ +, Common; +, uncommon; −, absent.

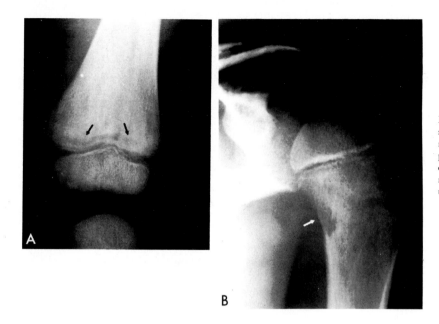

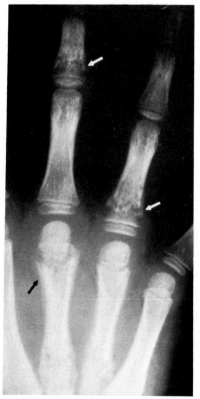

Figure 57–1. Acute childhood leukemia: Metaphyseal abnormalities. A Observe a transverse band of radiolucency (arrows) in the metaphysis of the distal part of the femur. Adjacent minimal sclerosis and epiphyseal radiolucency are evident. B The radiograph reveals lysis in the medial aspect of the metaphysis of the humerus (arrow). Diaphyseal periostitis also is seen.

zones in the metaphysis can lead to fracture or epiphyseal displacement.

Radiodense metaphyseal bands may be noted adjacent to the areas of increased radiolucency, reflecting altered osteogenesis. Parallel radiodense growth recovery lines may be observed in 50 per cent of children with leukemia.

Transverse radiolucent bands may also be observed under the vertebral endplates. Growth disturbances in the spine may lead to platyspondyly, brachyspondyly, and wedge-shaped vertebrae.

Osteolytic Lesions (30 to 50 Per Cent) (Figs. 57–2 and 57–3). Multiple (or solitary) radiolucent lesions related to bone destruction are encountered in tubular and flat bones. Similar lesions are seen in the cranial vault, pelvis, ribs, and shoulder girdle. The medial cortex of the proximal portion of the humerus is a characteristic site of involvement.

Periostitis (10 to 35 Per Cent) (Figs. 57–2 and 57–3). Periosteal bone formation can be associated with lytic lesions. Proliferating leukemic cells in the marrow invade the cortex via haversian canals and extend to subperiosteal locations, causing elevation of the periosteal membrane. Periostitis is particularly prominent in the long bones.

Osteosclerosis (5 to 10 Per Cent). Osteosclerosis is particularly prominent in the metaphyses of long bones.

OTHER SKELETAL ABNORMALITIES. Sutural diastasis is common in infants and children with leukemia (Fig. 57–4). It is produced by an increase in intracranial pressure owing to leukemic cell infiltration or intracerebral hemorrhage.

COURSE OF THE SKELETAL LESIONS. There is poor correlation between the extent of bone lesions and the progress of leukemia. During treatment, resolution of lytic defects is observed. Skeletal lesions may or may not reappear during relapse.

ARTICULAR ABNORMALITIES. The joint manifestations of acute leukemia are due to intraarticular leukemic cell infiltration and hemorrhage and more commonly to periarticular bone lesions. Soft tissue swelling, effusion, and juxtaarticular osteoporosis are occasionally seen.

Patients with acute leukemia often develop hyperuricemia, and a few individuals may reveal findings of secondary gout. This complication appears more frequent in chronic leukemia.

Epiphyseal osteonecrosis may occur in some patients, particularly those treated with steroid medication. Septic arthritis and osteomyelitis also can complicate the acute leukemias both in children and in adults.

Figure 57–2. Acute childhood leukemia: Dactylitis. Soft tissue swelling, lytic foci, and periosteal bone formation are observed in the metacarpals, metatarsals, and phalanges (arrows).

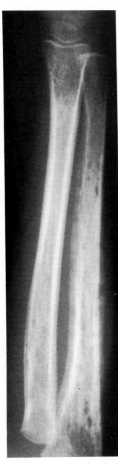

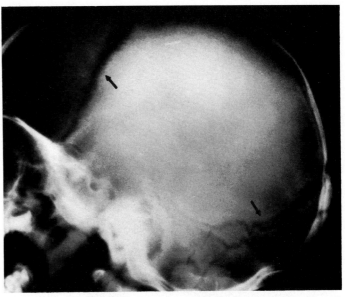

Figure 57–4. Acute childhood leukemia: Sutural diastasis. In an infant with leukemia, observe widening of the sutures in both the frontal and the occipital regions (arrows).

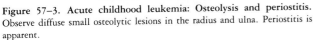

Figure 57–3. Acute childhood leukemia: Osteolysis and periostitis. Observe diffuse small osteolytic lesions in the radius and ulna. Periostitis is apparent.

DIFFERENTIAL DIAGNOSIS. Metaphyseal radiolucency is a nonspecific finding that may also be encountered in systemic childhood illnesses, including transplacental infections (toxoplasmosis, rubella, cytomegalic inclusion disease, herpes, syphilis), scurvy, juvenile chronic polyarthritis, healing rickets, and neuroblastoma. Osteolysis and periostitis, observed in acute leukemia, also are evident in sickle cell anemia, skeletal metastasis (especially from retinoblastoma and embryonal rhabdomyosarcoma), infection, and syphilis.

Acute Adult Leukemia

As a general rule, clinical and radiologic evidence of skeletal involvement in leukemia is less common in adults than in children. Acute leukemia in adults may be associated with bone pain and tenderness, however. Skeletal pain and tenderness are most frequent in the vertebral column and ribs.

The radiographic features in the skeleton in acute adult leukemia are diffuse osteopenia, discrete osteolytic lesions, and metaphyseal radiolucency. Lytic lesions (50 to 60 per cent) may be evident in the skull, pelvis, and proximal long bones. Metaphyseal radiolucent bands are not so frequent as in children with acute leukemia. Rare radiologic findings are large destructive lesions, periostitis, and focal or diffuse osteosclerosis.

Chronic Leukemia

The osseous and articular manifestations of chronic leukemia are less common and less severe than those of acute leukemia. Marrow hyperplasia in some patients may become evident as nonspecific diffuse osteopenia, particularly in the axial skeleton. Discrete osteolytic lesions are observed in fewer than 3 per cent of persons, particularly in the femur and the humerus (Fig. 57–5). Occasionally larger lesions may be encountered. Rarely, widespread or multifocal bone sclerosis is evident, perhaps related to diffuse marrow fibrosis. Soft tissue accumulation of masses of leukemic cells (chloromas) can produce subjacent osseous erosion.

In adults (and in children), leukemic involvement of the small bones of the hand may be associated with soft tissue edema, clubbing, and bone destruction. This combination of findings is termed leukemic acropachy or dactylitis (Fig. 57–2).

Articular findings in chronic leukemia have received little attention. Polyarticular involvement is more frequent than monoarticular involvement. Clinical findings commonly are a late manifestation of the disease and show a predilection for the knees, the shoulders, and the ankles. Osteopenia and soft tissue swelling may be evident on radiographs. As in acute leukemia, leukemic cellular infiltration of the synovium may be seen.

Secondary gout is a well known complication of chronic leukemia. Septic arthritis and osteomyelitis also may be evident.

Special Types of Leukemia

HAIRY CELL LEUKEMIA. This disorder, which is also termed leukemic reticuloendotheliosis, is responsible for approximately 2 per cent of all cases of leukemia. Its name

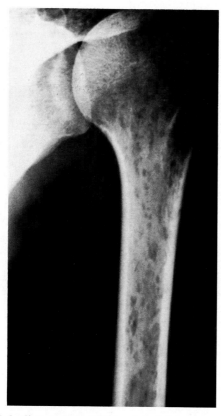

Figure 57–5. Chronic leukemia: Osteolytic lesions. Note small focal radiolucent lesions of the proximal portion of the humerus.

reflects the presence of numerous short villi, resembling hairs, about the membrane of the lymphocytes. The major clinical consequences of the disease relate to depressed bone marrow function and hypersplenism.

Hairy cell leukemia typically develops in adults in the fourth, fifth, and sixth decades of life. Men are affected more commonly than women. An insidious onset is characterized by fatigue, weakness, infectious episodes, abdominal pain, splenic rupture, and a pathologic fracture of bone. Splenomegaly, hepatomegaly, and lymphadenopathy are present, in order of decreasing frequency. The disease is slowly progressive, but most patients die in the first 5 years. The most frequent complication and primary source of morbidity and mortality is infection.

Bone involvement is an infrequent feature of hairy cell leukemia. Solitary or, less commonly, multiple osteolytic lesions are typical, with predilection for the spine and proximal portion of the femora. Bone sclerosis is rare. Spontaneous fracture is a recognized complication of such lesions. Infrequent manifestations are osteoporosis and ischemic necrosis of the femoral head. Radiation therapy and chemotherapy can lead to a decrease in symptoms and regression of the osteolytic process.

ACUTE MEGAKARYOBLASTIC LEUKEMIA. In this rare disorder, also termed malignant myelofibrosis, children and adults are affected with an acute clinical onset and a progressive course characterized by anemia, pancytopenia, and diffuse marrow fibrosis. The proliferating cells in the bone marrow are variable in type, immature, and dominated by megakaryocytes.

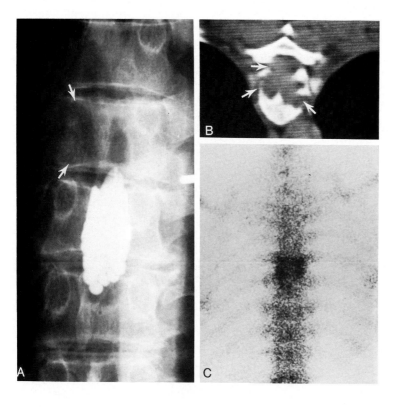

Figure 57–6. Granulocytic sarcoma (chloroma). A frontal radiograph of the thoracic spine after a myelogram (**A**) reveals osteolysis in a midthoracic vertebral body and destruction of a pedicle (arrows). A partial obstruction to the flow of the contrast material is evident. In **B**, a computed tomographic image (accomplished with the patient in the prone position) shows the degree of bone destruction and intraspinal extension (arrows). Accumulation of the bone-seeking radiopharmaceutical agent is evident (**C**).

Table 57–2. CLASSIFICATION OF LYMPHOMAS

New System	Old System
Non-Hodgkin's lymphoma	
Lymphocytic type	Lymphosarcoma
Histiocytic type	Reticulum cell sarcoma
Mixed lymphocytic-histiocytic type	Mixed lymphoma
Pleomorphic (undifferentiated) type	Stem cell lymphoma
Burkitt's tumor	Stem cell lymphoma
Hodgkin's disease	
Mycosis fungoides	

In children, radiolucency in the metaphyseal regions of tubular bones, periostitis, and osteolytic lesions are seen. In adults, focal or diffuse bone sclerosis is observed.

GRANULOCYTIC SARCOMA (CHLOROMA). Granulocytic sarcoma represents a localized tumor mass composed of immature cells of the granulocyte series. The term chloroma stems from the frequently observed greenish color of the tumor. Granulocytic sarcoma is associated most commonly with acute leukemia of the myeloid type, especially in children, although it is also observed in adults (Fig. 57–6) and in patients with additional varieties of leukemia, with other myeloproliferative disorders, or without obvious bone marrow dysfunction.

Granulocytic sarcomas may be single or multiple. Frequent sites of involvement are bone, periosteum, soft tissue, orbit, lymph node, and skin. Lytic lesions characterize intraosseous involvement, which is especially prominent in the skull, spine, ribs, and sternum. Soft tissue tumors can lead to masses that may erode the neighboring bone.

LYMPHOMAS
General Features

A variety of diseases are grouped together as lymphoreticular neoplasms, including non-Hodgkin's lymphoma, Hodgkin's lymphoma, Burkitt's lymphoma, and mycosis fungoides. The classification of such diseases is complicated and debated (Table 57–2).

The distribution of lymphoreticular tumors in the body's tissues and organ systems is highly variable. Some of these neoplasms arise in extraskeletal sites, appearing as single or multiple tumors in the lymph nodes, spleen, or gastrointestinal tract. From these locations, abnormal cells may circulate in the blood and lodge in distant sites, such as the bone marrow. Lymphomatous involvement of the skeleton may result from such dissemination. Alternatively, lymphoreticular neoplasms may arise as a primary process of bone, an occurrence that accounts for approximately 5 per cent of all primary malignant osseous tumors. The majority of cases originating in bone result from diffuse histiocytic lymphoma, and the disease is observed in older patients and in men more frequently than in women.

Skeletal abnormalities may be identified in 5 to 50 per cent of cases. In general, it has been observed that the more immature the cell composing the lesion, the greater the frequency of bone involvement.

As the prognosis of lymphoreticular neoplasms is intimately related to the extent of disease, evaluation must include a search for sites of involvement, a process called staging, using clinical and laboratory examinations supplemented with imaging and nonimaging techniques. The precise role of computed tomography and magnetic resonance imaging in this staging process is not yet clear, although both methods show promise in the detection of lympadenopathy. A truly primary bone lesion is considered stage I non-Hodgkin's lymphoma, whereas a bone lesion associated with disease in other sites is considered stage IV.

Skeletal Abnormalities

NON-HODGKIN'S LYMPHOMA. Involvement of bone in non-Hodgkin's lymphoma is more commonly a manifestation of diffuse disease than a primary lesion. Estimates of the prevalance of skeletal alterations in widespread non-Hodgkin's lymphoma are 10 to 20 per cent in adults and 20 to 30 per cent in children. In the disseminated form, abnormalities of the axial skeleton predominate. Hematogenous spread of tumor is responsible for most of these lesions, although alterations can develop as a result of osseous invasion from surrounding soft tissues and lymph nodes. Multiple osteolytic lesions with motheaten or permeative bone destruction are most common (Fig. 57–7). Periostitis is less frequent and severe than in Hodgkin's disease. On rare occasions, localized or diffuse osteosclerosis is evident.

Primary non-Hodgkin's lymphoma occurs at any age and affects men more frequently than women. The lesions predominate in the bones of the appendicular skeleton (Fig. 57–8). An osteolytic lesion with poorly defined margins in the metaphyseal region of a tubular bone is most typical. Pathologic fractures and soft tissue masses are common.

HODGKIN'S DISEASE. Skeletal involvement in Hodgkin's disease is quite common, being detectable on radiographs in 10 to 25 per cent of cases. Bone abnormalities are more common in adults than in children. Tumor may reach the osseous tissue through either hematogenous dissemination or

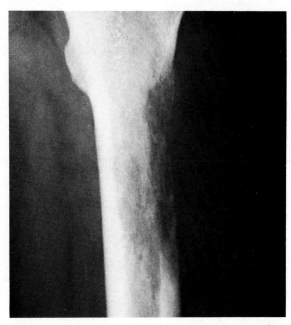

Figure 57–7. Non-Hodgkin's lymphoma: Histiocytic type—disseminated disease. Observe an eccentric diaphyseal lesion of the femur with motheaten bone destruction and cortical violation.

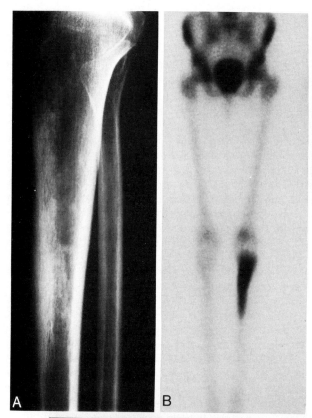

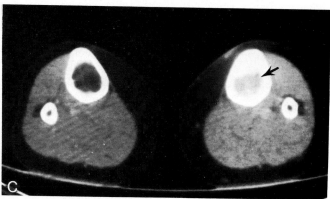

Figure 57–8. Non-Hodgkin's lymphoma: Histiocytic type—primary bone involvement. **A** A lateral radiograph shows a lesion with both osteolysis and osteosclerosis in the diaphysis of the tibia. **B** A bone scan documents increased accumulation of the radionuclide at the site of radiographic abnormality. **C** On a transverse section through the lesion, computed tomography shows increased radiodensity in the medullary canal of the affected tibia (arrow). Compare to the opposite side. **D, E** Magnetic resonance imaging with both T1 and T2 weighted coronal displays shows the proximal extent of the tumor (arrows). Biopsy confirmed the presence of histiocytic lymphoma. No other organ systems were involved. (Courtesy of G. Greenway, M.D., Dallas, Texas.)

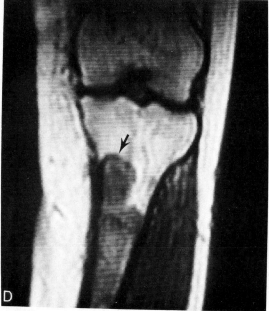

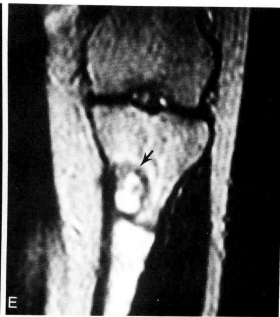

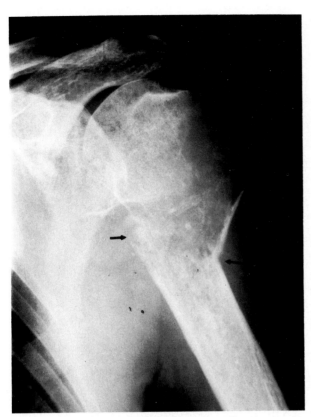

Figure 57–9. Hodgkin's disease: Extraspinal manifestations. A large osteolytic lesion of the proximal portion of the humerus has resulted in a pathologic fracture (arrows).

direct spread from contiguous involved lymph nodes. The most common sites of involvement are the spine, pelvis, ribs, femora, and sternum. Multiple lesions occur with a slightly greater frequency than solitary lesions.

Osteosclerosis alone, osteolysis alone, or osteosclerosis combined with osteolysis can be evident (Figs. 57–9 and 57–10). The reported frequency of sclerotic lesions varies from 14 per cent to 45 per cent. Diffuse sclerosis of the vertebral body, an ivory vertebra, is similar to that observed in other lymphomas, skeletal metastasis, and Paget's disease. Widespread osteosclerosis may result from an osseous response to extensive bone marrow involvement or bone marrow fibrosis.

The prognosis of Hodgkin's disease depends on its histologic type.

BURKITT'S LYMPHOMA. This disease is a stem cell lymphoma that is seen predominantly in children. It is the most common malignant disease of children in tropical Africa. Involvement of facial bones is particularly characteristic. Early radiographic changes include loss of the lamina dura and diminution and obscuration of trabeculae in the cancellous bone. With disruption of the cortex, a soft tissue mass may extend into the buccal cavity or maxillary antrum.

Lesions in the tubular bones and pelvis have been described but are less frequent. Osteolytic foci develop in the medullary portion of the bone, penetrate the cortex, produce periostitis, and lead to a soft tissue mass. They are commonly multiple and even symmetric in distribution.

MYCOSIS FUNGOIDES. Mycosis fungoides is considered an unusual form of malignant lymphoma with primary involvement of the skin. Its onset is in the fourth or fifth decade of life and it affects men more frequently than women. Cutaneous lesions may be associated with localized or generalized lymphadenopathy, and extracutaneous manifestations with visceral involvement may become evident. The lungs, spleen, liver, kidneys, thyroid gland, heart, brain, muscle and spinal cord may be affected. After dissemination, death commonly occurs within a few years.

Bone marrow involvement is rare. When present, bone lesions occur in the appendicular skeleton, with discrete or poorly defined medullary defects, cortical destruction, periostitis, and soft tissue swelling. Although the skeletal abnormalities are similar to other aggressive lesions such as metastasis and plasma cell myeloma, involvement of the peripheral skeleton including the hands may be a helpful clue in the diagnosis of mycosis fungoides.

The leukemic phase of this disease is termed Sézary syndrome. It is a malignant syndrome characterized by generalized erythroderma, splenomegaly, lymphadenopathy, and leukocytosis, which may lead to death within 5 years of its onset.

Rheumatologic Abnormalities

In the malignant lymphomas, joint symptoms referable to bone lesions are seldom prominent. Cellular infiltration in the synovium can lead to effusion and soft tissue swelling.

Secondary gout is observed in some patients with malignant lymphomas. Hypertrophic osteoarthropathy with its articular symptoms and signs may also be seen.

Effects of Therapy

The association of ischemic necrosis of bone and the treatment of lymphoma with combination chemotherapy regimens that include intermittent corticosteroids has been reported on numerous occasions. The frequency of this complication in treated patients is approximately 1 to 3 per cent in Hodgkin's disease and somewhat lower in non-Hodgkin's lymphoma. Typically, ischemic necrosis of bone occurs 1 to 3 years after the initiation of the therapy. The femoral head and, less commonly, the humeral head are preferred sites of involvement. The precise cause of ischemic necrosis in these individuals is not known.

A second complication of therapy in leukemia and, less typically, in lymphoma is related to the administration of methotrexate. Skeletal changes, which usually occur 6 to 18 months after institution of the therapy and which are termed methotrexate osteopathy, are characterized by pain, osteopenia, growth recovery lines, dense metaphyseal bands, and fractures. The clinical and radiologic findings subside after withdrawal of the chemotherapeutic agent. The cause of methotrexate osteopathy is not known, although it may be related to the drug's interference with folic acid metabolism.

Other Lymphomas and Lymphoproliferative Disorders

GIANT FOLLICLE LYMPHOMA (BRILL-SYMMERS DISEASE). Brill-Symmers disease was originally described as a benign form of lymphoma leading to enlarged lymph nodes. Subsequently, it has become apparent that malignant transformation may occur, leading to the patient's demise. Although skeletal involvement is infrequent in the early stage of the process, unusual osseous abnormalities have been

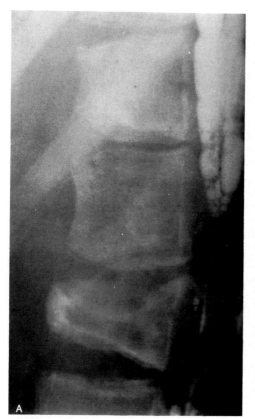 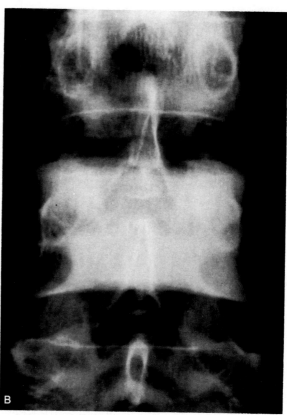

Figure 57–10. Hodgkin's disease: Spinal manifestations. A On a lateral radiograph of the thoracolumbar junction, observe patchy sclerosis and lucency of multiple vertebral bodies with destruction and collapse. A myelogram had been accomplished previously. **B** In a different patient, a frontal radiograph reveals an ivory vertebra. Note the homogeneous increase in radiodensity of the vertebral body without osseous enlargement.

described later in its course. Grossly destructive osteolytic lesions are seen, especially in the hands and feet (Fig. 57–11).

SJÖGREN'S SYNDROME
General Features

The classic triad of Sjögren's syndrome is keratoconjunctivitis sicca (dry eyes), xerostomia (dry mouth), and rheumatoid arthritis. The diagnosis is established by the presence of two of the three major components.

Clinical Abnormalities

The disease is more common in women than in men. The average age at the time of presentation is 40 to 50 years. Clinical manifestations of eye involvement include pain, a gritty sensation, redness, fatigue, photosensitivity, dryness, itching, decreased vision, and difficulties in moving the eyelids. Oral and salivary gland involvement leads to dryness of the lips and mouth, difficulty with mastication and swallowing, ulcerations of the buccal membranes, lips, and tongue, and poor dentition. Parotid gland enlargement is evident in approximately 50 per cent of patients.

Articular symptoms and signs may or may not be present. When apparent, the clinical manifestations are almost invariably those of rheumatoid arthritis. Subcutaneous nodules are apparent in approximately 60 per cent of patients with arthritis.

Additional manifestations of Sjögren's syndrome include Raynaud's phenomenon (20 per cent), splenomegaly and leukopenia suggestive of Felty's syndrome, infections, vasculitis, peripheral neuropathy, glomerulonephritis, and purpura.

Radiologic Abnormalities

The major articular findings are those of rheumatoid arthritis with soft tissue swelling, periarticular osteoporosis, marginal erosions, joint space narrowing, and intraarticular cystic lesions (Fig. 57–12). Typical target sites of rheumatoid arthritis are affected.

Pathologic Abnormalities

Pathologic examination reveals lymphocyte and plasma cell infiltration of salivary and lacrimal glands and other tissues, including muscle, and the mucous glands of the respiratory tract, oral cavity, and upper esophagus. In joints, the findings are similar to those of rheumatoid arthritis.

SYSTEMIC MASTOCYTOSIS
General Features

Systemic mastocytosis is a rare proliferative disorder of mast cells, affecting both men and women and beginning in

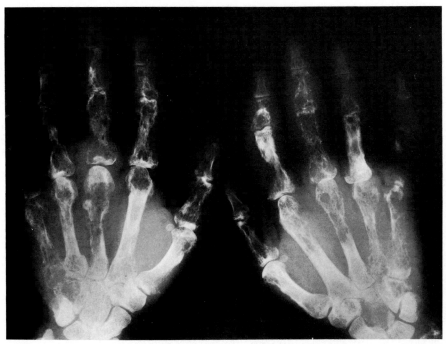

Figure 57–11. Giant follicle lymphoma (Brill-Symmers disease). In this unusual example, diffuse involvement in both hands is characterized by osteolysis, bone expansion, and soft tissue swelling. The findings resemble those of sarcoidosis. (Courtesy of R. Reichman, M.D., Los Angeles, California.)

adult life. Multiple organ systems may be altered, including the liver, the spleen, the lymph nodes, and the skeleton, although it is cutaneous involvement that is most common and characteristic. Skin or mucous membrane lesions resemble urticaria pigmentosa of childhood. This latter disease usually develops in infancy or early childhood, whereas systemic mastocytosis generally has an onset after puberty.

The clinical features relate, in part, to histamine release with local urticaria, flushing, shock-like episodes, diarrhea, and vomiting. In more severe cases, weight loss, weakness, malaise, hepatosplenomegaly, lymphadenopathy, and peptic ulcer disease are encountered. Hematologic abnormalities include anemia, leukopenia, thrombocytopenia, and eosinophilia. Hemorrhagic tendencies reflect the presence of both thrombocytopenia and prothrombin deficiency. Hepatic dysfunction occurs owing to mast cell proliferation and periportal fibrosis. The prognosis is variable, depending on the extent of systemic involvement. With extensive abnormalities of the reticuloendothelial system, death may occur within a few years.

Skeletal Abnormalities

Mast cell proliferation in skeletal tissue may be clinically silent, although pain, tenderness, soft tissue mass, and deformity secondary to pathologic fracture can be observed. Mast cell infiltration into the bone marrow stimulates fibroblastic activity and granulomatous reaction, which lead to trabecular destruction and replacement with adjacent new bone formation. This infiltration accounts for significant radiographic abnormalities, which can be classified into two types: osteopenia and bone destruction; and osteosclerosis

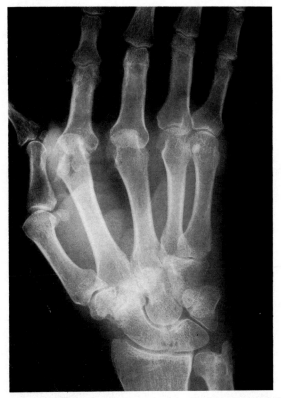

Figure 57–12. Sjögren's syndrome: Associated rheumatoid arthritis. Typical abnormalities of the hand and wrist indicate the presence of rheumatoid arthritis. Observe marginal erosions in the wrist and the metacarpophalangeal and proximal interphalangeal joints of the hand. Soft tissue swelling and subluxations are also evident.

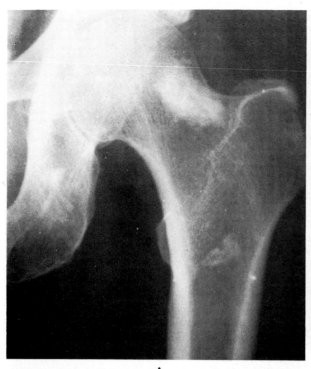

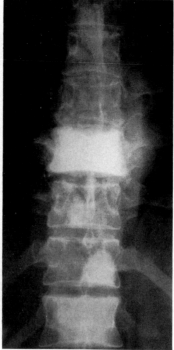

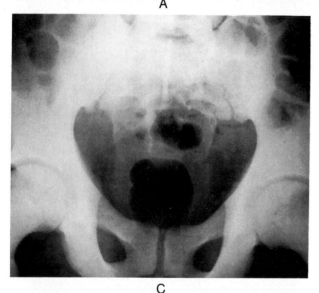

A

B

C

Figure 57–13. Mastocytosis: Radiographic abnormalities. A note radiodense foci of variable size in the proximal femur and ischium. B A frontal radiograph of the thoracic spine delineates focal osteosclerotic lesions of the vertebrae with paravertebral swelling. An ivory vertebra has resulted. C Diffuse osteosclerosis of the entire pelvis and proximal femora is evident. Note the chalk-like appearance.

(Fig. 57–13). In either type, a focal or diffuse distribution may be seen. Diffuse lesions predominate in the axial skeleton, whereas focal lesions occur in both the axial and the appendicular skeleton.

OSTEOPENIA AND BONE DESTRUCTION. Diffuse osteopenia or multiple lytic lesions may be observed in systemic mastocytosis. Generalized rarefaction simulates the appearance of osteoporosis and is most frequent in the skull, the pelvis, the spine, and the ribs. It may relate to the effects of heparin or prostaglandin, known by-products of mast cells. Discrete lytic lesions represent areas of osseous resorption, perhaps related to pressure atrophy of trabeculae from adjacent mast cell accumulations. They tend to be small in size, poorly or well defined, and surrounded by a "halo" of sclerosis. These circumscribed lytic defects are most common in the pelvis, the skull, and the tubular bones.

OSTEOSCLEROSIS. Focal or diffuse bone sclerosis is another radiographic pattern in systemic mastocytosis, which may appear in combination with osteolysis. Focal sclerotic lesions may be misinterpreted as skeletal metastases. Diffuse osteosclerosis may resemble that seen in myelofibrosis, fluorosis, sickle cell anemia, Paget's disease, and skeletal metastasis.

Differential Diagnosis

The skeletal manifestations of systemic mastocytosis are nonspecific (Table 57–3). Diffuse osteopenia in this disease is almost identical to that in osteoporosis, osteomalacia, hyperparathyroidism, and plasma cell myeloma. Diffuse cystic lesions in systemic mastocytosis can simulate the appearance of osteoporosis, sickle cell anemia, Gaucher's disease, and plasma cell myeloma. Diffuse osteosclerosis is observed not only in systemic mastocytosis but also in myelofibrosis, skeletal metastasis, fluorosis, Paget's disease, and renal osteodystrophy, as well as numerous other conditions. Multiple focal osteosclerotic lesions in systemic mastocytosis resemble the findings in skeletal metastasis and tuberous sclerosis.

POLYCYTHEMIA VERA
General Features

Polycythemia vera (primary polycythemia) is a disease of unknown cause that is characterized by hyperplasia of all of the cellular elements in the bone marrow, resulting in elevated red blood cell count, leukocytosis, and thrombocytosis. Polycythemia vera occurs in middle-aged or elderly patients, predominantly men. Clinical complaints include headache, dizziness, weakness, fatigue, paresthesias, dyspnea, and visual disturbances. On physical examination, a ruddy complexion,

Table 57–3. DIFFERENTIAL DIAGNOSIS OF OSTEOSCLEROSIS*

	Skeletal Metastasis	Mastocytosis	Myelofibrosis	Lymphomas	Paget's Disease	Fluorosis	Renal Osteo-dystrophy	Axial Osteo-malacia
Distribution	Axial > appendicular	Axial > appendicular	Axial > appendicular	Axial > appendicular	Axial > appendicular	Axial > appendicular	Axial > appendicular	Axial
Diffuse sclerosis	+	+	+	+	+	+	+	+
Focal sclerosis	+	+	−	+	+	−	−	−
Osteopenia or bone lysis	+	+	+	+	+	−	+	−
Bone enlargement	−	−	−	−	+	−	−	−
Osteophytosis, ligament ossification	−	−	−	−	−	+	−	−
Splenomegaly	−	+	+	+	−	−	−	−

*+, Common; −, uncommon or rare.

hepatosplenomegaly, and systolic hypertension are seen. Vascular thrombosis and bleeding are recognized complications of the disease. The disorder is compatible with many years of life.

Musculoskeletal Abnormalities

There are few musculoskeletal manifestations of this disease. Vascular thrombosis can lead to osteonecrosis, and generalized marrow hyperplasia can produce patchy radiolucent lesions. Myelofibrosis is associated with generalized increased radiodensity of the skeleton.

Hyperuricemia is not infrequent in (primary) polycythemia vera or in secondary polycythemia. Gouty arthritis has been estimated to occur in 5 to 8 per cent of all cases.

MYELOFIBROSIS
General Features

Myelofibrosis is an uncommon disease associated with fibrotic or sclerotic bone marrow and extramedullary hematopoiesis. A variety of names have been applied to this syndrome, including agnogenic myeloid metaplasia and myelosclerosis. The cause of the disorder has not been precisely determined.

It has been popular to divide myelofibrosis into two forms: primary or idiopathic and secondary. The basic pathologic finding in either form is fibrosis of the bone marrow. Focal or diffuse areas of hypercellular marrow may be combined with trabecular thickening and overgrowth. Simultaneously, proliferation of potential bone marrow elements occurs in the spleen, the liver, the lymph nodes, and the long bones (as well as the kidneys, the lungs, and other organs).

Clinical Abnormalities

Myelofibrosis generally is an insidious disease of middle-aged and elderly men and women. Symptoms include weakness, fatigue, weight loss, abdominal pain, anorexia, nausea, vomiting, and dyspnea. Physical signs may include abdominal swelling, hepatosplenomegaly, and purpura. Hematologic evaluation frequently reveals anemia, an increased number of nucleated red blood cells, leukocytosis or leukopenia, abnormal white blood cells, and elevated, normal, or low platelet counts. The diagnosis is established by bone marrow biopsy. The prognosis of the disease is variable. Some patients expire within a few months of the initial diagnosis, whereas others survive for a prolonged period of time.

Musculoskeletal Abnormalities

The radiographic picture reflects the presence of marrow fibrosis at sites of active hematopoiesis. In some instances, normal or osteopenic bone and osteolytic lesions are observed, but, in general, osteosclerosis is the predominant radiographic pattern, evident in both the axial skeleton and the proximal portions of the long bones (Fig. 57–14). The bones most commonly altered are the spine, the pelvis, the skull, the ribs, and the proximal ends of the humerus and femur. The osseous structures may be uniformly dense or demonstrate small areas of relative radiolucency. In the long bones, cortical thickening can be observed, owing predominantly to endosteal sclerosis. This results in obliteration of the normal demarcation between cortical and medullary bone. Periostitis is not prominent. In the spine, increased radiodensity or condensation of bone at the superior and inferior margins of the vertebral body (sandwich vertebrae) can be encountered. Focal or diffuse sclerosis in the skull may be evident.

Extramedullary hematopoiesis in this condition can create lobulated, paravertebral intrathoracic masses. Spinal cord compression from this abnormal tissue has been identified.

Articular Abnormalities

Bone and joint pain in both spinal and extraspinal sites can be evident. Hemarthrosis has been described in association with myeloproliferative disease and can be its presenting manifestation.

Fifty to 80 per cent of patients with myelofibrosis reveal elevated serum or urinary uric acid levels. Secondary gout, which may antedate the diagnosis of myelofibrosis, occurs in 5 to 20 per cent of patients.

Differential Diagnosis

The radiographic diagnosis of myelofibrosis should be suggested when axial skeleton osteosclerosis is combined with splenomegaly in a middle-aged or elderly patient (Table 57–3). Although lymphoma and leukemia can lead to splenomegaly, the extent of bone sclerosis is less in these conditions than in myelofibrosis. Systemic mastocytosis can produce diffuse or focal osteosclerosis and hepatosplenomegaly, and it may be difficult to differentiate from myelofibrosis.

Increased radiodensity of bone without splenic enlargement can be seen in some patients with myelofibrosis and is apparent in patients with this disorder who have had splenectomies.

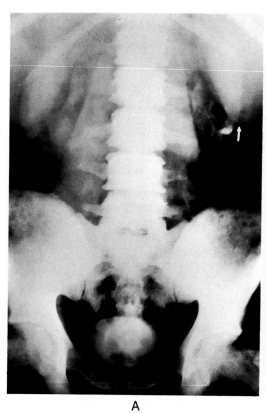

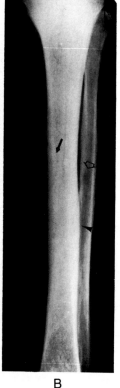

A   B

Figure 57–14. Myelofibrosis: Radiographic abnormalities.
A Observe widespread and uniform sclerosis of the pelvis and spine on an abdominal radiograph obtained during intravenous pyelography. The renal function is obviously diminished and the spleen is enlarged (arrow). **B** An anteroposterior radiograph of the tibia and fibula outlines increased radiodensity of bone caused predominantly by endosteal sclerosis (arrow), although there is evidence of periostitis as well (arrowhead). Focal lucent areas are also apparent (open arrow).

This combination of findings can be evident in other processes, including skeletal metastasis, fluorosis, Paget's disease, axial osteomalacia, and renal osteodystrophy. In general, the sclerosis observed in metastatic disease of the bone is less generalized, less symmetric, and more frequently associated with osteolytic lesions. In fluorosis, spinal osteophytosis, ligament calcification and ossification, and periostitis can be noted. In renal osteodystrophy, other changes, including those of hyperparathyroidism, are evident. In Paget's disease there is a characteristic coarsened trabecular pattern, whereas axial osteomalacia is confined to the axial skeleton and is associated with very prominent cervical spine abnormalities.

FURTHER READING

Bloch KJ, Buchanan WW, Whol MJ, Bunim JJ: Sjögren's syndrome. A clinical, pathological and serological study of sixty-two cases. Medicine 44:187, 1965.

Braunstein EM, White SJ: Non-Hodgkin lymphoma of bone. Radiology 135:59, 1980.

Coles WC, Schulz MD: Bone involvement in malignant lymphoma. Radiology 50:458, 1948.

Dalinka MK: Primary lymphoma of bone: Radiographic appearance and prognosis. Radiology 147:288, 1983.

Demanes DJ, Lane N, Beckstead JH: Bone involvement in hairy-cell leukemia. Cancer 49:1697, 1982.

Ferris RA, Hakkai HG, Cigtay OS: Radiologic manifestations of North American Burkitt's lymphoma. AJR 123:614, 1975.

Glatt W, Weinstein A: Acropachy in lymphatic leukemia. Radiology 92:125, 1969.

Leigh TF, Corley CC Jr, Huguley CM Jr, Rogers JV Jr: Myelofibrosis. The general and radiologic findings in 25 proven cases. AJR 82:183, 1959.

McKenna MJ, Frame B: The mast cell and bone. Clin Orthop 200:226, 1985.

Neiman RS, Barcos M, Berard C, Bonner H, Mann R, Rydell RE, Bennett JM: Granulocytic sarcoma: A clinicopathologic study of 61 biopsied cases. Cancer 48:1426, 1981.

Nixon GW, Gwinn JL: The roentgen manifestations of leukemia in infancy. Radiology 107:603, 1973.

Olson DO, Shields AF, Scheurich CJ, Porter BA, Moss AA: Magnetic resonance imaging of the bone marrow in patients with leukemia, aplastic anemia, and lymphoma. Invest Radiol 21:540, 1986.

O'Reilly GV, Clark TM, Crum CP: Skeletal involvement in mycosis fungoides. AJR 129:741, 1977.

Parker BR, Marglin S, Castellino RA: Skeletal manifestations of leukemia, Hodgkin disease and non-Hodgkin lymphoma. Semin Roentgenol 15:302, 1980.

Pettigrew JD, Ward HP: Correlation of radiologic, histologic and clinical findings in agnogenic myeloid metaplasia. Radiology 93:541, 1969.

Phillips WC, Kattapuram SV, Doseretz DE, Raymond AK, Schiller AL, Murphy G, Wyshak G: Primary lymphoma of bone: Relationship of radiographic appearance and prognosis. Radiology 144:285, 1982.

Poppel MH, Gruber WF, Silber R, Holder AK, Christman RO: The roentgen manifestations of urticaria pigmentosa (mastocytosis). AJR 82:239, 1959.

Rafii M, Firooznia H, Golimbu C, Balthazar E: Pathologic fracture in systemic mastocytosis. Radiographic spectrum and review of the literature. Clin Orthop 180:260, 1983.

Schabel SI, Tyminski L, Holland RD, Rittenberg GM: The skeletal manifestations of chronic myelogenous leukemia. Skel Radiol 5:145, 1980.

Schwartz AM, Leonidas JC: Methotrexate osteopathy. Skel Radiol 11:13, 1984.

Simmons CR, Harle TS, Singleton EB: The osseous manifestations of leukemia in children. Radiol Clin North Am 6:115, 1968.

Silbiger ML, Peterson CC Jr: Sjögren's syndrome. Its roentgenographic features. AJR 100:554, 1967.

Talbott JH: Gout and blood dyscrasias. Medicine 38:173, 1959.

Chapter 58

Bleeding Disorders

Donald Resnick, M.D.

The skeletal abnormalities associated with hemophilia and other bleeding diatheses result from hemorrhage in soft tissue, muscle, subperiosteal, intraosseous, and intraarticular locations. In involved joints, typical findings are radiodense effusions, regional or periarticular osteoporosis, subchondral bone erosions and cysts, and joint space narrowing. Hyperemia may lead to epiphyseal overgrowth in a child affected by these disorders. Tumor-like lesions may occasionally be encountered owing to massive subperiosteal, osseous, or soft tissue hemorrhage with erosion and distortion of adjacent bone. The differential diagnosis generally is not difficult when both clinical and radiologic features are studied.

Hemophilia is a term applied to a group of disorders characterized by an anomaly of blood coagulation resulting from a deficiency of a specific plasma clotting factor. This anomaly leads to easy bruising and prolonged and excessive bleeding. Of this group of disorders, two are associated most commonly with intraosseous and intraarticular bleeding: classic hemophilia (hemophilia A), in which there is a functional deficiency of antihemophilic factor (AHF), factor VIII; and Christmas disease (hemophilia B), in which there is a functional deficiency of plasma thromboplastin component (PTC), factor IX. These two types of hemophilia are X-linked recessive disorders that are manifested clinically in men and carried by women. Rarely, other disorders of blood coagulation may become manifest as bone and joint abnormalities. Furthermore, additional diseases, including the Klippel-Trenaunay-Weber and Kasabach-Merritt syndromes, may lead to osteoarticular manifestations that simulate those of hemophilia.

HEMOPHILIA

Clinical Abnormalities

Classic hemophilia occurs in approximately 1 in every 10,000 males in the United States. Christmas disease occurs about one tenth as often as classic hemophilia. Although both forms are confined almost exclusively to males, reports exist of significant clinical abnormalities appearing in female patients. The severity of the clinical manifestations of either form of hemophilia varies. In mild forms of disease, excessive bleeding may be apparent only during surgery. With moderate or severe forms of the disease, bleeding episodes also may occur spontaneously or after minor trauma. The diagnosis is established by performing appropriate laboratory tests to detect defects in blood coagulation.

Hemarthrosis occurs in approximately 75 to 90 per cent of patients with hemophilia. It is not uncommon for the first episode of joint hemorrhage to occur between the ages of 2 and 3 years. The most commonly altered joints are the knee, the elbow, the ankle, the hip, and the shoulder, in descending order of frequency. One episode of hemarthrosis predisposes the affected joint to another episode. Usually a single joint is involved in each episode, although eventually, multiple articulations are affected in this disease.

Clinical manifestations of hemophilic arthropathy can be divided into three types: acute, subacute, and chronic hemarthrosis.

1. *Acute hemarthrosis.* Joint bleeding may occur rapidly, producing a swollen and tender joint. Fever and leukocytosis are found. Symptoms decrease quickly after administration of appropriate clotting factor.

2. *Subacute hemarthrosis.* After two or more acute episodes, complete recovery of the joint is not evident. Periarticular swelling, restricted joint motion, muscle atrophy, and contractures become evident.

3. *Chronic hemarthrosis.* After subacute hemarthrosis has been present for 6 months to 1 year, severe and persistent contractures may be found, particularly in the elbow and the knee. Approximately 50 per cent of hemophilic patients develop permanent changes in the peripheral articulations, and only rarely do patients escape persistent deformity of any kind.

Articular bleeding may be accompanied by hemorrhage into muscles, fascial planes, and bones. Soft tissue bleeding can lead to fixed joint deformities and soft tissue necrosis. Volkmann's contractures relate to massive hemorrhage into the volar muscles of the forearm. Femoral neuropathy may be the result of hemorrhage into the iliopsoas muscle, and bleeding into the soleus or gastrocnemius muscle may lead to talipes equinus deformity. Common peroneal nerve entrapment in hemophilia has also been described. Hemorrhage in and around the spinal cord can lead to neurologic abnormalities. Subperiosteal and intraosseous bleeding can induce trabecular destruction, and large expansile lesions (hemophilic pseudotumors) may simulate neoplasm.

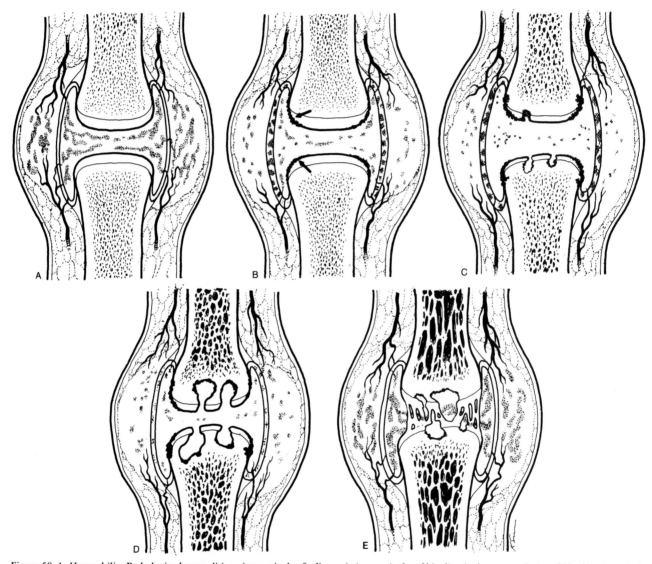

Figure 58–1. Hemophilia: Pathologic abnormalities—intraarticular findings. A Acute episodes of bleeding lead to accumulation of blood in the articular cavity and periarticular soft tissues. **B** After numerous bleeding episodes, absorption of blood is incomplete from the articular cavity and soft tissues. Brownish discoloration of the synovial membrane is associated with hypertrophy and hyperemia. Synovial inflammatory tissue or pannus appears at the margins of the articular cartilage (arrows). **C** At a later stage, periarticular osteoporosis and focal areas of cartilage and osseous destruction become apparent. Cystic lesions are evident, which generally communicate with the joint cavity. Note areas of relatively normal cartilage and bone. **D** Continued destruction of cartilage and bone leads to enlarging cystic lesions, surface irregularities, osteoporosis, and joint space narrowing. **E** In late stages of the disease, fibrous adhesions extend across the articular space. New episodes of bleeding occur.

Table 58–1. HEMOPHILIA: RADIOGRAPHIC-PATHOLOGIC CORRELATION

Pathology	Radiology
Recurrent intraarticular hemorrhage with hemosiderin-laden hypertrophied synovial membrane	Radiodense joint effusions
Synovial inflammation and pannus formation; hyperemia	Osteoporosis; epiphyseal overgrowth; accelerated skeletal maturation
Cartilaginous erosion; subchondral trabecular resorption and collapse	Bone erosions and cysts
Cartilaginous denudation	Joint space narrowing
Bone proliferation	Sclerosis and osteophytosis
Soft tissue, subperiosteal, and intraosseous hemorrhage	Pseudotumors

Pathologic Abnormalities

Characteristic pathologic abnormalities occur in hemophilia (Table 58–1) (Fig. 58–1). After an acute episode of intraarticular bleeding, blackish fluid containing clots is apparent in the articular cavity, embedded in the synovial membrane or adherent to the joint capsule and periarticular tissues. In the interval before the second bleed, these hemorrhagic collections may disappear. With each recurring episode of bleeding, resorption of blood is less complete.

Brownish discoloration of the synovial membrane is due to absorption of blood pigment. As a result of this absorption of hemosiderin, the synovial membrane demonstrates hypertrophy, hyperplasia, and increased vascularity. The altered synovial membrane appears as inflammatory tissue or pannus, which extends over the margins of the cartilage. Marginal cartilaginous erosion appears adjacent to synovial pannus, whereas more central defects may occur away from obvious synovial tissue. In either location, cartilaginous denudation may expose subchondral bone.

Subsequently, loss of the subchondral bone plate occurs. Trabecular thinning and resorption lead to enlarging marrow spaces, which may appear cystic. Subchondral cysts also represent sites of intraosseous hemorrhage. Osseous cystic lesions frequently are multiple and of varying size. Productive changes may appear, with sclerotic trabeculae and osteophytes.

Massive periosteal or intraosseous hemorrhage creates neoplastic-like lesions called hemophilic pseudotumors (Fig. 58–2). In subperiosteal locations, the periosteal membrane is lifted from the parent bone, and hemorrhage may extend into the adjacent soft tissues. Periosteal bone formation follows, creating expanded and irregular osseous contours. In intraosseous locations, large defects with well-defined bone destruction may be evident.

Radiographic Abnormalities

GENERAL FEATURES. It is convenient to divide the radiographic abnormalities of hemophilia into five stages on the basis of their severity: soft tissue swelling, osteoporosis, osseous lesions, cartilage destruction, and joint disorganiza-

tion. This division of the radiographic changes does not imply that all cases follow this sequence of events. In some patients, articular involvement may never progress beyond the first or second stage; in other patients, despite appropriate medical or surgical therapy, severe arthropathy develops.

DISTRIBUTION OF ABNORMALITIES. The knee, the ankle, and the elbow are the joints involved most frequently. Intraarticular bleeding distal to the elbows and the ankles is rare. Bilateral involvement is common.

Knee (Figs. 58–3 and 58–4). The knee is the joint affected most commonly in hemophilia. Dense joint effusions are common. Periarticular osteoporosis and irregularity of the articular surface of the femoral condyles, the tibial plateaus, and the posterior surface of the patella may become apparent. Multiple subchondral cysts are frequent.

Abnormalities of osseous shape have been emphasized in the diagnosis of hemophilia. Overgrowth of the distal femoral and proximal tibial epiphyses is seen. The distal condylar surface may appear flattened, and the intercondylar notch of the femur commonly is widened. The patella may demonstrate an abnormal "square" shape. It should be emphasized, however, that squaring of the patella is not specific for hemophilia, being a recognized manifestation of juvenile chronic arthritis. In fact, many of the distinctive alterations of the hemophilic knee are evident in patients with juvenile chronic arthritis.

Ankle (Fig. 58–5). Ankle abnormalities also are common in this disease. The radiographic findings are similar to those in other involved joints, including soft tissue swelling, osteoporosis, marginal and central osseous erosions, and joint

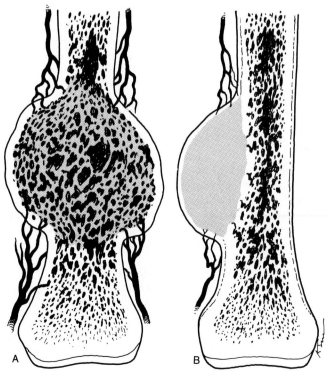

Figure 58–2. Hemophilia: Pathologic abnormalities. Intraosseous (A) and subperiosteal (B) hemorrhage. These types of hemorrhage can lead to hemophilic pseudotumors, with destruction and deformity of bone.

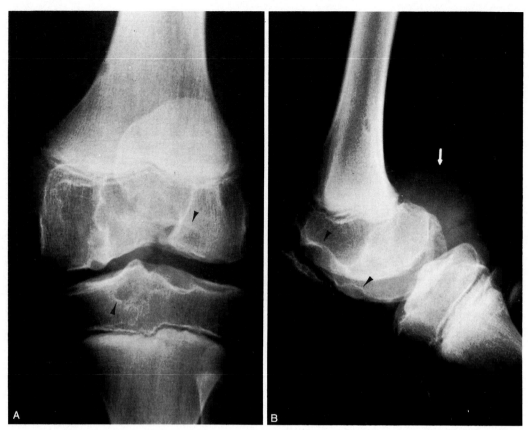

Figure 58–3. Hemophilia: Knee joint abnormalities. Frontal and lateral radiographs demonstrate characteristic findings of hemophilia. The bones are mildly osteoporotic and the epiphyses are enlarged. Note the well-defined or "etched" erosions of subchondral bone (arrowheads), the radiodense joint effusion (arrow), and the widened intercondylar notch of the femur.

space narrowing. In this articulation, tibiotalar slanting may be observed. This finding, which presumably is related to abnormal growth, is not specific, being observed in epiphyseal dysplasias, juvenile chronic arthritis, and perhaps sickle cell anemia.

Elbow (Fig. 58–6). Radiodense effusion, osteoporosis, and cartilaginous and osseous destruction are evident in the elbow in hemophilia. The trochlear and radial notches of the ulna are frequently widened and the radial head may be enlarged.

Other Joints. Typical hemophilic abnormalities can be apparent in other joints, including the hip, the glenohumeral joint, and the small articulations of the hand and foot. In the hip, unusual findings include severe bone resorption and spontaneous dislocation. In the hand and foot, predilection for the metacarpophalangeal, metatarsophalangeal, and subtalar joints exists.

ADDITIONAL ABNORMALITIES

Osteonecrosis (Fig. 58–7). Epiphyseal fragmentation and collapse in hemophilia are most frequent in the hip and ankle. They appear to be related to intraosseous bleeding with subsequent collapse of bone or intracapsular bleeding with elevation of intraarticular pressure, vascular occlusion, and subsequent osteonecrosis. These changes are particularly common in the femoral head and talus.

Ectopic Ossification (Fig. 58–8). Ossification may appear in periarticular soft tissues. This complication is apparent

most frequently in the pelvis, at which site ossification extending from the lateral aspect of the ilium or ischium to the proximal portion of the femur may be observed. Ossification may relate to traumatic tearing of the adjacent periosteum and intermuscular bleeding around the iliac, iliopsoas, and adductor muscles.

Fractures. In hemophilia, fractures may occur spontaneously or after minor trauma. This is not surprising in view of the presence of osteoporosis, joint contracture, and muscle imbalance in this disease. Fracture healing in hemophilic patients proceeds normally.

Hemophilic Pseudotumor (Fig. 58–9). Hemophilic pseudotumor of bone and soft tissue is a relatively uncommon manifestation of the disease, probably occurring in fewer than 2 per cent of cases. The bones that are implicated most frequently, in descending order of frequency, are the femur, the components of the osseous pelvis, the tibia, and the small bones of the hands. Pseudotumors may be intraosseous or subperiosteal or may occur within the soft tissues. It is probable that they arise from hemorrhage.

The radiographic appearance of a hemophilic pseudotumor is variable. Medullary bone destruction may produce small or large central or eccentric radiolucent lesions that are fairly well demarcated. Cortical violation and periosteal bone formation sometimes reach considerable proportions. A large soft tissue mass may be encountered.

Mild, moderate, or massive bleeding may occur in subperiosteal locations. Cortical atrophy owing to abnormal pressure, subperiosteal bone formation, and soft tissue extension are evident. Tumors arising in the soft tissue enlarge slowly, develop a fibrous capsule, and distort the subjacent osseous tissue by pressure erosion.

The differential diagnosis of hemophilic pseudotumors includes several other disorders. Initially, a subperiosteal hematoma in hemophilia produces periostitis that can simulate malignancy (Ewing's sarcoma, skeletal metastases) or infection. An intraosseous hematoma leading to osteolytic lesions of varying size simulates primary and secondary neoplasms, tumor-like lesions, and infection. In many patients, accurate diagnosis relies on knowledge of the patient's underlying disease.

Other Articular Manifestations. Chondrocalcinosis has been described in patients with hemophilia. Septic arthritis has also been recorded. In hemophilia, joint contractures may complicate intraarticular destruction or soft tissue hemorrhage, with impingement on vessels and nerves.

Scintigraphy

The evaluation of patients with hemophilia using bone-seeking radionuclide agents has been advocated. The radionuclide examination lacks specificity, however.

Computed Tomography

The major application of computed tomography to the evaluation of patients with hemophilia is assessing the extent of pseudotumors, soft tissue hemorrhage, or neurovascular compromise.

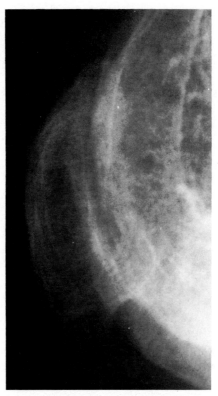

Figure 58–4. Hemophilia: Patellar abnormalities. Patellar size and shape are extremely variable in hemophilia. This bone may appear elongated and thin, as shown here. Abnormalities of the patellofemoral compartment are common in this disease. Osteoporosis, joint space narrowing, and osteophytes are evident.

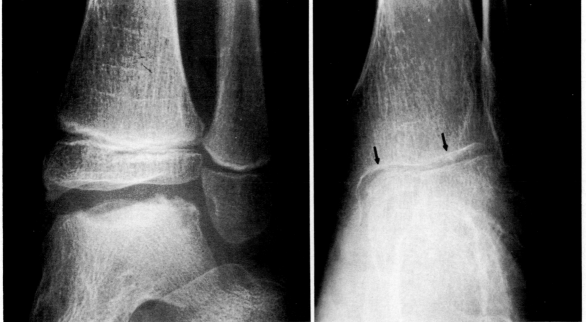

Figure 58–5. Hemophilia: Ankle joint abnormalities. A Radiograph demonstrates flattening and erosion of the superior surface of the talus. These osseous abnormalities may be related to collapse of weakened subchondral bone or osteonecrosis. The bones are osteoporotic, and horizontal radiodense areas in the tibia represent growth recovery lines. Mild perositis is also seen. The joint space is preserved. **B** More extensive abnormalities in the ankle include osteoporosis, osseous erosions and irregularity, and joint space narrowing. Note the tibiotalar slant with an angular joint surface (arrows).

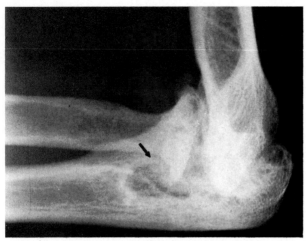

Figure 58-6. Hemophilia: Elbow joint abnormalities. Observe sclerosis, flattening, and deformity of the bones. The radial head is widened. Note the enlargement of the radial fossa (arrow).

Magnetic Resonance Imaging

The remarkable ability of magnetic resonance imaging to define soft tissue abnormalities and, specifically, hematomas, indicates its promising potential in the evaluation of intra- and extraarticular hemorrhagic manifestations of hemophilia (Fig. 58-10).

Pathogenesis of Hemophilic Arthropathy

It is generally assumed that arthropathy in hemophilia results from intra- and periarticular hemorrhage. In the synovial membrane, hypertrophy and inflammation, subsynovial fibrosis, and hemosiderin deposition are known responses

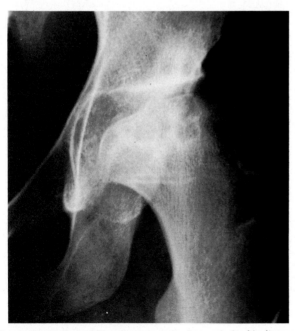

Figure 58-7. Hemophilia: Osteonecrosis. Intra-articular bleeding can produce osteonecrosis of the femoral head. Findings include considerable flattening of the femoral head, subchondral cysts, mild joint space narrowing, and acetabular deformity.

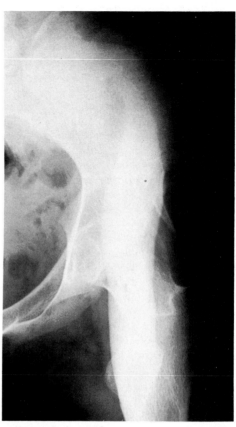

Figure 58-8. Hemophilia: Ectopic ossification. A large band of ossification extends from the lateral aspect of the ilium to the proximal portion of the femur. (Courtesy of M. Dalinka, M.D., Philadelphia, Pennsylvania.)

to experimental hemarthrosis. These same pathologic aberrations have been noted in hemophilia and posttraumatic hemarthrosis in humans. Cartilaginous abnormalities occurring after experimental hemarthrosis are less constant.

The osseous abnormalities in hemophilic joints may result from elevation of intraarticular pressure (owing to hemarthrosis) and intramarrow pressure (owing to focal destruction of weight-bearing surfaces). Hyperemia may account for epiphyseal overgrowth and osteoporosis in hemophilia.

The role of intraarticular iron deposits in the pathogenesis of hemophilic arthropathy is not clear.

Differential Diagnosis

Hemarthrosis is not confined to hemophilic arthropathy. It is frequent after trauma and in other articular and nonarticular disorders, such as scurvy or myeloproliferative disease, or after excessive administration of anticoagulant medication. The radiographic findings associated with hemarthrosis are not specific, consisting mainly of soft tissue swelling, although after traumatic hemarthrosis, a distinctive fat–blood fluid level detectable on cross-table radiographs of the involved joint may be associated with obvious fracture.

Articular abnormalities of hemophilia most resemble changes of juvenile chronic arthritis (Table 58-2). It frequently is impossible to distinguish between these two disorders on the basis of radiographic abnormalities in a single joint. For example, osteoporosis, overgrowth of the distal femoral and proximal tibial epiphyses, osseous irregularity, numerous subchondral cysts, joint space narrowing, widening

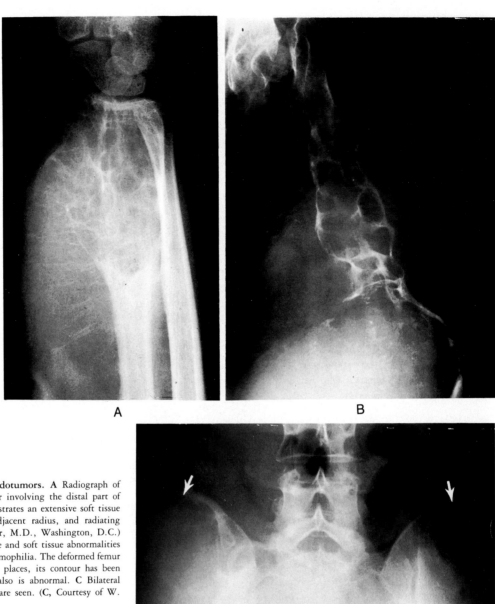

Figure 58–9. Hemophilia: Pseudotumors. A Radiograph of the forearm reveals a pseudotumor involving the distal part of the radius. The radiograph demonstrates an extensive soft tissue mass, scalloped erosion of the adjacent radius, and radiating trabeculae. (Courtesy of A. Brower, M.D., Washington, D.C.) **B** An example of the striking bone and soft tissue abnormalities that may accompany bleeding in hemophilia. The deformed femur has a "cystic" appearance and, in places, its contour has been completely obliterated. The hip also is abnormal. **C** Bilateral pseudotumors of the ilia (arrows) are seen. (**C,** Courtesy of W. Murray, M.D., Boise, Idaho.)

of the intercondylar notch, and squaring of the inferior pole of the patella may be observed in the knee in both hemophilia and juvenile-onset rheumatoid arthritis. Rather, it is the distribution of articular abnormalities in hemophilia and juvenile-onset rheumatoid arthritis (and other forms of juvenile chronic arthritis) that permits accurate radiographic diagnosis: In hemophilia, the knee, the ankle, and the elbow are the most commonly altered; in juvenile-onset rheumatoid arthritis, the joints of the hands and the wrists as well as the larger joints and spine may be affected.

In some articulations, the findings of hemophilia may simulate those of pigmented villonodular synovitis (Fig. 58–11) or infection. These latter disorders most characteristically are monoarticular in distribution, whereas joint involvement in hemophilia generally is polyarticular. Articular and skeletal alterations accompanying neuromuscular diseases, such as cerebral palsy, muscular dystrophy, and poliomyelitis, also may resemble those of hemophilia. On rare occasions, intraarticular bleeding in association with certain hemorrhagic diatheses may lead to an arthropathy identical to that of hemophilia. Two of these diatheses are discussed subsequently. Additional disorders leading to intraarticular, in-

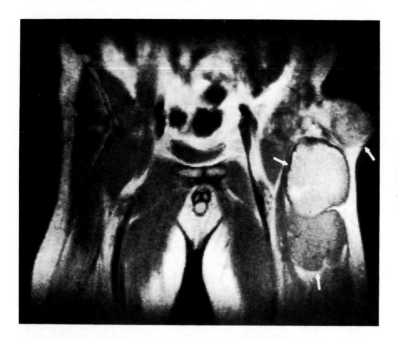

Figure 58–10. Hemophilia: Use of magnetic resonance imaging. A coronal image display reveals hemophilic pseudotumors (arrows). Note that the lesions vary in intensity and the masses are inhomogeneous, findings that relate to the varying duration of the soft tissue hemorrhages. (Courtesy of J. Tsurada, M.D., Los Angeles, California.)

traosseous, or soft tissue hemorrhage include Glanzmann's thrombasthenia (rare autosomal recessive disorder with platelet abnormality), congenital hereditary abnormalities of fibrinogen, von Willebrand's disease, and thrombocytopenic purpura (Table 58–3).

BLEEDING DIATHESES AND HEMANGIOMAS
General Features

Hemangiomas are vascular tumors, most frequently located in the skin, that appear in the early postnatal period. Their occurrence in other tissues, including the synovial membrane, is well known. Hemangiomas may be associated with unusual syndromes, some of which produce hematologic abnormality.

The association of varicose veins, soft tissue and bone hypertrophy, and cutaneous hemangiomas is known as the *Klippel-Trenaunay syndrome*. When an arteriovenous fistula occurs in this syndrome, the term *Parke-Weber syndrome* commonly is employed. Additional variants have included cutaneous lymphangiomas, facial hemihypertrophy, cavernous hemangiomas of the colon, and varicosities of the pulmonary veins.

With regard to the clinical manifestations of the Klippel-Trenaunay syndrome, both sexes are affected. A nevus is usually present at birth, and varices appear, typically in the first few years of life. Bone and soft tissue hypertrophy also is evident in early life but becomes more obvious during the adolescent growth spurt. Generally, only one lower limb is involved. The natural history of the Klippel-Trenaunay syndrome is variable, although worsening of venous insufficiency is the rule. The progressive nature of the condition commonly results in a shortened life span.

The *Kasabach-Merritt syndrome* consists of papillary hemangiomas and extensive purpura. Hematologic abnormalities in this syndrome have included thrombocytopenia, deficiencies of factors V, VII, VIII, and IX, prothrombin depression, hypofibrinogenemia, and microangiopathic hemolytic anemia. A consumption coagulopathy attributable to intravascular coagulation within the hemangioma makes these patients susceptible to hemorrhage.

Articular Abnormalities

Arthropathies are not commonly reported in either the Klippel-Trenaunay syndrome or the Kasabach-Merritt syndrome. Rarely, an arthropathy of the knee resembling hemophilia has been observed in association with either syndrome (Fig. 58–12).

Table 58–2. HEMOPHILIA VERSUS JUVENILE-ONSET RHEUMATOID ARTHRITIS (JRA)

	Hemophilia	JRA
Common articular sites	Knee, ankle, elbow	Knee, ankle wrist, hand
Soft tissue swelling	+	+
Osteoporosis	+	+
Joint space narrowing	±	±
Bone ankylosis	−	+
Epiphyseal overgrowth	+	+
Growth inhibition	−	+
Epiphyseal collapse or osteonecrosis	+	+
Periostitis	±	+
Pseudotumors	+	−
Spondylitis	−	+

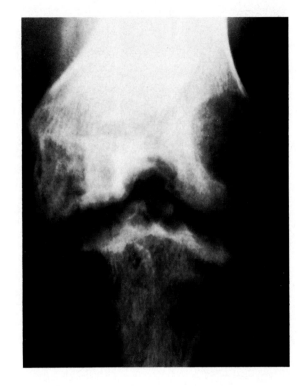

Figure 58–11. Pigmented villonodular synovitis. A radiograph of the knee outlines hemophilia-like changes with osteoporosis, joint space narrowing, and subchondral bone irregularity and cyst formation. (Courtesy of H. Griffiths, M.D., Toronto, Ontario, Canada.)

Table 58–3. HERITABLE DISORDERS OF BLOOD COAGULATION

Disorder	Heredity	Hemorrhagic Tendency	Hemarthrosis
Classic hemophilia (factor VIII deficiency)	X-linked	Mild to severe	Common
Christmas disease (factor IX deficiency)	X-linked	Mild to severe	Common
Von Willebrand's diseae (factor VIII deficiency, platelet abnormalities)	Autosomal dominant	Mild to severe	Uncommon
Plasma thromboplastin antecedent (PTA, factor IX) deficiency	Autosomal recessive	Mild	Rare
Hageman trait (deficiency of Hageman factor, factor XII)	Autosomal recessive	None to mild	Usually absent
Fletcher trait (deficiency of plasma prekallikrein)	Autosomal recessive	None	Absent
Fitzgerald trait (deficiency of high molecular weight kininogen)	Autosomal recessive	None	Absent
Parahemophilia (factor V deficiency)	Autosomal recessive	Moderate	Rare
Stuart factor deficiency (factor X deficiency)	Autosomal recessive	Severe	Variable
Factor VII deficiency	Autosomal recessive	Mild to moderate	Variable
Hereditary hypoprothrombinemia (prothrombin deficiency)	Autosomal recessive	Mild to severe	Variable
Congenital deficiency of fibrinogen	Autosomal recessive	Severe	Variable
Congenital dysfibrinogemia (structural abnormality of fibrinogen)	Autosomal dominant	None to mild	Variable
Congenital deficiency of fibrin-stabilizing factor (factor XIII deficiency)	Unknown	Severe	Rare

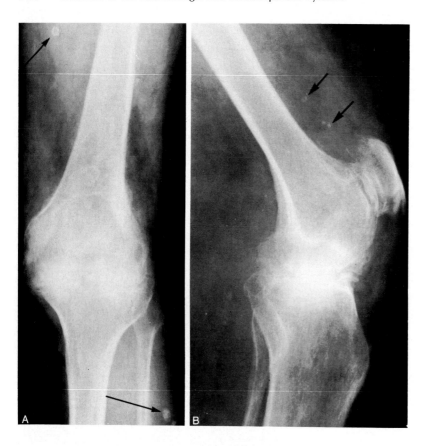

Figure 58–12. Arthropathy in association with hemangiomas and bleeding diatheses. This middle-aged man had a vascular malformation of the left lower extremity, extending from the buttock to the foot. Radiographs of the left knee reveal extensive osteoporosis, joint space narrowing, and sclerosis. The epiphyses appear enlarged in relation to the constricted diaphyses. Note the numerous phleboliths (arrows) in the soft tissues.

Table 58–4. RADIOGRAPHIC FEATURES OF ARTHROPATHY ASSOCIATED WITH HEMANGIOMAS

Soft tissue swelling
Osteoporosis
Epiphyseal overgrowth
Subchondral bone erosions and cysts
Calcifications (phleboliths)

The most likely explanation for the pathogenesis of the arthropathy resembling that accompanying hemophilia which occurs in some patients with the Klippel-Trenaunay or Kasabach-Merritt syndrome would involve recurrent episodes of intraarticular bleeding. This possible pathogenesis gains support from the appearance of this same arthropathy in patients with synovial hemangiomas without either of these syndromes. The diagnosis of the precise cause for the radiographic findings is based on the appearance of calcified circular radiodense lesions (phleboliths) in soft tissue and periarticular locations in combination with abnormalities resembling those of hemophilia, including soft tissue swelling, osteoporosis, epiphyseal overgrowth, irregularities of subchondral bone, and widening of the intercondylar notch of the femur (Table 58–4).

FURTHER READING

Arnold WD, Hilgartner MW: Hemophilic arthropathy. Current concepts of pathogenesis and management. J Bone Joint Surg [Am] 59:287, 1977.

Brant EE, Jordan HH: Radiologic aspects of hemophilic pseudotumors in bone. AJR 115:525, 1972.

deValderrama JAF, Matthews JM: The haemophilic pseudotumor or haemophilic subperiosteal haematoma. J Bone Joint Surg [Br] 47:256, 1965.

Johnson JB, Davis TW, Bullock WH: Bone and joint changes in hemophilia. Radiology 63:64, 1954.

Jordan HH: Hemophilic Arthropathies. Springfield, Ill, Charles C Thomas, 1958.

Kasabach HH, Merritt KK: Capillary hemangioma with extensive purpura. Report of a case. Am J Dis Child 59:1063, 1940.

Kontras SB: The Klippel-Trenaunay-Weber syndrome. Birth Defects 10:177, 1974.

Pettersson H, Gilbert MS: Diagnostic Imaging in Hemophilia. Berlin, Springer-Verlag, 1985.

Pettersson H, Ahlberg A, Nilsson IM: A radiologic classification of hemophilic arthropathy. Clin Orthop 149:153, 1980.

Phillips GN, Gordon DH, Martin EC, Haller JO, Casarella W: The Klippel-Trenaunay syndrome: Clinical and radiological aspects. Radiology 128:429, 1978.

Resnick D, Oliphant M: Hemophilia-like arthropathy of the knee associated with cutaneous and synovial hemangiomas. Report of 3 cases and review of the literature. Radiology 114:323, 1975.

Richardson ML, Helms CA, Vogler JB III, Genant HK: Skeletal changes in neuromuscular disorders mimicking juvenile rheumatoid arthritis and hemophilia. AJR 143:893, 1984.

Vaz W, Cockshott WP, Martin RF, Pai MK, Walker I: Myositis ossificans in hemophilia. Skel Radiol 7:27, 1981.

Weber FP: Hemangiectatic hypertrophy of limbs—congenital phlebacteriectasis and so-called congenital varicose veins. Br J Child Dis 15:13, 1918.

Wilson DA, Prince JR: MR imaging of hemophilic pseudotumors. AJR 150:349, 1988.

INFECTIOUS DISEASES

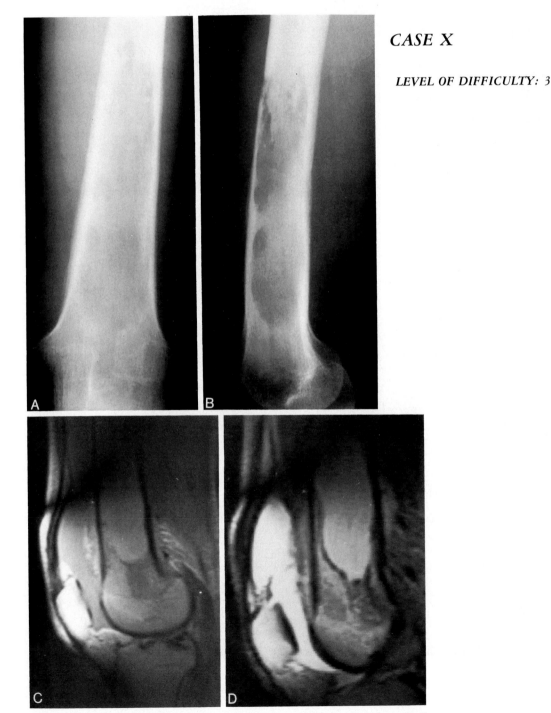

CASE X

LEVEL OF DIFFICULTY: 3

A 23 year old man had a 4 month history of pain in the knee and thigh. On physical examination, an effusion in the knee and a tender, firm mass in the thigh were observed.

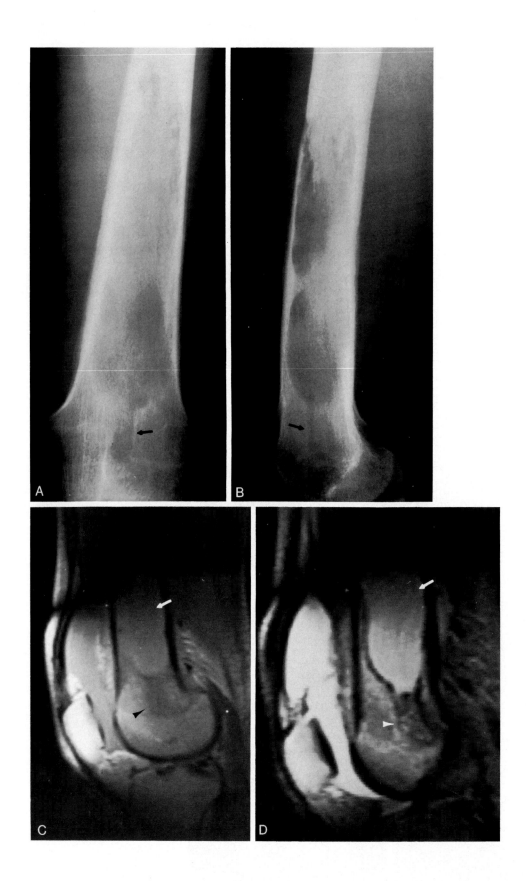

Frontal (A) and lateral (B) radiographs show a large destructive lesion involving the distal portion of the diaphysis and metaphysis of the femur. There is a motheaten pattern of osteolysis, cortical erosion and disruption, and linear periosteal reaction. Medial soft tissue fullness is evident; a large soft tissue mass was better demonstrated with computed tomography (not shown). Within the area of osteolysis, no radiographically visible calcification or ossification is apparent, although superiorly, irregular bone destruction has led to patchy radiodense areas. Inferiorly, a channel-like zone of osteolysis (arrows) extends from the metaphysis to the region of the physeal scar.

Proton density (C) and T2 weighted (D) sagittal magnetic resonance images reveal abnormalities of bone and soft tissue. In C, the majority of the osseous lesion has intermediate signal intensity (arrow) with an area of diminished signal intensity in the region of the channel-like zone (arrowhead). In D, there is increased signal intensity within the diaphysis and metaphysis (arrow), areas of similar intensity in the posterior soft tissues, and regions of both high and low signal intensity in the area of the channel-like defect (arrowhead). A large joint effusion is apparent.

The radiographic abnormalities are consistent with an aggressive process in the femur, leading to widespread bone destruction, cortical erosion, periostitis, and a soft tissue mass. Several malignant tumors of bone are realistic diagnostic possibilities. Of these, round cell neoplasms, especially Ewing's sarcoma, are most likely when both the age of the patient and the extent of bone abnormality are considered. Ewing's sarcoma generally is diametaphyseal in location and is accompanied by motheaten or permeative osteolysis, periostitis, and a soft tissue mass. In many instances, the pattern of periosteal reaction in Ewing's sarcoma is more exuberant than that shown in A and B. Lymphoma represents a second type of round cell tumor that could produce these abnormalities. Indeed, other types of malignant tumors, including osteosarcoma, fibrosarcoma, chondrosarcoma, and malignant fibrous histiocytoma, also must be considered.

Subacute or chronic osteomyelitis occasionally may lead to extensive areas of osteolysis, simulating the appearance of a neoplasm. The possibility of infection in the test case is strengthened by the occurrence of a channel-like region in the distal portion of the lesion. Such channels or serpentine-like tracts, indeed, are an extremely valuable sign of osteomyelitis. In the adolescent, these tracts classically extend from a metaphyseal focus of infection to the nearby physeal plate; in the adult, they may reach the articular cavity. These channels usually are associated with a pyogenic process, being uncommon in tuberculosis.

The abnormalities delineated by magnetic resonance imaging in C and D are not pathognomonic of infection, but they are certainly consistent with that diagnosis. Bone destruction resulting from osteomyelitis as well as from most tumors usually is accompanied by areas of intermediate signal intensity on T1 weighted images and high signal intensity on T2 weighted images. In instances of indolent infection, bone reaction in the form of a shell or rim produces a zone of diminished signal intensity at the periphery of the osseous lesion. The cause of the signal characteristics of the channel-like region in the test case is not entirely clear, although it is evident that the features on magnetic resonance imaging in this area differ from those in the remainder of the lesion. The presence of a joint effusion is not uncommon when an infectious (or neoplastic) process extends to the end of a tubular bone.

An open biopsy of the femur was performed in the patient illustrated in case X. The medullary cavity was found to contain creamy white fluid. Histologic examination revealed a mixed inflammatory cellular infiltrate, and cultures of the lesion led to the recovery of coagulase-positive *Staphylococcus aureus*.

FINAL DIAGNOSIS: Osteomyelitis.

FURTHER READING

Pages 735 and 736 and the following:

1. Bonakdarpour A, Gaines VD: The radiology of osteomyelitis. Orthop Clin North Am 15:21, 1983.
2. Unger E, Moldofsky T, Gatenby R, Hartz W, Broder G: Diagnosis of osteomyelitis by MR imaging. AJR 150:605, 1988.

(Case X, courtesy of G. Greenway, M.D., Dallas, Texas.)

Chapter 59

Osteomyelitis, Septic Arthritis, and Soft Tissue Infection: Mechanisms and Situations

Donald Resnick, M.D.
Gen Niwayama, M.D.

A thorough understanding of regional anatomy is fundamental to the accurate interpretation of clinical, radiologic, and pathologic characteristics of infections of bone, joint, and soft tissue. In most persons with such infections, a specific mechanism of contamination can be recognized; infection may be derived from hematogenous seeding, spread from a contiguous source, direct implantation, or operative contamination. The radiographic findings of osteomyelitis (including abscess, involucrum, sequestration), septic arthritis (including joint space loss, marginal and central osseous erosions), and soft tissue suppuration (including swelling, radiolucent streaks, periostitis) generally are delayed for a variable period after the clinical onset of infection. Other diagnostic techniques, including scintigraphy and magnetic resonance imaging, allow accurate diagnosis at an earlier stage of the process.

The manifestations of musculoskeletal infection are varied and depend on the site of involvement, the initiating event, the infecting organism, and the acute or chronic nature of the illness. Fundamental to any description of the radiographic and pathologic features of such infection is an analysis of the mechanisms by which the organisms reach the osseous and articular structures, the pathogenesis of the infective process itself, and any specific situations or circumstances that can influence the frequency and pattern of such contamination.

TERMINOLOGY

The term *osteomyelitis* implies an infection of bone and marrow. *Infective (suppurative) osteitis* indicates contamination of the bone cortex. Infective osteitis can occur as an isolated phenomenon or, more frequently, as a concomitant to osteomyelitis. Radiographic and pathologic differentiation of osteitis and osteomyelitis can be extremely difficult; furthermore, osteitis is not confined to infectious processes, as inflammation of the cortex can be observed in numerous other conditions, such as ankylosing spondylitis, psoriasis, and Reiter's syndrome. *Infective (suppurative) periostitis* implies contamination of the periosteal cloak that surrounds the bone. In this situation, a subperiosteal accumulation of organisms frequently leads to infective osteitis and osteomyelitis, to interruption of periosteal blood supply to the cortex, producing necrosis, or to disruption of the periosteum and the accumulation of pus in the soft tissues. Periostitis can be noted in the absence of infection, being evident in neoplastic, metabolic, inflammatory, and traumatic disorders. *Soft tissue infection* indicates contamination of cutaneous, subcutaneous, muscular, fascial, tendinous, ligamentous, or bursal structures. This may be seen as an isolated condition, as a forerunner to infective periostitis, osteitis, or osteomyelitis, or as a complication of periosteal, osseous, marrow, or articular infection. Soft tissue infection can lead to inflammation of adjacent periosteal tissue (periostitis) without necessarily implying that the periosteum is contaminated. *Articular infection* implies a septic process of the joint itself. Septic arthritis can occur as an isolated condition that may soon spread to the neighboring bone or as a complication of adjacent osteomyelitis.

The clinical stages of osteomyelitis frequently are designated *acute*, *subacute*, and *chronic*. This does not imply that all cases of osteomyelitis progress through each of these phases. The transition from acute to subacute and chronic osteomyelitis can indicate that inadequate therapeutic measures have been employed or that the organisms are especially resistant to accepted modes of therapy. Viable organisms can persist in small abscesses or fragments of necrotic bone. At intervals of months or even years, the residual organisms can produce flare-ups of osteomyelitis.

Descriptive terms have been applied to certain radiographic and pathologic characteristics that are encountered during the course of osteomyelitis. A *sequestrum* represents a segment of necrotic bone that is separated from living bone by granulation tissue. Sequestra may reside in the marrow for protracted periods of time, harboring living organisms that have the capability of evoking an acute flare-up of the infection. An *involucrum* denotes a layer of living bone that has formed about the dead bone. It can surround and eventually merge with the parent bone, or it can become perforated by *tracts* through which pus may escape. An opening in the involucrum is termed a *cloaca*; through it the granulation tissue and sequestra can be discharged. Tracts leading to the skin surface from the bone are termed *sinuses*. A *bone abscess* (Brodie's abscess) is a sharply delineated focus of infection that represents a site of active infection. It is lined by granulation tissue and frequently is surrounded by eburnated bone. Occasionally, a sclerotic nonpurulent form of osteomyelitis exists, which is termed *Garré's sclerosing osteomyelitis*. This term should be reserved for those cases in which intense proliferation of the periosteum leads to bone deposition and in which there is no necrosis or purulent exudate and little granulation tissue.

OSTEOMYELITIS
Routes of Contamination

There are four principal routes by which osseous (and articular) structures can be contaminated.

1. Hematogenous spread of infection. Infection can reach the bone (or the joint) via the bloodstream.

2. Spread from a contiguous source of infection. Infection can extend into the bone (or the joint) from an adjacent contaminated site. Cutaneous, sinus, and dental infections are three important examples of such contaminated sites.

3. Direct implantation. In certain situations (e.g., after puncture and penetrating wounds) there is direct implantation of infectious material into the bone (or the joint).

4. Postoperative infection. Although examples of this type of infection relate to direct implantation, spread from a contiguous septic focus, or hematogenous contamination of the bone (or the joint), infection after surgery is so important that it deserves special emphasis.

Hematogenous Spread of Infection
General Clinical Features

Traditionally, hematogenous osteomyelitis has been regarded as a disease of childhood. Neonatal and adult osteomyelitis is also well known, however. There are major differences in the presentation and course of hematogenous osteomyelitis in the child, the infant, and the adult. Childhood osteomyelitis can be associated with a sudden onset of high fever, a toxic state, and local signs of inflammation. In the infant, hematogenous osteomyelitis often leads to less dramatic findings; in this age group, contaminated indwelling umbilical venous and arterial catheters can become the source of septicemia, resulting in osteomyelitis at multiple sites. The adult form of hematogenous osteomyelitis may have a more insidious onset. Most series indicate that in children,

boys are affected more frequently than girls. A similar male dominance is observed in adults. In infancy, boys and girls are affected with approximately equal frequency. In the younger age groups, the long tubular bones of the extremities are especially vulnerable to infection; in adults, osteomyelitis of the vertebral column is not infrequent.

Although the list of potential organisms that can cause hematogenous osteomyelitis is long, *Staphylococcus aureus* is responsible for the vast majority of cases. Gram-negative, mycobacterial, and fungal organisms, and, less commonly, *Haemophilus influenzae* and *Streptococcus pneumoniae* are among the responsible agents.

Vascular Anatomy

OVERVIEW. The vascular supply of a tubular bone is derived from several points of arterial inflow, which become complicated sinusoidal networks within the bone (Fig. 59–1). In tubular bones, one or two diaphyseal nutrient arteries pierce the cortex and divide into ascending and descending branches. As they extend to the ends of the bones, they are joined by the terminals of metaphyseal and epiphyseal arteries. The arteries within the bone marrow form a series of cortical branches that connect with the fenestrated capillaries of the haversian systems. At the bone surface, the cortical capillaries form connections with overlying periosteal plexuses. Therefore, the cortices of the tubular bones derive nutrition from both the periosteal and the medullary circulatory systems. Exuberant anastomoses between the two systems allow blood to flow in either direction according to physiologic conditions.

The central arterioles drain into a thin-walled venous sinus, which subsequently unites with veins that retrace the course of the nutrient arteries, piercing the cortex at various points and joining larger and larger venous channels.

Joints receive blood vessels from periarterial plexuses that pierce the capsule to form a vascular plexus in the deeper part of the synovial membrane. The blood vessels of the synovial membrane terminate at the articular margins as looped anastomoses (circulus articularis vasculosus). The epiphysis and the adjacent synovium share a common blood supply.

THE THREE VASCULAR PATTERNS OF THE TUBULAR BONES. The radiologic and pathologic features of osteomyelitis differ in the child, the infant, and the adult, which is related in large part to peculiarities of the vascular anatomy of the tubular bones in each of these three age groups (Figs. 59–2 and 59–3; Table 59–1).

Childhood Pattern. Between the ages of approximately 1 year and the time when the open cartilaginous growth plates fuse, a childhood vascular pattern can be recognized in the ends of the tubular bones (Fig. 59–2A). Apart from those vessels in a narrow fringe at the periphery of the cartilage, the capillaries on the metaphyseal side of the growth plate are the terminal ramification of a nutrient artery. It is here in the metaphysis that the vessels turn in acute loops to join large sinusoidal veins, and that blood flow is slow and turbulent. The epiphyseal blood supply is distinct from that on the metaphyseal aspect of the plate. This anatomic characteristic explains, in part, the peculiar predilection of hematogenous osteomyelitis to affect metaphyses in the child.

Infantile Pattern. A fetal vascular arrangement may persist in some tubular bones up the age of 1 year with local

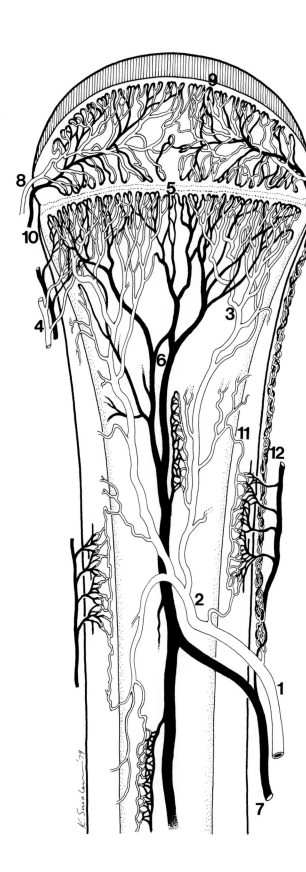

Figure 59–1. Normal osseous circulation to a growing tubular bone. Nutrient arteries (1) pierce the diaphyseal cortex and divide into descending and ascending (2) branches. These latter vessels continue to divide, becoming fine channels (3) as they approach the end of the bone. They are joined by metaphyseal vessels (4) and, in the subepiphyseal (growth) plate region, they form a series of end-arterial loops (5). The venous sinuses extend from the metaphyseal region toward the diaphysis, uniting with other venous structures (6) and eventually piercing the cortex as a large venous channel (7). At the ends of the bone, nutrient arteries of the epiphysis (8) branch into finer structures, passing into the subchondral region. At this site, arterial loops (9) are again evident, some of which pierce the subchondral bone plate before turning to enter the venous sinusoid and venous channels of the epiphysis (10). At the bone surface, cortical capillaries (11) form connections with overlying periosteal plexuses (12). Note that in the growing child, distinct epiphyseal and metaphyseal arteries can be distinguished on either side of the cartilaginous growth plate. Anastomoses between these vessels either do not occur or are infrequent.

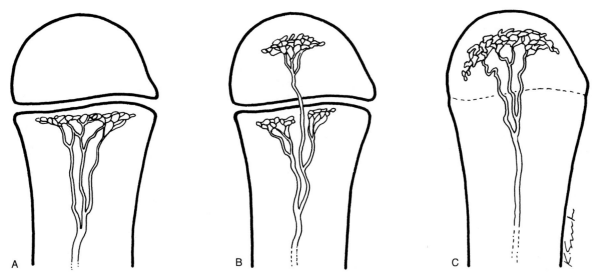

Figure 59–2. Normal vascular patterns of a tubular bone in the child, the infant, and the adult. A In the child, the capillaries of the metaphysis turn sharply, without violating the open growth plate. **B** In the infant, some metaphyseal vessels may penetrate or extend around the open growth plate, ramifying in the epiphysis. **C** In the adult, with closure of the growth plate, a vascular connection between metaphysis and epiphysis can be recognized.

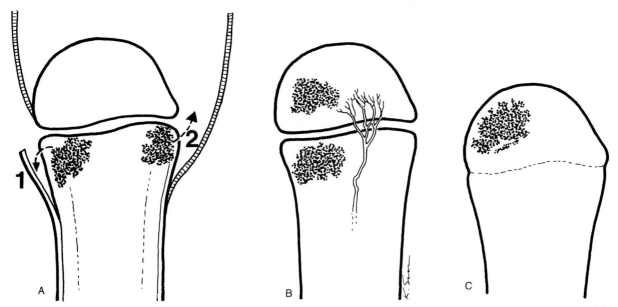

Figure 59–3. Sites of hematogenous osteomyelitis of a tubular bone in the child, the infant, and the adult. A In the child, a metaphyseal focus is frequent. From this site, cortical penetration can result in a subperiosteal abscess in those locations in which the growth plate is extraarticular (1) or in a septic joint in those locations in which the growth plate is intraarticular (2). **B** In the infant, a metaphyseal focus may be complicated by epiphyseal extension owing to the vascular anatomy in this age group. **C** In the adult, a subchondral focus in an epiphysis is not unusual, owing to the vascular anatomy in this age group.

Table 59–1. VASCULAR PATTERNS OF TUBULAR BONES

Pattern	Age	Characteristics
Infantile pattern	0–1 year*	Diaphyseal and metaphyseal vessels may perforate open growth plate
Childhood pattern	1–16 years†	Diaphyseal and metaphyseal vessels do not penetrate open growth plate
Adult pattern	>16 years	Diaphyseal and metaphyseal vessels penetrate closed growth plate

*Upper age limit depends on specific local anatomic variations in the appearance and growth of the ossification center.
†Upper age limit is related to the time at which the open growth plate closes.

variations corresponding to the time of complete maturation of the epiphyseal bone nucleus (Fig. 59–2B). In the terminal stages of intrauterine life and in the first 6 to 12 months after birth, when the growth cartilage is established but not yet limited by bone on its epiphyseal side, some vessels at the surface of the metaphysis penetrate the preexisting growth plate, ramifying in the epiphysis. After termination, they form large venous lakes not dissimilar to metaphyseal sinusoids. This arrangement affords a vascular connection between the metaphysis and epiphysis.

Adult Pattern. With closing of the physeal growth plate, metaphyseal vessels progressively penetrate the diminishing cartilaginous structure, reestablishing a vascular connection between the metaphysis and the epiphysis (Fig. 59–2C). Blood within the nutrient vessels can then reach the surface of the epiphysis through large anastomosing channels.

Hematogenous Osteomyelitis in the Child (Table 59–2)

Metaphyseal location of hematogenous osteomyelitis in the child (Fig. 59–4) is related to (1) the peculiar anatomy of the vascular tree (see previous discussion); (2) the inability of vessels to penetrate the open physeal plate; (3) the slow rate of blood flow in this region; (4) a decrease in phagocytic ability of neighboring macrophages; or (5) secondary thrombosis of the nutrient artery. Atypical localizations for the infectious process certainly exist, however, including primary involvement of an epiphysis or secondary extension across the physis to an epiphysis.

Inflammation in the adjacent bone of the metaphysis is characterized by vascular engorgement, edema, cellular response, and abscess formation. Transudates extend from the marrow to the adjacent cortex. A rise in intramedullary pressure encourages infectious fluid to enter the cortical bone and extend across it by way of the haversian and Volkmann's canals. The inflammatory process soon reaches the outer surface of the cortex, lifting the periosteum and disrupting the periosteal blood supply to the external cortical surface. Elevation of the periosteum is prominent in the immature skeleton because of its relatively loose attachment to the subjacent bone. The elevated periosteum lays down bone in the form of an involucrum that partially surrounds the infected bone. Infection may penetrate the periosteal membrane,

producing cloacae, and extend into the adjacent soft tissues, leading to abscesses.

Cortical sequestration can subsequently appear. Necrosis is facilitated by deprivation of blood supply to the inner portion of the cortex owing to thrombosis of the metaphyseal vessels and by interruption of periosteal blood supply to the outer portion of the cortex as a result of lifting of the periosteum.

Hematogenous osteomyelitis of the child is not confined to tubular bones. In flat or irregular bones, such as the calcaneus, the clavicle, and the bones of the pelvis, childhood osteomyelitis may show predilection for metaphyseal-equivalent osseous locations adjacent to an apophyseal cartilaginous plate and epiphyseal-equivalent locations adjacent to articular cartilage. In these areas, vascular anatomy is similar to that of the metaphyses of the tubular bones.

Hematogenous Osteomyelitis in the Infant (Table 59–2)

In the infant, as some of the vessels in the metaphysis penetrate the growth plate, a suppurative process of the metaphysis may extend into the epiphysis (Figs. 59–3B and 59–5). Epiphyseal infection can then result in articular contamination and damage the cells on the epiphyseal side of the growth cartilage, leading to arrest or disorganization of growth and maturation. Articular involvement is also facilitated by the frequent localization of infantile osteomyelitis to ends of the bone in which the growth plate is intraarticular (e.g., hip), allowing direct contamination of the joint space from a metaphyseal septic focus (see discussion later in this chapter).

Profuse involucrum formation is characteristic of osteomyelitis in the infant, reflecting the ease with which the immature periosteum is lifted and the extreme richness of the periosteal vessels in infancy.

Infantile osteomyelitis also is associated with cortical sequestration and soft tissue alterations such as edema or abscess formation. Sinus tracts are relatively rare in infantile osteomyelitis.

Hematogenous Osteomyelitis in the Adult (Table 59–2)

Hematogenous osteomyelitis of the spine, pelvis, and small bones is more common in the adult patient than is infection

Table 59–2. HEMATOGENOUS OSTEOMYELITIS OF TUBULAR BONES

	Infant	Child	Adult
Localization	Metaphyseal with epiphyseal extension	Metaphyseal	Epiphyseal
Involucrum	Common	Common	Not common
Sequestration	Common	Common	Not common
Joint involvement	Common	Not common	Common
Soft tissue abscess	Common	Common	Not common
Pathologic fracture	Not common	Not common	Common*
Sinus tracts	Not common	Variable	Common

*In neglected cases.

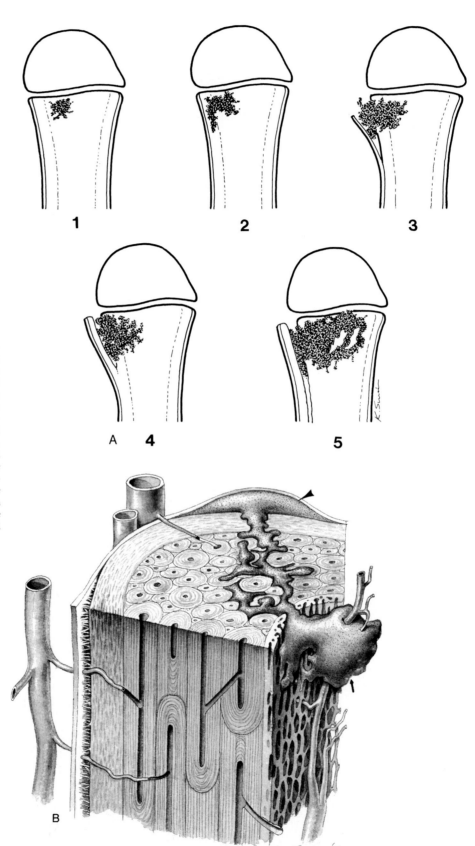

Figure 59–4. Hematogenous osteomyelitis of a tubular bone in the child. A Sequential steps in the initiation and progression of infection. 1, A metaphyseal focus is common; 2, the infection spreads laterally, reaching and invading the cortical bone; 3, cortical penetration is associated with subperiosteal extension and elevation of the periosteal membrane; 4, subperiosteal bone formation leads to an involucrum or shell of new bone; 5, the involucrum may become massive with continued infection. **B** A diagram of the manner in which an infectious process in the medullary canal (arrow) permeates the cortex and collects beneath the periosteal membrane (arrowhead).

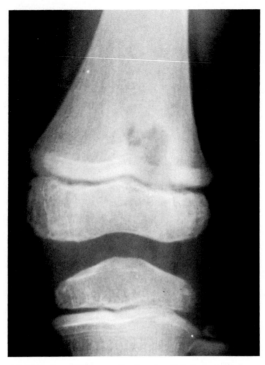

Figure 59–4 *Continued* **C** Two weeks after the clinical onset of osteomyelitis, a lytic metaphyseal focus in the femur is readily apparent. It extends to the growth cartilage.

of tubular bones. When tubular bones become infected, free communication of the metaphyseal and epiphyseal vessels through the closed growth plate allows infection to localize in the subchondral regions of the bone (Figs. 59–3*C* and 59–6). Joint contamination can complicate this epiphyseal location.

The fibrous and firm attachment of the periosteum to the cortex in the adult resists displacement and, therefore, subperiosteal abscess formation, extensive periostitis, and involucrum formation are relatively unusual in this age group. Furthermore, the intimacy of the periosteum and cortex in the adult ensures adequate cortical blood supply in most persons; extensive sequestration is not a common feature of adult-onset osteomyelitis. Rather, infection leads to cortical atrophy and predisposes the bone to pathologic fracture.

Acute Hematogenous Osteomyelitis: Radiographic and Pathologic Abnormalities (Table 59–3)

Radiographic evidence of significant osseous destruction in hematogenous pyogenic (nontuberculous) osteomyelitis is delayed for a period of days to weeks. Subtle radiographic changes in the soft tissues may appear within 3 days of bacterial contamination of bone, however. Soft tissue swelling results in displacement of the lucent tissue planes from the underlying bone. Muscle swelling and obliteration of the soft tissue planes then can be observed.

In pyogenic infection, radiographically evident bone de-

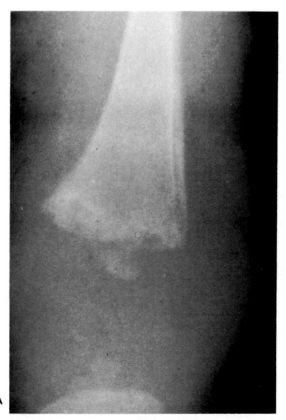

A

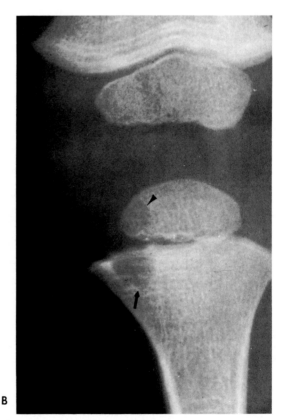

B

Figure 59–5. Hematogenous osteomyelitis of a tubular bone in the infant. A In this infant with acute staphylococcal osteomyelitis, metaphyseal and epiphyseal involvement of the distal part of the femur is associated with periostitis and joint involvement. **B** In an older infant or young child, transphyseal extension of metaphyseal infection (arrow) into the epiphysis (arrowhead) can be seen. (**B**, Courtesy of P. Sprague, M.D., Perth, Australia.)

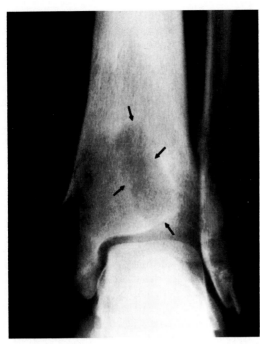

Figure 59–6. Hematogenous osteomyelitis of a tubular bone in the adult. An epiphyseal localization is not infrequent in this age group. Observe the lytic lesion (abscess) with surrounding sclerosis extending to the subchondral bone plate (arrows). Metaphyseal and diaphyseal sclerosis is evident. The elongated shape of the lesion is typical of infection.

struction and periostitis can be delayed for 1 to 2 weeks after intraosseous lodgment of the organisms. In the child, osseous lesions appear as enlarging, poorly defined lucent shadows of the metaphysis, extending to the growth plate. In the infant, the epiphyses are unossified or only partially ossified, so that radiographic recognition of epiphyseal destruction can be extremely difficult. Metaphyseal lucent lesions, periostitis, and a joint effusion are helpful radiographic clues. In the adult, epiphyseal, metaphyseal, and diaphyseal osseous destruction creates radiolucent areas of varying size, which are associated with mild periostitis. Cortical resorption can be identified as endosteal scalloping and intracortical lucent regions.

Subacute and Chronic Hematogenous Osteomyelitis: Radiographic and Pathologic Abnormalities

BRODIE'S ABSCESS. Single or multiple radiolucent abscesses, termed Brodie's abscesses, can be evident during subacute or chronic stages of osteomyelitis. These abscesses appear as circumscribed lesions showing predilection for (but not confinement to) the ends of tubular bones; they are characteristically found in subacute pyogenic osteomyelitis, usually of staphylococcal origin. Brodie's abscesses are especially common in children, in whom they typically appear in the metaphysis, particularly that of the distal or proximal portion of the tibia. Less frequently, they occur in other tubular, flat, or irregular bones, and are diaphyseal in location. Rarely, they traverse the open growth plate or are epiphyseal in location. Abscesses vary from less than 1 cm to over 4 cm in diameter. The wall of the abscess is lined by inflammatory granulation tissue that is surrounded by spongy bone eburnation.

Radiographs outline radiolucency with adjacent sclerosis (Fig. 59–7). This lucent region commonly is located in the metaphysis, where it may connect with the growth plate by a tortuous channel. Radiographic detection of this channel is important, ensuring the diagnosis of osteomyelitis. In the diaphysis, the radiolucent abscess cavity can be located in central or subcortical areas of the spongiosa or in the cortex itself and may contain a central sequestrum. In an epiphysis, a circular, well-defined osteolytic lesion is seen. When an abscess is located in the cortex, its radiographic appearance, consisting of a lucent lesion with surrounding sclerosis and periostitis, simulates that of an osteoid osteoma or a stress fracture. A circular or elliptical radiolucent lesion without calcification that is smaller or larger than 2 cm is characteristic of a cortical abscess; a circular lucent area with or without calcification smaller than 2 cm is typical of an osteoid osteoma; and a linear lucent shadow without calcification is characteristic of a stress fracture.

SEQUESTRATION. One or more areas of osseous necrosis, or sequestration, commonly are situated in the medullary aspect of a tubular bone, where they create radiodense bone spicules (Fig. 59–8). The increased density is related primarily to the fact that a sequestrum does not possess a blood supply and does not participate in the hyperemia and resulting osteoporosis of the adjacent living bone. The sequestrum frequently is sharply marginated as it rests in a space surrounded by granulation tissue, and it varies in size from minute fragments to long necrotic segments. Sequestra may extrude through cortical breaks, extending into the adjacent soft tissues, where they may eventually be discharged through draining sinuses.

Table 59–3. HEMATOGENOUS OSTEOMYELITIS: RADIOGRAPHIC-PATHOLOGIC CORRELATION

Pathologic Abnormality	Radiographic Abnormality
Vascular changes and edema of soft tissues	Soft tissue swelling with obliteration of tissue planes
Infection in medullary space with hyperemia, edema, abscess formation, and trabecular destruction	Osteoporosis, bone lysis
Infection in haversian and Volkmann's canals of cortex	Increasing lysis, cortical lucency
Subperiosteal abscess formation with lifting of the periosteum and bone formation	Periostitis, involucrum formation
Infectious penetration of periosteum with soft tissue abscess formation	Soft tissue swelling, mass formation, obliteration of tissue planes
Localized cortical and medullary abscesses	Single or multiple radiolucent cortical or medullary lesions with surrounding sclerosis
Deprivation of blood supply to cortex due to thrombosis of metaphyseal vessels and interruption of periosteal vessels, cortical necrosis	Sequestration
External migration of dead pieces of cortex with breakdown of skin and subcutaneous tissue	Sinus tracts

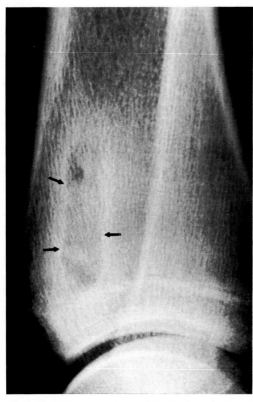

Figure 59–7. Hematogenous osteomyelitis: Brodie's abscess. A lateral radiograph outlines a typical appearance of an abscess of the distal part of the tibia caused by staphylococci. Observe the elongated radiolucent lesion with surrounding sclerosis extending to the closing growth plate (arrows). The channel-like shape of the lesion is important in the accurate diagnosis of this condition.

SCLEROSING OSTEOMYELITIS. In the subacute and chronic stages of osteomyelitis, periosteal bone formation and thickened trabeculae may lead to considerable radiodensity and contour irregularity of the affected bone (Fig. 59–9). Cystic changes may occur within the sclerotic area, but sequestra are uncommon. The radiographic findings resemble those of osteoid osteoma, fibrous dysplasia, and Ewing's sarcoma.

Spread from a Contiguous Source of Infection
General Clinical Features

Bone (and joint) contamination can result from spread from a contiguous source of infection. In most of the cases of osteomyelitis (and septic arthritis) arising from such a contiguous source, soft tissue infections are implicated (postoperative infection is discussed separately). The contamination of bone from an adjacent soft tissue infection is particularly significant in the hands, the feet, the mandible or maxilla, and the skull. The importance of osteomyelitis of the mandible and maxilla in individuals with poor dental hygiene and of the frontal portion of the skull and face in individuals with chronic sinusitis is undeniable. Pott's puffy tumor refers to an indolent soft tissue swelling of the scalp that is due to subperiosteal infection or an osteomyelitis of the frontal bone resulting from frontal sinusitis.

Soft tissue infections that lead to bone and joint contamination are frequent after animal and human bites and puncture wounds. Procedures such as venipuncture and catheterization can lead to secondary infection of soft tissue and bone. Irradiation and burns are other important sources of soft tissue and osseous contamination.

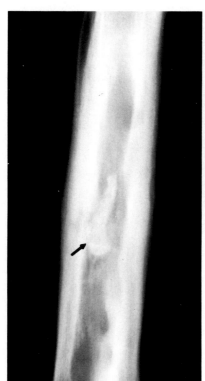

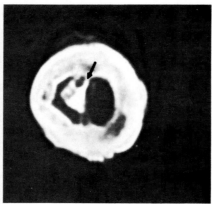

B

A

Figure 59–8. Chronic osteomyelitis: Sequestration. Conventional (**A**) and computed (**B**) tomography can be used to identify sequestered bone (arrows), as in this femur. (Courtesy of U.S. Naval Hospital, San Diego, California.)

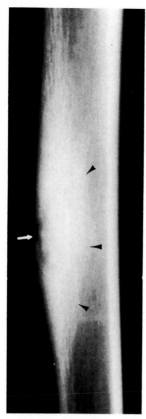

Figure 59–9. Chronic sclerosing osteomyelitis. Chronic osteomyelitis can be associated with considerable new bone formation. In this patient, a cortical abscess contains a sequestrum (arrow) and is surrounded by sclerosis (arrowheads). The appearance is reminiscent of that of an osteoid osteoma.

General Radiographic and Pathologic Features (Table 59–4)

Whereas the direction of contamination in hematogenous osteomyelitis is from the bone outward into the soft tissue, the direction of contamination in osteomyelitis resulting from adjacent sepsis is from the soft tissues inward into the bone (or joint) (Fig. 59–10). Organisms within soft tissues encroach on fascial planes, form abscesses, and disrupt the periosteum. Displacement of the periosteum is more marked in children because of its looser attachment. Resulting periosteal bone formation commonly is the initial radiographic manifestation of osteomyelitis. With further accumulation of pus, subperiosteal resorption of bone and cortical disruption ensue. Infection then may spread in the marrow, producing lytic osseous defects on the radiograph. Later radiographic and pathologic abnormalities are identical to those occurring in neglected hematogenous infections.

Specific Locations

HAND

Pathways of Spread of Infection. There are three distinct routes available to organisms that become lodged in the soft tissues of the hand; infection may disseminate via tendon sheaths, fascial planes, or lymphatics.

Synovial sheaths surround the flexor tendons of each digit of the hand; they extend from the terminal phalanges in a proximal direction to the palm. In the first and fifth digits, connection with the radial and ulnar bursae, two synovial sacs on the volar aspect of the wrist, frequently is apparent. The extensor tendon sheaths extend in six compartments beneath the dorsal carpal ligament on the dorsum of the wrist.

Infective digital tenosynovitis can result from a puncture wound. A sheath infection may perforate into an adjacent bone or joint in the finger (Fig. 59–11). Infection within the volar sheaths of the first and fifth digits may spread quickly to the ulnar and radial bursae and from these latter areas into the wrist.

There are two important fascial planes of the hand. The midpalmar space extends in a triangular fashion along the ulnar aspect of the hand from the third metacarpal to the hypothenar eminence; the thenar space extends along the radial aspect of the hand from the third metacarpal bone to the thenar eminence. Infection in the midpalmar space may result from direct implantation during injury or by extension from suppurative sheaths. Palmar swelling, semiflexion of the fingers, and bone destruction are the accompanying clinical and radiologic manifestations of neglected infection. Infection of the thenar space can also lead to osteomyelitis, especially of the metacarpal bones (Fig. 59–12).

Lymphangitis may result from superficial injuries. In intense cases, complications, including tenosynovitis, septicemia, osteomyelitis, and septic arthritis, may be noted.

Specific Entities. A *felon* results from infection in the terminal pulp space. Bone involvement is not infrequent in neglected cases (Fig. 59–13). In addition to osteomyelitis, soft tissue edema adjacent to the bone can produce ischemia and bone necrosis.

Subcuticular abscesses of the nail fold are termed *paronychia*. On rare occasions, osseous destruction of a terminal phalanx may be evident.

The frequency of hand infection in drug addicts is noteworthy; infections commonly follow local injections with contaminated needles. Bilateral swelling of the dorsum of the hand in addicts, the puffy-hand syndrome, however, can relate not to infection but to lymphedema resulting from lymphatic destruction and fibrosis of the subcutaneous tissues.

Table 59–4. OSTEOMYELITIS DUE TO SPREAD FROM A CONTIGUOUS SOURCE OF INFECTION: RADIOGRAPHIC-PATHOLOGIC CORRELATION

Pathologic Abnormality	Radiographic Abnormality
Soft tissue contamination and abscess formation	Soft tissue swelling mass formation, obliteration of tissue planes
Infectious invasion of the periosteum with lifting of the membrane and bone formation	Periostitis
Subperiosteal abscess formation and cortical invasion	Cortical erosion
Infection in haversian and Volkmann's canals of corterx	Cortical lucency and destruction
Contamination and spread in marrow	Bone lysis

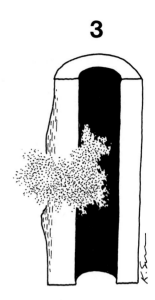

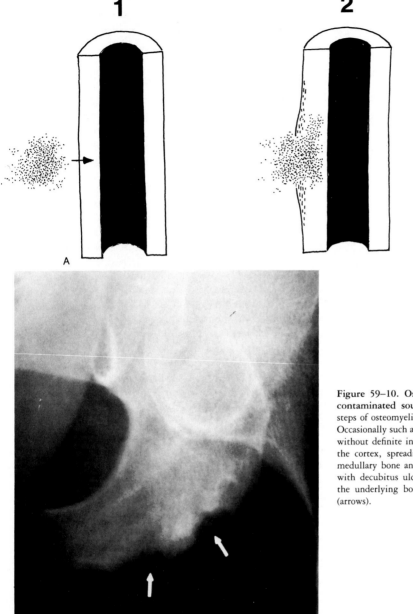

Figure 59–10. **Osteomyelitis resulting from spread from a contiguous contaminated source. A** A diagrammatic representation of the sequential steps of osteomyelitis. *1*, Initially, a soft tissue focus of infection is apparent. Occasionally such a focus can irritate the underlying bone, producing periostitis without definite invasion of the cortex. *2*, The infection subsequently invades the cortex, spreading via haversian and Volkmann's canals. *3*, Finally, the medullary bone and marrow spaces are affected. **B** In an immobilized patient with decubitus ulcerations, soft tissue infection has led to contamination of the underlying bone. Observe erosion and reactive sclerosis of the ischium (arrows).

FOOT

Pathways of Spread of Infection. The plantar aspect of the foot is especially vulnerable to soft tissue infection. Foreign bodies, puncture wounds, or skin ulceration from weight-bearing can represent the portal of entry for various organisms. Three plantar muscle compartments (medial, lateral, and intermediate) serve as avenues within the soft tissues in the foot that allow dissemination of localized infection.

Specific Entities

Puncture Wounds. Puncture wounds of the plantar aspect of the foot can lead to osteomyelitis and septic arthritis (Fig. 59–14). These injuries are especially prominent in children who walk barefoot, exposing the unprotected foot to nails,

glass, splinters, and other sharp objects. The infective organisms can vary, but gram-negative agents such as *Pseudomonas aeruginosa* frequently are implicated. Typically, local pain and swelling appear within days after a puncture wound. After a delay of 1 to 3 weeks, the radiographs reveal typical abnormalities of osteomyelitis or septic arthritis.

Osteomyelitis of the os calcis is a recognized complication of repeated heel punctures in the neonate. The mechanism of infection usually relates to the spread of soft tissue suppuration to the neighboring bone; subsequently, hematogenous dissemination with multifocal osteomyelitis may appear.

Foot Infections in Diabetes Mellitus. Clinical, radiologic, and pathologic characteristics of osteomyelitis (and septic arthritis) complicating foot infections in diabetic patients are

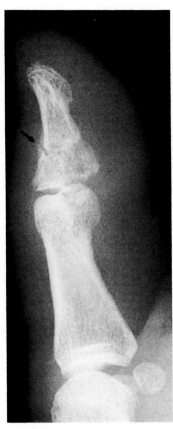

Figure 59–11. Spread of infection in the hand: Digital flexor tenosynovitis. A neglected infected flexor tenosynovitis of the thumb has led to osteomyelitis and a pathologic fracture (arrow) of the terminal phalanx in addition to soft tissue swelling.

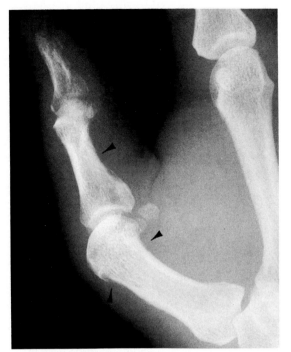

Figure 59–12. Spread of infection in the hand: Thenar space infection. Osseous resorption and contamination of the metacarpal bone and proximal phalanx can be seen (arrowheads). The source of the infection, the soft tissues of the tip of the thumb, is evident on the film. (From Resnick D: Osteomyelitis and septic arthritis complicating hand injuries and infections: Pathogenesis of roentgenographic abnormalities. J Can Assoc Radiol 27:21, 1976. Used with permission.)

modified by the associated problems of these individuals, including vascular insufficiency and neurologic deficit. Local symptoms and signs dominate, including pain, swelling, erythema, and diminished peripheral pulses. The radiographic picture usually reveals significant soft tissue swelling and mottled osteolysis (Fig. 59–15). Osteosclerosis, fragmentation, and periostitis may be seen. Radiolucent areas within the soft tissues also are commonly identified. This finding can relate to the presence of air owing to dissection around open wounds or after local débridement or to the presence of gas in clostridial or nonclostridial infections.

Infection and neuroarthropathy of the midfoot and forefoot frequently coexist in diabetic patients. The presence of poorly defined osseous contours is the most helpful radiologic clue to osteomyelitis.

PELVIS

Breakdown of soft tissue that occurs in debilitated persons who maintain a single position for long periods of time is referred to as a pressure sore, decubitus ulcer, or bedsore. It is most commonly seen in patients with spinal cord injury or other neurologic defects. Although other sites, such as the heels, may be affected, most pressure sores develop about the pelvis, especially near the sacrum, ischial tuberosities, trochanteric regions, and buttocks.

Local soft tissue infection and bacteremia commonly are associated with decubitus ulcers. Although bacteremia implies an attendant risk for hematogenous spread of infection to

distant bones, osteomyelitis most commonly is observed in the innominate bones and proximal portions of the femora, areas subjacent to sites of skin breakdown.

The accurate diagnosis of osteomyelitis complicating pressure sores is difficult, owing to a number of other conditions

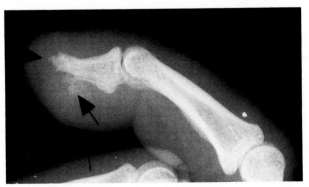

Figure 59–13. Spread of infection in the hand: Felon. An infection in the pulp space has produced considerable soft tissue swelling (open arrows). Extension into the tuft and diaphysis of the terminal phalanx is apparent (solid arrows). Shrapnel from a previous injury can be seen. (From Resnick D: Osteomyelitis and septic arthritis complicating hand injuries and infections: Pathogenesis of roentgenographic abnormalities. J Can Assoc Radiol 27:21, 1976. Used with permission.)

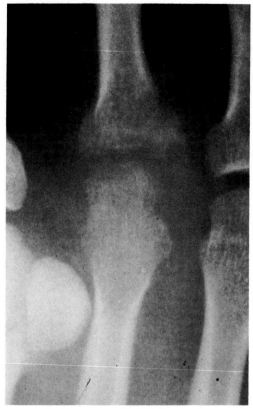

Figure 59–14. Spread of infection in the foot. Puncture wounds. After a puncture wound from a nail, osseous destruction of the metatarsal head and proximal phalanx, joint space narrowing, and soft tissue swelling became evident.

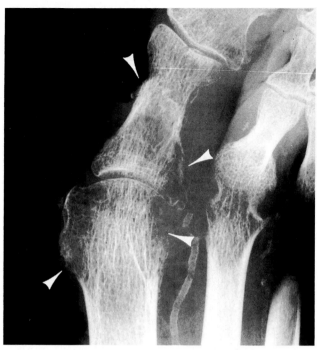

Figure 59–15. Spread of infection in the foot: Diabetes mellitus. A radiograph reveals a soft tissue infection about the first metatarsophalangeal joint with ulcerations and with erosion of bone (arrowheads). Observe vascular calcification and alterations at the second and third metatarsophalangeal joints.

that may become evident in the immobilized or paralyzed patient. Pressure related changes in bone are not infrequent, leading to flattening and sclerosis of bone prominences, such as the femoral trochanters and ischial tuberosities. Heterotopic ossification further complicates early diagnosis of osteomyelitis.

Direct Implantation
General Clinical Features

Puncture wounds of the hand and the foot can lead to osteomyelitis (and septic arthritis) by contaminating adjacent soft tissues or directly inoculating the bone or joint (Fig. 59–16). This latter complication is especially prevalent in the foot, at which site nails, splinters, or glass can lead to deep puncture wounds, producing immediate bone (and joint) contamination; in the hand, at which site a human bite received during a fist-fight can directly injure osseous and articular structures; and in any site after animal bites.

General Radiographic Features

The features of bone (and joint) involvement after direct implantation of an infectious process are virtually identical to those occurring after spread of infection from a contiguous contaminated source. Commonly, osseous destruction and proliferation lead to focal areas of lysis, sclerosis, and periostitis. Soft tissue swelling is common.

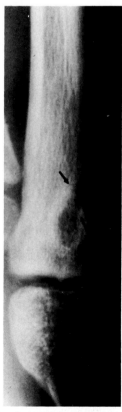

Figure 59–16. Infection due to direct implantation: Puncture wounds. After a puncture wound, an abscess of the distal part of the fibula owing to staphylococci developed. Note the tract running from the cortex to the lesion (arrows), indicating the nature of the original injury.

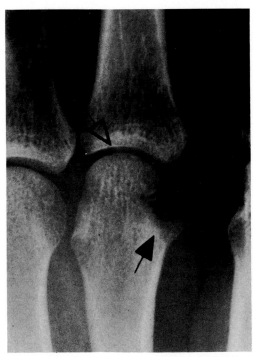

Figure 59–17. Infection due to direct implantation: Human bites. Progressive destruction of the third metacarpal head (solid arrow) and a narrowed metacarpophalangeal joint (open arrow) resulted from infection following a fist-fight. (From Resnick D: Osteomyelitis and septic arthritis complicating hand injuries and infections: Pathogenesis of roentgenographic abnormalities. J Can Assoc Radiol 27:21, 1976. Used with permission.)

Specific Entities

HUMAN BITES. Although human bites occur in a variety of situations, the most common cause of injury is a fist-blow to the mouth resulting in laceration of the dorsum of the metacarpophalangeal joint. Joint infection is more common than bone infection in these cases. *Staphylococcus aureus* or Streptococcus species is the usual implicated organism. The radiographic findings include peculiar fractures, tooth fragments, and osseous and articular destruction (Fig. 59–17).

ANIMAL BITES. Superficial animal bites or scratches can inoculate local soft tissues, later leading to infection of underlying bones and joints; and deep animal bites can introduce organisms directly into both osseous and articular structures. Dog bites account for approximately 90 per cent of these injuries and cat bites for about 10 per cent. The infecting organisms vary, but *Pasteurella multocida* commonly is implicated. Animal bites predominate in the hand, the arm, and the leg (Fig. 59–18).

OPEN FRACTURES AND DISLOCATIONS. Whenever a fracture or dislocation is complicated by disruption of the overlying skin, direct inoculation of bones and joints can occur. This problem is especially relevant to injuries of the tibia.

Postoperative Infection

Postoperative osteoarticular infections may occur as a result of contamination of bones and joints from adjacent infected soft tissues, direct inoculation of osseous and articular tissue at the time of surgery, or, less frequently, hematogenous spread to an operative site from a distant location. Clinically, considerable delay in diagnosis is not infrequent. Routine radiography, tomography, sinography, and arthrography can all be helpful in establishing the diagnosis; increasing osseous and cartilaginous destruction, periostitis, soft tissue swelling, and exaggerated lucency about cemented metallic prostheses can be recognized (see Chapter 20).

One special type of postoperative infection relates to pin tracts. This complication is particularly troublesome after transcutaneous insertion of pins into bone, its reported frequency varying from almost zero to 4 per cent. Radiographs reveal progressive osteolysis about the metal or, after removal of the pin, a ring sequestrum (Fig. 59–19). In the latter instance the central circular radiolucent area created by the pin itself is surrounded by a ring of bone, which, in turn, is surrounded by an area of osteolysis.

Complications
Severe Osteolysis

Some patients with osteomyelitis do not receive early or adequate treatment, and in these patients, severe osteolysis may ensue. Large foci of destruction can eventually lead to disappearance of long segments of tubular or flat bones.

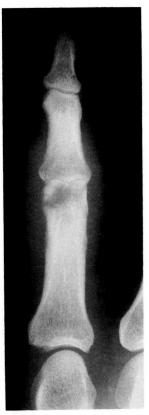

Figure 59–18. Infection due to direct implantation: Animal bites. After a cat bite, this patient developed Pasteurella osteomyelitis and septic arthritis. Observe soft tissue swelling, osseous destruction of the proximal and middle phalanges, and joint space narrowing and flexion at the proximal interphalangeal joint.

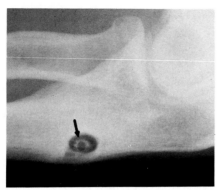

Figure 59–19. Postoperative infection: Pin-hole ring sequestrum. Percutaneous pins were used to treat a fracture about the wrist in this 27 year old man. Purulent drainage occurred, requiring removal of the pins. Note the classic radiographic findings of a ring sequestrum (arrow).

Epiphyseal Growth Disturbance

In the infant, infection that has spread to the epiphysis of a tubular bone can produce significant damage. Injury to the cartilage cells on the epiphyseal side of the growth plate is irreparable, and subsequent growth disturbances are to be expected. Even with severe epiphyseal disintegration, however, some regeneration of the epiphysis can occur after eradication of the infection.

Neoplasm

Epidermoid carcinoma arising in a focus of chronic osteomyelitis may be evident in at least 0.5 per cent of patients with long-term draining infections of bone. The latent period between the onset of osteomyelitis and the appearance of neoplasm varies, although a time span of 20 to 30 years is typical. Neoplasm most frequently arises adjacent to the femur and the tibia, being evident clinically as pain, increasing drainage, onset of a foul odor from the sinus tract, a mass, and lymphadenopathy; radiographically it appears as progressive destruction of bone (Fig. 59–20). The prognosis is guarded, as distant metastasis is not infrequent.

Although epithelial carcinoma is the most common neoplasm that is encountered in osteomyelitis, fibrosarcoma, angiosarcoma, rhabdomyosarcoma, histiocytic lymphoma, adenocarcinoma, basal cell carcinoma, and plasmacytoma have also been noted.

Modifications and Difficulties in Diagnosis
Antibiotic Modified Osteomyelitis

In the modern era of sophisticated chemotherapeutic techniques, the infective process often is interrupted at a relatively early stage. If therapy is adequate, complete healing of the osseous abnormalities can occur. During the early healing phase of osteomyelitis, bone resorption continues as damaged osseous tissue is removed. Thus, radiographically evident increased destruction can occur at a time when the clinical picture is improving.

"Active" and "Inactive" Chronic Osteomyelitis

Differentiation of active and inactive chronic osteomyelitis by radiographic techniques can be extremely difficult (Table 59–5). The extensive osteolytic and osteosclerotic changes of

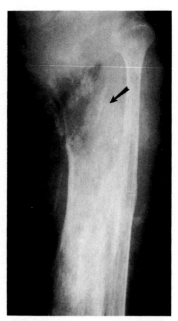

Figure 59–20. Complications of osteomyelitis: Neoplasm. Superimposed on the radiographic changes of chronic infection of the tibia is a lytic lesion of the proximal aspect of the bone (arrow), which represented an epidermoid carcinoma arising in a sinus tract and invading the osseous tissue.

a chronic osteomyelitic process that is dormant can obscure the changes of reactivation for a period of time. There are, however, certain indications on the radiograph that do allow documentation of active chronic osteomyelitis: new areas of bone destruction; periostitis that is thin and linear and separated from the subjacent bone; poorly defined periosteal excrescences extending into the adjacent soft tissues; and sequestration.

Differential Diagnosis

The combination of clinical and radiologic characteristics in osteomyelitis usually ensures correct diagnosis. Occasionally, aggressive bone destruction combined with periostitis and soft tissue swelling simulates the changes in malignant neoplasms, especially Ewing's sarcoma or osteosarcoma in the child, histiocytic lymphoma in the young adult, and skeletal metastasis in the older person.

The identification in a child of a metaphyseal radiolucent lesion abutting on the growth plate or connecting with it by a channel certainly suggests the presence of an abscess. Although osteosarcoma typically is metaphyseal in location and Ewing's sarcoma may be metaphyseal, the osteolytic foci in these tumors are more poorly marginated, and with osteosarcoma considerable neoplastic bone production may be evident. In an adult, osteolytic foci within an infected

Table 59–5. RADIOGRAPHIC SIGNS OF ACTIVITY IN CHRONIC OSTEOMYELITIS

Change from previous radiograph
Poorly defined areas of osteolysis
Thin, linear periostitis
Sequestration

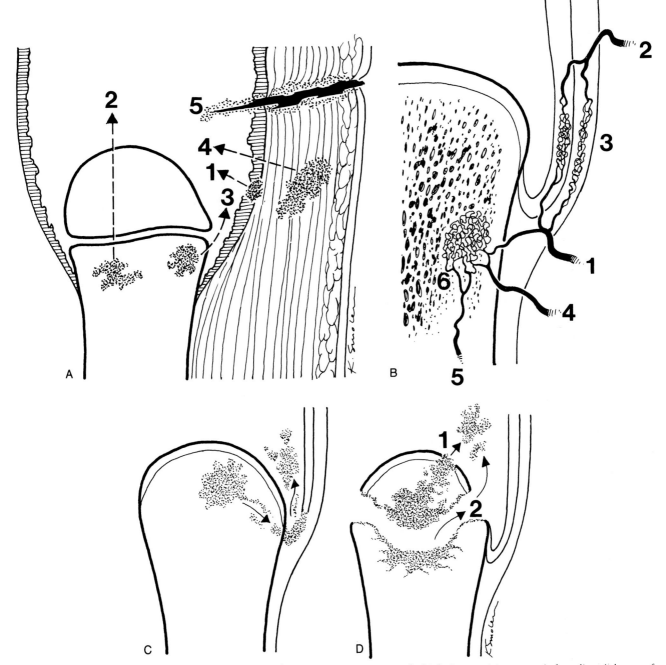

Figure 59–21. Septic arthritis: Potential routes of contamination. A Hematogenous spread of infection to a joint can result from direct lodgment of organisms in the synovial membrane (1) or, as illustrated in **B,** direct vascular continuity between an infected epiphysis and the synovial membrane. Spread into the joint from a contiguous source can occur from a metaphyseal focus that extends into the epiphysis and from there into the joint (2); from a metaphyseal focus with extension into the joint when the growth plate is intraarticular (3); or from a contiguous soft tissue infection (4). Direct implantation following a penetrating wound (5) can also lead to septic arthritis. **B, C** Hematogenous spread of infection to a joint can occur owing to vascular continuity between the epiphysis and synovial membrane. In **B** the vessels shown include arterioles (1), venules (2), and capillaries (3) of the capsule, periosteal vessels (4), the nutrient artery (5), and metaphyseal-epiphyseal anastomoses (6). In this fashion, the synovial membrane may become infected from an osseous focus before the joint fluid is contaminated. In **C,** this sequence of events is diagrammed. **D** Spread from a contiguous osseous surface can result from penetration of the cartilage (1) or pathologic fracture with articular contamination (2). In this situation, synovial fluid may become infected before the synovial membrane.

epiphysis can simulate the appearance of a giant cell tumor, intraosseous ganglion, or subchondral cyst.

Cortical lucent lesions can indicate an abscess, osteoid osteoma, or stress fracture. The nature of the lesion and the surrounding bone eburnation generally allow differentiation among these conditions (see earlier discussion).

In some cases of osteomyelitis, exuberant bone formation produces widespread sclerosis. The resulting radiographic picture can simulate malignant bone tumors (such as osteosarcoma, Ewing's sarcoma, histiocytic lymphoma, and chondrosarcoma), osteonecrosis, fibrous dysplasia, or Paget's disease.

Soft tissue prominence is a common finding in infectious and neoplastic conditions. In general, tumors are associated with circumscribed soft tissue masses that displace surrounding soft tissue planes and frequently contain visible tumor matrix. Infections lead to infiltration and obscuring of soft tissue planes.

SEPTIC ARTHRITIS
Articular Manifestations of Infection

Septic arthritis is but one of several processes that can cause articular disease in patients with infection. An infectious agent may trigger a sterile synovitis at a site distant from the primary infective focus, as the joint reacts to its presence in the form of an inflammatory, hypersensitivity, or immune-mediated response. Classic examples of reactive arthritis include acute rheumatic fever occurring as a complication of streptococcal throat infection, Reiter's syndrome, intestinal bypass surgery, and hepatitis. Clinical characteristics common to reactive arthritides include a symptom-free interval between the inciting infection and the rheumatic reaction; a self-limited course in which cartilage or bone destruction is rare; a characteristic clinical presentation that includes acute migratory polyarthritis and an elevated erythrocyte sedimentation rate; a tendency in some patients toward involvement of the heart; and a negative serologic test for rheumatoid factor. Inciting infections commonly reach the body through one of three portals of entry: the oronasopharynx and respiratory tract, the urogenital tract, and the intestinal tract. The existence of reactive arthritis in patients with infection underscores the importance of joint aspiration and attempts at isolation of the causative organisms in all cases of suspected septic arthritis.

Routes of Contamination

The potential routes of contamination of joints can be divided into four categories (Fig. 59–21).

1. Hematogenous spread of infection. Hematogenous seeding of the synovial membrane results from either direct transport of organisms within the synovial vessels or spread from an adjacent epiphyseal focus of osteomyelitis by means of vascular continuity between the epiphysis and the synovial membrane.

2. Spread from a contiguous source of infection. A joint may become contaminated by intraarticular extension of osteomyelitis from an epiphyseal or metaphyseal focus or of neighboring suppurative soft tissue processes.

3. Direct implantation. Inoculation of a joint can occur during aspiration or after a penetrating wound.

4. Postoperative infection. An intraarticular suppurative process can occur after any type of joint surgery.

Hematogenous Spread of Infection

Hematogenous spread of infection to a joint indicates that organisms are transported within the vasculature of the synovial membrane directly from a distant infected source or indirectly from an adjacent bone infection. In either case, infection of the synovial membrane precedes contamination of the synovial fluid. The reaction of the synovial tissue to the contained organisms varies according to the local and general resistance of the patient and the number, type, and virulence of the infecting agents.

General Clinical Features

Septic arthritis affects men and women of all ages, although it predominates in the young. Monarticular involvement is the major pattern of presentation. The knee, particularly in children, infants, and adults, and the hip, especially in children and infants, are frequently affected. With pyogenic infection, an acute onset with fever and chills is typical, and local pain, tenderness, redness, heat, and soft tissue swelling are common. Leukocytosis and positive blood and joint cultures are important laboratory parameters of pyogenic arthritis. The bacterium most commonly implicated is *Staphylococcus aureus*.

Radiographic-Pathologic Correlation (Table 59–6)

In response to bacterial infection, the synovial membrane becomes edematous, swollen, and hypertrophied. Increased amounts of cloudy synovial fluid are produced. After a few days, frank pus accumulates in the articular cavity and destruction of cartilage begins (Fig. 59–22). Prominent cartilaginous abnormality may appear at the margins or central portions of articulations, accompanied by growth of the inflamed synovium across the surface of the cartilage or between cartilage and bone. The capsule then becomes distended, surrounding soft tissue edema is evident, and osseous abnormalities ensue. Superficial marginal and central bone erosions may progress to extensive destruction of large segments of the articular surface. Fibrous or bone ankylosis can eventually occur.

Radiographically evident soft tissue swelling accompanies synovial hypertrophy (Fig. 59–23). Interosseous space narrowing reflects disruption of the chondral surface. Osseous ero-

Table 59–6. SEPTIC ARTHRITIS: RADIOGRAPHIC-PATHOLOGIC CORRELATION

Pathologic Abnormality	Radiographic Abnormality
Edema and hypertrophy of synovial membrane with fluid production	Joint effusion, soft tissue swelling
Hyperemia	Osteoporosis
Inflammatory pannus with chondral destruction	Joint space loss
Pannus destruction of bone	Marginal and central osseous erosion
Fibrous or bone ankylosis	Bone ankylosis

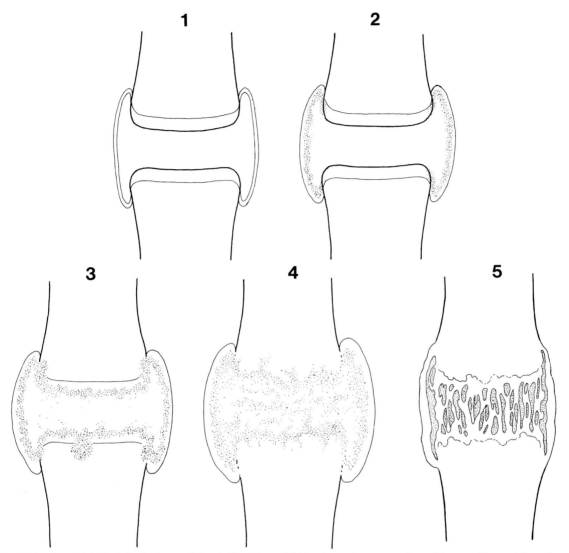

Figure 59–22. Septic arthritis: Pathologic abnormalities. 1, Normal synovial joint; 2, an edematous swollen and hypertrophic synovial membrane becomes evident; 3, 4, accumulating inflammatory pannus leads to chondral destruction and to marginal and central osseous erosions; 5, bone ankylosis can eventually result.

sions at the edges of the articulation lead to marginal defects that are similar to those of rheumatoid arthritis. Subchondral extension of pannus destroys the bone plate, leading to gaps in the subchondral "white" line on the radiograph. Further destruction of bone becomes evident and, in late stages, bone ankylosis of the articulation may be seen.

These pathologic and radiographic abnormalities are modified in accordance with the infecting organism. Rapid destruction of bone and cartilage is characteristic of bacterial arthritis, whereas in tuberculosis and fungal diseases, articular changes occur more slowly. In tuberculosis, marginal osseous erosions with preservation of joint space and periarticular osteoporosis can be prominent. In all varieties of septic arthritis, poorly defined bone destruction and periostitis are seen.

Rarely, gas formation within a joint can complicate septic arthritis. Much more frequently, the appearance of radiolucent collections in an infected joint indicates that a prior arthro-

centesis has been performed or that an open wound exists with communication between the joint and the skin surface.

Spread from a Contiguous Source of Infection

In certain age groups, osteomyelitis can lead to contamination of the adjacent joint. In the infant the presence of vascular communication between metaphyseal and epiphyseal segments of tubular bones allows organisms within nutrient vessels to localize in the epiphysis and subsequently extend into the joint. This may occur via the common vascular pathways of the epiphysis and synovial membrane (hematogenous spread of infection) or as a result of transchondral extension directly into the articular cavity (spread from a contiguous source). In the adult, vascular connections between the epiphysis and metaphysis allow hematogenous osteomyelitis to affect the epiphysis. Once again, subsequent joint contamination can occur.

A second situation is related to adjacent soft tissue infection

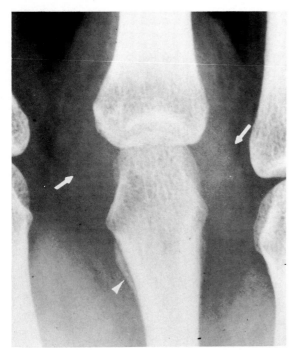

Figure 59–23. Septic arthritis: Radiographic abnormalities. Soft tissue swelling. A radiograph of an infected metacarpophalangeal joint demonstrates soft tissue edema (arrows), osteoporosis, and periostitis (arrowhead). (Courtesy of J. Weston, M.D., Lower Hutt, New Zealand.)

or, more rarely, nearby visceral infection (e.g., vesicoacetabular or enteroacetabular fistulae) (Fig. 59–24). Predisposing factors include pelvic trauma, surgical manipulation, and diverticulitis.

A third situation in which joint infection develops as a result of extension from a surrounding process occurs in those locations (e.g., hip and glenohumeral joint) in which the growth plate has an intraarticular location. Because of this anatomic arrangement, osteomyelitis localized to the metaphysis can enter the joint by extending laterally without violating the growth plate. With penetration of the thin metaphyseal cortex, organisms can extend directly into the synovium or the articular cavity.

Radiographic-Pathologic Correlation

Generally, there is radiographic evidence that the infective process originates outside the joint. This evidence may include soft tissue deficit, swelling, or gas formation; osteomyelitis with typical epiphyseal or metaphyseal destruction; and diverticulitis or cystitis with fistulization. In certain situations, however, joint effusion and cartilaginous and subchondral osseous destruction are the first radiographic clues to infection. In the infant in whom the epiphysis is unossified or only partially ossified, detection of primary osteomyelitis can be extremely difficult, and an effusion and displacement of the ossified epiphyseal nucleus may be the first evidence of sepsis.

Once the joint has been violated, the radiographic and pathologic abnormalities of the infection are virtually identical to those associated with hematogenously derived suppurative joint disease. Soft tissue swelling, diffuse loss of joint space, poorly defined marginal and central osseous defects, periostitis, fragmentation, and calcification can be observed.

Specific Entities

SEPTIC ARTHRITIS OF THE HIP IN INFANCY AND CHILDHOOD. Neonatal septic arthritis most frequently affects the hip, and *Staphylococcus aureus* is the most commonly implicated organism. In this age group, infection can reach this joint by spreading from a metaphyseal focus of osteomyelitis either directly into the joint (the growth plate is intraarticular) or to the epiphysis by way of vascular channels that cross the growth plate, and, from there, into the joint. Clinically, infants with septic arthritis of the hip may reveal irritability, loss of appetite, and fever. Local symptoms and signs may be absent, although swelling and a hip held in flexion, abduction, and external rotation are helpful clues. Initial radiographs of the hip frequently are unremarkable. Soft tissue swelling and a positive obturator sign, however, may be evident (Fig. 59–25), and subluxation or dislocation of the femoral head can occur.

Displacement of the femoral head or metaphysis also occurs in infants with congenital dislocation of the hip, neurologic deficits, and traumatic epiphyseal separations. Thus, aspiration of the joint is mandatory in firmly establishing the diagnosis of septic arthritis. Without early antibiotic administration, deformities, including coxa magna, complete dissolution of the femoral head and neck, or persistent dislocation of the femoral head or femoral shaft, may appear (Fig. 59–26).

Septic arthritis of the hip also is frequent in the child. It may be associated with fever, pain, swelling, and limping. On radiographs, accumulation of intraarticular fluid may produce soft tissue swelling, capsular distention, and subtle lateral displacement of the ossified epiphysis (Fig. 59–27). Concentric loss of joint space, subchondral osseous defects, and lytic foci of the femoral metaphysis can be evident. Abnormalities may be mistaken for those associated with juvenile chronic arthritis or Legg-Calvé-Perthes disease. Although the prognosis of septic arthritis of the hip for a child is far better than that for an infant, osteonecrosis of the femoral head is a very important complication of the disease.

Direct Implantation

Arthrocentesis accomplished for evaluation of synovial contents or used for arthrography can introduce bacteria. Similarly, penetrating injury, such as occurs in a fist-fight (see earlier discussion) or from a bullet, knife, nail, or other sharp object, can lead to septic arthritis.

Postoperative Infection

Articular surgery in the form of an arthrotomy, arthrodesis, arthroplasty, or other procedure can be complicated by joint infection in the postoperative period. Infections occurring soon after the procedure usually are related to direct inoculation of the joint during the operation or to intraarticular spread from an adjacent contaminated focus (e.g., soft tissue abscess). Joint infection occurring long after surgery frequently is associated with hematogenous spread to the joint from a distant infectious process.

Complications

Several potential complications of septic arthritis, such as epiphyseal destruction and osteonecrosis, have already been discussed. Occasionally, sepsis in a joint may become evident as distention and contamination of a communicating cyst.

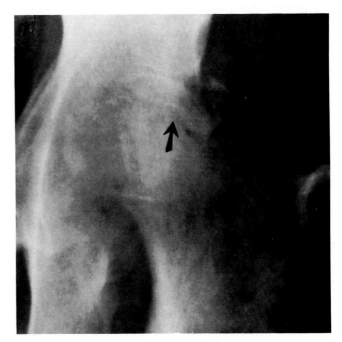

Figure 59–24. Septic arthritis: Contamination from a contiguous source of infection. This man with rheumatoid arthritis had undergone a laparotomy and bowel resection with a colostomy for sigmoid diverticulitis. A tract developed between the bowel, left hip, and skin, which was related to *Escherichia coli* infection. A radiograph of the hip outlines the narrowed joint space and bony destruction. A radiolucent fracture line can be seen in the femoral head (arrow). (From Resnick D: Pyarthrosis complicating rheumatoid arthritis: Report of 5 patients and a review of the literature. Radiology 114:581, 1975. Used with permission.)

Septic arthritis also can result in disruption of adjacent capsular, tendinous, and soft tissue structures. In cases of infection in the glenohumeral joint, arthrography may indicate intraarticular synovial inflammation, tears of the rotator cuff, and soft tissue abscess formation.

Partial or complete osseous fusion may represent the residual findings of septic arthritis. This complication is not frequent, however.

Significant destruction of articular cartilage can lead to incongruity of apposing articular surfaces and, later, to changes of secondary degenerative joint disease.

Modifications and Difficulties in Diagnosis

When infection is superimposed on a previous articular disorder such as rheumatoid arthritis, calcium pyrophosphate dihydrate crystal deposition disease, or osteoarthritis, the clinical and radiographic abnormalities can be hidden or changed by the underlying disease process. In the septic

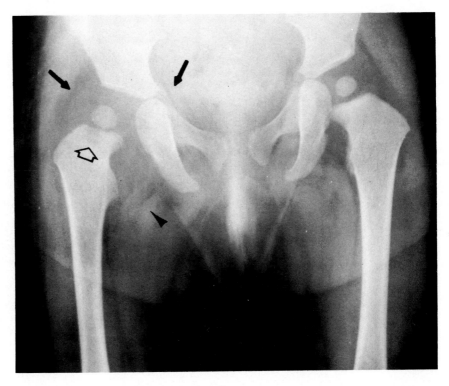

Figure 59–25. Septic arthritis of the hip: Infancy. Note displacement of the "capsular" and obturator fat planes (solid arrows), obliteration of the iliopsoas fat plane (arrowhead), and a metaphyseal focus of infection (open arrow). The femoral head is displaced laterally and is slightly enlarged. (Courtesy of J. Weston, M.D., Lower Hutt, New Zealand.)

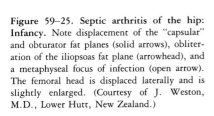

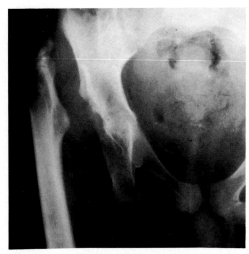

Figure 59–26. Septic arthritis of the hip: Infancy. Subsequent to infection, femoral dislocation, acetabular shallowness, and absence of epiphyseal ossification became evident. (Reproduced with permission from Freiberger RH, et al: Hip Disease of Infancy and Childhood. In RD Moseley Jr, et al: Current Problems in Radiology. Copyright 1973 by Year Book Medical Publishers, Inc, Chicago.)

rheumatoid joint, for example, the findings of soft tissue swelling, joint space narrowing, and osseous destruction related to the suppurative process are difficult to differentiate from those of rheumatoid arthritis (see Chapter 22).

Differential Diagnosis

Although numerous disorders such as pigmented villonodular synovitis, idiopathic synovial osteochondromatosis, juvenile chronic arthritis, and even adult-onset rheumatoid arthritis can be associated with monoarticular changes, infection must be considered the prime diagnostic possibility in cases of monoarthritis until appropriate aspiration and culture document its absence.

Of all the radiographic features of infection, it is the poorly defined nature of the bone destruction that is most characteristic. Osseous erosions or cysts are more sharply marginated in gout, rheumatoid arthritis, seronegative spondyloarthropathies, osteoarthritis, pigmented villonodular synovitis, idiopathic synovial osteochondromatosis, hemophilia, and calcium pyrophosphate dihydrate crystal deposition disease. Furthermore, concentric loss of interosseous space is typical in infection. A similar pattern of joint space loss accompanies rheumatoid arthritis, the seronegative spondyloarthropathies, calcium pyrophosphate dihydrate crystal deposition disease, chondrolysis, and chondral atrophy, but asymmetric diminution of the articular lumen, as noted in osteoarthritis, and relative preservation of articular space, as seen in gout, pigmented villonodular synovitis, idiopathic synovial osteochondromatosis, and hemophilia, are rare in pyogenic infection.

Marginal erosions of bone are frequent in processes associated with significant synovial inflammation, such as sepsis, rheumatoid arthritis, and the seronegative spondyloarthropathies. They may also be observed in gout and, less commonly, in pigmented villonodular synovitis and idiopathic synovial osteochondromatosis. Centrally located erosions and cysts are seen in many disorders, including septic arthritis. Similarly, periarticular osteoporosis can be encountered in rheumatoid arthritis, Reiter's syndrome, juvenile chronic arthritis, hemophilia, and nonpyogenic infections, such as tuberculosis or fungal disease. Intraarticular bone ankylosis can represent the end stage of septic arthritis, the seronegative spondyloarthrop-

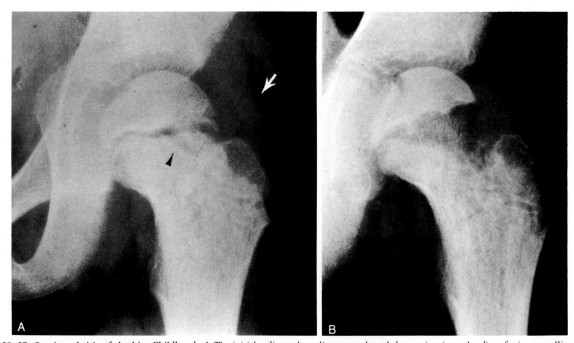

Figure 59–27. Septic arthritis of the hip: Childhood. A The initial radiograph outlines metaphyseal destruction (arrowhead), soft tissue swelling (arrow), and subtle lateral displacement of the femoral head. B Subsequently, progressive osteomyelitis and septic arthritis have produced increased intraarticular fluid and osteonecrosis of the femoral head manifested as increased radiodensity.

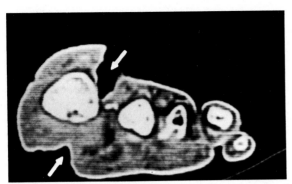

Figure 59–28. Soft tissue infection: Diabetes mellitus. This patient had a plantar infection confined to the medial compartment. A coronal computed tomographic scan at the level of the base of the first proximal phalanx reveals plantar and dorsal cutaneous ulcerations (arrows). (From Sartoris DJ, et al: Plantar compartmental infection in the diabetic foot. The role of computed tomography. Invest Radiol 20:772, 1985. Used with permission.)

athies, and, in some locations, rheumatoid arthritis and juvenile chronic arthritis.

Any joint can be the site of an infectious process. In children and infants, the joints of the appendicular skeleton, especially the knee and the hip, commonly are affected in hematogenous infections; in children and adults, the joints of the axial skeleton, particularly the sacroiliac joint and those in the spine, are not uncommonly involved. In the drug abuser, the sacroiliac, sternoclavicular, and acromioclavicular joints and the spine are common sites of involvement. In the patient with rheumatoid arthritis, any articulation affected by the primary disease process represents a potential site of infection. In the diabetic patient with infection, articulations of the foot commonly are altered.

SOFT TISSUE INFECTION
Routes of Contamination

Infection of soft tissue structures commonly results from direct contamination after trauma. Any process that disrupts the skin surface can potentially lead to secondary infection, particularly in the person with a debilitating illness (e.g., diabetes mellitus) (Fig. 59–28) or one who is being treated with immunosuppressive agents; furthermore, nonpenetrating trauma can lead to soft tissue infection, although the exact mechanism for this complication is not entirely clear. Hematogenous spread is less important as a mechanism in soft tissue contamination than in osteomyelitis and septic arthritis.

Radiographic-Pathologic Correlation

Swelling with obliteration of adjacent tissue planes is characteristic of soft tissue infection. Radiolucent streaks within the contaminated area can relate to collections of air derived from the adjacent skin surface or gas formation by various bacteria (Fig. 59–29). Erosion of bone owing to pressure from an adjacent soft tissue mass is much more frequent when the mass is neoplastic rather than infectious in origin. When osseous abnormalities appear after soft tissue contamination, infective periostitis, osteitis, or osteomyelitis usually is present. Occasionally, periostitis of the underlying bone may represent irritation rather than true suppuration.

A well-defined soft tissue mass is less typical of infection than of neoplasm. The edema of an infectious process usually leads to infiltration of surrounding soft tissues rather than displacement.

Complications

Although there are several complications of soft tissue infection, the most important in terms of the musculoskeletal structures is contamination of underlying osseous and articular tissues.

Specific Entities
Septic Subcutaneous Bursitis

There are numerous subcutaneous bursae in the human body. Afflictions of these structures have led to such well-known terms as housemaid's knee (prepatellar bursitis), miner's elbow (olecranon bursitis), and weaver's bottom (ischial bursitis). In addition, bursal swelling often is apparent in rheumatoid arthritis and gout, as well as after trauma.

Septic bursitis usually localizes to the olecranon, the prepatellar and, less frequently, the subdeltoid regions (Fig. 59–30). A history of recent injury, occupational trauma, or puncture frequently is present. Clinical manifestations include cellulitis, painful swelling localized to the involved bursa, a normal range of joint motion, and fever in approximately 40 per cent of cases. Complications include septic arthritis and osteomyelites.

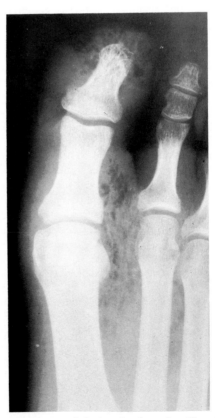

Figure 59–29. Soft tissue infection: Gas formation. Note the "bubbly" radiolucent collections in the foot.

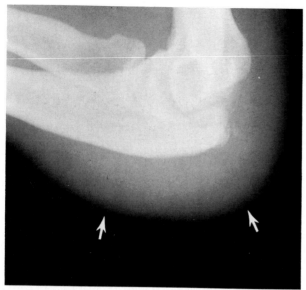

Figure 59–30. Septic olecranon bursitis. Note olecranon swelling (arrows) and soft tissue edema. Previous surgery and trauma are the causes of the adjacent bone abnormalities.

Septic Periarticular Bursitis

Infection of bursae that are located about joints (e.g., popliteal) usually is related to extension of an infective process within the joint.

Septic Tenosynovitis

Septic processes originating from a distant or local focus or occurring after trauma can lead to tenosynovitis. Soft tissue swelling and surface erosion of underlying bone may be evident.

Infectious Myositis

Inflammation of muscle may occur in a variety of infectious disorders caused by viruses, bacteria, protozoa, and parasites. In some instances, as in viral myositis, the precise mechanism leading to muscle inflammation is not clear, whereas in others, direct involvement of the muscle by the infectious agent is implicated.

Pyogenic myositis (pyomyositis) is a well-recognized and serious infection affecting children and young adults in tropical regions (tropical pyomyositis) and, less frequently, in other locations as well. Children and young adults are affected. The clinical findings are pain and tenderness of the muscle, induration of the overlying skin, and lymphadenopathy. Musculature in the lower extremity is affected more frequently than that in the upper extremity or trunk. Pyomyositis is related to *Staphylococcus aureus* infection in about 90 per cent of cases.

Clostridial myonecrosis, or gas gangrene, is a rare disease resulting from the presence of *Clostridium perfringens* or *C. septicum* (see Chapter 61). Gas within the soft tissues and muscles is an important diagnostic sign.

SPECIFIC SITUATIONS
Chronic Granulomatous Disease of Childhood

This heterogeneous disorder is a hereditary condition, usually transmitted as an X-linked recessive trait, which occurs in male children. The syndrome is characterized by purulent granulomatous and eczematoid skin lesions, granulomatous lymphadenitis with suppuration, hepatosplenomegaly, recurrent and persistent pneumonias, and chronic osteomyelitis (25 to 35 per cent); it frequently is fatal (40 per cent). In its classic form, chronic granulomatous disease is manifested as infections early in life, sometimes within the first week but usually during the first year. A fatal outcome before adolescence is common. Virtually every organ or tissue is vulnerable to infection in this disorder. A defect has been noted in the ability of the polymorphonuclear leukocytes and monocytes to adequately destroy certain pathogenetic organisms. Thus, although the leukocytes can phagocytize bacteria normally, they are incapable of killing them, especially certain strains of relatively low virulence.

Certain clinical and radiologic peculiarities characterize the osteomyelitis of chronic granulomatous disease of childhood.

1. The disease lacks the usual early clinical signs and symptoms of osteomyelitis, so that initial radiographs frequently reveal considerable bone involvement.

2. The causative organisms usually are of low virulence.

3. The most frequent site of involvement is the small bones of the hands and the feet.

4. The radiographic abnormalities are characterized by extensive osseous destruction with minimal reactive sclerosis. Sequestrum formation is unusual.

5. The osteomyelitis may develop in new areas despite continuous therapy.

6. The osteomyelitis eventually responds to long-term antibiotic therapy, so that operative intervention rarely is necessary.

Chronic Symmetric Plasma Cell Osteomyelitis (*Chronic Recurrent Multifocal Osteomyelitis*)

Chronic symmetric plasma cell osteomyelitis is a variety of subacute and chronic osteomyelitis of unknown cause that occurs in childhood and that frequently reveals multiple and symmetric alterations. It has also been referred to as condensing osteitis of the clavicle in childhood, chronic recurrent multifocal osteomyelitis, plasma cell osteomyelitis, and primary chronic osteomyelitis. The usual age of onset of the disease is 5 to 10 years. Pain, tenderness, and swelling are common initial clinical manifestations. The metaphyses of the bones of the lower extremity and the medial ends of the clavicles are particularly vulnerable (Fig. 59–31). Osteolysis with intense sclerosis may be noted. In certain locations, the bone may become massive and a diagnosis of fibrous dysplasia, Paget's disease, or sarcoma is suggested. Laboratory analysis generally is nonspecific, and cultures of the blood or of the bone after biopsy may be nonrewarding. Histologic evaluation is reported to be relatively specific, characterized in many instances by the predominance of plasma cells in the center of the osteolytic foci.

The peculiar features of this variety of osteomyelitis include a protracted clinical course, a striking degree of symmetric bone involvement, a predilection for the metaphyseal regions of the lower extremity (especially in the tibia and femur), common involvement of the clavicle, difficulty in implicating specific organisms from blood or bone, and histologic evidence of plasma cells. The radiographic features may simulate those of other types of osteomyelitis, chronic granulomatous disease of childhood, infantile cortical hyperostosis, vitamin D–resistant rickets, or bone infarction.

Selective hyperostosis of the clavicle, as noted in this condition, may also be seen in two additional disorders. Osteitis condensans of the medial end of the bone has been reported, especially in young women (see Chapter 53). A second disorder, sternocostoclavicular hyperostosis, leads to painful swelling of the sternum, clavicles, and upper ribs. Men and women are both affected, and the usual age of onset is in the fifth and sixth decades of life (see Chapter 83). The relationship of plasma cell osteomyelitis to these other conditions is not clear. That all three involve the clavicle may represent only a coincidence; however, a peculiar pustular lesion in the hands and feet, pustulosis palmaris et plantaris, is observed both in sternocostoclavicular hyperostosis and plasma cell osteomyelitis. Pustular skin disease, lesions of tubular bones, and sclerotic changes in the manubrium sterni and spine of young and elderly women have also been described, and histologic analysis of the manubrial lesion in some of these patients has documented plasma cell infiltration.

Osteomyelitis and Septic Arthritis in Drug Abusers

An increased frequency of infectious disease has been noted in drug abusers. The mechanisms for this association are not entirely known. Leukocyte dysfunction, use of contaminated narcotics or needles, colonization of the skin during previous hospitalizations, and alterations of the bacterial flora by pretreatment with antibiotics are potential mechanisms that may explain an increased frequency of infection in drug abusers.

Hematogenous osteomyelitis and septic arthritis in drug users are characterized by unusual localization and organisms. Although staphylococcal infection may be seen, Pseudomonas, Klebsiella, and Serratia commonly are implicated. Furthermore, the axial skeleton frequently is affected, especially the spine, the sacroiliac joint, and the sternoclavicular articulation, with less common involvement of the manubriosternal joint, the acromioclavicular joint, the hip, the pubic symphysis, the ribs, and the ischial tuberosities (Fig. 59–32).

Additional musculoskeletal manifestations in drug abusers include lymphedema, thrombophlebitis, subcutaneous fat necrosis, atrophy and calcification, myonecrosis, tenosynovitis, and chemical inflammation of the synovium owing to direct intraarticular administration of the drug. Furthermore, introduction of bacteria directly into the periosteum of the bones (radius, ulna) in the nondominant arm during injection of the drug may lead to osteomyelitis with extensive periostitis.

OTHER DIAGNOSTIC TECHNIQUES
Magnification Radiography

The early alterations of osteomyelitis, infective osteitis or periostitis, and septic arthritis may be readily apparent on magnification studies when conventional radiographs are equivocal or negative. The detection of small osteolytic foci in osteomyelitis, minor disruption of the subchondral bone plate in infectious arthritis, and slight periosteal proliferation in infective osteitis, periostitis, or osteomyelitis may be possible with this technique. Magnification radiography may

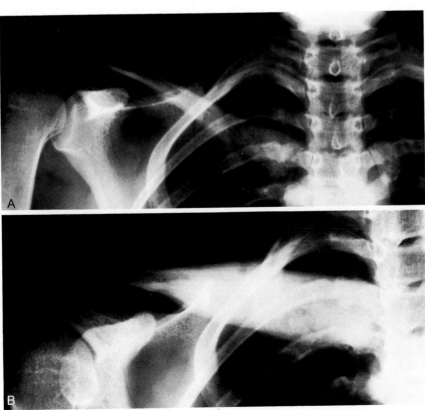

Figure 59–31. Chronic symmetric plasma cell osteomyelitis. Radiographs obtained 8 months apart reveal a process that is associated initially with permeative bone destruction and subsequently with massive enlargement of the clavicle. (Courtesy of G. Greenway, M.D., Dallas, Texas.)

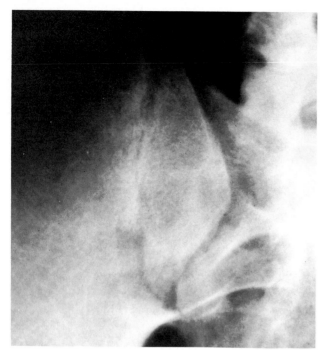

Figure 59–32. Hematogenous osteomyelitis and septic arthritis in the drug abuser. A common site of involvement is the sacroiliac joint. Note loss of joint space and poorly defined bone erosion.

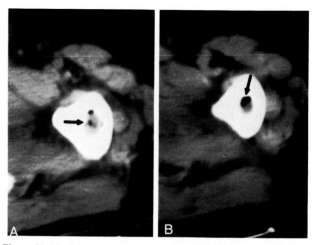

Figure 59–33. Acute osteomyelitis: Role of computed tomography. In a patient with osteomyelitis of the hip and the femur, two transaxial computed tomographic images at the level of the proximal portion of the femur reveal intramedullary gas collections (arrows). (Courtesy of V. Vint, M.D., San Diego, California.)

show definite bone disruption, indicating infection, in the diabetic patient in whom osseous structures are obscured on routine radiography by the presence of soft tissue gas or calcification. In chronic osteomyelitis, the documentation of poorly defined periosteal bone formation with magnification techniques implies existence of active infection.

Conventional Tomography

The major role of conventional tomography in infectious disorders is the detection of sequestra in a patient with chronic osteomyelitis. Occasionally, conventional tomographic examination outlines definite destruction of the subchondral bone plate, indicating the likely presence of septic arthritis rather than simple osteoporosis (which usually produces a thin but otherwise intact plate).

Computed Tomography

The primary applications of computed tomography to the evaluation of infections of the musculoskeletal system are the delineation of the osseous and soft tissue extent of the disease process, especially in areas of complex anatomy such as the vertebral column, and the monitoring of percutaneous aspiration and biopsy procedures, particularly of the spine, retroperitoneal tissues, and sacroiliac joints (see Chapter 60). Regarding the specificity of computed tomographic abnormalities in osteomyelitis, an increased attenuation value in the medullary canal, destruction of cortical bone, new bone formation, and a soft tissue mass are abnormalities common to both infectious and neoplastic disorders. The detection of gas within the medullary canal is an infrequent but reliable diagnostic sign of osteomyelitis (Fig. 59–33). Fat-fluid levels within the medullary canal or in the adjacent joint also are reported in osteomyelitis and septic arthritis.

Defining the proximal extent of an infection in a tubular bone is possible with computed tomography owing to the increased attenuation values that are characteristic of the inflammatory reaction of the bone marrow. This finding, however, also is evident in tumorous replacement of the bone, myelofibrosis, and fractures.

Computed tomographic evaluation in patients with subacute or chronic osteomyelitis may reveal cortical sequestration, cloacae, and soft tissue abscesses (Fig. 59–34).

Although metallic fragments are well shown on plain film radiography, particles of wood or glass within the soft tissues commonly escape detection. Computed tomography has been used successfully in this clinical situation.

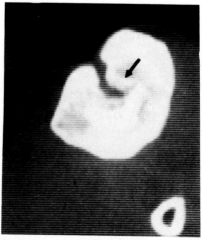

Figure 59–34. Chronic osteomyelitis: Role of computed tomography. A transaxial computed tomographic image through the tibia reveals a sequestered fragment (arrow), cortical erosion, and soft tissue changes. (Courtesy of P. Seron, D.C., Denver, Colorado)

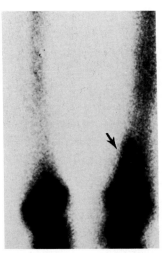

Figure 59–35. Acute osteomyelitis: Role of scintigraphy—bone scanning. A technetium phosphate bone scan documents increased accumulation of the radiopharmaceutical agent in the distal portion of the tibia (arrow). Compare to the opposite (normal) side. (Courtesy of G. Greenway, M.D., Dallas, Texas.)

Sinography

Opacification of a sinus tract will define the course and extent of the sinus tract and its possible communication with an underlying bone or joint.

Arthrography

The principal reason for performing a joint puncture in the clinical setting of infection is to obtain fluid for bacteriologic examination. After removal of the joint contents, however, contrast opacification of the joint will outline the extent of the synovial inflammation and the presence of capsular, tendinous, and soft tissue injury. This is especially helpful in those joints such as the hip and the glenohumeral articulation that are relatively inaccessible to direct clinical examination because of their deep location.

Radionuclide Examination

The role of this examination in the evaluation of bone, joint, and soft tissue infectious processes is firmly established (see Chapter 16). Technetium phosphate bone scans become abnormal within hours to days of the onset of bone infection and days to weeks before the disease becomes manifest on conventional radiographs. The scintigraphic abnormality may initially be evident as a photodeficient area ("cold" spot), but, within a few days, increased accumulation of the radioisotope ("hot" spot) is typical (Fig. 59–35). Occasional difficulty in interpreting the bone scan in younger patients arises from an inability to differentiate between normal and abnormal activity in the metaphyseal region. Although use of higher resolution gamma cameras and magnification techniques may diminish this difficulty, using gallium scans in this situation may allow more accurate interpretation of the metaphyseal activity.

The rationale for the use of gallium as an adjunct to technetium phosphates in evaluating inflammatory lesions of bone is based on several considerations. As technetium accumulation is related to the integrity of the vascular tree, increased intramedullary pressure accompanying osteomyelitis can partially prevent both augmented blood flow and significant accumulation of the radionuclide. Gallium, being less dependent on the vascular flow, might still localize at the site of infection. Thus, in the presence of a clinical suspicion of bone or joint infection and a negative bone scan, a gallium study could be useful. Unfortunately, as gallium accumulation occurs also with soft tissue infection, differentiation of cellulitis and osteomyelitis is usually not possible with this agent.

A gallium scan can be obtained in conjunction with a technetium scan in the same patient, and the information that is obtained may be even more useful than that of either examination alone (Table 59–7). Gallium scans may reveal abnormal accumulation in patients with active osteomyelitis when technetium scans reveal decreased activity ("cold" lesions) or perhaps normal activity (transition period between "cold" and "hot" lesions). Furthermore, gallium accumulation appears to correlate more closely with activity in cases of osteomyelitis than does technetium uptake, and it may be superior in determining the response of acute osteomyelitis and chronic osteomyelitis to various therapeutic regimens. Increased accumulation of gallium in sites of cellulitis can be helpful in establishing the presence of soft tissue infection.

The changing patterns of scintigraphic activity on initial and subsequent images after injection of bone-seeking radiopharmaceutical agents underscore the inaccuracy in interpretation that may occur during the analysis of single phase bone images alone. Although a definitely negative delayed bone image appears to be quite specific in excluding infection, a positive finding during the delayed static phase of the examination lacks specificity for infection. Furthermore, as noted earlier, the differentiation of cellulitis, osteomyelitis, and even septic arthritis may be difficult or impossible on the basis of alterations in this phase of the study. These problems have stimulated considerable interest in "three phase" examinations in patients with musculoskeletal infection: Serial images are obtained during the first minute following the bolus injection of the technetium compound (angiographic phase); a postinjection image is then obtained at the end of

Table 59–7. RADIONUCLIDE EVALUATION OF OSSEOUS AND SOFT TISSUE INFECTION

Agent	Cellulitis	Acute Osteomyelitis	Chronic Osteomyelitis
Technetium phosphates	Early scans show increased uptake; later scans are normal	Early and late scans show increased uptake (scans in early acute osteomyelitis may reveal "cold" spots)	Scans may remain positive even in inactive disease
Gallium	Increased uptake	Increased uptake	Increased uptake in areas of active disease

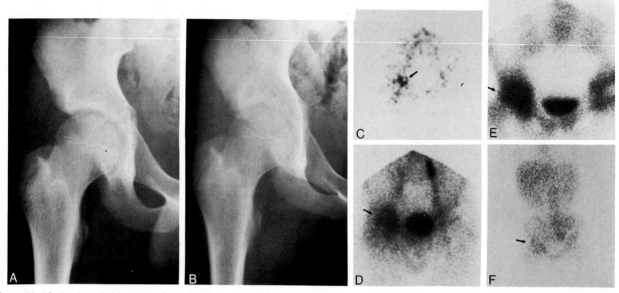

Figure 59–36. Septic arthritis: Role of scintigraphy—"three-phase" bone scanning. A, B Radiographs obtained 6 days apart show progressive joint space narrowing and osteopenia. **C–E** A three-phase technetium phosphate study documents increased flow (arrow) in the angiographic phase **(C)**, diffuse hyperemia about the hip (arrow) in the blood-pool stage **(D)**, and increased uptake of the radiopharmaceutical agent (arrow) in the delayed image **(E)**. The findings indicate septic arthritis. **F** A gallium scan is also abnormal, with increased scintigraphic activity about the hip (arrow). (Courtesy of G. Greenway, M.D., Dallas, Texas.)

the first minute or several minutes (blood pool phase); and further images are obtained 2 or 3 hours later (delayed phase). If increased accumulation of the radionuclide within the bone is observed in all three phases of the examination, the diagnosis of osteomyelitis is highly likely. Soft tissue infections are characterized by delayed images that either are normal or reveal minimally increased tracer accumulation within the bone, blood pool images that reveal diffuse hyperemia, and radionuclide angiograms that show soft tissue hyperemia. Septic arthritis usually is accompanied by increased uptake of the radiopharmaceutical agent in juxta-articular bone in the delayed images, moderate and diffuse blood pool hyperemia, and, on the radionuclide angiogram, increased flow to the joint space (Fig. 59–36).

The accumulation of leukocytes at sites of abscess formation has led to attempts to isolate and label autologous leukocytes with radioactive tracers. Of the potential agents that have been studied, indium-111, with a half-life of 67 hours, appears to be the most suitable, providing reasonable images as early as 4 to 6 hours following injection of the labeled leukocytes. The success of ^{111}In leukocyte labeling in the identification of septic foci requires the migration of the leukocytes to the site of infection. The technique is better applied to acute infections associated with vigorous leukocyte infiltration, as opposed to chronic infections in which such migration may be insufficient. In general, ^{111}In labeled leukocyte scintigraphy is less sensitive in detecting bone infections than soft tissue infections and leads to difficulty in differentiating osteomyelitis and septic arthritis. Furthermore, positive leukocyte images are encountered in musculoskeletal conditions other than infection.

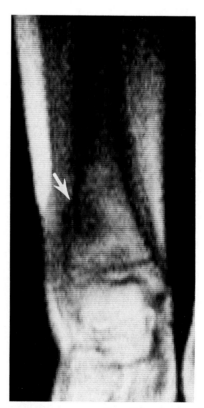

Figure 59–37. Recurrent osteomyelitis: Role of magnetic resonance imaging. A coronal magnetic resonance image reveals an area of diminished signal (arrow) in the medullary cavity of the tibia. Note the adjacent soft tissue swelling and disruption of the bright signal of subcutaneous fat laterally. (From Fletcher BD, et al: Osteomyelitis in children: Detection by magnetic resonance. Work in progress. Radiology 150:57, 1984. Used with permission.)

Magnetic Resonance Imaging

In the presence of osteomyelitis, an inflammatory response leads to increased water content in the marrow space, a change that can be detected as a less intense marrow signal on magnetic resonance images with enhanced T1 tissue characteristics (Fig. 59–37). The sensitivity of magnetic resonance imaging to the detection of acute osteomyelitis is greater than that of plain film radiography and computed tomography, although the technique lacks specificity (see Chapter 11). Magnetic resonance imaging also has been applied, with some success, to the diagnosis of infections of the axial skeleton, including the spine (see Chapter 60).

FURTHER READING

Azouz EM: Computed tomography in bone and joint infections. J Can Assoc Radiol 32:102, 1981.

Bonakdar-pour A, Gaines VD: The radiology of osteomyelitis. Orthop Clin North Am 14:21, 1983.

Bressler EL, Conway JJ, Weiss SC: Neonatal osteomyelitis examined by bone scintigraphy. Radiology 152:685, 1984.

Butt WP: The radiology of infection. Clin Orthop 96:20, 1973.

Butt WP: Radiology of the infected joint. Clin Orthop 96:136, 1973.

Capitanio MA, Kirkpatrick JA: Early roentgen observations in acute osteomyelitis. AJR 108:488, 1970.

Curtiss PH Jr: The pathophysiology of joint infections. Clin Orthop 96:129, 1973.

Davis LA: Antibiotic modified osteomyelitis. AJR 103:608, 1968.

Fitzgerald RH, Brewer NS, Dahlin DC: Squamous-cell carcinoma complicating chronic osteomyelitis. J Bone Joint Surg [Am] 58:1146, 1976.

Fletcher BD, Scoles PV, Nelson AD: Osteomyelitis in children: Detection by magnetic resonance. Work in progress. Radiology 150:57, 1984.

Gilday DL, Paul DJ, Paterson J: Diagnosis of osteomyelitis in children by combined blood pool and bone imaging. Radiology 117:331, 1975.

Goldberg JS, London WL, Nagel DM: Tropical pyomyositis: A case report and review. Pediatrics 63:298, 1979.

Green NE, Beauchamp RD, Griffin PP: Primary subacute epiphyseal osteomyelitis. J Bone Joint Surg [Am] 63:107, 1981.

Handmaker H, Leonards R: The bone scan in inflammatory osseous disease. Semin Nucl Med 6:95, 1976.

Hofer P: Gallium and infection. J Nucl Med 21:484, 1980.

Kaye JJ: Bacterial infections of the hips in infancy and childhood. Curr Probl Radiol 3:17, 1973.

Kido D, Bryan D, Halpern M: Hematogenous osteomyelitis in drug addicts. AJR 118:356, 1973.

Kemp HBS, Lloyd-Roberts GC: Avascular necrosis of the capital epiphysis following osteomyelitis of the proximal femoral metaphysis. J Bone Joint Surg [Br] 56:688, 1974.

McAfee JG, Subramanian G, Gagne G: Technique of leukocyte harvesting and labeling: Problems and perspective. Semin Nucl Med 14:83, 1984.

Mendelson EB, Fisher MR, Deschler TW, Rogers LF, Hendrix RW, Spies S: Osteomyelitis in the diabetic foot: A difficult diagnostic challenge. RadioGraphics 3:248, 1983.

Miller WB, Murphy WA, Gilula LA: Brodie abscess: Reappraisal. Radiology 132:15, 1979.

Mok PM, Reilly BJ, Ash JM: Osteomyelitis in the neonate. Clinical aspects and the role of radiography and scintigraphy in diagnosis and management. Radiology 145:677, 1982.

Murray SD, Kehl DK: Chronic recurrent multifocal osteomyelitis. A case report. J Bone Joint Surg [Am] 66:1110, 1984.

Resnick D: Osteomyelitis and septic arthritis complicating hand injuries and infections: Pathogenesis of roentgenographic abnormalities. J Can Assoc Radiol 27:21, 1976.

Resnick D, Pineda CJ, Weisman MH, Kerr R: Osteomyelitis and septic arthritis of the hand following human bites. Skel Radiol 14:263, 1985.

Rosenbaum DM, Blumhagen JD: Acute epiphyseal osteomyelitis in children. Radiology 156:89, 1985.

Solheim LF, Paus B, Liverud K, Stoen E: Chronic recurrent multifocal osteomyelitis. Acta Orthop Scand 51:37, 1980.

Trueta J: Studies of the Development and Decay of the Human Frame. Philadelphia, WB Saunders Co, 1968.

Unger E, Moldofsky P, Gatenby R, Hartz W, Broder G: Diagnosis of osteomyelitis by MR imaging. AJR 150:605, 1988.

Waldvogel FA, Vasey H: Osteomyelitis: The past decade. N Engl J Med 303:360, 1980.

Wolfson JJ, Kane WJ, Laxdal SD, Good RA, Quie PG: Bone findings in chronic granulomatous disease of childhood. A genetic abnormality of leukocyte function. J Bone Joint Surg [Am] 51:1573, 1969.

Wood BP: The vanishing epiphyseal ossification center: A sequel to septic arthritis of childhood. Radiology 134:387, 1980.

Chapter 60

Osteomyelitis, Septic Arthritis, and Soft Tissue Infection: Axial Skeleton

Donald Resnick, M.D.
Gen Niwayama, M.D.

The routes of contamination of the spine, the sacroiliac joint, and other axial skeletal sites are identical to those of the appendicular skeleton. In the spine, early loss of intervertebral disc space is characteristic of pyogenic infection and is associated with lysis and sclerosis of neighboring bone. These findings can simulate those of other disorders, such as rheumatoid arthritis, intervertebral (osteo)chondrosis, and conditions complicated by cartilaginous node formation. Sacroiliac joint infection typically is unilateral in distribution, a feature that allows differentiation from many other articular processes. Additional locations in the axial skeleton are not uncommonly infected in drug abusers and in patients after trauma, surgery, or diagnostic or therapeutic procedures.

The distribution of osteomyelitis and septic arthritis is dramatically influenced by the age of the patient, the specific causative organism, and the presence or absence of any underlying disorder or situation. In the child and the infant, frequent involvement of the bones and the joints of the appendicular skeleton is evident, whereas in the adult, localization of infection to the osseous and articular structures of the vertebral column is common. Pyogenic (nontuberculous) organisms can affect axial or extraaxial sites and commonly are implicated in hematogenous osteomyelitis of the tubular bones in children and infants. Tuberculous organisms can also select appendicular or axial skeletal sites, although the occurrence of tuberculous spondylitis is especially well known. In specific circumstances, infection may also show predilection for certain musculoskeletal locations. Examples of such predilection include osteomyelitis and septic arthritis of the spine and the sacroiliac and sternoclavicular joints in the drug addict, of the foot in the diabetic patient, of the diaphyses of tubular bones in individuals with sickle cell anemia, and of altered articular sites in various arthritides. This chapter delineates the radiographic and pathologic characteristics of infection in important axial skeletal locations, especially the spine and the sacroiliac joint.

SPINAL INFECTIONS

Routes of Contamination

HEMATOGENOUS SPREAD OF INFECTION. Organisms may reach the vertebrae in several fashions. Hematogenous spread via arterial and venous routes (Batson's paravertebral venous system) can result in lodgment of organisms in the bone marrow of the vertebrae. The basic arrangement of the nutrient vessels is similar in the cervical, the thoracic, and the lumbar spine; a vertebral, intercostal, or lumbar artery lying closely apposed to the vertebral body supplies minute vessels to the nearby bone, which penetrate the cortex and ramify within the marrow. In addition, at each intervertebral foramen, a posterior spinal branch enters the vertebral canal and divides into an ascending and a descending branch, which anastomose with similar branches from the segments above and below and from the other side, creating an arterial network on the dorsal or posterior surface of each vertebral body. Three or four nutrient arteries are derived from this network and enter the vertebral body through a large dorsal, centrally placed nutrient foramen.

The venous drainage of the vertebral body is treelike in configuration. Minute tributaries drain from the peripheral

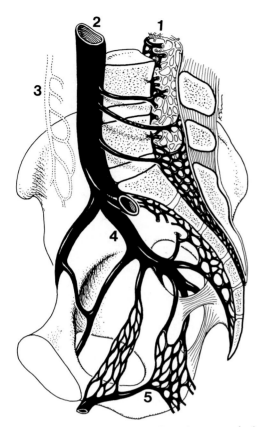

Figure 60–1. Anatomic considerations: Batson's paravertebral venous system. This valveless, plexiform set of veins lies outside the thoracoabdominal cavity, anastomosing with the cavitary veins at each segmental level. Thus, communication exists between the pelvic and vertebral venous system, femoral and iliac veins, inferior vena cava and superior vena cava, and other important venous structures. 1, Paravertebral venous plexus; 2, inferior vena cava; 3, inferior mesenteric vein; 4, internal iliac vein; 5, pelvic plexus. (After Vider M, et al: Significance of the vertebral venous (Batson's) plexus in metastatic spread in colorectal carcinoma. Cancer 40:67, 1977.)

osteomyelitis in the subchondral region of the vertebral body, an area richly supplied by nutrient arterioles, is consistent with an arterial route of contamination. Furthermore, the role of hematogenous spread of infection directly into the intervertebral disc has stimulated great interest (see later discussion).

SPREAD FROM A CONTIGUOUS SOURCE OF INFECTION. Vertebral or intervertebral discal infection can result from contamination by an adjacent soft tissue suppurative focus. This mechanism is not common, as many paravertebral abscesses dissect away from the spine along normal and abnormal soft tissue planes. Tuberculous and fungal infection, however, can extend from the spine to the neighboring tissue, dissect along the subligamentous areas for a considerable distance, and then reenter the vertebral body or intervertebral disc. Furthermore, examples of osteomyelitis and infective discitis as a complication of visceral perforation,

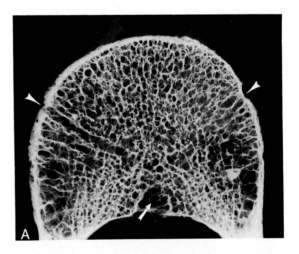

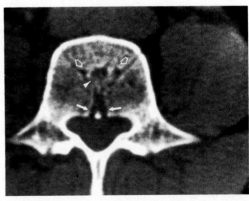

Figure 60–2. Anatomic considerations: Intraosseous venous drainage. A Normal anatomy of the basivertebral veins in the transaxial plane. A specimen radiograph illustrates a Y-shaped configuration of the major basivertebral venous channels, with a flared posterior channel (solid arrow) forming the base and the more anterior channels (open arrows) constituting the limbs. Note the anterolateral cortical fenestrations (arrowheads). **B** On the transaxial computed tomographic image of a normal lumbar vertebra, a Y-shaped configuration composed of paired posterior channels (solid arrows) and anterior channels (open arrows) is observed. A prominent central confluence of vessels (arrowhead) is evident.

portion of the vertebral body to its center, the blood being collected by a large valveless venous channel that emerges from the central dorsal nutrient foramen and drains into an extensive loose plexus lining the vertebral canal. The branching tributaries of the vertebral body are connected by channels that perforate the cortex and enter veins lying on the lateral and anterior surfaces of the vertebrae. This represents the paraspinal and spinal venous plexus of Batson (Fig. 60–1). Within the vertebral body, the ramification of blood vessels at the subchondral superior and inferior limits is reminiscent of the vascular arrangement in the childhood metaphysis and adulthood epiphysis of tubular bones. The intraosseous venous anatomy is well depicted on the transaxial sections afforded by computed tomography (Fig. 60–2).

This vascular arrangement allows two direct routes for the hematogenous spread of infection: via the nutrient arteries and via the paravertebral venous system. The contribution of each system to cases of spinal osteomyelitis is a matter of debate. The importance of the venous plexus is supported by many well-recognized pelvic precursors of vertebral osteomyelitis; alternatively, the common localization of early foci of

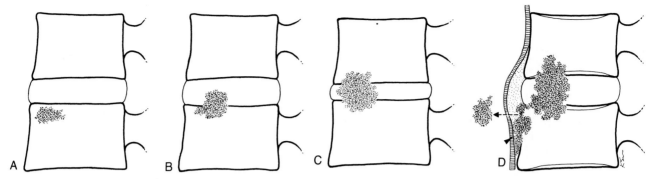

Figure 60–3. Spinal infection: Sequential stages. A An anterior subchondral focus in the vertebral body is typical. **B** Infection may then perforate the vertebral surface, reaching the intervertebral disc space. **C** With further spread of infection, contamination of the adjacent vertebral body and narrowing of the intervertebral disc space are recognizable. **D** With continued dissemination, infection may spread in a subligamentous fashion, eroding the anterior surface of the vertebral body (arrowhead), or perforating the anterior ligamentous structures (arrow).

fistulous communication with a pelvic abscess, arteritis (due to Salmonella infection), and dental extractions have been reported. In such cases, soft tissue abnormalities are followed by sequential invasion of the periosteum, cortex, and marrow of the vertebrae or of the ligaments, anulus fibrosus, and nucleus pulposus of the intervertebral disc.

DIRECT IMPLANTATION. Organisms can be implanted directly into the intervertebral disc (and far less commonly into the vertebra) during attempted punctures of the spinal canal, paravertebral and peridural tissues, or aorta or in penetrating injuries.

POSTOPERATIVE INFECTION. Laminectomy, diskectomy, instrumentation, and fusion can each be complicated by osteomyelitis or discal infection. The localization of osseous or articular contamination depends on the precipitating surgical event; infection may involve the vertebral body, the posterior osseous elements, the intervertebral disc, or even the spinal canal in any region of the vertebral column.

Clinical Abnormalities

The reported frequency of osteomyelitis and disc space infection (together these will be termed infective spondylitis)

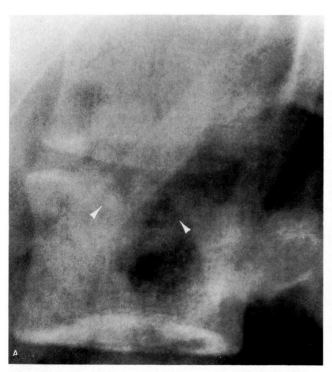

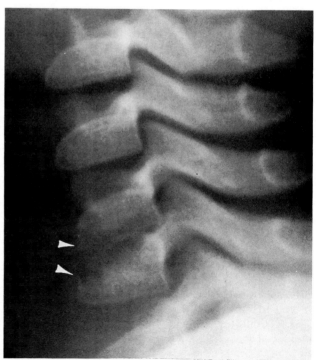

Figure 60–4. Spinal infection: Early and later radiographic abnormalities. A Observe loss of definition of the superior aspect of a lumbar vertebral body (arrowheads) with narrowing of the adjacent intervertebral disc space. This appearance (in a middle-aged man with pyogenic infection) conforms to the stage in Figure 60–3B. **B** In this young child, a staphylococcal infection has led to destruction of two adjacent vertebral bodies (arrowheads) and narrowing of the intervening intervertebral disc. A soft tissue mass is apparent. This appearance corresponds to the stage in Figure 60–3D.

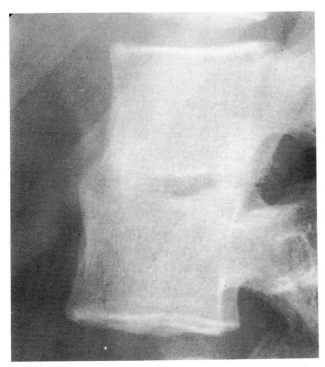

Figure 60–5. **Spinal infection: Bony fusion.** After a pyogenic infection, partial (or complete) bone ankylosis can result. Such bone fusion also can accompany trauma or congenital disorders, although the lack of hypoplasia of the vertebral bodies suggests that the process did not occur prior to the cessation of growth.

has risen dramatically in recent years. Men are affected more commonly than women. The highest frequency of septic spondylitis occurs in the fifth and sixth decades of life; the lumbar spine is the most typical site of involvement, followed by the thoracic spine, with sacral and cervical abnormalities about equal in frequency. The usual location of infection is the vertebral body.

A history of recent primary infection (urinary tract, respiratory, or skin infection), instrumentation (catheterization, cystoscopy), or diagnostic or surgical procedure (myelography, discography, or bowel, urinary, or back operations) is common. The most frequently encountered (80 to 90 per cent) pyogenic organism is *Staphylococcus aureus*, although other gram-positive (Streptococcus, pneumococcus) and, less typically, gram-negative (*Escherichia coli*, Pseudomonas, Klebsiella, and Salmonella) agents may be implicated. Nonpyogenic organisms accounting for infective spondylitis include tuberculous and syphilis organisms and various fungi.

Clinical manifestations include fever, malaise, anorexia, and weight loss. Back pain is a common initial local manifestation. With accompanying soft tissue abscess formation, hip contracture can occur (psoas muscle irritation). Paraplegia is evident in fewer than 1 per cent of cases. Appropriate culture of the blood can identify the causative organism in some cases, although more drastic methods, such as needle biopsy or aspiration, may be necessary.

Radiographic–Pathologic Correlation

Hematogenous spread of infection frequently leads to a focus in the anterior subchondral regions of the vertebral body

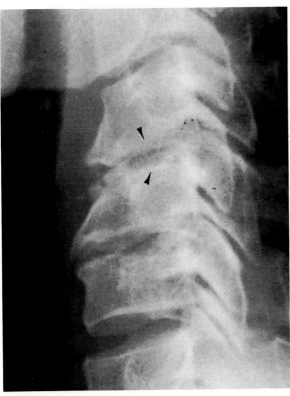

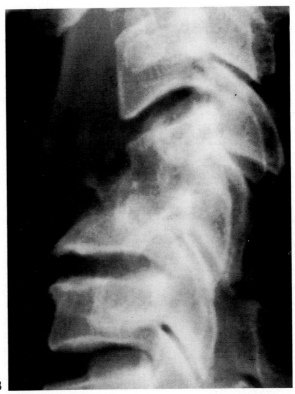

Figure 60–6. **Spinal infection: Residual deformity.** This patient developed Klebsiella spondylitis in the cervical region. **A** Initial radiograph reveals minimal bone indistinctness and destruction (arrowheads) at the C4-C5 level. Considerable degenerative disease of the intervertebral discs has resulted in disc space narrowing and osteophytes at multiple sites. **B** Five weeks later, angulation and subluxation are apparent. Soft tissue swelling is again seen.

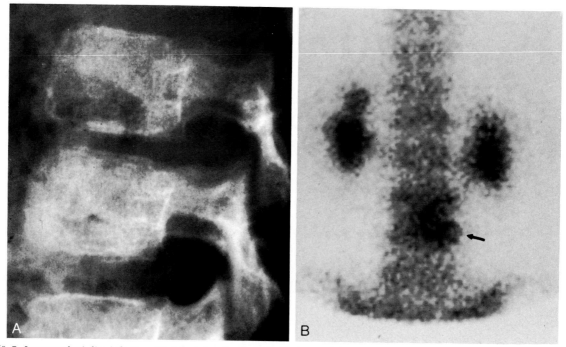

Figure 60–7. Intervertebral disc infection: Discitis. A lateral radiograph **(A)** shows subtle narrowing of the disc space between the third and the fourth lumbar vertebral bodies, which, on bone scan **(B)**, is associated with increased accumulation of the radionuclide (arrow). (Courtesy of T. Goergen, M.D., San Diego, California.)

adjacent to the intervertebral disc (Fig. 60–3). Extension to the intervertebral disc soon ensues. At this stage, radiographs may be entirely normal. Soon (1 to 3 weeks), however, a decrease in height of the intervertebral disc is accompanied by loss of normal definition of the subchondral bone plate and enlarging destructive foci within the neighboring vertebral body (Fig. 60–4). The combination of rapid loss of intervertebral disc height and adjacent lysis of bone is most suggestive of an infectious process. With further spread of infection, the process soon contaminates the adjacent vertebra. Such involvement of two contiguous vertebral bodies is associated almost uniformly with transdiscal infection.

After a variable period (10 to 12 weeks), regenerative changes appear in the bone with sclerosis or eburnation. The osteosclerotic response has been used in the past as a helpful sign in differentiating pyogenic from tuberculous infection. Although such sclerosis is indeed common in pyogenic (non-tuberculous) spondylitis, it may also be evident in tuberculosis, particularly in black patients. More helpful in this differentiation is a combination of findings that strongly indicates tuberculous spondylitis, including the presence of a slowly progressive vertebral process with preservation of intervertebral discs, large and calcified soft tissue abscesses, and the absence of severe bone eburnation.

Soft tissue extension of infection can be observed in approximately 20 per cent of cases of pyogenic spondylitis. In the lumbar spine, such extension can lead to displacement of the psoas margin; in the thoracic spine, a paraspinal mass can be encountered; and in the cervical spine, retropharyngeal swelling can lead to displacement and obliteration of adjacent prevertebral fat planes.

With early and proper treatment, reconstitution can result, with production of a radiodense (ivory) vertebra, a relatively

intact or ankylosed intervertebral disc, and surrounding osteophytosis (Fig. 60–5). Without such treatment, complete bony lysis and collapse, discal obliteration, deviation and deformity of the vertebral column (Fig. 60–6), and massive soft tissue abscesses can appear.

Special Types of Spinal Infection

INTERVERTEBRAL DISC INFECTION ("DISCITIS"). Most infections of the intervertebral disc occur as an extension of vertebral osteomyelitis or direct inoculation during diagnostic or surgical procedures. In children, however, a hematogenous route to the disc still exists, which may persist until the age of 20 or 30 years. Thus, certainly in children, hematogenous contamination of the discal tissue is possible, although organisms are not always isolated in cases of childhood discitis. Clinical manifestations generally are mild. When positive, blood or bone biopsy culture most typically reveals *Staphylococcus aureus*.

Radiologic abnormalities of discitis in children commonly are delayed (several weeks), although scintigraphy may reveal increased accumulation of bone-seeking pharmaceutical agents at a relatively early stage. Intervertebral disc space narrowing is later accompanied by erosion of the subchondral bone plate and osseous eburnation (Fig. 60–7). Antibiotic therapy usually is administered on an empirical basis, and reconstitution, although not complete, of the intervertebral disc commonly results. Rarely, psoas abscesses, interbody fusion, kyphosis, scoliosis, vertebral magna or wedging, and intraspinal extension may be noted.

The occurrence of hematogenous spread of infection to the adult intervertebral disc has also been proposed, although further documentation of this entity is required before its existence is truly established.

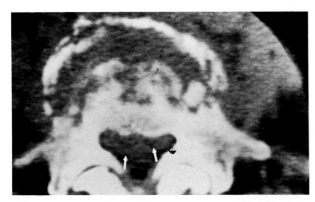

Figure 60–8. Spinal infection: Role of computed tomography. In this man with a spinal infection in the lower lumbar region, a transaxial computed tomographic image documents the extent of spinal destruction with a soft tissue mass in paraspinal and intraspinal locations (arrows).

Other Diagnostic Techniques

As at other sites of infection, a variety of diagnostic techniques in addition to routine radiography can be employed in cases of infective spondylitis. Especially important is the role of *radionuclide studies* in establishing the presence of spinal infection at a stage when radiographs are entirely normal. Technetium and gallium radiopharmaceutical agents can be used in this regard; the value of ^{111}In-labeled leukocytes in the early diagnosis of spinal infections is not clear.

Computed tomography can also be used in the investigation of patients with infective spondylitis. The examination will define the extent of osseous and discal destruction and of paravertebral and intraspinal involvement (Fig. 60–8). The intravenous injection of contrast material aids in the separation of abnormal and normal soft tissues. Gas may be identified in the infected soft tissues or, rarely, in the intervertebral disc itself.

Hypodensity of the intervertebral disc on computed tomograms has been reported as a reliable indicator of infection. The cause of the decreased radiodensity appears to be related to the edema and inflammatory exudate present within the granulation tissue.

Computed tomography can be especially helpful during attempts to aspirate fluid or tissue from sites of vertebral infection.

Magnetic resonance imaging also is quite useful in the early diagnosis of spinal infection. Typically, the signal intensity derived from the infected disc and bone is decreased on the T1 weighted images and markedly increased on the T2 weighted images (Fig. 60–9). Magnetic resonance imaging can be used to identify paravertebral soft tissue involvement in the infective process.

Differential Diagnosis

The radiographic hallmark of infective spondylitis is intervertebral disc space narrowing, frequently accompanied by lysis or sclerosis of adjacent vertebrae (Table 60–1). A similar radiographic pattern can be encountered in various articular

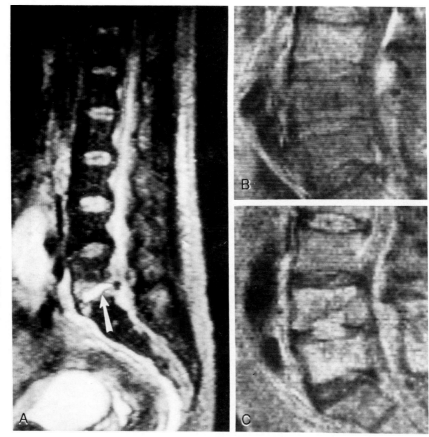

Figure 60–9. Spinal infection: Role of magnetic resonance imaging. A A T2 weighted sagittal image shows the bright signal (arrow) derived from the infected lumbosacral intervertebral disc. The normal intranuclear cleft, shown at the upper lumbar levels, is obliterated at the infected level, and the disc has protruded into the spinal canal. In the intervertebral disc between the fourth and fifth lumbar vertebral bodies, intervertebral (osteo)chondrosis explains the decrease in signal intensity. (Courtesy of M. Modic, M.D., Cleveland, Ohio.) **B, C** In a different patient, a T1 weighted sagittal magnetic resonance image (**B**) shows decreased signal intensity in the fourth and fifth lumbar vertebrae and intervening disc. On a T2 weighted image (**C**), these same areas show increased signal intensity. The findings are consistent with spinal infection. (Courtesy of M. Solomon, M.D., San Jose, California.)

disorders such as rheumatoid arthritis, the seronegative spondyloarthropathies, calcium pyrophosphate dihydrate crystal deposition disease, alkaptonuria, and neuroarthropathy, but in each of these disorders, clinical and additional radiographic features usually ensure accurate differential diagnosis. Sarcoidosis can occasionally be associated with disc space narrowing and bone eburnation at one or more levels of the spine.

Diminution of intervertebral disc height and bone sclerosis are associated with cartilaginous node formation (Schmorl's node). In general, the poor definition of the subchondral bone plate is less in cases of cartilaginous nodes than in infection.

Intervertebral (osteo)chondrosis also produces intervertebral disc space narrowing and reactive sclerosis of the neighboring bone (see Chapter 36). In this disorder, the vertebral endplates usually are smooth and well defined. Of particular diagnostic significance is the presence of one or more vacuum phenomena within the nucleus pulposus. Their detection makes the diagnosis of infection quite unlikely. In rare occasions, infections with gas-forming bacteria may lead to vacuum-like phenomena.

In general, primary or metastatic tumor in the spine does not lead to significant loss of intervertebral disc space; the combination of widespread lysis or sclerosis of a vertebral body and an intact adjacent intervertebral disc is much more characteristic of tumor than of infection. Certain neoplasms such as plasma cell myeloma and chordoma can extend across or around the intervertebral disc to involve the neighboring vertebra, however. Furthermore, neoplastic disruption of the subchondral bone can produce osseous weakening, allowing intraosseous discal displacement with some degree of disc space narrowing.

Paraspinal masses occur in infective spondylitis and traumatic and neoplastic disorders. Infection is likely if such masses contain gas. Intervertebral disc space ossification leading to bridging of vertebral bodies is encountered as a sequela of infective spondylitis. It may also be seen in congenital disorders and after surgery or trauma.

The accurate radiographic differentiation of pyogenic infective spondylitis from granulomatous infections (tuberculosis and fungal disorders) can be difficult. Rapid loss of intervertebral disc height, extensive sclerosis, and the absence of calcified paraspinal masses are findings that are more typical of pyogenic infection.

SACROILIAC JOINT INFECTIONS
Routes of Contamination

The sacroiliac joint may become infected by the hematogenous route, by contamination from a contiguous suppurative focus, by direct implantation, or after surgery.

The subchondral circulation of the ilium is slow, resembling the situation in the metaphysis of long bones in children. Thus, hematogenous implantation at this site is to be expected; the ilium is the most frequently infected flat bone of the body. From this location, extension of infection into the sacroiliac or hip joint can occur. Similarly, the association of sacroiliac joint infection with suppurative conditions of the pelvis or previous pelvic surgical procedures may indicate the importance of hematogenous spread via the paravertebral venous system of Batson.

Contamination of the sacroiliac joint or neighboring bone can occur from an adjacent infection. Thus, vaginal, uterine, ovarian, bladder, and intestinal processes can lead to iliac or sacral osteomyelitis and sacroiliac joint suppuration by contiguous contamination (as well as by hematogenous spread via Batson's plexus). Pressure sores related to prolonged immobilization are not infrequent in the sacral region and can lead to subsequent articular and osseous infection. Even infective conditions of the spine can spread beneath the spinal ligaments into the pelvis and sacroiliac articulations.

Direct implantation of organisms during or after diagnostic or surgical procedures represents another, although uncommon, source of sacroiliac joint infection.

Clinical Abnormalities

Pyogenic infection of the sacroiliac joint can lead to severe clinical manifestations, especially in children and adolescents. Unilateral alterations predominate. Fever, local or distant pain and tenderness, and a limp can be evident. Discharged

---

Table 60–1. DIFFERENTIAL DIAGNOSIS OF SOME DISORDERS PRODUCING DISC SPACE NARROWING

Disorder	Discovertebral Margin	Sclerosis	Vacuum Phenomena	Osteophytosis	Other Findings
Infection	Poorly defined	Variable[1]	Rare[2]	Absent	Vertebral lysis, soft tissue mass
Intervertebral osteochondrosis	Well defined	Prominent	Present	Variable	Cartilaginous nodes
Rheumatoid arthritis	Poorly or well defined with "erosions"	Variable	Absent	Absent or mild	Apophyseal joint abnormalities, subluxation
Calcium pyrophosphate dihydrate crystal deposition disease	Poorly or well defined	Prominent	Variable	Variable	Fragmentation, subluxation
Neuroarthropathy	Well defined	Prominent	Variable	Prominent	Fragmentation, subluxation, disorganization
Trauma	Well defined	Prominent	Variable	Variable	Fracture, soft tissue mass
Sarcoidosis	Poorly or well defined	Variable, may be prominent	Absent	Absent	Soft tissue mass

[1]Usually evident in pyogenic infections and in tuberculosis in the black patient.

[2]Vacuum phenomena may initially be evident when intervertebral osteochondrosis is also present or, rarely, when a gas-forming microorganism is responsible for the infection.

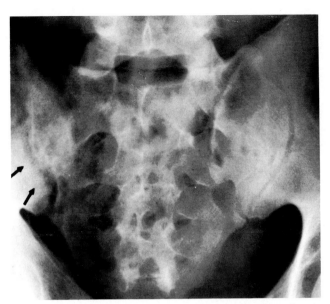

Figure 60–10. Sacroiliac joint infection: Early abnormalities. A male heroin addict developed Pseudomonas osteomyelitis and septic arthritis. The radiograph reveals the changes in the right sacroiliac joint, consisting of subchondral osseous erosion, poorly defined articular margins, and widening of the joint space (arrows).

purulent material may follow the iliac fossa, track along the iliopsoas muscle to the hip or thigh, follow the tendons of the short external rotators to the buttock, ascend into the lumbar region or along the crest of the ilium, or penetrate the pelvic floor to be discharged through the vagina or rectum. Delay in accurate diagnosis in cases of septic sacroiliitis is frequent.

Staphylococci, streptococci, pneumococci, Proteus, Klebsiella, Pseudomonas, Brucella, mycobacteria, and fungi can be implicated. Gram-negative bacterial agents are especially common in pyogenic arthritis of the sacroiliac joint in drug abusers.

Radiographic–Pathologic Correlation

In pyogenic arthritis, radiographic findings generally occur in 2 or 3 weeks, characterized by blurring and indistinctness of the subchondral osseous line and narrowing or widening of the interosseous space. The most extensive findings commonly are evident about the inferoanterior aspect of the joint. Progressive changes are accompanied by erosions, which usually are predominant in the lower ilium (Fig. 60–10). Surrounding condensation of bone is variable in frequency and degree. With treatment, intraarticular osseous fusion may be encountered.

Other Diagnostic Techniques

Conventional tomography may detect early erosive alterations when initial radiographs are normal; scintigraphy, using technetium phosphate or gallium agents, or both, may outline increased accumulation of radionuclide at a time when findings on routine radiographs and conventional tomograms are unimpressive. Abnormal unilateral uptake of isotope in the sacroiliac joint indicates infection until proved otherwise.

Although computed tomography (Figs. 60–11 and 60–12) has been used in the early diagnosis of septic sacroiliitis, it is better applied to the detection of soft tissue extension of the infection and as an aid to aspiration and biopsy techniques.

Differential Diagnosis

It is the unilateral nature of infective sacroiliac joint disease that is its most useful diagnostic feature. Bilateral symmetric or asymmetric articular changes are characteristic of ankylosing spondylitis, psoriasis, Reiter's syndrome, osteitis conden-

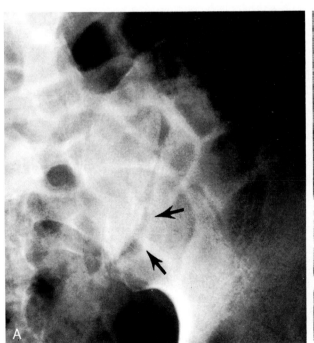

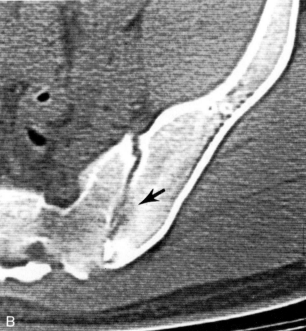

Figure 60–11. Sacroiliac joint infection: Role of computed tomography. An infected left sacroiliac joint has led to subtle radiographic abnormalities (**A**) consisting of osteopenia and superficial erosion of bone (arrows). A transaxial computed tomographic image (**B**) at the level of the lower part of the articulation shows the bone destruction to better advantage (arrow).

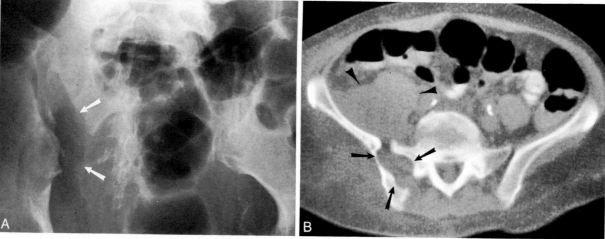

Figure 60–12. Sacroiliac joint infection: Role of computed tomography. Although the plain film shows the destruction of ilium and sacrum (arrows) that accompanies this infection, a computed tomographic image further documents this destruction (arrows) and reveals a large soft tissue mass (arrowheads).

Table 60–2. TYPICAL SITES OF INFECTION IN THE DRUG ABUSER

Spine
Sacroiliac joint
Sternoclavicular joint
Symphysis pubis
Acromioclavicular joint
Manubriosternal joint

sans ilii, and hyperparathyroidism. Unilateral changes can be encountered in rheumatoid arthritis, gout, Reiter's syndrome, and psoriasis. They may also appear on the paralyzed side in hemiplegic patients (owing to chondral atrophy) and on the contralateral side in patients with osteoarthritis of the hip. Unilateral sacroiliac joint disease characterized by blurring or

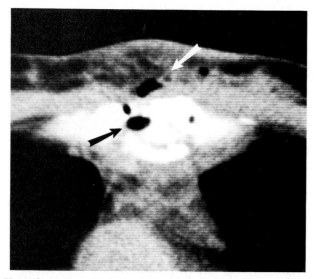

Figure 60–13. Sternal infection. This man developed group B streptococcal septicemia resulting in infections in the hip, spine, and sternum. In a transaxial image, computed tomography shows a destroyed sternum and an anterior soft tissue mass, both containing gas (arrows), and mediastinal adenopathy.

poor definition of subchondral bone and loss of joint space is virtually diagnostic of infection.

INFECTION AT OTHER AXIAL SITES

Infection can involve almost any additional site in the axial skeleton. In the drug abuser, osteomyelitis and septic arthritis of the sternoclavicular and acromioclavicular joints in addition to the spine and sacroiliac joint can be evident (Table 60–2). After urologic procedures, osteomyelitis of the symphysis pubis may be difficult to differentiate from osteitis pubis. Infection of the sternum and manubriosternal joint can result from direct hematogenous inoculation (Fig. 60–13) or secondary contamination owing to local injury, surgery, or diagnostic or therapeutic procedure (subclavian vein catheterization).

FURTHER READING

Allen EH, Cosgrove D, Millard FJC: The radiological changes in infections of the spine and their diagnostic value. Clin Radiol 29:31, 1978.

Batson OV: The vertebral vein system. AJR 78:195, 1957.

Brant-Zawadzki M, Burke VD, Jeffrey RB: CT in the evaluation of spine infection. Spine 8:358, 1983.

Fernandez-Ulloa M, Vasavada PJ, Hanslits ML, Volarich DT, Elgazzar AH: Diagnosis of vertebral osteomyelitis: Clinical radiological and scintigraphic features. Orthopedics 8:1141, 1985.

Goldin RH, Chow A, Edwards JE Jr, Louie JS, Guze LB: Sternoarticular septic arthritis in heroin users. N Engl J Med 289:616, 1973.

Jamison RC, Heimlich EM, Miethke JC, O'Loughlin BJ: Non-specific spondylitis of infants and children. Radiology 77:355, 1961.

Larde D, Mathieu D, Frija J, Gaston A, Vasile N: Vertebral osteomyelitis: Disk hypodensity on CT. AJR 139:963, 1982.

Lewkonia RM, Kinsella TD: Pyogenic sacroiliitis. Diagnosis and significance. J Rheumatol 8:153, 1981.

Modic MT, Feiglin DH, Piraino DW, Boumphrey F, Weinstein MA, Duchesneau PM, Rehm S: Vertebral osteomyelitis: Assessment using MR. Radiology 157:157, 1985.

Pinckney LE, Currarino G, Higgenboten CL: Osteomyelitis of the cervical spine following dental extraction. Radiology 135:335, 1980.

Rosenberg D, Baskies AM, Deckers PJ, Leiter BE, Ordia JI, Yablon IG: Pyogenic sacroiliitis. An absolute indication for computerized tomographic scanning. Clin Orthop 184:128, 1984.

Sartoris DJ, Moskowitz PS, Kaufman RA, Ziprkowski MN, Berger PE: Childhood diskitis: Computed tomographic findings. Radiology 149:701, 1983.

Wiley AM, Trueta J: The vascular anatomy of the spine and its relationship to pyogenic vertebral osteomyelitis. J Bone Joint Surg [Br] 41:796, 1959.

Chapter 61

Osteomyelitis, Septic Arthritis, and Soft Tissue Infection: Organisms

Donald Resnick, M.D.
Gen Niwayama, M.D.

Bacteria, mycobacteria, spirochetes, fungi, viruses, rickettsiae, protozoa, and worms are all capable of affecting the musculoskeletal system. In many instances, radiographic features, although typical of an infection, do not allow
diagnosis of a specific causative agent; in some cases, the distribution and the morphology of the lesions are sufficiently characteristic to suggest a single infectious process.

Although the skeleton can react in only a limited number of ways to infection or other insult, certain characteristics of its response to a particular infectious agent may differ, at least subtly, from the changes that are encountered in the presence of a different agent. Thus, certain organisms produce rapid and destructive osseous or articular disease, whereas others are associated with a more indolent process. Furthermore, some agents show predilection for certain anatomic regions of the skeleton.

BACTERIAL INFECTION
Gram-Positive Cocci
Staphylococcal Infection

Staphylococci (especially *Staphylococcus aureus*) are responsible for the majority of cases of acute osteomyelitis and nongonococcal infectious arthritis. Staphylococcal osteomyelitis is primarily a disease of children under the age of 12 or 13 years. Localization of the infection to the metaphysis of tubular bones of children is typical, and Brodie's abscesses may be seen (Fig. 61–1). Staphylococci (*S. aureus* and *S. epidermidis*) are responsible also for many of the deep infections that occur after bone or joint surgery; the foot infections in diabetic persons; cases of osteomyelitis and septic arthritis seen in hemodialysis patients with infected shunts, in drug addicts, and in patients with rheumatoid arthritis; and the osseous, articular, and soft tissue suppurative processes that follow penetrating or open wounds. *Staphylococcus aureus* is implicated in most cases of pyomyositis.

Streptococcal Infection

In infants, hemolytic streptococcal agents have been recognized as an important etiologic factor in neonatal or infantile osteomyelitis. Typically, the disease is discovered in the first few weeks of life. Infection of a single bone is most frequent, and predilection for humeral involvement has been noted. Lytic lesions with mild or absent sclerosis and periostitis can be seen.

The joints may be infected by streptococcal organisms either by extension from a neighboring site of osteomyelitis or cellulitis or directly, although the prevalence of such articular infection appears to be declining.

PNEUMOCOCCAL INFECTION. Formerly termed *Diplococcus pneumoniae*, the pneumococcus is now referred to as *Streptococcus pneumoniae*, as it shares many characteristics with streptococci. Pulmonary infections and those of the upper respiratory tract predominate. Pneumococcal arthritis is not frequent. Children or adults may be affected, and the knee appears to be the most commonly involved site. Soft tissue swelling, joint space narrowing, osseous erosions, periostitis, and periarticular calcification are encountered.

Pneumococcal osteomyelitis is rare. Sickle cell anemia may be an underlying problem.

Gram-Negative Cocci
Meningococcal Infection

Meningococcal infection, related to the presence of *Neisseria meningitidis*, occurs almost exclusively in persons who have no

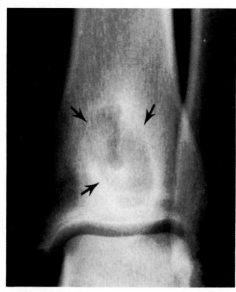

Figure 61–1. Staphylococcal osteomyelitis. A well-defined lucent lesion surrounded by a sclerotic margin at the end of the tubular bone (arrows) is typical of a Brodie's abscess.

measurable antimeningococcal antibody. It varies remarkably in its severity, appearing as a benign and asymptomatic illness in some persons and as a fulminant and fatal disorder in others.

Meningococcemia leads to the rapid development of fever, shaking chills, skin eruption, petechiae, myalgias, and neurologic manifestations. In fulminant cases (Waterhouse-Friderichsen syndrome), hypotension, confusion, tachypnea, and peripheral cyanosis develop, and disseminated intravascular coagulation with a consumptive coagulopathy produces diffuse bleeding from mucosal surfaces and the skin. Disseminated

intravascular coagulation is associated with occlusion of small blood vessels and subsequent necrosis in the skin, brain, kidneys, adrenal glands, and other tissues. In children, months or years after recovery from the acute illness, characteristic skeletal abnormalities have been described in which localized premature fusion of part of several physes is seen, usually in a bilateral and relatively symmetric distribution (Fig. 61–2). Subsequently, bowing and angular deformities appear, especially in the legs. Although the cause is not precisely known, a vascular insult is the most likely etiologic factor for the metaphyseal alterations.

Meningococcal arthritis is not a common condition. Three forms are recognized: an acute transient polyarthritis; a purulent arthritis involving one or more joints; and arthritis occurring after serum therapy, a variety that is not seen currently. The frequency of purulent arthritis in cases of meningococcal infection is 5 to 10 per cent. Rapid resolution of the joint disease is typical, although radiologic evidence of cartilaginous and osseous destruction occasionally is evident.

Gonococcal Infection

CLINICAL ABNORMALITIES. Gonorrhea is produced by the microorganism *Neisseria gonorrhoeae*, which infects the mucous membranes of the urethra, cervix, rectum, and pharynx. The disease is transmitted almost exclusively through sexual contact. Gonorrhea is more frequent in women than in men. The disease also may become evident in homosexual men, during pregnancy, and after gonococcal vulvovaginitis in children and in the neonate.

Only a minority of gonococcal infections eventually disseminate. Gonococcemia leads to skin rash, fever, and arthritis, the latter occurring in approximately 75 per cent of disseminated cases. Polyarticular findings are frequent. The affected joints, in decreasing order of frequency, are the knee, the ankle, the wrist, and the joints of the shoulder, foot, and

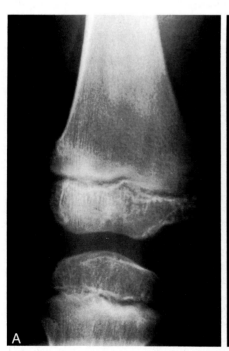
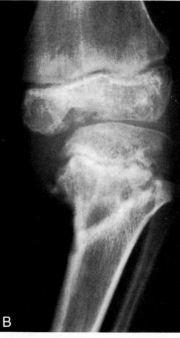

Figure 61–2. Meningococcemia with skeletal deformities. This boy demonstrates the skeletal deformities that can follow meningococcemia with intravascular coagulation. Findings in the knees include metaphyseal sclerosis, epiphyseal irregularity and deformity, subluxation, and, in one tibia, a previous fracture. (Courtesy of M. Dalinka, M.D., Philadelphia, Pennsylvania.)

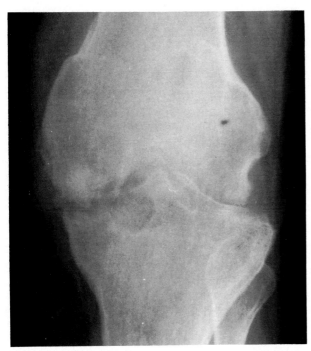

Figure 61–3. Gonococcal arthritis. Observe joint space loss, poorly defined marginal and central osseous erosions, and soft tissue swelling. The lack of osteoporosis is impressive. Bone proliferation is evident along the distal medial portion of the femur.

spine (Fig. 61–3). In approximately 50 to 70 per cent of cases, acute asymmetric tenosynovitis or periarthritis is evident.

PATHOLOGIC ABNORMALITIES. A reliable diagnosis of gonococcal arthritis depends on recovery of the bacteria from the blood, the synovial tissue, the synovial fluid, the genitourinary tract, or the skin. This is accomplished in 50 to 60 per cent of suspected cases. The appearance of the synovial membrane is typical of that of pyogenic articular processes. The articular cartilage and subchondral bone may become involved in later stages of joint infection or in early stages when hematogenous implantation has produced a primary osteomyelitis.

RADIOLOGIC ABNORMALITIES. When antibiotic treatment is instituted at an early stage, the only significant radiographic features are soft tissue swelling and osteoporosis. If treatment is delayed, more prominent radiographic findings are encountered, including joint space narrowing, marginal and central osseous erosions, lytic destruction of adjacent metaphyses and epiphyses, and periostitis (Fig. 61–3). Healing can be associated with intraarticular osseous fusion. The appearance of abnormalities at multiple joints and tenosynovitis are helpful clues to a specific diagnosis of gonococcal infection.

DIFFERENTIAL DIAGNOSIS. The accurate differentiation of gonococcal joint disease and that related to other pyogenic (nontuberculous) organisms usually is not possible radiographically. Furthermore, differentiating the radiographic features of gonococcal pyarthrosis and Reiter's syndrome can be extremely difficult. Gonococcal arthritis and Reiter's syndrome both produce soft tissue swelling, osteoporosis, joint space narrowing, osseous erosion, and periostitis in one or more joints, particularly in the lower extremity. Helpful features in accurately diagnosing Reiter's syndrome include (1) involvement of the joints of the foot, the calcaneus, the spine, and the sacroiliac articulation; (2) the presence of poorly defined periosteal proliferation about the involved joints; and (3) the absence of fuzzy or frayed central osseous margins.

Enteric Gram-Negative Bacilli

The terminology related to this group of bacteria is not constant; however, these gram-negative bacilli are responsible for as many as 25 per cent of skeletal infections.

Coliform Bacterial Infection

The coliform bacteria are gram-negative bacilli that normally inhabit the human intestinal tract. The best-known organisms in this group are *Escherichia coli* and *Enterobacter (Aerobacter) aerogenes*. Articular and osseous infections with these agents are rare except in the drug abuser, the person with preexisting joint disease, and the patient with a chronic debilitating disorder. Monarticular involvement, especially of the knee, is typical.

Proteus Infection

Proteus mirabilis infection of a joint is rarely observed. Urinary tract abnormalities may coexist. Osteomyelitis related to this microorganism also is rare.

Figure 61–4. Pseudomonas osteomyelitis and septic arthritis. In this drug abuser, osteomyelitis of the distal clavicle and septic arthritis of the acromioclavicular joint with osseous destruction and periostitis were related to Pseudomonas infection.

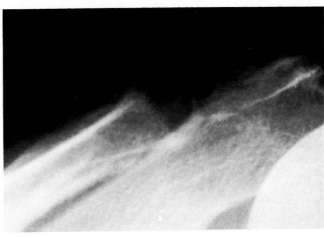

Pseudomonas Infection

Serious infection with Pseudomonas is almost invariably associated with diminished resistance of the host or damage to local tissues (Fig. 61–4). Premature infants, children with congenital anomalies, drug abusers, patients with myeloproliferative disorders or those receiving immunosuppressive agents, and geriatric patients with debilitating diseases are among those who may develop osteomyelitis or septic arthritis due to *Pseudomonas aeruginosa*. The peculiar proclivity of drug abusers to develop Pseudomonas osteomyelitis and septic arthritis and the common localization of such disease within the central skeleton are interesting but unexplained observations. Pseudomonas osteomyelitis also is a recognized complication of puncture wounds. No specific radiographic features characterize skeletal involvement with this organism.

Klebsiella Infection

Rarely, *Klebsiella pneumoniae* results in osteomyelitis and septic arthritis in a host with diminished resistance.

Salmonella Infection

Salmonella typhi produces a systemic infection, typhoid fever. Before the advent of antibiotics, bone infection was encountered in approximately 1 per cent of patients with typhoid fever; more recently, such cases have indeed become rare. Involvement can occur in extraspinal or spinal locations. In the latter site, the radiographic picture resembles that in tuberculosis.

An association exists between Salmonella infection and sickle cell anemia or other hemoglobinopathies, as well as leukemia, lymphoma, bartonellosis, cirrhosis of the liver, and systemic lupus erythematosus. The basis for the unusual propensity of persons with sickle cell anemia to develop Salmonella infection is not known. It has been postulated that multiple bowel infarcts allow the organisms to leave the colon and enter the blood stream, and that Salmonella organisms are well suited for survival in areas of medullary bone infarction. Salmonella osteomyelitis frequently originates in the medullary cavity of a tubular bone. In tubular bones, Salmonella infection may be characterized by a symmetric distribution, a combination of lysis and sclerosis, and periostitis, findings that are difficult to differentiate from infarction alone.

Shigella Infection

Two to 3 weeks after an episode of acute bacillary dysentery, a noninfectious polyarthritis showing predilection for the knees, the elbows, the wrists, or the fingers can be evident.

Yersinia Infection

Two types of bone or joint affliction can occur in association with infection caused by *Yersinia enterocolitica*. A nonsuppurative, self-limited polyarthritis can appear approximately 3 weeks after the onset of the illness. This articular manifestation may be complicated by sacroiliitis and the presence of the HLA-B27 antigen. The second type of affliction relates to the presence of *Y. enterocolitica* septicemia, particularly in patients with underlying abnormalities. Septic arthritis or osteomyelitis may appear in this setting.

Serratia Infection

Serratia marcescens can cause infection of the musculoskeletal system, especially in persons with underlying disorders such as diabetes mellitus, systemic lupus erythematosus, neutrophil dysfunction syndromes, and rheumatoid arthritis, or after trauma; intravenous, arterial, or urinary catheter placement; ischemic necrosis of bone; or drug abuse. Radiographic features of septic arthritis and osteomyelitis are entirely nonspecific.

Other Gram-Negative Bacilli
Haemophilus Infection

Acute septic arthritis due to *Haemophilus influenzae* is more frequent in children than in adults (Fig. 61–5). In fact, this microorganism appears to be the leading cause of pyarthrosis in children in the first 2 years of life. Hematogenous spread is the usual mechanism of joint infection. Single or, less commonly, multiple joints may be affected.

Brucella Infection

Brucellosis (undulant fever) can result from human infection with one of a variety of organisms, including *Brucella abortus*, *Brucella melitensis*, and *Brucella suis*. The disease is transmitted to humans from lower animals such as the goat, the cow, and the hog through the ingestion of milk or milk products containing viable bacteria or through contact of skin with infected tissues or secretions. The invading organisms localize in tissues of the reticuloendothelial system, such as the liver, the spleen, the lymph nodes, and the bone marrow.

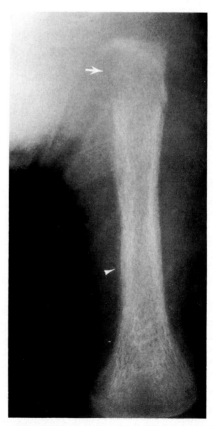

Figure 61–5. Haemophilus osteomyelitis and septic arthritis. This infant developed osteomyelitis of the proximal metaphysis and diaphysis of the humerus with glenohumeral joint involvement owing to Haemophilus. Observe metaphyseal erosion (arrow), permeative bone destruction, and periostitis (arrowhead).

Involvement of joints, bones, and bursae is relatively uncommon, although an inflammatory process in any one of these sites in a farmer or meathandler should arouse suspicion of brucellosis. Arthritis is usually monarticular, with the hip and knee being involved most frequently. Sacroiliac joint abnormalities also are common. Alterations of bursae may be especially characteristic.

Osteomyelitis frequently is chronic in nature. Brucellar spondylitis typically affects the lumbar spine and is associated with an acute clinical onset and rapid progression of radiologic findings (Fig. 61–6). Abnormalities include destruction of vertebrae and intervertebral discs, sclerosis, paravertebral abscess formation, and healing with intraosseous fusion and osteophytosis. Osteoporosis, large soft tissue abscesses, and paraspinal calcification may be somewhat less common in brucellosis than in tuberculosis.

Pasteurella Infection

Typical pathogens in animals, pasteurellae can produce human infections, including cutaneous abscesses, septicemia, endocarditis, osteomyelitis, and septic arthritis. *Pasteurella multocida* frequently is isolated from both wild and domestic animals, especially cats, dogs, swine, and rats, explaining the association of human infections with animal exposure, bites, or scratches. Cutaneous and subcutaneous abscesses, cellulitis, and lymphangitis can be followed by septicemia and involvement of distant sites. Localization of infection in the knee is common. Bone and joint contamination in the hand or foot commonly is related to direct inoculation of organisms or

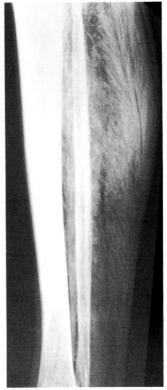

Figure 61–7. Clostridial soft tissue infection. Linear and circular collections of gas in the subcutaneous and muscular tissues reflect the presence of clostridial myositis and cellulitis.

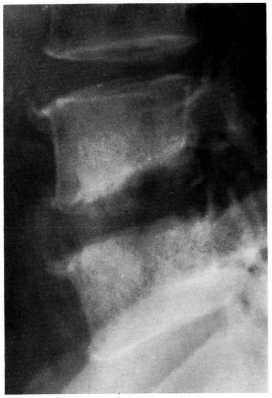

Figure 61–6 Brucellar spondylitis. Lumbar spine involvement is characterized by irregular destruction of the osseous surfaces of two adjacent vertebrae with reactive sclerosis.

spread of infection from involved soft tissues owing to the injury itself. Osteolysis, periostitis, and soft tissue swelling are observed.

Other Bacteria
Clostridial Infection

GAS GANGRENE. Wounds that are contaminated by gas gangrene may contain a mixture of clostridial organisms, including *Clostridium tetani, C. perfringens, C. septicum,* and *C. novyi*. These organisms are anaerobic and are capable of producing extensive tissue destruction with gas formation at the site of invasion. Soft tissue contamination with gas gangrene develops in devitalized tissues in which arterial blood supply has been compromised.

Clinical manifestations of clostridial myonecrosis may become evident within 6 to 8 hours of injury and include severe pain and an edematous, pulseless, and gangrenous limb. The clinical manifestations of cellulitis caused by clostridia are less striking.

On radiographs, radiolucent collections may appear within the subcutaneous or muscular tissues (Fig. 61–7). In the former location, they produce linear or net-like lucent areas, whereas in the muscular tissues, circular collections of varying size are evident. It should be emphasized, however, that soft tissue gas is not specific for clostridial infections, being evident in some cases related to infections with *E. coli,* other coliform bacteria, streptococci, and *Bacteroides* species. Nonbacterial mechanisms responsible for gas in the soft tissues include visceral rupture, skin lacerations and open fractures, explosive-type injuries, cutaneous ulcerations, and chemical exposures.

ARTHRITIS. *Clostridium perfringens* can be introduced into an articulation by contamination from a penetrating injury. Monarticular disease is typical. In addition to joint space narrowing and osseous defects, radiographs may delineate gas in the adjacent soft tissues or articulation itself.

Clostridial organisms may rarely cause infective spondylitis, which may be associated with intradiscal gas.

Bacteroides and Related Anaerobic Infection

Some non–spore-forming obligate anaerobes may cause clinically evident infections when breaks in the mucosa or skin allow the normal microflora to become displaced into deeper tissues and to reach the blood stream. Crepitant cellulitis, necrotizing fasciitis, and myonecrosis are typical musculoskeletal expressions of anaerobic infections related primarily to contamination of contiguous tissue. Septic arthritis and osteomyelitis are rare and may be manifestations of hematogenous dissemination. Gas formation in infected tissues aids in precise radiographic diagnosis.

Mycobacteria
Tuberculous Infection

FREQUENCY AND PATTERN. The frequency of tuberculosis has changed dramatically since the advent of appropriate chemotherapy for this disease. Currently, the frequency of tuberculosis in general, and of skeletal tuberculosis in particular, has diminished, although the use of modern therapeutic techniques, including BCG vaccination, has produced examples of iatrogenic infection (see discussion later in this chapter). Furthermore, the pattern of osteoarticular tuberculosis has changed over the years. Initially, the disease was usually encountered in children and young adults; currently, patients of all ages are affected. Persons with underlying disorders, those receiving corticosteroid medication, alcoholic patients, drug abusers, and immigrants are not infrequent hosts for this disease. In the past, there have been two modes of infection: inhalation and ingestion. The latter mechanism has been largely eradicated.

Tuberculous spondylitis has been the most typical form of the disease. In recent years, however, articular changes in extraspinal sites have been more prominent. Tuberculous dactylitis, multiple sites of involvement, and tendon sheath abnormalities are also commonly encountered.

CLINICAL ABNORMALITIES. Skeletal tuberculosis can affect persons of all ages. The vertebral column, the hip, and the knee are the most frequent sites of involvement. Tuberculous arthritis can lead to pain, swelling, weakness, muscle wasting, and a draining sinus, and a history of local trauma may be obtained in 30 to 50 per cent of cases. Tuberculous spondylitis is accompanied by the insidious onset of back pain, stiffness, local tenderness, and possibly fever and neurologic abnormalities. Paralysis is encountered as a result of spinal cord compression from abscesses, granulation tissue or bone fragments, arachnoiditis, ischemia of the cord resulting from endarteritis, or intramedullary granulomas. Spinal involvement in tuberculosis is associated most clearly with pulmonary disease. Tuberculous dactylitis usually appears as painless swelling of the hand or the foot. Tuberculous tenosynovitis and bursitis can produce soft tissue swelling and

tenderness in the ulnar or radial bursa, the fingers, and the toes.

Positive findings on the skin test for tuberculosis are of little help in the diagnosis of this disease, although a negative result usually excludes the diagnosis. Negative findings on chest radiograph in the adult patient does not exclude the possibility of skeletal tuberculosis. In a child, such a radiograph makes tuberculosis an unlikely cause of bone abnormalities. Presence of the disorder is confirmed by the demonstration of the tubercle bacilli in smear or culture; this may require aspiration of joint contents or biopsy of the synovial

Table 61–1. DISEASES ASSOCIATED WITH BONE MARROW GRANULOMA

Infectious Diseases
  Bacterial Infections
    Mycobacterial diseases
      Tuberculosis
      BCG vaccination
      Leprosy
    Brucellosis
    Tularemia
    Glanders
  Fungal Infections (Disseminated)
    Histoplasmosis
    Cryptococcosis
    Paracoccidioidomycosis
    Coccidioidomycosis
    Saccharomyces cerevisiae infection
  Viral Infections
    Infectious mononucleosis
    Cytomegalovirus infection
    Viral hepatitis
  Parasitic Infections
    Toxoplasmosis
    Leishmaniasis
  Other
    Rocky Mountain spotted fever
    Q-fever
    Mycoplasma pneumoniae infection

Malignant Diseases
  Hodgkin's disease
  Non-Hodgkin's lymphoma
  Metastatic carcinoma
  Acute lymphocytic leukemia

Drugs
  Chlorpropamide
  Phenylbutazone (oxyphenbutazone)
  Allopurinol
  Procainamide
  Ibuprofen
  Phenytoin

Autoimmune or Allergic Diseases
  Rheumatoid arthritis (Felty's syndrome)
  Systemic lupus erythematosus
  Primary biliary cirrhosis
  Farmer's lung

Miscellaneous
  Syndrome of marrow and lymph node granuloma, uveitis, and reversible renal failure
  Berylliosis
  Sarcoidosis

(From Bodem CR, et al: Granulomatous bone marrow disease. A review of the literature and clinicopathologic analysis of 58 cases. Medicine 62:372, 1983. ©1983, The Williams & Wilkins Co, Baltimore. Used with permission.)

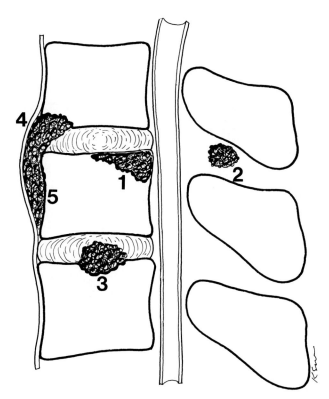

Figure 61–8. Tuberculous spondylitis: Sites of involvement. Tuberculous lesions can localize in the vertebral body (1) or, more rarely, the posterior osseous or ligamentous structures (2). Extension to the intervertebral disc (3) or prevertebral tissues (4) is not infrequent. Subligamentous spread (5) can lead to erosion of the anterior vertebral surface.

membrane in cases of tuberculous arthritis and closed or open biopsy of bone in cases of tuberculous osteomyelitis.

PATHOGENESIS. It is generally accepted that skeletal involvement in tuberculosis occurs mainly by the hematogenous route. Hematogenous seeding of the skeleton may arise from a primary infection of the lung, particularly in children, or, at a later date, from a quiescent primary site or an extraosseous focus. With healing of the primary complex, there is a tendency toward resolution of skeletal foci. Occasionally, reactivation of bone and joint tuberculosis is evident.

The frequency of associated visceral disease in patients with skeletal tuberculosis is considerable. Pulmonary involvement may be evident in 50 per cent of cases; urogenital lesions may coexist with skeletal involvement in 20 to 45 per cent of cases.

GENERAL PATHOLOGIC CONSIDERATIONS. The typical response of the tissue to tuberculosis is the formation of tubercles. Around a central zone are clusters of epithelioid cells. In the central part of the tubercle are multinucleated giant cells, whereas at the periphery of the tubercle is a mantle of lymphocytes. Central caseating necrosis is characteristic of these tubercles. It should be emphasized, however, that granulomatous disease, including that of the bone marrow, is a nonspecific response to a persistent antigenic stimulus and has been identified in a wide range of illnesses (Table 61–1).

TUBERCULOUS SPONDYLITIS

Frequency and Distribution. It is currently estimated that the vertebral column is affected in 25 to 60 per cent of cases of skeletal tuberculosis. The first lumbar vertebra is affected most commonly and the frequency of involvement decreases equally in either direction from this level. The disease is relatively infrequent in the cervical and sacral segments of the vertebral column, although sacroiliac joint tuberculosis is not rare. Solitary lesions are not uncommon, but typically more than one vertebra is affected. The vertebral body is involved more commonly than the posterior elements (Fig. 61–8). In the vertebral body, an anterior predilection is striking.

It is generally accepted that tuberculous spondylitis results from hematogenous spread of infection. A debate has existed, however, whether the primary vascular pathway is supplied by the arterial route or the paravertebral venous plexus of Batson.

Radiographic-Pathologic Correlation

Discovertebral Lesion. In most cases, tuberculous spondylitis begins as an infectious focus in the anterior aspect of the vertebral body adjacent to the subchondral bone plate (Fig. 61–9). Subsequently, infection may spread to the adjacent intervertebral discs. This may occur if the bacilli extend beneath the anterior longitudinal ligament or posterior longitudinal ligament to violate the peripheral discal tissue; if the organisms penetrate the subchondral bone plate and overlying cartilaginous endplate to enter the intervertebral disc; or if an intraosseous lesion weakens the vertebral body to such a degree that it produces a discal displacement (cartilaginous node), contamination of invading discal tissue, and subsequent spread through the defect into the intervertebral disc. The combination of vertebral body and discal destruction in tuberculosis is similar to that occurring in pyogenic spondylitis, although the tuberculous process usually is not rapidly progressive. Only rarely does vertebral body tuberculosis extend into the pedicles, laminae, or transverse or spinous processes.

In long-standing disease, involvement of neighboring vertebral bodies and intervertebral discs may become evident, and eventually, long segments of the spine can be affected.

Paraspinal Extension. Extension of tuberculosis from vertebral and discal sites to the adjacent ligaments and soft tissues is frequent. This extension usually occurs anterolaterally; rarely, it is observed posteriorly in the peridural space. Subligamentous extension of a tuberculous abscess can allow osseous and discal invasion at distant sites.

Burrowing abscesses can extend for extraordinary distances before perforating an internal viscus or the body surface. In the lumbar region, pus collecting beneath the fascia of the psoas muscle produces a psoas abscess, which can extend into the groin and the thigh. Among the organs and tissues that have been penetrated by paravertebral abscesses are the esophagus, the bronchus, the lung, the mediastinum, the liver, the kidney, the intestine, the urinary bladder, the rectum, the vagina, and the aorta.

Abscess formation in tuberculosis can produce soft tissue swelling on radiographs that appears out of proportion to the degree of osseous and discal destruction. The swelling commonly is bilateral and associated with scalloping of the anterior

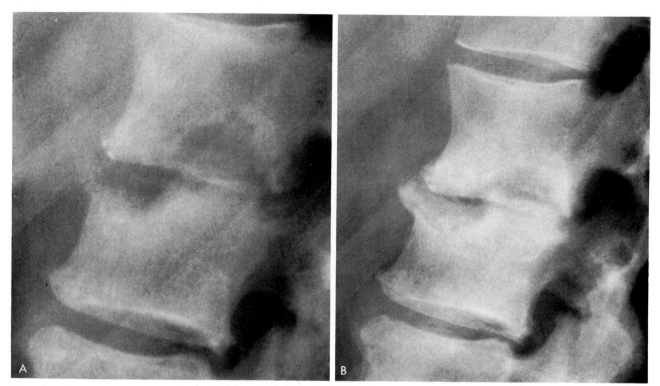

Figure 61–9. Tuberculous spondylitis: Discovertebral lesion. A The initial radiograph reveals subchondral destruction of two vertebral bodies with mild surrounding eburnation and loss of intervertebral disc height. The appearance is identical to that in pyogenic spondylitis. **B** Several months later, osseous reponse is evident. Note the increased sclerosis. Osteophytosis and improved definition of the osseous margins can be seen.

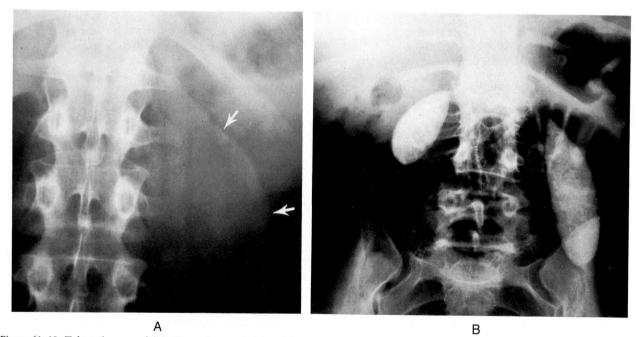

Figure 61–10. Tuberculous spondylitis: Psoas abscess. A A large left noncalcified psoas abscess (arrows) can be seen. **B** Diffusely calcified psoas abscesses are noted in association with spinal abnormalities.

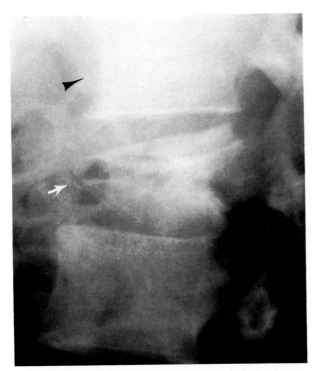

Figure 61–11. Tuberculous spondylitis: Solitary vertebral involvement. A collapsed vertebral body (arrow) represents the site of tuberculous involvement in this adult patient. Note anterior scalloping of the vertebral body above this level (arrowhead), indicating subligamentous spread of infection.

and lateral aspects of the vertebral bodies. Psoas abscesses may contain calcification (Fig. 61–10). Nontuberculous psoas abscesses rarely calcify.

Other diagnostic methods, including ultrasonography and computed tomography, can provide important information in patients with psoas or paraspinal abscesses. Computed tomographic findings indicative of abscess include an abnormal mass of low attenuation number, displacement of surrounding structures, obliteration of normal fascial planes, a "rind" sign, consisting of a rim of increased tissue attenuation, and abnormal gaseous collections. None of these findings is specific for infection, as hematomas and tumors produce similar alterations.

Posterior Element Lesions. Occasionally, the posterior elements may be the initial spinal site of tuberculosis. In these instances, radiographic findings include pediculate or laminal destruction, erosion of the posterior cortex of the vertebral body and adjacent ribs, a large paraspinal mass, and relative sparing of the intervertebral discs. With involvement of the pedicles, paraplegia is frequent owing to granulomatous extension into the spinal canal.

Other Spinal Lesions. Rarely, tuberculosis leads to isolated involvement of a single vertebral body (Fig. 61–11). In children, vertebra plana can appear, simulating the appearance of eosinophilic granuloma (Fig. 61–12).

Collapse of partially destroyed vertebral bodies during the course of tuberculous spondylitis can lead to severe deformities. Typically, an angulated posterior projection appears at the site of maximum spinal involvement, leading to tuberculous kyphosis or gibbus deformity. Angulation is more acute in the thoracic spine than in the cervical or lumbar

region. Radiography indicates destroyed vertebral bodies in the area of angulation and, in some cases of thoracic kyphosis, a remarkable increase in height of the vertebral bodies in the lordotic lumbar area. Although not so frequent as kyphosis, scoliosis also can occur in tuberculous spondylitis.

Healing in tuberculous spondylitis can be associated with osseous fusion of vertebral bodies. Not uncommonly, four to eight vertebrae are coalesced into a large osseous mass.

Increased radiodensity of the vertebral body in tuberculosis can lead to an ivory vertebra. This phenomenon usually is evident in the lumbar region.

Tuberculosis involving the upper cervical spine is a rare but important manifestation of the disease. Clinical features include pain and decreased range of motion in the neck, dysphagia, and weakness in one or more extremities. Radiographic abnormalities include occipitoatlantoaxial subluxation, bone erosion, and a prevertebral soft tissue mass (Fig. 61–13). Identical abnormalities are seen in occasional cases of fungal infection.

In rare circumstances, tuberculosis leads to an extradural granulomatous lesion in the absence of bone involvement. This manifestation is more common in the dorsal epidural space and in the thoracic segment.

Differential Diagnosis. The differential diagnosis of tuberculous spondylitis includes a wide variety of other infectious disorders of the spine. Differentiation of tuberculous and pyogenic vertebral osteomyelitis can be extremely difficult. Clinical data that favor a diagnosis of tuberculosis are an insidious onset of symptoms, a typical tuberculous pulmonary infiltrate, and a normal erythrocyte sedimentation rate. Radiographic features favoring tuberculosis are involvement of one or more segments of the spine, a delay in destruction of intervertebral discs, a large and calcified paravertebral mass, and absence of sclerosis. It should be noted, however, that sclerosis is encountered in tuberculosis, particularly in the black race.

Tuberculous spondylitis may simulate tumor. Intervertebral disc space destruction is more characteristic of infectious lesions of the spine. Scalloping of the anterior surface of the

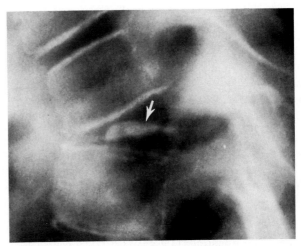

Figure 61–12. Tuberculous spondylitis: Vertebra plana and kyphosis. In this child, a wafer-like remnant of the infected vertebral body can be seen (arrow). Abnormal kyphosis is present. The adjacent vertebrae appear normal. (Courtesy of A. D'Abreu, M.D., Porto Alegre, Brazil.)

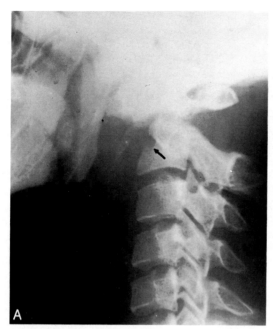
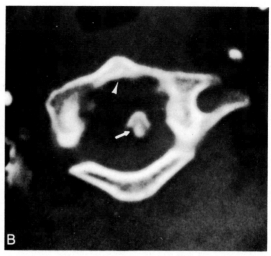

Figure 61–13. Tuberculous spondylitis: Atlantoaxial destruction. A A lateral radiograph of the cervical spine documents a large anterior soft tissue mass displacing the pharynx. Atlantoaxial subluxation is seen, the odontoid process is poorly visualized, and there is an erosion of the anterior portion of the axis (arrow). **B** A computed tomographic image at the level of the atlas confirms the presence of atlantoaxial subluxation. Note the increased space between the anterior arch of the atlas (arrowhead) and the odontoid process (arrow). Observe that the latter is displaced laterally, indicating rotation between the two bones. Osseous erosion of both the odontoid process and the atlas is evident. (From Dowd CF, et al: Case report 344. Skel Radiol *15*:65, 1986. Used with permission.)

vertebral bodies, evident in tuberculosis with subligamentous spread, can also be seen with paravertebral lymphadenopathy due to metastasis, myeloma, or lymphoma. Sarcoidosis can produce multifocal lesions of vertebrae and intervertebral discs with paraspinal masses, findings identical to those of tuberculosis.

TUBERCULOUS OSTEOMYELITIS

Frequency and Distribution. Tuberculous osteomyelitis is almost uniformly related to hematogenous dissemination. It can remain localized to bone or involve adjacent joints. Virtually any bone can be affected, including those of the pelvis, the phalanges and metacarpals (tuberculous dactylitis), the long bones, the ribs, the sternum, the skull, the patella, and the carpal and tarsal regions.

In the long tubular bones, tuberculosis usually originates in one of the epiphyses and soon spreads into the neighboring joint (Fig. 61–14). Metaphyseal foci in the child can occasionally violate the growth plate (Fig. 61–14). This feature deserves emphasis, as pyogenic infections arising in the metaphyseal segment of a child's tubular bone do not generally extend across the physis.

Radiographic-Pathologic Correlation. The pathologic process is initiated by tubercle formation in the marrow with secondary infection of the trabeculae. With caseation, an abscess cavity is created containing pus and small granules of bone termed "bone sand." On radiographs, foci of osteolysis are accompanied by varying amounts of eburnation and periostitis. Sequestrum formation can be encountered. The initial radiographic appearance in tuberculous osteomyelitis is similar to that in other types of osteomyelitis and even in aggressive neoplasm.

Special Types of Tuberculous Osteomyelitis

Cystic Tuberculosis. A rare variety of tuberculosis, more frequent in children than in adults, is associated with cystic lesions of one or multiple bones (Fig. 61–15). In children, these lesions usually affect the peripheral skeleton, may be symmetric in distribution, are of variable size, and generally are unaccompanied by sclerosis. In adults, the skull, the shoulder and pelvic girdles, and the axial skeleton are involved. The radiographic characteristics of cystic tuberculosis, which include well-defined osseous lesions with or without surrounding sclerosis, resemble those of eosinophilic granuloma, sarcoidosis, cystic angiomatosis, plasma cell myeloma, fungal infections, metastases, and other conditions.

Tuberculous Dactylitis. Tuberculous involvement of the short tubular bones of the hands and feet is termed tuberculous dactylitis. This form of tuberculosis is especially frequent in children; the reported frequency of dactylitis in cases of childhood tuberculosis has ranged from 0.5 to 14 per cent. Although involvement of one bone of the hand or the foot is common, multiple osseous foci can be identified in 25 to 35 per cent of cases.

Soft tissue swelling usually is the initial manifestation. Periostitis of phalanges, metacarpals, or metatarsals also may be evident (Fig. 61–16). Expansion of the bone with cystic quality is termed spina ventosa and is especially common in childhood. Similar expansion rarely can be evident in the radius, ulna, and humerus.

Tuberculous dactylitis can be imitated by other infectious disorders of bacterial or fungal origin. Syphilitic dactylitis in infants and children produces bilateral and symmetric involvement; in this disease, periostitis is more exuberant and soft

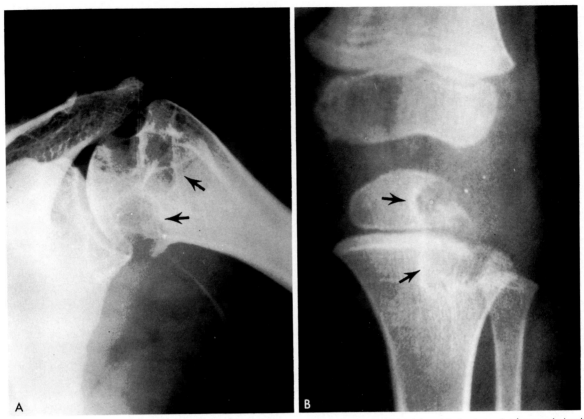

Figure 61–14. Tuberculous osteomyelitis: Radiographic abnormalities. A In this patient, an initial epiphyseal lesion (arrows) subsequently involved the glenohumeral joint. The lesions are well circumscribed, and the glenoid and acromion also are affected. **B** Observe the violation of the growth plate with adjacent metaphyseal and epiphyseal alterations (arrows).

Figure 61–15. Cystic tuberculosis. A Note the well-defined lytic lesions of the medullary and cortical areas of the metaphysis and diaphysis of the humerus. The proximal epiphysis is also affected. Sclerosis is absent, although periostitis can be seen. **B** Similar lesions are present in the tibia and fibula. Some of these are central, whereas others are eccentric or peripheral in location.

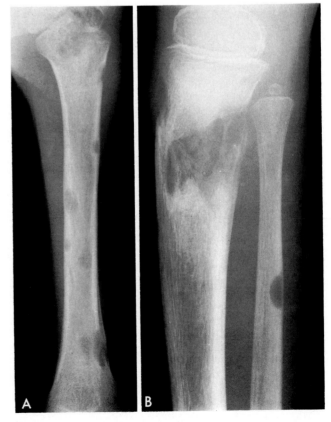

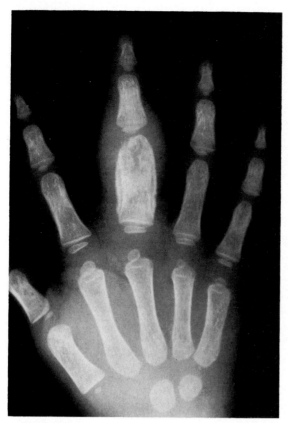

Figure 61–16. Tuberculous dactylitis. Radiographic findings in this child include soft tissue swelling of multiple digits, lytic lesions of several middle and proximal phalanges and metacarpals, and exuberant periostitis and enlargement of the proximal phalanx of the third finger.

tissue swelling is less prominent than in tuberculous dactylitis. Fibrous dysplasia, hyperparathyroidism, leukemia, sarcoidosis, and sickle cell anemia may produce phalangeal, metacarpal, and metatarsal changes.

Differential Diagnosis. Differentiation of tuberculous osteomyelitis and pyogenic osteomyelitis is difficult. Osteoporosis, bone lysis and sclerosis, and periostitis are evident in both conditions. Acute pyogenic osteomyelitis has a more rapid course and less frequently extends across the physis or to the neighboring joint than does tuberculous osteomyelitis. The latter condition is associated with radiographic findings that are virtually identical to those of fungal skeletal infections.

TUBERCULOUS ARTHRITIS

General Features. Tuberculous arthritis most typically affects large joints such as the knee and the hip. Monarticular disease is the rule. The majority of joint lesions are secondary to adjacent osteomyelitis. Most patients are middle-aged or elderly, and many have underlying disorders or have received intraarticular injections of steroids. Tuberculous joint disease may persist with chronic pain and only minimal signs of inflammation. Delay in diagnosis is frequent; correct diagnosis requires synovial fluid and tissue for culture and histologic studies.

Pathologic Abnormalities. An enlarging joint effusion and inflammatory thickening of the periarticular connective tissue and fat contribute to soft tissue swelling. The synovial membrane thickens and is covered with heavy layers of fibrin. On microscopic examination, richly vascular tuberculous granulation tissue is found to contain necrotic and fibrin-like material, caseous areas, and collections of leukocytes and mononuclear phagocytes.

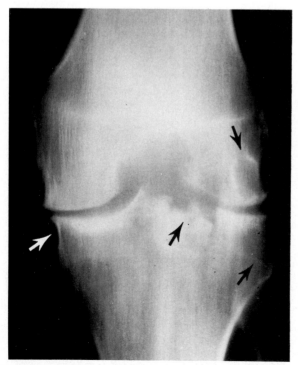

Figure 61–17. Tuberculous arthritis: Knee. On a conventional tomogram, typical marginal and central osseous erosions (arrows) accompany tuberculous arthritis. Osteoporosis is not prominent.

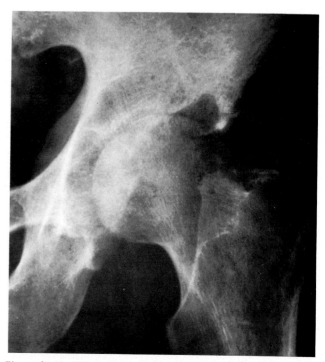

Figure 61–18. Tuberculous arthritis: Hip. Bone erosion of the femoral head and acetabulum, joint space loss, and osteoporosis are evident.

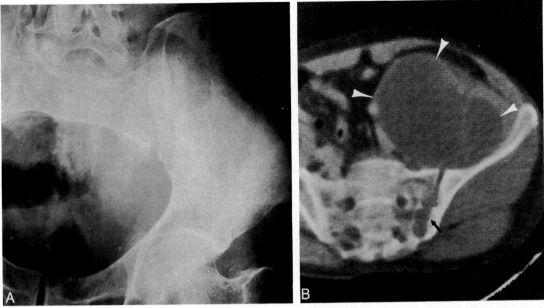

Figure 61-19. Tuberculous arthritis: Sacroiliac joint. A The plain film shows a large soft tissue mass and a widened sacroiliac joint with bone erosion, especially in the sacrum. **B** A computed tomographic scan better delineates the degree of osseous erosion in the lower portion of the joint (arrow) and the extent of the soft tissue mass (arrowheads). (Courtesy of J. Costello, M.D., Madrid, Spain.)

The granulation tissue spreads insidiously onto and erodes the cartilage. The erosive process is not evenly distributed. Rather, focal areas of cartilaginous destruction may be intermixed with areas of relatively normal-appearing chondral elements. Granulation tissue also insinuates itself between the cartilage and subchondral bone, especially in articulations (e.g., hip, ankle) in which the articular cartilages are in close contact. Detached cartilage may become necrotic, the osseous surface can be exposed, and destruction of the subchondral bone plate and trabeculae can ensue. Osseous erosion may be especially marked at the periphery of the joint.

Radiographic Abnormalities. A triad of radiographic findings (Phemister's triad) is characteristic of tuberculous arthritis: juxtaarticular osteoporosis, peripherally located osseous erosions, and gradual narrowing of the interosseous space (Figs. 61–17 to 61–20). Initially, soft tissue swelling and osteoporosis may dominate the radiographic picture. Marginal erosions are especially characteristic of tuberculosis

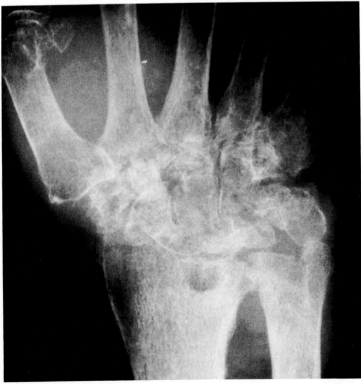

Figure 61-20. Tuberculous arthritis: Wrist. A Abnormalities include soft tissue swelling, osteoporosis, small and large osseous erosions throughout the carpus, metacarpal bones, ulna, and radius, and joint space narrowing.

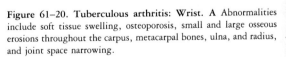

**Table 61–2. COMPARISON OF TUBERCULOUS
AND PYOGENIC ARTHRITIS**

	Tuberculous Arthritis	Pyogenic Arthritis
Soft tissue swelling	+	+
Osteoporosis	+	±
Joint space loss	Late	Early
Marginal erosions	+	+
Bone proliferation (sclerosis, periostitis)	±	+
Bone ankylosis	±	+
Slow progression	+	−

+ = Common; ± = infrequent; − = rare or absent.

in "tight" or weight-bearing joints, such as the hip, the knee, and the ankle. They produce corner defects simulating the erosions of other synovial processes, such as rheumatoid arthritis. The combination of regional osteoporosis, marginal erosions, and relative preservation of joint space is highly suggestive of tuberculous arthritis.

Bone proliferation generally is not so exuberant in tuberculous arthritis as it is in pyogenic arthritis. Similarly, periostitis can be evident, although its frequency and extent are not so great in tuberculosis as in pyogenic infection. Sequestered pieces of bone appear as dense, triangular collections at the edges of the joint.

The eventual result in tuberculous arthritis is usually fibrous ankylosis of the joint. Bone ankylosis is seen occasionally, but this sequela is more frequent in pyogenic arthritis.

Differential Diagnosis. The appearance of periarticular osteoporosis, marginal erosions, and absent or mild joint space narrowing is most helpful in the accurate diagnosis of tuberculous arthritis. In rheumatoid arthritis, osteoporosis and marginal erosions are accompanied by early loss of articular space. In gout, osteoporosis is mild or absent, although marginal erosions and preservation of interosseous space can be observed. In regional osteoporosis, marginal osseous defects are not evident, and the joint space is maintained.

A monarticular process must be regarded as infection until proved otherwise. Slow progression of disease, significant osteoporosis, and mild sclerosis are more prominent in tuberculosis and fungal disease than in pyarthrosis (Table 61–2). Accurate diagnosis mandates synovial fluid aspiration or synovial membrane biopsy, however. Other monarticular processes, such as pigmented villonodular synovitis and idiopathic synovial osteochondromatosis, can also simulate tuberculosis. In pigmented villonodular synovitis, a nodular soft tissue mass, preservation of joint space, and absence of osteoporosis are typical; in idiopathic synovial osteochondromatosis, calcified and ossified intraarticular bodies commonly are evident.

TUBERCULOUS BURSITIS AND TENOSYNOVITIS. The synovial membrane of bursae and tendon sheaths may be involved in tuberculosis (Fig. 61–21). Typical sites include the radial and ulnar bursae of the hand, the flexor tendon sheaths of the fingers, the bursae about the ischial tuberosities, and the subacromial (subdeltoid) and subgluteal bursae. Soft tissue swelling and osteoporosis eventually may be accompanied by bone destruction. Dystrophic calcification may appear.

BCG Vaccine-Induced Infection

BCG (bacille Calmette-Guérin) is a vaccine of an attenuated bovine tubercle bacillus that has been used for immunization against tuberculosis. Although complications are unusual, generalized BCG infection and bone and joint infection have been identified after vaccination. Bone and joint infection results from hematogenous spread of the BCG infection to the skeleton and has a favorable prognosis.

BCG osteomyelitis involves boys and girls between the ages of 5 months and 6 years. It usually affects the metaphyses and the epiphyses of the tubular bones, the ribs, the sternum, or the small bones of the hands and the feet. Spinal involvement is uncommon. Solitary lesions predominate and are characterized by well-defined lytic foci with only minor degrees of sclerosis or periostitis.

There is wide variation in the duration of the interval between the time of vaccination and the diagnosis of osteomyelitis. Although the diagnosis commonly is established in the first 6 or 12 months after vaccination, intervals of as long as 12 years are reported.

Atypical Mycobacterial Infection

Acid-fast bacteria that are morphologically similar to tubercle bacilli were long regarded as important in clinical medicine only because they might be mistaken for *Mycobacterium tuberculosis* (or *M. leprae*) on histologic examination. It is now recognized that many of these bacteria are pathogenic for humans. Although skin and pulmonary disease are the most recognized clinical manifestations of infection with these organisms, bone and joint alterations may also be noted. The mechanisms of the musculoskeletal alterations include hematogenous spread and contamination after injury or surgery. The atypical mycobacteria can lead to osteomyelitis, septic arthritis, tenosynovitis, and bursitis.

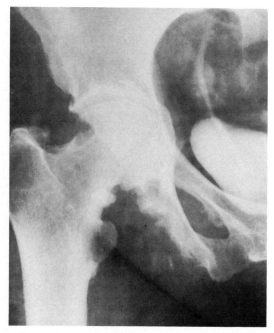

Figure 61–21. Tuberculous bursitis. Observe erosion of the ischial tuberosity with soft tissue calcification. The latter finding is typical of tuberculous bursitis. (Courtesy of J. Jimenez, M.D., Oviedo, Spain.)

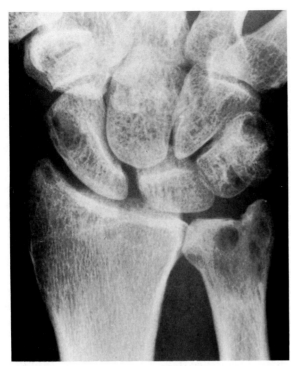

Figure 61–22. Atypical mycobacterial infection: Septic arthritis due to Mycobacterium avium. The radiograph shows cystic areas in the ulna, radius, scaphoid triquetrum, and pisiform bones. The joint spaces are preserved. (Courtesy of J. Scavulli, M.D., San Diego, California.)

Radiographically, multiple lesions predominate over solitary lesions; metaphyses and diaphyses of long bones commonly are affected; discrete lytic areas may contain sclerotic margins; osteoporosis may not be so striking as in tuberculous infection; abscesses and sinus tracts tend to develop; and articular disease can simulate tuberculosis or rheumatoid arthritis (Fig. 61–22). Information regarding specific occupational history or recreational activities is important for accurate diagnosis. For example, fishermen or aquarium workers may develop infections from *M. marinum*, as these organisms grow in fresh or salt water.

Leprosy (Hansen's Disease; Mycobacterium leprae Infection)

GENERAL FEATURES. Leprosy is an infectious disease caused by *Mycobacterium leprae*. Despite its infrequent occurrence in the United States, it is not uncommon in areas of Africa, South America, and the Orient. Leprosy is characterized by a lengthy incubation period and a chronic course with involvement of the skin, the mucous membranes, and the peripheral nervous system.

The lesions of leprosy have been divided into four principal types according to their microscopic appearance: lepromatous, tuberculoid, dimorphous, and indeterminate. The clinical manifestations vary among these types of leprosy.

CLINICAL ABNORMALITIES. It appears probable that the infection enters the body through the skin or mucous membranes. The organisms are disseminated via the blood stream and the lymphatics and localize in the skin, the nerves, and, in advanced cases, many of the viscera. The incubation period has been estimated to be 3 to 6 years. Men are affected more commonly than women, and the disease commonly is manifested prior to 20 years of age. Prodromal symptoms and

signs include malaise, fever, drowsiness, rhinitis, and profuse sweating. Lymphadenopathy is seen in all types of leprosy, although it is most striking in the lepromatous variety. Lepromatous granulation tissue may appear in and around the nerves, leading to tenderness and thickening of these structures, numbness, and tingling. Pruritus, anesthesia, or hyperesthesia may be evident. Muscle atrophy and contractions appear, and eventually extensive mutilation and secondary infection are noted.

Laboratory abnormalities may include positive results on lepromin skin test, an elevated erythrocyte sedimentation rate, and positive findings on serologic test for syphilis. The diagnosis is established by demonstration of the bacilli in typical histologic lesions.

MUSCULOSKELETAL ABNORMALITIES. The musculoskeletal abnormalities include (1) those directly related to presence of the bacilli, in which granulomatous lesions appear in the osseous tissue (direct or specific effects); and (2) those that involve the skeleton indirectly owing to neural abnormalities (indirect or nonspecific effects).

Leprous Periostitis, Osteitis, and Osteomyelitis. The reported frequency of direct involvement of the skeleton in leprosy has varied from 3 to 5 per cent among hospitalized patients. The changes usually are confined to the small bones of the face, the hands, and the feet. In these cases, osseous involvement usually results from extension of the infection from overlying dermal or mucosal areas; initially the periosteum is contaminated (leprous periostitis), and subsequently the cortex, spongiosa, and marrow (leprous osteitis and osteomyelitis) become involved. Less commonly, widespread

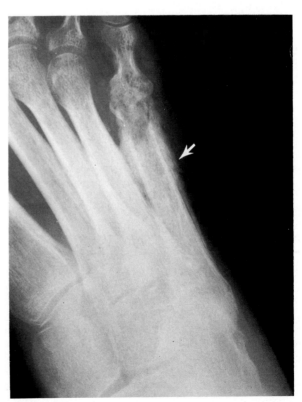

Figure 61–23. Leprous osteomyelitis and septic arthritis. Note destruction of the metatarsal bone with exuberant periostitis (arrow). The fifth metatarsophalangeal joint is obliterated. The soft tissues are abnormal as a result of adjacent infection.

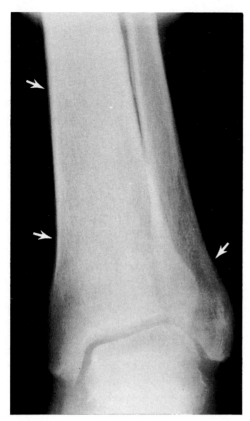

Figure 61–24. Leprous periostitis: "Red leg." A radiograph reveal periostitis of the tiba and fibula (arrows). The opposite side was affected similarly.

hematogenous spread of infection to the bone can occur. Pathologically, intraosseous lesions are characterized by granulomatous tissue reactions that lead to trabecular destruction.

In the face, nasal and maxillary destruction is most characteristic. In the hands and the feet, soft tissue swelling, osteoporosis, endosteal thinning, enlargement of the nutrient foramina, and osseous destruction with a cystic or honeycombed appearance are evident (Fig. 61–23). Pathologic fractures and epiphyseal collapse may appear.

Symmetric periostitis of the tibia, the fibula, and the distal portion of the ulna may be noted (Fig. 61–24), related to subperiosteal infiltration with *Mycobacterium leprae*. The constellation of erythematous skin lesions, pain, and periostitis involving the lower extremity has been called "red leg."

Leprous Arthritis. Specific leprous arthritis is rare. Joint involvement results from intraarticular extension of an osseous or periarticular infective focus or, less commonly, from hematogenous contamination of the synovial membrane.

Neuropathic Musculoskeletal Lesions. The skeletal abnormalities occurring on a neurologic basis are much more frequent and severe than those produced by direct leprous infiltration of the bone, being evident in 20 to 70 per cent of hospitalized patients. They result from sensory or motor nerve impairment, or both. Repeated injuries and secondary infections subsequently lead to considerable osseous and articular destruction. The bones of the hands and the feet are especially susceptible to this form of leprosy, and findings

include absorption of cancellous bone and the development of concentric bone atrophy. The result is a tapered appearance to the end of the bone, termed the "licked candy stick" (Fig. 61–25). In the foot, progressive resorption of the metatarsals and proximal phalanges occurs. In the hand and the foot, distal phalangeal resorption also is encountered. Furthermore, tarsal disintegration is not infrequent (Fig. 61–26). In extreme cases, dissolution of the midfoot results, and the tibia is driven downward, becoming weight-bearing.

The histologic characteristics of involved joints in leprous patients with neurologic deficit are similar to those in other neuroarthropathies. The radiographic appearance of neuroarthropathy in leprosy resembles that in syphilis, diabetes mellitus, congenital insensitivity to pain, and syringomyelia.

Secondary Infection. Ulceration followed by secondary infection and pyogenic osteomyelitis is common in the anesthetic feet of patients with leprosy. Septic arthritis also is seen.

Vascular Lesions. The frequency, nature, and importance of vascular lesions in leprosy are debated. It has been suggested that bone resorption occurs because of interference with the mechanism controlling vasoregulation owing to involvement of the nerves in the vascular reflex arch.

Soft Tissue Calcification. Rarely, linear calcification of involved nerves can be seen on radiographs (Fig. 61–27).

Soft Tissue Neoplasm. As in chronic osteomyelitis with soft tissue sinuses, leprosy with cutaneous ulcerations may be complicated by the development of secondary neoplasia, specifically squamous cell carcinoma in the skin.

Spirochetes and Related Organisms
Syphilis

GENERAL FEATURES. Syphilis is a chronic systemic infectious disease caused by *Treponema pallidum*. It is transmitted by intimate contact with moist infectious lesions of

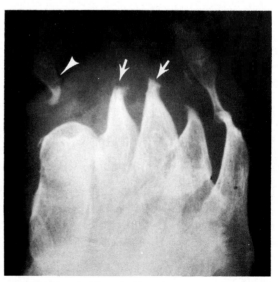

Figure 61–25. Leprosy: Neuropathic lesions. An example of concentric bone atrophy in the foot illustrates the tapered osseous surfaces (arrows) with isolation of distal bone fragments (arrowhead).

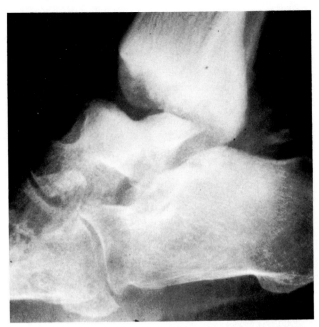

Figure 61–26. Leprosy. Neuropathic lesions. Fragmentation and collapse of the talar, tibial, and calcaneal surfaces can be seen. The appearance is similar to that in tabes dorsalis.

the skin and mucous membranes. Thus, infection is spread during sexual contact, although less commonly the disease may be contracted during biting or kissing. The appearance of the disorder traceable to these mechanisms is termed *acquired syphilis*. In addition, the fetus may be infected by transmission of the organism through the placenta; this is termed *congenital syphilis*. Once the spirochete has violated the epithelium, it enters lymphatics and reaches the regional

lymph nodes in a period of hours. Subsequently, the treponema may enter the blood stream, leading to dissemination of infection throughout the body.

Approximately 3 to 6 weeks after the organism has entered the body, a primary ulcerating lesion, the *chancre*, develops at the site of inoculation. About 6 weeks later, a generalized skin eruption known as *secondary syphilis* develops. After healing of both primary and secondary manifestations, the patient may be without symptoms for a protracted period of time, a stage termed *latent syphilis*. Cardiovascular syphilis or neurosyphilis may become manifest 10 to 30 years later, although approximately 50 per cent of affected persons never develop tertiary manifestations of syphilis. In those patients with significant later alterations, large destructive lesions or *gummas* can be evident in almost any organ of the body, particularly the skin and the bones.

CONGENITAL SYPHILIS

Frequency and Pathogenesis. Although earlier studies indicated that congenital syphilis might occur in 2 to 5 per cent of infants, modern techniques designed to improve the recognition of this disease in pregnant women have led to an impressive reduction in the number of cases of congenital syphilis. The disorder originates from transplacental migration of the treponema and invasion of the perichondrium, periosteum, cartilage, bone marrow, and sites of active endochondral ossification. The spirochetes inhibit osteogenesis and lead to degeneration of osteoblasts.

The infected fetus may be aborted or die shortly after birth. Early and late lesions may be identified in those infants who survive. In children, the hutchinsonian triad, consisting of Hutchinson's teeth, interstitial keratitis, and nerve deafness, may appear. Additional manifestations include fissuring about the mouth and anus (rhagades), anterior bowing of the lower leg (saber shin), collapse of the nasal bones (saddle nose), and perforation of the palate.

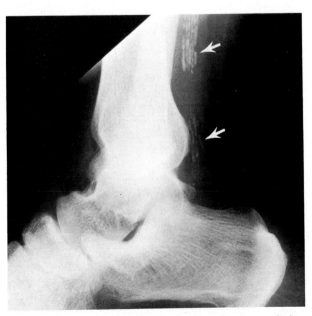

Figure 61–27. Leprosy: Calcification of nerves. The linear radiodense regions (arrows) represent calcification of nerves. This finding, although rare, is suggestive of the diagnosis of leprosy but must be distinguished from vascular calcification. (Courtesy of M. Dalinka, M.D., Philadelphia, Pennsylvania.)

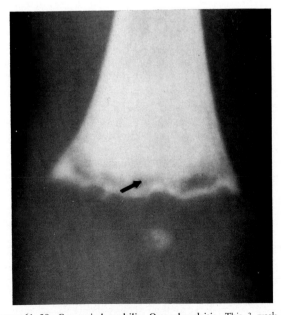

Figure 61–28. Congenital syphilis: Osteochondritis. This 3 week old infant reveals a lucent band in the metaphysis (arrow) owing to a disturbance in endochondral ossification. The appearance is similar to that in leukemia or neuroblastoma.

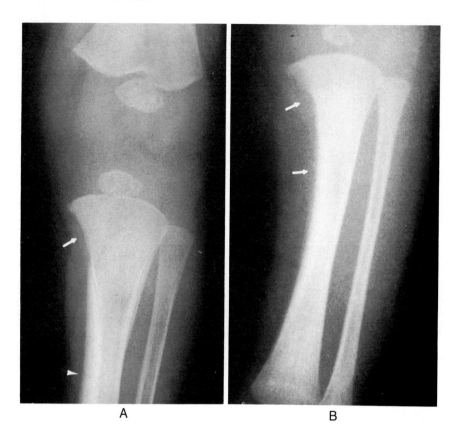

Figure 61–29. Congenital syphilis: Osteochondritis and osteomyelitis. In two different infants, the tibial alterations are well shown. Initially (A), defects in the medial tibial metaphysis (arrow) are characteristic, frequently associated with periostitis (arrowhead). Subsequently (B), the degree of osseous destruction may be more exaggerated (arrows). The predilection for the medial tibial metaphysis is noteworthy.

A   B

Early Osseous Lesions. In the fetus, the neonate, and the very young infant, bone abnormalities include (1) osteochondritis; (2) diaphyseal osteomyelitis (osteitis); and (3) periostitis.

Syphilitic osteochondritis usually results in symmetric involvement of sites of endochondral ossification. The epiphyseal-metaphyseal junction of tubular bones, the costochondral regions, and, in severe cases, the flat and short tubular bones and the centers of ossification of the sternum and vertebrae are affected. In the growing metaphyses of the long bones, widening of the provisional calcification zone, serrations, and adjacent osseous irregularity are seen. Radiographs (Fig. 61–28) outline broad horizontal radiolucent bands reminiscent of those that are identified in leukemia or metastasis from neuroblastoma.

If the process continues, metaphyseal irregularities appear (Fig. 61–29), presumably induced by the toxic effects of degenerating spirochetes. The medial surface of the proximal tibial shaft is a particularly characteristic site of erosion, a finding that is termed Wimberger's sign. Epiphyseal separation can result from the metaphyseal destruction.

The lesions of osteochondritis generally heal quickly with specific therapy. Growth retardation and osseous deformity are unusual.

Diaphyseal osteomyelitis (osteitis) can appear in infants with congenital syphilis who have not received therapy or in whom treatment has been inadequate or inappropriate. Osteolytic lesions with surrounding bone eburnation and overlying periostitis can be encountered on radiographs of involved tubular bones (Fig. 61–29).

Periostitis is a less frequent manifestation of congenital syphilis than is osteochondritis. It may relate to periosteal infiltration by syphilitic granulation tissue (Fig. 61–29).

Late Osseous Lesions. The early manifestations of congenital syphilis generally regress in the first few years of life, even in the absence of adequate therapy. Exacerbation of disease may appear in the young child or adolescent, however. Although the evolving skeletal lesions occurring late in the course of congenital syphilis may rarely resemble those of early congenital syphilis, they more typically resemble the changes observed in acquired syphilis (see later discussion). Osteomyelitis and periostitis in late congenital syphilis can involve the tubular bones, the flat bones, and even the cranium.

Gummatous or nongummatous osteomyelitis or periostitis results in diffuse hyperostosis of the involved bone. In the tibia, a typical saber shin may be encountered, with anterior bending of the bone. Its radiographic appearance may resemble that of Paget's disease, although the syphilitic hyperostosis may not extend to the epiphysis (Fig. 61–30).

Abnormalities of the skull and mandible include destruction of the nasal bones, calvarial gumma, and Hutchinson's teeth, characterized by peg-shaped, notched, and hypoplastic dental structures. In older syphilitic children, bilateral painless effusions, especially of the knee, have been termed Clutton's joints.

ACQUIRED SYPHILIS

Frequency. The frequency of osseous lesions in acquired syphilis has decreased dramatically owing to improvement in diagnosis and treatment of this disease. When present, the bone and joint manifestations usually appear in the latent or tertiary phase of syphilis.

Early Acquired Syphilis. A spirochetemia appearing 1 to 3 months after the documentation of a primary lesion can lead to dissemination of organisms throughout the body. A proliferative periostitis is the most common osseous lesion in

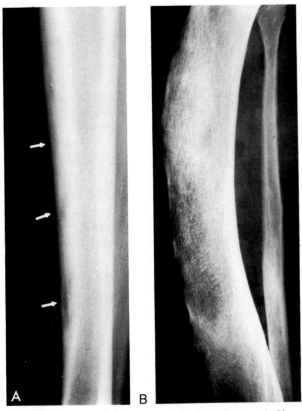

Figure 61–30. Congential syphilis: Late osseous changes. A Observe radiolucent foci within the anterior cortex of the tibia (arrows) with periostitis and endosteal proliferation. B A typical saber shin deformity of the tibia is associated with anterior bowing of the bone. The fibula also is involved.

early acquired syphilis. It may be especially prominent in the tibia, the skull, the ribs, and the sternum. New bone formation can become extensive, leading to considerable thickening of the cortex and simulating the appearance of an osteosarcoma. Bilateral tibial or clavicular periostitis in the adult frequently is syphilitic in origin.

Destructive bone lesions, which relate to osteomyelitis and infective osteitis, occur much less commonly than periostitis in early syphilis. Involvement of the skull is particularly characteristic (Fig. 61–31). At this site, irregular areas of bone lysis are observed with a moth-eaten or permeative pattern of destruction and periostitis. Nasal bone destruction also may be evident. In the long tubular bones, osteolytic foci, cortical sequestration, periostitis, and epiphyseal separation can be noted (Fig. 61–31).

Late Acquired Syphilis. Osseous lesions occurring during the later stages of acquired syphilis can be related to gummatous or nongummatous inflammation. A gumma represents an area of variable size containing caseous necrotic material. These areas of necrosis generally are related to the effects of the toxic products of spirochetal degeneration, although the organisms themselves usually are not demonstrable within the lesions. Resorption of cortical bone owing to the inflammatory reaction about a gumma is frequently termed *caries sicca*. If the necrotic osseous area enlarges and becomes detached from the adjacent tissue, the term *caries necrotica* is used. The sequestered piece of cortex may become displaced into the gumma itself and may be recognized on radiographic examination. Typically, however, cortical sequestration in syphilis is limited in extent. More frequent radiographic findings of gummatous lesions are lytic and sclerotic areas of bone and

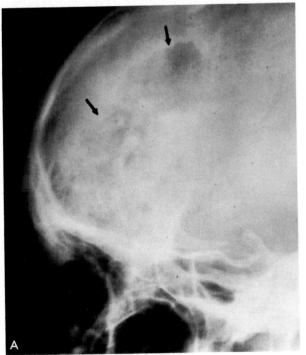

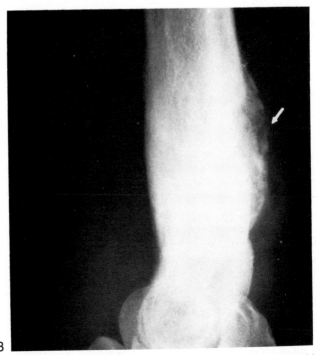

Figure 61–31. Acquired syphilis: Osteitis, osteomyelitis, and periostitis. A Lytic lesions of the frontal region of the skull (arrows) are accompanied by reactive sclerosis. B Note extreme bone proliferation of the distal portion of the humerus with soft tissue swelling (arrow) owing to a gummatous lesion.

adjacent periostitis. When large, the lesions may be associated with a pathologic fracture.

Nongummatous syphilitic periostitis, osteitis, or osteomyelitis can occur independently or in conjunction with gummas in the bone marrow. Nongummatous syphilitic osteomyelitis usually is limited in extent and is associated with infiltration of the marrow spaces with vascular and cellular connective tissue. Radiographs reveal destructive and productive bone changes associated with periostitis. Differentiation of these findings from those associated with gummas is better left to the pathologist.

Gummatous and nongummatous skeletal lesions can be delineated in many sites. Involvement of the cranial vault, nasal bones, maxilla, mandible, tubular bones of the appendicular skeleton, spine, and pelvis has been noted. The degree of periosteal proliferation can become extreme, and the resultant radiographic and pathologic features resemble those in the late stages of congenital syphilis, including the saber shin deformity. Dactylitis, which is not infrequent in congenital syphilis, is less typical of acquired disease.

ARTICULAR INVOLVEMENT

General Abnormalities. The frequency of articular involvement in syphilis is low. Joint abnormalities may occur in either congenital or acquired forms of the disease. In congenital syphilis, articular changes predominate in the late phases of the disorder; in acquired syphilis, joint manifestations appear in the tertiary or, less frequently, the secondary stage of the disorder.

Pathogenesis. Joint disease appearing during the course of congenital or acquired syphilis can relate to a variety of mechanisms:

1. *Spread from a contiguous source of infection.* In either congenital or acquired disease, syphilitic inflammation of periarticular bone can be complicated by joint involvement.

2. *Direct involvement of the synovial membrane.* In either congenital or acquired syphilis, the luetic process can originate in the synovial or parasynovial tissues. Although the articular findings in these cases are related primarily to infection, it is frequently difficult to identify spirochetes in the synovial membrane or synovial fluid.

3. *Sympathetic effusions.* In many cases of syphilis with synovitis, organisms are not identified in the articular cavity. In some of these cases, sympathetic effusion may relate to periosteal irritation from a neighboring intraosseous focus.

4. *Neuroarthropathy.* Neurosyphilis can be associated with neuroarthropathy, with consequent fragmentation and dissolution of one or more joints of the axial and appendicular skeleton (see Chapter 69).

Radiographic and Pathologic Abnormalities. In cases of noninfectious arthralgia or arthritis, radiographic and pathologic features may be lacking. Syphilitic infectious arthritis is associated with an effusion and capsular distention. Synovial inflammation with pannus can lead to cartilaginous and osseous destruction. On radiographs, osteoporosis, joint space narrowing, bone destruction, sclerosis, and intraarticular osseous fusion can be encountered.

Yaws

Yaws represents an infectious disorder caused by *Treponema pertenue*. Yaws occurs in tropical climates and is prevalent in Africa, South America, the South Pacific islands, and the West Indies. It generally is acquired before puberty by contact with open lesions containing the spirochetes. The transmission of the disease is rarely associated with sexual contact.

Within a period of weeks after inoculation, a granulomatous primary lesion appears, referred to as mother yaw. Nontender regional adenopathy and spirochetemia occur. Approximately 1 to 3 months later, a generalized papular skin eruption occurs; after several years, late destructive lesions may become evident in the cutaneous and osseous tissues.

The tubular bones of the extremities, the pelvis, the skull, and the facial bones may become the sites of periostitis or osteitis (Fig. 61–32). Saber shin deformities, dactylitis, and nasal destruction may be encountered. Localized expansile lesions in the epiphyses of tubular bones may simulate neoplasms. Destructive changes in the fingers and toes may resemble abnormalities of leprosy or psoriatic arthritis. The radiographic changes in the skeleton in patients with yaws also are similar to those of syphilis.

Bejel

Bejel, an infectious disease caused by a spirochete, is believed to be transferred by kissing or sharing eating utensils. Its manifestations include skin ulcerations on the lips and mouth, lymphadenopathy, osteitis, and periostitis. Destruction of facial bones, including the nose, may be detected.

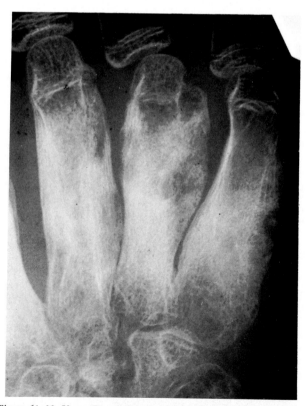

Figure 61–32. Yaws. Dactylitis is characterized by lytic lesions surrounded by florid periosteal proliferation. Note the enlarged and sclerotic osseous contours. (Courtesy of W. P. Cockshott, M.D., Hamilton, Ontario, Canada.)

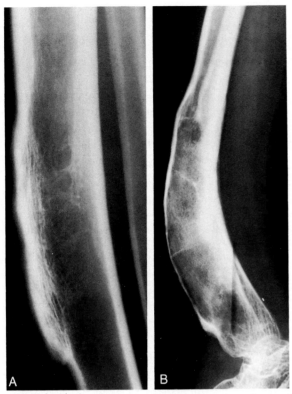

Figure 61–33. Tropical ulcer. A The anterior surface of the tibia reveals a broad-based excrescence and an ivory osteoma. The bone is bowed, and the thickened trabeculae in the medullary bone indicate a response to altered stress. **B** In a different patient, bowing of the tibia underscores the chronicity of the process. The bone is osteopenic and markedly expanded. (Courtesy of S. Bohrer, M.D., Winston-Salem, North Carolina.)

Tropical Ulcer

Tropical ulcers are seen in patients of all ages in Central and East Africa. Painful swellings appear in the lower limbs and spread rapidly. As the ulcer erodes muscles and tendons, it may reach the underlying bone. The favored target area is the middle third of the tibia; less frequent is involvement of the distal portion of the fibula. Periostitis leads to broad-based excrescences resembling osteomas (Fig. 61–33). In chronic cases, bowing deformities appear. Flexion deformities of the knee and foot deformities also are typical. In approximately 25 per cent of cases, epidermoid carcinomas of the involved skin appear. Cultures of tropical ulcers frequently isolate Vincent's types of fusiform bacilli, spirochetes, and staphylococci.

Another type of skin ulceration seen in the tropics is the Buruli ulcer, related to infection with *Mycobacterium ulcerans*.

Lyme Disease

Lyme disease, named after the town in Connecticut in which it was first described, is now recognized in approximately 15 states and in Europe and Australia. Both children and adults are affected. The illness characteristically begins in the summer in the form of a distinctive skin lesion, erythema chronicum migrans. In some cases, fatigue, chills,

fever, headache, stiff neck, and lymphadenopathy also are noted. Approximately 2 to 6 months later, a monarticular, oligoarticular, or polyarticular inflammatory process appears that is of sudden onset, of short duration, most frequent in the knees, and associated with recurrence. Radiographic characteristics of the joint involvement are soft tissue swelling and effusions.

Infrequently, a chronic arthritis develops that is associated with persistent joint swelling. In such cases, juxtaarticular osteoporosis, cartilage loss, osteophytes, and marginal bone erosions may appear (Fig. 61–34). Histologic inspection shows pannus formation similar to that in rheumatoid arthritis.

Lyme disease is transmitted by *Ixodes dammini* or related ixodid ticks and is caused by a newly recognized spirochete that spreads hematogenously to many different sites. The clinical and radiologic features of Lyme disease resemble those of juvenile chronic arthritis, Reiter's syndrome, and granulomatous infections such as tuberculosis.

FUNGAL AND HIGHER BACTERIAL INFECTION
Actinomycosis
General Features

Actinomycosis is a noncontagious suppurative infection that is caused by higher bacteria, resembling mycobacteria, that frequently are misclassified as fungi. Actinomycosis may develop in debilitated persons or in devitalized tissues. The infections are especially frequent in the face and the neck, which is probably explained by the prevalence of these organisms within the oral and nasal cavities. From infective foci in the face, lung, or bowel, hematogenous dissemination of organisms can lead to contamination of subcutaneous tissues, liver, spleen, kidneys, brain, bones, and joints.

Musculoskeletal Abnormalities

The skeleton usually becomes contaminated from an adjacent infected soft tissue focus; less commonly, hematogenous seeding of osseous or articular tissues occurs. The mandible, the flat bones of the axial skeleton, and the major joints of the appendicular skeleton are affected most commonly: Mandibular and maxillary bone involvement may follow trauma or extraction of a tooth; actinomycosis of the bones of the hands can occur after a human bite.

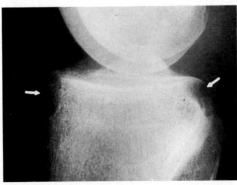

Figure 61–34. Lyme disease. Note bone erosions (arrows) in the anterior and posterior margins of the tibia. (Courtesy of J. Lawson, M.D., New Haven, Connecticut.)

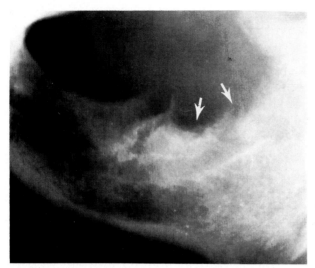

Figure 61–35. Actinomycosis. Note erosion and sclerosis of a segment of the mandible (arrows).

Osseous involvement is characterized by a combination of lysis and sclerosis (Fig. 61–35). In the ribs, the combination of severe osseous eburnation, cutaneous sinus tracts, and pleuritis is suggestive of actinomycosis. In the vertebral column, infection can originate from adjacent mediastinal or retroperitoneal foci. Several vertebrae commonly are affected, and the posterior elements often are involved. Paravertebral abscesses may appear, but they usually are smaller than those in tuberculosis and do not calcify. Additionally, collapse of the vertebrae and angulation of the spine are less frequent in actinomycosis than in tuberculosis. In the mandible and innominate bone, a mixed lytic and sclerotic response predominates.

Nocardiosis

Nocardia species are members of the aerobic actinomycetes. Introduction of organisms occurs via the respiratory tract, gastrointestinal tract, or skin after trauma. Persons with underlying chronic diseases, such as malignancy and pulmonary alveolar proteinosis, and those who are immunosup-

pressed are vulnerable to this infection. Osteomyelitis most commonly accompanies nearby skin infection or pleural disease. Hematogenous spread to bones or joints also is possible.

Cryptococcosis (Torulosis)
General Features

Cryptococcosis has a worldwide distribution and is caused by *Cryptococcus neoformans*, an organism that demonstrates unusual predilection for the central nervous system. This fungus can be recovered from the soil, pigeon droppings, fruit, and human intestinal tract and skin. The disease generally is acquired by the respiratory route through inhalation of aerosolized spores. Cryptococci subsequently can be detected in the brain, the meninges, the lungs, other viscera, and the bones and joints. Neurologic manifestations of the disease predominate, and many patients die within a few months.

The disease may be seen in association with leukemia, lymphoma, Hodgkin's disease, sarcoidosis, tuberculosis, and diabetes mellitus as well as in persons with acquired immune deficiency syndrome (AIDS) and those receiving steroid medications. Patients who have undergone renal transplantation are particularly susceptible.

Musculoskeletal Abnormalities

Osseous involvement usually is a manifestation of disseminated cryptococcosis, appearing in 5 to 10 per cent of such cases. Adults are affected far more frequently than children. The skeletal sites involved most commonly are the spine, the pelvis, the ribs, the skull, the tibia, and the knees. Bone prominences may be affected, a peculiarity that is also evident in coccidioidomycosis. Osteolytic lesions predominate, with discrete margins, mild surrounding sclerosis, and little or no periosteal reaction (Fig. 61–36). Eccentric cortical lesions, involvement of bone prominences and, in the skull, alterations of both tables, a soft tissue mass, and epidural extension are clues to correct diagnosis.

Arthritis related to cryptococcosis is quite uncommon and almost invariably is the result of intraarticular extension of organisms from an adjacent osseous focus. Rarely, extradural cryptococcal granulomas in the cervical, thoracic, or lumbar spine can lead to myelopathy or a cauda equina syndrome.

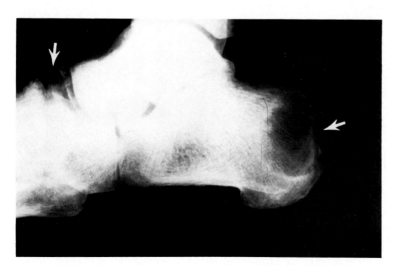

Figure 61–36. Cryptococcosis (torulosis). Discrete osteolytic foci with surrounding sclerosis are seen (arrows). The involvement of bone protuberances such as the calcaneus is not unexpected in this disease.

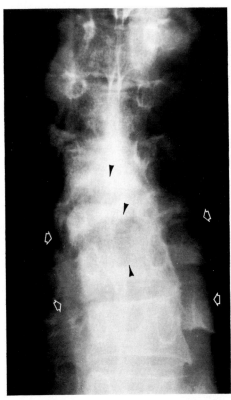

Figure 61–37. **North American blastomycosis.** Note vertebral body and intervertebral disc destruction (arrowheads) accompanied by a paravertebral mass (open arrows). (Courtesy of A. Brower, M.D., Washington, D.C.)

North American Blastomycosis

General Features

This fungal disease is produced by *Blastomyces dermatitidis.* In the United States, its frequency is highest in the Ohio and Mississippi River valleys and in the Middle Atlantic states. The skin or respiratory tract appears to be the portal of entry in some cases. Abscesses develop beneath the epidermis or in the lungs. Infection can subsequently spread to other viscera, lymph nodes, and bones. The disease predominates in persons between the ages of 20 and 50 years.

Musculoskeletal Abnormalities

Skeletal abnormalities, observed in as many as 50 per cent of patients with disseminated disease, can occur from hematogenous seeding or by direct extension from overlying cutaneous lesions; they predominate in the vertebrae, the ribs, the tibia, and the carpus and tarsus (Fig. 61–37). In the carpal and tarsal areas, cystic foci or diffuse, moth-eaten bone destruction can be seen, associated with osteoporosis and periostitis. In the tubular bones of the extremities, eccentric saucer-shaped erosions may be detected beneath cutaneous abscesses. The lesions frequently possess sclerotic margins and are surrounded by periostitis. Extension from the infected foci to soft tissues or articulations is not unusual. Draining sinuses and cortical sequestration may appear in neglected cases. In the spine, blastomycosis resembles tuberculosis; a thoracolumbar predilection, anterior vertebral erosion with extension into adjacent structures, osseous collapse, paraspinal masses, alteration of posterior elements, and intervertebral disc space destruction are common in both diseases. Rarely, blastomy-

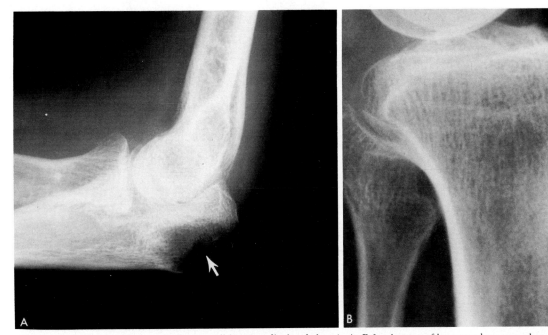

Figure 61–38. **Coccidioidomycosis: Osteomyelitis (appendicular skeleton). A, B** Involvement of bone protuberances such as the ulnar olecranon (arrow) and tibial tuberosity (arrowhead) is frequent. Discrete lesions with surrounding sclerosis are evident. (**B,** From Armbuster TG, et al: Utility of bone scanning in disseminated coccidioidomycosis: Case report. J Nucl Med *18*:450, 1977. Used with permission.)

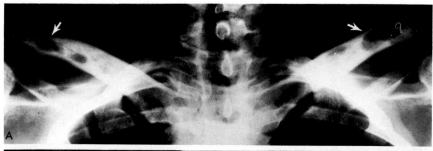

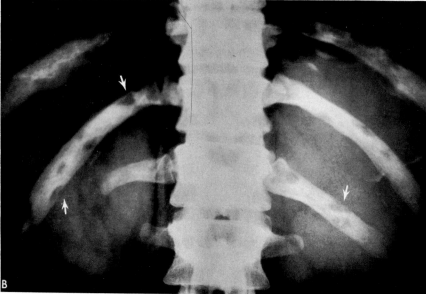

Figure 61–39. Coccidioidomycosis: Osteomyelitis (axial skeleton). Radiographs outline lytic lesions with surrounding sclerosis involving ribs and clavicles. (From Armbuster TG, et al: Utility of bone scanning in disseminated coccidioidomycosis: Case report. J Nucl Med *18*:450, 1977. Used with permission.)

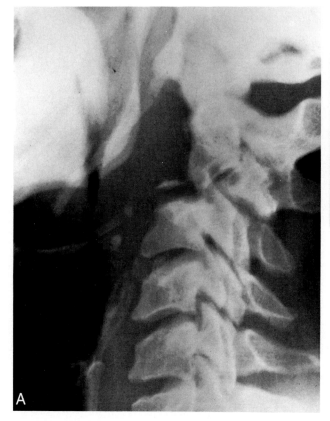

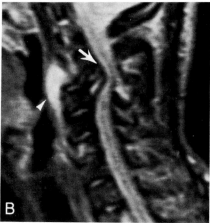

Figure 61–40. Coccidioidomycosis: Spondylitis. A In this adult patient, the third cervical vertebral body is destroyed, with only a small piece of bone evident. The axis and the remaining portions of the third cervical vertebra are displaced posteriorly with respect to the fourth cervical vertebra. A large soft tissue mass is apparent. B A T2 weighted magnetic resonance image in the sagittal plane shows extrinsic compression on the spinal cord (arrow) by the displaced bone. The high intensity signal (arrowhead) anterior to the vertebrae represents a soft tissue abscess. (Courtesy of J. Mall, M.D., San Francisco, California.)

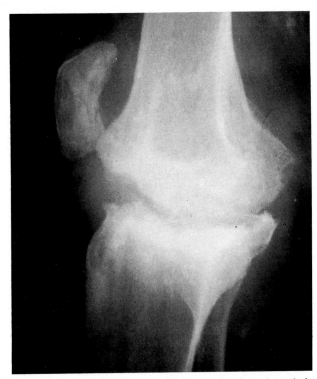

Figure 61–41. Coccidioidomycosis: Septic arthritis. Extensive articular destruction of the knee is apparent. Note the degree of reactive sclerosis and the large joint effusion.

cosis leads to dactylytis, producing findings that are reminiscent of tuberculosis.

Articular involvement usually is related to extension from an adjacent site of osteomyelitis. Rarely, however, joint destruction can occur in the absence of osseous disease. Evidence of pulmonary or cutaneous disease aids in the correct evaluation of the joint disease.

South American Blastomycosis (Paracoccidioidomycosis)

The fungal disorder termed South American blastomycosis, caused by the organism *Blastomyces (Paracoccidioides) brasiliensis*, occurs only in South America and in areas of Mexico and Central America. The infective agents invade the pharynx, presumably after inhalation, and from there spread locally or are disseminated throughout the body. Nasopharyngeal ulceration and local lymphadenopathy may antedate clinical findings in other locations. Hematogenous spread of infection to the lungs, spleen, other abdominal viscera, and bones can occur. In general, the features of musculoskeletal involvement are similar to those in North American blastomycosis.

Coccidioidomycosis
General Features

Coccidioidomycosis results from inhalation of the fungus *Coccidioides immitis* in endemic areas of the Southwestern portion of the United States, in Mexico, and in some regions of South America. After being inhaled, the organisms lodge in the terminal bronchioles and alveoli of the lungs where an inflammatory reaction may ensue. In some persons, disseminated disease may develop, with spread of infection to the

liver, spleen, lymph nodes, skin, kidney, meninges, pericardium, and bones. Men and women are affected equally, although the disseminated form is more common in men. Blacks are especially susceptible. Clinical manifestations vary in accordance with the distribution of the lesions, and in cases of wide dissemination, the mortality rate is high.

Musculoskeletal Abnormalities

Although an acute, self-limited arthritis ("desert rheumatism") may develop in 33 per cent of cases of coccidioidomycosis, only 10 to 20 per cent of patients develop granulomatous lesions in the bones and the joints. In most cases, bone alterations relate to hematogenous spread, although cutaneous infection can lead to contamination of subjacent bones. Involvement of the spine, the ribs, and the pelvis predominates. Symptoms and signs can be prominent.

Radiographs frequently reveal multiple osseous lesions in the metaphyses of long tubular bones and in bone prominences (patella, tibial tuberosity, calcaneus, ulnar olecranon) (Fig. 61–38). Well-demarcated lytic foci of the spongiosa are typical. Periostitis can be seen, but bone sclerosis and sequestration are unusual. Lesions involving the ribs can be associated with prominent extrapleural masses (Fig. 61–39). Abnormalities of one or more vertebral bodies with paraspinal masses and contiguous rib changes are typical. There is relative sparing of the intervertebral discs, and vertebral collapse is uncommon (Fig. 61–40).

Joint involvement is most common in the ankle and the knee (Fig. 61–41). In general, articular changes result from extension of an osteomyelitic focus, although, rarely, direct hematogenous implantation of the organisms into a joint can occur. Radiographic findings (osteoporosis, effusion, joint

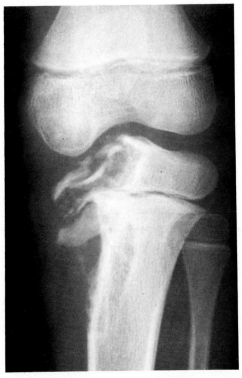

Figure 61–42. Histoplasma capsulatum var. duboisii osteomyelitis. Extensive lesions of the tibial epiphysis and metaphysis have produced collapse of the articular surface, with sclerosis and mild periostitis. The extension across the growth cartilage is not unusual in fungal infections.

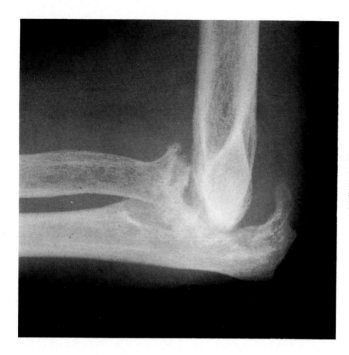

Figure 61–43. Sporotrichosis: Septic arthritis. An example of elbow involvement. Note soft tissue swelling, joint space loss, and irregularity and poor definition of subchondral bone, with large osseous erosions. The changes are identical to those in other forms of septic arthritis. (Courtesy of A. Brower, M.D., Washington, D.C.)

space narrowing, bone destruction) are similar to those in other granulomatous articular infections. Coccidioidal bursitis and tenosynovitis of the hand and wrist also have been reported.

Biopsy of skeletal or articular foci in this disease reveals granulomatous lesions similar to those of tuberculosis.

Histoplasmosis
General Features

Histoplasmosis is caused by the dimorphic fungus *Histoplasma capsulatum*, which is present in many areas of the United States, particularly the Mississippi River Valley region. A similar organism, *Histoplasma capsulatum* var. *duboisii*, can also lead to disease, especially in Africa. The disorder results from exposure to soil containing the spores of this fungus. The portal of entry usually is the respiratory tract. Diffuse disease can result, and the fungus proliferates most extensively in cells of the reticuloendothelial system. Involvement of the brain, lymph nodes, spleen, adrenal gland, lung, bowel, and bone marrow is most typical.

Musculoskeletal Abnormalities

Skeletal involvement may occur in association with *H. capsulatum* or, more frequently, *H. duboisii* infection. In histoplasmosis due to *H. capsulatum*, the pelvis, the skull, the ribs, and the small tubular bones most typically are affected. Joint alterations have also been noted, leading to clinical, radiologic, and pathologic findings similar to those of sarcoidosis and tuberculosis.

In histoplasmosis due to *H. duboisii*, granulomatous ulcerating and papular lesions of the skin can be associated with osseous and articular changes in as many as 80 per cent of patients. Multiple bone foci predominate in the flat bones, although the spine and tubular bones can also be affected (Fig. 61–42).

Sporotrichosis
General Features

Sporotrichosis is caused by *Sporothrix schenckii* and is characterized by suppurating nodular lesions of the skin and the subcutaneous tissues. The fungus resides on vegetation and can invade the human body through a wound of the skin; the disease is not uncommon after cutaneous puncture with thorns and is a recognized occupational hazard of florists and farmers. Human disease has also resulted from animal contact. After inoculation, a painless, ulcerating cutaneous lesion develops, and the organisms spread locally. Rarely, disseminated disease can evolve, perhaps by a gastrointestinal or respiratory portal of entry; bone and joint changes may appear in 80 per cent of such cases, and death can occur rapidly.

Musculoskeletal Abnormalities

Osseous and articular involvement can occur from hematogenous dissemination of infection or from extension of a contaminated cutaneous or subcutaneous focus. Joint abnormalities predominate in the knee, the wrist and hand, the ankle, the elbow, and the metacarpophalangeal joints. Soft tissue swelling, effusion, joint space loss, and destruction of subchondral bone margins are seen (Fig. 61–43). Synovial biopsy reveals granulomatous inflammation. Tendon and tendon sheath involvement has been recorded.

Bone changes may take several forms. Eccentric erosions beneath subcutaneous lesions can be encountered but are more typical of blastomycosis. Conversely, single or multiple lytic areas in bone can appear. The tibia, fibula, femur, humerus, and short tubular bones of the hand and foot are involved most commonly. Osteolysis predominates and periostitis usually is absent.

The radiographic features of osseous and articular involvement in sporotrichosis simulate those of tuberculosis, other

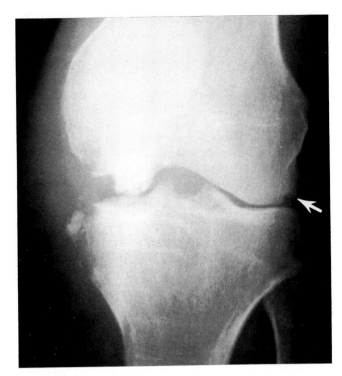

Figure 61–44. Candidiasis: Septic arthritis. Observe massive soft tissue swelling, marginal osseous erosions (arrow), bone collapse and fragmentation, and joint space narrowing.

fungal disorders, or pigmented villonodular synovitis. Involvement of the small joints of the hands and feet appears to be more characteristic of this fungal disease than of the others.

Candidiasis (Moniliasis)
General Features

Of the various Candida species, *Candida albicans* is associated most commonly with human disease. Candida organisms normally reside on the mucous membranes. Abnormal proliferation on these membranes is especially characteristic in debilitated children or adults, in patients receiving broad-spectrum antibiotics, in those with diabetes mellitus, and in patients with intravenous or Foley catheters. Rarely, a widespread infection can occur.

Musculoskeletal Abnormalities

Bone involvement in cases of disseminated candidiasis is relatively rare. Such involvement can result from direct hematogenous seeding of the bone, hematogenous involvement of a joint with spread to the periarticular bone, or extension from an overlying soft tissue abscess. Infants, children, or adults can be affected. Osteomyelitis in any age group can occur in one or more sites, including the tubular bones of the extremities; the flat bones, such as the pelvis, sternum, and scapula; the ribs; and the spine.

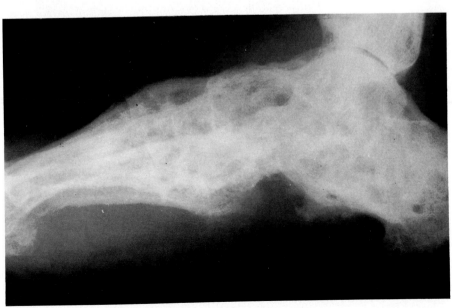

Figure 61–45. Maduromycosis: Madura foot. A lateral radiograph delineates the osseous and articular effects of chronic involvement of the foot. Bone destruction and widespread intraarticular osseous fusion can be noted.

Septic arthritis also is observed in candidiasis. As in the case of Candida osteomyelitis, debilitation and underlying disorders are frequent in Candida arthritis. Typically, infection predominates in large weight-bearing joints; the knee is the most common site of involvement. The pathogenesis of articular infection can relate to hematogenous contamination of the synovium or extension from an adjacent infected osseous or soft tissue structure. Radiographic findings include soft tissue swelling, joint space narrowing, irregularity of subchondral bone, and more widespread changes of osteomyelitis (Fig. 61–44). The diagnosis is confirmed by aspiration of synovial fluid or biopsy of synovial membrane with isolation of Candida.

Mucormycosis

Mucormycosis is a rare, serious, and commonly fatal infection caused by several types of fungus in the class Phycomycetes. It appears in association with debilitating illnesses, as well as after massive corticosteroid therapy. The usual portal of entry of the fungus appears to be the paranasal sinuses, from which site infection can reach the retroorbital tissues and cerebrum. In the brain, arterial and venous thrombosis leads to multiple infarcts, and hematogenous spread of mucormycosis produces infective foci, especially in the lungs and intestines. The clinical varieties of mucormycosis are frequently termed rhinocerebral, pulmonary, alimentary, or disseminated.

Osseous abnormalities generally are confined to the skull and the face. Sinusitis can be complicated by destruction of the adjacent bone walls. Although localized osteolysis predominates, more extensive dissolution of some of the facial structures may ensue. The differential diagnosis includes other varieties of osteomyelitis and neoplasm.

Aspergillosis

Aspergillus normally is a harmless inhabitant of the upper respiratory tract. Uncommonly, in patients with low resistance or in those who have received an overwhelming inoculum, a chronic localized pulmonary infection may result. Spinal involvement can rarely be evident, generally owing to contiguous spread from a pulmonary focus. The radiographic features resemble those of tuberculosis. Similarly, extension of infection into the orbital bones and ribs also can be encountered. Rarely, the tubular bones of the extremities are affected.

Maduromycosis (Mycetoma)

Maduromycosis, a chronic granulomatous fungal disease, affects the feet (Madura foot). It may be observed throughout the world but is especially prevalent in India. In the United States, a variety of organisms can cause Madura foot. The infection results from posttraumatic soft tissue invasion of organisms that are normal inhabitants of soil. The organisms then may penetrate the underlying muscles, tendons, bones, and joints. Sinus tracts arising from the infected osseous tissues are common. The course of maduromycosis usually is progressive.

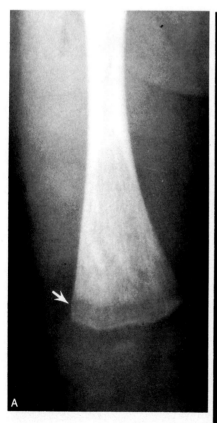
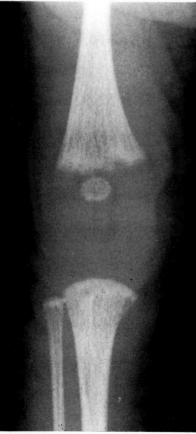

Figure 61–46. Intrauterine rubella infection. A A radiolucent metaphyseal band (arrow) in the distal femur of this infant is associated with relative sclerosis of the diaphysis. B In a different infant, longitudinal striations have produced the characteristic "celery stalk" appearance. Periostitis is absent.

The radiographic findings vary with the virulence of the invading organism. In some cases, single or multiple localized osseous defects are evident; in others, extensive soft tissue and bone disruption occurs, with associated periostitis and sclerosis. Intraarticular osseous fusion may appear (Fig. 61–45), leading to an appearance that is termed "melting snow."

VIRAL INFECTION
Rubella Infection (German Measles)

Rubella is a contagious disease of viral origin. Although it generally is a benign disorder in the adult, maternal infection in the first half of pregnancy can lead to serious skeletal and nonskeletal alterations in the fetus.

Postnatal Rubella Infection

In the adult patient, rubella arthritis may occur within a few days of the skin rash. Articular findings are most common in the small joints of the hands and wrists, the knees, and the ankles. After live, attenuated rubella virus became available for active immunization, episodes of acute arthritis also were noted in children injected with the virus. Recovery of the wild or attenuated rubella virus has been accomplished from the synovial fluid after natural rubella infection or vaccination, respectively.

A chronic arthropathy has also been associated with rubella vaccination. In this arthropathy radiography may document the presence of nonspecific destructive and reactive changes. The fact that the arthropathy resembles juvenile chronic arthritis is of interest, as reports have indicated that rubella antibody levels are elevated not only in rubella vaccine arthritis but also in a significant proportion of persons with juvenile chronic arthritis.

Intrauterine Rubella Infection

Radiographically evident osseous lesions attributable to intrauterine rubella infection consist of metaphyseal lesions in long bones characterized by the presence of symmetry, linear areas of radiolucency, and increased bone density, producing a longitudinally oriented striated pattern (celery stalk appearance), and the absence of periostitis (Fig. 61–46). With healing, beak-like exostoses can be noted at the metaphyses. Although positive cultures for rubella can be obtained from the bone marrow, histologic evidence of osteomyelitis generally is lacking. Indeed, it is generally believed that the metaphyseal and diaphyseal lesions of rubella are related to alterations in bone formation.

These osseous alterations, which may occur in as many as 45 per cent of cases of intrauterine rubella, can simulate those that are noted in other viral disorders (see discussion later in this chapter). They usually are transient in nature, disappearing after several weeks.

Cytomegalic Inclusion Disease

Intrauterine infection related to cytomegalic inclusion disease can lead to intracranial calcifications and rubella-like abnormalities of the skeleton (Fig. 61–47). Metaphyseal osteopenia, irregularity of the growth plate, and a striated pattern parallel to the long axis of the bone (characterized by alternating lucent and sclerotic bands) are noted. Spontaneous pathologic fractures have also been observed in infants with cytomegalic inclusion disease. The metaphyseal changes usually are evident in the first few days of life and then disappear completely within a period of days to weeks. They generally are attributed to a disturbance in endochondral bone formation, and these changes can be confused with findings of intrauterine rubella, erythroblastosis fetalis, congenital syphilis, and hypophosphatasia.

Varicella (Chickenpox)

Varicella is a common benign disorder, usually evident in children, in which skeletal alterations are rarely encountered.

Herpes Zoster

Herpes zoster, related to reactivation of latent varicella-zoster virus, is associated with nerve involvement. Although disease dissemination is observed occasionally, musculoskeletal manifestations are rarely reported.

Herpes Simplex

Herpes simplex virus types 1 and 2 can cause a variety of clinical syndromes. Infants can acquire the infection at birth, owing to the presence of the virus in the mother's cervix. Nonspecific skeletal abnormalities of the metaphyseal regions of tubular bones, similar to those seen in other congenital viruses, are observed.

Mumps

Arthritis is a well-recognized manifestation of mumps. This complication usually is seen in young adult men, approximately 10 to 14 days after the parotitis. A migratory polyarthritis affects predominantly the large joints.

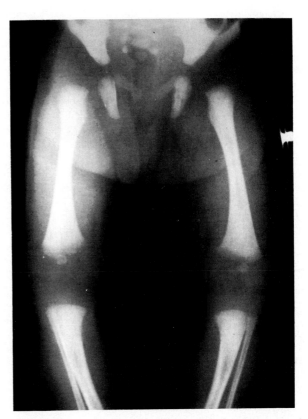

Figure 61–47. Cytomegalic inclusion disease. Metaphyseal changes consist of irregularity of the growth plate and osseous fragmentation, most evident in the distal femora. (Courtesy of F. N. Silverman, M.D., Palo Alto, California.)

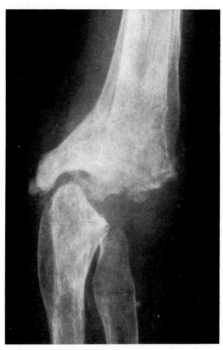

Figure 61–48. Variola osteomyelitis and septic arthritis: Elbow involvement. Note irregularity of the articular surfaces, osteolysis, and periostitis. (Courtesy of W. P. Cockshott, M.D., Hamilton, Ontario, Canada.)

Variola (Smallpox)

Osteomyelitis and septic arthritis are well-known complications of smallpox. Infection may originate in the bone, in the joint, or in both; most typically, osseous and articular changes occur together. Symmetric involvement is frequent, and articular infection reveals an unusual affinity for the elbow (80 per cent of patients).

Three types of bone and joint lesions have been described:

1. A nonsuppurative osteomyelitis, probably attributable to the smallpox virus itself, commonly involves the diaphyses of long tubular bones, leading to epiphyseal contamination, with destruction and deformity.

2. A suppurative arthritis related to contamination of the joint is probably the result of secondary infection of a pustule.

3. A nonsuppurative arthritis may appear 1 to 4 weeks after the initial infection. It may be followed by secondary infection of the joint and articular deformities.

During the acute stage of osteomyelitis variolosa, findings simulate those of pyogenic osteomyelitis. Juxtametaphyseal destruction, epiphyseal extension, periostitis, involucrum formation, and articular contamination are seen. The elbow (Fig. 61–48), the glenohumeral joint, the knee, the hip, and the small joints of the hand, wrist and foot can be altered. During the later stages of the disease, osseous destruction with or without loose bodies, bone or fibrous ankylosis, subluxation, growth retardation, and secondary osteoarthritis can be encountered.

Although radiographic characteristics of osseous and articular involvement in smallpox simulate those of pyogenic infection, certain differences can be seen. Symmetric changes, epiphyseal extension and destruction, predilection for the elbow, extensive osteoperiostitis of diaphyses of tubular bones, and peculiar deformities suggest the diagnosis of osteomyelitis variolosa.

Vaccinia

A viremia may occur after vaccination for smallpox, but osseous and articular complications are indeed unusual. With bone involvement, periostitis and hyperostosis coupled with soft tissue swelling or nodules can lead to an erroneous radiographic diagnosis of infantile cortical hyperostosis (Caffey's disease). In some instances of vaccinia, bone lysis and involucrum formation are consistent with the radiographic findings of osteomyelitis, whereas in others, metaphyseal irregularity may represent a virus-related growth disturbance.

PROTOZOAN INFECTION

Toxoplasmosis

Toxoplasmosis is an infectious disorder caused by an intracellular protozoan parasite, *Toxoplasma gondii*. Human infections with Toxoplasma may be either congenital or acquired. In the congenital variety of toxoplasmosis, an infant may be stillborn at term or be born prematurely with active infection characterized by fever, rash, hepatosplenomegaly, mental retardation, chorioretinitis, and convulsions. Osseous lesions are unusual, although metaphyseal alterations in tubular bones may simulate those of rubella, cytomegalic inclusion disease, or syphilis. Cerebral calcification may be evident.

The acquired variety of the disease can occur at any age and may display rash, lymphadenopathy, ocular changes, myositis, and widespread vascular alterations. Periarticular swelling and tenosynovitis also can be apparent.

INFECTION PRODUCED BY WORMS (HELMINTHS) (TABLE 61–3)

Hookworm Disease

Hookworm disease is produced by *Ancylostoma duodenale* or *Necator americanus*. Anemia and its complications are the major clinical manifestations of this disorder. Musculoskeletal abnormalities are indeed rare; they include joint swelling and osteolytic bone lesions.

Loiasis

Loiasis is prevalent in West and Central Africa and is produced by the filaria *Loa loa* (African eye worm). Infective larvae are deposited in the victim's skin by the bite of the mango fly. The larvae burrow into the deeper subcutaneous tissue, where they mature to adult worms over a period of 6 months or longer. Localized areas of allergic inflammation in the subcutaneous tissue, particularly in the forearm, produce Calabar swellings, named after the Nigerian town in which the disease is rampant. The dead worms cause abscesses or undergo calcification, or both (Fig. 61–49) (Table 61–4).

Onchocerciasis

Onchocerciasis is a form of filariasis produced by *Onchocerca volvulus* and transmitted by flies. It is prevalent in Africa and Central and South America. Soft tissue calcifications, similar to those in loiasis, may be detected.

Filariasis

Filariasis is produced by the adult worms of the species *Wuchereria bancrofti* or *Brugia malayi*, which locate in the

Table 61–3. MAJOR HELMINTHIC INFECTIONS OF HUMANS

Nematodes (Roundworms)		Trematodes (Flatworms)		Cestodes (Tapeworms)	
Intestinal	*Tissue*	*Tissue*	*Intravascular*	*Pathogenic Form: Adult*	*Pathogenic Form: Larva*
Ancylostoma duodenale	Wuchereria bancrofti	Clonorchis sinensis	Schistosoma mansoni	Diphyllobothrium latum	Echinococcus granulosus
Necator americanus	Brugia malayi	Fasciola hepatica	Schistosoma japonicum	Taenia saginata	Echinococcus multilocularis
Ascaris lumbricoides	Onchocerca volvulus	Fasciolopsis buski	Schistosoma haematobium	Taenia solium	Taenia solium
Enterobius vermicularis	Loa loa	Paragonimus westermani		Hymenolepis nana	Hymenolepis nana
Trichuris trichiura	Trichinella spiralis				
	Toxocara canis				
	Dracunculus medinensis				

From Korzeniowski OM: Diseases due to helminths. *In* JH Stein (Ed): Internal Medicine. Boston, Little, Brown, 1983, p 1455. Used with permission.

lymphatic and soft tissues of the human body. The disease is predominant in tropical areas of Asia, Africa, South America, Australia, and the South Pacific islands. Filariasis can lead to massive lymphedema or elephantiasis, especially of the legs and the scrotum. Radiographs show an affected limb to be greatly enlarged, with soft tissue thickening, blurring of subcutaneous fat planes, and a linear striated pattern. Soft tissue calcification also has been noted. The calcifications are smaller than those in loiasis and occur predominantly in the lymphatic channels of the scrotum, thighs, and legs (Table 61–4).

Dracunculiasis (Guinea Worm Disease)

The guinea worm, *Dracunculus medinensis*, may cause human disease, particularly in parts of Africa, the Middle East, South America, India, and Pakistan. The disorder is contracted when the larvae in contaminated water are ingested by a water flea (Cyclops) that is, in turn, swallowed in the drinking water by humans. The larvae eventually enter the circulation and mature within the human subcutaneous tissues. When the female parasites die, they may calcify, producing long, curled radiodense shadows in the lower extremities and hands (Fig. 61–50). The deposits may become fragmented because of the action of adjacent musculature. If a migratory guinea worm dies adjacent to a joint, severe cellular reaction can apparently lead to joint effusion and secondary bacterial infection.

Cysticercosis

The relationship between humans and the pork tapeworm, *Taenia solium*, is twofold: Humans are the only definitive host of the adult tapeworm, the parasite inhabiting the intestine; and humans may serve as an intermediate host (the usual intermediate host is the hog), harboring the larval stage, *Cysticercus cellulosae*. In this latter case, deposits of the larval form of the tapeworm may appear in subcutaneous and muscular tissues and in a variety of viscera. When the larvae die, a foreign body reaction may ensue, followed, over a period of years, by necrosis, caseation, and calcification.

On radiographs, linear or oval elongated calcifications appear in the soft tissues and musculature. The long axis of the calcified cysts lies in the plane of the surrounding muscle bundles (Fig. 61–51).

Echinococcosis

Echinococcosis is produced principally by the larval stage of *Echinococcus granulosus* and is most prevalent in sheep- and cattle-raising areas of North and South Africa, South America, Central Europe, Australia, and Canada; less commonly, *E. multilocularis* is the causative agent. In humans, *E. granulosus* is contracted by ingestion of the eggs, which are contained in the feces of the dog (sheep dog). After ingestion, the embryos escape from the eggs, traverse the intestinal mucosa, and are disseminated via venous and lymphatic channels. Cysts may develop in various viscera, particularly the liver and the lungs. These may calcify, producing irregular curvilinear radiodense areas.

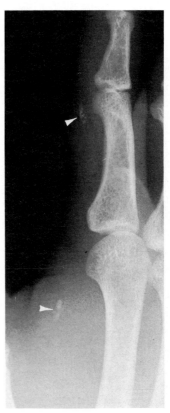

Figure 61–49. Loiasis (African eye worm disease). Soft tissue calcifications (arrowheads) are evident in the hand. (Courtesy of M. Dalinka, M.D., Philadelphia, Pennsylvania.)

Table 61–4. SOME HELMINTHS (WORMS) ASSOCIATED WITH CALCIFICATIONS

Helminth (Disease)	Frequency of Radiologic Calcification	Typical Location of Calcification	Typical Appearance of Calcification
Loa loa (loiasis)	Common	Widespread; subcutaneous tissues	Extended or coiled, linear or beaded, variable in size
Onchocerca volvulus (river blindness)	Rare	Legs, trunk, head; subcutaneous nodules	Extended or coiled, linear or beaded, small
Wuchereria bancrofti; Brugia malayi (filariasis)	Rare	Thighs, legs, scrotum; subcutaneous tissues	Straight or coiled, small
Dracunculus medinensis (guinea worm disease)	Common	Extremities	Extended or coiled, long
Taenia solium (cysticercosis)	Common	Widespread; muscular tissues	Numerous, linear or oval, variable in size, lie in plane of muscle
Echinococcus granulosus (echinococcosis)	Common	Liver, lungs, other organs	Curvilinear, cystic, eggshell
Sarcocystis lindemanni (sarcosporidiosis)	Common	Extremities; muscular and subcutaneous tissues	Numerous, linear or oval, variable in size and orientation
Armillifer armillatus, Porocephalida, Pentastomomida (porocephalosis)	Variable	Abdomen, thorax	Multiple, crescent-shaped or oval
Schistosoma haematobium (schistosomiasis)	Variable	Bladder, urinary tract	Linear, nodular

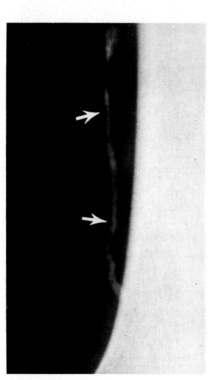

Figure 61–50. Dracunculiasis (guinea worm disease). Observe the long linear calcification (arrows) adjacent to the lower tibia owing to the presence of a dying female worm.

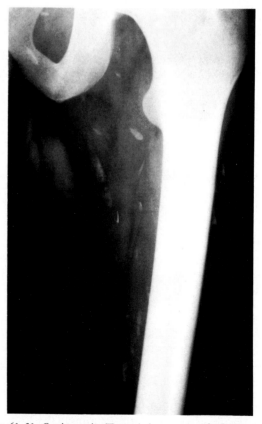

Figure 61–51. Cysticercosis. The typical appearance of soft tissue calcification in this disorder consists of elongated linear or oval dense lesions oriented in the plane of the surrounding muscle bundles.

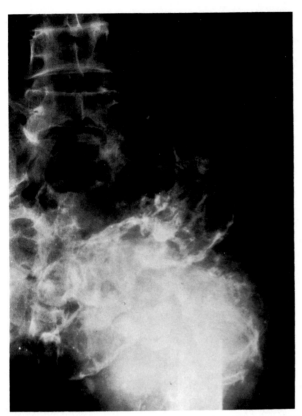

Figure 61–52. Echinococcosis. The expansile, "bubbly" lytic lesions of the pelvis, sacrum, and proximal portion of the femur are associated with deformity, osseous fragmentation, and soft tissue swelling.

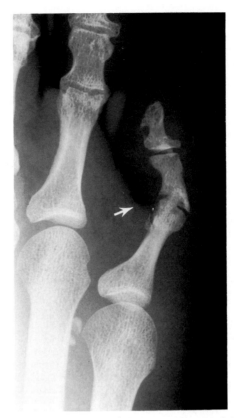

Figure 61–53. Ainhum. Note the soft tissue groove (arrow) and the osseous resorption, especially on the medial aspect of the proximal and middle phalanges of the fifth toe. Periostitis is absent.

Bone lesions are reported in 1 to 2 per cent of cases of echinococcosis. Although hematogenous seeding of the skeleton in echinococcosis can conceivably occur in any site, one bone, a few adjacent bones, or one skeletal region usually is affected; the vertebral column, the pelvis, the long bones, the thorax, and the skull are involved most commonly.

Radiographs may reveal single or multiple expansile cystic osteolytic lesions containing trabeculae (Fig. 61–52). These may be associated with cortical violation and soft tissue mass formation, with calcification. The radiographic characteristics are similar to those of fibrous dysplasia, plasmacytoma, giant cell tumor, cartilaginous neoplasms, skeletal metastases, a brown tumor of hyperparathyroidism, angiosarcoma, or a hemophilic pseudotumor.

Complications of osseous involvement in echinococcosis include pathologic fracture, secondary infection, rupture into the spinal canal with neural problems, transarticular extension, intrapelvic extension, and cranial lesions with involvement of the dura and arachnoid membranes.

ADDITIONAL DISORDERS OF POSSIBLE INFECTIOUS CAUSE
Ainhum

Ainhum (dactylolysis spontanea) is a self-limited dermatologic disorder that is characteristically found in African blacks. In West Africa, it may be seen in 2 per cent of the population. Ainhum is occasionally encountered in patients in the United States. Most typically, the fifth toe on one or both feet is affected, although other toes and even the fingers can be involved. Most patients are men in the fourth and fifth

decades of life. A deep soft tissue groove is evident initially along the medial aspect of the fifth toe and deepens and encircles the toe. Bone resorption begins on the medial aspect of the distal portion of the proximal phalanx or the middle phalanx of the fifth toe (Fig. 61–53). As more bone is resorbed, fracture and autoamputation are seen.

The cause of ainhum is not clear. Traumatic and infectious factors appear most likely.

Tietze's Syndrome

Tietze's syndrome, the costosternal syndrome, and costochondritis are terms that are used to describe pain, tenderness, and swelling at the costosternal joints. Tietze's syndrome is common, benign, and self-limited. Typically, painful swelling of one or more costosternal junctions is observed in a patient in the second to fourth decades of life.

Radiographs commonly are not revealing, although soft tissue swelling, calcification, and periostitis are encountered rarely. Increased activity may be demonstrated on bone scans. The cause is unknown.

FURTHER READING

Alexander GH, Mansuy MM: Disseminated bone tuberculosis (so-called multiple cystic tuberculosis). Radiology 55:839, 1950.

Allen JH Jr: Bone involvement with disseminated histoplasmosis. AJR 82:250, 1959.

Barre PS, Thompson GH, Morrison SC: Late skeletal deformities following meningococcal sepsis and disseminated intravascular coagulation. J Pediatr Orthop 5:584, 1985.

Beggs I: The radiology of hydatid disease. AJR 145:639, 1985.

Bertcher RW: Osteomyelitis variolosa. AJR 76:1149, 1956.

Bonakdarpour A, Zadeh YFA, Maghssoudi H, Shariat S, Levy W: Costal echinococcosis. Report of six cases and review of the literature. AJR 118:371, 1973.

Braithwaite PA, Lees RF: Vertebral hydatid disease: Radiological assessment. Radiology 140:763, 1981.

Brown JS, Middlemiss JH: Bone changes in tropical ulcer. Br J Radiol 29:213, 1956.

Chang AC, Destouet JM, Murphy WA: Musculoskeletal sporotrichosis. Skel Radiol 12:23, 1984.

Chapman M, Murray RO, Stoker DJ: Tuberculosis of the bones and joints. Semin Roentgenol 14:266, 1979.

Chilton SJ, Aftimos SF, White PR: Diffuse skeletal involvement of streptococcal osteomyelitis in a neonate. Radiology 134:390, 1980.

Comstock C, Wolson AH: Roentgenology of sporotrichosis. AJR 125:651, 1975.

Cremin BJ, Fisher RM: The lesions of congenital syphilis. Br J Radiol 43:333, 1970.

Dalinka MK, Dinnenberg S, Greendyke WH, Hopkins R: Roentgenographic features of osseous coccidioidomycosis and differential diagnosis. J Bone Joint Surg [Am] 53:1157, 1971.

de Roos A, van Meerten ELVP, Bloem JL, Bluemm RG: MRI of tuberculous spondylitis. AJR 146:79, 1986.

Duran H, Ferrandez L, Gomez-Castresana F, Lopez-Duran L, Mata P, Brandau D, Sanchez-Barba A: Osseous hydatidosis. J Bone Joint Surg [Am] 60:685, 1978.

Ehrlich I, Kricun ME: Radiographic findings in early acquired syphilis: Case report and critical review. AJR 127:789, 1976.

Enna CD, Jacobson RR, Rausch RO: Bone changes in leprosy: A correlation of clinical and radiographic features. Radiology 100:295, 1971.

Faget GH, Mayoral A: Bone changes in leprosy: A clinical and roentgenological study of 505 cases. Radiology 42:1, 1944.

Fang D, Leong JCY, Fang HSY: Tuberculosis of the upper cervical spine. J Bone Joint Surg [Br] 65:47, 1983.

Feldman F, Auerbach R, Johnston A: Tuberculous dactylitis in the adult. AJR 112:460, 1971.

Fetterman LE, Hardy R, Lehrer H: The clinico-roentgenologic features of Ainhum. AJR 100:512, 1967.

Gelman MI, Everts CS: Blastomycotic dactylitis. Radiology 107:331, 1973.

Goldblatt M, Cremin BJ: Osteo-articular tuberculosis: Its presentation in coloured races. Clin Radiol 29:669, 1978.

Goldenberg DL: "Postinfectious" arthritis. New look at an old concept with particular attention to disseminated gonococcal infection. Am J Med 74:925, 1983.

Green WH, Goldberg HI, Wohl GT: Mucormycosis infection of the craniofacial structures. AJR 101:802, 1967.

Harverson G, Warren AG: Tarsal bone disintegration in leprosy. Clin Radiol 30:317, 1979.

Hook EW, Campbell CG, Weens HS, Cooper GR: Salmonella osteomyelitis in patients with sickle cell anemia. N Engl J Med 257:403, 1957.

Jacobs P: Osteo-articular tuberculosis in coloured immigrants: A radiological study. Clin Radiol 15:59, 1964.

Jaffe HL: Metabolic, Degenerative and Inflammatory Diseases of Bones and Joints. Philadelphia, Lea & Febiger, 1972.

Keats TE: Cysticercosis: A demonstration of its roentgen manifestations. Mo Med 58:457, 1961.

Kelly PJ, Martin WJ, Schirger A, Weed LA: Brucellosis of the bones and joints. Experience with 36 patients. JAMA 174:347, 1960.

Lawson JP, Steele AC: Lyme arthritis: Radiologic findings. Radiology 154:37, 1985.

Lewall DB, Ofole S, Bendl B: Mycetoma. Skel Radiol 14:257, 1985.

Lewis R, Gorbach S, Altner P: Spinal Pseudomonas chondro-osteomyelitis in heroin users. N Engl J Med 286:1303, 1972.

Lifeso RM, Harder E, McCorkell SJ: Spinal brucellosis. J Bone Joint Surg [Br] 67:345, 1985.

McGahan JP, Graves DS, Palmer PES, Stadalnik RC, Dublin AB: Classic and contemporary imaging of coccidioidomycosis. AJR 136:393, 1981.

McLaughlin GE, Utsinger PD, Trackat WF, Resnick D, Moidel RA: Rheumatic syndromes secondary to guinea worm infestation. Arthritis Rheum 27:694, 1974.

Merten DF, Gooding CA: Skeletal manifestations of congenital cytomegalic inclusion disease. Radiology 95:333, 1970.

Mertz LE, Wobig GH, Duffy J, Katzmann JA: Ticks, spirochetes, and new diagnostic tests for Lyme disease. Mayo Clin Proc 60:402, 1985.

Mortensson W, Eklöf O, Jorulf H: Radiologic aspects of BCG-osteomyelitis in infants and children. Acta Radiol (Diagn) 17:845, 1976.

Patriquin HB, Trias A, Jeoquier S, Marton D: Late sequelae of infantile meningococcemia in growing bones of children. Radiology 141:77, 1981.

Rabinowitz JG, Wolf BS, Greenberg EI, Rausen AR: Osseous changes in rubella embryopathy (congenital rubella syndrome). Radiology 85:494, 1965.

Reeder MM: Tropical diseases of the foot. Semin Roentgenol 5:378, 1970.

Rehm-Graves S, Weinstein AJ, Calabrese LH, Cook SA, Boumphrey FRS: Tuberculosis of the greater trochanter bursa. Arthritis Rheum 26:77, 1983.

Sachdev M, Bery K, Chawla S: Osseous manifestations in congenital syphilis: A study of 55 cases. Clin Radiol 33:319, 1982.

Samuel E: Roentgenology of parasitic calcification. AJR 63:512, 1950.

Sengupta S: Musculoskeletal lesions in yaws. Clin Orthop 192:193, 1985.

Silverman FN: Virus diseases of bone. Do they exist? AJR 126:677, 1976.

Steinbach HL: Infections of bone. Semin Roentgenol 1:337, 1966.

Weaver P, Lifeso RM: The radiological diagnosis of tuberculosis of the adult spine. Skel Radiol 12:178, 1984.

Woolfitt R, Park H-M, Greene M: Localized cryptococcal osteomyelitis. Radiology 120:290, 1976.

Yousefzadeh DK, Jackson JH: Neonatal and infantile candidal arthritis with or without osteomyelitis: A clinical and radiographical review of 21 cases. Skel Radiol 5:77, 1980.

SECTION XI

TRAUMATIC, IATROGENIC, AND NEUROGENIC DISEASES

CASE XI   LEVEL OF DIFFICULTY: 2

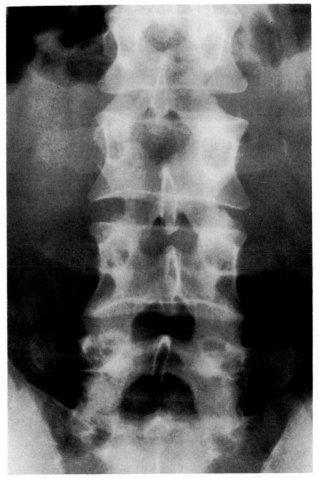

A 37 year old man complained of nonradiating back pain that was exacerbated by prolonged sitting and participation in sports activities. The pain had been present for 3 years. There was no history of spinal injury.

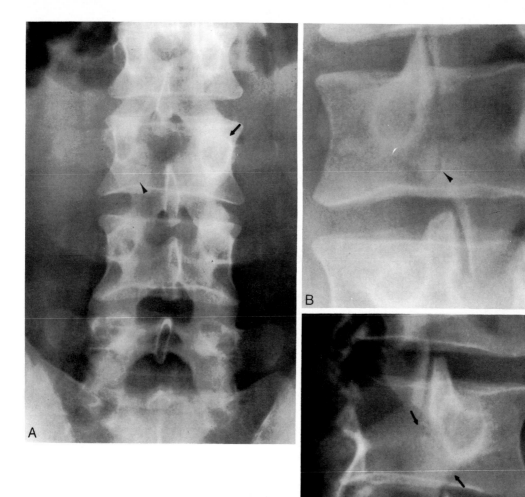

The frontal radiograph of the spine (A) reveals abnormalities of the third lumbar vertebra. The left pedicle of this vertebra is prominent (arrow) and somewhat radiodense in appearance. The adjacent lamina is osteosclerotic and enlarged. The pedicle and lamina on the opposite side are smaller, and there is diminished height of the right side of the third lumbar vertebral body. The remainder of the osseous and soft tissue structures are normal, and there is no evidence of scoliosis.

An osteoid osteoma is an important cause of back pain and osteosclerosis of the posterior elements of a vertebra in patients in the first, second, or third decade of life. Approximately 5 to 10 per cent of osteoid osteomas arise in the vertebral column. These lesions predominate in the lumbar region of the spine, and they usually arise in the transverse process, lamina, or pedicle. Classically, the accompanying pain is prominent, especially at night, and an abnormality of spinal curvature, particularly scoliosis, is typical. The lesion usually is located on the concave aspect of the scoliotic curve, near its apex, and osteosclerosis is the dominant radiographic abnormality. The absence of scoliosis in the test case militates against the diagnosis of an osteoid osteoma, although this diagnosis is still possible.

The clue to the correct interpretation of A lies in the detection of abnormalities in the right side of the third lumbar vertebra. The pedicle appears small and the adjacent portion of the vertebral body is diminished in height. Although a subtle radiolucent area is visible in the region of the pars interarticularis (arrowhead), it is more evident in the right posterior oblique projection (arrowhead in B). This confirms the diagnosis of spondylolysis. Hypertrophy and

reactive sclerosis of the contralateral pedicle and lamina, which are well shown in the left posterior oblique projection (arrows in C), occur as a physiologic response to an unstable neural arch created by a unilateral spondylolysis. Similar bone hypertrophy may be evident contralateral to a congenitally absent pedicle, lamina, or articular facet.

FINAL DIAGNOSIS: Unilateral spondylolysis of the third lumbar vertebra with contralateral hypertrophy of the lamina and pedicle.

FURTHER READING
Pages 812 to 815 and the following:

1. Sherman FC, Wilkinson RH, Hall JE: Reactive sclerosis of a pedicle and spondylolysis in the lumbar spine. J Bone Joint Surg [Am] 59:49, 1977.
2. Downey EF Jr, Whiddon SM, Brower AC: Computed tomography of congenital absence of posterior elements in the thoracolumbar spine. Spine 11:68, 1986.

(Case XI, courtesy of J.R. Grilliot, D.C., Toronto, Ontario, Canada.)

Chapter 62

Physical Trauma

Donald Resnick, M.D.
Thomas G. Goergen, M.D.
Gen Niwayama, M.D.

Physical trauma may lead to a variety of radiographic abnormalities in addition to such complications as the reflex sympathetic dystrophy syndrome, osteolysis, osteonecrosis, many of the osteochondroses, neuroarthropathy, heterotopic bone formation, and infection. In this chapter, radiologic characteristics of fractures and dislocations in the various skeletal sites are explained on the basis of biomechanical principles. Special types of injuries include pathologic, stress, greenstick, torus, bowing, and transchondral frac-
tures and osseous infractions accompanying subluxations and dislocations. Trauma to synovial joints may lead to synovitis, hemarthrosis, and lipohemarthrosis; trauma to symphyses may result in intraosseous cartilaginous displacements; trauma to synchondroses may cause variable patterns of growth plate injury; and trauma to supporting structures may lead to tendinous and ligamentous disruption, avulsion, and diastasis. Characteristic skeletal abnormalities also appear in the abused child.

Physical injury contributes to a wide variety of alterations in the bones, the joints, and the soft tissues. In addition to fractures, dislocations, subluxations, and capsular, tendinous, and ligamentous tears, trauma can affect the growth plate of the immature skeleton as well as the hyaline cartilaginous and fibrocartilaginous articular structures. Further complications of trauma include the reflex sympathetic dystrophy syndrome (see Chapter 47), osteolysis (see Chapter 84), osteonecrosis (see Chapter 70), many of the osteochondroses (see Chapter 71), neuroarthropathy (see Chapter 69), infection (see Chapters 59 to 61), and heterotopic bone formation (see Chapter 85). Trauma has also been implicated in the development of certain neoplasms, such as aneurysmal bone cysts. Nonmechanical trauma to the musculoskeletal system can result from thermal and electrical injury (see Chapter 63), irradiation (see Chapter 64), and chemical substances (see Chapters 65 to 67).

AVAILABLE DIAGNOSTIC TECHNIQUES

The sensitivity as well as the availability of conventional radiography has led to its routine use in the delineation of skeletal injuries. Specialized radiographic techniques such as conventional tomography (see Chapter 9) and magnification radiography (see Chapter 6) generally are not necessary for proper diagnosis in cases of skeletal trauma. Occasionally such techniques can identify subtle fracture lines when initial radiographs are normal, as in fractures of the carpal scaphoid bone, tibial plateaus, and femoral neck (Figs. 62–1 and 62–2). Xeroradiography (see Chapter 8) and low KV radiography (see Chapter 7) also can be helpful in the evaluation of trauma, especially when a soft tissue injury is suspected. Stereoradiography, too, may be of aid.

The role of computed tomography in the area of skeletal trauma is summarized in Chapter 10. In general, this tech-

nique is able to define the presence and extent of certain fractures or dislocations, to detect intraarticular abnormalities, including cartilage damage and osteocartilaginous bodies, and to assess the nearby soft tissues. Its application to traumatic abnormalities in regions of complicated anatomy, such as the spine and the bones in the face and pelvis, is especially noteworthy (Fig. 62–3). The fact that plaster casts do not cause significant deterioration of the image quality also is important.

The excellent contrast resolution provided by magnetic resonance imaging (see Chapter 11) allows analysis of the spinal cord and many soft tissue structures, including cartilage, intra- and periarticular ligaments, and muscles (Fig. 62–4). This feature, when combined with others such as the absence of radiation exposure and the capability of obtaining direct coronal, sagittal, or transaxial images, ensures that magnetic resonance imaging will be increasingly used to evaluate acutely traumatized patients.

After trauma to the musculoskeletal system, the important indication for arteriography is the identification of vascular abnormalities, including disruption and occlusion of major vessels, arteriovenous fistulae, and aneurysms, in patients whose physical examination indicates signs such as ischemia, pulse deficit, or bleeding that are compatible with a significant injury to the blood vessels. With regard to the extremities, the vessels that are injured most commonly are in close proximity to a bone and held in a relatively fixed position by fascial or muscular attachment: the subclavian artery may be injured by the distal fragment of a clavicular fracture; the axillary artery may be damaged in shoulder dislocations owing to the injury itself or to attempts at reduction of the humeral head; the brachial artery may be injured by a fracture of the humerus or a dislocation of the elbow; the radial or ulnar artery may be lacerated by fractures of the radius and ulna;

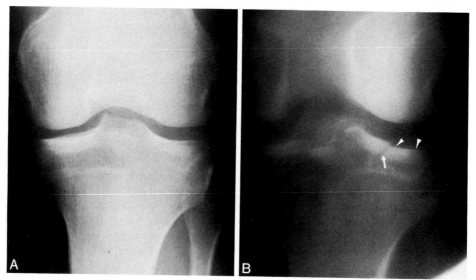

Figure 62–1. Physical trauma: Use of conventional tomography. The fracture line (arrow) and the slight depression of the articular surface (arrowheads) are evident only on the conventional tomogram.

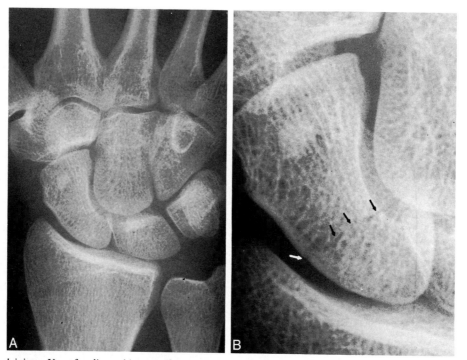

Figure 62–2. Physical injury: Use of radiographic magnification. Although both the conventional radiograph and the magnified projection reveal a scaphoid fracture, its extent (arrows) is better determined with magnification.

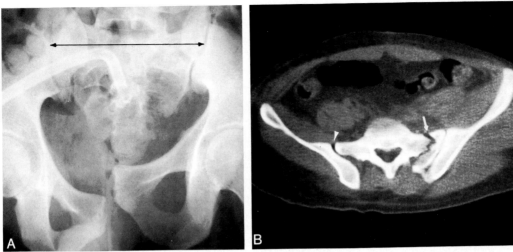

Figure 62–3. **Physical trauma: Use of computed tomography.** Double-headed arrows indicate the approximate level of the transaxial scan. Although the initial radiograph (**A**) shows symphyseal diastasis and a fracture of the sacrum, the latter (**arrow**) is better demonstrated with computed tomography (**B**) which also reveals diastasis of the contralateral sacroiliac joint with a vacuum phenomenon (**arrowhead**).

the femoral artery in the adductor canal and the popliteal artery throughout its course are vulnerable in fractures or dislocations of contiguous bones; the anterior tibial artery or, less commonly, the posterior tibial artery may be compromised by fractures of the tibia; and the posterior tibial and dorsalis pedis arteries may be affected in fractures or dislocations of the ankle or foot. The mechanisms leading to the vascular injury include a tear resulting from the presence of a sharp bone fragment, compression related to a hematoma or swelling within a tight fascial compartment, a shearing type of injury, and entrapment in the fracture fragments with angulation and occlusion.

Scintigraphy is also useful in the evaluation of patients with skeletal trauma. This role is perhaps best exemplified in the diagnosis of stress fractures (see later discussion), although scintigraphy may be helpful in detecting subtle acute fractures when radiographs are normal or in excluding fractures in the presence of significant clinical findings. The vast majority of fractures are detected by bone scintigraphy within hours of the injury, with some delay in scintigraphic abnormality (24 hours) encountered in older patients, particularly those with osteoporosis. Difficulty arises in determining the age of a fracture because of considerable variability in the time required for fracture sites to return to normal on bone scintigraphy. The minimal time required for the bone scan to return to normal after fracture appears to be about 5 to 7 months, and in 90 per cent of cases the scan is normal by 2 years after the injury.

A knowledge of the scintigraphic patterns that are characteristic of normal fracture healing is required for the accurate diagnosis of delayed healing or nonunion by radionuclide techniques. Nonunion of a fracture, which is particularly common in the tibia, femur, and, to a lesser extent, humerus, radius, ulna, and clavicle, has been divided into two types according to the amount of metabolic activity at the fracture site: an atrophic nonunion in which there is a diminution of radioactivity at the fracture site when compared with the expected intensity of radiotracer concentration, and a reactive nonunion in which the radionuclide concentration is normal or increased. In instances of atrophic nonunion, a generalized

decrease in radioactivity may be accompanied by a focal zone of photopenia, indicative of a pseudarthrosis, interposition of soft tissues, a region of avascularity, or infection.

Scintigraphy also has been used to delineate early avascularity of bone after fracture, especially in the proximal portion of the femur (see Chapter 70).

FRACTURES
Epidemiology

The likelihood as well as the location and configuration of a fracture occurring after an injury depends on a number of factors, including the age and sex of the person, the type and mechanism of the injury, and the presence of any predisposing factors that might alter the bones or soft tissues of the musculoskeletal system. Birth-related trauma in the newborn, sports-related activities in the adolescent or young adult, occupation-related stresses in the mature adult, and normal

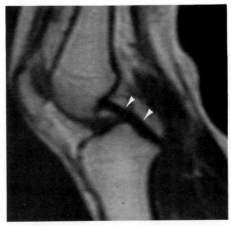

Figure 62–4. **Physical trauma: Use of magnetic resonance imaging.** Normal posterior cruciate ligament (**arrowheads**) of the knee (sagittal image, TE, 25 ms; TR, 0.6 s) is seen.

activities in the elderly are typical situations leading to skeletal injury. In men, the frequency of fractures is greatest in the second and third decades of life and in old age; in women the frequency is less than that in men until the age of approximately 45 or 50 years, after which fractures become more common in women than in men.

Fractures of the small bones of the hands and feet, the tubular bones of the extremities (tibia and humerus), and the clavicle predominate in adolescents and young adults owing to their participation in recreational or occupational activities; fractures of the proximal portions of the femur and humerus, the distal portion of the radius, and the pelvis are especially common in elderly persons, particularly women, reflecting the locations vulnerable to trauma in a skeleton weakened by metabolic diseases, such as osteoporosis. The physeal and metaphyseal regions in children, the epiphyses in teenagers, the diaphyses in young adults, and the epiphyses and metaphyses in elderly individuals are sites in the tubular bones that are often injured. Such site selection relates to changing patterns of skeletal strength and weakness as well as mechanisms of injuries. Even an identical type of injury, such as a fall on the outstretched hand, will lead to musculoskeletal consequences that differ among the various age groups, however: a supracondylar fracture of the humerus in the young child; a metaphyseal fracture of the distal portion of the radius in the older child; an epiphyseal separation of the radius in the adolescent; a carpal injury in the young adult; a Colles' type fracture of the distal portion of the radius in the middle-aged person; and a fracture of the surgical neck of the humerus in the elderly patient.

Terminology

A *fracture*, in its most simple definition, is a break in the continuity of bone or cartilage, or both. Every fracture is associated with soft tissue injury. A *transchondral fracture* is one that involves a cartilaginous surface. If the cartilage alone is involved, the term *chondral fracture* is used; a fracture involving cartilage and subjacent bone is termed an *osteochondral fracture*.

In a *closed (simple) fracture* the skin is intact, which prevents communication between the fracture and the outside environment. An *open fracture* allows communication between the fracture and the outside environment owing to disruption of the skin. Findings indicating an open fracture may be apparent on the radiographs (Table 62–1). Open fractures have a higher

Table 62–1. RADIOGRAPHIC SIGNS OF OPEN FRACTURES

Soft tissue defect
Bone protruding beyond soft tissues
Subcutaneous or intraarticular gas
Foreign material beneath skin
Absent pieces of bone

rate of disturbances in healing, in part related to an increased frequency of infection.

A *complete fracture* occurs when the entire circumference (tubular bone) or both cortical surfaces (flat bone) of a bone have been disrupted. In an *incomplete fracture* a break in the cortex does not extend completely through the bone. Incomplete fractures occur in the resilient elastic bones of children and young adults. They may be further classified into various types, including bowing, greenstick, and torus fractures (see later discussion). The descriptive nomenclature of fractures may be further amplified by the use of terms denoting the direction of the fracture line with reference to the shaft (long bones) or cortex (irregular bones). The direction of the fracture line reflects the vector of the applied force (see later discussion). Four basic types of linear fractures involving the shaft of a tubular bone may be recognized: *transverse, oblique, oblique-transverse,* and *spiral*. A *comminuted fracture* is one with more than two fracture fragments, regardless of the total number of such fragments. In general, the greater the applied force and the more rapid its application, the greater is the energy absorption by the bone and the severity of comminution.

A *butterfly fragment* (Fig. 62–5) is a wedge-shaped fragment arising from the shaft of a long bone at the apex of the force input. The most common sites of butterfly fragments are the femoral and humeral diaphyses. A *segmental fracture* (Fig. 62–6) is one in which the fracture lines isolate a segment of the shaft of the tubular bone. Segmental fractures have special implications regarding adequacy of the blood supply and healing rate.

A tubular bone may be divided roughly into thirds, and a fracture may be described as arising in the proximal, middle, or distal third or at the junction of the proximal and middle or middle and distal thirds. A fracture approximately equidistant from the ends of a bone may be called a midshaft fracture.

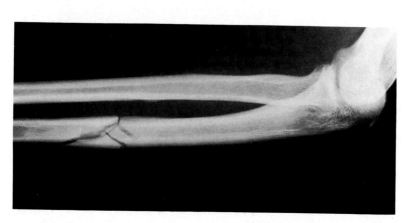

Figure 62–5. Butterfly fracture fragment. A comminuted fracture of the midportion of the shaft of the ulna contains a wedge-shaped butterfly fragment.

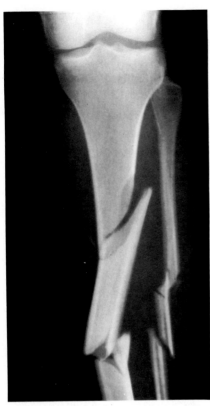

Figure 62–6. Segmental fracture. A segment of the shaft of the tibia and a portion of the fibula have been isolated in this injury.

The *alignment* of a fracture refers to the longitudinal relationship of one fragment to another. If there is no significant angulation, the fracture is said to be in anatomic or near anatomic alignment. By convention, angulation of the distal fragment is described in relationship to the proximal one. Such angulation may be medial or lateral, dorsal or ventral, or, in the forearm, radial or ulnar. The terms *varus* and *valgus* are often used. By current convention, varus refers to angulation of the distal fracture fragment toward the midline of the body; valgus refers to angulation of the distal fracture fragment away from the midline of the body (Fig. 62–7). Alternatively, terms describing the angulation at the fracture site may be used. *Anterior angulation* at the fracture site means that the apex of the fracture is directed anteriorly (ventrally). Conversely, *posterior angulation* at the fracture site indicates that the apex of the fracture site is directed posteriorly (dorsally).

Fracture position is the relationship of the fracture fragments, exclusive of angulation. Deviation from anatomic position is called displacement; terminology descriptive of displacement includes apposition and rotation. *Apposition* considers the degree of bone contact at the fracture site. A fracture with complete apposition is usually described as *undisplaced*. If the fracture surfaces are separated, the amount of *distraction* may be measured. Overlapping fracture surfaces with resultant shortening are described as a bayonet deformity (Fig. 62–8).

Radiographic evaluation of *rotatory displacement* of a fracture (i.e., rotation about the long axis of a bone) is facilitated by including the joints both proximal and distal to the fracture on the film (Fig. 62–9).

An *avulsion fracture* occurs when an osseous fragment is pulled from the parent bone by a tendon or ligament (Fig. 62–10). Such fractures often are located at sites of bone prominences.

An *impaction fracture* results when one fragment of bone is driven into an apposing fragment. Two specific types of impaction fractures are recognized. A *depression fracture* results when impacting forces occur between one hard bone surface

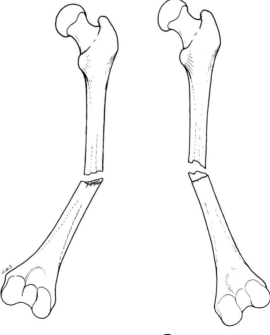

Figure 62–7. Varus and valgus angulation. A Varus angulation. The distal fragment is angulated toward the midline. B Valgus angulation. The distal fragment is angulated away from the midline.

A   B

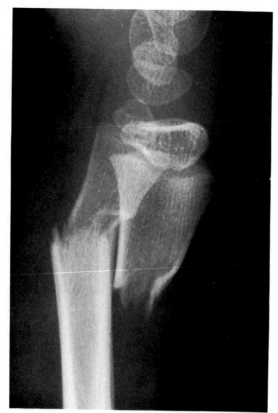

Figure 62–8. Bayonet deformity. Observe fractures of the distal portions of the radius and ulna. The radial fragment is displaced dorsally with overriding, a bayonet deformity.

and an apposing softer surface (Fig. 62–11). A *compression fracture* is a type of impaction fracture characteristically involving vertebral bodies. Forceful flexion of the spine may result in depression of the endplate(s) within the spongy bone of the vertebral centrum (Fig. 62–12).

Fracture Healing

After a fracture occurs, as shown in Figure 62–13, a remarkable series of events takes place that leads to osseous healing in the majority of cases. Many local factors can modify the healing process, however:

- the degree of trauma (retarded healing is expected in fractures associated with extensive osseous and soft tissue injury)
- the degree of bone loss (retarded healing occurs when the bone loss is substantial)
- the type of bone involved (cancellous bone unites rapidly at sites of osseous contact, whereas cortical bone may unite with or without extensive external callus, depending on the degree of apposition of the fragments)
- the extent of immobilization (improper immobilization may lead to delayed union or nonunion)
- the presence of infection (retarded bone healing occurs when infection is present)
- the presence of an underlying pathologic process (neoplastic, metabolic, and other disorders delay the healing process)
- use of radiation therapy (irradiated bone unites at a slower rate)

- the presence of extensive osteonecrosis (avascular bone impedes fracture healing)
- and the occurrence of intraarticular extension (fibrinolysins in the synovial fluid may destroy the initial clot, producing a delay in fracture union)

Systemic factors such as the age of the patient (healing is more rapid in the immature skeleton) and the presence of abnormal serum levels of certain hormones (corticosteroids inhibit fracture healing) can also be influential in fracture repair.

In some instances, the healing process is markedly slowed (*delayed union*) or arrested altogether (*nonunion*). There is no uniformly accepted definition of delayed union. Nonunion generally indicates that the fracture site has failed to heal completely during a period of approximately 6 to 9 months after the injury and that a typical pseudarthrosis (consisting of a synovium-lined cavity and synovial fluid) or a fibrous union has developed. Nonunion of a tibial or femoral fracture is encountered most commonly, whereas nonunion after a fracture of the humerus, radius, ulna, and clavicle is less frequent. The causes of nonunion include open, comminuted, segmental, or pathologic fractures, insufficient immobilization of the osseous fragments, infection, interposition of soft tissue between the edges of the fractured bone, inadequate blood supply, poor nutritional status, and metabolic bone disease.

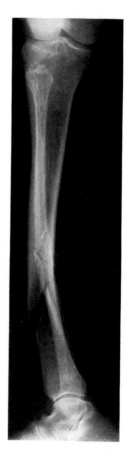

Figure 62–9. Rotatory displacement. This radiograph of the lower portion of the leg reveals that the knee is in an oblique position and the ankle is in a lateral attitude. There are fractures of the shafts of the tibia and fibula, with marked lateral rotation of the distal fragments.

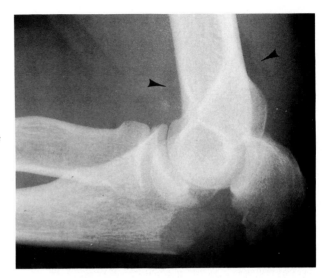

Figure 62–10. **Avulsion fracture.** The triceps tendon is attached to the large fracture fragment. A joint effusion is noted (arrowheads).

Special Types of Fractures

PATHOLOGIC FRACTURES. A pathologic fracture is one in which the bone is disrupted at a site of preexisting abnormality, frequently by a stress that would not have fractured a normal bone. The most common underlying abnormalities are tumors and osteoporosis. Of the tumorous causes of pathologic fractures, skeletal metastasis predominates, followed, in order of frequency, by benign lesions (such as simple bone cysts, enchondromas, and giant cell tumors) and primary osseous malignancies (including plasma cell myeloma, histiocytic lymphoma, Ewing's sarcoma, and osteo-

sarcoma). It is generally believed that the size of the lesion and the extent of cortical destruction are fundamental factors influencing the likelihood of pathologic fracture.

The radiographic distinction between a pathologic and a nonpathologic fracture is not always easy. When a small lesion is present, the fracture itself may obscure the area of lysis or sclerosis. The absence of a history of trauma or fracture pain and the presence of preexisting findings, such as angular deformity, painless swelling, or generalized bone pain, are clinical aids to the diagnosis of a pathologic fracture. A transverse fracture line is a radiographic clue (Fig. 62–14). Diagnostic difficulty may be encountered in the patient who

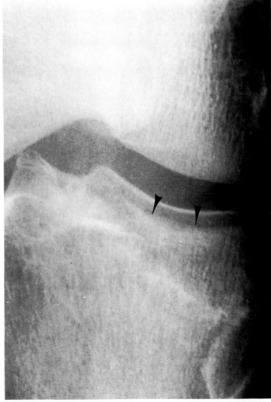

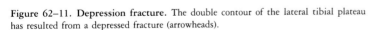

Figure 62–11. **Depression fracture.** The double contour of the lateral tibial plateau has resulted from a depressed fracture (arrowheads).

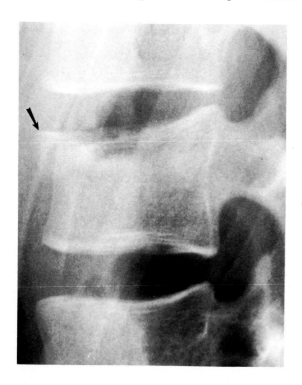

Figure 62–12. Compression fracture. A compression fracture of the superior surface of the second lumbar vertebral body is present, with a small comminuted corner fragment (arrow).

has a nonpathologic fracture that is days to weeks old, as resorption, osteolysis, or rotation about the fracture site may create the illusion of an underlying lesion.

STRESS FRACTURES. Stress fractures can occur in normal or abnormal bone that is subjected to repeated cyclic loading, with the load being less than that which causes acute fracture of bone. Two types of stress fractures can be recognized: a *fatigue fracture*, resulting from the application of abnormal stress to a bone with normal elastic resistance; and an *insufficiency fracture*, occurring when normal stress is placed

on a bone with deficient elastic resistance. Fatigue fractures frequently share the following features: The activity is new or different for the person; the activity is strenuous; and the activity is repeated with a frequency that ultimately produces symptoms and signs. Typical examples are the fatigue fractures that occur in the metatarsal bones of military recruits ("march" fractures), and in the lower extremities in athletes, joggers, and dancers. The causes of insufficiency fractures include rheumatoid arthritis, osteoporosis, Paget's disease, osteomalacia or rickets, hyperparathyroidism, renal osteodys-

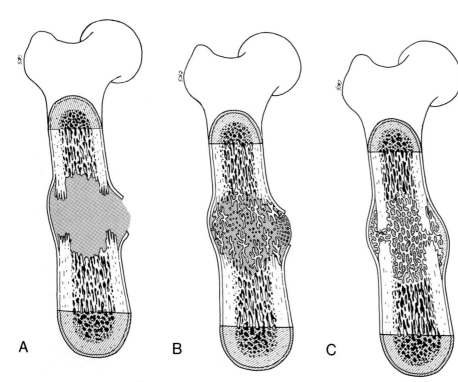

A　　　　　B　　　　　C

Figure 62–13. Normal fracture healing. **A** After the injury, bleeding is related to osseous and soft tissue damage. A hematoma followed by clot formation develops within the medullary canal between the fracture ends and beneath the periosteal membrane, which itself may have been torn. **B** Callus formation takes place, consisting of external bridging callus at the periosteal surface, intramedullary callus, and primary callus at the ends of the fracture fragments. **C** The callus rapidly envelops the bone ends, producing increasing stability at the fracture site.

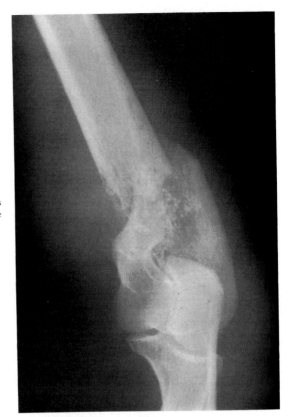

Figure 62–14. **Pathologic fracture.** A transverse fracture line through a metastatic focus from bronchogenic carcinoma can be detected in the distal portion of the humerus. Note the osteolysis, cortical irregularity, and soft tissue swelling.

trophy, osteogenesis imperfecta, osteopetrosis, fibrous dysplasia, and irradiation. In rheumatoid arthritis, predisposing factors include disuse, corticosteroid therapy, angular deformities in the extremities, and arthroplasties allowing new physical activities; the insufficiency fractures predominate in the bones of the legs. In osteoporosis, such fractures usually occur in the sacrum, pubic rami, and lower extremities (Fig. 62–15). In Paget's disease, the convex aspect of the tubular bones, especially the femur, is affected (Fig. 62–16). Fatigue and insufficiency fractures are not infrequent after surgical procedures, such as bunion surgery, that result in altered stress or an imbalance of muscular force.

The radionuclide examination provides a means of early detection of stress fractures. The stressed bone undergoing accelerated remodeling reveals poorly defined areas of increased accumulation of bone-seeking pharmaceutical agents that are observed in the absence of radiographic findings. Appropriate modification of the physical activity may allow osseous "healing" without the appearance of cortical infraction. If the strenuous activity continues, a true stress fracture develops in which focal fusiform, sharply marginated areas of increased radionuclide activity can be associated with radiolucent cortical areas and periosteal and endosteal thickening on the radiograph (Fig. 62–17).

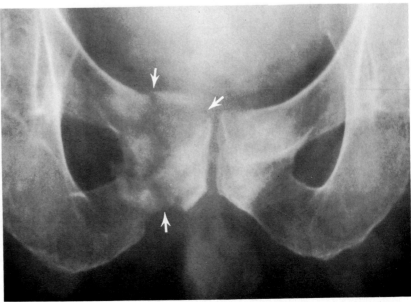

Figure 62–15. **Insufficiency fractures: Rheumatoid arthritis and osteoporosis.** In parasymphyseal bone, such fractures (arrows) are accompanied by osteolysis, osteosclerosis, and bone fragmentation.

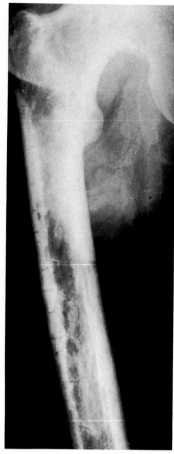

Figure 62–16. Insufficiency fractures: Paget's disease. Multiple radiolucent fracture lines are seen in the lateral aspect of the diaphysis. Note osseous thickening in the endosteal margin of the cortex at the sites of fracture. (Courtesy of C. Wackenheim, M.D., and Y. Dirheimer, M.D., Paris, France.)

Scintigraphy may be used to investigate other stress injuries. In patients with shin splints, radionuclide angiograms and blood pool images are normal, whereas on delayed images, a longitudinally oriented area of increased radionuclide accumulation is seen in the posteromedial cortex of the tibia (Fig. 62–18). This pattern of abnormality differs from that typically seen in an acute stress fracture (in which all phases of the radionuclide examination are abnormal and a more fusiform area of augmented activity is apparent) and is consistent with the belief that shin splints represent periosteal disruptions, possibly caused by rupture of the Sharpey's fibers that extend from the muscle through the periosteum into the cortex. Abnormal excursion of the soleus muscle may be responsible for the clinical manifestations.

The clinical findings of stress fractures include activity-related pain that is relieved by rest. The radiographic abnormalities are influenced by the location of the fracture and the interval between the time of injury and that of the radiographic examination. In the diaphysis of a tubular bone, a linear cortical radiolucent area (or areas) is frequently associated with periosteal and endosteal cortical thickening (Fig. 62–19). The abnormality can be differentiated from that of an osteoid osteoma (circular or elliptical cortical radiolucent area with or without calcification in an area of sclerosis) and an abscess (circular or oval radiolucent area without calcification with surrounding sclerosis). In an epiphyseal or metaphyseal location, focal sclerosis representing condensation of trabeculae is the typical finding, and periostitis is not prominent (Fig. 62–20).

Stress fractures are most frequent in the bones of the lower extremity, but they can occur almost anywhere (Table 62–2). Examples include the following.

1. *Calcaneal or other tarsal stress fracture.* Fatigue fracture of the calcaneus is not uncommon in military recruits, and insufficiency fractures in this site can accompany rheumatoid

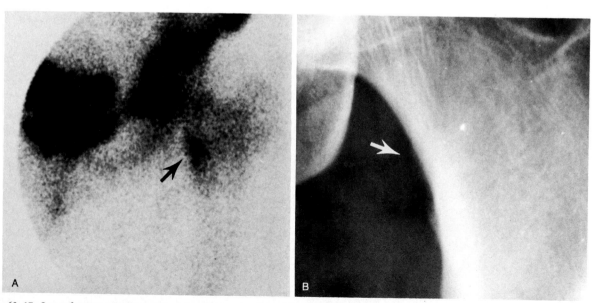

Figure 62–17. Stress fractures: Radionuclide abnormalities. A radionuclide examination (**A**) reveals a focal, sharply marginated area of increased activity in the femoral neck (arrow). A radiograph (**B**) of the hip delineates a minimal amount of indistinct new bone formation along the medial aspect of the femoral neck (arrow).

Table 62–2. LOCATION OF STRESS FRACTURE BY ACTIVITY

Location	Activity or Event
Sesamoids of metatarsal bones	Prolonged standing
Metatarsal shaft	Marching; stamping on ground; prolonged standing; ballet; after bunionectomy
Navicular	Stamping on ground; marching; long distance running
Calcaneus	Jumping; parachuting; prolonged standing; recent immobilization
Tibia: Mid and distal shaft	Long distance running
Proximal shaft (children)	Running
Fibula: Distal shaft	Long distance running
Proximal shaft	Jumping; parachuting
Patella	Hurdling
Femur: Shaft	Ballet; long distance running
Neck	Ballet; marching; long distance running; gymnastics
Pelvis: Obturator ring	Stooping; bowling; gymnastics
Lumbar vertebra (pars interarticularis)	Ballet; lifting heavy objects; scrubbing floors
Lower cervical, upper thoracic spinous process	Clay shoveling
Ribs	Carrying heavy pack; golf; coughing
Clavicle	Postoperative radical neck
Coracoid of scapula	Trap shooting
Humerus: Distal shaft	Throwing a ball
Ulna: Coronoid	Pitching a ball
shaft	Pitchfork work; propelling wheelchair
Hook of hamate	Holding golf club, tennis racquet, baseball bat

Modified from Daffner RH: Stress fractures: Current concepts. Skel Radiol 2:221, 1978. Used with permission.

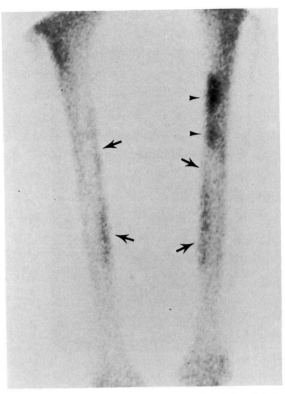

Figure 62–18. Stress changes: Shin splints. On a frontal view of the lower legs during the delayed portion of a bone scan, longitudinally oriented areas of increased tracer accumulation are apparent in the medial cortex of the midportion of the tibiae (arrows). Two localized areas of increased radionuclide activity in the left tibia (arrowheads) may represent true stress fractures.

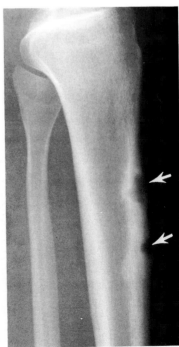

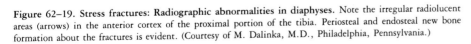

Figure 62–19. Stress fractures: Radiographic abnormalities in diaphyses. Note the irregular radiolucent areas (arrows) in the anterior cortex of the proximal portion of the tibia. Periosteal and endosteal new bone formation about the fractures is evident. (Courtesy of M. Dalinka, M.D., Philadelphia, Pennsylvania.)

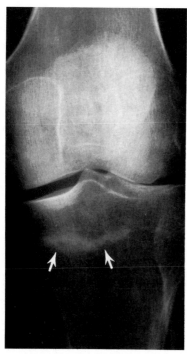

Figure 62–20. Stress fractures: Radiographic abnormalities in metaphyses and epiphyses. Band-like focal sclerosis (arrows) is typical of a stress fracture in the proximal portion of the tibia.

arthritis, neurologic disorders, and other diseases (Fig. 62–21). Stress fractures in other tarsal bones are less common. Those in the tarsal navicular bone have been observed in physically active persons, especially in basketball players and runners (Fig. 62–22).

2. *Fibular stress fracture.* Changing muscular stresses can result in the "runner's fracture" of the fibula. Jumping can also produce fibular stress fractures; classically, the proximal portion of the bone is affected in jumping, whereas the distal portion may be altered in running.

3. *Tibial stress fracture.* Stress fracture of the proximal diaphysis of the tibia can occur during running, and stress fracture of the middle and distal tibial diaphysis can take place during long-distance running, marching, and ballet dancing.

4. *Femoral stress fracture.* Stress fracture of the shaft or neck of the femur can result from long-distance running, ballet dancing, and marching. Two types of stress fracture are seen: a transverse type, appearing as a radiolucent area in the superior aspect of the femoral neck and becoming displaced in some situations; and a compression type (Fig. 62–23), appearing as a haze of callus in the inferior aspect of the neck, and being stable in most cases.

5. *Metatarsal stress fracture.* Stress fractures of the metatarsal bones may accompany marching, ballet dancing, prolonged standing, and surgical resection of adjacent metatarsal bones (Fig. 62–24). The middle and distal portions of the shafts of the second and third metatarsal bones are affected most often.

6. *Pubic rami stress fracture.* Stress fractures of the pubic arch are encountered in joggers, long-distance runners, or marathoners, in patients with osteoarthritis of the hip, in those who have undergone hip arthroplasty, and in association with osteoporosis and rheumatoid arthritis.

7. *Upper extremity stress fracture.* These fractures are far less frequent than stress fractures in the bones of the lower extremity. Typical sites include the ribs in golfers, rowers, and tennis players; the coracoid process of the scapula in trapshooters; the ulna of tennis players, baseball pitchers, volleyball players, weightlifters, and patients using wheelchairs; the hook of the hamate in tennis players, golfers, and baseball players; and the olecranon process in baseball pitchers and javelin throwers.

8. *Stress fracture of bones in the thorax.* Stress fractures of the ribs (related to physical activity or coughing), the clavicle, and the sternum (related to osteoporosis, thoracic kyphosis, and pulmonary disease) have been described.

9. *Stress fracture of the neural arch of the vertebra (spondylolysis).* Spondylolysis represents a defect in the pars interarticularis of the vertebra (Fig. 62–25). It may or may not be associated with a slippage of one vertebral body onto the adjacent one,

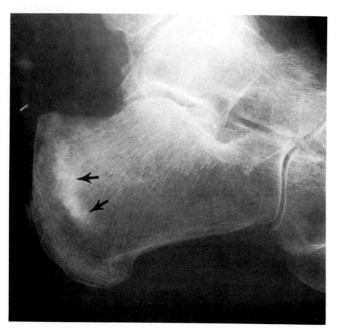

Figure 62–21. Calcaneal stress fracture. Note the vertically oriented radiodense band (arrows).

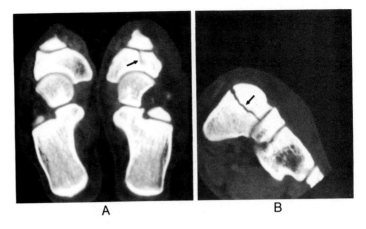

Figure 62–22. **Tarsal navicular stress fracture.** In a professional basketball player, direct transverse (**A**) and coronal (**B**) computed tomograms show a stress fracture in the tarsal navicular bone that has progressed to a complete fracture (arrows). (Courtesy of L. Rogers, M.D., Chicago, Illinois.)

the slippage being termed spondylolisthesis. Spondylolysis is most frequently observed in the lumbar region of the spine. In the cervical spine, the defect occurs most typically at the sixth vertebral level, usually is bilateral, and commonly is accompanied by spina bifida, suggesting a congenital predisposition or cause. In the lower portion of the spine, the fifth lumbar vertebra is affected most commonly (approximately 67 per cent), and the frequency of spondylolysis diminishes on proceeding cephalad in the lumbar region. Symptoms and signs may be absent, although pain, tenderness, gait abnormality, and neurologic deficits can be observed.

It has been estimated that 3 to 7 per cent of vertebral columns reveal at least one area of spondylolysis. Most series demonstrate a male predominance. Typically, spondylolysis is discovered in childhood or early adulthood. The frequency of these defects rises precipitously between the ages of 5 and 7 years.

The cause of lumbar spondylolysis has long been debated; however, the current consensus strongly supports an acquired traumatic lesion originating sometime between infancy and early adult life. It seems probable that spondylolysis results most frequently from a fatigue fracture occurring after repeated trauma rather than from an acute fracture following a single traumatic episode. Radiographic and scintigraphic abnormalities have been detected in the area of the pars interarticularis in athletes, presumably related to chronic stress. Genetic influences also are important in this condition. A familial history of the condition and an increased frequency of nearby congenital anomalies of the spine, such as transitional vertebrae and spina bifida, are recognized.

Lumbar spondylolysis and spondylolisthesis have been classified into five types:

Type 1: Dysplastic, with associated congenital abnormality of the upper sacrum and the arch of the lumbar vertebra.

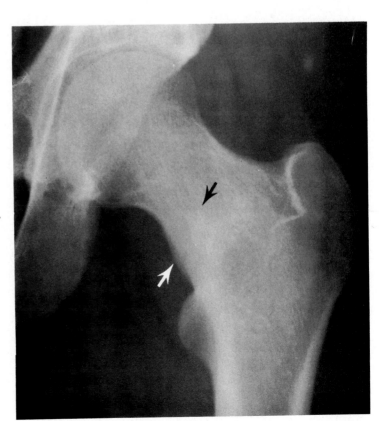

Figure 62–23. **Femoral stress fracture.** In the femoral neck, observe buttressing and sclerosis (arrows).

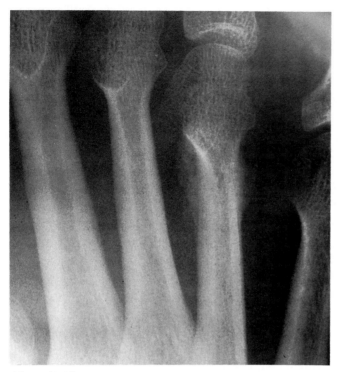

Figure 62–24. Metatarsal stress fracture. Note considerable periostitis about the distal portion of the metatarsal shaft.

Type II: Isthmic, with a defect in the pars interarticularis that may be (a) a fatigue fracture, (b) an elongated but intact pars, or (c) an acute fracture.

Type III: Degenerative, resulting from long-standing intersegmental instability.

Type IV: Traumatic, caused by fractures in areas of the posterior elements other than the pars interarticularis.

Type V: Pathologic, owing to generalized or localized bone disease.

Radiographic alterations of spondylolysis are diagnostic (Fig. 62–25). Spondylolysis is usually evident in the lateral radiographic projection; however, oblique views are particularly helpful. The spine has a "Scottie dog" appearance on oblique projections. A unilateral or bilateral radiolucent area (with or without sclerosis) through the neck of the "Scottie dog" is well demonstrated. On frontal radiographs, laminar fragmentation may be seen. Spondylolisthesis may be encountered in some cases. In cases of unilateral spondylolysis, hypertrophy of the contralateral pedicle and lamina may be detected as a physiologic response to the presence of an unstable neural arch (Fig. 62–26). This appearance may simulate that of an osteoid osteoma. Furthermore, similar hypertrophy occurs contralateral to a congenitally absent pedicle, lamina, or articular facet.

Scintigraphy can be a helpful diagnostic method in cases of low back pain of obscure cause. It has been suggested that

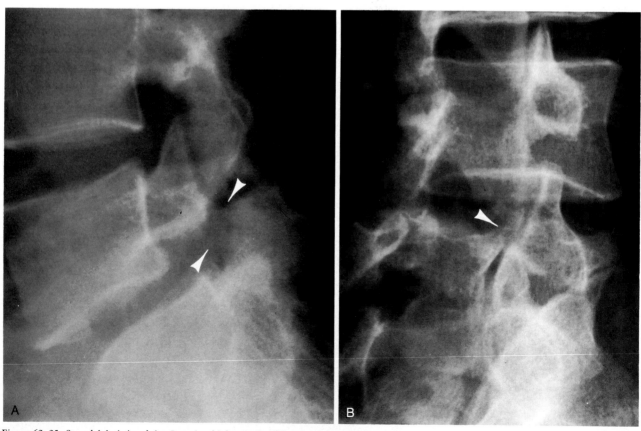

Figure 62–25. Spondylolysis in adults. Lateral and left posterior oblique projections reveal a defect through the pars interarticularis (arrowheads). The spine has a "Scottie dog" appearance on oblique views. The resulting lucent lesion has produced a break in the "neck" of the "Scottie dog" on the oblique projection. A grade I spondylolisthesis of L5 on S1 can be noted on the lateral radiograph.

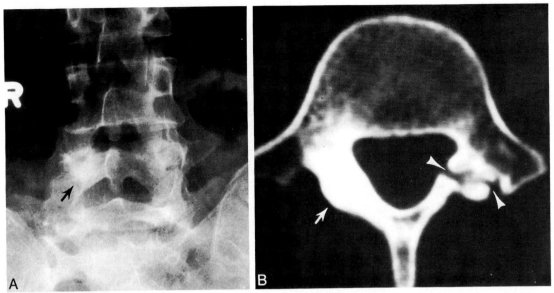

Figure 62–26. Unilateral spondylolysis with contralateral bone hypertrophy and reactive sclerosis. A The predominant abnormality on the frontal radiograph of the lumbar spine is osteosclerosis in the region of the right pedicle of the fifth lumbar vertebra (arrow). The left transverse process of this vertebra is smaller than that on the right. **B** A transaxial computed tomographic scan of this vertebra reveals spondylolysis (arrowheads) and contralateral bone hypertrophy (arrow). (Courtesy of J. A. Amberg, M.D., San Diego, California.)

scintigraphy allows the detection of more recently acquired and symptomatic spondylolyses, as such defects will accumulate the bone-seeking radiotracer, whereas older and non-symptomatic spondylolyses will not.

Computed tomography represents a further imaging technique that has been used to delineate areas of spondylolysis and associated foraminal encroachment and indentation of the neural canal from callus formation. Computed tomography also allows detection of other clefts in the neural arch that are rarer than those in the pars interarticularis (Fig. 62–27).

It is difficult to predict which patients with spondylolysis will develop spondylolisthesis. Progressive slippage in association with spondylolysis can potentially occur at any time but generally is seen prior to the age of 16 years and typically is asymptomatic. Rather, spondylolisthesis usually is demonstrable at about the same time that spondylolysis is discovered. A variety of methods of measurement of the degree of spondylolisthesis have been proposed (Fig. 62–28).

GREENSTICK, TORUS, AND BOWING FRACTURES. In the immature skeleton, fractures that do not completely penetrate the entire shaft of a bone are not infrequent. The main types of incomplete fractures, in addition to stress fractures, are greenstick, torus, and bowing fractures.

A *greenstick (hickory stick, willow) fracture* is one that perforates one cortex and ramifies within the medullary bone (Fig. 62–29). Greenstick fractures commonly become converted to complete fractures because of the exaggeration of the deformity as the bone continues to grow. Typical locations of greenstick fractures are the proximal metaphysis or diaphysis of the tibia and the middle third of the radius and ulna. In the healing stage of these fractures, well-defined subperiosteal defects may be observed.

A *torus (buckling) fracture* results from an injury insufficient in force to create a complete discontinuity of bone but sufficient to produce a buckling of the cortex (Fig. 62–30).

Torus fractures are common in metaphyseal regions and in patients with osteoporosis. Follow-up examination may reveal transverse bands of increased radiodensity, indicating osseous impaction. A combination of the greenstick and torus fractures is termed the *lead pipe* fracture.

Bowing fractures are a plastic response, usually to longitudinal stress in a bone. They are virtually confined to children and are most typically apparent in the radius and the ulna, although their presence in adults and involvement of other

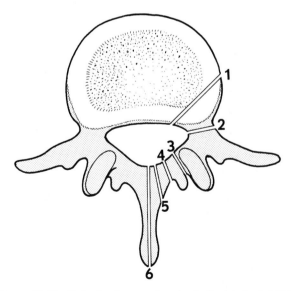

Figure 62–27. Clefts in the neural arch. 1, Persistent neurocentral synchondrosis; 2, pediculate or retrosomatic cleft; 3, pars interarticularis cleft, or spondylolysis; 4, retroisthmic cleft; 5, paraspinous cleft; 6, spinous cleft. (From Johansen JG, et al: Retrosomatic clefts: Computed tomographic appearance. Radiology *148*:447, 1983. Used with permission.)

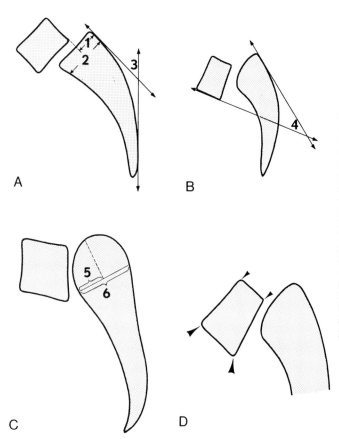

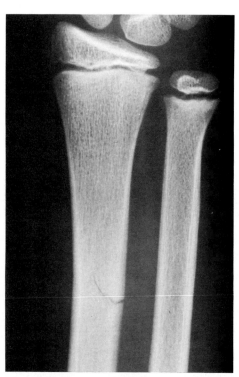

Figure 62–28. Spondylolisthesis: Methods of measurement. A The degree of anterior displacement of the fifth lumbar vertebra with respect to the sacrum is expressed as the percentage obtained by dividing the amount of displacement (1) by the maximum anteroposterior diameter of the first sacral vertebra (2) and multiplying this value by 100. Sacral inclination is calculated by drawing a line along the posterior border of the first sacral vertebra and measuring the angle created by this line intersecting a true vertical line (angle at 3). B Sagittal rotation is determined by extending a line along the anterior border of the body of the fifth lumbar vertebra until it intersects a line drawn along the posterior border of the first sacral vertebra. The angle of intersection of these lines (4) is measured. C Percentage of rounding of the top of the sacrum is determined from a series of radiographs by dividing line 5 by line 6 and multiplying by 100. D The degree of wedging of the slipped vertebra is expressed as a percentage determined by dividing the posterior height of the vertebral body (between small arrowheads) by the anterior height (between large arrowheads) and multiplying this value by 100. (From Wiltse LL, Winter RB: Terminology and measurement of spondylolisthesis. J Bone Joint Surg [Am] 65:768, 1983. Used with permission.)

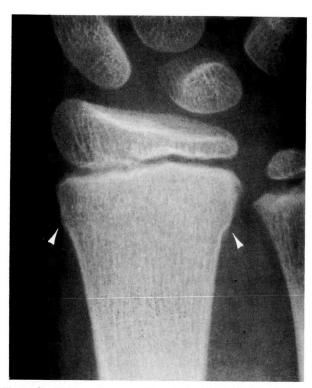

Figure 62–29. Greenstick fractures. Observe that the fracture involves one side of the radius and extends incompletely through the bone.

Figure 62–30. Torus fractures. Note the buckling of the cortex (arrowheads).

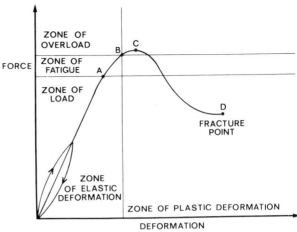

Figure 62–31. Graphic relationship of bone deformation (bowing) and force (longitudinal compression). The linear response in the zone of elastic deformation and the weakening of bone in the zone of plastic deformation are demonstrated. (From Borden S IV: Roentgen recognition of acute plastic bowing out of the forearm in children. AJR *135*:524, 1975. Copyright 1975, American Roentgen Ray Society. Used with permission.)

areas, such as the clavicle, tibia, humerus, fibula, and femur, also are encountered.

After the application of longitudinal compression, an initial zone of elastic deformation of bone is characterized by bowing that disappears with release of the offending force (Fig. 62–31). With greater force, plastic deformation occurs, which results in permanent bowing of the bone. Still further increase in stress will lead to fracture.

Radiographic analysis of bowing deformities reveals lateral or anteroposterior bending of the affected bone (Fig. 62–32). Sequential radiographs usually reveal no evidence of periostitis, although thickening of the involved cortex may be detected. Scintigraphy may identify increased uptake of bone-seeking pharmaceutical agents. A bowed bone generally remains bowed, resists attempts at reduction, holds an adjacent fracture in angulation, and prevents relocation of an adjacent dislocation.

TRANSCHONDRAL FRACTURES (OSTEOCHONDRITIS DISSECANS). Osteochondritis dissecans indicates fragmentation and possible separation of a portion of the articular surface. The age of onset varies from childhood to middle age, but an onset in adolescence is most frequent. Patients may be entirely asymptomatic; however, pain aggravated by movement, limitation of motion, clicking, locking, and swelling may be apparent. Single or multiple sites can be affected.

Despite the existence of reports that emphasize genetic factors or growth disturbances in the pathogenesis of osteochondritis dissecans, osteochondral fractures generally are believed to be the result of shearing, rotatory, or tangentially aligned impaction forces. Acute injuries can produce fragments consisting of cartilage alone (chondral fractures) or cartilage and underlying bone (osteochondral fractures). Obviously, a purely cartilaginous fragment creates no direct radiographic abnormalities, whereas one containing calcified cartilage and bone becomes apparent owing to a varying degree of radiodensity. Secondary radiographic signs consisting of soft tissue swelling and a joint effusion can be apparent. Arthrography with or without conventional or computed tomography may be used to define the nature and location of the fracture more accurately.

After the injury, the detached portion of the articular surface can remain in situ, be slightly displaced, or become loose within the joint cavity (Figs. 62–33 and 62–34). In

many cases, the osteocartilaginous fragments attach to the synovial lining at a distant site and become reabsorbed. If a fragment maintains some attachment to its site of origin, it can undergo revascularization and new bone formation. Free chondral or osteochondral fragments may become more visible with time owing to proliferation of new cartilage and bone or secondary degenerative calcification.

The radiographic identification of osteocartilaginous bodies requires a careful search of the dependent portions of the joint, such as the olecranon fossa in the elbow, the axillary and subscapular recesses in the glenohumeral joint, and the

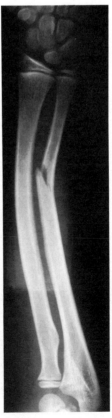

Figure 62–32. **Bowing deformities of bone.** Note the bowing of the radius associated with a fracture of the adjacent ulna.

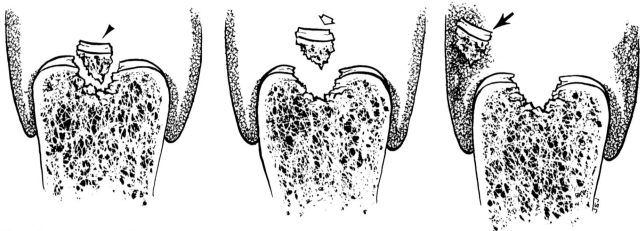

Figure 62–33. Transchondral fractures (osteochondritis dissecans): Fate of fragments. Chondral or osteochondral fragments can remain in situ (arrowhead), be slightly displaced or loose in the articular cavity (open arrow), or become embedded at a distant synovial site, evoking a local inflammatory reaction (solid arrow).

posterior regions in the knee. The detection of osteocartilaginous bodies should stimulate a search for their site of origin. Single or multiple chondral or osseous bodies can accompany idiopathic synovial (osteo)chondromatosis and articular disorders such as neuroarthropathy, crystal-induced arthropathy, degenerative joint disease, and osteonecrosis. Typically, in idiopathic synovial (osteo)chondromatosis, multiple opaque areas of approximately equal size are scattered throughout the articular cavity, and there is no evidence of an underlying articular disorder or trauma.

Femoral Condyles. The most typical location of osteochondritis dissecans is the condylar surfaces of the distal portion of the femur. Men are affected more frequently than women, and the average age at onset of symptoms (pain, swelling) is 15 to 20 years. Unilateral changes predominate.

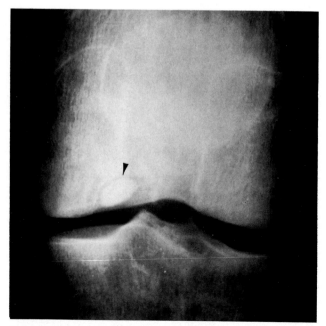

Figure 62–34. Transchondral fractures (osteochondritis dissecans). Fragment remaining in situ: Note the osseous dense area (arrowhead), indicating a fragment that remains in its bed in the medial femoral condyle.

A history of knee trauma can be elicited in about 50 per cent of cases. The medial condyle is affected in approximately 85 per cent of cases and the lateral condyle in 15 per cent of cases (Fig. 62–35). A defect on the inner (lateral) aspect of the medial femoral condyle is most frequent (Fig. 62–36).

The pathogenesis of osteochondritis dissecans of the femoral condyles is not agreed on. Although a juvenile form of the disease, characterized by a familial history, involvement of multiple sites, and irregularities of ossification, has been described (Fig. 62–37), bone necrosis may be recognized on histologic evaluation of the lesions in most cases. The cause of the osteonecrosis and the role of trauma have been debated, however.

With regard to the radiographic characteristics of osteochondritis dissecans, a linear radiolucent fracture line in the subchondral bone rarely may be observed in acute cases. More commonly, a small osseous lesion may be separated from the normal or sclerotic base of the femoral defect by a radiolucent crescentic zone. Fragmentation and collapse of the partially separated body can be recognized. Displacement of the osteochondral fragment produces a loose or synovium-embedded intraarticular osseous body (Fig. 62–38). The site of origin on the femur may gradually be remodeled, although a slightly flattened or irregular articular surface can frequently be detected for decades.

The major disorder for consideration in the differential diagnosis for the radiographic features of condylar osteochondritis dissecans is spontaneous osteonecrosis of the knee. This lesion occurs in older persons, is associated with the sudden onset of clinical manifestations, and almost invariably involves the weight-bearing portion of the medial femoral condyle (see Chapter 70). Osteochondritis dissecans of the knee must also be differentiated from the fragmentation that may accompany neuroarthropathy and from the normal grooves that appear on the medial and lateral femoral condyles on lateral radiographs.

Patella. Osteochondritis dissecans of the patella is rare. Unilateral involvement predominates, and the age of clinical onset is usually between 15 and 20 years. The typical site of the lesion is the medial facet of the patella. Involvement of the lateral facet occurs in approximately 30 per cent of cases. The middle or lower portion of the bone is affected almost universally. Although a history of an injury may not be

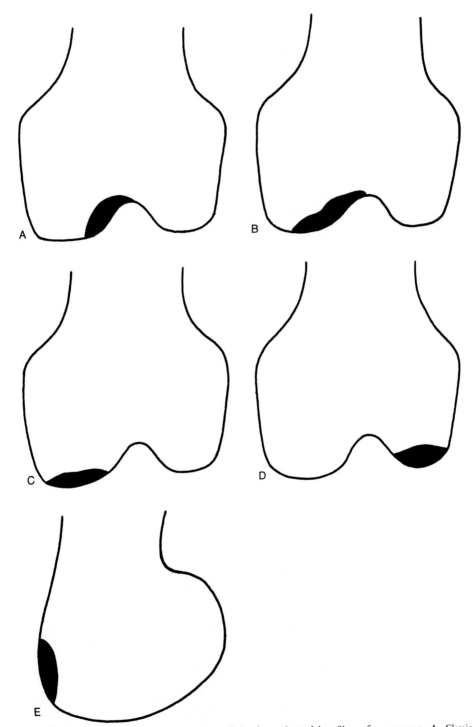

Figure 62–35. Transchondral fractures (osteochondritis dissecans) of the femoral condyles: Sites of occurrence. **A,** Classic (medial condyle); **B,** extended classic (medial condyle); **C,** inferocentral (medial condyle); **D,** inferocentral (lateral condyle); **E,** anterior (lateral condyle).

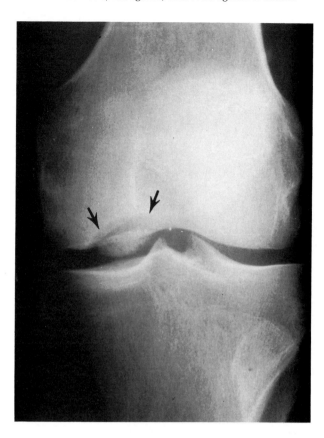

Figure 62–36. Transchondral fractures (osteochondritis dissecans) of the femoral condyles. Classic defect of medial condyle (arrows).

elicited, it is well recognized that the articular surface of the patella is exposed repeatedly to trauma, and a tangential shearing force may be responsible for the lesion. The lesions are optimally identified on lateral and axial radiographs, appearing as osseous defects near the convexity between the condylar articular surfaces of the patella (Fig. 62–39).

The major disorders to be ruled out in the differential diagnosis are chondromalacia patellae, dorsal defect of the patella, and osteochondral fractures related to direct injury or recurrent dislocation. Chondromalacia patellae usually is confined to the cartilaginous layer of the bone, and radiographs are entirely normal. The dorsal defect of the patella is a benign, well-defined lytic defect in the superolateral aspect of the bone. This defect may be bilateral and is asymptomatic. Dislocation of the patella is associated with an osteochondral fracture at the medial side of the patella and, less frequently,

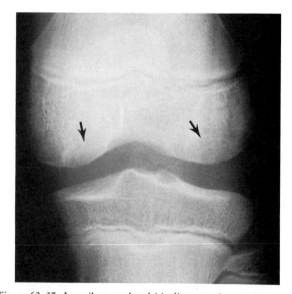

Figure 62–37. Juvenile osteochondritis dissecans. Symmetric abnormalities in both knees were evident on radiographic examination of this child. The frontal radiograph of one knee shows irregularities in both the medial and the lateral femoral condyles (arrows). (Courtesy of J. Eglehoff, M.D., and R. Towbin, M.D., Cincinnati, Ohio.)

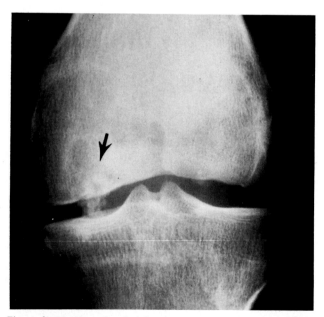

Figure 62–38. Transchondral fractures (osteochondritis dissecans) of the femoral condyles. Note the healed defect in the medial femoral condyle (arrow) and osseous bodies in the joint.

at the lateral margin of the lateral femoral condyle (Fig. 62–40).

Talus. Osteochondral fractures are also recognized in the talar dome, especially the middle third of the lateral border of the talus and the posterior third of the medial border. Men are affected more often than women, and the patients are usually in the second to fourth decades of life. Clinical findings are variable. The lateral talar lesion appears to relate to an inversion injury of the ankle (Fig. 62–41). This osteochondral fragment may remain in place, invert or rotate, or be displaced. The medial talar dome lesion may be related to plantar flexion of the foot with inversion, followed by rotation of the tibia on the talus (Fig. 62–42). The medial talar fracture is frequently larger than the lateral talar lesion. Although unilateral alterations predominate, bilateral changes involving the medial talar dome, the lateral talar dome, or both domes are encountered.

Anteroposterior, lateral, internal, and external oblique projections should be obtained to evaluate this lesion. These views may be supplemented by radiographs taken with the ankle in stress and with varying degrees of plantar and dorsiflexion of the ankle, and by fluoroscopy and conventional or computed tomography.

Other Sites. Posttraumatic osteochondral fractures, osteochondritis dissecans, and necrosis can be identified at other sites (see Chapter 71), including other tarsal bones and the tibia, the humeral head, the elbow (Fig. 62–43), and the wrist. In fact, osteochondral fractures can accompany a variety of joint dislocations, a typical example of which is the Hill-Sachs deformity that complicates anterior dislocation of the humeral head (see later discussion).

Fractures of the Shafts of the Long Tubular Bones

BIOMECHANICS. It is the application of an abnormal force to a bone, a process termed loading, that results in an injury. The ability of bone to absorb energy varies with the

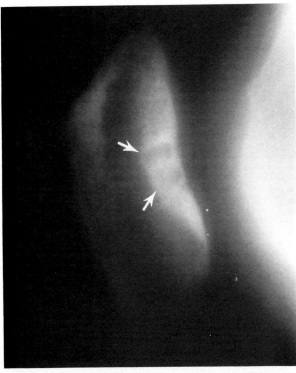

Figure 62–39. Transchondral fractures (osteochondritis dissecans) of the patella. A lateral tomogram identifies the site of injury, appearing as a cystic area with surrounding sclerosis (arrows).

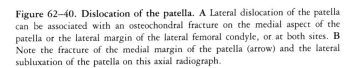

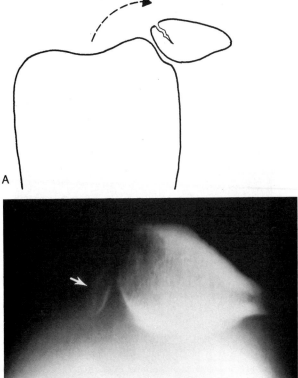

Figure 62–40. Dislocation of the patella. A Lateral dislocation of the patella can be associated with an osteochondral fracture on the medial aspect of the patella or the lateral margin of the lateral femoral condyle, or at both sites. **B** Note the fracture of the medial margin of the patella (arrow) and the lateral subluxation of the patella on this axial radiograph.

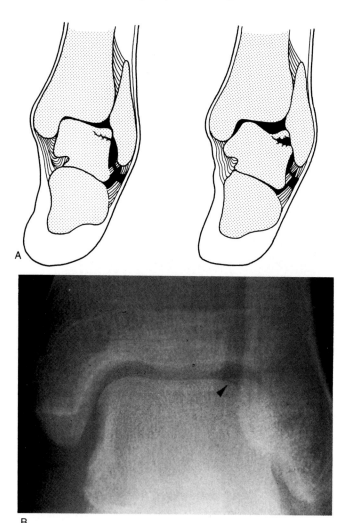

A

B

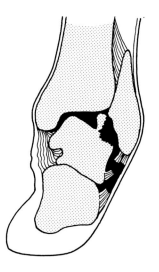
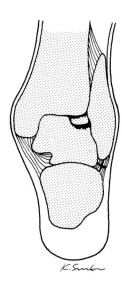

Figure 62–41. Transchondral fractures (osteochondritis dissecans) of the talus: Lateral lesion. A As the foot is inverted, the lateral border of the talar dome is compressed against the face of the fibula. Although initially the adjacent ligaments may remain intact, further inversion can produce rupture of these ligaments, with avulsion of the osteochondral fragment. This fragment may remain in situ, become inverted, or be displaced. (After Berndt AL, Harty M: Transchondral fracture (osteochondritis dissecans) of the talus. J Bone Joint Surg [Am] 41:988, 1959. Used with permission.) B An example of the lateral talar transchondral fracture. Note the oblique fracture line (arrowhead).

person's age, sex, and metabolic status and the integrity of surrounding tissues. The bones of children are more plastic than the more brittle bones of adults, a fact that contributes to the occurrence of incomplete and bowing fractures in the pediatric age group. Additional factors that contribute to the production of a fracture are the presence of a preexisting lesion and a previous surgical procedure. Cortical bone graft donor sites and pin tracts are at risk for fracture.

There are four basic types of load that can be applied to an object such as a long tubular bone: *tension* (or traction) forces act perpendicular to the cross section of the bone, pulling apart trabeculae; *compression* forces act in a similar perpendicular direction, pressing together trabeculae; *torsion* (or rotational) forces are twisting in nature; and *bending* forces lead to angulation. Of these types of force, compression, torsion, and bending working independently or in combination are common causes of bone injury; tension forces usually result in soft tissue rather than osseous alterations.

The fracture configuration or pattern depends on the interaction of a particular load and a specific bone (Fig. 62–44; Table 62–3):

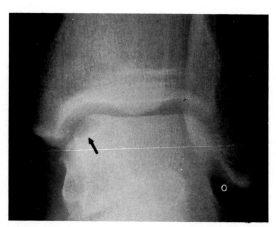

Figure 62–42. Transchondral fractures (osteochondritis dissecans) of the talus: Medial lesion. Note the lucent lesion of the medial talar dome (arrow), the site of an osteochondral fragment.

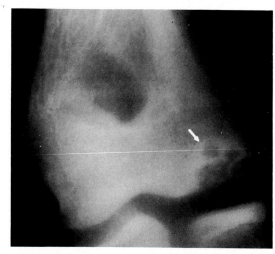

Figure 62–43. Transchondral fractures (osteochondritis dissecans) of the capitulum of the humerus. Note cystic and sclerotic changes (arrow).

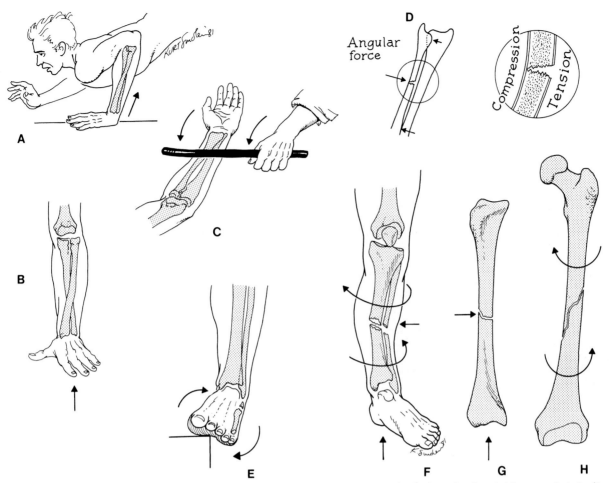

Figure 62–44. Biomechanics of fractures in long tubular bones. A, B Application of longitudinal compression force (axial compression). Loading of a long bone in this manner may cause an incomplete (bowing or torus) fracture in a child or an impaction of the diaphysis into the metaphysis in an adult (e.g., an intercondylar fracture of the distal portion of the humerus or femur.) C, D Application of angular force (bending). This may result in a greenstick fracture in a child or a transverse fracture in an adult. Cortical bone is stronger in compression than in tension, so that the bone fails initially on the tension side (opposite to the input force) and the fracture propagates transversely to the long axis of the bone. The periosteum may be preserved on the side of the input force. E Traction force (tension) at the site of a tendon or ligament insertion may result in a transverse (avulsion) fracture. F The oblique fracture configuration results from a combination of multiple forces, including longitudinal compression and angular and rotational forces. G An oblique-transverse fracture results from a combination of angular and axial compression forces. The direction of the fracture line is determined by the relative magnitude of the two forces: When axial compression force predominates, the oblique component is larger; conversely, a predominantly angular force results in a more transverse fracture configuration. The oblique fragment may separate in a butterfly configuration. H A spiral fracture results from rotational forces. The fracture line approximates an angle of 40 to 45 degrees, and the direction of the spiral denotes that of the rotational forces.

Table 62–3. BIOMECHANICS OF FRACTURES IN LONG TUBULAR BONES

Fracture Pattern	Mechanism of Injury	Location of Soft Tissue Hinge	Energy Load	Common Sites
Transverse	Bending	Concavity	Low	Diaphyses
Oblique	Compression, bending, and torsion	Concavity (often destroyed)	Moderate	Radius, ulna, tibia, fibula
Oblique-transverse	Compression and bending	Concavity or side of butterfly fragment	Moderate	Femur, tibia, humerus
Spiral	Torsion	Vertical segment	Low	Tibia, humerus
Diaphyseal impaction	Compression	Variable	Variable	Humerus, femur, tibia
Comminuted	Variable	Destroyed	High	Variable

From Gozna ER, Harrington IJ: Biomechanics of Musculoskeletal Injury. © 1982, Williams & Wilkins Co, Baltimore, pp 2, 21. Used with permission.

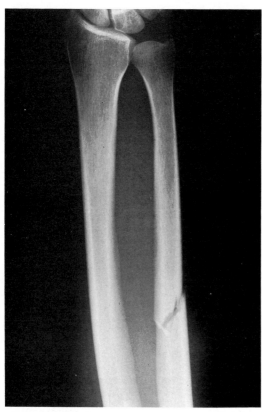

Figure 62–45. Oblique fracture. An oblique fracture of the midshaft of the ulna has resulted from a direct blow. The radius is intact.

1. *Transverse fracture* (mechanism: bending, or angular, forces in long bones; tensile, or traction, forces in short bones). A transverse fracture line, occurring at a right angle to the shaft, usually is the result of a bending force. There is tensile failure of the bone on its convex side (opposite to the input force) with subsequent compressive failure of bone on its concave side. Often, the cortex on the compressive side fails before the transverse fracture is complete, resulting in cortical splintering. A soft tissue hinge may be preserved on the side of the input force. Transverse fractures may also be caused by traction forces at sites of tendon or ligament insertion in bone.

2. *Oblique fracture* (mechanism: a combination of compression, bending, and torsion forces). Combined forces consisting of compression and torsion and, to a lesser extent, bending typically lead to an oblique fracture (Fig. 62–45). Such a fracture resembles a spiral fracture superficially, although it has a higher frequency of nonunion. In an oblique fracture, the ends of the bones are short and blunt, a vertical segment is not identified, and a clear space may be seen. In a spiral fracture, long, sharp, and pointed ends and a vertical segment are characteristic, and, unless the fracture is distracted, no clear space is evident. An oblique fracture most commonly involves the paired bones of either the forearm or the lower leg.

3. *Oblique-transverse fracture* (mechanism: a combination of axial compression and bending forces). An oblique-transverse fracture (Fig. 62–46) is a common fracture configuration, particularly in the tibia, femur, and humerus. A butterfly fragment may be an added component of this fracture pattern. This fragment occurs on the compression side of the bone on

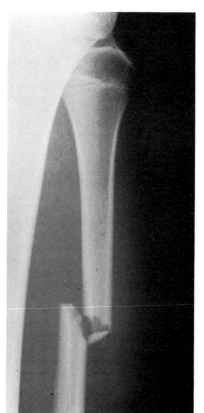

Figure 62–46. Oblique-transverse fracture. This fracture of the fibula is slightly comminuted.

which the force impacts. Such fragments commonly are identified in fractures of the tubular bones of the lower extremity in pedestrians injured by automobiles.

4. *Spiral fracture* (mechanism: torsion force). Spiral fractures, which are relatively uncommon, are usually observed in the humerus and the tibia (Fig. 62–47). The short, straight longitudinal portion of a spiral fracture represents the initial site of bone failure, which subsequently propagates both proximally and distally.

5. *Diaphyseal impaction fracture* (mechanism: axial compression force). In certain locations such as the humerus, femur, and tibia, an axially applied load will drive the diaphyseal bone, with its thick and rigid cortex, into the thin metaphyseal bone; examples of this injury are the supracondylar fracture of the femur and the comminuted fracture of the tibial plateaus.

6. *Comminuted fracture* (mechanism: variable). Indirect or direct application of force, usually of high energy, leads to multiple osseous fragments of varying size.

SPECIFIC SITES. Some of the important characteristics of fractures of the shafts of the humerus, radius, ulna, femur, tibia, and fibula are contained in Tables 62–4 to 62–7.

DISLOCATIONS
Terminology

A *dislocation* results when there is complete loss of contact between two osseous surfaces that normally articulate. A *subluxation* represents a partial loss of this contact. A closed subluxation or dislocation exists when the skin and soft tissues remain intact over the injured joint; an open dislocation or

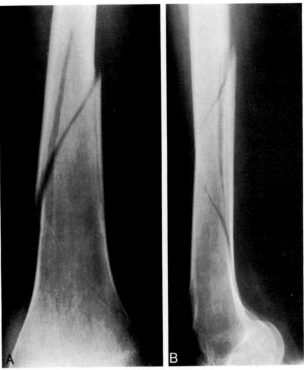

Figure 62–47. Spiral fracture. Anteroposterior (**A**) and lateral (**B**) radiographs reveal the fracture of the femoral diaphysis.

Table 62–4. FRACTURES OF THE HUMERAL METAPHYSES AND SHAFT

Site	Characteristics	Complications
Proximal	Middle-aged and elderly adults	Lipohemarthrosis
	Classified as one-part to four-part based on the degree and the location of displacement	Drooping shoulder related to hemarthrosis, capsular tear, muscle or nerve injury
		Osteonecrosis, especially with displaced fractures of humeral neck and four-part fractures
		Osteoarthritis
		Heterotopic ossification
		Rotator cuff tear
		Brachial plexus and, less commonly, axillary artery injury
		Painful arc of motion
Middle	Adults > children	Delayed union or nonunion when fracture is transverse or distracted
	Most common at junction of distal and middle thirds	Radial nerve injury in 5 to 15 per cent of cases
	Associated fractures in 25 per cent of cases (ulna, clavicle, or humerus)	Brachial artery injury
	Characteristic displacements related to sites of muscular attachment	
Supracondylar	Children >> adults	Brachial artery injury
	Extension (95 per cent) and flexion (5 per cent) types	Median, ulnar, or radial nerve injury
	Paradoxic posterior fat pad sign	Alignment abnormalities
	Supracondylar process may fracture	Heterotopic ossification
		Volkmann's ischemic contracture

Table 62–5. FRACTURES OF THE RADIAL AND ULNAR SHAFTS

Site	Characteristics	Complications
Ulna (alone)	*"Nightstick" fracture*: direct blow to forearm, distal ulna > middle ulna > proximal ulna	Displacement at fracture site (uncommon)
	Monteggia injury:	Injury to branches of radial nerve (approximately 20 per cent of cases)
	Type I: Fracture of middle or upper third of ulna with anterior dislocation of radial head (65 per cent)	
	Type II: Fracture of middle or upper third of ulna with posterior dislocation of radial head (18 per cent)	
	Type III: Fracture of ulna just distal to coronoid process with lateral dislocation of radial head (16 per cent)	
	Type IV: Fracture of upper or middle third of ulna with anterior dislocation of radial head and fracture of proximal portion of the radius (1 per cent)	
Radius (alone)	*Proximal and middle segments*: Uncommon as usually associated with ulnar fracture	
	Galeazzi's injury: Fracture of the radial shaft with dislocation or subluxation of inferior radioulnar joint, caused by direct blow or fall on the outstretched hand with pronation of forearm, variable degrees of displacement at fracture site	Angulation
		Entrapment of extensor carpi ulnaris tendon (rare)
		Delayed union or nonunion
Radius and ulna	Closed or open	Delayed union or nonunion (especially of ulna)
	Nondisplaced or displaced (displacement more common in adults than in children)	Infection, especially in open fractures
		Nerve and vascular injuries, especially in open fractures and those with severe displacement
		Compartment syndromes
		Synostosis between radius and ulna (rare)

Table 62–6. FRACTURES OF THE FEMORAL SHAFT

Site	Characteristics	Complications
Any level	Major violence with associated injuries of femur, tibia, patella, acetabulum, hip, and knee	Refracture
	Open or closed	Peroneal nerve injury owing to skeletal traction
	Spiral, oblique, or transverse fracture with possible butterfly fragment and comminution	Vascular injury (femoral artery)
		Thrombophlebitis
		Nonunion (1 per cent of cases), malunion, or delayed union
		Infection
		Fat embolization (approximately 10 per cent of cases)
Proximal	Associated with osteoporosis and Paget's disease	Malalignment
	Less common than midshaft fractures	Nonunion
	Commonly extend into subtrochanteric region	
Middle	Most common site	
	Transverse fracture is most typical	
Distal and supracondylar	Less common than midshaft fractures	Malalignment
		Arterial injury

Table 62–7. FRACTURES OF THE TIBIAL AND FIBULAR SHAFTS

Site	Characteristics	Complications
Tibia	Direct or indirect trauma	Delayed union (no osseous union at 20 weeks) in 5 to 15 per cent of cases
	Associated fractures of the fibula especially in direct and severe trauma	Nonunion (no osseous union at 6 months to 1 year) is most common in the distal third of tibia
	Transverse or comminuted fracture in direct trauma; oblique or spiral fracture in indirect trauma; sometimes segmental fractures	Infection with or without nonunion
	Middle and distal thirds > proximal third	Vascular injury (to anterior tibial artery or, less commonly, posterior tibial artery)
	Minor, moderate, or major categories of injury, the last associated with comminuted and open fractures	Compartment syndrome (anterior > posterior or lateral compartments)
	Prognosis related to amount of displacement, degree of comminution, open or closed fracture, and infection	Nerve injury (uncommon, peroneal and posterior tibial nerves)
		Refracture (especially in athletes)
	Childhood fractures:	Leg shortening
	Toddler fracture—spiral fracture, undisplaced	Osteoarthritis (if fracture extends into joint)
	Proximal metaphyseal fracture—associated with genu valgum deformity	Reflex sympathetic dystrophy syndrome
		Fat embolism
Fibula	Isolated fractures are rare, related to direct injury	Related to those of the associated tibial or ankle injury
	Associated fractures of the tibia and ankle injuries	

subluxation exists if there is associated soft tissue injury that exposes the joint to the outside environment (Fig. 62–48).

Many traumatic dislocations and subluxations are associated with fractures of a neighboring bone. Indeed, characteristic fractures in periarticular bone can confirm the presence of a previous dislocation in patients in whom spontaneous reduction of the injury has occurred. Typical examples of such fractures are the Hill-Sachs lesion of the humeral head occurring after an anterior dislocation of the glenohumeral joint and the medial patellar fracture following lateral dislocation of the patella. Furthermore, these fractures may predispose the joint to future dislocations.

An accurate description of a dislocation or subluxation varies with the anatomic complexity of the involved joint. When the joint is composed of two bones, the joint injury derives its name from that articulation (e.g., dislocation of the hip, glenohumeral, or interphalangeal joint). When the joint comprises more than two bones, the dislocation is still

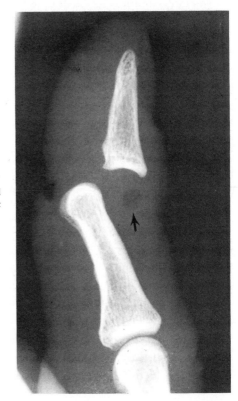

Figure 62–48. Open dislocation. Dorsal dislocation of the terminal phalanx at the interphalangeal joint of the thumb is associated with a soft tissue defect in the volar surface of the finger and soft tissue air (arrow).

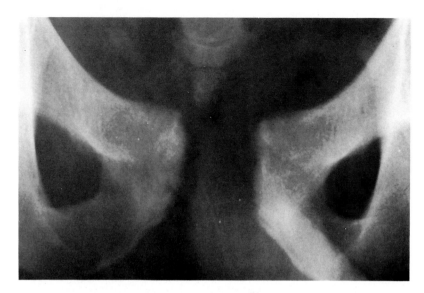

Figure 62–49. Diastasis. Abnormal widening of the symphysis pubis is apparent.

named after the involved articulation if it affects the two major bones. If the smaller bone of the three is dislocated, the injury is named after that bone (e.g., a dislocation of the patella).

A third type of joint derangement is termed a *diastasis* (Fig. 62–49). This term refers to abnormal separation of a joint that is normally only slightly moveable (e.g., the distal tibiofibular syndesmosis, the symphysis pubis, or the sacroiliac joint).

Biomechanics

Conventional classification schemes define four types of joint motion: gliding and angular movements, circumduction, and rotation. The precise characteristics of joint movement are governed principally by the shape of the articular surfaces (Table 62–8). In general, increasing freedom of movement is achieved at the expense of joint stability.

The stability of a joint can be influenced by both intrinsic factors (the shape of the apposing articular surfaces) and

extrinsic factors (the strength of surrounding ligaments and muscles). Closely fitted articular surfaces, such as exist in the hip, are inherently stable; poorly fitted articular surfaces, such as exist in the knee, are inherently unstable and depend on the stability provided by the strong ligaments and muscles that connect their components. Although trauma may produce a dislocation of any joint, the most commonly involved sites are the glenohumeral joint, elbow, ankle, hip, and interphalangeal joints.

SOME SPECIFIC SITES OF FRACTURE AND DISLOCATION
Shoulder

GLENOHUMERAL JOINT DISLOCATION. The glenohumeral joint is relatively unstable, the stability being provided in large part by surrounding capsular and ligamentous structures. Therefore, dislocations of this joint occur often. These dislocations can be classified into anterior, posterior, superior, and inferior types. *Anterior dislocation* is by far the most frequent, representing over 95 per cent of such injuries (Fig. 62–50). Anterior dislocations are further classified as subcoracoid (the most common type), subglenoid (second in frequency), and subclavicular and intrathoracic (rare types of anterior dislocation). Anterior dislocations (as well as posterior dislocations of the glenohumeral joint) are best evaluated radiographically by the inclusion of a lateral scapular projection or an axillary projection, or both, in addition to the standard frontal views of the shoulder.

Anterior dislocations are associated with a compression fracture, the Hill-Sachs lesion, on the posterolateral aspect of the humeral head that is produced by impaction of the humerus against the anterior rim of the glenoid fossa. It has been detected in approximately 25 per cent of acute anterior dislocations and 75 per cent of recurrent anterior dislocations. It frequently is larger in those cases that are dislocated for a considerable period of time, those that are recurrent, and those in which the direction of dislocation is anteroinferior rather than purely anterior. Films obtained in various degrees of internal rotation are mandatory for radiographic diagnosis of the Hill-Sachs lesion, as such rotation of the humerus will

Table 62–8. MORPHOLOGIC CLASSIFICATION OF SYNOVIAL JOINTS

Type of Joint	Motion	Examples
Plane	Uniaxial	Intermetatarsal, intercarpal
Hinge	Uniaxial	Humeroulnar, interphalangeal
Pivot	Uniaxial	Proximal radioulnar, median atlantoaxial
Bicondylar	Uniaxial (minimal movement also in a second axis)	Knee, temporomandibular
Ellipsoid	Biaxial	Radiocarpal, metacarpophalangeal
Sellar	Biaxial	First carpometacarpal, ankle, calcaneocuboid
Spheroidal	Triaxial	Hip, glenohumeral

Adapted from Williams PL, Warwick R: Gray's Anatomy, 36th British Ed. Philadelphia, WB Saunders Co, 1980, p 430. Used with permission.

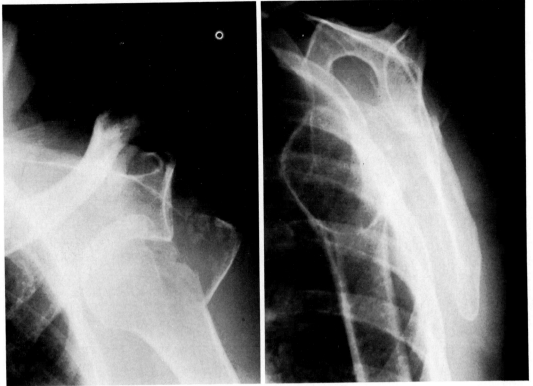

Figure 62–50. Glenohumeral joint: Anterior dislocation. A standard frontal radiograph (**A**) shows medial displacement of the humeral head and a fracture of the greater tuberosity. The tangential scapular projection (**B**) reveals the abnormal position of the humeral head, which is located in front of the glenoid cavity.

produce a tangential view of the osseous lesion (Fig. 62–51). The radiographic detection of a Hill-Sachs lesion confirms the nature of a shoulder injury that may be obscure clinically, implies a propensity for recurrent dislocation, and influences

the necessity for and choice of a surgical procedure (Table 62–9).

A second type of fracture accompanying anterior dislocation of the humeral head involves the glenoid fossa and is called the Bankart lesion (Fig. 62–52). When osseous fragmentation of the anterior glenoid rim occurs, the abnormality may be apparent on plain film radiographs in frontal or axillary projections. Specialized radiographic projections such as the Didiee and the West Point views are of further diagnostic help. The fracture may include only the cartilaginous surface of the bone, however, and conventional or computed arthro-

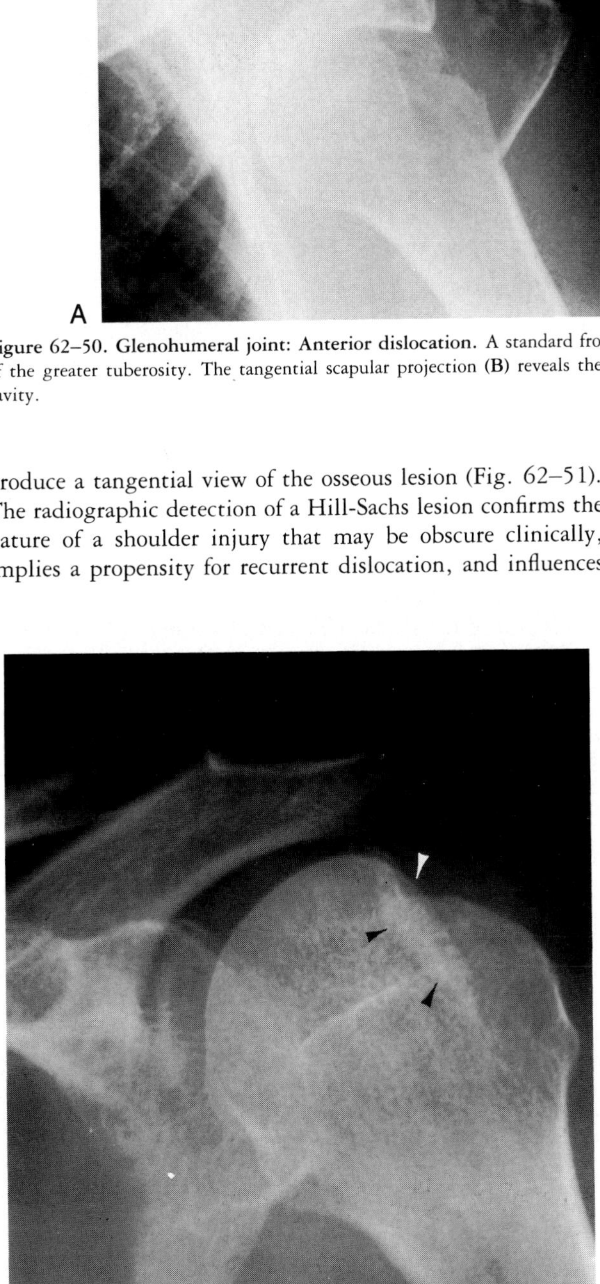

Figure 62–51. Glenohumeral joint: Anterior dislocation—Hill-Sachs lesion. The internal rotation view reveals the extent of the Hill-Sachs lesion (arrowheads).

Table 62–9. SOME TYPES OF SURGICAL PROCEDURES USED FOR RECURRENT ANTERIOR GLENOHUMERAL JOINT DISLOCATIONS

Procedure	Technique
Bankart	Repair of anterior capsular mechanism using drill holes and sutures
Putti-Platt	Shortening of the anterior capsule and subscapularis muscle
Magnuson-Stack	Transfer of the subscapularis tendon from lesser tuberosity to greater tuberosity
Eden-Hybbinette	Bone graft to anterior glenoid region
Oudard	Bone graft to coracoid process
Trillat	Osteotomy with displacement of coracoid process
Bristow-Helfet	Transfer of coracoid process with its attached tendons to neck of the scapula

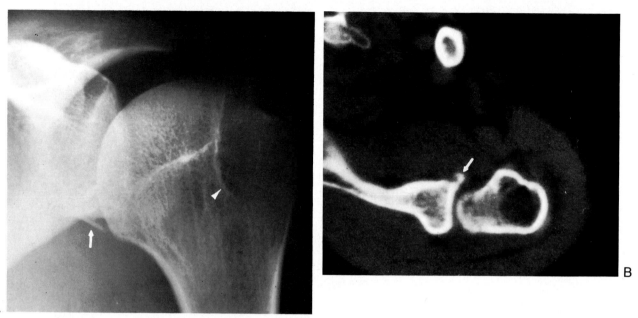

A

B

Figure 62–52. Glenohumeral joint: Anterior dislocation—Bankart lesion. A Disruption of the anterior margin of the glenoid fossa is seen (arrow). A Hill-Sachs lesion also is seen (arrowhead). B Computed tomography (transaxial scan) shows a typical osseous Bankart lesion (arrow).

tomography may be necessary to detect the changes (see Chapter 14).

Posterior dislocation of the glenohumeral joint constitutes approximately 2 to 4 per cent of all shoulder dislocations. Specific types of posterior dislocation include the subacromial (the most common type) and the subglenoid and subspinous (rare injuries) varieties. Many cases of posterior dislocation result from convulsions. Physical examination reveals a posteriorly displaced humeral head that is held in internal rotation. Associated injuries include fracture of the posterior aspect of the glenoid rim, an avulsion fracture of the lesser tuberosity of the humerus, and a stretched or detached subscapularis tendon.

The routine radiographic examination must include a lateral view of the scapula (Fig. 62–53) or an axillary view of the shoulder, or both. On an anteroposterior radiograph, posterior dislocation of the humeral head distorts the normal elliptical radiodense area created by the overlapping of the head and the glenoid fossa (Fig. 62–54). The posterior displacement of the humeral head may create a space between the anterior rim of the glenoid and the humeral head that frequently is greater than 6 mm ("vacant" glenoid cavity). In addition, the normal parallel pattern of the articular surfaces of the glenoid concavity and the humeral head convexity is lost. Other radiographic signs of posterior dislocation on frontal radiographs include a fixed position of internal rotation of the humerus and a second cortical line, the trough line, parallel and lateral to the subchondral articular surface of the humeral head. This line represents the margin of a trough-like impaction fracture of the humeral head created when this structure contacts the posterior glenoid rim during the dislocation.

Computed tomography also can be used to evaluate patients with acute (or chronic) dislocations of the glenohumeral joint (Fig. 62–55).

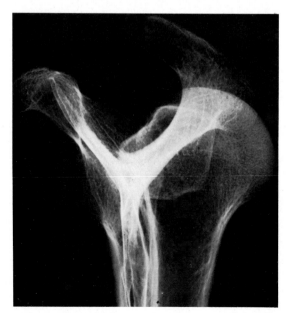

Figure 62–53. Glenohumeral joint: Posterior dislocation—use of lateral scapular projection (specimen radiograph). The lateral projection of the scapula outlines the posterior position of the humeral head, which is located beneath the acromion process. The degree of humeral displacement in cases of posterior glenohumeral joint dislocation is variable; in many instances, it is subluxed rather than truly dislocated. (From Greenway GD, et al: The painful shoulder. Med Radiogr Photogr 58:22, 1982. Used with permission.)

Superior dislocation of the glenohumeral joint is rare (Fig. 62–56). An extreme forward and upward force on the adducted arm can produce extensive damage to the rotator cuff, capsule, biceps tendon, and surrounding musculature and fracture of the acromion, clavicle, coracoid process, or humeral tuberosities. *Inferior dislocation* of the glenohumeral joint (luxatio erecta) is also rare (Fig. 62–57). After this injury, the superior aspect of the articular surface of the humeral head is directed inferiorly and does not contact the inferior glenoid rim. As a result, the arm is held over the patient's head, the inferior aspect of the capsule is torn, and associated injuries, including a fracture of the greater tuberosity of the humerus, of the acromion process, or of the inferior glenoid margin, may be seen.

A special type of inferior displacement of the humeral head is termed the *drooping shoulder* (Fig. 62–58). It can be associated with uncomplicated fractures of the surgical neck of the humerus. Relaxation or stretching of the supporting musculature, detachment of the capsule, and hemarthrosis have each been proposed as possible mechanisms. Recognition of this condition will eliminate erroneous diagnosis of fracture-dislocation of the proximal humerus, and conservative therapy will lead to disappearance of the drooping shoulder over a period of weeks.

ACROMIOCLAVICULAR JOINT DISLOCATION.
Subluxation or dislocation of the acromioclavicular joint represents approximately 10 per cent of all dislocations involving the shoulder. Injury to the acromioclavicular joint can result from indirect or direct forces. Such injury is classified in several ways, according to the extent of ligamentous damage (Fig. 62–59). Type I injuries are diagnosed clinically rather than radiographically, although there may be soft tissue swelling and minimal widening of the acromioclavicular joint. The radiographic diagnosis of type II and type III injuries is based on the detection of displacement of the

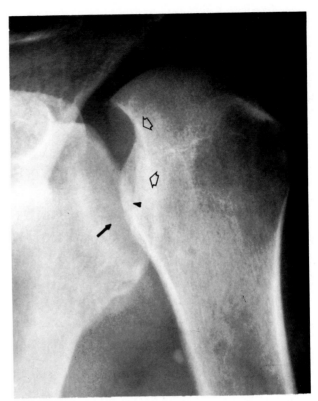

Figure 62–54. Glenohumeral joint: Posterior dislocation. An anteroposterior radiograph in a patient with a posterior glenohumeral joint dislocation. Findings include distortion of the normal elliptical radiodense region created by overlying of the humeral head and glenoid fossa (arrowhead), a "vacant" glenoid cavity (solid arrow), loss of parallelism between the articular surfaces of the glenoid cavity and humeral head, internal rotation of the humerus, and an impaction fracture (open arrows).

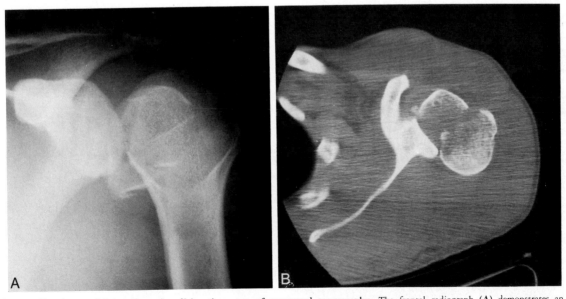

Figure 62–55. Glenohumeral joint: Posterior dislocation—use of computed tomography. The frontal radiograph (**A**) demonstrates an abnormal relationship of the humeral head and glenoid fossa, an empty glenoid cavity, and avulsion and fragmentation of the lesser tuberosity of the humerus. A transaxial computed tomographic scan (**B**) shows a posterior dislocation of the glenohumeral joint and the avulsed tuberosity.

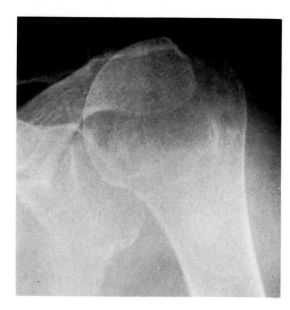

Figure 62–56. Glenohumeral joint: Superior dislocation. Note the elevation of the humeral head with respect to the glenoid cavity.

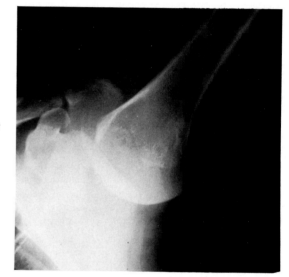

Figure 62–57. Glenohumeral joint: Inferior dislocation. The arm is held over the head.

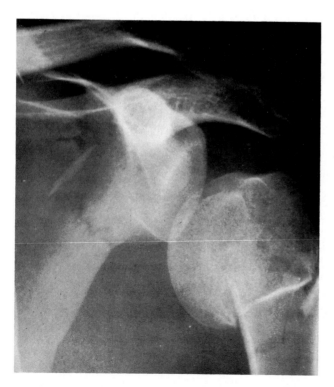

Figure 62–58. Glenohumeral joint: Drooping shoulder. A fracture of the surgical neck of the humerus is associated with inferior subluxation of the head with respect to the glenoid cavity. Observe an associated scapular fracture.

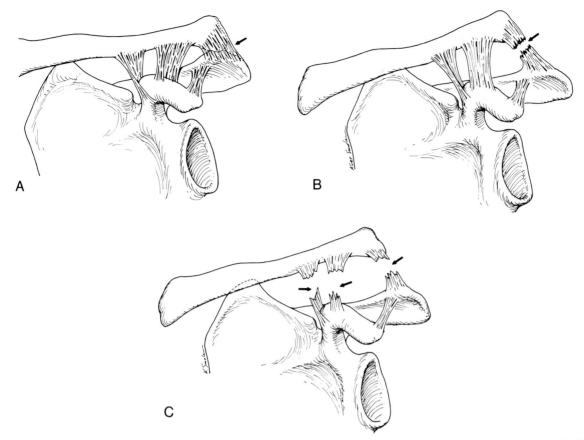

Figure 62–59. Acromioclavicular joint: Classification of injuries. A Type I injury. Stretching or tearing of the fibers of the acromioclavicular ligaments (arrow) constitutes a mild sprain. The relationship between the distal portion of the clavicle and the acromion remains normal. **B** Type II injury. Disruption of the acromioclavicular ligaments (arrow) constitutes a part of this injury, which is classified as a moderate sprain. The coracoclavicular ligament may be strained but otherwise is intact. Minor elevation of the distal portion of the clavicle or widening of the acromioclavicular joint, or both, is the anticipated radiographic abnormality. **C** Type III injury. This is a severe sprain and is characterized by disruption of both the acromioclavicular and the coracoclavicular ligaments (arrows) with dislocation of the acromioclavicular joint.

distal portion of the clavicle with relation to the acromion and on the degree of displacement that is evident (Fig. 62–60). Special radiographs may be required, including films obtained with weight held in the hand (stress radiographs).

Certain complications can be noted after subluxation or dislocation of the acromioclavicular joint. Coracoclavicular ligamentous ossification may occur within a period of weeks after the traumatic episode and can be prominent in as many as 70 per cent of cases (Fig. 62–61). Posttraumatic osteolysis of the distal portion of the clavicle is another complication of acute or repetitive injury to the acromioclavicular joint or adjacent bones (see Chapter 84), and osteoarthritis of the acromioclavicular joint represents a further complication of dislocation or subluxation.

STERNOCLAVICULAR JOINT DISLOCATION. Sternoclavicular joint injuries represent only about 2 to 3 per cent of all shoulder dislocations and result from direct or indirect force of great magnitude. Anterior dislocations predominate over posterior (retrosternal) dislocations. Radiographic analysis is facilitated by a variety of special projections (see Chapter 3) and may be supplemented with conventional or computed tomography. Prompt recognition of the less common posterior sternoclavicular joint dislocation (Fig. 62–62) is required because the displaced clavicle may impinge on the trachea, the esophagus, the great vessels, or the major

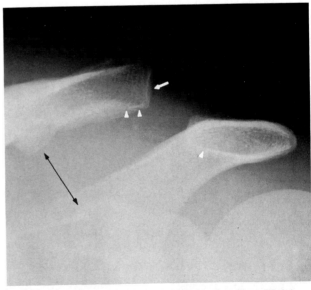

Figure 62–60. Acromioclavicular joint dislocation: Type III injury. Observe superior displacement of the clavicle (arrow) with respect to the acromion. The inferior margin of the clavicle no longer is aligned with the inferior margin of the acromion (arrowheads). There is widening of the acromioclavicular joint and an increased distance between the clavicle and the coracoid process (double-ended arrow.)

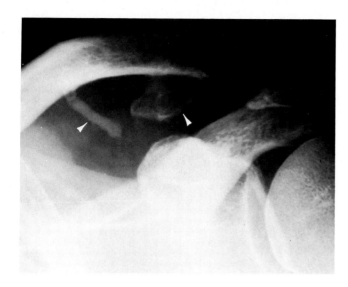

Figure 62–61. Acromioclavicular joint dislocation: Coracoclavicular ligament ossification. Observe ligamentous ossification (arrowheads) in a patient who had a type III injury of the acromioclavicular joint.

nerves in the superior mediastinum, leading to vascular compromise, cough, dysphagia, and dyspnea.

An additional injury of the medial end of the clavicle is an epiphyseal fracture or separation. The growth plate at this site is among the last to become obliterated during skeletal maturation, disappearing at approximately 25 years of age. Before the medial clavicular epiphysis ossifies at the age of about 18 years, it is extremely difficult to differentiate between a dislocation of the sternoclavicular joint and a fracture through the growth plate.

FRACTURES OF THE PROXIMAL PORTION OF THE HUMERUS. Fractures of the proximal portion of the humerus typically are seen in middle-aged and elderly patients. They are more frequent in women than in men, and—in common with fractures of the vertebral bodies, proximal portion of the femur, and distal portion of the radius—their likelihood of occurrence after injury is very much dependent on the severity of osteopenia.

The classification of fractures of the proximal region of the humerus is based on the presence or the absence of significant displacement of one or more of the four major osseous segments of this part of the humerus (Fig. 62–63). These segments are the articular segment containing the anatomic neck; the greater tuberosity; the lesser tuberosity; and the shaft and surgical neck. Approximately 80 per cent of fractures of the proximal portion of the humerus are undisplaced. A displaced fracture exists if any of the four segments is separated by more than 1 cm from its neighbor or is angulated more than 45 degrees. Nondisplaced fractures or fractures with minimal displacement that do not meet these criteria are considered one-part fractures. A two-part fracture is one in which only a single segment is displaced in relation to the other three; two-part fractures represent approximately 15 per cent of all fractures of the proximal portion of the humerus. A three-part fracture, representing approximately 3 or 4 per cent of humeral fractures, occurs when two segments are displaced with relationship to the other two parts, and a four-part fracture, occurring in approximately 3 or 4 per cent of cases, exists when all the humeral segments are displaced. The term fracture-dislocation indicates that the articular segment of the humerus is displaced beyond the joint space (Fig. 62–64).

Several patterns of intraarticular fracture of the humeral head may be encountered. Impaction of the articular surface

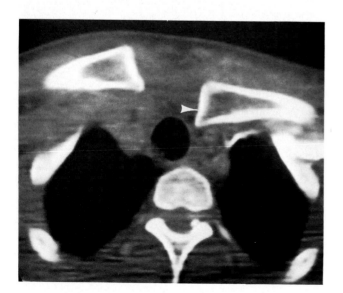

Figure 62–62. Sternoclavicular joint: Posterior dislocation. A transaxial computed tomographic scan reveals the posterior position of the injured clavicle (arrowhead) and its relationship to the trachea.

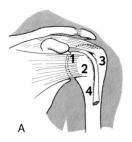

A

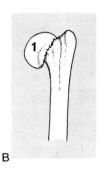

B

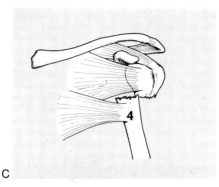

C

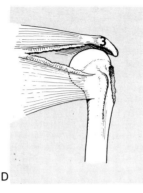

D

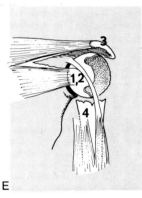

E

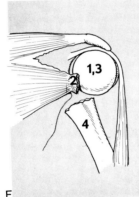

F

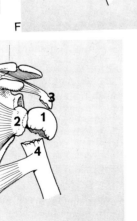

G

Figure 62–63. Fractures of the proximal portion of the humerus: System of classification. A Normal situation. Four major segments of the proximal portion of the humerus are identified: 1, humeral head; 2, lesser tuberosity; 3, greater tuberosity; 4, humeral shaft. B Two-part fracture. In this example, a fracture of the anatomic neck has led to displacement of the humeral head (1). Ischemic necrosis may complicate this rare injury. C Two-part fracture. In this example, displacement of the humeral shaft (4) relates to the pull of the pectoralis major muscle. The rotator cuff is intact and holds the humeral head in a neutral position. Variations of this fracture pattern relate to the extent of impaction, angulation, and comminution. D Two-part fracture. In this example, displacement of the greater tuberosity (3) occurs owing to the forces generated by a portion of the rotator cuff musculature. Retraction of more than 1.0 cm of the entire greater tuberosity or one of its facets is pathognomonic of a longitudinal tear of the rotator cuff. The fragment tends to be large in younger patients and small in older individuals. A complication of this injury is impaired motion of the shoulder. E Three-part fracture. In this injury, the greater tuberosity (3) is displaced and the subscapularis rotates the humeral head (1,2) so that its articular surface faces posteriorly. The diaphysis (4) is displaced relative to the rotated head owing to the action of the pectoralis major muscle. F Three-part fracture. In this type of injury, the lesser tuberosity (2) is detached and displaced by the action of the subscapularis muscle, and the supraspinatus and external rotators cause the articular surface of the humeral head (1,3) to face anteriorly. 4, Humeral shaft. G Four-part fracture. The articular segment (1) is detached from the tuberosities (2,3) and from its circulation and is displaced laterally (as shown), anteriorly, or posteriorly, losing contact with the glenoid cavity. The tuberosities are usually retracted by the attached musculature. (From Neer CS II, Rockwood CA Jr: Fractures and dislocations of the shoulder. In CA Rockwood, DP Greene [Eds]: Fractures in Adults. 2nd Ed. Philadelphia, JB Lippincott Co, 1984, p 675. Used with permission.)

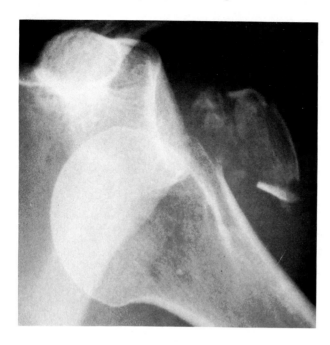

Figure 62–64. Fracture-dislocation of the shoulder. An anterior (subcoracoid) dislocation of the glenohumeral joint is associated with a displaced and comminuted fracture of the greater tuberosity of the humerus.

against the anterior or posterior rim of the glenoid cavity in cases of anterior or posterior glenohumeral joint dislocation has been considered earlier in this chapter. More severe fragmentation or comminution can accompany central impaction of the humeral head against the glenoid cavity. Complications of fractures of the articular head of the humerus include lipohemarthrosis, production of intraarticular osteocartilaginous fragments, inferior displacement of the humeral head (drooping shoulder), and osteoarthritis.

Lipohemarthrosis, with the release of fat and blood into the articular cavity, can follow intracapsular fractures of the humerus (as well as similar fractures at other sites). The source of the fat within the joint space is assumed to be the bone marrow. Radiographic demonstration of lipohemarthrosis is facilitated by the inclusion of radiographs obtained with horizontal beam technique.

Inferior displacement of the humerus, producing the drooping shoulder, may accompany intraarticular or extraarticular fractures (Fig. 62–58). The findings should not be misinterpreted as a true dislocation of the glenohumeral joint, as the condition is self-limited. Factors important in its development may include hemarthrosis, detachment of the joint capsule, stretching of the support musculature, or injury to the brachial plexus.

Delayed union or nonunion can accompany any type of fracture of the proximal portion of the humerus. *Osteonecrosis* is associated with fractures of the humeral head and neck that lead to loss of the blood supply from both the muscular insertions and the arcuate branch of the internal humeral circumflex artery. This complication, which is reported in 7 to 50 per cent of cases, is most typical of displaced fractures of the anatomic neck of the humerus and a severe fracture or fracture-dislocation of the bone (four-part fracture).

Fractures involving the articular surface of the humeral head may be complicated by *osteoarthritis* with joint space narrowing, sclerosis, and osteophytosis. Fracture-dislocations of the proximal portion of the humerus can also be associated with *heterotopic bone formation* in pericapsular regions. Humeral fractures associated with considerable retraction of the greater

tuberosity or the lesser tuberosity are characterized by tears in the *rotator cuff* (see later discussion).

Anterior fracture-dislocation of the proximal portion of the humerus can lead to injury of the nearby *brachial plexus* and, less commonly, the *axillary artery*.

FRACTURES OF THE CLAVICLE. It is the subcutaneous location of the clavicle that is responsible, at least in part, for the high frequency of fractures of this bone. With regard to the analysis of these fractures, it is convenient to divide the bone into three functional segments: a distal or interligamentous segment consisting of the outer 25 to 30 per cent of the bone, the region about and distal to the coracoclavicular ligament; an intermediate segment consisting of the middle 40 to 50 per cent of the bone; and an inner segment consisting of the medial 25 per cent of the bone. Approximately 75 to 80 per cent of clavicular fractures involve the middle segment of the bone, 15 to 20 per cent involve the distal segment, and 5 per cent affect the inner segment. Nonunion is frequent in cases of fracture distal to the coracoclavicular ligament, whereas this complication is rare in cases of fracture of the medial segment of the bone.

Fractures of the middle segment of the clavicle usually result from a fall onto the outstretched hand or a fall on the shoulder. The radiographic findings permit prompt and accurate diagnosis (Fig. 62–65).

Fractures of the distal portion of the clavicle, related to a force applied on the shoulder driving the humerus and scapula downward, are divided into two types: type I fractures, in which the coracoclavicular ligaments are intact; and type II fractures, in which the coracoclavicular ligaments are severed (Fig. 62–66). Type II fractures have a poorer prognosis related to more significant displacement at the fracture site and to nonunion. Associated fractures of the coracoid process and ribs may be evident (Fig. 62–67).

Direct trauma accounts for the majority of fractures of the medial end of the clavicle. When the costoclavicular ligament remains intact and attached to the outer fragment, displacement does not occur.

In children, clavicular fractures heal rapidly without sig-

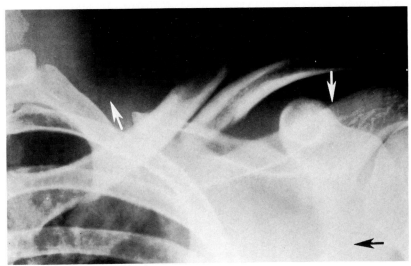

Figure 62–65. Clavicular fracture: Intermediate segment. The typical configuration of such a fracture is illustrated. Note that the medial portion of the clavicle is pulled upward by the sternocleidomastoid muscle; the lateral portion is pulled downward by the weight of the arm and inward by the pectoralis major and latissimus dorsi muscles. Arrows indicate the direction of these forces. The result is a bayonet deformity at the fracture site.

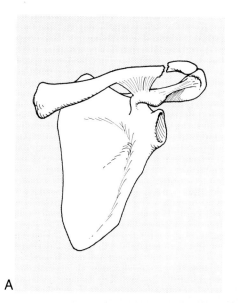

A

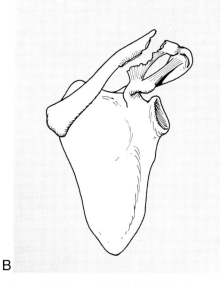

B

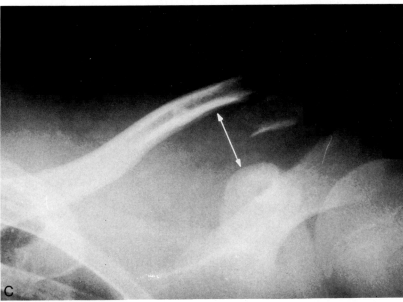

C

Figure 62–66. Clavicular fracture: Distal segment—types of injury. A Type I injury. The coracoclavicular ligaments remain intact. B Type II injury. The coracoclavicular ligaments are severed. C Type II injury. Note the widening of the coracoclavicular distance (double-ended arrow), indicating disruption of the coracoclavicular ligaments. This finding may be better evaluated with the patient holding 5 or 10 pounds of weight in the ipsilateral hand or with this weight tied to the ipsilateral wrist.

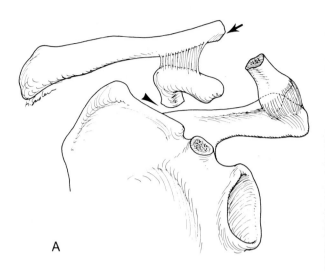

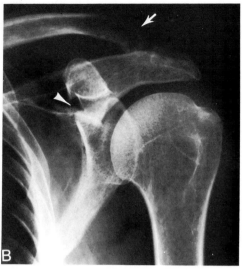

Figure 62–67. Clavicular fracture: Associated fracture of the coracoid process. A displaced fracture of the lateral segment of the clavicle (arrows) with intact coracoclavicular ligaments is accompanied by avulsion of the coracoid process (arrowheads).

nificant sequelae. In adults, resultant deformities secondary to extensive callus formation may be observed. Nonunion of a clavicular fracture is uncommon; when nonunion is present, a posttraumatic pseudarthrosis of the clavicle must be differentiated from a congenital pseudarthrosis.

FRACTURES OF THE SCAPULA. Scapular fractures constitute approximately 1 per cent of all fractures and 5 to 7 per cent of those about the shoulder. They commonly are associated with additional injuries, including fractures of the ribs, clavicle, and skull. Scapular fractures may involve one or more of the following anatomic regions: glenoid fossa and articular surface, neck, body, spinous process, acromion process, and coracoid process (Fig. 62–68). They are found most frequently in the scapular body, followed by the neck and the other regions of the bone.

A fracture of the rim of the glenoid cavity occurs in approximately 20 per cent of traumatic glenohumeral joint dislocations. Either the anterior glenoid rim (in anterior glenohumeral joint dislocations) or the posterior glenoid rim (in posterior glenohumeral joint dislocations) may be affected. Larger portions of the glenoid fossa may be fractured when the humeral head is driven against the glenoid cavity by a direct force.

A fracture in the neck of the scapula typically occurs after a direct blow on the shoulder (Fig. 62–69). The fracture line extends from the supraclavicular notch above to the coracoid process below.

Approximately 50 to 70 per cent of scapular fractures involve the body of the bone (Fig. 62–69). The typical mechanism of injury is a direct force, which may also result in fractures of neighboring ribs and pneumothorax. Radiographs will reveal the vertical or horizontal nature of the fracture line or its comminution. Displacement of the osseous fragment is unusual.

Isolated fractures of the spinous process of the scapula are infrequent. Fractures of the acromion process generally follow direct trauma; depression of the shoulder and contralateral flexion of the neck occurring after these fractures predispose to injuries of the brachial plexus.

Fractures of the coracoid process relate to a direct injury from a dislocating humeral head, a direct force on the tip of the coracoid itself, or an avulsion owing to traction on the coracoclavicular ligament (in association with acromioclavicular joint dislocation), the short head of the biceps, or the coracobrachialis. Isolated fractures of the coracoid process are observed in athletes as a result of an avulsion injury or in trapshooters related to repetitive stress from the impact of the recoiling rifle.

Traumatic lateral displacement of the scapula, scapulothoracic dissociation, is rare and is accompanied by partial or complete amputation through the soft tissue and injuries to the brachial plexus and the subclavian artery and vein.

FRACTURES OF THE FIRST AND SECOND RIBS. Fractures of the first or second rib indicate major trauma to the thorax or shoulder. Associated abnormalities include rupture of the apex of the lung or of the subclavian artery, aneurysm of the aortic arch, tracheoesophageal fistula, pleurisy, hemothorax, cardiac alterations, neurologic injury, and additional fractures. The detection of a fracture of the first rib, therefore, requires a careful evaluation of intrathoracic structures.

Elbow

ELBOW DISLOCATION. Dislocation of the elbow is a relatively frequent injury. In cases of dislocation involving both the radius and the ulna, a posterior dislocation (Fig. 62–70) is most frequent (approximately 80 to 90 per cent of all elbow dislocations). In adults, this injury may be complicated by fracture of the coronoid process of the ulna or the radial head, and in children and adolescents, the medial epicondylar ossification center is frequently avulsed and may become entrapped during reduction. Medial and lateral dislocations of the elbow are not common. Anterior dislocation also is unusual. Divergent dislocation of the elbow in which the radius and ulna move in different directions is rare.

Isolated dislocation of the ulna at the elbow is unusual. Similarly, isolated radial head dislocation without an associ-

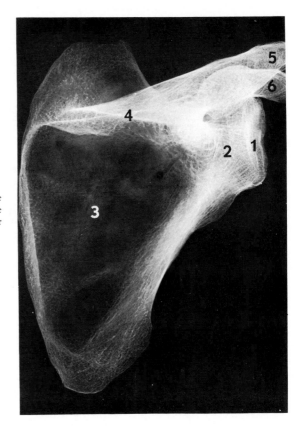

Figure 62–68. Scapular fracture: Sites of injury. Fractures of the scapula may involve the glenoid fossa and articular surface (1), the neck (2) or body (3) of the bone, or the spinous (4), acromion (5), or coracoid (6) process. They are most common in the scapular body and neck.

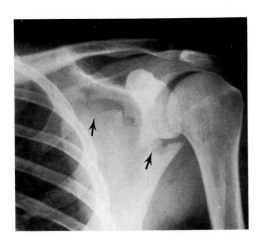

Figure 62–69. Scapular fracture: Injuries of the scapular body and neck. A horizontal fracture involves the body and neck of the bone (arrows).

Figure 62–70. Elbow: Posterior dislocation of both the radius and the ulna. The trochlea of the humerus and the coronoid process of the ulna contact each other (arrow), resulting in fracture of the articular surfaces.

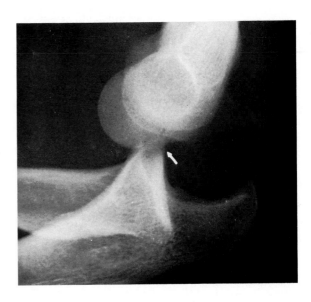

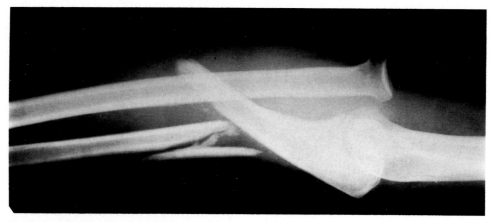

Figure 62–71. Monteggia fracture-dislocation (type I). Note the fracture of the upper one third of the ulna with anterior angulation at the fracture site and anterior dislocation of the radial head.

ated fracture in the ulna is rare in adults. In the child, subluxation of the radial head, which is usually transient in nature, is termed nursemaid's elbow.

The combination of an ulnar fracture and radial head dislocation is termed a Monteggia fracture-dislocation (Fig. 62–71). Various types of Monteggia fracture-dislocations are recognized:

1. Type I: fracture of the middle or upper third of the ulna with anterior dislocation of the radial head and anterior angulation of the ulna.

2. Type II: fracture of the middle or upper third of the ulna with posterior dislocation of the radial head and posterior angulation of the ulna.

3. Type III: fracture of the ulna just distal to the coronoid process with lateral dislocation of the radial head.

4. Type IV: fracture of the upper or middle third of the ulna with anterior dislocation of the radial head and fracture of the upper third of the radius below the bicipital tuberosity.

Type I injuries are most frequent (approximately 65 per cent), followed by type II (approximately 18 per cent), type III (approximately 16 per cent), and type IV (approximately 1 per cent). As the Monteggia fracture-dislocation is a common injury in adults, multiple views of the elbow should be obtained in all patients who demonstrate fractures of the proximal half of the ulna.

Complications of elbow dislocations include heterotopic calcification and ossification and neural and vascular injury. Damaged structures include the brachial artery and the median and ulnar nerves.

INTRAARTICULAR FRACTURES OF THE DISTAL PORTION OF THE HUMERUS. The following discussion pertains principally to injuries in the mature skeleton; those occurring in children and adolescents are discussed later in this chapter.

Intraarticular fractures of the distal portion of the humerus can be classified as transcondylar, intercondylar, condylar, epicondylar, transchondral, and miscellaneous in type. *Transcondylar fractures* resemble supracondylar fractures but are intraarticular in location. The fracture line traverses both condylar surfaces in a horizontal direction. Two types are described: an extension type and a flexion type (Fig. 62–72).

Intercondylar fractures of the distal portion of the humerus (Fig. 62–73) result in comminuted and complex fracture lines that generally include one component that traverses the supracondylar region of the humerus in a transverse or oblique fashion and a second component, vertical or oblique in nature, that enters the articular lumen. These fractures are relatively rare and typically are observed in patients over the age of 50 years. They usually are produced by direct trauma to the elbow in which the ulnar articular surface is driven against the articular surface of the distal portion of the humerus. Complications of intercondylar fractures include soft tissue injury, instability, and loss of elbow function.

The condylar portions of the humerus are separated into medial and lateral structures by the capitulotrochlear sulcus. Each condyle contains an articular and a nonarticular portion. The lateral condyle is composed of the nonarticular lateral epicondyle and the articular capitulum; the medial condyle is composed of the nonarticular medial epicondyle and the trochlea. Condylar fractures imply that the fracture line separates both the articular and the nonarticular portions of one condyle with or without an attached segment of the opposite condyle.

Condylar fractures are relatively uncommon, occurring predominantly in children. Fractures involving the lateral condyle are more frequent than those of the medial condyle (Fig. 62–74). Each can be associated with significant disability, especially if the fracture fragment is large. A classification system has been devised on the basis of the size of the fragment and the presence or absence of disruption of the lateral trochlear ridge. This structure, separating the trochlea and capitulum, is important in providing medial and lateral stability to the elbow. Disruption of this ridge allows translocation of the radius and the ulna in a mediolateral direction, resulting in a fracture-dislocation.

Fractures of the capitulum are rare and involve only the articular surface of the lateral condyle (Fig. 62–75). The mechanism of injury is considered to be a direct force, applied through the radial head. Anteroposterior radiographs may appear surprisingly normal, so that accurate assessment usually depends on the review of optimal lateral radiographs. A semicircular radiopaque shadow representing the displaced

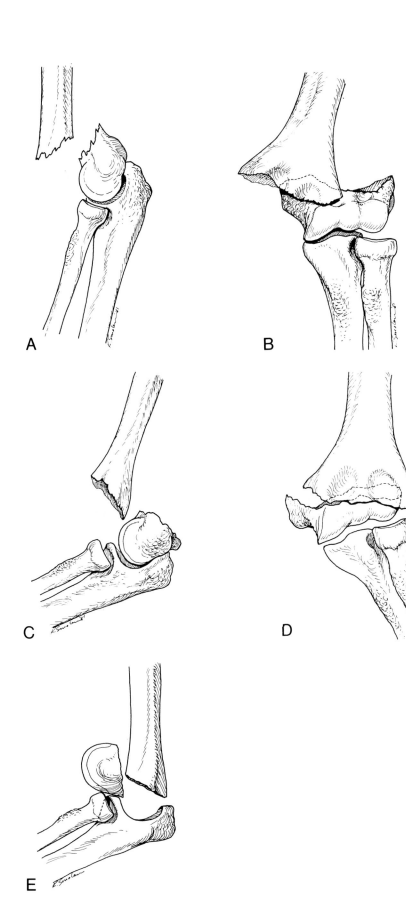

A

B

C

D

E

Figure 62–72. Humeral fractures: Supracondylar and transcondylar. A, B Supracondylar fracture (extension type). A fall on the outstretched hand with the elbow in extension is the probable mechanism of this fracture. On the lateral view (A), the fracture line extends obliquely upward from a more distal point anteriorly to a more proximal point posteriorly. Posterior and proximal displacement of the distal fragment results, in part, from the force of the triceps muscle attaching to the ulna. Observe the sharp margin of the proximal fragment, which projects into the antecubital fossa, accounting for the associated injuries to the brachial artery and median nerve. On the anteroposterior view (B) the fracture line generally is transverse in configuration. Displacement and angulation at the fracture site are of variable degree. C, D Transcondylar fracture (extension type). The fracture line passes through the condyles of the humerus and is intracapsular in location. On the lateral view (C), posterior displacement of the distal fragment predominates. On the frontal view (D), the fracture line is commonly transverse and inferior to that of a supracondylar fracture. E Transcondylar fracture (Posadas type). Note anterior displacement of the condylar fragment and dislocation of the radius and ulna posteriorly, with the coronoid process wedged between the condyles and the humeral shaft. (E, From DeLee JC, et al: Fractures and dislocations of the elbow. In CA Rockwood Jr, DP Greene [Eds]: Fractures in Adults. 2nd Ed. Philadelphia, JB Lippincott Co, 1984, p 573. Used with permission.)

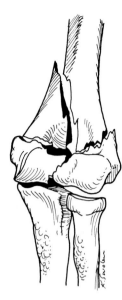

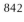

Figure 62–73. Humeral fractures: Intercondylar. In this example, a comminuted fracture has led to separation of the trochlear and capitular fragments. Rotation at the fracture site and incongruity of the articular surface are potential complications.

Figure 62–74. Humeral fractures: Condylar. A Fracture of the medial condyle. **B** Fracture of the lateral condyle.

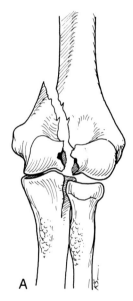

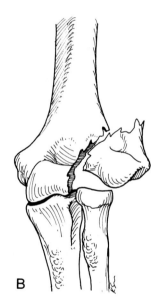

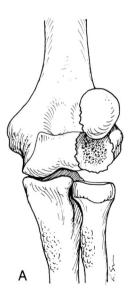

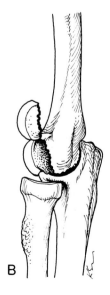

Figure 62–75. Humeral fractures: Capitular. Note the coronal orientation of the fracture line and the characteristic pattern of displacement.

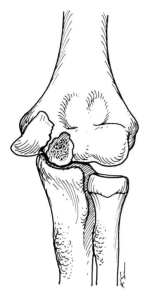

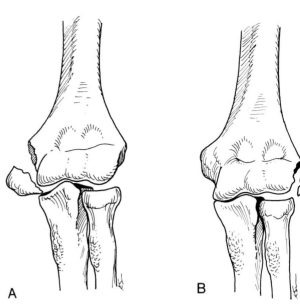

Figure 62–76. Humeral fractures: Trochlear. These fractures are rare and of variable configuration, and they may involve portions of the medial epicondyle.

Figure 62–77. Humeral fractures: Epicondylar. **A** Fracture of the medial epicondyle. **B** Fracture of the lateral epicondyle.

capitulum is apparent, usually anterior to the distal portion of the humerus within the radial fossa.

The articular surface of the medial condyle, the *trochlea*, rarely is fractured as an isolated event. The trochlear fragment with or without a portion of the medial epicondyle is displaced along the medial portion of the joint (Fig. 62–76).

The *epicondyles* are injured more frequently in the child or adolescent than in the adult (Fig. 62–77). In the mature skeleton, the medial epicondyle is fractured more commonly than the lateral epicondyle. Radiographs reveal a fracture fragment that is displaced in a distal or anterior direction by the action of the forearm flexor muscles. Injury to the adjacent ulnar nerve may also be apparent.

FRACTURES OF THE OLECRANON AND CORONOID PROCESSES OF THE ULNA. Fractures of the olecranon process result from direct or indirect injury. The pull of the triceps muscle accounts for displacement of the fragment(s). The complications of olecranon fractures include a decreased range of elbow motion, osteoarthritis, and non-union (the last occurring in approximately 5 per cent of

olecranon fractures). Ulnar nerve damage is evident in approximately 10 per cent of patients.

Isolated fractures of the coronoid process of the ulna are rare.

FRACTURES OF THE HEAD OF THE RADIUS. Radial head fractures represent a common injury in adults, resulting principally from indirect trauma. The radiographic abnormalities may be subtle; the diagnostic importance of a positive "fat pad sign" as well as that of specialized radiographic projections (see Chapter 1) is well recognized (Fig. 62–78). Complications occurring after radial head fractures are infrequent, consisting of a limited range of motion, osteoarthritis, and, in cases of more severe injuries, heterotopic ossification.

Wrist

FRACTURES OF THE DISTAL PORTIONS OF THE RADIUS AND ULNA. The most common mechanism of injury to the wrist is a fall on the outstretched hand causing dorsiflexion of the joint. Metaphyseal fractures of the radius

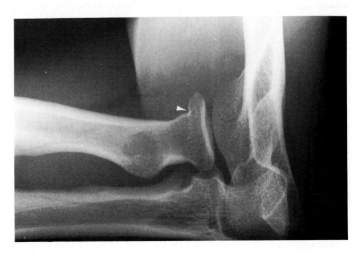

Figure 62–78. Radial fractures: Head of the radius. A specialized radiographic projection is used in the demonstration of a radial head fracture (arrowhead).

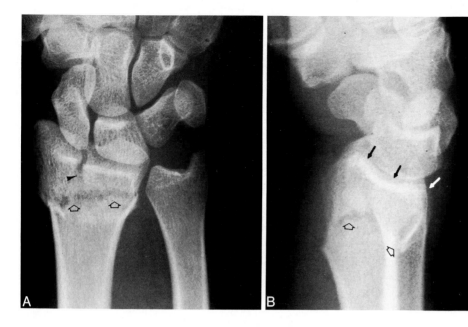

Figure 62–79. Wrist fractures: Colles' fracture. Observe the transverse fracture of the distal portion of the radius (open arrows) with extension into the radiocarpal joint (arrowhead). In the lateral projection, dorsal angulation of the articular surface of the radius is apparent (solid arrows) owing to the compaction of bone dorsally. The ulnar styloid process is intact, and there is no evidence of subluxation of the distal portion of the ulna.

and ulna in young children, physeal separations of the radius in adolescents, scaphoid fractures in young adults, and fractures of the distal portion of the radius or radius and ulna in middle-aged and elderly patients typically follow this type of fall. Fractures of the distal regions of the radius and ulna are approximately 10 times more frequent than those of the carpal bones.

Many eponyms are used to describe the fractures of the distal ends of the radius and ulna. Examples include Colles' fracture (fracture of the distal portion of the radius with dorsal displacement), Smith's fracture (fracture of the distal portion of the radius with palmar displacement), Barton's fracture (fracture of the dorsal rim of the radius), and Hutchinson's fracture (fracture of the radial styloid process). The major

characteristics of these fractures are described in Table 62–10 and illustrated in Figures 62–79 to 62–81.

DISLOCATION OF THE INFERIOR RADIOULNAR JOINT. Although isolated dislocations of the inferior radioulnar joint are seen infrequently, dislocation or subluxation of this articulation may occur in association with a fracture of the radius. This combination of findings is termed a Galeazzi fracture-dislocation (Fig. 62–82). Most commonly, the fracture occurs at the junction of the middle and distal thirds of the radius, and the distal radial fragment is displaced in an ulnar direction. Dislocation of the ulna usually occurs in a distal, dorsal, and medial direction.

CARPAL INJURIES. Two important concepts regarding the radiographic anatomy of the wrist should be emphasized.

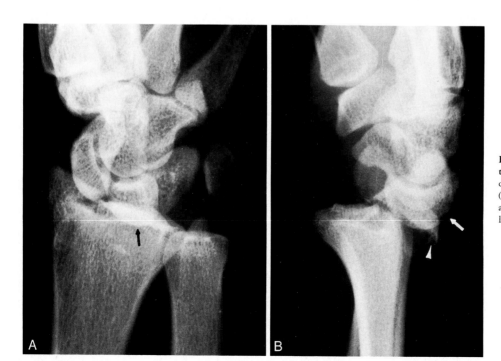

Figure 62–80. Wrist fractures: Barton's fracture. The dorsal rim of the distal portion of the radius is fractured (arrowhead). It is displaced proximally and posteriorly, and there is dorsal subluxation of the carpus (arrows).

Table 62–10. FRACTURES OF THE DISTAL PORTIONS OF THE RADIUS AND ULNA

Fracture	Mechanism	Characteristics	Complications
Colles' (Pouteau's)	Dorsiflexion	Fracture of distal portion of radius with dorsal displacement	Deformity related to radial shortening and angulation
		Classification system based on extra-articular versus intraarticular location, presence or absence of ulnar fracture	Subluxation or dislocation of inferior radioulnar joint
		Varying amounts of radial displacement, angulation, and shortening	Reflex sympathetic dystrophy syndrome
			Injury to median or, less commonly, radial or ulnar nerve
		Ulnar styloid fracture in about 50 to 60 per cent of cases	Osteoarthritis
			Tendon rupture
		Associated injuries to carpus, elbow, humerus, and femur (in osteoporotic patients), inferior radioulnar joint	
Barton's	Dorsiflexion and pronation	Fracture of dorsal rim of radius with intra-articular extension	Similar to those of Colles' fracture
Radiocarpal fracture-dislocation	Dorsiflexion	Uncommon and severe injury	Entrapment of ulnar nerve and artery, tendons
		Associated fractures of dorsal rim and styloid process of radius, ulnar styloid process	
		May be irreducible	
Hutchinson's (Chauffeur's)	Avulsion by radial collateral ligament	Fracture of styloid process of radius	Scapholunate dissociation
		Usually nondisplaced	Osteoarthritis
			Ligament damage
Smith's (reverse Colles')	Variable	Fracture of distal portion of radius with palmar displacement	Similar to those of Colles' fracture
		Less common than Colles' fracture	
		Varying amounts of radial comminution, articular involvement	
		Associated fracture of ulnar styloid process	
Ulnar styloid process	Dorsiflexion or avulsion by ulnar collateral or triangular ligament	Usually associated with radial fractures, rarely isolated	Nonunion
		Usually nondisplaced	

On the posteroanterior view, three smooth carpal arcs define the normal intercarpal relationships. Arc 1 follows the proximal surfaces of the scaphoid, lunate, and triquetrum; arc 2 is located along the distal surfaces of these same carpal bones; and arc 3 defines the curvature of the proximal surfaces of the capitate and hamate. In the normal situation, these curvilinear arcs are roughly parallel, without disruption, and the interosseous spaces are approximately equal in size. Second, on a lateral radiograph of the normal wrist (in neutral position), a continuous line can be drawn through the longitudinal axes of the radius, lunate, and capitate, and this line will intersect a second line through the longitudinal axis of the scaphoid, creating an angle of 30 to 60 degrees (Fig. 62–83). Alterations in these relationships (as well as others) indicate carpal instability, which, in most instances, is related to trauma.

Several characteristic and distinct patterns of carpal instability have been recognized. The first pattern relates principally to abnormalities in the central column, consisting of the lunate and the capitate, but affects the lateral carpus as well. Two varieties of this pattern are emphasized (Fig. 62–83): *dorsal intercalary segment carpal instability* (DICI, DISI, dorsiflexion carpal instability), in which the lunate is tilted dorsally, the scaphoid is flexed, and the scapholunate angle is greater than 70 degrees, is the more common of the two; *volar intercalary segment carpal instability* (VICI, VISI, palmar

flexion carpal instability) occurs when the lunate is tilted in a palmar direction and the scapholunate angle is decreased below the normal value of approximately 47 degrees. Dorsiflexion instability commonly occurs after scaphoid fractures with scapholunate separation, or dissociation, as well as after fractures of the proximal portion of the radius; palmar flexion instability may be seen after disruption of the lunotriquetral interosseous membrane, excision of the triquetrum, and sprains of the midcarpal joint that attenuate the extrinsic ligaments. Similar patterns of instability are seen in various articular disorders, including rheumatoid arthritis and calcium pyrophosphate dihydrate crystal deposition disease.

A second pattern of instability is termed *triquetrohamate dissociation or instability.* Abnormal motion between the triquetrum and the hamate is observed during fluoroscopy. Another type of medial carpal instability is termed *triquetrolunate dissociation*, indicating abnormal motion at the intervening articulation.

Ulnar translocation occurs when the carpus shifts in an ulnar direction, which may follow severe capsular injury or articular disorders such as rheumatoid arthritis. *Dorsal carpal translocation* is usually associated with malunited fractures involving the dorsal rim of the radius and the radial styloid process. *Palmar carpal translocation* accompanies Barton's fractures or disruptions of the volar rim of the radius.

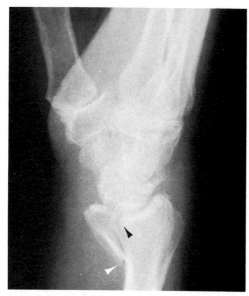

Figure 62–81. Wrist fractures: Smith's fracture. A fracture of the distal portion of the radius (arrowheads) involves the volar surface. Note the mild volar and proximal displacement of the fracture fragment and the carpus.

Scapholunate dissociation (rotatory subluxation of the scaphoid) is suggested when the distance between the scaphoid and lunate is 2 mm or wider (Terry-Thomas sign) (Fig. 62–84). This finding implies that an abnormality exists in the scapho-

lunate interosseous ligament. Rotatory subluxation of the scaphoid also is associated with palmar tilting of the scaphoid, a ring produced by the cortex of the distal pole of the scaphoid, and a foreshortened scaphoid. Degenerative joint disease of the radiocarpal and midcarpal compartments may complicate this condition.

Virtually any of the carpal bones may be dislocated following an injury. Because the lunate and the proximal scaphoid are protected to some extent by the distal radius, a common pattern of injury is a perilunate or transscaphoid perilunate dislocation (Fig. 62–85). In a perilunate dislocation, the lunate remains aligned with the distal portion of the radius, and the other carpal bones dislocate, usually dorsally. A fall on the hyperextended hand is the usual mechanism of injury. With continued hyperextension force, the capitate may force the lunate ventrally, thus converting the perilunate dislocation

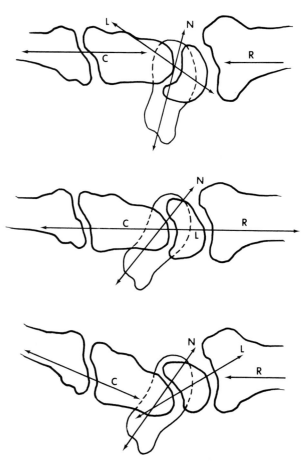

Figure 62–83. Wrist: Normal and abnormal alignment. Lateral projection. Line drawings of longitudinal axes of third metacarpal, navicular (N) or scaphoid, lunate (L), capitate (C), and radius (R) in dorsiflexion instability (upper drawing), in normal situation (middle drawing), and in palmar flexion instability (lower drawing). When the wrist is normal, a continuous line can be drawn through the longitudinal axes of the capitate, the lunate, and the radius, and this line will intersect a second line through the longitudinal axis of the scaphoid, creating an angle of 30 degrees to 60 degrees. In dorsiflexion instability, the lunate is flexed toward the back of the hand and the scaphoid is displaced vertically. The angle of intersection between the two longitudinal axes is greater than 60 degrees. In palmar flexion instability, the lunate is flexed toward the palm and the angle between the two longitudinal axes is less than 30 degrees. (From Linscheid RL, et al: Traumatic instability of the wrist. Diagnosis, classification, and pathomechanics. J Bone Joint Surg [Am] *54*:1612, 1972. Used with permission.)

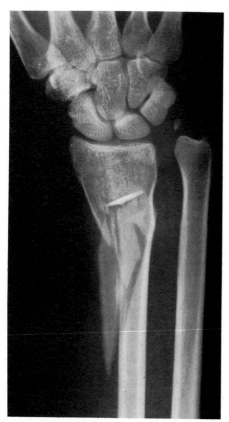

Figure 62–82. Galeazzi fracture-dislocation. Observe an oblique fracture of the distal portion of the radial diaphysis, a fracture of the ulnar styloid, and dorsomedial dislocation of the ulna.

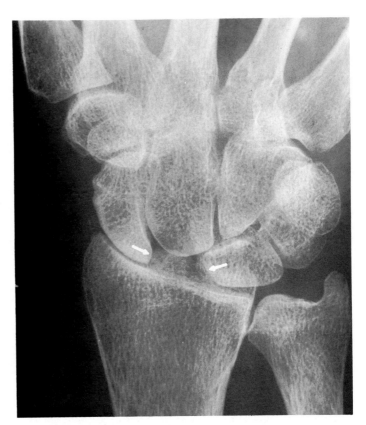

Figure 62–84. Scapholunate dissociation (rotary subluxation of the scaphoid). Observe the gap or widening in the scapholunate space (arrows). The radiocarpal and midcarpal joints are narrowed.

into a lunate dislocation in which the lunate is displaced in a palmar direction and the capitate appears to be aligned with the distal portion of the radius.

Closer inspection of the functional anatomy of the wrist and the patterns of injury has indicated that a predictable sequence of events generally occurs after trauma (Fig. 62–86). These injuries usually commence on the radial side of the wrist. Four stages in the resulting abnormalities are defined. The stage I injury represents scapholunate dissociation with rotary subluxation of the scaphoid; the stage II injury is characterized by perilunar instability owing to failure of the radiocapitate ligament or a fracture of the radial styloid process and leads to a perilunate dislocation; the stage III injury creates ligamentous disruption at the triquetrolunate joint related to partial or complete failure or avulsion of the volar radiotriquetral ligament and dorsal radiocarpal ligaments and may be accompanied by radiographically evident triquetral malrotation, triquetrolunate diastasis, or triquetral fracture; the final stage IV injury is associated with disruption of the dorsal radiocarpal ligaments, freeing the lunate and

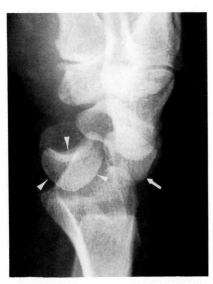

Figure 62–85. Perilunate dislocation. Observe the alignment of the lunate (arrowheads) with the distal radius and dorsal displacement of the capitate (arrow) and the rest of the carpal bones.

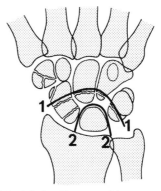

Figure 62–86. Wrist injuries: Greater and lesser arcs. The locations of the greater (1) and lesser (2) arcs are shown, as are the common sites of carpal fractures that can be produced experimentally. A pure greater arc injury consists of a transscaphoid, transcapitate, transhamate, transtriquetral fracture-dislocation; a pure lesser arch injury is a perilunate or lunate dislocation. Various combinations of these injury patterns are seen clinically. (From Johnson RP: The acutely injured wrist and its residuals. Clin Orthop 149:33, 1980. Used with permission.)

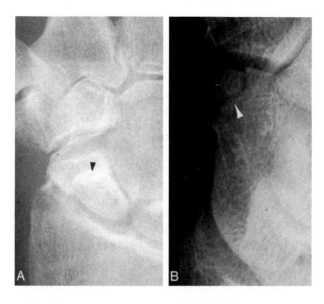

Figure 62–87. Carpal scaphoid fractures. **A** Scaphoid waist. A fracture line possessing sclerotic margins is identified (arrowhead). **B** Scaphoid tuberosity. An acute fracture is seen (arrowhead).

allowing it to become volarly displaced (lunate dislocation). This series of events affecting ligaments and joint spaces takes place about the circumference of the lunate and is termed a *lesser arc injury. Greater arc injuries* represent fracture-dislocation patterns as this arc passes through the scaphoid, capitate, hamate, and triquetrum.

Dislocations about the common carpometacarpal joint are rare injuries, most typically involving the ulnar aspect of the wrist. They commonly involve two or more of the metacarpals. Dorsal dislocation predominates. Recognized complications include injuries to the ulnar nerve or median nerve, rupture of extensor tendons, and fractures of one or more metacarpals. Dislocation of the first carpometacarpal articulation may be combined with fractures of the base of the first metacarpal (Bennett's fracture-subluxation).

Fractures of the carpal bones are observed most frequently in the scaphoid (Fig. 62–87). Fractures of the scaphoid are classified principally according to their location (proximal pole, waist, distal body, tuberosity, and distal articular). In general, the prognosis of distal fractures is better than that

of proximal fractures because of more rapid osseous healing and less extensive vascular interruption. The most frequent scaphoid fracture occurs in the waist (approximately 70 per cent) or proximal pole (approximately 20 per cent) of the bone, although in children, avulsion fractures of the distal portion of the scaphoid are typical. The frequency of delayed union or nonunion is greatest in fractures of the proximal pole of the bone. Radiographic abnormalities of scaphoid nonunion, which occurs in approximately 5 per cent of cases, include bone sclerosis, cyst formation, and resorption, and, subsequently, osteoarthritis. The frequency of ischemic necrosis following scaphoid fractures is approximately 10 to 15 per cent; this frequency rises to 30 to 40 per cent in case of nonunion. Owing to the vascular anatomy of the scaphoid, the proximal portion of the bone is the site of osteonecrosis.

Isolated fractures of the other carpal bones are less frequent than those of the scaphoid. It is the dorsal surface of the triquetrum that typically is fractured (Fig. 62–88). Fractures of the hook of the hamate may occur in athletes involved in sports that use racquets, bats, or clubs. Accurate diagnosis is

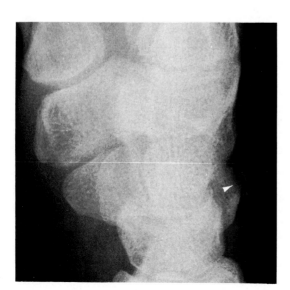

Figure 62–88. Carpal fractures: Dorsal surface of triquetrum (arrowhead).

difficult, and computed tomography may be required (Fig. 62–89). Complications of fractures of the hook of the hamate include nonunion, injuries to the ulnar or median nerve, and tendon rupture.

Hand

METACARPOPHALANGEAL AND INTERPHALANGEAL JOINT DISLOCATION. Dislocation of a metacarpophalangeal joint (excluding the thumb) results from a fall on the outstretched hand that forces the joint into hyperextension. Dorsal dislocation predominates. Radiographs may reveal a widened joint space, indicating interposition of the volar plate within the joint.

Dislocation of the proximal interphalangeal joint can occur in a posterior or, more rarely, an anterior direction. Radiographs reveal the abnormal position of the phalanx and, in many cases, small avulsed fragments of bone. Posterior dislocation of a distal interphalangeal joint or the interphalangeal joint of the thumb can also be encountered. Such dislocations may be irreducible owing to interposition of the volar plate or flexor tendon.

A Bennett's fracture-dislocation is a relatively common intraarticular injury that occurs at the base of the first metacarpal (Fig. 62–90A). An oblique fracture line separates the major portion of the bone from a small fragment of the volar lip. The base of the metacarpal is pulled dorsally and radially. A second intraarticular injury, the Rolando's fracture, represents a Y- or T-shaped comminuted fracture (Fig. 62–90B).

Dislocations and collateral ligament injuries of the first metacarpophalangeal joint are important complications of trauma. One type relates to a sudden valgus stress applied to the metacarpophalangeal joint of the thumb, the gamekeeper's thumb. Initially described as an occupational hazard in English gamewardens, the injury is now recognized to occur in various settings, including skiing. Attenuation or disrup-

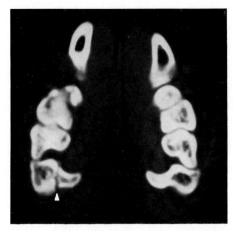

Figure 62–89. Carpal fractures: Hook of the hamate. Note the fracture line (arrowhead). Compare with the opposite normal side. (Courtesy of G. Greenway, M.D., Dallas, Texas.)

tion of the ligamentous apparatus along the ulnar aspect of the thumb is seen. Initial radiographs can be negative, although small avulsed fragments from the base of the proximal phalanx can be delineated in some instances (Fig. 62–91). Radiographs obtained with radial stress applied to the first metacarpophalangeal joint can reveal subluxation, and arthrography may outline leakage of contrast material from the joint.

FRACTURES OF THE METACARPAL BONES AND PHALANGES. Fractures of the metacarpal bones are classified according to anatomic location: metacarpal head, metacarpal neck, metacarpal shaft, and metacarpal base. Typical locations of fractures include the shaft and neck of the fifth metacarpal (boxer's fracture), the shaft of the third or fourth metacarpal, and the articular surface of the second metacarpal (Fig. 62–92). Displacement, angulation, or rotation is commonly encountered.

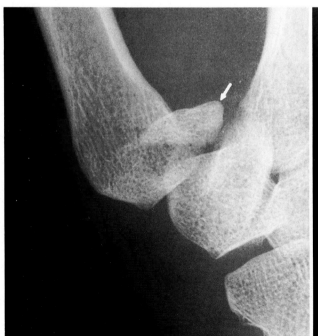
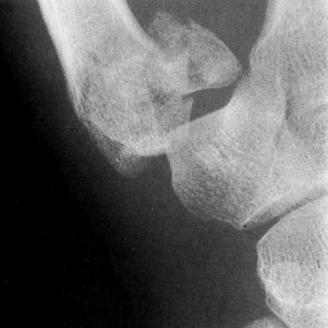

Figure 62–90. Fractures and dislocations of the base of the first metacarpal bone. A Bennett's fracture-dislocation. Observe the typical oblique fracture of the volar lip of the first metacarpal bone (arrow). **B** Rolando's fracture. A comminuted fracture of the metacarpal base is evident.

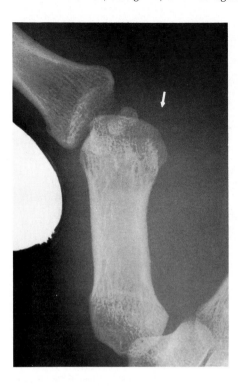

Figure 62–91. Gamekeeper's thumb. A radiograph obtained during radial stress reveals subluxation of the phalanx on the metacarpal bone. Fracture fragments are identified (arrow).

Phalangeal fractures are more frequent than those of the metacarpals and most typically involve the distal phalanges. Important varieties include the mallet fracture (in which an avulsion injury at the base of the dorsal surface of the terminal phalanx is produced by damage to the extensor mechanism), the volar plate fracture (in which a dorsal dislocation of a proximal interphalangeal joint may be associated with an avulsion fracture in the middle phalanx at the site of attachment of the volar plate), any fracture with intraarticular extension or significant rotational deformity, a fracture of the shaft of the proximal or middle phalanx (whose volar surface

forms the floor of the flexor tendon sheath so that accurate reduction is desirable), a fracture of the base of the proximal phalanx (in which angulation is easily overlooked owing to superimposition of other bones on the lateral radiograph), and, in the immature skeleton, a physeal separation at the base of the distal phalanx (the nailbed injury, in which an open skin surface leads to secondary infection) (Fig. 62–93).

Hip

HIP DISLOCATION. Dislocation of the femoral head with or without an acetabular fracture is an injury that usually

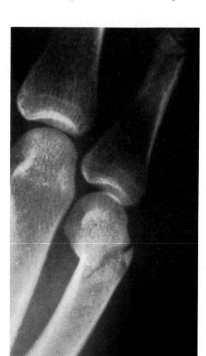

Figure 62–92. Metacarpal bone fractures: Neck of the fifth metacarpal.

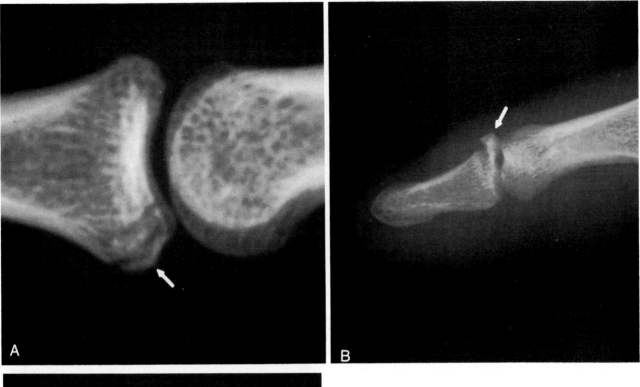

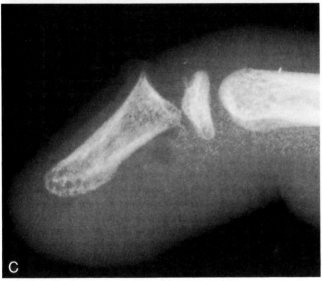

Figure 62–93. Phalangeal fractures. A, B Small avulsion fractures (arrows) near the proximal interphalangeal or distal interphalangeal joint can result from traction on the volar plate (**A**) or extensor tendons (**B**). Dislocations may also be evident. **C** This physeal separation at the base of the distal phalanx, the nailbed injury, is open to the environment with the risk of infection.

follows considerable trauma. Dislocations are classified as anterior, posterior, and central in type.

Anterior dislocation of the hip, due to forced abduction, represents 5 to 10 per cent of all hip dislocations. On frontal radiographs, an anteriorly displaced femoral head typically moves inferomedially with the femur abducted and externally rotated, and a posteriorly displaced femoral head is usually located superolaterally with the femur adducted and internally rotated. Fractures of the femoral neck or, more commonly, femoral head may accompany anterior dislocations (Fig. 62–94).

Posterior dislocation of the hip, representing 80 to 85 per cent of all hip dislocations, may result when the flexed knee strikes the dashboard during a head-on automobile collision.

The leg is shortened, internally rotated, and adducted. Associated problems include knee trauma, femoral head or shaft fractures, and sciatic nerve injury. The frequent occurrence of posterior acetabular rim fractures after posterior dislocation of the hip requires careful analysis of routine radiographs and use of oblique and lateral projections (Fig. 62–94). Additional complications of this injury are periarticular soft tissue calcification, intraarticular fragments, acetabular labrum tears, osteonecrosis of the femoral head, and osteoarthritis.

Central acetabular fracture-dislocation usually results from a force applied to the lateral side of the trochanter and pelvis. Acetabular fractures, pelvic hemorrhage, and osteoarthritis are complications of this injury.

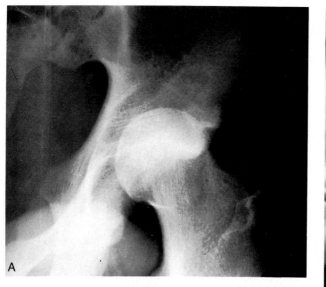

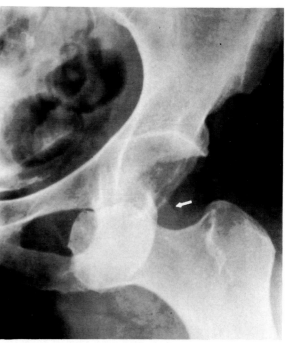

Figure 62–94. Hip dislocation. A Posterior dislocation. The radiograph reveals a posterosuperior dislocation of the femoral head. A large osseous fragment of the posterior acetabular rim was present. **B** Anterior dislocation. Plain film reveals an inferomedial position of the dislocated femoral head and a fracture fragment of the lateral portion of the head (arrow).

FRACTURES OF THE PROXIMAL PORTION OF THE FEMUR. Although evident as a stress fracture in the young athlete and as a pathologic fracture in individuals with skeletal metastasis, Paget's disease, and other disorders, it is the occurrence of fractures of the proximal portion of the femur in elderly persons with osteopenia that has received the greatest attention. Two major mechanisms of injury have been proposed in the production of femoral neck fractures: a fall producing a direct blow on the greater trochanter; and lateral rotation of the extremity.

Anatomic designations, including subcapital, transcervical, basicervical, intertrochanteric, and subtrochanteric, frequently are used to define the location of the femoral fracture and can be modified to include intracapsular fractures (those in the subcapital and transcervical regions) and extracapsular fractures (those in the basicervical and trochanteric regions) (Fig. 62–95). Intracapsular fractures, which are approximately twice as frequent as those in the trochanteric region, may also be classified according to the direction of the fracture angle or the degree of displacement of the fracture fragments.

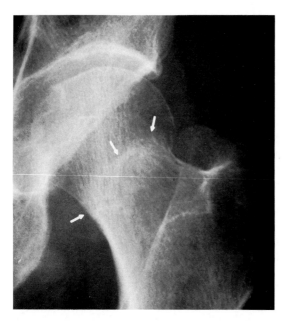

Figure 62–95. Fractures of the femoral neck: Intracapsular fracture. An example of a subtle intracapsular fracture (arrows) is shown. Observe the band of increased radiodensity.

Classification of intracapsular fractures according to the degree of displacement on prereduction radiographs commonly is referred to as the Garden system. Four types of fractures are identified: Type I fractures are incomplete or impacted in nature; type II fractures are complete without osseous displacement; type III fractures are also complete but with partial displacement of the fracture fragments; and type IV fractures are complete with total displacement of the fracture fragments.

Delayed union and nonunion of intracapsular fractures are not uncommon. Factors predisposing to nonunion (which occurs in approximately 5 to 25 per cent of cases) include advanced age of the patient, osteoporosis, posterior comminution of the fracture, inadequate reduction, and poor internal fixation technique. The frequency of ischemic necrosis of the femoral head varies from 10 to 30 per cent. The vascular insult to the femoral head may occur not only at the time of fracture but also after attempts at reduction.

Intertrochanteric fractures also predominate in osteopenic, elderly patients. Direct or indirect force(s) resulting from a fall constitutes the typical mechanism of injury. Fracture comminution is common. Systems of classification of intertrochanteric fractures are based on stability versus instability or the ease by which fracture reduction can be accomplished. A stable fracture (approximately 50 per cent of cases) is characterized by the absence of comminution of the medial cortices of the proximal and distal fragments and of displacement of the lesser trochanter. Unstable intertrochanteric fractures include fractures in which there is absence of contact between the proximal and distal fragments owing to comminution or medial and posterior displacement of fracture fragments. Complications of intertrochanteric fractures include varus displacement both in nonsurgically treated injuries and in those associated with failure of internal reduction, nonunion (which is uncommon), and ischemic necrosis of the femoral head (which appears in less than 1 per cent of cases).

Isolated fractures of the greater trochanter in adults are infrequent and generally occur in elderly patients after a fall (Fig. 62–96). Similar fractures of the lesser trochanter may represent the initial manifestation of skeletal metastasis.

Fractures of the femur that commence immediately below the trochanter are considered subtrochanteric. Those subtrochanteric fractures that occur more distally are associated with a greater frequency of nonunion or delayed union and implant failure. Approximately 5 to 30 per cent of fractures of the proximal portion of the femur are subtrochanteric. These fractures occur in older patients with relatively minor injuries and in younger persons with major trauma.

FRACTURES OF THE ACETABULUM. Although the classic descriptions of acetabular fractures used complete radiographic examinations, including oblique projections, computed tomography currently plays an important role in their evaluation. With any imaging system, the delineation of four bone landmarks remains fundamental to proper assessment of the extent of injury: the anterior acetabular rim, the posterior acetabular rim, the iliopubic (anterior) column, and the ilioischial (posterior) column. With computed tomography, the integrity of the acetabular dome and quadrilateral surface as well as the presence of intraarticular osseous fragments and associated fractures of the osseous pelvis also can be readily determined (Fig. 62–97).

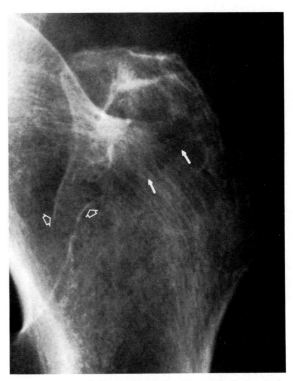

Figure 62–96. Fractures of the proximal portion of the femur: Isolated fractures of the greater trochanter. Observe the fracture (solid arrows) with interruption of the intertrochanteric line (open arrows). These injuries should not be misinterpreted as fractures of the femoral neck.

Acetabular fractures result from the impact of the femoral head against the central regions of the acetabulum or its rims, especially the posterior rim in association with a posterior dislocation of the hip. Fractures may involve the anterior or posterior column alone, or a transverse fracture may involve both of these columns. Although displacement of fracture fragments is not uncommon, nondisplaced or occult fractures of the acetabulum present diagnostic difficulties. The complications of acetabular fractures include osteoarthritis of the hip, ischemic necrosis of the femoral head (in cases in which there is an associated posterior dislocation of the hip), and hemorrhage as well as urinary tract and peripheral nerve injury.

Knee

FRACTURES OF THE DISTAL PORTION OF THE FEMUR. These fractures can be classified as supracondylar, intercondylar, or condylar in type. Most of these injuries result from axial loading combined with varus or valgus stress and rotation. *Supracondylar fractures* commonly are transverse or oblique in configuration, with varying degrees of displacement and comminution of the fracture fragments. Injury to the popliteal artery may occur. These supracondylar fractures may be accompanied by a vertical fracture line extending into the knee, leading to *intercondylar fractures. Condylar fractures* display sagittal or coronal fracture lines that are isolated to a single condyle (Fig. 62–98).

FRACTURES OF THE PATELLA. These fractures result from direct or indirect forces, the latter related to contraction

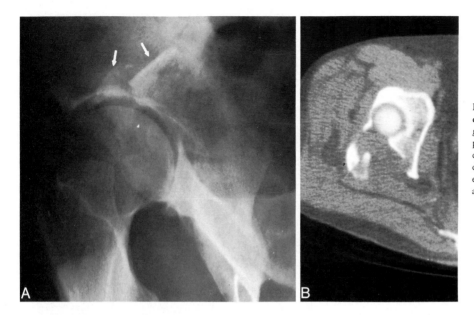

Figure 62–97. Acetabular fractures: Use of computed tomography. An oblique radiograph (A) reveals an obvious fracture involving principally the acetabular dome (arrows). A computed tomographic scan (B) shows the comminuted nature of the fracture and the extent of involvement of the acetabular roof and posterior rim.

of the quadriceps muscles. Transverse fractures represent approximately 50 to 80 per cent of all patellar fractures, and they generally are the product of indirect force (Fig. 62–99). Longitudinal (25 per cent) and stellate or comminuted (20 to 35 per cent) fractures are less frequent and usually result from direct injury, such as striking the dashboard of an automobile. Osteochondral fractures occur in combination with patellar dislocation (see later discussion). Fractures should be differentiated from bipartite patellae, in which separate ossification centers develop in the superolateral aspect of the bone.

Fragmentation and separation of the lower pole of the patella is referred to as Sinding-Larsen-Johansson disease (see Chapter 71).

FRACTURES OF THE PROXIMAL PORTION OF THE TIBIA. These fractures may be extraarticular or intraarticular. Oblique and horizontal-beam projections and conventional or computed tomography (Fig. 62–100) frequently are required for accurate assessment of these injuries, and the tomographic techniques allow further analysis of the extent of displacement and depression of the articular segment. Tibial plateau fractures may be accompanied by injuries to the cruciate or collateral ligaments of the knee. Important considerations related to tibial fractures include the detection of lipohemarthrosis, avulsion fractures and sites of ligamentous detachment (femoral condyles, fibular head, and intercondylar eminence), meniscal injuries, abnormal widening of the joint space during the application of stress, and disruption of the

articular surface. Recognized complications of these injuries include peroneal nerve involvement, ruptures of the popliteal artery, residual varus or valgus angulation, and osteoarthritis.

Fractures of the tibial spine are indicative of possible damage to the cruciate ligaments of the knee. Either the anterior tibial spine or, less commonly, the posterior tibial spine is affected.

FRACTURES OF THE PROXIMAL PORTION OF THE FIBULA. Isolated fractures of the head or neck of the fibula are distinctly uncommon; the detection of a fracture in these regions should prompt a search for a ligamentous injury or fracture of the knee or ankle. Additional complications of fractures of the proximal portion of the fibula include contusion of the biceps tendon, injury to the anterior tibial artery or peroneal nerve, and avulsion of the fibular head with intraarticular entrapment.

KNEE DISLOCATION. This is a rare but serious injury owing to the neurovascular insult that may result from popliteal artery and peroneal nerve damage. Anterior (the most common type), posterior, lateral, medial, and rotatory types of dislocation are recognized (Fig. 62–101). After any type of dislocation, capsular, cruciate, and ligamentous injury can be seen. Arteriography should be employed to delineate the status of the popliteal artery.

PATELLAR DISLOCATION. Traumatic dislocation of the patella can be produced by a direct blow or an exaggerated contraction of the quadriceps mechanism. Abnormalities pre-

A   B   C   D

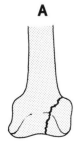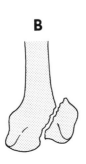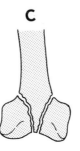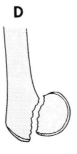

Figure 62–98. Fractures of the distal portion of the femur: Condylar fractures—classification system. Such fractures may be undisplaced (A) or displaced (B-D), involve one (A, B) or both (C, D) condyles, and be oriented principally in the sagittal (A-C) or coronal (D) plane. (From Hohl M, et al: Fractures and dislocations of the knee. In CA Rockwood Jr, DP Greene [Eds]: Fractures in Adults. 2nd Ed. Philadelphia, JB Lippincott Co, 1984, p 1444. Used with permission.)

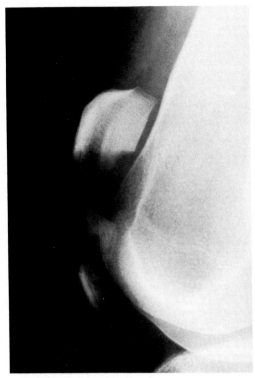

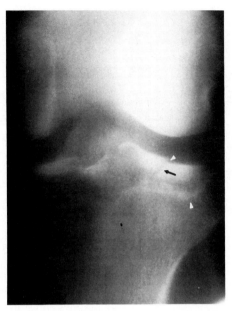

Figure 62–100. **Fractures of the proximal portion of the tibia.** Conventional tomography is used to identify a subtle fracture (arrow) of the lateral plateau and the degree of osseous compression (arrowheads).

Figure 62–99. **Patellar fractures.** Transverse patellar fracture with comminution and displacement on lateral radiograph.

disposing to displacement may include an abnormally high patella (patella alta), deficient height of the lateral femoral condyle, shallowness of the patellofemoral groove, genu valgum or recurvatum, and excessive tibial torsion. Lateral dislocation predominates. Recurrent dislocation and osteochondral fractures of the medial patellar facet and lateral femoral condyle are common (Fig. 62–102).

PROXIMAL TIBIOFIBULAR JOINT DISLOCATION. Although rare, proximal tibiofibular joint dislocation may be seen in parachuting, hang-gliding, sky-diving, and horseback riding injuries. Anterior or, less frequently, posterior dislocation of the fibular head can be noted. Peroneal nerve injury can appear after a posterior dislocation of this joint. In cases of anterior dislocation, the fibular head also is displaced laterally; in posterior dislocation, the fibular head is displaced medially. Radiographic findings may be subtle, however.

Ankle

FRACTURES ABOUT THE ANKLE. Stability of the ankle joint depends on the integrity of a ring formed by the tibia, fibula, and talus, united by surrounding ligaments (Fig. 62–103). Two or more breaks in the ring, whether fractures or a fracture in combination with a ruptured ligament, will allow abnormal talar motion (Fig. 62–104). The application of stress to the ankle during the radiographic examination can be of considerable diagnostic importance (Fig. 62–105).

Grouping of ankle injuries according to mechanism of injury is possible on the basis of radiographic abnormalities. Within each grouping are stages of injury, designated by Roman numerals; the higher the number, the greater the

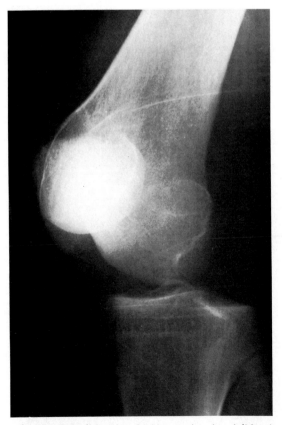

Figure 62–101. **Knee dislocation.** In this example, a lateral dislocation of the tibia with respect to the femur is seen. Abnormal rotation between the two bones is also evident.

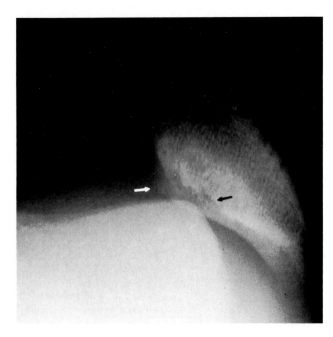

Figure 62–102. Patellar dislocation. An axial radiograph reveals lateral dislocation of the patella with fragmentation and erosion of a portion of the patellar articular surface (arrows).

Figure 62–103. Ankle: Stable and unstable characteristics. A The stability of the ankle joint is determined by the status of a ring comprising the mortise and surrounding ligaments. The latter include the deep and superficial deltoid ligaments (1), the anterior (2) and posterior (not shown) talofibular ligaments, the calcaneofibular ligament (3), the anterior (4) and posterior (not shown) tibiofibular ligaments, the inferior transverse ligament (not shown), and the interosseous membrane and ligament (not shown). **B** A single break in this ring will not allow displacement. **C** Two or more breaks in the ring allow displacement of the mortise.

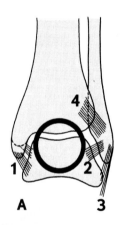
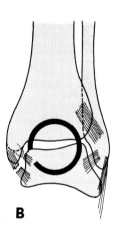
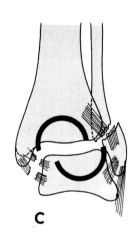

A   **3**   **B**   **C**

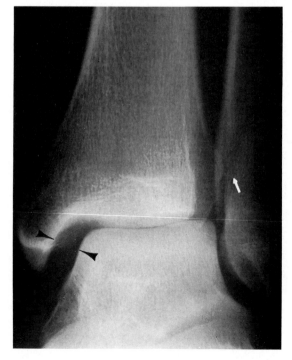

Figure 62–104. Ankle instability: Routine radiography. Direct lateral displacement of the talus with respect to the tibia results in widening of the medial "clear" space (arrowheads) indicative of rupture of the deep deltoid ligament. The superficial deltoid ligament may also be torn. There is a fibular fracture (arrow), which allows the talus to move laterally.

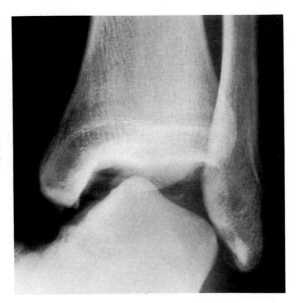

Figure 62–105. Ankle instability: Stress radiography. An anteroposterior varus (inversion) stress view (with the foot in neutral position) shows obvious widening of the lateral portion of the joint, indicating some degree of ligamentous disruption. The tibiotalar angle measured 34 degrees. Small fracture fragments are evident.

applied force and resultant damage. Each of the groups is designated by two characteristic terms. The first term is either *pronation* or *supination* and refers to the position of the foot at the time of injury. The foot is pronated when there is outward rotation and eversion of the forefoot with abduction of the hindfoot. Supination represents inward rotation and inversion of the forefoot with adduction of the hindfoot. The second term reflects the direction in which the talus is displaced or rotated relative to the mortise formed by the distal regions of the tibia and fibula. There are five possible directions of talar displacement: external rotation (in which the talus is displaced externally or laterally); internal rotation (in which the talus is displaced internally or medially); abduction (in which the talus is displaced laterally without significant rotation); adduction (in which the talus is displaced medially without significant rotation); and dorsiflexion (in which the talus is dorsiflexed on the tibia).

1. *Supination–external rotation fracture* (SER stages I, II, III, and IV). The SER category constitutes almost 60 per cent of all ankle fractures (Figs. 62–106 and 62–107). External rotation of the foot forces the talus against the fibula, commonly resulting in rupture of the anterior tibiofibular ligament (stage I). As the mechanism of injury continues, a short oblique fracture of the distal portion of the fibula will occur (stage II). The next stage of injury is a fracture of the posterior aspect of the tibia of varying size (stage III). The final stage (stage IV) is characterized by a fracture of the medial malleolus or a rupture of the deltoid ligament.

2. *Supination-adduction fracture* (SAD stages I and II). The SAD category constitutes about 20 per cent of all ankle fractures (Figs. 62–108 and 62–109). Supination causes tension on the lateral ligaments and, with adduction, either a lateral ligament rupture or transverse fracture of the distal portion of the fibula occurs (SAD stage I). Continued pressure from the medially directed talus results in a fracture of the medial malleolus or a rupture of the deltoid ligament (SAD stage II). The malleolar fracture is often oblique or nearly vertical.

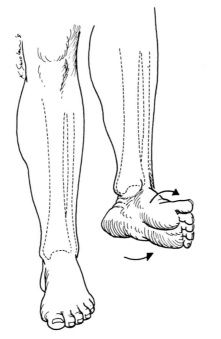

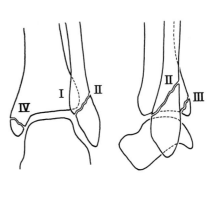

Figure 62–106. Ankle injuries: Supination–external rotation fracture. External rotation forces applied to the supinated foot result initially in a rupture of the anterior tibiofibular ligament (stage I). As the forces continue, a short oblique fracture of the distal portion of the fibula occurs (stage II). The next stage of the injury is a fracture of the posterior aspect of the tibia (stage III). The final stage of the injury is a fracture of the medial malleolus (stage IV).

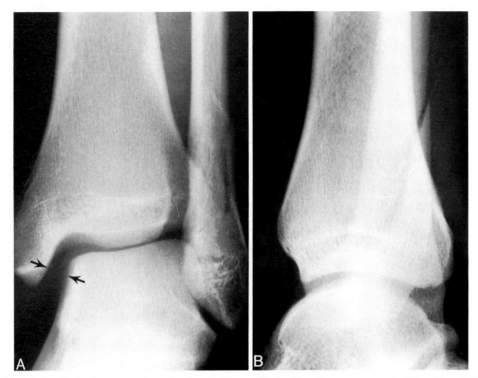

Figure 62–107. Ankle injuries: Supination–external rotation fracture—stage IV. In this patient, anteroposterior (**A**) and lateral (**B**) radiographs reveal disruption of the deltoid ligament (manifested by widening of the medial clear space [arrows]) in addition to the fibular fracture.

3 and 4. *Pronation–external rotation fracture* (PER stages I, II, III, and IV); *pronation–abduction fracture* (PAB stages I, II, and III). The PER (Figs. 62–110 and 62–111) and PAB (Fig. 62–112) fractures constitute about 20 per cent of all fractures occurring about the ankle. Fractures of the PER stages I and II, and PAB stages I and II cannot be distinguished radiographically. Forceful pronation of the foot and external rotation or abduction of the talus result in either deltoid ligament rupture (60 per cent) or fracture of the medial malleolus (40 per cent) (PER or PAB stage I). In a PER or PAB stage II lesion, a rupture of the distal tibiofibular syndesmosis also occurs. This latter injury may be purely ligamentous or may be an avulsion fracture arising from either the anterior or the posterior tubercle, or from both. PAB stage III fractures imply, in addition, a transverse supramalleolar fibular fracture. PER stage III injuries include a short

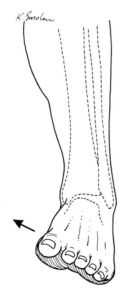

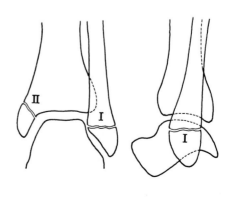

Figure 62–108. Ankle injuries: Supination-adduction fracture. Adduction forces applied to the supinated foot initially result in a traction or avulsion fracture of the distal portion of the fibula or rupture of the lateral ligaments (stage I). As forces continue, a fracture of the medial malleolus or a rupture of the deltoid ligament occurs (stage II). The fibular fracture typically is transverse and that of the medial malleolus is oblique or nearly vertical.

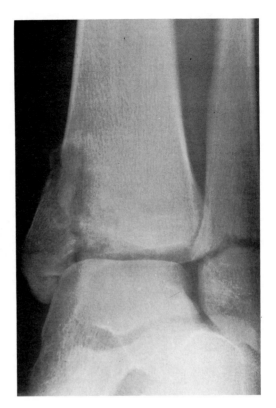

Figure 62–109. Ankle injuries: Supination-adduction fracture—stage II. Note the transversely oriented fibular fracture and the nearly vertical fracture of the medial malleolus.

spiral fracture of the fibula more than 2.5 cm above the tibiotalar joint. Associated rupture of the syndesmosis ligaments and interosseous membrane occurs. PER stage IV fractures include also a fracture of the posterior tibial margin.

5. *Pronation-dorsiflexion fracture* (PDF stages I, II, III, and IV). These injuries, produced by axial loading, constitute less than 0.5 per cent of all ankle fractures. Their mechanism is forced dorsiflexion of the pronated foot which forces the talus into the ankle mortise (Fig. 62–113). The important radiographic features of PDF fractures are the intraarticular anterior lip fracture of the stage II injury and the comminution of the tibia of the stage IV injury.

A fracture of the posterior tibial margin occurs rarely as an isolated lesion or, more commonly, in combination with other injuries. It may be overlooked on the true lateral view of the

ankle; its detection is facilitated by the use of an off-lateral projection achieved by slight external rotation of the patient's foot. An isolated fracture of the anterior margin of the distal portion of the tibia also is an uncommon lesion.

ANKLE DISLOCATION. Dislocations of the ankle commonly are associated with fracture of the adjacent malleolar surfaces. Posterior dislocation is more frequent than anterior dislocation (Fig. 62–114).

Foot

FRACTURES AND DISLOCATIONS OF THE TALUS. The talus has functional importance in transmitting the body's weight and allowing motion between the lower leg and foot; it also has unique anatomic characteristics that include a tenuous blood supply (see Chapter 70), which increases its

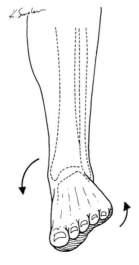
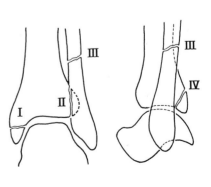

Figure 62–110. Ankle injuries: Pronation-external rotation fracture. Forces of external rotation applied to the pronated foot result initially in rupture of the deltoid ligament or a fracture of the medial malleolus (stage I). As forces continue, there is rupture of the anterior tibiofibular ligament (stage II). A high fibular fracture (stage III) and a fracture of the posterior tibial margin (stage IV) are the final stages in this mechanism of injury.

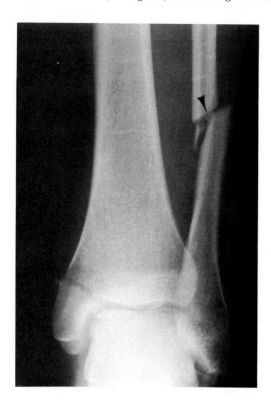

Figure 62–111. Ankle injuries: Pronation-external rotation fracture: Stage III injury. Findings include a fracture of the medial malleolus and an oblique fracture of the fibula (arrowhead), well above the level of the ankle joint.

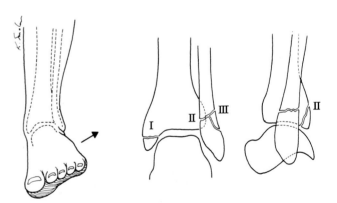

Figure 62–112. Ankle injuries: Pronation-abduction fracture. The first two stages of this injury are identical to those of the pronation-external rotation fracture complex. Stage III is a transverse supramalleolar fibular fracture that may be comminuted laterally.

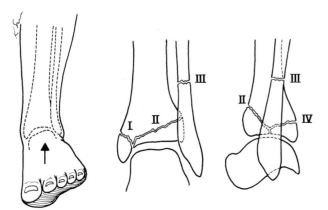

Figure 62–113. Ankle injuries: Pronation-dorsiflexion fracture. Initially, a fracture of the medial malleolus occurs (stage I). Subsequent injuries include a fracture of the anterior tibial margin (stage II), a supramalleolar fracture of the fibula (stage III), and a transverse fracture of the posterior aspect of the tibia, which connects with the anterior tibial fracture (stage IV).

susceptibility to posttraumatic ischemic necrosis, and lack of muscular attachments, which increases the likelihood of dislocation. It is second only to the calcaneus as a site of tarsal fracture. Such fractures (originally termed "aviator's astragalus") are seen today after sudden hyperextension of the forefoot (e.g., during sudden application of the brakes of an automobile to avoid an accident). Avulsion fractures predominate; most such fractures are produced by a twisting or rotational force combined with flexion or extension stresses (Fig. 62–115).

Fractures of the head of the talus are rare and are probably related to a longitudinal compression force combined with plantar flexion of the foot. Associated injuries of the tarsal navicular and talonavicular joint are encountered.

Fractures of the talar neck are second in frequency to avulsion injuries of the bone (Fig. 62–116). Dorsiflexion related to a force from below or, more rarely, a direct blow to the talus produces this fracture. Displaced fractures combined with subluxation or dislocation of the subtalar joint or both the subtalar and the ankle joints are indicative of considerable injury. Complications of talar neck fractures include delayed union or nonunion, infection, osteoarthritis of adjacent joints, and ischemic necrosis, the latter occurring in as many as 80 to 90 per cent of cases of displaced fractures. It is the proximal portion of the bone that is affected in ischemic necrosis.

Fractures of the body of the talus are infrequent. Varying amounts of displacement of the fragments and adjacent joints are observed. Complications include ischemic necrosis, osteoarthritis, and delayed union.

Subluxations or dislocations of the talus generally are accompanied by fractures of the bone. They are usually classified as subtalar (peritalar) dislocations and total talar dislocations (Fig. 62–117). The first pattern indicates simultaneous disruption of the talocalcaneal and talonavicular joints. Medial subtalar dislocations are most frequent, an

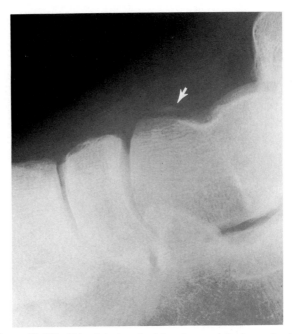

Figure 62–115. Talar injuries: Avulsion fracture of talar neck. An example of this relatively common injury is shown (arrow).

injury that occurs most typically in basketball games. Total dislocation of the talus is an extremely infrequent and serious injury. Ischemic necrosis of the talus and infection are two important complications.

FRACTURES OF THE CALCANEUS. The calcaneus is the most common site of tarsal fracture. Although accurate diagnosis commonly is provided by routine radiographs, especially if attention is directed at Bohler's angle (Fig. 62–118), computed tomography is a technique that ideally displays the extent of injury. Fractures of the calcaneus can

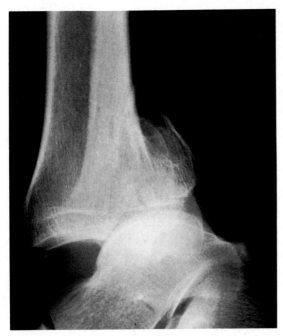

Figre 62–114. Ankle injuries: Tibiotalar dislocation. A large posterior tibial fracture is associated with the talar dislocation.

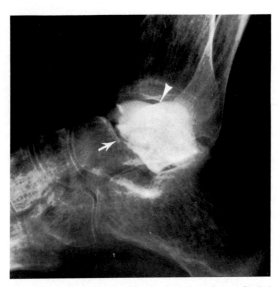

Figure 62–116. Talar injuries: Fracture of the talar neck. Ischemic necrosis (arrowhead) of the proximal half of the talus, leading to a relative increase in radiodensity of the bone owing to adjacent widespread osteoporosis, is the result of a fracture of the talar neck (arrow).

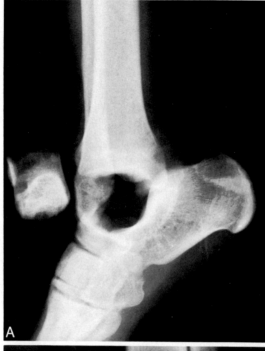

Figure 62–117. Talar injuries: Dislocation. A Total dislocation of the talus. (Courtesy of J. Hembree, M.D., Palo Alto, California.) **B, C** Medial subtalar dislocation. Note the dislocation of the anterior talocalcaneonavicular and posterior subtalar joints and a relatively normal alignment of the calcaneocuboid joint.

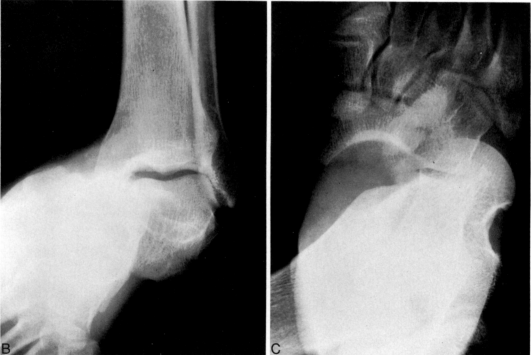

be classified broadly into those that are intraarticular (approximately 75 per cent) and those that are extraarticular (approximately 25 per cent of cases); the former are associated with a poorer prognosis. Intraarticular fractures generally occur as a result of a vertical fall; this mechanism of injury explains the frequency (10 per cent) of bilateral calcaneal fractures as well as the simultaneous occurrence of spinal injuries. Extraarticular calcaneal fractures (Fig. 62–119) result principally from twisting forces. They may localize to the anterior or medial processes, the sustentaculum tali, the body, or the tuberosity.

Comminution and displacement after intraarticular fractures are common. It is here that computed tomography is most useful in defining not only the acute injury but also its sequelae, including osteoarthritis of the subtalar joints, malunion, and peroneal tendon entrapment between the calcaneus and the fibula.

FRACTURES OF OTHER TARSAL BONES. Fractures elsewhere in the tarsus are infrequent. Typical sites of injury in the tarsal navicular bone are its dorsal surface near the talonavicular space and the tuberosity and body of the bone. Isolated fractures of the cuboid and the cuneiforms are rare.

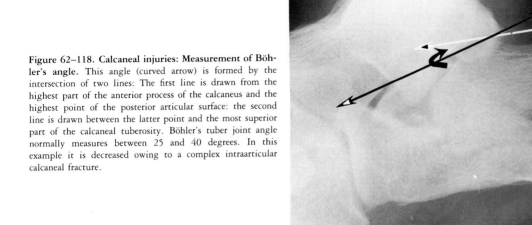

Figure 62–118. Calcaneal injuries: Measurement of Böhler's angle. This angle (curved arrow) is formed by the intersection of two lines: The first line is drawn from the highest part of the anterior process of the calcaneus and the highest point of the posterior articular surface: the second line is drawn between the latter point and the most superior part of the calcaneal tuberosity. Böhler's tuber joint angle normally measures between 25 and 40 degrees. In this example it is decreased owing to a complex intraarticular calcaneal fracture.

TARSAL DISLOCATION. The Lisfranc's fracture-dislocation of the tarsometatarsal joints (Fig. 62–120) is an important injury. Normally, the heads of the metatarsal bones are joined by transverse ligaments, and the bases of most of the metatarsal bones reveal ligamentous connections. An oblique ligament extends between the medial cuneiform and the second metatarsal base, anchoring the base of this recessed metatarsal bone. Injuries of the tarsometatarsal joints can result from direct or indirect trauma. Violent abduction of the forefoot can lead to lateral displacement of the four lateral metatarsal bones with or without a fracture at the base of the second metatarsal bone and the cuboid bone (Fig. 62–120). Accompanying dorsal displacement is more frequent than plantar displacement. The first metatarsal bone may dislocate in the same direction as or in the opposite direction to the other metatarsal bones.

Proper recognition of abnormal alignment in the tarsometatarsal joints requires knowledge of normal radiographic anatomy. Normally, the medial edge of the base of the second metatarsal bone aligns with the medial edge of the second cuneiform on the frontal and oblique views of the foot. Disruption of the alignment of the second metatarsal bone and second cuneiform with a step-off between the bones is diagnostic of an injury. The normal alignment of the bases of the fourth and fifth metatarsal bones with the cuboid and that of the base of the first metatarsal bone with the medial cuneiform are more variable.

Other varieties of tarsal subluxation and dislocation are rare.

METATARSOPHALANGEAL AND INTERPHALANGEAL JOINT DISLOCATION. Dislocations at the metatarsophalangeal joints can occur in any direction and commonly involve the first digit. Similarly, dislocation of interphalangeal joints predominates in the hallux.

FRACTURES OF THE METATARSAL BONES AND PHALANGES. Metatarsal fractures, which may result from direct or indirect forces, may be transverse, oblique, spiral, or comminuted in configuration. Those of the shaft and neck of the bone commonly result from a heavy object falling on the foot; fractures of the metatarsal head are uncommon.

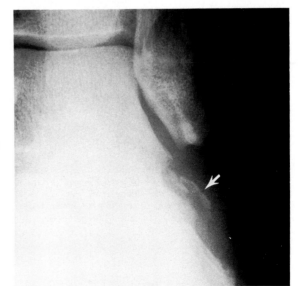

Figure 62–119. Calcaneal injuries: Extraarticular fractures. Fracture at the origin of the extensor digitorum brevis muscle (arrow).

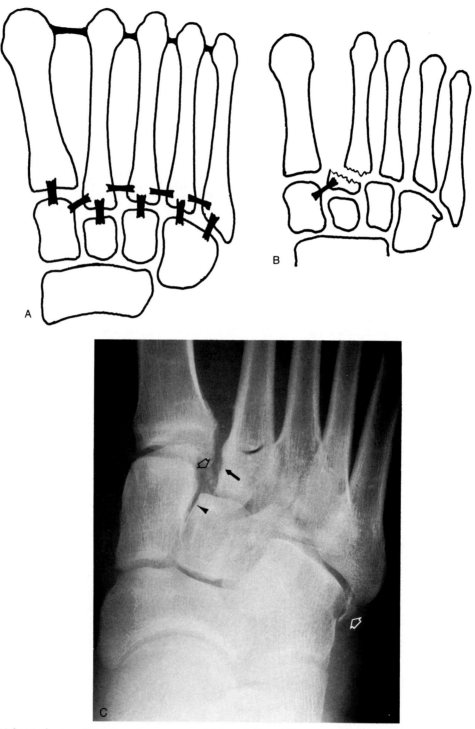

Figure 62–120. Lisfranc's fracture-dislocation of tarsometatarsal joints. A Normal ligamentous anatomy (see text). **B** Lateral dislocation of the second through fifth metatarsal bones may be associated with fractures of the base of the second metatarsal bone and cuboid. **C** In this patient, note subtle displacement of the second through fifth metatarsal bases. The medial edge of the second metatarsal base (solid arrow) is not aligned with the medial edge of the second cuneiform (arrowhead). Fractures of the base of the second metatarsal bone and cuboid are evident (open arrows). (**A, B,** From Wiley JJ: The mechanism of tarso-metatarsal joint injuries. J Bone Joint Surg [Br] 53:474, 1971. Used with permission.)

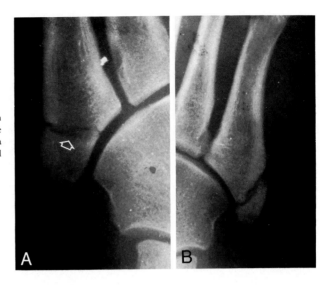

Figure 62–121. Metatarsal bone fractures: Fracture at the base of the fifth metatarsal bone. A The fracture line (open arrow) is identified entering the space between the metatarsal base and the cuboid. B On the opposite side, a normal apophysis is present. The radiolucent line between it and the metatarsal bone does not enter the joint.

Two major types of fractures of the fifth metatarsal bone exist: an avulsion fracture of the tuberosity and a transverse fracture of the proximal portion of the diaphysis. The latter injury is termed a Jones fracture; it is associated with delayed union or nonunion and refracture. Avulsion of a portion of the tuberosity of the fifth metatarsal bone results from an indirect injury associated with sudden inversion of the foot. The fracture line is usually transverse and may enter the cuboid-metatarsal joint space. Differentiation of the fracture from a normal-appearing apophysis of the fifth metatarsal bone in children can be difficult; the latter is oriented in a longitudinal direction and the radiolucent line that exists between it and the parent bone does not enter the cuboid-metatarsal space (Fig. 62–121). Normal sesamoid bones (including the os peroneum and os vesalianum) that occur in this region are smooth and round, differing in appearance from bone fragments seen with an avulsion fracture.

Fractures of the phalanges of the toes are common and create few diagnostic problems. Of particular importance are displaced intraarticular fractures and, in children, physeal injuries of the distal phalanx (the stubbed great toe, which may be open and accompanied by osteomyelitis).

Pelvis

FRACTURES AND DISLOCATIONS OF THE PEL-
VIS. The bony pelvis is intimate with vital internal organs and it is the evaluation of these organs that becomes mandatory in cases of injury. Hemorrhage owing to vascular injury of arteries (e.g., hypogastric and superior gluteal arteries and their branches) or veins, injury of the urinary tract (e.g., bladder and urethra), compression of peripheral nerves (e.g., the sacral plexus, sciatic nerve and lumbosacral nerve roots), and disruption of viscera (e.g., liver and spleen) are among the significant complications of pelvic fractures and dislocations. Furthermore, as the osseous pelvis as a whole is a ring-like structure and, indeed, some of its components are also rings (e.g., pubic rami), it is common to encounter more than a single injury (in the form of a fracture, subluxation, or dislocation).

The major forces acting on the pelvic ring are external rotation, lateral compression (internal rotation), vertical shear,

and complex forces. The resultant injuries are summarized in Figure 62–122. In this scheme, stability of the pelvic ring is considered to depend primarily on the integrity of its ligamentous structures, especially those located posteriorly. Instability is most characteristic of injuries resulting from vertical shear and complex forces. In other classification systems, stable fractures generally are considered to be those that either do not disrupt the osseous ring or disrupt it only in one place, and unstable fractures are those that disrupt the ring in two or more places (Table 62–11; Fig. 62–123).

1. *Type I injuries.* Type I injuries, which do not lead to disruption of the pelvic ring, constitute approximately 30 per cent of all injuries that involve the bony pelvis. Avulsion fractures occur at sites of muscular and tendinous insertions (see later discussion).

Unilateral fractures of a single ramus are quite common in elderly patients after a fall and occur in the form of a stress

Table 62–11. INJURIES OF THE OSSEOUS PELVIS

Injuries without Disruption of the Pelvic Ring
Avulsion fracture
Fracture of the pubis or ischium
Fracture of the iliac wing
Fracture of the sacrum
Fracture or dislocation of the coccyx

Injuries with Single Break in the Pelvic Ring
Fractures of two ipsilateral rami
Fracture near, or subluxation of, the symphysis pubis
Fracture near, or subluxation of, the sacroiliac joint

Injuries with Double Breaks in the Pelvic Ring
Double vertical fractures or dislocations of the pubis (straddle fractures)
Double vertical fractures or dislocations of the pelvis (Malgaigne fractures)
Multiple fractures

Injuries of the Acetabulum
Undisplaced fractures
Displaced fractures

From Kane WJ: Fractures of the pelvis. *In* CA Rockwood Jr, DP Green (Eds): Fractures in Adults. 2nd Ed. Philadelphia, JB Lippincott Co, 1984, p 1112. Used with permission.

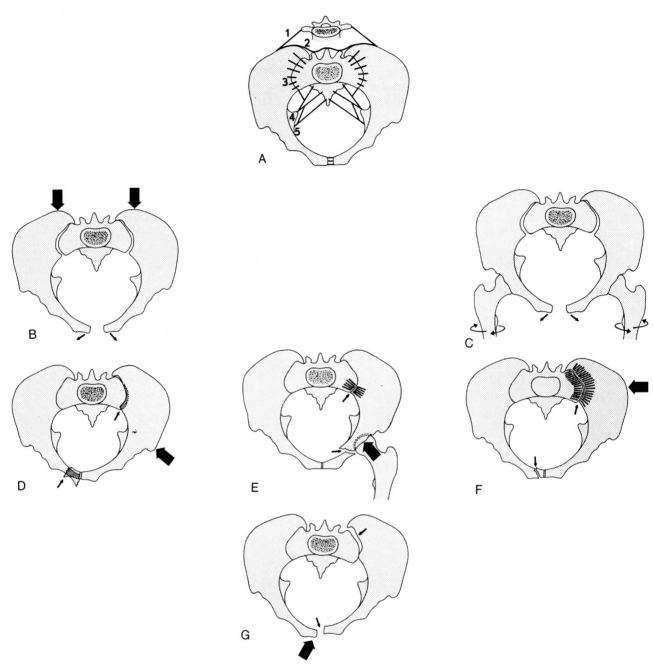

Figure 62–122. Fractures and dislocations of the pelvis: Biomechanical principles. A Normal situation. Schematic representation of the major ligamentous structures is shown. These include the iliolumbar ligaments (1), posterior (2) and anterior (3) sacroiliac ligaments, sacrospinous ligaments (4), and sacrotuberous ligaments (5). **B** External rotation forces. A direct blow to the posterior superior iliac spines (large arrows) leads to opening of the symphysis pubis (small arrows). Without the addition of a shearing force, the posterior ligamentous complex remains intact. **C** External rotation forces. External rotation of the femora (curved arrows) or direct compression against the anterior superior iliac spines also produces springing of the symphysis pubis (small arrows). Without the addition of a shearing force, the posterior ligamentous complex remains intact. **D** Lateral compression forces. A lateral compression force against the iliac crest (large arrow) causes the hemipelvis to rotate internally. The anterior portions of the sacrum and pubic rami (small arrows) are injured. **E** Lateral compression forces. A direct force against the greater trochanter (large arrow) leads to similar injuries to the pubic rami and ipsilateral sacroiliac joint ligamentous complex (small arrows). **F** Lateral compression forces. A force (large arrow) directed parallel to the trabeculae about the sacroiliac joint may produce impaction of bone posteriorly and disruption of the pubic rami (small arrows). **G** Vertical shearing forces. A shearing force (large arrow) crosses perpendicular to the main trabecular pattern, and causes both anterior and posterior injuries (small arrows). (From Tile M: Fractures of the Pelvis and Acetabulum. Copyright 1984, Williams & Wilkins Co, Baltimore, p 22. Used with permission.)

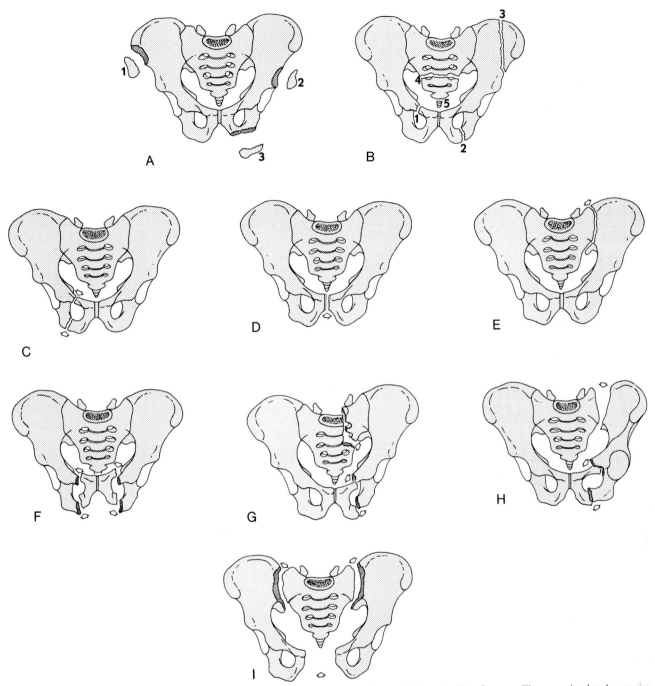

Figure 62–123. Fractures and dislocations of the pelvis: Classification system. A Type I injury: Avulsion fractures. These may involve the anterior superior iliac spine (1), the anterior inferior iliac spine (2), or the ischial tuberosity (3) **B** Type I injury: Fractures of a single pubis ramus or iliac wing (Duverney fracture). A single break in the superior or inferior pubic ramus (1, 2), certain fractures of the ilium (3), or some types of fractures of the sacrum (4) or coccyx (5) do not lead to disruption of the pelvic ring. **C** Type II injury: Ipsilateral fractures of the pubic rami. Such fractures (open arrows) lead to a single break in the pelvic ring. **D** Type II injury: Diastasis of the symphysis pubis. This injury (open arrow), or an isolated fracture of parasymphyseal bone, also leads to a single break in the pelvic ring. **E** Type II injury: Subluxation of the sacroiliac joint. This subluxation (open arrow), or an isolated fracture near the sacroiliac joint, is an additional example of a single break in the pelvic ring. **F** Type III injury: Straddle fracture. Note disruption of the pelvis in two places owing to bilateral vertical fractures involving both pubic rami (open arrows). **G** Type III injury: Malgaigne fracture. Vertical fractures of both pubic rami on one side combined with a sacral fracture (open arrows) lead to disruption of the pelvic ring in two places. **H** Type III injury: Malgaigne fracture. Similar vertical fractures of both pubic rami on one side combined with dislocation of the sacroiliac joint (open arrows) again produce disruption of the pelvic ring in two places. **I** Complex injury: "Sprung" pelvis. Disruptions of the pelvic ring relate to bilateral dislocations of the sacroiliac joint and diastasis of the symphysis pubis (open arrows).

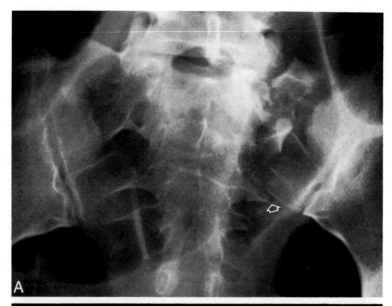

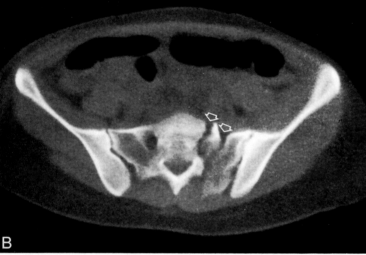

Figure 62–124. Fractures and dislocations of the pelvis: Types II and III fractures of the sacrum. Vertical fractures of the sacrum disrupt the arcuate lines (open arrow), as depicted on frontal radiographs (A). Computed tomography (B) is better able to define the extent of injury (open arrows).

fracture in athletes. These fractures may be associated with subsequent osteolysis simulating that of a malignant tumor (see Chapter 84).

A fracture of the iliac wing, the Duverney fracture, follows a direct injury and rarely is displaced. An isolated transverse fracture of the sacrum is rare and is easily overlooked on radiographic examination. Disruption of sacral nerve roots represents a complication of this fracture. These injuries should be distinguished from vertical fractures (Fig. 62–124) of the sacrum (which may be associated with additional osseous and ligamentous injuries) and from insufficiency stress fractures (which occur in the osteopenic skeleton). A fracture or dislocation of the coccyx represents an additional example of a type I pelvic injury.

2. *Type II injuries.* Because the pelvis is a ring-like structure, in many instances of an apparently isolated pelvic fracture, a second region of abnormality exists. As the bony pelvis is not a truly rigid structure, however, a single break in the pelvic ring (type II injury) may be encountered. Ipsilateral fractures of both pubic rami, a fracture of the symphysis itself, subluxation of the sacroiliac joint or symphysis pubis, and a fracture near the sacroiliac joint are

examples of type II pelvic injuries. The greater the degree of joint diastasis or the more extensive the displacement at the fracture site, the more likely is the occurrence of a second break in the pelvic ring (type III pattern). Diastasis of the symphysis pubis by more than 15 mm should raise the strong suspicion of disruption of the posterior aspect of the pelvic ring as well.

3. *Type III injuries.* Examples of these injuries, which represent double breaks in the pelvic ring (Fig. 62–125), include straddle fractures and Malgaigne fractures.

Straddle injuries are characterized by disruption of the anterior portion of the pelvis in two places (e.g., bilateral vertical fractures involving both pubic rami or a unilateral fracture of both rami). These injuries represent 20 per cent of all pelvic fracture patterns, and are accompanied by urethral or visceral damage in about 30 to 40 per cent of cases.

The term Malgaigne fracture generally is applied to injuries that disrupt the anterior and posterior regions of the pelvic ring. The forms of this injury include (1) a vertical fracture of both pubic rami combined with either a dislocation of the sacroiliac joint or a fracture of the ilium or sacrum and (2) symphyseal dislocation combined with either a dislocation of

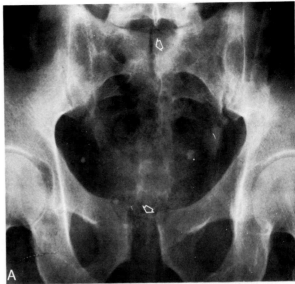

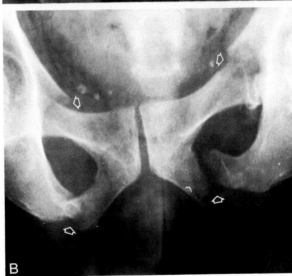

Figure 62–125. Fractures and dislocations of the pelvis: Type III injuries. A In this example, symphyseal diastasis and a vertical fracture of the sacrum (open arrows) have led to disruption of the pelvic ring in two locations. B A straddle injury with bilateral vertical fractures of both pubic rami (open arrows) is apparent.

the sacroiliac joint or a fracture of the ilium or sacrum. Malgaigne fractures represent approximately 15 per cent of all injuries of the osseous pelvis.

More extensive disruptions of the pelvis result from massive crushing injuries (Fig. 62–126).

4. *Type IV injuries.* Fractures of the acetabulum are considered earlier in this chapter.

Excessive bleeding that accompanies many of these fractures, particularly type III injuries, requires blood transfusions in almost 50 per cent of cases. Injuries to the urinary tract are associated most typically with symphyseal diastasis or fractures of the pubic rami. Hematuria after a pelvic fracture deserves immediate attention and may require retrograde urethrography, cystography, or intravenous pyelography. Damage to the peripheral nerves occurs in approximately 10 per cent of patients after injuries to the osseous pelvis, and this frequency increases in those with sacral fractures.

Thoracic Cage

FRACTURES AND DISLOCATIONS OF THE STERNUM. The usual mechanism leading to fractures or disloca-

tions of the sternum is direct trauma, and associated injuries of the anterior portion of the ribs and costocartilages are common. Aortic, tracheal, cardiac, and pulmonary injuries represent serious complications of direct sternal trauma.

FRACTURES OF THE RIBS. Such fractures result from direct injuries owing to blows to the chest or falls and generally are of lesser significance than that of simultaneous injuries in the nearby lung. Soft tissue emphysema implies that there has been violation of the lung and should prompt a careful search for a pneumothorax. Fractures of the first and second ribs generally imply severe trauma and may be associated with vascular disruptions.

Spine

FRACTURES AND DISLOCATIONS OF THE SPINE. Such injuries can occur at any level in the lumbar, thoracic, or cervical segments. In the *cervical spine*, 12 significant signs of trauma have been formulated, related to abnormalities of soft tissues (widened retropharyngeal space, widened retrotracheal space, displacement of the prevertebral fat stripe, and tracheal deviation or laryngeal dislocation); of vertebral align-

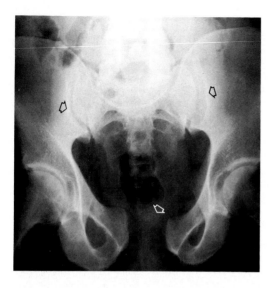

Figure 62–126. Fractures and dislocations of the pelvis: Complex injuries. A "sprung" pelvis is characterized by subluxations or dislocations of both sacroiliac joints and symphyseal diastasis (open arrows).

ment (loss of lordosis, acute kyphotic angulation, torticollis, widened interspinous space, and rotation of vertebral bodies); and of joints (widened median anterior atlantoaxial joint, alteration of intervertebral disc, and widening of apophyseal joints). Classification of the specific traumatic conditions of the cervical spine is usually accomplished according to the mechanisms of injury (Table 62–12).

Atlantooccipital Dislocation. Atlantooccipital dislocation, a rare injury, is almost universally fatal. Extreme hyperextension with a distractive force applied to the head is one proposed mechanism of trauma. Anterior movement of the cranium with respect to the cervical spine is typical, and accurate radiographic diagnosis depends on certain measurements indicative of the relative position of the occiput and the atlas. On a lateral radiograph, the ratio of the length of a line drawn from the basion (midline anterior margin of the

foramen magnum) to the anterior margin of the spinous process of the atlas (arch-canal line) to that of a second line drawn from the opisthion (midline posterior margin of the foramen magnum) to the midpoint of the posterior surface of the anterior arch of the atlas is calculated. If this ratio is less than 1, no anterior atlantooccipital dislocation exists; if it is greater than 1, such a dislocation is present. This calculation does not allow the identification of the less frequent posterior atlantooccipital dislocation.

Atlantoaxial Rotary Fixation. The principal motion that occurs at the atlantoaxial articulations is rotation. Self-limited and completely reversible rotation at the atlantoaxial junction is especially frequent in children with torticollis and may follow trivial trauma. Occasionally, the abnormal displacement persists and the condition is termed rotary fixation. Rotary fixation may occur as an isolated injury or in combi-

---

Table 62–12. CLASSIFICATION OF INJURIES OF THE CERVICAL SPINE

Hyperflexion Injuries
  Disruptive hyperflexion
    Hyperflexion sprain (momentary dislocation)
    Hypeflexion-dislocation (locked facets)
      Bilateral
      Unilateral (with associated rotational force)
    Spinous process fracture
  Compressive hyperflexion
    Wedge-like compression of vertebral body
    Comminuted (teardrop) fracture of vertebral body
    Hyperflexion fracture-dislocation (type IV)
  Hyperflexion or shearing forces
    Anterior atlantooccipital dislocation(?)
    "Pure" anterior atlantoaxial dislocation (without associated fracture)
    Anterior fracture-dislocation of the dens

Hyperextension Injuries
  Disruptive hyperextension
    Horizontal fracture of the anterior arch of C1
    Hangman's fracture (traumatic spondylolisthesis of C2)
    Anteroinferior margin of the body of the axis (C2)
    Hyperextension sprain (momentary dislocation)
    Spinous process fracture

  Compressive hyperextension
    Posterior arch of the atlas fracture
    Vertebral arch fracture (articular pillar, pedicle, lamina)
    Hyperextension fracture-dislocation (types IV-V)
  Hyperextension or shearing forces
    Posterior fracture-dislocation of the dens
    "Pure" posterior atlantoaxial dislocation (without associated fracture)

Hyperrotation Injuries
  Rotary atlantoaxial dislocation
  Anterior and posterior ligament disruption

Lateral Hyperflexion Injuries
  Fracture of transverse process
  Uncinate process fracture
  Lateral fracture-dislocation of the dens
  Brachial plexus avulsion associated with cervical fractures or dislocations, or both
  Lateral wedge-like compression of vertebral body

Axial Compressive Injuries
  Isolated fracture of the lateral mass of the atlas
  Burst fracture of Jefferson (C1)
  Vertical and oblique fractures of the axis body
  Burst fracture of a vertebral body

From Gehweiler JA Jr, Osborne RL Jr, Becker RF: The Radiology of Vertebral Trauma. Philadelphia, WB Saunders Co, 1980, p 107. Used with permission.

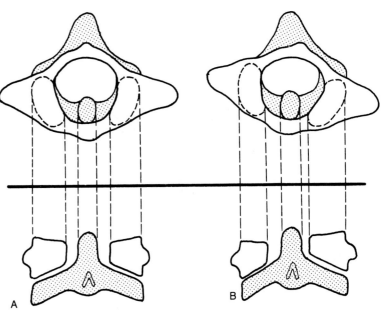

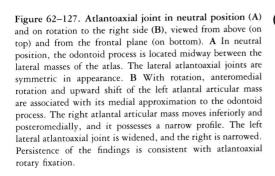

Figure 62–127. Atlantoaxial joint in neutral position (A) and on rotation to the right side (B), viewed from above (on top) and from the frontal plane (on bottom). **A** In neutral position, the odontoid process is located midway between the lateral masses of the atlas. The lateral atlantoaxial joints are symmetric in appearance. **B** With rotation, anteromedial rotation and upward shift of the left atlantal articular mass are associated with its medial approximation to the odontoid process. The right atlantal articular mass moves inferiorly and posteromedially, and it possesses a narrow profile. The left lateral atlantoaxial joint is widened, and the right is narrowed. Persistence of the findings is consistent with atlantoaxial rotary fixation.

nation with a transverse ligament rupture or fracture of the atlas or the axis. The patient holds the head tilted to one side and rotated to the opposite side with slight flexion.

The correct diagnosis can be established on a carefully performed radiographic examination if the physician is cognizant of the normal shifts of alignment between the atlas and axis that occur with rotation and lateral bending of the neck (Fig. 62–127). In patients with atlantoaxial rotary fixation, a persistent asymmetry of the odontoid process in its relationship to the articular masses of the atlas is seen that is not corrected by changes in head position (Fig. 62–128). Documentation of this abnormal situation is provided by a radiographic study that includes five open-mouth views of the odontoid process: anteroposterior (AP) view in neutral position; AP views with the head tilted 10 degrees to either side; and AP views with the head rotated 10 degrees to either side. Normally, the relative position of the odontoid process and lateral masses of the atlas will vary among these views; in the presence of atlantoaxial rotary fixation, no change in alignment is apparent. If rotary fixation is complicated by rupture or attenuation of the transverse ligament of the atlas, the distance between the atlas and the dens will be increased on lateral radiographs obtained during neck flexion. Furthermore, the transverse images provided by computed tomography will identify whether the odontoid process or one lateral articular process is serving as the pivot.

Atlantoaxial Subluxation and Dislocation. Traumatic subluxation of the atlas and the axis is almost always accompanied by a fracture of the odontoid process. Isolated atlantoaxial subluxation (without fracture) indicates abnormality of the transverse ligament that may be related to trauma, inflammation, or congenital anomaly; underlying inflammatory disease processes include rheumatoid arthritis, juvenile chronic arthritis, ankylosing spondylitis, pharyngitis, and tonsillitis, processes that presumably lead to ligament laxity owing to hyperemia. With isolated atlantoaxial subluxation, the atlas almost always slides anteriorly, increasing the distance between the anterior arch of the atlas and the dens.

This distance is best measured on carefully obtained lateral radiographs during neck flexion. Normally, it may reach 2.5 to 3.0 mm in adults and 3.5 to 4.5 mm in children.

Fracture of the odontoid process with atlantoaxial subluxation can result from either a hyperflexion or a hyperextension injury (Fig. 62–129). In hyperflexion injuries, the dens is displaced anteriorly with the atlas; in hyperextension injuries, it is displaced posteriorly.

Fractures of the Atlas. Five types of atlas fractures have been identified: burst fracture of Jefferson, horizontal fracture of the anterior arch, unilateral or bilateral fractures of the posterior arch, fracture of the lateral mass, and fracture of the transverse process. Of these, the first three are encountered more commonly.

Jefferson fractures result from an axial compressive force applied to the vertex of the skull with the head erect (Fig. 62–130). The atlas is caught between the occipital condyles. Fractures of the anterior and posterior arches of the atlas occur, allowing displacement of the lateral masses and creating an offset between these masses and those of the axis on frontal radiographs of the cervical spine (open-mouth projections). These fractures can occasionally be simulated by congenital clefts. Displacement of the lateral masses of the atlas of more than 6.9 mm relative to the axis usually is indicative of a tear in the transverse ligament of the atlas. Neurologic deficits are infrequent in cases of Jefferson fracture owing to the increases in the transverse and sagittal diameters of the spinal canal that characterize this injury.

Horizontal fractures of the anterior arch of the atlas are usually associated with additional injuries in the cervical spine, including fractures of the odontoid process. Fractures of the posterior arch of the atlas (Fig. 62–131) are probably related to a combination of axial compression and hyperextension in which the posterior arch is crushed between the spinous process of the axis and the basiocciput.

Fractures of the Odontoid Process of the Axis. Fractures of the odontoid process represent approximately 10 per cent of all injuries of the cervical spine. In cases of fracture-

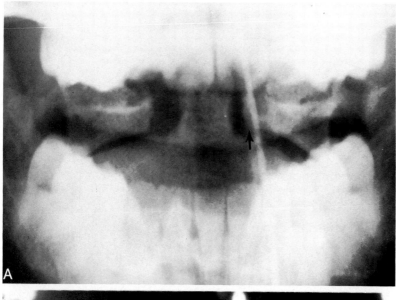

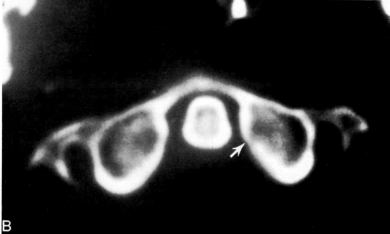

Figure 62–128. Atlantoaxial rotary fixation: Use of computed tomography. A The open-mouth radiographic projection, obtained with the head in a neutral position, shows an asymmetric location of the odontoid process between the lateral masses of the atlas. The left lateral mass (arrow) is closer to the midline and higher than the right lateral mass. These findings indicate that the lateral mass on the left has moved forward. **B** A transaxial computed tomographic scan at this level confirms anterior movement of the left lateral mass (arrow) of the atlas. Note the narrowing of the distance between this mass and the odontoid process. The fact that the right lateral mass has moved backward an equal amount would suggest that rotary fixation occurred, with the point of rotation at the odontoid process. In other instances, the point of rotation occurs elsewhere, such as at one of the lateral masses itself, a pattern that indicates probable rupture of the transverse ligament of the atlas.

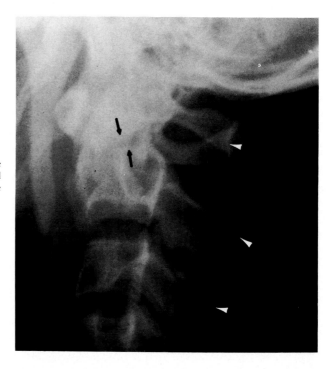

Figure 62–129. Odontoid fracture with atlantoaxial subluxation. Note the odontoid fracture (arrows) with anterior displacement of the atlas and odontoid with respect to the remainder of the axis. Note also the malalignment of the spinolaminar lines (arrowheads), indicating the degree of subluxation.

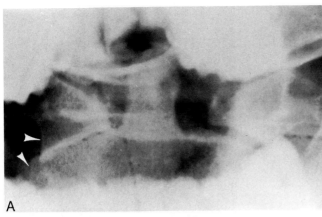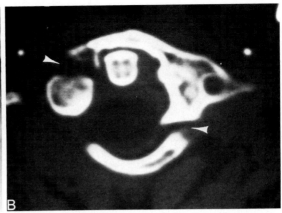

Figure 62–130. Cervical spine injury: Jefferson fracture. The initial open-mouth radiograph **(A)** shows an asymmetric position of the odontoid process between the lateral masses of the atlas. The right lateral atlantoaxial joint is obliterated, and there is offset in the position of the lateral borders of the right lateral mass of the atlas and of the axis (arrowheads). Computed tomography **(B)** reveals two fractures of the atlas (arrowheads). Identification of such fractures requires analysis of multiple contiguous transaxial scans.

dislocation, the direction of displacement (i.e., anterior, posterior, or lateral) depends on the precise type of injury. Odontoid fractures are generally classified into three categories: Type I fractures occur at the top of the odontoid process; type II fractures are located at the base of the process; and type III fractures occur through the body of the axis (Fig. 62–132). Type I fractures always unite and type III fractures nearly always unite; type II fractures, which represent the most common pattern of injury, have the highest rate of nonunion (approximately 30 to 40 per cent of cases). This feature relates to the intrinsically unstable nature of type II fractures and their tendency to become displaced at the fracture site. On radiographs, a type III odontoid fracture will disrupt a normal elongated ring-like shadow that is superimposed on the body of the axis in the lateral cervical radiograph.

Osteolysis following fracture can produce a separate ossicle above the base of the odontoid (Fig. 62–133), the os odontoideum.

Fractures of the odontoid process must be differentiated from pseudofractures caused by Mach bands, an optical illusion that leads to the appearance of a radiolucent line across the base of the dens.

Other Fractures of the Axis. Bilateral disruption of the arch of the axis generally is referred to as the "hangman's fracture" after the trauma produced by judicial hanging, in which a sudden submental force jerks the head backward. Neurologic compromise and other life-threatening sequelae occurring after this injury of the axis generally are considered to be infrequent. Vertical or oblique fracture lines usually occur through the pedicles of the axis close to the vertebral body with or without subluxation or dislocation at the C2-

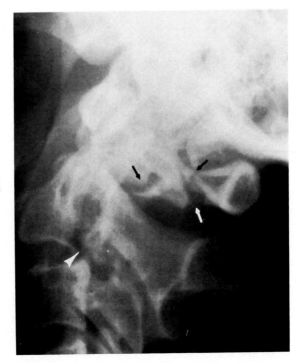

Figure 62–131. Cervical spine injury: Fracture of the posterior arch of the atlas. In this example, bilateral comminuted fractures are evident (arrows). An associated fracture of the axis is seen (arrowhead).

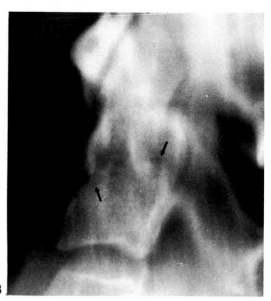

Figure 62–132. Cervical spine injury: Odontoid fractures. A Type II odontoid fracture. This open-mouth radiographic projection shows the fracture (arrows) at the base of the odontoid process. **B** Type III odontoid fracture. A lateral tomogram reveals the fracture line (arrows).

C3 spinal level (Fig. 62–134). The odontoid process and the transverse ligament of the atlas characteristically are intact.

Subaxial Fractures and Dislocations in the Cervical Spine. The categorization of traumatic abnormalities is best attempted according to the mechanism of injury (Table 62–12). Some typical fracture patterns of the vertebral body include the following:

1. *Anterior teardrop fracture (hyperflexion).* Hyperflexion, probably combined with compression, leads to splitting of the vertebral body into two fragments, a smaller anteroinferior triangular fragment (the teardrop fragment) and a larger posterior fragment (Fig. 62–135). The latter commonly is displaced into the spinal canal, whereas the triangular fragment is displaced anteriorly. Additional fractures of the vertebral body (e.g., sagittal fractures) and posterior osseous elements also are encountered.

2. *Sagittal fracture (axial compression).* A vertical fracture of

the cervical vertebral body in the sagittal plane may represent the sequela of a downward compressive force. Laminar fractures may accompany this injury. Conventional or computed tomography may be used to establish the diagnosis (Fig. 62–136).

3. *Anterior avulsion fracture (hyperextension).* A hyperextension force leads to disruption of the anterior components of the spine, including the anterior longitudinal ligament and intervertebral disc. A small avulsion fracture of the anterior surface of the vertebral body may occur at the site of discal or ligamentous attachment (Fig. 62–137). It is smaller in size than the flexion teardrop fracture and may be accompanied by widening of the intervertebral disc, indicating that hyperextension was the mechanism of injury.

4. *Comminuted (burst) fracture (axial compression).* A vertical force applied to the erect head may lead to a severely comminuted fracture of the vertebral body.

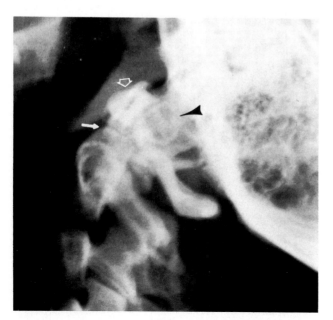

Figure 62–133. Nonunion of an odontoid fracture with separate ossicle. The findings include an amputated axis (solid arrow), posterior displacement of the anterior arch of the atlas (open arrow), and a separate ossific dense area (arrowhead).

5. *Uncinate process fracture (lateral hyperflexion).* Fractures of the uncinate process occur either in isolation or in combination with fractures of the undersurface of the vertebral body.

In hyperextension, excessive stress on the articular or spinous processes, laminae, and pedicles explains the occurrence of posteriorly located alterations in addition to the anterior ones that have already been noted; similarly, in hyperflexion, fractures, subluxations, dislocations, or ligamentous disruptions of the posterior spinal structures may complicate the injury to the vertebral body.

1. *Perched or locked articular facets (hyperflexion).* This injury relates to disruptive hyperflexion and usually occurs in the lower portion of the cervical spine. The unilateral or bilateral nature of the process, the extent of forward motion, and the presence or absence of associated vertebral fractures depend on the precise magnitude of the forces. If a total loss of contact of the apposing articular processes exists, the inferior processes of the vertebra above become locked in front of the superior processes of the vertebra below; if a partial loss of this contact occurs, the inferior processes of the superior vertebra become perched on those below (Fig. 62–138).

In cases of unilateral locking of the facets, there is rotation of the vertebrae above the level of injury such that they are seen in an oblique attitude in the lateral radiograph, whereas those below the level of injury are seen in the usual lateral attitude (Fig. 62–138). In the frontal projection in such cases, the spinous process will be deviated from the midline toward the side of the lock. With bilateral locking of the facets, no abnormal vertebral rotation occurs, but there is anterior subluxation of the upper cervical vertebra with respect to the lower, and the distance between the spinous processes of these vertebrae will increase (Fig. 62–138).

2. *Vertebral arch fracture (variable mechanisms).* Fractures of the articular pillars predominate in the lower cervical region.

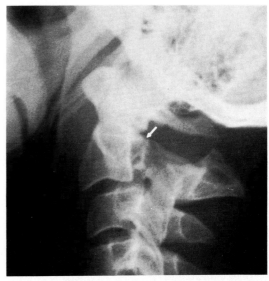

Figure 62–134. Cervical spine injury: "Hangman's fracture" of the axis. Bilateral vertical fractures (arrow) of the pedicles of the axis close to the vertebral body are accompanied by anterior subluxation of the atlas and the body of the axis with regard to the remainder of the cervical spine.

Fractures of the pedicles below the level of the axis are uncommon and those of the laminae usually are observed in the lower portion of the cervical spine.

3. *Spinous process fracture (variable mechanisms).* Direct or indirect violence and chronic stress represent the principal mechanisms of fracture of the spinous processes of the cervical vertebrae (Fig. 62–139). Those in the lowest cervical and upper thoracic regions are termed the clay-shoveler's fracture in recognition of their occurrence in men who shovel heavy soil or clay. These latter fractures are believed to result from

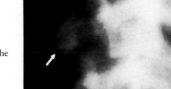

Figure 62–135. Cervical spine injury: Hyperflexion (with compression) injury. Observe the anterior osseous fragment (arrow) and the posterior displacement of the fractured vertebra.

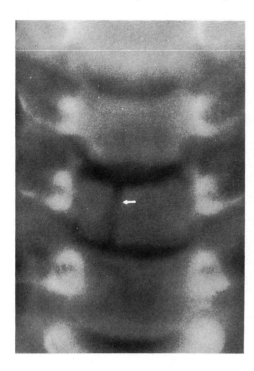

Figure 62–136. Cervical spine injury: Axial compression (with lateral flexion). The sagittally oriented fracture (arrow) is detected with conventional tomography. Loss of vertical height of the right side of the fractured vertebral body suggests lateral flexion as an additional mechanism of injury.

repeated stress caused by the pull of the trapezius and rhomboid muscles on the spinous processes. As injuries of these processes may also accompany hyperflexion and hyperextension fracture-dislocations, careful radiographic evaluation of other cervical regions should be accomplished in such cases.

Certain injuries of the cervical spine are limited to or dominated by ligamentous rather than osseous abnormalities.

The *hyperflexion sprain* represents an important example of this phenomenon (Fig. 62–140). Subtle radiologic alterations include widening of the distances between adjacent spinous processes, minor intervertebral subluxation, asymmetric widening of the apophyseal joints, narrowing of the anterior portion of the intervertebral disc, and irregularity of the anterior surface of the vertebral body. These alterations may

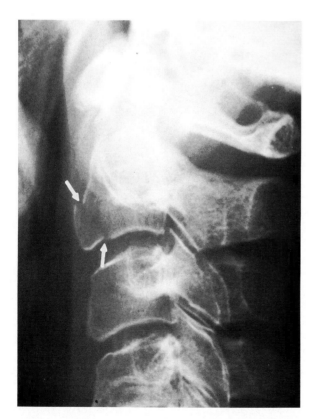

Figure 62–137. Cervical spine injury: Hyperextension. Disruptive hyperextension is the probable mechanism accounting for the fracture (arrows) at the anteroinferior margin of the body of the axis.

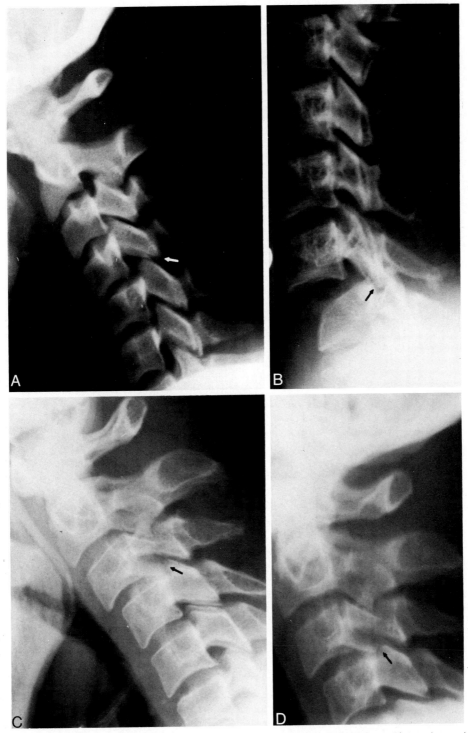

Figure 62–138. Cervical spine injury: Hyperflexion with perched or locked articular facets. A Perched facets. Observe the anterior displacement of the articular pillars of the fourth cervical vertebra with respect to those of the vertebra below (arrow). The degree of displacement is not great enough to produce locked articular facets. **B** Bilateral locked articular facets. In the lower cervical spine, note considerable anterior displacement of the sixth cervical vertebra with respect to the seventh. Bilateral facet locks are evident (arrow). A fracture of the anterior surface of the seventh vertebral body is also seen. **C, D** Unilateral locked articular facets. The important clue to the correct diagnosis of this abnormality is the identification of the articular pillars of the fourth, fifth, and sixth cervical vertebrae in a lateral projection and those above in an oblique projection. This combination of findings indicates abnormal spinal rotation. The locked facets themselves can also be seen (arrows).

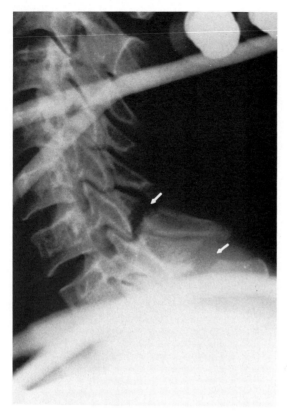

Figure 62–139. Cervical spine injury: Spinous process fracture. The spinous processes of the sixth and seventh cervical vertebrae are fractured (arrows).

become more exaggerated on lateral radiographs obtained with flexion of the neck. When the injury is left untreated, it can lead to increasing vertebral displacement and neurologic sequelae.

Fractures and Dislocations in the Thoracolumbar Spine. In the thoracolumbar spine, acute injuries have traditionally been classified on the basis of a two-column system consisting of an anterior portion (the intervertebral discs and vertebral bodies with their adjacent ligaments) and a posterior portion (the posterior osseous elements of the vertebrae and their surrounding ligaments). More recently, three functional columns of this portion of the spine have been defined.

1. Anterior column, composed of the anterior longitudinal ligament, the anterior portion of the anulus fibrosus, and the anterior part of the vertebral body.

2. Middle, or intermediate, column, composed of the posterior longitudinal ligament, the posterior portion of the anulus fibrosus, and the posterior wall of the vertebral body.

3. Posterior column, containing the posterior osseous complex (neural arch) and the posterior ligamentous structures (supraspinous and interspinous ligaments, ligamentum flavum, and capsule of the apophyseal joints).

Injuries of the thoracolumbar spine can be divided first into major and minor categories; the former affect one or more of the three spinal columns and lead to instability, and the latter involve a part of a single column and are considered stable.

Four specific types of major injuries are encountered (Table 62–13).

1. *Compression fracture.* A single compression fracture, usually related to anterior flexion of the spine, leads to failure of the anterior column with an intact middle column acting as a hinge. Radiographic abnormalities include loss of vertical height of the anterior portion of the vertebral body, but the posterior surface of the vertebral body remains intact (Fig. 62–141). Subluxation of the vertebral bodies is absent, although angulation leads to an increase in the interspinous distance. Compression typically is less than 50 per cent of the height of the vertebral body. The usual compression fracture with failure of the anterior column alone has no propensity for further progression of spinal deformity or for neurologic injury.

2. *Burst fracture.* A burst fracture results from an axial load with compression of both the anterior and the middle columns. Radiographs reveal loss of height of the vertebral body with involvement of its posterior cortex. Fragments may be displaced into the spinal canal (Fig. 62–142). Associated findings include an increase in the interpediculate distance, splaying of the posterior joints, and vertical fracture or fractures of the anterior cortex of the lamina. The posterior ligamentous structures remain intact. Neurologic compromise is evident in approximately 50 per cent of cases. Burst fractures usually affect the lower thoracic and upper lumbar vertebrae.

3. *Seat-belt injury.* These injuries, also termed Chance fractures, are characterized by failure of the posterior and middle spinal columns under tension forces and, potentially, failure of the anterior column under compression. Seat-belt injuries result from acute flexion occurring on an axis that classically is located on the anterior abdominal wall (i.e., the position of the lap seat-belt). Radiographic features include three patterns: a disruption of the posterior spinous ligaments,

Table 62–13. MAJOR FRACTURES AND DISLOCATIONS OF THE THORACOLUMBAR SPINE

Type of Injury	Site of Injury		
	Anterior Column	*Middle Column*	*Posterior Column*
Compression fractures	Compression	None	None or distraction
Burst fracture	Compression	Compression	None
Seat-belt injury	None or compression	Distraction	Distraction
Fracture-dislocation	Compression, rotation, shear	Distraction, rotation, shear	Distraction, rotation, shear

From Denis F: The three column spine and its significance in the classification of acute thoracolumbar spinal injuries. Spine 8:817, 1983. Used with permission.

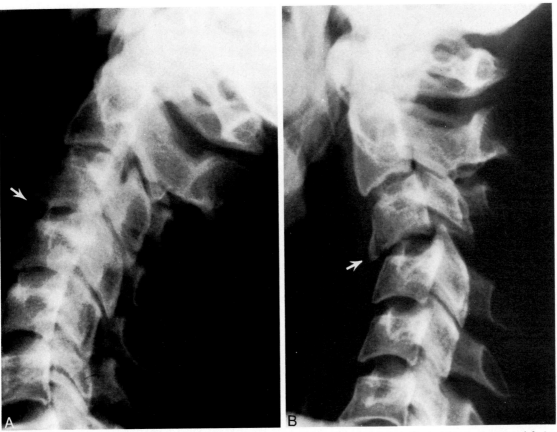

Figure 62–140. Cervical spine injury: Hyperflexion sprain. Lateral radiographs of the cervical spine are obtained with extension (**A**) and flexion (**B**) of the neck. In (**A**), vertebral alignment appears normal. A subtle fracture of the third vertebral body is seen (arrow). In **B**, anterior displacement of the third vertebral body with respect to the fourth is obvious. Note the narrowing of the anterior aspect of the intervening intervertebral disc, and widening of the apophyseal joints and interspinous distance at this level. The fracture is again evident (arrow).

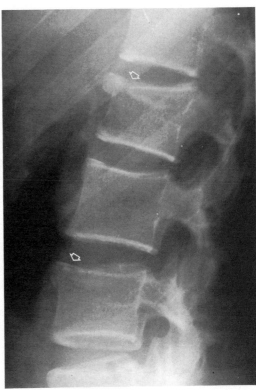

Figure 62–141. Thoracolumbar spine injury: Compression fracture. Acute compression fractures of the first and third lumbar vertebral bodies are evident. At both levels, it is the anterior portion of the superior surface of the vertebral body that is predominantly affected (open arrows). The posterior part of these vertebral bodies is normal in height.

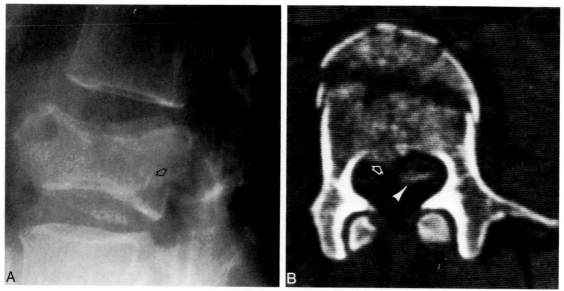

Figure 62–142. Thoracolumbar spine injury: Burst fracture. The lateral radiograph (**A**) reveals loss of vertical height of a lumbar vertebral body with involvement of the posterior cortex (open arrow). With computed tomography (**B**), the comminuted fracture lines and posterior cortical involvement (open arrow) are evident. Observe the fragment of bone in the spinal canal (arrowhead).

articular facets, and intervertebral discs with or without an associated avulsion of an articular facet or the posteroinferior aspect of the vertebral body; a transverse fracture involving the posterior elements (one or both pedicles, transverse processes, articular facets and laminae, and the spinous process) with or without extension into the posterosuperior or posteroinferior aspect of the vertebral body; and a transverse fracture of the posterior elements with an associated transverse fracture of the vertebral body (Fig. 62–143). Typically, the upper lumbar level is affected. Neurologic sequelae are infrequent.

4. *Fracture-dislocation.* Spinal instability results from failure of all three columns under compression, tension, rotation, or shear. Three basic injury types have been defined: flexion-rotation fracture-dislocation, in which there is complete rupture of the posterior and middle columns under tension and rotation and of the anterior column in rotation or varying combinations of compression and rotation; shear fracture-dislocation, in which the force is applied in a posteroanterior or, less frequently, an anteroposterior direction and all three columns, including the anterior longitudinal ligament, are violated; and the flexion-distraction fracture-dislocation,

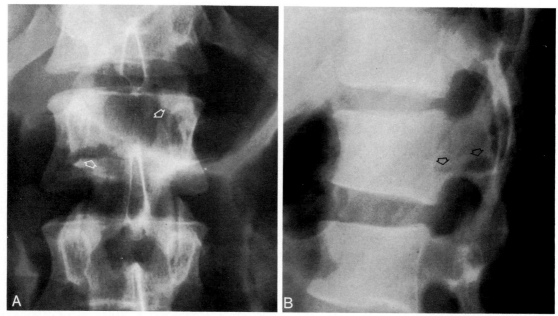

Figure 62–143. Thoracolumbar spine injury: Seat-belt injury. Frontal (**A**) and lateral (**B**) radiographs reveal a horizontal fracture (open arrows) involving laminae, articular processes, pedicles, and the posterior portion of the first lumbar vertebral body. Note the widening of the distance between the twelfth thoracic and first lumbar spinous processes.

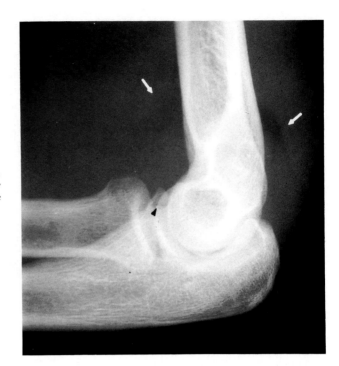

Figure 62–144. Traumatic synovitis, hemarthrosis, and soft tissue edema. Displacement of the anterior and posterior fat pads (arrows) about the elbow after trauma usually indicates intraarticular fluid or blood. Note the fracture of the coronoid process of the ulna (arrowhead).

which is similar to but more severe than a seat-belt injury, resulting in disruption of the anterior hinge (anterior longitudinal ligament and anterior fibers of the anulus fibrosus) as well. In all three types, subluxation or dislocation in the spine is evident. In addition to a variety of fractures, findings may include widening of the interpediculate distance, disruption of the apophyseal joints (the "naked" facet), locked facets, and an increase in interspinous distance. Neurologic damage is frequent.

Isolated minor injuries of the transverse, spinous, or articular processes or pars interarticularis relate to direct trauma or extreme muscle pull. Neurologic compromise is absent.

Fractures of a transverse process require great force and may be associated with disruption of abdominal viscera, paraspinal hemorrhage, and scoliosis.

TRAUMA TO SYNOVIAL JOINTS
Traumatic Synovitis and Hemarthrosis

Bloody or nonbloody effusions occurring after trauma are associated with radiographic findings that are related to displacement of intraarticular fat pads and edema of extraarticular fat planes. Typical examples of these findings are widening of the suprapatellar pouch in cases of knee trauma; displacement of the fat pads about the distal portion of the humerus (Fig. 62–144) in cases of elbow trauma; displacement and obliteration of the fat plane overlying the pronator quadratus muscle and about the carpal scaphoid in cases of wrist trauma; and "bulging" of the "capsular" fat in cases of hip trauma in children. Widening of the articular space owing to accumulation of fluid can follow intraarticular trauma.

Lipohemarthrosis

The discovery of bloody synovial fluid containing fat droplets and bone marrow spicules is reliable evidence of an intraarticular fracture, the fat being released from the marrow after cortical violation. Frequently, however, a hemorrhagic effusion containing fat may be observed in patients without fracture, probably related to significant cartilaginous or ligamentous injury.

Radiographic examination using horizontal beam technique may demonstrate a fat-blood fluid level following injury to the joint (Fig. 62–145). This finding usually is seen in a knee or a shoulder; in the knee, subtle tibial plateau fractures may be the source of the fat.

TRAUMA TO SYMPHYSES

Traumatic insult to symphyses (symphysis pubis, manubriosternal joint, and intervertebral disc) is not infrequent. Subluxation or dislocation of the symphysis pubis leads to a single break in the pelvic ring and, as indicated previously, commonly is combined with a second injury with pelvic disruption. Minor degrees of instability in this location may be discovered during radiographic examination performed with the patient standing first on one leg, then on the other. Subluxation or dislocation of the manubriosternal joint may be seen after automobile accidents in which the chest strikes the steering wheel.

Trauma to the discovertebral junction can result from obvious or occult injury. In either situation, violation of the cartilaginous endplate and subchondral bone plate of the vertebral body may allow intraosseous displacement of discal material (cartilaginous or Schmorl's nodes) (Fig. 62–146). With axial loading of the spine, there is an increase in nuclear pressure. Fracture of the cancellous bone of the vertebral body and disruption of the cartilaginous endplate allow discal material to enter the vertebral body. Invading discal tissue may split the vertebral body, producing a burst fracture of the vertebra (see earlier discussion).

Another type of injury of the discovertebral junction occurs at the site of firm attachment of the anulus fibrosus to the rim of the vertebral body. In the developing skeleton, this union is far more solid than that between the cartilage in the

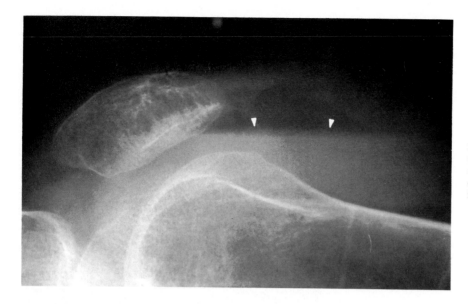

Figure 62–145. Lipohemarthrosis. On a cross-table lateral radiograph, a straight radiodense fluid line (arrowheads) at a fat-blood interface can be a helpful clue to an underlying yet subtle fracture.

vertebral rim and the ossified portion of the vertebral body. Thus, in the young patient, anterior or posterior prolapse of the contiguous intervertebral disc can lead to displacement of the ossified portion of the vertebral rim owing to separation of the osteocartilaginous junction between the rim and the remaining vertebral body (Fig. 62–147).

TRAUMA TO SYNCHONDROSES (GROWTH PLATES)
Mechanisms and Classification

The growth plate of the immature skeleton is especially vulnerable to injury; approximately 6 to 15 per cent of fractures of the tubular bones in children under the age of 16 years involve the growth plate and neighboring bone. Forces that produce ligamentous tear or joint dislocation in the adult may lead to growth plate injury in the child and adolescent. Four types of stress may produce growth plate injury: shearing or avulsive forces account for approximately 80 per cent of injuries, and splitting or compressive stresses account for the remainder. Sites that are affected most typically are the distal tibial, fibular, ulnar, and radial growth plates and the proximal humeral growth plate. Subtle clinical and radiographic findings may follow the traumatic insult.

It is the hypertrophic zone of the growth plate that is most vulnerable to shearing and avulsive injuries (Fig. 62–148). The vulnerability of the blood supply varies with the specific region of the body that is traumatized (Fig. 62–149). In certain locations, such as the proximal portion of the femur, the growth plate is situated intraarticularly, and the vascular supply to the epiphysis is applied closely to the periphery of the plate, increasing its susceptibility to injury and to subsequent growth disturbance. The younger the patient, the greater the potential for future deformity.

Although there are several proposed classification systems of growth plate injuries, that of Salter and Harris is accepted

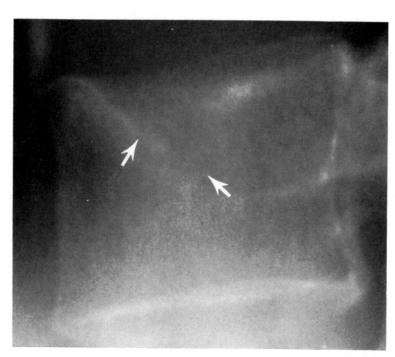

Figure 62–146. Discovertebral trauma: Acute compression fracture. After an injury with axial loading of the spine, intraosseous displacement of discal material (cartilaginous node) (arrows) can be seen.

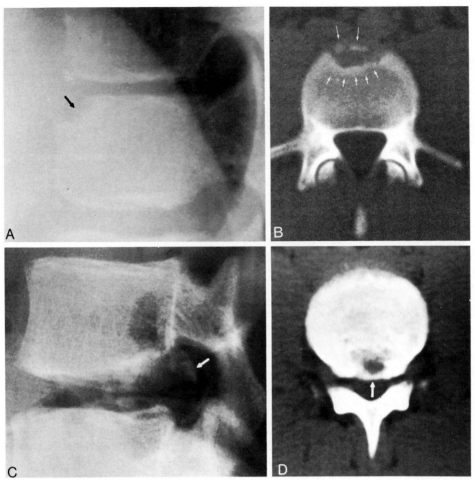

Figure 62–147. Cartilaginous nodes: Anterior and posterior prolapse. A, B Anterior prolapse leading to limbus vertebra. On a radiograph (A) in this young child, a radiolucent area in the vertebral body (arrow) has resulted from a cartilaginous node. This finding in combination with loss of height of the intervertebral disc simulates infection. (Courtesy of A. D'Abreu, M.D., Porto Alegre, Brazil.) In a different patient, computed tomography (B) shows the characteristics of a limbus vertebra. A radiolucent area is accompanied by bone spicules anteriorly, representing a portion of the ossified vertebral rim, and bone sclerosis posteriorly (arrows). (Courtesy of R. Yagan, M.D., Cleveland, Ohio.) **C, D** Posterior prolapse leading to intraspinal bone displacement. A lateral radiograph (C) shows displacement of a portion of the ring apophysis (arrow) into the spinal canal. Computed tomography (D) reveals the location of the displaced bone (arrow). (Courtesy of G. Greenway, M.D., Dallas, Texas.)

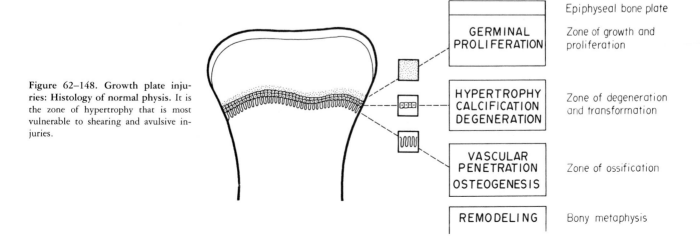

Figure 62–148. Growth plate injuries: Histology of normal physis. It is the zone of hypertrophy that is most vulnerable to shearing and avulsive injuries.

Epiphyseal bone plate

GERMINAL PROLIFERATION — Zone of growth and proliferation

HYPERTROPHY CALCIFICATION DEGENERATION — Zone of degeneration and transformation

VASCULAR PENETRATION OSTEOGENESIS — Zone of ossification

REMODELING — Bony metaphysis

A   **B**

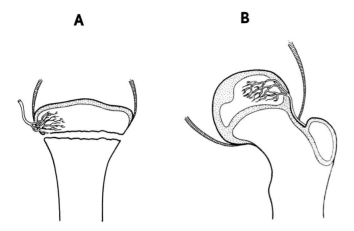

Figure 62–149. Growth plate injuries: Anatomy of normal blood supply to epiphysis. In most locations (A), the articular capsule inserts directly into the epiphysis so that the growth plate is extraarticular. The epiphyseal vessels penetrate the periosteum of the epiphysis at a site remote from the growth plate. Less commonly (B), the physis is intraarticular owing to the attachment of the joint capsule to the metaphysis. The epiphyseal vessels enter the epiphysis after crossing the edge of the growth plate and are at risk for injury when growth plate disruption occurs.

most widely. This system separates the lesions into five types according to their radiographic appearance (Fig. 62–150).

TYPE I (6 PER CENT). Type I represents a pure epiphyseal separation, with the fracture isolated to the growth plate itself (Fig. 62–151A). A shearing or avulsion force causes a cleavage through the zone of hypertrophic cells. This type of injury has a favorable prognosis; it is especially frequent under the age of 5 years and as a result of birth injury. The proximal portions of the humerus and femur and distal portion of the humerus are the sites most commonly affected. Radiographic recognition of this injury is not difficult when the growth plate is wide and when the epiphysis remains displaced. In many instances, however, spontaneous reduction of the separation takes place, and the radiographic diagnosis is more difficult. Helpful signs are soft tissue swelling and minimal widening or irregularity of the growth plate.

TYPE II (75 PER CENT). Type II, the most common type of growth plate injury, results from a shearing or avulsion force that splits the growth plate for a variable distance before entering the metaphyseal bone, separating a small fragment of the bone, the Thurston Holland or "corner sign" (Fig. 62–151B). The periosteum on the side of the metaphyseal fracture remains intact, but that on the opposite side is disrupted. Because of the intact periosteum, the fracture fragment usually is easily reduced, and the eventual prognosis generally is favorable. The usual age of injury is 10 to 16 years, and the common sites of involvement are the distal portions of the radius, tibia, fibula, and femur, and the ulna, in order of decreasing frequency. A relatively common variation of the type II lesion results when a thin layer of the metaphysis that lies parallel to the growth plate is fractured with or without the usual triangular metaphyseal fragment. This pattern of injury is common in the phalanges of the hands.

TYPE III (8 PER CENT). In the type III variety of injury, the fracture line extends vertically through the epiphysis and growth plate to the hypertropic zone and then horizontally across the growth plate itself, usually on one side or the other (Fig. 62–151C). Type III injuries are especially common in children between the ages of 10 and 15 years and in the distal part of the tibia, with less frequent involvement of the proximal part of the tibia and distal portion of the femur. Displacement generally is minimal, and if care is exercised in the reduction of the fracture, growth arrest and deformities are rare.

TYPE IV (10 PER CENT). A vertically oriented splitting force can produce a fracture that extends across the epiphysis, the growth plate, and the metaphysis, producing a fragment that consists of a portion of both the epiphysis and the metaphysis (Fig. 62–151D). This injury is encountered most frequently in the distal portions of the humerus and tibia. In younger children in whom the epiphysis is unossified or only partially ossified, the injury may be mistaken for a type II growth plate fracture. When there is radiographic evidence of a triangular metaphyseal fracture fragment in a location in which the epiphyseal ossific center is small, a type IV lesion should be suspected. A type IV injury may require open reduction and careful realignment so that growth arrest and joint deformity are not encountered at a later date.

TYPE V (1 PER CENT). A crushing or compressive injury to the end of a tubular bone can lead to the rare type V growth plate fracture. Injury to the vascular supply in the germinal cells of the plate occurs without any immediate radiographic signs. Subsequent radiographic examination may indicate focal areas of diminished bone growth, which can lead to angular deformity. This injury is more prominent in older children and adolescents. The physes of the distal portions of the femur and tibia are more typically affected.

Several additional types of injury to the growth plate or neighboring bone have been emphasized.

TYPE VI. An injury to the perichondrium can produce reactive bone formation external to the growth plate. The resultant osseous bridge may act as a barrier to growth of the adjacent portion of the plate so that progressive osseous angulation may appear.

TYPE VII. Type VII, a relatively common type of injury, is associated with epiphyseal alterations in the absence of involvement of the growth plate or metaphysis. Transchondral fractures (osteochondritis dissecans) are examples of type VII injuries.

TYPE VIII. A type VIII injury affects metaphyseal growth and remodeling mechanisms in the immature skeleton, related primarily to effects on the blood supply.

TYPE IX. An injury to the periosteum of the diaphysis may, in rare circumstances, result in disruption of normal diaphyseal growth and remodeling.

Approximately 25 to 30 per cent of patients with growth plate injuries develop some degree of growth deformity, and in 10 per cent of persons, this deformity is quite significant. In general, the younger the patient at the time of injury, the

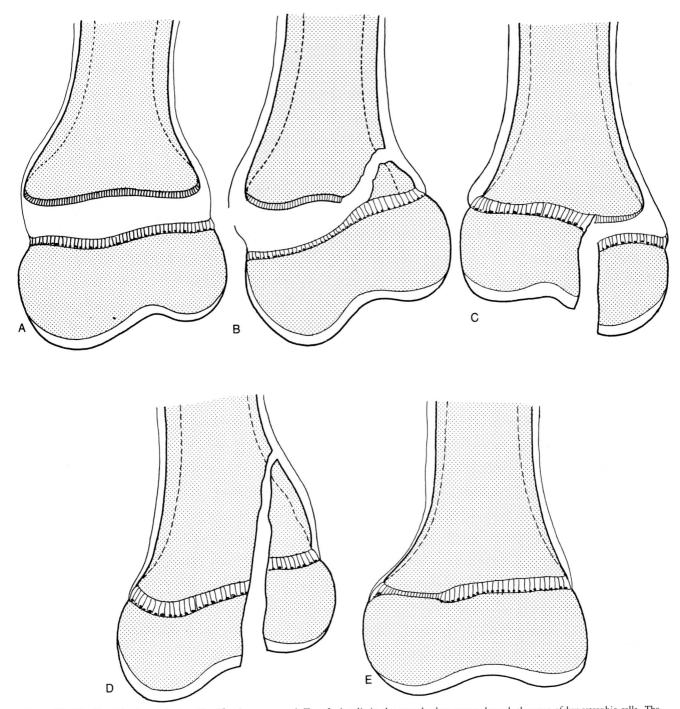

Figure 62–150. Growth plate injuries: Classification system. A Type I: A split in the growth plate occurs through the zone of hypertrophic cells. The periosteum is intact. **B** Type II: The growth plate is split and the fracture enters the metaphyseal bone, creating a triangular fragment. The periosteum about the fragment is intact, whereas that on the opposite side may be torn. **C** Type III: A vertical fracture line extends through the epiphysis to enter the growth plate. It then extends transversely across the hypertrophic zone of the plate. **D** Type IV: A fracture extends across the epiphysis, growth plate, and metaphysis. Note the incongruity of the articular surface and the violation of the germinal cells of the growth plate. **E** Type V: Compression of portion of the growth plate may be unassociated with immediate radiographic abnormalities.

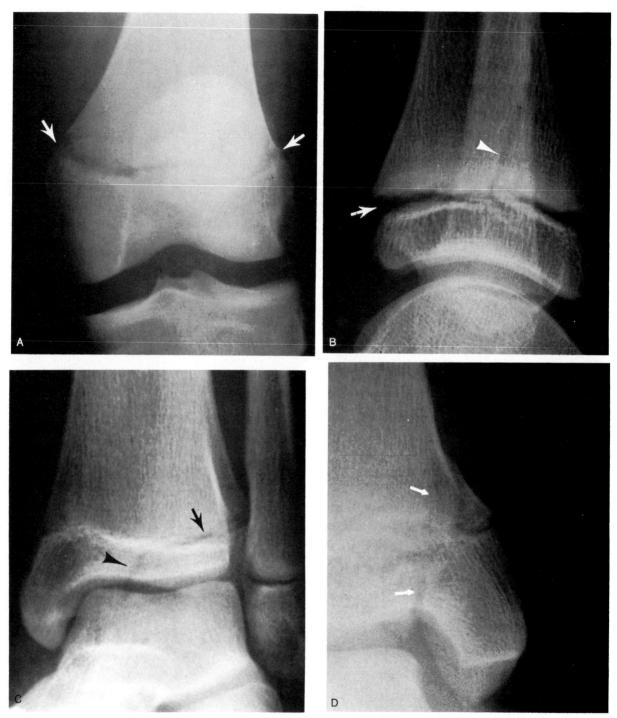

Figure 62–151. Growth plate injuries: Different types of fractures. A Type I: Note the widening (arrows) of the growth plate of the distal femur. **B** Type II: Observe the widening of the growth plate (arrow) and the metaphyseal fracture (arrowhead). **C** Type III: The epiphyseal fracture line (arrowhead) and growth plate violation (arrow) can be recognized. **D** Type IV: Observe the fracture line extending vertically through the epiphysis and metaphysis (arrows).

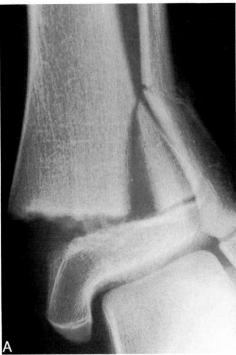 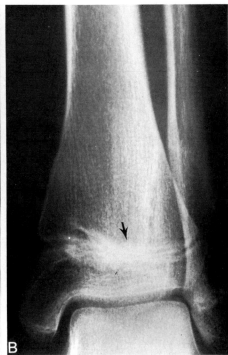

Figure 62–152. Growth plate injuries: Premature partial arrest of growth. Initially (A), a type II physeal injury in the distal portion of the tibia (as well as a fibular fracture) is seen. Subsequently (B), a bone bar (arrow) has led to premature closure of a portion of the tibial physis.

poorer the prognosis for residual deformity. Types I, II, and III injuries have a relatively good prognosis, whereas type IV injuries carry a guarded prognosis, and types V and VI injuries carry a poor prognosis. Late sequelae include growth impairment, premature growth plate fusion, epiphyseal malposition and rotation, and osteonecrosis.

Premature partial arrest of growth is produced by a bridge of bone, or bone bar, that extends from the metaphysis to the epiphysis across a portion of the physis (Fig. 62–152). The remaining portion of the physis continues to grow, resulting in increasing angular deformity. Central closure of the growth plate leads to "cupping" of the metaphysis. Although acute physical trauma is a typical cause of a bone bar, thermal injury, irradiation, infection, neoplasm, and iatrogenic events as well as chronic stress (e.g., Blount's disease) are additional causes. It is the type IV injury that most characteristically leads to closure of a portion of the physis; a type V injury may result in premature closure of the entire growth plate. The majority of bone bars are located in the proximal portion of the tibia and the distal portion of the femur, and accurate diagnosis often requires the use of conventional or computed tomography as a supplement to routine radiography.

Specific Injuries

SLIPPED CAPITAL FEMORAL EPIPHYSIS. Slippage of the capital femoral epiphysis is observed most typically between the ages of 10 and 17 years in boys and 8 and 15 years in girls. Boys are affected more frequently than girls, and the frequency is greater in black patients than in whites, and in overweight children. About 25 per cent of patients with slipped capital femoral epiphysis have bilateral involvement.

A variety of contributing factors have been emphasized in the pathogenesis of slipped capital femoral epiphysis.

1. *Trauma.* Although trauma is an important precipitating event in slipped epiphyses in infants and young children, it appears to have only a minor contributing role in older persons.

2. *Adolescent growth spurt.* The association of slipped capital femoral epiphysis with the adolescent growth spurt is well recognized. The vulnerability of the growth plate during periods of rapid growth is accentuated by its change in configuration from a horizontal to an oblique plane, increasing the shearing stresses.

3. *Hormonal influences.* The relationship of slipped capital femoral epiphysis to periods of rapid growth has led to speculation regarding the influence of various hormones in the pathogenesis of this condition. The list of endocrine diseases that have been associated with this femoral disorder includes hypothyroidism, hypoestrogenic states, acromegaly, gigantism, cryptorchidism, and pituitary and parathyroid tumors.

4. *Weight and activity.* One of the most striking characteristics of patients with slipped capital femoral epiphysis is a tendency to be overweight. Obesity increases the shearing stress on the growth plate and can lead to slippage even during usual activity. It also has been suggested that the alignment of the proximal femoral growth plate in obese persons may favor the occurrence of epiphyseal slipping.

The stresses about the hip that are most likely to produce growth plate shear are those of abduction and external rotation. With the exception of the adductor group, the musculature about this joint inserts laterally into the region below the greater trochanter and thus pulls the femoral shaft laterally and anteriorly in external rotation. The femoral head is located in a posterior and medial direction with respect to the remainder of the femur. Although a posteromediioinferior "slippage" of the capital femoral epiphysis is typical, other directions in which the epiphysis can "move" are anteriorly and superiorly or in a valgus orientation.

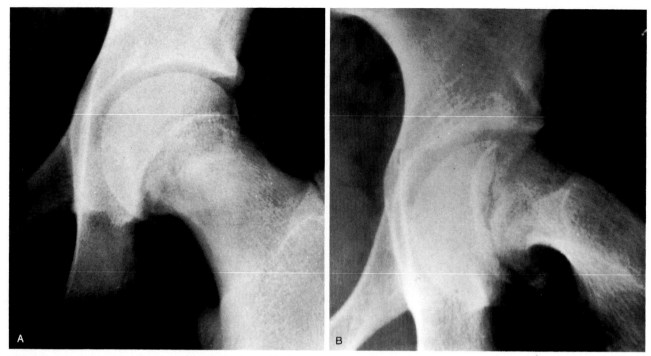

Figure 62–153. Slipped capital femoral epiphysis: Radiographic abnormalities. A Anteroposterior view. Subtle findings include mild osteoporosis of the proximal femur and indistinct metaphyseal margin. **B** Frog-leg view. The degree of posterior slippage is readily apparent. Note the widened growth plate.

Both anteroposterior and frog-leg or lateral radiographic projections are mandatory in the diagnosis of slipped capital femoral epiphysis; abnormalities on the frontal projection alone may be quite subtle. Comparison radiographs of the opposite side also can be very useful. In acute or subacute stages of this disorder, several radiographic signs may be apparent. On the anteroposterior view, osteoporosis of both the femoral head and the femoral neck is common (Fig. 62–153A). The margin of the metaphysis may appear indistinct, and the growth plate may appear increased in width. The epiphyseal height frequently is reduced. A tangential line along the lateral border of the femoral neck may fail to intersect any of the epiphysis or may cross only a small portion of it. The metaphysis may appear to be displaced from the acetabulum so that no overlap exists between the medial third of the metaphysis and the posterior margin of the acetabulum. On the frog-leg view, the degree of epiphyseal displacement is usually quite easy to ascertain (Fig. 62–153B).

In chronic stages of slipped capital femoral epiphysis, reactive bone formation appears along the medial and posterior portions of the femoral neck. Premature fusion of the growth plate may result in femoral shortening.

Sequelae of slipped capital femoral epiphysis include severe varus deformity, shortening and broadening of the femoral neck, osteonecrosis, chondrolysis, and degenerative joint disease. Osteonecrosis has been described in 6 to 15 per cent of patients with this disorder. This complication is accentuated after acute severe slippage, closed or delayed manipulation, open reduction, and a femoral neck osteotomy. Chondrolysis may be observed in as many as 40 per cent of patients with epiphyseal slippage and is more frequent in black than in white patients, in women than in men, and in persons with severe slippage. It usually occurs within 1 year of the slippage, may be evident in untreated or treated individuals, and may appear in conjunction with osteonecrosis (see Chapter 84). Radiographs outline osteoporosis, concentric narrowing of the interosseous space, and eburnation and osteophytosis of apposing osseous margins. Some recovery in the joint space may be seen after a period of months in approximately one third of persons. The cause of chondrolysis is unknown.

GROWTH PLATE INJURIES ABOUT THE KNEE. Growth plate trauma in the distal portion of the femur may be related to birth, athletic, or automobile injuries. An example is the clipping injury of adolescent football players. Type II and type III Salter-Harris injuries are especially common.

Injury to the proximal tibial physis is relatively rare, as the collateral ligaments attach distal to the growth plate. Serious complications include growth arrest and neurovascular compromise.

GROWTH PLATE INJURIES ABOUT THE ANKLE. Injuries to the growth plate in the distal portion of the tibia are common. The type II injury is most frequent, followed in order of decreasing frequency by types III, IV, and I lesions. Ten to 12 per cent of physeal injuries in this site are followed by growth disturbances.

The triplane fracture of the distal portion of the tibia represents approximately 5 to 10 per cent of all injuries in this location. It typically is seen in adolescents when physiologic closure of the distal tibial physis is occurring. This closure is initiated at the anterolateral aspect of the circumference of the medial malleolus and spreads posteriorly and laterally; the anterolateral quadrant of the physis is the last

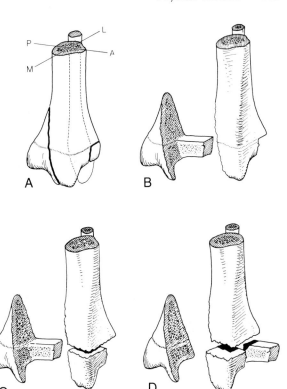

Figure 62–154. Growth plate injuries: Ankle—triplane fracture. A, B Two-part triplane fracture in place (A), and separated (B) as viewed from the medial side. (A, anterior; P, posterior, M, medial; L, lateral.) C Three-part triplane fracture. D Four-part triplane fracture.

to be obliterated. The resulting injury has several variations (Fig. 62–154), including a two-plane fracture pattern (Tillaux or Kleiger fracture, which involves only the epiphysis) or three-plane fracture patterns (in which an additional metaphyseal fracture is present).

Radiographically, a triplane fracture presents the appearance of two different types of Salter-Harris injuries (a type III lesion on the anteroposterior radiograph and a type II lesion on the lateral radiograph), although, in reality, it represents a variation of a type IV injury pattern (Fig. 62–155). Two,

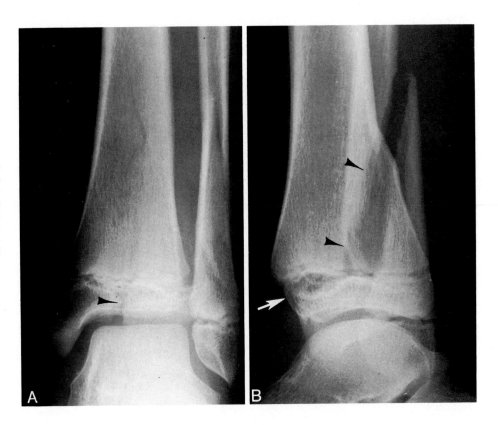

Figure 62–155. Growth plate injuries: Ankle—triplane fracture. A The anteroposterior radiograph shows an injury that has the appearance of a type III lesion (arrowhead). B On the lateral radiograph, a type II lesion is apparent (arrowheads). Note posterior displacement of the distal tibial epiphysis (arrow) and an oblique fibular fracture.

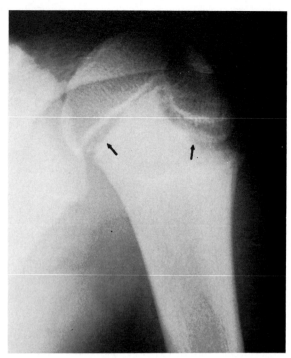

Figure 62–156. Growth plate injury: Shoulder—Little League shoulder syndrome. Note widening and irregularity of the humeral physis (arrows) on the left side in a left-handed baseball pitcher. This is a type I growth plate injury. (Courtesy of G. Greenway, M.D., Dallas, Texas.)

three, or four fragments may result. Computed tomography represents an excellent technique for delineating the site and extent of involvement. Although early closure of the traumatized physis is expected, significant shortening of the involved limb is infrequent.

An isolated vertical fracture of the distal tibial epiphysis (type I or III injury) is also evident in the adolescent age group.

GROWTH PLATE INJURIES ABOUT THE SHOULDER. Disruption of the epiphysis and physis in the proximal portion of the humerus is relatively infrequent. It usually is observed in boys between the ages of 11 and 16 years. Its occurrence in adolescent baseball pitchers as an epiphysiolysis is termed the Little League shoulder syndrome (Fig. 62–156).

The epiphysis of the inner margin of the clavicle is the last one in the body to merge with the adjacent shaft of the bone. This epiphysis ossifies at approximately 18 to 20 years of age and, with the closure of the growth plate, merges with the shaft of the clavicle at approximately 25 years of age. Injury to the medial end of the clavicle in the immature skeleton can produce an epiphyseal separation that may be misdiagnosed as a sternoclavicular joint dislocation.

GROWTH PLATE INJURIES ABOUT THE ELBOW. The accurate diagnosis of elbow injury in the immature skeleton requires that the physician know the time and the pattern of ossification of the multiple ossification centers (Fig. 62–157). At birth, the entire distal portion of the humerus is cartilaginous. The first distal humeral ossification center to appear is the capitulum, which ossifies during the first year of life. The medial epicondyle appears at approximately 5 to 7 years of age, followed by the trochlea at ages 9 to 10 years and, finally, by the lateral epicondyle at ages 9 to 13 years. These centers fuse with the shaft between the ages of 14 and 16 years, except for the medial epicondyle, which may not fuse until 18 or 19 years of age. The ossification center of the radial head appears at ages 3 to 6 years, and the olecranon center of the ulna appears at ages 6 to 10 years. An acronym that may be used as an aid in remembering the sequence of appearance of some of these ossification centers is CRIT: C,

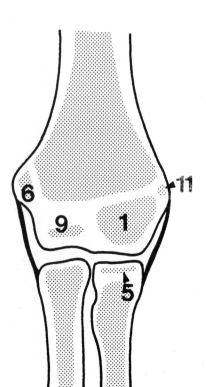

Figure 62–157. Normal pattern of ossification about the elbow. Numbers indicate approximate age in years at which the center begins to ossify (see text).

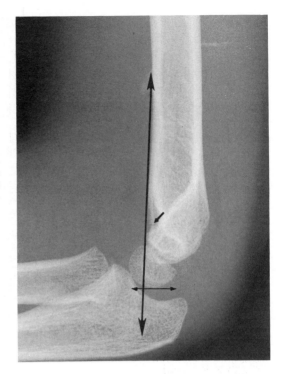

Figure 62–158. Elbow injuries: Supracondylar fracture of the humerus. On the lateral radiograph, elevation of the intracapsular fat pads and a subtle supracondylar fracture line (arrow) are seen. A line drawn along the anterior cortex of the humerus intersects the anterior third of the capitular ossification center. This indicates minimal posterior displacement at the fracture site.

capitulum; R, radial head; I, internal or medial epicondyle; T, trochlea.

Normally, the metaphysis of the distal portion of the humerus and the capitulum are anteverted about 140 degrees relative to the shaft of the humerus. A line drawn along the anterior cortex of the humerus on the lateral radiograph, the anterior humeral line, should intersect the middle third of the capitular ossification center. In the presence of supracondylar fractures of the humerus, the most common fracture of the elbow in children, posterior displacement or angulation of the distal fragment will allow the anterior humeral line to pass through the anterior third of the ossification center or even anterior to the capitulum (Fig. 62–158).

Many types of epiphyseal injuries affect the child's elbow.

A fracture of the lateral condyle is frequent and represents a Salter-Harris type IV injury. Separation of the medial epicondyle ossification center represents approximately 10 per cent of all elbow injuries. In some instances, the epicondyle may become entrapped within the joint (Fig. 62–159). In this situation, the displaced epicondylar ossification center can simulate a normal trochlear center; however, the appearance of a "trochlear" center without a medial epicondylar center is inconsistent with the normal sequence of ossification about the distal portion of the humerus.

Separation with or without fracture of the entire distal humeral epiphysis may be mistaken for a fracture of the lateral humeral condyle or a dislocation of the elbow (Fig. 62–160). In most cases, a Salter-Harris type I or II injury is

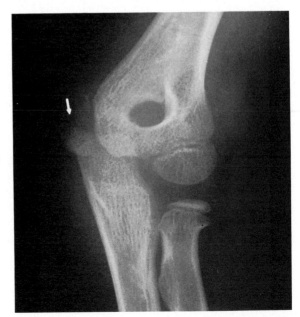

Figure 62–159. Injuries of the medial epicondyle of the humerus. Note the position of the avulsed epicondyle (arrow).

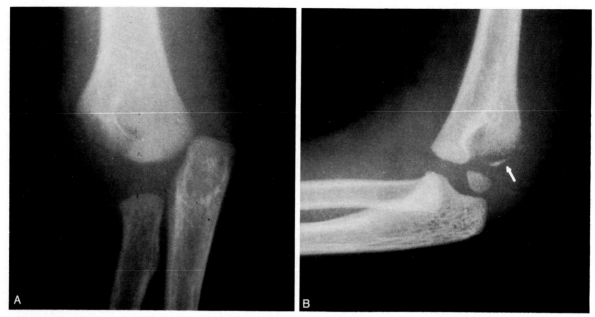

Figure 62–160. Growth plate injury of the distal portion of the humerus. Although the anteroposterior radiograph (**A**) appears to delineate a dislocation of the elbow with medial displacement of the ulna and the radius, the lateral radiograph (**B**) identifies the metaphyseal ossific flake (arrow) and the normal alignment of the radius and capitulum, indicating that a separation of the distal humeral growth plate has occurred.

present. Differentiation between these two types of epiphyseal displacement requires visualization of the metaphyseal osseous fragment that accompanies the type II injury. Anteroposterior and lateral radiographs usually reveal a normal alignment of the radius and ulna and malalignment of these bones with the humerus.

OTHER GROWTH PLATE INJURIES. The relative frequency of some physeal injuries is indicated in Table 62–14.

TRAUMA TO SUPPORTING STRUCTURES, SYNDESMOSES, AND ENTHESES
Tendon and Ligament Injury and Healing

Tendon tears or ruptures can appear at virtually any site in the body. Typical examples are injuries of the tendons in the hands and feet and of the patellar, triceps, peroneal, quadriceps, rotator cuff, and Achilles tendons (Fig. 62–161). In most cases, significant trauma initiates the tendon injury, although spontaneous ruptures have been documented, especially in patients with rheumatoid arthritis and systemic lupus erythematosus and in those receiving local corticosteroid injection. Soft tissue swelling, changes in tendon contour, and bone displacement (Fig. 62–162) may be detected on radiographs. Xeroradiography, magnetic resonance imaging, and arthrography also can be helpful diagnostically.

Ligament tears are particularly noteworthy about the wrist, ankle, elbow, and knee. Plain film radiography may require supplementation with stress radiography and arthrography. Stress radiographs can outline displacement or tilting of the apposing articular surfaces, especially in the ankle and knee.

Avulsion Injuries

Abnormal stress on ligaments and tendons may lead to characteristic avulsions at their sites of attachment to bone. For example, avulsion of a portion of the calcaneus, the patella, or the ulnar olecranon may accompany exaggerated pull of the Achilles, quadriceps, or triceps tendon, respectively (Fig. 62–161). Avulsion may also accompany cruciate ligament injuries and spinal trauma (e.g., clay-shoveler's fracture).

Several avulsion injuries about the pelvis and the hips in young athletes have characteristic radiographic features (Fig.

Table 62–14. RELATIVE FREQUENCY OF SOME PHYSEAL INJURIES*

	Frequency (Per Cent)	Typical Age† (Years)	Age Range (Years)
Distal portion of radius	49.9	9–14	
Distal portion of humerus‡	16.7	birth–5§	
		6 ‖	3–10
Distal portion of tibia	11.0	12	8–13
Distal portion of fibula	9.1		
Distal portion of ulna	5.7		
Proximal portion of radius	4.2	9–10	8–13
Proximal portion of humerus	3.1	14–15	10–16
Distal portion of femur	1.2	11–12	10–15
Proximal portion of ulna	0.7		
Proximal portion of tibia	0.5	13–15	
Proximal portion of femur	0.1	2–6 12–15	
Other	0.8		

*From Shapiro F: Epiphyseal growth plate fracture-separations. A pathophysiologic approach. Orthopedics 5:720, 1982. Used with permission.

†Girls, owing to earlier skeletal maturity and advanced skeletal age relative to boys, have injuries at an average age 1 to 2 years younger than boys.

‡The majority of these fractures are lateral condyle lesions.

§Distal humeral fracture-separations.

‖ Lateral humeral condyle fracture-separations.

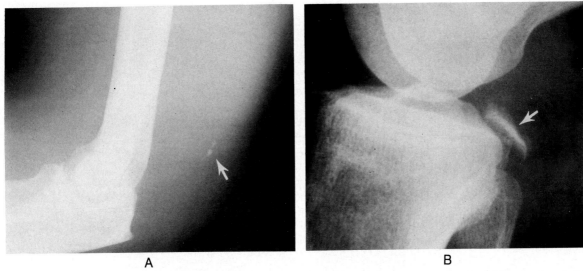

Figure 62–161. Tendon and ligament injuries. A Triceps tendon avulsion. Note massive soft tissue swelling and avulsion of fragment (arrow) of the ulnar olecranon. **B** Cruciate ligament avulsion. Observe the posterior bony fragment (arrow), resulting from an old posterior cruciate injury.

62–163). These include (1) avulsion injuries of the anterior superior iliac spine, which occur in sprinters as the result of stress at the origin of the tensor fasciae femoris or the sartorius muscle; (2) avulsion injuries of the anterior inferior iliac spine and of a groove just above the superior aspect of the acetabular rim, which relate to stress at the origins of the straight and reflected heads of the rectus femoris muscle; (3) avulsion injuries of the apophysis of the lesser trochanter owing to stress of the psoas major muscle during strenuous hip flexion; (4) avulsion injuries of the apophysis of the ischial tuberosity owing to violent contraction of the hamstring muscles, often occurring in hurdlers; (5) avulsion injuries of the greater trochanter of the femur produced by gluteal muscle contraction; (6) avulsion of the apophysis of the iliac crest owing to severe contraction of the abdominal muscles associated with running; and (7) avulsion injuries near the symphysis pubis related to adductor muscle insertion sites. Radiographs reveal irregularity at the site of avulsion and displaced pieces of bone. Follow-up radiographs may reveal considerable new bone formation with incorporation of the fragment into the parent bone (Fig. 62–164).

Rotator Cuff Tear

The rotator cuff, composed of the teres minor, infraspinatus, supraspinatus, and subscapularis muscles, is a common site of acute or chronic tears. The location of the injury in a tendinous area of relative avascularity may indicate the importance of ischemia in the production of the lesion. Inflammation or degeneration of the cuff accentuates its vulnerability to rupture. The torn tendon retracts and becomes ineffective in its normal action as an antagonist to the upward pull of the deltoid muscle; the humeral head eventually becomes juxtaposed to the undersurface of the acromion process (Fig. 62–165). Radiographic manifestations that accompany chronic rotator cuff injuries include the following.

1. *Narrowing of the acromiohumeral space.* This interosseous

space may measure less than the lower limit of normal, 0.6 to 0.7 cm.

2. *Reversal of the normal inferior acromial convexity.* Straightening and concavity of the undersurface of the acromion may become evident.

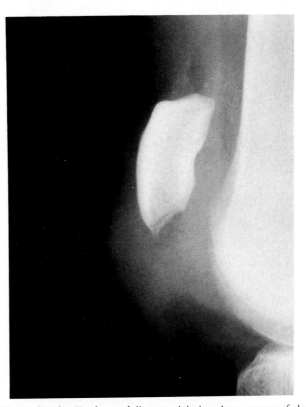

Figure 62–162. Tendon and ligament injuries. Acute rupture of the infrapatellar tendon is associated with soft tissue swelling, loss of the normal tendinous contour, and superior displacement of the patella.

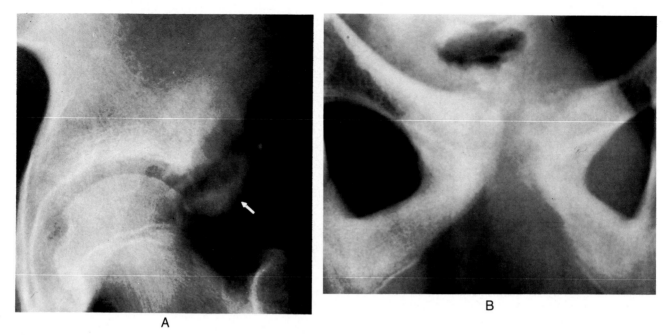

A

B

Figure 62–163. Avulsion injuries of the pelvis. A Anterior inferior iliac spine. The avulsed fragment (arrow) is related to stress at the origin of the rectus femoris muscle. **B** Symphysis pubis and inferior pubic ramus. Example of the type of osseous irregularity that may result from avulsion injuries due to stress in the adductor brevis, adductor longus, and gracilis muscles. **B,** From Schneider R, et al: Adductor avulsive injuries near the symphysis pubis. Radiology, *120:*567, 1976. Used with permission.)

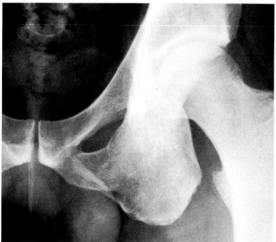

Figure 62–164. Avulsion injuries of the pelvis: Ischial tuberosity. Observe osseous enlargement that simulates the appearance of an osteochondroma.

Figure 62–165. Rotator cuff tears: Radiographic abnormalities. Note elevation of the humeral head with respect to the glenoid, contact of the humeral head and the acromion, concavity of the inferior surface of the acromion, and sclerosis and cyst formation on apposing surfaces of acromion and humeral head.

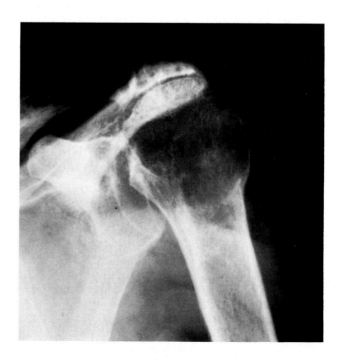

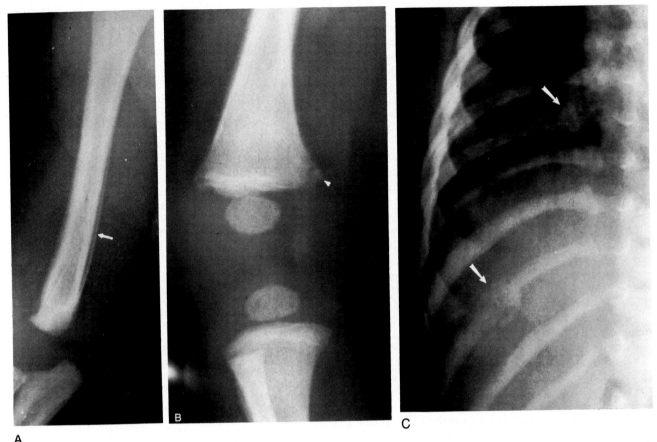

A

B

C

Figure 62–166. Abused child syndrome: Radiographic abnormalities. A Periostitis (arrow) is a delayed radiographic sign of trauma. **B** Metaphyseal irregularity and corner fractures (arrowhead) are more immediate clues to child abuse. **C** Rib fractures (arrows) are frequent in the abused child. (Courtesy of D. Edwards, M.D., San Diego, California.)

3. *Cystic lesions and sclerosis of the acromion and humeral head.* Small cystic lesions surrounded by a thin rim of sclerosis can be noted along the inferior aspect of the acromion and within the greater tuberosity.

Several limitations of these radiographic findings must be noted. Acute tears of the rotator cuff in younger patients may be unaccompanied by significant radiographic changes; the diagnosis in these persons is better established by arthrography. Second, apparent elevation of the humeral head with malalignment of the humerus and glenoid and narrowing of the acromiohumeral space can be an artifact of the x-ray technique related to incident beam angulation. Third, severe atrophy of the rotator cuff without tear can lead to many of the same abnormalities that are noted in association with chronic tears of the rotator cuff.

Complications of disruption of the rotator cuff include lesions of the bicipital tendon or acromioclavicular joint capsule, dissecting synovial cysts, interposition of the torn cuff in the glenohumeral joint, and osteoarthritis.

Rotator cuff tear can complicate a variety of articular diseases, such as rheumatoid arthritis, ankylosing spondylitis, and septic arthritis. In these processes, synovial inflammation may lead to erosion of the undersurface of the cuff and subsequent disruption. Disruption of the rotator cuff also has been associated with the shoulder impingement syndrome and calcium hydroxyapatite crystal deposition disease.

Diastasis

The term diastasis implies a separation of normally joined bone elements; it is frequently applied to injuries of the ligaments that extend between the lower tibia and the lower fibula. Radiographs may reveal fractures and abnormal separation of the tibia and fibula in which the space (la ligne claire) between the medial cortex of the fibula and the posterior edge of the peroneal groove is greater than 5.0 to 5.5 mm in the anteroposterior radiograph. Soft tissue ossification may occur subsequently.

TRAUMATIC ABUSE OF CHILDREN (ABUSED CHILD SYNDROME)

As many as 200,000 incidents of deliberate child abuse are reported each year in the United States. Boys and girls are affected in equal numbers, and most children are younger than 6 years of age. Radiographic abnormalities can be detected in 50 to 70 per cent of cases. Although these abnormalities may involve multiple systems in the body, it is the skeletal alterations that have received a great deal of emphasis.

Traumatic insult to the child's skeleton can produce elevation of the periosteal membrane, which is loosely attached to the diaphysis of tubular bones. Although the resultant periostitis is a delayed radiographic finding (Fig. 62–166A), it has repeatedly been emphasized that the firm attachment of the periosteal membrane to the metaphyses of the tubular bones can lead to an immediate radiographic abnormality—single or multiple metaphyseal bone fragments (Fig. 62–166B). The resultant fragments consist of a disc of bone and calcified cartilage. Reactive bone formation with sclerosis can be a prominent change associated with periostitis and metaphyseal fracture. Physeal injuries may also occur.

The proper work-up of a child suspected of having been physically abused includes a radiographic survey of all of the long bones, the pelvis, the spine, the ribs, and the skull. Scintigraphy with bone-seeking pharmaceutical agents may also be a useful adjunct to the radiographic examination. Radiographic findings include single or multiple fractures, especially in the ribs (Fig. 62–166C), but also involving, in order of descending frequency, the humerus, the femur, the tibia, the small bones of the hand and foot, and the skull. Diaphyseal or metaphyseal fractures can be seen in various stages of healing. "Unusual" fractures such as those of the sternum, the lateral aspect of the clavicle, the scapula, and the vertebrae should arouse suspicion of abuse. Other clues to correct diagnosis include overabundant callus formation, bilateral acute fractures, and fractures in the lower extremities in infants and young children who are not walking.

Extraosseous alterations may include cutaneous lesions, myositis, malnutrition, pulmonary contusion and pneumothorax, gastrointestinal hemorrhage, pancreatitis, hepatic and renal injuries, mucosal alterations in the mouth and palate, ocular lesions, and intracranial and subdural hematomas.

Disorders that must be differentiated from this syndrome are the normal periostitis of infancy, osteogenesis imperfecta, types of congenital insensitivity to pain, and infantile cortical hyperostosis. Metaphyseal avulsion fractures may also accompany abnormal copper metabolism in the kinky hair syndrome (Menkes' syndrome). Metaphyseal changes in scurvy may resemble those in the abused child syndrome.

FURTHER READING

Amato M, Totty WH, Gilula LA: Spondylolysis of the lumbar spine: Demonstration of defects and laminal fragmentation. Radiology 153:627, 1984.

Arndt JH, Sears AD: Posterior dislocation of the shoulder. AJR 94:639, 1965.

Bayliss AP, Davidson JK: Traumatic osteonecrosis of the femoral head following intracapsular fracture: Incidence and earliest radiological features. Clin Radiol 28:407, 1977.

Berndt AL, Harty M: Transchondral fracture (osteochondritis dissecans) of the talus. J Bone Joint Surg [Am] 41:988, 1959.

Bledsoe RC, Izenstark JL: Displacement of fat pads in disease and injury of the elbow: A new radiographic sign. Radiology 73:717, 1959.

Bloomberg TJ, Nuttall J, Stoker DJ: Radiology in early slipped femoral capital epiphysis. Clin Radiol 29:657, 1978.

Bostrom A: Fracture of the patella. A study of 422 patellar fractures. Acta Orthop Scand (Suppl)143:5, 1972.

Borden S IV: Roentgen recognition of acute plastic bowing of the forearm in children. AJR 125:524, 1975.

Brant-Zawadski M, Jeffrey RB, Minagi H, Pitts LH: High resolution CT of thoracolumbar fractures. AJR 138:699, 1982.

Bruce HE, Harvey JP Jr, Wilson JC Jr: Monteggia fractures. J Bone Joint Surg [Am] 56:1563, 1974.

Cancelmo JJ Jr: Clay-shoveler's fracture. A helpful diagnostic sign. AJR 115:540, 1972.

Chessare JW, Rogers LF, White H, Tachdjian MO: Injuries of the medial epicondylar ossification center of the humerus. AJR 129:49, 1979.

Cisternino SJ, Rogers LF, Stufflebam BC, Kruglik GD: The trough line: A radiographic sign of posterior shoulder dislocation. AJR 130:951, 1978.

Clanton TO, DeLee JC: Osteochondritis dissecans. History, pathophysiology and current treatment concepts. Clin Orthop 167:50, 1982.

Cone RO III, Nguyen V, Flournoy JG, Guerra J Jr: Triplane fracture of the distal tibial epiphysis: Radiographic and CT studies. Radiology 153:763, 1984.

Cooper KL, Beabout JW, Swee RG: Insufficiency fractures of the sacrum. Radiology 156:15, 1985.

Crowe JE, Swischuk LE: Acute bowing fractures of the forearm in children: A frequently missed injury. AJR 128:981, 1977.

Currarino G, Pinckney LE: Genu valgum after proximal tibial fractures in children. AJR 136:915, 1981.

Daffner RH: Stress fractures: Current concepts. Skel Radiol 2:221, 1978.

Daffner RH, Riemer BL, Lupetin AR, Dash N: Magnetic resonance imaging in acute tendon ruptures. Skel Radiol 15:619, 1986.

Denis F: The three column spine and its significance in the classification of acute thoracolumbar spinal injuries. Spine 8:817, 1983.

DeOliveira JC: Barton's fractures. J Bone Joint Surg [Am] 55:586, 1973.

Deutsch AL, Resnick D, Mink JH, Berman JL, Cone RO III, Resnik CS, Danzig L, Guerra J Jr: Computed tomography of the glenohumeral joint: Normal anatomy and clinical experience. Radiology 153:603, 1984.

Devas M: Stress Fractures. London, Churchill Livingstone, 1975.

Dias JJ, Stirling AJ, Finlay DBL, Gregg PJ: Computerised axial tomography for tibial plateau fractures. J Bone Joint Surg [Br] 69:84, 1987.

Downey EF Jr, Curtis DJ, Brower AC: Unusual dislocations of the shoulder. AJR 140:1207, 1983.

Dussault RG, Beauregard G, Fauteaux P, Laurin C, Boisjoly A: Femoral head defect following anterior hip dislocation. Radiology 135:627, 1980.

El-Khoury GY, Yousefzadeh DK, Mulligan GM, Moore TE: Subtalar dislocation. Skel Radiol 8:99, 1982.

Elliott JM Jr, Rogers LF, Wissinger JP, Lee JF: The hangman's fracture. Fractures of the neural arch of the axis. Radiology 104:303, 1972.

Essex-Lopresti P: The mechanism, reduction technique, and results in fractures of the os calcis. Br J Surg 39:395, 1952.

Fernbach SK, Wilkinson RH: Avulsion injuries of the pelvis and proximal femur. AJR 137:581, 1984.

Fielding JW, Hawkins RJ: Atlanto-axial rotatory fixation. (Fixed rotatory subluxation of the atlanto-axial joint.) J Bone Joint Surg [Am] 59:37, 1977.

Fisher MR, Rogers LF, Hendrix RW: Systematic approach to identifying fourth and fifth carpometacarpal joint dislocations. AJR 140:319, 1983.

Fisher RG, Ward RE, Ben-Menachem Y, Mattox KL, Flynn TC: Arteriography and the fractured first rib: Too much for too little? AJR 138:1059, 1982.

Foster SC, Foster RR: Lisfranc's tarsometatarsal fracture-dislocation. Radiology 120:79, 1976.

Fredrickson BE, Baker D, McHolick WJ, Yuan HA, Lubicky JP: The natural history of spondylolysis and spondylolisthesis. J Bone Joint Surg [Am] 66:699, 1984.

Freiberger RH, Kotzen LM: Fracture of the medial margin of the patella, a finding diagnostic of lateral dislocation. Radiology 88:902, 1967.

Freiberger RH, Wilson PD Jr, Nicholas JA: Acquired absence of the odontoid process. A case report. J Bone Joint Surg [Am] 47:1231, 1965.

Gehweiler JA Jr, Osborne RL Jr, Becker RF: The Radiology of Vertebral Trauma. Philadelphia, WB Saunders Co, 1980.

Gehweiler JA Jr, Duff DE, Martinez S, Miller MD, Clark WM: Fractures of the atlas vertebra. Skel Radiol 1:97, 1976.

Gelberman RH, Cohen MS, Shaw BA, Kasser JR, Griffin PP, Wilkinson RH: The association of femoral retroversion with slipped capital femoral epiphysis. J Bone Joint Surg [Am] 68:1000, 1986.

Gilley JS, Gelman MI, Edson M, Metcalf RW: Chondral fractures of the knee. Arthrographic, arthroscopic, and clinical manifestations. Radiology 138:51, 1981.

Gilmer PW, Herzenberg J, Frank JL, Silverman P, Martinez S, Goldner JL: Computerized tomographic analysis of acute calcaneal fractures. Foot Ankle 6:184, 1986.

Gilula LA, Weeks PM: Post-traumatic ligamentous instabilities of the wrist. Radiology 129:641, 1978.

Giustra PE, Killoran PJ, Furman RS, Root JA: The missed Monteggia fracture. Radiology 110:45, 1974.

Goergen TG, Resnick D, Greenway G, Saltzstein SL: Dorsal defect of the patella (DDP): A characteristic radiographic lesion. Radiology 130:333, 1979.

Goiney RC, Connell DG, Nichols DM: CT evaluation of tarsometatarsal fracture-dislocation injuries. AJR 144:985, 1985.

Harley JD, Mack LA, Winquist RA: CT of acetabular fractures: Comparison with conventional radiography. AJR 138:413, 1982.

Harris JH, Harris WH: The Radiology of Emergency Medicine. Baltimore, Williams & Wilkins Co, 1975.

Harris JH Jr, Burke JT, Ray RD, Nichols-Hosteter S, Lester RG: Low (type III) odontoid fracture: A new radiographic sign. Radiology 153:353, 1984.

Hawkins LG: Fractures of the neck of the talus. J Bone Joint Surg [Am] 52:991, 1970.

Hill HA, Sachs MD: The grooved defect of the humeral head. A frequently unrecognized complication of dislocations of the shoulder joint. Radiology 35:690, 1940.

Hiller HG: Battered or not—a reappraisal of metaphyseal fragility. AJR 114:241, 1972.

Holdsworth F: Fractures, dislocations, and fracture-dislocations of the spine. J Bone Joint Surg [Am] 52:1534, 1970.

Horne JG, Tanzer TL: Olecranon fractures: A review of 100 cases. J Trauma 21:469, 1981.

Hudson TM, Caragol WJ, Kaye JJ: Isolated rotatory subluxation of the carpal navicular. AJR 126:601, 1976.

Ingram AJ, Clarke MS, Clark CS Jr, Marshall WR: Chondrolysis complicating slipped capital femoral epiphysis. Clin Orthop 165:99, 1982.

Jackson H, Kam J, Harris JH Jr, Harle TS: The sacral arcuate lines in upper sacral fractures. Radiology 145:35, 1982.

Johansen JG, McCarty DJ, Haughton VM: Retrosomatic clefts: Computed tomographic appearance. Radiology 148:447, 1983.

Jones R: Fractures of the base of the fifth metatarsal bone by indirect violence. Ann Surg 35:697, 1902.

Judet R, Judet J, Letournel E: Fracture of the acetabulum: Classification and surgical approaches for open reduction. J Bone Joint Surg [Am] 46:1615, 1964.

Kattan KR: Trauma to the bony thorax. Semin Roentgenol 13:69, 1978.

Keller RH: Traumatic displacement of the cartilaginous vertebral rim: A sign of intervertebral disc prolapse. Radiology 110:21, 1974.

Kirks DR: Radiological evaluation of visceral injuries in the battered child syndrome. Pediatr Ann 12:888, 1983.

Kleinman PK, Marks SC, Blackbourne B: The metaphyseal lesion in abused infants: a radiologic-histopathologic study. AJR 146:895, 1986.

Kogutt MS, Swischuk LE, Fagan CJ: Patterns of injury and significance of uncommon fractures in the battered child syndrome. AJR 121:143,1974.

Kotzen LM: Roentgen diagnosis of rotator cuff tear. Report of 48 surgically proven cases. AJR 112:507, 1971.

Laskin RS, Schreiber S: Inferior subluxation of the humeral head: The drooping shoulder. Radiology 98:585, 1971.

Lauge-Hansen N: Fractures of the ankle: Genetic roentgenologic diagnosis of fractures of the ankle. AJR 71:456, 1954.

Lee C, Kim KS, Rogers LF: Triangular cervical vertebral body fractures: Diagnostic significance. AJR 138:1123, 1982.

Levinsohn EM, Bunnell WP, Yuan HA: Computed tomography in the diagnosis of dislocations of the sternoclavicular joint. Clin Orthop 140:12, 1979.

Linscheid RL, Dobyns JH, Beckenbaugh RD, Cooney WP III, Wood MB: Instability patterns of the wrist. J Hand Surg 8:682, 1983.

MacNealy GA, Rogers LF, Hernandez R, Poznanski AK: Injuries of the distal tibial epiphysis: Systematic radiographic evaluation. AJR 138:683, 1982.

Mayfield JK, Johnson RP, Kilcoyne RK: Carpal dislocations: Pathomechanics and progressive perilunar instability. J Hand Surg 5:226, 1980.

McGahan JP, Rab GT, Dublin A: Fractures of the scapula. J Trauma 20:880, 1980.

Merten DF, Radkowski MA, Leonidas JC: The abused child: A radiological reappraisal. Radiology 146:377, 1983.

Mickelson MR, El-Khoury GY, Cass JR, Case KJ: Aseptic necrosis following slipped capital femoral epiphysis. Skel Radiol 4:129, 1979.

Milgram JW: Radiological and pathological manifestations of osteochondritis dissecans of the distal femur. A study of 50 cases. Radiology 126:305, 1978.

Milgram JW, Rogers LF, Miller JW: Osteochondral fractures: Mechanisms of injury and fate of fragments. AJR 130:651, 1978.

Miller MD, Gehweiler JA, Martinez S, Charlton OP, Daffner RH: Significant new observations on cervical spine trauma. AJR 130:659, 1978.

Montana MA, Richardson ML, Kilcoyne RF, Harley JD, Shuman WP, Mack LA: CT of sacral injury. Radiology 161:499, 1986.

Murray WT, Meuller PR, Rosenthal DI, Jauernek RR: Fracture of the hook of the hamate. AJR 133:899, 1979.

Nance EP Jr, Kaye JJ, Milek MA: Volar plate fractures. Radiology 133:61, 1979.

Neer CS II: Displaced proximal humeral fractures. Part I. Classification and evaluation. J Bone Joint Surg [Am] 52:1077, 1970.

Newberg AH, Greenstein R: Radiographic evaluation of tibial plateau fractures. Radiology 126:319, 1978.

Newberg AH, Seligson D: The patellofemoral joint: 30°, 60°, and 90° views. Radiology 137:57, 1980.

Newberg A, Wales L: Radiographic diagnosis of quadriceps tendon rupture. Radiology 125:367, 1977.

Nicoll EA: Fractures of the tibial shaft. A survey of 705 cases. J Bone Joint Surg [Br] 46:373, 1964.

O'Callaghan JP, Ullrich CG, Yuan HA, Kieffer SA: CT of facet distraction in flexion injuries of the thoracolumbar spine: The "naked" facet. AJR 134:563, 1980.

Ogden JA: Subluxation and dislocation of the proximal tibiofibular joint. J Bone Joint Surg [Br] 56:145, 1974.

Ogden JA, Gossling HR, Southwick WO: Slipped capital femoral epiphysis following ipsilateral femoral fracture. Clin Orthop 110:167, 1975.

Ozonoff MB: Pediatric Orthopedic Radiology. Philadelphia, WB Saunders Co, 1979.

Pavlov H, Freiberger RH: Fractures and dislocations about the shoulder. Semin Roentgenol 13:85, 1978.

Peirce CB, Eaglesham DC: Traumatic lipohemarthrosis of the knee. Radiology 39:655, 1942.

Pfister-Goedek L, Braune M: Cyst-like cortical defects following fractures in children. Pediatr Radiol 11:93, 1981.

Pennell RG, Maurer AH, Bonakdarpour A: Stress injuries of the pars interarticularis: Radiologic classification and indications for scintigraphy. AJR 145:763, 1985.

Peterson HA: Partial growth plate arrest and its treatment. J Pediatr Orthop 4:246, 1984.

Phemister DB: Fractures of the neck of the femur, dislocation of the hip and obscure vascular disturbances producing aseptic necrosis of the head of the femur. Surg Gynecol Obstet 59:415, 1934.

Pinckney LE, Currarino G, Kennedy LA: The stubbed great toe: A cause of occult compound fracture and infection. Radiology 138:375, 1981.

Rang M: Children's Fractures. Philadelphia, JB Lippincott Co, 1974.

Reckling FW: Unstable fracture-dislocations of the forearm (Monteggia and Galeazzi lesions). J Bone Joint Surg [Am] 64:857, 1982.

Reckling FW, Peltier LF: Acute knee dislocations and their complications. J Trauma 9:181, 1969.

Resnick D, Niwayama G: Intravertebral disk herniations: Cartilaginous (Schmorl's) nodes. Radiology 126:57, 1978.

Resnik CS, Gelberman RH, Resnick D: Transscaphoid, transcapitate, perilunate fracture dislocation (scaphocapitate syndrome). Skel Radiol 9:192, 1983.

Ring EJ, Athanasoulis C, Waltman AC, Margolies MN, Baum S: Arteriographic management of hemorrhage following pelvic fracture. Radiology 109:65, 1973.

Roberts N, Hughes R: Osteochondritis dissecans of the elbow joint: A clinical study. J Bone Joint Surg [Br] 32:348, 1950.

Rockwood CA, Green DP: Fractures in Adults. 2nd Ed. Philadelphia, JB Lippincott Co, 1984.

Rogers LF: The radiography of epiphyseal injuries. Radiology 96:289, 1970.

Rogers LF: The roentgenographic appearance of transverse or Chance fractures of the spine: The seat belt fracture. AJR 111:844, 1971.

Rogers LF: Fractures and dislocations of the elbow. Semin Roentgenol 13:97, 1978.

Rogers LF: Radiology of Skeletal Trauma. New York, Churchill Livingstone, 1982.

Rogers LF, Campbell RE: Fractures and dislocations of the foot. Semin Roentgenol 13:157, 1978.

Rogers LF, Jones S, Davis AR, Dietz G: "Clipping injury" fracture of the epiphysis in the adolescent football player: An occult lesion of the knee. AJR 121:69, 1974.

Rogers LF, Malave S Jr, White H, Tachdjian MO: Plastic bowing, torus and greenstick supracondylar fractures of the humerus: Radiographic clues to obscure fractures of the elbow in children. Radiology 128:145, 1978.

Rogers LF, Novy SB, Harris NF: Occult central fractures of the acetabulum. AJR 124:96, 1975.

Rogers LF, Rockwood CA Jr: Separation of the entire distal humeral epiphysis. Radiology 106:393, 1973.

Roub LW, Gumerman LW, Hanley EN Jr, Clark MW, Goodman M, Herbert DL: Bone stress: A radionuclide imaging perspective. Radiology 132:431, 1979.

Rupani HD, Holder LE, Espinola DA, Engin SI: Three-phase radionuclide bone imaging in sports medicine. Radiology 156:187, 1985.

Salter RB, Harris WR: Injuries involving the epiphyseal plate. J Bone Joint Surg [Am] 45:587, 1963.

Schatzker J, Rorabeck CH, Waddell JP: Fractures of the dens (odontoid process). An analysis of thirty-seven cases. J Bone Joint Surg [Br] 53:392, 1971.

Schneider R, Kaye JJ: Insufficiency and stress fractures of the long bones occurring in patients with rheumatoid arthritis. Radiology 116:595, 1975.

Schneider R, Kaye JJ, Ghelman B: Adductor avulsive injuries near the symphysis pubis. Radiology 120:567, 1976.

Seinsheimer F: Subtrochanteric fractures of the femur. J Bone Joint Surg [Am] 60:300, 1978.

Seinsheimer F III: Fractures of the distal femur. Clin Orthop 153:169, 1980.

Shapiro R, Youngberg AS, Rothman SLG: The differential diagnosis of traumatic lesions of the occipito-atlanto-axial segment. Radiol Clin North Am 11:505, 1973.

Smith GR, Loop JW: Radiologic classification of posterior dislocations of the hip: Refinement and pitfalls. Radiology 119:569, 1976.

Smith WS, Kaufer H: Patterns and mechanisms of lumbar injuries associated with lap seat belts. J Bone Joint Surg [Am] 51:239, 1969.

Stener B: Displacement of the ruptured ulnar collateral ligament of the metacarpophalangeal joint of the thumb. A clinical and anatomical study. J Bone Joint Surg [Br] 44:869, 1962.

Tachdjian MO: Pediatric Orthopedics. Philadelphia, WB Saunders Co, 1972.

Tile M: Fractures of the Pelvis and Acetabulum. Baltimore, Williams & Wilkins Co, 1984.

Waddell JP, Johnston DWC, Neidre A: Fractures of the tibial plateau: A review of ninety-five patients and comparison of treatment methods. J Trauma 21:376, 1981.

Watson-Jones R: Dislocations and fracture-dislocations of the pelvis. Br J Surg 25:773, 1938.

Wesenberg RL, Gwinn JL, Barnes GR Jr: Radiological findings in the kinky-hair syndrome. Radiology 92:500, 1969.

Whitehouse GH: Radiological aspects of posterior dislocation of the hip. Clin Radiol 29:431, 1978.

Williams TG: Hangman's fracture. J Bone Joint Surg [Br] 57:82, 1975.

Wiltse LL, Newman PH, Macnab I: Classification of spondylolysis and spondylolisthesis. Clin Orthop 117:23, 1976.

Yeager BA, Dalinka MK: Radiology of trauma to the wrist: Dislocations, fracture dislocations, and instability patterns. Skel Radiol 13:120, 1985.

Chapter 63

Thermal and Electrical Injuries

Donald Resnick, M.D.

A variety of radiographic alterations may be found in the skeleton after thermal and electrical injuries. Epiphyseal abnormalities are common in frostbite, especially in the distal phalanges. Osteoporosis and periarticular calcification and ossification are prominent after thermal burns. With electrical burns, severe or even fatal injuries may occur; various types of fractures and osteonecrosis are among the findings.

Exposure of the human body to extremes in temperature or to electricity can lead to significant and varied abnormalities (Table 63–1). Osseous and articular structures may participate in the body's response to such insult, and the changes that are induced may be irreparable.

FROSTBITE
Terminology and General Abnormalities

Local damage can follow nonfreezing (immersion foot) and freezing (frostbite) injuries. *Immersion foot* occurs in soldiers (trench foot) and in survivors of shipwrecks. Tissue injury relates to prolonged exposure to cold and dampness, immobility and dependency of the extremities, semistarvation, dehydration, and exhaustion. These factors cause decreased blood flow to the affected body part. Plasma escapes through the injured capillary wall, producing edema, which further compromises the integrity of the vascular supply to nerve and muscle tissue. Although gangrene and necrosis of skin are frequent, and induration and fibrosis of subcutaneous tissue may be seen for several years after the injury, complete recovery from immersion foot is common.

Frostbite differs from immersion foot in that blood vessels are severely or irreparably injured, the circulation of blood ceases, and the vascular beds within the frozen tissue are

Table 63–1. RADIOGRAPHIC FINDINGS ASSOCIATED WITH THERMAL AND ELECTRICAL INJURIES

Soft tissue swelling, loss, or contracture

Osteoporosis

Acroosteolysis

Periostitis

Epiphyseal injury and growth disturbance

Articular abnormalities

Periarticular calcification and ossification

Osteolysis, osteosclerosis, and fracture

occluded by thrombi and cellular aggregates. Once the freezing process has been initiated, it progresses rapidly, and superficially located tissue, such as that in the ears, nose, and digits, is increasingly damaged by the formation of tiny crystals of ice.

Musculoskeletal Abnormalities

During the period of exposure, vascular spasm in the involved extremities is evident. With thawing of the injured parts, vasodilation leads to increased permeability of the vascular wall, transudation of fluid, perivascular edema, and intravascular stasis, with agglutination of erythrocytes and deposition of fibrin.

Bone and joint manifestations of frostbite are related to cellular injury from the freezing process itself or from the vascular insufficiency it produces. Findings are most marked in the hands and the feet.

Early radiographic manifestations include soft tissue swelling and loss of tissue, especially at the tips of the digits; osteoporosis and periostitis may occur at a slightly later stage. In the hand, sparing of the thumb is characteristic and can be attributed to clenching of the fist with the thumb clasped in the palm during the exposure to cold.

Late skeletal manifestations are variable (Fig. 63–1). In children, epiphyseal injuries involve primarily the distal phalanges, although other phalangeal epiphyses and, rarely, metacarpal (or metatarsal) epiphyses can be affected. Fragmentation, destruction, and disappearance of epiphyseal centers are seen. Premature epiphyseal fusion is also noted, resulting in brachydactyly. Secondary infection of bone or joint can develop. Interphalangeal joint abnormalities, which relate to injury to articular cartilage, may eventually simulate those of osteoarthritis (Fig. 63–2). Tuftal resorption of terminal phalanges can be traced to loss of overlying soft tissue structures.

Frostbite injury of the ears can become manifest as calcification and ossification of the pinna, simulating that occurring with mechanical trauma, hyperparathyroidism, calcium py-

899

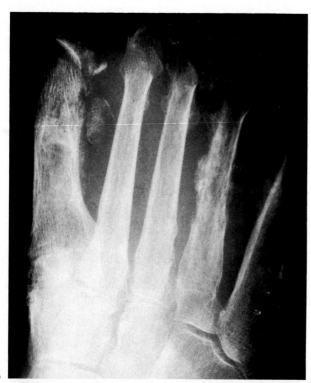

A

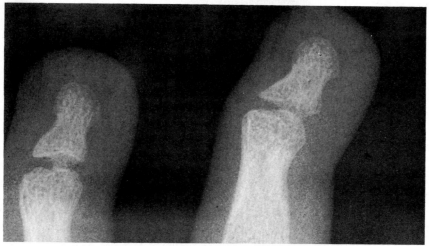

B

Figure 63–1. Frostbite: Late changes. A The changes on this radiograph include soft tissue swelling, acroosteolysis, and poorly defined destruction of the metatarsals with periostitis. **B** Epiphyseal destruction and disappearance can occur after frostbite in children. (Courtesy of M. Dalinka, M.D., Philadelphia, Pennsylvania.)

rophosphate dihydrate crystal deposition disease, gout, Addison's disease, alkaptonuria, and acromegaly.

Other Diagnostic Techniques

The role of arteriography in the diagnosis and treatment of frostbite is noted in Chapter 15. The uptake of a bone-seeking radionuclide in the region of frostbite depends on the integrity of the vascular tree; absence of such uptake indicates bone that lacks vascular perfusion. Persistent perfusion defects indicate nonviable tissue, whereas reperfusion, which may be evident on studies performed weeks after the injury, indicates tissue viability.

Differential Diagnosis

In Thiemann's disease, swelling of the fingers is associated with epiphyseal irregularity, sclerosis, and fragmentation. The distribution of epiphyseal abnormalities (changes predominate in proximal and middle phalanges, especially in the

third finger, with sparing of the distal phalanges) differs from that in frostbite.

Ungual tuftal resorption can occur in a variety of conditions other than frostbite, including collagen disease, epidermolysis bullosa, neuroarthropathy, hyperparathyroidism, and psoriatic arthritis.

THERMAL BURNS
General Abnormalities

Thermal injury results in coagulative tissue necrosis, and an inflammatory response is evoked. In both second and third degree burns, massive outpouring of protein-rich fluid is due to both endothelial capillary damage and interference with normal lymphatic absorption. Secondary bacterial invasion may contribute to ischemic necrosis of tissue.

Musculoskeletal Abnormalities

Thermal burns can produce significant skeletal and soft tissue abnormalities, which generally are more frequent and

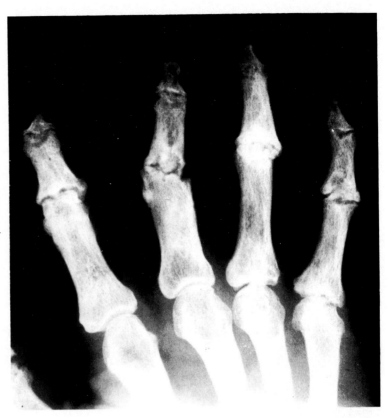

Figure 63–2. Frostbite: Interphalangeal joint abnormalities. In addition to acroosteolysis, osseous and cartilaginous destruction is evident in the proximal interphalangeal, distal interphalangeal, and, to a lesser extent, metacarpophalangeal joints. Subchondral erosion and collapse, sclerosis, osteophytosis, and joint space narrowing with or without intraarticular bone ankylosis simulate the findings of inflammatory (erosive) osteoarthritis. (Courtesy of M. Dalinka, M.D., Philadelphia, Pennsylvania.)

severe in children than in adults; the pathogenesis of many of the findings is not clear.

Early radiographic alterations include soft tissue loss, osteoporosis, and periostitis; late alterations include articular and periarticular changes and growth disturbances.

Osteoporosis is the most frequent bone response to thermal burns (Fig. 63–3). The pathogenesis of such osteoporosis probably includes immobilization and disuse, a reflex vasomotor response, or a metabolic reaction to tissue destruction.

Periosteal bone formation usually appears within a period of months after the injury in those bones that underlie severely burned area. It represents a local response to periosteal irritation.

The appearance of irregular periarticular calcification is not infrequent within 1 month or more after thermal injury. The deposits create poorly defined radiodense areas that are separate from the underlying bone. They are found most commonly about the elbow. Calcified deposits can become incorporated into enlarging areas of soft tissue ossification.

Periarticular ossification is encountered most commonly about the hip, the elbow, and the glenohumeral joint (Fig. 63–4). Such ossification usually becomes evident in the second or third month after injury. Heterotopic bone is intimately associated with the surrounding musculature, and the bone ridges commonly attach to the adjacent osseous structure.

The pathogenesis of heterotopic calcification and ossification occurring after burns is unknown. Although the deposits may be prominent in proximity to the area of burn, calcification and bone formation can also be observed in the contralateral unburned extremity. Thus, superimposed mechanical trauma,

immobility, and vascular alterations may be important causative factors.

Acromutilation with partial or complete loss of phalanges can be a prominent finding when the hand or the foot is burned (Fig. 63–5).

Progressive destruction of one or more joints with eventual fibrous or bone ankylosis may be evident after thermal burns. Destruction may appear within a period of a few weeks, and ankylosis may appear within a few months. These changes can occur either close to the initial site of injury or at a remote site. The elbow, the hip, the ankle, and the articulations of the hand are affected most typically. Thermal injury, mechanical trauma, infection, neuroarthropathy, and immobilization have all been considered as possible factors in the pathogenesis of these articular changes.

Contractures attributable to soft tissue and muscular changes in the burn patient are frequent, especially about the elbow and the hand. Joint malalignment, subluxation, and dislocation as well as disuse osteoporosis may be evident (Fig. 63–6).

Differential Diagnosis

The radiographic features of osteoporosis, periarticular calcification and ossification, joint space loss, intraarticular bone ankylosis, and contracture that are encountered in burn patients may also be seen after paralysis (or immobilization). Accurate differential diagnosis often depends on appropriate clinical history.

Phalangeal tuftal resorption or destruction occurring after thermal burns must be differentiated from similar changes

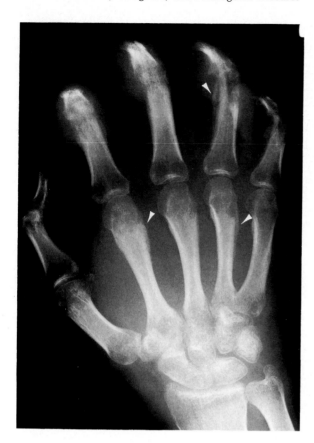

Figure 63–3. Thermal burn: Early changes. The early radiographic findings include diffuse soft tissue swelling, soft tissue and bone loss in the digits, severe periarticular osteoporosis, and periostitis, especially of the phalanges and metacarpals (arrowheads).

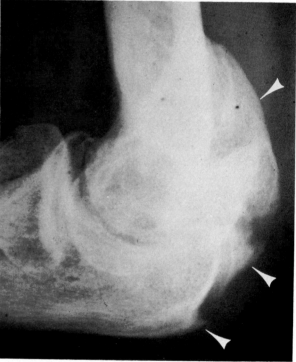

Figure 63–4. Thermal burn: Soft tissue ossification. Several months after a thermal burn, local ossification (arrowheads) appears along the posterior surface of the humerus and ulna.

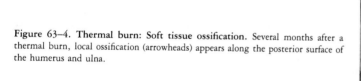

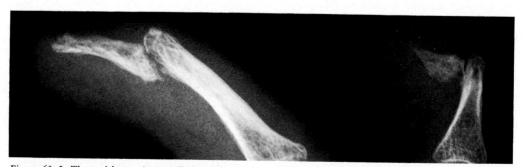

Figure 63–5. Thermal burn: Acromutilation. Observe the terminal phalangeal destruction of two burned digits. Joint destruction and subluxation also are evident.

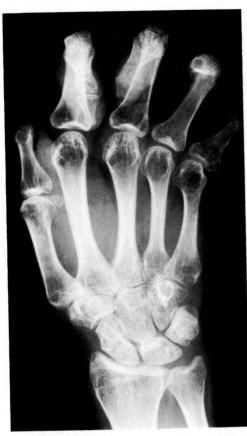

Figure 63–6. Thermal burn: Contractures. Flexion contractures of the digits, osteolysis, and osteoporosis represent the sequelae of a burn that had occurred many years previously.

relate to the effects of heat, mechanical trauma from accompanying uncoordinated muscle spasm, neural and vascular tissue damage, infection, disuse or immobilization, and, perhaps, a specific effect of the electricity itself.

Initial radiographic features include loss of cutaneous, subcutaneous, and osseous tissues owing to tissue charring. Other findings are soft tissue hematomas; compression fractures of the spine, dislocation of joints, and avulsions at tendinous insertions related to muscle spasm; and various fractures due to accompanying falls (Fig. 63–7). Small radiodense osseous lesions resembling wax drippings (attributable to melting of the bone), microfractures with a zigzag contour, and periostitis are also encountered.

Delayed musculoskeletal alterations are related predominantly to ischemia. Osteonecrosis may be attributed to periosteal stripping or damage to the vascular wall with thrombosis. Medullary lucent areas in the tubular bones, endosteal resorption, cystic rarefactions, cortical sequestration, and epiphyseal collapse and fragmentation can be evident. Accelerated bone growth and premature fusion of damaged epiphyses may follow electrical injury in children. Osteomyelitis and septic arthritis, nonunion of pathologic fractures, neuroarthropathy, periarticular ossification, and contracture with joint subluxation have also been described.

Differential Diagnosis

The radiographic findings occurring after this type of injury represent a combination of thermal, mechanical, and electrical effects on bones and joints. They are complicated by vascular and neurologic damage and secondary infection. Some of the radiographic abnormalities are identical to those accompany-

seen in association with frostbite, collagen disorders, and articular diseases.

ELECTRICAL BURNS
General Abnormalities

Electricity can produce severe injury or death. The extent of bodily harm depends on the type of electricity, the voltage, the water content of tissues, and the points of entry and exit of the charge. Electrical injury associated with a relatively short route from a point of entry in an arm to a point of exit in a finger is associated with less tissue damage than an injury in which the electricity enters the head and exits at the foot. With alternating currents, muscular contraction after injury may prevent the person's releasing the source of electricity, leading to more prolonged and severe tissue damage.

Electrical energy is converted to heat in traversing the skin. Resulting burns are accentuated by vascular spasm. Death from low voltage electrical injury is usually attributable to ventricular fibrillation; death related to high voltage electricity results from inhibition of the respiratory center in the brain.

Musculoskeletal Abnormalities

Severe injury induced by electricity is much more common in adults than in children. The hand, because of its grasping function, is the most commonly affected area in the body. Severe skin burns are encountered at the points of entry and exit of the electrical charge. Osseous and articular changes

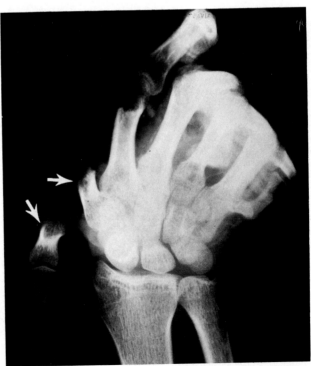

Figure 63–7. Electrical burn. This man developed changes in the hand after touching a high tension wire. The severe alterations in the hand resulted from sustained grasping of the wire. They include contracture, soft tissue injury, subluxation, dislocation, and fracture (arrows).

ing trauma from any cause, whereas others resemble those of septic arthritis, neuroarthropathy, osteoporosis, thermal burns, frostbite, and neurologic deficit.

FURTHER READING

Brinn LB, Moseley JE: Bone changes following electrical injury. Case report and review of literature. AJR 97:682, 1966.

Carrera GK, Kozin F, Flaherty L, McCarty DJ: Radiographic changes in the hands following childhood frostbite injury. Skel Radiol 6:33, 1981.

Evans EB, Smith JR: Bone and joint changes following burns. A roentgenographic study—preliminary report. J Bone Joint Surg [Am] 41:785, 1959.

Gralino BJ, Porter JM, Rosch J: Angiography in the diagnosis and therapy of frostbite. Radiology 119301, 1976.

Ogden JA, Southwick WO: Electrical injury involving the immature skeleton. Skel Radiol 6187, 1981.

Reed MH: Growth disturbances in the hands following thermal injuries in children. 2. Frostbite. J Can Assoc Radiol 39:95, 1988.

Salimi Z, Vas W, Tang-Barton P, Eachempati RG, Morris L, Carron M: Assessment of tissue viability in frostbite by ^{99m}Tc pertechnetate scintigraphy. AJR 142:415, 1984.

Schiele HP, Hubbard RB, Bruck HM: Radiographic changes in burns of the upper extremity. Radiology 104:13, 1972.

Selke AC Jr: Destruction of phalangeal epiphyses by frostbite. Radiology 93:859, 1969.

Tishler J: The soft tissue and bone changes in frostbite injuries. Radiology 102:511, 1972.

Chapter 64

Radiation Changes

Murray K. Dalinka, M.D.
Lawrence M. Neustadter, D.O.

Exposure to irradiation, whether accidentally or from diagnostic or therapeutic procedures, may produce diverse effects on the skeleton. Among the changes are disruption of normal bone growth and maturation, scoliosis, osteonecrosis, and development of both benign and malignant neoplasms. Frequently the changes are dose- and age-related, and various regions of the body respond in characteristic ways to radiation injury.

As early as 6 months after the initial discovery of the X ray by Roentgen, such precancerous effects as pigmentation, telangiectasia, fibrosis, alopecia, scarring, ulceration, and dermatitis were noted. More serious was the finding several years later that malignant lesions could be induced by exposure to diagnostic and therapeutic irradiation as well as to radioactive agents such as radium and thorium.

RADIUM

Radium was used therapeutically, both orally and intravenously, in the treatment of many ailments between 1910 and 1930. It also had commercial application as a component of the luminous paint used for watchdials, and many workers who pointed their paint brushes with their tongues, thus ingesting radium, later developed radium jaw (a type of osteomyelitis), severe aplastic anemia, and neoplasms.

Radium taken into the body becomes deposited, like calcium, in the bone. It accumulates mainly in the outer cortex of bone, with an irregular and generalized distribution. It can be leached back into the bloodstream, becoming bound to other tissues and causing deleterious effect wherever it becomes deposited. When large quantities of radium have been bound in bone for more than 20 years, the bone loses its normal physiologic function and consists largely of dead osteoid tissue. Large resorption cavities are formed as a result of constant alpha particle bombardment. These cavities contain gelatinous material with an osteoid-like matrix and appear as sharply defined bone lesions resembling those of multiple myeloma (Fig. 64–1). Other abnormal findings include metaphyseal sclerosis similar to that of Paget's disease, although the bone is of normal size; large areas of osteonecrosis; pathologic fractures; osteosarcomas; and fibrosarcomas.

THORIUM

Thorium dioxide in dextran (Thorotrast) was introduced as a contrast agent in 1928 and was widely used in the United States between 1930 and the early 1950s. Its clinically inert properties and high atomic number made it the agent of choice for hepatolienography, peripheral and cerebral angiography, and the opacification of body cavities.

Extravasation of Thorotrast at the site of injection leads to continuous alpha particle irradiation, resulting in an expanding cicatricial mass (Thorotrastoma), which invades contiguous structures; extraskeletal chondrosarcomas and osteosarcomas also have been described at the extravasation sites.

Thorotrast is a colloidal suspension that is phagocytized by the reticuloendothelial system; hence, the liver, spleen, and bone marrow are subjected to continuous low-dose alpha radiation and are at risk for radiation-induced neoplasia,

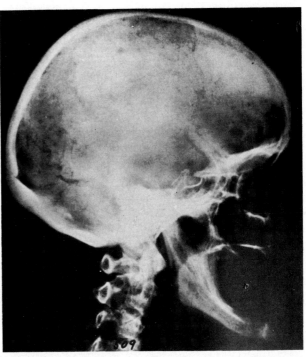

Figure 64–1. Radiation changes from radium. Skull of radium dial worker demonstrating multiple small lucent areas within the calvarium, mainly in the parietal region, simulating the lesions in multiple myeloma. (From Dalinka MK, et al: Complications of radiation therapy: Adult bone. Semin Roentgenol 9:29, 1974. Used with permission.)

including hemangioendothelial sarcoma of the liver, osteosarcoma, and fibrosarcoma. Furthermore, in bone, irradiation leads to sclerosis adjacent to the endosteum, probably secondary to vascular ischemia, bone marrow aplasia, and osteomalacia. The injection of Thorotrast into children may produce growth arrest and give rise to a "bone within bone" or "ghost vertebra" appearance (Fig. 64–2).

EFFECTS OF RADIATION THERAPY

The effects of radiation on bone depend on dosage, quality of the x-ray beam, age of the patient, method of fractionation, length of time after therapy, specific bone or bones involved, and the coexistence of trauma or infection. These effects include disruption of normal growth and maturation, scoliosis, osteonecrosis, and neoplasms.

Bone Growth Disturbances

Radiation effects on growth of bones differ depending on which portions of the bone are irradiated. When the entire bone is included in the field, a decrease in overall size and diameter is seen, simulating osteogenesis imperfecta. Irradiation of only the epiphysis results in growth deformity with a decrease in width reminiscent of achondroplasia. Irradiation of only the metaphysis leads to a bowing deformity, and irradiation of only the diaphysis causes a narrow shaft with normal cortical diameter.

The epiphysis (including the region of the growth plate) has been found to be most sensitive to radiation. Any bone capable of growth that is exposed to 2000 cGy or more will show growth disturbance. Decreased growth, however, may occur with exposure to only 400 cGy. Microscopic changes may be observable as early as 2 to 4 days after therapy and with a dose as low as 300 cGy. Histologic recovery occurs rapidly when low doses of 600 to 1200 cGy are given. With doses larger than 1200 cGy, damage is more extensive and

takes 6 months or longer to appear. Late changes, including premature cartilage degeneration and bone marrow atrophy, occur as a result of cellular injury.

Widening of the growth plate has also been described as early as 1 to 2 months after radiotherapy. In mild cases, the plate returns to normal in about 6 months. Metaphyseal changes may be irreversible and include irregularity, fraying, and sclerosis, which may resemble rickets superficially (Fig. 64–3). A broad band of increased density may appear in the metaphysis, possibly indicating repair; its absence may predict substantial limb shortening.

In humans, the diaphysis is relatively resistant to radiation, and periosteal new bone formation is affected less than enchondral bone formation. Osteoporosis is a frequent and nonspecific finding.

A slipped capital femoral epiphysis may occur after radiation therapy when the femoral head is included in the field of therapy (Fig. 64–4). Radiation-induced slipped epiphyses usually occur at an earlier age than the idiopathic variety. Concomitant chemotherapy may help weaken the growth cartilage and contribute to slippage. Ischemic necrosis and osteosarcomas have also been seen. Prophylactic percutaneous pinning in patients with a widened physeal plate and metaphyseal sclerosis may be attempted to prevent a slipped epiphysis.

Cartilage Abnormalities

Articular cartilage is relatively radioresistant. Severe cartilaginous destruction can occasionally be seen with joint space narrowing and productive osteophyte formation. This may represent secondary degenerative arthritis caused by destructive changes with collapse of the subchondral bone. However, it also may be a direct effect of radiation therapy.

Scoliosis

Irradiation to the spine may lead to loss of vertebral height and destruction of the adjacent bone marrow. Scoliosis most likely results from a combination of factors, including "fall off" at the edge of the x-ray beam, changes in the small blood vessels, and fibrosis of the overlying soft tissues. Radiation effects on the growing spine are dose- and age-related, being more severe in children treated before the age of 2 years.

Patients receiving less than 1000 cGy show no radiologic abnormalities, and those receiving between 1000 and 2000 cGy develop changes secondary to growth arrest. These changes occur 9 to 12 months after treatment and consist of horizontal lines of increased density occurring parallel to the vertebral endplates and occasionally a "bone within bone" appearance. The changes are not confined to the treatment field but instead are related to the general effect on bone growth. When doses between 2000 and 3000 cGy are given, irreversible changes confined to the irradiated area become evident; these include irregularity and scalloping of the vertebral endplates, decreased vertebral height, and abnormal bone contour. A mild, nonprogressive scoliosis is common (Fig. 64–5).

Although some investigators have believed that irradiation of the entire vertebral body would prevent the development of scoliosis, many times this has not proved to be the case, even though asymmetric radiation is associated with more frequent deformities and more severe curvature.

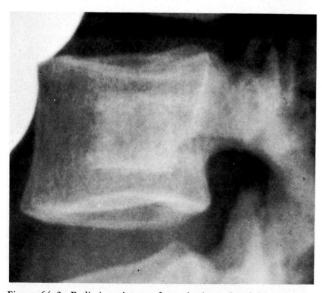

Figure 64–2. Radiation changes from thorium. Coned-down view of lumbar vertebra showing "bone within bone" appearance in patient injected with Thorotrast at the age of 3 years. (From Teplick JG, et al: Ghost infantile vertebra and hemi-pelves within adult skeleton from Thorotrast administration in childhood. Radiology 129:657, 1978. Used with permission.)

Figure 64–3. **Metaphyseal changes and periostitis after irradiation.** This patient was irradiated approximately 2 years prior to this film for leukemia and knee pain. The treated field included most of the tibia as well as the knee. There is a fracture through the midshaft of the tibia with periosteal reaction about it. Periosteal reaction also is noted about the midshaft of the fibula. There is metaphyseal irregularity of the distal portion of the femur, with deformity secondary to radiation therapy. Diffuse osteopenia is also present. (Courtesy of P. Borns, M.D., Wilmington, Delaware.)

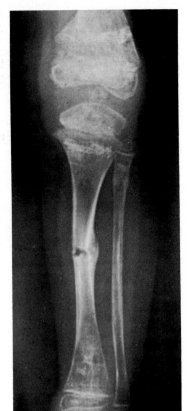

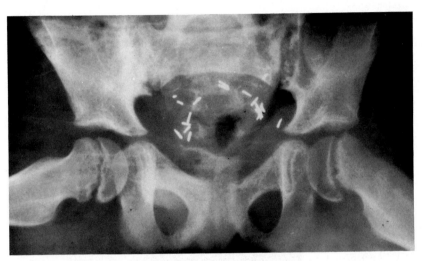

Figure 64–4. **Slipped capital femoral epiphysis after radiation therapy.** Frog-leg lateral view of the pelvis in an 8 year old child following radiation therapy for an embryonal rhabdomyosarcoma. The pelvis was treated with 5940 centigrays (cGy) with a femoral shield added at 4500 cGy. Note the slipped epiphysis on the left side. The right sacroiliac joint has sclerotic margins also secondary to the radiation therapy. (Courtesy of A. Newburg, M.D., Boston, Massachusetts.)

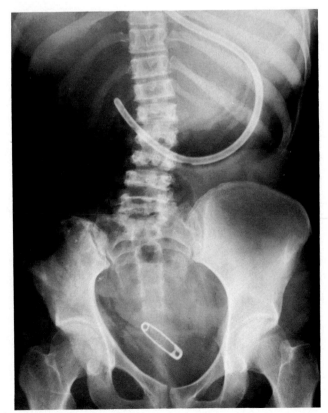

Figure 64–5. **Spinal changes after irradiation.** This patient was irradiated for a right-sided Wilms' tumor in childhood. Note the severe decrease in the height of the vertebral bodies and a slight scoliosis convex to the left. The ribs and iliac crest on the right side are also hypoplastic. The tube is present because of intestinal obstruction, which later was shown to be secondary to radiation enteritis.

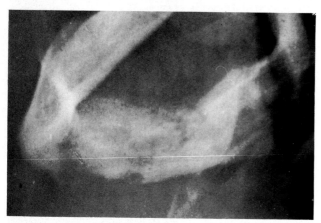

Figure 64–6. Radiation necrosis of the mandible in a patient previously treated for carcinoma of the floor of the mouth. There is a poorly defined destructive lesion in the body of the mandible, with a pathologic fracture. There is no discernible soft tissue mass.

Because radiation-induced spinal deformity is thought to progress with skeletal growth, children who are irradiated should be followed until skeletal maturity. Preventive measures include limiting the size of the radiation field to one as small as possible, irradiating the entire vertebral body, and shielding the iliac crest apophysis, which is responsible for 40 per cent of the growth of the ilium.

Radiation Necrosis

The effects of radiation in bone are mainly on the osteoblasts, with the primary event being decreased matrix production. Immediate or delayed cell death, injury with recovery, arrest of cellular division, abnormal repair, or neoplasia may occur. These changes may be seen secondary to either internal or external sources of radiation.

"Radiation osteitis" is a term used to describe osseous abnormalities that include temporary cessation of growth, periostitis, bone sclerosis with increased fragility, ischemic necrosis, and infection. The contribution of vascular injury to the pathogenesis of radiation osteitis is debated. Furthermore, some investigators maintain that radiation leads to bone atrophy and that true necrosis requires the presence of superimposition of infection. Radiation osteitis is accompanied by a mottled appearance with a mixture of osteoporosis, increased density, and coarse trabeculation on radiographs. Fractures, which heal normally, also are evident. These bone abnormalities are dose-dependent; the threshold of radiation changes in bone is believed to be 3000 cGy, with cell death occurring at 5000 cGy. Furthermore, radiation abnormalities of bone are influenced also by the quality of the x-ray beam and the size of the treatment field. Different bones develop changes at varying lengths of time after therapy. Mandibular osteonecrosis frequently appears within a year after therapy, whereas in most other sites the latent period is longer.

Regional Effects

MANDIBLE. Osteonecrosis is considerably more common in the mandible than in the maxilla because of its compact bone and poor blood supply. Owing to its superficial location, the mandible also receives a larger dose of radiation during therapy. Osteonecrosis varies in frequency with the treatment method and location of the lesions; it is least common with parallel opposing fields and more common when the tumor

involves or is adjacent to bone. The necrosis is usually of a mild and temporary nature, and it may be aseptic or septic.

Mandibular osteonecrosis may be difficult to differentiate from tumor recurrence. Recurrence and osteoradionecrosis both usually occur within 1 year after therapy. Pain, ulceration, bleeding, and weight loss are common to both. Mandibular necrosis frequently becomes manifest as a poorly defined destructive lesion without sequestration (Fig. 64–6). The absence of a soft tissue mass helps differentiate necrosis from tumor recurrence, but an inflammatory mass may be present with osteonecrosis. The necrosis, which is confined to the treated area, may progress slowly or heal with vigorous conservative therapy. Hyperbaric oxygenation and intraoral mandibular surgery are sometimes necessary.

SKULL. Radiation injury to the calvarium may occur after a minimum of 3600 cGy absorbed dose. Typically there is a mixed region of lysis and sclerosis that radiates outward from the epicenter of the radiation portal (Fig. 64–7). Osteomyelitis may occur if soft tissue necrosis accompanies the calvarial changes.

SHOULDER. Radiation changes in the shoulder girdle occurring after therapy for breast carcinoma have been reported in 1 to 3 per cent of patients. Osteopenia is common after such therapy and is frequently associated with a coarse, disorganized trabecular pattern, which may superficially resemble Paget's disease. Rib fractures also are common. The fractures frequently are multiple (Fig. 64–8), and the edges

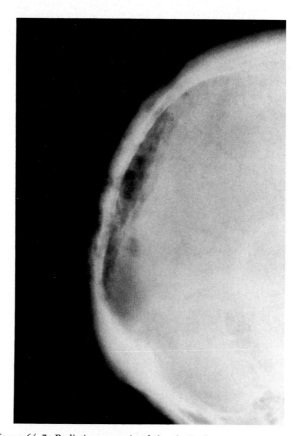

Figure 64–7. Radiation necrosis of the skull after treatment of basal cell carcinoma. Note that the edges of the lesion are sharp and that the area of necrosis is well-defined and relatively superficial. (Reprinted with permission from Dalinka MK, Mazzeo VP Jr: Complications of radiation therapy. CRC Crit Rev Diagn Imaging 23:235, 1985. Copyright CRC Press, Inc, Boca Raton, FL. Used with permission.)

of the fracture fragments may show sclerotic or pointed ends. Progressive bone resorption or spontaneous fracture healing may be evident.

Clavicular fractures are commonly associated with rib fractures. Scapular fractures can be associated with rib and clavicular fractures.

Radiation necrosis of the humerus (Fig. 64–8) can be seen 7 to 10 years after therapy. Changes may include resorption cavities, fractures, and ischemic necrosis of the humeral head. Slipped proximal humeral epiphyses are a rare complication of irradiation. The relative infrequency of this lesion in comparison to its femoral counterpart is attributable to the lack of weight-bearing and decreased stress in the upper extremities compared to the lower extremities.

PELVIS. Fractures of the femoral neck following radiation therapy to the pelvis (Fig. 64–9) occur in approximately 2 per cent of patients treated with pelvic radiation. The fractures are usually subcapital and may be unilateral or bilateral. Fractures of the femoral neck have been reported following as little as 1540 cGy and as early as 5 months after therapy. Sclerotic changes in the femoral neck with increased trabecular density frequently are present prior to fracture. The fractures heal normally, with adequate callus formation. Ischemic necrosis of the femoral head also may be evident (Fig. 64–10).

The sacroiliac joints may be wide and irregular, with sclerosis about the joint margins (Fig. 64–11). This sclerosis, which is often bilateral and symmetric, may extend from the region of the joint to the ilium, simulating osteitis condensans ilii.

Fractures of the pelvic bones also are noted after radiation therapy. These may be isolated in the sacrum or extend through portions of the innominate bone in a unilateral or bilateral distribution (Fig. 64–12). Changes in the symphysis pubis simulating osteitis pubis also can occur, as may fractures about the pubic rami or ischium.

Protrusio acetabuli has been reported after irradiation (Fig. 64–13). The mechanism of acetabular protrusion in these patients may be related to remodeling of weakened, previously irradiated bone. Associated calcification in the peritoneum may be evident.

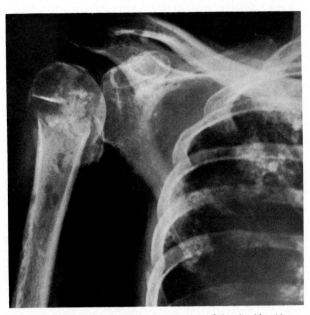

Figure 64–8. Radiation necrosis. Examination of the shoulder 10 years after radiation for carcinoma of the breast reveals pathologic fractures of the right humerus and multiple ribs. The lucent lesions in the proximal humeral shaft are also secondary to radiation necrosis. (From Dalinka MK, et al: Complications of radiation therapy: Adult bone. Semin Roentgenol 9:29, 1974. Used with permission.)

STERNUM. Sternal changes after radiation therapy are best explained by damage to microvascular structures similar to that which occurs in sickle cell disease with infarction. Mild changes consist of osteoporosis, abnormal trabeculae, and localized bone necrosis with sclerosis. Moderate changes include the development of localized pectus excavatum and necrosis involving more than one sternal segment. Severe changes are characterized by complete osseous necrosis of one or more sternal segments with deformity.

MISCELLANEOUS SITES. Well-defined lucent shadows within the field of therapy can occur in normal bone following therapy for a soft tissue lesion (Fig. 64–14) or in bone

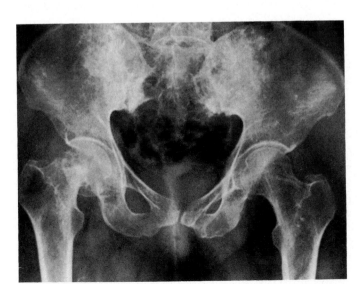

Figure 64–9. Fracture of the right femoral neck 4 years after therapy for carcinoma of the cervix. The patient was treated with 2500 cGy external radiation plus two applications of radium. There are sclerotic changes about sacroiliac joints with adjacent calcification.

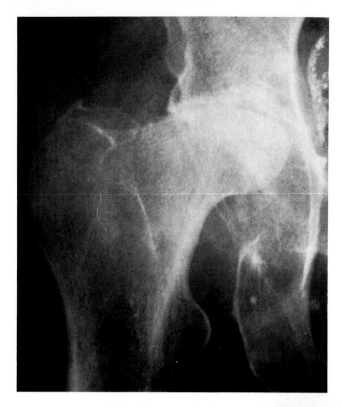

Figure 64–10. Radiation necrosis following treatment for carcinoma of the cervix. Nine months after therapy, the femoral head is collapsed and there is marked narrowing of the hip joint.

Figure 64–11. Radiation changes about the sacroiliac joint after therapy for carcinoma of the cervix. Note the irregular sclerotic areas near the sacroiliac joints and the wavy periosteal new bone along the arcuate (iliopubic) lines of the pelvis. Radiation changes in the bladder were also evident. (Reprinted with permission from Dalinka MK, Mazzeo VP Jr: Complications of radiation therapy. CRC Crit Rev Diagn Imaging *23*:235, 1985. Copyright CRC Press, Inc, Boca Raton, FL. Used with permission.)

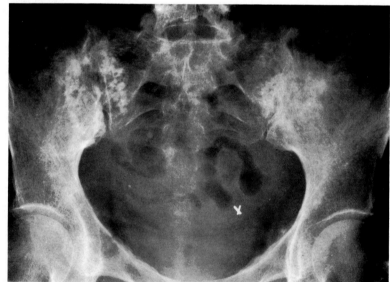

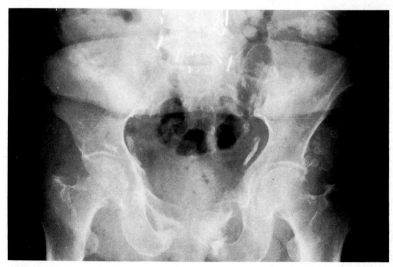

Figure 64–12. Multiple pelvic fractures after radiation therapy and surgery for carcinoma of the cervix. Note the bilateral fractures about the symphysis pubis and the symmetric fractures of the iliac wings.

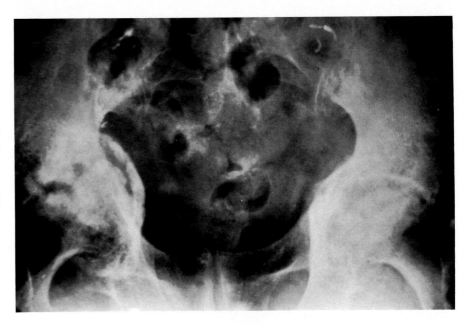

Figure 64–13. Protrusio acetabuli following treatment of prostatic carcinoma with 7000 cGy. There is a considerable degree of protrusio acetabuli on the right side with an acetabular fracture and loss of the joint space. Mild protrusio acetabuli is present on the left. (From Hasselbacher P, Schumacher HR: Bilateral protrusio acetabuli following pelvic irradiation. J Rheumatol 41:189, 1977. Used with permission.)

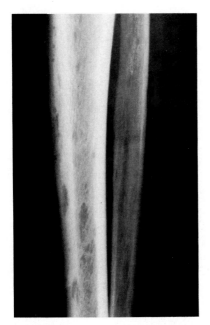

Figure 64–14. Radiation changes in the tibia and fibula after treatment for varicose veins. Approximately 50 years after this therapy, radiolucent lesions are observed in these long bones. (Courtesy of G. Beauregard, M.D., Montreal, Quebec, Canada.)

Figure 64–15. Ewing's tumor followed by late radiation necrosis. A Oblique view of femur demonstrating destructive diaphyseal lesion with saucerization, perpendicular periosteal new bone formation, and a large soft tissue mass. Codman's triangles are present at both edges of the lesion. B Same patient 31 years later, revealing multiple well-defined lucent areas in the shaft of the femur secondary to radiation necrosis.

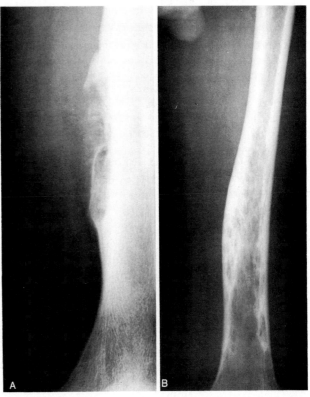

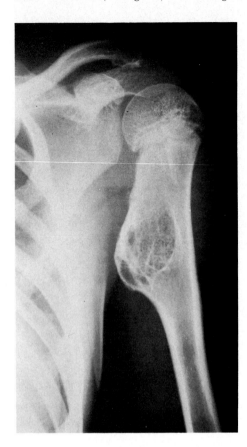

Figure 64–16. Radiation-induced exostosis in the proximal humerus after radiation therapy. This appearance is identical to that of a spontaneously occurring osteochondroma. (Courtesy of W. E. Berdon, M.D., New York, New York.)

previously treated for an osseous lesion (Fig. 64–15). Secondary infection of the bone may be evident.

Radiation-Induced Neoplasms

BENIGN NEOPLASMS. Benign radiation-induced neoplasms occur almost exclusively in patients who are treated during childhood, especially those who were younger than 2 years of age at treatment. Osteochondromas (exostoses) are the most common benign radiation-induced tumors reported in humans. They can be seen in any bone in the irradiated field (Fig. 64–16), usually within 5 years after the radiation therapy.

Radiation-induced exostoses are histologically and radiologically identical to spontaneously occurring osteochondromas, but to date there has been no well-documented case of malignant degeneration. Such exostoses usually are seen with doses ranging from 1600 to 6425 cGy.

MALIGNANT NEOPLASMS. Malignant tumors are a well-recognized complication of radiation therapy (Figs. 64–17 and 64–18). In most series osteosarcoma (Fig. 64–18) is the most common radiation-induced sarcoma, but in some series, fibrosarcoma is the most common. Malignant fibrous histiocytoma and chondrosarcoma also have occurred as a consequence of radiotherapy. Radiation-induced neoplasms form in the areas that receive radiation sufficient to induce mutation, but not enough to destroy the regenerating capacity of the bone. Sarcomas have been reported with doses as little as 800 cGy for the treatment of bursitis, but radiation-

induced sarcomas usually require a dose of at least 3000 cGy. In children, a higher frequency of radiation-induced tumors would be expected because of the longer potential period at risk, although the latent period does not seem to differ for children and adults. The latent period for radiation-induced tumors varies from 4 to 42 years, with an average of 11 years. Osteosclerotic changes frequently precede the development of the sarcoma (Fig. 64–17), and radiation osteitis often is present adjacent to radiation-induced tumors.

Criteria for diagnosis of radiation-induced sarcoma are as follows:

1. The condition for which therapy was instituted must show microscopic or radiologic evidence of being nonmalignant.

2. The sarcoma must arise within the irradiated field.

3. A latent period of at least 4 years must occur.

4. There must be histologic proof of sarcoma.

It has also been suggested that a malignant tumor of different histologic type from the primary lesion should likewise be considered proof of a radiation-induced neoplasm.

Radiation necrosis can usually be differentiated from sarcoma arising in irradiated bone, although occasional cases may cause difficulty. Both necrosis and sarcoma occur within the field of radiation and often have long latent periods. The presence of pain and a soft tissue mass favors the diagnosis of neoplasm, whereas their absence favors radiation necrosis. The relative lack of progression on serial radiographs also favors the diagnosis of radiaton necrosis.

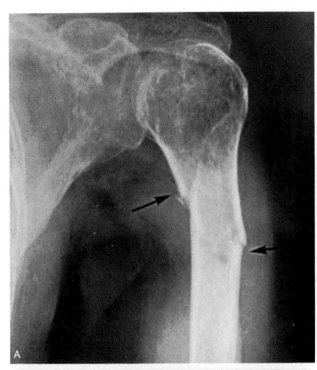

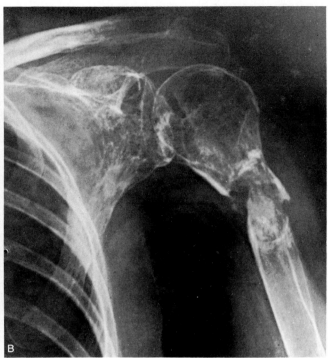

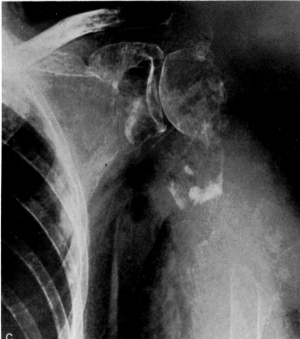

Figure 64–17. Sarcoma arising in irradiated bone. **A** Pathologic fracture (arrows) of proximal humerus 6 years after radiation therapy for carcinoma of the breast. **B** Same patient 2 years later, revealing pseudarthrosis of the humerus with radiation changes in the scapula and humerus. **C** Same patient 6 years following **B**, with an undifferentiated radiation-induced sarcoma of the humerus. (**A, C,** From Dalinka MK, et al: Complications of radiation therapy: Adult bone. Semin Roentgenol 9:29, 1974. Used with permission.)

Figure 64–18. Radiation-induced neoplasm. Anteroposterior view of pelvis with osteosarcoma of left iliac wing 17 years after therapy for cervical carcinoma. (From Dalinka MK, et al: Complications of radiation therapy: Adult bone. Semin Roentgenol 9:29, 1974. Used with permission.)

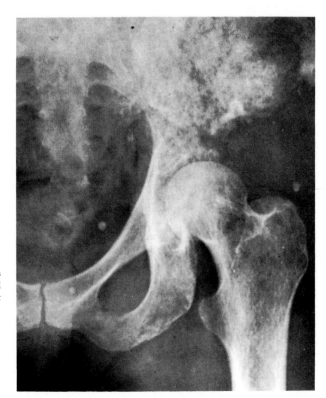

FURTHER READING

Arlen M, Higinbotham NL, Huvos AG, Marcove RC, Miller T, Shah IC: Radiation induced sarcoma of bone. Cancer 28:1087, 1971.

Bonfiglio M: The pathology of fractures of the femoral neck following irradiation. AJR 70:449, 1953.

Brady LW: Radiation induced sarcomas of bone. Skel Radiol 41:72, 1979.

Bragg DG, Shidnia H, Chu FCH, Higinbotham NL: The clinical and radiographic aspects of radiation osteitis. Radiology 97:103, 1970.

Chapman JA, Deakin DP, Green JH: Slipped upper femoral epiphysis after radiotherapy. J Bone Joint Surg [Br] 62:337, 1980.

Cohen J, D'Angio GJ: Unusual bone tumors after roentgen therapy of children. AJR 86:502, 1961.

Cooper KL, Beabout JW, Swee RG: Insufficiency fractures of the sacrum. Radiology 156:15, 1985.

Dalinka MK, Edeiken J, Finkelstein JB: Complications of radiation therapy: Adult bone. Semin Roentgenol 9:29, 1974.

Deleeuw HW, Pottenger LA: Osteonecrosis of the acetabulum following radiation therapy. J Bone Joint Surg [Am] 70:293, 1988.

DeSmet AA, Kuhns LR, Fayos JV, Holt JF: Effects of radiation therapy on growing long bones. AJR 127:935, 1976.

Glazer HS, Lee JKT, Levitt RG, Heiken JP, Ling D, Totty WG, Balfe DM, Emani B, Wasserman TH, Murphy WA: Radiation fibrosis: Differentiation from recurrent tumor by MR imaging—work in progress. Radiology 156:721, 1985.

Gondos B: Late clinical and roentgen observations following Thorotrast administration. Clin Radiol 24:195, 1973.

Hall FM, Mauch PM, Levene MB, Goldstein MA: Protrusio acetabuli following pelvic irradiation. AJR 132:291, 1979.

Howland WJ, Loeffler RK, Starchman DE, Johnson RG: Post irradiation atrophic changes of bone and related complications. Radiology 117:677, 1975.

Kim JH, Chu FCH, Woodard HQ, Melamed MR, Huvos A, Cantin J: Radiation induced soft tissue and bone sarcoma. Radiology 129:501, 1978.

Libshitz HI, Cohen MA: Radiation induced osteochondromas. Radiology 142:643, 1982

Neuhauser EBD, Wittenborg MH, Berman CZ, Cohen J: Irradiation effects of roentgen therapy on the growing spine. Radiology 59:637, 1952.

Paling MR, Herdt JR: Radiation osteitis: A problem of recognition. Radiology 137:339, 1980.

Phillips TL, Sheline GE: Bone sarcomas following radiation therapy. Radiology 81:992, 1963.

Rubin P, Probhasawat D: Characteristic bone lesions in post irradiated carcinoma of the cervix—metastases versus osteonecrosis. Radiology 76:703, 1961.

Chapter 65

Disorders Caused by Medications and Other Chemical Agents

Donald Resnick, M.D.

A survey of some of the musculoskeletal manifestations associated with certain medications and chemical substances indicates that at times the therapeutic regimen may indeed be more detrimental than the disease. Corticosteroids and other anti-inflammatory agents can produce osteoporosis, osteonecrosis, and neuropathic-like alterations. Osteosclero-sis, periostitis, osseous excrescences, ligamentous calcification, and dental abnormalities can accompany fluorosis. Soft tissue calcification may appear after calcium gluconate injection or milk and alkali ingestion. New bone formation is seen in some patients receiving prostaglandins or isotretinoin.

Significant musculoskeletal changes can result from medications and other chemical agents. In this chapter, consideration is given to the musculoskeletal alterations that may accompany administration of corticosteroids and other anti-inflammatory agents, fluorine, calcium gluconate, milk-alkali, prostaglandins, and retinoic acid.

CORTICOSTEROIDS AND OTHER ANTI-INFLAMMATORY AGENTS

The complications of cortisone therapy can become manifest in almost all systems of the body, including the skeleton (Table 65–1).

Osteoporosis

The occurrence of generalized osteoporosis in patients receiving systemic corticosteroids has been noted by many observers (see also Chapter 47). Stress (insufficiency) fractures occur that heal with extensive callus formation. Collapse of vertebral bodies with condensation of bone at the superior and inferior surfaces (Fig. 65–1) and infractions of ribs are particularly characteristic. The radiologic diagnosis of insufficiency fractures related to corticosteroid therapy frequently is difficult, owing to the associated generalized osteopenia, the presence of skeletal alterations of the underlying process (such as rheumatoid arthritis) for which the medication was administered, a lack of clinical manifestations, and, in some cases, the involvement of skeletal sites (such as the sacrum) that are suboptimally visualized on radiographs. Bone scintigraphy and computed tomography are especially useful in detecting such fractures, particularly in anatomically complex regions, such as the sacrum (see Chapter 47).

Steroid-induced osteoporosis may be more significant in patients who are elderly, in women, and in those receiving larger cumulative doses and may be uninfluenced by the exact schedule of the therapeutic regimen. The exact mechanism by which corticosteroids lead to bone loss is not known.

Currently, it is believed that two primary mechanisms are involved in glucocorticoid-induced osteopenia: direct inhibition of bone formation and indirect stimulation of bone resorption resulting from increased parathyroid hormone secretion secondary to diminished intestinal absorption of calcium.

Osteonecrosis

The true frequency of steroid-induced osteonecrosis is difficult to determine. In patients receiving corticosteroids after renal transplantation, the frequency appears to be approximately 10 per cent; this complication is probably less common in other conditions. In many reviews of patients with osteonecrosis, steroid medications have been implicated in 20 to 35 per cent of cases. In general, the frequency of ischemic necrosis in association with corticosteroid therapy is greater when (1) divided rather than single daily doses are used; (2) long-term (greater than 6 months) rather than short-term treatment is employed; (3) high dose rather than low dose therapy is used; and (4) an associated disorder is present that itself causes avascular necrosis.

The onset of symptoms and signs related to osteonecrosis usually is delayed for a period of 2 to 3 years after adminis-

Table 65–1. MUSCULOSKELETAL ABNORMALITIES ASSOCIATED WITH CORTICOSTEROID MEDICATION

Osteoporosis
Osteonecrosis
Neuropathic-like arthropathy
Osteomyelitis (septic arthritis)
Tendinous injury or rupture
Soft tissue atrophy
Intraarticular calcification
Periarticular calcification
Accumulation of fat

915

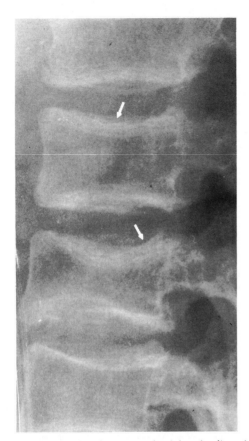

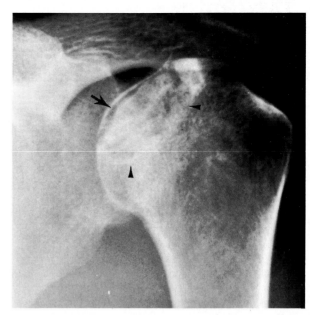

Figure 65–2. Steroid-induced osteonecrosis: Proximal humerus. Abnormalities consist of flattening of the humeral head with a subchondral radiolucent line (crescent sign) (arrow), surrounding osteolysis and osteosclerosis (arrowheads), and relative preservation of joint space.

Figure 65–1. Steroid-induced osteoporosis. A lateral radiograph of the lumbar spine reveals biconcave deformities of multiple vertebral bodies with bone condensation at the superior and inferior aspects of each vertebra (arrows). This appearance can be seen with exogenous or endogenous hypercortisolism.

tration of the drug. Single or multiple osseous sites can be affected; the femoral head, the humeral head, the distal portion of the femur, and the proximal portion of the tibia, in decreasing order of frequency, are most commonly altered. There is a tendency for widespread abnormalities to appear over a period of time. In general, however, changes in the diaphyses and metaphyses of tubular bones are encountered less frequently than epiphyseal alterations.

Radiographic and pathologic characteristics of epiphyseal osteonecrosis attributable to corticosteroids are not unique, being evident in cases of bone necrosis from other causes (see Chapter 70). Osteoporosis, patchy osteosclerosis, subchondral radiolucent lines (crescent sign), osseous collapse, and fragmentation are recognized (Figs. 65–2 and 65–3). Preservation of joint space is also typical during the early stages of the process.

Figure 65–3. Steroid-induced osteonecrosis: Distal femur. Frontal (A) and lateral (B) tomograms demonstrate fragmentation of the osseous surface with the creation of multiple intraarticular bone pieces (arrows).

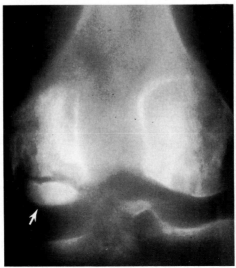

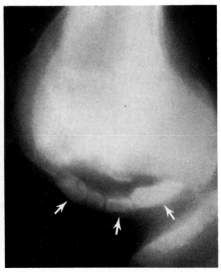

A

B

As observed in ischemic necrosis in general, bone scanning is more sensitive than plain film radiography in detecting sites of osseous necrosis in patients receiving corticosteroids. Findings include an initial "cold" stage with decreased accumulation of the bone-seeking radiopharmaceutical agent, followed by a stage in which there is increased uptake of the radionuclide. Other techniques, including magnetic resonance imaging and computed tomography, are also helpful in diagnosis (see Chapter 70).

The pathogenesis of steroid-associated osteonecrosis is not clear (Table 65–2). Osteoporosis leading to microfractures and eventual bone collapse (mechanical factors) and vascular compromise owing to compression from marrow accumulation of adjacent fat cells, fat embolization, vasculitis, or hyperviscosity (vascular factors) are frequently proposed mechanisms for this complication. Of interest, additional analgesics may be associated with drug-induced arthropathy and osteonecrosis. These medications include phenylbutazone and indomethacin. The pathogenesis of the articular abnormalities that are evident after treatment with nonsteroidal anti-inflammatory agents is presumed to be similar to that occurring with corticosteroid administration.

Osteonecrosis of vertebral bodies in association with administration of steroid medications has been recognized. Radiolucent linear shadows in the subchondral bone reflect fractures of necrotic bone (Fig. 65–4). The phenomenon is termed the vacuum vertebral body. Although it is not universally associated with ischemic necrosis of bone, it is most suggestive of that diagnosis, and the finding almost completely eliminates the alternative diagnoses of infection and neoplasm.

Neuropathic-like Articular Destruction

A neuropathic-like, rapidly progressive joint disease characterized by severe osseous and cartilaginous destruction represents one variety of steroid arthropathy that appears most typically after intraarticular injection of the drug (Table 65–3). Although any joint can be affected, it is the hip and the knee that are most frequently involved. The rapidity of the process may be remarkable; eventually significant osseous collapse and fragmentation are found (Fig. 65–5). The pathogenesis of the process is not certain.

Osteomyelitis and Septic Arthritis

Bone and joint infections can complicate steroid therapy, although such complications are rare. Septic arthritis in one or more joints can appear after oral, intravenous, or intraarticular administration. Similarly, osteomyelitis can appear,

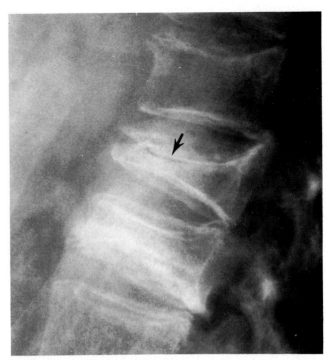

Figure 65–4. Steroid-induced osteonecrosis: Vertebral bodies. Observe collapse of multiple osteoporotic lumbar vertebral bodies, reactive sclerosis of endplates, and a radiolucent line or crescent within the bone (arrow). The latter finding differs from a vacuum intervertebral disc, in which the radiolucent collection is located over the disc itself.

either alone or in conjunction with septic arthritis. The initiation and spread of infection are promoted by the medication's interference with normal host defense mechanisms.

Tendinous Injury

Tendinous rupture has been described in association with systemically or locally administered corticosteroids, but it is not certain if the complication relates to the effect of steroids or the disease process for which the steroids are being used. It appears likely that steroids, particularly when administered locally, accelerate degeneration and rupture of a tendon that is already the site of a pathologic process.

Intraarticular and Periarticular Calcification

Numerous reports have documented a definite association of calcification in the synovial membrane, joint capsule, periarticular tissue, and, perhaps, cartilage in patients receiv-

Table 65–2. PATHOGENESIS OF STEROID-INDUCED OSTEONECROSIS

Theory	Possible Mechanisms
Mechanical	Osteoporosis leading to microfractures and osseous collapse
Vascular	Vascular compression from marrow accumulation of fat
	Fat embolization following steroid-induced fatty liver
	Vasculitis
	Hyperviscosity

Table 65–3. STEROID-INDUCED NEUROPATHIC-LIKE ALTERATIONS

Possible Pathogenesis	Characteristics
Neuroarthropathy due to sensory loss induced by medication	Usually evident after intra-articular administration of drug
	Predilection for the hip and the knee
	Rapid onset and progression
Osteonecrosis	Osseous defects ("bites"), collapse, and fragmentation
	Cartilaginous destruction

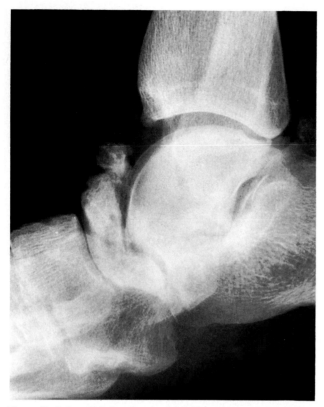

Figure 65–5. Steroid-induced neuropathic-like arthropathy. This patient with rheumatoid arthritis had had repeated injections of corticosteroids into the talonavicular space. A radiograph reveals fragmentation of the talus and navicular bone. The findings resemble neuropathic changes.

ing intraarticular corticosteroid injections, especially if multiple injections are given for a period of years. The responsible crystal is calcium hydroxyapatite, which itself can cause joint inflammation, and the typical radiographic findings are cloud-like radiodense collections within the joint and curvilinear and punctate calcifications in the articular capsule and surrounding soft tissues.

Accumulation of Fat

Endogenous or exogenous excess of corticosteroids leads to abnormal accumulations of fat. Mediastinal lipomatosis represents one manifestation of this phenomenon. Similarly, paraspinal localization of fat produces characteristic radiographic findings consisting of widening of the paraspinal lines and a lobulated or mass-like contour, simulating the abnormalities of lymphoma, metastatic disease, or neurogenic tumor. Computed tomography documents the fatty nature of the abnormal accumulations of tissue. Epidural lipomatosis in patients receiving corticosteroid therapy (as well as those with Cushing's disease) may produce neurologic complications.

FLUORINE

Chronic fluorine intoxication, fluorosis, arises when the drinking water contains fluoride in concentrations higher than 4 parts per million (ppm). Fluorosis may also appear in industrial workers who are exposed to fluorine compounds over a period of years, in laboratory personnel who have inhaled fluorine vapors, in patients receiving medications containing high doses of fluorine, and in persons who habit-

Table 65–4. RADIOGRAPHIC ABNORMALITIES IN FLUOROSIS

Hypoplasia and irregularity of dental structures
Osteosclerosis
Vertebral osteophytosis
Ligamentous calcification
Periostitis

ually drink fluorine-containing wine. Bone changes also are recognized in patients with osteoporosis who are treated with sodium fluoride. Approximately 50 per cent of the absorbed fluoride is excreted, mainly in the urine, and approximately 99 per cent of the fluoride retained in the body is deposited in the calcified tissue. With cessation of the exposure to fluoride and with continued metabolism of bone tissue, excretion of fluoride can lead to an improvement in the pulmonary and skeletal manifestations of the disease.

Clinical manifestations of acute fluoride exposure include nausea, vomiting, constipation, loss of appetite, and toxic nephritis; manifestations in more prolonged cases of exposure include joint pain and restriction of motion, back stiffness, restriction of respiratory movements, functional dyspnea, dental alterations, paraplegia, and palpable thickening of the bones, including the clavicle, tibia, and ulna.

Dental Fluorosis

Mottled enamel is an early dental sign of fluoride intoxication. Progression of the dental changes leads to depressions of variable size and discoloration. Radiographs outline hypoplasia, irregular dental roots, and periapical sclerosis.

Skeletal Fluorosis

RADIOGRAPHIC ABNORMALITIES. Involvement of the axial skeleton is characteristic (Table 65–4) (Figs. 65–6 and 65–7). Osteosclerotic changes are most marked in the

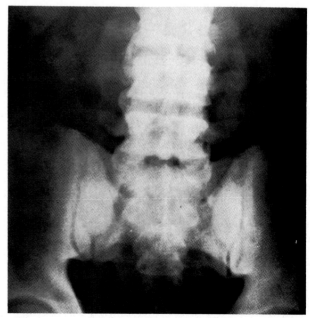

Figure 65–6. Fluorosis: Axial skeletal abnormalities. Osteosclerosis and vertebral osteophytosis are evident. Note the bone eburnation about the sacroiliac joints.

spine, the pelvis, and the ribs. Increasing trabecular condensation eventually creates a chalky appearance throughout the thorax, vertebral column, and pelvis with obscuration of bone architecture. The skull and tubular bones of the appendicular skeleton are relatively spared in this sclerotic process.

Vertebral osteophytosis can lead to encroachment on the spinal canal and intervertebral foramina. In the axial skeleton, hyperostosis and bone excrescences develop at sites of ligamentous attachment, especially in the iliac crests, ischial tuberosities, and inferior margins of the ribs. Calcification of paraspinal ligaments as well as sacrotuberous and iliolumbar ligaments can be noted.

In the appendicular skeleton, periosteal thickening (periostitis deformans), calcification of ligaments, and excrescences at ligamentous and muscular attachments to bone can be seen at one or more sites, particularly near the interosseous membranes of the forearm and leg, the calcaneus, the posterior surface of the femur, the tibial tuberosity, and the proximal portion of the humerus. Fluorosis can lead to undulating periosteal bone, which may surround the humeri, femora, ulnae, radii, tibiae, fibuli, metatarsals, metacarpals, and phalanges.

PATHOLOGIC ABNORMALITIES. Accelerated bone formation and resorption may occur simultaneously in fluorosis. Irregular laying down of periosteal bone may be associated with an increased rate of resorption, as indicated by cancellization of the cortex, the presence of enlarged haversian canals, and an increased number of lacunae. It has been suggested that the concomitant increase in bone formation and resorption in skeletal fluorosis is caused by overactivity of parathyroid hormone. The fluoroapatite crystals, which are large, may be less reactive in surface exchange reactions, increasing the resistance of bone to the actions of parathyroid hormone and inciting parathyroid stimulation.

COMPLICATIONS. Advanced stages of fluorosis can lead to kyphosis, restricted spinal and chest motion, and contractures and deformities of extraspinal articulations. A high frequency of genu valgum deformity has been noted. Neurologic complications include paresthesias, muscular weakening and wasting, sensory disturbances, and paralysis.

REVERSIBILITY OF SKELETAL ABNORMALITIES. The identification of less striking radiographic abnormalities of the skeleton in retired workers who had been exposed to fluoride while employed is consistent with the concept that such abnormalities are reversible. Extensive fading of the sclerotic changes in the pelvis, ribs, and vertebrae is seen. The resulting radiographic appearance resembles that of Paget's disease.

FLUORIDE TREATMENT OF OSTEOPOROSIS. Sodium fluoride has been used in the treatment of osteoporosis for approximately 30 years. The rationale for its use is the ability of fluoride to stimulate new bone formation and to depress bone resorption through the deposition of relatively stable fluoroapatite. The first detectable radiographic changes occur at least 1 year after the start of the fluoride therapy (Fig. 65–8). Findings include pronounced bone radiodensity, cortical thickening, coarsening of the trabecular pattern, and partial obliteration of the medullary space, which are observed principally in the axial skeleton. Ligamentous calcification is not a feature of iatrogenic fluorosis. The abnormalities simulate those of Paget's disease, myelofibrosis, and renal osteodystrophy.

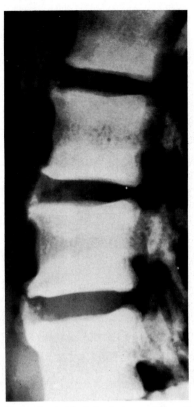

Figure 65–7. Fluorosis: Axial skeletal abnormalities. Note radiodense vertebrae and spinal osteophytes. (Courtesy of G. Beauregard, M.D., Montreal, Quebec, Canada.)

Although the radiographic appearance of osteoporotic bone in patients receiving sodium fluoride is one of progressive osteosclererosis, it is not clear if a commensurate increase in bone strength occurs. In fact, fractures of tubular bones are reported during fluoride treatment. The femoral neck is a common site of fracture in this situation. These findings suggest that the sclerotic bone is not so strong as it looks but is probably stronger than it was before treatment began.

DIFFERENTIAL DIAGNOSIS. The combination of findings noted on radiographs of patients with skeletal fluorosis is virtually diagnostic. Osteosclerosis, osteophytosis, and ligamentous calcification represent a useful triad of abnormalities that are evident on pelvis and spine radiographs. Osteosclerosis alone, however, is not diagnostic of fluorosis, being evident in skeletal metastasis, myelofibrosis, mastocytosis, certain hemoglobinopathies, renal osteodystrophy, Paget's disease, and congenital disorders. Likewise, vertebral osteophytes or similar outgrowths can accompany many diseases, including fluorosis, spondylosis deformans, diffuse idiopathic skeletal hyperostosis, ankylosing spondylitis, the spondylitis of psoriasis, Reiter's syndrome, inflammatory bowel disorders, acromegaly, neuroarthropathy, and alkaptonuria. Proliferative changes at ligamentous and tendinous insertions in bones are apparent not only in fluorosis but also in diffuse idiopathic skeletal hyperostosis, hypoparathyroidism, X-linked hypophosphatemic osteomalacia, and certain plasma cell dyscrasias. Periostitis similar to that which may be seen in fluorosis can be detected in hypertrophic osteoarthropathy, pachydermoperiostosis, and thyroid acropathy.

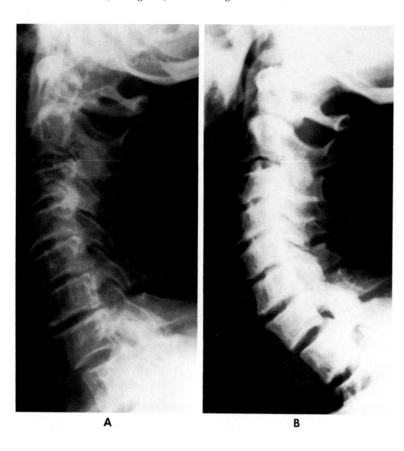

A   **B**

Figure 65–8. Fluoride treatment of osteoporosis. Radiographs obtained 5 years apart of a 70 year old woman with osteoporosis who began receiving sodium fluoride at the time the initial study (**A**) was obtained. At this time, osteoporosis is evident. Five years later (**B**), note the increase in skeletal radiodensity and the coarsened trabecular pattern. (Courtesy of V. Vint, M.D., San Diego, California.)

CALCIUM GLUCONATE

Intravenous administration of calcium gluconate has been used in the treatment of neonatal tetany and neonatal asphyxia. Subcutaneous masses of calcification at sites of recent or previous injections can appear. Clinical findings include erythema and bulla formation, which may be followed by skin sloughing and secondary infection. Calcification, which is related to tissue necrosis, can be noted within 4 or 5 days or as late as 3 weeks after injection (Fig. 65–9). With healing, clinical and radiologic manifestations may disappear. The radiographic changes simulate those in subcutaneous fat necrosis and hematomas occurring after trauma.

MILK-ALKALI

The milk-alkali syndrome was initially described in patients with chronic peptic ulcer disease and renal insufficiency in whom excessive intake of milk and alkali (for a few to many years) led to metastatic calcification. These patients revealed hypercalcemia without hypercalciuria or hypophosphatemia, normal serum alkaline phosphatase levels, azotemia, and mild alkalosis. The radiographic manifestations of this syndrome include unilateral or bilateral periarticular calcific deposits, which are amorphous and vary in size from small nodules to bulky tumors (Fig. 65–10). Widespread calcification in blood vessels, kidneys, ligaments, and falx cerebri is also observed, and the osseous tissues are normal.

The milk-alkali syndrome occurs principally in middle-aged men who are ingesting milk and calcium carbonate, or calcium carbonate alone, for abdominal pain or heartburn. Although hypercalcemia, alkalosis, and renal impairment represent the classic triad of the syndrome, the clinical characteristics are variable. It is the chronic pattern of the

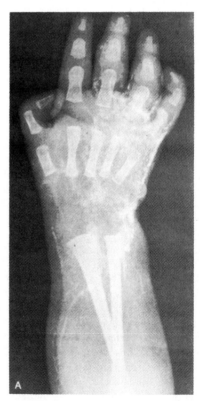

Figure 65–9. Calcium gluconate extravasation. This infant received an infusion of calcium gluconate into a vein in the dorsum of the hand that subsequently infiltrated into the soft tissues. A radiograph taken approximately 1 week later reveals extensive linear and plate-like subcutaneous deposits with vascular calcification. (From Berger PE, et al: Extravasation of calcium gluconate as a cause of soft tissue calcification. AJR *121*:109, 1974. Copyright 1974, American Roentgen Ray Society. Used with permission.)

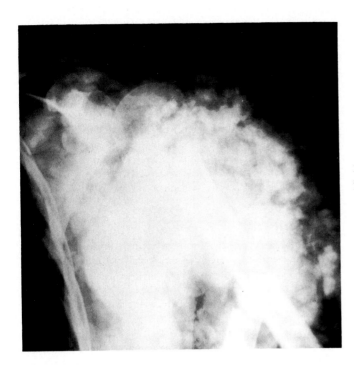

Figure 65–10. Milk-alkali syndrome. Bizarre calcific collections about the shoulder are seen. (Courtesy of M. K. Dalinka, M.D., Philadelphia, Pennsylvania.)

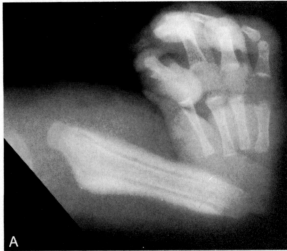

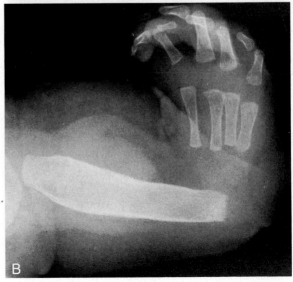

Figure 65–11. Prostaglandin periostitis. This male infant was noted to have multiple congenital abnormalities at birth, including tetralogy of Fallot. An infusion of prostaglandin E$_1$ was begun when the patient was 3 weeks of age and maintained for 7 weeks. Bone changes were observed initially in the ribs and clavicle at 20 days of therapy. **A** A radiograph of the forearm, obtained when the infant was 43 days of age, reveals extensive periosteal elevation in the ulna. Note the absence of the radius, a finding of the VATER syndrome. **B** At 6 months of age, the periosteal bone has been incorporated into the diaphysis of the ulna. (From Poznanski AK, et al: Bone changes from prostaglandin therapy. Skel Radiol *14*:20, 1985. Used with permission.)

syndrome that is associated with major metabolic consequences consisting of renal failure with hyperphosphatemia, alkalosis, and hypercalcemia, and with diffuse calcification in the soft tissues, kidneys, eyes, and other regions. After a period in which some of these consequences are reversible, irreversible renal disease and soft tissue calcification appear. The ingestion of calcium and absorbable alkali is fundamental to the occurrence of the milk-alkali syndrome, although questions remain as to the precise pathogenesis of the syndrome.

The differential diagnosis of periarticular calcific deposits accompanying the milk-alkali syndrome includes collagen disorders, hyperparathyroidism, renal osteodystrophy, hypervitaminosis D, and idiopathic tumoral calcinosis.

PROSTAGLANDINS

Prostaglandin E_1 is commonly used to maintain the patency of the ductus arteriosus in neonates with ductus-dependent congenital heart disease, including interruption or coarctation of the aortic arch, pulmonary atresia complex, and tetralogy of Fallot. Although the duration of prostaglandin E_1 administration is usually confined to the period of time that is required to allow stabilization of the infant's condition prior to surgical intervention, longer periods of infusion occasionally are required. Complications that have been encountered during and after prostaglandin E_1 therapy include damage of the ductus, hypotension, hyperthermia, diarrhea, apnea, bradycardia, and flushing and edema of the skin. One further complication is new bone formation appearing as periostitis and cortical thickening.

Periosteal bone formation is characteristic of long-term (40 days or more) prostaglandin E_1 infusion. Affected sites include the ribs, tubular bones, and, to a lesser extent, the mandible, clavicle, scapula, and pelvis. Periostitis varies in intensity from subtle osseous deposits to widespread and severe alterations leading to enlargement of the bone (Fig. 65–11). Generally the process is self-limited; complete resolution is commonly seen over a 6 month to 1 year period.

The differential diagnosis of the osseous alterations includes physiologic periostitis, trauma, Caffey's disease, congenital syphilis, hypervitaminosis A, scurvy, hypertrophic osteoarthropathy, leukemia, and skeletal metastasis.

ISOTRETINOIN

Natural and synthetic forms of vitamin A, known collectively as retinoids, have been employed in the treatment of various dermatologic disorders. Reports indicate that the long-term use of some of the agents, such as isotretinoin (Accutane) and etretinate, is associated with skeletal hyperostosis resembling that seen in chronic vitamin A intoxication. Both axial and appendicular skeletal sites are affected. Vertebral alterations predominate in the cervical region, although thoracic and lumbar spinal changes also are evident. The findings consist of pointed excrescences arising from the anterior and posterior margins of the vertebral bodies, which, with time, progress to larger osteophytic outgrowths (Fig. 65–12). In the appendicular skeleton, point-like hyperostosis is seen at the promontories of bones, such as the tarsal navicular and calcaneus. Clinical manifestations are absent or mild.

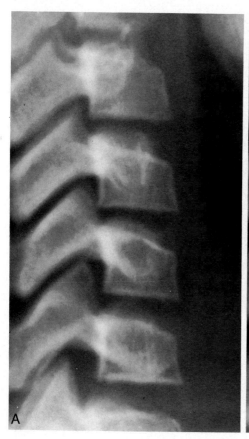
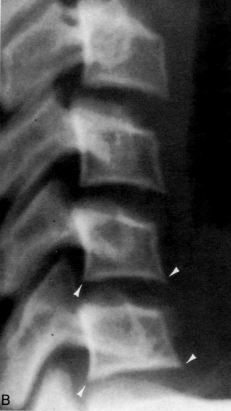

Figure 65–12. Isotretinoin hyperostosis. In this patient, a lateral radiograph of the cervical spine obtained prior to therapy (**A**) and another after 1 year of therapy (**B**) are shown. A definite interval change can be noted. In B, observe "pointing" of the bone at the anteroinferior and posteroinferior portions of the vertebral bodies (arrowheads). (From Pennes DR, et al: AJR *142*:979, 1984. Used with permission.)

A   B

ADDITIONAL CHEMICALS

Phenytoin (Dilantin) has been associated with calvarial thickening and enlargement of the heel pad. Dilantin, along with heparin, alcohol, and methotrexate, can lead to skeletal osteopenia. With long-term methotrexate therapy for childhood neoplasms, severe osteopenia and multiple fractures in the tubular bones of the extremities are seen; additional findings include growth recovery lines and radiodense areas in the metaphyses and epiphyses, simulating the changes of scurvy.

FURTHER READING

Abiteboul M, Arlet J: Retinol-related hyperostosis. AJR *144*:435, 1985.

Berger PE, Heidelberger KP, Poznanski AK: Extravasation of calcium gluconate as a cause of soft tissue calcification in infancy. AJR *121*:109, 1974.

Burnett CH, Commons RR, Albright F, Howard JE: Hypercalcemia without hypercalcuria or hypophosphatemia, calcinosis, and renal insufficiency. N Engl J Med *240*:787, 1949.

Conklin JJ, Alderson PO, Zizic TM, Hungerford DS, Densereaux JY, Gober A, Wagner HN: Comparison of bone scan and radiograph sensitivity in the detection of steroid-induced ischemic necrosis of bone. Radiology *147*:221, 1983.

Dalinka MK, Stewart V, Bomalaski JS, Halpern, M, Kricun ME: Periarticular calcifications in association with intra-articular corticosteroid injections. Radiology *153*:615, 1984.

DiGiovanna JJ, Helfgott RK, Gerber LH, Peck GL: Extraspinal tendon and ligament calcification associated with long-term therapy with etretinate. N Engl J Med *315*:1177, 1986.

El-Khoury GY, Moore TE, Albright JP, Huang HK, Martin RK: Sodium fluoride treatment of osteoporosis: Radiologic findings. AJR *139*:39, 1982.

Grandjean P, Thomsen G: Reversibility of skeletal fluorosis. Br J Indust Med *40*:456, 1983.

Halpern AA, Horowitz BG, Nagel DA: Tendon ruptures associated with corticosteroid therapy. West J Med *127*:378, 1977.

Harris V, Ramamurthy RS, Pildes RS: Late onset of subcutaneous calcifications after intravenous injections of calcium gluconate. AJR *123*:845, 1975.

Kattan KR: Calvarial thickening after Dilantin medication. AJR *110*:102, 1975.

Kilcoyne RF, Cope R, Cunningham W, Nardella FA, Denman S, Franz TJ, Hanifin J: Minimal spinal hyperostosis with low-dose isotretinoin therapy. Invest Radiol *21*:41,1986.

Maldague B, Noel H, Malghem J: The intravertebral vacuum cleft: A sign of ischemic vertebral collapse. Radiology *129*:23, 1978.

Miller WT, Restifo RA: Steroid arthropathy. Radiology *86*:652, 1966.

Murray RO: Radiological bone changes in Cushing's syndrome and steroid therapy. Br J Radiol *33*:1, 1960.

Murray RO: Iatrogenic lesions of the skeleton. AJR *126*:5, 1976.

Orwoll ES: The milk-alkali syndrome: Current concepts. Ann Intern Med *97*:242, 1982.

Pennes DR, Ellis CN, Madison KC, Voorhees JJ, Martel W: Early skeletal hyperostosis secondary to 13-cis-retinoic acid. AJR *141*:979, 1984.

Poppel MH, Zeitel BE: Roentgen manifestations of milk drinker's syndrome. Radiology *67*:195, 1956.

Poznanski AK, Fernbach SK, Berry TE: Bone changes from prostaglandin therapy. Skel Radiol *14*:20, 1985.

Quint DJ, Boulos RS, Sanders WP, Mehta BA, Patel SC, Tiel RL: Epidural lipomatosis. Radiology *169*:485, 1988.

Ringel RE, Brenner JI, Haney PJ, Burns JE, Moulton AL, Berman MA: Prostaglandin-induced periostitis: A complication of long-term PGE₁ infusion in an infant with congenital heart disease. Radiology *142*:657, 1982.

Sackler JP, Liu L: Heparin-induced osteoporosis. Br J Radiol *46*:548, 1973.

Schnitzler CM, Solomon L: Trabecular stress fractures during fluoride therapy for osteoporosis. Skel Radiol *14*:276, 1985.

Schwartz AM, Leonidas JC: Methotrexate osteopathy. Skel Radiol *11*:13, 1984.

Singh A, Dass R, Hayreh SS, Jolly SS: Skeletal changes in endemic fluorosis. J Bone Joint Surg [Br] *44*:806, 1962.

Soriano M, Manchon F: Radiological aspects of a new type of bone fluorosis, periostitis deformans. Radiology *87*:1089, 1966.

Stevenson CA, Watson AR: Fluoride osteosclerosis. AJR *78*:13, 1957.

Tondreau RL, Hodes PJ, Schmidt ER Jr: Joint infections following steroid therapy: Roentgen manifestations. AJR *82*:258, 1959.

Chapter 66

Hypervitaminosis and Hypovitaminosis

Donald Resnick, M.D.

Deficiencies and excesses of certain vitamins may have a pronounced effect on the musculoskeletal system. In addition to vitamin D deficiency leading to rickets, hypervitaminosis A and D and hypovitaminosis C (scurvy) are examples of vitamin-related disorders that affect the osseous, articular, or soft tissue structures.

Vitamins are biologically active organic compounds that are essential to but not synthesized by the body and are obtained from exogenous sources, mainly the diet. Vitamins are either fat soluble (vitamins A, D, E, and K) or water soluble (vitamins B_1, B_2, niacin, B_6 or pyridoxine, folic acid, cyanocobalamin, C or ascorbic acid, biotin, and pantothenic acid). Musculoskeletal manifestations accompany deficiencies and excesses of certain vitamins. As an example, rickets is caused by a deficiency in vitamin D or its active metabolites (Chapter 48). In addition, excessive levels of the vitamins D and A and depressed levels of the vitamins A and C can produce characteristic changes in the skeleton.

HYPERVITAMINOSIS A

Vitamin A poisoning appears in both children and adults. Its clinical and radiologic manifestations are influenced by the acute or chronic nature of the vitamin abuse.

Acute Poisoning

After a massive dose of vitamin A, acute clinical findings can develop. Nausea, vomiting, headache, drowsiness, and irritability are noted in adults with acute hypervitaminosis A. Children develop drowsiness and vomiting from accidental overdose of vitamin drops. Bulging of the fontanelles can appear within 12 hours after vitamin ingestion, usually disappearing after 36 to 48 hours. Although skull films can reveal widening of the sutures, the finding is transient.

Subacute and Chronic Poisoning

In both children and adults, anorexia and itching represent nonspecific early findings of chronic vitamin A poisoning. After a period of weeks or months, hard and tender soft tissue nodules appear in the extremities. Additional manifestations include dry scaly skin, coarse and sparse hair, hepatosplenomegaly, and digital clubbing. An elevated serum vitamin A level is diagnostic in this clinical setting, and rapid disappearance of the symptoms and signs follows withdrawal of vitamin A intake.

Radiographic signs are characteristic, and they are virtually confined to children, usually appearing near the end of the first year of life. Cortical thickening of the tubular bones is a constant finding and is usually related to the areas in which soft tissue nodules are present. Typically, hyperostosis is observed in the ulnae and metatarsal bones, producing a wavy diaphyseal contour (Fig. 66–1). The clavicles, tibiae, and fibulae are not uncommonly affected; changes in the mandible are rarely observed. Scintigraphy, using bone-seeking radiopharmaceutical agents, further documents this characteristic distribution of abnormalities.

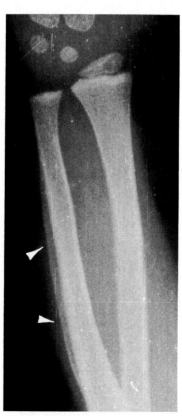

Figure 66–1. Hypervitaminosis A: Periostitis. Note periosteal bone formation in the diaphysis of the ulna (arrowheads). (Courtesy of F. Silverman, M.D., Stanford, California.)

Additional findings in the epiphyseal and metaphyseal segments of tubular bones may lead to crippling deformities. The distal femora are altered most commonly. Cupping, shortening, and splaying of the metaphyses, narrowing of the cartilaginous growth plates, and hypertrophy and premature fusion of the epiphyseal ossification centers can be noted (Fig. 66–2). Although cortical hyperostosis may disappear after removal of the excess vitamin A, the damage to the epiphyseal cartilage may be irreversible. Flexion contractures, short stature, and leg length discrepancies may ensue.

Increased intracranial pressure has been noted in association with chronic hypervitaminosis A. Cranial findings include widening of the sutures, hyperostosis in the occipital and the temporal bones, and ventricular dilatation.

The condition that produces skeletal changes that most resemble those of chronic hypervitaminosis A is infantile cortical hyperostosis (Caffey's disease) (Table 66–1). In vitamin A intoxication, cortical hyperostosis usually becomes manifest no earlier than the end of the first year of life (whereas infantile cortical hyperostosis may produce changes in the first 6 months of life), mandibular and facial involvement is unusual (whereas these areas typically are affected in infantile cortical hyperostosis), metatarsal alterations are frequent (whereas these bones generally are spared in infantile cortical hyperostosis), and biochemical analysis of the blood reveals marked elevation of vitamin A concentration.

HYPOVITAMINOSIS A

Chronic vitamin A deficiency in infancy, childhood, or adulthood produces a variety of epithelial alterations; in infancy, additional manifestations include a susceptibility to infection, anemia, cranial nerve injury, and growth retardation. Increased intracranial pressure is observed in this condition. Vitamin A deficiency also may have a dramatic effect on dental development.

HYPOVITAMINOSIS C (SCURVY)

A long-term deficiency of dietary vitamin C (ascorbic acid) results in scurvy.

Infantile Scurvy

Infantile scurvy occurs in babies who are fed pasteurized or boiled milk; the process of heating the milk leads to disruption of vitamin C. Disease develops after deficiency of the vitamin has existed for 4 to 10 months; thus, it is exceedingly unusual to detect this disorder in infants below the age of 4 months, the manifestations generally becoming apparent at 8 to 14 months of age. Prior to the appearance of hemorrhagic tendencies, infants with scurvy can develop a failure to thrive and digestive alterations. Later, findings include pale skin with petechial hemorrhages, ulcerated gums, palatal petechiae, hematuria, melena, hematemesis, and secondary infections. This hemorrhagic tendency may be related to a lack of intercellular cement substance in the endothelial layer of the capillaries. Additional clinical findings include soft tissue swelling owing to edema and hemorrhage, and costochondral tenderness and prominence.

METAPHYSEAL CHANGES. Skeletal alterations result from a depression of normal cellular activity, which is most marked in areas of active endochondral bone growth (ends of tubular bones and costochondral junctions). Disorganization of the growth zone is evident (Fig. 66–3). Extensive resorption of cortical and spongy bone contributes to a tendency to

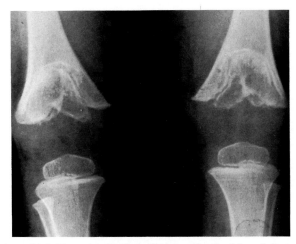

Figure 66–2. Hypervitaminosis A: Metaphyseal and epiphyseal changes. Observe the striking splaying and cupping of the distal femoral metaphyses, with narrowing of the cartilaginous growth plates and hypertrophy and invagination of the epiphyses.

fracture through this zone. The abnormal marrow in the junctional area is termed "Gerüstmark," and the entire zone consists of detritus ("Trümmerfeldzone"). Lateral extension of the heavy provisional zones of calcification in conjunction with elevation and stimulation of the adjacent periosteal membrane produces small excrescences of the metaphysis.

A radiograph of the end of an involved tubular bone will reveal several zones (Table 66–2) (Fig. 66–4). A radiodense line borders on the growth plate, representing the sclerotic provisional zone. On its metaphyseal side between the provisional zone of calcification and the heavy spongiosa deeper in the shaft is a transverse band of diminished density, the "scurvy" line. Small beak-like outgrowths of the metaphysis, incomplete or complete separation of the plate from the shaft

Table 66–1. HYPERVITAMINOSIS A VERSUS INFANTILE CORTICAL HYPEROSTOSIS (CAFFEY'S DISEASE)

	Hypervitaminosis A	Infantile Cortical Hyperostosis
Age of onset	End of first year of life	First 6 months of life
Findings	Soft tissue nodules Periostitis and hyperostosis Metaphyseal changes Growth disturbances Increased intracranial pressure	Soft tissue nodules Periostitis and hyperostosis Growth disturbances
Sites of hyperostosis (descending order of frequency)	Ulnae Metatarsals Clavicles Tibiae Fibulae Metacarpals Other tubular bones Ribs	Mandible Clavicles Scapulae Ribs Tubular bones
Etiology	Vitamin A poisoning	Unknown; possibly a viral disease

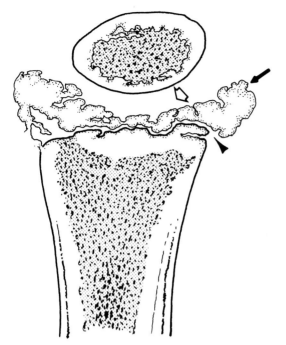

Figure 66–3. Hypovitaminosis C (scurvy): Pathologic abnormalities. The changes in the ends of tubular bones consist of an irregular arrangement of cartilage cells in the proliferating zone of the growth plate (open arrow), a metaphyseal area containing a latticework of calcified cartilage that is free of osseous tissue (solid arrow), and a decrease in trabeculae, fracture, and detritus in the junctional area (arrowhead). Metaphyseal excrescences can develop.

owing to subepiphyseal marginal clefts and infractions, extensive physiolysis, and periosteal new bone formation attributable to subperiosteal hemorrhage complete the distinctive radiographic picture of scurvy. These changes are most marked in areas of active endochondral bone formation.

EPIPHYSEAL CHANGES. In the epiphyses of tubular bones and in the carpus and tarsus, similar but less marked alterations are seen. Thickening of the provisional zone of calcification produces a radiodense shell around the ossification center (Wimberger's sign of scurvy).

DIAPHYSEAL CHANGES. Atrophy of spongiosa in the shafts of tubular bones accounts for a nonspecific decreased radiodensity. Cortical diminution is common, yet fracture of the shafts is unusual. Subperiosteal hemorrhage is most frequent in the larger tubular bones. Radiographically, soft tissue masses of increased density, displacement of adjacent bones, and shells of periosteal bone are observed.

ARTICULAR CHANGES. Hemarthrosis is a rare manifestation of scurvy, demonstrating a predilection for the large weight-bearing joints of the lower extremities.

DENTAL CHANGES. Cyst formation in the enamel and interruptions of the lamina dura may be dental manifestations of scurvy in humans.

GROWTH DISTURBANCES. Permanent growth disturbances after scurvy are unusual. Central metaphyseal cupping can lead to intrusion of the epiphysis into the exaggerated concavity of the metaphysis and early fusion of the growth plate. The degree of limb shortening, however, may be minimal. Similar cupping may be observed after trauma, infection, irradiation, immobilization, and vitamin A poison-

ing, as well as in sickle cell anemia and hereditary bone disorders.

EFFECTS OF THERAPY. With treatment of the disease, thickening of the cortex, increased density of the radiolucent zone of the metaphysis, transverse dense areas within the shaft, subperiosteal bone formation, spontaneous shifting of the diaphysis to realign with the displaced epiphysis, and increased density of the epiphysis can all be observed.

DIFFERENTIAL DIAGNOSIS. The appearance of a radiolucent metaphyseal band in scurvy is not pathognomonic. Other chronic illnesses, such as leukemia and neuroblastoma, can produce bone atrophy in this region. The identification of radiodense lines at the metaphysis and about the epiphysis, metaphyseal fractures, osseous beaks, epiphyseal displacements, and diaphyseal periostitis allows an accurate diagnosis of scurvy. Leukemia can lead to periostitis and diaphyseal destruction in combination with band-like metaphyseal radiolucency, but fracture and epiphyseal separation are not identified. Syphilis produces symmetric destructive foci in the metaphyses, particularly in the proximal portion of the tibia. Metaphyseal changes can also accompany rubella, cytomegalic inclusion disease, toxoplasmosis, and a variety of traumatic and dysplastic disorders.

Adult Scurvy

Currently, scurvy is rarely encountered in adults, although it may be observed in severely malnourished persons. Weakness, anorexia, weight loss, and fatigue generally antedate the more diagnostic hemorrhagic manifestations.

Hemarthrosis and bleeding at synchondroses can be observed in adult scurvy. Osteoporosis is prominent in the axial and appendicular skeleton. Biconcave deformities of vertebral bodies and condensation of bone at the vertebral margins are identical to changes of osteoporosis accompanying a wide spectrum of disorders; in the extremities, cortical thinning can be associated with mild periosteal proliferation.

Table 66–2. HYPOVITAMINOSIS C (SCURVY): RADIOGRAPHIC-PATHOLOGIC CORRELATION

Radiographic Finding	Pathologic Finding
Transverse metaphyseal line of increased density	Prominent thickened provisional zone of calcification
Transverse metaphyseal line of decreased density ("scurvy" line)	Decrease in trabeculae and detritus in junctional area of metaphysis ("Trümmerfeldzone")
Metaphyseal excrescences or beaks	Lateral extension of the heavy provisional zone of calcification with periosteal elevation and stimulation
Subepiphyseal infractions ("corner" or "angle" sign)	Decrease and brittleness of trabeculae in junctional area with fracture and hemorrhage
Periostitis	Subperiosteal hemorrhage with elevation and stimulation of periosteum
Epiphyseal shell of increased density with central lucency (Wimberger's sign of scurvy)	Prominent thickened provisional zone of calcification with atrophy of central spongiosa

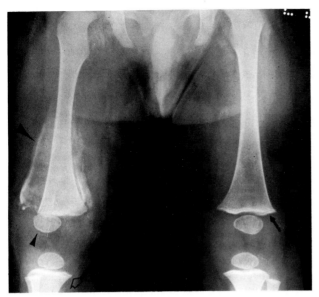

Figure 66–4. Hypovitaminosis C (scurvy): Radiographic abnormalities. At the ends of tubular bones, osteoporosis, a thick sclerotic metaphyseal line beneath which is a radiolucent line ("scurvy line") (solid arrow), small beak-like excrescences (open arrow), epiphyseal displacement (small arrowhead), and subperiosteal hemorrhage with periostitis (large arrowhead) can be noted. (Courtesy of F. Silverman, M.D., Stanford, California.)

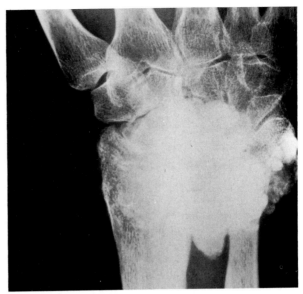

Figure 66–5. Hypervitaminosis D: Soft tissue abnormalities. Note massive soft tissue calcification about the wrist.

HYPERVITAMINOSIS D

Excessive intake of vitamin D can be associated with manifestations in both children and adults.

Musculoskeletal Abnormalities

Vitamin D poisoning can be acute or chronic. Acute clinical manifestations may appear within days after massive doses of the vitamin and include vomiting, fever, dehydration, abdominal cramps, bone pain, convulsions, and coma. With chronic poisoning, lassitude, thirst, anorexia, and polyuria are followed by vomiting, abdominal pain, and diarrhea. Laboratory analysis indicates albuminuria, hematuria, hypercalciuria, and hypercalcemia.

In infants and in children, metaphyseal bands of increased density, reflecting calcification of the matrix of the proliferating cartilage alternating with areas of increased lucency, are evident. Cortical thickening may be observed, and osteoporosis may be evident at other locations. Widespread osteosclerosis also has been noted. Metastatic calcification of viscera, blood vessels, periarticular structures, muscles, laryngeal and tracheal cartilage, the falx cerebri, and the tentorium cerebelli can be noted.

In adults, hypervitaminosis D can lead to osteoporosis. The bones of the appendicular skeleton, the spine, the pelvis, and even the skull reveal varying degrees of bone loss. Massive soft tissue calcification can become apparent. Lobulated masses of calcium are evident in periarticular regions, bursae, tendon sheaths, joint capsules, and intraarticular cavities (Fig. 66–5). On pathologic evaluation, calcium hydroxyapatite is identified, and an inflammatory reaction can be seen.

Metastatic soft tissue calcification accompanies a variety of disorders, including hypervitaminosis D, milk-alkali syndrome, hyperparathyroidism, plasma cell myeloma, and skeletal metastasis. Furthermore, soft tissue calcinosis can be evident in various collagen disorders, and dystrophic calcification can occur after tissue injury or devitalization from any cause. Periarticular deposits are most characteristic of hypervitaminosis D, milk-alkali syndrome, hyperparathyroidism, renal osteodystrophy, collagen disorders, and idiopathic tumoral calcinosis.

Chronic Idiopathic Hypercalcemia

The major clinical manifestations of idiopathic infantile hypercalcemia include a peculiar facies, anorexia, hypotonia, mental and physical retardation, and vomiting. Radiographically, a generalized increase in skeletal density is observed. The disease may relate to the excessive ingestion of vitamin D over prolonged periods by infants who are slightly sensitive to this vitamin.

Infants with a facies similar to that of patients with idiopathic hypercalcemia may reveal supravalvular aortic stenosis and mental retardation (Williams' syndrome). Additional vascular manifestations include stenosis of the branches of the aorta, the peripheral pulmonary vessels, or the carotid arteries, and aortic hypoplasia.

FURTHER READING

Caffey J: Chronic poisoning due to excess of vitamin A. Description of the clinical and roentgen manifestations in seven infants and young children. Pediatrics 5:672, 1950.

Caffey J: Traumatic cupping of the metaphyses of growing bones. AJR 108:451, 1970.

Christensen WR, Liebman C, Sosman MC: Skeletal and peri-articular manifestations of hypervitaminosis D. 65:27, 1951.

Holman CB: Roentgenologic manifestations of vitamin D intoxication. Radiology 59:805, 1952.

Joffe N: Some radiological aspects of scurvy in the adult. Br J Radiol 34:429, 1961.

Keating JP, Feigin RD: Increased intracranial pressure associated with probable vitamin A deficiency in cystic fibrosis. Pediatrics 46:41, 1970.

Miller JH, Hayon II: Bone scintigraphy in hypervitaminosis A. AJR 144:767, 1985.

Shiers JA, Neuhauser EBD, Bowman JR: Idiopathic hypercalcemia. AJR 78:19, 1957.

Singleton EB: The radiographic features of severe idiopathic hypercalcemia of infancy. Radiology 68:721, 1957.

Sprague PL: Epiphyseo-metaphyseal cupping following infantile scurvy. Pediatr Radiol 4:122, 1976.

Chapter 67

Heavy Metal Poisoning and Deficiency

Donald Resnick, M.D.

In some cases of heavy metal poisoning, radiodense lines may appear in the metaphyses of tubular bones and within flat or irregular bones. The resulting radiographic findings, which are observed most characteristically in lead, phosphorus, and bismuth poisoning, must be differentiated from *normal variants, stress lines of Park or Harris, and changes in various metabolic, endocrine, and infectious disorders. Significant radiographic abnormalities are also observed in the aluminum accumulation that accompanies dialysis and in nutritional or inherited deficiencies of copper.*

Poisoning with or deficiency of certain heavy metals can produce characteristic musculoskeletal alterations. One of the most well-recognized changes associated with ingestion, inhalation, or injection of lead or other heavy metals is the appearance of radiodense lines at the ends of tubular bones or along the contours of flat and irregular bones. These lines must be differentiated from the transverse radiodense areas that are commonly observed at some of these locations in persons who have not been poisoned with metals.

TRANSVERSE OR STRESS LINES (OF PARK OR HARRIS)

The appearance of opaque transverse lines that extend across the metaphyses of tubular bones is a common radiographic phenomenon that may be observed in children and adults (Fig. 67–1). They are often referred to as Park or Harris lines and as transverse or growth arrest lines. Investigations of these lines have indicated that they are recognized in both healthy and sick individuals, that similar lines are encountered in patients who have been poisoned with a variety of heavy metals, and that the lines may be used as a determinant of growth potential. These transverse radiodense lines can be evident at birth or during infancy; they do not appear after growth has ceased but once formed, they persist into adult life. Similar lines can appear in both the appendicular and the axial skeleton (Fig. 67–2). The radiodense lines are more frequent and prominent at sites of rapid bone growth. Although the causation of the dense lines is not certain, it is the close proximity and similarity between the lines and the growth plate that have suggested that the bands are related to a disturbance of normal growth patterns. They are more properly termed "recovery" lines, as they indicate periods of renewed growth, presumably following a period of inhibited growth of the bone. Anatomically, the transverse bands consist of horizontally oriented trabeculae that partially or completely cross the medullary cavity. With regard to pathogenesis, during the initial stage of growth arrest, the osteoblasts form a thin transverse bone template beneath the zone of proliferative cartilage. With resurgence of growth during the recovery phase, cartilaginous proliferation and increased osteoblastic activity contribute to the thickening and metaphyseal migration of the transverse line.

Transversely or obliquely oriented radiodense lines also are encountered regularly in the tubular bones of adults with osteopenia. These lines, which are termed reinforcement lines, are discussed in Chapter 47.

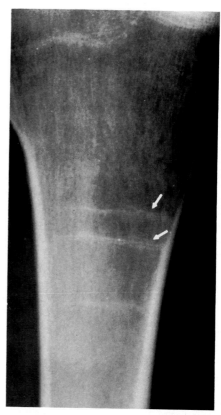

Figure 67–1. Transverse or stress lines: Appendicular skeleton. In the proximal tibia, multiple transverse radiodense lines extend almost completely across the medullary cavity (arrows).

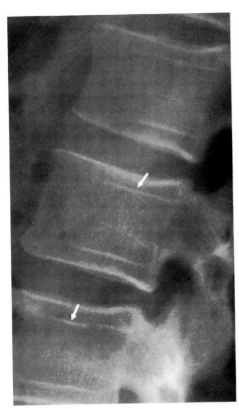

Figure 67–2. Transverse or stress lines: Axial skeleton. In multiple vertebral bodies, observe radiodense lines paralleling the superior and inferior osseous margins (arrows), creating a bone-within-bone appearance.

LEAD POISONING
General Abnormalities

Lead poisoning results from prolonged ingestion of lead-containing materials, such as paint; inhalation of fumes from burning storage batteries or similar substances; or, rarely, absorption of the material from bullets or buckshot that is contained within a serous cavity after a wound. Lead poisoning may also appear in the fetus of a mother exposed to lead; delayed dental and skeletal development, lead lines, and osteosclerosis may be evident in infants with congenital lead poisoning.

The onset of symptoms and signs after chronic lead poisoning may be abrupt. Abdominal pain, encephalopathy with convulsions, delirium, coma or death, peripheral neuritis, and anemia are clinical manifestations of the disorder. Examining the urine for porphyrin is a useful screening test for establishing the diagnosis.

Musculoskeletal Abnormalities in Infants and Children

Lead poisoning is associated with the appearance of thick transverse radiodense lines in the metaphyses of growing tubular bones. Deposition of calcium is the basis of the lead lines; even though lead is deposited in the metaphysis, it is in very minute amounts relative to the content of calcium.

The lead lines are not an early manifestation of the process and are, therefore, of little diagnostic aid. The radiodense zones are especially prominent in the bones about the knees (Fig. 67–3); identification of density in the proximal fibular metaphysis may be particularly helpful in establishing a radiographic diagnosis of lead poisoning, as similar changes

in the distal portion of the femur and proximal part of the tibia can be seen in apparently healthy children. Other bones, even those in the axial skeleton, may be affected, however (Fig. 67–4). In the absence of continued lead poisoning, the migrating lead lines decrease in radiodensity and disappear in approximately 4 years.

An additional manifestation of plumbism is failure of normal modeling of the tubular bones, which is most prominent in the femora. Widening of the metaphyses can resemble the changes in Pyle's disease.

Lead poisoning can be associated with signs of increased intracranial pressure. Widening of the cranial sutures may be evident in as many as 10 per cent of cases of chronic lead poisoning.

Musculoskeletal Abnormalities in Adults

Lead intoxication may relate to retained lead missiles within the body. Bullets, shrapnel, and buckshot are potential sources of the lead, and the resulting clinical findings may be intermittent in nature and delayed for as long as 50 years after the injury. As metallic lead is insoluble, lead intoxication is a rare complication of retained lead missiles, however. The absorption of lead from the missile generally requires that it be located in a cystic cavity, typically a synovium-lined joint. Synovial inflammation and fibrosis and discrete particles of lead in the synovial membrane and in the articular cartilage are the pathologic findings. Localized or systemic manifestations rarely are associated with lead missiles that are retained in soft tissues, bursal sacs, bones, and spinal tissues. Radiographic evidence of dissolution of lead missiles is provided by progressive fragmentation, enlargement, and migration of the radiodense foci.

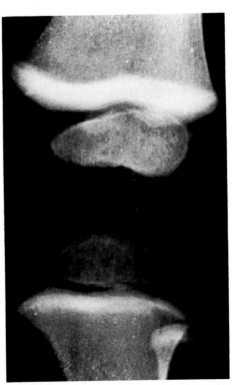

Figure 67–3. Lead poisoning: Knee. Observe the transverse radiodense bands of the metaphyses of femur, tibia, and fibula.

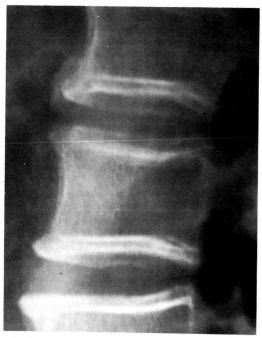

Figure 67–4. Lead poisoning: Spine. Radiodense lines are evident in the vertebral bodies. (Courtesy of A. Brower, M.D., Washington, D.C.)

Saturnine gout is also termed the "moonshine malady" because of the appearance of the condition in moonshiners whose home-brewed liquor contained an appreciable quantity of lead. Saturnine gout appears to be an expression of renal injury from lead in which a tubular defect leading to uric acid retention becomes evident.

Differential Diagnosis

Radiodense lines in the metaphyses of tubular bones can be seen as a normal variant, as an indication of previous stress, in heavy metal poisoning, including lead poisoning, and in the healing stages of leukemia, rickets, and scurvy (Table 67–1). Similar findings may accompany hypothyroidism, hypervitaminosis D, and transplacental infections (rubella, cytomegalic inclusion disease, herpes, toxoplasmosis, and syphilis). Metaphyseal flaring or widening is seen not only in lead poisoning but also in various anemias (sickle cell anemia, thalassemia), storage disorders (Gaucher's disease, Niemann-Pick disease), and congenital syndromes (Pyle's disease, multiple familial exostoses, osteopetrosis, Ollier's disease), and as a normal variant.

Table 67–1. SOME CAUSES OF RADIODENSE METAPHYSEAL LINES

Stress lines of Park or Harris
Heavy metal poisoning
Leukemia
Rickets
Scurvy
Hypothyroidism
Hypoparathyroidism
Hypervitaminoses
Transplacental infections

PHOSPHORUS POISONING

Phosphorus poisoning had previously been seen in rachitic and tuberculous children who were being treated with phosphorized cod liver oil; it is rarely encountered today. Single or multiple bands of increased radiodensity are seen in the ends of growing tubular bones and within flat or irregular bones and persist for many years.

BISMUTH POISONING

In the pregnant woman with syphilis, injected bismuth may cross the placenta and enter the fetal circulation to be deposited in the skeleton. Single or multiple radiodense bands or lines in the metaphyses of the tubular bones in cases of bismuth poisoning are similar to those that appear in cases of lead poisoning. The radiographic findings may resemble syphilitic osteochondritis, and differentiation of this condition from bismuth poisoning in the fetus of a syphilitic mother who has received bismuth during pregnancy can be difficult. In adults, radiographic abnormalities simulating those of osteonecrosis also have been described in cases of bismuth poisoning.

ALUMINUM TOXICITY

The oral or parenteral administration of aluminum compounds may lead to its deposition in the body's tissues, and in some sites—such as the brain and bones—it may cause toxic effects. This situation can arise in nonuremic adults, some with peptic ulcer disease, who are ingesting large amounts of aluminum carbonate; in uremic patients who ingest aluminum salts as phosphate binders and whose renal clearance of aluminum is reduced or who are undergoing hemodialysis in which the tap water is contaminated or aluminum hydroxide is present in the Redy sorbant cartridge; and in patients who have lost small bowel function and are maintained on chronic total parenteral nutrition.

The toxic effects of aluminum on the brain and bone have been well studied in patients with chronic renal failure who are maintained on regular hemodialysis or, rarely, peritoneal dialysis (see Chapter 52). Accumulation of aluminum appears to play a major role in dialysis encephalopathy. Furthermore, bone toxicity, manifested clinically as pain, tenderness, and deformity, is accompanied by the accumulation of aluminum in osseous tissue.

Osteopenia (related to osteomalacia), rickets-like changes, Looser's zones (insufficiency fractures), periostitis, and complete fractures are the principal radiographic manifestations of aluminum-induced osteopathy. Histologic analysis documents the presence of excessive amounts of lamellar osteoid and the deposition of aluminum mainly at the interface between mineralized bone and excessive osteoid. The precise mechanism by which aluminum alters mineralization of bone is not known, however.

COPPER DEFICIENCY

A human disorder associated with hypocupremia has been reported in infants who are malnourished, those receiving long-term parenteral nutrition, or those who were born prematurely and are maintained on diets low in copper. Radiographic findings include osteopenia, periostitis, metaphyseal radiodense lines and spurs, fractures, and physeal disruptions with malalignment of the epiphysis and metaphysis. Reversal of the osseous abnormalities occurs when copper supplementation is employed.

Menkes' syndrome (kinky hair syndrome) is an X-linked inherited disorder that relates to a defect in copper absorption from the gut. Obliteration or tortuosity of arteries occurs in the brain and in other tissues. Radiographic findings are similar to those in nutritional copper deficiency. The changes resemble those of rickets and the abused child syndrome. The early introduction of copper supplementation may improve the prognosis of this syndrome.

FURTHER READING

Andreoli SP, Smith JA, Bergstein JM: Aluminum bone disease in children: Radiographic features from diagnosis to resolution. Radiology 156:663, 1985.

Ashkenazai A, Levin S, Djaldetti M, Fisherl E, Benvenisti D: The syndrome of neonatal copper deficiency. Pediatrics 52:525, 1971.

Blickman JG, Wilkinson RH, Graef JW: The radiologic "lead band" revisited. 146:245, 1986.

Danks DM, Campbell PE, Stevens BJ, Mayne V, Cartwright E: Menkes' kinky hair syndrome. An inherited defect in copper absorption with widespread effects. Pediatrics 50:188, 1972.

Follis RH Jr, Park EA: Some observations on bone growth with particular respect to zones and transverse lines of increased density in the metaphysis. AJR 68:709, 1952.

Garrett P, McWade M, O'Callaghan J: Radiological assessment of aluminum-related bone disease. Clin Radiol 37:63, 1986.

Garn SM, Silverman FN, Hertzog KP, Rohmann CG: Lines and bands of increased density. Their implication to growth and development. Med Radiogr Photogr 44:58, 1968.

Klinenberg JR: Saturnine gout—a moonshine malady. N Engl J Med 280:1238, 1969.

Leonard MH: The solution of lead of synovial fluid. Clin Orthop 64:255, 1969.

Leone AJ Jr: On lead lines. AJR 103:165, 1968.

Park EA: The imprinting of nutritional disturbances on the growing bone. Pediatrics 33:815, 1964.

Pearl M, Boxt LM: Radiographic findings in congenital lead poisoning. Radiology 136:83, 1980.

Pease CN, Newton GG: Metaphyseal dysplasia due to lead poisoning in children. Radiology 79:233, 1962.

Sebes JI, Pinstein ML, Massie JD, Scott RL, Palmieri GM, Williams JW, Acchiardo SR: Radiographic manifestations of aluminum-induced bone disease. AJR 142:424, 1984.

Sachs HK: The evolution of the radiologic lead line. Radiology 139:81, 1981.

Sclafani SJA, Vuletin JC, Twersky J: Lead arthropathy: Arthritis caused by retained intra-articular bullets. Radiology 156:299, 1985.

Wesenberg RL, Gwinn JL, Barnes GR Jr: Radiological findings in the kinky hair syndrome. Radiology 92:500, 1969.

Chapter 68

Neuromuscular Disorders

Donald Resnick, M.D.

The musculoskeletal abnormalities accompanying neuromuscular disorders include osteoporosis, soft tissue atrophy, growth disturbances, deformities, growth plate injuries, infection, heterotopic ossification, cartilage atrophy, synovitis, clubbing, joint capsule alterations, and neuroarthropathy. Typical radiographic changes are encountered. Although the pathogenesis of some of the findings is clear, that of heterotopic ossification and sacroiliac joint alterations is unknown.

Some specific types of neuromuscular disease lead to characteristic clinical and imaging findings. Of particular importance, entrapment neuropathies occur at vulnerable sites along the course of the peripheral nerves as well as in plexuses. Hereditary neuropathies of sensory neurons produce neuroarthropathy, which is discussed further in Chapter 69.

Although the specific response of the musculoskeletal system depends to some degree on the nature of the disorder, certain general abnormalities are evident in many neuromuscular diseases. These alterations include osteoporosis, soft tissue atrophy or hypertrophy, growth disturbances and deformities attributable to altered muscular forces, growth plate and epiphyseal changes, soft tissue, bone, and joint infections, heterotopic ossification, cartilage and muscle atrophy, synovitis, and capsular abnormalities (Table 68–1). Neuroarthropathy, which may also accompany neurologic disorders, is described in Chapter 69.

GENERAL ABNORMALITIES

Osteoporosis

Profound osteoporosis accompanies immobilization, disuse, or paralysis. It can affect the entire skeleton or a portion of it, according to the cause or the circumstances (Fig. 68–1). The pathogenesis of osteoporosis is not clear, although alterations in bone circulation in neuromuscular disorders can modify cellular function. Initially, osteoclastic activity may be stimulated and osteoblastic activity may be reduced. The contribution of each cortical envelope as well as trabecular bone to osseous resorption is influenced by the nature of the underlying disorder.

The radiographic counterpart of the altered cellular dynamics is osteopenia in both the axial and appendicular skeletons. A generalized or localized, uniform or patchy, diffuse or periarticular decrease in spongy bone density is associated with diminution of the cortex and accentuation of stress trabeculae. Muscle weakness leads to frequent episodes of falling or stumbling, resulting in fractures of tubular bones. Fractures also accompany seizures (as a result of a fall or violent muscle contraction) and predominate in the spine, proximal portion of the femur, acetabulum, and shoulder region. Insufficiency (stress) fractures also may be encountered. Excessive callus formation can appear in the healing phase, probably the result of continued active or passive motion at the fracture site (Fig. 68–2). Furthermore, focal areas of

cortical resorption can develop, such as in the ribs, owing to pressure erosion from apposing bone or muscle atrophy with loss of normal mechanical stress.

Soft Tissue and Muscle Atrophy and Hypertrophy

Soft tissue atrophy with muscle wasting and fatty infiltration accompanies most neuromuscular disorders. In Duchenne muscular dystrophy and congenital myotonia, however, the actual bulk of the musculature is increased.

Computed tomography has been used to document the extent of muscle abnormality that occurs in neuromuscular disorders. Neural diseases generally are manifested as initial atrophy of muscle and a subsequent decrease in radiodensity; primary muscle disorders are characterized by decreased radiodensity followed by atrophy. In some specific situations, muscle hypertrophy occurs alone or in combination with atrophy. In all instances, computed tomographic abnormalities parallel in distribution the pathologic aberrations of the individual neuromuscular disorder.

Growth Disturbances and Deformities Caused by Altered Muscular Forces

Activity is essential to the normal growth and development of bones. With inactivity from any cause, muscle contraction diminishes or is lost, and, in the immature skeleton, the

Table 68–1. MUSCULOSKELETAL ABNORMALITIES IN PARALYSIS

Osteoporosis
Soft tissue atrophy or hypertrophy
Osseous deformities
Growth disturbances
"Stress" fragmentation of bone
Epiphyseal and metaphyseal fracture or fragmentation
Infection
Heterotopic ossification
Cartilage atrophy
Synovitis
Abnormalities of joint capsule
Reflex sympathetic dystrophy syndrome

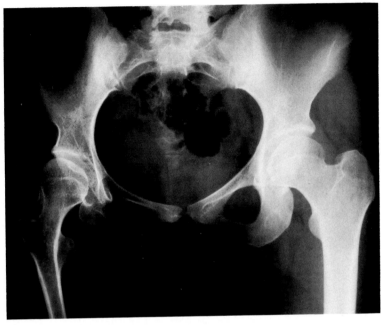

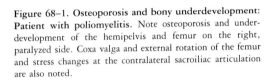

Figure 68–1. Osteoporosis and bony underdevelopment: Patient with poliomyelitis. Note osteoporosis and underdevelopment of the hemipelvis and femur on the right, paralyzed side. Coxa valga and external rotation of the femur and stress changes at the contralateral sacroiliac articulation are also noted.

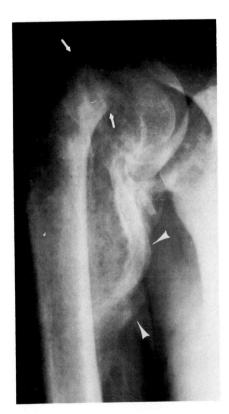

Figure 68–2. Osteoporosis and fracture. Observe the displaced fracture of the proximal portion of the humerus (arrows) and excessive callus formation (arrowheads).

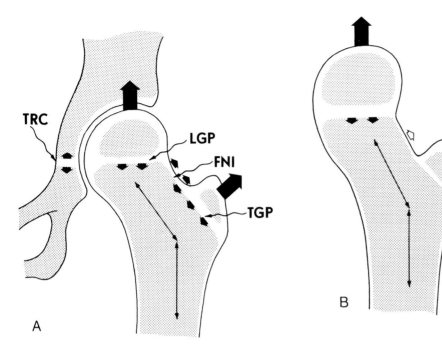

Figure 68–3. Pathogenesis of coxa valga. A Normal. The growth zones in this region are the articular cartilage, the longitudinal growth plate (LGP), the femoral neck isthmus (FNI), and the trochanteric growth plate (TGP). The triradiate cartilage (TRC) is present on the acetabular side of the joint. The direction of growth is indicated by small and large bold arrows. The double-headed arrows indicate the normal neck-shaft angle. B Coxa valga. A weakness in the abductor musculature reduces the growth stimulus to the trochanteric growth plate and the femoral neck isthmus (open arrows). The horizontally oriented longitudinal growth plate continues to lengthen the femoral neck in line with the femoral shaft (small and large bold arrows). A valgus angulation results (double-headed arrows). (Modified from Siffert RS: Patterns of deformity of the developing hip. Clin Orthop 160:14, 1981. Used with permission.)

growth cartilage is damaged. Neonates with muscle hypotonia and inactive children who spend most of their time in a horizontal position can reveal vertebral bodies with increased vertical dimensions and narrowed intervertebral discs. Similarly, an increase in the neck-shaft angle of the femur, producing coxa valga (Figs. 68–1 and 68–3), can result from muscular imbalance or a decrease in weight-bearing, particularly in very young children. In severe cases, subluxation or dislocation of the hip may occur (Fig. 68–4). In cases of subluxation of the femoral head, an osseous notch may be observed in the superolateral aspect of the femoral head, presumably related to bone molding produced by the superior portion of the joint capsule.

Coxa vara deformity is also reported in children with sensory-deficient neuromuscular disorders, such as spina bifida. It is accompanied by spontaneous separation of the femoral metaphysis and epiphysis owing to disruption of the longitudinal growth plate and fragmentation of the femoral neck.

Additional examples of the effects of altered muscular activity on neighboring bone can easily be identified (Fig. 68–5). In the child with cerebral palsy, scoliosis, lordosis, and pelvic obliquity (see Chapter 75) may result from unbalanced spine and hip muscle contraction and spasticity; external rotation of the upper femur with a prominent lesser trochanter results from the exaggerated pull of the iliopsoas muscle; and flexion contractures of the hips and the knees with abnormal stress in the quadriceps mechanism may lead to patella alta, an elongated patellar shape, and fragmentation of the lower pole of the patella. An exaggerated pull of the flexor muscles of the leg relative to the extensors can produce equinus at the ankle. In the child with poliomyelitis or peroneal muscle atrophy, a pes cavus deformity is attributable to altered muscle function and stress.

Growth Plate and Epiphyseal Changes

Premature closure of the growth plate, particularly in the metatarsals and knees, is noted in patients with poliomyelitis

(Fig. 68–6). The fourth metatarsal is affected most frequently. The altered epiphyses in the foot or the knee can be buried in the adjacent metaphyses (ball-and-socket epiphyses), and, after physeal fusion, the involved bone is shortened.

Premature physeal closure can become evident in other neuromuscular diseases, and it may be associated with epiphyseal overgrowth, findings resembling those of hemophilia or juvenile chronic arthritis.

Epiphyseal and metaphyseal trauma is a recognized manifestation in patients with certain neurologic disorders (menin-

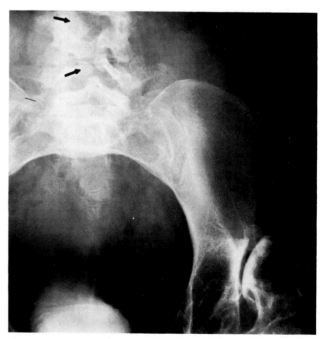

Figure 68–4. Dislocation of the hip. In a paraplegic patient with spina bifida (arrows) and meningomyelocele, note the dislocated left femoral head, which is flattened and sclerotic. A neurogenic bladder is also apparent.

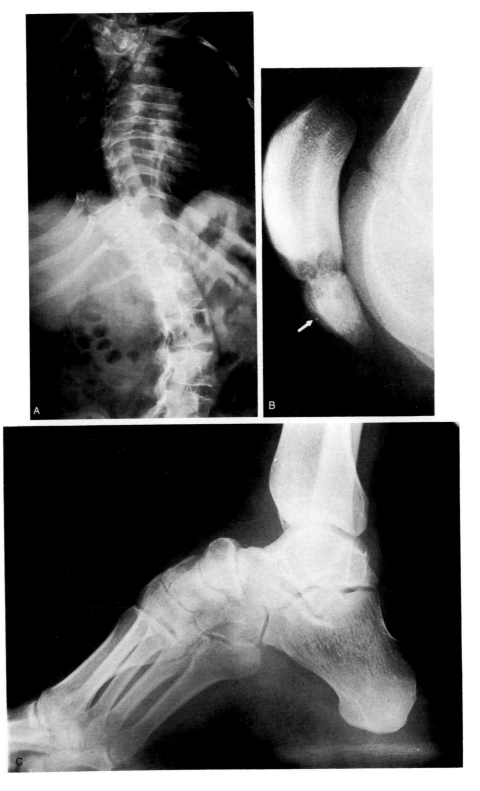

Figure 68–5. Additional osseous effects related to altered muscular activity. A Scoliosis in cerebral palsy. Note the prominent scoliotic curvatures, which were associated with considerable pelvic obliquity. **B** Patellar fragmentation in cerebral palsy. Observe the large fragment of the inferior pole of the patella (arrow) caused by altered stress in the quadriceps mechanism. **C** Pes cavus deformity in poliomyelitis. Observe the exaggerated arch of the foot, soft tissue atrophy, and osteoporosis.

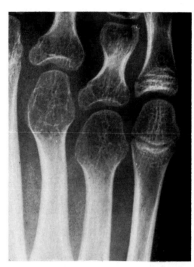

Figure 68–6. Premature closure of the growth plate in a patient with poliomyelitis. Closure of the growth plate of the third and fourth metatarsal bones has produced shortening of these digits.

gomyelocele and congenital insensitivity to pain) owing to their sensory deficiency, osteoporosis, and musculoligamentous laxity (see Chapter 69).

Osseous, Articular, and Soft Tissue Infection

Skin breakdown over pressure points is a common problem in immobilized persons, and infection may reach the underlying bones and joints. The ischial tuberosities, the femoral trochanters, the hips, and other bone protuberances are most typically affected.

Heterotopic Ossification

Heterotopic new bone formation is a well-documented complication of central nervous system and spinal cord disorders. It is reported most commonly in association with paraplegia secondary to spinal cord trauma. Less frequently, heterotopic ossification is evident after acute anoxia, head injury, cerebrovascular accident, encephalomyelitis, poliomyelitis, multiple sclerosis, neoplastic disease, and tetanus. It occurs in both flaccid and spastic forms of paralysis.

In general, ossification appears 2 to 6 months after injury. Single or multiple sites may be affected. The areas most typically involved are the hip (Fig. 68–7), the knee, and the shoulder (Fig. 68–8); less commonly, the elbow and the small joints of the hand and the foot are altered. Ossification is almost always seen in a paralyzed limb or limbs. Many patients have no symptoms or signs in addition to those of the primary neurologic disorder itself. Others develop pain, swelling, and restricted joint motion, simulating the findings of an acute arthritis.

Radiographic examination delineates initially poorly defined periarticular radiodense areas that enlarge, demonstrating trabecular architecture. Eventually, complete periarticular osseous bridging may result.

Scintigraphic examination may also be used to determine the evolution and maturity of this process. This determination is important, as surgical removal of immature new bone frequently is followed by recurrence of the abnormal deposits,

whereas excision of mature ossification is not associated with such recurrence. Images obtained with bone-seeking pharmaceutical agents reveal an acute phase with increased radionuclide activity occurring as early as 2 weeks after the neurologic insult; a subacute phase with a rapid increase in activity; a chronic active immature phase with a steady state of increased activity; a chronic active maturing phase with decreased activity; and a chronic mature phase with a return of the normal scan.

The cause of the ectopic bone formation is unknown. The common factor in heterotopic ossification in neurologic disorders is immobilization. The deposition of calcium and bone may relate to vascular stasis, perhaps in Batson's paravertebral plexus, but the exact pathogenesis of such ossification and why it is present in some persons and absent in others remain mysteries.

Heterotopic ossification of soft tissues is not confined to patients with neuromuscular disease. Burns, mechanical trauma, and venous stasis (varicosities) can lead to similar changes. In addition, a progressive form of ossification of unknown cause, myositis (fibrodysplasia) ossificans progressiva, also is recognized.

Cartilage Atrophy

Articular cartilage is nourished predominantly by diffusion of synovial fluid (Fig. 68–9). The diffusion into cartilage of nutrients from the synovial fluid and subchondral bone depends on a pumping action that develops during normal activity. Immobilization leads to significant changes in cartilaginous nutrition. The radiographic counterpart of the chondral changes is a loss of interosseous (joint) space in the patient with neurologic disease (Fig. 68–10). Changes are

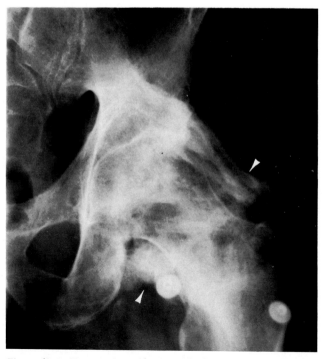

Figure 68–7. Heterotopic ossification: The hip. The deposits begin as poorly defined opaque areas and progress to radiodense lesions of considerable size possessing trabecular pattern (arrowheads).

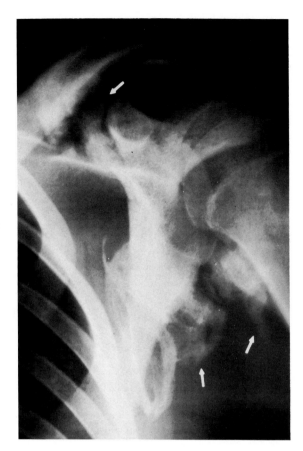

Figure 68–8. Heterotopic ossification: The shoulder. Deposits of varying size can also be noted about the shoulder (arrows).

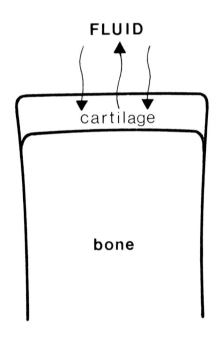
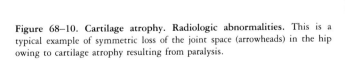

Figure 68–9. Normal cartilage nutrition. The predominant mechanism of cartilage nutrition is derived from a pumping action in which synovial fluid diffuses into and out of the chondral substance. A subchondral route of nutrition is present but of less magnitude.

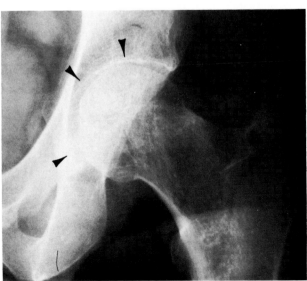

Figure 68–10. Cartilage atrophy. Radiologic abnormalities. This is a typical example of symmetric loss of the joint space (arrowheads) in the hip owing to cartilage atrophy resulting from paralysis.

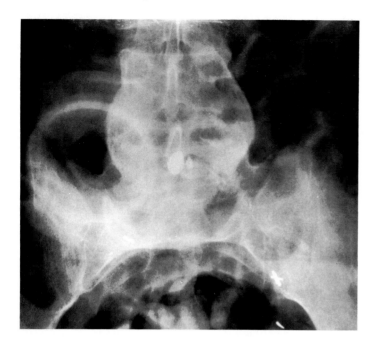

Figure 68–11. Sacroiliac joint and spinal abnormalities. Bilateral sacroiliac joint changes consisting of narrowing of the interosseous space are combined with peculiar spinal outgrowths at the discovertebral junction that resemble syndesmophytes. Previous surgery and myelography had been accomplished.

especially characteristic in the hip, the knee, and the sacroiliac joint. Characteristically, in the hip, diffuse loss of interosseous space is evident with axial migration of the femoral head. In the sacroiliac joint, abnormalities consist of periarticular osteoporosis and joint space narrowing, which, in some cases, progresses to intraarticular bone ankylosis. The sacroiliac joint abnormalities appear to be more frequent and severe in patients with paralysis of longer duration. Rarely, they are combined with changes in the spine, including syndesmophytes, interspinous ossification, osteophytes, and intervertebral disc calcification (Fig. 68–11).

Joint Capsule Abnormalities

Fibrosis in the joint capsule, especially about the glenohumeral joint, may explain the association of adhesive capsulitis and neurologic injury, particularly hemiparesis. Inferior subluxation of the humeral head with respect to the glenoid region of the scapula, the drooping shoulder, is a second manifestation of paralysis. It should be differentiated from true dislocations of the glenohumeral joint, as no surgical manipulation is required. The drooping shoulder also occurs in hemophilia and after capsular injury. In paralysis, the drooping shoulder is produced by loss of muscular tone leading to subluxation produced by the weight of the dependent upper extremity. With progressive displacement, the glenohumeral joint space widens.

Miscellaneous Abnormalities

Significant digital clubbing may be encountered in paralyzed patients. The reflex sympathetic dystrophy syndrome also has been observed in paralyzed patients.

SPECIFIC TYPES OF NEUROMUSCULAR DISEASE
Peripheral Neuropathies

Peripheral neuropathies represent primary disorders of peripheral motor, sensory, and autonomic neurons and are accompanied by muscle weakness, muscle atrophy, sensory change, or autonomic dysfunction. They can be further classified as mononeuropathy, multiple mononeuropathies, and polyneuropathies (Table 68–2).

ENTRAPMENT NEUROPATHIES. Peripheral nerve entrapment syndromes involve the compression of a short segment of a single nerve at a specific site, frequently as a result of the vulnerability of that nerve as it passes through a fibroosseous tunnel or an opening in fibrous or muscular tissue. Clinical manifestations, consisting of motor and sensory abnormalities, vary according to the specific nerve that is affected. Entrapment neuropathies typically involve the median, ulnar, radial, musculocutaneous, suprascapular, dorsoscapular, or brachial plexus nerves in the upper extremities and the sciatic, common peroneal, posterior tibial, femoral, saphenous, lateral femoral cutaneous, obturator, ilioinguinal, or genitofemoral nerve in the lower extremity (Table 68–3).

Median Nerve. Entrapment of the *median nerve* occurs most frequently in the wrist as the carpal tunnel syndrome, but it may also develop in the region of the distal portion of the humerus or proximal portion of the forearm.

Ligament of Struthers. In approximately 1 per cent of limbs, the ligament of Struthers connects an anomalous bone excrescence (the supracondylar process), arising from the anterior surface of the distal portion of the humerus and extending to the medial epicondyle of the humerus (Fig. 68–12). Compromise of the median nerve is a possible complication.

Pronator Syndrome. An entrapment neuropathy of the median nerve can occur in the antecubital area where the nerve passes between the two heads of the pronator teres muscle and then under the edge of the flexor digitorum sublimis muscle.

Anterior Interosseous Nerve Syndrome (Kiloh-Nevin Syndrome). The anterior interosseous nerve is the largest branch of the median nerve and is purely motor. Its compression leads to weakness of the thumb and index finger and occurs on an idiopathic basis, after radial or supracondylar humeral fractures, or as a result of aberrant fibrous bands.

Carpal Tunnel Syndrome. The most frequent entrapment syndrome of the median nerve occurs as the nerve passes

Table 68–2. CLASSIFICATION OF PERIPHERAL NEUROPATHIES

Type	Characteristics	Pathophysiology	Common Causes
Mononeuropathy	Involves one cranial or peripheral nerve or nerve root	Trauma Compression Entrapment Infarction	Common peroneal palsy Carpal tunnel syndrome Diabetes mellitus
Multiple mononeuropathy	Involves several nerves 　Contiguous nerves	Neoplastic invasion	Invasion of the brachial plexus by cancer
		Infarction	Diabetes mellitus
	Noncontiguous nerves	Infarction	Diabetes mellitus Vasculitis
Polyneuropathy	Involves the longest nerves first; distal, symmetric	Toxic-metabolic	Alcohol-nutritional Diabetes mellitus Uremia Systemic cancer
		Inflammatory or immune (or both)	Guillain-Barré syndrome

From Sherman DG: Peripheral neuropathies. *In* JG Stein (Ed): Internal Medicine. Boston, Little, Brown, 1983, p 872. Used with permission.

Table 68–3. SOME NERVE ENTRAPMENT SYNDROMES

Nerve	Site (Syndrome)	Causes or Findings
Median	Distal portion of the humerus	Supracondylar spur, ligament of Struthers
	Elbow (pronator syndrome)	Abnormality of pronator teres, flexor digitorum sublimis, or biceps
	Elbow (anterior interosseous nerve syndrome, Kiloh-Nevin syndrome)	Fracture of humerus or radius, fibrous band, or idiopathic
	Wrist (carpal tunnel syndrome)	Systemic and local factors or idiopathic
	Wrist (sublimis syndrome, pseudo–carpal tunnel syndrome)	Sublimis muscle belly
Ulnar	Elbow (cubital tunnel syndrome, tardy ulnar palsy)	Fracture, arthritis, cubitus valgus, trochlear hypoplasia
	Wrist (ulnar tunnel syndrome, Guyon's canal syndrome)	Fracture, ganglion, arthritis, ulnar artery abnormalities
Radial	Axilla (Saturday night palsy, sleep palsy)	Alcoholism, drug addiction, prolonged sleep with abnormal position of arm
	Distal portion of the humerus	Fracture involving spiral groove
	Elbow (posterior interosseous nerve syndrome)	Fracture, dislocation, rheumatoid arthritis, tumor, fibrous band
Suprascapular	Shoulder	Scapular fracture, glenohumeral joint dislocation, ganglion, tumor
Plantar and interdigital	Foot (Morton's metatarsalgia)	Digital nerve compression and ischemia, digital neuroma
Posterior tibial	Ankle (tarsal tunnel syndrome)	Sprain, fracture, arthritis, tumor, ganglion, venous tortuosity
Common peroneal	Knee	Sprain, fracture, use of casts, surgery, ganglion, fabella, popliteal cyst
Lateral femoral cutaneous	Anterior superior iliac spine (meralgia paresthetica)	Trauma, pelvic fracture, pelvic tilt
Femoral	Inguinal region	Trauma, tumor, abscess, aneurysm, bleeding
Obturator	Obturator canal	Hernia, inflammation
Sciatic	Sciatic foramen (including piriformis syndrome)	Hip surgery, gluteal injection, tumor
	Knee	Popliteal cyst
Brachial plexus	Neck and shoulder (thoracic outlet syndrome, scalenus anticus syndrome)	Fracture, dislocation, tumor, infection, surgery, injection, cervical rib

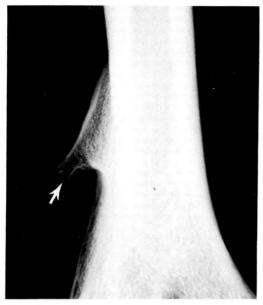

Figure 68–12. Entrapment of the median nerve: Supracondylar process. This bone outgrowth (arrow) arises from the anterior surface of the distal portion of the humerus. The ligament of Struthers may extend from its tip to the medial epicondyle of the humerus, leading to compromise of the median nerve.

through the narrow tunnel that exists between the carpal bones and the inelastic transverse carpal ligament. Although the carpal tunnel view allows analysis of the osseous components of this passageway, delineation of the other structures within the canal requires computed tomography or magnetic resonance imaging (Fig. 68–13).

Causes of the carpal tunnel syndrome are many (Fig. 68–14) (Table 68–4), although frequently the disorder occurs on an idiopathic basis. Most patients are between the ages of 35 and 65 years. Women are affected more frequently than men. Clinical findings include sensory and motor deficits, and physical examination documents a positive Tinel's sign (paresthesias occurring after percussion of the nerve in the volar aspect of the wrist) and reproduction of symptoms with the Phalen maneuver, accomplished by flexing the patient's hand at the wrist for longer than 1 minute.

Sublimis Syndrome (Pseudo–Carpal Tunnel Syndrome). Compromise of a more proximal portion of the median nerve may relate to its compression by the lateral border of the sublimis muscle belly.

Ulnar Nerve. Entrapment of the *ulnar nerve* occurs most commonly near the elbow or wrist and rarely in the forearm.

Cubital Tunnel Syndrome. Ulnar nerve entrapment is seen most frequently at the level of the cubital tunnel, where the nerve extends through a canal formed by the medial epicondyle and an aponeurotic band bridging the dual origin of the flexor carpi ulnaris muscle. Typical causes of compression of the ulnar nerve in the cubital tunnel are trauma and progressive cubitus valgus deformity (tardy ulnar nerve palsy); additional causes include nerve subluxation, osteoarthritis, rheumatoid arthritis, flexion deformity of the elbow, anomalous muscles, trochlear hypoplasia, and masses as well as idiopathic entrapment. Clinical findings are weakness of the flexor carpi ulnaris muscle, flexor digitorum profundus muscle of the fourth and fifth fingers, and intrinsic hand muscles. A

positive Tinel's sign follows percussion of the ulnar nerve at the level of the elbow, and the nerve itself may be enlarged and tender. Axial radiographs may reveal medial trochlear osteophytes or medial incongruity of the elbow joint, or both.

Guyon's Canal Syndrome (Ulnar Tunnel Syndrome). An entrapment neuropathy of the ulnar nerve may occur in the wrist where the nerve enters the palm through the canal of Guyon, the ulnar tunnel (Fig. 68–15). The walls of the canal consist of the pisiform bone medially and the hook of the hamate laterally. The floor of the canal is composed of the flexor retinaculum and the origin of the hypothenar muscles, and the roof is composed of the volar carpal ligament, palmaris brevis, and fibers from the palmar fascia.

The most frequent causes of ulnar verve entrapment in Guyon's canal are ganglia and accidental, occupational, or recreational (bicycling) trauma. Fractures of the hook of the hamate may also lead to such entrapment.

Double Crush Syndrome. The double crush syndrome refers to entrapment of the ulnar nerve occurring concomitantly with disease of the lower cervical spine or the thoracic outlet syndrome.

Radial Nerve. Entrapment of the *radial nerve* may occur in the axilla, elbow, or proximal portion of the forearm.

Saturday Night Palsy. Individuals who sleep with pressure exerted on the proximal medial aspect of the extremity may develop radial nerve dysfunction owing to its compression in the axilla or spiral groove of the humerus. This type of sleep palsy is particularly common in alcoholics and drug abusers and in patients using crutches.

Entrapment in the Spiral Groove of the Humerus. Compression of the radial nerve, usually related to fractures, may occur where it winds around the humerus in close proximity to the bone.

Posterior Interosseous Nerve Syndrome. Compression of the posterior interosseous nerve occurs just distal to the elbow as the nerve passes into the supinator muscle. Causes of this neuropathy include dislocations of the elbow, fractures, rheumatoid arthritis, soft tissue tumors, and fibrous bands.

Suprascapular Nerve. Entrapment of the *suprascapular nerve* occurs most commonly as it passes through the suprascapular notch. Potential causes of this entrapment include a scapular fracture or glenohumeral joint dislocation, stress (as in weight-lifting), ganglia, tumors, and developmental anomalies of the notch.

Medial or Lateral Plantar Nerves. Entrapment of the *medial or lateral plantar nerves* of the foot occurs as a result of injury near the transverse intertarsal ligament. In this location, a neuroma may develop, especially between the third and fourth toes (Morton's neuroma).

Posterior Tibial Nerve. Compression of the *posterior tibial nerve* at the medial aspect of the ankle results in the tarsal tunnel syndrome (Fig. 68–16). The tarsal tunnel is located behind and below the medial malleolus; its floor is osseous and its roof is formed by the flexor retinaculum. Tissue scarring occurring after an ankle sprain or osseous deformity following a calcaneal fracture is a common cause of this neuropathy. Additional causes are synovial inflammation, foot deformities, benign tumors, and dilated veins.

Common Peroneal Nerve. Compression of the *common peroneal nerve or its branches* occurs near the knee (Fig. 68–17). Entrapment of the common peroneal nerve typically occurs as it winds around the neck of the fibula; causes of such

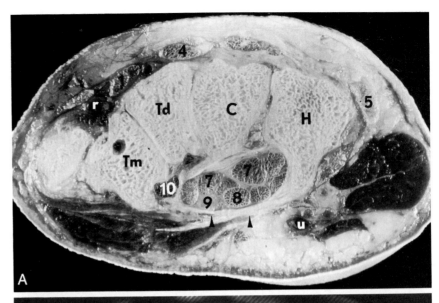

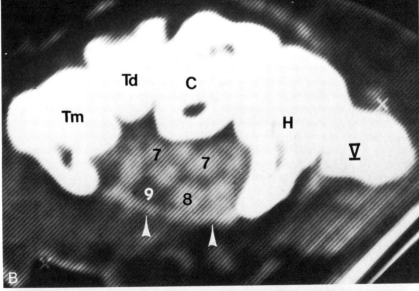

Figure 68–13. Entrapment of the median nerve: Carpal tunnel syndrome—normal sectional anatomy. Photograph (**A**), computed tomogram (**B**), and magnetic resonance image (**C**) at the level of the hook of the hamate. Observe the position of the median nerve (9) and the transverse carpal ligament (arrowheads). H, Hamate; C, capitate; Td, trapezoid; Tm, trapezium; 4, digital extensors; 5, extensor carpi ulnaris; 7, flexor digitorum profundus; 8, flexor digitorum superficialis; 10, flexor carpi radialis; u, ulnar artery; r, radial artery; V, base of fifth metacarpal. (**A, B,** From Cone RO, et al: Computed tomography of the normal soft tissues of the wrist. Invest Radiol *18*:546, 1983. Used with permission.)

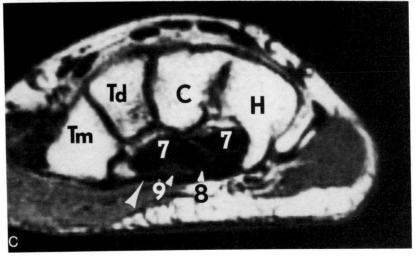

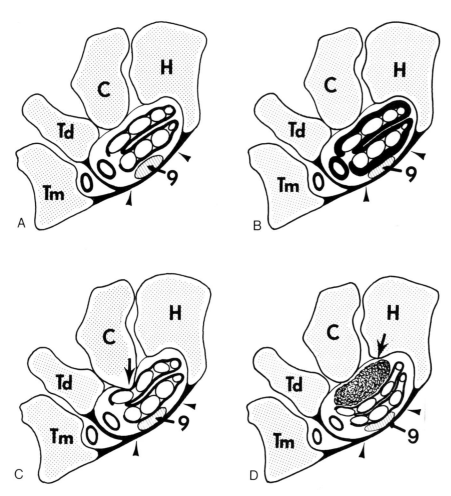

Figure 68–14. Entrapment of the median nerve: Carpal tunnel syndrome—potential causes. A Normal. The median nerve (9) and transverse carpal ligament (arrowheads) are indicated. H, Hamate; C, capitate; Td, trapezoid; Tm, trapezium. B Tenosynovitis. C Osseous spur (arrow). D Mass (arrow). (From Lipscomb TR: J Musculoskel Med 1:35, 1984. Carpal tunnel syndrome: Guide to office diagnosis. Used with permission.)

entrapment are injury, popliteal cysts, total knee arthroplasty, tight casts, ganglia, and the fabella. Clinical findings include impaired dorsiflexion and eversion of the foot and impaired extension of the toes, resulting in a footdrop.

Sciatic Nerve. The *sciatic nerve,* the largest in diameter in the body, is derived from the sacral plexus, which is formed from the fourth and fifth lumbar and first and second sacral roots. As a single trunk, it exits the pelvis by traversing the greater sciatic foramen, below the piriformis muscle, and then descends between the greater trochanter of the femur and the ischial tuberosity, deep to the gluteus maximus muscle. In the back of the thigh, above the popliteal fossa, it divides into two large branches, the tibial nerve and the common peroneal nerve.

The proximal portion of the sciatic nerve is infrequently compressed. Slightly more distally, compression neuropathy of the sciatic nerve may be produced by immobility, prolonged squatting, intramuscular injections, and hip surgery. Below the sciatic foramen, a piriformis syndrome represents a distinct pattern of nerve compression in which symptoms and signs resemble those of discal herniation. The lower portion of the sciatic nerve in the region of the knee may be compressed by synovial cysts in the popliteal fossa.

Plexus Neuropathies. Tumors, infections, trauma, surgical and diagnostic procedures, and injections can involve all or some of the branches of the brachial plexus, leading to thoracic outlet, scalenus anticus, costoclavicular, and other syndromes. Anatomic variations, such as a cervical rib, may contribute to these neuropathies.

HEREDITARY NEUROPATHIES. Slowly progressive peripheral neuropathies that are hereditary in nature can be differentiated according to the specific type of neurons that are affected predominantly: sensory neurons, motor neurons, and autonomic neurons. Classification of these disorders is complicated, as many of the diseases affect more than one type of neuron. These disorders differ in their mode of inheritance, age of onset, natural history and prognosis, distribution of abnormalities, and pathologic alterations. Some, such as those with prominent sensory loss, produce neuroarthropathy, the features of which are discussed in Chapter 69.

Friedreich's Ataxia

Friedreich's ataxia is one form of spinocerebellar degeneration. It is usually a recessive disorder that begins in childhood or adolescence, becoming manifest as progressive ataxia, dysarthria, and nystagmus with impairment of vibratory and position sensation and diminished or absent reflexes. Cardiomyopathy may lead to the patient's death. Specific causes of this disease (Friedreich's syndrome) include inborn errors of metabolism, disorders of lipid or oxidative metabolism, aminoacidurias, and the partial deficiency of hypoxanthine phosphoribosyltransferase. Orthopedic complications include severe scoliosis, coxa valga deformity, subluxation of the hips, instability of the knees and ankles, and pes cavus.

Muscle Diseases

Diseases of muscle can be classified as congenital or genetic, metabolic, inflammatory or infectious, traumatic, neoplastic, and of miscellaneous type. Many of these are considered elsewhere in this textbook. Diseases of muscle are better evaluated with computed tomography or magnetic resonance imaging than with routine radiography.

Table 68–4. SOME CAUSES OF THE CARPAL TUNNEL SYNDROME

Synovitis
  Rheumatoid arthritis
  Scleroderma
  Systemic lupus erythematosus
  Dermatomyositis
  Seronegative spondyloarthropathies
  Granulomatous and nongranulomatous infections
  Hemophilia
  Crystal deposition diseases

Infiltrative Diseases
  Amyloidosis
  Myxedema
  Acromegaly
  Mucopolysaccharidoses

Trauma
  Fractures and dislocations
  Repetitive and prolonged stress

Tumors and Tumor-like Lesions
  Neuromas
  Lipomas
  Synovial cysts
  Ganglia
  Multiple myeloma

Anatomic Factors
  Small carpal canal
  Thick transverse carpal ligament
  Anomalous nerves, muscles, bursae

Medical and Surgical Procedures
  Arteriovenous fistulae
  Artery punctures, catheterizations

Miscellaneous
  Diabetes mellitus
  Polymyalgia rheumatica
  Hemorrhage
  Hypoparathyroidism
  Pregnancy
  Use of oral contraceptives
  Gynecologic surgery
  Osteoarthritis
  Pyridoxine deficiency
  Paget's disease
  Idiopathic

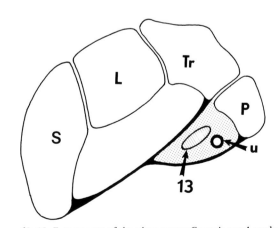

Figure 68–15. Entrapment of the ulnar nerve: Guyon's canal syndrome (ulnar tunnel syndrome)—normal sectional anatomy. Observe the ulnar nerve (13) and ulnar artery (u). S, scaphoid; L, lunate; Tr, triquetrum; P, pisiform. (From Grundberg AB: Ulnar tunnel syndrome. J Hand Surg [Br] 9:72, 1984. Used with permission.)

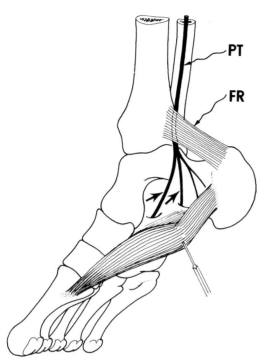

Figure 68–16. Entrapment of the posterior tibial nerve: Tarsal tunnel syndrome—normal anatomy. The posterior tibial nerve (PT) passes beneath the flexor retinaculum (FR), and then divides into various nerves, including the medial and lateral plantar nerves (arrows). (Reprinted by permission from Kopell HP, Thompson WAL: Peripheral entrapment neuropathies of the lower extremity. N Engl J Med 262:56, 1960.)

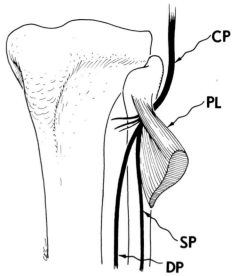

Figure 68–17. Entrapment of the common peroneal nerve and its branches: Normal anatomy. On this posterior view, observe that the common peroneal nerve (CP) winds around the back of the fibula in intimate association with the peroneus longus muscle (PL) and then divides into the deep peroneal nerve (DP) and the superficial peroneal nerve (SP). (Reprinted by permission from Kopell HP, Thompson WAL: Peripheral entrapment neuropathies of the lower extremity. N Engl J Med 262:56, 1960.)

MUSCULAR DYSTROPHIES. The universal clinical finding in the inherited myopathies is weakness, and the pathologic abnormalities are limited to the skeletal musculature (and, rarely, the cardiac musculature). In these myopathies, necrosis and regeneration of muscle fibers and their replacement with fibrous connective tissue and fat are observed.

The muscular dystrophies can be separated into several forms on the basis of their genetic patterns and such clinical manifestations as age of onset of the disease, distribution of muscle involvement, and the presence or absence of muscle hypertrophy (Table 68–5). Of these forms, *Duchenne muscular dystrophy* is the most common and has the greatest relevance to the musculoskeletal system. Findings include foot deformities (pes planus and equinovarus), spinal deformities (scoliosis and kyphosis), and knee and hip contractures.

Table 68–5. CLASSIFICATION OF HUMAN MUSCULAR DYSTROPHIES

	Duchenne Dystrophy	Facioscapulohumeral Dystrophy	Limb-Girdle Dystrophy	Myotonic Dystrophy
Genetic pattern	X-linked recessive	Autosomal dominant	Autosomal recessive	Autosomal dominant
Age at onset	Before age 5 years	Adolescence	Adolescence	Early or late
First symptoms	Pelvic	Shoulders	Pelvic	Distal; hands or feet
Pseudohypertrophy	+	−	−	−
Predominant early weakness	Proximal	Proximal	Proximal	Distal
Progression	Relatively rapid; incapacitated in adolescence	Slow	Variable	Slow
Facial weakness	−	+	−	Occasional
Ocular, oropharyngeal weakness	−	−	−	Occasional
Myotonia	−	−	−	+
Cardiomyopathy	− or late	−	−	Arrhythmia, conduction block
Associated disorders	None (?mental retardation)	None	None	Cataracts; testicular atrophy and baldness in men
Serum enzyme levels	Very high	Slight or no increase	Slight or no increase	Slight or no increase

From Rowland LP: Diseases of muscle and neuromuscular junction. In PB Beeson, W McDermott, JB Wyngaarden (Eds): Cecil Textbook of Medicine. 15th Ed. Philadelphia, WB Saunders Co, 1979, p 916. Used with permission.

FURTHER READING

Abel MS: Sacroiliac joint changes in traumatic paraplegics. Radiology 55:235, 1950.

Bhate DV, Pizarro AJ, Seitam A, Mak EK: Axial skeletal changes in paraplegics. Radiology 133:55, 1979.

Currarino G: Premature closure of epiphyses in the metatarsals and knees. A sequel of poliomyelitis. Radiology 87:424, 1966.

Daher YH, Lonstein JE, Winter RB, Bradford DS: Spinal deformities in patients with Friedreich ataxia: A review of 19 patients. J Pediatr Orthop 5:553, 1985.

Dyck PJ, Thomas PK, Lambert EH: Peripheral Neuropathy. 2nd Ed. Philadelphia, WB Saunders Co, 1984.

Houston CS: The radiologist's opportunity to teach bone dynamics. J Can Assoc Radiol 29:232, 1978.

Houston CS, Zaleski WA: The shape of vertebral bodies and femoral necks in relation to activity. Radiology 89:59, 1967.

Howard CB, Williams LA: A new radiological sign in the hips of cerebral palsy patients. Clin Radiol 35:317, 1984.

Kaye JJ, Freiberger RH: Fragmentation of the lower pole of the patella in spastic lower extremities. Radiology 101:97, 1971.

Kopell HP, Thompson WAL: Peripheral Entrapment Neuropathies. 2nd Ed. Huntington, New York, RE Krieger, 1976.

Lanzieri CF, Hilal SK: Computed tomography of the sacral plexus and sciatic nerve in the greater sciatic foramen. AJR 143:165, 1984.

Lev-Toaff AS, Karasick D, Rao VM: "Drooping shoulder"—nontraumatic causes of glenohumeral subluxation. Skel Radiol 12:34, 1984.

Major P, Resnick D, Greenway G: Heterotopic ossification in paraplegia: A possible disturbance of the paravertebral venous plexus. Radiology 136:797, 1980.

McIvor WC, Samilson RL: Fractures in patients with cerebral palsy. J Bone Joint Surg [Am] 44:858, 1966.

Middleton WD, Kneeland JB, Kellman GM, Cates JD, Sanger JR, Jesmanowicz A, Froncisz W, Hyde JS: MR imaging of the carpal tunnel: Normal anatomy and preliminary findings in the carpal tunnel syndrome. AJR 148:307, 1987.

Muheim G, Donath A, Rossier AB: Serial scintigrams in the course of ectopic bone formation in paraplegic patients. AJR 118:865, 1973.

Nakano KK: Entrapment neuropathies. In WN Kelley, ED Harris Jr, S Raddy, CB Sledge (Eds): Textbook of Rheumatology. 2nd Ed. Philadelphia, WB Saunders Co, 1985, p 1754.

Pech P, Haughton V: A correlative CT and anatomic study of the sciatic nerve. AJR 144:1037, 1985.

Pool WH Jr: Cartilage atrophy. Radiology 112:47, 1974.

Richardson ML, Helms CA, Vogler JB III, Genant HK: Skeletal changes in neuromuscular disorders mimicking juvenile rheumatoid arthritis and hemophilia. AJR 143:893, 1984.

Rosin AJ: Ectopic calcifications around joints of paralysed limbs in hemiplegia, diffuse brain damage, and other neurological diseases. Ann Rheum Dis 34:499, 1975.

Sauser DD, Hewes RC, Root L: Hip changes in spastic cerebral palsy. AJR 146:1219, 1986.

Schwentker EP, Gibson DA: The orthopaedic aspects of spinal muscular atrophy. J Bone Joint Surg [Am] 58:32, 1976.

Seigel RS: Heterotopic ossification in paraplegia. Radiology 137:259, 1980.

Seybold ME, Sherman DC: Muscle diseases. In JH Stein (Ed): Internal Medicine. Boston, Little, Brown, 1983, p 874.

Termote J-L, Baert A, Crolla D, Palmers Y, Bulcke JA: Computed tomography of the normal and pathologic muscle system. Radiology 137:439, 1980.

Thomas PK: Inherited neuropathies. Mayo Clin Proc 58:476, 1983.

Woodlief RM: Superior marginal rib defects in traumatic quadriplegia. Radiology 126:673, 1978.

Chapter 69

Neuroarthropathy

Donald Resnick, M.D.

The effect of the deprivation of sensory feedback on the musculoskeletal system can be profound. The anesthetized joint that is subject to continuing stress deteriorates progressively, leading to specific radiographic abnormalities. These changes, which include joint space narrowing, bone eburnation, osteophytosis, fragmentation, fracture, and subluxation, can accompany a variety of disorders but are most common in tabes dorsalis, diabetes mellitus, and syringomyelia. When severe, the resulting radiographic picture is diagnostic, although in earlier stages the findings may resemble those of osteoarthritis, calcium pyrophosphate dihydrate crystal deposition disease, calcium hydroxyapatite crystal deposition disease, osteonecrosis, or, in the spine, intervertebral (osteo)chondrosis.

In 1868, Charcot described an apparent cause-and-effect relationship between primary lesions of the central nervous system and certain arthropathies. Although his description was virtually confined to patients with tabes dorsalis, the name "Charcot joint" has become synonymous with all articular abnormalities related to neurologic deficits, regardless of the nature of the primary disease. Other terms applied to this articular disorder are neuroarthropathy and neurotrophic and neuropathic joint disease.

ETIOLOGY AND PATHOGENESIS

Central (upper motor neuron) and peripheral (lower motor neuron) lesions can lead to neuroarthropathy. Central lesions that may produce neuroarthropathy include syphilis, syringomyelia, meningomyelocele, trauma, multiple sclerosis, Charcot-Marie-Tooth disease, congenital vascular anomalies, and other causes of cord compression, injury, or degeneration. Peripheral causes include diabetes mellitus, alcoholism, amyloidosis, infection (tuberculosis, yaws, leprosy), pernicious anemia, trauma, and intraarticular or systemic administration of corticosteroids. Additionally, specific syndromes leading to congenital insensitivity to pain and dysautonomia produce similar alterations.

There is no uniform agreement on the pathogenesis of the articular changes. Two fundamental theories of pathogenesis initially arose. The "French theory" held that joint changes were the result of damage to the central nervous system trophic centers, which controlled nutrition of the bones and the joints, leading to atrophy of osseous and articular structures. The "German theory" proposed that unusual mechanical stresses about a weight-bearing joint in an ataxic individual led to recurrent subclinical trauma. Although additional theories exist, the current consensus supports the prominent role of abuse of insensitive joints in this arthropathy (Fig. 69–1). Loss of the protective sensations of pain and proprioception leads to relaxation of the supporting structures and chronic instability of the joint. Cumulative injury leads to progressive disorganization of the articulation. The radiographic and pathologic features reflect the joint disorganization. Productive changes commonly are associated with central spinal cord lesions and with diseases that often spare the sympathetic nervous system, such as tabes dorsalis and syringomyelia; destructive manifestations typically are linked to peripheral nerve injuries and related to trauma, alcoholism, and diabetes, which presumably affect postganglionic nerve segments carrying sympathetic vasoconstrictive as well as sensory and motor fibers.

The existence in neuroarthropathy of a neurally mediated vascular reflex leading to increased bone resorption in hyperemic areas that are devoid of vasoconstrictive impulses has been emphasized by some investigators. Proponents of this neurovascular cause indicate that osteoclastic resorption due to hyperemia could explain all of the radiographic changes of this joint disease. This mechanism is supported by angiographic and histologic evidence of hypervascularity of bone as well as radiologic evidence of nontraumatic osteolysis and fracture at involved sites.

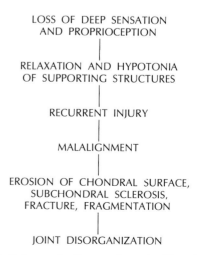

LOSS OF DEEP SENSATION
AND PROPRIOCEPTION

|

RELAXATION AND HYPOTONIA
OF SUPPORTING STRUCTURES

|

RECURRENT INJURY

|

MALALIGNMENT

|

EROSION OF CHONDRAL SURFACE,
SUBCHONDRAL SCLEROSIS,
FRACTURE, FRAGMENTATION

|

JOINT DISORGANIZATION

Figure 69–1. Pathogenesis of neuroarthropathy. The probable sequential steps in the development of the joint disease are indicated.

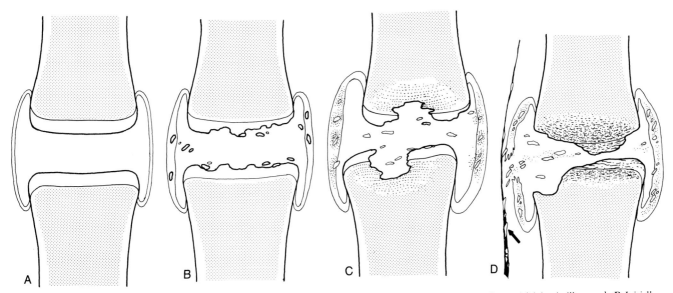

Figure 69–2. General radiographic and pathologic abnormalities: Stages of neuroarthropathy. **A** A normal synovial joint is illustrated. **B** Initially, cartilaginous fibrillation and fragmentation can be observed; some of the cartilaginous debris remains attached to the chondral surface, some is displaced into the articular cavity, and some becomes embedded in the synovial membrane. **C** Subsequently, osseous and cartilaginous destruction becomes more extensive, the embedded pieces of cartilage and bone producing local synovial irritation. Bone eburnation and subluxation are also evident. **D** Eventually, large portions of the chondral coat are lost, sclerosis is extreme, capsular rupture can occur, and shards of bone can dissect along the soft tissue planes (arrow).

GENERAL RADIOGRAPHIC AND PATHOLOGIC ABNORMALITIES

Early features of neuroarthropathy may simulate those of osteoarthritis (Fig. 69–2). Thus, cartilage loss and bone production are evident. The presence of an enlarging effusion, subluxation, fracture, and fragmentation should alert the radiologist to the possibility of neuroarthropathy; similarly, the finding of cartilaginous and osseous debris within the synovial membrane (detritic synovitis) should suggest to a pathologist that the changes may indeed represent neuropathic joint disease (Table 69–1). These early changes may show rapid progression (Fig. 69–3); indeed, acute subluxations or dislocations may be encountered.

In more advanced disease, depression, absorption, and shattering of subchondral bone, significant sclerosis and osteophytosis, intraarticular osseous fragments, subluxation, massive soft tissue enlargement and effusion, and fracture of neighboring bones become evident (Fig. 69–4). Pathologically, the capsule is thickened, and the synovial membrane is indurated and contains fragments of cartilage and bone. Embedded and metaplastic osteocartilaginous bodies in the synovium produce radiographically detectable calcific lesions, which may eventually become far removed from the joint itself (Fig. 69–5). Malalignment, angular deformity, subluxation or dislocation, and gross fractures may be observed (Fig. 69–6). In some patients, pseudarthrosis develops at sites of fracture or, after healing, refracture occurs.

In long-standing neuroarthropathy, the resulting sclerosis, osteophytosis, and fragmentation are greater than in any other process. Yet, the irregular articular surfaces in neuroarthropathy generally are well defined and sharp. Poorly marginated bone contours, as occur in septic arthritis, are not evident unless infection has become superimposed on the neuropathic process, a complication that is not infrequent, especially in diabetic patients and in those joints that are superficially located (e.g., metatarsophalangeal joints). Intraarticular bone fusion is an uncommon manifestation of neuroarthropathy at any site, with the exception of the spine.

SPECIFIC DISORDERS

It is now known that neuroarthropathy can accompany many disorders that lead to sensory disturbances. Although some motor function is fundamental in the pathogenesis of the articular lesions, patients with both sensory and motor loss can develop neuroarthropathy, presumably related to vigorous physical therapy.

Although the radiographic and pathologic features of neuroarthropathy generally are similar in these various disorders, certain subtle differences can be evident. Furthermore, the distribution of the articular abnormalities varies among these disorders (Table 69–2).

Tabes Dorsalis

It is estimated that 5 to 10 per cent of patients with tabes dorsalis will reveal neuroarthropathy. The joints of the lower extremity are affected in 60 to 75 per cent of cases. The knee, the hip, the ankle, the shoulder, and the elbow are altered, in descending order of frequency (Figs. 69–3, 69–4, 69–6, and 69–7). Other involved sites include the joints of the forefoot, midfoot, vertebral column, and fingers, and the temporomandibular and sternoclavicular joints. Monarticular

Table 69–1. SOME CAUSES OF DETRITIC SYNOVITIS

Neuroarthropathy
Osteonecrosis
Calcium pyrophosphate dihydrate crystal deposition disease
Psoriatic arthritis
Osteoarthritis
Osteolysis with detritic synovitis

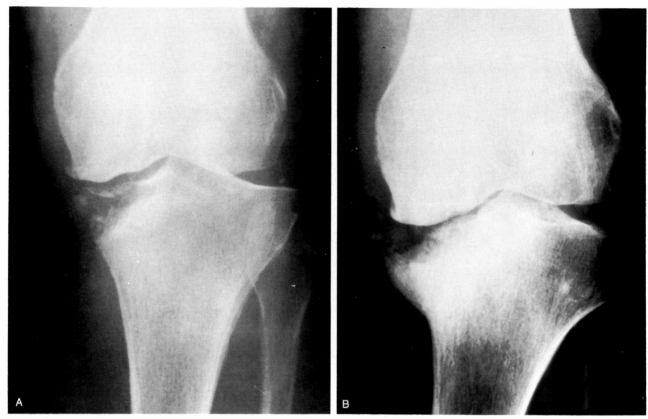

Figure 69–3. General radiographic and pathologic abnormalities of neuroarthropathy: Rapid progression of disease. The appearance and progression of articular destruction can occur rapidly. Initial foci of chondral and osseous destruction can lead to fragmentation and collapse in a period of weeks. This is a patient with tabes dorsalis.

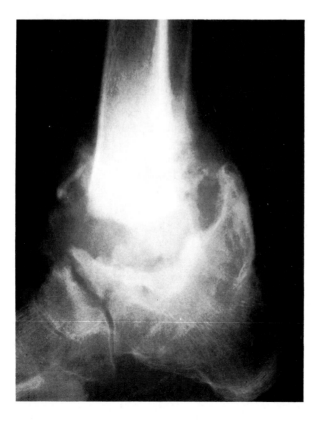

Figure 69–4. General radiographic and pathologic abnormalities of neuro-arthropathy: Advancing lesions. Note soft tissue swelling and considerable fragmentation and resorption of the talus, tibia, and fibula with extreme sclerosis, osteophytosis, and intraarticular osseous bodies.

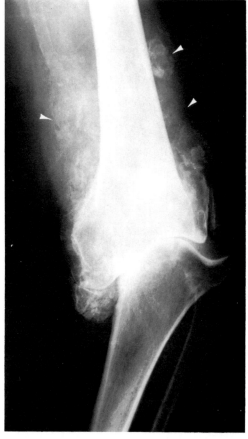

Figure 69–5. General radiographic and pathologic abnormalities of neuroarthropathy: **Migration of bone shards.** In this patient with syphilis, numerous fragments of bone originating from the destroyed articular surfaces have moved into the far recesses of the joint or migrated along adjacent tissue planes (arrowheads).

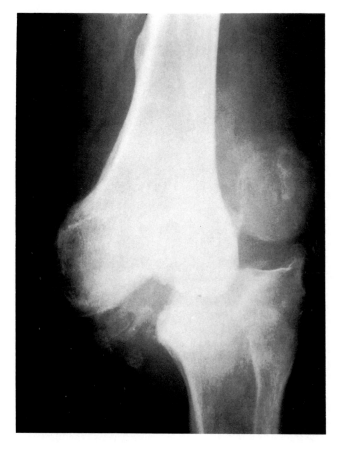

Figure 69–6. General radiographic and pathologic abnormalities of neuroarthropathy: **Fractures and subluxations.** Gross disorganization of the joint in a tabetic patient is characterized by lateral subluxation of the tibia on the femur, lateral patellar dislocation, soft tissue swelling, osseous fragmentation and sclerosis, and periostitis.

**Table 69–2. COMMON SITES OF INVOLVEMENT
IN NEUROARTHROPATHY**

Disease	Sites of Involvement
Tabes dorsalis	Knee, hip, ankle, spine
Syringomyelia	Glenohumeral joint, elbow, wrist, spine
Diabetes mellitus	Metatarsophalangeal, tarsometatarsal, intertarsal joints
Alcoholism	Metatarsophalangeal, interphalangeal joints
Amyloidosis	Knee, ankle
Meningomyelocele	Ankle, intertarsal joints
Congenital sensory neuropathy, hereditary sensory radicular neuropathy	Knee, ankle, intertarsal, metatarsophalangeal, interphalangeal joints
Idiopathic	Elbow

involvement predominates but polyarticular alterations are not unusual.

Most typically, painless swelling, deformity, and instability are evident. Affected joints may indeed be painful, however. The radiographs reveal typical features of neuroarthropathy, including exuberant eburnation and fragmentation. Scintigraphy accomplished with bone-seeking radiopharmaceutical agents shows areas of increased accumulation of the radionuclide. Abnormalities in certain laboratory parameters, such as the *Treponema pallidum* immobilization (TPI) test, the fluorescent treponemal antibody absorption (FTA-ABS) test, the Venereal Disease Research Laboroatory (VDRL) test, and the Automated Reagin Test (ART) provide important diagnostic clues.

Axial neuroarthropathy is not uncommon in tabes. It is seen most frequently in the lumbar spine, less commonly in the thoracic spine, and rarely in the cervical spine. One or more vertebrae can be affected. Axial neuroarthropathy often is symptomatic. Clinical signs include abnormal spinal curvature (kyphosis or scoliosis) and motor and sensory disturbances. Rarely, paraplegia is evident.

Radiographic features of tabetic axial neuroarthropathy may be productive or destructive in nature. The productive alterations of neuroarthropathy generally are more exaggerated than those of degenerative joint disease; eburnation may be florid, intervertebral disc space narrowing may be complete, osteophytes can be huge, and apophyseal joint subluxation with neighboring bone sclerosis can be profound (Fig. 69–8). Fracture and malalignment can also be evident. The resulting radiographic findings are unique to this disorder (Table 69–3).

Less commonly, destructive changes predominate in axial neuroarthropathy. These can appear acutely and progress rapidly. The appearance of this lytic variety of neuroarthropathy can resemble that in infection or skeletal metastasis.

Syringomyelia

It has been estimated that 20 to 25 per cent of patients with syringomyelia develop neuroarthropathy. Neuroarthropathy in syringomyelia is common in the joints of the upper extremity (Fig. 69–9). Less frequently, changes appear in the joints of the lower extremity, the spine (especially the cervical region), or, rarely, elsewhere, such as the sternoclavicular joint. Bilateral symmetric changes are not so common as in tabes. Generally, neuroarthropathy occurs during the later phases of syringomyelia, although occasionally joint findings may be the initial manifestation of the disease.

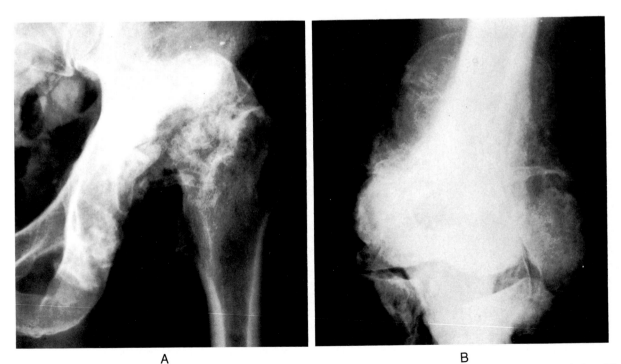

A   B

Figure 69–7. Tabes dorsalis: Neuroarthropathy of the appendicular skeleton. Examples of neuropathic joint disease of the hip (**A**) and elbow (**B**) are shown. Sclerosis and fragmentation are prominent, and dislocation of the hip is evident.

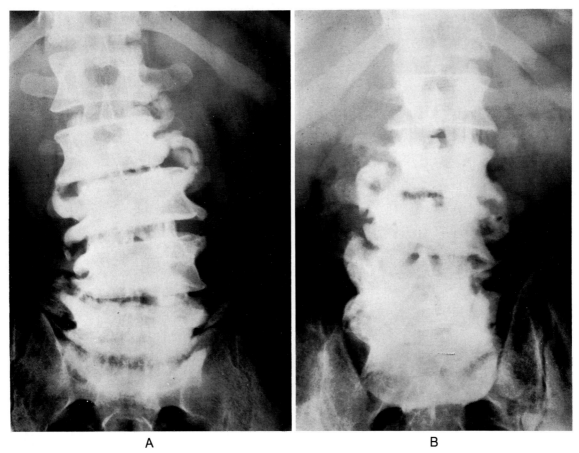

Figure 69–8. Tabes dorsalis: Neuroarthropathy of the axial skeleton. Two examples of widespread abnormalities in the lumbar spine consisting of loss of height of multiple intervertebral discs, extreme sclerosis, osteophytes, subluxation, and vertebral angulation are shown.

Table 69–3. AXIAL NEUROARTHROPATHY AND ITS DIFFERENTIAL DIAGNOSIS

	Neuroarthropathy	Intervertebral (Osteo)Chondrosis	Infection	CPPD Crystal Deposition Disease[1]
Sites of involvement	One or more levels Predominates in thoracolumbar spine[2]	Frequently widespread Cervical, thoracic, or lumbar spine	Frequently one level Predominates in thoracolumbar spine	Widespread Cervical, thoracic, or lumbar spine
Intervertebral disc spaces	Narrowed or obliterated	Narrowed	Narrowed or obliterated	Calcification; narrowed
Bone sclerosis	May be extreme	Usually mild to moderate	Variable[3]	Variable[5]
Osteophytosis	May be massive	Absent or moderate in size	Usually absent	Variable
Bone fragmentation	May be extreme	Absent or minimal	Usually absent	Variable[6]
Subluxation, angulation	Common	Rare	Variable[4]	Variable
Paravertebral mass	Usually absent	Absent	Common	Absent

[1]CPPD, Calcium pyrophosphate dihydrate.
[2]Influenced by the specific underlying disorder.
[3]Sclerosis is more typical in pyogenic spondylitis and in black patients with tuberculous spondylitis.
[4]In tuberculosis, kyphosis may become prominent.
[5]Discal calcification may appear without sclerosis, or disc space loss may be combined with moderate or severe sclerosis.
[6]In some patients, fragmentation and deformity may be severe, especially in the cervical spine.

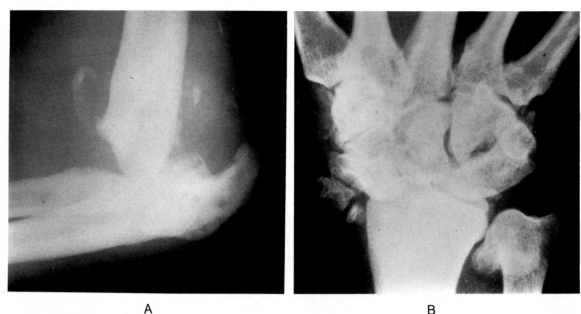

A

B

Figure 69–9. Syringomyelia. A The classic features of neuroarthropathy consist of soft tissue swelling, subluxation of the radius and ulna with relation to the humerus, extensive osseous resorption and fragmentation, sclerosis, and adjacent bone debris. **B** Note the resorption, flattening, and sclerosis of the distal portions of the radius and ulna, fragmentation, and carpal malalignment.

The clinical, radiographic, and pathologic alterations of neuroarthropathy in syringomyelia are similar to those in tabes.

Diabetes Mellitus

Countless descriptions of "neuropathic," "neuroarthropathic," "osteoarthropathic," "osteopathic," "neurogenic," and "atrophic" articular changes in this disease have appeared, and the wide variation of terms applied to the alterations reflects a continuing debate as to their pathogenesis. Loss of pain and loss of proprioceptive sensation appear to be of major importance in diabetic neuroarthropathy. The role of ischemia also may be important, although adequate blood supply is a prerequisite for the occurrence of osteolysis. Infectious processes commonly are superimposed on neuropathic changes in the diabetic patient.

Diabetes mellitus has overtaken both syphilis and syringomyelia as the leading cause of neuroarthropathy. Typically, diabetic neuroarthropathy appears in a middle-aged man or woman with long-standing diabetes mellitus. Changes in younger and older patients, however, can occur. The joints of the forefoot and midfoot are altered most commonly, although the ankle, the knee, the spine, and the joints of the upper extremity, in descending order of frequency, can be affected. Mono- or polyarticular involvement can occur.

Destructive or resorptive bone abnormalities can predominate, depending on the location of the neuroarthropathy. In the intertarsal or tarsometatarsal joints, osseous fragmentation, sclerosis, and subluxation or dislocation can be prominent (Fig. 69–10). Talar disruption and dorsolateral displacement of the metatarsals in relation to the cuneiforms and cuboid bone are characteristic, and the resulting radiographic picture may resemble that observed in an acute Lisfranc's fracture-dislocation (Fig. 69–11). At the metatarsophalangeal joints, osseous resorption is frequent, leading to partial or complete disappearance of the metatarsal heads and proximal phalanges with tapering or "pencil-pointing" of phalangeal and metatarsal shafts (Fig. 69–12). Flattening and fragmen-

tation of the metatarsal heads are particularly characteristic (Fig. 69–13). Progressive resorption of the phalanges and dorsiflexion and foreshortening of the toes may appear. Concomitant ulceration of soft tissues leads to osteomyelitis or septic arthritis.

Changes in the joints of the upper extremities are infrequent. Although fragmentation may be less prominent about the joints of the upper limbs, patients with severe bone fracture, eburnation, and dissolution are seen occasionally.

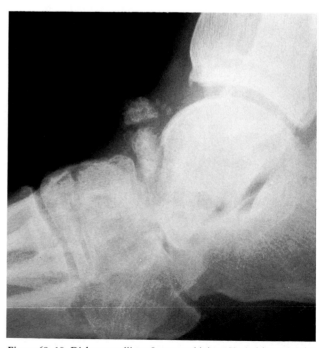

Figure 69–10. Diabetes mellitus: Intertarsal joints. Typical fragmentation and sharply defined osseous debris characterize the involvement of the dorsal aspect of the talus and the entire navicular bone in this patient without signs of infection.

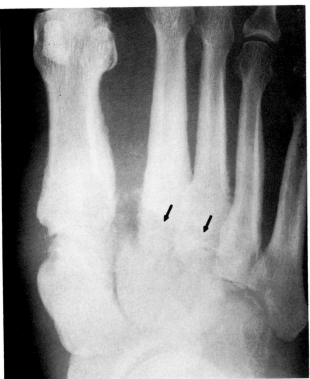

Figure 69–11. Diabetes mellitus: Tarsometatarsal joints. Note the lateral displacement of the bases of the metatarsals (arrows) with respect to the tarsals. This finding, combined with soft tissue swelling and fragmentation, resembles a Lisfranc's fracture-dislocation.

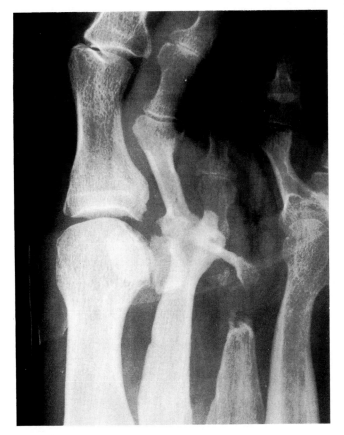

Figure 69–12. Diabetes mellitus: Metatarsophalangeal and interphalangeal joints. Neuroarthropathy and infection in the forefoot of a diabetic patient can combine to produce bizarre abnormalities consisting of osteolysis of distal metatarsals and proximal phalanges, with tapering of the osseous contours.

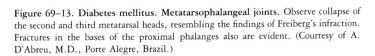
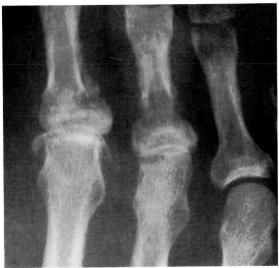

Figure 69–13. Diabetes mellitus. Metatarsophalangeal joints. Observe collapse of the second and third metatarsal heads, resembling the findings of Freiberg's infraction. Fractures in the bases of the proximal phalanges also are evident. (Courtesy of A. D'Abreu, M.D., Porte Alegre, Brazil.)

Diabetic axial neuroarthropathy may be generalized or localized in distribution. The resulting radiographic changes, which include destruction of vertebral bodies, sclerosis, osteophytosis, fragmentation, bone ankylosis, and spinal angulation, resemble those in tabes or syringomyelia (Fig. 69–14).

The pathologic aberrations accompanying neuroarthropathy in the diabetic patient are not significantly different from those in other neurologic disorders.

Alcoholism

Although peripheral neuropathy may be evident in as many as 30 per cent of alcoholic patients who are examined at a hospital, reports of neuroarthropathy in these persons are infrequent. When present, changes typically are evident in the feet and resemble those of diabetes mellitus.

Amyloidosis

Neuropathy, which is encountered in certain variants of amyloidosis, is not commonly associated with neuroarthropathy. Occasionally, patients with amyloidosis with or without additional plasma cell dyscrasias will develop neuropathic joint disease. The knee and the ankle appear to be the predominant sites of involvement.

Congenital Indifference to Pain

Indifference or insensitivity to pain is a feature common to several distinct hereditary sensory neuropathies that differ in their patterns of inheritance, precise clinical manifestations, and prognosis. In most of these syndromes, the neurologic deficit can be recognized in infancy or childhood. A decreased or absent reaction to pain, scars on the tongue or finger related to burns or infections, corneal opacities resulting from unnoticed foreign bodies, and self-mutilation with amputation of fingers and toes are encountered. Radiographic abnormalities include fractures of the metaphysis and diaphysis of long

bones, epiphyseal separations, neuroarthropathy, and soft tissue ulcerations. These changes are more frequent in the lower extremity than in the upper extremity (Fig. 69–15). Epiphyseal separations are the result of chronic trauma or stress; widening and irregularity of the growth plate, lysis and sclerosis of the metaphysis, periostitis and callus, and variable degrees of epiphyseal displacement are recognized. Neuroarthropathy is especially common in the ankle and tarsal areas.

It should be emphasized that overt neurologic symptoms and signs may be absent in children and adolescents with some types of congenital insensitivity to pain, although careful and detailed clinical examination often will detect subclinical sensory neuropathy. Therefore, the presence of unusual fractures and physeal abnormalities on radiographs should stimulate a search for subtle neurologic deficit. Virtually identical skeletal abnormalities are seen in all of the syndromes of congenital insensitivity to pain, such as familial dysautonomia or the Riley-Day syndrome, congenital sensory neuropathy with anhidrosis, congenital sensory neuropathy without anhidrosis, and hereditary sensory radicular neuropathy (acrodystrophic neuropathy).

Meningomyelocele (Spinal Dysraphism)

Skeletal abnormalities are detected in patients with various types of spinal dysraphism. Sensory impairment resulting from spina fibida and meningomyelocele is the most frequent underlying cause of neuropathic arthropathy in childhood, affecting principally the ankle and the tarsal joints. In active children, changes may appear in the first 3 years of life and are identical to those in the syndromes of congenital indifference to pain (Fig. 69–16). Coxa valga deformity is a common finding in neuromuscular disease, owing to muscular imbalance. In spinal dysraphism, however, coxa vara deformity develops as a sequel to disruption of the physis in the femoral neck.

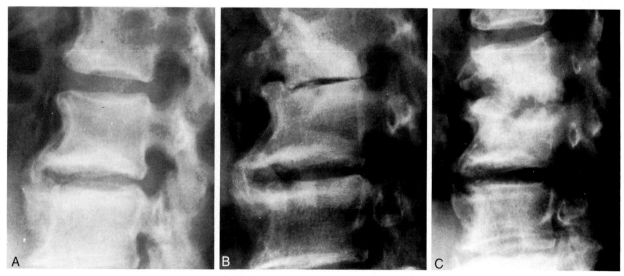

Figure 69–14. Diabetes mellitus: Spine. Progressive deterioration of the lumbar spine is apparent during a 3 year period of observation. Initially (**A**), the changes at the lower lumbar level resemble degenerative disc disease. Subsequently (**B, C**), this level deteriorates very slowly but, one level above, rapid destruction of the intervertebral disc and bone is evident. The vacuum phenomenon in the upper disc as well as the well-defined and sclerotic bone in **B** makes infection unlikely. In **C**, the pattern of discal destruction is identical to that of infection, although the latter was not apparent clinically. (Courtesy of U.S. Naval Hospital, San Diego, California.)

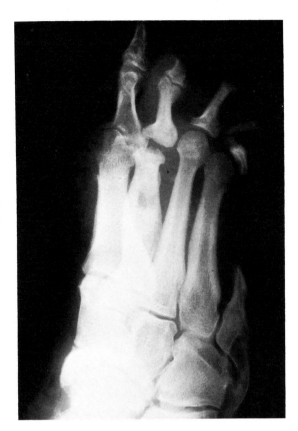

Figure 69–15. **Syndrome of congenital indifference to pain.** Observe the resorption and tapering of metatarsals and phalanges of the foot, with periostitis, sclerosis, and fragmentation. (Courtesy of M. Pallayew, M.D., Montreal, Quebec, Canada.)

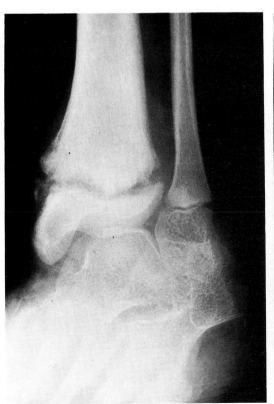

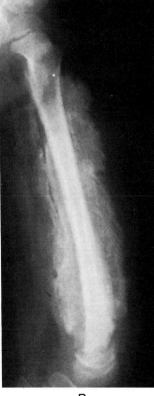

Figure 69–16. **Meningomyelocele (spinal dysraphism).** A Note an epiphyseal separation of the distal portion of the tibia, with a widened and irregular growth plate, sclerosis, and periostitis. B Lateral radiograph of the femur reveals an irregular and widened distal femoral growth plate, fracture and fragmentation, and exuberant periostitis. (Courtesy of J. E. L. Desautels, M.D., Calgary, Alberta, Canada.)

A   B

Other Diseases

Other causes of neuropathic skeletal alterations include spinal cord or peripheral nerve injury, myelopathy of pernicious anemia, Charcot-Marie-Tooth disease, arachnoiditis, intraspinal tumors, degenerative spinal disease, paraplegia, familial interstitial hypertrophic polyneuropathy of Dejerine and Sottas, leprosy, and yaws. An idiopathic variety of neuroarthropathy of the elbow has also been identified.

DIFFERENTIAL DIAGNOSIS

When severe, neuroarthropathy is associated with radiographic changes that are virtually pathognomonic. Bone eburnation, fracture, subluxation, and joint disorganization can be more profound in this disorder than in any other athropathy. In the joints of the appendicular skeleton, joint space loss, sclerosis, and fragmentation in early stages of neuroarthropathy, however, can resemble changes in osteoarthritis. Flattening and deformity of the articular surfaces, numerous intraarticular bodies, and increasing sclerosis and osteophytosis suggest the diagnosis of neuroarthropathy. In calcium pyrophosphate dihydrate crystal deposition disease, neuropathic-like changes can appear. The identification of articular and periarticular calcification; the involvement of specific areas of the joint, such as the radiocarpal compartment of the wrist and the patellofemoral compartment of the knee; and the variability of osteophyte formation are helpful clues to the accurate diagnosis of pyrophosphate arthropathy. Intraarticular deposition of calcium hydroxyapatite crystals may lead to progressive destruction of a joint, especially in the shoulder, with fracture and dissolution of bone. Bone fragmentation and collapse are also manifestations of osteonecrosis, posttraumatic osteoarthritis, intraarticular steroid arthropathy, neglected infection, and alkaptonuria.

In the joints of the axial skeleton, early findings of neuroarthropathy, such as intervertebral disc space narrowing and vertebral sclerosis, resemble those of intervertebral osteochondrosis, infection, or alkaptonuria. With the appearance of significant fragmentation, sclerosis, and osteophytosis, the diagnosis of axial neuropathic disease is not difficult (see Table 69–3).

Once the radiographic findings are interpreted as those of neuroarthropathy, the identification of the underlying disorder usually depends on the location of the changes. Tabes typically produces changes in the hip, the knee, the ankle, and the spine; diabetes mellitus leads to alterations in the midfoot and forefoot; syringomyelia affects the joints of the upper extremity and cervical spine; and the syndromes of congenital indifference to pain and meningomyelocele commonly localize in the joints of the lower extremity. The presence of metaphyseal and growth plate destruction in the immature skeleton is especially characteristic of congenital indifference to pain and meningomyelocele.

FURTHER READING

Bjorkengren AG, Weisman M, Pathria MN, Zlatkin MB, Pate D, Resnick D: Neuroarthropathy associated with chronic alcoholism. AJR 151:743, 1988.

Blanford AT, Keane SP, McCarty DJ, Albers JW: Idiopathic Charcot joint of the elbow. Arthritis Rheum 21:723, 1978.

Brower AC, Allman RM: Pathogenesis of the neurotrophic joint. Neurotraumatic versus neurovascular. Radiology 139:349, 1981.

Campbell WL, Feldman F: Bone and soft tissue abnormalities of the upper extremity in diabetes mellitus. AJR 124:7, 1975.

Citron ND, Paterson FWN, Jackson AM: Neuropathic osteonecrosis of the lateral femoral condyle in childhood. A report on four cases. J Bone Joint Surg [Br] 68:96, 1986.

Clouse ME, Gramm HF, Legg M, Flood T: Diabetic osteoarthropathy: Clinical and roentgenographic observations in 90 cases. AJR 121:22, 19794.

Eichenholtz SN: Charcot Joints. Springfield, Ill. Charles C Thomas, 1966.

El-Khoury GY, Kathol MH: Neuropathic fractures in patients with diabetes mellitus. Radiology 134:313, 1980.

Feldman F, Johnson AM, Walter JF: Acute axial neuroarthropathy. Radiology 111:1, 1974.

Forrester DM, Magre G: Migrating bone shards in dissecting Charcot joints. AJR 130:1133, 1978.

Giesecke SB, Dalinka MK, Kyle GC: Lisfranc's fracture-dislocation: A manifestation of peripheral neuropathy. AJR 131:139, 1978.

Goldman AB, Freiberger RH: Localized infectious and neuropathic diseases. Semin Roentgenol 14:19, 1979.

Gondos B: The pointed tubular bone. Its significance and pathogenesis. Radiology 105:541, 1972.

Hodgson J, Pugh D, Young H: Roentgenologic aspects of certain lesions of bone: Neurotropic or infectious? Radiology 50:65, 1948.

Katz I, Rabinowitz JG, Dziadiw R: Early changes in Charcot's joints. AJR 86:965, 1961.

Kirkpatrick RH, Riley CR: Roentgenographic findings in familial dysautonomia. Radiology 68:654, 1957.

Meyer GA, Stein J, Poppel MH: Rapid osseous changes in syringomyelia. Radiology 69:415, 1957.

Norman A, Robbins H, Milgram JE: The acute neuropathic arthropathy—a rapid severely disorganizing form of arthritis. Radiology 90:1159, 1968.

Pogonowska MJ, Collins LC, Dobson HL: Diabetic osteopathy. Radiology 89:265, 1971.

Schneider R, Goldman AB, Bohne WH: Neuropathic injuries to the lower extremities in children. Radiology 128:713, 1978.

Siegelman S, Heimann WG, Manin MC: Congenital indifference to pain. AJR 97:242, 1966.

Silverman FN, Gilden JJ: Congenital insensitivity to pain; a neurologic syndrome with bizarre skeletal lesions. Radiology 72:176, 1959.

SECTION XII

OSTEONECROSIS AND OSTEOCHONDROSIS

CASE XII   *LEVEL OF DIFFICULTY: 3*

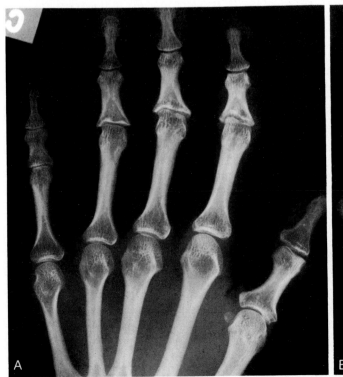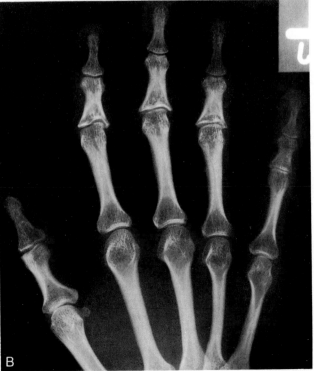

A 34 year old woman had painless swelling about the proximal interphalangeal joints of the hands and deformity of the fingers. She stated that the abnormalities began when she was a teenager. No other skeletal sites were affected.

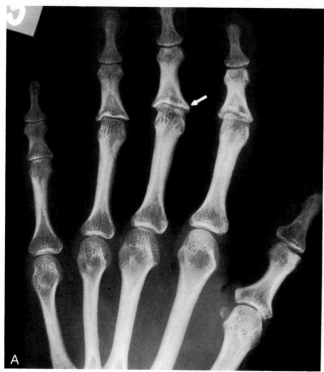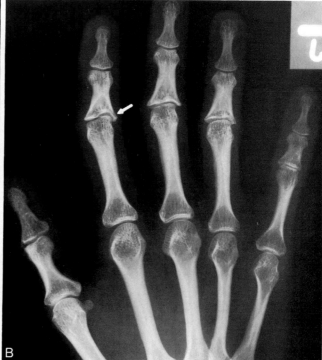

Posteroanterior radiographs of the hands (Case XII) reveal bilateral and relatively symmetric abnormalities affecting the proximal interphalangeal joints. The findings include periarticular soft tissue prominence, especially in the second, third, and fourth fingers in both hands, deformity of the bases of the middle phalanges, and shortening of the phalanges. Observe that the phalangeal bases are flattened and enlarged and, in some locations, adjacent osteophytes are evident (arrows). The proximal interphalangeal joints are slightly narrowed. Although osteoporosis is seen about many of the articulations of the hand, additional abnormalities in the distal interphalangeal and metacarpophalangeal joints are absent. The proximal phalanges in the thumb are minimally shortened, but the adjacent joints appear normal.

Several diagnostic possibilities could explain the abnormalities noted in Case XII. Certain types of juvenile chronic arthritis commonly involve the hands, and residual deformity and shortening of the fingers are potential complications of this disease. Typically, prominent joint abnormalities and more widespread involvement of the hand would be expected in juvenile chronic arthritis, and additional joints in the upper extremity and lower extremity, or both, and the spine usually are affected.

Infection or physical trauma can be accompanied by growth disturbance leading to deformity and shortening of the digits. Involvement of multiple interphalangeal joints of the hand in a bilateral and symmetric distribution would not be expected, however.

Thermal injury, especially frostbite, must be considered as a possible cause for the radiographic abnormalities illustrated in Case XII. Bone and joint manifestations of frostbite relate to either cellular necrosis or vascular insufficiency (or both) that accompanies the freezing process. In the hand, findings classically predominate in the four medial digits, with relative sparing of the thumb. Frostbite injury to the epiphysis in the immature skeleton can be followed by partial or complete osteolysis and, subsequently, by premature physeal fusion, leading to brachydactyly. Indeed, interphalangeal joint abnormalities may resemble those of osteoarthritis. Additional alterations, including osteolysis of the phalangeal tufts, may aid in the correct diagnosis of frostbite.

Although frostbite cannot be eliminated as a diagnostic choice, the most likely cause of these radiographic abnormalities is Thiemann's disease. This disorder generally begins in the second decade of life as painless swelling of the proximal interphalangeal joints of the hands and digital deformities. A familial history is evident in the majority of cases, and the pathogenesis of the disease is probably related to vascular insufficiency with osteonecrosis. The characteristic radiographic alterations include predilection for the middle digits of the hand and the proximal interphalangeal joints and, initially, epiphyseal sclerosis and fragmentation. Subsequently, premature physeal closure produces short and deformed middle phalanges. As in the test case, the phalangeal bases may be broad and irregular, and adjacent joint space loss may be evident.

Other types of congenital disorders, such as acrodysostoses, may produce radiographic abnormalities that are virtually identical to those of the test case.

FINAL DIAGNOSIS: Thiemann's disease.

FURTHER READING

Page 988 and the following:

1. Rubinstein HM: Thiemann's disease: A brief reminder. Arthritis Rheum 18:357, 1975.
2. Schantz K, Rasmussen F: Thiemann's finger or toe disease. Follow-up of seven cases. Acta Orthop Scand 57:91, 1986.

(Case XII, courtesy of B. Howard, M.D., Toronto, Ontario, Canada.)

Chapter 70

Osteonecrosis

Donald Resnick, M.D.
Gen Niwayama, M.D.
Donald E. Sweet, M.D.
John E. Madewell, M.D.

Osteonecrosis can accompany many diverse disease processes, such as trauma, hemoglobinopathy, exogenous or endogenous hypercortisolism, alcoholism, pancreatitis, dysbaric conditions, and Gaucher's disease. It may also become evident without any recognizable disease or event (primary or spontaneous osteonecrosis). Posttraumatic osteonecrosis is most frequent in the femoral and humeral heads, scaphoid, and talus. Dysbaric osteonecrosis can produce widespread skeletal alterations of epiphyseal, metaphyseal, or diaphyseal segments of tubular bones. Spontaneous osteonecrosis is recognized most commonly about the hip and the knee. Possible complications of bone necrosis are secondary degenerative joint disease, formation of intraarticular osseous and cartilaginous bodies, and cystic or sarcomatous transformation.

The causes of osteonecrosis are varied. Important etiologic factors include trauma, hemoglobinopathies, exogenous or endogenous hypercortisolism, renal transplantation, alcoholism or pancreatitis, dysbaric conditions, small vessel disease, Gaucher's disease, gout and hyperuricemia, irradiation, and synovitis with elevation of intraarticular pressure (infection, hemophilia) (Table 70–1). In some of these conditions, the exact pathogenesis of osteonecrosis has not been defined despite the accumulation of a great deal of clinical and experimental data. There is also a group of persons in whom no underlying causative disorder can be detected. In this situation, the term primary, idiopathic, or spontaneous osteonecrosis is used.

PRINCIPLES OF INFARCTION

Ischemic necrosis of bone, like infarction in other organ systems, results from a significant reduction in or obliteration of the affected area's blood supply. In each case of ischemic necrosis of bone, one or more of the following phenomena can usually be demonstrated or inferred as impeding blood flow: (1) intraluminal obstruction (e.g., thromboembolic disorders, sludging of blood cells, or stasis): (2) vascular compression (e.g., external mechanical pressure or vasospasm); or (3) physical disruption of the vessel (e.g., trauma).

Cell death from "anoxia" is not immediate, but rather occurs through progressive stages of ischemic injury: Stage 1, interruption of intracellular enzyme systems; stage 2, alteration or cessation of intracellular metabolic activity at a chemical level; stage 3, disruption or dissolution of intracellular nuclear and cytoplasmic ultrastructure. Dissolution of intracellular structural integrity is irreversible and results in cell death.

The production of ischemic injury or necrosis and the rapidity with which cell death occurs depend on the sensitivity of the individual cell type as well as the degree and duration of anoxia. The sensitivity of the cellular elements of bone and marrow to anoxia varies. It is generally acknowledged that the hematopoietic elements are the first to undergo anoxic death (in from 6 to 12 hours), followed by bone cells (osteocytes, osteoclasts, and osteoblasts) (in 12 to 48 hours) and, subsequently, marrow fat cells (48 hours to 5 days). The variation in cell sensitivity of the different cellular constituents of bone and the marrow cavity makes it possible for temporary anoxia to result in the death of hematopoietic elements without necessarily being sufficient to cause osteocytic or marrow fat cell death. Once ischemic marrow fat cell death occurs, the involved segment of bone and marrow can clearly be labeled infarcted.

Infarcts, including those in bone, are three-dimensional and can be subdivided into four zones: a central zone of cell death surrounded by successive zones of ischemic injury,

Table 70–1. SOME CAUSES OF OSTEONECROSIS

Trauma (fracture or dislocation)
Hemoglobinopathies (sickle cell anemia, sickle cell variant states)
Exogenous or endogenous hypercortisolism (corticosteroid medication, Cushing's disease)
Renal transplantation
Alcoholism
Pancreatitis
Dysbaric conditions (caisson disease)
Small vessel disease (collagen disorders)
Gaucher's disease
Gout and hyperuricemia
Irradiation
Synovitis with elevation of intraarticular pressure (infection, hemophilia)

active hyperemia, and finally normal tissue. The ischemic zone reflects a gradation of hypoxic injury ranging from severe cell damage immediately adjacent to the central zone of cell death to marginal cellular alterations adjacent to the hyperemic zone. Bone infarcts occurring in the metadiaphyseal intramedullary cavity will have a central core of dead marrow and bone surrounded by zones of ischemically injured marrow and bone, active hyperemia, and viable marrow and bone. Those infarcts occurring within an epiphysis or small, round bone will demonstrate a similar three-dimensional pattern, except that one surface will almost always be covered by compact subchondral bone and articular cartilage. Articular cartilage receives the bulk of its nourishment from the synovial fluid, and its viability therefore usually is not significantly affected initially by the underlying osteonecrosis, except for the cartilage cells below the tidemark, which may die. Because the osteonecrotic segment is by definition avascular, repair begins along its outer perimeter at the junction between the ischemic zone surrounding the dead area and the viable area with an intact circulation (the hyperemic zone). This reparative response results in the progressive development of a reactive margin (interface) between the dead zone and adjacent viable tissues.

Bone structure is initially unaltered as a direct result of osteocyte death or osteonecrosis. The x-ray absorbing quality of bone (density) is based on attenuation of the x-ray beam by the total amount of bone matrix and mineral content (especially calcium), not on cellular viability. Therefore, any alteration in bone density—either a real increase or a decrease in radiographic density—is an indication of viability requiring osteoblastic or osteoclastic cell activity, respectively, and will be initially perceived in the viable bone and marrow surrounding the osteonecrotic segment.

MARROW CAVITY

The medullary cavity is an admixture of cancellous bone, hematopoietic marrow, fatty marrow, and sinusoidal vascular bed confined by a nonexpandable shell of cortical bone. Radiographic observations indicate that ischemic necrosis of bone is most commonly encountered within the epiphyseal (especially the femoral and humeral heads) and metadiaphyseal marrow cavities of adult long tubular bones. Occasional involvement of the distal femoral condyles, of the small, round bones of the wrist and ankle, and of other sites is seen.

The extensive arterial supply to adult long tubular bones includes the nutrient artery with its ascending and descending diaphyseal branches, the penetrating metaphyseal and epiphyseal (retinacular) arteries, and the superficial periosteal vessels and the diffuse intramedullary sinusoidal vascular bed; these vessels provide excellent collateral circulation. Venous outflow is also extensive, as evidenced by numerous perforating channels exiting from the cortex.

Despite the extensive circulation available to the metadiaphyseal cortex and intramedullary cavity, the epiphyseal ends of long bones have limited arterial access and venous outflow because much of their surface is covered by articular cartilage. Arterial access to the epiphysis is further compromised in the growing skeleton, in which the epiphysis is separated from the metaphysis by the growth plate. Although occasional small arterioles penetrate the physeal growth plate (physis), little or no significant collateral circulation exists between a developing epiphysis and its adjacent metaphysis. In the absence of collateral circulation, the likelihood that a single or dominant artery will supply an entire epiphysis or a significant segment of an epiphysis is increased. The small carpal and tarsal bones are also covered to a great extent by articular cartilage. In many respects, their ossification centers are analogous to the developing epiphyses of a long bone with regard to blood supply. Compromise of a dominant artery supplying a developing epiphysis or small round bone ossification center is a possible mechanism for Legg-Calvé-Perthes disease (femoral head), Köhler's disease (tarsal navicular), and Kienböck's disease (lunate bone).

The relative amounts and localization of hematopoietic or fatty marrow depend primarily on hematopoietic demand. The marrow cavities of all bones in the newborn infant and young child are actively engaged in hematopoiesis. As the total marrow volume increases with skeletal growth, normal hematopoietic demand can eventually be satisfied by the marrow capacity of the axial skeleton. Therefore, the marrow cavities of the adolescent and adult appendicular skeleton normally contain predominantly fatty marrow, unless some special circumstance requires increased hematopoiesis. Both radiographic and anatomic observations indicate that ischemic necrosis of bone occurs almost invariably within areas of predominantly fatty marrow. The converse is equally true; ischemic necrosis in areas of normal active hematopoiesis is distinctly unusual except in sickle cell disease and related hemoglobinopathies or after complete traumatic disruption of the arterial blood supply. Ischemic necrosis of cortical bone is relatively rare and occurs only when there is extensive interruption of the arterial blood supply, as in osteomyelitis.

DIAGNOSTIC TECHNIQUES
Radiography

The plain film radiographic findings of osteonecrosis of an epiphysis, metaphysis, or diaphysis in a tubular bone or of a flat or irregular bone are characteristic. Arc-like subchondral radiolucent lesions, patchy lucent areas and sclerosis, osseous collapse, and preservation of the joint space in an epiphyseal region (Fig. 70–1); lucent shadows with a peripheral rim of sclerosis and periostitis in a diametaphyseal region (Fig. 70–2); and patchy lucent areas and sclerosis with bone collapse in a flat or irregular bone (Fig. 70–3) are typical radiographic signs of osteonecrosis. Unfortunately, these abnormalities do not appear for several months after the onset of clinical manifestations in many persons and, therefore, do not represent a sensitive indication of early disease (Fig. 70–4).

Radiographs obtained during the application of traction may accentuate the curvilinear radiolucent shadow that is evident in an osteonecrotic epiphysis, perhaps owing to the release of gas in the zone of subchondral separation with the induction of a vacuum by traction. The failure of intraarticular gas to be released during this procedure can indicate the presence of joint fluid.

Conventional Tomography

Conventional tomography is indicated occasionally for the accurate diagnosis of osteonecrosis. The technique may reveal angular or wedge-shaped lesional margins and subtle collapse of the osseous surface, allowing a precise diagnosis of bone necrosis (Fig. 70–5).

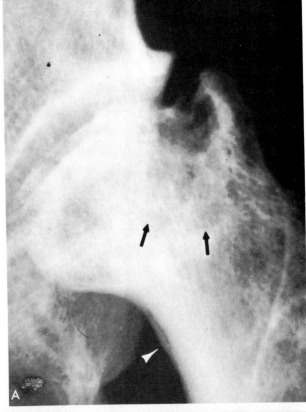

Figure 70–1. Osteonecrosis: Epiphysis—radiographic-pathologic correlation. A The preoperative radiograph outlines extensive collapse of the articular surface of the femoral head with cystic lucent areas (arrows), patchy sclerosis, buttressing (arrowhead), and preservation of joint space. **B, C** Sectional radiograph and photograph show displaced cartilage and subchondral bone plate (arrowheads), subjacent osseous resorption (solid arrows), reactive bone formation, and buttressing. Osteophytic lipping is observed (open arrows).

Illustration continued on following page

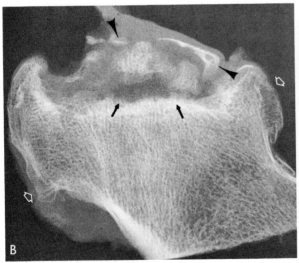

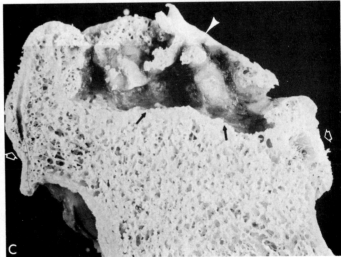

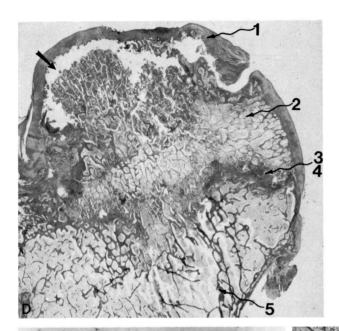

Figure 70–1 *Continued* **D** A photomicrograph (2 ×) shows a superficial zone of detached articular cartilage and subarticular trabeculae (1), with subjacent curvilinear area of bone separation (arrow) representing a fracture. Note also a large zone of bone necrosis (2), zones of vascular granulation tissue and new bone formation (3, 4), and deep zone of normal cancellous bone (5). **E** A photomicrograph (20 ×) reveals the superficial zone of detached viable articular cartilage and subarticular trabeculae (1), an area of bone separation or fracture (arrow), and a zone of bone necrosis (2). **F** In another area, fibrosis of the marrow space and neovascularization can be identified (20 ×). (**A-D**, From Resnick D, et al: Subchondral cysts (geodes) in arthritic disorders: Pathologic and radiographic appearance of the hip joint. AJR 128:799, 1977. Copyright 1977. American Roentgen Ray Society. Used with permission.)

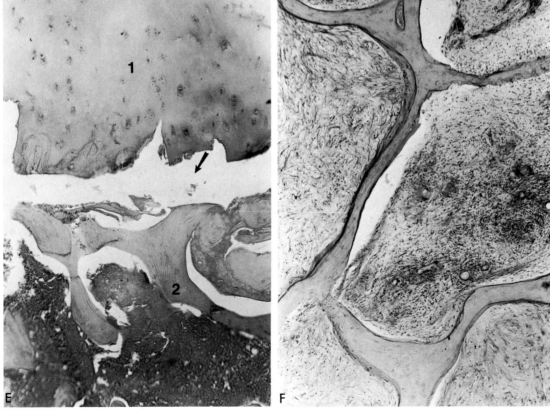

Figure 70–2. Osteonecrosis: Diametaphysis—radiographic-pathologic correlation. **A** A radiograph of the lower half of the left femur demonstrates a bone infarction. Observe the typical shell-like calcification of the lesion. **B** A photograph of the cut surface of the lower half of the left femur demonstrates necrotic spongy bone and marrow, which are walled off by calcified collagenous fibrous tissue, which varies in thickness from place to place and is serpentine in configuration. In some of the resultant locules, there are residual areas of necrotic spongiosa and fatty marrow. (From Jaffe HL: Ischemic necrosis of bone. Med Radiogr Photogr *45*:58, 1969. Used with permission.)

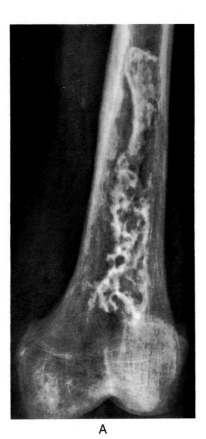

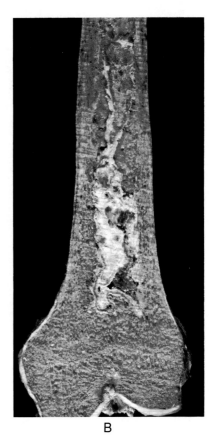

A

B

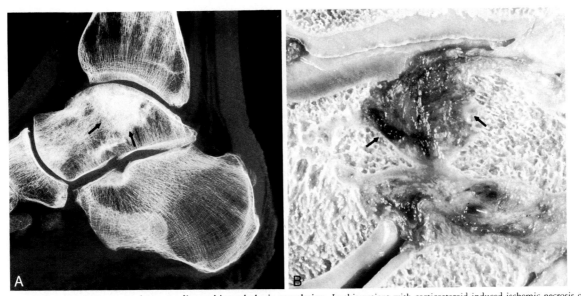

Figure 70–3. Osteonecrosis: Irregular bone—radiographic-pathologic correlation. In this patient with corticosteroid-induced ischemic necrosis of bone, observe the sclerotic zone in the talus (as well as the calcaneus), corresponding in position to an irregular hemorrhagic area of infarction (arrows).

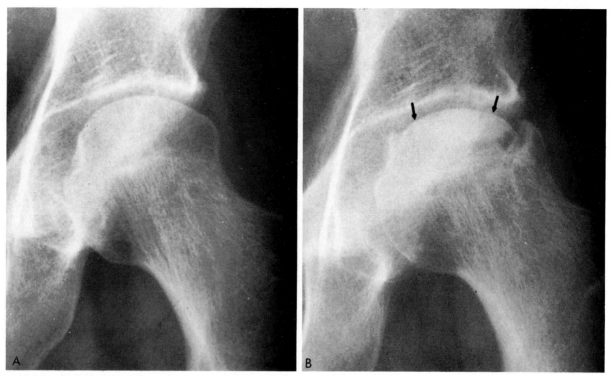

Figure 70–4. Osteonecrosis: Inadequacy of radiographic examination. This 35 year old man had had hip pain at the time of his initial radiographic examination, which progressed over the subsequent 6 to 9 months. **A** The initial radiograph was interpreted as normal. A bone scan was not accomplished. **B** Seven months later, significant collapse of the superolateral aspect of the femoral head is identified (arrows). The joint space is not narrowed.

Computed Tomography

The goals of computed tomographic evaluation of ischemic necrosis of bone (especially in the femoral head) are twofold: to allow early diagnosis of the condition; and to identify the

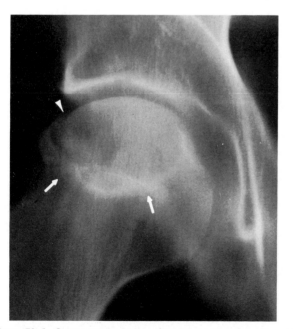

Figure 70–5. Osteonecrosis: Value of conventional tomography. Although the lesion of the femoral head resembles a bone neoplasm, such as a chondroblastoma, typical signs of ischemic necrosis are the curvilinear zone of bone sclerosis (arrows) and the subtle depression of the articular surface (arrowhead). (Courtesy of P. VanderStoep, M.D., Saint Cloud, Minnesota.)

presence and extent of bone collapse. Although the advantages of computed tomography over other methods in early diagnosis of ischemic necrosis are questionable, previous reports have demonstrated the application of computed tomography to the initial diagnosis of osteonecrosis in the femoral head. Subtle changes in the trabecular architecture are observed (Fig. 70–6). In patients with more advanced changes of osteonecrosis of the femoral head, transverse computed tomographic scans reveal centrally or peripherally located circular areas of decreased attenuation. At this stage, reformation of the computed tomographic data in a sagittal or coronal plane depicts subchondral fractures and collapse of the articular surface (Fig. 70–7). The latter finding has therapeutic significance, as the presence of bone collapse indicates a more advanced stage of the process (Table 70–2) and limits the number of orthopedic procedures (Table 70–3) that can be employed successfully.

Scintigraphy

Although intraosseous phlebography or pressure readings may reveal elevated intraosseous pressure in the initial stages of osteonecrosis (see later discussion), the radionuclide examination is considered one of the most effective techniques for early diagnosis of this disorder. Scintigraphy may be especially useful in studying the contralateral "silent" hip in cases of apparent unilateral osteonecrosis of the femoral head.

Immediately after interruption of the osseous blood supply, bone scans can reveal an area of decreased or absent uptake, a "cold" lesion (Fig. 70–8A). Only a few other processes, including infection, plasma cell myeloma, skeletal metastasis,

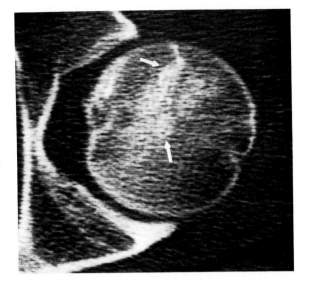

Figure 70–6. Osteonecrosis: Value of computed tomography—abnormal asterisk sign. Both early and later stages of ischemic necrosis are characterized by modifications (arrows) of the normal asterisk. The normal asterisk is an area of condensation of bone formed by the primary compressive group of trabeculae and a portion of the primary tensile group of trabeculae in the femoral head. In ischemic necrosis, the radiodense zone of crossing trabeculae reaches the articular surface of the femoral head.

and irradiation, lead to localized regions of diminished radiotracer uptake. After weeks or months, reparative processes in the surrounding bone are associated with revascularization and increased accumulation of the radioisotope, a "hot" lesion (Fig. 70–8B). At some point between these two stages, the radionuclide examination can be normal.

Bone marrow scans with ^{99m}Tc-sulfur colloid have also been used to evaluate osteonecrosis (Fig. 70–9). A decrease in osseous accumulation is suggestive of deficient circulation.

Magnetic Resonance Imaging

Magnetic resonance imaging represents the noninvasive technique of choice in the early diagnosis of this condition. Although the initial event after interruption of blood supply is death of the hematopoietic cells, the population of such cells is small compared with that of the fat cells, so that the first alteration detectable with magnetic resonance imaging appears to coincide with death of the latter cells (12 to 48 hours). A decrease in normal marrow signal intensity is characteristic and may be observed when bone scintigraphic findings are normal (Fig. 70–10). The finding is not specific, however, being evident also with other marrow replacing processes, including neoplasms and storage diseases. An additional abnormality seen with magnetic resonance imaging in patients with ischemic necrosis of the femoral head is an effusion.

Other Techniques

Measurement of the *pressure in the bone marrow* in the femoral head can be accomplished with a cannula placed in the intertrochanteric region; pressure values above 30 mm Hg are regarded as abnormal. *Oxygen saturation* of greater than 85 per cent in a specimen of blood removed through the cannula is indirect evidence of circulatory failure.

Intramedullary phlebography is accomplished by the injection of contrast material directly into the intertrochanteric region of the femur. The normal venogram is characterized by the absence of pain and the presence of rapid opacification of efferent vessels, without any diaphyseal reflux or stasis; in ischemic necrosis of the femoral head, a painful injection is followed by reflux in the diaphysis and intramedullary stasis for 15 minutes after the procedure.

To obtain a *core biopsy,* a hollow trephine is introduced into the femoral neck from an opening in the greater trochanter and advanced into the subchondral regions of the femoral head; a second channel is made with a smaller trephine in a different direction.

POSTTRAUMATIC OSTEONECROSIS

After a fracture, bone death of variable extent on either side of the fracture line is common. Necrosis of a large segment of bone occurring after fracture or dislocation,

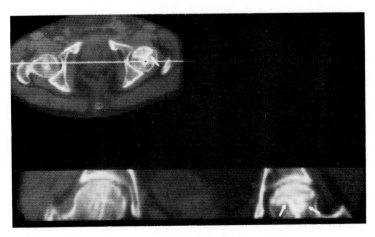

Figure 70–7. Osteonecrosis: Value of computed tomography—more advanced changes. A transaxial computed tomographic image (top) and a coronal reconstruction (bottom) illustrate a curvilinear zone of sclerosis (arrows) diagnostic of ischemic necrosis of the femoral head. No collapse of the articular surface is evident.

Table 70–2. STAGING OF ISCHEMIC NECROSIS OF THE FEMORAL HEAD

Stage	Findings
0	Suspected necrosis but no clinical findings and normal radiographs and bone scan
I	Clinical findings, normal radiographs, and abnormal bone scan
II	Osteopenia, cystic areas, and bone sclerosis on radiographs
III	Crescent sign and subchondral collapse without flattening of the femoral head on radiographs
IV	Flattening of the femoral head and normal joint space on radiographs
V	Joint space narrowing and acetabular abnormalities on radiographs

however, generally is restricted to those sites that possess a vulnerable blood supply, such as the femoral head, the body of the talus, the humeral head, and the carpal scaphoid. Additional characteristics common to each of these areas are an intraarticular location of necrotic bone and a limited attachment of soft tissue. The necrotic bone may appear radiodense as a result of compression of trabeculae, reaction accompanying the healing process, or lack of participation of the bone in the hyperemia and osteoporosis of neighboring viable bone.

Femoral Head

Osteonecrosis of the femoral head is a well-recognized complication of femoral neck fractures and dislocations. The principal blood supply to the adult femoral head is via the circumflex femoral branches of the profunda femoris artery (Fig. 70–11). A second supply of blood is derived from the vessels of the ligamentum teres, which enter the bone of the fovea capitis. A third (less important) vascular pathway is the nutrient artery supplying blood to the proximal femoral metaphysis. The superior (lateral) retinacular vessels represent the most important source of blood to the femoral head.

A fracture of the femoral neck that traverses the entry site of the superior retinacular vessels into the epiphysis can lead to osteonecrosis. This complication is more frequent in intracapsular fractures (subcapital, transcervical) than in extracapsular fractures (intertrochanteric) (Fig. 70–12). With intracapsular fractures, injury to the superior retinacular arteries is frequent. The frequency of necrosis may increase with displacement and an exaggerated valgus position at the site of fracture, with fractures that involve the superolateral portion of the femoral neck or head, in late reduction, and after use of hardware that is positioned near the fovea. The radiographic features may include increased density of the necrotic segment, osseous collapse, and fragmentation.

Scintigraphy has frequently been applied to the patient with a fracture of the femoral neck to assess the viability of the femoral head and to predict the likelihood of delayed collapse of the head. Although not uniformly successful, bone scintigraphy can identify decreased vascularity in the femoral head shortly after the injury, and such deficient vascular supply indicates a propensity for later osseous collapse.

Other traumatic causes of osteonecrosis of the femoral head include dislocation of the hip and slipped capital femoral epiphysis. Osteonecrosis has been reported in as many as 25 per cent of patients with dislocation, especially if it is complicated by fracture of the acetabulum, a delay in diagnosis and treatment, and early weight-bearing. After a slipped capital femoral epiphysis, a frequency rate of osteonecrosis of less than 5 per cent in patients with minimal displacements can rise to 40 per cent in patients with severe slips in whom aggressive orthopedic manipulations have been undertaken.

Osteonecrosis of the femoral head has also been recorded in as many as 68 per cent of patients after congenital dislocation of the hip. Extreme positions of abduction during immobilization may lead to obstruction of the nearby vascular structures or excessive mechanical pressure on the femoral head. Indeed, osteonecrosis may be observed in the normal hip after immobilization of both sides in cases of unilateral congenital dislocation of the hip.

Talus

Osteonecrosis of the talus is a recognized and disabling complication of various fractures and injuries. The talar blood supply is derived mainly from branches of the posterior tibial, peroneal, and dorsalis pedis arteries; the artery of the tarsal sinus and that of the tarsal canal are the two most important branches. Free anastomoses among the intraosseous vascular branches exist. Because of these anastomosing channels, a

Table 70–3. SOME SURGICAL METHODS OF TREATMENT OF ISCHEMIC NECROSIS OF THE FEMORAL HEAD

Method	Rationale
Drilling or forage	Multiple drill holes in the femoral head and neck to establish channels for revascularization
Core decompression	Coring device to create large and small channels from trochanteric region to femoral head, allowing decompression of elevated intraosseous pressure
Free bone grafts with cancellous or cortical bone	Placement of cortical bone (for mechanical support) or cancellous bone (for rapid incorporation) into channels in the femoral head and neck
Vascularized bone grafts with attached muscle pedicle	Same as last except living rather than dead bone is used
Osteochondral allograft	Replacement of collapsed portion of the articular surface with allograft
Osteotomy: Varus or valgus	Shift of femoral head in acetabulum to provide new weight-bearing area
Rotational	Rotation of femoral head in acetabulum to provide new weight-bearing area
Electrical stimulation	Use of electrical current to induce bone formation
Arthroplasty	Replacement of abnormal femoral head (and acetabulum) with prosthesis

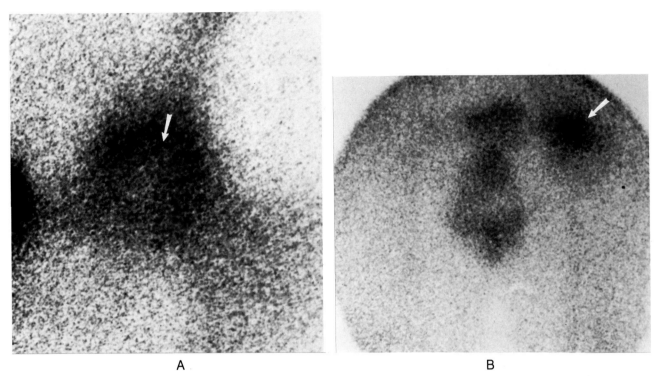

Figure 70–8. Osteonecrosis: Value of radionuclide examination—bone scan. A This scan of the hip using technetium pyrophosphate depicts a central area of diminished uptake surrounded by a zone of augmented activity (arrow). **B** In a different patient with osteonecrosis, the scan with technetium pyrophosphate demonstrates an area of increased uptake of isotope in the left hip (arrow). Note the activity in the bladder.

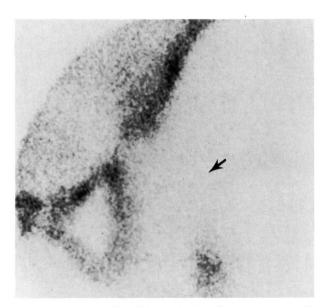

Figure 70–9. Osteonecrosis: Value of radionuclide examination—bone marrow scan. The sulfur colloid bone marrow scan reveals no uptake in the proximal portion of the femur (arrow), indicative of necrosis. (Courtesy of V. Vint, M.D., San Diego, California.)

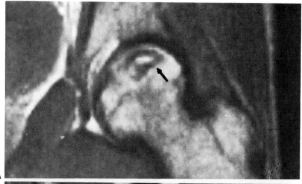

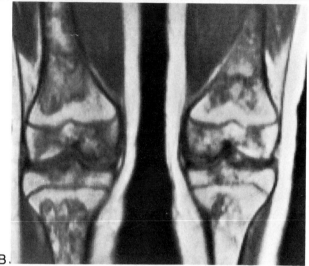

Figure 70–10. Osteonecrosis: Value of magnetic resonance imaging. A In this patient with sickle cell anemia, a peripheral region of decreased signal intensity and a central region of increased signal intensity (arrow) are noted on the coronal display. (Courtesy of L. Rogers, M.D., Chicago, Illinois.) B In a patient with systemic lupus erythematosus being treated wth corticosteroid preparations, observe bilateral areas of osteonecrosis in the diaphyses and epiphyses of the femora and tibiae. The abnormal regions are manifested as zones of decreased signal intensity. (Courtesy of L. Bassett, M.D., Los Angeles, California.)

severe soft tissue injury must occur for osteonecrosis to be initiated. The body of the talus is more prone to necrosis than the talar head and neck, and this complication is especially prevalent after fracture of the neck.

The radiographic diagnosis of osteonecrosis of the talus usually is delayed until osteoporosis of the surrounding viable bone creates a relatively increased density of the talar body. This finding can be apparent within 1 to 3 months after injury and may be combined with collapse of the articular surface (Fig. 70–13). The presence of a subchondral radiolucent band in the proximal portion of the talus, the Hawkins sign, represents bone resorption and can be a useful radiographic sign of an intact vascular supply.

Humeral Head

The blood supply of the head of the humerus is derived from three major sources: a branch of the anterior circumflex humeral artery, the arcuate artery, which enters the bone in the bicipital groove; branches of the posterior circumflex

humeral artery, which enter the base of the neck; and vessels in the rotator cuff, which enter at the tendinous insertion to the bone (Fig. 70–14). Osteonecrosis of the humeral head occurs if a fracture leads to loss of blood supply from both the muscular insertions and the arcuate branch of the anterior circumflex humeral artery; this may result after a displaced fracture of the anatomic neck or a severe fracture or fracture-dislocation of the bone. The radiographic findings parallel those in the femoral head (Fig. 70–15), although osseous collapse is less prominent in the humeral head.

Scaphoid

Osteonecrosis of the proximal pole of the carpal scaphoid is a well-documented complication after injury to this bone. Osteonecrosis is most likely to occur when a scaphoid fracture involves the proximal pole of the bone; with more distal infractions, the interruption of blood supply is less constant or severe. With rare exceptions, it is the proximal aspect of the bone that undergoes necrosis. The frequency of this complication following scaphoid injuries is approximately 10 to 15 per cent. The radiographic diagnosis depends on a relative increase in density of the devitalized portion of the scaphoid in comparison with the osteoporotic viable bone (Fig. 70–16), an appearance that is delayed for a period of 4 to 8 weeks and that may be associated with delayed union or nonunion of the fracture, collapse of the necrotic segment, and, eventually, secondary degenerative joint disease of the radiocarpal compartment of the wrist (Fig. 70–17). Bone scans may be useful shortly after the injury to identify decreased vascularity of the proximal pole of the scaphoid.

Capitate

Ischemic necrosis of the capitate occurs after accidental or occupational trauma or on an idiopathic basis. It is the proximal pole of the capitate that is the site of ischemic necrosis.

Osteonecrosis of this bone is a recognized complication of a transscaphoid, transcapitate, perilunate fracture-dislocation (scaphocapitate syndrome). This injury may be associated with 180 degree rotation of the proximal pole of the capitate. Delay in diagnosing the nature of the capitate injury increases the likelihood of subsequent ischemic necrosis as well as of osteoarthritis.

Vertebral Body

Posttraumatic collapse of vertebral bodies that is delayed for a period of weeks to years after an injury is termed Kümmell's disease. The vertebral collapse probably occurs owing to a vascular insult leading to secondary bone necrosis; the presence of an intraosseous vacuum phenomenon within the collapsed vertebral body is a finding that is consistent with ischemic necrosis.

Kümmell's disease is not uncommon. Affected patients generally are middle-aged or elderly men or women, and the lower thoracic and upper lumbar vertebral bodies are involved principally (Fig. 70–18).

Other Sites

Following significant injury or prolonged stress, ischemic necrosis can appear in the lunate, tarsal navicular, patella, glenoid region of the scapula, odontoid process of the axis, and even metatarsal and metacarpal heads.

Text continued on page 973

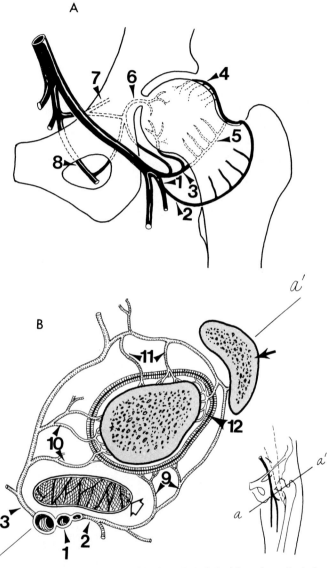

Figure 70–11. Femoral head: Vascular supply in adults. A The major blood supply is derived from the profunda femoris artery (1), from which arise the lateral (2) and the medial (3) circumflex arteries. (The medial and lateral circumflex arteries may arise from the femoral artery rather than the profunda femoris artery in some individuals.) As these latter vessels pass anterior and posterior to the femur to anastomose at the level of the trochanters, they send off small branches beneath the capsule of the hip joint. These branches, including the superior retinacular (lateral epiphyseal) arteries (4) and the inferior retinacular (inferior metaphyseal) arteries (5), raise the synovial membrane into folds or retinacula. A second supply of blood is derived from the vessels of the ligamentum teres. Here, the foveal (medial epiphyseal) arteries (6) can be noted. Additional regional vessels are the inferior gluteal artery (7) and the obturator artery (8). (After Graham J, Wood S: In JK Davidson: Aseptic Necrosis of Bone. New York, American Elsevier Publishing Co., 1976, p 101. Used with permission.) **B** A cross section of the proximal femur at the base of the neck better delineates the nature of the blood supply. The greater trochanter (arrow) and iliopsoas muscle (open arrow) are indicated. Note the profunda femoris artery (1) and the lateral (2) and medial (3) circumflex arteries. From the lateral circumflex arteries are derived the anterior ascending cervical arteries (9). From the medial circumflex artery are derived the medial (10), posterior (11), and lateral (12) ascending cervical arteries, which, in combination with the anterior ascending cervical arteries, form a subsynovial anastomotic ring on the surface of the femoral neck at the margin of the articular cartilage. The inset shows the plane of section (line a-a′). (After Chung SM: The arterial supply of the developing proximal end of the human femur. J Bone Joint Surg [Am] 58:961, 1976. Used with permission.)

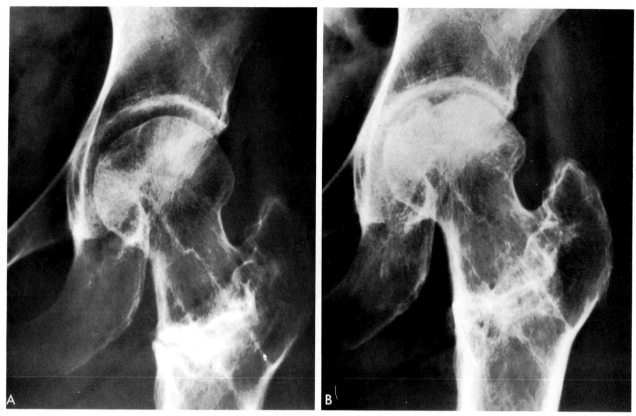

Figure 70–12. Posttraumatic osteonecrosis: Femoral head. Intertrochanteric fracture. Films obtained 2½ years apart reveal evidence of a previous intertrochanteric fracture treated with a Richards nail (that has been removed) and progressive osteonecrosis of the femoral head. This complication is less frequent in intertrochanteric fractures than in subcapital fractures.

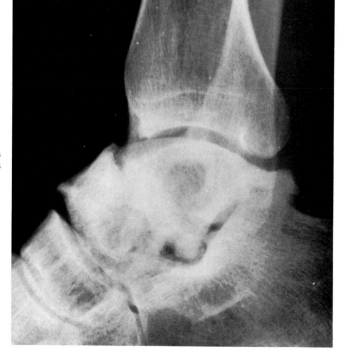

Figure 70–13. Posttraumatic osteonecrosis: Talus. In a person with a nonunion of a midtalar fracture, extensive necrosis is associated with sclerosis and cyst formation.

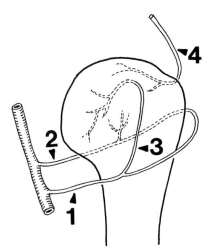

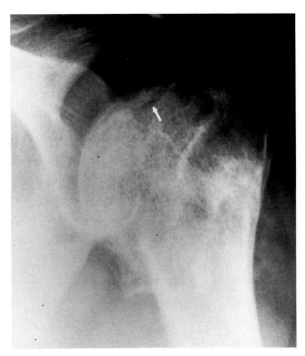

Figure 70–14. Humeral head: Vascular supply. Vessels include the anterior circumflex humeral artery (1), the posterior circumflex humeral artery (2), the arcuate artery (3), and the vessels of the rotator cuff (4). (After Graham J, Wood S: In JK Davidson: Aseptic Necrosis of Bone. New York, American Elsevier Publishing Co, 1976, p 101. Used with permission.)

Figure 70–15. Posttraumatic osteonecrosis: Humeral head. Although the fracture of the anatomic neck of the humerus is healed in this 61 year old man, observe the small and flattened humeral head and subchondral radiolucent area (arrow), indicative of ischemic necrosis.

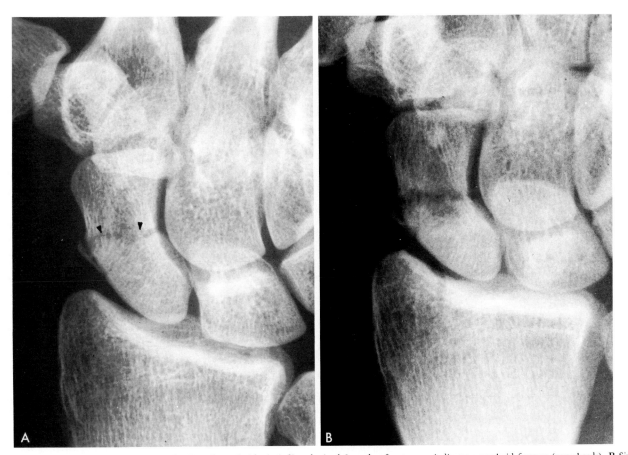

Figure 70–16. Posttraumatic osteonecrosis: Carpal scaphoid. A A film obtained 2 weeks after trauma indicates a scaphoid fracture (arrowheads). **B** Six weeks after **A**, increased radiodensity of the proximal half of the scaphoid is accentuated by osteoporosis of the distal half of the bone, indicating the presence of osteonecrosis and reparative bone formation.

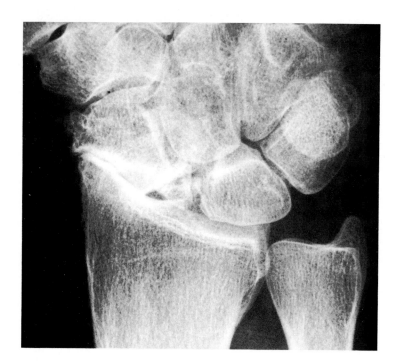

Figure 70–17. Posttraumatic osteonecrosis: Carpal scaphoid. Nonunion and secondary degenerative joint disease. A remote fracture of the scaphoid is associated with nonunion, collapse of the necrotic proximal pole, and joint space narrowing, sclerosis, and osteophytes of the radiocarpal and midcarpal compartments.

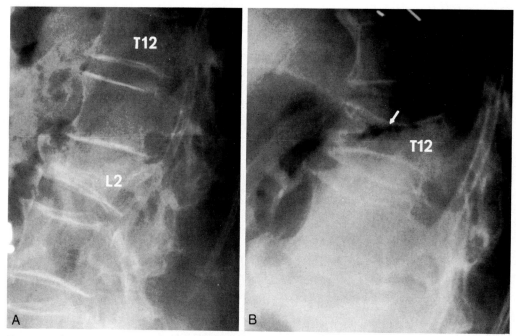

Figure 70–18. Posttraumatic osteonecrosis: Vertebral body (Kümmell's disease). This 89 year old woman was involved in a motor vehicle accident approximately 1 year previously. **A** An initial lateral radiograph shows an old fracture of the second lumbar vertebra (L2), with considerable collapse of the vertebral body. The remaining vertebral bodies are normal. **B** Seven days after **A**, a repeat lateral radiograph of the thoracolumbar spine shows a new collapse of the twelfth thoracic vertebral body (T12). Observe the intraosseous vacuum within the body (arrow), probably indicating ischemic necrosis.

DYSBARIC OSTEONECROSIS

Exposure of humans to high pressure environments, as occurs in scuba diving, underwater and space exploration, and off-shore oil drilling, subsequently may lead to osteonecrosis; this phenomenon has been designated as dysbaric osteonecrosis, caisson disease, pressure-induced osteoarthropathy, and barotraumatic osteoarthropathy.

The term decompression sickness indicates the acute consequences of the liberation of gas bubbles, principally nitrogen, in the blood and the tissues of a person who has undergone decompression too rapidly after a period of exposure to a hyperbaric environment. Ventilation may allow dispersion of the excess of oxygen and carbon dioxide, but the released nitrogen may produce bubbles within the vascular tree that partially or completely occlude vessels at one or more sites. Nitrogen accumulation is greatest in tissues rich in fat, and the fatty marrow does not escape this accumulation.

The association of decompression sickness and dysbaric osteonecrosis is not clear. It generally is assumed, however, that gas bubbles initiate the manifestations of decompression sickness and that they likely represent the cause of osteonecrosis as well. The frequency of dysbaric osteonecrosis appears to be exaggerated in patients with repeated exposures, exposures to greater pressures, a rapid rate of exposure, and obesity. In compressed-air workers, the reported frequency has varied from almost zero to 75 per cent, most estimates being in the 10 to 20 per cent range. The reported prevalence of osteonecrosis in divers has varied from 4 to 65 per cent. In both compressed-air workers and divers, a delay of 4 to 12 months between the first exposure to the increased atmospheric pressure and the onset of radiologically evident skeletal alterations is typical.

Radiographic and Pathologic Abnormalities

The radiographic and pathologic abnormalities of dysbaric osteonecrosis include two major changes: juxtaarticular lesions occurring most frequently in the head of the humerus and femur (Figs. 70–19 and 70–20) and diaphyseal and metaphyseal lesions situated at a distance from the articulation (Fig. 70–21). Juxtaarticular alterations consist of radiodense areas varying between 3 and 20 mm in diameter, which are slightly less discrete than bone islands, spherical opaque areas that may eventually produce a "snow-capped" configuration, radiolucent subcortical bands (crescent sign), and osseous collapse and fragmentation; diaphyseal and metaphyseal abnormalities consist of poorly defined radiodense foci and irregular calcified areas with a shell-like configuration. Bilateral or unilateral alterations can be seen. The distal shaft of the femur, the humeral head, the femoral head, and the tibial shaft, in descending order of frequency, are the most typical sites of involvement. Scintigraphy using bone-seeking radiopharmaceutical agents allows accurate analysis of the distribution of the alterations.

Pathologic examination reveals necrotic subchondral bone surrounded by collagenous fibrous tissue and thickened, spongy trabeculae. One or more fracture lines can extend through the cartilage, creating osteochondral fragments. Cartilaginous abnormalities are relatively mild in comparison to the severity of the osseous alterations until secondary osteoarthritis supervenes.

Differential Diagnosis

The radiographic findings associated with dysbaric osteonecrosis generally are indistinguishable from those associated with osteonecrosis of other causes, such as sickle cell anemia, Gaucher's disease, and steroid medication. Although diaphyseal calcification in an infarct may simulate that in an enchondroma, a shell-like calcific pattern in infarction differs from the punctate and central calcification in an enchondroma. Small, dense foci in dysbaric osteonecrosis are virtually identical to bone islands, and only those that are larger and more numerous may allow accurate diagnosis of this condition.

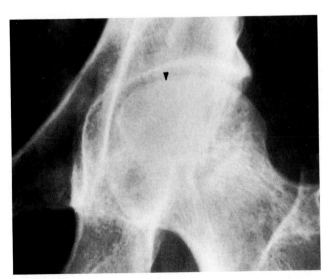

Figure 70–19. Dysbaric osteonecrosis: Juxtaarticular lesions. This middle-aged man had worked in a decompression chamber for 20 years. A radiograph reveals patchy lucency and sclerosis of the femoral head, with subtle flattening of the articular surface, a subchondral radiolucent crescent or fracture (arrowhead), and buttressing of the femoral neck. The opposite hip was affected similarly.

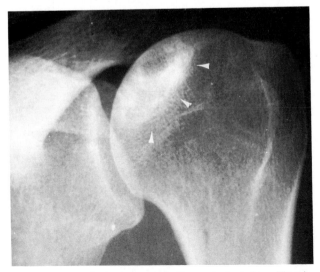

Figure 70–20. Dysbaric osteonecrosis: Juxtaarticular lesions. The sclerosis or "snow-capped" appearance of the humeral head (arrowheads) is typical of dysbaric osteonecrosis but may be evident in other varieties of necrosis as well.

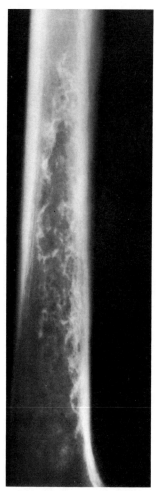

Figure 70–21. Dysbaric osteonecrosis: Diaphyseal lesion. In this deep sea diver and astronaut, the irregular calcific deposits in the femur with a shell-like configuration are typical of a bone infarct.

IDIOPATHIC (PRIMARY OR SPONTANEOUS) OSTEONECROSIS

Osteonecrosis may appear in certain locations in the absence of any recognizable underlying disorder or event. Most characteristically, it is the femoral head or femoral condyles that are involved, although, rarely, spontaneous osteonecrosis can appear at other sites.

Spontaneous Osteonecrosis of the Femoral Head in Adults

Idiopathic or spontaneous osteonecrosis of the femoral head in adults is sometimes designated Chandler's disease. It affects men more frequently than women and usually is seen between the fourth and seventh decades of life. Unilateral or bilateral involvement may be detected. The radiographic features vary with the stage of the disorder. Initially, a femoral head of normal osseous contour may reveal radiodense areas scattered throughout its anterosuperior region with a faint curvilinear band of diminished density in the anterior subchondral bone, the crescent sign. As the disease progresses, a focus of increased radiodensity or a lucent zone with a peripheral rim of increased radiodensity and flattening of the femoral contour are observed. Osteoarthritis may eventually occur.

The pathologic findings are virtually identical to those in other varieties of osteonecrosis.

Spontaneous Osteonecrosis About the Knee in Adults

Although osteonecrosis about the knee may be observed in association with steroid therapy, sickle cell anemia, other hemoglobinopathies, and renal transplantation, it may also occur in a spontaneous or idiopathic fashion. This disorder, which is distinct from osteochondritis dissecans occurring in adolescence (Table 70–4), is characterized by the onset, in an older patient (usually over 60 years of age), of abrupt pain in the knee, almost always confined to the medial aspect of the joint. Localized tenderness and stiffness, an effusion, and restricted motion may be apparent. Unilateral involvement predominates. Initially radiographs are normal, and it is not until a period of weeks or months has passed that subtle flattening and sclerosis of the weight-bearing articular surface of the medial femoral condyle are seen (Fig. 70–22) (the lateral condyle is infrequently affected). A radiolucent lesion in the condyle can be detected over the ensuing weeks; within this lesion, a radiodense line consisting of cartilage and subchondral bone plate can frequently be identified. If untreated, further depression of the bone margin, intraarticular osseous bodies, progressive sclerosis, and periostitis of the distal femur can be encountered on later examination. Secondary osteoarthritis subsequently may appear, leading to speculation that a significant number of cases of degenerative joint disease of the knee have their origin in an ischemic event.

In the vast majority of cases, it is the weight-bearing surface of the medial femoral condyle that is involved. Spontaneous ischemic necrosis is occasionally observed in the tibial plateau or in the lateral femoral condyle, alone or in combination with changes in the medial condyle of the femur (Fig. 70–22).

Scintigraphic examination using bone-seeking radiopharmaceutical agents (Fig. 70–23) may reveal focal accumulation of radionuclide long before radiographic changes appear. The results of both scintigraphy and radiography can be used to group the affected patients into categories reflecting the subsequent clinical course of the disease. Those with scintigraphic abnormalities alone have a good prognosis and respond to conservative treatment; those with positive radionuclide findings and small and stable radiographically evident lesions also do well with conservative therapy; and those with abnormal bone scans and considerable radiographic alterations generally require surgical intervention.

The cause and pathogenesis of this condition are not clear. The dominant opinion implicates vascular insufficiency leading to infarction of bone. A prominent role of meniscal injury in the pathogenesis of spontaneous osteonecrosis has also been proposed. Meniscal tears have been reported in association with this condition, and the impact of the articular surface against a fragmented meniscus during everyday activity could result in local ischemia of the medial femoral condyle.

The other entities that enter into the differential diagnosis of the radiographic changes in spontaneous osteonecrosis about the knee are osteonecrosis from additional causes, osteochondritis dissecans, calcium pyrophosphate dihydrate crystal deposition disease, transient osteoporosis, stress fracture, and neuroarthropathy.

Table 70–4. SPONTANEOUS OSTEONECROSIS VERSUS OSTEOCHONDRITIS DISSECANS (ABOUT THE KNEE)

	Spontaneous Osteonecrosis	Osteochondritis Dissecans
Age of onset	Middle-aged and elderly	Adolescent
Symptoms	Pain, tenderness, swelling, restricted motion	Variable; may be lacking
Typical location	Weight-bearing surface of medial femoral condyle	Non–weight-bearing surface of medial femoral condyle
Probable pathogenesis	Trauma, perhaps related to meniscal tear; or vascular insult	Trauma
Sequelae	Degenerative joint disease; intraarticular osteocartilaginous bodies	Intraarticular osteocartilaginous bodies

COMPLICATIONS
Cartilaginous Abnormalities

One of the striking pathologic features of osteonecrosis is the intactness of the chondral surface despite the presence of adjacent severe osseous abnormality. This finding, which has its radiographic counterpart in preservation of the joint space, supports the commonly held impression that articular cartilage in mature adults derives most, if not all, of its nutrition from synovial fluid. In those cases in which osteonecrosis leads to significant collapse of the articular surface, secondary degenerative joint disease may appear (Fig. 70–24).

Intraarticular Osseous Bodies

Infrequently, one or more chondral or osteochondral fragments can appear in osteonecrosis. They may exist free in the articular cavity, in situ in the depressed bone area, or embedded in the synovium at a distant site.

Cyst Formation

Cystic degeneration in areas of bone infarction predominates in the diaphyses of tubular bones, especially the tibia (Fig. 70–25) and the humerus. An expanding osteolytic area that erodes the cortex is seen, usually at a single site. As it

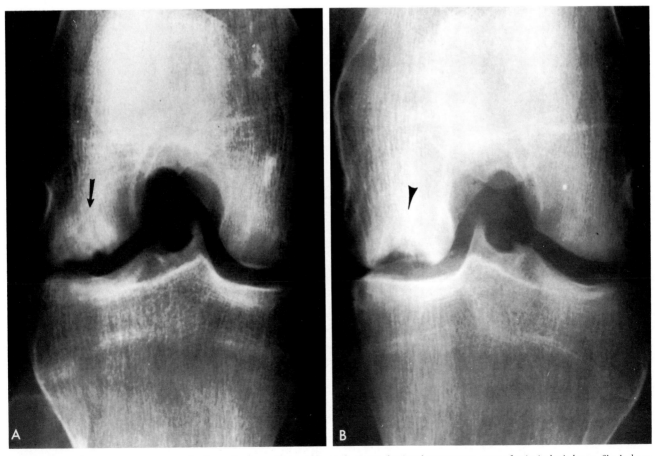

Figure 70–22. Spontaneous osteonecrosis about the knee. This middle-aged woman developed spontaneous onset of pain in both knees. She had not received corticosteroids. Observe osseous depression, irregularity and sclerosis of the lateral condyle of the right femur (arrow) and the medial condyle of the left femur (arrowhead).

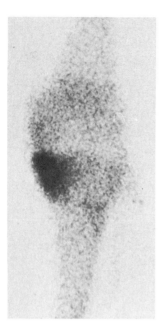

Figure 70–23. Spontaneous osteonecrosis about the knee: Medial tibial plateau. Increased accumulation of the bone-seeking radionuclide in the medial aspect of the tibia is consistent with spontaneous necrosis. A radiograph (not shown) was normal.

evolves, the cyst becomes sharply marginated. This feature and the absence of cortical disruption suggest the correct diagnosis, although differentiation of a cyst and malignant degeneration of an osseous infarct may be difficult.

Malignant Degeneration

Sarcoma arising in areas of bone infarction has been documented in both idiopathic cases and those related to caisson disease or other disorders. Men are affected more commonly, and the patient usually is in the fifth to seventh decades of life. Multiple bone infarcts commonly are present. Typically the distal portion of the femur (Fig. 70–26) or proximal portion of the tibia is the site of neoplasm, although other areas may be affected. The lesions may be interpreted as fibrosarcoma, malignant fibrous histiocytoma, or, more rarely, osteosarcoma. A long latent period between bone infarction and malignant transformation is evident. Although the prognosis in patients with bone infarction and sarcoma is guarded and disseminated metastasis and death commonly appear in a short period of time, the rarity of the complication should be emphasized. The radiographic diagnosis is not difficult, as a soft tissue mass and osseous destruction appear at a site of obvious infarction. Occasionally, the radiographic appearance of dissolution of bone and adjacent calcification may resemble a chondrosarcoma, with or without dedifferentiation, occurring in the absence of osteonecrosis.

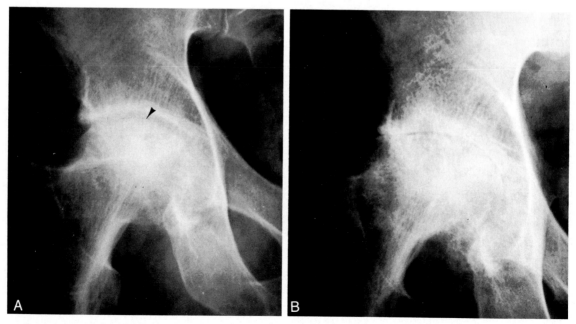

Figure 70–24. Osteonecrosis: Complications—cartilaginous abnormalities. Radiographs obtained 6 years apart reveal initially (**A**) collapse of the articular surface of the femoral head (arrowhead) and, subsequently (**B**), secondary osteoarthritis with considerable narrowing of the joint space. In cases such as these, it is difficult to state with certainty that the changes in **B** do not represent osteoarthritis alone unless the sequence of radiographs is available for examination.

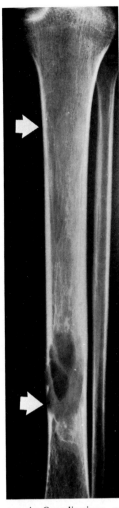

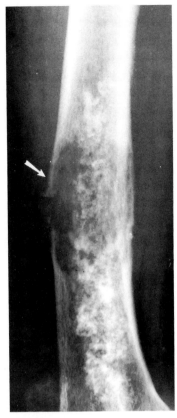

Figure 70–26. Osteonecrosis: Complications—malignant degeneration. A fibrosarcoma has developed at the site of bone necrosis in the femur. In addition to the typical calcification of a bone infarct, observe the osteolytic destruction (arrow) with a pathologic fracture. (Courtesy of V. Vint, M.D., San Diego, California.)

Figure 70–25. Osteonecrosis: Complications—cyst formation. Observe a bone infarct (upper arrow) in the shaft of the tibia. A cystic area (lower arrow) has led to erosion of the endosteal margin of the cortex. (From Norman A, Steiner GC: Radiographic and morphological features of cyst formation in idiopathic bone infarction. Radiology 146:335, 1983. Used with permission.)

FURTHER READING

Ahlbäck S, Bauer GCH, Bohne WH: Spontaneous osteonecrosis of the knee. Arthritis Rheum 11:705, 1968.

Barquet A: Natural history of avascular necrosis following traumatic hip dislocation in childhood. A review of 145 cases. Acta Orthop Scand 53:815, 1982.

Bell ALL, Edson GN, Hornick N: Characteristic bone and joint changes in compressed air workers: A survey of symptomless cases. Radiology 38:698, 1913.

Brower AC, Downey EF Jr: Kümmell disease: Report of a case with serial radiographs. Radiology 141:363, 1981.

Burt RW, Matthews TJ: Aseptic necrosis of the knee: Bone scintigraphy. AJR 138:571, 1982.

Catto M: A histological study of avascular necrosis of the femoral head after transcervical fracture. J Bone Joint Surg [Br] 47:749, 1965.

Davidson JK: Dysbaric osteonecrosis. In JK Davidson (Ed): Aseptic Necrosis of Bone. Amsterdam, Excerpta Medica, 1976, p 147.

Davidson JK, Hanison JAB, Jacobs P, Hilditch TE, Catto M, Hendry WT: The significance of bone islands, cystic areas and sclerotic areas in dysbaric osteonecrosis. Clin Radiol 28:381, 1977.

Dihlmann W: CT analysis of the upper end of the femur: The asterisk knee. Investigation by radionuclide scintimetry and radiography. J Bone Joint Surg [Br] 52:605, 1970.

Gelberman RH, Menon J: The vascularity of the scaphoid bone. J Hand Surg 5:508, 1980.

Glimcher MJ, Kenzora JE: The biology of osteonecrosis of the human femoral head and its clinical implications. II. The pathological changes in the femoral head as an organ and in the hip joint. Clin Orthop 139:283, 1979.

Gohel VK, Dalinka MK, Edeiken J: Ischemic necrosis of the femoral head simulating chondroblastoma. Radiology 107:545, 1973.

Houpt JB, Alpert B, Lotem M, Greyson ND, Pritzker KPH, Langer F, Gross AE: Spontaneous osteonecrosis of the medial tibial plateau. J Rheumatol 9:81, 1982.

Jaffe HL: Ischemic necrosis of bone. Med Radiogr Photogr 45:57, 1969.

Lotke PA, Ecker ML: Osteonecrosis-like syndrome of the medial tibial plateau. Clin Orthop 176:148, 1983.

Maldague BE, Noel HM, Malghem JJ: The intravertebral vacuum cleft: A sign of ischemic vertebral collapse. Radiology 129:23, 1978.

Mankin HJ, Brower TD: Bilateral idiopathic aseptic necrosis of the femur in adults: "Chandler's disease." Bull Hosp Joint Dis 23:42, 1962.

Martel W, Poznanski AK: The effect of traction on the hip in osteonecrosis. A comment on the "radiolucent crescent line." Radiology 94:505, 1970.

Mirra JM, Bullough PG, Marcove RC, Jacobs B, Huvos AG: Malignant fibrous histiocytoma and osteosarcoma in association with bone infarcts. Report of four cases, two in caisson workers. J Bone Joint Surg [Am] 56:932, 1974.

Mitchell DG, Kressel HY, Arger PH, Dalinka M, Spritzer CE, Steinberg ME: Avascular necrosis of the femoral head: Morphologic assessment by MR imaging with CT correlation. Radiology 161:739, 1986.

Mitchell DG, Rao V, Dalinka M, Spritzer CE, Gefter WB, Axel L, Steinberg M, Kressel HY: MRI of joint fluid in the normal and ischemic hip. AJR 146:1215, 1986.

Morris HD: Aseptic necrosis of the talus following injury. Orthop Clin North Am 5:177, 1974.

Mulfinger GL, Trueta J: The blood supply of the talus. J Bone Joint Surg [Br] 52:160, 1970.

Nellen JR, Kindwall EP: Aseptic necrosis of bone secondary to occupational exposure to compressed air: Roentgenologic findings in 59 cases. AJR *115*:512, 1972.

Norman A, Baker ND: Spontaneous osteonecrosis of the knee and medial meniscal tears. Radiology *129*:653, 1978.

Norman A, Steiner GC: Radiographic and morphological features of cyst formation in idiopathic bone infarction. Radiology *146*:335, 1983.

Ohta Y, Matsunaga H: Bone lesions in divers. J Bone Joint Surg [Br] *56*:3, 1974.

Patterson RJ, Bickel WH, Dahlin DC: Idiopathic avascular necrosis of the head of the femur. A study of fifty-two cases. J Bone Joint Surg [Am] *46*:267, 1964.

Totty WG, Murphy WA, Ganz WI, Kumar B, Daum WJ, Siegel BA: Magnetic resonance imaging of the normal and ischemic femoral head. AJR *143*:1273, 1984.

Vance RM, Gelberman RH, Evans EF: Scaphocapitate fractures. J Bone Joint Surg [Am] *62*:271, 1980.

Vogler JB III, Murphy WA: Bone marrow imaging. Radiology *168*:679, 1988.

Williams JL, Cliff MM, Bonakdarpour A: Spontaneous osteonecrosis of the knee. Radiology *107*:15, 1973.

Chapter 71

Osteochondroses

Donald Resnick, M.D.

The osteochondroses are a heterogeneous group of disorders that are usually characterized by fragmentation and sclerosis of an epiphyseal or apophyseal center in the immature skeleton. Reossification and reconstitution of osseous contour can be evident in some cases. These disorders can be divided into three major categories: (1) conditions characterized by *primary or secondary osteonecrosis; (2) conditions related to trauma or abnormal stress, without evidence of osteonecrosis; and (3) conditions that represent variations in normal patterns of ossification. In some cases, a definite pathogenesis has not been identified.*

The designation "osteochondrosis" has traditionally been used to describe a group of disorders that share certain features: predilection for the immature skeleton; involvement of an epiphysis, apophysis, or epiphysioid bone; and a radiographic picture that is dominated by fragmentation, collapse, sclerosis, and, frequently, reossification with reconstitution of the osseous contour. The radiologic and pathologic features of the osteochondroses were initially interpreted as evidence of a primary impairment of local arterial supply that led to osteonecrosis. With further investigation of these disorders, it became apparent that dissimilarities among them were considerable, and that the osteochondroses were a heterogeneous group of unrelated lesions (Table 71–1). It is now recognized that osteonecrosis is not apparent on histologic examination in some of the osteochondroses and that, in others, ischemic bone necrosis is not a primary event but appears to follow a fracture or other traumatic insult. Indeed, certain of the osteochondroses are not disorders at all but appear to represent variations in normal ossification. In this

chapter, the osteochondroses are grouped according to their probable pathogenesis rather than their site of involvement.

GENERAL CHARACTERISTICS

Many of the osteochondroses become apparent in the first decade of life at a time when the developing bone still contains a cartilaginous model. The rapidly ossifying central nucleus of bone within the cartilage anlage of the epiphysis is vulnerable to mechanical pressures superimposed on hormonal or nutritional changes, explaining the appearance of certain of these conditions during the "midgrowth" spurt of childhood; others, such as Scheuermann's disease and Osgood-Schlatter disease, occur during the adolescent growth spurt of puberty. Almost all of the osteochondroses are more frequent in boys than in girls. Although a single and unilateral distribution predominates, examples of involvement of multiple and bilateral sites are not uncommon. The concept that generalized factors may initiate or aggravate some of the osteochondroses is supported by their occurrence in several

Table 71–1. OSTEOCHONDROSES

Disorder	Site	Age (Years)	Probable Mechanism
Legg-Calvé-Perthes disease	Femoral head	4–8	Osteonecrosis, perhaps due to trauma
Freiberg's infraction	Metatarsal head	13–18	Osteonecrosis due to trauma
Kienböck's disease	Carpal lunate	20–40	Osteonecrosis due to trauma
Köhler's disease	Tarsal navicular	3–7	Osteonecrosis or altered sequence of ossification
Panner's disease	Capitulum of humerus	5–10	Osteonecrosis due to trauma
Thiemann's disease	Phalanges of hand	11–19	Osteonecrosis, perhaps due to trauma
Osgood-Schlatter disease	Tibial tuberosity	11–15	Trauma
Blount's disease	Proximal tibial epiphysis	1–3 (infantile)	Trauma
		8–15 (adolescent)	Trauma
Scheuermann's disease	Discovertebral junction	13–17	Trauma
Sinding-Larsen-Johansson disease	Patella	10–14	Trauma
Sever's disease	Calcaneus	9–11	Normal variation in ossification
Van Neck's disease	Ischiopubic synchondrosis	4–11	Normal variation in ossification

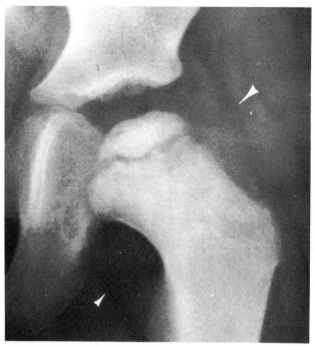

Figure 71–1. Legg-Calvé-Perthes disease: Radiographic abnormalities. A radiograph reveals soft tissue distortion (arrowheads), a sclerotic femoral ossification center that is laterally displaced and contains radiolucent fissures, and metaphyseal irregularity.

members of a single family and in children who have a delay in skeletal maturation. Furthermore, the changes at some sites resemble those of hypothyroidism and sickle cell anemia. The importance of trauma as an initiating event or common pathway in most of these disorders cannot be denied, however.

Although the radiologic features of the osteochondroses have been well described, it should be remembered that irregularity of endochondral ossification is regarded as a normal variation at certain sites, such as the calcaneus and the tarsal navicular bone. Nevertheless, the identification of irregularity on radiographs of sites that normally ossify in a uniform fashion and of necrosis, granulation tissue, disorderly ossification, bone absorption, and reparative osteogenesis on histologic inspection supports the belief that some of the osteochondroses should not be regarded as variations of normal.

DISORDERS CHARACTERIZED BY PRIMARY OR SECONDARY OSTEONECROSIS
Legg-Calvé-Perthes Disease

CLINICAL ABNORMALITIES. Legg-Calvé-Perthes disease affects children, particularly those between the ages of 4 and 8 years. The disorder is much more frequent in boys than in girls. Bilateral abnormalities are detected in about 10 per cent of cases; when both hips are involved, the two hips are usually affected successively, not simultaneously. Bilateral symmetric fragmentation of the capital femoral epiphyses should suggest the presence of other diseases, such as hypothyroidism. Legg-Calvé-Perthes disease is rare among blacks. A family history of the condition may be detected in approximately 6 per cent of cases.

The principal clinical signs are limping, pain, and limitation of joint motion. These manifestations may persist for only a few days or weeks. At other times, prolonged signs and atrophy of the soft tissues of the thigh, muscle spasm, and contracture are recognized. A history of trauma can be observed in approximately 25 per cent of cases.

The possibility of Legg-Calvé-Perthes disease must be considered in a child with acute or chronic manifestations in the hip. The acute onset of pain in the hip, groin, or knee combined with a limp and limitation of motion in a child has been referred to as the observation hip, the irritable hip, and transient synovitis of the hip. Although the clinical manifestations generally resolve in a period of days and radiographs are usually normal, reports of more persistent findings and radiologic sequelae have appeared, suggesting that this type of acute syndrome may represent one pattern of clinical presentation of Legg-Calvé-Perthes disease. The cause of transient synovitis of the hip as well as its relationship to Legg-Calvé-Perthes disease is, however, not clear.

RADIOGRAPHIC ABNORMALITIES. The early radiographic abnormalities include the following (Fig. 71–1).

1. *Soft tissue swelling on the lateral side of the joint.* Capsular bulging with displacement of the capsular fat pad relates to accumulation of intraarticular fluid.

2. *Smallness of the femoral ossification nucleus.* A diminutive ossification center may be apparent in as many as 50 per cent of patients. It may relate to retardation of bone growth.

3. *Lateral displacement of the femoral ossification nucleus.* The ossific nucleus may be displaced laterally 2 to 5 mm, producing an enlargement of the medial portion of the joint space. This change, which may occur in as many as 85 per cent of cases, may be due either to synovitis with intraarticular fluid accumulation or to cartilaginous hypertrophy.

4. *Fissuring and fracture of the femoral ossific nucleus.* This important radiographic sign may be detected only on radiographs obtained in the frog-leg position. Linear radiolucent shadows commence in the anterior margin of the epiphysis and extend posteriorly, and the fracture fragment may remain in situ or be slightly displaced.

5. *Flattening and sclerosis of the femoral ossific nucleus.* Flattening of the epiphyseal nucleus predominates near the fracture lines on the anterolateral superior segment of the femoral head. This finding is preceded by, or occurs simultaneously with, the development of fissures in the bone. On the anteroposterior view, the entire femoral head may appear radiodense, whereas in the frog-leg position, a segmental location is evident. Sclerosis is a secondary phenomenon caused by compression of trabeculae and revascularization, with deposition of new bone on necrotic trabeculae.

6. *Intraepiphyseal gas.* A vacuum phenomenon, caused by release of gas into the clefts and gaps in the subchondral trabeculae, accentuates the exaggerated radiolucent appearance in this area.

Although the progression and extent of disease are highly variable, further compression, disintegration, fragmentation, and sclerosis of the epiphysis, together with metaphyseal changes, can be seen (Fig. 71–2).

1. *Metaphyseal "cysts."* Radiolucent lesions of the metaphysis are a characteristic part of the radiographic picture of Legg-Calvé-Perthes disease, although their pathogenesis is debated, with alternative theories supporting osteonecrosis or a disturbance in endochondral ossification. The resulting radiolucent area of the metaphysis may simulate an abscess or tumor.

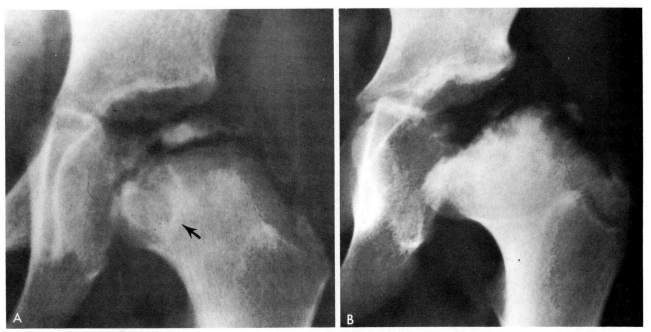

Figure 71–2. **Legg-Calvé-Perthes disease: Metaphyseal abnormalities. A** Metaphyseal "cysts." Observe the large cystic lesion of the medial metaphysis of the femur (arrow), which is associated with a fragmented, sclerotic, and laterally placed ossific nucleus. **B** In another child, note the broad and short femoral neck containing multiple radiolucent lesions. Most of the epiphyseal ossification center is destroyed.

2. *Widening and shortening of the femoral neck.* Widening and irregularity of the growth plate and broadening of the metaphysis are additional manifestations of this disorder. As the greater trochanter possesses a separate blood supply and can continue to develop despite growth disturbance in the adjacent bone, it eventually may appear disproportionately large in comparison to the shortened femoral neck.

PATHOLOGIC ABNORMALITIES. The fundamental pathologic aberration of the femoral head in this disease is necrosis of trabeculae and marrow, which eventually is accompanied by structural failure of the femoral head, resulting in flattening and collapse. As in other varieties of osteonecrosis, the chondral surfaces are remarkably well preserved during the early and intermediate stages of Legg-Calvé-Perthes disease. As opposed to the situation in other forms of osteonecrosis, however, separation of articular cartilage and underlying necrotic bone even in late stages of Legg-Calvé-Perthes disease is unusual.

COURSE OF DISEASE. The course of Legg-Calvé-Perthes disease is variable. The degree of reconstitution of the ossific nucleus and the ultimate shape of the femoral head depend on the amount of necrosis, its exact location, and the magnitude of forces across the joint. In some instances, the eventual radiographic appearance of the involved femoral head may be indistinguishable from that of its uninvolved counterpart, whereas in others, coxa plana, shortening and widening of the femoral neck, osteochondroma-like lesions of the femoral neck, degenerative joint disease, and intraarticular osseous bodies may be identified (Figs. 71–3 and 71–4). One interesting residual of this disease is a radiodense curvilinear shadow at the base of the femoral neck, termed the sagging rope sign (Fig. 71–4D). This sign probably represents the radiodense shadow cast by the anterior or lateral edge of a severely deformed femoral head.

In most cases of Legg-Calvé-Perthes disease, changes are isolated to or predominantly involve one hip. In those instances in which bilateral abnormalities are encountered, symmetric involvement is exceedingly rare, a feature that serves to distinguish Legg-Calvé-Perthes disease from other disorders, such as hypothyroidism and epiphyseal dysplasias, that affect the hip. Some investigators have noted mild radiographic changes of unclear cause in the "normal" hip in children with "unilateral" Legg-Calvé-Perthes disease.

A detached osteochondral fragment (osteochondritis dissecans) can be seen in approximately 3 per cent of patients with this disease (Fig. 71–5). It is observed almost exclusively in male patients. The average interval between the diagnosis of Legg-Calvé-Perthes disease and the presentation of an intra-articular osteocartilaginous body is about 8 years. The pathogenesis of osteochondritis dissecans in this condition is not clear; it may be due to persistence of an ununited fragment or to fragmentation of a femoral head that is weakened by revascularization during the healing process.

Although recurrent episodes of infarction may be essential to the development of Legg-Calvé-Perthes disease, cases demonstrating clinical and radiographic evidence of recurrent disease are unusual.

PROGNOSIS. It is the variability in the course of Legg-Calvé-Perthes disease that stimulated investigations into the predictive value of certain radiographic or clinical signs in the eventual outcome of the disorder. In general, a better prognosis is observed in boys and in younger patients. Other prognostic signs relate to the radiographic characteristics of the affected hip, which have been separated into four groups (Table 71–2).

Group I. The anterior part of the epiphysis is the only affected site. Collapse and sequestration are not evident. Metaphyseal changes are unusual. Radiographically, the

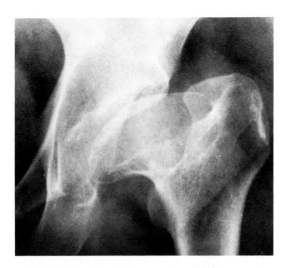

Figure 71–3. Legg-Calvé-Perthes disease: Coxa plana and coxa magna. Note the smoothly flattened femoral head, the prominent greater trochanter, and the flattened acetabular margin.

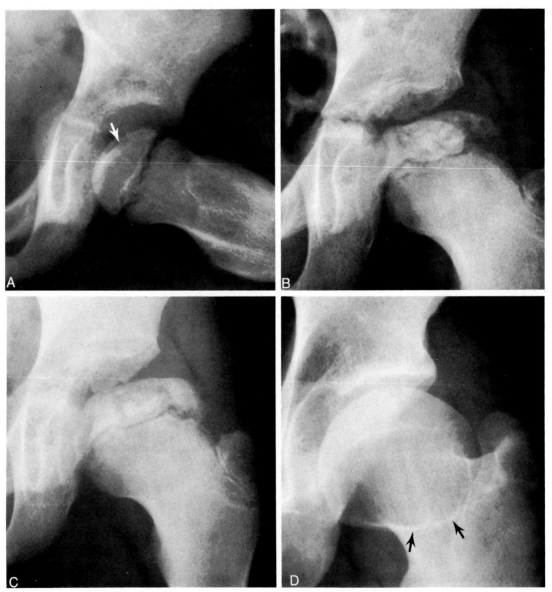

Figure 71–4. Legg-Calvé-Perthes disease: Sagging rope sign. Sequential radiographs of the left hip indicate the course of the disease over a 16 year period. A Age 7 years (phase of disease onset). On this frog-leg view, note the radiolucent crescent sign (arrow). B Age 8 years (phase of fragmentation). The lateral two thirds of the femoral head is collapsed and fragmented, and the lateral portion of the head is not covered by the acetabulum. C Age 9 years (phase of healing). The medial aspect of the epiphysis is larger and there is an increase in the amount of bone that is present laterally. The femoral head is not completely covered. D Age 22 years (residual phase). The femoral head is slightly flattened and large. Note the radiodense curved line, the sagging rope sign (arrows). (Courtesy of P. VanderStoep, M.D., Saint Cloud, Minnesota.)

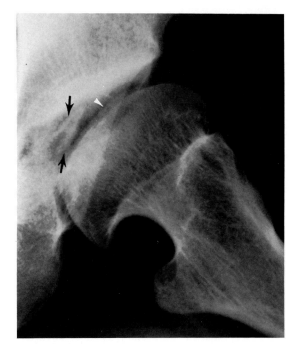

Figure 71–5. Legg-Calvé-Perthes disease: Osteochondral fragment. A frog-leg view reveals a flattened femoral head, acetabular deformity, and an osseous body (arrows) within the joint, highlighted by the spontaneous release of gas into the joint. The presence of gas also permits the identification of a thinned cartilaginous surface (arrowhead).

course of the disease is characterized by absorption of the involved segment, followed by regeneration commencing from the periphery.

Group II. Greater involvement is apparent. Collapse and sequestration are followed by absorption and healing.

Group III. Only a small portion of the epiphysis is not sequestered. Anteroposterior radiographs reveal a "head within a head" appearance, and collapse of a centrally placed sequestrum is identified. Subsequent broadening of the femoral neck is common. The course of the disease is similar to that in group II, although metaphyseal changes are more generalized.

Group IV. The whole epiphysis is affected. Total epiphyseal collapse and metaphyseal changes are evident. Epiphyseal displacement occurs, and a mushroom-like appearance of the head can be identified.

In general, patients in groups III and IV have a relatively poor prognosis, whereas those in groups I and II do better. These generalizations are not without exception, however. Furthermore, it is difficult to recognize which pattern is present at an early phase of the disease. Early radiographic changes that may indicate a capital femoral epiphysis "at risk" for collapse are the following: (1) Gage's sign (a small, osteoporotic segment that forms a transradiant "V" on the lateral side of the epiphysis); (2) calcification lateral to the epiphysis (reflecting the presence of extruded cartilage); (3)

lateral subluxation of the femoral head; and (4) a transverse epiphyseal line.

It is evident that no simple radiologic observation is indicative of a good or poor result, and that a combination of findings must be used for prognostic accuracy. Most patients are symptom-free 30 to 40 years later, although persistent roentgenographic alterations are usually evident.

OTHER DIAGNOSTIC METHODS. In the early stages of Legg-Calvé-Perthes disease, *arthrography* can reveal subtle flattening of the cartilage at the site of osseous fissuring and an increase in width of both the femoral and the acetabular cartilage. In later stages, arthrography frequently indicates a smooth cartilaginous surface despite the presence of considerable ossific fragmentation. Flattening and lateral extrusion of the chondral coat can be identified in some instances. As arthrography identifies the abnormal femoral head more accurately than does plain film radiography, it may be a useful guide for the orthopedic surgeon who is interested in knowing what percentage of the head is contained within the acetabulum.

Radionuclide examination with bone-seeking radiopharmaceutical agents can identify an area of deficient uptake in the early phase of the disease, owing to impairment of the blood supply. This defect is seen most frequently in the anterolateral aspect of a femoral head with partial necrosis and across the

Table 71–2. GRADES OF FEMORAL INVOLVEMENT IN LEGG-CALVÉ-PERTHES DISEASE (Catterall Classification)

	Grade			
	I	*II*	*III*	*IV*
Site of epiphyseal involvement	Anterior part	Anterior part	Almost whole epiphysis	Whole epiphysis
Sequestrum	No	Yes	Yes	Yes
Crescent sign	No	Anterior	Anterior and extends posteriorly	Anterior and posterior
Collapse	No	Yes	Yes	Yes
Metaphyseal abnormalities	No	Localized	Diffuse	Diffuse

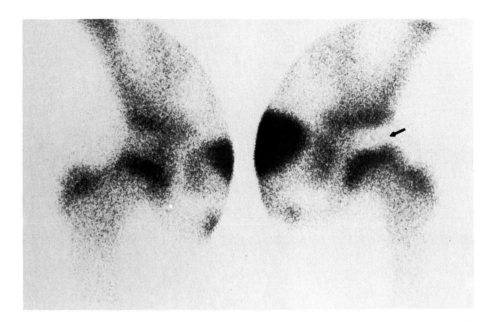

Figure 71–6. Legg-Calvé-Perthes disease: Radionuclide abnormalities. Note the characteristic "cold" area (arrow) in the left femoral head on the bone scan. The opposite hip is normal. (Courtesy of V. Vint, M.D., San Diego, California.)

entire width of the epiphysis in a head with total necrosis (Fig. 71–6). With the appearance of regeneration, the photodeficient areas may return to normal or be replaced by areas of augmented activity.

Ultrasonography has been used to define the presence of an effusion and joint space widening in the hips of patients with Legg-Calvé-Perthes disease.

Angiography has been employed as an investigative technique in some patients with Legg-Calvé-Perthes disease. *Intraosseous venography* also has been used to identify venous patterns of drainage in patients with Legg-Calvé-Perthes disease.

Magnetic resonance imaging is ideally applied to the evaluation of ischemic necrosis of bone and has been used to identify infarction of the femoral head in Legg-Calvé-Perthes disease. This method has the added advantage of delineating the cartilaginous surface of the femoral head, perhaps eliminating the need for arthrography.

ETIOLOGY AND PATHOGENESIS. It is generally held that vascular insufficiency to the femoral head triggers the radiographic and pathologic findings in Legg-Calvé-Perthes disease, although the factors leading to deficiency of blood supply have not been identified precisely. Some investigators, however, favor a traumatic cause in which direct compression of the femoral head by the adjacent acetabular roof leads to the characteristic radiographic features of the disease. Indeed, a general retardation of bone development can be identified in patients with this disease, suggesting that concomitantly retarded supporting connective tissues about the hip might not be able to provide adequate support for the normal heavy stresses in this location.

The role of synovitis and raised intraarticular pressure in the pathogenesis of Legg-Calvé-Perthes disease also has been emphasized. A history of synovitis or the presence of thickening and sclerosis of the capsular and synovial tissues on pathologic examination in persons with this disease could indicate that the obliteration of blood supply to the femoral head is caused by vascular compression from accumulation of intraarticular fluid. Alternatively, such fluid may lead to

venous obstruction and an increase in intraosseous pressure in the femoral neck.

Finally, the delayed skeletal maturation of persons with this disease and the reported higher frequency of congenital anomalies in extraskeletal sites have suggested to some investigators that genetic and developmental factors may be important.

DIFFERENTIAL DIAGNOSIS. Fragmentation and collapse of the femoral head (Table 71–3) can be seen in hypothyroidism and in osteonecrosis from other causes. The appearance of femoral head necrosis in a black patient should lead to hemoglobin analysis before the changes are ascribed to Legg-Calvé-Perthes disease. Similarly, bilateral symmetric alterations should be interpreted cautiously, as they may indicate hypothyroidism, sickle cell anemia, Gaucher's disease, and multiple epiphyseal and spondyloepiphyseal dysplasias.

Meyer's dysplasia of the femoral head is characterized by retarded skeletal maturation, mild clinical signs, and femoral bone nuclei that appear late and are small and granular. The abnormal femoral head epiphyses are usually apparent by the age of 2 years and are gradually transformed over the ensuing

Table 71–3. SOME CAUSES OF FEMORAL HEAD IRREGULARITY AND COLLAPSE IN INFANTS AND CHILDREN

Disease	Distribution
Legg-Calvé-Perthes disease	Unilateral or bilateral
Meyer's dysplasia	Unilateral or bilateral
Hypothyroidism	Bilateral
Epiphyseal dysplasia	Bilateral
Spondyloepiphyseal dysplasia	Bilateral
Sickle cell anemia	Unilateral or bilateral
Gaucher's disease	Unilateral or bilateral
Infection	Unilateral
Eosinophilic granuloma	Unilateral
Hemophilia	Unilateral or bilateral

2 to 4 years by growth and coalescence into enlarging, normal-appearing ossification centers. Sclerosis and metaphyseal changes are not evident in Meyer's dysplasia. The earlier age of onset, the bilateral nature of the changes, the absence of prominent radiographic abnormalities, and the lack of progression are all features that allow differentiation of Meyer's dysplasia from Legg-Calvé-Perthes disease.

Freiberg's Infraction

Freiberg's infraction typically is accompanied by involvement of the head of the second metatarsal, although it is recognized that the third and fourth metatarsal heads also can be affected (Fig. 71–7). Unilateral changes are characteristic, although bilateral involvement and alterations of more than one digit can be encountered.

Women predominate among patients affected with this disease. The disease usually is seen in adolescents between the ages of 13 and 18 years. Clinical features consist of local pain, tenderness, and swelling and limitation of motion of the corresponding metatarsophalangeal joint.

Radiographic abnormalities include, initially, subtle flattening, increased radiodensity, and cystic lucent lesions of the metatarsal head and widening of the metatarsophalangeal joint (Fig. 71–7); and, subsequently, an osteochondral fragment with progressive flattening and sclerosis of the metatarsal head and periostitis with increased cortical thickening of the adjacent metaphysis and diaphysis of the bone (Fig. 71–8). Premature closure of the growth plate, intraarticular osseous bodies, deformity of the metatarsal head, and secondary degenerative joint disease are recognized complications of the process (Fig. 71–9).

The pathogenesis of the disease process remains speculative. Prevailing opinion suggests that trauma represents the primary event in Freiberg's infraction. The high rate of occurrence of the disorder in women could conceivably be related to the wearing of high heeled shoes. Repeated injury at this site may then lead to disruption of the articular cartilage, ischemic necrosis of subchondral bone, compression fracture, collapse, and fragmentation.

The radiographic features of Freiberg's infraction are virtually pathognomonic, as they indicate osteonecrosis at a characteristic site, the metatarsal head. Occasionally other disorders, such as systemic lupus erythematosus, can produce bone necrosis at this location. Additional diseases leading to fragmentation of metatarsal heads with articular abnormality include rheumatoid arthritis, calcium pyrophosphate dihydrate crystal deposition disease, diabetes mellitus, and gout. In some persons, a mild degree of normal flattening of the articular surface of the metatarsal head can resemble Freiberg's infraction.

Kienböck's Disease

Kienböck's disease of the carpal lunate is most commonly observed in patients between the ages of 20 and 40 years. Bilateral abnormalities occur but are less frequent than unilateral changes. A history of trauma may be elicited but is not constant. Progressive pain, swelling, and disability can be apparent.

Radiographic changes are distinctive. Initially, the lunate may have a normal architecture and density, but a linear or compression fracture can be delineated. Subsequently, an

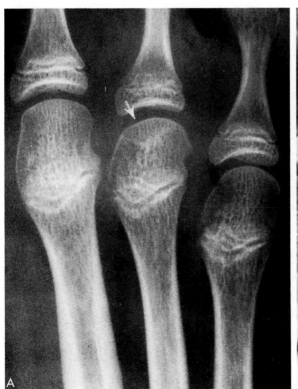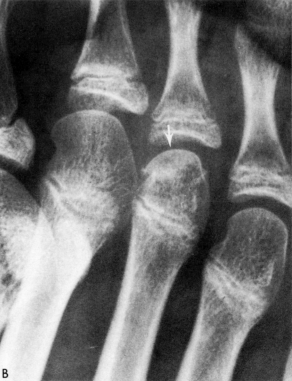

Figure 71–7. Freiberg's infraction: Early radiographic abnormalities. A An initial radiograph reveals minimal increased radiodensity of the head of the third metatarsal bone (arrow). **B** Two weeks later, the depression of the articular surface of the metatarsal head and the sclerosis are more apparent (arrow).

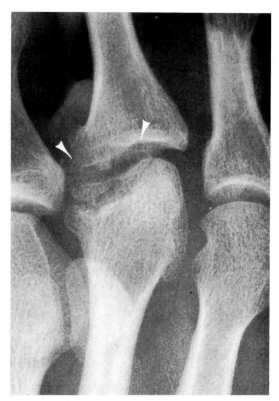

Figure 71–8. **Freiberg's infraction: Later radiographic abnormalities.** Note the flattened metatarsal head with two osteochondral fragments (arrowheads), osteophytosis, joint space narrowing, and widening of the phalangeal base.

increased density of the lunate bone is noted, followed by evidence of altered shape and diminished size of the bone (Fig. 71–10). Eventually the entire lunate may collapse and fragment. Complications include scapholunate separation, ulnar deviation of the triquetrum, and secondary degenerative joint disease in the radiocarpal and midcarpal compartments of the wrist.

The cause of the condition is not clear. Pathologic descriptions emphasize the occurrence of both fracture and osteonecrosis. Certain anatomic features may predispose the lunate to injury and subsequent osteonecrosis. These features include (1) a vulnerable blood supply, and (2) a fixed position in the wrist, resulting in forces that may be greater than those on neighboring carpal bones. Mechanical forces may be accentuated by the presence of a short ulna (ulna minus variant), a finding that can be encountered in as many as 75 per cent of cases.

In cases in which increased radiodensity and collapse of the lunate are observed, the radiographic features are easily differentiated from other conditions affecting the wrist.

Köhler's Disease

Köhler's disease of the tarsal navicular is relatively rare, although its exact frequency is difficult to determine because the symptoms and signs may not be of sufficient magnitude to require radiography, and it is impossible to distinguish the radiographic abnormalities from those that occur as a normal variation of growth. The disorder is more frequent in boys. Complaints, when present, are noted most commonly

between the ages of 3 and 7 years. Unilateral involvement is evident in approximately 75 to 80 per cent of cases.

Radiographs at an early stage can reveal patchy increase in density, nodularity, and fragmentation with multiple ossific nuclei (Fig. 71–11A). Soft tissue swelling may be evident. The bone may be diminished in size and flattened, yet the interosseous space between the navicular and neighboring bones can be normal (Fig. 71–11B). Over a period of 2 to 4 years the bone may regain its normal size, density, and trabecular structure. It is the self-limited and reversible nature of the process that has led to speculation that the "disease" is, in reality, an altered sequence of tarsal ossification. An apparent overlap with normal patterns of ossification leads to considerable difficulty in diagnosis, and certain criteria must be used in establishing the presence of Köhler's disease: (1) changes are detected in a previously normal navicular bone; (2) alterations consisting of resorption and reossification must be compatible with those of osteonecrosis. Furthermore, clinical manifestations should be present if the diagnosis is to be considered seriously.

There is evidence that Köhler's disease may have a mechanical basis. The location of the tarsal navicular at the apex of the longitudinal arch of the foot may lead to concentration of forces on this bone during normal locomotion. Compression of the bone nucleus at a critical phase of growth could result in altered ossification and osteonecrosis.

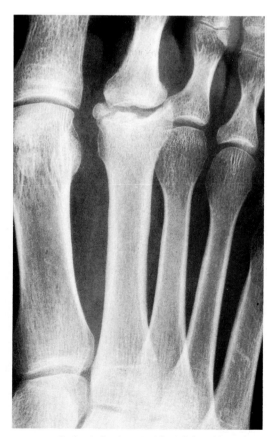

Figure 71–9. **Freiberg's infraction: Residual deformities.** Note residual flattening of the second metatarsal head, narrowing of the adjacent joint space, intraarticular osseous bodies, expansion of the phalangeal base, and widening of the second metatarsal with cortical thickening.

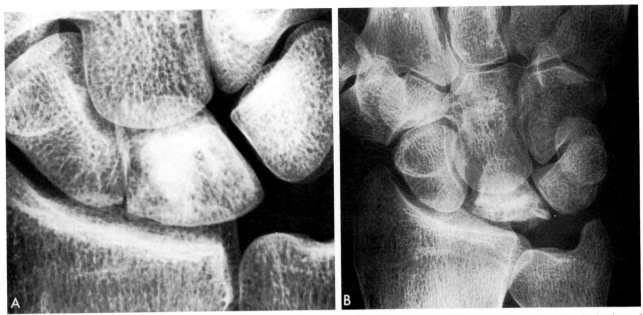

Figure 71–10. Kienböck's disease. A A magnification radiograph demonstrates patchy increased density of the lunate without alterations in the shape of the bone. **B** In a different patient, observe the collapse of a sclerotic lunate bone.

Panner's Disease

Panner's disease, or osteochondrosis of the capitulum of the humerus, is a rare disease that usually appears between the ages of 5 and 10 years. Boys are affected almost exclusively, and the condition commonly is linked to a history of trauma. It is sometimes termed "little-leaguer's elbow" because of its frequency in young baseball pitchers. Bilateral involvement is rare.

The clinical manifestations typically are mild, and complete recovery is frequent. Pain, tenderness, and restricted range of motion of the elbow are seen. Radiographs reveal fissuring and increased density of the capitulum, with fragmentation and resorption (Fig. 71–12). Regeneration of the capitulum is observed subsequently, and in most cases no residual deformity or disability is seen.

The detection of a subchondral radiolucent band in the capitulum in the early stages of the disorder is reminiscent of findings in Legg-Calvé-Perthes disease. It probably indicates that osteonecrosis has occurred as a secondary event related to a traumatic insult. The disease is differentiated from osteo-

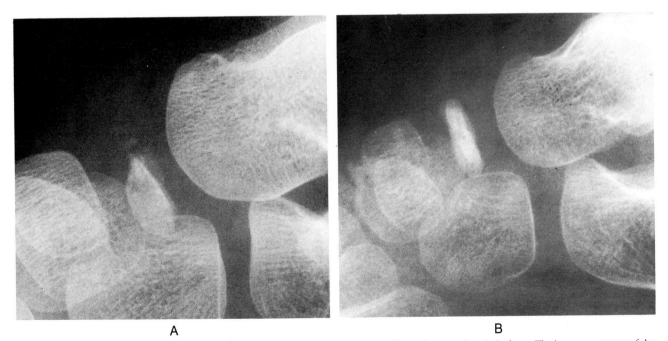

A   B

Figure 71–11. Köhler's disease. A A lateral radiograph reveals the small fragmented and slightly dense tarsal navicular bone. The interosseous spaces of the tarsus are not disturbed. **B** A wafer-like radiodense tarsal navicular bone is identified in a different child. Again, the neighboring joint spaces are not diminished in width.

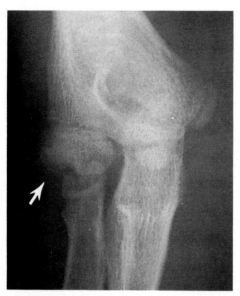

Figure 71–12. Panner's disease. Findings include fissuring and fragmentation of the capitulum (arrow) and deformity of the adjacent radial head in this child with elbow pain and swelling. (Courtesy of V. Vint, M.D., La Jolla, California.)

chondritis dissecans of the elbow principally on the basis of the age of the patient. Osteochondritis dissecans typically occurs in adolescents or adults at a time when ossification of the capitulum has been completed.

Thiemann's Disease

The principal clinical manifestations of Thiemann's disease are an onset in the second decade of life, a predilection for boys, painless swelling of proximal interphalangeal joints of the fingers, digital shortening, and deformity. Involvement of the metacarpophalangeal and tarsometatarsal joints and the interphalangeal articulations of the toes also has been noted in some cases. The disease usually is familial. A relationship to trauma has also been suggested, and the pathogenesis of the disease appears to be an osteonecrosis.

Radiographs reveal irregularity of the epiphyses of the phalanges, especially in the middle fingers. The epiphyses appear sclerotic and fragmented and may contain medial and lateral osseous excrescences (Fig. 71–13). Eventually, the joint space becomes narrowed, the base of the phalanx thickens, and phalangeal shortening is seen.

The differential diagnosis of the phalangeal alterations of Thiemann's disease includes trauma, infection, thermal injury, such as frostbite, other disorders associated with ischemic necrosis of bone, and additional congenital diseases.

DISORDERS RELATED TO TRAUMA OR ABNORMAL STRESS WITHOUT EVIDENCE OF OSTEONECROSIS

Osgood-Schlatter Disease

Osgood-Schlatter disease of the tibial tuberosity occurs in adolescents, usually between the ages of 11 and 15 years. Boys are affected more frequently than girls. Although the disease generally is unilateral in distribution, bilateral alterations are detected in approximately 25 per cent of cases. Clinically, patients usually have local pain and tenderness.

Soft tissue swelling and firm masses can be palpated in the involved region.

Radiographic abnormalities are well known. Initially, soft tissue swelling in front of the tuberosity results from edema of the skin and subcutaneous tissue (Fig. 71–14). The margins of the patellar tendon may be indistinct. If the tuberosity is entirely cartilaginous in structure, no change will be detected in it initially, but examination 3 or 4 weeks later may show ossific collections in the avulsed fragment (Fig. 71–15). In the older child in whom the ossification center has begun to develop, one or more foci of radiopacity can be recognized in the vicinity of the tubercle.

After the acute stage, soft tissue swelling diminishes, and displaced pieces of bone may increase in size or may reunite with each other and the underlying tibial tuberosity. Eventually, the radiographic appearance may revert to normal, although persistent ossific fragments frequently mark the site of previous disease.

The accurate diagnosis of this condition is based on both the radiographic and the clinical findings. A fragmented tuberosity, in the absence of current or previous symptoms, may indicate only a normal ossification pattern. Soft tissue swelling is fundamental to the radiographic diagnosis of Osgood-Schlatter disease.

In the past, Osgood-Schlatter disease was considered by some investigators to be an osteonecrosis. More recent studies, however, have indicated that the findings in this condition are most consistent with a traumatically induced disruption somewhere along the site of attachment of the patellar ligament to the tibial tuberosity. The normal tuberosity growth plate is not affected. Thus, premature closure of the physis of the tibial tuberosity with genu recurvatum is rare in this disease. Other reported complications of Osgood-Schlatter disease include nonunion of the bone fragment, patellar subluxation, chondromalacia, and avulsion of the patellar tendon.

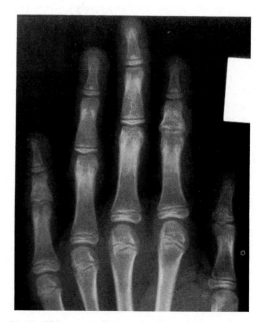

Figure 71–13. Thiemann's disease. A radiograph shows physeal closure and shortened middle phalanges in the second and fifth finger. The opposite side was similarly affected. (From Gewanter H, Baum J: Thiemann's disease. J Rheumatol 12:150, 1985. Used with permission.)

Blount's Disease

Blount's disease, tibia vara, or osteochondrosis deformans tibiae is a local disturbance of growth of the medial aspect of the proximal tibial epiphysis. The condition is classified into two types, an infantile type in which deformity is noted in the first few years of life, and an adolescent type in which deformity appears in children between the ages of 8 and 15 years (Table 71–4). The infantile type is approximately five to eight times more frequent than the adolescent variety.

INFANTILE TIBIA VARA. Infantile tibia vara appears to develop when normal physiologic bowing, rather than disappearing progressively to a straight leg or slight valgus position, persists and worsens when the growing child becomes heavier and begins to put weight on the knee joint. Mechanical factors that may contribute to infantile tibia vara include excessive body weight, walking at an early age, peculiarities in the manner in which children are carried on their mothers' backs, and abnormal articular laxity. Altered mechanical forces in the proximal tibia from various primary causes could result in a change of direction of weight-bearing forces on the upper tibial epiphysis and a tendency to displace the tibial epiphysis in a lateral direction.

Histologic examination confirms the absence of changes of infection or osteonecrosis. The microscopic findings are consistent with the effects of persistent abnormal pressure on the growth plate.

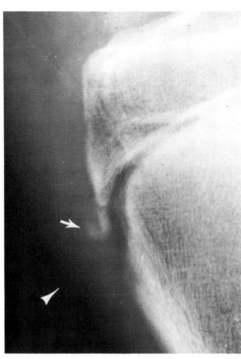

Figure 71–15. Osgood-Schlatter disease: Osseous abnormalities. Observe soft tissue swelling (arrowhead) and an avulsed osseous fragment of the tibial tuberosity (arrow).

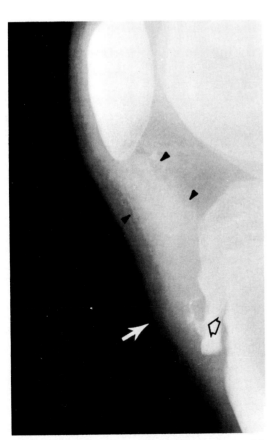

Figure 71–14. Osgood-Schlatter disease: Soft tissue abnormalities. Low KV radiography indicates soft tissue edema over the tibial tuberosity (solid arrow). Note indistinctness of the infrapatellar tendon (arrowheads) and osseous irregularity of the tuberosity (open arrow). (Courtesy of J. Weston, M.D., Lower Hutt, New Zealand.)

Clinically, progressive bilateral (60 per cent) or unilateral (40 per cent) bowing of the leg during the first year of life is difficult to differentiate from physiologic changes. The tibia may be angulated acutely inward just below the knee. Pain is not evident. Associated findings are obesity, shortening of the leg, tibial torsion, and pronated feet.

Radiographic abnormalities simulate those of physiologic bowing but are more severe. Furthermore, altered alignment in Blount's disease occurs in the proximal portion of the tibia, not between the femur and the tibia, as seen in physiologic bowing. In Blount's disease, the tibia is in varus position owing to angulation of the metaphysis, and the tibial shaft is adducted without intrinsic curvature. A depressed medial tibial metaphysis with an osseous excrescence or spur is seen. The changes have been divided into six stages (Figs. 71–16 and 71–17).

Stage I (2 to 3 Years). A progressive increase in the degree of varus deformity of the tibia is associated with irregularity of the entire growth plate. The medial part of the metaphysis protrudes with a medial and distal beak.

Stage II (2½ to 4 Years). A lateromedial depression of the ossification line of the medial portion of the metaphysis and a wedge-shaped medial end of the epiphysis are observed. Complete healing of the lesion is possible at this stage.

Stage III (4 to 6 Years). The cartilage-filled depression in the metaphyseal beak deepens. The medial part of the bone epiphysis remains wedge-shaped and is less distinct. Small calcific foci may be evident beneath the medial border.

Stage IV (5 to 10 Years). With increasing bone maturation, the cartilaginous growth plate is reduced to a narrow plate, and the bone epiphysis occupies an increasing part of the end of the bone. The medial margin of the epiphysis

Table 71–4. INFANTILE VERSUS ADOLESCENT TIBIA VARA

	Infantile	Adolescent
Age of onset	1–3 years	8–15 years
Distribution	Bilateral: 50–75%	Unilateral: 90%
Clinical findings	Obesity	Normal body weight
	Absent pain, tenderness	Pain and tenderness
	Prominent deformity	Mild deformity
	Slight leg shortening	Moderate, severe leg shortening
Etiology or pathogenesis	Trauma	Trauma
	Growth arrest or dysplasia	Growth arrest

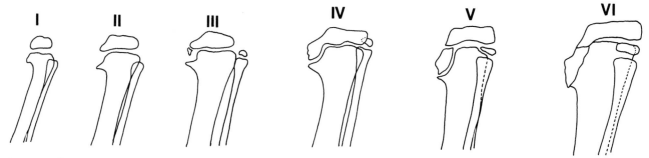

Figure 71–16. Blount's disease: Infantile tibia vara. Six stages of the disease (see text for details). (After Langenskiold A: Tibia vara. Osteochondrosis deformans tibiae. A survey of 23 cases. Acta Chir Scand *103*:1, 1952. Used with permission.)

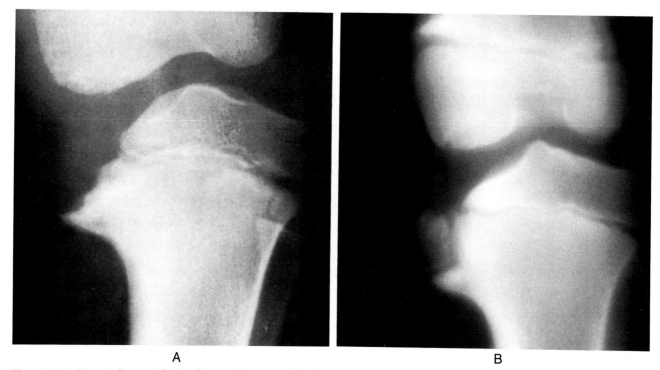

Figure 71–17. Blount's disease: Infantile tibia vara. Two stages of the disease are well illustrated in this child. **A** Stage II, at age 4 years. **B** Stage IV, at age 8½ years. (Courtesy of L. Danzig, M.D., Santa Ana, California.)

shows definite irregularity. Even at this stage, restoration of a relatively normal epiphysis can occur.

Stage V (9 to 11 Years). The bone epiphysis and the corresponding articular surface are greatly deformed. The epiphysis is separated in two portions by a clear band, extending medially from the lateral portion of the growth plate to the articular cartilage.

Stage VI (10 to 13 Years). The branches of the medially located double growth plate ossify, whereas growth continues in the normal lateral part. Stages V and VI represent phases of irreparable structural damage.

Lateral widening of the growth plate of the proximal tibia and, less frequently, the distal femur has been identified in infantile tibia vara; it may result from the chronic stress of the genu varum on the growth plates in the area of the knee.

ADOLESCENT TIBIA VARA. The less frequent adolescent form develops in children between the ages of 8 and 15 years. The cause is not clear, although an arrest of epiphyseal growth is suspected. A history of trauma or infection is elicited occasionally, and conventional tomography may indicate an osseous bridge between the epiphysis and metaphysis.

Unilateral alterations occur in approximately 90 per cent of cases. Leg shortening and mild to moderate varus deformity may be associated with pain and tenderness. Radiographs outline a proximal tibia that is angled about 10 to 20 degrees. The proximal tibial epiphysis reveals medial wedging, and the medial tibial growth plate is diminished in height (Fig. 71–18).

DIFFERENTIAL DIAGNOSIS. The radiographic abnormalities in infantile and adolescent tibia vara are usually diagnostic. Some difficulty is occasionally encountered in differentiating the infantile type from physiologic bowed legs, and serial radiographs may be necessary (Fig. 71–19). Metaphyseal alterations and bowing in Blount's disease may also simulate findings in rickets.

Scheuermann's Disease

Scheuermann's disease is a disorder of the spine, leading to lower thoracic kyphosis. On the basis of irregularities involving the rims of the vertebral bodies, early investigators suggested that the disease was related to osteonecrosis; considerable disagreement as to the cause and pathogenesis of this disorder subsequently developed, however. Debate also existed regarding the criteria necessary for the diagnosis of Scheuermann's disease. Currently used criteria frequently require the presence of abnormalities of at least three contiguous vertebrae, each with wedging of 5 degrees or more. Such criteria are not ideal, as they exclude those cases of Scheuermann's disease that are associated predominantly with vertebral irregularity without wedging.

Because of the discrepancies in the criteria used to diagnose juvenile kyphosis, a precise rate of occurrence is difficult to define. Most affected persons are between the ages of 13 and 17 years; the disorder is unusual before the age of 10 years.

CLINICAL ABNORMALITIES. Clinical manifestations are highly variable. In some persons the disease is totally asymptomatic; in others fatigue, defective posture, aching pain aggravated by physical exertion, and tenderness to palpation are encountered. Kyphotic deformity, which may be associated with mild scoliosis, predominates in the thoracic region (75 per cent of patients), although it may be observed

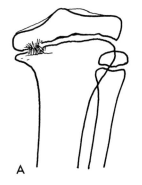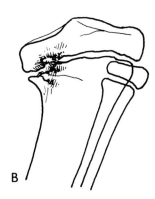

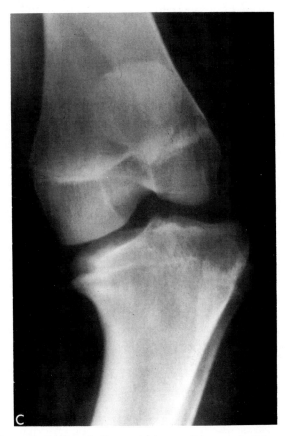

Figure 71–18. Blount's disease: Adolescent tibia vara. A, B Stages of the process. Observe fusion of the medial aspect of the growth plate with progressive sclerosis and varus deformity. (After Langenskiold A: Tibia vara. Osteochondrosis deformans tibiae. A survey of 23 cases. Acta Chir Scand 103:1, 1952. Used with permission.) C An example of adolescent tibia vara. Note varus deformity, depression of the articular surface of the medial tibial plateau, sclerosis, and osteophyte formation.

in the thoracolumbar or lumbar segments. A dorsal kyphosis is frequently combined with an exaggerated lumbar and cervical lordosis. The deformity may be correctable initially, but it may become progressively more fixed in position. Neurologic complaints are not common.

RADIOGRAPHIC AND PATHOLOGIC ABNORMALITIES. On radiographs, an undulant superior and inferior surface of affected vertebral bodies is associated with intraosseous radiolucent zones of variable size (cartilaginous or Schmorl's nodes), with surrounding sclerosis (Figs. 71–20

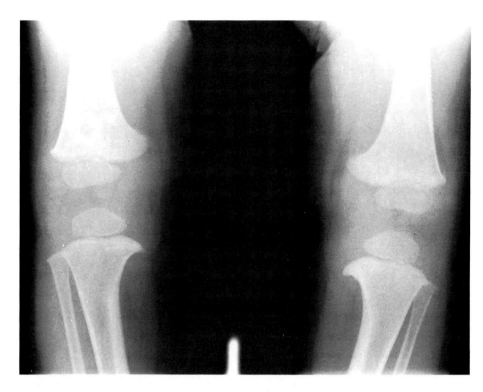

Figure 71–19. **Physiologic bowed legs.** Note the gradual varus curvature of the knees in this child. There is no evidence of a proximal tibial step-off or varus deformity.

and 71–21). The degree of osseous irregularity is variable, but when severe can be accompanied by loss of intervertebral disc height and wedging of the anterior portion of the vertebral bodies. The degree of thoracic kyphosis also is variable; the kyphotic curvature usually develops slowly.

Anteriorly extruded disc material may extend beneath the apophyseal centers of ossification. Under these circumstances, a portion of the proximal or distal ring-like apophyseal centers of ossification may be separated from the vertebral body, producing a limbus vertebra (Fig. 71–21*B*). Furthermore, discal tissue beneath the anterior longitudinal ligament can produce pressure erosion on the adjacent anterior surface of the vertebral body. Ossification of the anterior portions of the intervertebral disc can lead to synostosis of one vertebral body with its neighbor.

In addition to thoracic kyphosis, scoliosis located at approximately the same level as the kyphosis may be observed. A second pattern of scoliosis occurs in regions of compensatory lordosis situated above or below the kyphosis.

ETIOLOGY AND PATHOGENESIS. Cartilaginous node formation is fundamental to the disease process. The precise cause of these nodes, however, is not clear. It has been suggested that congenital weakness of the endplates predisposes certain persons to intraosseous discal prolapse during periods of excessive physical stress. It has been further suggested that the cartilaginous node is simply an endplate fracture resulting from failure under dynamic load in compression or shear, at a time when the plate and the metaphysis are vulnerable as a result of rapid growth. A familial occurrence of the disease may reflect genetically determined defects in vertebral strength.

DIFFERENTIAL DIAGNOSIS. Cartilaginous nodes can accompany any disease process that weakens the cartilaginous endplate or subchondral bone of the vertebral body, allowing intraosseous discal displacement. A partial list of such processes includes trauma, neoplasm, metabolic disorders (hyper-

parathyroidism, osteoporosis, Paget's disease), infection, intervertebral osteochondrosis, and articular disorders (rheumatoid arthritis). Accurate radiographic diagnosis of these conditions is based on additional spinal and extraspinal manifestations. The combination of kyphosis, cartilaginous nodes, and irregular vertebral outlines is virtually pathognomonic of Scheuermann's disease. Kyphosis of other causes, such as tuberculosis, and postural, osteoporotic, and senile kyphosis can be eliminated by the absence of these characteristic radiologic findings. Occasionally the spinal abnormalities in certain congenital or inherited disorders, such as the mucopolysaccharidoses and Turner's syndrome, can simulate those of Scheuermann's disease.

Sinding-Larsen-Johansson Disease

Sinding-Larsen-Johansson disease occurs most commonly in an adolescent between 10 and 14 years of age, and consists of tenderness and soft tissue swelling over the lower pole of the patella, accompanied by radiographic evidence of osseous fragmentation. The lesion is probably related to a traction phenomenon in which contusion or tendinitis in the proximal attachment of the patellar tendon can be followed by calcification and ossification, or in which patellar fracture or avulsion produces one or more distinct ossification sites. The association of fragmentation of the inferior portion of the patella with spastic paralysis is consistent with this traction phenomenon. Similar findings are observed in athletes, in whom the term "jumper's knee" has been applied.

In Sinding-Larsen-Johansson disease, radiographs reveal small bone fragments adjacent to the distal surface of the patella with overlying soft tissue swelling (Fig. 71–22). The radiodense areas may subsequently become incorporated into the patella, eventually yielding a normal radiographic appearance. The natural duration of the disease is approximately 3 to 12 months.

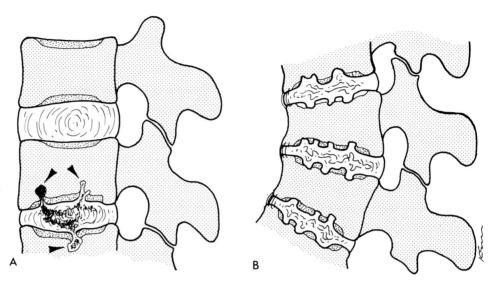

Figure 71–20. Scheuermann's disease. The underlying abnormality relates to intraosseous displacement of disc material (cartilaginous nodes) through the cartilaginous endplates (arrowheads). This produces radiolucent lesions of the vertebral bodies with surrounding sclerosis, intervertebral disc space narrowing, and irregularity of vertebral contour. Kyphosis may appear.

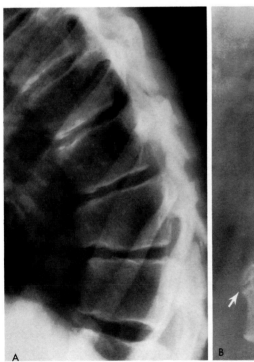

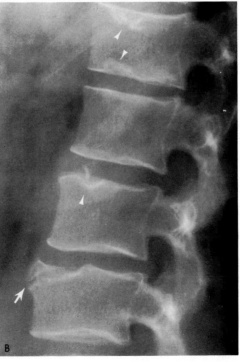

Figure 71–21. Scheuermann's disease. A Thoracic spine. Findings include irregularity of vertebral contour, reactive sclerosis, intervertebral disc space narrowing, anterior vertebral wedging, and kyphosis. B Lumbar spine. Observe the cartilaginous nodes (arrowheads) creating surface irregularity, lucent areas, and reactive sclerosis. An anterior discal displacement (arrow) has produced an irregular anterosuperior corner of a vertebral body, the limbus vertebra.

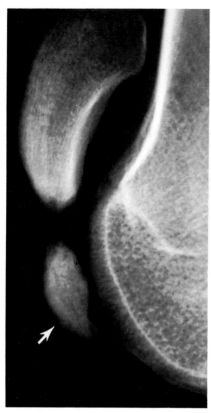

Figure 71–22. Sinding-Larsen-Johansson disease. In this patient with spastic paralysis, observe fragmentation of the lower pole of the patella (arrow) related to abnormal stress.

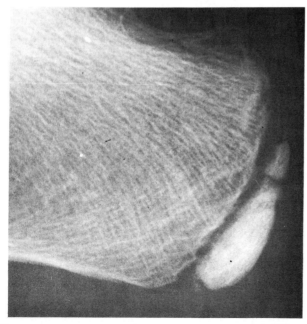

Figure 71–23. Sever's disease. An example of sclerosis of the secondary calcaneal ossification center is illustrated. This is a normal consequence of weight-bearing.

Patellar fragmentation may also represent a normal variation of ossification or the presence of accessory ossification centers.

"DISORDERS" DUE TO VARIATIONS IN OSSIFICATION

Sever's Disease

Irregularity of the secondary calcaneal ossification center is a normal variation unrelated to the painful heels of adolescents. Indeed, fragmentation and sclerosis of the secondary ossification center of the calcaneus (Fig. 71–23) are the result of proper weight-bearing. Such osseous changes may be absent in patients who are immobilized as a result of neurogenic disease or fracture.

Ischiopubic Osteochondrosis

A lesion consisting of rarefaction and swelling of the ischiopubic synchondrosis and the neighboring bone was originally described as an osteochondritis. This condition is now regarded as a common, normal pattern of ossification. The time of closure of the synchondrosis is somewhat variable; it usually takes place between the ages of 9 and 11 years.

Table 71–5. THE OSTEOCHONDROSES

Year Reported	Investigator(s)	Location of Lesion
1887	Koenig	Osteochondritis dissecans
1903	Osgood; Schlatter	Tibial tubercle
1908	Köhler	Primary patellar center
1908	Haglund	Os tibiale externum
1908	Köhler	Tarsal navicular
1909	Thiemann	Phalangeal bases
1910	Legg; Calvé; Perthes	Femoral epiphysis
1910	Kienböck	Carpal lunate
1911	Preiser	Carpal scaphoid
1912	Sever	Calcaneal apophysis
1912	Iselin	Fifth metatarsal base
1914	Freiberg	Second metatarsal head
1921	Hass	Head of humerus
1921	Burns	Lower ulna
1921	Scheuermann	Vertebral apophysis
1921	Sinding-Larsen	Secondary patellar center
1922	Mandl	Greater trochanter
1924	Friedrich	Medial end of clavicle
1924	Van Neck	Ischiopubic synchondrosis
1925	Calvé	Vertebral body
1927	Panner	Capitulum of humerus
1927	Mauclaire	Heads of metacarpals
1927	Buchman	Iliac crest
1928	Diaz	Talus
1929	Pierson	Symphysis pubis
1932	Dietrich	Heads of metacarpals
1937	Blount	Medial proximal tibia
1945	Caffey	Entire carpus bilaterally
1950	Liffert and Arkin	Distal tibial center
1953	Milch	Ischial apophysis
1956	Caffey	Tibial spines

After Brower AC: The osteochondroses. Orthop Clin North Am 14:99, 1983. Used with permission.

The differential diagnosis of this normal variant includes a stress fracture, posttraumatic osteolysis, and infection.

MISCELLANEOUS DISORDERS

Osteochondroses have been described in almost every epiphysis and apophysis in the body (Table 71–5). In most cases, boys are affected more frequently than girls, alterations rarely develop before the age of 3 years or after the age of 12 years, and developmental irregularities in ossification can be encountered at many of the same skeletal sites. Other sites of osteochondroses include the primary ossification center of the patella, greater trochanter, acetabular roof, proximal tibial epiphysis, distal tibial epiphysis, talus, os tibiale externum, cuneiforms, epiphysis of the fifth metatarsal bone, proximal epiphysis of the hallux, humeral head, trochlea, ulnar olecranon process, distal ulnar epiphysis, heads of the metacarpals, radial head, iliac crest, ischial apophysis, and symphysis pubis. In many instances, the pathogenesis of the osseous fragmentation and sclerosis is not clear, although alterations owing to stress or variations of normal ossification appear likely at certain locations.

FURTHER READING

Alexander CJ: Scheuermann's disease. A traumatic spondylodystrophy? Skel Radiol 1:209, 1977.

Arie E, Johnson F, Harrison MHM, Hughes JR, Small P: Femoral head shape in Perthes' disease. Is the contralateral hip abnormal? Clin Orthop 209:77, 1986.

Bateson EM: The relationship between Blount's disease and bow legs. Br J Radiol 41:107, 1968.

Braddock GTF: Experimental epiphyseal injury and Freiberg's disease. J Bone Joint Surg [Br] 41:154, 1959.

Caffey J: The early roentgenographic changes in essential coxa plana; their significance in pathogenesis. AJR 103:620, 1968.

Caffey J, Ross SE: The ischiopubic synchondrosis in healthy children: Some normal roentgenologic findings. AJR 76:488, 1956.

Catterall A: The natural history of Perthes' disease. J Bone Joint Surg [Br] 53:37, 1971.

Catterall A: Legg-Calvé-Perthes Disease. Edinburgh, Churchill Livingstone, 1982.

Christensen F, Soballe K, Ejsted R, Luxhoj T: The Catterall classification of Perthes' disease: An assessment of reliability. J Bone Joint Surg [Br] 68:614, 1986.

Clarke NMP, Harrison MHM, Keret D: The sagging rope sign: A critical appraisal. J Bone Joint Surg [Br] 65:285, 1983.

Cullen JC: Thiemann's disease. Osteochondrosis juvenilis of the basal epiphyses of the phalanges of the hand. Report of two cases. J Bone Joint Surg [Br] 52:532, 1970.

Freiberg AH: Infraction of the second metatarsal bone; a typical injury. Surg Gynecol Obstet 19:191, 1914.

Gelberman RH, Salamon PB, Jurist JM, Posch JL: Ulnar variance in Kienböck's disease. J Bone Joint Surg [Am] 57:674, 1975.

Goldman AB, Hallel T, Salvati EM, Freiberger RH: Osteochondritis dissecans complicating Legg-Perthes disease. A report of four cases. Radiology 121:561, 1976.

Herring JA, Lundeen MA, Wenger DR: Minimal Perthes' disease. J Bone Joint Surg [Br] 62:25, 1980.

Hulting B: Roentgenologic features of fracture of the tibial tuberosity (Osgood-Schlatter's disease). Acta Radiol 48:161, 1957.

Kaye JJ, Freiberger RH: Fragmentation of the lower pole of the patella in spastic lower extremities. Radiology 101:97, 1971.

Klein EW: Osteochondrosis of the capitulum (Panner's disease). Report of a case. AJR 88:466, 1952.

Langenskiöld A, Riska EB: Tibia vara (osteochondrosis deformans tibiae). J Bone Joint Surg [Am] 46:1405, 1964.

McCauley RGK, Kahn PC: Osteochondritis of the tarsal navicula. Radioisotopic appearances. Radiology 123:705, 1977.

Melo-Gomes JA, Melo-Gomes E, Viana-Queiros M: Thiemann's disease. J Rheumatol 8:462, 1981.

Murphy RP, Marsh HO: Incidence and natural history of "head at risk" factors in Perthes' disease. Clin Orthop 132:102, 1978.

Ogden JA: Radiology of postnatal skeletal development. X. Patella and tibial tuberosity. Skel Radiol 11:246, 1984.

Osgood RB: Lesions of the tibial tubercle occurring during adolescence. Boston Med Surg J 148:114, 1903.

Ozonoff MB: Pediatric Orthopedic Radiology. Philadelphia, WB Saunders Co, 1979.

Panner HJ: An affection of the capitulum humeri resembling Calvé-Perthes disease of the hip. Acta Radiol 8:617, 1927.

Rush BH, Bramson RT, Ogden JA: Legg-Calvé-Perthes disease: Detection of cartilaginous and synovial changes with MR imaging. Radiology 167:473, 1988.

Schmorl G, Junghanns H: The Human Spine in Health and Disease. Translated by EF Besemann. 2nd Ed. New York, Grune & Stratton 1971.

Scoles PV, Yoon YS, Makley JT, Kalamchi A: Nuclear magnetic resonance imaging in Legg-Calvé-Perthes disease. J Bone Joint Surg [Am] 66:1357, 1984.

Shopfner CE, Coin CG: Effect of weight-bearing on the appearance and development of the secondary calcaneal epiphysis. Radiology 86:201, 1966.

Siffert RS: Classification of the osteochondroses. Clin Orthop 158:10, 1981.

Silverman FN: Lesions of the femoral neck in Legg-Perthes disease. AJR 144:1249, 1985.

Sinding-Larsen MF: A hitherto unknown affection of the patella in children. Acta Radiol 1:171, 1921.

Spragge JW: Legg-Calvé-Perthes disease. In RH Freiberger et al (Eds): Hip Disease of Infancy and Childhood. Curr Probl Radiol 3:30, 1973.

Ståhl F: On lunatomalacia (Kienböck's disease). A clinical and roentgenological study, especially on its pathogenesis and the late results of immobilization treatment. Acta Chir Scand Suppl 126:1, 1947.

Wolinski AP, McCall IW, Evans G, Park WM: Femoral neck growth deformity following the irritable hip syndrome. Br J Radiol 57:773, 1984.

SECTION XIII

CONGENITAL DISORDERS

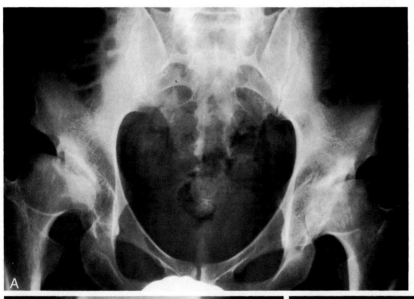

CASE XIII

LEVEL OF DIFFICULTY: 2

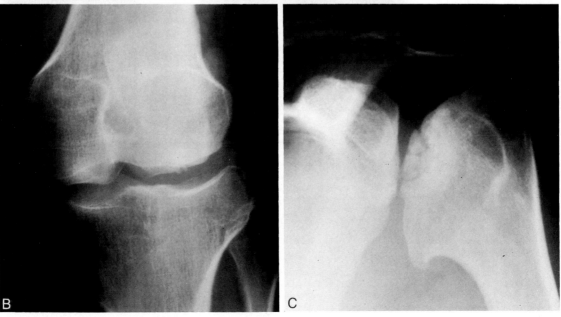

This 26 year old man had pain and restricted motion of multiple joints that had begun in late childhood or adolescence and had progressed in recent years. Physical examination revealed short stature, normal intelligence, and a waddling gait.

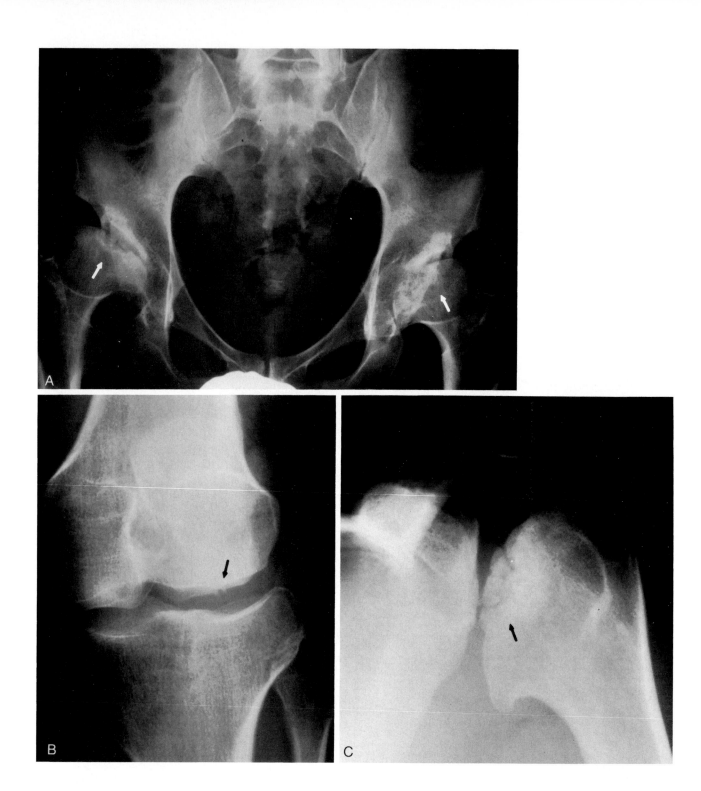

Radiographs of the pelvis (A), knee (B) and shoulder (C) reveal abnormalities of multiple epiphyses, consisting of osseous flattening and fragmentation (arrows). The femoral heads are deformed, and the acetabula are shallow and irregular. The articular surfaces of the femur and tibia also are irregular, with osseous hypoplasia, particularly in the lateral aspect of the articulation. Depression and fragmentation of the humeral head are accompanied by bone sclerosis and osteophyte formation, and the scapular neck appears hypoplastic. The joint spaces themselves are remarkably preserved in most locations.

The occurrence of abnormalities of multiple joints that begin in childhood or adolescence requires that juvenile chronic arthritis or hemophilia be given diagnostic consideration. In certain types of juvenile chronic arthritis, involvement of large joints of the appendicular skeleton can be prominent, and an irregular or crenated appearance of the epiphyses is encountered. Joint space narrowing usually is more prominent in long-standing juvenile chronic arthritis than is demonstrated in the test case, however, and osteoporosis and epiphyseal overgrowth frequently are prominent. Hemophilia most typically involves the knees, ankles, and elbows. Although hip and glenohumeral joint abnormalities resembling those shown in the test case are seen, such abnormalities are infrequent, and hypoplasia and deformity of periarticular bone, as in the scapula and acetabula, would not be expected.

Careful attention to the morphology of the altered epiphyses in the test case reveals findings consistent with ischemic necrosis of bone, particularly in the femoral and humeral epiphyses. Although sickle cell anemia and other hemoglobinopathies and Gaucher's disease may lead to osteonecrosis in young patients, additional skeletal abnormalities would be expected. Classically, in osteonecrosis, isolated involvement of a portion of the epiphyseal surface, such as the superolateral aspect of the femoral head, is evident, and abnormalities of the entire epiphysis, as seen in the humeral head, would not be expected.

Hypothyroidism may lead to maldevelopment of multiple epiphyses, a process termed epiphyseal dysgenesis. Patients with hypothyroidism are mentally retarded, however, and osteoporosis and a widened femoral neck may be seen. Additional diagnostic considerations include the mucopolysaccharidoses, Stickler's syndrome, and other dysplasias. Many of these conditions are accompanied by clinical and laboratory features that ensure accurate diagnosis.

The radiographic features illustrated in Case XIII are most compatible with the diagnosis of dysplasia epiphysealis multiplex, or multiple epiphyseal dysplasia. These terms are used to describe a heterogeneous group of disorders in which defective bone formation becomes evident in the secondary ossification centers of the tubular bones and sometimes the vertebrae. Epiphyseal dysplasias may affect many different regions of the skeleton or one or two sites, leading to difficulties in accurate classification and diagnosis.

Dysplasia epiphysealis multiplex is considered the prototype of the epiphyseal dysplasias, although it is characterized by genetic heterogeneity, with examples of autosomal dominant or autosomal recessive inheritance, as well as spontaneous mutation. Typically, it occurs in boys and girls with approximately equal frequency and has its onset in childhood. The most frequent sites of involvement are the hips, shoulders, knees, ankles, and wrists. Pain, disturbances of gait, and restricted motion are common clinical manifestations. The patients are of short stature and have normal intelligence.

Radiographic abnormalities become evident in the first few years of life. The distribution and extent of involvement are extremely variable, however. The secondary centers of ossification appear late and ossify in an irregular fashion. They may be small in size or flattened. Incongruity of apposing articular surfaces leads to maldevelopment, as in the acetabula and scapula, and premature osteoarthritis eventually may become evident.

In certain stages of the disease, the radiographic abnormalities resemble those of ischemic necrosis of bone, with fragmented and irregular epiphyseal centers and intraarticular osseous bodies. A symmetric distribution, predominant involvement of the hips, knees, wrists, and ankles, and evidence of hypoplasia of bone are useful diagnostic features. Spinal alterations, which resemble those of Scheuermann's disease, are evident in approximately two thirds of cases and differ from the more severe abnormalities that become apparent in spondyloepiphyseal dysplasias.

FINAL DIAGNOSIS: Dysplasia epiphysealis multiplex (multiple epiphyseal dysplasia).

FURTHER READING

Pages 1027–1030 and the following:

1. Koslowski K, Lipska E: Hereditary dysplasia epiphysealis multiplex. Clin Radiol *18*:330, 1967.
2. Berg PK: Dysplasia epiphysealis multiplex. AJR 97:31, 1966.

(Case XIII, courtesy of V. Vint, M.D., San Diego, California.)

Chapter 72

Congenital Dysplasia of the Hip

David J. Sartoris, M.D.
John A. Ogden, M.D.

Congenital deformity of both sides of the hip joint (dysplasia) may be present at birth or become apparent months to years later. Early diagnosis and treatment are crucial in preventing severe long-term structural abnormalities. Three patterns of subluxation or dislocation are seen. Diagnostic methods include the Ortolani and Barlow maneuvers in newborn infants and analysis of radiologic lines drawn on anteroposterior views of the hip and pelvis. Conventional tomography, contrast arthrography, ultrasonography, computed tomography, and magnetic resonance imaging also are valuable for the evaluation of this disease.

Congenital dysplasia of the hip (CDH) is a disease with extremely variable morphologic patterns. Although detection of CDH at birth by appropriate neonatal clinical and radiographic examinations and immediate inception of treatment are desirable, the diagnosis is missed in many children, who subsequently come to medical attention for evaluation and treatment at several months to years of age. At any stage of initial diagnosis, regardless of age, the primary goal is to delineate the specific pathologic morphology to direct the most appropriate treatment.

Subluxation and dislocation of the developing hip represent arbitrary definitions of static stages within a spectrum of dynamic morphologic alterations that are often insidious in onset and subtle in initial clinical and radiographic presentation. External factors, whether antenatal or postnatal, may have a significant role in the progressive deformation that inexorably occurs if the condition is not recognized clinically and radiographically. Such factors may be breech presentation, anteversion of the femur, and contractures of the hip joint. Unfortunately, during the neonatal period, when prompt diagnosis should be accomplished, routine radiography of the chondroosseous hip has significant limitations.

ETIOLOGY

The cause and pathogenesis of CDH are controversial and not completely understood. Although commonly used terminology implies that the dislocation occurs prenatally, most dislocations probably occur after birth. The factors predisposing to this situation, however, are unquestionably present in utero. The complex of musculoligamentous, capsular, carti-laginous, and osseous alterations that follow the dislocation are thought to be secondary effects and not causative.

Some investigators contend that instability, partial dislocation (subluxation) and complete dislocation exist as a continuum, with one form passing to another under appropriate conditions, whereas other researchers maintain that subluxation and dislocation are discrete fixed entities. Pathophysiologically, abnormal laxity rather than structural abnormality is most likely responsible for CDH. Increased laxity of the hip and other joints is seen in many patients with CDH as well as otherwise normal members of their families. There may also be a hormonal effect induced by maternal estrogen that is not completely inactivated by the immature fetal liver.

Although in the great majority of cases no other family members besides the patient have the disease, heritable factors are important. The risk for normal parents of a child with CDH to have another affected child is about 6 per cent; if one parent is also affected, the risk increases to 36 per cent. The risk to a patient's own children is estimated to be 12 per cent.

The etiologic role of anatomic variation in the acetabulum or femoral neck is controversial. The acetabulum tends to become shallower and the femoral head more hemispherical during fetal life, a situation that could promote dislocation, and the parents of children with CDH are found to have diminished acetabular coverage. Of great importance is the role that the usual intrauterine position of hip flexion plays in maintaining proper position of the femoral head. Both extreme flexion with knee extension (assumed with some breech positions) and sudden extension during birth tend to

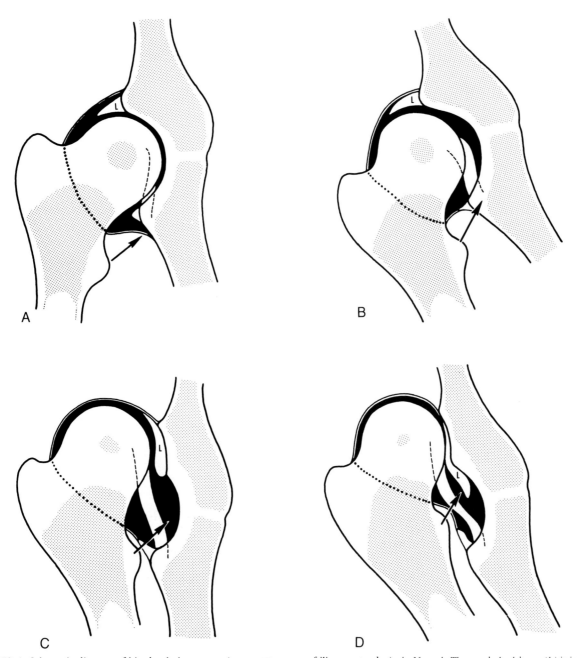

Figure 72–1. Schematic diagram of hip dysplasia patterns (arrows = course of iliopsoas tendon). A, Normal. The acetabular labrum *(L)* is in everted position. **B** Type 1. Positionally unstable or subluxatable hip. The pliable labrum *(L)* may be slightly deformed. **C** Type 2. Subluxated hip, with eversion of the fibrocartilaginous labrum *(L)* which may exhibit some inversion. This hip may be reduced relatively easily in flexion. **D** Type 3. Dislocated hip, with inversion and hypertrophy of the labrum *(L)*, which presents an impediment to reduction

promote femoral head dislocation. The hyperflexion of breech presentation leads also to shortening and contracture of the iliopsoas muscle, which tends to perpetuate femoral displacement.

Prenatal and postnatal pathologic patterns of the hip can be classified into three major groups (Fig. 72–1). Type 1 is the most common group and corresponds to the dislocatable, unstable hip. Anatomic alterations include a slight increase in femoral anteversion and mild marginal abnormalities in the acetabular cartilage with early labral eversion. Type 2 includes the partially dislocated or subluxed hip, characterized by loss of femoral head sphericity, increased femoral anteversion, early labral eversion with hypertrophy, and a shallow acetabulum. In type 3, accentuated flattening of the femoral head and acetabulum occur, with inward growth and hypertrophy of the labrum (so-called limbus formation). Conventional radiography is relatively insensitive to these changes until acetabular ossification is advanced.

The concept of the dislocatable or unstable (type 1) hip is important clinically. Such instability is estimated to occur in from 0.25 to 0.85 per cent of all newborn infants. More than 60 per cent of these hips, however, will become stable when reexamined by Ortolani or Barlow maneuvers within 1 week of birth, and 88 per cent are stable by the age of 2 months. Thus, the vast majority of hips noted to be dislocatable at birth will not be persistently dislocated. As it is not possible to predict which of these will become stable spontaneously, all are treated conventionally to prevent established dislocation.

Although most dislocations occur during the first 2 weeks after birth, occasionally a dislocation will occur up to 1 year of age in patients documented to be previously normal. There is also evidence that rare late initial dislocations occur during childhood.

EPIDEMIOLOGY

Female infants are affected by hip dislocation approximately eight times more frequently than male infants. Among affected infants, breech deliveries are six times more frequent than vertex presentations. CDH is significantly more common among white than among black newborns.

Nearly two thirds of infants with hip instability are firstborn, suggesting that the maternal uterus and abdominal wall in a primigravida are more confining and thus perpetuate abnormal stresses on the developing hip joint. The position of the fetus within the uterus and the relationship between the two legs may account for the 11:1:4 ratio of left to right to bilateral hip involvement.

CLINICAL DETECTION

The most reliable methods for diagnosing CDH in the neonatal period are clinical: the Ortolani and Barlow maneuvers. Basically the Ortolani test assesses proximal femoral reduction into the acetabulum by progressive abduction of the hip. The Barlow test is the reverse—the proximal portion of the femur is displaced by progressive adduction. These tests are positive for only a few days after birth. During the first year, certain clinical findings become more obvious in the child with undiagnosed CDH. Anatomically, the surrounding soft tissues and chondroosseous components gradually adapt to the abnormal relationship between the femoral head and the acetabulum. Reduction of the femoral head

becomes progressively more difficult, and results of the Ortolani and Barlow tests become negative. Major muscle groups become shortened and contracted; adductor muscle tightness becomes increasingly apparent.

DIAGNOSTIC IMAGING EVALUATION
Conventional Radiography

NEONATAL PERIOD. If the hip is unstable or has dislocated postnatally, conventional radiography in neutral and frog-leg projections will be unrevealing. Both of these positions may reduce a dislocatable hip and result in an erroneous impression of normality. The pelvis will similarly be normal as no secondary alterations in the osseous acetabulum will have occurred.

Radiologic confirmation of dislocation is not mandatory prior to initiation of treatment in clinically positive cases. A positive radiograph can, however, be obtained by applying a dislocating Ortolani or Barlow maneuver during the exposure (Fig. 72–2A). A dislocation-promoting position has also been described in which the legs are abducted to at least 45 degrees with simultaneous forced internal rotation. A line drawn along the axis of the femoral shaft in a nondislocated hip will pass through the upper edge of the acetabulum and cross the midline at the lumbosacral junction. In a dislocated hip, this line will intersect the anterosuperior iliac spine and traverse the midline in the lumbar region. The abduction–internal rotation position can on occasion lead to spontaneous hip reduction and a false negative finding (Fig. 72–2B, C). Assessment of the relationship of the femoral head to the acetabulum in the neonate is complicated by the fact that the ossification center is not yet visible, hence its position must be inferred from the orientation of the femoral metaphysis (Fig. 72–3). The femoral shaft should be located below a horizontal line drawn through the Y synchondroses, and the apex of the metaphysis should lie medial to the edge of the acetabulum. The cartilaginous femoral epiphysis is slightly larger than the neck segment on which it rests. Hence, if a circle with diameter equivalent to the width of the femoral metaphysis is drawn on the shaft, the position of the epiphysis relative to the acetabulum can be estimated. Fat planes along the labrum and the edge of the joint capsule also help to delineate the position of the cartilaginous epiphysis.

CHILDHOOD PERIOD. Secondary capsular, ligamentous, muscular, and cartilaginous changes occur soon after persistent dislocation has been established. These abnormalities are extremely important to therapeutic decision making and prognosis but are occult radiologically. Early positive conventional radiographic findings imply that substantial cartilage and soft tissue deformation has already occurred. The earliest time at which the radiologic changes of a typical dislocated hip on a single radiograph can be recognized reliably is approximately 6 weeks of age.

As the child grows, the adaptive changes of the hip joint and femur become more evident on the routine radiograph. The characteristic findings include (1) proximal and lateral migration of the femoral neck adjacent to the ilium, (2) a shallow, incompletely developed acetabulum (acetabular dysplasia), (3) development of a false acetabulum, and (4) delayed ossification of the femoral ossific nucleus (Fig. 72–3 to 72–5). Several radiologic lines have been described to distinguish between the normal and the dislocated hip (Fig. 72–6). The lines are drawn on an anteroposterior view of the pelvis and

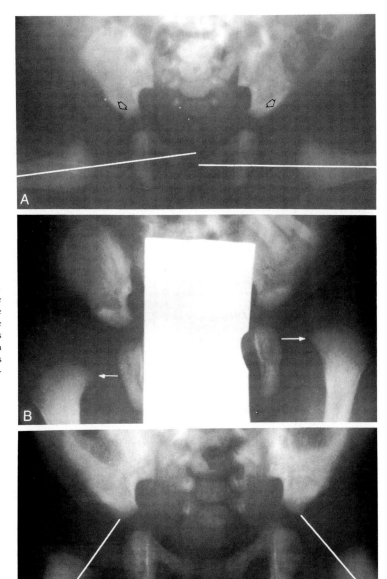

Figure 72–2 Bilateral type I congenital dysplasia of the hip. **A** On a radiograph with the hips in an Ortolani position, absence of femoral head ossification and shallow acetabula (arrows) are evident, as well as symmetric malalignment. White lines indicate femoral shaft axes. **B** Lateralization of both femora (arrows) is demonstrated with the joints in neutral position. **C** On an abduction–internal rotation (Von Rosen) view, alignment is normal (femoral shaft axes indicated by white lines pass symmetrically through the acetabula), indicating bilateral reduction.

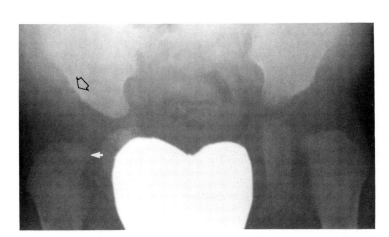

Figure 72–3. Type I congenital dysplasia of the hip. The right femur is slightly lateralized (white arrow), in association with subtle flattening of the lateral acetabular margin (black arrow).

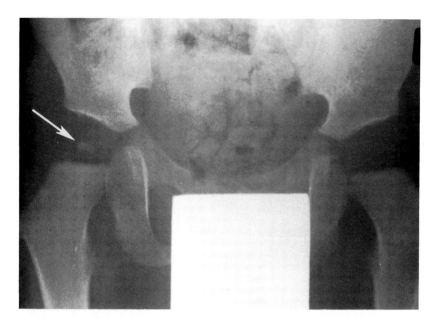

Figure 72–4. Type I congenital dysplasia of the hip. Delayed development of the left femoral head ossification center is evident by comparison to the normal right side (arrow).

hips. Accurate positioning is critical; the hips must be extended, with the lower extremities normally aligned and in neutral rotation. Abnormal position can considerably alter the diagnostic value of the lines.

The radiologic lines that have been found to be the most reliable and helpful in the diagnosis of CDH are summarized as follows:

1. The *acetabular index or angle* (Fig. 72–7) is a measurement of the apparent slope of the acetabular roof, which averages 27.5 degrees in newborn infants. The upper limit of normal is 30 degrees; a measurement greater than this strongly suggests acetabular dysplasia.

2. Lateral migration of the femoral head is measured by using the horizontal *line of Hilgenreiner* (through the triradiate

cartilage) and its intersection with *Perkin's line* (a vertical line drawn downward from the lateral rim of the acetabulum). The intersection of these two lines divides the hip joint into quadrants. The femoral ossific nucleus, if present, or medial beak of the femoral metaphysis is within the inner lower quadrant if the hip is normal, but in the upper outer quadrant if the hip is dislocated.

3. Proximal migration of the femur is measured by observing the shortening of the vertical distance from the femoral ossific nucleus or the femoral metaphysis to Hilgenreiner's line.

4. *Shenton's line* is drawn between the medial border of the neck of the femur and the superior border of the obturator foramen. In the normal hip this line is an even, continuous

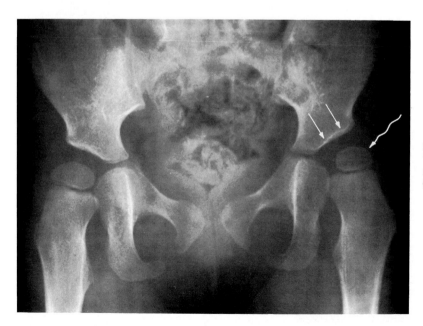

Figure 72–5. Type I congenital dysplasia of the hip. The left femoral head ossification center (wavy arrow) is relatively small, and the left acetabulum is shallow (straight arrows).

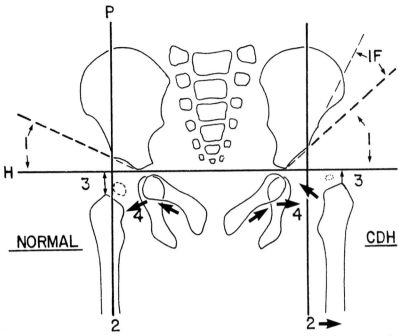

Figure 72–6. Radiographic indications of congenital dysplasia of the hip (left side is abnormal). *1*, Acetabular index; IF, additional index of false acetabulum; *2*, lateral migration; *H*; Hilgenreiner's line; *P*; Perkin's line; *3*, Superior migration; *4*, Shenton's line. (Courtesy of J. Ogden, M.D., Tampa, Florida.)

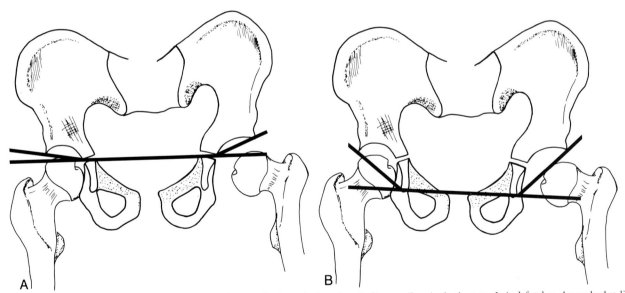

Figure 72–7. Acetabular index. A, Pediatric. The pediatric index is used when the triradiate cartilage is clearly open. It is defined as the angle that lies between a line connecting the superolateral margin of each triradiate cartilage (Y line) and a line drawn from the most superolateral ossified edge of the acetabulum to the superolateral margin of the triradiate cartilage. **B,** Adult. The angle that lies between a line connecting the teardrops on the inferior margin of the acetabula (Hilgenreiner's line) and a line drawn from the most superolateral ossified edge of the acetabulum to the teardrop constitutes the adult acetabuluar index *(AI)*. (Courtesy of David S. Marcus, M.D.)

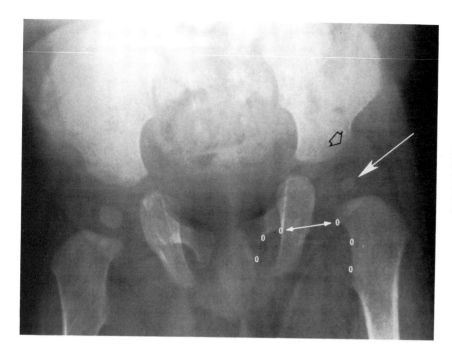

Figure 72–8. Type I congenital dysplasia of the hip. The left femur is displaced superiorly and has a relatively small secondary ossification center (white arrow) in association with a slightly shallow acetabulum (black arrow). Shenton's line (indicated by 0) is disrupted (white double-headed arrow).

arc, whereas in a dislocated hip with proximal displacement of the femoral head, it is broken and interrupted (Figs. 72–8 and 72–9).

These lines are helpful in the child with unilateral dislocation, when the abnormal side can be compared to the normal side, but they are of limited value in the child with bilaterally dislocated hips. It is important to recognize that the acetabular index may be normal despite significant dysplasia of the hip. Many of the changes associated with an increased acetabular index do not occur until the postnatal phase, when the hip gradually loses its intrauterine flexion contracture. Continued pressure from the femoral head even-

tually induces osteoclastic resorption and delayed endochondral bone formation at the lateral margin of the acetabular roof. The angle of acetabular acclivity relative to the pelvic baseline is variable; normally, at birth, it ranges from 18 to 36 degrees, and it decreases by 5 degrees during the ensuing 6 months. Measurement of this angle is thus of limited value unless it is markedly increased. It is more important to document the position of the femoral head relative to the acetabulum and to characterize the osseous acetabular margin.

Several additional measurements have been developed (Fig. 72–10). The normal acetabulum has a slight central concavity and a distinct lateral edge. Absence of either of these findings

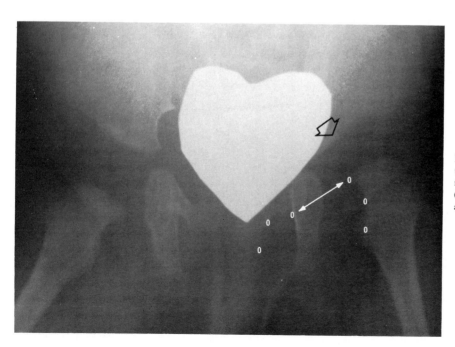

Fiture 72–9. Type II congenital dysplasia of the hip. Superolateral displacement of the left femur is evident, as well as a shallow acetabulum (black arrow) and disruption (white double-headed arrow) of Shenton's line (indicated by 0).

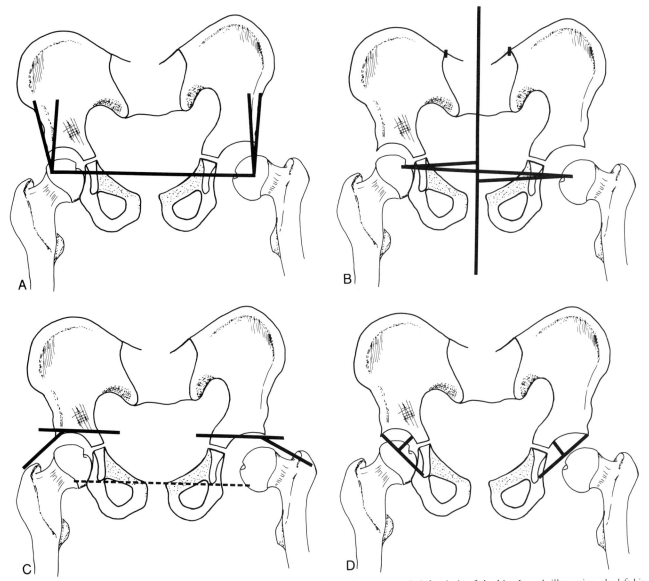

Figure 72–10. Additional measurements performed on conventional radiographs in congenital dysplasia of the hip. In each illustration, the left hip is dysplastic. **A** Center-edge (CE) angle. The CE angle lies between a line drawn from the center of the femoral head perpendicular to the line connecting the center of rotation of each femoral head and a line drawn from the center of the head to the superolateral ossified edge of the acetabulum. In a dislocated hip in which the center of the femoral head lies lateral to the superolateral ossified edge of the acetabulum, the CE angle will have a negative value. **B** Relative lateral displacement of femoral head from midline. The pelvic midline is formed by a line connecting the point that lies equidistant between the superolateral margin on each side of the sacrum and the point that lies directly in the middle of the symphysis pubis. The lateral displacement of each femoral head is indicated by the length of a line drawn perpendicular to the midline from the center of the head. **C** Slope of the lateral edge of the acetabulum. The angle formed between a line that is parallel to Hilgenreiner's line and tangent to the roof of the acetabulum and a line that is parallel to the lateral edge of the acetabulm is termed the slope. The normal acetabulum has a slope of the lateral edge that is defined as positive. **D** Acetabular depth. The greatest perpendicular distance between the medial articular surface of the acetabulum and a line drawn from the teardrop to the most superolateral ossified edge of the acetabulum is the acetabular depth. (Courtesy of David S. Marcus, M.D.)

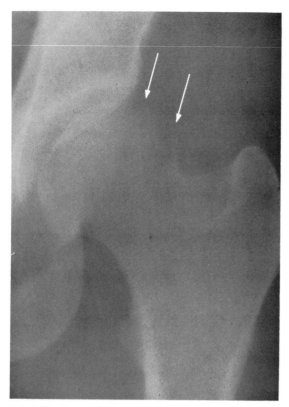

Figure 72–11. Untreated type I congenital dysplasia of the hip. The acetabulum is shallow in association with aspherical deformity and lateral uncovering (arrows) of the femoral head.

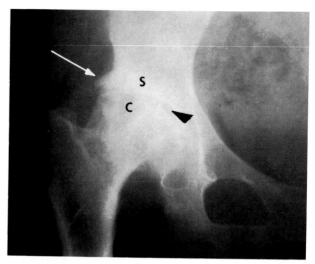

Figure 72–12. Degenerative joint disease secondary to untreated congenital dysplasia of the hip. Deformity of the right femoral head and acetabulum is associated with superimposed joint space narrowing (arrowhead), subchondral sclerosis (S), subarticular cyst formation (C), and osteophytosis (arrow).

and persistent accentuated obliquity of the acetabular margin indicate abnormal femoral-acetabular relationships. Abnormal sclerosis of the outer aspect of the acetabulum is an associated finding. If these acetabular alterations are observed in a newborn infant, prenatal dislocation is implied.

With appropriate early treatment, many of these alterations diminish or disappear completely. Ossification of a dislocated femoral head epiphysis generally lags behind that of a contralateral normal side, and disparity in size can persist for 6 to 12 months. Sequential radiographic examinations generally are performed at the time of clinical evaluation or cast change. The intervals between radiographic examinations should be as long as possible, and gonadal shielding is mandatory in both sexes. If the condition is not treated, the dysplastic alterations will progress to a point and then stabilize (Fig. 72–11). With persistent subluxation and associated instability, severe secondary degenerative abnormalities may occur at a young age and progress into adulthood (Fig. 72–12). In untreated type III dysplasia, progressive changes will create a false acetabulum incapable of withstanding prolonged use (Figs. 72–13 and 72–14).

Conventional Tomography

When visualization of the hip is impaired by a heavy cast, conventional tomography may be helpful. Restricting the arc of tube excursion or use of a book cassette can limit radiation exposure to an acceptable level, but in general tomography should not be performed unless absolutely necessary. This technique will demonstrate the femoral and acetabular margins more clearly.

Contrast Arthrography

Positive contrast arthrography is not indicated in the typical case of readily reducible neonatal hip instability, but it should be performed if concentric reduction is questionable or difficult to maintain. This procedure is indicated strongly when dislocation is discovered late or when sequential radiographic examinations do not document satisfactory therapeutic response.

Arthrography, which should be undertaken only after 2 to 3 weeks of traction to loosen soft tissue contracture, is done under a general anesthetic that will allow muscle relaxation and a proper assessment of reducibility. After sterile preparation of the skin, a narrow (20 gauge) spinal needle is introduced into the hip joint under fluoroscopic control. A trial injection ascertains whether the hip capsule is penetrated satisfactorily. A small amount of contrast material (1 to 2 ml) is then injected, again using fluoroscopy to determine

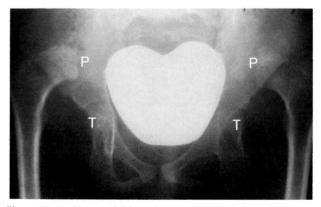

Figure 72–13. Untreated bilateral type III congenital dysplasia of the hip in a child. Marked superior displacement of both femora is evident, in association with underdevelopment of the true acetabula (T) and the formation of pseudoacetabula (P) within the iliac wings.

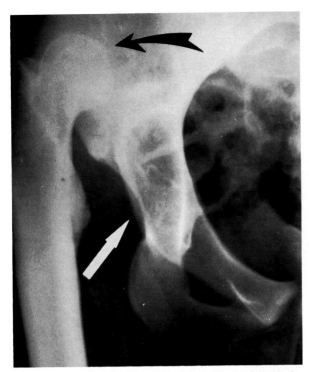

Figure 72–14. Untreated type II congenital dysplasia of the hip in an adult. The right femur is hypoplastic and markedly displaced superolaterally, articulating with the iliac wing via a pseudoacetabulum (black arrow). The true acetabulum (white arrow) is underdeveloped.

satisfactory filling of the joint. The contrast material should be dilute, as too dense a contrast medium will obscure the femoral head, as will too large a volume. The needle is removed and the hip is manipulated under fluoroscopy to determine reducibility and appropriate positions that maintain reduction. Spot films (anteroposterior views) are then taken in the following positions: (1) extension–external rotation, (2) extension–neutral rotation, (3) extension–internal rotation, (4) abduction–neutral rotation, (5) abduction–internal rotation, (6) abduction-flexion, (7) adduction, (8) adduction-push, and (9) adduction-pull.

On arthrographic images in *subluxation,* the femoral head lies lateral to and below the margin of the labrum. The labrum may be displaced superiorly by the head during stress maneuvers, but the head always remains below or lateral to its undersurface. The labrum may be elevated and flattened against the pelvis. The joint capsule generally is loose, and the articular cavity is more capacious than normal (Fig. 72–15). Although reduction of the femoral head is easy, maintenance frequently is difficult. The femoral head often lies medially in normal position and displaces only with lateral stress. Pooling of contrast material is then observed medial to the lateralized femoral epiphysis.

In *complete dislocation,* the femoral head lies superior and lateral to the margin of the acetabular labrum (Fig. 72–16). As the femoral head migrates proximally on the ilium, the capsule is pushed ahead, stretching out and narrowing behind the femoral head. The iliopsoas tendon compresses the isthmus of the capsule as the tendon passes toward its insertion on the lesser trochanter. The capsule is adherent to the labrum, and these fused structures (termed the limbus) are interposed

between the femoral epiphysis and the acetabulum. The portion of the capsule lying medial to the head is constricted in the form of an isthmus, resulting in a figure-of-eight capsular configuration. The ligamentum teres femoris frequently is thickened but occasionally is elongated and attenuated. The intraacetabular capsular space is constricted and contains hyperplastic synovium and fat, manifested as filling defects at its base. The limbus frequently is folded on itself (inverted) and lies within the acetabulum, with loss of the characteristic "rose thorn" appearance of the normal labrum. The capsular isthmus, interposed limbus, and tight iliopsoas muscle impede complete reduction, although the impression of the last on the contrast-filled capsule ("hourglass" configuration) generally is not identifiable. The hypertrophied intracapsular soft tissues or ligamentum teres femoris may also prevent complete medial seating of the femoral epiphysis.

The type 3 dislocation is not reducible, even when capsular laxity has been induced by preliminary traction. Arthrography overcomes the potential for a false impression of reduction on conventional radiographs owing to compression of the infolded labrum and capsule by the femoral head in this situation.

Ultrasonography

Real-time ultrasonography of the infant hip provides an accurate image of anatomic relationships as well as valuable information concerning function. The technique clearly images the cartilaginous femoral head and enables accurate assessment of its size, shape, and symmetry. The dynamic relationship of the cartilaginous head to the acetabulum is defined clearly, and instability, subluxation, and dislocation can be demonstrated. The size, shape, and position of the hip can be monitored with the infant in a spica cast, brace, or harness. Now that real-time ultrasonography is employed successfully to determine hip position in infancy, it also offers an alternative method for evaluating acetabular development. A sonographic technique for evaluating the ossification center of the infant's hip allows identification of the ossific nucleus before it can be visualized radiographically. Delay in ossification associated with pathologic conditions of the hip also can be recognized. Proper assessment of the size of the ossific nucleus requires scanning in orthogonal planes. Acoustic shadowing causes the growing ossification center to appear curved and may make the medial acetabulum and triradiate cartilage difficult to identify. Sonographic hip evaluation usually ceases to be reliable in children over 1 year of age.

Cross-Sectional Imaging Techniques

Computed tomography (CT) usually can provide accurate documentation of the adequacy of a reduction in CDH (Fig. 72–17). It should supplement other radiographic examinations when the status of a reduction is in question because the patient is wearing a plaster cast. CT provides a clear image of the reduction in the transverse plane, so that anterior or posterior subluxation of the femoral head can be detected easily. In addition, it allows direct measurement of acetabular anteversion, which previously had not been possible with noninvasive studies in the living patient. Acetabular anteversion is increased on the dislocated side and returns to normal as treatment progresses. Radiation exposure is less than that for conventional tomography. CT, particularly with three-dimensional analysis, is extremely useful in characterizing the abnormal acetabular morphology of untreated CDH.

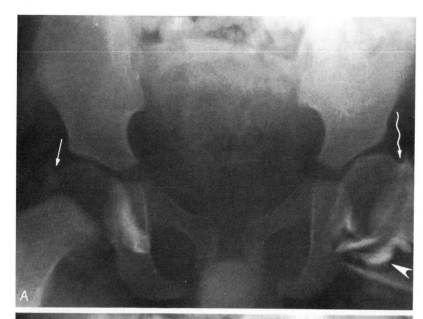

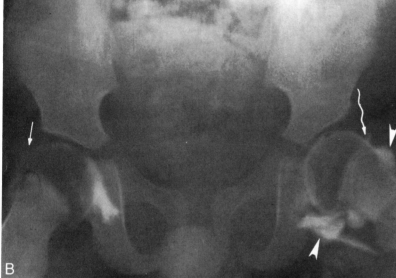

Figure 72–15. Arthrography in type I congenital dysplasia of the hip. In both the neutral (A) and abducted (B) positions, the left acetabular labrum (wavy arrows) remains in a completely everted configuration, similar to that (straight arrows) of the contralateral normal hip. The joint capsule is more redundant on the left (arrowheads).

Figure 72–16. Arthrography in bilateral type III congenital dysplasia of the hip. The acetabular labra (L) are totally inverted, effectively blocking reduction of the superolaterally displaced femoral heads (H). The ossified acetabula are shallow (arrows), and the joint capsules are capacious (arrowheads).

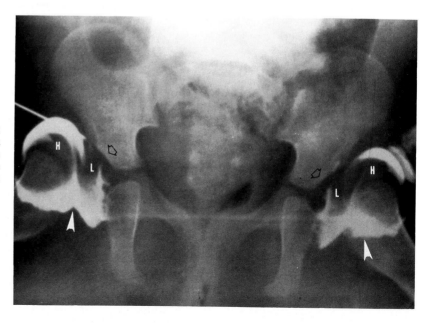

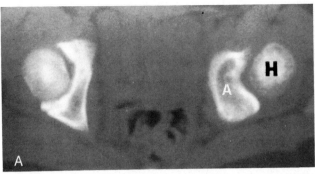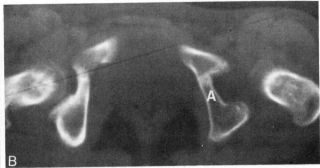

Figure 72–17. Computed tomography of untreated type II congenital dysplasia of the hip. Sequential scans (**A, B**) depict altered acetabular morphology (*A*) and deformity of the femoral head (*H*) on the left. The dysplastic femur is displaced superolaterally compared with the normal right side.

Magnetic resonance imaging offers great promise in the evaluation of CDH (Fig. 72–18), owing to its excellent depiction of unmineralized tissues, including cartilage, its direct multiplanar imaging capabilities, its freedom from exposure to ionizing radiation, and its high sensitivity in the early detection of ischemic necrosis.

TREATMENT

Early (preferably neonatal) diagnosis and reduction of CDH is directed toward reestablishing normal chondroosseous development of the hip. When instability or frank dislocation has been detected clinically using the Ortolani or Barlow maneuver, the infant generally is placed in a flexion–abduction–external rotation brace, splint, or cast. Sequential clinical and radiographic examinations subsequently document that satisfactory acetabular-femoral relationships are achieved in most patients. In the minority of conservative treatment failures, arthrography is indicated, possibly followed by surgical intervention for achievement of complete anatomic reduction. Congruent concentric reductions accomplished before the age of 4 years lead to normal hip relationships in over 95 per cent of patients.

A large number of surgical procedures on the pelvis or femur have been designed for late salvage of cases with persistent acetabular maldevelopment and hip instability. The common goals of such intervention are the provision of improved acetabular coverage, enhanced femoral head–acetabular congruence, decreased pressure loading of the femoral head, and increased efficiency of the hip musculature. These objectives can be achieved by many methods, the most commonly used of which include femoral varus osteotomy (Fig. 72–19), pelvic (Salter) or acetabular rotation (Figs. 72–19 and 72–20), increase in acetabular depth (Pemberton), or medialization of the femoral head (Chiari).

The innominate (Salter) osteotomy is the most frequently performed late surgical procedure. Indicated for persistent subluxation with mild to moderate acetabular dysplasia but a concentrically reduced hip, it reorients the acetabulum without changing its size or shape. The osteotomy is performed in a horizontal plane across the pelvis, just above the acetabulum (Figs. 72–19 and 72–20). All three pelvic components are rotated forward and laterally as a unit using the pubic symphysis as a hinge axis. A bone block is used to maintain the open wedge. Postoperative radiographs demonstrate marked asymmetry between the two iliac wings and obturator

foramina. Owing to pelvic flexibility, this disparity becomes progressively less pronounced with time.

The circumacetabular osteotomy (Pemberton) is a means of reducing acetabular size and increasing articular congruence in patients with moderate to severe CDH. A pericapsular osteotomy is performed around the periphery of the acetabulum, the margin of which is displaced inferiorly, wrapped around the femoral head, and held in position by a bone block. The osteotomy is hinged at the pelvic Y synchondrosis and thus cannot be used after early adolescence, when the flexibility of the synchondrosis diminishes. Both the Salter and the Pemberton procedures increase pressure on the femoral head, predisposing to ischemic necrosis as a complication.

The median displacement pelvic osteotomy (Chiari) medializes the femoral head and provides greater femoral head coverage by enlarging the acetabulum. The biomechanical effect of medial weight-bearing transfer is to unload the femoral head and increase the efficiency of the abductor musculature. The angle of osteotomy is 10 to 20 degrees relative to the plane of the upper acetabular margin, and the lower segment is displaced medially by approximately half its width. A false radiographic impression of adequate medial shift can be produced by rotation as opposed to displacement. When performed bilaterally, this procedure may lead to significant pelvic narrowing with possible obstetric complications in women who later have children.

Eventually in untreated or unsuccessfully treated cases, pain and disability secondary to residual deformity (Fig. 72–20) or osteoarthritis will probably necessitate reconstructive surgery at some time during adult life, although frequently not until the fifth or sixth decade. This is important to consider before embarking on any treatment when a child, particularly one who is over 1 year of age, has a unilateral or bilateral dislocation.

COMPLICATIONS OF THERAPY

Ischemic necrosis of the femoral head occurs in CDH only after treatment and can thus be considered an iatrogenic complication that may lead to severe radiographic changes and a painful dysfunctional hip in early adult life. The reported frequency has been as high as 73 per cent, and the condition can occur in the contralateral normal hip when both hips are immobilized. Lack of preliminary traction and rigid immobilization in extreme positions of abduction are important causative factors. Vascular occlusion may occur in

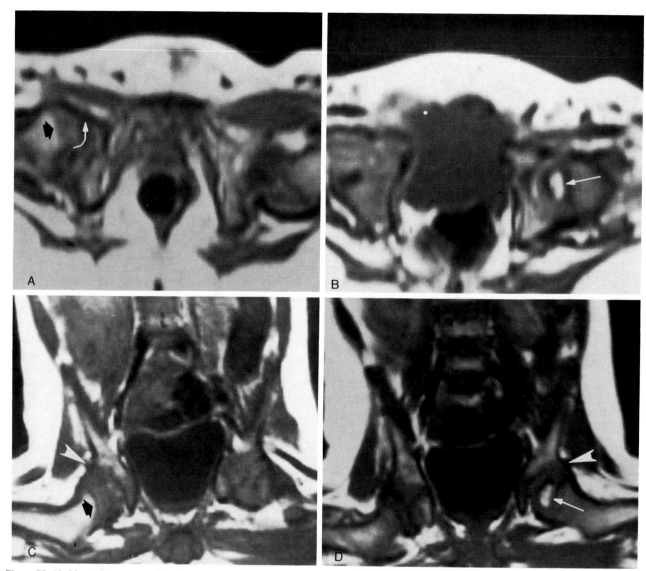

Figure 72–18. Magnetic resonance imaging in type I congenital dysplasia of the hip. On transaxial (**A, B**) and coronal (**C, D**) T1 weighted images with the hips in an abducted position, absence of marrow signal within the right femoral head (black arrows) indicates delayed development of its secondary ossification center. White arrows indicate the normal left side. The acetabular labrum (arrowheads) is everted bilaterally, and the right femur is displaced slightly anteriorly (curved arrow).

vessels along the femoral neck or the enchondral circulation. Identification of early ischemic necrosis is difficult by conventional radiography. Ossification of the cartilaginous head ensues soon after reduction and may be manifested as several granular foci rather than a single homogeneous center. This phenomenon may represent early ischemic necrosis or a transient growth disturbance that does not result in significant late deformity.

Failure of appearance or growth of the femoral ossification center during an interval of approximately 1 year after reduction is good evidence of necrosis. Characteristic signs of the process, such as broadening of the femoral neck, also may occur during this time or become evident later. Premature fusion of a physeal segment with secondary rotation of the epiphysis is a characteristic complication.

In the older child with initial late reduction, the radiographic appearance is that of Legg-Calvé-Perthes disease. The

sequelae, however, generally are more severe; femoral neck shortening and epiphyseal deformity occur with much higher frequency. Incomplete epiphyseal necrosis is more difficult to recognize radiographically and can occur despite preliminary traction, gentle reduction, and avoidance of extreme immobilization positions.

Developmental coxa vara has also been described as a rare late complication of treated CDH. Vascular impairment with diminished medial growth plate activity may be responsible.

DIFFERENTIAL DIAGNOSIS

INCOMPLETE FEMORAL HEAD COVERAGE. Inadequate acetabular coverage of the ossified femoral head epiphysis can be observed in a variety of conditions other than CDH. Lateral uncovering occurs in situations in which the acetabulum is developmentally small or the femoral head is enlarged (as in ischemic necrosis). Femoral neck valgus and anteversion tend to rotate the femoral head outward and contribute to poor coverage. The cause of deficient acetabular coverage may be evident on conventional radiographs (as in the pelvic tilt of cerebral palsy), although stress maneuvers or arthrography often are required for correct analysis.

INFLAMMATORY DISEASE. Hip subluxation, manifested as lateralization of the femoral metaphysis, occurs in pyogenic arthritis of infancy. Soft tissue swelling and thigh flexion increase the density of the hip region and provide an important clue to the correct radiologic diagnosis. Associated growth plate dissolution and epiphyseal slip are best demonstrated by contrast arthrography.

NEUROMUSCULAR DISEASE. Superior and lateral displacement of the femoral head is common in patients with meningomyelocele and may occur during infancy. The acetabulum may be shallow owing to prenatal onset of the disease, and evidence of spinal dysraphism should be present on pelvic radiographs. The hip subluxation of cerebral palsy and other spastic conditions rarely develops during infancy and is associated with severe femoral anteversion and neck-shaft valgus.

TRAUMATIC EPIPHYSEAL SLIP. This condition may occur in the setting of infantile abuse or birth trauma. If the epiphyseal ossification center is not yet mineralized, lateral shift of the femoral shaft can be misinterpreted as CDH rather than a shearing fracture.

CONGENITAL COXA VARA. Congenital coxa vara without femoral shortening is extremely rare and can be distinguished from CDH by clinical examination and arthrography during the neonatal period.

ABNORMAL JOINT LAXITY. Articular hypermobility is a feature of a variety of conditions other than CDH. Familial joint laxity is probably inherited as an autosomal dominant trait, and most affected individuals do not have significant orthopedic problems. Hypotonia and joint laxity occur in Down's syndrome, and recurrent hip dislocation can be observed. Cutaneous and articular hyperlaxity with inconstant spherical subcutaneous calcifications are part of the generalized connective tissue derangement seen in the Ehlers-Danlos syndrome.

In Larsen's syndrome, early joint laxity leads to multiple dislocations (particularly in the hips, elbows, and knees).

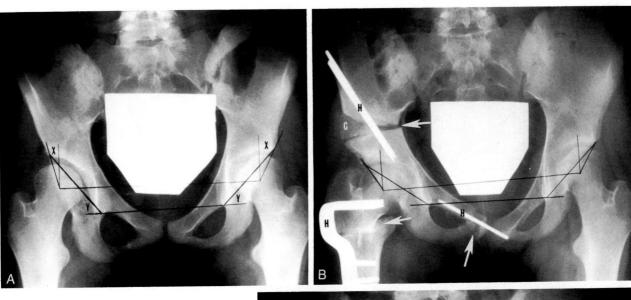

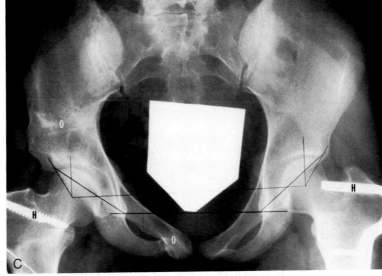

Figure 72–19. **Proximal femoral varus osteotomies and Salter procedure for bilateral congenital dysplasia of the hip. A** Preoperative radiograph depicts more severe femoral lateralization (smaller CE angle, *X*) and acetabular deformity (larger acetabular index, *Y*), on the right. **B** Osteotomy sites (arrows), internal fixation hardware *(H)*, and bone graft *(G)* are evident, as well as congruity between the right femoral head and acetabulum. Angle measurements appear symmetric. **C** Two years after the initial surgery, both hips appear well aligned. In the interval, the patient has undergone proximal femoral varus osteotomy on the left as well as a greater trochanteric advancement procedure on the right as indicated by new hardware *(H)*. The pelvic osteotomies *(O)* have healed with mild residual asymmetry.

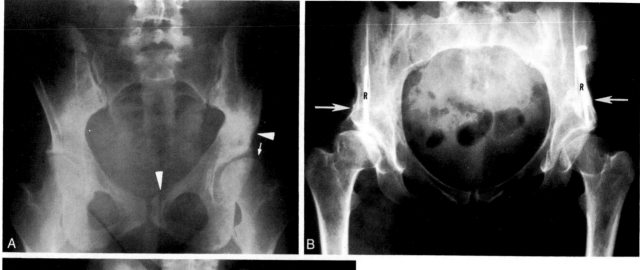

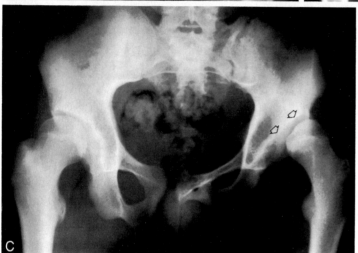

Figure 72–20. Surgically treated congenital dysplasia of the hip (Salter procedure.) **A** Healed pelvic osteotomy sites (arrowheads) are associated with mild lateral uncovering (arrow) of the deformed left femoral head. **B** Healed iliac osteotomy sites (arrows) and retained pins *(R)* are noted on both sides, in association with deformity and slight lateralization of both femoral heads. **C** In a patient with type II CDH, the left femoral head is small, deformed, and displaced superolaterally, and the left acetabulum is shallow (arrows) with underdevelopment of the left hemipelvis, related in part to previous surgery. The right hip is also mildly dysplastic (type I).

Other typical features include flat facies with a saddle nose deformity and a distinctive juxtacalcaneal ossification center.

Within the group of children with arthrogryposis multiplex congenita, recurrent dislocation of many joints or only mild hyperextensibility of the metacarpophalangeal, elbow, or knee joints may be observed. When hip dislocation occurs in this disease, it is readily reduced but difficult to maintain on cessation of immobilization. Conventional radiography reveals marked lateral femoral subluxation with relatively normal acetabula. Arthrography demonstrates prominent redundant and lax capsular structures within which the femoral heads can be moved readily. When factors external to the hip joint per se are present, particularly neuromuscular diseases such as meningomyelocele and arthrogryposis multiplex congenita, the term "teratologic hip" often is applied.

FURTHER READING

Boal DKB, Schwenkter EP: The infant hip: Assessment with real-time US. Radiology *157*:667, 1985.

Harcke HT, Lee MS, Sinning L, Clarke NMP, Borns PF, MacEwen GD: Ossification center of the infant hip: Sonographic and radiographic correlation. AJR *147*:317, 1986.

Lafferty CM, Sartoris DJ, Tyson R, Resnick D, Kursunoglu S, Pate D, Sutherland D: Acetabular alterations in untreated congenital dysplasia of the hip: Computed tomography with multiplanar re-formation and three-dimensional analysis. J Comput Assist Tomogr *10*:84, 1986.

Ozonoff MB: Pediatric Orthopedic Radiology. Philadelphia, WB Saunders Co, 1979.

Chapter 73

Collagen Diseases, Epiphyseal Dysplasias, and Related Conditions

Amy Beth Goldman, M.D.

Certain disorders of connective tissue can lead to significant radiologic alterations. The radiographic changes are diverse, ranging from joint incongruity with secondary degeneration to soft tissue calcification or ossification with or without osseous overgrowth. Although clinical and laboratory fea- *tures exist in some of these diseases that provide important clues to the correct diagnosis, an awareness of the radiographic alterations allows early and appropriate assessment in cases in which the diagnosis may be more obscure.*

Marfan's syndrome, homocystinuria, the Ehlers-Danlos syndrome, and osteogenesis imperfecta are all disorders of connective tissue synthesis. In varying degrees they involve the skin, ligaments, tendons, eyes, cardiovascular system, and skeleton.

MARFAN'S SYNDROME

Marfan's syndrome is a rare familial disorder of connective tissue that involves primarily the eye, the skeleton, and the cardiovascular system. It usually is an inherited autosomal dominant disorder with a high degree of penetrance. Fifteen per cent of cases are sporadic.

Pathology and Pathophysiology

The nature of the defect in the connective tissues of patients with Marfan's syndrome remains unknown, and it is uncertain whether the abnormality involves collagen, elastic fibers, or both.

Pathologic changes in the tunica media of the aorta are part of the characteristic findings of Marfan's syndrome and predispose these patients to aortic dissection and rupture. Medial necrosis of the main pulmonary artery segment and fibromyxomatous changes in the anulus, leaflets, and chordae tendineae of the aortic and mitral valves may be observed. Additional pathologic alterations include changes in the suspensory ligaments of the lens that lead to bilateral ectopia lentis and severe muscle hypotonia.

The cause and pathologic features of the skeletal changes are the most puzzling of all. None of the current theories concerning a defect in collagen synthesis can adequately explain the skeletal overgrowth that characterizes this disorder.

Clinical Findings

There is no sexual or racial predisposition for Marfan's syndrome. Patients characteristically are tall and thin. The limbs are disproportionately elongated in relation to the trunk, and arm span can exceed height. The increased length of the extremities is most exaggerated distally, particularly in the hands and feet, leading to arachnodactyly. Chest deformities (pectus carinatum or excavatum) and scoliosis accentuate the limb-trunk discrepancy. The subcutaneous fat and muscle are atrophic, the skull typically is dolichocephalic, the face elongated, the jaw prominent, and the palate high and arched. Manifestations of ligamentous laxity include angular deformities of the joints, pes planus, and kyphoscoliosis. Blue sclerae and poor dentition are sometimes present. Intelligence is normal. The most common ocular abnormalities are bilateral ectopia lentis and myopia. Cataracts occur late in the course of the disease.

The cardiac abnormalities are responsible for the shortened life expectancy of patients with Marfan's syndrome. Cystic medial necrosis of the aorta or pulmonary artery, aortic and mitral valve insufficiency, septal defects, and sinus of Valsava aneurysms also are associated with Marfan's syndrome.

The diagnosis can be established reliably if at least two of the three systems are affected (ocular, cardiovascular, skeletal) and if there is a family history of the disease. Two clinical tests and one radiographic test also have been advocated as a means of establishing the diagnosis. The first is the "thumb sign," in which the protrusion of the thumb beyond the confines of a clenched fist is observed. The second test relates to the distance from the pubic symphysis to the floor and the distance from the top of the head to the floor. In normal adults, the ratio of these two measurements is less than 0.85.

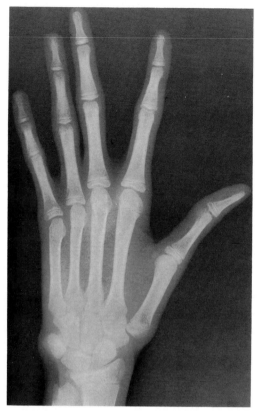

Figure 73–1. Marfan's syndrome. Posteroanterior view of the hand demonstrates absence of subcutaneous fat, elongation of phalanges and metacarpal bones, and normal bone density.

In patients with Marfan's syndrome, the ratio is increased. The third test is the metacarpal index. When the lengths of the metacarpals are divided by the respective width of each diaphysis, an increased value is observed in Marfan's syndrome.

Radiographic Findings

In the older child or adult with Marfan's syndrome, radiographs of the hands and feet demonstrate arachnodactyly (Fig. 73–1). Flexion deformity of one or both fifth digits of the hands may be evident. Bone age is normal or advanced. Other deformities in the hands and feet include hallux valgus, pes planus, hammer toes, clubfeet, calcaneal spurs, and carpal instability.

The extremities of patients with Marfan's syndrome demonstrate both muscular atrophy and sparse subcutaneous fat. The long bones are slender and gracile. Osteoporosis is not present. Joints are hypermobile, predisposing to deformities (genu recurvatum, patella alta), dislocations (patellae, hips, clavicles, mandible), and joint instability. The hyperlaxity is also responsible for premature degenerative joint disease.

Scoliosis occurs in 40 to 60 per cent of patients with Marfan's syndrome. The curve pattern is similar to that of idiopathic scoliosis, with an increased frequency of spondylolysis and spondylolisthesis (Fig. 73–2). The progressive scoliosis of Marfan's syndrome, however, begins earlier than the idiopathic form and does not have the female predominance of the idiopathic type. Posterior scalloping of the vertebral bodies, attributed to dural ectasia, is observed in Marfan's syndrome. A rare but serious complication is atlantoaxial subluxation, resulting in compression of the medulla and cerebellar tonsils.

Protrusio acetabuli deformities have also been associated with Marfan's syndrome. In the skull, findings include a longer, thicker, and, most significantly, taller osseous configuration than in normal persons, frontal bossing, and enlargement of the frontal sinuses.

"Marfanoid" skeletal changes occur in several other syndromes. Homocystinuria may simulate Marfan's syndrome (see following discussion); patients are mentally retarded, however, and the skeleton is osteoporotic. Congenital contractural arachnodactyly, another inherited disorder of connective tissue, also is characterized by long, thin limbs, scoliosis, and dolichostenomelia. The absence of eye and cardiac changes and the presence of joint contractures and deformed ears distinguish the two entities, however. Type I multiple endocrine neoplasia syndrome (parathyroid and pituitary tumors) and type IIb multiple endocrine neoplasia syndrome (mucosal neuromas, pheochromocytoma, medullary carcinoma of the thyroid) also are associated with marfanoid features, as is the Ehlers-Danlos syndrome. Lastly, Stickler's syndrome, a hereditary connective tissue disorder affecting ocular, skeletal, and orofacial structures, can be associated with marfanoid features. Its distinctive orofacial changes, however, establish the diagnosis.

HOMOCYSTINURIA

The term homocystinuria encompasses a group of disorders characterized by inborn defects in methionine metabolism. The best known of these disorders is the syndrome associated with a deficiency in the enzyme cystathionine synthetase. It is inherited on an autosomal recessive basis and affects the eye, skeleton, central nervous system, and vascular structures.

Pathology and Pathophysiology

The enzyme cystathionine synthetase catalyzes the conversion of serine and homocysteine to cystathionine. Cystathionine levels are decreased in the brain, skin, and liver. Homocysteine accumulates in the tissues, and excessive amounts are excreted in the urine. In some cases of homocystinuria, the clinical and chemical abnormalities can be altered by massive doses of vitamin B_6 (pyridoxine).

Homocystinuria is associated with a defect in collagen synthesis. It is currently postulated that high levels of homocysteine bind and interfere with the formation of the aldehyde cross-linkages that stabilize the collagen macromolecule.

Arterial and venous thromboses complicate the course of homocystinuria, perhaps related to an increase in platelet "stickiness." The thromboembolic phenomena are the most common cause of death in patients with homocystinuria. As in Marfan's syndrome, cystic medial necrosis and fragmentation of elastic fibers are found in the aortas of patients with homocystinuria. Unlike Marfan's syndrome, however, similar changes occur in the media of all elastic arteries and are uniquely accompanied by the presence of patchy intimal pads or ridges. In addition, despite thinning of the media, aortic dissections are not a characteristic feature of homocystinuria, as they are in Marfan's syndrome.

Mental retardation and seizures occur as a result of cystathionine synthetase deficiency. Approximately 30 per cent of patients have abnormally low intelligence. The most characteristic ocular abnormality of homocystinuria is bilateral dislocation of the lens.

Clinical Findings

Patients appear normal at birth and during infancy. Even in infants, however, the urine does contain increased levels of homocystine. In early childhood, motor development slows or even regresses. Patients with homocystinuria tend to have thin skin with large pores and prominent venous markings. Striae occur over the buttocks and shoulders. A malar flush frequently is present, and "cigarette paper" scars occur with minor trauma. Livedo reticularis can be present over the extensor surfaces of the extremities or the buttocks. Hair is thin and sparse. A high, arched palate and poor dentition are both characteristic of this disorder.

The most frequent physical finding is bilateral lens dislocations. Other, less frequent eye abnormalities include cataracts, optic atrophy, microphthalmus, and congenital glaucoma.

Spontaneous venous and arterial thromboses complicate the clinical course of homocystinuria and frequently are life-threatening. Common sites of arterial clotting are the intermediate-sized vessels, including the coronary, renal, and carotid arteries, and the other major branches of the aorta. Venous thromboses frequently involve the mesenteric vessels, the vena cava, the iliac vessels, and the pulmonary veins.

Twenty-five to 60 per cent of patients with homocystinuria have skeletal abnormalities that resemble those of Marfan's syndrome. Patients are tall, with disproportionately long extremities, a "duck-like" gait, scoliosis, pectus excavatum, and joint laxity. Several clinical findings differentiate the two disorders, however. First, mental retardation, the malar flush, and vascular thromboses are not found in Marfan's syndrome. Second, although both entities are characterized by bilateral lens dislocations, this sign can be detected in infancy in patients with homocystinuria. Third, in Marfan's syndrome, contractures occur only in the fifth digits of the hands, whereas in homocystinuria, contractures occur in multiple digits as well as in the elbows and knees. Fourth, the primary life-endangering vascular changes in Marfan's syndrome are related to the aorta, as opposed to homocystinuria, in which sudden death more frequently is the result of thromboembolic phenomena or rupture of medium-sized vessels. Lastly, unlike Marfan's syndrome, there are positive and specific laboratory findings in homocystinuria. The plasma levels of homocysteine, homocystine, and methionine are all elevated, and the urine contains abnormal amounts of homocysteine.

Radiographic Findings

Skeletal changes occur gradually during childhood. The skull can show a variety of changes, including enlargement of the sinuses, widening of the diploic space, extensive dural calcification, or prognathism. Examination of the spine can reveal generalized osteoporosis and scoliosis. The vertebral bodies have an increased anteroposterior diameter and may be biconcave in shape. Compression fractures are frequent. Posterior scalloping of the vertebral bodies and premature degenerative disc disease also have been described.

Changes in the extremities include dolichostenomelia, osteoporosis, and multiple growth recovery lines. Frequent deformities include flattening of the epiphyses, broad metaphyses, and varus deformities of the humeri. A characteristic stippled appearance can occur in the growth plates of the distal portions of the radii and ulnae. Abnormal laxity may result in genu valgum deformities and patella alta (Fig. 73–3). Flexion contractures occur in the digits, the elbows, and the knees. Characteristic radiographic changes in the hands include arachnodactyly and carpal deformities. Bone age may be normal, accelerated, or retarded.

The presence of osteoporosis, metaphyseal flaring, and multiple contractures should distinguish the radiographic appearance of dolichostenomelia in a patient with homocystinuria from that in a patient with Marfan's syndrome.

EHLERS-DANLOS SYNDROME

The Ehlers-Danlos syndrome is a familial disorder of connective tissue that is characterized by hyperelasticity and fragility of the skin, hyperlaxity of the joints, and a bleeding diathesis. The eye, the gastrointestinal tract, the bronchopulmonary tree, and the cardiovascular system may also be affected. The Ehlers-Danlos syndrome, however, is not a single homogeneous disorder but a group of related entities that share the same complex of clinical abnormalities. Although the majority of cases have an autosomal dominant pattern of inheritance, the Ehlers-Danlos syndrome is associ-

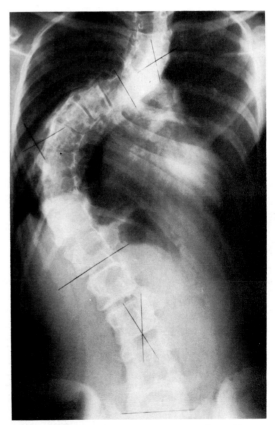

Figure 73–2. Marfan's syndrome: Scoliosis. The radiographic appearance is indistinguishable from that of idiopathic scoliosis.

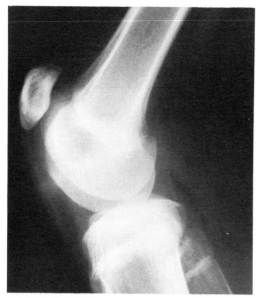

Figure 73–3. Homocystinuria. Patella alta is seen, and the bones are osteoporotic.

ated with variable inheritance patterns, extremely variable expression, and marked clinical heterogeneity. Indeed, nine distinct categories of the disorder have been identified. Type I is the full-blown clinical syndrome. Type II is a milder syndrome than type I, with minimal cutaneous and joint manifestations. Type III is characterized by the predominance of joint findings. These three types all are associated with an autosomal dominant mode of inheritance. Type IV is the most serious form of the disease and is dominated by vascular fragility. It is associated with both autosomal dominant and autosomal recessive modes of inheritance. Type IV (acrogeria) is accompanied by numerous skin folds in the face and extremities. Type V (an X-linked recessive form) is characterized by dramatic skin stretching. Type VI (autosomal recessive) is dominated by ocular abnormalities and rheumatologic symptoms. Type VII (autosomal recessive) is associated with short stature and congenital dislocations. Type VIII (autosomal dominant) is a rare syndrome associated with periodontal disease, skin fragility, and hypermobility. Type IX (X-linked recessive) is associated with abnormalities in copper metabolism, relating the Ehlers-Danlos syndrome to the fatal childhood disease Menkes' syndrome (steely hair or kinky hair syndrome). In addition, type IX is associated with specific skeletal changes (occipital "horns," deformed clavicles, bowed shafts of long bones). Approximately 50 per cent of cases lack the precise clinical findings necessary to fit them neatly into one of these nine clinical slots.

Pathology and Pathophysiology

The Ehlers-Danlos syndrome is primarily a genetic disorder of collagen synthesis related to Marfan's syndrome, osteogenesis imperfecta, and, possibly, Menkes' syndrome; the observed changes in the elastic fibers are a secondary phenomenon. Multiple specific defects in collagen formation have been defined and then related to the different clinical manifestations of the Ehlers-Danlos syndrome. The mesenchymal defect in the various types of Ehlers-Danlos syndrome involves the joint capsules, the ligaments, and the paravertebral supporting tissues. No primary osseous abnormality has been reported in clinical studies of this syndrome.

The molluscoid fibrous tumors, found predominantly on the pressure points of the body, are composed of proliferating connective tissue and degenerated fat. Subcutaneous spherules of necrotic fat are also found in the skin, perhaps related to subclinical trauma. The bleeding diathesis associated with the Ehlers-Danlos syndrome is ascribed to abnormalities in the vessel walls as well as to defects in the supporting perivascular tissues.

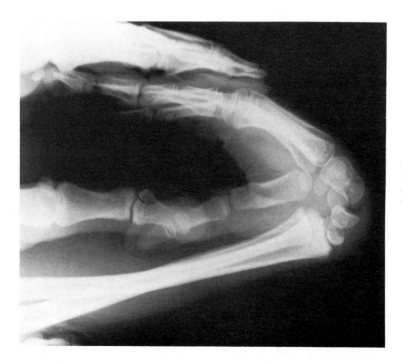

Figure 73–4. Ehlers-Danlos syndrome. Lateral view of the wrist shows a vacuum phenomenon in the lunate-capitate articulation secondary to joint laxity. Patient is able to touch the forearm with the thumb.

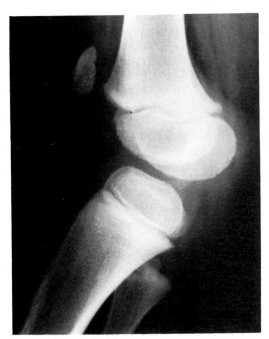

Figure 73–5. Ehlers-Danlos syndrome. Lateral view of the knee shows fibular head dislocation and genu recurvatum deformity.

Clinical Findings

The diagnosis of Ehlers-Danlos syndrome continues to rest on the clinical triad of skin fragility, hyperelasticity of joints, and vascular fragility. Molluscoid tumors and subcutaneous nodules formed at sites of fatty degeneration also are considered diagnostic criteria. The clinical expression of the syndrome is extremely variable, however.

The Ehlers-Danlos syndrome usually comes to medical attention during childhood. There is a male predominance. Dolichostenomelia can be present or absent. Typical facial characteristics include lop ears, redundant skin folds around the eyes, poor dentition, and a high, arched palate. Blue sclerae may be seen. Mental retardation is not present.

The skin is velvety, thin, and hyperelastic, and it can be raised in high folds. The skin is also easily bruised, with scarring. The appearance of these scars has been compared to "cigarette paper."

Hypermobility of joints in the Ehlers-Danlos syndrome has provided many a circus with an "India rubber man." Patients are able to (1) touch their thumbs to their forearms (Fig. 73–4), (2) passively dorsiflex their fifth fingers beyond 90 degrees, (3) hyperextend their elbows beyond 10 degrees, and (4) hyperextend their knees beyond 10 degrees (recurvatum). Spontaneous dislocations are frequent. Ligamentous laxity results in kyphoscoliosis, pes planus, and inguinal and hiatal hernias.

The fragility of the vessel walls can result in bleeding from the gastrointestinal tract, the bronchopulmonary tree, or the gums. Dissecting aneurysms of the aorta and spontaneous ruptures of the large vessels may result in death.

Ocular abnormalities include strabismus, ectopia lentis, and retinal detachments. Muscular weakness also is a feature of this syndrome.

Radiographic Findings

Calcification of fatty spherules produces multiple subcutaneous dense lesions that occur primarily in the forearms, shins, and extensor surfaces of the extremities. These calcifications usually have a dense rim and resemble phleboliths. Other soft tissue calcifications occur in molluscoid lesions, scars, or hematomas and in areas of myositis ossificans.

Joint findings include persistent effusions or hemarthroses. Olecranon and prepatellar bursitis may be evident. The joint spaces may widen with minor stress (Fig. 73–4). Lateral knee films can show varying degrees of recurvatum (Fig. 73–5).

Dislocations and subluxations frequently complicate the clinical course (Fig. 73–6). Affected sites are the digits, the shoulder joints, the patellofemoral joints, the hips, the temporomandibular joints, the radial heads, and the sternoclavicular and acromioclavicular joints. Precocious osteoarthritis is the sequela of the repetitive minor trauma associated with capsular laxity. Eventually contractures can occur.

Ligamentous laxity also results in pes planus deformities and abnormalities of the axial skeleton. The thorax can be asymmetric, with pectus carinatum and prominence of the costochondral junctions. The upper ribs may slant sharply downward. A kyphoscoliosis frequently is present at the thoracolumbar junction. Severe spondylolysis and spondylolisthesis have been reported (Fig. 73–7). As in neurofibromatosis, posterior scalloping of the vertebral bodies (secondary to dural ectasia) has been reported. If there is an associated Raynaud's disease, acroosteolysis may be present.

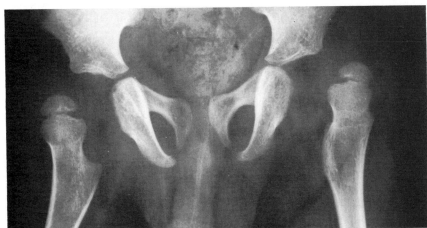

Figure 73–6. Ehlers-Danlos syndrome. Bilateral hip dislocations.

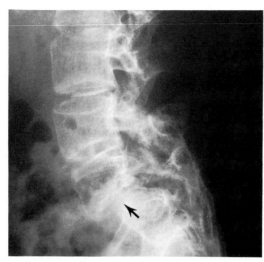

Figure 73–7. Ehlers-Danlos syndrome. Lateral view of the lumbar spine shows a spondylolysis and spondylolisthesis (arrow).

Congenital abnormalities in Ehlers-Danlos syndrome include arachnodactyly, triphalangeal thumbs, radioulnar synostoses, clubfeet, supernumerary teeth, delayed cranial ossification, elongation of the ulnar styloid, a short fifth proximal phalanx, and posterior radial head dislocations.

The radiographic differential diagnosis of joint laxity includes Marfan's syndrome, Larsen's syndrome, cachexia, Down's syndrome, and neuromuscular disorders. The soft tissue calcifications of the Ehlers-Danlos syndrome may be confused with cysticercosis, vascular tumors, phleboliths, or collagen diseases.

OSTEOGENESIS IMPERFECTA

Osteogenesis imperfecta is an inherited disorder of connective tissue that affects the skeleton, ligaments, skin, sclerae, and dentin. It is thought to be characterized by the abnormal maturation of collagen in both mineralized and nonmineralized tissues. The four major clinical criteria are (1) osteoporosis with abnormal fragility of the skeleton, (2) blue sclerae, (3) dentinogenesis imperfecta, and (4) premature otosclerosis. The presence of two of these abnormalities confirms the diagnosis. Other features are ligamentous laxity, episodic diaphoresis with abnormal temperature regulation, easy bruisability, constipation, hyperplastic scars, premature vascular calcifications, and inappropriate euphoria.

Osteogenesis imperfecta originally was subclassified into two forms on the basis of the age at the time of the first fracture: the congenita form, which has a high infant mortality rate, and the tarda form, which has a normal life expectancy. The terms congenita and tarda now refer to the presence or absence of osseous deformities. Bowing of the long bones is a useful guide to the severity of the disorder because it correlates with both the number of fractures and the probability of ambulation. Most patients with the tarda form have a family history consistent with an autosomal dominant mode of inheritance. The less common (10 per cent) congenita form of the disease is more often the result of spontaneous mutations or an autosomal recessive pattern of inheritance.

It is as yet uncertain whether osteogenesis imperfecta is a single disorder or a group of related entities. Four groups of the disease have been defined by some investigators. Group 1

(autosomal dominant with variable penetrance) is the most frequent form of osteogenesis imperfecta and includes most patients with the tarda form. It is characterized by fractures of varying severity, blue sclerae, dentinogenesis imperfecta, and premature otosclerosis. Group 2 (autosomal recessive) comprises a high proportion of the congenita cases and is associated with severe neonatal fractures and blue sclerae. Most patients in this group die in the perinatal period. Group 3 (mostly sporadic cases but also recessive and dominant cases) is associated with blue sclerae and severe progressive skeletal deformities; over two thirds of patients have fractures at birth. If patients in group 3 survive, they have the most dramatic dwarfed type of osteogenesis imperfecta. Group 4 (autosomal dominant) has variable skeletal findings. The sclerae are normal.

Pathology and Pathophysiology

Osteogenesis imperfecta is a generalized connective tissue disorder characterized by the abnormal synthesis or quality of fibrillar collagen. The clinical abnormalities are present in tissues with high type I collagen content (e.g., ligaments, tendons, fasciae, sclerae, teeth, and bones).

The pathologic and histologic changes in the osseous tissue in osteogenesis imperfecta are characterized by a primary defect in extracellular bone matrix. Periosteal bone formation is decreased. Osteoblastic activity is slowed, and there is a failure to replace fetal bone with normal lamellar bone, which leaves the cortex thinned and mechanically weakened. The number of osteoblasts and osteocytes, per unit matrix, actually is increased, however. Therefore, the decrease of bone synthesis per individual osteoblast is partly compensated for by an increase in the number of cells.

Abnormalities of the cartilage growth plate have been reported, but their origin remains controversial. It is uncertain whether these alterations represent a primary growth disturbance or whether they are secondary to trauma within the adjacent supporting bone.

Bone, skin, and dentin share similar extracellular matrix, and therefore it is predictable that defects described in fibroblast cultures and bone also occur in the teeth. Immature collagen and abnormal granular calcifications have been observed in the pulp of the teeth. The enamel itself is normal, but it fractures and separates from the deficient dentin.

The sclerae are thin and contain abnormal collagen. The blue translucency results from the brown choroid shining through the abnormal outer layer. The exact reason for premature otosclerosis in osteogenesis imperfecta is unknown.

Clinical Findings

Osteogenesis imperfecta occurs in all races. Some series report an equal sex distribution, whereas others have observed a slight female predominance. The congenita cases (10 per cent) have high intrauterine and infant mortality rates owing to the complications of intracerebral hemorrhage or a flail chest. The age at which the diagnosis is established depends on the pattern of inheritance, the severity of the clinical expression, and whether there is a known family history. Most cases are diagnosed at birth or, with the use of ultrasonography, in utero.

Facial characteristics include temporal bulging, flattening of the features, micrognathia, and hypertelorism. Blue sclerae

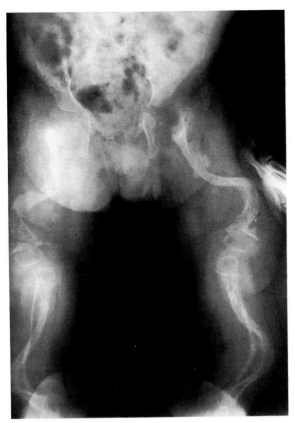

Figure 73–8. **Osteogenesis imperfecta.** Anteroposteror view of pelvis and lower extremities reveals a decrease in osseous density associated with thin, gracile long bones. Multiple fractures in various stages of healing are present. The long bones are bowed.

occur in over 90 per cent of cases. A small ring of sclera surrounding the cornea can retain a normal white color and is called a "Saturn's ring." Abnormal dentition with opalescent blue-gray or brown teeth is termed dentinogenesis imperfecta.

Growth retardation occurs in most cases. The short stature is related to defects in collagen synthesis, the gross fracture deformities, telescoping fractures, and fragmentation of the physeal plate. The limbs are more involved than the trunk, and the lower extremities are more shortened than the upper extremities. Skeletal deformities include kyphoscoliosis and bowing of the long bones. The spinal deformities can result in pain, paresthesias, difficulty in ambulating, and, in severe congenita cases, respiratory failure or paraplegia.

Multiple fractures are the predominant clinical finding in osteogenesis imperfecta. The frequency of the pathologic fractures appears to decrease after puberty. In both male and female patients, the frequency of fractures peaks in childhood and decreases in adolescence.

Otosclerosis can occur prior to the age of 40 years. Rarely, nerve conduction deafness may occur with associated vertigo and tinnitus.

The clinical abnormalities of osteogenesis imperfecta include thin skin, a tendency to form hyperplastic scars, premature vascular calcifications, joint laxity, a high frequency of hernias, and platelet abnormalities.

The central nervous system also can be affected. Basilar impression is associated with platybasia or the "tam-o'-shanter" skull. Once present, basilar impression can interfere with the flow of cerebrospinal fluid (hydrocephalus), disturb cerebellar function, and result in compression of the brain stem.

Radiographic Findings

The most characteristic radiographic finding of osteogenesis imperfecta is a diffuse decrease in osseous density (Figs. 73–8 and 73–9), which involves equally the axial and appendicular portions of the skeleton. The degree of osteopenia is highly variable, however, and in the tarda form, at the mildest end of the spectrum, patients can appear to have normal bone density on plain films.

On the basis of the radiographic appearance of the extremities, three categories of disease have been defined. The first category encompasses those cases with thin, gracile bones (Fig. 73–8). This is the most common expression of the disease and occurs in most patients with the tarda form. The second group includes the patients with short, thick limbs. This type of radiographic appearance occurs almost exclusively in patients with a congenita form of the disease and is associated with a poor prognosis. Third, and least frequent, is a group of cases with cystic changes in the extremities (Fig. 73–9). These occur in severely affected individuals, and the radiographic findings in this category are characterized by

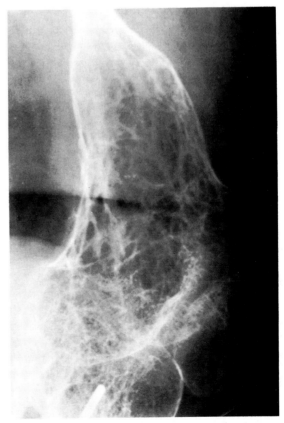

Figure 73–9. **Osteogenesis imperfecta.** Lateral view of knee demonstrating the rare cystic type of disease. The metaphyses are flared and honeycombed by thick, coarse trabeculae.

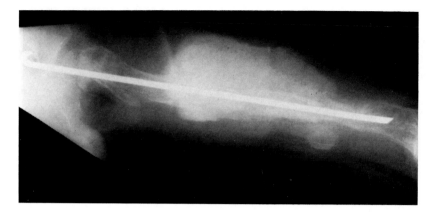

Figure 73–10. Osteogenesis imperfecta. Tumoral callus formation around Sofield osteotomies.

flared metaphyses, which are hyperlucent and traversed by a honeycomb of coarse trabeculae. As with the clinical and genetic categories, the radiographic classification is descriptive. Considerable variation exists within each category. The cortices of the long bones may be either abnormally thin or abnormally thick. The metaphyses may be flared or undermodeled, and the shafts can be straight or bowed.

The fractures that complicate the course of osteogenesis imperfecta occur most frequently in the lower extremities. Avulsion injuries and transverse fractures are common. Bowing deformities are the sequelae of multiple telescoping fractures. Fracture healing usually is normal, but tumoral callus (Fig. 73–10) and pseudarthroses may occur. The tumoral callus of osteogenesis imperfecta may mimic an osteosarcoma.

In children with severe osteogenesis imperfecta, the metaphyses or epiphyses of the long bones may contain multiple scalloped radiolucent areas with sclerotic margins (Fig. 73–11). The latter appearance is referred to as "popcorn calcifications," and it is thought to result from the traumatic fragmentation of the cartilage growth plate.

The joints of the extremities are affected by two separate processes, both of which lead to premature degenerative joint disease. First, fracture deformities distort the articular surfaces and result in incongruity. Second, ligamentous and capsular laxity produces repetitive minor trauma, which also results in damage to the hyaline cartilage.

Since 1959, use of the Sofield procedure, multiple osteotomies, and intramedullary rodding have changed the course of this disease. The intramedullary rods both correct the bowing deformities and protect the limb from further fractures.

Radiographs of the skull demonstrate enlargement of the frontal and mastoid sinuses and intrasutural bones (wormian bones) (Fig. 73–12). The presence of wormian bones is probably the sequela of abnormal skull development. Platybasia, with or without basilar impression, is a frequent deformity in osteogenesis imperfecta. Very rarely, thickening and not thinning of the calvarium has been observed in cases of severe osteogenesis imperfecta.

The spine studies show flattening of the vertebral bodies, which are either biconcave or wedge-shaped anteriorly (Fig. 73–13). Severe kyphoscoliosis occurs in approximately 40 per cent of patients with osteogenesis imperfecta. The multiple thoracic deformities, including fractured, beaded ribs, pectus

carinatum, and kyphoscoliosis, contribute to compromised respiratory function.

The pelvis is narrowed and frequently triradiate in shape (Fig. 73–14). Protrusion deformities of the acetabula and shepherd's crook deformities of the femora may be present.

In pregnant women with the disease, ultrasonography is currently being used in the detection of fetuses with congenita or severe osteogenesis imperfecta tarda. Detectable findings on ultrasonography include shortening of the femora, femoral fractures, disproportion of fetal body to head size, a poorly

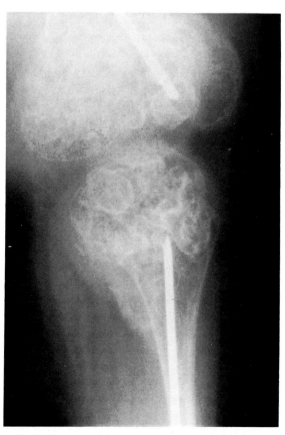

Figure 73–11. Osteogenesis imperfecta. Oblique view of the knee showing popcorn calcifications. These lucent areas with sclerotic margins are associated with absence of a normal horizontal growth plate and severe growth retardation. Sofield procedures have been performed.

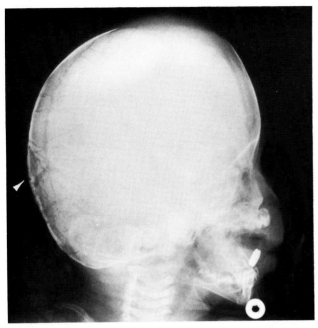

Figure 73–12. Osteogenesis imperfecta. Lateral view of the skull shows decreased osseous density, thinning of both tables, and multiple wormian bones (arrowhead).

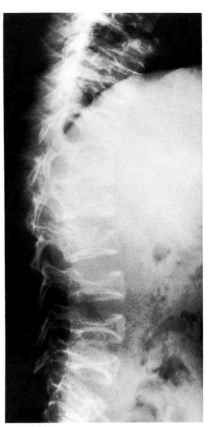

Figure 73–13. Osteogenesis imperfecta. Lateral view of the spine shows both biconcave vertebrae and vertebrae with anterior wedge deformities.

defined calvarium, and a narrow thorax that makes the heart and liver appear enlarged.

The differential diagnosis of osteogenesis imperfecta includes other entities with multiple fractures, such as the child abuse syndrome and congenital indifference to pain. The relatively normal bone density at uninvolved sites and the absence of eye or dental abnormalities should differentiate these latter disorders from fragilitas ossium. Hypophosphatasia is associated with lucent bones and bowing deformities of the extremities, but the metaphyseal changes of rickets

also are present, distinguishing it from osteogenesis imperfecta. The radiographic findings of idiopathic juvenile osteoporosis and Cushing's disease may be indistinguishable from those of osteogenesis imperfecta.

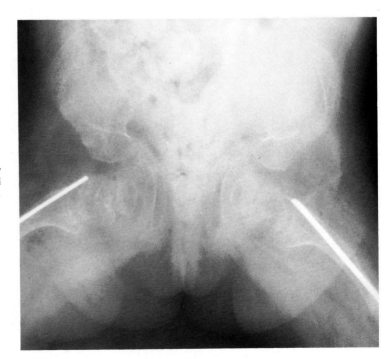

Figure 73–14. Osteogenesis imperfecta. Anteroposterior view of the pelvis showing a triradiate shape and protrusio acetabuli deformities. Sofield procedures have been performed in the femora.

MYOSITIS (FIBRODYSPLASIA) OSSIFICANS PROGRESSIVA

Myositis ossificans progressiva is a hereditary mesodermal disorder characterized by progressive ossification of striated muscles, tendons, ligaments, fasciae, aponeuroses, and occasionally skin. The pattern of inheritance remains unknown. Indeed, most reported cases are the result of spontaneous mutations. The disease is also called fibrogenesis ossificans progressiva or fibrodysplasia ossificans progressiva.

Pathology and Pathophysiology

The cause of myositis ossificans progressiva is unknown. There is a high association of congenital digital anomalies. Seventy-five to 90 per cent of patients with myositis ossificans progressiva (and 5 per cent of members of their families) have bilateral microdactyly of the first toes, often associated with synostosis of the phalanges (Fig. 73–15). The nature of the association between the digital anomalies and the heterotopic ossification remains obscure. Even the target tissue of the disease is uncertain. The prevailing theory postulates that the disease affects primarily the interstitial tissues and that muscle damage is secondary to pressure atrophy. Involvement of skin, tendons, and ligaments, which contain no muscle fibers, and the detectable localized increase in alkaline phosphatase and elevated urinary levels of collagen metabolites (hydroxyproline and hydroxylysine), support the concept of a fibrous defect.

The pathologic abnormalities that characterize the individual lesions are similar but not identical to those of myositis ossificans circumscripta. The earliest histologic changes are edema and an inflammatory exudate. Mesenchymal proliferation then results in the formation of multifocal interconnecting nodules. Gradually, the nodules coalesce to form large masses, the lesions become less cellular, the muscle fibers decrease in diameter, and the abnormal tissue is transformed into membranous bone. Eventually, the entire muscle or muscle group is replaced by columns or plates of lamellar bone.

Clinical Findings

Myositis ossificans progressiva is a rare disease. It has variously been reported to occur equally in both sexes or to occur more commonly in men. Although the onset of symptoms usually is in the first decade of life, ossification is rarely present at birth. The most frequent presenting symptom is torticollis resulting from a painful mass within the sternocleidomastoid muscle. The disease usually progresses from the shoulder girdle to the upper arms, spine, and pelvis. The distal portions of the extremities are involved late in the course of the disease. The heart, diaphragm, larynx, tongue, and sphincters are spared, as are all smooth muscle structures. The natural history of myositis ossificans progressiva is one of erratic remissions and exacerbations. Joint ankylosis occurs as the result of ossification of the surrounding soft tissues. Fusion of the hips is usually present by the third decade of life, leaving the patient wheelchair bound. Involvement of the temporomandibular joints limits nutrition.

Conductive hearing loss is another common complication of myositis ossificans progressiva. Other clinical findings observed in this disease include premature baldness and mental retardation.

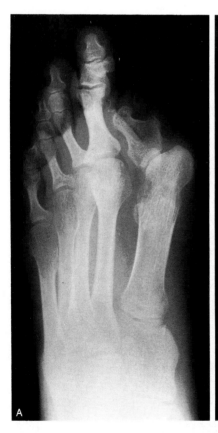 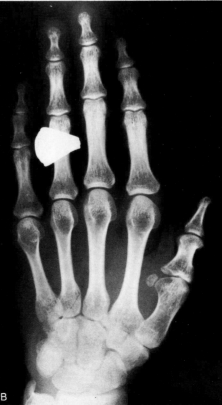

Figure 73–15. Myositis ossificans progressiva. Frontal views of the foot (A) and hand (B) demonstrating microdactyly of the first digits with hypoplasia and fusion of the phalanges.

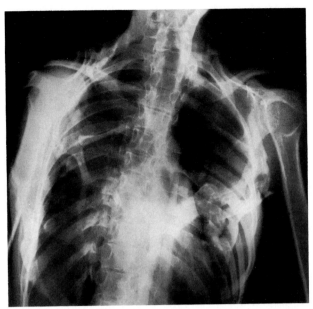

Figure 73–16. Myositis ossificans progressiva. An anteroposterior view of the thorax showing the early distribution of soft tissue ossification: shoulders, neck, and cervical spine.

Death from the disease is inevitable and may be secondary to respiratory failure with constriction of the chest wall and, in many cases, pneumonia, or it may result from starvation consequent to ossification of the masseter muscles.

Radiographic Findings

Digital abnormalities are present at birth, are symmetric, and usually precede the soft tissue ossification. The most common type of abnormality is microdactyly of the first toes, with hypoplasia or synostosis of the phalanges, or both (Fig. 73–15). The proximal phalanges of the great toes have an abnormal contour (broad and square) and are often fused to the distal phalanges. The first metatarsals are also abnormal. Fusion of the phalanges of all of the toes can also occur. Similar abnormalities to those described in the feet frequently involve the hands (Fig. 73–15B).

Other congenital anomalies of the skeleton associated with myositis ossificans progressiva are hallux valgus deformities, clinodactyly, broad femoral necks, bilateral thickening of the medial cortices of the tibiae, an abnormal carrying angle at the elbow, and an increased frequency of spina bifida.

After the onset of symptoms, the radiographic findings in the individual locations are similar to those of the traumatic form of myositis ossificans. The first such finding is a soft tissue mass. The lesion gradually shrinks in size and ossifies, and the final appearance of the lesion may be that of solid new bone replacing the entire muscle of the neck or extremities (Fig. 73–16). Pseudarthroses can occur within these masses of bone. Involvement of the insertions of fasciae, ligaments, and tendons produces "pseudoexostoses" (not true osteochondromas) (Fig. 73–17). Joint ankylosis results from ossification of the surrounding soft tissue structures.

Abnormalities in the spine occur as a result of loss of motion. In the majority of cases, ossification of the soft tissues is followed by fusion of the posterior osseous elements (Fig. 73–18) and finally, fusion of the vertebral bodies (Fig. 73–

19). The intervertebral discs become hypoplastic and calcified. The findings can mimic the appearance of ankylosing spondylitis. In the thoracic and lumbar regions, so-called "dog vertebrae," which are higher than they are wide, occur as a result of limited weight-bearing. Scoliotic deformities frequently are present. The sacroiliac joints, like other articulations, can become fused owing to extensive soft tissue ossification.

The radiographic differential diagnosis includes the causes of metastatic calcifications (e.g., idiopathic calcinosis universalis, dermatomyositis, idiopathic tumoral calcinosis, and disorders of calcium metabolism). In all of these conditions, however, the dense lesions remain calcific and do not mature into trabecular bone. Systemic diseases related to multicentric areas of myositis circumscripta, including tetany, paraplegia, and burns, can mimic myositis ossificans progressiva. In the cervical spine, other causes of fusion of the posterior elements (Klippel-Feil syndrome, Still's disease, ankylosing spondylitis) can resemble myositis ossificans progressiva. The presence of soft tissue ossification and digital anomalies in cases of myositis ossificans progressiva greatly simplifies interpretation, however.

PSEUDOXANTHOMA ELASTICUM

Pseudoxanthoma elasticum is an inherited disorder of unknown pathogenesis characterized by a defect in elastic fibers that involves the skin, eyes, and cardiovascular system. Most patients have a family history consistent with a recessive mode of inheritance, although dominant patterns also are recognized. The clinical expressions of pseudoxanthoma elasticum are protean; four variants of the disease have been described: dominant type I (typical peau d'orange rash, severe

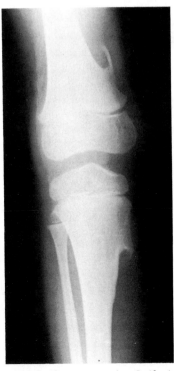

Figure 73–17. Myositis ossificans progressiva. Ossification of ligamentous insertions results in metaphyseal "exostoses."

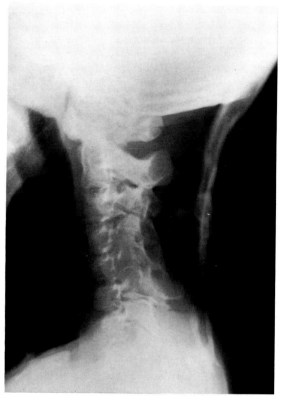

Figure 73–18. Myositis ossificans progressiva. Note ossification of the soft tissues and secondary fusion of the apophyseal joints.

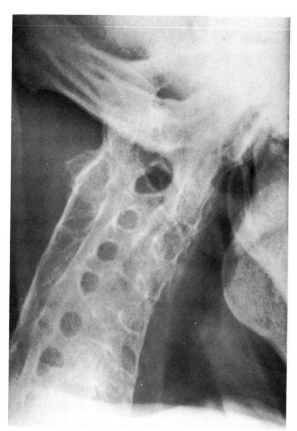

Figure 73–19. Myositis ossificans progressiva. Lateral view of the cervical spine showing the late changes of the disease with fusion of the soft tissues, apophyseal joints, and vertebral bodies.

vascular disease, early blindness), dominant type II (mild skin changes, mild retinal findings, mild vascular disease, blue sclerae, high arched palate, skin extensibility), recessive type I (typical skin changes, mild retinal and vascular abnormalities), and recessive type II (very severe changes in the elastic fibers of the skin, resulting in laxity and distensibility, no systemic symptoms).

Pathology and Pathophysiology

The primary tissue affected in pseudoxanthoma elasticum is a matter of controversy, and there is still doubt as to whether the disease involves the biosynthesis of collagen or elastin. Evidence against a primary abnormality of elastic fibers includes (1) sparing of the aorta, lungs, plantar fascia, and palmar fascia, all tissues rich in elastic fibers, and (2) the vascular changes of pseudoxanthoma elasticum that involve the walls of the muscular, not elastic, vessels.

The ocular changes are characterized by angioid streaks, which represent the fissuring and scarring of the membrane beneath the retina. Narrowing and occlusion of the large muscular arteries of the extremities, viscera, and central nervous system also are findings of pseudoxanthoma elasticum. The vascular calcifications in this disorder occur most frequently in the femoral arteries, involve the media of the vessel wall, and are uniform in distribution.

Clinical Findings

Pseudoxanthoma elasticum occurs in all races, and there is a slight female predominance. Skin abnormalities usually become apparent in the second decade of life. Changes involve primarily the neck, the face, the axillary and inguinal folds,

the cubital areas, and the periumbilical region. Also affected are the heart, the soft palate, and the mucosae of the mouth, gastrointestinal tract, and vagina. The earliest clinical findings are accentuation of the normal skin lines. Later, the skin becomes thickened, redundant, deeply grooved, and hyperextensible. The most characteristic clinical feature is the yellow papules that occur between the thickened folds, producing a "pebbly" texture or a peau d'orange appearance.

The angioid streaks that characterize the ocular findings of pseudoxanthoma elasticum also begin in the second decade of life. Angioid streaks also are seen in Paget's disease, sickle cell anemia, and the Ehlers-Danlos syndrome. Chorioretinitis, a more severe threat to vision, is a second ocular abnormality that may occur in pseudoxanthoma elasticum.

Involvement of the muscular arteries usually takes place in the third decade of life. Physical examination reveals weakening of the peripheral pulses. The vascular changes may result in claudication in the extremities, coronary insufficiency, abdominal angina, hypertension, and bleeding from almost every organ.

Radiographic Findings

Radiographs of the skull frequently demonstrate premature calcification of the falx, the tentorium, the choroid plexus, and the petroclinoid ligaments. Thickening of the calvarium and the base of the skull also has been reported. Films of the extremities may demonstrate calcifications in the dermis, within tendons and ligaments, around the metacarpophalangeal joints, the hip joints, or the elbow joints, and within both large peripheral veins and arteries. Angiography of the extremities demonstrates localized narrowing of large arteries as well as the formation of localized aneurysms and arteriovenous malformations. Resorption of the tufts of the distal phalanges may result from the vascular changes.

The radiographic differential diagnosis includes other entities with both soft tissue and vascular calcification. Both renal disease and collagen disease can produce calcifications in soft tissues as well as erosion of the distal tufts of the phalanges. The Ehlers-Danlos syndrome and parasitic disorders can also produce soft tissue calcifications.

FIBROGENESIS IMPERFECTA OSSIUM

Fibrogenesis imperfecta ossium is a rare disorder of collagen synthesis. The cause is unknown, and changes are limited to the skeleton.

Pathology and Pathophysiology

The characteristic pathologic abnormality of this disorder is the presence of abnormal collagen in the lamellar bones. Unlike normal collagen, the fibrils are not birefringent when viewed with the polarizing microscope. The collagen defect results in incomplete mineralization of the bone and in wide osteoid seams. Therefore, the pathologic and radiologic findings of this disease can superficially resemble those of osteomalacia.

There are no reports of radiographically apparent joint changes associated with this disease. The collagen of tissues other than bone and calcified cartilage is normal.

Clinical Findings

This disorder appears late in adult life. The onset of symptoms is heralded by spontaneous fractures. Changes are rapidly progressive, with eventual debilitation of the patient. Serum calcium and phosphorus levels are normal. There may, however, be elevation of the serum alkaline phosphatase level. The most characteristic laboratory abnormality is the excessive fecal excretion of calcium. The diagnosis is suggested on the basis of the radiographic changes and confirmed by collagen studies of biopsy material.

Radiographic Findings

The radiographic changes in fibrogenesis imperfecta ossium are found in the entire skeleton, with relative sparing of the skull. Two radiographic patterns have been described. First, and most typical, is the so-called fishnet appearance. There is a decrease in osseous density and in the number of trabeculae, but those that remain are coarse and dense. The thick, abnormal trabeculae follow the lines of stress. The size and contour of the bones remain normal. The vertebral endplates are dense, mimicking the rugger-jersey spine of renal osteodystrophy. The skull may show widening of the vault and homogeneous sclerosis of the base. The second, less common appearance of fibrogenesis imperfecta ossium is that of a generalized increase in osseous density with obliteration of the trabecular architecture. Both radiographic patterns can coexist in the same patient, and both are most marked in the axial skeleton or around joints.

Multiple pathologic fractures usually are present. In addition, pseudoexostoses of dense callus-like bone form around

the axial skeleton. Extensive calcification of ligamentous and tendinous insertions as well as diffuse periosteal new bone formation has been described.

The radiographic differential diagnosis includes advanced osteitis fibrosa cystica (hyperparathyroidism), Paget's disease, fluorosis, and atypical axial osteomalacia. Atypical axial osteomalacia produces radiographic changes almost identical to those of fibrogenesis imperfecta ossium. The principal differences are the abnormal collagen, which is found only in fibrogenesis imperfecta ossium, and the distribution of the radiographic changes. In fibrogenesis imperfecta ossium, the skeletal changes are generalized. In atypical axial osteomalacia, the changes occur only in the central skeleton.

MULTIPLE EPIPHYSEAL DYSPLASIAS

The epiphyseal dysplasias have been divided into two large categories: the spondyloepiphyseal dysplasias (with universal platyspondyly or beaking) and multiple epiphyseal dysplasias (with minimal or no spinal changes). The category of multiple epiphyseal dysplasias is far from homogeneous and contains isolated epiphyseal dysplasias, epiphyseal dysplasias associated with ocular, auditory, or endocrine abnormalities, and those that combine the findings of epiphyseal and metaphyseal dysostoses.

The entity referred to as dysplasia epiphysealis multiplex (multiple epiphyseal dysplasia tarda) is considered to be the prototype of the epiphyseal dysplasias. Most affected families have an inheritance pattern consistent with an autosomal dominant gene with high penetrance. Cases of spontaneous mutation and cases with autosomal recessive inheritance have also been reported, however.

Pathology and Pathophysiology

The primary defect in dysplasia epiphysealis multiplex appears to involve the epiphyseal chondrocyte. On gross specimens, the growth plate is found to be widened and to have an irregular metaphyseal margin. Tongues of cartilage extend into the osseous metaphysis, and there is irregularity of the peripheral trabeculae. Histologic specimens of the growth plate demonstrate a decrease in the number of chondrocytes in all zones, invasion of vessels into the cartilage, and loss of the normal columnar arrangement of the chondrocytes. There is excessive matrix as well as areas of degeneration and cleft formation. Bars of calcified fibrous tissue extend from the epiphysis to the metaphysis. The result of these abnormalities is delayed and disorderly ossification of the epiphyseal ends of the bones. Joint incongruity inevitably leads to secondary degenerative joint disease.

Clinical Findings

Dysplasia epiphysealis multiplex affects both sexes equally, and intelligence is normal. The most frequent sites of involvement are the hips, knees, shoulders, ankles, and wrists. The onset of symptoms usually is early in childhood, and common presenting complaints include articular pain and gait disturbances. In milder cases, symptoms may not occur until adulthood.

Physical examination reveals short stature, but only in severe cases is dwarfing present. The growth disturbance may lead to symmetric shortening of the skeleton. The hands and feet have a characteristic stubby appearance. Associated de-

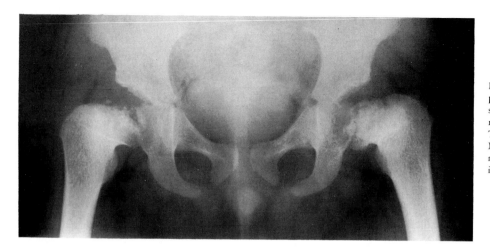

Figure 73–20. Multiple epiphyseal dysplasia. Anteroposterior view of the pelvis showing irregular femoral epiphyses and multiple epiphyseal ossification centers. There are bilateral coxa vara deformities. Mild irregularity of the metaphyses is also noted, and the acetabula show minimal irregularities.

formities include coxa vara, genu valgum, genu varum, or tibiotalar slants.

Radiographic Findings

Radiographic abnormalities appear in the second or third year of life and are most marked in the hips, knees, wrists, and ankles. Bone involvement is always bilaterally symmetric.

In young children, the epiphyseal centers of the long bones are late in appearing and slow in mineralizing, and when they begin to ossify they are irregularly fragmented (Figs. 73–20 to 73–22). The epiphyses frequently ossify from multiple centers and have a mulberry-like appearance. The secondary centers are small or flattened.

In older children, slipped epiphyses complicate the coxa vara deformities. The decrease in the neck-shaft angle rotates the growth plate into a more vertical alignment than normal and, in turn, increases the sheer stress on the cartilage. Incongruity results in premature osteoarthritis.

In adolescents, apparent improvement in the radiographic appearance has been reported to occur as the result of puberty. The smoother appearance of the ends of the bones is simply the result of the completion of skeletal growth and the fusion of the multiple centers of ossification, however. Even after puberty, the affected articular surfaces of the long bones remain irregular. The femoral heads and femoral condyles are flattened (Fig. 73–23). The proximal end of the tibia is square instead of biconcave. The talar articular surface also is flat. Differential growth rates within the same physeal plate result in wedge-shaped epiphyses and eventually deformities, which include coxa vara, genu valgum, genu varum, tibiotalar slant (Fig. 73–24), and V-shaped deformities of the wrist (Fig. 73–25). In most cases of multiple epiphyseal dysplasia, changes of secondary degenerative joint disease are present before the third or fourth decade of life (Fig. 73–26).

The spine is affected in two thirds of patients, and the radiographic changes are similar to those of Scheuermann's

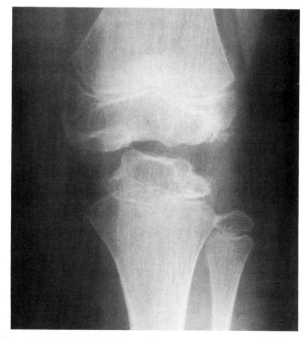

Figure 73–21. Multiple epiphyseal dysplasia. Note flattening of condyles and irregularity of the contours of the epiphyses.

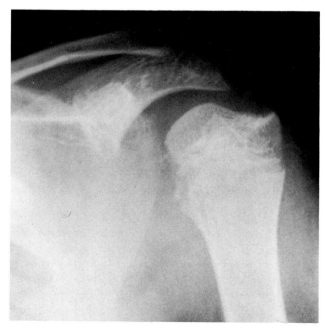

Figure 73–22. Multiple epiphyseal dysplasia. Anteroposterior view of a shoulder revealing an irregular contour and abnormal shape to the humeral head.

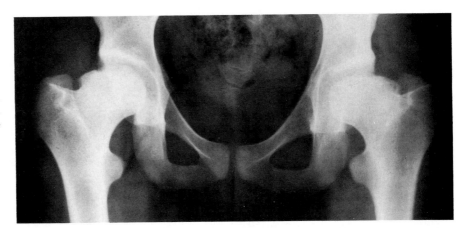

Figure 73–23. Multiple epiphyseal dysplasia. Anteroposterior view of the pelvis demonstrates flattening and irregularity of the surfaces of the femoral heads.

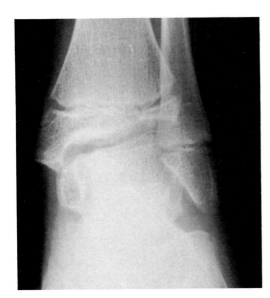

Figure 73–24. Multiple epiphyseal dysplasia. Anteroposterior view demonstrates tibiotalar slant with a wedge-shaped distal tibial epiphysis.

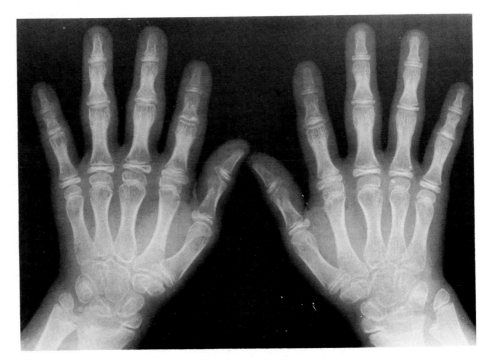

Figure 73–25. Multiple epiphyseal dysplasia. Frontal view of both hands showing the characteristic stubby phalanges and a V-shaped deformity of the wrists. The epiphyses of the radii and ulnae have an abnormal wedge shape.

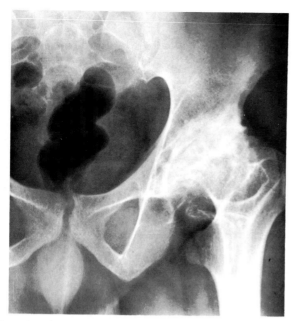

Figure 73–26. Multiple epiphyseal dysplasia. Anteroposterior view of the hip showing secondary degenerative changes complicating the epiphyseal dysplasia.

disease (Fig. 73–27). The frequency of spinal involvement does not correlate with the severity of the peripheral changes. The vertebral abnormalities associated with this entity include irregularity of the anterior aspects of the vertebral endplates, anterior wedging of the vertebral bodies, mild platyspondyly, and scoliosis.

The radiographic differential diagnosis includes other causes of irregular articular surfaces, such as inflammatory arthritides (e.g., Still's disease), osteonecrosis, cretinism, the mucopolysaccharidoses, Stickler's syndrome, and other dysplasias (see Chapter 84). Cretinism is associated with epiphyseal irregularities, but in addition there are retardation of bone age, generalized osteoporosis, wormian bones, and broad femoral necks. Stickler's syndrome has many features of an epiphyseal dysplasia, but they are combined with marfanoid osseous abnormalities and dislocation of the lens. The radiographic findings of spondyloepiphyseal dysplasias and the mucopolysaccharidoses are characterized by more severe spinal changes than those noted in epiphysealis dysplasia multiplex.

Chondrodysplasia Punctata

Chondrodysplasia punctata is a form of multiple epiphyseal dysplasia that is characterized by the calcification of the cartilaginous epiphyseal centers during the first year of life (Fig. 73–28). Also referred to as multiple epiphyseal dysplasia congenita, this entity is manifested at birth and has been divided into two syndromes. First is the rhizomelic form, which follows an autosomal recessive pattern of inheritance, is characterized by symmetric limb involvement, and is lethal early in childhood. Second is the Conradi-Hünermann syndrome, which is genetically heterogeneous, associated with asymmetric limb shortening, and usually consistent with a normal life expectancy. Most cases of Conradi-Hünermann syndrome are associated with an autosomal dominant mode of transmission or result from spontaneous mutations. This

syndrome can be the result of maternal use of warfarin sodium during the early months of pregnancy. Subgroups of Conradi-Hünermann syndrome are thought to be related to X-linked modes of transmission.

Pathologic findings in the epiphyseal centers include mucoid degeneration, cyst formation, and calcification. Calcifications, although present at birth, are resorbed during the first year of life, but during growth the epiphyses ossify in an irregular fashion.

The clinical findings include shortening of the extremities, scoliosis, a flattened face, wide-set eyes, and a saddle nose deformity. In the rhizomelic form of chondrodysplasia punctata, limb changes are symmetric and the spine is not abnormal on physical examination. This form is twice as common in females as in males. Findings include mental retardation, cataracts, cardiac anomalies, recurrent infections, joint contractures, alopecia, and ichthyosiform rashes. In the Conradi-Hünermann type of chondrodysplasia punctata, limb shortening is asymmetric and spinal deformities are prominent. Precise clinical abnormalities, however, vary according to the specific genetic subgroup that is being considered.

The radiographic changes differ in the two major syndromes. In the milder Conradi-Hünermann form, radiographs obtained in the first year of life demonstrate punctate or stippled calcifications at the ends of the long bones (Fig. 73–28), at the ends of the short tubular bones, in the vertebral endplates, in the cartilage rings of the trachea, and in the cartilage structures of the pharynx. Later in life, radiographic

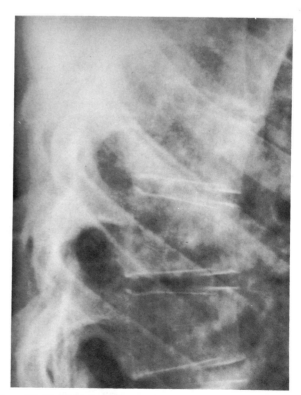

Figure 73–27. Multiple epiphyseal dysplasia. Lateral view of spine shows the mild changes that are associated with epiphyseal dysplasias. The vertebral bodies and intervertebral discs are wedge-shaped and there are minor irregularities of the vertebral endplates.

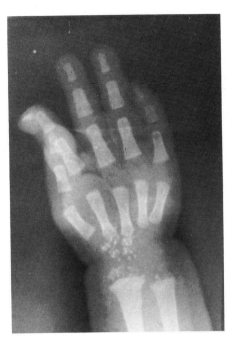

Figure 73–28. Chondrodysplasia punctata. Posteroanterior view of hand obtained at birth demonstrates stippling of cartilage epiphyses.

changes are variable. In some cases, the ossified skeleton is normal. More frequently, however, the early cartilage changes result in a diffuse asymmetric epiphyseal dysplasia (Fig. 73–29). The asymmetric limb involvement, brachydactyly, and scoliotic deformity of this syndrome should suggest the correct diagnosis.

In the severe recessive form of chondrodysplasia punctata, the stippled calcifications occur primarily in the hips and shoulders. Shortening of the extremities is symmetric and more severe proximally than distally. The metaphyses are flared, and the bones are bowed. The vertebral bodies show a characteristic coronal cleft. If the patient survives infancy, radiographs show irregularity of the cartilaginous growth plate and abnormal contours of the secondary ossification centers.

The radiographic differential diagnosis of chondrodysplasia punctata includes other causes of "stippled epiphyses," such as the gangliosidoses, infections, and the Fanconi-Albertini-Zellweger syndrome (cerebrohepatorenal syndrome).

Meyer's Dysplasia

Meyer's dysplasia represents either a mild localized epiphyseal dysplasia limited to the femoral capital epiphyses or a normal variant of ossification. Most cases are discovered as an incidental finding on radiographs that are obtained for other reasons. The most serious problem encountered is the risk of misdiagnosing the condition as Legg-Calvé-Perthes disease. Radiographic studies reveal delayed ossification of the femoral heads, which appear at approximately 2 years of age instead of at 6 months. As the femoral capital epiphyses begin to ossify, multiple irregular centers develop with an abnormal flattened appearance (Fig. 73–30). As growth continues, a return to the normal hemispheric shape of the femoral heads is observed. Unlike osteonecrosis, the changes are bilaterally symmetric, there is no predilection for the superior aspect of the femoral heads, and the density of the epiphyses is not increased.

MACRODYSTROPHIA LIPOMATOSA

Macrodystrophia lipomatosa is a rare form of localized gigantism characterized by a congenital and progressive overgrowth of all the mesenchymal elements of a digit, with a disproportionate increase in the fibroadipose tissue. It is classified as a developmental anomaly and is not hereditary.

Pathology and Pathophysiology

The cause of macrodystrophia lipomatosa remains obscure. Several authors have postulated that macrodystrophia lipomatosa is an expression of neurofibromatosis, but this conclusion is controversial.

The most dramatic pathologic finding is the increase in fibroadipose tissue, which involves the bone marrow, periosteum, muscles, nerve sheaths, and subcutaneous tissues.

Figure 73–29. Chondrodysplasia punctata. Anteroposteror view of hips shows epiphyseal dysplasia resulting from the Conradi-Hünermann syndrome.

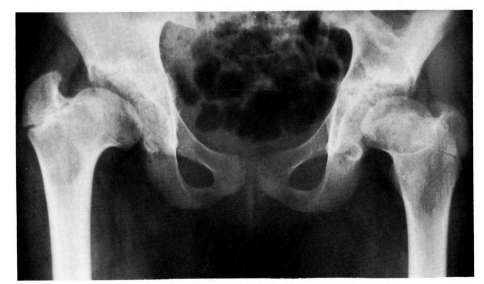

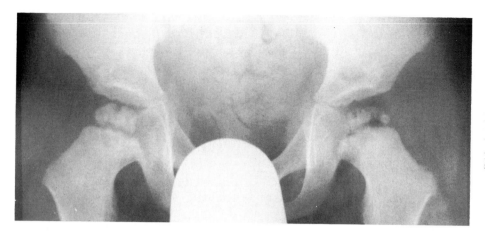

Figure 73–30. Meyer's dysplasia. Note irregular ossification of both femoral heads. The irregularity involves the entire epiphysis, and the changes are symmetric. The femoral heads are of normal density.

Neural enlargement may be prominent, most frequently involving the median nerve in the hand and the plantar nerve in the foot. The phalanges are enlarged by both endosteal and periosteal deposition of bone.

Clinical Findings

The localized gigantism associated with macrodystrophia lipomatosa is recognizable at birth. There is no known sexual predilection. Involvement is almost always unilateral. The lower extremity is involved more commonly than the upper extremity, and the second and third digits are the favored sites in both upper and lower extremities. The usual reason for seeking surgical correction is cosmetic. Mechanical problems are not encountered until adolescence, when secondary degenerative joint disease appears. Growth of the digit ceases at puberty.

Radiographic Findings

Radiographs of patients with macrodystrophia lipomatosa demonstrate abnormalities in both soft tissues and osseous structures (Figs. 73–31 and 73–32). The soft tissue overgrowth is most marked at the distal end of the digit and along its volar aspect. Small lucent areas reflecting overgrowth of fat are usually detectable within the soft tissues. The phalanges are long, broad, and often splayed at their distal ends. If more than one digit is involved, the digits are always adjacent to one another. The articular surfaces may slant, and, late in childhood, severe secondary degenerative joint disease supervenes. There is a high frequency of associated local anomalies, including syndactyly and polydactyly. Clinodactyly is almost invariably present.

The radiographic differential diagnosis of localized gigantism includes both acquired and congenital disorders. On the

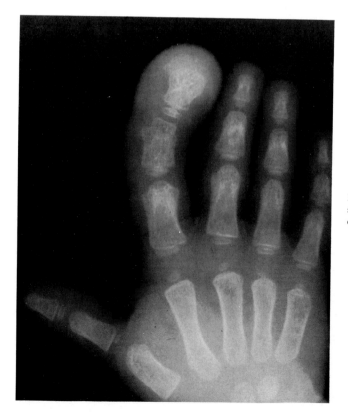

Figure 73–31. Macrodystrophia lipomatosa. Posteroanterior radiograph shows osseous and soft tissue enlargement, affecting predominantly the distal end of the second digit, and splaying of the ends of the phalanges.

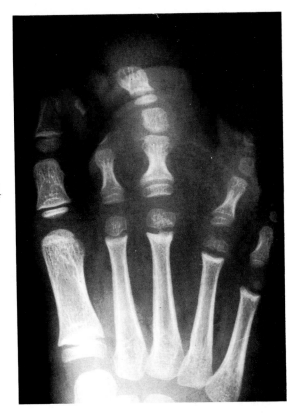

Figure 73-32. Macrodystrophia lipomatosa. Anteroposterior radiograph demonstrates soft tissue and osseous overgrowth with predominant involvement of the distal ends of the digits. Soft tissue lucent areas are apparent.

basis of the history, the acquired causes (dactylitis secondary to infection, trauma, infarction, or Still's disease, osteoid osteoma, melorheostosis) can be eliminated. The majority of congenital causes can also be excluded. Hyperemia secondary to tumorous overgrowth of hemangiomatous and lymphangiomatous elements produces soft tissue hypertrophy and symmetric overgrowth of the bones. The Klippel-Trenaunay syndrome has obvious cutaneous abnormalities. The absence of enchondromas eliminates the possibility of Ollier's disease.

The most difficult differential diagnosis involves neurofibromatosis (Fig. 73-33). Several radiographic findings can help to differentiate macrodystrophia lipomatosa from neu-

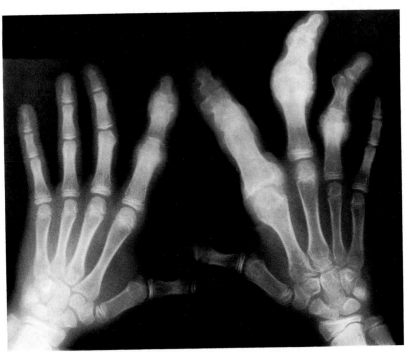

Figure 73-33. Neurofibromatosis. Bilateral macrodactyly can be evident in this disease. In addition, digital overgrowth is not most severe in the distal phalanges, there is premature fusion of the growth plates, and the cortices of the affected phalanges are dense and wavy. From Goldman AB, Kaye JJ: Macrodystrophia lipomatosa: Radiographic diagnosis. AJR 128:101, 1977. Copyright 1977, American Roentgen Ray Society. Used with permission.)

rofibromatosis, however. In neurofibromatosis, unlike macrodystrophia lipomatosa, the enlarged digits may be bilateral, involvement of one extremity does not necessarily involve contiguous digits, and the distal phalanges are not the most severely affected. Second, the hemangiomatous elements of the plexiform neurofibroma can produce premature fusion of the growth plates. Growth in a digit involved by macrodystrophia lipomatosa ceases with puberty. Third, the enlarged osseous structures in neurofibromatosis may have a wavy cortex and an elongated, sinuous appearance. The latter deformity is related to the periosteal abnormalities in neurofibromatosis. Last, the observation of soft tissue lucent areas has not been reported in patients with macrodactyly who have the neurocutaneous manifestations of neurofibromatosis.

FURTHER READING

Beals RK, Mason L: The Marfan skull. Radiology 140:723, 1981.

Berg PK: Dysplasia epiphysialis multiplex. AJR 97:31, 1966.

Bjerkreim I, Skogland LB, Trygstad O: Congenital contractural arachnodactyly. Acta Orthop Scand 47:250, 1976.

Brenton DP, Dow CJ: Homocystinuria and Marfan's syndrome. A comparison. J Bone Joint Surg [Br] 54:277, 1972.

Brill PW, Mitty JA, Gaull GE: Homocystinuria due to cystathionine synthetase deficiency: Clinical roentgenologic correlations. AJR 121:45, 1974.

Cremin B, Connor M, Beighton P: The radiological spectrum of fibrodysplasia ossificans progressiva. Clin Radiol 33:499, 1982.

Cremin B, Goodman H, Spranger J, Beighton P: Wormian bones in osteogenesis imperfecta and other diseases. Skel Radiol 8:35, 1982.

Golding FC: Fibrogenesis imperfecta. J Bone Joint Surg [Br] 50:619, 1968.

Goldman AB, Kaye JJ: Macrodystrophia lipomatosa: Radiographic diagnosis. AJR 128:101, 1977.

Goldman AB, Davidson D, Pavlov H, Bullough PG: "Popcorn calcifications." A prognostic sign of osteogenesis imperfecta. Radiology 136:351, 1980.

Holt JF: The Ehlers-Danlos syndrome. AJR 55:420, 1946.

Hulvey JT, Keats T: Multiple epiphyseal dysplasia. A contribution to the problem of spinal involvement. AJR 106:170, 1969.

Mason RC, Kozlowski K: Chondrodysplasia punctata. A report of 10 cases. Radiology 109:145, 1973.

McCall RE, Bax JA: Hyperplastic callus formation in osteogenesis imperfecta. Pediatr Orthop 4:361, 1984.

McKusick VA: Heritable Disorders of Connective Tissue. 4th Ed. St Louis, CV Mosby Co, 1972.

McKusick VA: The classification of heritable disorders of connective tissue. Birth Defects 11:1, 1975.

Mitchell GE, Lourie H, Berne AS: The various causes of scalloped vertebrae with notes on their pathogenesis. Radiology 89:67, 1967.

Prick JJG, Thijssen HDM: Radiodiagnostic signs in pseudoxanthoma elasticum generalisatum (dysgenesis elastofibrillaris mineralisans). Clin Radiol 28:549, 1977.

Rogers JG, Geho WB: Fibrodysplasia ossificans progressiva. A survey of forty-two cases. J Bone Joint Surg [Am] 61:709, 1979.

Rubin P: Dynamic Classification of Bone Dysplasias. Chicago, Year Book Medical Publishers, 1964.

Sartoris DJ, Luzzatti L, Weaver DD, MacFarlane JD, Hollister DW, Parker BR: Type IX Ehlers-Danlos syndrome. A new variant with pathognomonic radiologic features. Radiology 152:665, 1984.

Silengo MC, Luzzatti L, Silverman FN: Clinical and genetic aspects of Conradi-Hünermann disease. A report of three familial cases and review of the literature. J Pediatr 97:911, 1980.

Sillence D: Osteogenesis imperfecta: An expanding panorama of variants. Clin Orthop 159:11, 1981.

Sillence DO, Senn A, Danks DM: Genetic heterogeneity in osteogenesis imperfecta. J Med Genet 16:101, 1979.

Smith SW: Roentgen findings in homocystinuria. AJR 100:147, 1967.

Sofield HA, Millar EA: Fragmentation realignment and intramedullary rod fixation of deformities of the long bones in children. A ten year appraisal. J Bone Joint Surg [Am] 41:1371, 1959.

Stoddart PGP, Wickremaratchi T, Watt I: Fibrogenesis imperfecta ossium. Br J Radiol 57:744, 1984.

Thickman D, Bonakdar-pour A, Clancy M, Van Orden J, Steel H: Fibrodysplasia ossificans progressiva. AJR 139:935, 1982.

Chapter 74

Osteochondrodysplasias, Dysostoses, Chromosomal Aberrations, Mucopolysaccharidoses, and Mucolipidoses

William H. McAlister, M.D.

The number of skeletal dysplasias is large and continues to increase. Systems of nomenclature are complex and not agreed upon. A summary of only the more important dysplasias is contained in this chapter; certain other conditions, such as fibrous dysplasia, osteogenesis imperfecta, and melorheostosis, are discussed elsewhere in this book. Knowledge of the characteristic clinical and radiographic manifestations of these diseases is fundamental to accurate diagnosis and proper parental counseling.

OSTEOCHONDRODYSPLASIAS

Defects of Growth of Tubular Bones or Spine, or Both

ACHONDROGENESIS. Achondrogenesis, a type of dwarfism of neonates, is characterized by a disproportionately large head, short trunk, protuberant abdomen, severe micromelia, and hydrops. Two general types of achondrogenesis are recognized: type I (Parenti-Fraccaro type) and type II (Langer-Saldino type). Radiographic findings common to both types include severe lack of ossification of the vertebral bodies, small iliac bones, poor ossification of pubic and ischial bones, short tubular bones, and short ribs (Fig. 74–1). Milder forms of achondrogenesis, which may allow the patient to survive for months, have been termed hypochondrogenesis.

THANATOPHORIC DYSPLASIA. Thanatophoric or "death bearing" dysplasia is a well-recognized disorder (Fig. 74–2). Affected children are usually stillborn or die shortly after birth. There is marked short-limbed dwarfism, a large head with frontal bossing, and a depressed nasal bridge. The anteroposterior diameter of the chest is narrow, and the child has a relatively long trunk. Radiographic findings include marked shortening of the long tubular bones in a rhizomelic pattern of distribution, with metaphyseal flaring and osseous bowing and widening. The bowed femora resemble telephone receivers. Pronounced flattening of the vertebral bodies and wide intervertebral disc spaces are evident. The appearance of each vertebra on frontal radiographs resembles an inverted U or H. The thorax is slender owing to short ribs, and small, rectangular iliac bones, small sacrosciatic notches, and short and wide pubic and ischial bones are seen. The phalanges are short, relatively broad, and cupped. The base of the skull is short and the foramen magnum is small. A variety of extraskeletal malformations have been described, including a dysplastic temporal cortex and basal ganglia, megalocephaly, polymicrogyria, heart defects, and some degree of hydronephrosis.

SHORT RIB SYNDROMES (WITH OR WITHOUT POLYDACTYLY). Multiple syndromes are characterized by a narrow thorax with short ribs, micromelia, and frequent polydactyly. Early death occurs from pulmonary hypoplasia. Only three types will be noted here, and each demonstrates probable autosomal recessive inheritance.

In the *type I (Saldino-Noonan) syndrome*, the newborn infant appears hydropic and has extreme limb shortening, postaxial polydactyly, and a narrow thorax (Fig. 74–3). The tubular bones are extremely short, have irregular ends, and are sometimes pointed. The vertebral bodies are poorly ossified; coronal clefts are also present. The iliac bones are small, with flat acetabular roofs.

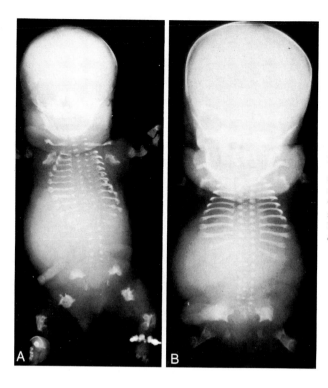

Figure 74–1. Achondrogenesis. A In the Type I syndrome, the vertebral bodies are poorly ossified; the tubular bones are bowed and short, with cupped and irregular ends; the iliac bones are deformed, with poor ossification; and the ribs are short, with multiple fractures and flared anterior ends. (Courtesy of C. S. Houston, M.D., Saskatoon, Saskatchewan, Canada.) **B** In the Type II syndrome, the ribs are short, the vertebral bodies are poorly ossified, the tubular bones are short with "mushroom-stem" femora, and the iliac bones have a crescent-shaped inner border.

In the *type II (Majewski) syndrome*, in addition to severe rib reduction and polydactyly, affected patients have hydrops, a small flat nose, low-set ears, and cleft lip or cleft palate.

In the *type III lethal thoracic dystrophy (Naumoff) syndrome*, a narrow thorax, short ribs, and short and squared scapulae and iliac bones are seen. Abnormalities resemble those in the type I syndrome.

CHONDRODYSPLASIA PUNCTATA. This dysplasia is discussed in Chapter 73.

CAMPTOMELIC DYSPLASIA. Camptomelic (meaning bent limbs) dysplasia describes a distinct entity separate from a number of other conditions that are accompanied by bending of the extremities. Affected newborns have a large head and a short trunk and short limbs. The anterolateral bowing of the limbs is most marked in the legs. Clubfeet, joint contractures, bowing of the bones in the forearm, small hands, and a short neck are seen. The calvarium is large, with a small face, depressed nasal root, low-set ears, small jaw, and cleft palate. The disease probably is of autosomal recessive inheritance and usually is fatal in infancy.

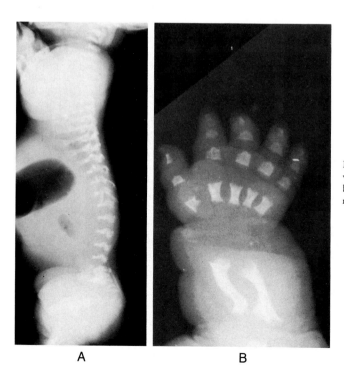

Figure 74–2. Thanatophoric dysplasia. Two patients are shown. A The vertebral bodies are markedly flattened with wide disc spaces. **B** The tubular bones of the hands are markedly shortened but relatively broad. Bowing and metaphyseal flaring are evident in the bones of the forearm.

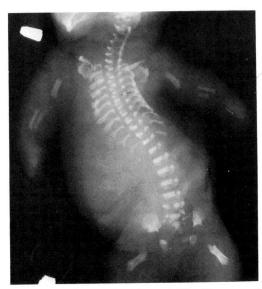

Figure 74–3. Short rib syndrome: Type I (Saldino-Noonan syndrome). The ribs are severely shortened, the scapulae are small, the tubular bones are short, with irregular ends, and the iliac bones are squared.

Radiographic findings (Fig. 74–4), which are most marked in the extremities, consist of anterolateral angulation of the femora, slightly above the middle third of the diaphysis. Tibial bowing occurs primarily in an anterior direction at the junction of the middle and distal thirds of the bone. The long tubular bones of the upper extremities are slightly shortened. Patients have small hands, with shortening of the middle and distal phalanges and clinodactyly of the fifth digit. The chest is bell-shaped; there are thin, wavy ribs and slender clavicles. Typical findings in the pelvis include the absence of the ala of the sacrum, narrow iliac bones, acetabular

hypoplasia, poor pubic ossification, and widely separated ischial bones. The hips frequently are dislocated. There is delayed ossification of the epiphyses about the knees, the talus, and the sternum. Vertebral anomalies are seen. The most characteristic radiographic findings are the curved femora and tibiae, small scapulae, and hypoplastic pedicles of the thoracic spine.

A variety of abnormalities of internal organs are seen in camptomelic dysplasia, including pulmonary hypoplasia, hydronephrosis, hydroureters, congenital heart disease, and hydrocephalus.

CLASSIC (HETEROZYGOUS) ACHONDROPLASIA. Classic achondroplasia, a relatively common type of dwarfism of autosomal dominant inheritance, relates to a disturbance in endochondral bone formation. It is evident at birth and is compatible with a long life span. Clinical manifestations include short limbs, especially of the proximal portions (rhizomelic micromelia), a large head with a prominent forehead and a depressed nasal bridge, thoracolumbar kyphosis in infancy, and exaggerated lumbar lordosis with prominent buttocks in children and adults. The hands are trident. Because of the constricted basicranium, foramen magnum, and spinal canal, compression of the spinal cord, lower brain stem, cauda equina, and nerve roots may develop in infants, children, or adults.

Radiographic findings include a large cranium with a small foramen magnum. The interpediculate distances of the lower lumbar vertebrae, which normally increase on proceeding distally, remain the same at all levels or decrease in the lower lumbar region (Fig. 74–5). The pedicles are short, the backs of the vertebral bodies are often concave, and the spinal canal is small (Fig. 74–6). The iliac bones are squared with small sacrosciatic notches and flat acetabular angles (Fig. 74–7). The proximal tubular bones are shortened and have metaphyseal flaring (Fig. 74–8). A V-shaped configuration of the distal femoral growth plate may be seen. The ribs and the tubular bones in the hands and feet also are shortened.

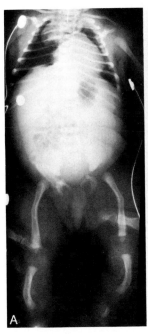
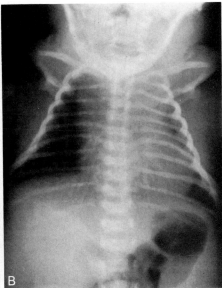

Figure 74–4. Camptomelic dysplasia. A In the lower extremity, the tubular bones reveal anterolateral bowing. The iliac bones, scapulae, fibulae, and lungs are hypoplastic, and the hips are dislocated. The 11 pairs of ribs and the clavicles are thin, and the pedicles of the thoracic spine are hypoplastic. **B** In another patient, hypoplasia of the vertebrae and scapulae and thin ribs are seen.

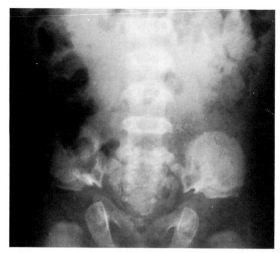

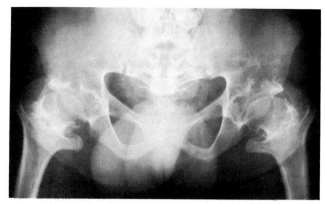

Figure 74–7. Classic (heterozygous) achondroplasia: Pelvis. In this adult patient, findings include spinal stenosis, lack of flaring of the iliac wings, which have rounded corners, and short femoral necks.

Figure 74–5. Classic (heterozygous) achondroplasia: Spine. The interpediculate distances in the lumbar vertebrae narrow distally. The iliac bones are squared, the sacrosciatic notches are small, and the ischial bones are shortened.

are found in this autosomal recessive disorder. The disease is characterized by short stature, progressive scoliosis, clubfeet, multiple contractures and dislocations, and distinctive abnormalities of the hands, feet, and ears. The thumbs and great toes are held in a hitchhiker's position. Although the prognosis is good, respiratory complications resulting from tracheal collapse can cause death in infancy.

Radiographic findings include marked shortening of the tubular bones with metaphyseal widening (Fig. 74–9). The epiphyses are delayed in appearance and deformed. The radial heads may be dislocated. The bones of the hands and feet are small, especially the first metacarpal, which may be round or oval in shape (Fig. 74–9). Femora may have broad intertrochanteric regions with short femoral necks. Scoliosis tends to

HOMOZYGOUS ACHONDROPLASIA. Homozygous achondroplasia is an extremely rare type of congenital short-limbed dwarfism that is lethal; an affected infant dies within the first days or weeks of life. The condition results when both parents are achondroplastic dwarfs. The changes are more severe than those in classic (heterozygous) achondroplasia.

DIASTROPHIC DYSPLASIA. The term diastrophic, which means "twisted" or "crooked," has been used to emphasize the twisted extremities and vertebral column that

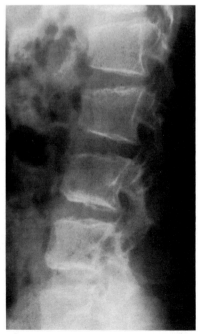

Figure 74–6. Classic (heterozygous) achondroplasia: Spine. The pedicles are short, with a small spinal canal, and the vertebral bodies have a posterior concavity.

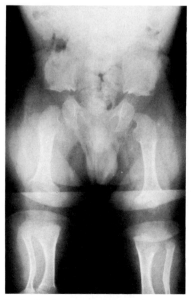

Figure 74–8. Classic (heterozygous) achondroplasia: Lower extremities. In a newborn, there is rhizomelic shortening of the tubular bones with metaphyseal flaring and medial slanting of distal femoral metaphyses.

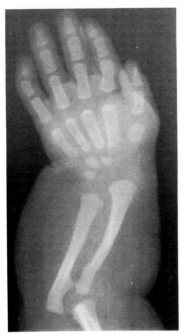

Figure 74–9. Diastrophic dysplasia. The tubular bones of the forearm are shortened, especially the distal portion of the ulna, and there is bowing of the distal portion of the radius. There is premature carpal ossification, a rounded first metacarpal, and clinodactyly of the fifth digit.

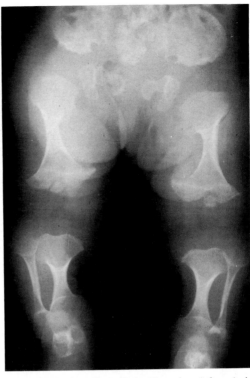

Figure 74–10. Metatropic dysplasia. In this newborn infant, the bones are shortened, with marked metaphyseal flaring and large femoral trochanters. The ilium is short, with curved lateral margins and small sacrosciatic notches.

be progressive and rigid. The cervical vertebrae may reveal defective development, and there is slight narrowing of the interpediculate distances distally in the lumbar spine.

METATROPIC DYSPLASIA. The term metatropic means "variable," indicative of the evolving stages of the disease. At birth, the ends of the bones are prominent in the extremities, and joint movement is limited. In infancy, the thorax appears to be long and narrow, and there may be a small soft tissue tail at the end of the spine. The hands and feet are initially long and slender but become relatively shortened later in life. There is progressive kyphoscoliosis.

The radiographic findings are dramatic. The tubular bones of the extremities are short and have marked metaphyseal widening, which resembles the appearance of a trumpet or dumbbell (Fig. 74–10). The trochanters are particularly large. The epiphyses are delayed in appearance and deformed. The vertebral bodies are flat or diamond-shaped in infancy. Although the vertebral bodies subsequently increase in size, they remain irregular and wedged anteriorly. Atlantoaxial instability may be present, leading to neurologic deficits. The pelvis is characterized by shortened ilia with curved lateral margins, flat acetabular roofs, and small sacrosciatic notches that resemble a battle ax (Fig. 74–11). In infancy the thorax is elongated and has a decreased anteroposterior diameter as a consequence of the short ribs; the development of kyphoscoliosis and sternal protrusion during childhood leads to a small thorax. The tubular bones of the hands and feet have metaphyseal expansion and delayed and irregular epiphyseal ossification.

The inheritance of this condition is uncertain, but both autosomal recessive and dominant patterns appear to exist.

CHONDROECTODERMAL DYSPLASIA (ELLIS–VAN CREVELD SYNDROME). The Ellis–van Creveld syndrome is characterized by ectodermal dysplasia, polydactyly, and congenital heart disease. It is inherited as an autosomal recessive trait and is manifested at birth. Short stature, distal shortening of limbs, polydactyly, hypoplastic fingernails or toenails, dysplastic teeth, and, less commonly, cardiac defects are clinical features of the disease. The radio-

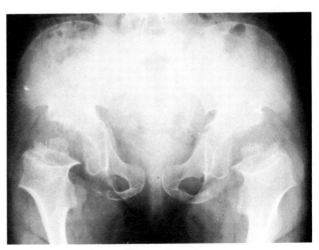

Figure 74–11. Metatropic dysplasia. Note the "battle axe" appearance of the iliac bones, with small sacrosciatic notches, deformed capital femoral epiphyses, and broad femoral necks.

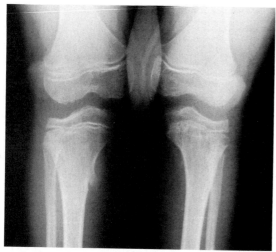

Figure 74–12. Chondroectodermal dysplasia. The tubular bones are shortened, with metaphyseal flaring. The lateral portion of the proximal tibial epiphyses is poorly developed. A medial diaphyseal spur is present on the tibia, and the patellae are dislocated.

graphic features include an elongated chest, shortened ribs, hypoplastic ilia, a trident pelvis, shortening of the tubular bones, polydactyly, carpal fusion, cone-shaped epiphyses, swelling of the proximal end of the ulna and distal end of the radius (drumstick appearance), anterior dislocation of the radial head, slanting proximal tibial metaphyses, medial tibial diaphyseal exostoses, and genu valgum (Figs. 74–12 and 74–13). The skull and spine usually are normal.

Death in childhood is common owing to cardiac and pulmonary complications.

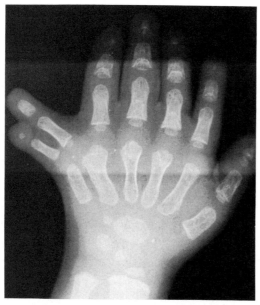

Figure 74–13. Chondroectodermal dysplasia. Postaxial polydactyly and shortening of the tubular bones (especially the distal phalanges) are apparent. Cone-shaped epiphyses are seen. The capitate and hamate are fused, and an extra carpal ossicle appears lateral to the hamate.

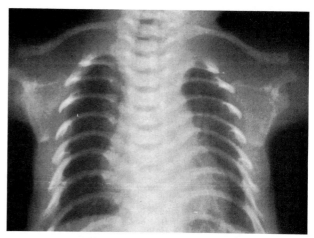

Figure 74–14. Asphyxiating thoracic dysplasia: Chest. Note the short ribs and handle-bar appearance of the clavicles.

ASPHYXIATING THORACIC DYSPLASIA (JEUNE'S SYNDROME). Initial reports of this autosomal recessive condition described infants with constricted chests who died from pulmonary hypoplasia. Later reports included patients with less severe respiratory symptoms. The striking radiographic features are a narrow thorax with short, horizontally oriented ribs (Fig. 74–14). The early pelvic findings are short iliac, pubic, and ischial bones. The acetabula are flat, with downward spike-like projections, the so-called triradiate acetabulum (Fig. 74–15). The pelvis becomes normal with age, however. In addition, the long tubular bones are slightly shortened. In infancy, there is mild digital shortening and inconstant polydactyly. Later, the epiphyses become cone-shaped and fuse prematurely, producing further shortening of phalanges. The skull and spine are normal.

Asphyxiating thoracic dystrophy differs from chondroectodermal dysplasia, being characterized by shorter ribs, progressive renal disease, hepatic fibrosis, absence of heart disease, less prominent nail changes, and inconstant polydactyly.

SPONDYLOEPIPHYSEAL DYSPLASIA CONGENITA. Spondyloepiphyseal dysplasia congenita, a short-trunk dwarfism, is distinguished by mild shortening of the limbs,

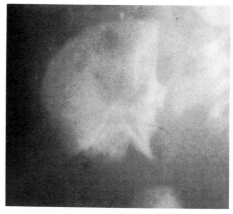

Figure 74–15. Asphyxiating thoracic dystrophy: Pelvis. Observe the three downward-projecting acetabular spikes.

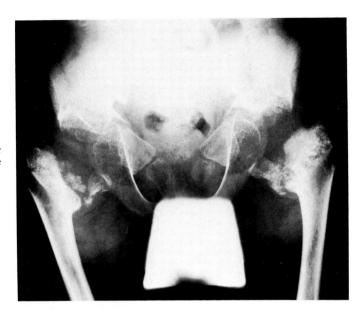

Figure 74–16. Spondyloepiphyseal dysplasia congenita. In an 11 year old patient, the femoral heads are small and inferiorly placed, and the femoral necks and pubic bones are poorly developed.

flat face, cleft palate, short neck, increased chest diameter, and joint restriction. During growth progressive kyphoscoliosis or lumbar lordosis occurs. Important additional features include myopia and retinal detachment, which can lead to blindness, and atlantoaxial instability (with a small odontoid process), which can result in spinal cord compression. The pattern of inheritance usually is autosomal dominant.

Radiographic findings include a decreased height of the vertebral bodies and, in infancy, pear-shaped vertebrae. In childhood, there is anterior wedging, irregularity, and generalized flattening of the vertebral bodies. Ossification of the pubic bones and proximal portion of the femora is delayed. The femoral heads often ossify from multiple centers, and a progressive coxa vara develops, with premature osteoarthritis (Fig. 74–16). The chest is bell-shaped, the scapula is malformed, and sternal ossification is delayed. The ends of the ribs flare anteriorly, and pectus carinatum is present. The long tubular bones have delayed ossification and variable metaphyseal flaring. The proximal carpal and tarsal bones also may reveal delayed ossification.

KNIEST DYSPLASIA. The clinical findings of Kniest dysplasia include a short trunk, prominent articulations, and a flattened face with a depressed nasal bridge. Ocular abnormalities, stiff joints, deafness, inguinal hernias, hip dislocations, delayed ambulation, cleft palate, and clubfeet occur. Marked dorsal kyphosis or kyphoscoliosis and lumbar lordosis develop.

Radiographic findings include shortening and flaring of the tubular bones and delayed development of epiphyses (Fig. 74–17). Swelling about the interphalangeal joints may be associated with enlargement similar to Heberden's and Bouchard's nodes. The spine demonstrates generalized osseous flattening. Kyphoscoliosis also may develop. In addition to a marked delay in ossification of the femoral capital epiphyses and pubic bones, pelvic abnormalities include broad and short femoral necks and hip contractures.

Histologic evaluation reveals hypertrophic cartilage cells and surrounding loose matrix containing large holes resembles Swiss cheese.

CLEIDOCRANIAL DYSPLASIA. This autosomal dominant disorder with high penetrance has a wide range of clinical manifestations. Mild shortening of stature may be seen. The head is large and brachycephalic, the sutures are wide, and their closure is delayed. Oral findings include a high, arched palate with delayed eruption of poorly formed and supernumerary teeth. Hearing loss is not uncommon. Genu valgum and short fingers can be seen.

Radiographic findings include poor ossification of the skull with wide sutures and multiple wormian bones. The foramen magnum may be deformed, and basilar impression may be evident. The mandible sometimes is broad. Although total clavicular absence is rare, any portion of the clavicle may be absent; the middle or outer portion is commonly affected most (Fig. 74–18). The scapula is hypoplastic, and the thorax

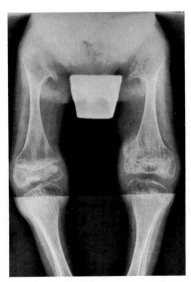

Figure 74–17. Kniest dysplasia. In the lower extremities, observe metaphyseal expansion and irregular epiphyseal ossification. Note the delay in appearance of ossification in the capital femoral epiphyses.

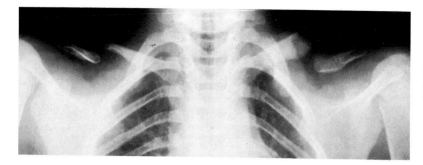

Figure 74–18. Cleidocranial dysplasia. Note clavicular defects at the junction of the outer and middle thirds of the bone.

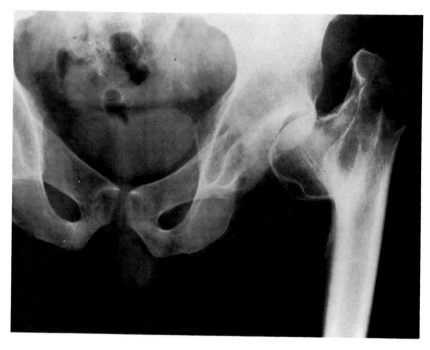

Figure 74–19. Cleidocranial dysplasia. Findings include acetabular malformation and hypoplasia of the pubic bones with widening of the symphysis pubis as well as coxa vara with broadening of the femoral head and enlargement of the greater trochanter. (Courtesy of R. Freiberger, M.D., New York, New York.)

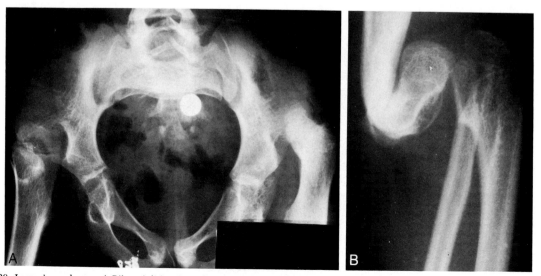

Figure 74–20. Larsen's syndrome. A Bilateral dislocations of the hip are seen. **B** A dislocation of the elbow with considerable osseous deformity is evident.

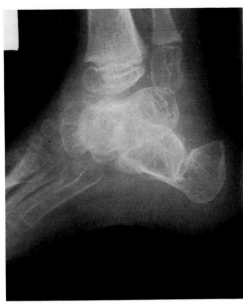

Figure 74–21. **Larsen's syndrome.** A clubfoot and partial fusion of two ossification centers in the os calcis are present.

may be bell-shaped. Pelvic alterations consist of a delay in ossification of the pubic bones, a wide symphysis pubis, and narrow iliac wings (Fig. 74–19). Although coxa valga is more frequent, coxa vara deformity may develop. Diaphyseal narrowing and expanded metaphyses of the tubular bones may be evident. Spinal changes consist primarily of spina bifida occulta. The findings in the hand include small distal phalanges, pseudoepiphyses in the metacarpal bones, somewhat large phalangeal epiphyses, and retarded ossification of the carpal and tarsal bones.

LARSEN'S SYNDROME. Larsen's syndrome is characterized by multiple dislocations, clubfeet, and a typical clinical appearance consisting of a recessed midface, widely spaced eyes, and a depressed nasal bridge. Additional findings in this syndrome include a cleft palate, broad thumbs, and spinal involvement that may lead to progressive neurologic impairment. Radiographs show dislocations, usually of the knees, hips, and elbows (Fig. 74–20). The carpal and tarsal bones may be supernumerary or possess an abnormal shape, and the calcaneus typically ossifies from two separate centers (Fig. 74–21). The tubular bones of the hands and feet may be broad and shortened, and pseudoepiphyses often are present in the metacarpals and the metatarsals. Abnormalities of the vertebral bodies consist of errors in segmentation or flattening and can be associated with kyphoscoliosis. Radiographs of the skull demonstrate hypertelorism, a small jaw, and brachycephaly.

Both autosomal dominant and autosomal recessive transmission patterns have been reported. Because the dislocations are difficult to treat, the patients may develop secondary degenerative changes.

DYSCHONDROSTEOSIS. Dyschondrosteosis refers to a mild mesomelic type of limb shortening with a Madelung's deformity of the forearm. The inheritance pattern is autosomal dominant, and the disease expresses itself more frequently and severely in female patients. Radiographic findings include a shortened radius that is bowed dorsally and laterally and a distal segment of the ulna that is often subluxed or dislocated dorsally (Fig. 74–22). The lack of development of the distal radial epiphysis with premature fusion on the medial side of the physis is the most characteristic finding in dyschondrosteosis. The carpal bones fit into the resulting V-shaped deformity of the radius and ulna. The radial head may be flattened and dislocated. Less shortening of the tibia and the fibula is seen, and a medial bone spicule may project from the proximal portion of the tibia. Coxa valga and ankle deformity also can occur.

METAPHYSEAL CHONDRODYSPLASIA. This term applies to a number of conditions in which the maximal disturbance occurs in the metaphyses; the epiphyses and diaphyses also may be abnormal, however.

Metaphyseal chondrodysplasia *type Jansen* is a rare, severe disorder characterized by marked dwarfism, swelling of the joints, and bowed forearms and legs. The face has typical features: frontonasal hyperplasia, hypertelorism, and a receding chin. The inheritance pattern is autosomal dominant. In infancy there is marked irregularity of the metaphyses, widening of the growth plates, and mild bowing. In this age group, subperiosteal bone resorption and fractures have led to diagnostic confusion with hyperparathyroidism. In childhood, the cupped metaphyses have zones of irregular calcification that eventually disappears as the growth plate closes. The resultant bones are bowed and have metaphyseal flaring. The spine shows minimal platyspondyly.

Metaphyseal chondrodysplasia *type Schmid* probably is the most common form of metaphyseal dysplasia. The genetic transmission of this disease is autosomal dominant. Patients have short stature of variable severity and bowed legs.

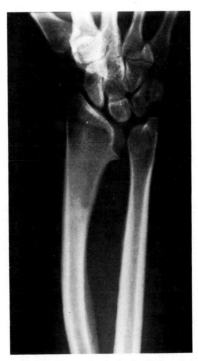

Figure 74–22. **Dyschondrosteosis.** A classic, V-shaped deformity of the radiocarpal joint is present.

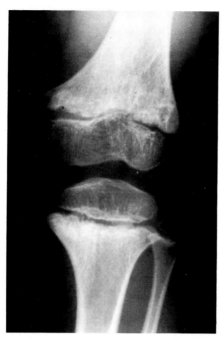

Figure 74–23. Metaphyseal chondrodysplasia: Type Schmid. In a 5 year old child, the tubular bones are short, and there are V-shaped metaphyseal irregularities, best observed in the femur.

Radiographically, the physes are widened and the metaphyses are irregular (Fig. 74–23). Coxa vara is a potential complication of the metaphyseal involvement. The femoral neck may be shortened. After physeal closure, osseous shortening and deformities may remain.

Metaphyseal chondrodysplasia *type McKusick,* of autosomal recessive inheritance, is often termed cartilage-hair hypoplasia. The patients are of normal intelligence and are short, with fine blond hair, small hands, bowed legs, and joint laxity. Because these patients may have lymphocyte dysfunction, there is an increased risk of lethal viral infections. Radiographic findings include minimal epiphyseal flattening and an irregular provisional zone of calcification, with metaphyseal irregularity, cupping, and flaring. Foot deformities and dislocation of the radial head are present occasionally. Spinal abnormalities include atlantoaxial subluxation, small vertebral bodies, and Schmorl's nodes.

Metaphyseal chondrodysplasia *with exocrine pancreatic insufficiency and cyclic neutropenia* (Schwachman-Diamond syndrome) is characterized by anemia, thrombocytopenia, growth retardation, ectodermal dysplasia, recurrent pulmonary infections, and malabsorption. Metaphyseal alterations are found more frequently in the lower extremities than in the upper extremities (Fig. 74–24). Coxa vara or a slipped capital femoral epiphysis may result. Osteopenia is frequent and probably secondary to the gastrointestinal disease.

SPONDYLOEPIPHYSEAL DYSPLASIA TARDA, X-LINKED RECESSIVE SYNDROME. The X-linked recessive condition occurs only in male patients and generally becomes evident between the ages of 5 and 10 years because of impaired spinal growth. Complaints of back and hip pain are common. Radiographic findings in the spine are quite characteristic, consisting of vertebral bodies that have a hump-shaped area of dense bone on the central and posterior portions of the endplates (Fig. 74–25). Degenerative spinal changes develop in early adulthood. There is mild flattening of the epiphyses about the major joints, especially the hips and the shoulders. Osteoarthritis, particularly in the hips, can eventually become disabling.

Disorganized Development of Cartilage and Fibrous Components of the Skeleton

DYSPLASIA EPIPHYSEALIS HEMIMELICA. Dysplasia epiphysealis hemimelica, also known as Trevor's disease or tarsoepiphyseal aclasis, is characterized by asymmetric

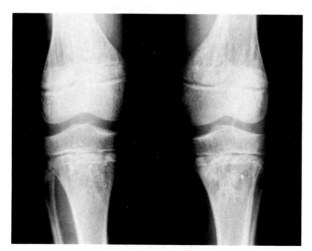

Figure 74–24. Metaphyseal chondrodysplasia with exocrine pancreatic insufficiency and neutropenia (Schwachman-Diamond syndrome). Multiple rounded, radiolucent areas are observed in the metaphyses about the knees.

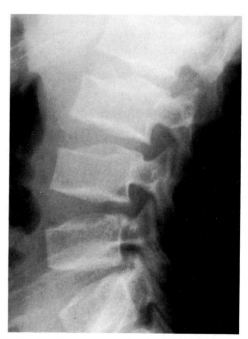

Figure 74–25. Spondyloepiphyseal dysplasia tarda, X-linked recessive syndrome. The characteristic osseous "humps" are evident in the central and posterior portions of the vertebral endplates. The disc spaces are narrow posteriorly and wide anteriorly.

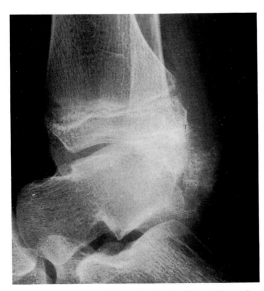

Figure 74–26. Dysplasia epiphysealis hemimelica. Note a bone mass arising from the posterior surface of the talus.

cartilaginous overgrowth (histologically identical to that of an osteochondroma) in one or more epiphyses or a tarsal or carpal bone. A painless bone swelling or deformity about a joint, usually in the lower extremities, becomes evident, typically when the patient is 2 to 4 years of age. Boys are affected more commonly than girls.

Characteristic radiographic features include the early appearance and excessive growth of the involved epiphysis, with a resultant irregularly calcified mass projecting from the epiphysis or the tarsal or carpal bone (Fig. 74–26). Although the irregular mass may initially appear distinct from the surrounding bone, it eventually fuses with the adjacent epiphysis. When the epiphyseal malformation involves the epiphyses on one side of the body, it may be associated with hemihypertrophy. Joint deformity may require surgical intervention.

MULTIPLE CARTILAGINOUS EXOSTOSES. The true frequency of this autosomal dominant condition, also called diaphyseal aclasis, is unknown, but it is a common disease, characterized by cartilage-capped exostoses that usually arise near the diaphyseal side of the physeal line (see also Chapter 78). The patients, usually boys, develop painless lumps near the ends of the long tubular bones and have mild shortness of stature.

The radiographic appearance of the exostoses is extremely variable (Fig. 74–27). Associated metaphyseal expansion may be evident adjacent to the base of the exostosis. Of great importance, growth of the osteochondromas can be apparent as long as endochondral ossification is proceeding in the adjacent physis but should cease when this normal ossification halts with closure of the growth plate.

With regard to abnormalities at specific sites, the bones of the forearm frequently are deformed owing to shortening of the distal portion of the ulna and bowing of the radius; dislocation of the radial head is not uncommon. The fibula also may be shortened, and lateral obliquity of the ankle joint occurs. Although the ends of the long tubular bones are involved most frequently, the ribs, scapula, and iliac bones often are affected. Vertebral involvement, although uncommon, can lead to spinal cord and nerve root compression.

Complications related to the osteochondromas are interference with growth, compression of surrounding structures, including vessels, nerves, and tendons, and malignant transformation, the last occurring in 3 to 25 per cent of cases. The radiographic findings that suggest malignant transfor-

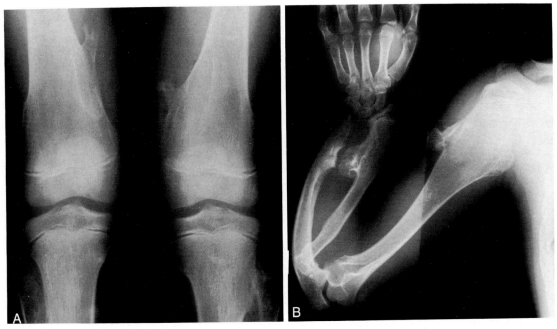

Figure 74–27. Multiple cartilaginous exostoses. A Observe multiple exostoses arising from expanded metaphyses. **B** Similar exostoses are seen in association with metaphyseal expansion and bowing of bones. The radial head is dislocated.

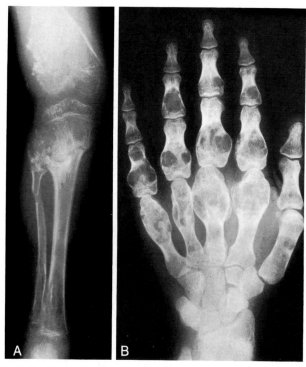

Figure 74–28. Enchondromatosis (Ollier's disease). A Radiolucent masses of varying shapes are present, containing calcifications that are best demonstrated in the femur and fibula. B Multiple expanded radiolucent lesions are evident.

mation are continued growth of the osteochondroma after cessation of normal growth, a changing appearance of calcifications in the cartilage cap, an irregular outline of the osteochondroma, and evidence of bone destruction at the base of the exostosis. Computed tomography, magnetic resonance imaging, and bone scintigraphy represent additional techniques that may be used to define malignant transformation of osteochondromas.

ENCHONDROMATOSIS (OLLIER'S DISEASE). Ollier's disease, a nonhereditary condition, results in multiple enchondromas in the tubular and flat bones of the body (see also Chapter 78). Clinical manifestations include masses that increase in size as the child grows, asymmetric limb shortening, and either genu varum or genu valgum deformities. The femur and tibia are the most commonly affected bones. Radiographically, the lesions consist of radiolucent or calcified masses of variable shape (Fig. 74–28). There may be considerable expansion of the tubular bones, and pathologic fractures may occur. Osseous shortening and angular deformity may be evident.

The enchondromas typically stabilize or even regress in adulthood. Malignant transformation is uncommon.

ENCHONDROMATOSIS WITH HEMANGIOMAS (MAFFUCCI'S SYNDROME). Maffucci's syndrome represents the combination of enchondromatosis and soft tissue hemangiomas (see also Chapter 78). The hemangiomas are detected at birth or shortly thereafter and are of variable size and number, whereas the enchondromas can produce large masses and distortion of bone growth, including scoliosis. The distribution of the hemangiomas does not correlate with

that of the enchondromas. In fact, hemangiomas may occur in other organs, including those of the gastrointestinal tract.

The radiographic features in this syndrome are similar to those of Ollier's disease with the addition of phleboliths and soft tissue masses (Fig. 74–29). Involvement of the hands and feet is frequent and severe. There is a higher frequency of malignant transformation in Maffucci's syndrome when compared to Ollier's disease.

Abnormalities of Diaphyseal Density or Metaphyseal Modeling, or Both

OSTEOPETROSIS. Osteopetrosis is a complex disease of at least four different types.

Osteopetrosis, Autosomal Recessive Lethal Type. The autosomal recessive, lethal form is also termed osteopetrosis with precocious manifestations. Clinical abnormalities include hepatosplenomegaly, hydrocephalus, and cranial nerve dysfunction, especially blindness and deafness. The obliteration of the marrow cavity by abnormal bone leads to anemia and thrombocytopenia and predisposes to recurrent infections with early patient demise.

The radiographic findings are characterized by generalized osteosclerosis. In the tubular bones, there is a failure of differentiation between the cortex and the medullary cavity (Fig. 74–30). Modeling in these bones is defective and, in infants, there may be a rickets-like configuration in the ends of the bones. The presence of "bone within bone" is an unusual but characteristic finding. Periostitis may be seen, and fractures, which generally heal, are common.

The entire skull is involved, but the base is affected most frequently and most severely (Fig. 74–31A). The mastoids and paranasal sinuses are poorly developed. The vertebral bodies tend to be uniformly radiodense, with a prominent anterior vascular notch (Fig. 74–31B).

Osteopetrosis, Intermediate Recessive Type. This milder, recessive form of osteopetrosis is distinct from both the more severe, recessive form of the disease that is seen in infants and the less severe, autosomal dominant form. Affected

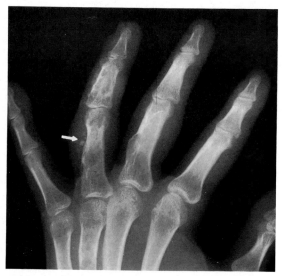

Figure 74–29. Enchondromatosis with hemangiomas (Maffucci's syndrome). In addition to multiple enchondromas, phleboliths with calcification are evident in the proximal portion of the fourth digit (arrow).

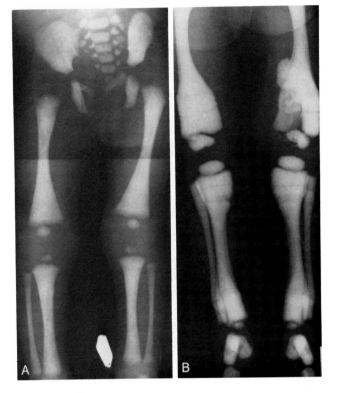

Figure 74–30. Osteopetrosis: Autosomal recessive lethal type. A In a newborn infant, diffuse osteosclerosis and slight metaphyseal expansion of the tubular bones are evident. **B** In a second patient, 16 months of age, marked osteosclerosis and bone expansion are seen. Note the transverse and horizontal radiolucent lines in the metaphyses and a pathologic fracture in the left femur.

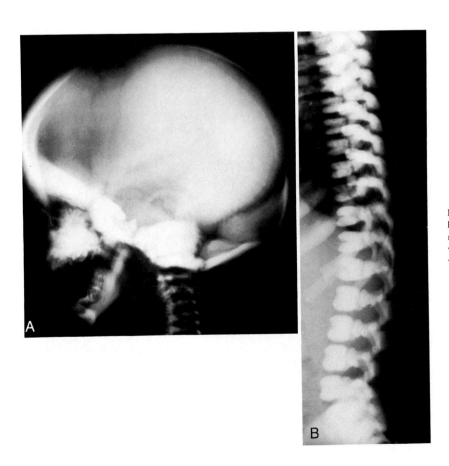

Figure 74–31. Osteopetrosis: Autosomal recessive lethal type. A Diffuse osteosclerosis of the skull, most marked at the base, is present. **B** Diffuse vertebral sclerosis and accentuation of the anterior vascular notches are evident.

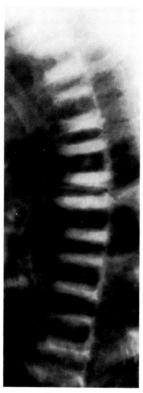

Figure 74–32. Osteopetrosis: Autosomal dominant type. Osteosclerosis in the superior and inferior portions of the vertebral bodies has produced a "sandwich" appearance.

patients often are of short stature, with pathologic fractures, anemia, and hepatomegaly. The radiographic findings are characterized by diffuse bone sclerosis, especially in the base of the skull, interference with normal bone modeling, and a "bone within bone" appearance. The facial bones also are involved.

Osteopetrosis, Autosomal Dominant Type. The autosomal dominant type of osteopetrosis is also designated Albers-Schönberg disease. Affected persons may be relatively asymptomatic, or the disease may be detected because of a pathologic fracture, problems occurring after tooth extraction, mild anemia, or cranial nerve palsies. The radiographic findings are similar to but less severe than those in the autosomal recessive form of the disease. The bones are diffusely osteosclerotic, with defective tubulation and a thickened cortex. The vertebral endplates become accentuated, especially with advancing age (Fig. 74–32). There can be a "bone within bone" appearance or radiolucent bands in the ends of the diaphyses (Fig. 74–33).

Osteopetrosis, Recessive Type with Tubular Acidosis. This form, also called "marble brain" disease, consists of osteopetrosis, renal tubular acidosis, and cerebral calcifications. The inheritance pattern is autosomal recessive, and the clinical course is compatible with long survival. Many of the patients, however, are mentally retarded. A deficiency in carbonic anhydrase has been identified in some affected persons. Typical clinical findings include a failure to thrive, symptoms related to renal tubular acidosis, muscle weakness, and hypotonia.

Radiographic findings include osteosclerosis, obliteration of the medullary cavity, and pathologic fractures. Progressive improvement in the radiographic abnormalities is more characteristic of this syndrome than of other forms of osteopetrosis.

PYKNODYSOSTOSIS. The syndrome of pyknodysostosis consists of osteosclerosis, short stature, frontal and occipital bossing, a small face with a receding chin, short broad hands, and hypoplasia of the nails. It is of autosomal recessive inheritance and is often accompanied by multiple fractures. Radiographic findings include generalized and uniform osteosclerosis (Fig. 74–34). In the tubular bones, metaphyseal modeling is only mildly abnormal, and the medullary cavities may be narrowed. The bones of the hands and feet are short, with hypoplasia or osteolysis of the distal phalanges. A marked delay in the closure of the cranial sutures is evident, and the anterior fontanelle may remain open. Wormian bones are common. A thickened and sclerotic base and, elsewhere, a thin vault without diploic markings represent additional cranial manifestations of the disease. The mastoids are poorly developed, the orbits are radiodense, the mandible is hypoplastic without normal angulation, the maxilla is small, and the teeth are malformed. In addition, the vertebral bodies are sclerotic, and there may be errors in vertebral segmentation.

DIAPHYSEAL DYSPLASIA (CAMURATI-ENGELMANN DISEASE). Camurati-Engelmann disease is a rare, autosomal dominant, generalized, bilaterally symmetric dysplasia of bone that is characterized by cortical thickening, increased diameter, and a narrowed medullary cavity in the diaphyses of the tubular bones with epiphyseal sparing. In some patients the presenting symptoms initially appear in the first decade of life, whereas in others the disease is discovered in the second to fourth decades of life. Characteristic radiographic features include cortical thickening and sclerosis of the diaphyses of the tubular bones (Fig. 74–35). In order of decreasing frequency, the tibia, the femur, the humerus, the ulna, the radius, and the bones of the hands and feet are

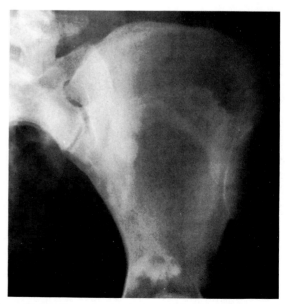

Figure 74–33. Osteopetrosis: Autosomal dominant type. The "bone within bone" appearance is seen in the ilium of an adult patient.

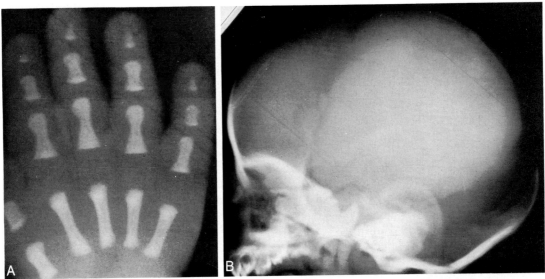

Figure 74–34. Pyknodysostosis. A In a newborn infant, diffuse osteosclerosis with hypoplasia of the distal phalanges is present. B In a 4 month old child, wide sutures and basal sclerosis represent the significant cranial abnormalities.

affected. Calvarial hyperostosis and sclerosis of the base of the skull also are encountered.

The course of this disease is variable. Progressive findings are common, but spontaneous improvement in adolescence also has been recognized.

ENDOSTEAL HYPEROSTOSIS. Three types of endosteal hyperostosis deserve emphasis.

Endosteal Hyperostosis, Autosomal Dominant Syndrome (Worth's Syndrome). The autosomal dominant form of endosteal hyperostosis may be detected incidentally on radiographs obtained for unrelated reasons; however, asymmetric enlargement of portions of the face and the presence of a palatal mass may be important clinical signs. Radiographic findings include endosteal thickening in the cortex of the tubular bones with encroachment on the medullary cavity. The bones are not expanded, and abnormal modeling is not seen. In the skull, osteosclerosis begins in the base and subsequently involves the facial bones, especially the mandible. In the spine, changes are most prominent in the spinous processes. The ribs and osseous pelvis are affected only mildly. Unlike the recessive form of the disease, the serum levels of alkaline phosphatase are normal, the basilar foramina are not affected, cranial nerve involvement is rare, and the clinical course is benign.

Endosteal Hyperostosis, Autosomal Recessive Syndrome (Van Buchem's Syndrome). Symptoms and signs occur at an earlier age in this disorder compared with the age of clinical onset in the autosomal dominant form of the disease and are characterized by more severe enlargement of the mandible and more frequent cranial nerve involvement, including facial nerve palsy and deafness. Affected patients also have a prominent forehead and widened nasal bridge, and the serum level of alkaline phosphatase may be elevated. Radiographic findings are similar to but more severe than those in the dominant form of the disease (Fig. 74–36). Specific abnormalities include periosteal excrescences in the tubular bones, osteosclerotic and enlarged ribs and clavicles, and increased radiodensity in the spine.

Endosteal Hyperostosis, Autosomal Recessive Syndrome (Sclerosteosis). This disorder usually becomes evident in infancy or early childhood. Clinical findings are excessive height and weight, peculiar facies, a broad, flat nasal bridge, ocular hypertelorism, mandibular prominence, deafness, facial palsy, syndactyly of the fingers, dysplastic nails, and radial

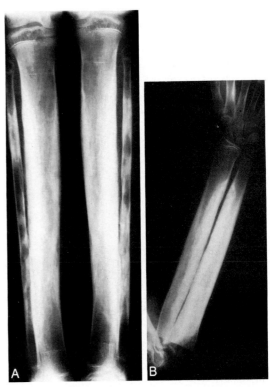

Figure 74–35. Diaphyseal dysplasia (Camurati-Engelmann disease). The tubular bones are wide, with thickened cortices and narrowed medullary canals. There are mottled areas of rarefaction, best observed in the fibulae.

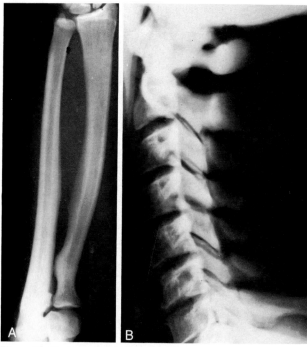

Figure 74–36. Endosteal hyperostosis: Autosomal recessive syndrome (Van Buchem's syndrome). A Note diffuse osteosclerosis and cortical thickening. B Osteosclerosis is especially marked in the neural arches and spinous processes.

calvarial hyperostosis, absent frontal sinuses, micrognathia, dental malformations, accentuated flare of the iliac bones, undertubulation of the metaphyses of the tubular bones, waviness and bowing of the tibiae and fibulae with genu valgum, tibia recurvatum, and elongation or widening of metacarpals and phalanges (Fig. 74–38). In older patients, progressive erosion and fusion of the carpus and tarsus have been noted, which may simulate the findings in juvenile chronic arthritis or various osteolytic syndromes.

The presence of prominent cranial abnormalities in this dysplasia allows its differentiation from Pyle's disease. Its features resemble those in craniometaphyseal dysplasia, although facial and occipital bone involvement and a normal pelvic contour in the latter condition allow separation of the two disorders.

CRANIOMETAPHYSEAL DYSPLASIA. The basic features of this disease in both its autosomal dominant and recessive forms are facial deformity, cranial hyperostosis, and failure of normal modeling of tubular bones. The recessive forms of the disease are accompanied by more severe facial involvement. Dental malocclusion, deafness, optic atrophy, and facial paralysis often occur. Life span usually is within normal limits.

Radiographically, progressive sclerosis of the base of the skull and about the cranial sutures, obliteration of the paranasal sinuses, and loss of the lamina dura about the teeth are seen. In infancy, osteosclerosis in the diaphysis of the tubular bones, similar to that observed in diaphyseal dysplasia, is evident; it subsequently disappears, being replaced by

deviation of the terminal phalanges. Radiographs outline hyperostosis of the skull and mandible and sclerosis of the cortices of the tubular bones and, perhaps, the pelvis and pedicles. There is a lack of normal diaphyseal constriction of the tubular bones. Pathologic fractures generally do not occur.

TUBULAR STENOSIS (KENNY-CAFFEY SYNDROME). Kenny-Caffey syndrome is characterized by a short stature, transient hypocalcemia (a consequence of hypoparathyroidism) that may lead to tetany, delayed closure of the anterior fontanelle, widening of the cranial sutures, ocular abnormalities, and stenosis of the medullary canal in multiple bones. The syndrome probably is of dominant inheritance. Radiographs show thinning of the shafts of the tubular bones (Fig. 74–37). The cortex is thickened, and the metaphyses are flared.

PACHYDERMOPERIOSTOSIS. The clinical and radiologic features of pachydermoperiostosis, which resemble, in part, those of secondary hypertrophic osteoarthropathy, are discussed in Chapter 83.

FRONTOMETAPHYSEAL DYSPLASIA. This dysplasia encompasses cranial hyperostosis, abnormal tubulation of cylindric bone, and additional skeletal and extraskeletal abnormalities. Clinical manifestations include childhood onset, prominent horn-like supraorbital ridges, micrognathia, defective dentition, a wide nasal bridge, a high, arched palate, hearing loss, visual disturbances, a short trunk with long extremities, elongated fingers with ulnar deviation of the hands, genu valgum, decreased joint mobility, and contractures. A dominant mode of inheritance or an X-linked disorder is likely.

Radiographic features are a prominent supraorbital ridge,

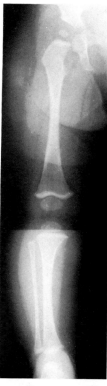

Figure 74–37. Tubular stenosis (Kenny-Caffey syndrome). The marked tubular stenosis is evident in the bones of the lower extremities in a 9 month old child.

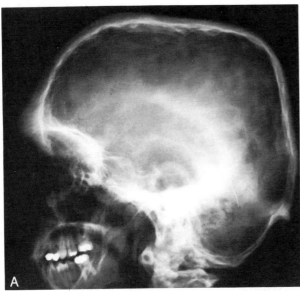

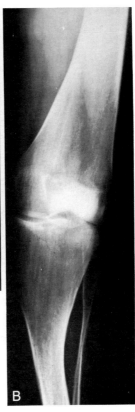

Figure 74–38. **Frontometaphyseal dysplasia. A** Marked thickening of the supraorbital ridges is evident. **B** The long tubular bones reveal metaphyseal splaying. (Courtesy of L. Langer, M.D., Minneapolis, Minnesota.)

metaphyseal expansion, cortical thinning, and club-shaped epiphyses.

METAPHYSEAL DYSPLASIA (PYLE'S DISEASE). Pyle's disease, a rare disorder that demonstrates either recessive or dominant transmission, becomes manifest at a variable age with mild clinical symptoms and signs, including joint pain, muscular weakness, scoliosis, genu valgum deformity, dental malocclusion, and bone fragility. The radiographic abnormalities are striking (Fig. 74–39). Marked expansion of the metaphyseal segments of tubular bones leads to an Erlenmeyer flask appearance, especially about the knee. Minor alterations in the skull include supraorbital prominence, an obtuse angle of the jaw, and mild sclerosis of the cranial vault. The bones of the pelvis and thoracic cage are expanded.

DYSOSTEOSCLEROSIS. Dysosteosclerosis is an autosomal recessive disorder manifested in early childhood as small stature, dental anomalies, increased bone fragility, and, occasionally, neurologic abnormalities. Although thickening and sclerosis of the cranial vault, base of the skull, ribs, clavicles, and tubular bones may resemble the findings in osteopetrosis, the presence of platyspondyly and lucency about expanded diametaphyseal segments of long bones allows differentiation of this syndrome (Fig. 74–40).

HEREDITARY HYPERPHOSPHATASIA. Hereditary hyperphosphatasia, which is also known as juvenile Paget's disease and osteoectasia with hyperphosphatasia, is a rare condition of infancy and childhood characterized by generalized cortical thickening of bones and chronic sustained ele-

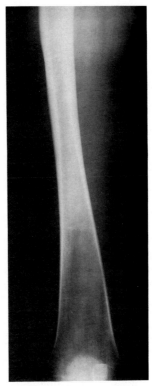

Figure 74–39. **Metaphyseal dysplasia (Pyle's disease).** The femur has an Erlenmeyer flask appearance.

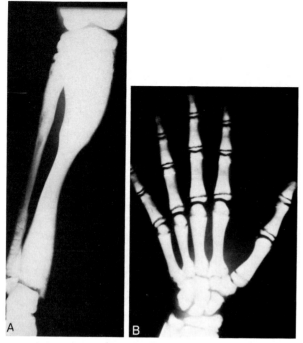

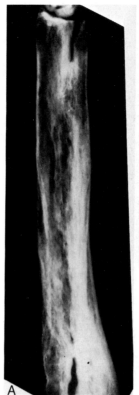

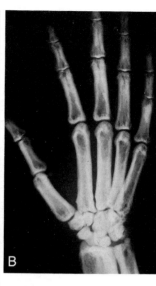

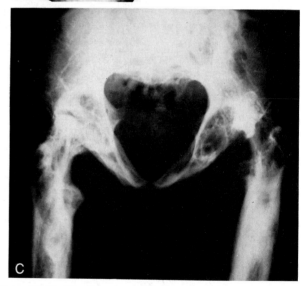

Figure 74–40. Dysosteosclerosis. **A** Note failure of normal tubulation and osteosclerosis with several radiolucent transverse zones. **B** Similar findings are present in the hand. (Courtesy of R. Lachman, M.D., Los Angeles, California.)

vation of the serum level of alkaline phosphatase. An autosomal recessive inheritance seems to exist. Involvement may be severe or mild. Overproduction of bone and bone collagen by osteocytes and failure of primitive fibrous tissue to mature into compact lamellar bone can be noted. Affected children have a small stature, large skull, fusiform swelling and bowing of the tubular bones, and a tendency toward fracture. Laboratory abnormalities, in addition to elevated levels of serum alkaline phosphatase, include raised serum levels of acid phosphatase, uric acid, and leucine aminopeptidase, and elevation of urinary peptide-bound hydroxyproline and uric acid levels. On radiographic analysis, virtually every bone is seen to be affected (Fig. 74–41). Calvarial thickening, osteopenia, and osseous bowing and widening are discovered. By the second and third decades of life, most patients are severely deformed and incapacitated.

DYSOSTOSES

Malformation of Individual Bones, Singly or in Combination

CRANIOSYNOSTOSIS. The term craniosynostosis implies premature fusion of one or more of the sutures in the skull. Premature closure of a suture results in local cessation of growth and distortion of the calvarial configuration. Accurate radiographic interpretation should be directed toward the identification of the affected suture(s) rather than toward the use of specific but, sometimes, confusing terminology that describes the abnormal shape of the skull. The affected suture can be identified by a straight rather than a serrated radiolucent line, osseous proliferation at the suture line, or frank osseous fusion. As a supplement to conventional radiog-

Figure 74–41. Hereditary hyperphosphatasia. **A** Cortical thickening in the radius and ulna is associated with loss of definition between the cortex and the medullary bone. **B** Similar findings are present in the hand. **C** In the pelvis, a pagetoid appearance is evident. There is subluxation of the left femoral head.

raphy, computed tomography may be used to delineate any associated abnormalities of the face and central nervous system.

Isolated closure of the sagittal suture accounts for more than 50 per cent of cases of craniosynostosis. Its closure results in an increased anteroposterior diameter of the skull and a decreased biparietal diameter (Fig. 74–42A,B). Synostosis of

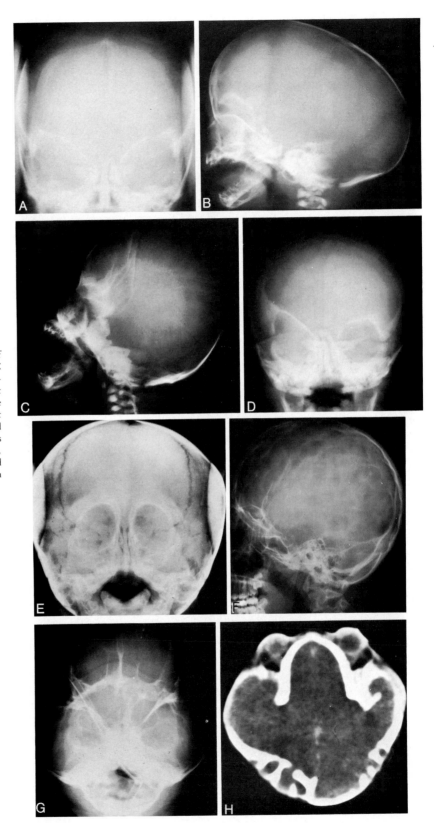

Figure 74–42. Craniosynostosis. A, B Closure of the sagittal suture. Dolichocephaly has occurred. **C** Closure of both coronal sutures. The skull is brachycephalic, with a small anterior fossa and a hypoplastic maxilla. **D** Closure of one coronal suture. Note the harlequin-shaped right orbit. **E** Closure of the metopic suture. Hypotelorism and a triangular-shaped forehead are observed. **F** Closure of all sutures. The skull is brachycephalic, with prominent digital markings. **G, H** Kleeblattschädel skull. Note osseous scalloping and a trilobed appearance of the cranial vault. The brain projects into the multiple bone channels.

Table 74–1. ACROCEPHALOSYNDACTYLY SYNDROMES

Eponym	Skull				Hands				Feet				Associated Features	Inheritance
	Acro-cephaly	Hypo-plastic Maxilla	Hypo-plastic Mandible	Asym-metry	Osseous Fusion	First Phalangeal Deformity	Hypoplasia (Aplasia) of Middle Phalanx	Key Features	Osseous Fusion	First Phalangeal Deformity	Hypoplasia (Aplasia) of Middle Phalanx	Key Features		
Acrocephalosyndactyly														
Apert	Severe	+	–	–	+	+	+	Mitten hand	+	+	+	Sock foot	Cervical spine fusion, joint ankylosis, subluxations	Autosomal dominant
Chotzen	Mild	+	–	+	–	–	–	Syndactyly 2 and 3	–	–	–	Syndactyly 2 and 3; brachy-meso-dactyly	Ptosis, short stature	Autosomal dominant
Pfeiffer	Mild	+	–	–	+	+	+	Broad thumb	+	+	+	Broad first toe with varus deformity	Cervical spine fusion, cone epiphyses	Autosomal dominant
Waardenburg	Moderate	–	+	+	–	+	+	Bifid distal phalanges 2 and 3	–	–	+	Absent first digit	Pointed nose, contractures, eye abnormalities	Not known
Summit	Mild	+	–	–	–	–	–	Syndactyly	–	–	–	Syndactyly	Obesity, genu valgum	Autosomal recessive
Acrocephalo-polysyndactyly														
Carpenter	Severe	+	+	–	–	+	+	Broad or duplicated thumb	–	+	–	Preaxial polydactyly	Genu valgum, obesity, hypogonadism, congenital heart disease	Autosomal recessive
Noack	Moderate	–	–	–	–	+	+	Broad thumb	–	+	–	Duplication of first toe	May not be distinct from Pfeiffer's syndrome	Autosomal dominant
Sakati	Severe	+	+	–	+	+	–	Brachy-dactyly	+	+	+	Duplication of first toe, preaxial polydactyly	Hypoplastic tibia, bowed femora, coxa valga, congenital heart disease	? Autosomal dominant

Adapted from Spranger JW, Langer LO, Wiedemann HR: Bone Dysplasias: An Atlas of Constitutional Disorders of Skeletal Development. Philadelphia, WB Saunders Co, 1974, p 262. Used by permission.

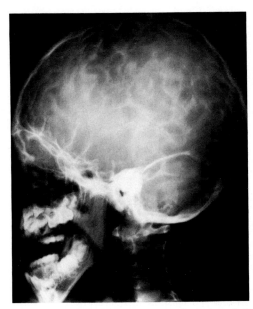

Figure 74–43. Craniofacial dysostosis (Crouzon's syndrome). The skull is brachycephalic, and there is slight maxillary hypoplasia. Abnorma osseous fusion in the cervical spine also was present.

calcification in the stylohyoid ligament, deviation of the nasal septum, and hypoplasia of the maxilla. Hypertelorism is common and hydrocephalus may occur. Spinal anomalies are seen in approximately one third of the patients. The absence of significant abnormalities of the hands and feet helps to distinguish Crouzon's disease from other syndromes accompanied by craniosynostosis.

Cor pulmonale, due to obstruction of the nasopharyngeal airway, is a recognized complication of this disease.

ACROCEPHALOSYNDACTYLY. Acrocephalosyndactyly encompasses a number of disorders, not all clearly distinct. Apert's syndrome, the most common, consists of craniosynostosis that typically involves the coronal sutures and anomalies of the hands and feet (Fig. 74–44). A brachycephalic skull, midface hypoplasia, hypertelorism, hydrocephalus, prominent eyes, down-slanting palpebral fissures, a

both coronal sutures produces a skull that is short in its anteroposterior diameter, often with a decrease in the depth of the orbits and maxillary hypoplasia (Fig. 74–42C). Unilateral closure of a coronal suture produces flattening of the orbit on the involved side; a classic harlequin-shaped orbit is identified (Fig. 74–42D). Isolated closure of the lambdoid suture leads to flattening of one side of the back of the head, or plagiocephaly. An isolated metopic synostosis creates a triangular forehead with hypotelorism (Fig. 74–42E). In cases of closure of multiple sutures, the skull is variable in shape, although generally brachycephalic, and digital markings in the cranium are quite prominent (Fig. 74–42F). The kleeblattschädel, or three-leaf clover, configuration of the skull is also associated with premature synostosis of multiple sutures (Fig. 74–42G,H), and it is frequently accompanied by hypoplasia of the midportion of the face, hydrocephalus, and mental retardation.

Craniosynostoses can be further classified as primary or secondary in type. Primary closures are sometimes an isolated phenomenon or occur in conjunction with other malformation syndromes. Secondary synostoses are evident in rickets, hypophosphatasia, thyroid disorders, and hypercalcemia. Certain patients with craniosynostosis have characteristic abnormalities of the limbs, and the specific combination of findings forms the basis of some common and recognizable syndromes (Table 74–1).

CRANIOFACIAL DYSOSTOSIS (CROUZON'S SYNDROME). Crouzon's syndrome is characterized by craniosynostosis, exophthalmos, and midface retrusion. It has an autosomal dominant mode of transmission. The skull is usually brachycephalic in shape, with fusion of the coronal and sagittal sutures (Fig. 74–43). Fusion of the lambdoid suture also is evident in 80 per cent of patients. Other findings include prominent digital markings in the skull,

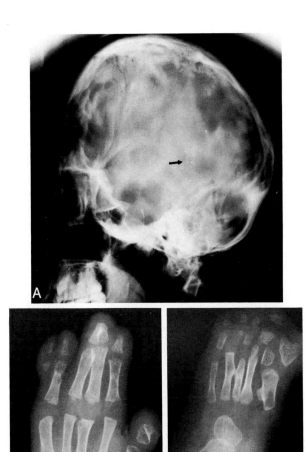

Figure 74–44. Acrocephalosyndactyly—Apert's syndrome. A Findings in the skull include brachycephaly, a hypoplastic anterior fossa, a prominent sella turcica, and choroid calcifications (arrow). Abnormalities in the cervical spine are also present in this adult. **B** In the hand of a child, symphalangism, osseous and soft tissue syndactyly, phalangeal deformity in the thumb, polydactyly, and carpal fusion are seen. **C** Similar abnormalities are observed in the foot.

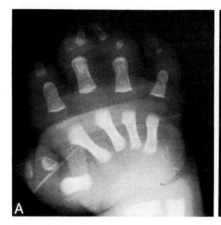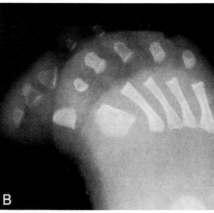

Figure 74–45. Acrocephalopolysyndactyly (Carpenter's syndrome). **A** Hand. Soft tissue syndactyly involves the third and fourth digits. The middle phalanges of the fingers are either absent or hypoplastic, and the proximal phalanx of the thumb is hypoplastic. **B** Foot. There is soft tissue syndactyly with preaxial polydactyly and some phalangeal deformities. The first metatarsal bone is short and broad.

"mitten hand," and a "sock foot" are among its characteristic clinical features. Radiographs demonstrate premature sutural closure, brachycephaly, a small anterior fossa, and severe maxillary hypoplasia. In the hands and feet, soft tissue and osseous syndactyly, progressive obliteration of the interphalangeal joints (symphalangism), carpal and tarsal fusions, and deformed thumbs are observed. Occasionally polydactyly can be seen. Osseous fusions may also be evident in other joints of the extremities.

Other acrocephalosyndactyly syndromes are summarized in Table 74–1.

ACROCEPHALOPOLYSYNDACTYLY (CARPENTER'S SYNDROME AND OTHER SYNDROMES). The basic features of the acrocephalopolysyndactyly syndromes are craniosynostosis and polysyndactyly. The best known of these disorders is Carpenter's syndrome, which is of autosomal recessive inheritance. Acrocephaly, obesity, hypogonadism, abdominal hernias, and congenital heart disease are among its many abnormalities. Mental retardation may be present. On radiographs, a relatively late closure of the coronal suture is seen, the tubular bones of the hands and feet are shortened, and syndactyly commonly occurs (Fig. 74–45). Coxa valga, flared iliac wings, genu valgum, and spinal anomalies can also be seen.

CHROMOSOMAL ABERRATIONS

Chromosomal abnormalities tend to result from genetic imbalances and involve either autosomal or sex chromosomes. Many are lethal, owing to severe defects in normal morphogenesis. They can be classified as trisomy conditions (in which three rather than the normal pair of chromosomes are present), translocations (in which part of a chromosome becomes transposed to another chromosome), and deletions (in which a portion of a chromosome is absent). Only a few of the more common chromosomal abnormalities are summarized here.

5p– SYNDROME. Deletion of the short arm of chromosome 5 results in this well-known syndrome named after the characteristics of the cry (cat cry or cri du chat syndrome) made by affected patients. Mental retardation is severe, growth is slow, and microcephaly, a round face, hypertelorism, epicanthal folds, and an antimongoloid slant of the palpebral fissures are seen. Nonspecific radiographic features include microcephaly, hypertelorism, abnormal development

of long bones, scoliosis, shortening of some metacarpal bones, and small iliac wings.

TRISOMY 8 SYNDROME. Patients with trisomy 8 syndrome have a large skull with a prominent bulging forehead, hypotelorism, a broad shallow nose, thick lips, a small mandible, and a short neck. The trunk appears long and narrow, and there are multiple joint contractures and clubfeet. Mental retardation is mild. Radiologically generalized osteopenia, multiple joint subluxations, hypoplastic iliac bones, small patellae, coxa valga, spinal anomalies, and metaphyseal flaring in the tubular bones are seen. Skeletal maturation is delayed. Cardiac and renal anomalies can also occur.

TRISOMY 13 SYNDROME. Affected infants have severe anomalies, with mental retardation, seizures, and apnea. A small skull, arhinencephaly, holoprosencephaly, abnormal eyes and ears, cleft lip and cleft palate, cutaneous hemangiomas, flexion deformities of fingers, and congenital heart disease are evident. The most common skeletal alterations are polydactyly, syndactyly, asymmetry of the thorax, prominence of the calcaneus, midline craniofacial anomalies, small first ribs, and rocker-bottom feet.

TRISOMY 18 SYNDROME. Affected infants are of low birth weight and possess a narrow head, prominent occiput, malformed ears, micrognathia, high, arched palate, finger deformities, hypertonicity, and hernias. Cardiac and renal anomalies are other features of this syndrome. Radiographs of the hand reveal adduction of the thumb, superimposition of the second and third fingers, and hypoplasia of the first metacarpal. Rocker-bottom feet, metatarsus varus, a shortened first toe, hypoplastic terminal phalanges of the toes, hypoplasia of ribs, clavicles, and sternum, and pelvic deformities complete the radiographic picture.

DOWN'S SYNDROME—TRISOMY 21. Patients with this syndrome are identified at birth by the ocular abnormalities (which include oblique palpebral fissures, epicanthal folds, cataracts, Brushfield spots, nystagmus, and strabismus), hypotonia, brachycephaly, mental retardation, and large tongue. Congenital hip dysplasia is evident in approximately 40 per cent of patients, and gastrointestinal abnormalities, including duodenal atresia, are well recognized.

Radiographs of the pelvis reveal flared iliac wings and flattened acetabular roofs (Fig. 74–46). Hypoplasia of the

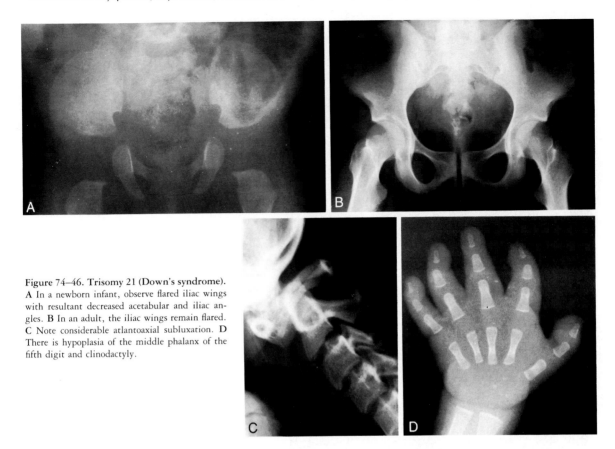

Figure 74–46. Trisomy 21 (Down's syndrome). A In a newborn infant, observe flared iliac wings with resultant decreased acetabular and iliac angles. B In an adult, the iliac wings remain flared. C Note considerable atlantoaxial subluxation. D There is hypoplasia of the middle phalanx of the fifth digit and clinodactyly.

middle phalanx of the fifth finger with clinodactyly, short and irregular metacarpals, accessory epiphyses, an extra manubrial ossification center, cuboid vertebral bodies, 11 pairs of ribs, microcephaly, a high, arched palate, delayed sutural closure, and sinus hypoplasia may be identified. Atlantoaxial instability and myelopathy can lead to significant neurologic deficits.

TURNER'S SYNDROME. Turner's syndrome is produced when a fetus has a normal complement of autosomes but only one sex chromosome, X (45,X). Most fetuses with this combination of chromosomes are aborted in the first trimester of pregnancy; rarely, a live infant is born, which has a female phenotype. In the newborn infant, edema of the hands and feet may be evident (Fig. 74–47), and large edematous masses about the neck occur. Secondary sex characteristics do not appear, primary amenorrhea is frequent, and the ovaries consist of fibrous tissue. Clinical manifestations include lymphedema of the lower extremities; loose skin about the neck; congenital anomalies of the heart, great vessels, and kidneys; short stature; and laterally displaced nipples on a shield-like chest.

There are many radiographic abnormalities that may be evident in this syndrome (Fig. 74–47). Osteoporosis is most pronounced in the spine, carpus, and tarsus. Epiphyseal fusion is delayed and may not occur until the third decade of life. Shortening of the metacarpals, especially the fourth, and of the metatarsals can be evident. Drumstick phalanges have been observed. Although a decrease in the carpal angle has been noted in this syndrome, it does not appear to be a useful radiographic sign. Deformities of the knees with flattening of

the medial tibial plateau, beaking of the proximal portion of the tibia, and enlargement of the medial femoral condyle are observed. Cubitus valgus, Madelung-like deformities, thin clavicles and ribs, vertebral body irregularities, and odontoid and atlas abnormalities have also been described. With regard to the skull and face, brachycephaly, small facial bones, mandibular prominence, enlarged sinuses, and calcification in the petroclinoid ligaments have been observed.

KLINEFELTER'S SYNDROME. Klinefelter's syndrome usually results from the presence of two or more X chromosomes and a Y chromosome, although a number of variant chromosomal patterns are also recognized, such as XXYY. Muscular weakness, mental retardation, delayed puberty, azospermia, and infertility are frequent. A variety of nonspecific radiographic changes have been outlined, including metacarpal shortening, clinodactyly, accessory epiphyses, a flattened ulnar styloid process, pointed phalangeal tufts, radioulnar synostosis, and retarded bone age.

PRIMARY METABOLIC ABNORMALITIES
Mucopolysaccharidoses (MPS) and Related Disorders

The term mucopolysaccharidosis (MPS) was first used to describe the histologic findings in patients with gargoylism, which included swollen collagen tissues filled with water-soluble material. Later studies indicated extensive amounts of certain mucopolysaccharides in the urine of affected patients. In the ensuing years, the detection of different chemical substances in the urine of patients with similar varieties of dwarfism led to the delineation of closely related but distinct

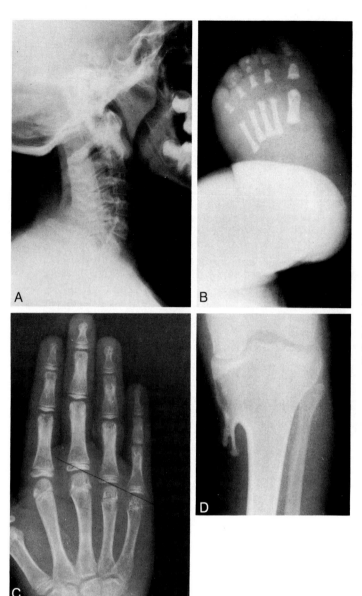

Figure 74–47. Turner's syndrome. A In an 8 year old patient, soft tissue abnormality, related to webbing of the neck, projects over the posterior portion of the vertebrae. Osteopenia is evident. **B** In a newborn infant, note soft tissue edema. **C** The fourth metacarpal bone is relatively short, and the phalanges are relatively long, with a drumstick configuration. **D** Findings include an exostosis projecting from the medial aspect of the tibia and prominence of the medial femoral condyle.

disorders (Table 74–2). Common to the MPS and mucolipidoses are certain clinical and radiographic characteristics: the radiographic abnormalities are designated dysostosis multiplex and are described in the following paragraph.

The *skull* is usually large and dolichocephalic, with premature closure of the sagittal suture (Fig. 74–48). The mastoids and paranasal sinuses are poorly developed. Commonly, an elongated J-shaped sella turcica, prominent adenoids, malformed teeth, flattened mandibular condyles, a large tongue, and a thick diploic space are seen. In the *spine*, there is defective development of the anterosuperior portion of the vertebral bodies at the thoracolumbar junction with gibbus formation owing to the presence of hook-shaped vertebrae (Fig. 74–49). The vertebral bodies are oval in shape or slightly diminished in height (Fig. 74–50). In the *pelvis*, there is underdevelopment of the superior acetabular region, resulting in a widened acetabular roof and large acetabular angle (Fig. 74–51). Coxa valga is frequent, and the femoral heads are dysplastic. In the *chest*, the ribs are widened but taper near their vertebral margins (Fig. 74–51). The clavicles are short and widened. The changes in the *long tubular bones* are greater in the upper extremities than in the lower extremities, with diaphyseal and metaphyseal expansion, delay in epiphyseal ossification, and cortical thinning. Constriction of the humeral and femoral necks with resultant varus deformities may occur. In the *hand*, diffuse osteopenia, cortical thinning, and proximal tapering of the second to fifth metacarpals (Fig. 74–52) are observed. The proximal and middle phalanges are short and wide, and the terminal phalanges are hypoplastic. The carpal bones are small and deformed. Similar but less dramatic changes also occur in the foot. The distal portion of the radius and ulna tapers, thus altering the carpal angle. In addition, cardiomegaly and hepatosplenomegaly, flexion contractures, and umbilical and inguinal hernias may be seen.

A more precise diagnosis of the mucopolysaccharidosis requires clinical information, including the pattern of genetic transmission, and biochemical data, including the pattern of

Table 74–2. MUCOPOLYSACCHARIDOSES AND MUCOLIPIDOSES

Designation	Eponym or Synonym	Excessive Urinary Mucopolysaccharide	Enzyme Deficient	Clinical Features
Mucopolysaccharidoses (MPS):				
MPS I-H	Hurler's syndrome	Dermatan sulfate Heparan sulfate	Alpha-L-iduronidase	Early clouding of cornea, mental retardation, heart disease, coarse facial features
MPS I-S	Scheie's syndrome	Dermatan sulfate Heparan sulfate	Alpha-L-iduronidase	Late onset, stiff joints, cloudy cornea, aortic valve disease, intelligence unaffected, mild facial dysmorphism
MPS I-H-S	Hurler-Scheie syndrome	Dermatan sulfate	Alpha-L-iduronidase	Intermediate between Hurler's and Scheie's syndromes
MPS II	Hunter's syndrome	Dermatan sulfate	Iduronate sulfatase	Mild somatic features, slow progression, no clouding of cornea
MPS III	Sanfilippo's syndrome (Types A, B, C, D)	Heparan sulfate	Multiple deficiencies	Severe mental retardation, very mild skeletal and somatic features
MPS IV	Morquio's syndrome (Types A and B)	Keratan sulfate	Multiple deficiencies	Severe dwarfism, short trunk and neck, knock-knees, corneal changes (seen with slit lamp), intelligence unaffected
MPS VI	Maroteaux-Lamy syndrome	Dermatan sulfate	Arylsulfatase B	Dwarfism, coarse facial features, corneal clouding, normal intelligence
MPS VII	Sly's syndrome	Dermatan sulfate	Beta-glucuronidase	Hepatosplenomegaly, variable mental retardation
Mucolipidoses (ML):				
ML I	Lipomucopoly-saccharidosis	None	N-acetyl-neuraminidase	Mild somatic features, progressive neuromuscular symptoms
ML II	I-cell disease	None	Multiple deficiencies	Exaggerated somatic features, marked gingival hyperplasia
ML III	Pseudo-Hurler's polydystrophy	None	Multiple deficiencies	Variable somatic features, stiff joints, corneal clouding, short stature
GM-1-gangliosidosis	GM₁ gangliosidosis	None	Beta-galactosidase	Severe to mild somatic features, onset in infancy

From Silverman FN: Caffey's X-Ray Diagnosis: An Integrated Imaging Approach. 8th Ed. Chicago, Ill, Year Book Medical Publishers, p 690. After McKusick VA: Heritable Disorders of Connective Tissue. 4th Ed. St Louis, CV Mosby Co, 1972, p 525. Used by permission.

increased urinary excretion of acid mucopolysaccharides (Table 74–2). Only Hurler's syndrome and Morquio's syndrome are discussed here.

MPS I (HURLER'S SYNDROME). Hurler's syndrome, an autosomal recessive disorder, is manifested in the first few years of life. Patients reveal distinctive facies, mental retardation, deafness, dwarfism, corneal opacities, hepatosplenomegaly, cardiomegaly, and cardiac murmurs. Laboratory analysis indicates increased urinary excretion of dermatan sulfate and heparan sulfate, abnormal mucopolysaccharide accumulation in the bone marrow and peripheral leukocytes, and low or absent activity of alpha-L-iduronidase in various tissues. Radiographs reveal macrocephaly, craniostenosis, a J-shaped sella turcica, widening of the anterior portion of the ribs, hypoplasia of vertebrae about the thoracolumbar junction, resulting in kyphosis, atlantoaxial subluxation, hypoplasia of the ilia, shortening and widening of the shafts of the long tubular bones, pointing of the proximal portions of the metacarpals, and osteoporosis (Figs. 74–48, 74–49, and 74–52). Mental retardation and skeletal deformities may be

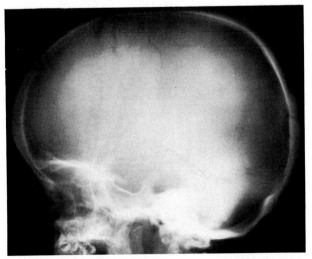

Figure 74–48. Dysostosis multiplex (MPS I, Hurler's syndrome). The skull is large, the mastoids are poorly developed, and the sella turcica is J-shaped.

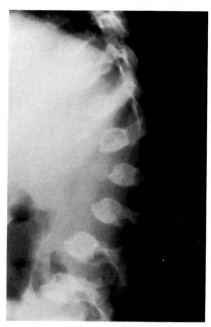

Figure 74–49. Dysostosis multiplex (MPS I, Hurler's syndrome). Note the hook-shaped vertebrae and a gibbus deformity at the thoracolumbar junction.

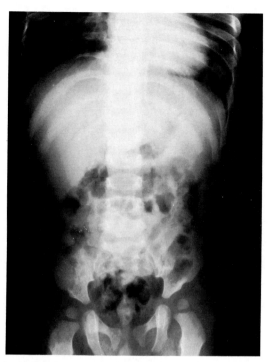

Figure 74–51. Dysostosis multiplex (MPS II, Hunter's syndrome). Underdevelopment of the superior acetabular region, wide femoral necks, coxa valga deformity, and wide ribs with posterior tapering are seen.

progressive. Death in the first decade of life may result from cardiac or pulmonary abnormalities.

MPS IV (MORQUIO'S AND RELATED SYN-DROMES). MPS IV includes a type A or Morquio's syndrome, related to a deficiency of N-acetyl-galactosamine-6-sulfate sulfatase, and a type B syndrome, attributable to a deficiency of beta-galactosidase. Clinical findings include severe dwarfism, spinal shortening and kyphoscoliosis, anterior bulging of the sternum, joint laxity, prominence of the lower face, hypoplasia of the enamel, a short neck, exaggerated lumbar lordosis, and flat feet. Corneal clouding, deafness, genu valgum, and degenerative hip disease also occur. Normal intelligence and a variable life span are additional features.

It is the abnormalities on spinal radiographs that are most helpful in the accurate diagnosis of MPS IV. In early infancy, the vertebral bodies are slightly rounded, with a small anterior beak. With subsequent growth, a central tongue appears,

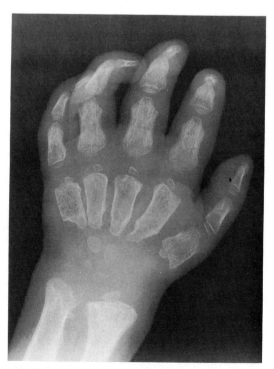

Figure 74–52. Dysostosis multiplex (MPS I, Hurler's syndrome). Osteopenia, pointing of the proximal portion of the metacarpals, widening of the proximal and middle phalanges, small carpal bones, and a V-shaped deformity of the distal portions of the radius and ulna are evident.

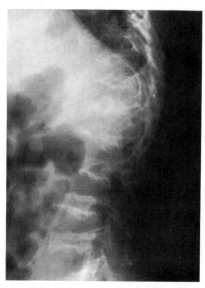

Figure 74–50. Dysostosis multiplex (MPS IV, Morquio's syndrome). The vertebral bodies are flattened and possess anterior tongues of bone.

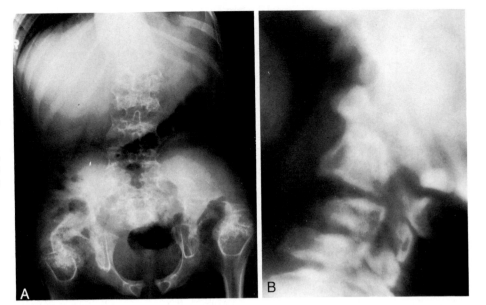

Figure 74–53. Morquio's syndrome (MPS IV). A In a 10 year old patient, marked platyspondyly, flared iliac wings, and severe changes about the hips are evident. **B** A lateral tomogram of the cervical spine shows odontoid hypoplasia and narrowing of the spinal canal.

protruding from the anterior surface of the vertebral bodies. In adulthood, the vertebrae are flat and irregular (Figs. 74–50 and 74–53A). The odontoid process is hypoplastic, and resulting atlantoaxial instability may lead to neurologic damage during anesthesia (Fig. 74–53B).

The anteroposterior diameter of the chest is increased. Anterior bowing of the prematurely fused sternum is associated with short, wide ribs. In the pelvis, increased obliquity in the lateral aspect of the acetabular roofs and considerable flaring of the iliac wings are observed. Coxa valga deformity and progressive dysplasia of the capital femoral epiphysis are also seen (Fig. 74–53A). Additional findings include deformity of the mandibular condyles, expansion of the metacar-

pals, with pointed proximal ends, small and irregular carpal bones, and slanting of the distal articular surface of the radius. The long tubular bones exhibit diminished growth, metaphyseal flaring, and epiphyseal deformity.

Menkes' Kinky Hair Syndrome

Menkes' syndrome is an X-linked disorder leading to defective copper absorption from the intestine. The typical patient is a male with sparse, light, kinky hair, failure to thrive, and progressive degeneration of the central nervous system. Radiographic findings, which include osteopenia and metaphyseal spurs, have been confused with child abuse syndrome and rickets (Fig. 74–54). Periosteal new bone formation is common, and wormian bones are identified in the lambdoid sutures. Thin tubular bones, a wooly appearance of certain ossification centers, flaring of the ends of the ribs, a small mandible, and scalloping of the posterior surface of the vertebral bodies are other radiographic features. Dramatic changes occur in the blood vessels, particularly in the brain. Cerebral atrophy, bladder diverticula, dilatation of portions of the urinary tract, and emphysema have been seen in this condition.

FURTHER READING

Azour EM, Slomic AM, Marton D, Rigault P, Finidori G: The variable manifestations of dysplasia epiphysealis hemimelica. Pediatr Radiol 15:44, 1985.

Baker DH, Berdon WE, Morishima A, Conte F: Turner syndrome and pseudo-Turner's syndrome. AJR 100:40, 1967.

Beighton P, Cremin BJ: Sclerosing Bone Dysplasias. New York, Springer-Verlag, 1980.

Beighton P, Emery AEH: Inherited Disorders of the Skeleton. New York, Churchill Livingstone, 1978.

Beligere N, Harris V, Pruzansky S: Progressive bone dysplasia in Apert syndrome. Radiology 139:593, 1981.

Bergsma D: Birth Defects Compendium. 2nd Ed. New York, Alan R Liss, 1973.

Caffey J: Congenital stenosis of the medullary spaces and tubular bones and calvaria in two proportionate dwarfs—mother and son; coupled with transient hypercalcemic tetany. AJR 100:1, 1967.

Carlson DH, Wilkinson RH: Variability of unilateral epiphyseal dysplasia (dysplasia epiphysialis hemimelica). Radiology 133:369, 1969.

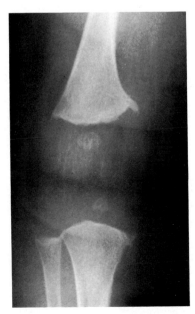

Figure 74–54. Menkes' kinky hair syndrome. Observe metaphyseal spurs in the femur and tibia in a 3 month old infant.

Carmel PW, Luken MG, Ascheri GF: Craniosynostosis: Computed tomographic evaluation of skull base and calvarial deformities and associated intracranial changes. Neurosurgery 9:366, 1981.

Cremin BJ: Sclerosteosis in children. Pediatr Radiol 8:173, 1979.

Elmore SM: Pycnodysostosis. A review. J Bone Joint Surg [Am] 49:153, 1967.

Engfeld B, Fajers CM, Lodin H, Pherson M: Studies of osteopetrosis. Roentgenological and pathologic-anatomical investigations on some of the bone changes. Acta Pediatr 49:391, 1960.

Gelman MI: Autosomal dominant osteosclerosis. Radiology 125:289, 1977.

Giedion A, Kesztler R, Muggiasca F: The widened spectrum multicartilaginous exostosis (MCE). Pediatr Radiol 3:93, 1975.

Gorlin RJ, Koszalk MS, Spranger J: Pyle's disease (familial metaphyseal dysplasia). A presentation of 2 cases and argument for its separation from craniometaphyseal dysplasia. J Bone Joint Surg [Am] 52:347, 1970.

Hall BD, Spranger JW: Campomelic dysplasia. Am J Dis Child 134:285, 1980.

Heselson NG, Raad MS, Hamersma H, Cremin BJ, Beighton P: Radiologic manifestations of metaphyseal dysplasia (Pyle's disease). Br J Radiol 52:431, 1979.

Holzgrave W, Grobe H, von Figura K, Kresse H, Beck H, Mattei JF: Morquio syndrome. Clinical findings of 11 patients with MPS IV-A and 2 patients with MPS IV-B. Hum Genet 57:360, 1981.

Hungerford GD, Akkaraju V, Rawe SE, Young GF: Atlanto-occipital and atlanto-axial dislocations with spine cord compression in Down's syndrome: A case report and review of the literature. Br J Radiol 54:758, 1981.

James AE, Belcourt CL, Atkins L, Janower ML: Trisomy 18. Radiology 92:37, 1969.

James AE, Adkins L, Feingold M, Janower ML: The cri-du-chat syndrome. Radiology 92:50, 1969.

Jarvis JL, Keats TE: Cleidocranial dysostosis. The review of 40 cases. AJR 121:5, 1974.

Kaufmann HJ (Ed): Intrinsic Diseases of Bones (Progress in Pediatric Radiology, Vol 4). Basel, S Karger, 1973.

Kosowicz J: The roentgen appearance of the hand and wrist in gonadal dysgenesis. AJR 93:354, 1965.

Kozlowski K, Beighton P: Gamut Index of Skeletal Dysplasias. New York, Springer-Verlag, 1984.

Kozlowski K, Butzler HO, Galatius-Jensen F, Tulloch A: Syndromes of congenital bowing of the long bones. Pediatr Radiol 7:40, 1978.

Kozlowski K, McCrossin R: Early osseous abnormalities in Menke's kinky hair syndrome. Pediatr Radiol 8:191, 1980.

Lachman RS, Rimoin DL, Hollister DW, Dorst JP, Siggers DC, McAlister WH, Kaufman RL, Langer LO: The Kniest syndrome. AJR 123:805, 1975.

Larsen LJ, Schottstaedt ER, Boist FC: Multiple congenital dislocations associated with a characteristic facial deformity. J Pediatr 37:574, 1950.

Langer LO: Spondyloepiphysial dysplasia tarda. Hereditary chondrodysplasia with characteristic vertebral configuration in the adult. Radiology 82:833, 1964.

Langer LO: Diastrophic dwarfism in early infancy. AJR 93:399, 1965.

Langer LO: Dyschondrosteosis of the inheritable bone dysplasia with characteristic roentgenographic features. AJR 95:178, 1965.

Langer LO, Baumann PA, Gorlin RJ: Achondroplasia. AJR 100:12, 1967.

Langer LO Jr: Thoracic-pelvic-phalangeal dystrophy. Asphyxiating thoracic dystrophy of the newborn, infantile thoracic dystrophy. Radiology 91:447, 1968.

Mainzer F, Minagi H, Steinbach HL: The variable manifestation of multiple enchondromatosis. Radiology 99:377, 1971.

McAlister WH: Enchondromatosis with hemangioma. Semin Roentgenol 8:230, 1973.

McAlister WH: Larsen's syndrome. Semin Roentgenol 8:246, 1973.

McAlister WH: Metatropic dwarfism. Semin Roentgenol 8:154, 1973.

McAlister WH: Thanatophoric dwarfism. Semin Roentgenol 8:158, 1973.

McClennan TW, Steinbach HL: Schwachman's syndrome—a broad spectrum of bony abnormality. Radiology 112:167, 1974.

Milgram JW, Jasty M: Osteopetrosis. A morphological study of twenty-one cases. J Bone Joint Surg [Am] 64:912, 1982.

Naveh Y, Kaftori JK, Alan V, Ben-Durd J, Berant M: Progressive diaphyseal dysplasia: Genetics and clinical and radiographic manifestations. Pediatrics 74:399, 1984.

Nazara Z, Hernandez A, Corona-Rivera E, Vaca G, Panduro A, Martinez-Basalo C, Cantu JM: Further clinical and radiological features in metaphyseal chondrodysplasia Jansen Type. Radiology 140:697, 1981.

Ohsawa T, Furuse M, Kikuchi Y, Suda Y, Tamiya T, Hikita M: Roentgenographic manifestation of Klienfelter syndrome. AJR 112:78, 1971.

Pavone L, Mollica F, Giovanni S, Sorge G: Metaphyseal chondrodysplasia Schmid Type. Am J Dis Child 134:699, 1980.

Roberts GM, Starey N, Harper P, Nuki G: Radiology of the pelvis and hips in adults with Down's syndrome. Clin Radiol 31:475, 1980.

Robinson LK, Jameds HE, Mubarak SJ, Allen EJ, Jones KL: Carpenter syndrome: Natural history and clinical spectrum. Am J Med Genet 20:461, 1985.

Silverman FN: Caffey's Pediatric X-Ray Diagnosis: An Integrated Imaging Approach. Chicago, Year Book Medical Publishers, 1985.

Spranger JW, Langer LO: Spondyloepiphyseal dysplasia congenita. Radiology 94:313, 1970.

Spranger JW, Langer LO, Wiedemann HR: Bone Dysplasias: An Atlas of Constitutional Disorders of Skeletal Development. Philadelphia, WB Saunders Co, 1974.

Taylor GA, Jordan CE, Dorst SK, Dorst JP: Polycarpaly and other abnormalities of the wrist in chondroectodermal dysplasia: The Ellis–van Creveld syndrome. Radiology 151:393, 1984.

Thomas SL, Childress MH, Quinton B: Hypoplasia of the odontoid with atlanto-axial subluxation in Hurler's syndrome. Pediatr Radiol 15:353, 1985.

Tishler JM, Martel W: Dislocation of the atlas in mongolism. A preliminary report. Radiology 84:904, 1965.

Whalen JP, Horwith M, Krook L, MacIntyre I, Mena E, Viteri F, Torun B, Nunez EA: Calcitonin treatment in hereditary bone dysplasia with hyperphosphatasemia. A radiographic and histologic study of bone. AJR 129:29, 1977.

Willich E, Fuhr U, Kroll W: Skeletal manifestations in Down's syndrome. Correlation between roentgenologic and cytogenetic findings. Ann Radiol 18:355, 1975.

Wynne-Davies R, Fairbank TJ: Fairbank's Atlas of General Affections of the Skeleton. New York, Churchill Livingstone, 1976.

Wynne-Davis R, Walsh WK, Gormley J: Achondroplasia and hypochondroplasia: Clinical variation and spinal stenosis. J Bone Joint Surg [Br] 63:4508, 1981.

Chapter 75

Spinal Anomalies and Curvatures

M. B. Ozonoff, M.D.

A great variety of congenital anomalies may affect the spine, and the causes and patterns of abnormal spinal curvature also are varied. Accurate diagnosis of these alterations relies on careful clinical evaluation supple-mented with imaging examinations that include routine radiography, conventional and computed tomography, ul-trasonography, myelography, and magnetic resonance imaging.

Congenital anomalies of the spine are frequent and varied. Some are discovered as incidental radiographic findings, whereas others lead to significant clinical manifestations. Certain important structural alterations and abnormal curvatures of the spine are summarized here.

CONGENITAL ANOMALIES OF THE SPINE

Structural Abnormalities

Many congenital vertebral anomalies are of such minor degree and resolve so quickly, as a result of skeletal growth and maturation, that they are properly considered normal developmental variants; a typical example of this would be the transient coronal cleft vertebra of infancy. Others are remnants of previous embryologic states that have failed to evolve completely but nevertheless have little or no clinical importance (e.g., nonfusion of lumbar or sacral neural arches). Many, such as meningomyelocele, are of major structural and clinical significance, however.

Some anomalies are restricted to skeletal structures, either isolated at one or two levels or part of larger complexes. Others are associated with neural tube defects (meningomye-locele, diastematomyelia, and congenital intraspinal tumors). Additionally, the skeletal and neural anomalies may be part of a multisystem abnormality, such as the VATER (vertebral-anorectal-tracheal-esophageal-renal-rectal) complex and numerous dysplasias and syndromes.

ANOMALIES OF THE VERTEBRAL BODY. The vertebral body develops originally from paired chondral centers and, at a later stage, from a single ossification focus that is transiently separated by the notochordal remnant into anterior and posterior centers. Total aplasia can be explained by failure of development of the mesoderm in the involved segment. Lack of development of one of the paired chondral centers produces a lateral hemivertebra, whereas if the failure occurs at the ossification stage, anterior agenesis will result in a posterior hemivertebra.

Hemivertebrae may vary in size, and the contralateral segment at the same level may be completely absent or hypoplastic (Fig. 75–1). The pedicle or rib on the side of the hemivertebra may be normal or enlarged, and its counterpart at the same level may be either absent or hypoplastic. The hemivertebra may exist in place of a normal vertebra, or it may be a supernumerary structure. In many cases, the anomaly that is present in the vertebral body is associated with fusion or segmentation defects in the neural arch.

The vertebral body occasionally is constricted centrally, most probably after incomplete fusion of the two chondral centers, with hypoplasia where they join (butterfly vertebra). Two or more vertebral somites also may be subject to nonsegmentation, in which case a block vertebra is formed. The intervertebral discs may be completely absent or may be represented by rudimentary, irregularly calcified structures. Often a waist-like constriction of the fused structure is found at the level of the intervertebral disc (causing an hourglass appearance), and the total height of the block vertebra is usually less than expected from the number of segments that are involved. In the cervical spine, it may be difficult to differentiate this congenital anomaly from abnormalities caused by juvenile chronic arthritis.

ANOMALIES OF THE VERTEBRAL ARCH. The same anomalies of formation, segmentation, and maturation may affect the neural arches. Each neural arch develops from a separate chondrification (and subsequently an ossification) center; these paired arches normally unite in the midline by the age of 2 years but frequently remain open at the L5 or S1 spinal level. The use of the term "spina bifida occulta" for these minor failures of fusion is to be strongly discouraged as the term implies significant clinical abnormalities, which generally are not present.

Abnormalities of the neural arch include total absence, underdevelopment with wide osseous separation, and failure of segmentation. When pedicle aplasia occurs, it is most

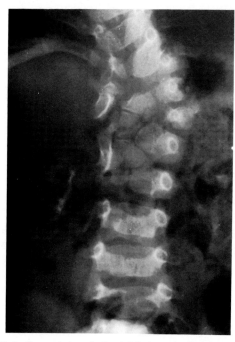

Figure 75–1. Congenital scoliosis. A left thoracolumbar scoliosis is associated wtih right upper lumbar pediculate bars and multiple supernumerary hemivertebrae on the left. (From Theros EG, Harris JH Jr [Eds]: American College of Radiology Bone Syllabus IV. American College of Radiology, in press. Used with permission.)

Occipitalization (assimilation) of the atlas is a normal variant that is asymptomatic in most cases. Typically, the anterior arch of the atlas is fused to the skull base, and other portions of the ring of the atlas reveal similar fusion in many cases. As many as one half of patients with occipitalization of the atlas also have vertebral fusion at the C2-C3 spinal level. Although the odontoid process is high, platybasia and basilar impression are uncommon.

SACRAL AGENESIS. Sacral agenesis is a well-known spinal anomaly that is discussed in Chapter 76. There is a significant rate of occurrence of this anomaly as part of the VATER and VACTEL (vertebral-anorectal-cardiac-tracheal-esophageal-limb) complexes.

Spinal Dysraphism Complexes

Dysraphism represents a failure of midline fusion that encompasses not only structural vertebral defects but also associated abnormalities of embryonic tissue in those organ systems developing at the same time as the neural tube, including the neurologic, gastrointestinal, and genitourinary systems. Dysraphic abnormalities are described as open (uncovered) or closed (covered or occult) lesions. Open defects, such as meningomyelocele, usually are clinically obvious at birth. Closed or occult lesions may have a cutaneous marker such as a nevus, hairy patch, hemangioma, or lipoma that signals the possible presence of an underlying abnormality;

common in the cervical and lumbar regions. The opposite pedicle at the same level frequently is hyperplastic. There may be hypoplasia of the ipsilateral articular facets. The spinous process at the affected level frequently tilts toward the abnormal side. Facet, laminar, or spinous process fusion may be an associated finding.

Failure of segmentation leads to linkage and fusion of adjacent laminae or pedicles, termed congenital vertebral bars. These abnormalities are usually unilateral and restrict growth on the side on which they lie.

Radiographically, pedicle bars appear as a discrete osseous line encircling the pedicles at two or more vertebral levels (Fig. 75–1).

KLIPPEL-FEIL SYNDROME. The Klippel-Feil syndrome and its associated abnormalities are discussed in Chapter 76.

CRANIOVERTEBRAL JUNCTION ABNORMALITIES. The craniovertebral junction is a developmentally unstable transitional region in which congenital anomalies are common. Many abnormalities of this region have been described. Abnormalities at other levels in the cervical spine are seen in two thirds of patients.

Odontoid aplasia, in which no extension of the dens above the body of the axis is present, may be an isolated congenital anomaly, or it may be associated with the mucopolysaccharidoses and other syndromes.

The os odontoideum is a well-defined ossicle that lies at the tip of the odontoid process and is about one half the size of a normal dens. There is strong evidence that this is an acquired lesion that follows trauma (see Chapter 62).

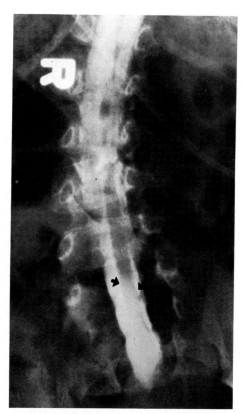

Figure 75–2. Meningomyelocele. The dysraphic abnormalities include a widened interpediculate distance at the L3 spinal level and distally. The myelogram demonstrates tethering of the spinal cord (arrows) in the sacral area.

in most of these cases, obvious vertebral anomalies are evident radiologically.

MENINGOMYELOCELE. As already stated, meningomyelocele is clinically evident at birth. The origin of this anomaly is not completely settled. The point at which widening of the interpediculate distance and vertebral body occurs is usually taken as the superior limit of the anomaly, but the upper extent of the lesion predicted radiologically may not correlate with the functional neurologic level.

The expanding neural and meningeal mass causes reorientation or displacement of the pedicles, laminae, and transverse processes (Fig. 75–2). Computed tomography, with or without the administration of contrast agents, or magnetic resonance imaging, is necessary to show some of the vertebral and neural abnormalities. Furthermore, the status of the urinary tract should be evaluated at standard intervals with cystography, urography, and ultrasonography.

Vertebral hypoplasia, hemivertebra, laminar and pediculate fusion, diastematomyelia (Fig. 75–3), and lipoma may all be associated with the meningomyelocele. Although no abnormality of spinal curvature is seen initially in about one third of patients, scoliosis is present at an early age in one half of all patients and in 80 per cent of those more than 10 years of age; kyphosis is present in about one fifth of patients.

Anterior sacral meningoceles are rarer than the typical posterior protrusions. They are usually associated with a unilateral, scimitar-like hemisacral osseous defect and a mass protruding through the defect that may be detectable on barium studies of the rectum or on computed tomography.

OCCULT SPINAL DYSRAPHISM. The basic pathogenic processes accompanying occult spinal dysraphism are identical to those causing open lesions: failure of midline fusion; duplication (diplomyelia, diastematomyelia); overgrowth of normal tissues (lipoma, dermoid); herniation of one germ layer through another (neurenteric cyst); and abnormalities attributable to differences in the growth patterns of neural and skeletal structures (tethered cord). Among the numerous solitary or combined lesions that may occur are abnormal or supernumerary nerve roots, dural and arachnoid adhesions, spinal cord angiomas and hamartomas, and failure of differentiation of the conus.

Occult dysraphism is twice as common in girls as in boys, whereas open lesions are seen with equal frequency in the two sexes. Approximately one half of these abnormalities have cutaneous markers; additional clinical manifestations include leg length and motor power discrepancy, foot deformities, gait abnormality, and neurogenic bladder.

Radiologic evaluation generally will reveal structural vertebral defects, although 15 per cent of patients may have no radiographic abnormalities. Neural arch anomalies are common. Interpediculate widening and enlargement of the spinal canal are often present, and the vertebral bodies may be deformed or scalloped.

The most common occult spinal dysraphic lesions are diastematomyelia, low conus (tethered filum), and congenital intraspinal tumors (lipomas and dermoids).

Diastematomyelia refers to a congenital longitudinal diastasis in the spinal cord, leading to two parts that are usually of unequal size. Although an osseous spur may be present between the two parts of the spinal cord, approximately one half of patients with this anomaly have no true septum.

Diastematomyelia occurs in 15 per cent of all patients with congenital scoliosis and is two times more common in girls than in boys. Skin changes are noted in about 80 per cent of patients. The septum is most common at the L1 to L4 spinal segment, with an abnormal radiologic density visible in about 75 per cent of cases (Fig. 75–3). Computed tomography can demonstrate nonosseous septa when intrathecal contrast material is employed. When a bone septum is present, it frequently extends from the neural arch forward, not necessarily being fused anteriorly to the vertebral body.

The most common radiologic finding in diastematomyelia is an intersegmental laminar fusion associated with a defect in the neural arch at the same or an adjacent level. An increased interpediculate distance and scoliosis are present in about two thirds of patients. In fewer than 10 per cent of patients, the spine is completely normal.

Myelography will show the perimedullary space surrounding the normal and the divided portions of the spinal cord. The length of the divided cord averages five vertebral segments, but it may be as long as 15 vertebrae. Computed tomography demonstrates that the two portions of the spinal cord are unequal in size.

The low conus (tethered conus) syndrome generally is believed to represent another manifestation of occult spinal

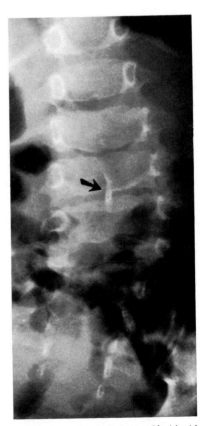

Figure 75–3. Diastematomyelia. This 2 year old girl with meningomyelocele has a well-defined bone spicule projecting over the third lumbar vertebra (arrow). Associated dysraphic changes include widened interpediculate distances, asymmetric development of the lower vertebral bodies, and undeveloped sacral neural arches.

dysraphism. Intraspinal dermoids, lipomas, congenital bands, and meningomyeloceles (Fig. 75-2) may all cause tethering of the conus, but in many cases no associated lesions are found. The conus medullaris is considered abnormally low when it lies below the L2-L3 spinal level at the age of 5 years. The low position of the conus causes the nerve roots to emerge more horizontally than usual. The dural sac usually is increased in volume. The filum terminale may be thickened, often owing to fatty infiltration.

Congenital intraspinal tumors are associated with vertebral changes, cutaneous manifestations, and clinical symptoms identical to those of other forms of occult spinal dysraphism. Of these congenital tumors, dermoids and lipomas constitute a large proportion. Lipomas may be intramedullary, intradural, or extradural in location and are frequently associated with open dysraphism in the form of lipomeningocele. Vertebral scalloping at the level of an intraspinal tumor is frequent. The conus may be low, and extradural abnormalities are seen, consisting of smooth compression or dural adhesions causing plication, with a sharply defined abnormality or an irregular deformity. Computed tomography is particularly useful in the evaluation of an extradural lipoma or lipomeningocele.

SPINAL CURVATURES

Scoliosis (Greek: curvature, crookedness) refers to lateral spinal curvature in the coronal plane. Scoliosis may be caused by congenital architectural imbalance or growth asymmetry; neoplastic, traumatic, or infectious damage; radiation; reflexive splinting owing to nerve irritation; bone dysplasias; or asymmetric neuromuscular control. The great majority of cases, however, are of unknown cause (idiopathic scoliosis).

Imaging Techniques in Evaluating Scoliosis

After clinical examination of the patient, plain film radiography should be employed. The initial radiologic examination should be a limited one, obtained to confirm the abnormal spinal curvature, estimate its magnitude and location, and detect any congenital anomalies. The entire spine is examined in the erect position with the patient standing without shoes. A lateral film is needed to evaluate accompanying kyphosis. Gonadal shielding is used in all patients. Every attempt should be made to reduce radiation exposure to the lowest level feasible. Posteroanterior rather than anteroposterior views are recommended for routine use, with the main advantage being reduction of radiation to the breast. It should be noted that measurement uncertainty in the range of 3 or 4 degrees, compared with a theoretical maximum progression rate of 1 degree per month, suggests that radiography repeated at intervals of less than 3 or 4 months may not be reliable.

Specialized imaging techniques are helpful in certain situations. As examples, bone scintigraphy is valuable in confirming the presence of osteoid osteomas, osteoblastomas, or pseudarthroses after surgery. Ultrasonography can evaluate the contents of the spinal canal in normal infants under 6 months of age and in other children, if there is an open neural arch or previous laminectomy. Myelography may be used to evaluate symptomatic patients with idiopathic scoliosis. In the presence of dysraphism, severe scoliosis, or scoliosis with neurologic abnormality, it may be helpful to supplement myelography with computed tomography. Eval-

uation of the genitourinary tract in patients with congenital scoliosis is indicated. This can be accomplished by ultrasonography or intravenous urography.

Maturity may be estimated roughly from the degree of development of the iliac crest apophyses. If a more reliable evaluation of maturity is needed, bone age analysis of the hand and wrist is indicated.

Radiologic Analysis of Scoliosis

On a frontal radiograph, the normal child's spine is straight, without curvature in the coronal plane. On a lateral radiograph, the newborn has a relatively straight spine but develops thoracic kyphosis and lumbar lordosis as he or she adopts an erect position. The median T5 to T12 thoracic kyphosis in normal older children is 27 degrees (ninetieth percentile, 40 degrees). The median L1 to L5 lumbar lordosis is normally 40 degrees (ninetieth percentile, 54 degrees). It should be noted that the lumbar lordosis is measured between L1 and L5, not to the superior surface of the sacrum.

The scoliotic curvature should be identified as nonstructural (flexible, with correction to linear alignment with lateral bending) or structural (curvature not completely corrected with lateral bending). Attempts to label the spinal curvatures as primary or secondary usually are futile. The curvature above or below the level of the major structural curve is usually considered to be compensatory and nonstructural in nature.

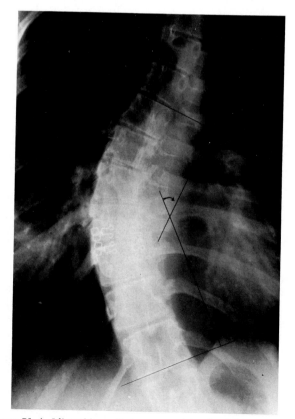

Figure 75-4. Idiopathic scoliosis measured by the Cobb technique. Lines drawn perpendicular to the axes of the endplates are measured (arrows). The vertebral bodies are normal with only minimal wedging caused by asymmetric growth.

The first task in the radiologic analysis of scoliosis is the identification of the vertebrae at either end of the curvature. The most laterally displaced and rotated vertebra is designated the apical vertebra and will be located between these two terminal vertebrae. The degree of rotation and displacement from the midline of the vertebrae above and below the apical vertebra will diminish progressively until the end vertebrae are reached, at which point the spine will straighten or a second curve in the opposite direction will be detected. The intervertebral disc adjacent to each end vertebra will be maximally wedged. The psoas margin on the concave side of a lumbar curve often is absent.

The curvature is measured by constructing lines along the superior endplate of the highest vertebra and along the inferior endplate of the lowest vertebra (Fig. 75–4). In the case of mild or moderate curvatures, lines drawn perpendicular to these endplate lines will ease the task of measuring the angle of scoliosis.

Rotation of the spine is greatest at the level of the apical vertebra but is quite variable from one patient to another. Scoliotic curves of the same magnitude in two patients may have much different degrees of vertebral rotation. In general, curves of less than 40 degrees are proportionately more rotated than larger ones. Normally, pedicles are placed symmetrically with respect to the vertebral edges; when spinal rotation occurs, the pedicle will move inward from the edge of the body. Vertebral rotation can be analyzed by computed tomography.

Kyphosis and lordosis are measured in the same manner by constructing lines along the vertebral endplates on the lateral radiograph. In severe scoliosis, the normal patterns of kyphosis and lordosis are diminished and the lateral profile of the spine is straightened.

Evaluation of the skeletal maturity is a helpful clinical tool as most mild or moderate spinal curvatures will no longer progress after the cessation of growth. Exceptions to this rule occur, and many severe spinal curvatures will increase throughout the life of the patient. Skeletal maturity can be determined by analysis of the development of the apophysis of the iliac crest; most curves will not increase after the appearance of complete ossification of the iliac apophysis (which occurs at an average age of 15 years 3 months in girls and about 6 months later in boys). In some patients, complete fusion of the iliac apophysis rather than its total ossification seems to correlate better with cessation of progression of the spinal curvature.

Congenital Scoliosis

Scoliosis initiated and perpetuated by a congenital anomaly of the spine is termed congenital scoliosis. It may be caused by failure of formation (wedge vertebra or hemivertebra), partial duplication (supernumerary hemivertebra), failure of segmentation (unilateral block vertebra, pedicle bar, neural arch fusion), or a combination of these lesions. The thoracolumbar region is most commonly affected.

Progression of congenital scoliosis is seen in about 75 per cent of patients, the poorest prognosis occurring in association with a unilateral bar and a contralateral hemivertebra. Associated rib abnormalities are common. The radiologic evaluation of congenital scoliosis should include spot and oblique radiographs of any area of abnormality detected during initial workup. Supplementation with computed tomography, myelography, and magnetic resonance imaging may be required.

Examination of the genitourinary tract is indicated in all patients with congenital anomalies of the spine. Investigations have shown that associated genitourinary tract abnormalities, especially unilateral renal agenesis, horseshoe kidneys, and renal duplications and ectopia, are frequent and unrelated to the level, side, or severity of the spinal changes. Other abnormalities associated with congenital scoliosis include congenital heart disease, undescended scapulae, and thumb anomalies.

Congenital Kyphosis and Lordosis

Congenital lordosis is uncommon and usually is limited to the thoracic region, where growth inhibition will lead to a severe restrictive thoracic dysplasia. The lordosis is caused by fusion of the posterior neural elements and continued anterior vertebral growth. Synostosis of the posterior portion of the ribs also may add to the growth inhibition.

Congenital kyphosis, which is much more frequent than congenital lordosis, is related to agenesis or underdevelopment of the anterior portion of the vertebral centrum, resulting in a posterior hemivertebra (Fig. 75–5); less commonly, it is related to failure of segmentation anteriorly with a congenital bar formed between the vertebral bodies. Genitourinary abnormalities are common. Some patients with congenital kyphosis will also have Klippel-Feil fusional anomalies in the cervical spine. Congenital kyphosis is common in meningomyelocele, diastrophic dwarfism, and certain other dysplasias.

The thoracolumbar spine is the area that is most typically involved. Anterior subluxation of the spine above the level of the anomaly may lead to displacement of the hypoplastic vertebral body into the neural canal (Fig. 75–5).

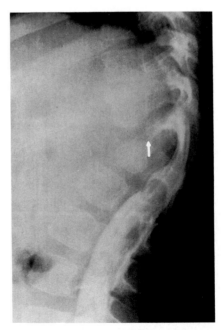

Figure 75–5. Congenital kyphosis associated with posterior hemivertebra. The upper spine is subluxed anteriorly at the level of a hypoplastic vertebral body (arrow). The resultant kyphosis narrows the contrast-filled thecal space.

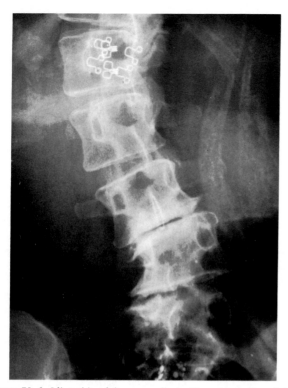

Figure 75–6. Idiopathic adolescent scoliosis. The residual effect of this condition is shown in a 43 year old woman. Disc space narrowing, osteophyte formation, vertebral sclerosis, and lateral vertebral subluxation are present.

the basis of age of the patient at the time the condition is recognized.

Infantile scoliosis is detected before the age of 4 years. Resolution of the spinal curvature occurs in 74 per cent of cases of infantile scoliosis; scoliotic curves that are greater than 50 degrees are the ones that usually progress. Associated plagiocephaly has been noted in 86 per cent of affected infants, with the skull depression invariably located on the convex side of the curve.

Juvenile scoliosis is that which is recognized between the ages of 4 and 10 years. About 13 per cent of all cases of scoliosis are discovered in this age period. In distinction to adolescent scoliosis, boys are affected predominantly when the diagnosis is established prior to the age of 6 years; between the ages of 7 and 10 years, girls are affected principally. Juvenile scoliosis almost invariably progresses with growth.

Adolescent scoliosis is detected between the ages of 10 years and the time of skeletal maturity and is by far the most common type of idiopathic scoliosis in the United States. The ratio of affected girls to boys ranges between 4 to 1 and 8 to 1.

EVOLUTION AND TREATMENT OF IDIOPATHIC SCOLIOSIS. As a general rule, spinal curvatures less than 20 degrees in magnitude are not actively treated unless they occur in preadolescent children and show evidence of rapid progression. With more severe curvature, thoracolumbar or-

Idiopathic Scoliosis

The frequency of idiopathic scoliosis in the normal population depends on the magnitude of the curvature being described. Scoliosis of more than 25 degrees has been documented in 1.5 per 1000 persons in the United States. Scoliosis seems to be more common in taller and heavier persons and in those with decreased skeletal maturation. Adolescent scoliosis is four to eight times more common in girls than in boys, but there is evidence that its frequency in the two sexes is more nearly equal at younger ages.

The ability to predict which curves will progress and which will regress or remain stable is obviously of great clinical importance. The reported frequency of progression of the spinal curvature has varied from 5 per cent to 79 per cent. Sixty per cent of curvatures in rapidly growing prepubertal children will progress. Curvatures less than 30 degrees generally will not progress after the child is mature, but severe curvatures will continue to increase at the rate of about 1 degree per year in adults. Marked tilting and lateral subluxation of vertebral bodies occur in older patients with severe idiopathic scoliosis (Fig. 75–6).

The cause(s) of idiopathic scoliosis remains elusive. Although there is some evidence for a dominant, X-linked inheritance pattern with incomplete penetrance and variable expressivity, most studies tend to favor a multifactorial inheritance pattern.

CLINICAL PATTERNS. Idiopathic scoliosis has been divided into three groups (infantile, juvenile, adolescent) on

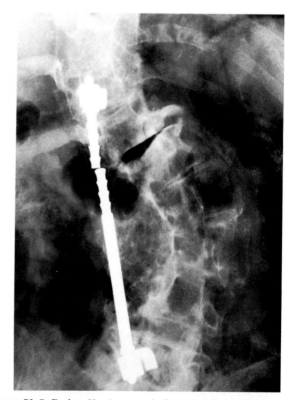

Figure 75–7. Broken Harrington rod after spinal fusion. Gas is present in the T12-L1 intervertebral disc with lateral subluxation, osteophytosis, and bone sclerosis. Although no pseudarthrosis is evident on this film, the presence of the broken rod and evidence of vertebral motion indicate that a pseudarthrosis must be present.

thotic braces are used. High thoracic curves occasionally require the use of a Milwaukee type brace. The purpose of such bracing is to restrict the degree of spinal curvature to that which was encountered when treatment was instituted. The braces are removed when spinal growth has been completed.

At least three types of operative stabilization procedures are now in use, with a common purpose of eliminating the progression of the spinal curvature. Stabilization of a posterior fusion site can be accomplished with Harrington rods (Fig. 75–7) or segmental (Luque) instruments. In certain situations in which the scoliosis is accompanied by neurologic problems, anterior fusion using the Dwyer cable-screw system is used to provide further stability. Complications of spinal fusion include breakage of wires or rods, loosening and migration of hooks, spondylolysis, pseudarthrosis, bronchial compression by the fusion mass, dislocation above the fusion site after trauma to the long lever arm of the ankylosed spine, gastric volvulus, aortic aneurysm, and retroperitoneal fibrosis.

Neuromuscular Scoliosis

Asymmetric innervation or unbalanced muscular function may lead to scoliosis. The typical neuromuscular curvature is a long, C-shaped scoliosis extending from the upper thoracic region to the pelvis. Pelvic obliquity is characteristic. In some

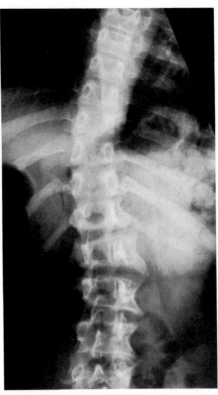

Figure 75–9. Neurofibromatosis. Scoliosis is associated with asymmetric development of the lumbar vertebral bodies, lateral vertebral scalloping, and coarse trabeculae.

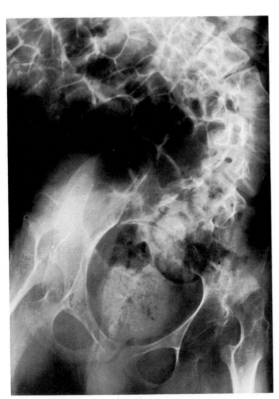

Figure 75–8. Neuromuscular scoliosis in cerebral palsy. Severe left lumbar scoliosis with marked rotation is present. The pelvis is oblique, with bilateral hip dislocations. (From Theros EG, Harris JH Jr [Eds]: American College of Radiology Bone Syllabus IV. Chicago, American College of Radiology, in press. Used with permission.)

instances, however, neuromuscular scoliosis may be indistinguishable from idiopathic scoliosis.

Cerebral palsy is the most common cause of neuromuscular scoliosis (Fig. 75–8). Additional features include pelvic obliquity and hip dislocation. Scoliosis is seen in as many as 70 per cent of patients with syringomyelia. Spinal cord tumors also may lead to scoliosis. Abnormal curvatures occurring after traumatic paraplegia or quadriplegia also are common.

Scoliosis after poliomyelitis is no longer a common occurrence. In spinal muscular atrophy, scoliosis occurs in more than 60 per cent of patients and usually develops between the ages of 3 and 6 years. It is seen in as many as 80 per cent of patients with Friedreich's ataxia, and it is frequent in familial dysautonomia, hypertrophic interstitial polyneuritis, and peroneal muscular atrophy. In the Duchenne type of muscular dystrophy, scoliosis does not usually develop until the child is older than 10 years and confined to a wheelchair.

Scoliosis Associated with or Secondary to Other Conditions

Although most cases of scoliosis are idiopathic in nature, others occur as part of many different syndromes or are associated with systemic disease, regional irritative foci, or fibromuscular change adjacent to or remote from the spine.

The scoliosis of neurofibromatosis has classically been described as one with sharp angulation and associated kyphosis but, in reality, most abnormal spinal curvatures in this disease resemble those of idiopathic scoliosis. When abrupt angulation of the spine, kyphosis, and adjacent rib dysplasia are

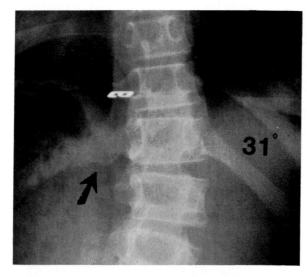

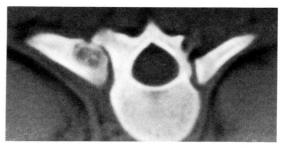

Figure 75–10. Scoliosis secondary to osteoid osteoma. **A** There is expansion of the head of the left twelfth rib at the apex of the thoracolumbar scoliosis (arrow). (Posteroanterior projection.) **B** Computed tomography demonstrates expansion and sclerosis of the proximal portion of the left twelfth rib. A central nidus is present. (The orientation of the computed tomogram has been inverted to correspond with that of the other image.)

evident, however, the radiologic diagnosis of neurofibromatosis is assured. Associated findings may include a paravertebral soft tissue mass, deformed transverse processes, enlarged vertebral foramina, marked rotation of the spinal curvature, and a coarsened and sclerotic trabecular pattern (Fig. 75–9).

Tumors in the vertebrae or adjacent ribs may be associated with scoliosis. In this situation, *osteoid osteomas* or osteoblastomas generally are located on the concave side of the spinal curvature at its apex (Fig. 75–10).

Scoliosis is seen in about 10 per cent of patients with intraspinal tumors. In over 50 per cent of such cases, there are radiologic changes in the pedicles, spinal canal, or paravertebral area.

The spinal curvature that results from significant leg length discrepancy is convex to the side of the shorter leg, characteristically involves the lumbar or thoracolumbar region, and is a functional rather than a structural scoliosis.

Radiation therapy employed in the treatment of malignant tumors of the kidney, thorax, or retroperitoneum will cause both clinical and radiologic spinal deformity. Although the abnormal curvature is most severe when only a portion of the spine is included in the radiation field, it nevertheless can result even when the entire spine is irradiated (see Chapter 64).

Scoliosis in Bone Dysplasias and Generalized Syndromes

Scoliosis is a common feature of many bone dysplasias and syndromes. Examples include achondroplasia, spondyloepiphyseal dysplasia congenita, diastrophic dwarfism, metatropic dwarfism, chondrodysplasia punctata, and the mucopolysaccharidoses (see Chapter 74).

FURTHER READING

Arredondo F, Haughton VM, Hemmy DC, Zelaya B, Williams AL: The computed tomographic appearance of the spinal cord in diastematomyelia. Radiology 13:685, 1980.

Bethem D, Winter RB, Lutter L, Moe JH, Bradford DS, Lonstein JE, Langer LO: Spinal disorders of dwarfism. Review of the literature and report of eighty cases. J Bone Joint Surg [Am] 63:1412, 1981.

Burrows FGO: Some aspects of occult spinal dysraphism: A study of 90 cases. Br J Radiol 41:496, 1968.

Chaglassian JH, Riseborough EJ, Hall JE: Neurofibromatous scoliosis. Natural history and results of treatment in thirty-seven cases. J Bone Joint Surg [Am] 58:695, 1976.

Dawson EG, Smith L: Atlanto-axial subluxation in children due to vertebral anomalies. J Bone Joint Surg [Am] 61:582, 1979.

De Smet AA: Radiology of Spinal Curvature. St Louis, CV Mosby, 1985.

DeSousa AL, Kalsbeck JE, Mealey J Jr, Campbell RL, Hockey A: Intraspinal tumors in children. A review of 81 cases. J Neurosurg 51:437, 1979.

Fitz CR, Harwood-Nash DC: The tethered conus. AJR 125:515, 1975.

Jeffries BF, Tarlton M, De Smet AA, Dwyer SJ, Brower AC: Computerized measurement and analysis of scoliosis. A more accurate representation of the shape of the curve. Radiology 134:381, 1980.

Kaplan JO, Quencer RM: The occult tethered conus syndrome in the adult. Radiology 137:387, 1980.

Luque ER: Current concepts review. The anatomic basis and development of segmental spinal instrumentation. Spine 7:256, 1982.

MacEwen GD, Conway JJ, Millet WT: Congenital scoliosis with a unilateral bar. Radiology 90:711, 1968.

McAlister WH, Shackelford GD: Classification of spinal curvatures. Radiol Clin North Am 13:93, 1975.

McAlister WH, Shackelford GD: Measurement of spinal curvatures. Radiol Clin North Am 13:113, 1975.

McMaster MJ, Ohtsuka K: The natural history of congenital scoliosis. A study of two hundred and fifty-one patients. J Bone Joint Surg [Am] 64:1128, 1982.

McRae DL: Bony abnormalities in the region of the foramen magnum: Correlation of the anatomic and neurologic findings. Acta Radiol 40:335, 1953.

Naidich TP, McLone DG, Mutluer S: A new understanding of dorsal dysraphism with lipoma (lipomyeloschisis): Radiologic evaluation and surgical correction. AJNR 4:103, 1983.

Propst-Proctor SL, Bleck EE: Radiographic determination of lordosis and kyphosis in normal and scoliotic children. J Pediatr Orthop 3:344, 1983.

Schwartz AM, Wechsler RJ, Landy MD, Wetzner SM, Goldstein SA: Posterior arch defects of the cervical spine. Skel Radiol 8:135, 1982.

Taybi H: Radiology of Syndromes and Metabolic Disorders. 2nd Ed. Chicago, Year Book Medical Publishers, 1983.

Tomsick TA, Lebowitz ME, Campbell C: The congenital absence of pedicles in the thoracic spine. Report of two cases. Radiology 111:587, 1974.

Winter RB, Lonstein JE, Leonard AS, Smith DE Jr: Congenital Deformities of the Spine. New York, Thieme-Stratton Inc, 1983.

Winter RB, Moe JH, Bradford DS, Lonstein JE, Pedras CV, Weber AH: Spine deformity in neurofibromatosis. A review of one hundred and two patients. J Bone Joint Surg [Am] 61:677, 1979.

Winter RB, Moe JH, Wang JF: Congenital kyphosis. Its natural history and treatment as observed in a study of one hundred and thirty patients. J Bone Joint Surg [Am] 55:223, 1973.

Chapter 76

Additional Congenital or Heritable Anomalies and Syndromes

Donald Resnick, M.D.

Many other congenital and inherited disorders in addition to the diseases discussed in earlier chapters also involve the skeleton. These diseases have varied clinical and radiographic manifestations and may sometimes simulate ac- *quired disorders. In some instances, radiographic features are entirely specific, whereas in others, they must be interpreted with knowledge of clinical abnormalities to arrive at a correct diagnosis.*

The separation of skeletal anomalies and skeletal variations is not accomplished uniformly with ease. An *anomaly* represents a marked deviation from normal standards, especially as a result of a congenital or hereditary defect, whereas a *variation* indicates a modification of some characteristics that are considered normal (variant of normal) or typical of a disease (variant of a disease). In some ways, then, the designation of a particular finding (or findings) as a skeletal anomaly or, alternatively, as a skeletal variation is arbitrary and accomplished on the basis of the presence and severity of accompanying clinical manifestations.

AREAS OF NORMAL AND ANOMALOUS TRABECULAR DIMINUTION OR PROMINENCE

It has been suggested that the trabecular architecture of bone coincides with routes of stress. Therefore, trabeculae are not uniformly distributed in the human skeleton. The radiographic consequence of this inhomogeneity is the appearance of radiolucent areas that are entirely normal yet easily misinterpreted as evidence of disease. Important examples include the normal areas of rarefaction in the femoral neck (Ward's triangle), the body of the calcaneus, and the proximal portion of the humerus adjacent to the greater tuberosity (Fig. 76–1). Alternatively, prominent trabeculae are normally encountered at many different sites, of which the distal portion of the humerus deserves emphasis.

The external surface of bone possesses normal sites of elevation, depression, and irregularity that may lead to difficulty during the interpretation of the radiographs. Important examples of such sites include the linea aspera in the posterior surface of the femoral shaft, the soleal line on the posterior surface of the proximal third of the tibia, and the deltoid tuberosity in the lateral surface of the midportion of the humerus.

Cystic areas and cortical irregularities in the posterior aspect of the femur at the site of attachment of tendinous fibers of the adductor magnus muscle present a real diagnostic challenge. Terms used to describe these findings include fibrous cortical defects; subperiosteal, periosteal, and cortical desmoids; and (benign) metaphyseal and avulsive cortical irregularities. The proximity of the extensor tendon of the adductor magnus muscle to the site of the typical femoral proliferative lesion is consistent with a traumatic pathogenesis (Fig. 76–2). A second area of rarefaction has been identified lateral to the medial supracondylar line and adductor tubercle, approximately 1 cm above the superior limit of the medial condyle, corresponding to the osseous attachment of the medial head of the gastrocnemius muscle. Radiolucent lesions also have been described at osseous sites of insertion of other muscles.

SKELETAL CANALS, APERTURES, AND FORAMINA

A channel that extends through a bone is termed a foramen or, when large, an aperture. When the channel is oriented obliquely and, therefore, is of considerable length, it is referred to as a canal. Nutrient canals, through which pass the nutrient arteries, extend in an oblique fashion from one or more foramina on the osseous surface (Fig. 76–3). Resulting radiolucent channels rarely lead to diagnostic difficulty, although, on occasion, they resemble a fracture line. In flat bones such as the scapula and ilium, nutrient canals create linear or branching radiolucent areas.

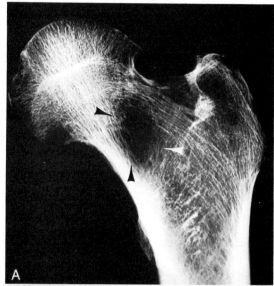

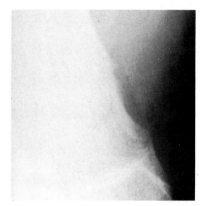

Figure 76–2. Normal sites of osseous irregularity: Avulsive (proliferative) cortical irregularity in the femur. Observe the normal cortical thickening and small periosteal excrescences extending into the soft tissue. The spongiosa is entirely normal and a soft tissue mass is not apparent.

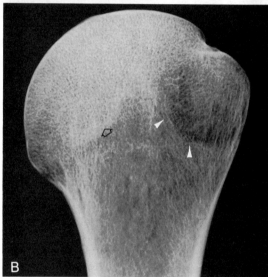

Figure 76–1. Normal sites of trabecular diminution. A Femoral neck. A radiolucent area in the femoral neck (arrowheads) represents Ward's triangle and is a normal occurrence. It is bordered by prominent tensile and compressive trabeculae. B Proximal portion of the humerus. The area of rarefaction adjacent to the greater tuberosity (arrowheads) is termed a humeral pseudocyst and is a normal finding. A fusion line, marking the site of closure of a portion of the physis, is faintly visible (arrow). (B, From Resnick D, Cone RO III: The nature of humeral pseudocysts. Radiology 150:7, 1984. Used with permission.)

and feet. Although, in the past, emphasis has been given to the differentiation of accessory ossicles or ossification centers from fractures, the possibility exists that some of these ossific foci are acquired after injury and that they may be associated with significant clinical manifestations. The os trigonum near the posterior surface of the talus, the os vesalianum adjacent to the cuboid and base of the fifth metatarsal, the os

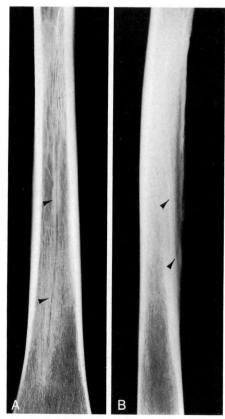

Figure 76–3. Normal nutrient canals. Femur. A frontal (A) and lateral (B) radiograph of two different femoral specimens indicate the position and configuration of the normal nutrient canal (arrowheads), which pierces the posterior cortex and extends proximally. It may simulate a fracture.

Sites of osseous thinning or true foramina are common in bones containing thin plates, such as the parietal and occipital bones of the skull, the sternum, and the scapula.

ACCESSORY OSSIFICATION CENTERS AND FRAGMENTED SESAMOID BONES

Although the appearance of more than one center of ossification during the development of an epiphysis can be a manifestation of disease (as in the epiphyseal dysgenesis that accompanies hypothyroidism), such centers are frequently encountered in asymptomatic children and adolescents and, as such, are generally regarded as a variation of normal. Accessory ossicles are also seen, especially in the hands, wrist,

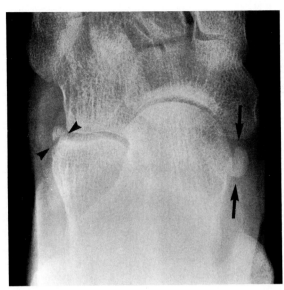

Figure 76–4. Accessory navicular bone: Type I (sesamoid bone in the posterior tibial tendon). In this 22 year old woman with pain over the lateral aspect of the foot following a fall, an anteroposterior radiograph of the foot shows a fracture of the anterolateral margin of the calcaneus (arrowheads). A well-defined oval ossicle (arrows) is noted adjacent to the posteromedial margin of the navicular bone. (From Lawson JP, et al: The painful accessory navicular. Skel Radiol 12:250, 1984. Used with permission.)

intermetatarsale between the bases of the first and second metatarsals, and the os supratrochleare dorsal in the olecranon fossa are examples of accessory ossicles that reportedly have been accompanied by pain. Although there are many additional ossicles that may have clinical significance, two deserve emphasis.

1. *Accessory navicular bone (os tibiale externum or naviculare secundarium).* Two distinct types of accessory navicular bones have been described: A separate ossicle may occur as a sesamoid bone in the posterior tibial tendon (type I); and an accessory ossification center may appear in the tubercle of the navicular bone (type II) (Figs. 76–4 and 76–5). Type I ossicles account for approximately 30 per cent of cases, generally are well defined, have a round or oval configuration, and are located up to 5 mm medial and posterior to the medial aspect of the navicular. Type II accessory ossification centers represent approximately 70 per cent of cases, are triangular or heart-shaped in configuration, and are located within 1 to 2 mm from the medial and posterior aspect of the navicular. It is the type II ossification center that has been associated with pain, which usually becomes evident in the second decade of life. Histologic analysis has revealed changes compatible with chronic stress-related injury.

2. *Carpal boss (os styloideum).* A commonly occurring bone protuberance on the dorsum of the wrist at the base of the second and third metacarpals adjacent to the capitate and trapezoid bones is termed a carpal boss or carpe bossu. It relates to either an osteophyte or an accessory ossification center, the os styloideum. Although generally asymptomatic, the carpal boss can occasionally lead to pain and limitation of hand motion.

The occurrence of multiple ossification centers in a sesamoid bone, of which the bipartite patella is the best example, has long been regarded as a normal variation without clinical significance; however, recent evidence suggests that local pain may accompany this patellar variation and, furthermore, the

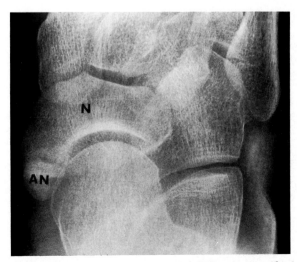

Figure 76–5. Accessory navicular bone: Type II (accessory ossification center in the tubercle of the navicular bone). This 12 year old girl developed progressive pain over the medial aspect of the foot, which was aggravated by gymnastics and skiing. A radiograph demonstrates the triangular, accessory navicular bone (AN) adjacent to the medial and posterior margin of the navicular (N). (From Lawson JP, et al: The painful accessory navicular. Skel Radiol 12:250, 1984. Used with permission.)

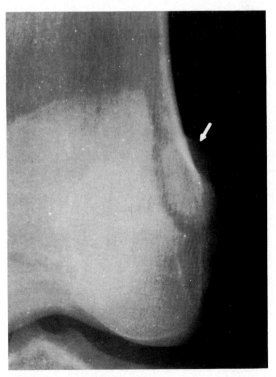

Figure 76–6. Bipartite patella. Localization to the superolateral aspect of the patella (arrow) is the most characteristic radiographic finding.

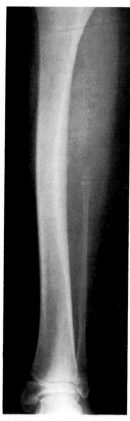

Figure 76–7. Hypoplasia: Fibula. Note severe hypoplasia of the fibula with medial bowing of the midshaft of the tibia.

alteration may relate to chronic tensile failure of the bone in skeletally immature persons. The predilection for the superolateral aspect of the bone (Fig. 76–6) remains the radiographic hallmark of the finding

SKELETAL APLASIA AND HYPOPLASIA

The entire bone or a portion thereof may fail to form in the normal fashion, producing a variety of congenital deficiencies. Of the major tubular bones, aplasia or hypoplasia most typically affects the fibula, radius, femur, ulna, and humerus in order of descending frequency.

Fibular Aplasia and Hypoplasia

Congenital absence or severe hypoplasia of the fibula can be combined with bowing of the companion tibia, an equinovalgus foot, absence of the lateral rays of the foot, tarsal aplasia or fusion, and retarded development or shortening of the ipsilateral femur (Fig. 76–7). Distal fibular hypoplasia may be associated with a valgus deformity of the ankle, whereas proximal fibular hypoplasia can be accompanied by valgus knee deformity and instability at the proximal tibiofibular articulation.

Radial and Ulnar Aplasia and Hypoplasia

Radial anomalies may include total or partial aplasia or hypoplasia. Bilateral abnormalities are common and may be combined with hypoplasia or absence of the thumb or radial carpal bones. Such radial lesions can be associated with the vertebral-anal-tracheal-esophageal-radial-renal syndrome (VA-

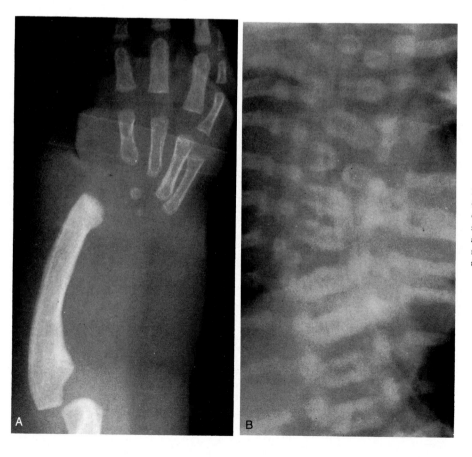

Figure 76–8. Vertebral-anal-tracheal-esophageal-radial-renal (VATER) syndrome. This 2½ year old child demonstrates radial aplasia, absence of the thumb, and severe spinal anomalies. Additional abnormalities included a tracheoesophageal fistula and renal and anal anomalies.

Table 76–1. CLASSIFICATION OF PROXIMAL FEMORAL FOCAL DEFICIENCY

Class	Head of Femur	Acetabulum	Femoral Segment	Relationship Among Components of Femur and Acetabulum at Skeletal Maturity
A	Present	Adequate	Short	Bone connection between components of femur; head in acetabulum; subtrochanteric varus, often with pseudarthrosis
B	Present	Adequate or moderately dysplastic	Short; usually proximal bone tuft	No osseous connection between head and shaft; head in acetabulum
C	Absent or represented by ossicle	Severely dysplastic	Short; usually proximally tapered	May be osseous connection between shaft and proximal ossicle; no osseous connection between femur and acetabulum
D	Absent	Absent; obturator foramen enlarged; pelvis squared in bilateral cases	Short, deformed	

From Levinson ED, Ozonoff MB, Royen PM: Proximal femoral focal deficiency [PFFD]. Radiology 125:197, 1977. Used with permission.

TER syndrome) (Fig. 76–8); cardiac abnormalities, including ventricular septal defect, atrial septal defect, pulmonary artery atresia, and patent ductus arteriosus; and thrombocytopenia with absent radius (TAR syndrome).

Deficiency of the ulna is less frequent and severe than that of the radius.

Proximal Femoral Focal Deficiency (PFFD)

Proximal femoral focal deficiency is the term applied to a spectrum of conditions characterized by partial absence and shortening of the proximal portion of the femur. Although some cases of PFFD are associated with other skeletal defects, it is usually an isolated occurrence, appearing in a unilateral fashion in 90 per cent of patients. A variety of classification systems have been suggested on the basis of presence and location of the femoral head and neck (Table 76–1) (Fig. 76–

9). Radiographs of a newborn infant demonstrate a short femur that is displaced superiorly, posteriorly, and laterally to the iliac crest. The distal end of the femur usually is normal. Ossification of the femoral capital epiphysis is invariably delayed. After the second year of life, affected children reveal either dysgenesis or absence of subtrochanteric ossification. At skeletal maturity, changes include subtrochanteric varus deformity or pseudarthrosis, a large unossified gap between the femoral capital epiphysis and dysplastic shaft, or ossification of only the distal femoral epiphysis. Secondary abnormalities of the pelvis and acetabulum are common. The major differential diagnosis is developmental coxa vara, in which familial and bilateral characteristics may be seen and in which abnormalities are less severe, delayed in appearance, progressive, and related to a true decrease in the neck-shaft angle as opposed to the subtrochanteric varus that appears in PFFD.

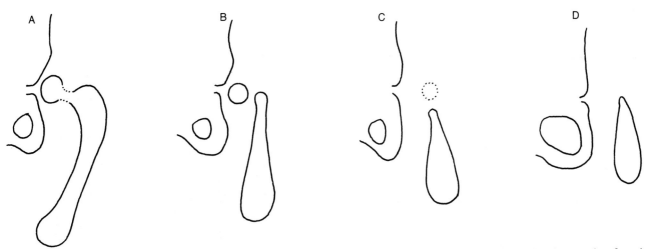

Figure 76–9. Proximal femoral focal deficiency (PFFD): Classification system. Classes A to D are described. In all classes, there is a very short femoral shaft. Dashed lines indicate structures that will (class A) or may (class C) ossify at a later date. (After Levinson ED, et al: Proximal femoral focal deficiency [PFFD]. Radiology 125:197, 1977. Used with permission.)

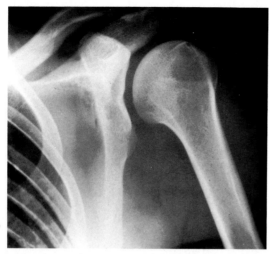

Figure 76–10. Hypoplasia (dysplasia) of the glenoid neck of the scapula. Hypoplasia of the scapular neck, an irregular notched glenoid articular surface, and widening of the lower portion of the joint space are evident. The opposite side was affected similarly. (From Resnick D, et al: Bilateral dysplasia of the scapular neck. AJR 139:387, 1982. Copyright 1982, American Roentgen Ray Society. Used with permission.)

Hypoplasia (Dysplasia) of the Glenoid Neck of the Scapula

This entity is also termed glenoid hypoplasia and dentated glenoid anomaly (Fig. 76–10). Men and women are affected with about equal frequency. The age at which the diagnosis is established varies. Shoulder pain and limitation of motion often are evident; less commonly, the condition may be discovered as an incidental finding.

Bilateral and relatively symmetric radiographic changes predominate, consisting of dysplasia of the scapular neck and irregularity of the glenoid surface. Additional findings may include hypoplasia of the humeral head and neck, varus deformity of the proximal portion of the humerus, and enlargement and bowing of the acromion and the clavicle. The glenohumeral joint appears widened, especially inferiorly.

The radiographic abnormalities associated with dysplasia of the neck of the scapula are virtually diagnostic. The absence of alterations in other epiphyses eliminates the diagnosis of multiple epiphyseal dysplasia. An injury to the brachial plexus occurring at birth can lead to an upper arm type of paralysis (Erb's paralysis) with subsequent radiographic abnormalities about the shoulder that might resemble dysplasia of the scapular neck.

Sacrococcygeal Agenesis (Caudal Regression Syndrome)

This well-known anomaly leads to absence of one or more segments of the sacrum, which may be combined with aplasia of the lower thoracic and upper lumbar spine (Fig. 76–11). Approximately 20 per cent of persons with this syndrome are the children of diabetic mothers. Associated abnormalities include neurogenic bladder and serious urologic problems, hip dislocations, flexion contractures of the knees and hips, and foot deformities. Complete sacral agenesis is combined

with deformed ilia that may articulate with each other or with the lowest vertebral body or that fuse in the midline. Partial agenesis may lead to a deformed and sickle-shaped sacrum through which an anterior meningocele may protrude. Central sacral defects may be combined with hereditary presacral teratoma.

The detection of associated skeletal and visceral abnormalities requires myelography, urography, cystography, and contrast studies of the gastrointestinal tract in addition to plain film radiography.

SKELETAL HYPERPLASIA

Congenital enlargement may involve a single bone, a portion of a limb, or the entire limb. Soft tissue hypertrophy generally accompanies the osseous abnormality. Although they usually are idiopathic, similar changes can be evident in neurofibromatosis, lipomatosis, macrodystrophia lipomatosa, hemangiomatosis, lymphangiomatosis, arteriovenous malformations, endocrine disorders, cerebral gigantism, Wilms' tumor, and neoplasms of the adrenal glands.

MALSEGMENTATIONS AND FUSIONS
Hyperphalangism and Polydactyly

Extra phalanges in humans are virtually confined to the thumb (Fig. 76–12). The triphalangeal thumb can occur as an isolated finding, or it may also be associated with poly-

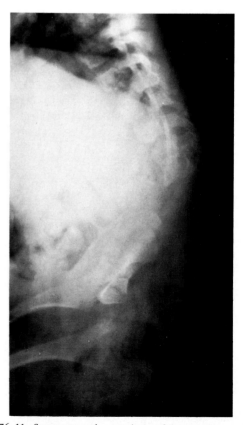

Figure 76–11. Sacrococcygeal agenesis (caudal regression syndrome). In this child of a diabetic mother, observe absence of much of the lumbar spine and all of the sacrum. Deformity of the ilia is evident.

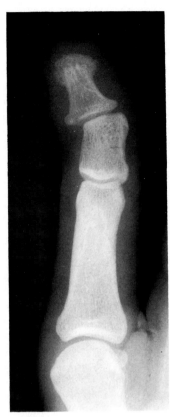

Figure 76–12. **Hyperphalangism: Thumb.** In this patient with the Holt-Oram syndrome, observe three separate phalanges in the thumb.

dactyly, duplications, the Holt-Oram syndrome, trisomy 13, and Blackfan-Diamond anemia. Accessory phalanges should be differentiated from pseudoepiphyses of the digits that may accompany cleidocranial dysostosis and hypothyroidism.

Polydactyly, representing an increased number of digits, can appear in the hand or the foot. Its appearance on the radial side of the hand is termed preaxial polydactyly, and its existence on the ulnar side of the hand is known as postaxial polydactyly. Preaxial polydactyly may be associated with acrocephalosyndactyly, brachydactyly B, acropectorovertebral dysplasia, Fanconi's syndrome, Holt-Oram syndrome, and other conditions; postaxial polydactyly can appear in the Ellis–van Creveld syndrome, Laurence-Moon-Biedl syndrome, trisomy 13, asphyxiating thoracic dystrophy, Goltz's focal dermal hypoplasia, and other diseases.

Syndactyly

Syndactyly, a common anomaly, relates to a lack of differentiation between two or more digits. It may be subdivided into cases with either soft tissue or osseous involvement. Most cases are inherited. A large number of syndromes have been associated with syndactyly. Included in this list is Poland's syndrome, in which there is syndactyly and absence of the pectoral muscles (Fig. 76–13).

Symphalangism

Symphalangism represents a fusion of one phalanx to another within the same digit. It is usually inherited as a dominant trait. Typical sites of involvement include the proximal interphalangeal joints of the fingers and the distal interphalangeal joints of the toes. The thumb is rarely affected. Associated syndromes include diastrophic dwarfism, Bell's brachydactyly types A and C, popliteal pterygium syndrome, and certain acrocephalosyndactyly syndromes.

It is important to differentiate this anomaly from acquired intraarticular fusions accompanying various arthritides, including juvenile chronic arthritis and psoriatic arthritis.

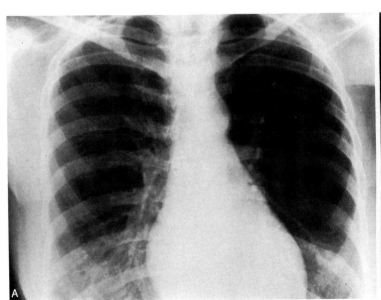

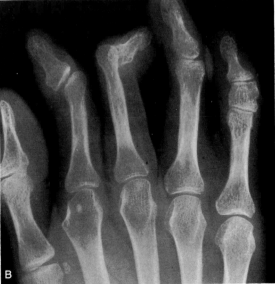

Figure 76–13. **Poland's syndrome. A** Note the absence of the left pectoral muscles, creating increased lucency of the left hemithorax. Elevation of the scapula and deformity of the ribs also are seen. **B** The involved hand reveals aplasia (second, third, and fourth digits) and hypoplasia (fifth digit) of the middle phalanges, partial soft tissue syndactyly between the fourth and fifth fingers and between the second and third fingers, and osseous deformities.

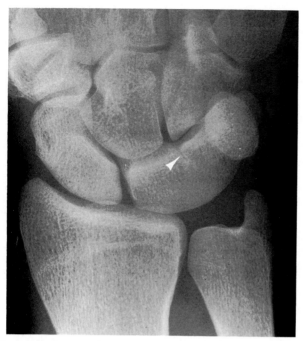

Figure 76–14. Carpal fusion (coalition). Note the bone fusion between the lunate and the triquetrum with a small cleft (arrowhead) at the site of ankylosis.

Carpal Fusion (Coalition)

Carpal coalition is a relatively common abnormality that may occur as an isolated phenomenon or as part of a generalized congenital malformation syndrome. As a rule, isolated fusions involve bones in the same carpal row (proximal or distal), whereas syndrome-related fusions may affect bones in different rows (proximal and distal).

The most common site of the isolated fusion is between the triquetrum and the lunate bones (Fig. 76–14). Less common isolated coalitions that may be encountered include capitate-hamate fusion, trapezium-trapezoid fusion, and pisi-form-hamate fusion. In most cases, symptoms are entirely lacking, although pain has been observed in association with partial coalitions and cystic changes in the adjacent bones.

Massive carpal fusion or fusion between bones of the proximal and distal carpal rows or between the carpal bones and radius or ulna generally is associated with additional malformations, such as acrocephalosyndactyly syndromes, arthrogryposis, diastrophic dwarfism, Ellis–van Creveld syndrome, hand-foot-uterus syndrome, Holt-Oram syndrome, otopalatodigital syndrome, Turner's syndrome, or symphalangism.

Accessory Carpal Bones

A number of extra ossification centers may appear in the wrist adjacent to the eight normal carpal bones. Although they produce no symptoms or signs, certain ossicles are associated with specific malformation syndromes. Accessory bones in the distal carpal row can accompany diastrophic dwarfism, Ellis–van Creveld syndrome, Larson's syndrome, otopalatodigital syndrome, and brachydactyly A-1. The os centrale can be noted in the hand-foot-uterus syndrome, Holt-

Oram syndrome, otopalatodigital syndrome, and Larsen's syndrome.

Radioulnar Synostosis

A common site of osseous fusion in the tubular bones of the extremities is between the proximal portions of the radius and ulna (Fig. 76–15). Two distinct types have been recognized: proximal radioulnar synostosis, in which the radius and ulna are smoothly fused at their proximal borders for a distance of about 2 to 6 cm; and a second variety, in which fusion just distal to the proximal radial epiphysis is associated with congenital dislocation of the radial head. In both types, there is interference with normal forearm supination. The condition is bilateral in distribution in approximately 60 per cent of patients. Sporadically occurring examples appear more often than familial cases.

Additional anomalies that may accompany radioulnar synostosis are clubfeet, congenital dislocation of the hip, knee anomalies, hypoplasia of the thumb, carpal fusion, symphalangism, and Madelung's deformity. Radioulnar synostosis may also appear as part of arthrogryposis, multiple hereditary exostoses, acrocephalopolysyndactyly, acrocephalosyndactyly, Holt-Oram syndrome, mandibulofacial dysostosis, Nievergelt-Pearlman syndrome, Klinefelter's syndrome, and other chromosomal aberrations. Furthermore, such synostosis can be acquired when osseous proliferation of one or both bones appears in the course of trauma, infection, or infantile cortical hyperostosis.

Tarsal Fusion (Coalition)

Tarsal coalition may be fibrous, cartilaginous, or osseous and may be congenital or acquired in response to infection, trauma, articular disorders, or surgery. Congenital tarsal coalition is of unknown cause. It appears, however, that familial factors are important in some cases, particularly those with massive tarsal fusions.

The association of congenital tarsal coalition and peroneal spastic flatfoot is well recognized. Typically, symptoms and

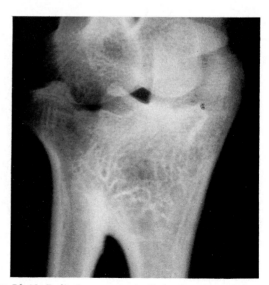

Figure 76–15. Radioulnar synostosis. Fusion has occurred just distal to the proximal border of the radius, and there is a congenital dislocation of the radial head.

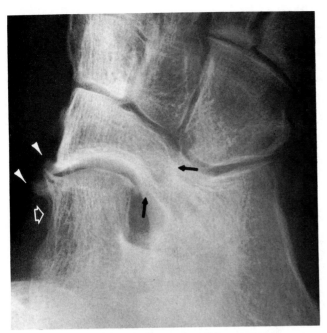

Figure 76–16. Calcaneonavicular tarsal coalition. A complete osseous coalition (solid arrows) is evident on the medial oblique view. Observe the bone excrescences at the talonavicular joint space (arrowheads) and hypoplasia of the distal aspect of the talus (open arrow).

Isolated tarsal coalitions can be classified according to the bones that are affected; calcaneonavicular, talocalcaneal, talonavicular, and calcaneocuboid fusions, in order of decreasing frequency, can be detected. Tarsal fusions accompanying multiple malformation syndromes may involve the entire tarsus. Tarsal fusions may accompany hereditary symphalangism, arthrogryposis, acrocephalosyndactyly (Apert's syndrome), the otopalatodigital syndrome, the hand-foot-uterus syndrome, and many other disorders.

CALCANEONAVICULAR COALITION. This type of coalition is one of the most frequent, is sometimes bilateral, and can be asymptomatic or associated with rigid flatfoot. Coalition is optimally identified on a 45 degree medial-oblique view of the foot (Fig. 76–16). The diagnosis is simplified by the presence of a solid bone bar extending between the calcaneus and the navicular bone. A close approximation of the contours of these two bones, especially if adjacent sclerosis is evident, should raise the possibility of a nonosseous coalition. A secondary radiographic sign of calcaneonavicular coalition is hypoplasia of the head of the talus. Talar "beaking" is uncommon. Other diagnostic techniques such as scintigraphy and computed tomography generally are not required.

TALOCALCANEAL COALITION. The talocalcaneal fusion represents the other common type of tarsal coalition. Almost all such fusions occur at the middle facet, between the talus and sustentaculum tali (Fig. 76–17); ankylosis of the posterior subtalar joint or of the anterior facets is far less frequent. The condition is more common in boys and is bilateral in 25 per cent of patients. Cartilaginous, fibrous, or osseous bridges may be identified, although a penetrated axial radiograph (Harris-Beath view) obtained with varying degrees of beam angulation, oblique radiographs, and conventional or computed tomograms may be necessary. In cases of

signs of tarsal coalition appear in the second or third decade of life. After minor trauma or unusual activity, the affected person complains of vague pain in the foot. Limited subtalar motion, pes planus, and shortening with persistent or intermittent spasm of the peroneal muscles are seen on physical examination.

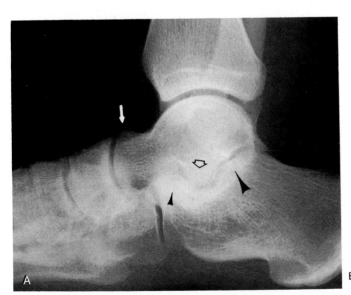

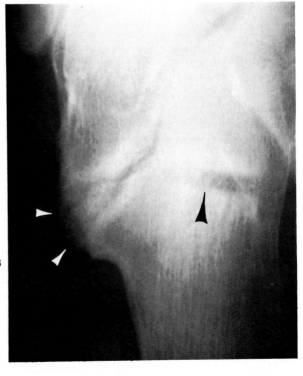

Figure 76–17. Talocalcaneal tarsal coalition: Middle facets. A A lateral radiograph reveals talar beaking (solid arrow), broadening of the lateral process of the talus (open arrow), narrowing of the posterior subtalar joint (large arrowhead), and absence of visualization of the space between the sustentaculum tali and talus (middle subtalar joint) (small arrowhead). B In a different patient, a Harris-Beath view outlines partial bone ankylosis (small arrowheads) between the sustentaculum tali and talus. Note the intact posterior subtalar joint (large arrowhead).

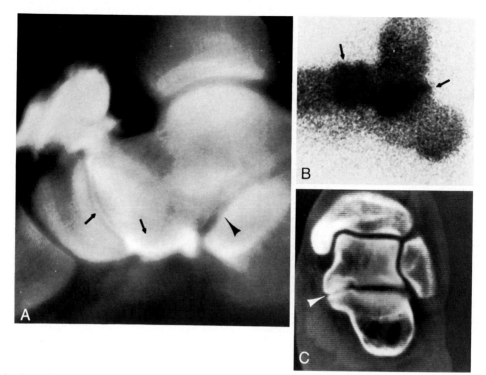

Figure 76–18. Talocalcaneal tarsal coalition: Use of arthrography, scintigraphy, and computed tomography. A Arthrography of the anterior talocalcaneonavicular joint followed by conventional tomography indicates opacification of the talonavicular space and anterior talocalcaneal space (arrows) but absence of contrast material in the area of the middle facets (arrowhead). Incidentally noted is extravasation of the contrast agent into the dorsal soft tissue. **B** Bone scintigraphy shows accumulation of the radionuclide about the anterior and posterior subtalar joints (arrows). **C** A direct coronal computed tomographic scan shows a fibrous or cartilaginous coalition (arrowhead) in the area of the middle facets. The normal interosseous space in this region is narrowed with adjacent bone sclerosis.

coalition, contrast medium introduced into the talonavicular space will fail to flow beneath the anterior aspect of the talus and over the sustentaculum tali (Fig. 76–18).

A number of secondary radiographic signs have been described in association with talocalcaneal coalition.

1. Talar beaking. Dorsal subluxation of the navicular bone leads to elevation of the periosteum below the talonavicular ligament and the production of a beak at the dorsal surface of the talar head adjacent to the talonavicular space (Fig. 76–19). This beak should be differentiated from a normal talar ridge on the dorsum of the bone; a similar beak may be identified in diffuse idiopathic skeletal hyperostosis and acromegaly.

2. Broadening of the lateral process of the talus. Broadening of this process (Fig. 76–17) is present in 40 to 60 per cent of patients and may occur in the absence of a talar beak.

3. Narrowing of the posterior subtalar joint. This finding can be evident in as many as 50 to 60 per cent of patients.

4. Concave undersurface of the talar neck and asymmetry of the talocalcaneonavicular joint.

5. Failure of visualization of the "middle" subtalar joint.

6. Ball-and-socket ankle joint. A rounded appearance of the proximal talar articular surface and a concomitant concave appearance of the distal portion of the tibia may accompany talocalcaneal coalition, presumably owing to an adaptation of the ankle joint to provide the inversion and eversion function that is restricted at the talocalcaneal joints (Fig. 76–20).

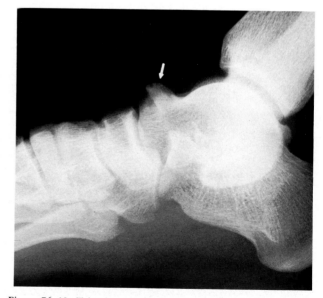

Figure 76–19. Talocalcaneal tarsal coalition: Talar beak. In a patient with a talocalcaneal coalition involving the middle facets, observe a large osseous excrescence (arrow) on the dorsal surface of the talus. (Reprinted from Sartoris DJ, Resnick D: Tarsal coalition. Arthritis Rheum 28:331, 1985. Copyright 1985. Used by permission of the American Rheumatism Association.)

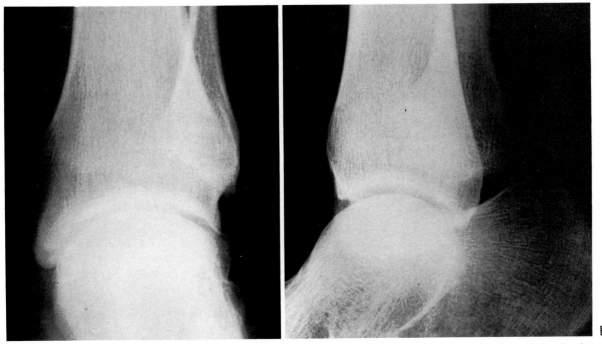

Figure 76–20. Tarsal coalition with ball-and-socket ankle joint (congenital coalition). Talocalcaneal coalition is associated with a ball-and-socket ankle joint and with a shortened fibula. (Courtesy of F. Brahme, M.D., San Diego, California.)

Although direct visualization of the bone bridge or identification of one or more of these secondary signs ensures accurate radiographic diagnosis of talocalcaneal coalition in many instances, the importance of bone scintigraphy as a screening examination and of computed tomography as a definitive examination should be understood. Abnormal uptake of the bone-seeking radionuclide occurs about the subtalar joints and in the dorsum of the foot; with regard to computed tomography, a coronal scanning plane appears to be best, and the technique allows assessment of both feet at the same time (Fig. 76–18).

TALONAVICULAR COALITION. This is an uncommon type of coalition. Patients may be asymptomatic or may have peroneal spasm. Radiography usually outlines the osseous bridge.

Rib Anomalies

Accessory *cervical ribs* may develop in a unilateral or bilateral distribution at the level of the seventh and, rarely, the sixth cervical vertebrae. The scalenus anticus syndrome is a recognized complication of this anomaly.

Intrathoracic ribs usually are supernumerary and are extremely rare (Fig. 76–21). These ribs are unilateral and are more common on the right side. Although they generally are asymptomatic, intrathoracic ribs may have a fibrous diaphragmatic attachment, which can restrict ventilation.

Pelvic ribs are also rare, being asymptomatic and discovered on radiographic examinations performed for incidental reasons. These ribs may arise as single or multiple radiodense areas, adjacent to the upper portion of the lumbar spine, ilium, acetabulum, sacrum, or coccyx.

Synostosis involving ribs may occur either as an isolated phenomenon, usually affecting the first and second ribs, or in association with abnormalities of spinal segmentation or the basal cell nevus syndrome (Gorlin's syndrome).

Klippel-Feil Syndrome

The term Klippel-Feil deformity was originally applied to a triad of signs: a short neck, a low posterior hairline, and a limitation of movement of the neck. As currently used, the designation of the Klippel-Feil syndrome indicates a congen-

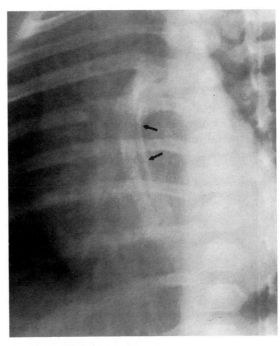

Figure 76–21. Intrathoracic rib. The supernumerary rib (arrows) arises from the posteroinferior margin of another rib and is projected over the inner portion of the lung field in this frontal radiographic projection. (Courtesy of S. Hilton, M.D., San Diego, California.

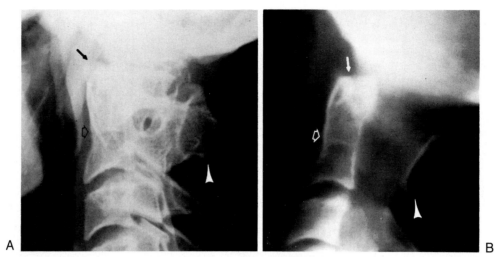

Figure 76–22. Klippel-Feil syndrome. Lateral radiography (**A**) and conventional tomography (**B**) indicate osseous fusion of cervical vertebrae. Note the incorporation of the odontoid process into the anterior arch of the atlas (solid arrows), the narrowed "waist" of the fused vertebral bodies (open arrows), and ankylosis of the posterior elements, including the spinous processes (arrowheads).

ital fusion of two or more cervical vertebrae; the classic triad is not apparent in more than 50 per cent of patients.

Congenital cervical vertebral fusion is equally frequent in men and women. The level and extent of cervical involvement are not constant. In most cases, fusion begins at the occiput and the first cervical vertebra, at the first and second cervical vertebrae, or at the second and third cervical vertebrae (Fig. 76–22). The joints of the second and third and of the fifth and sixth cervical vertebrae are altered most frequently. Occasionally, cases involve upper thoracic vertebrae as well.

Patients with a Klippel-Feil deformity usually do not reveal evidence of a familial history of disease. On clinical examination, the patient has a short neck with restricted neck motion and, possibly, torticollis. Neurologic abnormalities may include spasticity, hyperreflexia, pain, muscle atrophy, oculomotor disturbances, pyramidal tract findings, paralysis, anesthesia, and paresthesia.

Many associated malformations have been described.

1. Sprengel's deformity. Unilateral or bilateral elevation of the scapula is present in approximately 25 per cent of cases (Fig. 76–23). An omovertebral bone connecting the scapula and vertebrae is present in approximately 30 per cent of cases of fixed elevated scapula. It may consist of osseous, cartilaginous, or fibrous tissue.

2. Cervical ribs. Anomalous ribs are evident in approximately 10 per cent of cases.

3. Webbed neck (pterygium colli). Webbing of the soft tissues on each side may involve the skin, muscles, and fascia.

4. Hemivertebrae. A hemivertebra is present in approximately 15 per cent of cases.

5. Spina bifida. Anterior or posterior spina bifida is frequent in patients with cervical fusions.

6. Other anomalies. Kyphosis, scoliosis, spinal stenosis, fused, absent, or deformed ribs, basilar impression, cranial asymmetry, deformed dens, cleft palate, supernumerary lobes of the lung, patent foramen ovale, interventricular septal defect, renal anomalies, and enteric cysts represent some of the additional malformations that may be apparent.

On radiographs, the fusion may affect the vertebral bodies, the pedicles, the laminae, or the spinous processes (Fig. 76–22). With fusion of the vertebral bodies, small atrophic intervertebral discs may be apparent, which can contain calcification. The anteroposterior diameter of the vertebral bodies at the level of an affected discovertebral junction may

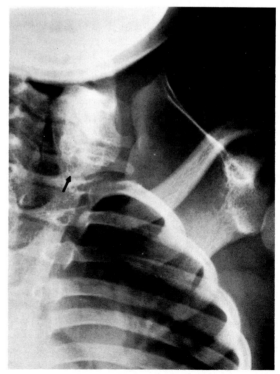

Figure 76–23. Klippel-Feil syndrome with Sprengel's deformity. Note the elevated position of the scapula, an omovertebral bone (arrow), and cervical spinal abnormalities.

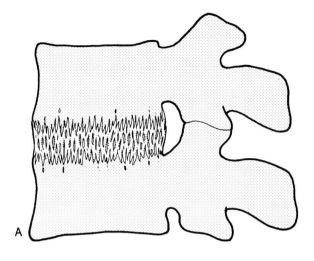

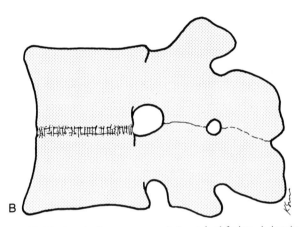

Figure 76–24. Acquired versus congenital vertebral fusion. A Acquired ankylosis. Note the absence of posterior element fusion. B Congenital ankylosis. A constricted appearance at the level of the intervertebral disc has produced a trapezoidal shape of the bone mass. The posterior elements are also ankylosed, and the intervertebral disc is atrophic.

be smaller than that at the superior and inferior limits of the vertebrae adjacent to uninvolved discs. The resulting trapezoidal shape of the vertebral body is very suggestive of a congenital fusion or at least one that has occurred at an early age, as it is related to the interference with normal growth at the site of fusion.

The radiographic features of a congenital fusion of cervical vertebral bodies must be distinguished from those in acquired cases of ankylosis (Fig. 76–24). Application of the guidelines illustrated in Figure 76–24 may allow differentiation of congenital fusion from other processes, particularly juvenile chronic arthritis. Furthermore, in this articular disease, abnormalities of other skeletal sites are apparent, and an elevated position of the scapula is not seen. In ankylosing spondylitis, ankylosis of vertebral bodies and apophyseal joints is noted, but the vertebrae and intervertebral discs are not diminutive in size.

Congenital Block Vertebrae

Congenital synostosis of vertebrae in the thoracic and lumbar spine also may be encountered (Fig. 76–25). The anomaly usually is limited in extent, affecting two adjacent vertebrae, and commonly is asymptomatic. The fusion typically affects the vertebral bodies, although the posterior elements can also be incorporated into an ossified mass. The intervening intervertebral disc is atrophic and calcified.

ARTICULAR ABNORMALITIES
Madelung's Deformity

Madelung's deformity represents a bowing of the distal end of the radius. Typically, the radial bowing occurs in a volar direction while the ulna continues to grow in a straight fashion. Thus, the ulna is relatively long in comparison to the radius, and the carpal angle, formed by the intersection of two lines (the first tangent to the proximal surfaces of the scaphoid and the lunate bones, the second tangent to the proximal margins of the triquetrum and the lunate bones), which normally is 130 to 137 degrees, is decreased (Table 76–2). Specific radiographic alterations in Madelung's deformity (Fig. 76–26) include the following.

1. Radial abnormalities. Dorsal and ulnar curvature, decreased length, triangularization of the distal radial epiphysis with unequal growth of the epiphysis, premature fusion of the medial half of the radial epiphysis, a localized area of

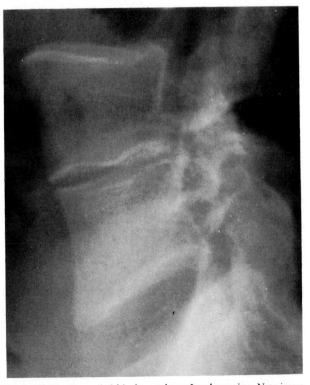

Figure 76–25. Congenital block vertebrae: Lumbar spine. Note incomplete fusion between the fourth and fifth lumbar vertebral bodies. The intervertebral disc is atrophic and the anteroposterior width of the vertebral bodies at the site of fusion is less than at the uninvolved portions of the bodies, creating a trapezoidal vertebral shape.

**Table 76–2. SYNDROMES ASSOCIATED WITH ABNORMALITY
OF THE CARPAL ANGLE**

Decreased	Increased
Madelung's deformity	Arthrogryposis
Dyschondrosteosis	Diastrophic dwarfism
Turner's syndrome	Epiphyseal dysplasias
Morquio's syndrome	Frontometaphyseal dysplasia
Hurler's syndrome	Otopalatodigital syndrome
	Pfeiffer's syndrome
	Spondyloepiphyseal dysplasia
	Trisomy 21

From Poznanski AK: The Hand in Radiologic Diagnosis. Philadelphia, WB Saunders Co, 1974, p 140. Used with permission.

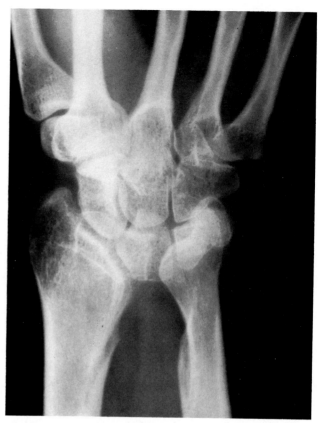

lucency along the ulnar border of the radius, osteophytosis along the inferior ulnar portion of the radius, and ulnar and volar angulation of the distal radial articular surface have been reported.

2. Ulnar abnormalities. Dorsal subluxation, enlargement and distortion of the ulnar head, and changes in length have been observed.

3. Carpal abnormalities. Wedging of the carpus between the deformed radius and protruding ulna, triangular configuration with the lunate at the apex, and arched curvature in the lateral projection as a direct continuation of the arch of posterior bowing of the radial epiphysis have occurred.

There has been much confusion regarding the cause of this deformity. Furthermore, a mesomelic variety of dwarfism known as dyschondrosteosis is accompanied by similar radiographic abnormalities of the wrist, although the lower legs also are short in this syndrome. The isolated variety of Madelung's deformity is more commonly bilateral than unilateral, is asymmetric, and is at least three to five times more common in female patients. Clinical manifestations usually become evident in the adolescent or young adult, in whom

Figure 76–26. Madelung's deformity. Abnormalities include increased width between the distal portions of the radius and ulna, a relatively long ulna compared to the length of the radius, a decreased carpal angle, triangularization of the distal radial epiphysis, osseous excrescences on apposing metaphyseal regions of radius and ulna, distortion of the ulnar head, and wedging of the carpus between the deformed radius and protruding ulna, with the lunate at the apex of the wedge.

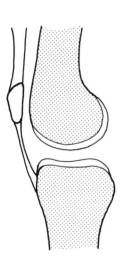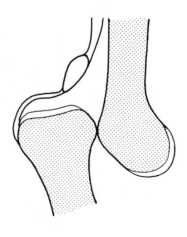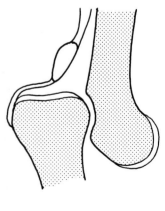

Figure 76–27. Congenital subluxation and hyperextension of the knee. Variable patterns can be encountered. Mild subluxation or frank dislocation with anterior femoral erosion may be seen.

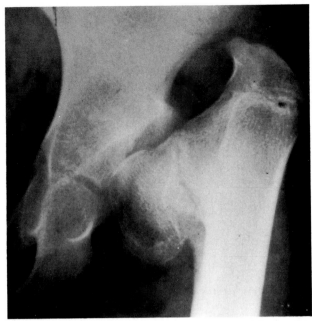

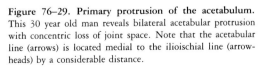

Figure 76–28. Infantile coxa vara. Note the severe varus deformity of the proximal portion of the femur, the vertically located and irregular growth plate, thickening of the medial cortex of the femoral neck, a prominent greater trochanter, and acetabular flattening.

visible deformity, pain, fatigue, and limited range of motion are noted. After several years of progressive symptoms and signs, the findings may become stationary.

Congenital Subluxation and Hyperextension of the Knee

Congenital subluxation and hyperextension of the knee is a rare congenital deformity in which the tibia and femur are abnormally related. There is a definite female preponderance. Hereditary factors appear to be important in some cases, and associated congenital deformities include dislocation of the hip, foot abnormalities, and dislocation of the elbow. The severity of the deformity is variable (Fig. 76–27). Hyperex-

tension can occur without tibial malposition, tibial subluxation or dislocation can appear without hyperextension, or both hyperextension and subluxation or dislocation may occur together.

This condition should be distinguished from genu recurvatum due to ligament laxity, acquired quadriceps contracture, and traumatic changes.

Congenital Dislocation of the Radial Head

Although it is a rare condition, congenital dislocation of the radial head represents the most common anomaly of the elbow region. It may occur as an isolated phenomenon or in association with other congenital abnormalities. A familial history of the anomaly may be evident. Clinical findings usually appear in infancy. Radiographic abnormalities include a relatively short ulna or long radius, hypoplasia or aplasia of the capitulum, a partially defective trochlea, prominence of the ulnar epicondyle, a dome-shaped radial head with an elongated radial neck, and grooving of the distal portion of the humerus. Unilateral or bilateral involvement is seen, and progressive subluxation or dislocation of the radial head usually proceeds in a posterior direction. Diagnostic difficulty is encountered in the differentiation of congenital versus traumatic dislocation of the radial head.

Infantile Coxa Vara

Normally, the angle of intersection of the axis of the femoral neck and that of the femoral shaft varies with age but is approximately 150 degrees at birth and 120 to 130 degrees in the adult. The term coxa vara indicates a neck-shaft angle that is less than 120 degrees. Coxa vara may accompany various processes, including proximal femoral focal deficiency, osteogenesis imperfecta, renal osteodystrophy, rickets, and fibrous dysplasia. Infantile or developmental coxa vara is a designation of a proximal femoral deformity that usually becomes apparent in the first few years of life. Boys and girls are affected with approximately equal frequency, and the condition is unilateral in 60 to 75 per cent of cases. Clinically, the affected child has an abnormal gait.

Radiographs reveal a decrease in the femoral shaft-neck angle and a medially located triangular piece of bone in the

Figure 76–29. Primary protrusion of the acetabulum. This 30 year old man reveals bilateral acetabular protrusion with concentric loss of joint space. Note that the acetabular line (arrows) is located medial to the ilioischial line (arrowheads) by a considerable distance.

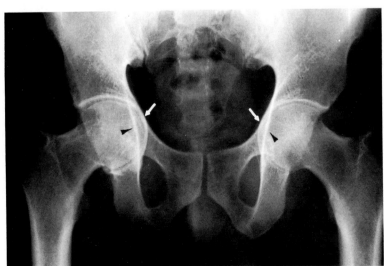

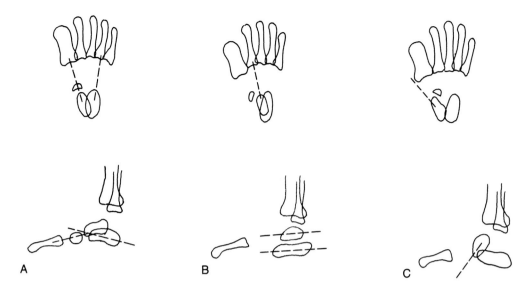

Figure 76–30. Foot: Normal and abnormal hindfoot and forefoot relationship. A Normal. On an anteroposterior radiograph, the talar axis intersects or points slightly medial to the first metatarsal bone, and the navicular bone is situated directly opposite the head of the talus. The calcaneus points toward the fourth metatarsal bone, creating a talocalcaneal angle of approximately 35 degrees in the adult and somewhat greater in the infant. On a lateral radiograph, the anterior portion of the talus is mildly flexed in a plantar direction, and the calcaneus is slightly dorsiflexed. An extended line through the longitudinal axis of the talus is directed along the axis of the first metatarsal bone. The talocalcaneal angle is approximately 35 degrees. **B Hindfoot varus deformity.** The anteroposterior radiograph reveals a decrease in the talocalcaneal angle as the two bones lie closely together and more parallel to each other. The navicular bone is displaced medially, and the talar axis points lateral to the first metatarsal base. In the lateral projection, the talus and the calcaneus are both more horizontal and parallel with each other. **C Hindfoot valgus deformity.** On the anteroposterior radiograph, the talocalcaneal angle is increased, with the navicular bone and remaining tarsal bones being located lateral to the talus. The talar axial line passes medial to the first metatarsal bone. On the lateral radiograph, the talus is oriented more vertically, and the long axis of the talus and that of the first metatarsal bone angulate in a plantar direction. (After Ozonoff MB: Pediatric Orthopedic Radiology. Philadelphia, WB Saunders Co, 1979. Used with permission.)

neck adjacent to the head that is bounded by two radiolucent bands traversing the neck and forming an inverted V. The growth plate itself is widened, and is vertical in alignment. With further growth, the varus deformity frequently progresses (Fig. 76–28).

The precise cause of this condition has not been delineated.

Primary Protrusion of the Acetabulum

Acetabular protrusion (protrusio acetabuli) refers to intrapelvic displacement of the medial wall of the acetabulum. It may be evident in many disorders, including rheumatoid arthritis, ankylosing spondylitis, septic arthritis, degenerative joint disease, osteomalacia, Paget's disease, neoplasm, and trauma, and as an effect of irradiation. Protrusio acetabuli can also appear in the absence of any recognizable cause, and, in such a case, it is termed primary acetabular protrusion. The primary variety is sometimes referred to as Otto pelvis.

The cause of primary acetabular protrusion is unknown. It usually affects both hips and is much more frequent in women. With progressive protrusion deformity, the femoral head assumes an intrapelvic location, and the joint space may be normal, narrowed, or obliterated.

Acetabular deformity in mild cases of primary protrusion must be distinguished from normal variations in acetabular depth. An abnormal situation exists in the adult pelvis when the distance between the medially located acetabular line and the laterally located ilioischial line is 6 mm or more in women and 3 mm or more in men (Fig. 76–29).

Foot Deformities

A brief summary of the major foot deformities is included here. Proper radiographic analysis requires both anteroposterior and lateral projections exposed during weight-bearing. The normal alignment of the foot is inferred from the information obtained on anteroposterior and lateral radiographs using, in large part, the relationship of the talus and the calcaneus (Figs. 76–30 and 76–31).

In *hindfoot (heel) valgus* (Fig. 76–30), an anteroposterior projection reveals an increase in the talocalcaneal angle. An extended line through the longitudinal axis of the talus will fall medial to the first metatarsal, and the navicular and other tarsal bones will be displaced laterally to the talus. On the lateral projection, the talus will be tilted more vertically than normal owing to the abduction of the calcaneus. The long axis of the talus and that of the first metatarsal will angulate in a plantar direction. In *hindfoot (heel) varus* (Fig. 76–30), on anteroposterior views, the long axis of the talus falls lateral to the base of the first metatarsal owing to the adduction of the anterior end of the calcaneus. The talocalcaneal angle is decreased. The navicular bone is displaced medially. On the lateral view, the calcaneus and talus are both more horizontal and parallel with each other. Hindfoot or heel valgus is present in flatfoot, metatarsus varus, congenital vertical talus, and certain congenital and neurologic deformities of the foot. Hindfoot or heel varus commonly is visible in talipes equinovarus and some paralytic deformities.

In *hindfoot equinus*, in the lateral projection, the calcaneus

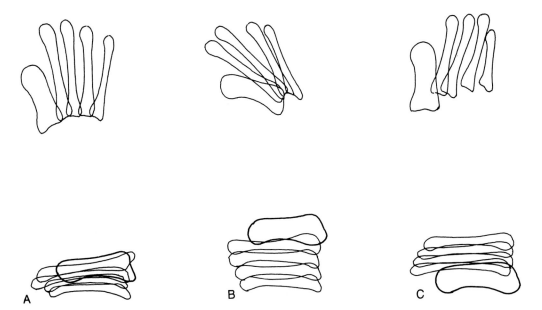

Figure 76–31. Foot: Normal and abnormal forefoot alignment. A Normal. On the anteroposterior radiograph, the metatarsal bones converge proximally with overlapping at their bases. On the lateral projection, the fifth metatarsal bone is in the most plantar position, with the other metatarsals being superimposed. **B** Forefoot varus deformity. On the frontal radiograph, the forefoot is narrowed, with increased convergence at the metatarsal bases, resulting in more overlap than normal. On the lateral radiograph, a ladder-like arrangement is seen, with the first metatarsal bone being most dorsal. **C** Forefoot valgus deformity. The forefoot is broadened, with the metatarsal bones being more prominent than normal and with decreased overlap at the metatarsal bases. In the lateral projection, a ladder-like arrangement can be noted in some cases, with the first metatarsal bone being in the most plantar position. (After Ozonoff MB: Pediatric Orthopedic Radiology. Philadelphia, WB Saunders Co, 1979. Used with permission.)

is flexed in a plantar direction so that the angle between the axes of the calcaneus and the tibia is greater than 90 degrees. This deformity accompanies talipes equinovarus and congenital vertical talus. In *calcaneal hindfoot deformity*, in the lateral projection, the calcaneus is abnormally dorsiflexed so that its anterior end has a more superior position, and the bone possesses a box-like appearance. Calcaneal positions (fixed dorsiflexion) of the calcaneus appear in association with cavus deformities of the foot.

The term *clubfoot* represents a condition associated with equinovarus foot deformity and hindfoot varus (Fig. 76–32). The clubfoot deformity is relatively common, occurs more frequently in male children, and can be unilateral or bilateral in distribution. Its exact cause is not clear. The accurate diagnosis of the clubfoot deformity relies on routine radiography, which may be supplemented with arthrography, conventional or computed tomography, and arteriography, and the diagnosis can be accomplished prenatally with ultrasonography.

After inadequate treatment of the clubfoot, certain deformities may remain. These include the rocker-bottom deformity, which is due to correction of the foot dorsiflexion before the equinus, and the flattop talus, which is due to flattening of the superior surface of the plantar flexed talus that is articulating with the tibia.

A *congenital vertical talus* (congenital flatfoot with talonavicular dislocation) can occur as an isolated condition or as part of a generalized malformation syndrome. The condition occurs with approximately equal frequency in boys and girls and in a unilateral or bilateral distribution. It frequently is associated with arthrogryposis or meningomyelocele. On the anteroposterior radiograph, severe heel valgus and forefoot abduction result in an increased talocalcaneal angle with the talar axis lying medial to the first metatarsal. On the lateral radiograph, an equinus heel with plantar flexion of both the calcaneus and the talus is evident (Fig. 76–33). The forefoot is dorsiflexed at the midtarsal level, resulting in a convex plantar surface of the foot, the rocker-bottom deformity. The navicular bone is dislocated dorsally, locking the talus into its plantar flexed position.

The *cavus foot deformity* is a frequent accompaniment of neurologic or muscular disorders, such as peroneal muscular atrophy, poliomyelitis, and meningomyelocele (Fig. 76–34).

The *flexible flatfoot deformity* is associated, on the anteroposterior view, with an increase in the talocalcaneal angle, heel valgus, and forefoot abduction. The midtarsal transverse arch is flattened, and the metatarsals are approximately parallel in their orientation. On the lateral projection, hindfoot valgus is again noted, with the talus in a more vertical attitude than normal. The calcaneus and the metatarsals are aligned horizontally, and the plantar arch is flattened. Although the resulting radiographic picture may superficially resemble that seen in congenital vertical talus, the flexible flatfoot deformity is not associated with equinus, and the navicular bone retains its normal position with regard to the distal surface of the talus.

Metatarsus adductus and metatarsus varus is a common deformity of unknown cause (Fig. 76–35).

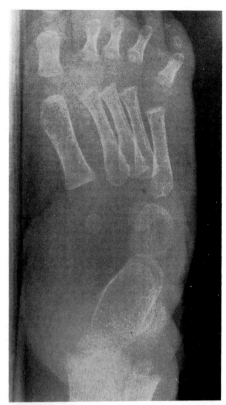

A

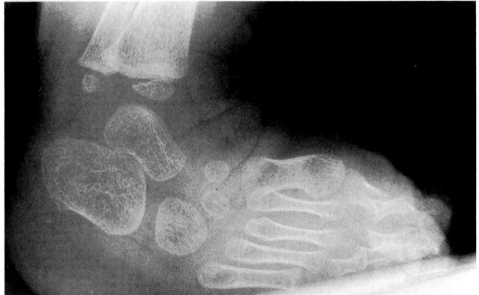

B

Figure 76–32. Clubfoot (equinovarus) deformity. A Anteroposterior projection. The hindfoot is in marked varus position, with superimposition of the talar and calcaneal centers. A line drawn through the talus will pass far laterally to the first metatarsal bone. The navicular is not ossified, but its abnormal position can be inferred from the location of the first metatarsal base and the first cuneiform center. The forefoot is narrowed, with increased overlap of the metatarsal bases. **B** Lateral projection. The talus and the calcaneus are more parallel than normal. The calcaneus is in equinus position, abnormally flexed in a plantar direction. Forefoot inversion with a ladder-like arrangement of the metatarsal bones is apparent. (From Ozonoff MB: Pediatric Orthopedic Radiology. Philadelphia, WB Saunders Co, 1979. Used with permission.)

MISCELLANEOUS SYNDROMES AND CONDITIONS

Osteoonychodysostosis

Osteoonychodysostosis, an autosomal dominant disorder, is also referred to as the nail-patella syndrome, hereditary osteoonychodysplasia (HOOD), and Fong's syndrome. It is characterized by dysplastic fingernails, hypoplastic or absent patellae, additional bone deformities, iliac horns, widespread soft tissue changes, and renal dysplasia. Renal osteodystrophy

and death can result from the kidney disease. Clinical manifestations are seen most frequently in the second and third decades of life. Hypoplasia of fingernails, palpable absence of the patellae, presence of iliac protuberances, increased carrying angle of the elbow, abnormal pigmentation of the iris, and proteinuria may be recognized on initial clinical examination.

In infancy, the demonstration of posterior iliac horns allows identification of this dysplasia. In the knee, absence or hypoplasia of the patella, asymmetric development of the

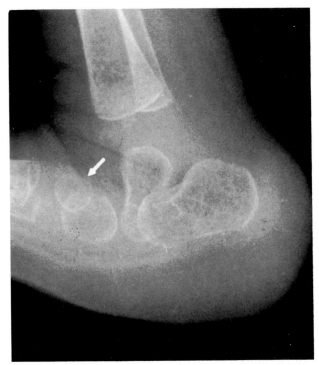

Figure 76–33. **Congenital vertical talus.** The talar axis is markedly vertical in orientation, and the calcaneus is in equinus position, producing an inferior convexity to the plantar surface of the foot. The navicular is unossified, but, because of the position of the ossified third cuneiform (arrow), it should be displaced dorsally, occupying the space between the cuneiform and the talus.

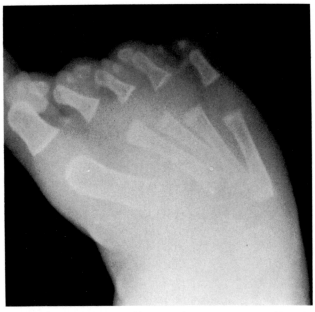

Figure 76–35. **Metatarsus adductus and metatarsus varus.** Note the adducted varus position of the forefoot, with a concave medial border and convex lateral border.

consist of dysplasia of the iliac wings and the presence of iliac horns (Fig. 76–37). Bilateral outgrowths from the posterior ilium are virtually pathognomonic of osteoonychodysostosis.

Additional bone changes can be evident in the shoulder, wrist, ankle, and subtalar joints.

femoral condyles, and a sloping tibial plateau with a prominent tibial tubercle are identified (Fig. 76–36). In the elbow, asymmetric development of the humeral condyles, hypoplasia of the capitulum, and subluxation or dislocation of the radial head are the major changes. Abnormalities of the pelvis

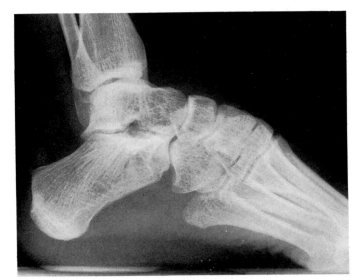

Figure 76–34. **Cavus foot.** After poliomyelitis, this 18 year old girl reveals an increased plantar arch with a calcaneus position of the os calcis and increased plantar flexion of the forefoot. (From Ozonoff MB: Pediatric Orthopedic Radiology. Philadelphia, WB Saunders Co, 1979. Used with permission.)

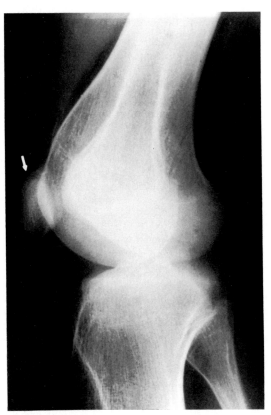

Figure 76–36. **Osteoonychodysostosis: Knee abnormalities.** Observe the hypoplastic patella (arrow). (Courtesy of A. Goldman, M. D., New York, New York.)

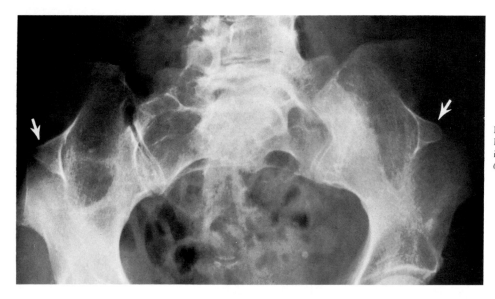

Figure 76–37. Osteoonychodysostosis: Pelvic abnormalities. Bilateral posterior iliac outgrowths or horns can be identified (arrows).

Progeria

Clinical manifestations of progeria become evident within the first few years of life. Dwarfism, alopecia, brown pigmentation of the trunk, atrophic skin, loss of subcutaneous fat, impaired extension at the hips and knees, a receding chin, a beaked nose, and exophthalmos are seen. Radiographic findings include hypoplastic facial bones and mandible, delay of cranial sutural closure, and coxa valga. Acroosteolysis of the terminal phalanges of the hands and feet and of the clavicles is a distinctive finding.

Arthrogryposis Multiplex Congenita

The term arthrogryposis is derived from two Greek words meaning curved joints, an appropriate name for this disorder. At birth, affected infants display multiple joint contractures. A "diamond deformity" of the lower extremities is typical, with the hips abducted, flexed, and rotated externally and with the knees flexed. Sensation is intact.

Radiographic features include decreased muscle mass and contractures. Equinovarus deformity of the foot, talocalcaneal coalition, clubhand in ulnar deviation, carpal fusion, and dislocation of the hips are frequent. Fractures are not unusual, and scoliosis can be detected in many individuals.

Werner's Syndrome

Werner's syndrome is similar to but distinct from progeria. Its principal clinical manifestations include retardation of growth, graying and loss of the hair, cataracts, skin ulcerations, and, in some cases, mild diabetes mellitus. Additional changes are vascular and soft tissue calcifications, generalized osteoporosis, atrophy of muscle and fat, and hypogonadism. Neoplasms, especially sarcomas and meningiomas, may complicate the clinical picture. The prognosis is guarded, as many patients succumb by the fourth or fifth decade of life to complications of cardiovascular involvement. Genetic studies in Werner's syndrome reveal findings compatible with an autosomal recessive mode of inheritance.

Radiographic evaluation reveals osteoporosis, arterial and cardiac valvular calcifications, and soft tissue calcification. The last finding predominates about the knees, feet, and hands. Soft tissue atrophy also may be apparent. Destructive osseous lesions relate to osteomyelitis and septic arthritis.

Congenital Pseudarthrosis

Congenital pseudarthrosis is an unusual condition associated with fracture followed by a nonunion. It is identified most typically in the tibia, although pseudarthroses may also be seen in the fibula, femur, clavicle, humerus, ulna, rib, and, rarely, other bones. In some patients, pseudarthroses are present at birth (true congenital pseudarthrosis), whereas in other patients, they develop in the first few years of life (infantile pseudarthrosis). Some affected persons may have stigmata of neurofibromatosis or fibrous dysplasia, although others do not. The precise relationships among congenital pseudarthrosis, neurofibromatosis, and fibrous dysplasia remain a mystery.

The more common infantile variety of the tibial lesion usually develops in the first or second year of life. Unilateral changes predominate. Initially, anterior bowing of the lower half of the tibia is recognized. At the apex of the curve, sclerosis, narrowing of the medullary canal, and cystic abnormality may indicate impending fracture and pseudarthrosis. Once the fracture appears, the margins of the adjacent bone ends taper further (Fig. 76–38). The prognosis for ultimate union at the fracture site varies with the age of the patient (fractures developing before 2 years of age carry a poor prognosis) and the pattern of radiographic abnormality (a cystic appearance may be associated with a better prognosis).

Congenital pseudarthrosis of the clavicle occurs almost exclusively on the right side of the body, although it may be bilateral in 10 per cent of cases. Adjacent vascular structures such as the subclavian artery may be important in the pathogenesis of this osseous defect. A familial occurrence of the disorder is noted occasionally. The lesion usually is discovered within the first few months of life owing to the presence of a painless lump over the middle one third of the clavicle. On radiographs, the medial end of the clavicle is seen to be superior to the lateral end, osseous discontinuity is evident, and callus formation is absent. It is the absence of pain and visible callus that usually allows differentiation from a posttraumatic pseudarthrosis.

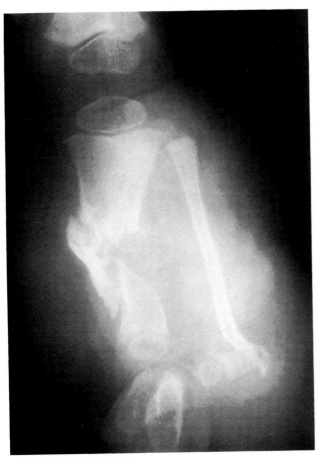

Figure 76–38. Congenital pseudarthrosis. Fractures with pseudarthroses are observed in the middle third of the tibia and the lower third of the fibula. Some of the ends of the fractured bones are tapered. Considerable soft tissue swelling and hypertrophy are evident, although this child had no clinical evidence of neurofibromatosis.

FURTHER READING

Alexander C: The aetiology of primary protrusio acetabuli. Br J Radiol 38:567, 1965.

Barnes JC, Smith WL: The VATER association. Radiology 126:445, 1978.

Beckly DE, Anderson PW, Pedegana LR: The radiology of the subtalar joint with special reference to talo-calcaneal coalition. Clin Radiol 26:333, 1975.

Boyd HB: Pathology and natural history of congenital pseudarthrosis of the tibia. Clin Orthop 166:5, 1982.

Brower AC, Culver JE Jr, Keats TE: Histologic nature of the cortical irregularity of the medial posterior distal femoral metaphysis in children. Radiology 99:389, 1971.

Brown GA, Osebold WR, Ponseti IV: Congenital pseudarthrosis of long bones. A clinical, radiographic, histologic, and ultrastructural study. Clin Orthop 128:228, 1977.

Caffey JP: Pediatric X-ray Diagnosis. 7th ed. Chicago, Year Book Medical Publishers, 1978.

Calhoun JD, Pierret G: Infantile coxa vara. AJR 115:561, 1972.

Carlson DH, O'Connor J: Congenital dislocation of the knee. AJR 127:465, 1976.

Conway JJ, Cowell HR: Tarsal coalition: Clinical significance and roentgenographic demonstration. Radiology 92:799, 1969.

Conway WF, Destouet JM, Gilula LA, Bellinghausen HW, Weeks PM: The carpal boss: An overview of radiographic evaluation. Radiology 156:29, 1985.

Cope JR: Carpal coalition. Clin Radiol 25:261, 1974.

Deutsch AL, Resnick D, Campbell G: Computed tomography and bone scintigraphy in the evaluation of tarsal coalition. Radiology 144:137, 1982.

Felman AH, Kirkpatrick JA Jr: Madelung's deformity: Observations in 17 patients. Radiology 93:1037, 1969.

Freiberger RH, Hersh A, Harrison MO: Roentgen examination of the deformed foot. Semin Roentgenol 5:341, 1970.

Goldman AB, Schneider R, Wilson PD Jr: Proximal focal femoral deficiency. J Can Assoc Radiol 29:101, 1978.

Greenspan A, Norman A: The "pelvic digit"—an unusual developmental anomaly. Skel Radiol 9:118, 1982.

Greenspan A, Norman A: The pelvic digit. Bull Hosp J Dis 44:72, 1984.

Hall JG, Levin J, Kuhn JP, Ottenheimer EJ, Van Berkum KAP, McKusick VA: Thrombocytopenia with absent radius (TAR). Medicine 48:411, 1969.

Hensinger RN, Lang JE, MacEwen GD: Klippel-Feil syndrome. A constellation of associated anomalies. J Bone Joint Surg [Am] 56:1246, 1974.

Hotston S, Carty H: Lumbosacral agenesis: A report of three new cases and review of the literature. Br J Radiol 55:629, 1982.

Jacobsen ST, Crawford AH: Congenital vertical talus. J Pediatr Orthop 3:306, 1983.

Jacobson HG, Rifkin H, Zucker-Franklin D: Werner's syndrome: A clinical-roentgen entity. Radiology 74:373, 1960.

Kelleher J, O'Connell DJ, MacMahon H: Intrathoracic rib: Radiographic features of two cases. Br J Radiol 52:181, 1979.

Lawson JP: Symptomatic radiographic variants in extremities. Radiology 157:625, 1985.

Lawson JP, Ogden JA, Sella E, Barwick KW: The painful accessory navicular. Skel Radiol 12:250, 1984.

Manashil G, Laufer S: Congenital pseudarthrosis of the clavicle: Report of three cases. AJR 132:678, 1979.

Margolin FR, Steinbach HL: Progeria. Hutchinson-Gilford syndrome. AJR 103:173, 1968.

McKusick VA: Heritable Disorders of Connective Tissue. St Louis, CV Mosby Co, 1972.

Miller JH, Bernstein SM: The roentgenographic appearance of the "corrected clubfoot." Foot Ankle 6:177, 1986.

Mital MA: Limb deficiencies: Classification and treatment. Orthop Clin North Am 7:457, 1976.

Ogden JA, McCarthy SM, Jokl P: The painful bipartite patella. J Pediatr Orthop 2:263, 1982.

Ogden JA, Conlogue GJ, Phillips SB, Bronson ML: Sprengel's deformity. Radiology of the pathologic deformation. Skel Radiol 4:204, 1979.

Ozonoff MB: Pediatric Orthopedic Radiology. Philadelphia, WB Saunders Co, 1979.

Ozonoff MB, Clemett AR: Progressive osteolysis in progeria. AJR 100:75, 1967.

Pate D, Kursunoglu S, Resnick D, Resnik CS: Scapular foramina. Skel Radiol 14:270, 1985.

Pavlov H, Goldman AB, Freiberger RH: Infantile coxa vara. Radiology 135:631, 1980.

Percy EC, Mann DL: Tarsal coalition: A review of the literature and presentation of 13 cases. Foot Ankle 9:40, 1988.

Poznanski AK: The Hand in Radiologic Diagnosis. Philadelphia, WB Saunders Co, 1974.

Poznanski AK, LaRowe PC: Radiographic manifestations of arthrogryposis syndrome. Radiology 95:353, 1970.

Preger L, Miller EH, Winfield JS, Choy SH: Hereditary onycho-osteo-arthrodysplasia. AJR 100:546, 1967.

Renshaw TS: Sacral agenesis: A classification and review of twenty-three cases. J Bone Joint Surg [Am] 60:373, 1978.

Resnick D, Cone RO III: The nature of humeral pseudocysts. Radiology 150:27, 1984.

Resnick D, Greenway G: Distal femoral cortical defects, irregularities, and excavations. A critical review of the literature with the addition of histologic and paleopathologic data. Radiology 143:345, 1982.

Resnick D, Walter RD, Crudale AS: Bilateral dysplasia of the scapular neck. AJR 139:387, 1982.

Resnik CS, Grizzard JD, Simmons BP, Yaghmai I: Incomplete carpal coalition. AJR 147:301, 1986.

Ritchie GW, Keim HA: A radiographic analysis of major foot deformities. Can Med Assoc J 91:840, 1964.

Rubin P: Dynamic Classification of Bone Dysplasias. Chicago, Year Book Medical Publishers, 1964.

Spranger JW, Langer LO Jr, Wiedemann HR: Bone Dysplasias. An Atlas of Constitutional Disorders of Skeletal Development. Philadelphia, WB Saunders Co, 1974.

Williams HJ, Hoyer JR: Radiographic diagnosis of osteo-onychodysostosis in infancy. Radiology 109:151, 1973.

TUMORS AND TUMOR-LIKE DISEASES

CASE XIV

LEVEL OF DIFFICULTY: 2

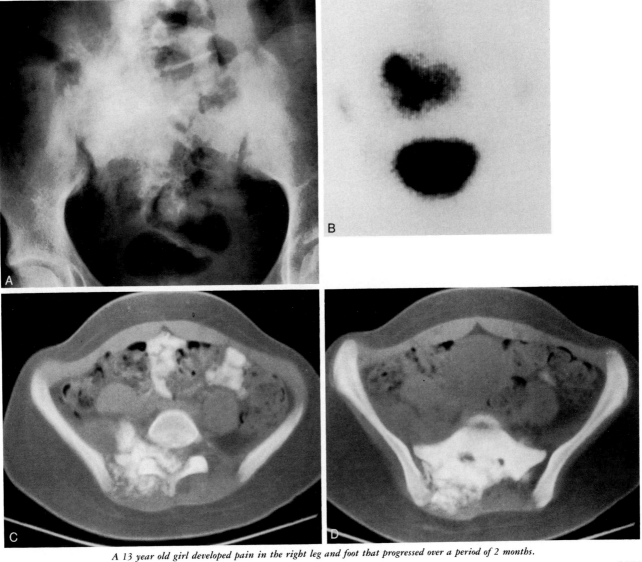

A 13 year old girl developed pain in the right leg and foot that progressed over a period of 2 months.

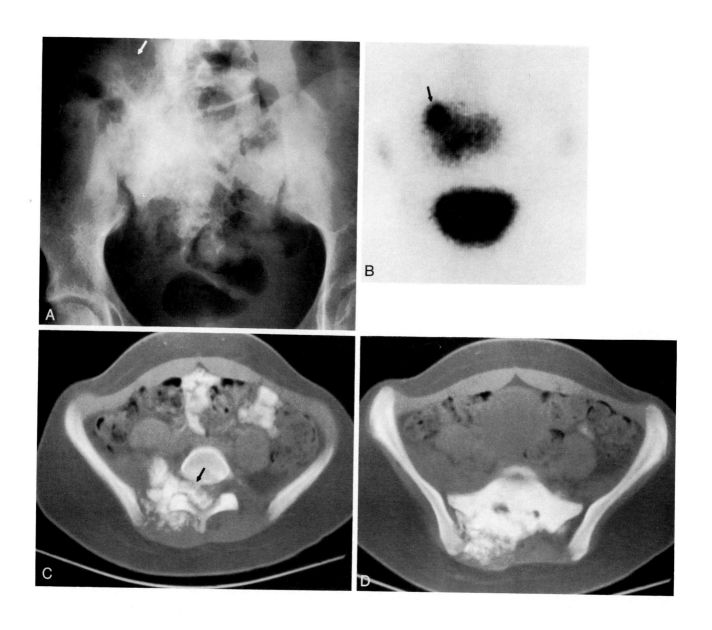

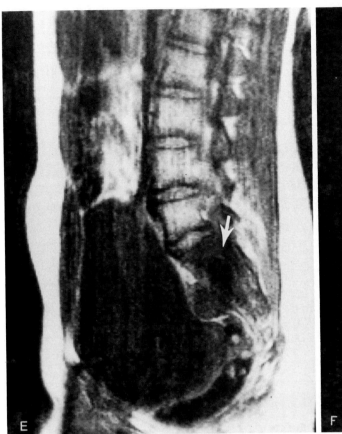

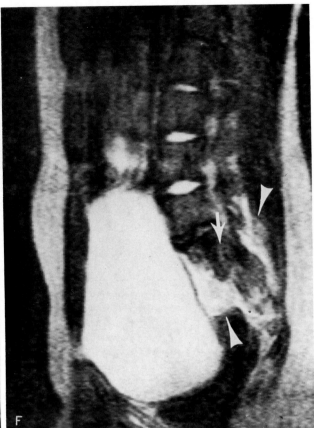

A frontal radiograph of the pelvis (A) reveals a predominantly osteosclerotic lesion involving the right side of the sacrum. A soft tissue mass is evident, especially adjacent to the right side of the fifth lumbar vertebra, and calcification or ossification is present within this mass (arrow). Scintigraphy with a bone-seeking radiopharmaceutical agent (B) shows intense accumulation of the isotope within the lesion (arrow). Myelography (not shown) documented a complete extradural block to the flow of contrast material at the level of the superior margin of the fifth lumbar vertebra. Transaxial computed tomograms (C,D) reveal the osteosclerotic lesion, which is extending into the retroperitoneum, the gluteal muscles, and the spinal canal (arrow). The ilium appears not to be involved. T1 weighted (E) and T2 weighted (F) sagittal magnetic resonance images demonstrate that the sacral portion of the lesion (arrows) has low signal intensity in both imaging sequences. On the T2 weighted sequence, however, the soft tissue component has increased signal intensity (arrowheads).

The imaging features are those of an aggressive tumor; the findings are not those of infection. Although Ewing's sarcoma would be considered a likely choice on the basis solely of the age of the patient and the location of the neoplasm, the imaging abnormalities are not characteristic of Ewing's sarcoma. Osteosclerosis is evident in approximately 40 per cent of patients with this tumor, but soft tissue calcification or ossification is apparent in fewer than 10 per cent of such patients. In the sacrum, osteolysis, cortical destruction, and a soft tissue mass are most characteristic of Ewing's sarcoma.

Chondrosarcoma is a reasonable diagnostic consideration, as this tumor can involve adjacent soft tissues and lead to extensive intraosseous and extraosseous calcification. Chondrosarcomas are observed most typically in the fourth to sixth decades of life, and children rarely are affected. Spinal or sacral involvement is evident in about 6 per cent of conventional chondrosarcomas.

Osteosarcoma is a common malignant tumor in young patients that classically is associated with bone formation in both the osseous and the extraosseous components of the tumor. Sacral involvement is evident in 2 to 3 per cent of cases. Computed tomography and magnetic resonance imaging are well suited to the evaluation of the extent of these tumors, particularly those that develop in sites of complex anatomy, such as the spine and sacrum. In the test case, computed tomography confirmed the soft tissue and intraspinal spread of tumor. Magnetic resonance imaging also revealed the extent of the neoplasm and indicated differing signal characteristics in various portions of the lesion. The intense osteosclerosis that was apparent in the sacral component of the tumor would explain persistent decreased signal intensity in both T1 and T2 weighted images. The higher signal intensity within the soft tissue portion of the tumor on the T2 weighted sequence indicates nonossified neoplastic tissue.

A needle biopsy of the sacral lesion confirmed the diagnosis of osteosarcoma.

FINAL DIAGNOSIS: Osteosarcoma.

FURTHER READING

Pages 1117 to 1126 and the following:

1. Patel DV, Hammer RA, Levin B, Fisher MA: Primary osteogenic sarcoma of the spine. Skel Radiol 12:276, 1984.
2. Shives TC, Dahlin DC, Sin FH, Pritchard DJ, Earle JD: Osteosarcoma of the spine. J Bone Joint Surg [Am] 68:66, 1986.

(Case XIV, courtesy of G. Greenway, M.D., Dallas, Texas.)

Chapter 77

Tumors and Tumor-Like Lesions of Bone: Radiographic Principles

Donald Resnick, M.D.

Conventional radiographic techniques remain of fundamental importance in the analysis of bone tumors and tumor-like lesions. The morphologic characteristics of the process provide important diagnostic information regarding the aggressive or nonaggressive behavior of the lesion. These characteristics, when combined with information related to the site or distribution of skeletal involvement, allow the formulation of a single diagnostic choice or several choices that are most likely in any individual patient. The addition of clinical information, including the age of the patient and, in some cases, histologic data, also is essential.

Owing to the great number of tumors and tumor-like lesions of bone, accurate diagnosis of a pathologic process on the basis of its radiographic characteristics or features on other imaging studies often is not possible. The radiographic findings, however, do provide reliable information regarding the aggressiveness or rate of growth of a lesion, and this information, coupled with data reflecting the site of the lesion and the age of the patient, allows the formulation of a reasonable diagnosis in most cases. Although aggressive lesions commonly are malignant and benign tumors commonly are nonaggressive, this is not uniformly true. Rapid osseous expansion, an aggressive characteristic, can occur in nonmalignant conditions such as an aneurysmal bone cyst. Similarly, a rim of bone sclerosis about a lesion is a nonaggressive characteristic that, in rare circumstances, becomes evident in malignant neoplasms. Furthermore, osteomyelitis frequently is associated with poorly demarcated osteolysis and periostitis, findings resembling those of a malignant tumor.

MORPHOLOGY
Pattern of Bone Destruction

The radiograph is not extremely sensitive in the detection of small amounts of bone destruction. Cortical lesions are more readily detected than those in cancellous bone (Fig. 77–1). In fact, the detection of a sharply marginated radiolucent area overlying the medullary portion of a tubular bone in a single radiographic projection almost always implies cortical involvement, which becomes readily apparent when a second projection is obtained.

Three radiographic patterns of bone destruction have been identified: geographic, motheaten, and permeative.

GEOGRAPHIC BONE DESTRUCTION (FIG. 77–2). The geographic pattern is the least aggressive one, as it generally is indicative of a slow-growing lesion. The margin of the lesion is well defined and easily separated from the surrounding normal bone. This margin may be smooth or irregular, and it may or may not be sclerotic. There is a short zone of transition from normal to abnormal bone. Although benign bone tumors usually demonstrate geographic bone destruction, malignant diseases (such as plasma cell myeloma and metastasis) and osteomyelitis (particularly granulomatous infections) also can demonstrate a similar pattern of bone destruction.

MOTHEATEN BONE DESTRUCTION (FIG. 77–3). The motheaten pattern is a more aggressive pattern, characteristic of a lesion that is more rapidly growing than one demonstrating geographic bone destruction. The motheaten pattern is associated with a less well defined lesional margin and with a longer zone of transition from normal to abnormal bone. Malignant bone tumors and osteomyelitis may demonstrate the motheaten pattern of bone destruction.

PERMEATIVE BONE DESTRUCTION (FIG. 77–4). The permeative pattern indicates an aggressive bone lesion with rapid growth potential. The lesion is poorly demarcated and not easily separated from the surrounding normal bone, creating a zone of transition that is very long. Certain malignant bone tumors, such as Ewing's sarcoma, may demonstrate permeative bone destruction.

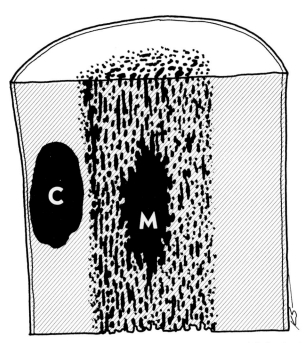

Figure 77–1. Cortical versus medullary involvement. A lesion in the medullary bone (M) may be more difficult to recognize than one in the cortical bone (C). In addition, a nonaggressive cortical lesion will produce a sharp interface with the surrounding bone, whereas such a lesion in the medullary bone may not.

Size, Shape, and Margin of Lesion

In general, primary malignant tumors of bone are larger than benign tumors and may be greater than 6 cm in size when first discovered. Although the shape of a lesion is a relatively poor guide to its nature, elongated lesions, in which the greatest lesional diameter is at least 1.5 times the least diameter, may be indicative of Ewing's sarcoma, histiocytic lymphoma, chondrosarcoma, and angiosarcoma.

The growth rate of a lesion is of great importance in assessing the aggressiveness of any skeletal process. Benign tumors usually grow more slowly than malignant tumors, or they may show no change in size over a long period of observation. Plasma cell myeloma occasionally is associated with slow growth, and histologically low grade or benign giant cell tumors may enlarge rapidly, however.

Slowly growing lesions can be associated with reactive sclerosis of the surrounding normal bone. The sclerotic margin can be of variable thickness and may partially or completely surround the bone lesion.

Presence and Nature of Visible Tumor Matrix

Certain tumors produce matrix that calcifies or ossifies. The resulting radiodense areas must be distinguished from calcification that may develop in regions of necrotic tissue, from callus formation that may indicate the presence of a pathologic fracture, and from a sclerotic response of non-neoplastic bone to the adjacent tumorous deposit.

Certain cartilage tumors are associated with matrix calcification (Fig. 77–5). These include chondromas, chondroblastomas, chondrosarcomas, and, less frequently, chondromyxoid fibromas. Cartilage matrix calcification frequently is centrally located and may appear as ring-like, flocculent, or fleck-like radiodense areas. Similar findings can be apparent within the cartilaginous cap of an osteochondroma.

Visible tumor matrix is also associated with neoplastic bone. Examples of neoplasms producing such tumor matrix are osteosarcomas, parosteal osteosarcomas, ossifying fibromas, osteomas, and osteoblastomas.

Certain lesions, such as fibrous dysplasia, can be accom-

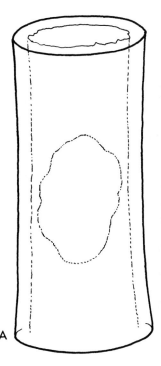

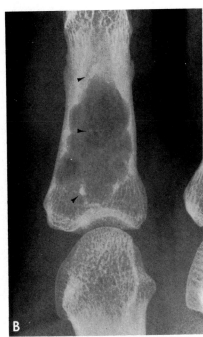

Figure 77–2. Geographic bone destruction. A This pattern of bone destruction is characterized by well-defined lesional margins and a short zone of transition from normal to abnormal bone. **B** The lesion in the proximal phalanx demonstrates geographic bone destruction, a central location, lobulated margins, and small foci of calcification (arrowheads). (Final diagnosis—enchondroma.)

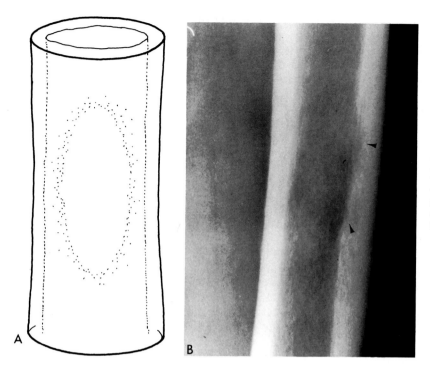

Figure 77–3. Motheaten bone destruction. A This pattern of bone destruction is associated with lesional margins that are less well defined and a longer zone of transition from normal to abnormal bone. **B** A lesion with motheaten bone destruction is identified in this femur. Note its poorly defined margins and its erosion of the endosteal margin of the cortex (arrowheads). (Final diagnosis—histiocytic lymphoma.)

panied by a uniform increase in radiodensity, an appearance that is called the ground-glass pattern.

Internal or External Trabeculation

Within or around the lesion, trabeculated shadows may be identified on the radiograph. In some instances, these reflect the location of residual trabeculae that have been displaced by the neighboring tumor. In other instances, the trabeculation represents new bone formation evoked as a response to the presence of a nearby neoplasm. The appearance of the trabeculation provides information regarding the nature of the neoplasm (Table 77–1) (Fig. 77–6).

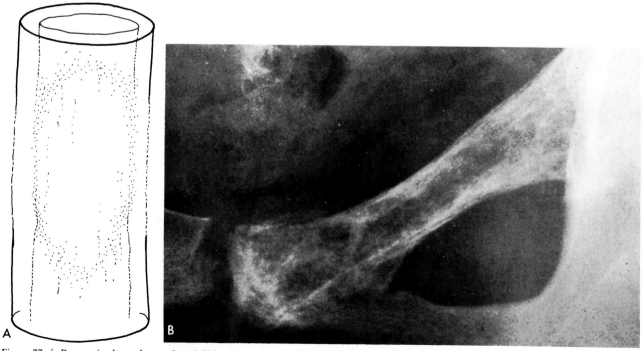

Figure 77–4. Permeative bone destruction. A This pattern of bone destruction is associated with very poorly defined lesional margins and a very long zone of transition from normal to abnormal bone. **B** The lesion in the superior pubic ramus reveals permeative bone destruction with cortical erosion, periostitis, and a soft tissue mass. (Final diagnosis—histiocytic lymphoma.)

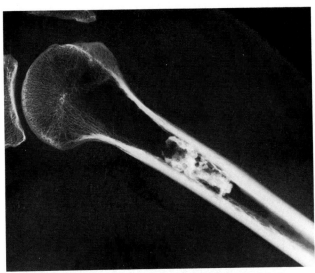

Figure 77–5. Matrix calcification. A sectional radiograph of the humerus reveals a centrally located tumor containing calcification. (Final diagnosis— enchondroma.)

Cortical Erosion, Penetration, and Expansion

The bone cortex can serve as an effective barrier to the further lateral growth of certain tumors, whereas in other instances, the neoplasm may partially or completely penetrate the cortex. Nonaggressive medullary lesions may provoke little change in the endosteal surface of the cortex. Other slow-growing lesions, such as enchondromas, can lead to lobulated erosion of the inner margin of the cortex, producing a scalloped endosteal margin. If progressive endosteal erosion is associated with periosteal bone deposition, an expanded osseous contour can be created. Certain tumors expand bone very slowly, and the accompanying periosteal response may eventually produce a surrounding cortical shell of such thickness that further expansion of the cortex is resisted. Other lesions, such as an aneurysmal bone cyst, expand bone very rapidly.

Aggressive bone lesions can penetrate the entire thickness of the cortex in one or more places. As the tumor reaches the outer aspect of the cortex, the periosteal membrane may be elevated, leading to a variety of patterns of periosteal new bone formation.

Periosteal Response (Fig. 77–7)

A slowly growing tumor that is eroding the cortex can evoke a periosteal response in which additional layers of new bone are added to the exterior, creating an expanded osseous contour. In these instances, the ultimate thickness of the surrounding cortical bone depends on the extent of endosteal erosion and periosteal proliferation. It can be of diminished or of normal thickness, or the new cortex can be thickened in a uniform or nonuniform fashion. If the interface between the normal and expanded cortex is "filled in" with bone, a buttressed pattern has evolved. With more rapid tumor growth, the periosteal response may be characterized by delicate layers of new bone. Single or multiple laminated bone formation may be identified. Multiple concentric layers

of periosteal new bone produce the onion-peel pattern, which can be identified in some cases of Ewing's sarcoma and osteosarcoma.

At the periphery of a neoplasm or an infective focus, a triangular elevation of the periosteum may be identified, termed a Codman's triangle. Usually, the subperiosteal area in the region of the Codman's triangle is itself free of tumor.

In some aggressive bone tumors, delicate rays of periosteal bone formation can form. In certain neoplasms, such as osteosarcoma, the rays extend away from the bone in a radiating or sunburst pattern; in other neoplasms, such as Ewing's sarcoma, the rays extend in a direction perpendicular to the underlying bone, creating a hair-on-end periosteal pattern.

Soft Tissue Mass

Soft tissue masses are not infrequently associated with primary malignant bone neoplasms and, less commonly, with skeletal metastasis. Osteomyelitis also is associated with a soft tissue mass or swelling. Radiographic characteristics that may separate an inflammatory mass from a neoplastic mass are not extremely reliable.

DISTRIBUTION IN A SINGLE BONE

The distribution of a solitary lesion within a tubular bone provides an important clue to the correct diagnosis.

Position of Lesion in Transverse Plane (Figs. 77–8 and 77–9)

The position of the center of a lesion can frequently be identified as of central, eccentric, cortical, juxtacortical (parosteal), or soft tissue location. This analysis is facilitated when the lesion is not of great size. Establishing the position of the center of a lesion is less reliable when a narrow tubular bone, such as the fibula, is the site of involvement, as eccentric lesions in narrow tubular bones soon appear central in location.

Some lesions characteristically lie close to the central axis of the bone (i.e., central lesions) within the medullary canal. These include enchondromas and simple bone cysts. Other lesions arise to one side of the central axis of the medullary bone (i.e., eccentric lesions) or within the cortex (i.e., cortical lesions). Eccentric lesions include giant cell tumor, osteosarcoma, chondrosarcoma, fibrosarcoma, and chondromyxoid fibroma. Cortical lesions include nonossifying fibromas and osteoid osteomas. Lesions arising adjacent to the outer surface of the cortex are parosteal or juxtacortical in location. Typical

Text continued on page 1106

Table 77–1. SOME TRABECULATED LESIONS

Lesion	Pattern
Giant cell tumor	Delicate, thin
Chondromyxoid fibroma	Coarse, thick
Nonossifying fibroma	Lobulated
Aneurysmal bone cyst	Delicate, horizontally oriented
Hemangioma	Striated, radiating

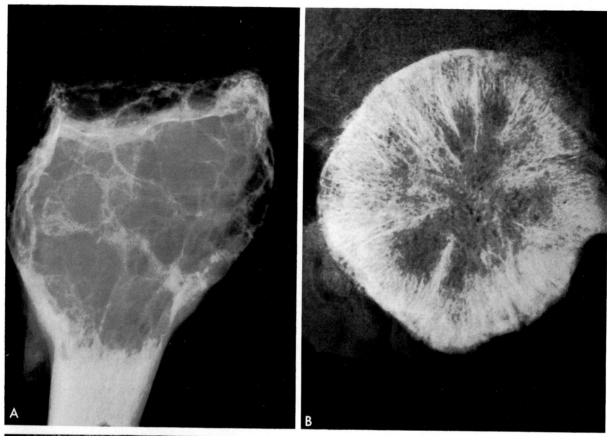

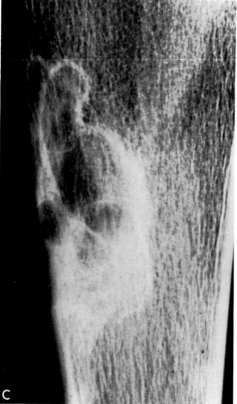

Figure 77–6. Trabeculation. A Giant cell tumor. Note delicate trabeculae that extend through and around this lesion of the distal portion of the radius (specimen radiograph). **B** Hemangioma. Observe the radiating pattern of trabeculation associated with this lesion of the cranial vault (specimen radiograph). **C** Nonossifying fibroma. A lobulated pattern of trabeculation characterizes this lesion of the proximal portion of the tibia (specimen radiograph).

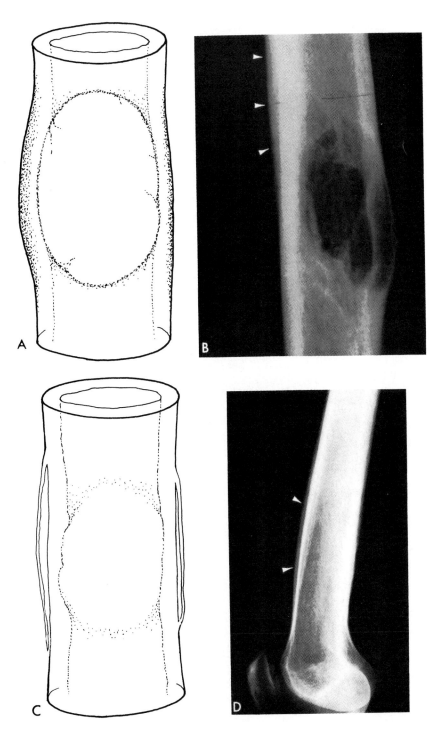

Figure 77–7. Periosteal response. A, B Periosteal buttressing. The diagram (**A**) indicates that periosteal bone formation in response to a lesion may merge with the underlying cortex, producing a buttressed appearance. On the radiograph (**B**), a thick single layer of periosteal bone (arrowheads) about this femoral lesion is still separated from the underlying cortex. The thickness of the periosteal response would indicate a relatively slow-growing lesion. (Final diagnosis—simple bone cyst.) **C, D** Single layer of periosteal bone. The diagram (**C**) demonstrates the appearance of a single thin layer of periosteal bone about a lesion, separated from the underlying bone. The radiograph (**D**) indicates a single layer of periosteal bone on both the anterior and posterior surfaces of the femur. Anteriorly, the periosteal layer is quite thick and still separated from the underlying bone (arrowheads). Posteriorly, the periosteal bone has merged with the femur. (Final diagnosis—hypertrophic osteoarthropathy.)

Illustration continued on following page

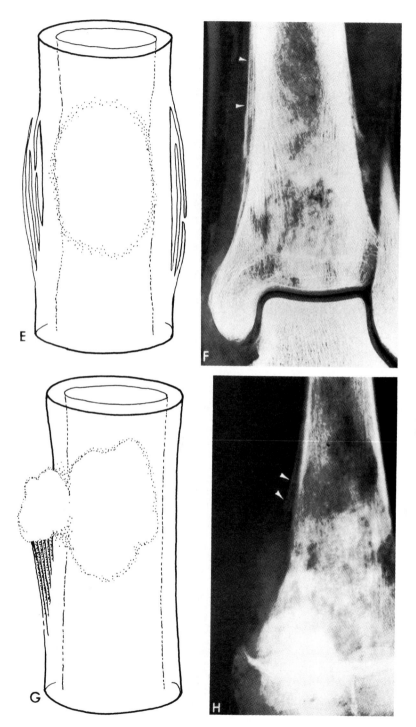

Figure 77–7 *Continued* **E, F** Multiple layers of periosteal bone: Onion-peel pattern. The diagram (**E**) indicates multiple concentric layers of periosteal bone about the lesion. The specimen radiograph (**F**) shows such a pattern along one side of the distal portion of the tibia (arrowheads). On the other side of the bone, a more complex pattern of periostitis is seen. The medullary lesion contains radiopaque foci. (Final diagnosis—osteosarcoma.) **G, H** Codman's triangle. The diagram (**G**) reveals triangular elevation of the periosteum beneath an aggressive lesion that is penetrating the cortex. The specimen radiograph (**H**) shows such a Codman's triangle (arrowheads). Note the medullary and cortical bone destruction, soft tissue mass, and radiodense foci within the lesion. (Final diagnosis—osteosarcoma.)

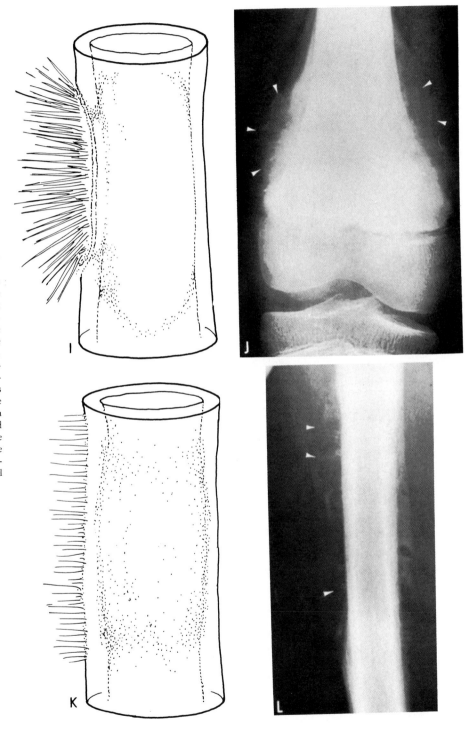

Figure 77–7 *Continued* **I, J** Radiating spicules of periosteal bone: Sunburst pattern. The diagram (**I**) shows radiating spicules that emanate from a single focus within the bone. The radiograph (**J**) indicates such a sunburst pattern of periosteal bone (arrowheads), which is intermixed with tumor bone formation. Note the radiodense lesion in the medullary bone and the Codman's triangle. (Final diagnosis—osteosarcoma.) **K, L** Radiating spicules of periosteal bone: Hair-on-end pattern. The diagram (**K**) demonstrates the parallel horizontal spicules that emanate from the underlying bone. The radiograph (**L**) indicates a femoral lesion characterized by a hair-on-end pattern (arrowheads). The individual striations of periosteal bone have created an inhomogeneous band of radiodensity on the opposite side of the bone. (Final diagnosis—Ewing's sarcoma.)

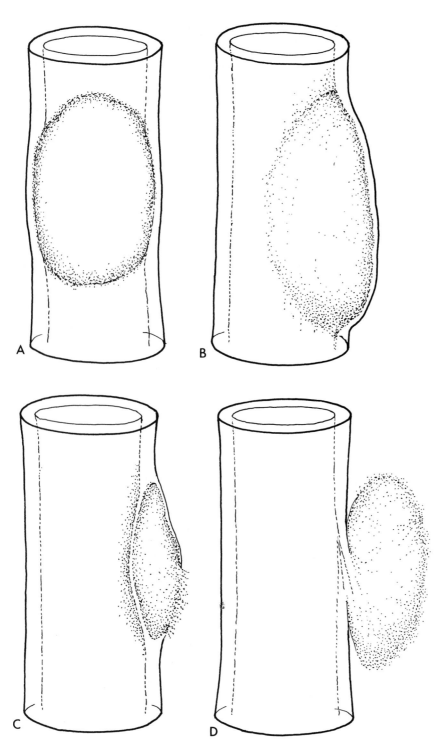

Figure 77–8. **Position of lesion in transverse plane.** Lesions may be central (**A**), eccentric (**B**), cortical (**C**), or parosteal (**D**). Identification of the precise position of the lesion requires that radiographs be obtained in more than one projection.

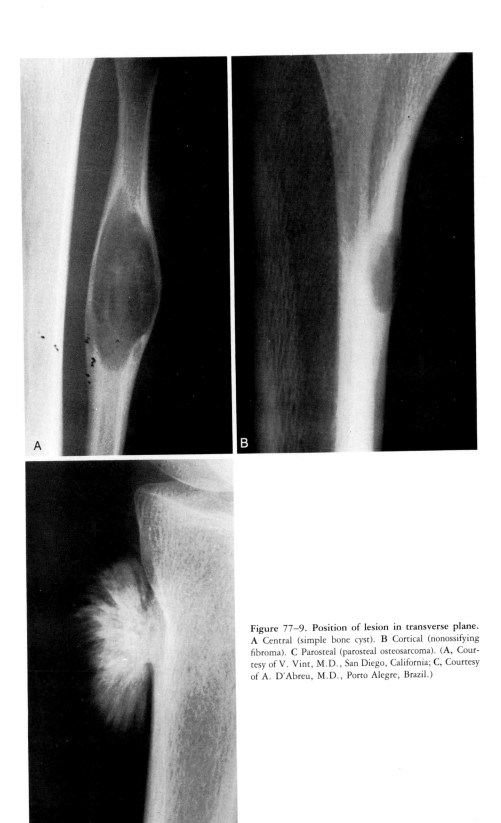

Figure 77–9. Position of lesion in transverse plane. A Central (simple bone cyst). B Cortical (nonossifying fibroma). C Parosteal (parosteal osteosarcoma). (A, Courtesy of V. Vint, M.D., San Diego, California; C, Courtesy of A. D'Abreu, M.D., Porto Alegre, Brazil.)

Table 77–2. MESENCHYMAL SARCOMA VERSUS ROUND CELL SARCOMA*

	Mesenchymal	Round Cell
Examples	Osteosarcoma, chondrosarcoma, fibrosarcoma	Ewing's sarcoma, leukemias
Location in tubular bones	Metaphyseal	Metadiaphyseal
Types of bone destruction	Motheaten pattern	Permeative pattern
Visible tumor matrix	Common (osteosarcoma, chondrosarcoma)	Rare
Periostitis	Sunburst, Codman's triangle	Onion-peel, hair-on-end, Codman's triangle

*Classic features are indicated for each type of sarcoma, although considerable variability can be evident.

examples are juxtacortical chondromas, osteochondromas, and parosteal osteosarcomas. Some kinds of lesions, such as osteosarcomas, chondrosarcomas, fibrosarcomas, and osteoblastomas, may arise from any one of these locations.

Position of Lesion in Longitudinal Plane

Certain solitary lesions in the tubular bones show a remarkable propensity to develop in specific anatomic locations, such as the epiphysis, metaphysis, and diaphysis. Examples of epiphyseal lesions include chondroblastoma and intraosseous ganglion. Although originating in the metaphysis, giant cell tumors quickly penetrate the closed growth plate, involving the epiphysis with extension to the subchondral bone adjacent to the joint. Metaphyseal lesions include nonossifying fibroma, chondromyxoid fibroma, simple bone cyst, osteochondroma, Brodie's abscess, and mesenchymal sarcomas, such as osteosarcoma and chondrosarcoma (Table 77–2). Lesions that may develop in a diaphysis include round cell tumors, such as Ewing's sarcoma. Nonaggressive lesions that may appear in the diaphysis of a tubular bone include nonossifying fibromas, simple bone cysts, aneurysmal bone cysts, enchondromas, osteoblastomas, and fibrous dysplasia. In flat bones, epiphyseal equivalent areas exist beneath the articular cartilage in the bones of the pelvic and shoulder girdles; lesions within these areas commonly are those that show predilection for the epiphyses in the tubular bones.

LOCATION IN THE SKELETON

Knowledge of typical locations of osseous neoplasms, although perhaps not entirely allowing a particular diagnosis, certainly permits the physician to better gauge diagnostic probabilities in any individual case.

Certain tumors predominate in areas of red, or hematopoietic, marrow, related either to their being derived from cells of the red marrow or to their being transported to such areas by the vasculature of the marrow. Metastatic disease, plasma cell myeloma, Ewing's sarcoma, and histiocytic lymphoma are among the tumors that localize primarily in hematopoietic marrow. The tendency for these neoplasms to involve both the appendicular and the axial skeleton in the young, and predominantly the axial skeleton in the aged, is consistent with the changing distribution of red marrow that takes place with advancing age.

Many primary osseous neoplasms develop in areas of rapid bone growth, especially the distal portion of the femur and the proximal portions of the tibia and the humerus. Furthermore, the vascular anatomy peculiar to these regions, consisting of looped vessels and sinusoidal channels, promotes sluggish blood flow and, with it, metastatic seeding of tumor (and infection).

Certain tumors, because of their derivation, predominate in one or more particular areas of the skeleton. A variety of neoplasms related to dentition are virtually confined to the mandible and maxilla. Chordomas, developing from the remnants of the primitive notochord, typically are seen at the cranial and caudal limits of the vertebral column. Epidermoid cysts, apparently occurring because of implantation of cells from superficial tissues, have a definite predilection for the terminal phalanges and calvarium. Neurilemomas occur most commonly in sites containing extensive intraosseous nerves, such as the mandible and the sacrum.

FURTHER READING

Kricun ME: Radiographic evaluation of solitary bone lesions. Orthop Clin North Am *14*:39, 1983.

Kricun ME: Red-yellow marrow conversion: Its effect on the location of some solitary bone lesions. Skel Radiol *14*:10, 1985.

Lodwick GS: The bones and joints. *In* PJ Hodes (Ed): Atlas of Tumor Radiology. Chicago, Year Book Medical Publishers, 1971.

Lodwick GS, Wilson AJ, Farrell C, Virtama P, Dittrich F: Determining growth rates of focal lesions of bone from radiographs. Radiology *134*:577, 1980.

Lodwick GS, Wilson AJ, Farrell C, Virtama P, Smeltzer FM, Dittrich F: Estimating the rate of growth in bone lesions: Observer performance and error. Radiology *134*:585, 1980.

Volberg FM Jr, Whalen JP, Krook L, Winchester P: Lamellated periosteal reactions: A radiologic and histologic investigation. AJR *128*:85, 1977.

Chapter 78

Tumors and Tumor-Like Lesions of Bone: Imaging and Pathology of Specific Lesions

Donald Resnick, M.D.
Michael Kyriakos, M.D.
Guerdon D. Greenway, M.D.

A large number of tumors and tumor-like lesions may involve bone. Because many of the findings are nonspecific and the lesions often are rare, accurate diagnosis requires close cooperation among the orthopedic surgeon, radiologist, and pathologist. The patient's age and the site of skeletal localization are fundamental to the proper interpretation of the abnormalities as detected with routine radiography and specialized imaging techniques. In many instances, however, a single diagnosis cannot be offered on the basis of such abnormalities, and careful histologic analysis is required.

The number of specific tumors that affect the skeleton is large and to select one from among this group of neoplasms as most likely on the basis of the radiographic findings can be extremely difficult. Although many imaging methods exist that can provide diagnostic help in many of these cases, the importance of complete clinical information cannot be overstated. In particular, knowledge of the age of the patient is fundamental to the correct interpretation of the imaging abnormalities (Table 78–1). Almost equal in diagnostic importance is knowledge of skeletal sites that characteristically are affected by each of these lesions (Table 78–2).

In Chapter 77, the principles fundamental to the interpretation of conventional radiographs in cases of tumor and tumor-like lesions of the skeleton are outlined. In the present chapter, further emphasis is placed on the imaging aberrations that characterize each of the important neoplastic lesions that affect the skeleton. Although some histologic characteristics also are addressed, a thorough discussion of the pathology of each of the lesions is beyond the scope of this book.

BONE-FORMING TUMORS
Benign Tumors
Osteoma

Osteomas, which are benign lesions that usually arise from membranous bones and are composed of dense, compact osseous tissue, are discussed in Chapter 83.

Enostosis (Bone Island)

The common lesions known as enostoses or bone islands also are discussed in Chapter 83.

Osteoid Osteoma

An osteoid osteoma is a benign osteoblastic lesion consisting of a central core of vascular osteoid tissue and a peripheral zone of sclerotic bone. The osteoid osteoma has been the subject of heated debate regarding, for example, its neoplastic or infectious origin and its precise relationship to a second lesion of bone, the osteoblastoma.

Clinical Abnormalities. Osteoid osteomas are observed most frequently in patients between the ages of 7 and 25 years. The ratio of male patients to female patients is approximately 3 to 1. Pain is the hallmark of the lesion and, without this symptom, the diagnosis is suspect. The pain typically is more dramatic at night and ameliorated when small doses of salicylates are used. In the immature skeleton, significant aberrations in growth, muscle atrophy, and skeletal deformity also are recognized complications of osteoid osteomas. Torticollis, spinal stiffness, and scoliosis are among the clinical characteristics of those lesions that develop in the vertebral column, whereas joint swelling, synovitis, and limitation of motion may represent the initial clinical manifestations of intraarticular osteoid osteomas.

Skeletal Location. The femur is the most common site of

Table 78–1. TUMORS AND TUMOR-LIKE LESIONS: TYPICAL AGES OF PATIENTS

AGE (Years)

TUMOR	0	10	20	30	40	50	60	70	80

MALIGNANT
- OSTEOSARCOMA
- PAROSTEAL OSTEOSARCOMA
- CHONDROSARCOMA
- FIBROSARCOMA
- FIBROUS HISTIOCYTOMA
- MALIGNANT GIANT CELL TUMOR
- EWING'S SARCOMA
- ADAMANTINOMA
- HEMANGIOENDOTHELIOMA
- HISTIOCYTIC LYMPHOMA
- CHORDOMA
- PLASMA CELL MYELOMA
- SKELETAL METASTASIS

BENIGN
- OSTEOMA
- OSTEOCHONDROMA
- ENCHONDROMA
- CHONDROBLASTOMA
- CHONDROMYXOID FIBROMA
- OSTEOID OSTEOMA
- OSTEOBLASTOMA
- NONOSSIFYING FIBROMA
- DESMOPLASTIC FIBROMA
- LIPOMA
- HEMANGIOMA
- GIANT CELL TUMOR
- NEURILEMOMA
- SIMPLE BONE CYST
- ANEURYSMAL BONE CYST

localization of an osteoid osteoma, followed by the tibia. These two bones together account for 50 to 60 per cent of the total cases, and these bones or other long bones are the site of origin in approximately 70 per cent of cases. The bones in the hands and feet are involved in 20 per cent of cases. In the hands, osteoid osteomas usually are found in a proximal phalanx or a metacarpal bone; of the carpal bones, the scaphoid is affected most frequently, whereas in the foot, the talus and the calcaneus are involved most commonly. Within long bones, osteoid osteoma usually is located in the diaphysis, but it may extend into the metaphysis. Epiphyseal and intraarticular osteoid osteomas are rare (see later discussion).

Vertebral osteoid osteomas usually arise from the posterior elements; the vertebral body is involved only rarely. The lumbar vertebrae are the sites most typically affected. Infrequent sites of localization of osteoid osteomas are the innominate bone, skull, mandible or maxilla, clavicle, scapula, ribs, and radius.

Radiographic Abnormalities. When present, the classic radiographic appearance of a centrally located, oval or round radiolucent area, measuring less than 1 cm in diameter, surrounded by a zone of uniform bone sclerosis is virtually diagnostic of this lesion. Unfortunately, this appearance is not present uniformly. As an example, an osteoid osteoma arising in the vertebral column, in a small bone in the wrist, hand, or foot, or within a joint reveals unique radiographic characteristics that differ from those associated with an osteoid osteoma in the diaphysis of a long tubular bone. Furthermore, this lesion may occur in the cortex, in the medullary or cancellous bone, or in a subperiosteal location, and the resulting radiographic abnormalities are not identical in these three locations.

Long Tubular Bones. Those osteoid osteomas that are *diaphyseal* in location (and some that are metaphyseal) typically are observed in the cortex, appearing as a radiolucent lesion, representing the nidus, that is surrounded by bone sclerosis with cortical thickening (Fig. 78–1). The nidus itself may be uniformly radiolucent or contain variable amounts of calcification. It usually is less than 1 cm in diameter and oval or round in configuration; these characteristics generally allow differentiation of an osteoid osteoma from a stress fracture (which is accompanied by a linear, radiolucent cortical area) and an osteoblastoma (which commonly is a larger lesion). In

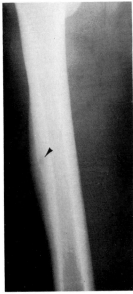

Figure 78–1. **Osteoid osteoma: Radiographic abnormalities—long tubular bones.** Femur. Note the radiolucent nidus (arrowhead) with surrounding endosteal and periosteal bone formation in the diaphysis of the femur.

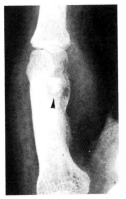

Figure 78–3. **Osteoid osteoma: Radiographic abnormalities—phalanges.** In the proximal phalanx of the fifth finger, the nidus (arrowhead) is partially calcified, and considerable soft tissue swelling is evident. (Courtesy of P. Major, M.D., Winnipeg, Manitoba, Canada.)

rare circumstances, a single osteoid osteoma may contain more than one nidus, or more than one osteoid osteoma, each with its own nidus, may be found in the same bone or neighboring bones. The nidus generally is located in the center of the sclerotic reaction, but its precise delineation may require conventional or computed tomography. Those osteoid osteomas that are subperiosteal in location may evoke more limited osseous proliferation immediately adjacent to or at a distance from the lesion.

Carpus, Tarsus, and Epiphyses. In these locations (Fig. 78–2), an osteoid osteoma usually arises in the medullary spongiosa and, radiographically, appears as a well-circumscribed lesion that is partially or completely calcified. Exten-

sive reactive sclerosis generally is absent. In the immature skeleton of children and adolescents, an osteoid osteoma arising in an epiphyseal ossification center can lead to growth abnormalities and osseous deformity.

Small Bones of the Hand and Foot. When located in the cortex of these small bones, osteoid osteomas generally provoke a periosteal response similar to that observed in the diaphysis of the long tubular bones. In subperiosteal sites, they produce scalloping of the adjacent cortical surface; and in the cancellous bone, a partially or totally calcified lesion is identified (Fig. 78–3). In any of these locations, soft tissue swelling may be prominent.

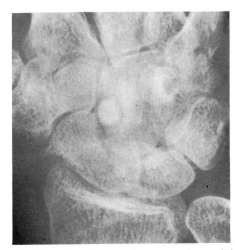

Figure 78–2. **Osteoid osteoma: Radiographic abnormalities—carpal bones.** This osteoid osteoma in the capitate is manifested as a partially calcified lesion with osteopenia in all of the carpal bones.

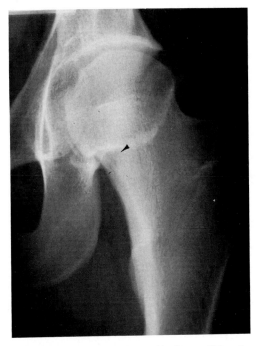

Figure 78–4. **Osteoid osteoma: Radiographic abnormalities—intraarticular location (hip).** An osteoid osteoma with a radiolucent nidus (arrowhead) in the femoral neck has produced extensive adjacent new bone formation, osteophytosis, and mild narrowing of the hip joint.

Table 78–2. TUMORS AND TUMOR-LIKE LESIONS: TYPICAL SITES OF SKELETAL LOCALIZATION

Tumor or Tumor-like Lesion (Number of Cases Evaluated)	Site*								
	Femur	Tibia	Fibula	Foot	Patella	Humerus	Radius	Ulna	Hand, Wrist
Enostosis (371)	25	7	1	5	<1	9	1	<1	9
Osteoid Osteoma (661)	32	24	4	11	<1	7	1	3	9
Osteoblastoma (Conventional) (298)	14	10	4	7	<1	3	1	2	3
Osteoblastoma (Aggressive) (47)	11	13	6	11		2			2
Osteosarcoma (Conventional) (3844)	46	21	3	1	<1	11	<1	<1	<1
Osteosarcoma (Telangiectatic) (191)	54	16	5	<1		14	<1	<1	<1
Osteosarcoma (Periosteal) (69)	44	41	4			7			
Osteosarcoma (Parosteal) (300)	64	11	3	2		15	2	1	<1
Chondroma (Enchondroma) (1028)	11	3	2	7	<1	7	2	<1	57
Chondroma (Periosteal) (130)	25	8	3	5		32	2	2	20
Chondroblastoma (642)	33	18	1	10	2	22	1		2
Chondromyxoid Fibroma (231)	17	38	8	16		1	3	3	2
Osteochondroma (Solitary) (1604)	31	18	4	6	<1	19	1	1	5
Chondrosarcoma (Conventional) (1937)	24	7	2	2	<1	10	1	1	3
Chondrosarcoma (Clear Cell) (64)	64	5				16		2	2
Chondrosarcoma (Mesenchymal) (92)	15	7	1	8		7		1	
Chondrosarcoma (Dedifferentiated) (107)	43	7				17			
Nonossifying Fibroma (833)	38	43	8	1		5	1	<1	1
Desmoplastic Fibroma (121)	12	8	2	2		10	8	2	1
Fibrosarcoma (621)	39	16	3	2		11	1	1	<1
Giant Cell Tumor (1949)	31	27	4	2	<1	6	10	3	4
Fibrous Histiocytoma (Malignant) (271)	44	21	2	2	1	9	1	1	
Lipoma (66)	15	14	20	15		9		2	
Hemangioma (Solitary) (195)	4	3	2	5	1	3	1	1	2
Hemangiopericytoma (48)	10		6	4		15	4	2	2
Hemangioendothelioma (151)	18	23	4	6	1	13	2		2
Neurofibroma (42)		7	5			2			
Neurilemoma (76)	7	4	1	3	3	4		5	8
Chordoma (503)									
Simple Bone Cyst (884)	27	6	5	1		56	1	1	1
Aneurysmal Bone Cyst (465)	14	15	7	8	<1	9	3	4	5
Adamantinoma (189)	3	81	3	1		6	1	4	1
Ewing's Sarcoma (1974)	22	11	9	3		10	2	1	1

*Numbers indicate percentages of the lesions that affect each of the skeletal sites based upon analysis of major reports containing the greatest number of cases. Percentages may not always total 100 per cent because numbers were rounded to nearest whole number.

Table 78–2. TUMORS AND TUMOR-LIKE LESIONS: TYPICAL SITES OF SKELETAL LOCALIZATION *Continued*

Tumor or Tumor-like Lesion (Number of Cases Evaluated)	Scapula	Clavicle	Sternum	Ribs	Vertebrae, Including Sacrum and Coccyx	Innominate Bone	Skull	Face	Mandible, Maxilla
Enostosis (371)	1	<1		12	2	25			
Osteoid Osteoma (661)	1			<1	6	2	<1		<1
Osteoblastoma (Conventional) (298)	1	<1		4	30	2	—4—		11
Osteoblastoma (Aggressive) (47)	4			2	23	13	11		2
Osteosarcoma (Conventional) (3844)	1	<1	<1	1	2	7	1	<1	4
Osteosarcoma (Telangiectatic) (191)	2			2		3	2		<1
Osteosarcoma (Periosteal) (69)				1		1			1
Osteosarcoma (Parosteal) (300)	<1					1			
Chondroma (Enchondroma) (1028)	1	<1	1	5	1	3	<1		
Chondroma (Periosteal) (130)				2	1	2			
Chondroblastoma (642)	2	<1	<1	2	1	4	1		<1
Chondromyxoid Fibroma (231)	1		<1	3	2	6	<1		
Osteochondroma (Solitary) (1604)	4	<1	<1	2	2	5	<1		
Chondrosarcoma (Conventional) (1937)	5	1	2	8	6	24	1	1	2
Chondrosarcoma (Clear Cell) (64)	2			3	3	2	2		2
Chondrosarcoma (Mesenchymal) (92)	2		1	12	11	12	8	1	14
Chondrosarcoma (Dedifferentiated) (107)	8		<1	4	1	22			
Nonossifying Fibroma (833)	<1	<1		1		1	<1		<1
Desmoplastic Fibroma (121)	3	2		2	3	11	1		33
Fibrosarcoma (621)	2	1	<1	1	4	10	1		7
Giant Cell Tumor (1949)	<1	<1	<1	1	7	4	1	<1	<1
Fibrous Histiocytoma (Malignant) (271)	1	1	<1	3	2	9	2		3
Lipoma (66)				8	5		5		9
Hemangioma (Solitary) (195)	2	1		9	25	3	29	2	8
Hemangiopericytoma (48)	2	4	4	8	15	11	2		10
Hemangioendothelioma (151)	3		1	5	10	8	3		2
Neurofibroma (42)					7			2	76
Neurilemoma (76)	1			3	16	1	3		42
Chordoma (503)					75		25		
Simple Bone Cyst (884)	<1	<1		<1		2			
Aneurysmal Bone Cyst (465)	2	3		3	14	9	2	<1	2
Adamantinoma (189)				1		1			
Ewing's Sarcoma (1974)	5	2	<1	8	6	18	1	<1	1

*Numbers indicate percentages of the lesions that affect each of the skeletal sites based upon analysis of major reports containing the greatest number of cases. Percentages may not always total 100 per cent because numbers were rounded to nearest whole number.

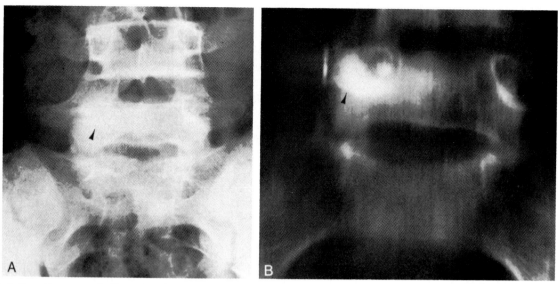

Figure 78–5. Osteoid osteoma: Radiographic abnormalities—spine. The increased density of the right pedicle in the fifth lumbar vertebra (arrowheads) reflects the presence of an osteoid osteoma.

Intraarticular Sites. Osteoid osteomas arising in an intra-articular location deserve special emphasis (Fig. 78–4). Clinical manifestations in such cases may be attributed falsely to a primary articular disorder. A synovial inflammatory response may lead to irreversible cartilaginous and osseous destruction. Osteopenia, uniform narrowing of the interosseous space, and periarticular subperiosteal bone apposition may be encountered, particularly in the hip. Eventually, hypertrophic changes similar to those in osteoarthritis may be seen.

Spine. When osteoid osteomas arise in the spine, pain commonly is prominent and usually is accompanied by an abnormality of spinal curvature, specifically scoliosis. Local tenderness and paraspinal muscle atrophy are additional clinical manifestations; neurologic abnormalities are relatively infrequent.

On radiographs, the lesion characteristically is located on the concave aspect of the scoliotic curve, near its apex. Osteosclerosis of a pedicle, lamina, articular process, or, less commonly, a transverse or spinous process is observed. A radiolucent nidus may be present, but its identification frequently requires conventional or computed tomography (Fig. 78–5).

Although an osteosclerotic focus in the posterior osseous elements represents an important diagnostic sign of an osteoid osteoma, a similar abnormality may occur in patients with skeletal metastasis and infection, such as tuberculosis, and as a response to a contralateral spondylolysis or hypoplastic neural arch.

Other Skeletal Sites. In the innominate bones of the pelvis (Fig. 78–6) and in the scapula, an osteoid osteoma most typically appears as a radiolucent or partially calcified lesion with limited surrounding bone sclerosis. In a rib, the lesion may be accompanied by a profound sclerotic reaction, which can extend to adjacent ribs and, rarely, by scoliosis.

Other Imaging Techniques. Scintigraphy (Fig. 78–7)

has been used in the preoperative and intraoperative evaluation of patients with osteoid osteoma. These lesions avidly accumulate bone-seeking radiopharmaceutical agents during the vascular, blood-pool, and delayed phases of the scintigraphic examination. The resulting abnormalities initially were considered to be quite sensitive but relatively nonspecific, although more recently, a distinctive pattern of abnormality, designated the double-density sign, has been observed in

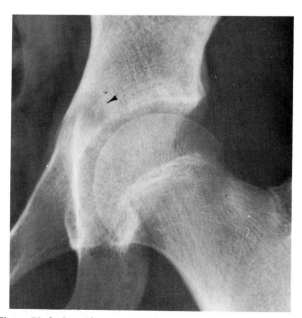

Figure 78–6. Osteoid osteoma: Radiographic abnormalities—innominate bone. An osteoid osteoma (arrowhead) is located in the acetabular region.

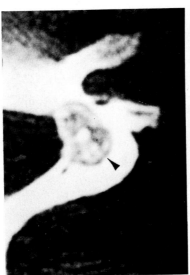

Figure 78–7. Osteoid osteoma: Scintigraphic abnormalities. As shown in this classic osteoid osteoma of the proximal portion of the femur, avid accumulation of a bone-seeking radionuclide (arrowhead) corresponds in location to the site of the radiographically evident lesion (A). Note that the region of most intense scintigraphic activity is surrounded by a zone of less intense but abnormal activity (B).

radionuclide bone scans in patients with osteoid osteoma. This sign is characterized by intense scintigraphic activity centrally in the region of the nidus and less intense accumulation of the radionuclide peripherally in the sclerotic bone.

Intraoperative radionuclide methods have also been used in patients with osteoid osteoma, particularly for precise localization of the nidus.

Computed tomography (Fig. 78–8) has largely replaced conventional tomography in the imaging evaluation of osteoid osteomas. The method is most valuable in defining osteoid osteomas in the spine, osseous pelvis, and femoral neck.

Pathologic Abnormalities. Microscopically, the nidus of an osteoid osteoma consists of bone in various stages of maturity within a highly vascular connective tissue stroma containing numerous dilated capillaries. Seams of osteoid are found that undergo calcification and form irregular trabeculae of woven or reticular bone.

Histologically, osteoid osteoma and osteoblastoma are essentially similar, although osteoblastomas may be more vascular and possess more osteoblasts, wider trabeculae, and less organization than osteoid osteomas.

Natural History. Surgical resection of the entire nidus is a prerequisite for an optimal clinical response. Recurrences are likely when surgical removal of the lesion is incomplete. True recurrences after complete resection of the nidus are indeed rare and, in some cases, relate to the presence of more than one nidus in a single osteoid osteoma or a second osteoid osteoma in the same bone or a different bone. It should be noted also that there exist reports in which lesions with clinical and radiologic characteristics of an osteoid osteoma have healed spontaneously.

Differential Diagnosis. In an intracortical location, a lesion containing a radiolucent center (with or without calcification) and peripheral bone sclerosis is almost certainly an

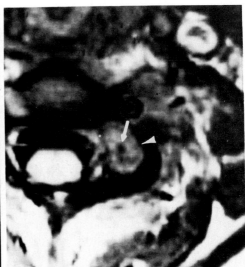

Figure 78–8. Osteoid osteoma: Computed tomographic and magnetic resonance imaging abnormalities. An osteoid osteoma (arrowheads) of the sixth cervical vertebra is shown by transaxial computed tomography (A) and magnetic resonance imaging (B). The partially calcified nidus (arrow) and the sclerotic bone have a low signal intensity in the T1 weighted image in B. (Courtesy of J. Tsurada, M.D., San Francisco, California.)

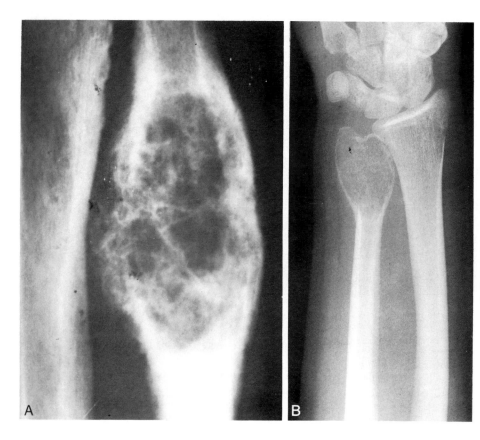

Figure 78–9. Osteoblastoma: Radiographic abnormalities—long tubular bones. A This aggressive lesion of the ulnar diaphysis is characterized by irregular osteolysis and osteosclerosis with cortical thickening and osseous expansion. (Courtesy of C. Resnik, M.D., Baltimore, Maryland.) B Epiphyseal localization, as in this case, is rare. The lesion is predominantly osteolytic, containing faint trabeculae, and the bone is expanded. A giant cell tumor or aneurysmal bone cyst is a reasonable alternative diagnosis. (Courtesy of H. Spjut, M.D., Houston, Texas.)

osteoid osteoma despite occasional reports in which an abscess or a bone tumor (i.e., hemangioma, osteosarcoma) has had a similar radiographic appearance. In a subperiosteal or intramedullary location or within a joint, the radiographic diagnosis of an osteoid osteoma is more difficult.

Osteoblastoma

Osteoblastoma can be further categorized into conventional and aggressive types.

CONVENTIONAL OSTEOBLASTOMA. Benign osteoblastoma is a relatively uncommon primary neoplasm of bone that is composed of a well-vascularized connective tissue stroma in which there occurs active production of osteoid and primitive woven bone.

Clinical Abnormalities. The lesion is observed most frequently in individuals under 30 years old, with approximately 70 per cent of cases appearing in the second or third decade of life. Male patients are affected more frequently than female patients, in a ratio of approximately 2 to 1. Local pain is a common manifestation of osteoblastoma, although generally it is mild. Accentuation of pain at night and its amelioration with salicylates are inconstant clinical features of osteoblastoma. Spinal lesions may be accompanied by muscle spasm, scoliosis, and neurologic manifestations.

Skeletal Location. Osteoblastomas occur in the vertebrae in approximately 30 per cent of cases and in the long tubular bones in about 35 per cent of cases. Fifteen per cent of tumors affect the skull, mandible, or maxilla, 5 per cent of tumors occur in the innominate bone, and 10 per cent of the osteoblastomas are localized in the bones of the hands and feet.

In the long tubular bones, approximately 75 per cent of osteoblastomas are situated in the diaphysis with the remainder in the metaphysis. Epiphyseal involvement is distinctly unusual. The femur is the long bone most typically affected by osteoblastoma. The thoracic and lumbar vertebrae are the most frequent spinal sites of involvement. Vertebral osteoblastomas arise mainly in the posterior osseous elements.

Radiographic and Pathologic Abnormalities. The radio-

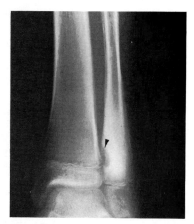

Figure 78–10. Osteoblastoma: Radiographic abnormalities—long tubular bones. Routine radiography reveals an osteolytic focus (arrowhead) with considerable sclerosis and periostitis, the latter affecting a long segment of the fibula and the adjacent surface of the tibia.

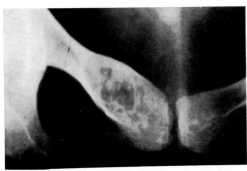

Figure 78–11. Osteoblastoma: Radiographic abnormalities—innominate bone. Considerable osteosclerosis and calcification are evident in this lesion. (Courtesy of P. Feldman, M.D., Toronto, Ontario, Canada.)

graphic features of osteoblastoma are, in most instances, nondiagnostic. Osteolysis alone, osteosclerosis alone, or a combination of both osteolysis and osteosclerosis may be observed. Expansion of bone, cortical thinning, and a soft tissue mass may accompany this lesion. When radiographs reveal an expansile, well-circumscribed, partially calcified lesion or one that resembles a large osteoid osteoma, the diagnosis of osteoblastoma should be considered.

In the long tubular bones, osteoblastomas may originate in the medullary or cortical bone (Figs. 78–9 and 78–10) or, rarely, in a subperiosteal location. These lesions are predominantly osteolytic, with areas of calcification or ossification, well marginated, and expansile. Bone sclerosis and periostitis may be exuberant. Similar radiographic alterations may accompany osteoblastomas in the small bones of the hands and feet and in the innominate bone (Fig. 78–11).

In the spine, a well-defined, expansile osteolytic lesion that is partially or extensively calcified or ossified, arising from the posterior osseous elements, should suggest the diagnosis of an osteoblastoma (Fig. 78–12). Occasionally, destruction of a vertebral body may occur alone or in combination with involvement of the dorsal osseous elements, a nidus may be seen similar to that of an osteoid osteoma, or a large and purely radiolucent osteoblastoma in the posterior arch may resemble an aneurysmal bone cyst (Fig. 78–13). Scoliosis may accompany spinal or rib osteoblastomas (Fig. 78–14).

Although osteoblastomas are infrequent in the skull, an oval radiolucent defect, with varying degrees of central calcification, involving both the inner and the outer tables of the skull, is typical of such lesions. Osteoblastomas are somewhat more frequent in the mandible than in the maxilla.

When sectioned, osteoblastomas are fairly well delineated, and a thin rim of limiting bone may be present on the medullary aspect of a tumor of cancellous bone. The neoplasms are hemorrhagic and have a gritty consistency with occasional softer cystic regions. Microscopically, the basic pattern of osteoblastoma is similar to that of osteoid osteoma, consisting of a well-vascularized connective tissue stroma in which there is active production of osteoid and primitive woven bone. Considerable variation may be seen in this pattern, however. With maturation of the tumor, there is progressive mineralization of the osteoid. The overall pattern of osteoblastoma

tends to be less well organized than that of osteoid osteoma. Some osteoblastomas have large tumor cells simulating the findings of osteosarcoma. Indeed, with small biopsy specimens, it may be impossible to distinguish between these two tumors. Cases are encountered in which foci of osteosarcoma coexist with areas of osteoblastoma, and, furthermore, osteoblastomas have recurred with "transformation" to osteosarcoma. Whether these phenomena are the result of initial misdiagnosis of an osteosarcoma or a true transformation of an osteoblastoma sometimes is unclear.

Differential Diagnosis. The radiographic abnormalities of osteoblastoma commonly do not allow a precise diagnosis, although those tumors in the posterior osseous elements of the vertebrae (which lead to an expansile, partially calcified area of osteolysis) or in the skull (which produce a sharply marginated radiolucent defect containing central calcification or ossification) may be identified accurately as osteoblastomas. In other sites, this neoplasm may have features suggestive of osteoid osteoma, aneurysmal bone cyst, eosinophilic granuloma, enchondroma, fibrous dysplasia, chondromyxoid fibroma, or solitary bone cyst.

AGGRESSIVE (MALIGNANT) OSTEOBLASTOMA. Although typical osteoblastomas are known to recur in as many as 10 per cent of cases, the documentation of recurrent osteoblastoma in which the histologic appearance is more aggressive than that of the original tumor indicates that osteoblastomas should not be regarded as uniformly benign. In general, the anatomic distribution of aggressive (malignant) osteoblastoma parallels that of conventional osteoblastoma. In all sites, the radiologic and macropathologic features of these lesions resemble the findings of typical osteoblastoma but with a greater likelihood of soft tissue involvement. The histologic characteristics of aggressive osteoblastoma include findings of conventional osteoblastoma as well as those suggestive of malignancy.

The major diagnostic problem is differentiating these aggressive or malignant osteoblastomas from osteosarcoma. It

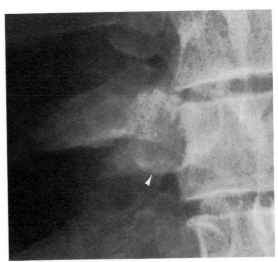

Figure 78–12. Osteoblastoma: Radiographic abnormalities—spine. An osteosclerotic lesion (arrowhead) is located primarily in the transverse process of a thoracic vertebra. (Courtesy of V. Vint, M.D., San Diego, California.)

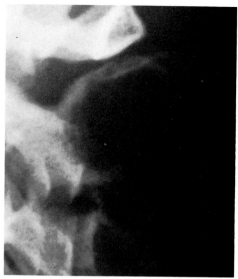

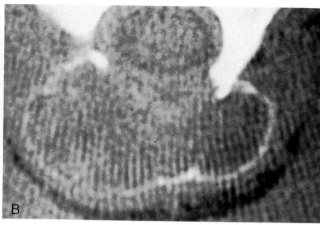

Figure 78–13. Osteoblastoma: Radiographic abnormalities—spine. A radiograph (A) and transaxial computed tomographic scan (B) reveal a large, expansile, osteolytic lesion with an osseous rim involving the spinous process of the axis. It resembles an aneurysmal bone cyst.

also is important to differentiate between aggressive osteoblastomas and conventional osteoblastomas, as the former tumors show a far greater likelihood to recur. In some instances, aggressive osteoblastomas have led to the patient's death.

Ossifying Fibroma

This fibroosseous lesion is closely related radiographically and pathologically to fibrous dysplasia. Most ossifying fibromas arise in the facial bones, although a similar tumor can appear in a tubular bone.

OSSIFYING FIBROMA OF FACIAL BONES. The ossifying fibromas of the jaws are well-circumscribed, slowly growing lesions affecting patients in the second, third, and fourth decades of life. Their similarity to fibrous dysplasia has been emphasized repeatedly.

In general, a painless expansion of the tooth-bearing portion of the mandible or, less commonly, the maxilla is observed on clinical examination. Radiographically, the lesion typically is 1 to 5 cm in diameter, although larger tumors are encountered. Well-defined unilocular or multilocular areas of osteolysis containing varying degrees of calcification are seen, and cortical thinning and expansion with displacement of adjacent teeth are additional radiographic abnormalities. Histologic findings include osseous products consisting of woven and lamellar trabeculae, spheroid products with nonpolarizable features or exhibiting Sharpey's fiber–like fringes, and a fasciculated or storiform stroma containing dystrophic calcification.

OSSIFYING FIBROMA OF TUBULAR BONES. Ossifying fibromas of the tubular bones are rare. These lesions have also been designated osteofibrous dysplasia. The majority

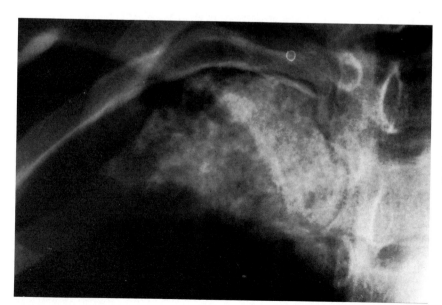

Figure 78–14. Osteoblastoma: Radiographic abnormalities—ribs. A large, expansile, heavily calcified lesion involves the posterior portion of the rib, extending to the costovertebral joints.

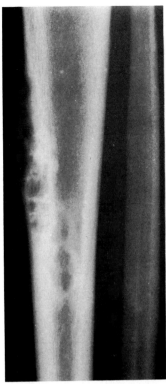

Figure 78–15. Ossifying fibroma: Radiographic abnormalities—tibia. A lateral radiograph reveals a sharply marginated, lobulated, eccentric lesion in the diaphysis, affecting mainly the anterior cortex. (From Goergen TG, et al: Long bone ossifying fibromas. Cancer 39:2067, 1977. Used with permission.)

of cases have consisted of lesions isolated to the tibia (Fig. 78–15); additional patterns of distribution have included involvement of the tibia and ipsilateral fibula (Fig. 78–16), of the fibula alone, and of both tibiae and fibulae. Exceptional sites of ossifying fibromas are the radius, humerus, and metatarsal and phalangeal bones. Diaphyseal localization in the tibia is typical, and involvement of the distal diaphyseal segment of the fibula also is characteristic. In the tibia, the lesion usually is located in the anterior aspect of the bone.

Ossifying fibromas of the tubular bones generally are seen in the first or second decade of life, in boys or girls with approximately equal frequency, leading to painless enlargement and bowing of the bone. Osseous deformity may be accentuated by pathologic fractures. Intracortical osteolysis clearly marginated by a band of sclerosis may be seen as a single confluent region or multiple, elongated, bubble-like areas. A hazy or ground-glass appearance similar to that of fibrous dysplasia or osteosclerosis alone may be evident. Although ossifying fibroma of the tubular bones usually is stable or may even regress spontaneously on serial radiographic examinations, progression of the lesion occasionally is observed, and tumor recurrence after curettage is well documented.

Histologically, ossifying fibroma consists of a fairly abundant well-vascularized fibrous stroma in which reside trabeculae of new bone. Woven bone lined by osteoblasts is typical. Some ossifying fibromas contain small foci of cartilage.

The radiographic features of ossifying fibromas in the tubular bones most resemble those of fibrous dysplasia. Tibial

involvement with predilection for the anterior cortex of the diaphysis, a unilocular or multilocular elongated lesion, osseous bowing, and, in some cases, associated abnormalities of the fibula are highly characteristic of ossifying fibroma. Monostotic fibrous dysplasia commonly affects patients in the second and third decades of life and, in addition to the tibia, frequently involves the rib, femur, facial bones, or skull. The major point of histologic difference between ossifying fibroma and fibrous dysplasia is the lack of osteoblastic rimming on the metaplastic trabeculae in the latter lesion. Adamantinoma represents a second lesion sharing many radiographic features with ossifying fibroma, including a propensity to affect the middle region of the tibia. Another potential source of diagnostic difficulty is distinguishing histologically between ossifying fibroma and well-differentiated intraosseous osteosarcoma.

Malignant Tumors
Osteosarcoma

Osteosarcoma, which has also been designated osteogenic sarcoma, is second in frequency only to plasma cell myeloma as a primary malignant neoplasm of bone. It is characterized histologically by proliferating tumor cells that, in most instances, produce osteoid or immature bone. Extensive modifications in the classification scheme of osteosarcomas have appeared in recent years. Currently available systems employ such features as the precise location of the tumor within the bone (intramedullary or central, intracortical, surface, perios-

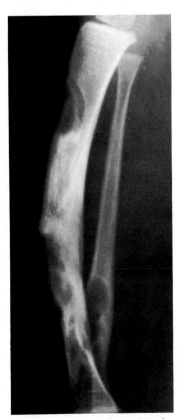

Figure 78–16. Ossifying fibroma: Radiographic abnormalities—tibia and fibula. Note the multiloculated, eccentric cortical lesion of the tibia with an additional lesion of the fibula. (Courtesy of J.E.L. Desautels, M.D., Calgary, Alberta, Canada.)

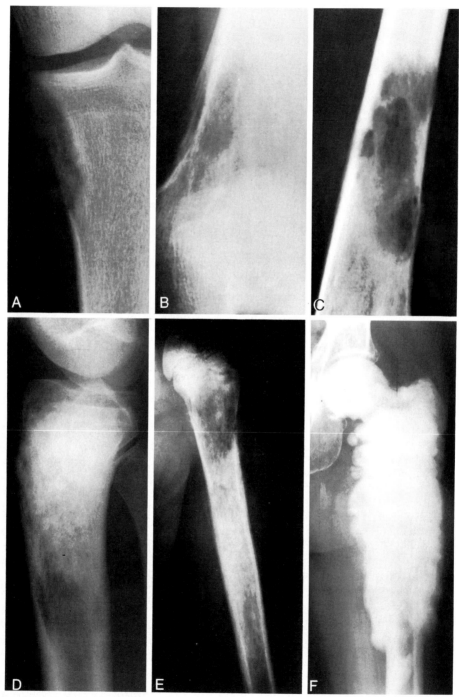

Figure 78–17. Conventional osteosarcoma: Radiographic abnormalities—basic patterns of osseous involvement. A Purely osteolytic pattern (metaphyseal and epiphyseal). **B** Purely osteolytic pattern (metaphyseal and diaphyseal). **C** Purely osteolytic pattern (diaphyseal). **D** Mixed osteolytic and osteosclerotic pattern (metaphyseal and diaphyseal). **E** Mixed osteolytic and osteosclerotic pattern (metaphyseal and diaphyseal). **F** Purely osteosclerotic pattern (epiphyseal, metaphyseal, and diaphyseal). (**F**, Courtesy of P. Major, M.D., Winnipeg, Manitoba, Canada.)

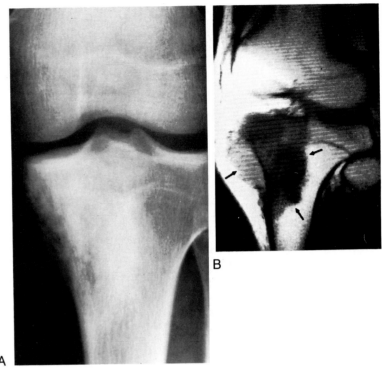

Figure 78–18. Conventional osteosarcoma: Radiographic abnormalities—purely osteosclerotic pattern. A conventional radiograph (A) shows the purely osteosclerotic lesion in the medial aspect of the metaphysis and epiphysis of the proximal portion of the tibia. In B, a coronal magnetic resonance image (TE, 30 ms; TR, 0.5 s) reveals low signal intensity in the intraosseous and extraosseous components of the tumor (arrows).

teal, or parosteal); the degree of cellular differentiation (high grade or low grade); the histologic composition (osteoblastic, chondroblastic, fibroblastic, fibrohistiocytic, telangiectactic, small cell); the number of foci of involvement (single or multicentric); and the status of the underlying bone (normal or the site of disease, injury, or another neoplasm).

CONVENTIONAL OSTEOSARCOMA. Conventional osteosarcoma generally is seen in the second and third decades of life. Men are affected more frequently than women. Clinical manifestations include pain and swelling, restriction of motion, warmth, and pyrexia. Frequently, the patient seeks medical assistance only after a traumatic episode, which may or may not result in a pathologic fracture.

Skeletal Location. The most typical sites of involvement are the tubular bones in the appendicular skeleton (80 per cent of cases), particularly the femur (40 per cent), the tibia (16 per cent), and the humerus (15 per cent). Fifty to 75 per cent of all cases develop in the osseous structures about the knee. Osteosarcomas are relatively infrequent in the fibula, innominate bone, mandible, maxilla, and spine and are rare in the skull, ribs, scapula, clavicle, sternum, radius, ulna, and small bones of the hands and feet. With regard to the long tubular bones, metaphyseal location predominates. Initial involvement of the diaphysis occurs in 2 to 11 per cent of cases. A primary epiphyseal origin is quite rare.

Radiographic Abnormalities. The radiographic pattern of involvement is variable, depending to a large extent on the amount of bone produced by the tumor (Fig. 78–17). A mixed pattern consisting of both osteolysis and osteosclerosis is most typical, with purely osteolytic or osteosclerotic lesions (Fig. 78–18) being encountered less frequently. Osteolysis is especially characteristic of the telangiectatic variety of osteosarcoma. In the tubular bones, conventional osteosarcoma usually is evident as a poorly defined, intramedullary, meta-

physeal lesion that has extended through the cortex and produced a sizeable soft tissue mass. Periosteal reaction in the form of a Codman's triangle or with a "sunburst" appearance and, rarely, a pathologic fracture are additional radiographic features. Osteosarcomas in the diaphysis of a tubular bone

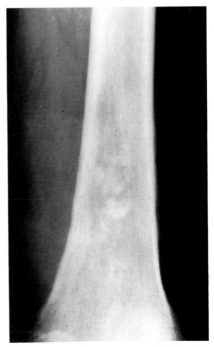

Figure 78–19. Conventional osteosarcoma: Radiographic abnormalities—tubular bones. Anteroposterior radiograph reveals an elongated osteolytic lesion containing calcification or ossification in the diaphysis of the femur. Periostitis is also evident.

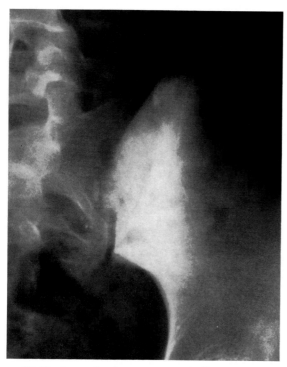

Figure 78–20. Conventional osteosarcoma: Radiographic abnormalities—ilium. An osteosclerotic lesion involves the bone about the sacroiliac joint.

is ideal in delineating soft tissue extension of this neoplasm (Fig. 78–18).

Pathologic Abnormalities. As most osteosarcomas occur in young children and adolescents, the neoplasm usually is noted to abut on an open physeal plate. Macroscopic or microscopic evidence of transphyseal extension is common. Osteosarcomas that involve the epiphysis may extend to the articular cartilage, but generally they do not penetrate the cartilage to enter the joint space. Areas of tumor that are separate from the main neoplasm ("skip" areas) have been observed in as many as 25 per cent of cases.

The microscopic pathology of conventional osteosarcoma has traditionally been subdivided into three categories, osteoblastic, chondroblastic, and fibroblastic, depending on the predominant differentiation of tumor cells. Approximately 50 per cent of these tumors produce osteoid in significant amounts to be considered osteoblastic osteosarcomas; 25 per cent of these neoplasms show predominant differentiation toward cartilage and are termed chondroblastic osteosarcomas; and the remaining 25 per cent of osteosarcomas reveal a spindle cell stroma with a herringbone pattern similar to that seen in fibrosarcoma and are designated fibroblastic osteosarcomas. Additional histologic types, such as fibrohistiocytic osteosarcomas, exist, however. In general, all conventional osteosarcomas contain pleomorphic stromal elements that are either spindle-shaped fibroblast-like cells or osteoblasts with irregular, hyperchromatic nuclei, and many contain multi-

(Fig. 78–19) may reveal only osteosclerotic foci and endosteal thickening.

The radiographic features of osteosarcoma in other skeletal sites are similar to those in the tubular bones and include varying degrees of osteolysis and osteosclerosis, cortical violation, periostitis, and a soft tissue mass (Fig. 78–20). Five to 10 per cent of osteosarcomas involve the flat bones, including those of the pelvis. Analysis of the rarely occurring spinal osteosarcomas indicates that the vertebral bodies are the preferred site of involvement. Rib lesions may be accompanied by large, extrapleural masses.

Other Imaging Techniques. Additional imaging methods are useful in defining the extent of the neoplasm and its relationship to surrounding neurovascular structures and in evaluating the response of the tumor to therapy. The radionuclide examination uniformly shows an increased accumulation of the bone-seeking radiopharmaceutical agent within the primary tumor itself and, less uniformly, at sites of skeletal or extraskeletal metastasis. An extended pattern of radionuclide accumulation beyond the true margin of the osteosarcoma, perhaps related to marrow hyperemia, medullary reactive bone, and periostitis, creates difficulty in accurate interpretation of the scintigraphic findings (Fig. 78–21). Angiography provides identification of the extraosseous component of the tumor and defines the degree of displacement (or invasion) of vessels. Computed tomography is useful in assessing the intramedullary and soft tissue extent of the neoplasm. An increase in the attenuation values of the tissue within the medullary canal generally is indicative of tumor extension or "skip" metastases. Magnetic resonance imaging

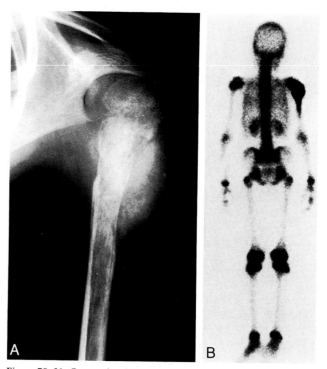

Figure 78–21. Conventional osteosarcoma: Scintigraphic abnormalities. The radiograph (**A**) reveals an osteosclerotic lesion in the metaphysis and diaphysis of the humerus. The epiphysis appears uninvolved. Note the soft tissue component of the neoplasm and the erosion of the external surface of the humerus. A bone scan (**B**) reveals an extended pattern of uptake involving the humeral epiphysis and scapula as well as the metaphysis and diaphysis of the humerus.

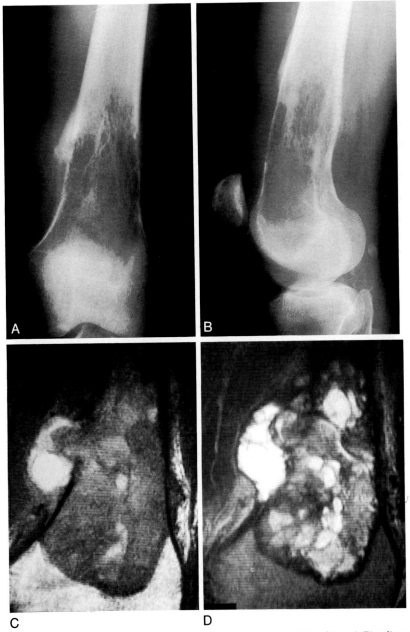

Figure 78–22. Telangiectatic osteosarcoma: Radiographic abnormalities. A, B Anteroposterior (A) and lateral (B) radiographs show an osteolytic lesion containing small and large areas of bone destruction in the femur. The cortex is thinned or perforated, and Codman's triangles and a large soft tissue mass are evident. **C, D** T1 (C) (TE, 30 ms; TR, 0.5 s) and T2 (D) (TE 120 ms; TR, 2.0 s) weighted coronal magnetic resonance images vividly demonstrate the extent of the tumor. In **C,** only the soft tissue component of the lesion has a high signal intensity; in **D,** the overall intensity of the tumor has increased.

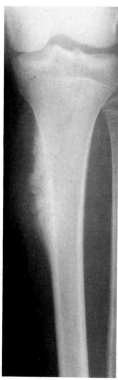

Figure 78–23. Periosteal osteosarcoma: Radiographic abnormalities. Observe the location of the lesion in the medial cortex of the tibia, cortical thickening, and radiating and cloud-like osseous proliferation in the external surface of the bone. The medullary portion is uninvolved.

nucleated tumor cells with grotesque shapes. The form and shape of the malignant osteoid are also highly variable.

Histologic grading of osteosarcomas, based on the degree of cellular differentiation, has been used by some investigators to separate the tumors into four categories, I to IV, with grade IV being the least differentiated. As the histologic characteristics of osteosarcomas may vary greatly from one area to another in the same tumor, and the grade of the tumor has not been shown to have prognostic importance, many pathologists do not use any such grading system.

Natural History. The application of new chemotherapeutic strategies as a supplement to surgery and irradiation has resulted in a dramatic increase in the number of patients who can be expected to survive for 5 years or more. Local recurrence and distant skeletal metastasis after amputation lead to osseous alterations that are similar to those of the primary tumor. Lymph node, soft tissue, or visceral metastases from osteosarcoma may appear as calcified or ossified lesions on the radiograph, and pulmonary metastatic foci can be associated with a spontaneous pneumothorax.

GNATHIC OSTEOSARCOMA. Compared with conventional osteosarcomas, gnathic osteosarcomas have a later age of onset and a decreased tendency for systemic metastases. Tumors arising in the mandible are slightly more frequent than those occurring in the maxilla. Gnathic osteosarcoma may be purely osteolytic or purely osteosclerotic or demonstrate a mixed pattern of osteolysis and osteosclerosis.

TELANGIECTATIC OSTEOSARCOMA. The presence in some osteosarcomas of microscopic features that include

large cystic cavities filled with blood has led to the segregation of a distinct variety of tumor that has been designated telangiectatic osteosarcoma. Such neoplasms represent as many as 11 per cent of all osteosarcomas. Telangiectatic osteosarcomas have a prognosis that is similar to or poorer than that for ordinary osteosarcomas.

Telangiectatic osteosarcoma is primarily a tumor of the long tubular bones; the metaphysis is the usual site of origin, but the tumor can extend into the epiphysis when the physeal plate is closed. Diaphyseal involvement occurs in approximately 10 per cent of cases.

It is the osteolytic nature of the process that is the radiographic hallmark of telangiectatic osteosarcoma (Fig. 78–22). A large, multilocular, expansile lesion often lacking periosteal bone production is characteristic. Pathologic fractures and soft tissue masses are also encountered.

Microscopically, telangiectatic osteosarcoma has features resembling those of an aggressive aneurysmal bone cyst. The dominant histologic pattern is that of large cystic blood spaces separated by thin fibrous septa. The neoplasms are quite vascular, and the amount of osteoid formed in these osteosarcomas is scant.

The radiographic and histologic features of telangiectatic osteosarcoma most resemble those of an aneurysmal bone cyst, giant cell tumor, or angiosarcoma.

SMALL CELL OSTEOSARCOMA. This neoplasm is usually seen in a patient of either sex in the second, third, or fourth decade of life. Pain and swelling of short duration are the typical clinical manifestations. Sites of involvement, in order of decreasing frequency, include the femur, humerus, tibia, and ilium. Lesions in the tubular bones predominate in the epiphysis and metaphysis. The prognosis of the tumor appears to be poorer than for conventional osteosarcoma.

Radiographically, a large, predominantly osteolytic lesion involving the medullary and cortical bone is accompanied by periostitis or a soft tissue mass, or both, in approximately 50 per cent of cases. Microscopically, small cell osteosarcoma is composed of small cells arranged in solid sheets or separated into lobules by dense fibrous septa; variable amounts of intercellular osteoid are evident.

INTRAOSSEOUS LOW GRADE OSTEOSARCOMA. Low grade or well-differentiated osteosarcomas arising within a bone are uncommon. Such tumors typically affect young or middle-aged adults and are located mainly in the tibia or femur. The clinical manifestations may be mild. Radiographs usually reveal a relatively large, metaphyseal lesion, which may be purely osteosclerotic or both osteolytic and osteosclerotic in appearance. Epiphyseal extension, cortical violation, osseous expansion, and soft tissue extension are features that are encountered inconsistently. Well-differentiated intraosseous osteosarcomas are composed of spindle cells arranged in interlacing fascicles separated by collagen fibers. Benign giant cells are evident in more than 50 per cent of cases. The amount of osteoid produced by the tumor is variable.

Intraosseous low grade osteosarcoma is associated with a better prognosis than conventional osteosarcoma.

INTRACORTICAL OSTEOSARCOMA. This tumor appears to represent the rarest form of osteosarcoma. Intracortical osteosarcoma arises within the confines of the cortex as an osteolytic lesion with surrounding cortical sclerosis and with-

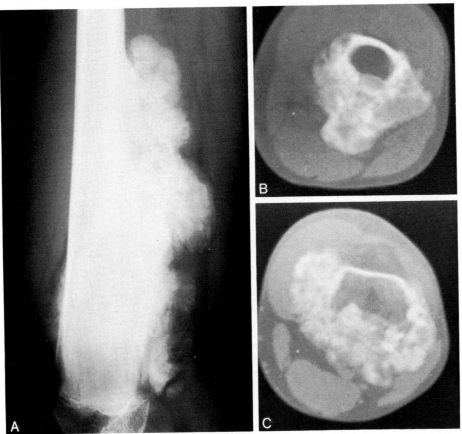

Figure 78–24. Parosteal osteosarcoma: Radiographic abnormalities. A An exuberant, densely ossified lesion involves the posterior metaphyseal and diaphyseal regions of the femur. It has wrapped itself around the femur, accounting for the radiodense shadows seen anterior to the bone. The lesion is lobulated and irregular in outline, and the underlying cortex is thickened. B, C Transaxial computed tomographic scans of diaphyseal (B) and metaphyseal (C) levels show the extent of the ossifying process, which involves not only the posterior surface of the bone but also the medial and lateral surfaces. The cortex is thickened and the medullary bone appears to be involved. (Courtesy of Regional Naval Medical Center, San Diego, California.)

out radiating osseous spicules. Typically affecting young adults, intracortical osteosarcoma is a diaphyseal lesion of the tibia or femur. A radiolucent focus containing osteoid and surrounded in part by a sclerotic margin usually is seen. Reactive thickening of the adjacent cancellous trabeculae may be evident. The majority of intracortical osteosarcomas reveal a microscopic pattern identical to that of a conventional osteoblastic osteosarcoma.

SURFACE HIGH GRADE OSTEOSARCOMA. Three types of osteosarcoma involve predominantly the surface of a bone: parosteal osteosarcoma, periosteal osteosarcoma, and high grade conventional osteosarcoma. Surface high grade osteosarcomas occur in male or female patients of various ages. Histologically, these tumors are identical to conventional osteosarcoma, and it is only their localization to the surface of the bone that represents a differentiating feature. The radiographic appearance of surface high grade osteosarcoma resembles that of periosteal osteosarcoma (see later discussion). The prognosis of this type of tumor appears to be identical to that of conventional high grade osteosarcoma and poorer than that of parosteal or periosteal osteosarcoma.

PERIOSTEAL OSTEOSARCOMA. Periosteal osteosarcoma is an infrequent neoplasm; the age range of affected patients is broad, with most reports indicating that the tumor predominates in the second and third decades of life. Involvement of the diaphysis of a long tubular bone, especially the femur or the tibia, is most typical. When a periosteal osteosarcoma is seen in the distal region of the femur, it is usually located in the anterior, lateral, or medial portion of the bone, differing from the posterior femoral involvement that characterizes a parosteal osteosarcoma.

Periosteal osteosarcomas are variable in size, appearing radiographically as a lesion on the surface of the bone. The tumor is limited to the cortex, which is thickened, and commonly is accompanied by radiating osseous spicules (Fig. 78–23). The medullary cavity, with rare exceptions, is uninvolved.

Histologically, periosteal osteosarcoma is relatively poorly differentiated and predominantly chondroblastic. It may not be possible on histologic analysis alone to differentiate between the periosteal and conventional varieties of osteosarcoma.

The prognosis of this tumor definitely is better than that of conventional osteosarcoma, although local recurrences or systemic metastases occur if surgical resection is inadequate.

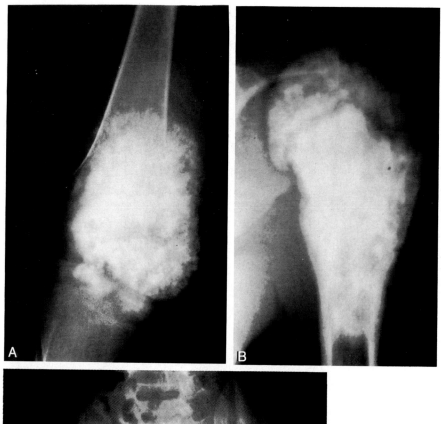

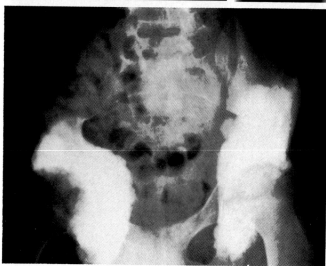

Figure 78–25. Multicentric osteosarcoma: Radiographic abnormalities. Skeletal radiographs reveal multiple foci of osteosarcoma involving the femur (A), humerus (B), and innominate bones (C). It is difficult in these cases to document whether the lesions arose simultaneously or metachronously and whether they represent multiple primary tumors or a single primary neoplasm and multiple metastatic foci.

PAROSTEAL OSTEOSARCOMA. This lesion is the third type of osteosarcoma arising on the surface of a bone. Affected patients generally are adults in the second to fifth decades of life. Symptoms and signs consist of pain, swelling, and a palpable mass; an enormous size of the tumor is often present at the time of initial clinical evaluation.

Skeletal Location. Parosteal osteosarcomas occur almost exclusively in the long tubular bones; the femur is the predominant site of involvement (approximately 65 per cent of cases), followed in order of frequency by the humerus (15 per cent), tibia (10 per cent), fibula (3 per cent), radius (2 per cent), and ulna (1 per cent). Other bones are rarely affected. Parosteal osteosarcomas are particularly common in the posterior surface of the distal portion of the femur and

proximal regions of the tibia, fibula, and humerus. These tumors characteristically arise in the metaphyseal region of a tubular bone.

Radiographic Abnormalities. A large, radiodense mass is evident (Fig. 78–24). Typically it is attached in a sessile fashion to the external cortex, and a thin radiolucent line may separate the remaining portion of the tumor from the underlying bone. It may later grow around the surface of the bone with obliteration of the radiolucent plane. Ossification within the tumor proceeds from the base of the lesion to its periphery. The pattern of ossification differs from that seen in posttraumatic heterotopic bone formation (myositis ossificans), in which the periphery of the lesion is the first to ossify. Medullary destruction is infrequent.

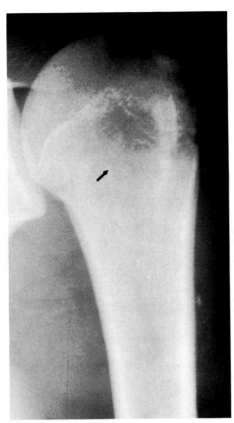

Figure 78–33. Chondroblastoma: Radiographic abnormalities—long tubular bones. An osteolytic lesion involves the proximal metaphysis of the humerus (arrow). Periostitis in the metaphysis and diaphysis is evident.

PERIOSTEAL (JUXTACORTICAL) CHONDROMA.

Periosteal chondroma, composed of hyaline cartilage, develops adjacent to the cortical surface, beneath the periosteal membrane. Periosteal chondromas are discovered in men more frequently than in women and occur in patients of all ages, although they predominate in persons under 30 years of age. Clinical manifestations include local swelling followed by mild to moderate pain. The long tubular bones, particularly the humerus and the femur, are affected in approximately 70 per cent of cases, and the bones in the hands or, less commonly, the feet are affected in approximately 25 per cent of cases. Metaphyseal localization predominates.

Radiographically, a soft tissue mass with erosion of the adjacent cortex is evident (Fig. 78–31). Periostitis may be seen. Calcification within the lesion is evident in approximately 50 per cent of cases. Microscopically, a periosteal chondroma is composed of lobules of hyaline cartilage that varies in cellularity. Some tumors are hypercellular, such that the diagnosis of low grade chondrosarcoma is suggested.

A periosteal chondroma must be differentiated from a periosteal, or juxtacortical, chondrosarcoma. Patients with periosteal chondrosarcoma usually are older than those with periosteal chondroma and the chondrosarcomas tend to be larger. If the lesion has an aggressive radiologic pattern with cortical destruction, a diagnosis of chondrosarcoma should be considered.

Chondroblastoma

Chondroblastoma is an uncommon, benign, cartilaginous neoplasm originating in bone.

Clinical Abnormalities. Chondroblastomas are most frequent in the second and third decades of life. Approximately 90 per cent of cases occur in persons between the ages of 5 and 25 years. Men are affected more commonly than women. Local pain, swelling, and tenderness are evident, varying in duration from several months to many years. Joint manifestations may simulate a primary synovial process.

Skeletal Location. Chondroblastomas generally arise in an epiphysis or apophysis of a long tubular bone. Metaphyseal extension of an epiphyseal tumor is not uncommon, however. The femur, the humerus, and the tibia are the most frequent sites of involvement. The bones in the lower extremity are affected more commonly than those in the upper extremity.

Approximately 10 per cent of chondroblastomas arise in the bones of the hands and feet, with particular predilection for the talus and the calcaneus. Although infrequent, tumors occurring in the innominate bone reveal a paraacetabular distribution. The skull, mandible, and maxilla are rare sites of chondroblastomas, as are the vertebrae, scapula, patella, and sternum.

Radiographic Abnormalities. The radiographic features of this neoplasm consist of an osteolytic lesion, eccentrically or centrally located in an epiphysis or apophysis, usually less than 5 or 6 cm in size, which is well defined and spheroid or ovoid in shape (Figs. 78–32 and 78–33). A thin sclerotic rim may separate the tumor from the adjacent normal bone. Extension of the lesion to subarticular bone (or, rarely, into the joint space) is well recognized; metaphyseal involvement occurs in 25 to 50 per cent of cases. Calcific foci within the lesion are documented in approximately 30 to 50 per cent of patients. Periostitis in the adjacent metaphysis or diaphysis

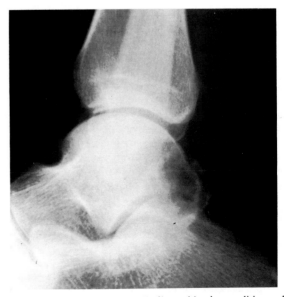

Figure 78–34. Chondroblastoma: Radiographic abnormalities—talus. Note an osteolytic area involving the posterior portion of the talus. It is well defined without calcification. (Courtesy of Regional Naval Medical Center, San Diego, California.)

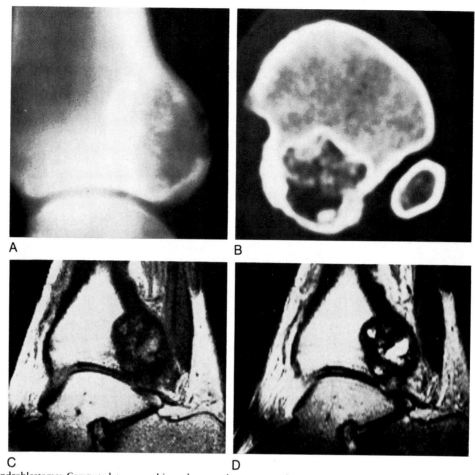

Figure 78–35. Chondroblastoma: Computed tomographic and magnetic resonance imaging abnormalities. A conventional tomogram (**A**) shows a lobulated radiolucent lesion in the posterior aspect of the tibia, adjacent to the joint. It is slightly expansile, contains calcification, and possesses a sclerotic margin. A transaxial computed tomogram (**B**) defines the extent of the lesion, as well as its central calcifications and sclerotic margin. The lesion has low signal intensity on a T1 weighted sagittal magnetic resonance image (**C**), and it has some regions of higher signal intensity on a T2 weighted sagittal magnetic resonance image (**D**).

is evident in approximately 30 per cent of cases. Soft tissue masses and pathologic fractures are rare.

In sites other than the tubular bones, the radiographic features of chondroblastomas are less specific (Fig. 78–34).

Other Imaging Techniques. Scintigraphy reveals avid accumulation of the bone-seeking radiopharmaceutical agent. In some instances, areas of calcification and metaphyseal extension are well delineated with conventional or computed tomography (Fig. 78–35). Magnetic resonance imaging may be used to further define the intraosseous extent of the tumor (Fig. 78–35).

Pathologic Abnormalities. Chondroblastomas vary in size from 1 to 19 cm, with most being between 3 and 5 cm. The larger tumors are found in the flat bones. Histologically, chondroblastoma is characterized by broad areas of round, oval, or polyhedral chondroblasts that have well-defined cytoplasmic borders. Multinucleated osteoclast-type giant cells are found dispersed among the chondroblasts or concentrated about areas of hemorrhage or necrosis. Hemorrhagic foci and cystic blood spaces that simulate those in an aneurysmal bone cyst are reported in 15 to 25 per cent of chondroblastomas. Foci of cellular necrosis associated with dystrophic calcification frequently are identified.

Natural History. Although intraosseous recurrences of chondroblastoma have occurred after curettage of the neoplasm, the vast majority of these tumors behave in a benign fashion. Occasionally, however, chondroblastomas pursue a more aggressive course, with invasion of joint spaces, soft tissues, or adjacent bones. In fact, metastatic foci of chondroblastoma have been identified in the lungs of patients, usually subsequent to some form of surgical therapy for the primary bone tumor. In these instances, removal of the pulmonary lesions has resulted in long-term survival, and the histologic appearance of the metastatic foci has been identical to that of a conventional chondroblastoma. The occurrence of pulmonary metastases may indicate that a benign osseous neoplasm has gained access to the vascular system owing to the surgical manipulation. A variety of chondroblastoma exists, however, that invades soft tissue structures (including neurovascular bundles and lymphatic channels, with extension into adjacent bones), or metastasizes, involving not only the lung but other organ systems as well. Whether this variety of tumor should be regarded as a malignant chondroblastoma or a chondroblastoma-like chondrosarcoma is not clear.

Differential Diagnosis. The radiographic features of chondroblastoma generally are easily differentiated from those

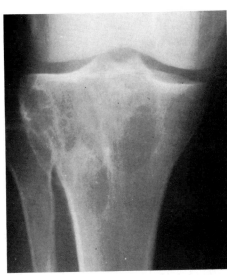

Figure 78–36. Chrondromyxoid fibroma: Radiographic abnormalities—tibia. An osteolytic, eccentric, slightly expansile lesion involves the metaphysis and epiphysis of the bone and extends to the subchondral region. Slight trabeculation is evident. The lesion is well defined and contains no calcification. Periostitis is absent. (Courtesy of O. J. Wollenman, M.D., Fort Worth, Texas.)

typical of a giant cell tumor (epiphyseal lesion without calcification in the mature skeleton) and chondromyxoid fibroma (metaphyseal lesion with coarse trabecular pattern); however, in occasional cases, radiographic differentiation among these tumors as well as among other lesions, such as an enchondroma, osteoblastoma, eosinophilic granuloma, infection, and chondrosarcoma, may be difficult. A significant problem in differential diagnosis arises owing to the recent descriptions of a specific type of chondrosarcoma, the clear cell chondrosarcoma, that shares many radiographic and histologic features with chondroblastoma (see later discussion).

Chondromyxoid Fibroma

This is the least common benign neoplasm of cartilage.

Clinical Abnormalities. This tumor is identified most typically in persons who are less than 30 years of age and is especially common in the second and third decades of life. The neoplasm may be slightly more frequent in men than in women. Slowly progressive pain, tenderness, swelling, and restriction of motion are observed.

Skeletal Location. Chondromyxoid fibroma is observed most frequently in the long tubular bones. Involvement of the tibia or femur is evident in approximately 55 per cent of patients. Favored sites for the tumor are the proximal end of the tibia, proximal and distal ends of the femur and fibula, and, less commonly, small bones of the foot. Involvement of the spine, ribs, sternum, scapula, skull, carpal bones, mandible, and maxilla is relatively rare. In a tubular bone, a metaphyseal focus is favored, with extension into the adjacent epiphysis or diaphysis. Primary localization in a diaphysis is rare.

Radiographic Abnormalities. Although the radiographic findings usually are indicative of a benign tumor, they are variable. When located in a long tubular bone, chondromyxoid fibromas generally are eccentrically situated, metaphyseal lesions that are radiolucent, of varying size, and elongated in shape (Fig. 78–36). Cortical expansion, exuberant endosteal sclerosis, and coarse trabeculation commonly are noted. Extensive periostitis and pathologic fractures are unusual, and calcification is rare. Larger lesions may lead to penetration of the cortex; the resulting osseous defect or "bite" is believed to be highly characteristic of a chondromyxoid fibroma.

In the flat and irregular bones, as well as the small bones of the hands and feet (Fig. 78–37), chondromyxoid fibromas lead to osteolysis, scalloped osseous erosions, bone expansion, and a coarse trabecular pattern.

Pathologic Abnormalities. The tumor usually has a scalloped, sclerotic medullary border. Its orientation is parallel to the long axis of the tubular bone, and classically it is eccentric in position. Chondromyxoid fibroma is characterized by several histologic patterns in which chondroid, myxomatous, and fibrous areas occur in varying proportions. Areas consisting of dilated vascular sinusoidal spaces lined by multinucleated giant cells and tumor cells also may be present, resembling the features of an aneurysmal bone cyst. Some chondromyxoid fibromas contain foci of hyaline cartilage, similar to but less extensive than those found in an enchondroma. Focal calcification in chondromyxoid fibroma occurs in 5 to 27 per cent of cases.

Natural History. Although there are reports that document the occurrence of locally aggressive behavior and tumor recurrence, the prevailing view is that chondromyxoid fibroma is a benign cartilaginous neoplasm and that its recurrence relates to inadequate local excision. Soft tissue involvement is rare and may indicate true tumor invasion or implantation of the neoplasm in the soft tissues at the time of surgery. Rare documented cases of malignant transformation of this neoplasm do exist.

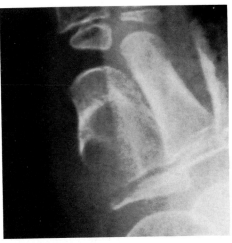

Figure 78–37. Chondromyxoid fibroma: Radiographic abnormalities—proximal phalanx of foot. An aggressive osteolytic lesion has led to cortical disruption. A sclerotic margin is apparent distally.

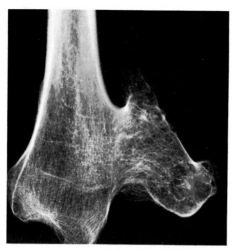

Figure 78–38. Solitary osteochondroma: Radiographic abnormalities—long tubular bones. The pedunculated osteochondroma arising from the distal metaphysis of the fibula contains spongiosa and cortex that are continuous with those of the parent bone. The metaphysis itself is slightly widened, a finding that is much more frequent and prominent in instances of multiple osteochondromas.

Differential Diagnosis. The radiographic signs of chondromyxoid fibroma are usually those of a nonmalignant process. Accurate diagnosis of a chondromyxoid fibroma is least difficult when the osteolytic lesion is localized to the metaphyseal region of a tubular bone and reveals an eccentric position, endosteal sclerosis, and cortical expansion or violation with a bite-like configuration. The presence of radiographically detectable calcification within this tumor is rare; this finding therefore should suggest alternative diagnoses, such as an enchondroma, chondroblastoma, or even fibrous dysplasia. The thick trabeculae that commonly are found in a chondromyxoid fibroma differ from the thin trabeculae of a giant cell tumor or nonossifying fibroma. In nontubular bones, a precise radiographic diagnosis of a chondromyxoid fibroma is more difficult, as such lesions can be large and expansile. Alternative diagnoses in these cases include fibrous dysplasia and giant cell tumor as well as other lesions.

Osteochondroma

An osteochondroma can be considered a cartilage-covered osseous excrescence that arises from a surface of a bone. Osteochondromas may be solitary or multiple (hereditary multiple exostoses) or occur spontaneously or after accidental or iatrogenic injury or irradiation (see Chapter 64).

SOLITARY OSTEOCHONDROMA. The solitary osteochondroma, or osteocartilaginous exostosis, is a relatively frequent lesion. Its precise cause is not clear; some investigators consider the osteochondroma to be a true neoplasm and others believe it is a developmental physeal growth defect. Osteochondromas develop in bones that form through the process of endochondral ossification and are intimately related to the physis.

Clinical Abnormalities. The majority of solitary osteochondromas are discovered in children and adolescents, with

approximately 70 to 80 per cent of lesions occurring in patients who are younger than 20 years of age. A painless, slowly growing mass represents the most characteristic clinical manifestation. Osteochondromas occasionally may lead to more significant symptoms and signs related to a fracture of the exostosis, damage of adjacent nerves or vessels, or spinal cord compression.

Skeletal Location. The long tubular bones, especially the femur, humerus, and tibia, are involved most frequently. A metaphyseal location is characteristic; osteochondromas are rare in the diaphysis, whereas those in the epiphysis, which are also rare, are considered to be indicative of Trevor's disease or dysplasia epiphysealis hemimelica (see later discussion). Specific sites of predilection of osteochondromas are the distal metaphysis of the femur and proximal metaphyses of the humerus, tibia, and fibula. These regions correspond to areas of rapid bone growth.

The small bones of the hand and foot are involved in approximately 10 per cent of cases, and the innominate bone is involved in approximately 5 per cent of cases. Spinal involvement (less than 2 per cent of cases) may lead to compression of the spinal cord. Vertebral osteochondromas predominate in the posterior osseous elements. Osteochondromas of the cranial bones usually affect the base of the skull. Scapular exostoses occur in approximately 4 per cent of cases and can lead to dysfunction of shoulder movement.

Radiographic Abnormalities. An osteocartilaginous exostosis is characterized radiographically by an osseous protuberance arising from the external surface of a long tubular bone and containing spongiosa and cortex that are continuous with those of the parent bone (Fig. 78–38). The outgrowths may be pedunculated (with a narrow stalk and bulbous tip) or sessile (with a broad, flat base) (Fig. 78–39). Commonly occurring in the metaphysis at osseous sites of tendinous or ligamentous attachment, osteochondromas typically point away from the nearby joint. The metaphysis of the tubular bone may be widened, although this finding is far more characteristic of multiple rather than solitary osteochondromas.

The tip of the osteochondroma is covered by a cap composed of hyaline cartilage. If the cap is small and well defined, with regular calcification, the appearance is most compatible with a benign outgrowth; if it is large and poorly defined and contains irregular calcification, malignant transformation must be considered. Additional diagnostic methods may be required in this differentiation (see later discussion).

Osteochondromas arising in the innominate bone (Fig. 78–40) frequently are large, and differentiation of a benign osteochondroma from one that has undergone malignant transformation is extremely difficult. In the ribs, osteochondromas (as well as enchondromas) are particularly frequent at the costochondral junction. Osteochondromas in the small tubular bones of the hand and foot lead to radiographic features that are similar to those evident in the long tubular bones. Those in the spine typically arise in the posterior osseous elements.

Other Imaging Techniques. It has been emphasized that computed tomography (Fig. 78–41) has a role in differentiating between an osteochondroma and a peripheral chondrosarcoma by providing information regarding the relation of the lesion to the underlying bone, the type of lesional matrix,

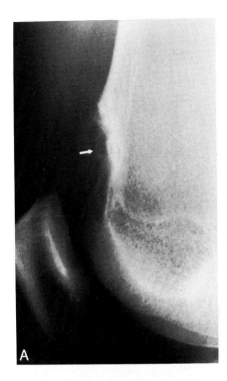

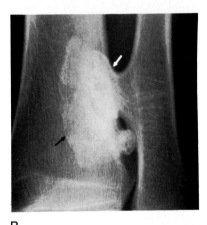

B

Figure 78–39. Solitary osteochondroma: Radiographic abnormalities—long tubular bones. A Femur. The sessile osteochondroma (arrow) on the anterior surface of the femur has produced osseous irregularity. There is no calcification in the cap of the osteochondroma. **B** Fibula. A large pedunculated osteochondroma arises from the posteromedial surface of the fibula. (**A,** Courtesy of S. Kursunoglu, M.D., San Diego, California.)

flat or irregular bones are usually larger. The cortex and periosteum of the bone from which the osteochondroma arises are continuous with those of the lesion. When sectioned, the usual osteochondroma is found to contain a cartilaginous cap beneath which is cancellous bone that is in direct continuity with that of the parent bone. In children and adolescents, in whom there is active bone growth, the cap may be as thick as 3 cm; in adults, the cap may be entirely absent. In adults, the occurrence of a cartilage cap that is thicker than 1 cm should raise the possibility of chondrosarcomatous transformation. Examination of the cap of the osteochondroma shows that its histomorphology is similar to that of a physeal growth plate.

Natural History. Osteochondromas may continue to increase in size in the immature skeleton. As such growth usually ceases at puberty with fusion of the adjacent growth plate, it has been emphasized repeatedly that osteochondromas that continue to enlarge after this time must be evaluated carefully for the possibility of malignant transformation. Alternatively, spontaneous resolution of an osteochondroma has been documented in children and adolescents.

Complications. Potential complications of an osteochondroma (or multiple exostoses) include fracture, osseous deformity, vascular injury, neurologic compromise, bursa formation, and malignant transformation.

Fracture. Fractures are not frequent. Those osteochondromas that are large or pedunculated are more likely to reveal fractures following an injury.

Osseous Deformity. Failure of normal tubulation may lead to a widened metaphysis and alterations in an adjacent articulation. Growth disturbances also may be identified (Fig. 78–42).

Vascular Injury. An osteochondroma may displace vessels, particularly those about the knee. More severe vascular com-

the pattern of mineralization within the outgrowth, and the thickness of the cartilaginous cap, although such analysis is not without difficulty (see later discussion). Scintigraphy with bone-seeking radiopharmaceutical agents also has been used for this differentiation (Fig. 78–41), but this method, too, is accompanied by diagnostic difficulty (see later discussion). Magnetic resonance imaging (Fig. 78–41) may be useful in defining the thickness of the cartilaginous cap.

Pathologic Abnormalities. The average size of osteochondromas arising in the long tubular bones is approximately 4 cm (in maximum dimension), whereas those occurring in the

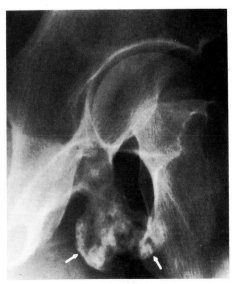

Figure 78–40. Solitary osteochondroma: Radiographic abnormalities—innominate bone. A pedunculated osteochondroma (arrows) arises from the pubic bone and contains a partially calcified cap.

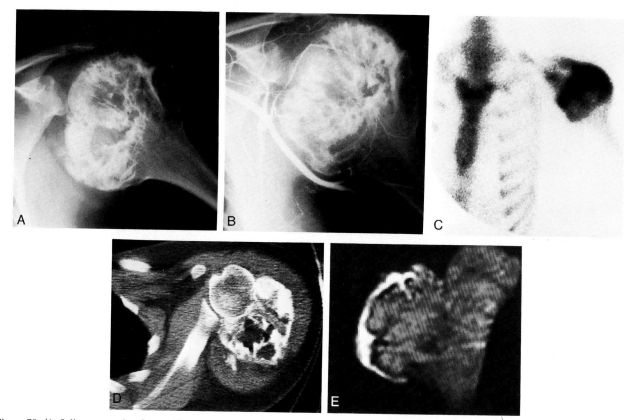

Figure 78–41. Solitary osteochondroma: Computed tomographic, scintigraphic, angiographic, and magnetic resonance imaging abnormalities. The conventional radiograph **(A)** shows a large, calcified lesion involving and extending from the proximal portion of the humerus. On an angiogram **(B)**, displacement of vessels is apparent, but there is no neovascularity. Intense uptake of the radionuclide at the site of the lesion is evident on a bone scan **(C)**. Computed tomography **(D)** confirms the extensive size of the calcified, posteriorly located lesion, which contains irregular radiolucent areas. Magnetic resonance imaging **(E)** following surgical removal of the specimen reveals a relatively smooth and thin cartilaginous cap.

plications, including arterial or venous stenosis and pseudo-aneurysms, are less frequent. Almost all the pseudoaneurysms complicating osteochondromas have arisen in the proximal portion of the popliteal artery. Such pseudoaneurysms tend to occur in the popliteal region for two reasons: (1) the most common locations for osteochondromas are the lower metaphysis of the femur and the upper metaphysis of the tibia; and (2) both the proximal and distal portions of the popliteal artery in this region are fixed in position. Correct diagnosis relies on arteriography.

Neurologic Compromise. Exostoses of the spine or, rarely, the head of a rib may lead to compression of the spinal cord or nerve roots or, in the case of lower spinal osteochondromas, the cauda equina.

Bursa Formation. A bursal compartment may surround the tip of an osteochondroma, especially when it is large. The bursa may subsequently become inflamed. Routine radiography may reveal a soft tissue mass, new areas of calcification, and irregularities in the osteochondroma, findings reminiscent of malignant transformation. Ultrasonography may document a cystic mass that may contain multiple intrabursal bodies. The latter reflect the presence of secondary synovial chondrometaplasia in the bursal lining with resultant osteocartilaginous nodules.

Malignant Transformation. Estimates of the risk of malignant transformation of an osteochondroma vary from 1 to

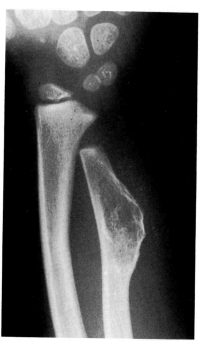

Figure 78–42. Solitary osteochondroma: Complications—osseous deformity. An osteochondroma in the distal portion of the ulna has led to shortening of the bone with deformity of the wrist.

25 per cent. The likelihood of such transformation is greater in patients with multiple osteochondromas, and the resulting malignant tumor most commonly is a chondrosarcoma, although examples of malignant fibrous histiocytoma and osteosarcoma occurring in this setting are documented. It appears likely that a more accurate estimate of the risk of malignant transformation of a solitary osteochondroma is about 1 per cent.

Although there are clinical guidelines (such as pain, swelling, and a soft tissue mass) and routine radiologic findings (such as the growth of a previously stable osteochondroma, bone erosion, and irregular or scattered calcification) that aid in the identification of such malignant transformation, they are not entirely reliable. Bone scintigraphy represents an effective method for defining those osteochondromas that are active metabolically (Fig. 78–43) but does not allow differentiation of the endochondral ossification occurring in a benign osteochondroma and the osteoblastic reaction occurring in a peripheral chondrosarcoma. A normal bone scan, however, virtually excludes the diagnosis of malignant transformation of an exostosis. Computed tomography (Fig. 78–43) has met with variable success in differentiation of a benign from a malignant osteochondroma. The reliability of this method to determine the thickness of the cartilage cap is inconsistent. This is unfortunate as peripheral chondrosarcomas generally possess a cartilage cap that is thicker than 1 cm and commonly greater than 2 cm, whereas in benign exostoses, the thickness is usually less than 1 cm. Variations in the thicknesses of the cartilage cap in both the benign and the malignant lesions, however, have been reported.

Differential Diagnosis. The radiographic features of a solitary osteochondroma usually are easily differentiated from findings associated with an osteoma, osteophyte, enthesophyte, heterotopic ossification, and parosteal osteosarcoma. Osteochondromas or osteochondroma-like lesions are encountered occasionally in systemic disorders, such as pseudohypoparathyroidism, pseudopseudohypoparathyroidism, and myositis (fibrodysplasia) ossificans progressiva, and in various congenital diseases (see Chapter 74).

The major difficulty in differential diagnosis arises in distinguishing between a benign osteochondroma and a peripheral chondrosarcoma. The entire spectrum of peripheral chondrosarcoma will be addressed in a subsequent portion of this chapter.

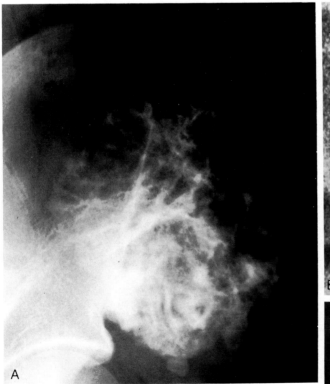
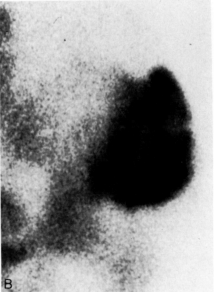
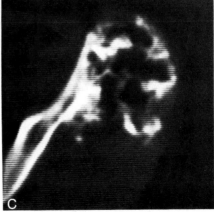

Figure 78–43. Solitary osteochondroma: Complications—malignant transformation. A The routine radiograph shows a large sessile outgrowth arising from the ilium. **B** A bone scan reveals nonuniform increased accumulation of the radionuclide in the lesion. **C** Transaxial computed tomography shows that the posteriorly located lesion is irregular in outline and contains multiple regions of low attenuation. Biopsy confirmed the presence of a chondrosarcoma.

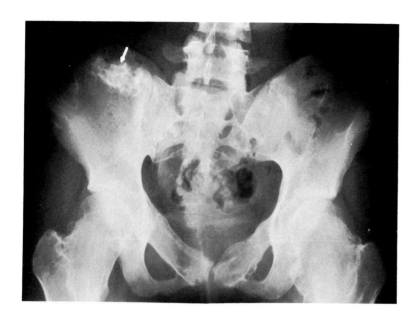

Figure 78–44. Hereditary multiple exostoses: Radiographic abnormalities. The radiograph reveals bilateral coxa valga deformity, widening of the femoral metaphyses, and multiple osteochondromas in the femora and innominate bones. Observe a large lesion (arrow) arising from the ilium.

HEREDITARY MULTIPLE EXOSTOSES. Hereditary multiple exostoses, an autosomal dominant disorder that is also discussed in Chapter 74, leads to clinical abnormalities in the first or second decade of life, including palpable osseous protuberances, shortening and bowing of bones, and joint restriction. Typical sites of osteochondromas are the distal and proximal portions of the femur, tibia, and fibula and the proximal portion of the humerus. It is virtually impossible to establish the diagnosis of this disease if exostoses are not present in the bones about the knee. Compared with the distribution of solitary osteochondromas, there is a greater tendency for involvement of the scapula, innominate bone (Fig. 78–44), and ribs in cases of multiple exostoses.

Highly characteristic of this disease is the occurrence of defects in normal modeling of bone and osseous deformities (Figs. 78–44 and 78–45). Of particular note is the presence of bilateral coxa valga and widening of the proximal femoral metaphysis (Fig. 78–44), and, in the wrist, of ulnar deviation, relative shortening of the ulna, bowing of the bones of the forearm, and shortening of the forearm. Clearly, an effective radiographic survey designed to delineate some of the more dramatic findings of hereditary multiple exostoses would include frontal radiographs of the knees (to demonstrate the osteochondromas), the pelvis (to define the metaphyseal changes in the femora), and the wrist (to document the presence of osseous deformities).

The complications associated with hereditary exostoses are identical in scope to but generally more frequent than the complications that accompany solitary osteochondromas and include (in addition to the osseous deformity) fracture, vascular injury, neurologic compromise, bursa formation, and malignant transformation (Fig. 78–46). The frequency of the last complication is probably about 5 per cent and is certainly greater than the frequency of malignant transformation in solitary osteochondromas. The resulting chondrosarcomas are especially frequent in the femur, humerus, tibia, and innominate bone.

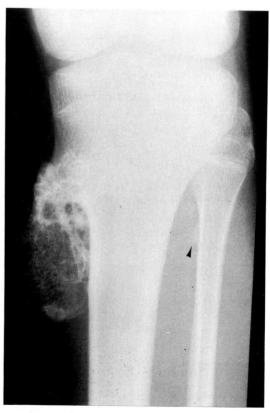

Figure 78–45. Hereditary multiple exostoses: Radiographic abnormalities. A radiograph shows widening of the tibial metaphysis, a small osteochondroma (arrowhead) in the fibula, and a large outgrowth arising from the proximal portion of the tibia.

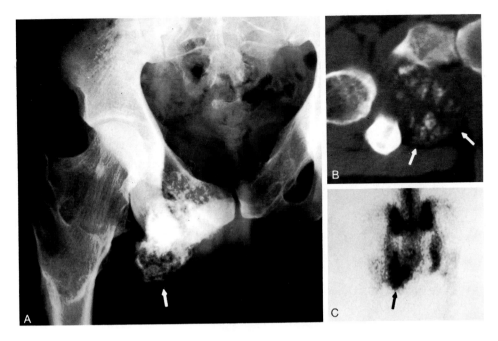

Figure 78–46. Hereditary multiple exostoses: Complications—malignant transformation. A Observe multiple exostoses of the femur and innominate bones and widening of the femoral neck. A large and irregular lesion (arrow) is seen adjacent to the ischium. **B** Transaxial computed tomography documents the size of the lesion (arrows) and internal calcification. **C** The bone scan shows increased scintigraphic activity at the site of the lesion (arrow). A chondrosarcoma was the final histologic diagnosis. (Courtesy of T. Broderick, M.D., Orange, California.)

DYSPLASIA EPIPHYSEALIS HEMIMELICA (TREVOR'S DISEASE). Dysplasia epiphysealis hemimelica (see Chapter 79) usually becomes evident in children and young adults and is more common in men than in women. Typical clinical manifestations include swelling, pain, and deformity, which usually are localized to one side of the body. Lower extremity involvement is far more frequent than upper extremity involvement. The talus, distal portion of the femur, and distal and proximal regions of the tibia are principal sites of abnormality. Multiple bones (in a single extremity) are affected in 60 to 70 per cent of cases. Dysplasia epiphysealis hemimelica involves primarily one side of an epiphysis.

The radiographic findings are characteristic. In an infant or young child, irregular ossifications are seen adjacent to one side of an ossifying epiphysis (or carpal or tarsal bone). The adjoining metaphysis may be widened. Subsequently, the ossifications become confluent with the adjacent bone, eventually appearing as a lobulated osseous mass protruding from the epiphysis (or carpal or tarsal bone). The final appearance resembles that of an osteochondroma with the affected area (or areas) remaining large and irregular. In severe cases, muscle wasting, growth disturbance, and joint deformity are identified.

The histologic features of the lesion are identical to those of an osteochondroma.

OTHER OSTEOCHONDROMAS OR OSTEOCHONDROMA-LIKE LESIONS. A *subungual exostosis* is an uncommon, benign bone tumor arising in the distal phalanx of a digit, near the nailbed. It usually occurs in patients who are in the second or third decade of life. Clinical manifestations include pain, swelling, and ulcerations of the nailbed. The great toe is involved in 70 to 80 per cent of cases. Radiographically, the lesion is approximately 1 cm in diameter and projects from the dorsomedial aspect of the distal portion of a terminal phalanx (Fig. 78–47). Histologically, the lesion consists of a base of trabecular bone with a proliferating fibrocartilaginous cap, features that differ from those of a

typical osteochondroma. Subungual exostoses are uniformly benign and local excision is the treatment of choice.

A *turret exostosis* is an infrequent osseous excrescence that typically arises on the dorsal surface of a proximal or middle phalanx in a finger. A traumatic event is followed by pain and soft tissue swelling or a lump. The mass may grow for a period of months and lead to loss of flexion of joints distal to the exostosis. Radiographs reveal soft tissue swelling and, subsequently, a broad-based bone protuberance on the dorsal surface of the affected phalanx. It is likely that a turret exostosis represents an ossifying, subperiosteal hematoma.

A *supracondylar (supracondyloid) process* of the humerus represents an outgrowth of bone that occurs on the antero-

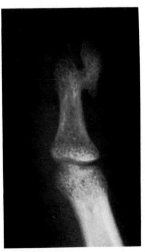

Figure 78–47. Subungual exostosis: Radiographic abnormalities. Note the osseous protuberance extending beneath the nail.

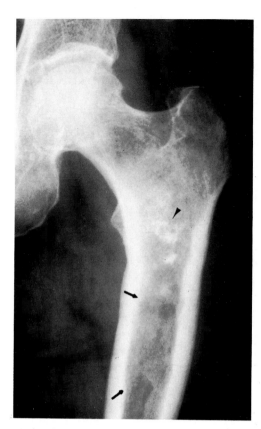

Figure 78–48. Conventional chondrosarcoma, central type: Radiographic abnormalities—long tubular bones. The routine radiograph reveals an elongated, central lesion of the diaphysis of the femur. Proximally it contains calcification (arrowhead), whereas distally osteolysis is evident without calcification (between arrows). Note endosteal erosion of the cortex.

medial surface of the distal portion of the humerus, approximately 5 to 7 cm above the medial epicondyle. It is believed to represent a phylogenetic vestige of the supracondyloid foramen found in reptiles and some mammals. The supracondylar process is variable in size, and it may afford insertion to a persistent part of the coracobrachialis muscle as well as an anomalous origin of the pronator teres muscle. A band of fibrous tissue, the ligament of Struthers, may join the tip of the supracondylar process and the medial epicondyle. Compression of the median nerve is one of the complications of this process.

Malignant Tumors
Chondrosarcoma

Malignant cartilage tumors may be categorized according to their precise location within the bone (central, peripheral, and juxtacortical chondrosarcomas); their occurrence as an initial (de novo) lesion (primary chondrosarcoma) or as a lesion superimposed on a preexistent process, such as an osteochondroma or enchondroma (secondary chondrosarcoma); their degree of cellular differentiation (low grade, medium grade, and high grade chondrosarcomas); the presence of unusual histologic characteristics (clear cell and mesenchymal chon-

drosarcomas); and the occurrence of changes in these histologic characteristics (dedifferentiated chondrosarcoma).

CONVENTIONAL CHONDROSARCOMA. In this category can be considered those malignant tumors that arise within the medullary cavity either de novo or as a secondary complication of a preexisting enchondroma (central chondrosarcoma) and those that arise near the surface of the bone (peripheral chondrosarcoma). Peripheral chondrosarcomas are sometimes divided further into two groups: those developing from a preexisting osteochondroma (exostotic chondrosarcomas) and those originating from the periosteal membrane (juxtacortical or periosteal chondrosarcomas).

Clinical Abnormalities. Conventional chondrosarcomas occur more frequently in men than in women. The average age of persons with chondrosarcoma is approximately 40 to 45 years; patients with this tumor generally are between the ages of 30 and 60 years. Pain of 1 or 2 years' duration is the most characteristic presenting symptom of a chondrosarcoma. A pathologic fracture is the initial manifestation in approximately 3 per cent of patients.

Skeletal Location. The long tubular bones are the sites of involvement in approximately 45 per cent of cases, with the femur being the most commonly affected bone. Other common locations of these tumors are the innominate bone (25 per cent of cases) and the ribs (8 per cent of cases). Less frequent sites of involvement are the vertebrae, scapula, and sternum, and rarely affected sites include the skull, mandible, maxilla, fibula, radius, ulna, clavicle, patella, and small bones of the hand and foot. Most chondrosarcomas in the long tubular bones are located in the metaphysis, but, with closure of the physis, tumor extension into the epiphysis is encountered. Excluding hematologic tumors, chondrosarcomas are the most frequent malignant neoplasm of the scapula, ribs, sternum, and small bones of the hand. Chondrosarcomas in the ribs or sternum typically arise near the costochondral junction.

Radiographic Abnormalities. The precise radiographic diagnosis of chondrosarcoma depends on a number of characteristic features, the most important of which is tumoral calcification. Other changes, including the patterns of bone destruction, cortical violation, and periostitis, are more variable. Radiographic alterations that imply tumor aggressiveness relate to the pattern of calcification, the nature of the tumoral margin, and the size of the soft tissue mass. Well-organized calcific rings within cartilage usually signify a low grade tumor. High grade chondrosarcomas frequently are associated with large areas of noncalcified tumor matrix. Furthermore, when calcification occurs within high grade chondrosarcomas, it typically is amorphous, scattered, or irregular. A poorly defined boundary with a long zone of transition between the abnormal and normal portions of the bone is indicative of an aggressive or high grade chondrosarcoma. The size and nature of the soft tissue component of the tumor are less useful predictors of its malignant potential.

Central Chondrosarcoma. Central chondrosarcomas occur in both the tubular bones (particularly the femur and the humerus) and the flat and irregular bones (especially those in the pelvis). With involvement of the appendicular skeleton, radiographs typically reveal an elongated, slightly expansile, multilobulated osteolytic lesion accompanied by periosteal bone formation, cortical thickening, endosteal bone erosion,

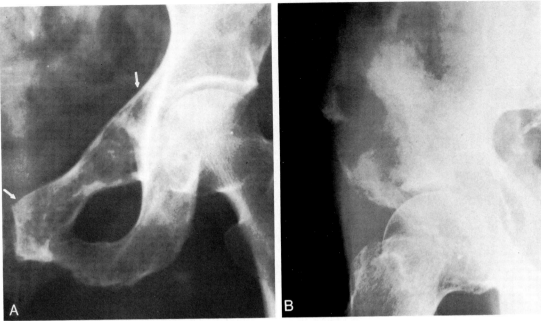

Figure 78–49. Conventional chondrosarcoma, central type: Radiographic abnormalities—innominate bone. A The elongated osteolytic lesion (between arrows) contains focal calcification. Note erosion of the cortex. B In a second case, a large, mixed osteolytic and osteosclerotic lesion in the ilium is associated with articular involvement and a pathologic fracture.

and, in 60 to 70 per cent of cases, scattered stippled or irregular calcification (Fig. 78–48). The pattern of bone destruction is variable. In some cases, obvious features of aggressive behavior, such as poorly defined osteolysis, cortical violation, and a soft tissue mass, are observed; however, more frequently, the radiographic abnormalities are those of a slowly evolving process. In the flat and irregular bones (Fig. 78–49), chondrosarcomas reveal similar radiographic features, although soft tissue involvement may be more pronounced.

Peripheral Chondrosarcoma. Peripheral chondrosarcomas most commonly arise from a preexisting osteochondroma or, rarely, from the periosteal membrane in the form of a juxtacortical chondrosarcoma (see later discussion), and they may occur in flat, irregular, or tubular bones (Fig. 78–43). In distinguishing between a benign osteochondroma and one that has undergone malignant transformation, features suggestive of malignancy are a bulky cartilaginous cap, an irregular or indistinct surface to the calcified tissue beneath the cartilaginous cap, scattered calcifications in the cartilaginous part of the tumor, focal areas of radiolucency in the interior of the osteochondroma, a significant soft tissue mass, and destruction or pressure erosion of the adjacent bone. The presence of a soft tissue mass, scattered and irregular calcification, and rapid growth of an osteochondroma are strong indicators of malignant transformation.

Other Imaging Techniques. In the evaluation of central chondrosarcomas, increased accumulation of the bone-seeking radionuclide at the site of tumor is uniformly present. In cases of peripheral chondrosarcoma, bone scanning allows documentation of those osteochondromas that are metabolically active but is unreliable in differentiating between those tumors that are benign and those that are malignant. Absence

of uptake of the bone-seeking agent virtually eliminates the possibility of malignant transformation of an osteochondroma.

Computed tomography has also been used in the analysis of central and peripheral chondrosarcomas (Fig. 78–50). Eccentric, lobular growth of a soft tissue mass generally indicates a low grade tumor; high grade chondrosarcomas more characteristically extend in all directions within the soft tissue and do not respect anatomic boundaries. In peripheral chondrosarcomas, computed tomography has been used with varying degrees of success to define the thickness of the cartilage cap of the underlying osteochondroma. Magnetic resonance imaging also is invaluable in assessing the osseous and soft tissue extent of both central and peripheral chondrosarcomas (Fig. 78–50).

Angiography can be used to define preoperatively the extent of the tumor and its relationship to adjacent vasculature.

Pathologic Abnormalities. Chondrosarcomas tend to be relatively bulky tumors, particularly in the flat and irregular bones. Central chondrosarcomas frequently erode the cortex and extend into the soft tissue. The cartilaginous caps of peripheral chondrosarcomas commonly are greater than 2 cm in thickness; such caps in a benign osteochondroma in an adult are usually less than 1 cm thick, whereas in children and adolescents, the thickness of the cartilaginous cap of a benign exostosis may be as great as 2.5 or 3 cm.

Chondrosarcomas usually are classified histologically into four grades, I to IV, with the lower numbers indicating the better differentiated or less aggressive tumors; most chondrosarcomas are classified as grade I or II. In general, chondrosarcomas contain many round to oval cells with plump nuclei with a distinct chromatin pattern, numerous binucleated cells, and giant tumor cells with single or multiple large nuclei.

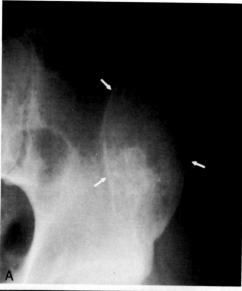

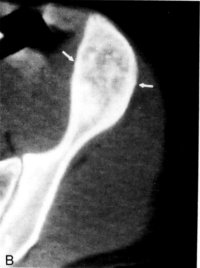

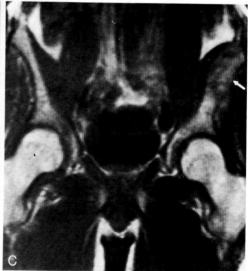

Figure 78–50. Conventional chondrosarcoma, central type: Computed tomographic and magnetic resonance imaging abnormalities. **A** A radiograph reveals a large lesion of the ilium (arrows) with a hazy interior and calcification. **B** Transaxial computed tomography shows the calcification within the lesion and osseous expansion (arrows). **C** A coronal magnetic resonance image (TE, 30 ms; TR, 0.55 s) documents that the iliac lesion has decreased signal intensity (arrow). A low signal intensity also was present on the T2 weighted images. A biopsy and subsequent excision of the lesion confirmed the presence of a low grade chondrosarcoma.

The usual criteria for the diagnosis of a chondrosarcoma do not apply to the cartilaginous tumors in the bones of the hands and feet. Enchondromas in these sites may have the cellular features of a grade II chondrosarcoma.

Chondrosarcomas usually are composed of lobules of cartilage. Low grade, well-differentiated chondrosarcomas contain an abundance of hyaline-like cartilage. Well-differentiated chondrosarcomas also possess areas of calcification and degeneration; such calcification is less frequent in the poorly differentiated neoplasms.

Natural History. It is well recognized that chondrosarcomas have the potential to be locally infiltrative and, in some cases, to metastasize through the blood stream to distant organs. Locally aggressive manifestations of chondrosarcoma include intraosseous extension, transarticular spread, and soft tissue invasion. These manifestations as well as systemic metastasis increase in frequency with higher grades of neoplasms. Tumor recurrence is also correlated with histologic

grade and adequacy of treatment; an increase in malignant potential is observed in approximately 10 per cent of such recurrences, accompanied by dedifferentiation of the tumor into a high grade spindle cell sarcoma (see later discussion). The reported overall rate of survival for a period of 10 years following treatment has varied from 30 to 70 per cent.

Differential Diagnosis. The differentiation of a central chondrosarcoma and an enchondroma in a tubular bone may be extremely difficult, although poorly defined osteolysis, a soft tissue mass, and the absence of calcification in a part of the lesion are radiographic findings more compatible with a chondrosarcoma. Similarly, the differentiation of a peripheral chondrosarcoma and a simple osteochondroma commonly is not possible on the basis of the conventional radiographic examination.

In the flat or irregular bones, a large osteolytic lesion with a soft tissue mass in an adult patient is compatible with a chondrosarcoma, plasmacytoma, lymphoma, solitary skeletal

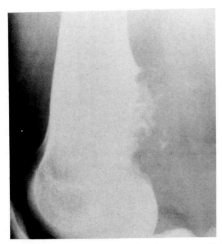

Figure 78–51. Juxtacortical (periosteal) chondrosarcoma: Radiographic abnormalities. A lateral radiograph reveals calcification adjacent to the posterior surface of the distal metaphysis of the femur with cortical thickening and a Codman's triangle. (Courtesy of S. Kursunoglu, M.D., San Diego, California.)

larger lesions, tumor extension into the metaphysis is frequent; primary involvement of the metaphysis is unusual and that of the diaphysis is exceedingly rare. This pattern of distribution is similar to that of a chondroblastoma. The most common site of involvement is the proximal portion of the femur, followed in order of decreasing frequency by the proximal portions of the humerus and the tibia.

Radiographic Abnormalities. Clear cell chondrosarcomas are predominantly osteolytic and slightly expansile. The margin of the tumor may be either poorly defined or well defined, with a sclerotic border. The reported frequency of calcification has varied, although in some cases the calcification is prominent. Endosteal erosion, cortical violation, pathologic fracture, and a soft tissue mass represent additional radiographic findings that are evident in some cases.

The radiographic features as well as the typical epiphyseal location in a tubular bone (Fig. 78–52) are identical to those of a chondroblastoma, and differentiation of these two neoplasms on the basis of radiographic abnormalities may be extremely difficult. The presence of metaphyseal involvement and the absence of periostitis are findings that favor the diagnosis of a clear cell chondrosarcoma.

focus of metastasis, and even an unusual infection, such as echinococcosis. More specific in such cases is the identification of calcification, although its differentiation from ossification, as might be seen in an osteosarcoma, may not be accomplished easily.

JUXTACORTICAL (PERIOSTEAL) CHONDROSARCOMA. A juxtacortical (periosteal) chondrosarcoma has a clinical and radiologic appearance similar to that of a periosteal osteosarcoma, leading many investigators to the conclusion that they are identical neoplasms. A long tubular bone, especially the femur, typically is affected, and the radiographic alterations include a small lesion on the osseous surface accompanied by spotty calcification, radiating bone spicules, and a typical Codman's triangle (Fig. 78–51).

Microscopically, chondroblastic elements are the dominant abnormality, with tumor osteoid and bone being conspicuously absent; however, the production of osteoid by a periosteal osteosarcoma may be very limited, and the ultimate classification of the neoplasm as a periosteal osteosarcoma or juxtacortical chondrosarcoma depends on the manner in which the cartilaginous and osseous tissue is interpreted. The prognosis of juxtacortical chondrosarcoma is favorable.

CLEAR CELL CHONDROSARCOMA. This rare low grade cartilaginous neoplasm possesses a distinctive histologic appearance, being termed a clear cell chondrosarcoma on the basis of its constituent tumor cells.

Clinical Abnormalities. Clear cell chondrosarcoma occurs more frequently in men; it may be evident at any age but usually is seen in the third, fourth, or fifth decade of life. Symptoms include localized pain and limited range of motion in the adjacent joint. Pathologic fractures occur in approximately 25 per cent of cases.

Skeletal Location. Clear cell chondrosarcomas predominate in the long tubular bones (approximately 85 per cent of cases), particularly the femur and the humerus. In the tubular bones, epiphyseal localization is the rule, although, with

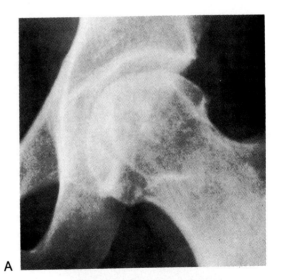

A

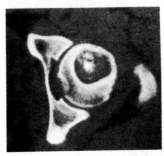

B

Figure 78–52. Clear cell chondrosarcoma: Radiographic and computed tomographic abnormalities. **A** A routine radiograph delineates a large, well-defined osteolytic lesion involving the femoral head and extending into the femoral neck. It contains central calcification and a peripheral sclerotic margin and has led to subtle collapse of the articular surface. **B** A transaxial computed tomographic scan shows the calcified lesion in the femoral head.

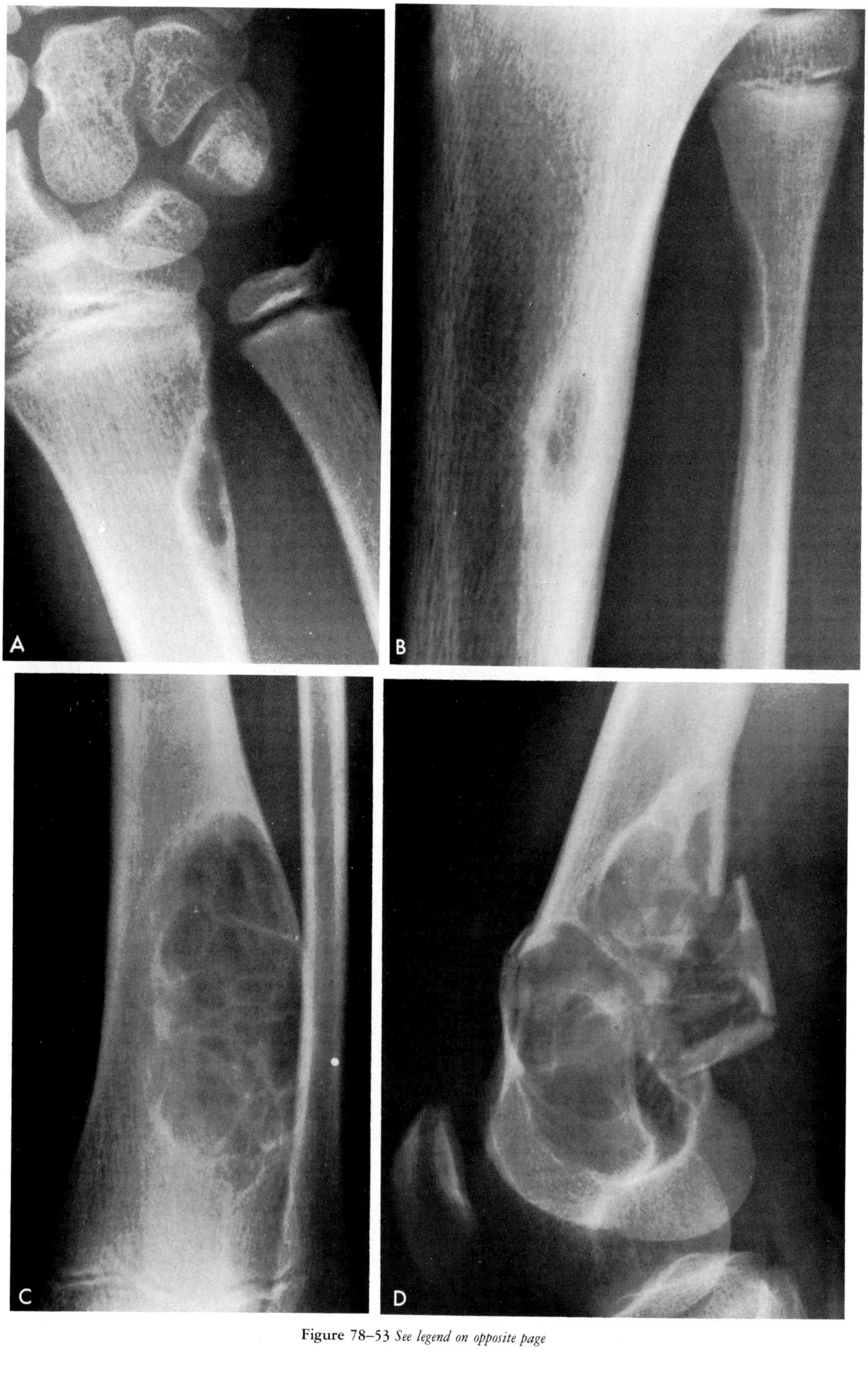

Figure 78–53 *See legend on opposite page*

Pathologic Abnormalities. The cells in this tumor have an abundant clear, glycogen-rich cytoplasm with distinct borders. In some cases, however, the histologic features of clear cell chondrosarcoma resemble those of other neoplasms. In fact, regions of conventional chondrosarcoma are found in approximately 50 per cent of these tumors. In clear cell chondrosarcomas, thin strands of calcium may be evident between the cartilage cells, creating a chicken-wire pattern, as is evident in chondroblastoma, or seams of lace-like osteoid are identified, as in an osteosarcoma.

Natural History. Clear cell chondrosarcomas are relatively slow growing, low grade malignant tumors with a much better prognosis than that of conventional chondrosarcomas. Local extension, tumor recurrence, or disseminated metastases may be seen, however.

Differential Diagnosis. Bone lesions that radiographically may resemble clear cell chondrosarcoma are chondroblastoma, aneurysmal bone cyst, osteoblastoma, giant cell tumor, plasmacytoma, skeletal metastasis, and the brown tumor of hyperparathyroidism. It is the differentiation of clear cell chondrosarcoma and chondroblastoma that is most difficult; an older age of onset, the presence of metaphyseal involvement, and the absence of periostitis are more characteristic of the former tumor. Although malignant transformation of a chondroblastoma has been described (see previous discussion), the resulting tumor has histologic features that resemble those of a conventional chondrosarcoma rather than a clear cell chondrosarcoma.

MESENCHYMAL CHONDROSARCOMA. Although relatively rare, mesenchymal chondrosarcomas represent one of the few primary malignant tumors of bone that not infrequently also arise in the soft tissues (30 to 75 per cent of cases).

Clinical Abnormalities. Men and women are affected in approximately equal numbers; the majority of affected patients are in the second, third, and fourth decades of life. Patients with mesenchymal chondrosarcomas typically are younger than those with conventional chondrosarcomas and similar in age to those with conventional osteosarcomas. Pain, swelling, a soft tissue mass, and stiffness are the most typical clinical manifestations.

Skeletal Location. The most frequent sites of involvement are the femur, ribs, and spine, followed in order of decreasing frequency by the skull, maxilla, innominate bone, humerus, tibia, mandible, calcaneus, and other bones.

Radiographic Abnormalities. Osteolysis, a permeative pattern of bone destruction, an irregular outline, bone sclerosis, periostitis, and intralesional calcification are among the most characteristic of the varied radiographic features of this neoplasm. All of the radiographic abnormalities resemble those of a typical chondrosarcoma; it is the relatively young age of the patient that may allow a more specific diagnosis of a mesenchymal chondrosarcoma.

Pathologic Abnormalities. Soft tissue and skeletal mesenchymal chondrosarcomas have an identical histomorphology. An accurate microscopic diagnosis depends on the presence of two components: undifferentiated stromal cells and islands of cartilage.

Natural History. Mesenchymal chondrosarcomas represent an aggressive variant of chondrosarcoma characterized by a poor prognosis. The tendency of this tumor to metastasize to regional and distant lymph nodes and to other bones is quite uncharacteristic of ordinary chondrosarcoma.

Differential Diagnosis. Radiographically, it generally is not possible to differentiate this neoplasm from a conventional chondrosarcoma.

DEDIFFERENTIATED CHONDROSARCOMA. Chondrosarcoma with dedifferentiated foci represents a variant of conventional chondrosarcoma of bone in which a highly anaplastic sarcoma is associated with a borderline or low grade malignant cartilage tumor. The importance of recognizing this dedifferentiated neoplasm relates to its frequency of occurrence (approximately 10 per cent of all chondrosarcomas), its locally aggressive behavior, and, ultimately, its poor prognosis.

Clinical Abnormalities. Men and women in the fifth, sixth, and seventh decades of life generally are affected. Pain is the most frequent symptom. Soft tissue swelling or a mass and pathologic fractures are additional, common clinical manifestations.

Skeletal Location. Dedifferentiated chondrosarcomas reveal a similar distribution to that of conventional chondrosarcomas. The femur, humerus, and innominate bone account for the majority of cases.

Radiographic Abnormalities. Typically, an osteolytic lesion with motheaten bone destruction is observed; the lesion is partially calcified, although, in one region, such calcification is sparse or entirely absent. These noncalcified areas commonly reveal the most aggressive bone destruction, with erosion and penetration of the cortex, soft tissue swelling, and, in some cases, a pathologic fracture.

The accurate radiographic diagnosis of a dedifferentiated chondrosarcoma relies on the identification within the lesion of two characteristic patterns. The first is indicative of a low grade chondrosarcoma; the second is indicative of the dedifferentiated and more aggressive portion of the tumor. The second diagnostic possibility of a sarcoma developing in an area of osteonecrosis also must be considered.

Pathologic Abnormalities. Histologically, dedifferentiated chondrosarcomas contain evidence of a low grade con-

Figure 78–53. Nonossifying fibroma: Radiographic abnormalities—spectrum of changes. A This eccentric, radiolucent lesion in the radius possesses a sclerotic inner margin. It is located a short distance from the physis. **B** Nonossifying fibromas (or fibrous cortical defects) are identified in the proximal portions of the tibia and the fibula. Note their eccentric location and the geographic bone destruction. The nonossifying fibroma of the fibula is located a short distance from the neighboring growth plate. **C** A large, nonossifying fibroma of the distal portion of the tibia has produced deformity of the adjacent fibula. Note the eccentric location, geographic bone destruction, radiolucent lesion with lobulated trabeculation, internal sclerotic border, and cortical expansion. This lesion, too, is located a short distance from the neighboring physis. **D** This large nonossifying fibroma of the distal portion of the femur has led to a spontaneous fracture. Its upper border indicates its eccentric location.

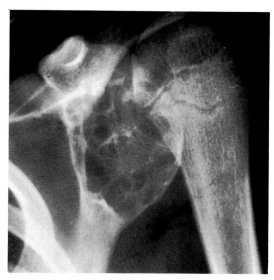

Figure 78–54. Nonossifying fibroma: Radiographic abnormalities—flat bone. An expansile, trabeculated, osteolytic lesion of the scapula is associated with osseous expansion. In addition to a nonossifying fibroma, an aneurysmal bone cyst and a chondroblastoma would represent diagnostic possibilities.

ventional chondrosarcoma and, in juxtaposition, an anaplastic sarcoma. The specific characteristics of the primitive or anaplastic tissue may be indicative of a fibrosarcoma, osteosarcoma, malignant fibrous histiocytoma, angiosarcoma, or rhabdomyosarcoma, in order of decreasing frequency.

TUMORS ARISING FROM OR FORMING FIBROUS CONNECTIVE TISSUE
Benign Tumors
Nonossifying Fibroma

Nonossifying fibroma and the related fibrous cortical (fibrocortical) defect are common lesions composed histologically of whorled bundles of connective tissue cells. The former designation is more appropriately applied to a larger lesion, whereas the latter designation is more suited for the description of a smaller, asymptomatic osseous abnormality.

An unrecognized traumatic insult to the periosteum, resulting in focal hemorrhage and edema, is consistent with both the natural history of fibrous cortical defects and their propensity to occur at osseous sites of muscular attachment. Evidence for an inflammatory or neoplastic cause is less compelling.

Clinical Abnormalities. Small, cortical fibrous lesions in the tubular bones are encountered regularly during radiographic examination of healthy children. Generally, the lesions are silent clinically. Their rarity in children less than 2 years of age is consistent with the belief that muscle pull during weight-bearing and walking is important in their pathogenesis, and their infrequency in adults supports the concept that most lesions heal by being replaced by normal bone. Some become quite large and may lead to pathologic fracture, however.

Skeletal Location. It is generally believed that the anatomic locations of fibrous cortical defects are very similar or identical to those of nonossifying fibromas. The smaller lesions (fibrous cortical defects), however, may occur at either a single site or in multiple locations in one or more bones, whereas the larger lesions (nonossifying fibromas) are far less commonly multifocal. Symmetry of involvement is characteristic of a bilateral distribution.

The long tubular bones are affected predominantly (approximately 90 per cent of cases). The tibia and the femur are the most frequent sites of involvement. Fibrous cortical defects and nonossifying fibromas in the bones of the upper extremity are uncommon. Involvement of the radius, ulna, ribs, innominate bone, clavicle, skull, mandible, scapula, and small bones of the hand and foot is rare.

In the tubular bones, fibrous cortical defects and nonossifying fibromas are predominantly metaphyseal lesions arising close to the physeal plate. If they do not involute during skeletal growth, they may extend into the diaphysis. Epiphyseal localization is distinctly unusual. In the femur, the vast majority of lesions affect the distal metaphyseal region. The bones about the knee account for about 55 per cent of all lesions. Fibrous cortical defects and nonossifying fibromas usually arise from the posterior wall of the tubular bone and affect the medial (rather than the lateral) osseous surface far more frequently.

Radiographic Abnormalities. Fibrous cortical defects and small nonossifying fibromas produce focal, shallow radiolucent areas in the cortex with normal or sclerotic adjacent bone and, in some instances, a blister-like peripheral osseous shell (Fig. 78–53). The lesions are oval and are not accompanied by significant periostitis. Characteristically, they arise in the metaphysis at a short distance from the physis or, less commonly, adjacent to the physeal plate. With growth of the tubular bone, apparent shaftward migration of the lesion may be accompanied by segmental sclerosis within a portion of the osseous defect. Larger lesions are more elongated, with a multiloculated appearance; cortical thinning or slight expansion may be evident.

These radiographic abnormalities are virtually diagnostic of a fibrous cortical defect or nonossifying fibroma. Other tumors and tumor-like lesions can generally be excluded, including an osteoid osteoma (a smaller radiolucent area in the cortex with more extensive cortical thickening), bone abscess (a lesion in the medullary or cortical bone with a thicker rim of sclerosis), periosteal chondroma (an eccentrically placed lesion leading to erosion of the external surface of the cortex and, perhaps, possessing calcification), chondromyxoid fibroma (a larger, trabeculated lesion abutting on the metaphysis that may extend into the epiphysis or diaphysis), avulsive cortical irregularity, or periosteal desmoid (a saucer-like radiolucent defect in the cortex with adjacent sclerosis and periostitis), desmoplastic fibroma (an aggressive osteolytic lesion with destruction of medullary bone, cortical erosion and expansion, and trabeculation), and aneurysmal bone cyst (a more expansile osteolytic lesion). In the flat and irregular bones (Fig. 78–54), nonossifying fibromas are more difficult to diagnose on the basis of the radiographic findings alone.

Pathologic Abnormalities. Fibrous cortical defects and nonossifying fibromas have an identical histomorphology. They are composed of uniform, spindle-shaped fibroblasts that are arranged in intersecting bands. Scattered within this fibrous stroma are multinucleated giant cells.

Natural History. Fibrous cortical defects and nonossifying fibromas are benign processes. In many instances, an orderly sequence of evolution and involution occurs. The initially small radiolucent lesions arising in the metaphysis may enlarge, migrate shaftward, shrink, develop sclerotic borders, and finally disappear. The relative infrequency of fibrous cortical defects and nonossifying fibromas in the mature skeleton compared with those in the immature skeleton, however, supports their typically self-limited nature. It is generally accepted that fibrous cortical defects and nonossifying fibromas do not appear for the first time in adults.

Complications. Although infrequent, several potential complications of fibrous cortical defects and nonossifying fibromas should be noted.

Pathologic Fracture. Pathologic fractures through larger nonossifying fibromas may be seen after minor trauma and are observed most frequently in the bones of the lower extremity (Fig. 78–53D). Such fractures generally heal in a normal fashion.

Osteomalacia and Rickets. As indicated in Chapter 48, hypophosphatemic vitamin D–refractory rickets and osteomalacia have been associated with a variety of soft tissue and osseous neoplasms. Nonossifying fibroma represents one of the bone neoplasms that can lead to these conditions. Hypophosphatemia is believed to be caused by a humoral substance elaborated by the tumor that decreases the threshold for renal resorption of phosphorus. The findings of rickets or osteomalacia disappear after removal of the tumor.

Extraskeletal Anomalies (Jaffe-Campanacci Syndrome). This syndrome consists of multiple nonossifying fibromas and extraskeletal congenital anomalies, including café-au-lait spots, mental retardation, hypogonadism or cryptorchidism, ocular abnormalities, and cardiovascular malformations. Radiographically, large, osteolytic lesions are observed in the long tubular bones; the natural history of the skeletal abnormalities is characterized by spontaneous resolution. A relationship of this condition to neurofibromatosis and giant cell reparative granulomas has been suggested.

Periosteal (Juxtacortical) Desmoid

As discussed in Chapter 76, a periosteal desmoid represents a tumor-like alteration of the periosteum, usually apparent in patients between the ages of 15 and 20 years. Almost all cases are localized to the posteromedial cortex of the distal end of the femur, adjacent to the femoral condyle. Most patients are asymptomatic. A history of local trauma is frequent. The radiographic characteristics include soft tissue swelling and a saucer-like defect of the cortex with adjacent sclerosis and periostitis; in some cases, the lesion may be mistaken for a malignant tumor. The periosteal desmoid, however, is not a neoplasm but a reaction to trauma occurring at the musculotendinous insertion site of the adductor magnus muscle.

Desmoplastic Fibroma

This is a rare benign neoplasm of bone that is characterized by abundant collagen formation and the absence of both significant cellularity and pleomorphism.

Clinical Abnormalities. Desmoplastic fibromas are most common in the second and third decades of life. Men and women are affected with equal frequency. Pain and swelling of weeks to months in duration are the major clinical manifestations.

Skeletal Location. Desmoplastic fibromas most typically arise in the mandible, long tubular bones (femur, humerus, tibia, and radius), and innominate bone (ilium). In the tubular bones, a central location in the metaphysis is most characteristic.

Radiographic Abnormalities. Desmoplastic fibromas are osteolytic lesions with a trabeculated, soap-bubble, or honeycomb pattern (Fig. 78–55). Endosteal erosion and limited periosteal bone formation may be accompanied by osseous expansion, with an appearance that may resemble that of nonossifying fibroma, chondromyxoid fibroma, giant cell tumor, aneurysmal bone cyst, or fibrous dysplasia. Desmoplastic fibromas occasionally become large and possess a more aggressive appearance; the possibility of a malignant tumor (e.g., fibrosarcoma, skeletal metastasis from thyroid or renal carcinoma) may be considered in these instances on the basis of the radiographic alterations.

Pathologic Abnormalities. Histologically, desmoplastic fibroma may be considered to be the intraosseous counterpart of the soft tissue desmoid tumor. A typical lesion is composed of uniform, small, spindle-shaped fibroblasts that have oval or elongated nuclei. The cells are separated by an abundant, collagenized stroma in which dense collagen bands may be arranged in intersecting patterns.

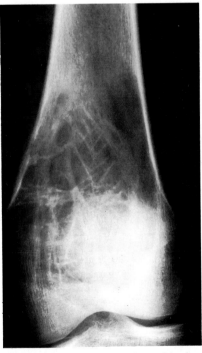

Figure 78–55. Desmoplastic fibroma: Radiographic abnormalities. A radiograph of the femur reveals a large, trabeculated, osteolytic lesion in the metaphysis and diaphysis of the bone. The endosteal margin of the cortex is eroded, and there is minimal periosteal response. The relatively central location of this lesion is more compatible with desmoplastic fibroma than with nonossifying fibroma or chondromyxoid fibroma.

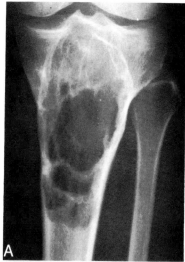

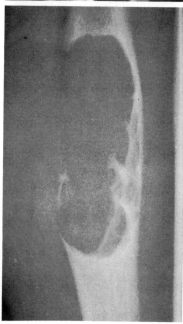

B

Figure 78–56. Fibrosarcoma: Radiographic abnormalities—long tubular bones (tibia). Two examples are shown. The epiphyseal and metaphyseal segments (**A**) or the diaphyseal segment (**B**) is affected. The lesions are osteolytic and in these cases possess a pattern of geographic bone destruction. Note the relative absence of periostitis. In **B**, observe a large tissue mass. (**A**, Courtesy of D. Wheeler, M.D., Flint, Michigan.)

Natural History. Although tumor recurrence may be evident after conservative surgery, wide resection of the lesion is usually curative.

Malignant Tumors

Fibrosarcoma

Fibrosarcoma, a rare malignant tumor of bone, is characterized histologically by poorly differentiated to well-differentiated fibrous tissue proliferation that is not associated with the production of cartilage, osteoid, or bone. Fibrosarcomas in bone can occur de novo or as a secondary phenomenon in

areas of Paget's disease, osteonecrosis, or chronic osteomyelitis, after irradiation, or related to dedifferentiation of other neoplasms, especially chondrosarcoma. An additional malignant tumor of bone, malignant fibrous histiocytoma (see later discussion) has only recently been differentiated from fibrosarcoma of bone.

Clinical Abnormalities. Fibrosarcomas of bone are observed in men and women with approximately equal frequency and are most common in the third through sixth decades of life. Clinical manifestations include local pain, swelling, and limitation of motion. Pathologic fractures are present at the time of the initial evaluation in approximately 33 per cent of patients.

Skeletal Location. The long tubular bones are involved in 70 per cent of cases; specific sites of involvement, in order of decreasing frequency, are the femur, tibia, humerus, fibula, radius, and ulna. The small bones of the hands and feet are rarely affected, and the osseous pelvis is involved in approximately 9 per cent of cases. The mandible and the maxilla are uncommon sites of fibrosarcomas.

In the tubular bones, a metaphyseal or metadiaphyseal location is the preferred site. Epiphyseal extension of a metaphyseal tumor is not infrequent.

Radiographic Abnormalities. Fibrosarcomas are characterized radiographically by (1) osteolytic foci with a geographic, motheaten, or permeative pattern of bone destruction, and (2) little osteoclerosis or periostitis (Fig. 78–56). Cortical destruction and soft tissue masses are seen. Visible tumor matrix is not evident, although dystrophic calcification and sequestered bone fragments may be encountered.

The radiographic abnormalities of fibrosarcomas of bone are not specific. Rather, they generally indicate an aggressive or malignant process. The absence of tumoral calcification or ossification in fibrosarcomas assumes diagnostic importance as

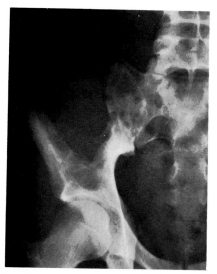

Figure 78–57. Fibrous histiocytoma: Radiographic abnormalities. A large, osteolytic lesion of the ilium is associated with sclerosis in the inferior aspect of the bone adjacent to the sacroiliac joint. The radiographic findings are not specific. (Courtesy of H. F. Holman, M.D., Maryville, Illinois.)

Table 78–3. DIFFERENTIAL DIAGNOSIS OF GIANT CELL LESIONS OF BONE

	Most Common Age Group	Location in Bone	Radiologic Appearance	Gross Features	Microscopic Features	
					Giant Cells	*Stromal Cells*
Giant cell tumor	Third and fourth decades	Epiphysis or metaphysis	Eccentric expanded radiolucent area	Fleshy soft tissue	Abundant number uniformly distributed	Plump and polyhedral cells with abundant cytoplasm
Nonossifying fibroma	First decade	Metaphysis	Eccentric oval defects	Fleshy soft tissue	Focal distribution, small with few nuclei	Slender and spindly cells with little cytoplasm; whorled pattern
Aneurysmal bone cyst	First and second decades	Vertebral column or metaphysis of long bone	Eccentric blow-out "soap bubble" appearance	Cavity filled with blood	Focal around vascular channels or hemorrhage	Large vascular channels; slender to plump cells with hemosiderin granules; metaplastic bone
Brown tumor of hyperparathyroidism	Any age	Anywhere in bone	Subperiosteal, subchondral, and subligamentous resorption of bone	Fleshy tissue or cystic spaces	Focal around hemosiderin pigment or hemorrhage	Fibrous stroma with slender spindle cells
Simple bone cyst	First and second decades	Metaphysis	Trabeculations in radiolucent area	Cyst filled with clear fluid	Focal around cholesterol clefts	Cyst wall of fibrous tissue; metaplastic bone
Chondroblastoma	Second decade	Epiphysis	Radiolucency with spotty opacities	Firm to fleshy tissue	Few and focal	Plump, and round or ovoid cells with pericellular calcifications
Fibrous dysplasia	First and second decades	Metaphysis	Ground-glass appearance	Firm and gritty	Few and focal	Woven bone and whorled fibrous tissue; no osteoblasts
Giant cell reparative granuloma	Second and third decades	Maxilla and mandible	Radiolucent focus	Soft fleshy tissue	Focal around hemosiderin pigment or hemorrhage	Slender or plump spindle cells
Ossifying fibroma	Second and third decades	Maxilla and mandible	Radiopaque	Firm and gritty	Few and focal	Lamellar bone trabeculae in fibrous tissue; osteoblastic rimming
Osteosarcoma	Second and third decades	Metaphysis	Radiolucent	Soft, firm, or hard	Focal distribution	Malignant cells with direct osteoid formation
Chondromyxoid fibroma	Second and third decades	Metaphysis	Eccentric with expanded cortex	Soft to firm	Focal distribution	Chondroid, myxoid, and fibrous lobules
Osteoblastoma	Second and third decades	Vertebral column; diaphysis of long bone	Radiolucent or dense	Hemorrhagic, gritty	Focal distribution	Abundant osteoid trabeculae with osteoblasts

Modified from Ghandur-Mnaymneh L, Mnaymneh WA: Bone lesions with giant cells: Problems in differential diagnosis. J Med Liban 25:91, 1972. Used with permission.

such findings are evident in chondrosarcomas and conventional osteosarcomas. Malignant fibrous histiocytoma, telangiectatic osteosarcoma, lymphoma, plasma cell myeloma, desmoplastic fibroma, and skeletal metastasis remain reasonable differential diagnostic possibilities in many cases of fibrosarcoma, however.

Pathologic Abnormalities. Fibrosarcomas are large, destructive, and infiltrating tumors. Histologically, they may be categorized as well-differentiated, moderately differentiated, or poorly differentiated neoplasms. The majority of fibrosarcomas are either moderately or poorly differentiated.

Well-differentiated fibrosarcomas are composed of elongated and spindle-shaped tumor cells with small and uniform tapered nuclei. The tumor cells characteristically are arranged in intersecting fascicles, producing a herringbone pattern. In less well differentiated fibrosarcomas, there is increased cellularity, and the herringbone pattern is less evident.

Natural History. Osseous fibrosarcomas are aggressive tumors with a tendency for one or more recurrences. Fibro-

sarcomas of bone carry a poorer prognosis than those of soft tissue and are similar in behavior to malignant fibrous histiocytomas.

HISTIOCYTIC OR FIBROHISTIOCYTIC TUMORS
Benign Tumors
Fibrous Histiocytoma

Fibrous histiocytoma (fibroxanthoma) (Fig. 78–57) is a term that has been used to describe a benign tumor of bone that histologically is similar or identical to nonossifying fibroma. Fibrous histiocytomas usually occur in patients older than 20 years of age, and many are accompanied by pain, localize in the sacrum or ilium, and involve epiphyseal and diaphyseal segments of the tubular bones; nonossifying fibromas are virtually confined to patients younger than 20 years of age, are painless, and predominate in the metaphyseal regions of tubular bones.

Fibrous histiocytomas are most frequent in the innominate and long tubular bones, ribs, and clavicle. The radiographic findings are not diagnostic; osteolysis, trabeculation and bone sclerosis are seen, and the resulting radiographic pattern may resemble that in nonossifying fibroma, fibrous dysplasia, enchondroma, eosinophilic granuloma, osteoblastoma, and chondromyxoid fibroma.

The lesion may behave in an aggressive fashion, with a potential for local spread and distant dissemination.

Locally Aggressive Tumors
Giant Cell Tumor*

This relatively common and locally aggressive lesion is composed of connective tissue, stromal cells, and giant cells, which vary in amount and appearance. It is the giant cell itself from which the name of this lesion is derived, but such cells are not specific for a giant cell tumor, being observed in a large number of neoplastic and nonneoplastic skeletal disorders (Table 78–3).

Clinical Abnormalities. Giant cell tumors usually are discovered in the third and fourth decades of life, although they may appear in older patients and in younger persons who have not yet ceased growing. The frequency of all types of giant cell tumors is approximately the same in men and women.

Pain is the most common symptom, followed in order of frequency by local swelling and limitation of motion in the adjacent articulation. The pain generally is of several months' duration. A pathologic fracture may be evident at the time of clinical presentation in approximately 10 per cent of patients. Neurologic symptoms may accompany spinal or sacral lesions.

Skeletal Location. Giant cell tumors predominate in the long tubular bones (75 to 90 per cent of all cases), especially the femur (approximately 30 per cent of cases), tibia (25 per cent of cases), radius (10 per cent of cases), and humerus (6 per cent of cases). The bones about the knee are affected in 50 to 65 per cent of giant cell tumors.

The spine (7 per cent of cases) and innominate bone (4 per cent of cases) are occasionally involved. In the vertebral column, it is the sacrum that is the most typical site of localization; giant cell tumors arising at spinal levels above the sacrum are uncommon.

Giant cell tumors are relatively rare in the skull. In the skull and the facial bones, giant cell tumors may be accompanied by Paget's disease (see Chapter 49) and, furthermore, in these locations, the identification of a giant cell tumor is complicated by the occurrence of a similar lesion, the giant cell reparative granuloma (see later discussion).

Approximately 5 per cent of giant cell tumors localize in the bones of the hands or, less commonly, the feet. Rarely, giant cell tumors occur in the ribs, scapula, patella, clavicle, and sternum.

In the tubular bones, giant cell tumors had long been considered an epiphyseal lesion, although, more recently, a metaphyseal origin has been emphasized. The vast majority of giant cell tumors occur in patients who are skeletally mature, with closed physeal plates; uncommonly, these tumors occur in the immature bones of the child or adolescent.

*The discussion of giant cell tumor is placed here arbitrarily, as the precise origin of this lesion is not clear.

In these instances, metaphyseal localization has repeatedly been documented. Despite the controversy regarding the epiphyseal or metaphyseal origin of giant cell tumors, the importance of epiphyseal involvement with extension to subchondral bone in the accurate diagnosis of these tumors is undeniable. The localization of giant cell tumors in subchondral regions in flat or irregular bones, such as the sternum, clavicle, scapula, ribs, and innominate bone, can also provide a decisive diagnostic clue.

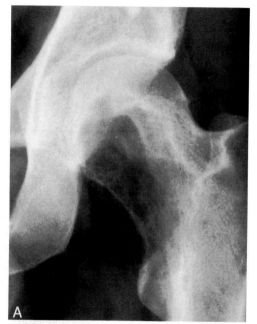
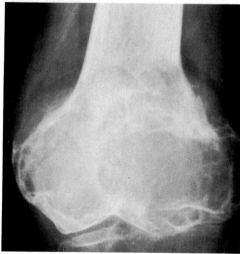

Figure 78–58. Giant cell tumor: Radiographic abnormalities—long tubular bones (femur). **A** The routine radiograph reveals an eccentric, osteolytic lesion involving the metaphysis and epiphysis in the proximal portion of the femur. At this time, it does not extend to the subchondral bone. **B** Note a large, trabeculated, osteolytic lesion involving the metaphysis and epiphysis of the distal portion of the femur. It extends to the subchondral region. The bone is expanded, and there is collapse of the articular surface.

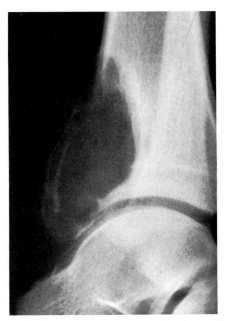

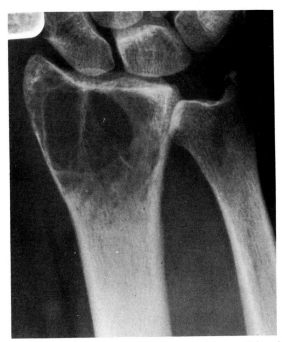

Figure 78-59. Giant cell tumor: Radiographic abnormalities—long tubular bones (tibia). The lateral radiograph shows an expansile, faintly trabeculated, eccentric osteolytic lesion in the distal portion of the tibia extending to subchondral bone and accompanied by minor periostitis. (Courtesy of R. Richley, M.D., San Diego, California.)

Figure 78-60. Giant cell tumor: Radiographic abnormalities—long tubular bones (radius). The tumor is osteolytic, eccentric, trabeculated, and metaphyseal and epiphyseal in location with extension to subchondral bone.

Multicentric giant cell tumors also are well documented.

Radiographic Abnormalities. In a long tubular bone (Figs. 78-58 to 78-60), an eccentric osteolytic lesion extending to the subchondral bone is seen, producing cortical thinning and expansion, and possessing a delicate trabecular pattern. The margins of the lesion may be well or poorly defined, although an extensive sclerotic rim and periostitis generally are not evident. Involvement of a portion of the metaphysis also is characteristic. The aggressive nature of giant cell tumors is underscored not only by their potentially large intraosseous components but also by their violation of the cortical surface and spread into the adjacent soft tissues. It should be emphasized, however, that the radiographic characteristics generally are a poor guide to the histologic composition and clinical behavior of the lesion.

In the short tubular bones of the hands (Fig. 78-61) and feet, the radiographic features of giant cell tumors are similar to those in the long tubular bones. Epiphyseal involvement, subchondral extension, osteolysis, delicate trabeculae, and osseous expansion are among the characteristics of such neoplasms. Involvement of the head of a metacarpal bone or the base of the proximal phalanx in the hand should be emphasized.

There is less uniformity in the radiographic characteristics of giant cell tumors of flat and irregular bones. Sternal and sacral lesions are osteolytic and, owing to a large size and a soft tissue component, may simulate the appearance of a malignant neoplasm. In the innominate bone, the region adjacent to the sacroiliac or hip joint commonly is affected. In the spine (Fig. 78-62), destruction of a vertebral body is more frequent than that of the posterior osseous elements; the neoplasm may lead to vertebral collapse or extend into the intervertebral disc, adjacent vertebral body, spinal canal, or paraspinal soft tissues.

Other Imaging Techniques. Although bone scintigraphy has been used to evaluate patients with giant cell tumors, an extended pattern of activity beyond the true limits of the tumor and the failure to define reliably the soft tissue extension of the process limit the usefulness of this technique.

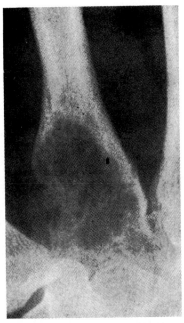

Figure 78-61. Giant cell tumor: Radiographic abnormalities—short tubular bones. Note the slightly expansile, trabeculated, osteolytic lesion of the second metacarpal bone that extends to its base.

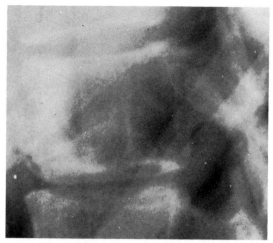

Figure 78–62. Giant cell tumor: Radiographic abnormalities—spine. Osteolysis affects the posterior two thirds of a thoracic vertebral body. There is increased radiodensity in the anterior one third of the body. (Courtesy of Regional Naval Medical Center, San Diego, California.)

Computed tomography allows evaluation of the extraosseous and, to a lesser degree, the intraosseous extent of the tumor and its relationship to major vessels and nerves. The identification with computed tomography (as well as with magnetic resonance imaging) of a fluid level within a giant cell tumor (Fig. 78–63) is a nonspecific finding.

The role of angiography in patients with giant cell tumors includes the preoperative evaluation of tumor extent into the soft tissues and of regional vascular anatomy and, perhaps, transcatheter arterial embolization using Gelfoam particles in instances of unresectable neoplasm. Angiography usually does not provide a specific diagnosis, however.

Magnetic resonance imaging may be extremely useful in

delineating the precise intraosseous and extraosseous components of the tumor (Fig. 78–64).

Pathologic Abnormalities. Giant cell tumors are fairly large; their maximum dimension in a long tubular or flat bone may exceed 12 cm, and an entire small tubular bone in the hand or foot may be involved. In unusual circumstances, the joint space may contain tumor tissue, and the neoplasm may extend to adjacent bones. Soft tissue extension is detected in 20 to 50 per cent of cases. Pathologic fracture, observed in 10 to 35 per cent of cases, may contribute to the soft tissue or articular tumor component.

Giant cell tumors typically contain an abundant number of homogeneously distributed giant cells mixed with ovoid, round, and spindle-shaped stromal cells. Vascular sinuses frequently are evident that may be either plugged or lined with the tumor cells; such vascular invasion has no prognostic significance. Additional findings may include recent and old stromal hemorrhage and nests of lipid-laden, foamy macrophages. Areas with features of an aneurysmal bone cyst are not uncommon, especially in larger tumors. Bands of fibrous tissue are evident in most giant cell tumors. Osteoid foci are also evident in 20 to 50 per cent of cases.

Natural History. Local extension, regional and systemic tumor implantation, and malignant transformation with widespread metastases are among the reported manifestations of these neoplasms that are indicative of their aggressive and unpredictable nature. Although the histologic appearance of a giant cell tumor represents the most important indicator of its behavior, analysis of additional data provided by the clinical and radiographic examinations and the gross pathologic features of this neoplasm is essential for appropriate management of the patient.

The rate of recurrence of a giant cell tumor is about 40 to 60 per cent. Recurrent tumors generally are observed within the first 2 years after treatment of the neoplasm, usually at the site of the primary giant cell tumor.

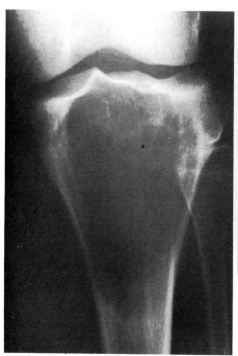

A

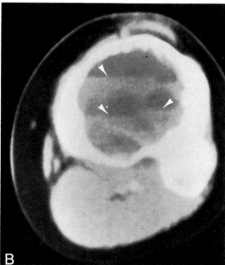

B

Figure 78–63. Giant cell tumor: Computed tomographic abnormalities—fluid level. Routine radiography (A) reveals a large osteolytic lesion of the tibia. A transaxial computed tomographic scan (B) through the lesion with the patient in a supine position shows multiple fluid levels (arrowheads). (Courtesy of P. Kaplan, M.D., Omaha, Nebraska.)

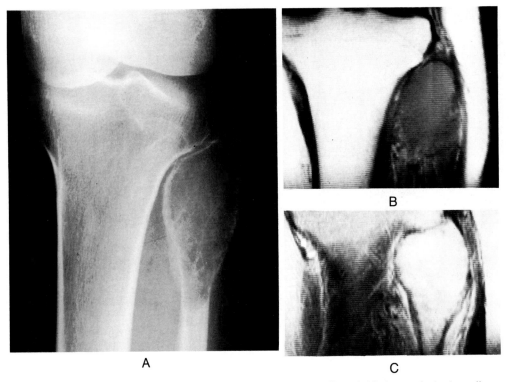

Figure 78–64. Giant cell tumor: Magnetic resonance imaging abnormalities. The routine radiograph **(A)** shows a classic giant cell tumor in the proximal portion of the fibula. A coronal T1 weighted magnetic resonance image (TE, 32 ms; TR, 0.5 s) **(B)** indicates low signal intensity within the lesion. A coronal T2 weighted magnetic resonance image (TE, 60 ms; TR, 2.0 s) **(C)** shows increased signal intensity in the tumor.

The radiographic abnormalities associated with recurrent giant cell tumors are characteristic (Fig. 78–65). With regard to intraosseous recurrence, osteolysis adjacent to the area of surgical resection or delayed resorption of a bone graft may be evident. Soft tissue implants may remain radiographically invisible, although they also may appear as enlarging masses with peripheral ossification in the form of a radiodense thin shell or thick rind.

Tumor implantation at distant sites, typically the lungs, occurs in patients with benign giant cell tumors. This phenomenon relates to simple vascular transport of neoplastic tissue from the primary musculoskeletal site to a remote location rather than true malignant metastasis. The pulmonary lesions are identical histologically to the primary giant cell tumor; they generally do not lead relentlessly to the demise of the patient.

The estimated frequency of malignant giant cell tumor (or malignant transformation of a benign giant cell tumor) is 5 to 10 per cent. The vast majority of malignant giant cell tumors develop after irradiation of the original giant cell tumor and reveal a histologic pattern consistent with fibrosarcoma, osteosarcoma, or, less commonly, malignant fibrous histiocytoma. Such neoplasms are best considered radiation-induced sarcomas rather than malignant giant cell tumors.

Multicentric Involvement. The presence of more than one primary giant cell tumor in the same patient occurs in 0.5 to 5 per cent of cases of giant cell tumor. Multifocal involvement in some cases may be a manifestation of metastasis rather than indicative of more than one independent tumor. The additional possibility of implantation of tissue

from one giant cell tumor to a second contiguous osseous site must also be considered. Furthermore, careful analysis of the patient is required to exclude the presence of hyperparathyroidism (with brown tumors) whenever the diagnosis of multiple giant cell tumors is being considered.

Multicentric giant cell tumors may appear simultaneously or metachronously. Although the clinical, radiographic, and histologic features of each giant cell tumor in patients with multifocal involvement generally are similar to those of a typical giant cell tumor, the bones of the hand are affected more frequently in multicentric disease than in solitary giant cell tumors. There is also an increased propensity for metaphyseal involvement in patients with multifocal lesions.

Differential Diagnosis. Although chondroblastoma, intraosseous ganglion, and a variety of cystic lesions can affect the epiphysis, clinical and radiologic characteristics usually allow the differentiation of a giant cell tumor from these other entities. Chondroblastoma typically occurs in the immature skeleton of a child or adolescent and may contain calcifications. An intraosseous ganglion is observed most frequently in the medial malleolus of the tibia, in the carpal bones, or in periarticular regions such as the hip (Fig. 78–66). It may be multilocular in appearance, with a sclerotic margin, and accompanied by a soft tissue ganglion. Although a variety of articular processes can lead to subchondral cysts, including rheumatoid arthritis, gout, calcium pyrophosphate dihydrate crystal deposition disease, hemophilia, and pigmented villonodular synovitis, such cysts commonly are multiple, communicate with the joint, and are associated with additional articular abnormalities. Further differential

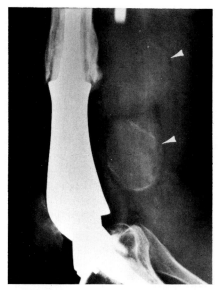

Figure 78–65. Giant cell tumor: Natural history—extraosseous recurrence. This 36 year old man had a giant cell tumor of the distal portion of the femur that was treated by curettage and grafting. Five months later, further curettage was required, and the lesion was packed with methylmethacrylate. A pathologic fracture later developed, requiring resection of bone and a custom total knee arthroplasty. A soft tissue tumor deposit was found in one of the surgical scars at the time of the arthroplasty. Two years following this surgical procedure, as shown on the lateral radiograph, ossified soft tissue masses (arrowheads) were present. (From Cooper KL, et al: Giant cell tumor: Ossification in soft-tissue implants. Radiology *153*:597, 1984. Used with permission.)

in the facial bones appears as a round or oval, radiolucent lesion that may be trabeculated and expansile and that may contain ossification.

These lesions may also affect the appendicular skeleton, particularly the bones of the hands and feet. Giant cell reparative granulomas (also designated giant cell reactions) arising in the hands and feet occur more commonly in women than in men. The age range of affected patients is wide (6 to 53 years of age). A history of trauma is infrequent. Clinical manifestations include pain, discomfort, swelling, and tenderness. The phalanges of the hand are the most common site of involvement, followed in order of decreasing frequency by the metacarpal, metatarsal, carpal, and tarsal bones and the phalanges of the foot. Multifocal osseous involvement is encountered. Radiographically, the lesions are osteolytic, trabeculated, and slightly expansile and involve the metaphysis and diaphysis, although they may extend to the epiphysis and subchondral bone (Fig. 78–68). Cortical violation and periostitis are rare. Recurrence of the lesion is seen if initial surgery is inadequate.

diagnostic considerations in patients with giant cell tumors include aneurysmal bone cyst, fibrous dysplasia, eosinophilic granuloma, the brown tumor of hyperparathyroidism (Fig. 78–67), and giant cell reparative granuloma. The problem of differentiating a giant cell tumor from a giant cell reparative granuloma can be considerable (see later discussion).

In the innominate bone, giant cell tumors may possess radiographic abnormalities that are sufficient for accurate diagnosis, especially when a lesion extends to the subchondral bone about the hip or sacroiliac joint. In fact, sacral giant cell tumors may violate the articular space and involve a contiguous portion of the ilium. In the spine, the predilection for involvement of the vertebral body is a feature of giant cell tumors that differs from the localization in the posterior vertebral elements that characterizes an osteoblastoma or aneurysmal bone cyst.

The *giant cell reparative granuloma* is an uncommon bone lesion that has slightly different histologic characteristics and a more benign clinical course than a giant cell tumor. Reports of giant cell granulomas have indicated their proclivity to affect the facial bones and sinuses and only an incidental relationship to trauma. Giant cell reparative granulomas represent less than 10 per cent of all benign tumors of the jaw and, in this location, demonstrate a female preponderance, a tendency to affect young patients, and a variety of clinical manifestations, including localized swelling, pain, headache, diplopia, and epistaxis. The giant cell reparative granuloma

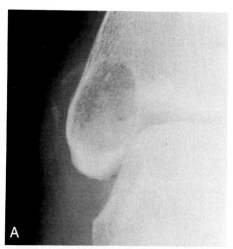

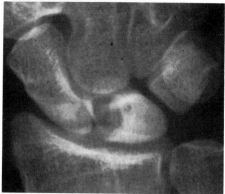

Figure 78–66. Intraosseous ganglion: Differential diagnosis of single or multicentric giant cell tumor. A A radiograph reveals a well-defined osteolytic lesion, with sclerotic margins in the medial malleolus of the tibia. Observe soft tissue swelling containing small osseous spicules. (Courtesy of J. Scavulli, M.D., San Diego, California). **B** Several cystic lesions in the lunate, accompanied by bone sclerosis, are shown. The large lunate lesion communicates with the radiocarpal joint.

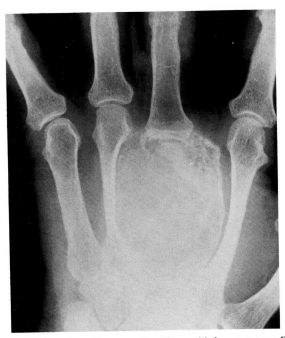

Figure 78–67. **Primary hyperparathyroidism with brown tumor: Differential diagnosis of single or multicentric giant cell tumor.** The lesion of the third metacarpal bone is expansile and trabeculated. Subtle phalangeal bone resorption is seen. (Courtesy of F. Heuck, M.D., Stuttgart, West Germany.)

far more frequently than those in the upper extremity. The femur, tibia, and humerus are the most common sites of tumor localization. Within the long tubular bones, metaphyseal localization is the rule, with frequent extension of the tumor into the epiphysis or diaphysis. The innominate bone is affected in approximately 10 per cent of cases; other sites of involvement are the skull and facial bones, ribs, and, less frequently, fibula, spine, scapula, and clavicle.

Radiographic Abnormalities. Osteolysis with a moth-eaten or permeative pattern of bone destruction, cortical erosion, limited periostitis, and a soft tissue mass represent the most characteristic radiographic abnormalities of a malignant fibrous histiocytoma (Fig. 78–69). The lesions may extend from the epiphysis to the diaphysis of a tubular bone, throughout the innominate bone, or between the body and posterior osseous elements of the vertebra. Osseous expansion is unusual.

In addition to malignant fibrous histiocytoma, osseous metastasis (especially from carcinoma of the lung or breast), plasmacytoma, lymphoma, osteolytic osteosarcoma, and fibrosarcoma are lesions that produce such radiographic abnormalities. Osteosarcoma usually is evident in younger persons. Furthermore, the presence of a pathologic fracture and the absence of extensive periostitis are more compatible with a malignant fibrous histiocytoma than with an osteosarcoma. A most difficult diagnostic problem arises in attempting to differentiate between malignant fibrous histiocytoma and fibrosarcoma of bone. It has been suggested that malignant fibrous histiocytomas are the more aggressive and rapidly growing of the two lesions.

Giant cell reparative granulomas do not calcify (as opposed to enchondromas) and usually occur after closure of the physeal plate (which is not a typical characteristic of an aneurysmal bone cyst). Their differentiation, however, from giant cell tumors may be impossible solely on the basis of the radiographic features. Histologically, giant cell reparative granulomas generally can be differentiated from true giant cell tumors, although they are indistinguishable from the brown tumors of hyperparathyroidism.

Malignant Tumors

Malignant Fibrous Histiocytoma

Malignant fibrous histiocytoma of bone can occur de novo, in association with other osseous abnormalities, including bone infarction and Paget's disease, and after radiation therapy.

Clinical Abnormalities. Malignant fibrous histiocytoma of bone occurs in men more frequently than in women and in patients of any age, although the majority of affected individuals are in the fifth, sixth, and seventh decades of life. Pain, tenderness, and an enlarging mass usually develop slowly over a period of months or even years. A pathologic fracture may eventually occur in 30 to 50 per cent of patients. A palpable mass is the most common physical finding associated with malignant fibrous histiocytoma of bone.

Skeletal Location. The skeletal distribution of malignant fibrous histiocytoma is similar to that of osteosarcoma, with the long tubular bones chiefly affected (approximately 75 per cent of cases). The bones in the lower extremity are involved

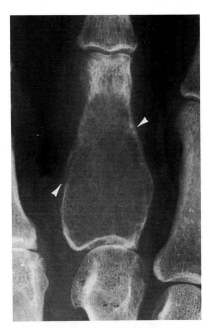

Figure 78–68. **Giant cell reparative granuloma: Differential diagnosis of single or multicentric giant cell tumor.** A radiograph shows an expansile, trabeculated lesion involving the proximal three quarters of the proximal phalanx of a finger. There appears to be a subtle pathologic fracture (arrowheads). The radiographic appearance is similar to that of a giant cell tumor.

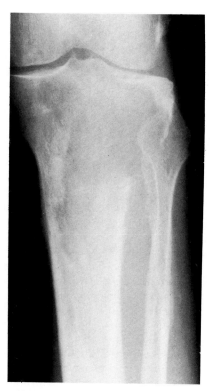

Figure 78–69. Malignant fibrous histiocytoma: Radiographic abnormalities—tibia. Observe motheaten bone destruction in the diaphysis, metaphysis, and epiphysis of the proximal portion of the tibia. The cortex is eroded, and a soft tissue mass and scalloped deformity of the adjacent fibula are seen. Limited periositis is evident. (Courtesy of I.S. Tolod, M.D., Alton, Illinois.)

Pathologic Abnormalities. Macroscopically, malignant fibrous histiocytoma usually is located centrally within the bone, producing little or no osseous expansion. Cortical destruction with extension of the tumor into the soft tissue is found in 80 to 100 per cent of cases.

Although malignant fibrous histiocytomas do not have a uniform histologic pattern, they all share common light microscopic features marked by the presence, in varying amounts, of cells with fibroblastic or histiocytic characteristics, or both. The spindle-shaped fibroblasts that are evident in the fibrous regions of a malignant fibrous histiocytoma are not arranged in the classic herringbone pattern of a fibrosarcoma. In highly fibrous tumors, extensive fibrous foci create an overall mat-like or storiform appearance. The histiocytic areas of malignant fibrous histiocytoma are more diverse histologically than the fibroblastic regions. Additional histologic findings encountered in malignant fibrous histiocytomas include inflammatory cells, foam cells, siderophages, and benign osteoclast-type giant cells. Thin bands of collagen that simulate osteoid may course between the tumor cells, making difficult the differentiation of a malignant fibrous histiocytoma and an osteosarcoma.

Natural History. The aggressive nature of malignant fibrous histiocytoma in bone is underscored by the frequency of local recurrence (as high as 80 per cent of tumors) and of metastasis to regional lymph nodes and distant sites. The reported rate of 5 year survival in patients with this neoplasm has varied from zero to approximately 70 per cent.

TUMORS OF FATTY DIFFERENTIATION
Benign Tumors
Lipoma

Lipomas are among the most common of soft tissue lesions but among the more unusual of osseous lesions. The infrequency of lipomas of bone may be explained, in part, by the classification of osseous lipomas as other processes, including ischemic necrosis, simple (unicameral) or aneurysmal bone cysts, or fibrous dysplasia on the basis of their radiographic or histologic characteristics. In fact, the true nature of the osseous lipoma is unclear. It has been considered either a neoplasm or a degenerative phenomenon related to trauma, infection, or vascular compromise.

Lipomas can be categorized according to their location in the bone as intraosseous, cortical, or parosteal lesions. The reader should refer to Chapters 79 and 85 for information related to soft tissue lipomas and to Chapter 56 for an analysis of membranous lipodystrophy.

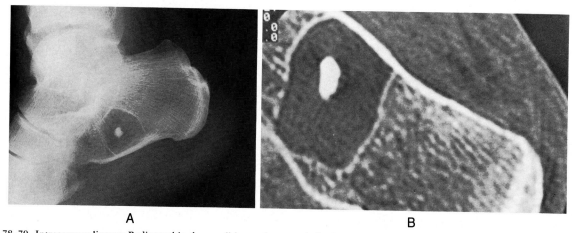

Figure 78–70. Intraosseous lipoma: Radiographic abnormalities—calcaneus. A classic lipoma is shown with radiography (**A**) and computed tomography (**B**). The lesion is well defined, radiolucent, and surrounded by a thin sclerotic margin, and it contains a central radiodense focus. The documentation of fat in the lesion can be accomplished with measurements of attenuation derived from computed tomography data. (Courtesy of J. Castello, M.D., Madrid, Spain.)

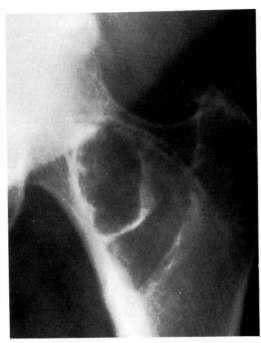

Figure 78–71. Intraosseous lipoma: Radiographic abnormalities—proximal portion of the femur. Note ossification involving principally the margin of this large osteolytic lesion located in the femoral neck above the intertrochanteric line.

INTRAOSSEOUS LIPOMA

Clinical Abnormalities. Intraosseous lipomas are observed in men and women with about equal frequency and in patients of all ages. These lesions may be entirely asymptomatic; however, approximately two thirds of patients with intraosseous lipomas have localized pain and soft tissue swelling.

Skeletal Location. Intraosseous lipomas occur most commonly in the long tubular bones, especially the fibula (20 per cent of cases), femur (15 per cent), and tibia (13 per cent), and in the calcaneus (15 per cent). Other reported sites have included the ribs, skull, sacrum, coccyx, thoracolumbar spine,

mandible, maxilla, the bones in the hands and feet, and the bones about the shoulders and elbows. In the tubular bones, a metaphyseal localization is characteristic.

Radiographic Abnormalities. Intraosseous lipomas typically appear as osteolytic lesions that are surrounded by a thin, well-defined sclerotic border. Internal osseous ridges are frequently present, and bone expansion may be evident. Cortical destruction and periosteal reaction are notably absent.

The aforementioned radiographic features are not entirely specific, but in two locations—the calcaneus and the proximal portion of the femur—the constellation of radiographic alterations is virtually diagnostic. In the calcaneus, intraosseous lipomas invariably occur in the triangular area between the major trabecular groups, in the same location as simple cysts (Fig. 78–70). An osteolytic area with sclerotic margins and, often, a central calcified nidus is evident. In the proximal portion of the femur (Fig. 78–71), an intraosseous lipoma is characterized by marked ossification involving a large portion of the lesional margin. In this site, lipomas most typically occur near the trochanters.

The radiographic features of an intraosseous lipoma in locations other than the calcaneus and proximal portion of the femur resemble those of other benign lesions. The major alternative diagnostic possibilities when considering intraosseous lipomas of the calcaneus are variations in the normal trabecular pattern and a simple bone cyst; in the proximal portion of the femur, intraosseous lipomas must be differentiated from fibrous dysplasia and a simple bone cyst.

Other Imaging Techniques. Computed tomography is able to identify the fatty component of an intraosseous (or parosteal) lipoma definitively owing to the characteristic low attenuation value of such tissue (Fig. 78–70). Other lesions, such as those containing histiocytes laden with fat vacuoles or areas of fatty degeneration resulting from infarction, may yield comparably low computed tomographic values, however.

Magnetic resonance imaging represents an additional method that is capable of demonstrating fatty tissue exquisitely, although it has been applied principally to the evaluation of soft tissue lesions. Benign lipomas and normal adipose tissue yield signals of comparable intensity regardless of the TR and TE times that are selected (Fig. 78–72).

Figure 78–72. Intraosseous lipoma: Magnetic resonance imaging abnormalities. Focus of fat within a cervical vertebral body is shown in sagittal magnetic resonance images. The lesion (arrows) is brighter in a T1 weighted image (TE, 40 ms; TR, 0.5 s), as in **A**, and is less bright in a T2 weighted image (TE, 80 ms; TR, 1.5 s), as in **B**. (Courtesy of M. Solomon, M.D., San Jose, California.)

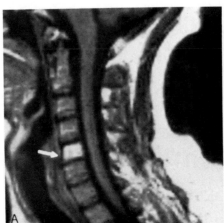
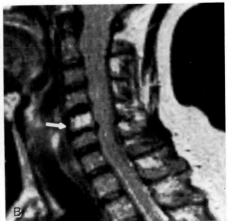

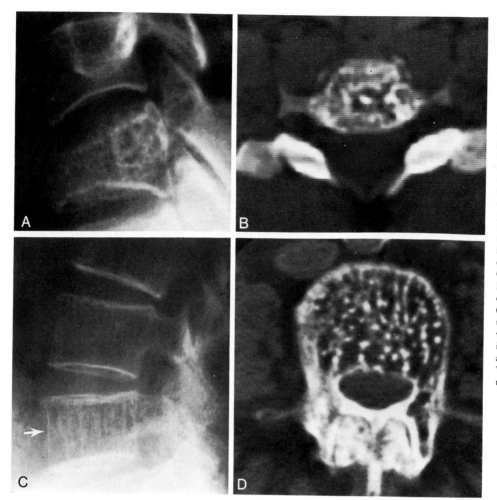

Figure 78–73. Hemangioma: Radiographic and computed tomographic abnormalities—spine. **A, B** Cervical spine. A radiograph (**A**) shows the characteristic coarse trabecular pattern of a hemangioma. Note that, in this case, the involved vertebral body is partially collapsed. Computed tomography (**B**) shows the thick vertical trabeculae, appearing as radiodense foci, in the vertebral body. (Courtesy of R. Linovitz, M.D., San Diego, Calironia.) **C, D** Lumbar spine. A lateral radiograph (**C**) shows osteopenia of the fifth lumbar vertebral body (arrow) and pedicles. The computed tomographic scan (**D**) through this vertebra documents hemangiomatous involvement of the vertebral body and at least the left pedicle. (Courtesy of V. Vint, M.D., San Diego, California.)

Pathologic Abnormalities. Intraosseous lipomas usually are pale or bright yellow and appear well demarcated. The lesions are divided into lobules of various sizes by delicate fibrous septa. Central areas of the lesion may contain white calcified foci. The basic histomorphology of an intraosseous lipoma is identical to that of an extraosseous lipoma. Nearby trabeculae may appear necrotic or normal.

INTRACORTICAL LIPOMA. The intracortical lipoma appears to represent the rarest of all osseous lipomas. A nonspecific radiolucent lesion is seen within the cortex. The differential diagnosis includes an osteoid osteoma and an abscess.

PAROSTEAL LIPOMA. Parosteal lipomas show no specific age or sex predilection and generally are asymptomatic. Usually a long tubular bone is affected. The diagnosis of this lesion can be suggested on the basis of the radiographic findings when a radiolucent mass (of fat density) is adherent to the external osseous surface in combination with cortical hyperostosis or periostitis (see Chapter 85). Additional radiographic abnormalities include bowing of the bone and cortical erosion.

Malignant Tumors
Liposarcoma

Liposarcoma rarely arises in bone. The tumor appears to be slightly more frequent in men than in women and may be seen in patients of all ages. Liposarcomas almost invariably occur in the long tubular bones. The diaphysis, metaphysis, or epiphysis may be affected. Radiographically, a nonspecific, well-defined or poorly defined area of osteolysis is observed. Microscopically, pleomorphic and myxoid varieties of liposarcoma have been observed.

To establish a firm diagnosis of an intraosseous liposarcoma, the tumor must have the histologic features of liposarcoma, and a soft tissue origin or metastatic neoplasm (e.g., renal cell carcinoma) must be excluded.

TUMORS OF MUSCLE DIFFERENTIATION
Benign Tumors
Leiomyoma

This neoplasm of smooth muscle is well recognized in extraskeletal sites. It may also occur in the superficial soft

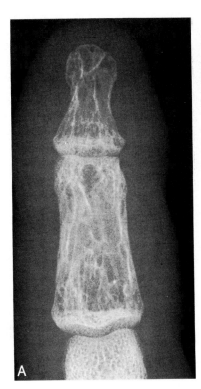

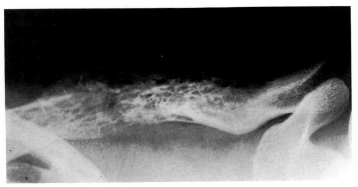

Figure 78–75. Hemangioma: Radiographic abnormalities—other osseous sites. **A** Phalanges of the hand. Note osteopenia of the middle and distal phalanges of a finger with a web-like trabecular pattern. Hemangiomas in the adjacent soft tissues have led to swelling. **B** Clavicle. An elongated lesion of the midportion of the clavicle is associated with osseous expansion and a lattice-like trabecular pattern. (**B** Courtesy of J. Knickerbocker, M.D., Vancouver, British Columbia, Canada.)

accompanied by a peripheral sclerotic rim. Polyostotic fibrous dysplasia can lead to skeletal abnormalities that closely resemble those of cystic angiomatosis.

Pathologic Abnormalities. The lesions of cystic angiomatosis do not differ histologically from cavernous or capillary hemangiomas or even from lymphangiomas. Blood or eosinophilic, proteinaceous fluid is evident within the cystic lesions. In the latter instance, the distinction between a hemangioma and a lymphangioma may be impossible. The rib provides the highest diagnostic yield in establishing a histologic diagnosis.

Lymphangioma and Lymphangiomatosis

Lymphangioma of bone can appear as one or more isolated lesions or in a more diffuse form as part of the spectrum of either cystic angiomatosis or massive osteolysis (Gorham's disease). Localized intraosseous lymphangiomas are rare and are most frequent in children or adolescents. The most typical sites of involvement are the tibia, humerus, ilium, skull, mandible, vertebrae, and small bones in the hand. Pain and swelling may be prominent, and neurologic findings may accompany spinal lesions. A nonspecific osteolytic lesion arising in the medullary portion of the bone is evident.

Multiple intraosseous lymphangiomas can occur in several situations: involvement of two or more widely separated bones (Fig. 78–77), involvement of two or more bones in one region of the body (e.g., shoulder girdle or spine), or diffuse involvement of many bones. Predilection exists for both the long tubular bones and the flat or irregular bones. Additional lymphangiomatous lesions may be evident in the soft tissues or viscera and may lead to a variety of findings, including chylothorax, chylopericardium, hepatosplenomegaly, lymph-

edema, and cystic hygromas. These extraosseous manifestations can cause an early demise. The bone lesions are again primarily osteolytic and septate but may be associated with involvement of the adjacent soft tissues. A specific diagnosis can be provided by lymphangiography owing to the accumulation of the contrast material in the intraosseous lymphangiomas.

Microscopically, the features of a lymphangioma are similar to those of a cavernous hemangioma, consisting of widely patent, thin-walled vascular spaces that are lined by flat endothelial cells. Hemangioma, lymphangioma, cystic angiomatosis, hemangiomatosis, and even massive osteolysis (Gorham's disease) are sometimes considered part of the spectrum of a single disease process despite attempts to sort out features that allow differentiation among these disorders.

Glomus Tumor

Although rare, the glomus tumor (angioglomoid tumor) has characteristic clinical manifestations and a typical location in the tips of the fingers. The lesion arises from the neuro-myoarterial glomus, which is located normally in some of the internal organs of the body and in the dermis and subcutaneous tissues in the extremities, particularly the palmar and plantar areas and the fingertips. Glomus tumors are far more common as extraosseous lesions than as intraosseous lesions. They may be encountered in the stomach, mediastinum, penis, eyelid, nasal fossa, and even the synovial membrane. In the extremities, glomus tumors most frequently are evident in the region of the fingertips or nailbeds. Bone involvement is usually related to invasion by a soft tissue glomus tumor, with rare exceptions in which a true intraosseous lesion exists.

Clinical Abnormalities. Glomus tumors can be observed

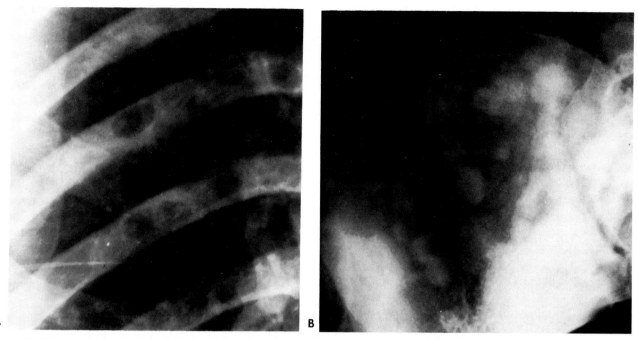

Figure 78–76. Cystic angiomatosis: Radiographic abnormalities. In this adult patient, note widespread skeletal lesions. Within the ribs (**A**), the lesions are well defined and osteolytic in nature, surrounded by a rim of sclerotic bone. In the pelvis (**B**), the circular lesions appear more radiodense but possess a central radiolucent zone.

in patients of any age. The tumors typically are small lesions in the soft tissues that are not palpable or visible on physical examination. Characteristically, aching pain and exquisite point tenderness are present. Exposure to cold or minimal trauma may induce severe paroxysmal attacks of pain. This lesion is benign, although incomplete removal of the tumor can result in local recurrence.

Skeletal Location. Secondary involvement of a bone adjacent to a soft tissue glomus tumor or primary intraosseous glomus tumors are characteristically observed in the hand, particularly in a distal phalanx but rarely in a proximal or middle phalanx or a metacarpal bone, or even in a long tubular bone.

Radiographic Abnormalities. Soft tissue glomus tumors

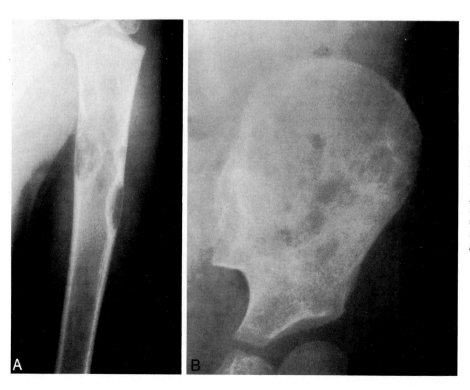

Figure 78–77. Lymphangioma and lymphangiomatosis: Radiographic abnormalities. This 3 year old boy had a neck mass, which on biopsy represented a cystic hygroma. Radiographs of the humerus (**A**) and ilium (**B**) show flame-shaped osteolytic lesions of variable size situated in both the medullary and cortical bone. Sclerotic margins are evident about some of the lesions.

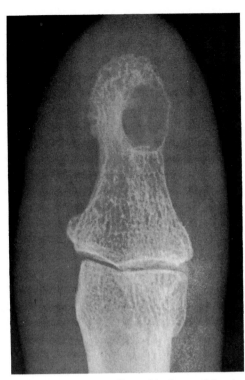

Figure 78–78. Glomus tumor: Radiographic abnormalities. An eccentric, osteolytic lesion of the distal phalanx in a finger is characterized by geographic bone destruction. This is the typical appearance of a glomus tumor originating in or involving bone.

produce shallow, well-marginated erosions in the subjacent bone, usually in the tuft of a terminal phalanx. A sclerotic margin may be apparent about the erosion. In some instances, a partial shell of bone extends into the soft tissue. Primary intraosseous tumors appear as a well-defined, noncalcified, osteolytic region, again usually in a terminal phalanx. The resulting radiographic appearance resembles that of an inclusion cyst (Fig. 78–78). Intraosseous glomus tumors in other phalanges or the metacarpal bones lead to radiographic alterations that are similar to those in an aneurysmal bone cyst or enchondroma. Additional diagnostic considerations are sarcoidosis, aneurysmal bone cyst, giant cell tumor, and tuberous sclerosis.

Pathologic Abnormalities. Glomus tumors usually are composed of various-sized vascular channels lined by flat or cuboidal endothelial cells that are cuffed by masses of polyhedral tumor (glomus) cells. The stroma varies from one that is loose, fibrillar, or hyalinized to one with a predominantly myxoid pattern.

Benign or Malignant Tumors
Hemangiopericytoma

The hemangiopericytoma is an uncommon tumor with a propensity to involve soft tissues and to behave in an erratic or unpredictable fashion. Hemangiopericytomas arising in bone are rare.

Clinical Abnormalities. Most affected patients are men or women who are middle-aged or elderly. Nonspecific symptoms and signs include local pain and swelling.

Skeletal Location. Involvement of the axial skeleton or proximal long bones is most characteristic; the long tubular bones are involved in approximately 40 per cent of cases, and

the innominate bone is involved in approximately 10 per cent of cases. Within the tubular bones, a diaphyseal or metaphyseal location is the preferred site. Less frequently, the ribs, clavicle, sternum, scapula, skull, and small bones of the hand and foot are affected. A solitary skeletal focus is typical of a hemangiopericytoma.

Radiographic Abnormalities. The nonspecific radiographic appearance of hemangiopericytoma of bone is characterized by osteolysis, delicate trabeculation, mild osseous expansion, and, in tumors of the sternum, spine, and calcaneus, significant bone sclerosis. Periostitis is exceedingly rare. More aggressive radiographic characteristics occasionally are seen.

Pathologic Abnormalities. Hemangiopericytoma of bone or soft tissue is characterized by the presence of abundant, ramifying thin-walled blood vessels surrounded by closely packed, plump, round to spindle-shaped stromal cells. The absolute diagnosis of an intraosseous hemangiopericytoma may rest with the identification of pericytes with electron microscopy, owing to the lack of specificity of the light microscopic studies and the existence of similar histologic alterations in a variety of other sarcomas.

Natural History. Hemangiopericytomas of bone, as well as their soft tissue counterparts, reveal a broad spectrum of behavioral features, and predicting the subsequent course of any single tumor on the basis of its radiographic (or histologic) characteristics is difficult. Radiographic abnormalities that include cortical violation or destruction and a soft tissue mass usually are indicative of a more malignant hemangiopericytoma of bone. Tumor recurrence or metastasis may develop years after initial therapy of hemangiopericytoma.

Malignant Tumors
Hemangioendothelioma (Angiosarcoma)

Hemangioendothelioma, a rare malignant tumor of bone, is composed of irregular anastomosing vascular channels lined by one or several layers of atypical endothelial cells. Hemangioendotheliomas of bone have also been referred to as angiosarcomas and hemangioendothelial sarcomas.

Clinical Abnormalities. Osseous hemangioendotheliomas are more frequent in men than in women. The lesions are observed in patients of all ages, although the majority of affected persons are in the third, fourth, or fifth decade of life. Local pain and, less commonly, swelling are the two most characteristic clinical findings. Cranial or spinal hemangioendotheliomas are associated with severe headaches, back pain, or neurologic manifestations. Pathologic fractures are observed in approximately 10 per cent of patients.

Skeletal Location. Hemangioendotheliomas predominate in the long tubular bones, especially those in the lower extremity. Preferential involvement of the tibia, femur, and humerus is noted. A metaphyseal or diaphyseal location is typical. Of the flat bones, those in the pelvis and skull are altered most commonly. The ribs are affected in approximately 5 per cent of cases, and the vertebrae are involved in approximately 10 per cent of cases. Unusual sites of involvement are the ribs, scapula, clavicle, sternum, radius, patella, and the small bones of the hand and foot.

One of the characteristic features of hemangioendothelioma is synchronous or metachronous multicentric disease, a phenomenon that is observed in 20 to 50 per cent of cases. Multiple lesions may occur in a single bone, or one or more

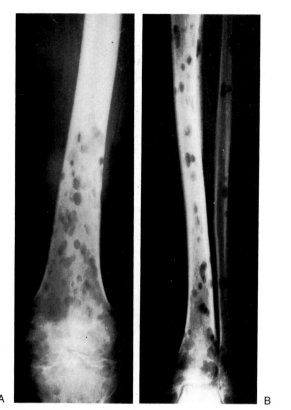

Figure 78–79. Hemangioendothelioma (angiosarcoma): Radiographic abnormalities—long tubular bones. Note multiple, well-defined, small osteolytic lesions scattered throughout the tibia, fibula, and femur. This type of regional distribution represents one of the characteristic patterns of hemangioendothelioma. (Courtesy of H. J. Spjut, M.D., Houston, Texas.)

tumor foci may be apparent in multiple bones in a single extremity or throughout the skeleton. A regional pattern of involvement of the tubular bones of an extremity should be emphasized as one important diagnostic sign of this neoplasm.

Hemangioendotheliomas may develop in bones with preexisting abnormalities, such as chronic osteomyelitis, osteonecrosis, or other neoplasms.

Radiographic Abnormalities. The principal radiographic pattern is one of osteolysis that, uncommonly, is accompanied by osteosclerosis. The lesions are variable in size, may localize in the cortex or the medullary bone, and possess either well-delineated or poorly defined margins. Cortical thinning and mild or moderate osseous expansion are additional radiographic features, and periostitis is infrequent.

Multifocal involvement may be manifested as two or more osteolytic lesions involving a long segment of a single bone or osteolysis in contiguous bones (Fig. 78–79). Radiographically, multiple foci in the cortical bone or spongiosa, perhaps leading to osseous expansion, without periostitis, in a tubular bone (or bones) of a lower extremity is highly characteristic. Other diagnostic considerations include skeletal metastasis, plasma cell myeloma, cystic angiomatosis, histiocytosis, Kaposi's sarcoma, and fungal or tuberculous osteomyelitis. In the flat or irregular bones, a similar osteolytic pattern may be demonstrated. In the spine, osteolysis in contiguous

vertebral bodies with narrowing of the intervening intervertebral disc(s) simulates the appearance of infection.

Pathologic Abnormalities. The two fundamental histologic criteria that are required for the diagnosis of a hemangioendothelioma are (1) the formation of atypical endothelial cells in greater numbers than would be required to line vessels with a simple endothelial membrane; and (2) the formation of vascular tubes and channels that possess a delicate framework of reticulin fibers and have a marked tendency to anastomose. Very well differentiated angiosarcomas usually contain numerous blood vessels whose endothelial cells show only minimal nuclear atypia. In more poorly differentiated tumors, spindle-shaped cells that clearly are pleomorphic may be evident.

The accurate diagnosis of hemangioendothelioma has been complicated somewhat by recent data that support the concept of an additional neoplasm, a *histiocytoid hemangioma*, characterized by an apparently histologically distinct population of endothelial cells. An analysis of reported cases of histiocytoid hemangioma indicates the following features: involvement of the tubular or flat bones, rare multicentric disease, associated skin lesions, and radiographically evident poorly marginated and occasionally expansile regions. Low grade or well-differentiated hemangioendotheliomas of bone that are associated with a more favorable prognosis may represent, in reality, histiocytoid hemangiomas.

Natural History. Well-differentiated neoplasms are associated with a more favorable prognosis; patients do well after surgical excision of such lesions. High grade hemangioendotheliomas of bone must be treated aggressively, although the prognosis for long-term survival in these cases remains grave.

TUMORS OF NEURAL DIFFERENTIATION

The designation of schwannoma has been applied by some investigators to both of the major benign neural tumors, neurilemoma and neurofibroma, whereas others use schwannoma as a synonym for neurilemoma alone. The malignant counterpart of these lesions has been designated a neurogenic sarcoma or malignant schwannoma.

Benign Tumors
Solitary Neurofibroma

Although multiple neurogenic tumors are well recognized as part of neurofibromatosis (see Chapter 82), solitary neurofibromas are uncommon. These lesions generally occur in individuals between the ages of 25 and 45 years, originating from the cranial, peripheral, and sympathetic nerves. When occurring adjacent to a bone, these tumors as well as those arising in the periosteum or at the outer portion of the osseous neurovascular foramina may lead to eccentric bone erosion. True intraosseous neurofibromas are indeed rare. Clinical manifestations include local pain, swelling, and tenderness.

The mandible is the bone that is affected most typically, being involved in approximately two thirds of cases; other sites of involvement, in order of decreasing frequency, include the maxilla, vertebral column (especially the sacrum), tibia, fibula, and humerus. Osteolytic lesions may result in cortical destruction and periosteal reaction. Intraosseous neurofibromas can be associated with neurofibromatosis as well as with congenital bowing of a tubular bone (see Chapter 76).

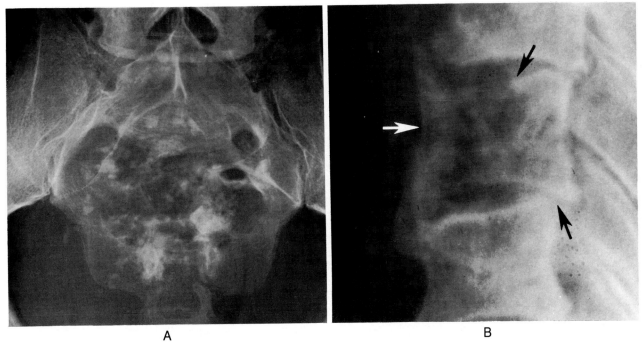

A   B

Figure 78–80. Chordoma: Radiographic abnormalities. A Sacrococcygeal tumor. Within the sacrum, this large chordoma had led to osteolysis with prominent calcification. **B** Vertebral tumor. This chordoma of a cervical vertebral body is associated with osteolysis (arrows). The adjacent intervertebral discs appear slightly narrowed.

Histologically, neurofibromas of bone are similar to those of soft tissues, being composed of spindle-shaped or stellate cells. Diffusely distributed collagen bundles or fibers are evident.

Neurilemoma

Neurilemomas, which arise from a nerve sheath, rarely originate in bone. Men and women of all ages are affected. Clinical manifestations include pain, swelling, and, less frequently, impairment of sensory and motor function. Rarely, the presenting symptoms and signs relate to a pathologic fracture.

The most frequent sites of involvement are the mandible, sacrum, maxilla, femur, and humerus, in order of descending frequency. It is of interest that the mandible and sacrum represent bones that normally contain lengthy nerve segments, perhaps explaining the predilection of neurilemomas (and neurofibromas) to affect these sites.

The radiographic characteristics of neurilemomas are not specific. Three modes of presentation are encountered: central involvement characterized as a cystic osteolytic focus with a sclerotic margin; localization to the nutrient canal with production of a dumbbell lesion; and periosteal involvement leading to cortical erosion or excavation.

Classically, neurilemomas are composed of compact cellular areas in combination with loosely arranged hypocellular regions, the former being termed Antoni A areas and the latter Antoni B areas. In the Antoni A areas, spindle cells are aligned in either interweaving fascicles or palisading patterns. In Antoni B areas, tumor cells are separated by a watery type of matrix. Neurilemomas are vascular lesions.

Malignant Tumors
Neurogenic Sarcoma (Malignant Schwannoma)

Neurogenic sarcomas are unusual lesions that have a variable histologic appearance, perhaps related to the versatility of Schwann cells, which, through metaplasia, can produce cartilage, bone, fat, and muscle. The malignant schwannoma of bone usually appears in a patient in the third, fourth, or fifth decade of life as a poorly defined osteolytic process with soft tissue extension. It may be seen in patients with generalized neurofibromatosis.

TUMORS OF NOTOCHORD ORIGIN
Locally Aggressive or Malignant Tumors
Chordoma

Chordoma is a rare lesion of notochord origin characterized by a lobular arrangement and composed of highly vacuolated (physaliferous) cells and mucoid intercellular material. It is a locally aggressive tumor that grows slowly, invades surrounding soft tissue structures, and metastasizes infrequently. Diagnosis is often delayed, such that the lesions commonly are large when first discovered.

Clinical Abnormalities. Chordomas can become evident in men and women of all ages, although most patients are in the fourth through seventh decades of life. Sacrococcygeal lesions arise in men more commonly than in women; sphenooccipital chordomas have an equal sex distribution.

Chordomas arising in the sacrococcygeal region produce gradually progressive perineal pain and numbness. Additional manifestations depend on the pressure exerted by the tumor on surrounding structures, including the rectum, the bladder, and the emerging nerve roots.

Sphenooccipital chordomas lead to an increase in intracranial pressure and may become manifest as headaches, blurred vision, diplopia, weakness, memory loss, emotional instability, amenorrhea, sterility, loss of libido, and visual disturbances.

Vertebral chordomas involve the adjacent spinal cord and nerve roots progressively, resulting in pain, numbness, motor weakness, and, eventually, paralysis.

Skeletal Location. Favored locations of chordomas are the sacrococcygeal region (50 to 60 per cent of cases), sphenooccipital region (25 to 40 per cent), and remaining portions of the vertebral column (15 to 20 per cent); of the vertebrae above the sacrum, those in the cervical region are affected most commonly.

Although cranial chordomas predominate in the sphenooccipital region, especially in the clivus, these lesions rarely may occur in the nasopharynx, maxilla, or paranasal sinuses. Sacrococcygeal tumors develop as retrorectal masses that frequently extend into the buttocks. Spinal chordomas generally arise in the vertebral body, although they may extend into the posterior osseous elements of the vertebra.

Radiographic and Other Imaging Abnormalities. Osteolysis with or without calcification, cortical violation, and a soft tissue mass are the predominant radiographic findings.

Sacrococcygeal Tumors. The fundamental radiographic features of these chordomas are irregular destruction of bone, osseous expansion, and an anterior soft tissue mass. Calcification (50 to 70 per cent of cases) and osteosclerosis are additional abnormalities (Fig. 78–80A). Computed tomography may define the extent of the tumor, particularly its soft tissue component, and detect calcification in as many as 90 per cent of cases. Such calcification is amorphous and predominates in the periphery of the tumor. Magnetic resonance imaging also delineates the osseous and soft tissue components of chordomas. The neoplasms appear bright on T2 weighted images.

With regard to the differential diagnosis of the radiographic features, an expansile lesion of the sacrum may also indicate a giant cell tumor, plasmacytoma, chondrosarcoma, neurogenic tumor, or skeletal metastasis.

Sphenooccipital Tumors. Destruction of the clivus and sella turcica, osseous expansion, a soft tissue mass, and extension of tumor to the petrous and sphenoid bones as well as the nasopharynx may be evident. Calcifications within the lesion are detected in 20 to 70 per cent of cases. A specific variety of chordoma, the chondroid chordoma, exhibits cartilaginous features, represents approximately one third of all chordomas in this region, and is accompanied by a better prognosis. Computed tomography, angiography, and magnetic resonance imaging are additional methods that allow further evaluation of sphenooccipital chordomas.

The differential diagnosis of these tumors includes craniopharyngioma, meningioma, osteochondroma, pituitary neoplasms, aneurysm, optic glioma, nasopharyngeal carcinoma, and metastasis.

Vertebral Tumors. Initially, destruction of the vertebral body is unaccompanied by loss of height of the adjacent intervertebral disc (Fig. 78–80B). Subsequently, osteosclerosis and soft tissue abnormalities may become prominent, and contiguous vertebral bodies may be affected, with involvement of the intervertebral discs. Calcification in an anterior soft tissue mass occurs in approximately 30 per cent of cases. Vertebral collapse, radiodense vertebral bodies (ivory vertebrae), and enlarged neural foramina are additional manifestations of this lesion. Intraspinal extension is readily apparent during myelography.

Spinal chordomas produce radiographic findings that are also evident in skeletal metastasis, plasma cell myeloma, lymphoma, chondrosarcoma, giant cell tumor, and infection.

Pathologic Abnormalities. Chordomas of the sacrococcygeal region may be enormous, measuring more than 30 cm in maximum dimension. Sphenooccipital chordomas may be as small as 2 or 3 mm or large enough to fill the entire middle cranial fossa. Vertebral chordomas are small or moderate in size.

The most prominent histologic feature of a chordoma is its abundant production of intracellular and extracellular mucin. Most chordomas have a distinct lobular pattern. These lobules consist of either solid masses of tumor cells or pools of mucin in which reside fragments of the neoplasm and individual tumor cells. As intracellular mucin accumulates, the cytoplasmic vacuoles become larger and more numerous, creating a signet-ring appearance. Larger cells, termed physaliferous cells, also are characteristically found in chordomas.

Natural History. The prognosis of a chordoma is variable. Unfortunately, many chordomas are massive when evaluated initially and have infiltrated adjacent structures. In these instances, palliative surgery is the only option. In recurrent tumors or in those that have been irradiated, large areas of sarcomatous-appearing cells may develop similar to those of malignant fibrous histiocytoma, fibrosarcoma, chondrosarcoma, or osteosarcoma.

Hematogenous metastases may eventually be evident in 10 to 40 per cent of chordomas. This phenomenon is far more frequent in cases of chordoma of the sacrococcygeal region or spine than of the base of the skull.

TUMORS OF HEMATOPOIETIC ORIGIN
Malignant Tumors
Non-Hodgkin's Lymphomas, Hodgkin's Disease, Leukemias

The skeletal manifestations of these tumors are discussed in Chapter 57.

PLASMA CELL DYSCRASIAS
Locally Aggressive or Malignant Tumors
Plasmacytoma, Multiple Myeloma

These and other plasma cell dyscrasias are discussed in Chapter 55.

TUMORS AND TUMOR-LIKE LESIONS OF MISCELLANEOUS OR UNKNOWN ORIGIN
Benign Tumors
Simple (Solitary or Unicameral) Bone Cyst

The simple bone cyst is a common lesion of unknown cause and pathogenesis. Recent evidence has supported the importance of venous obstruction and of the blocking of drainage of interstitial fluid in a rapidly growing and remodeling area of cancellous bone in the pathogenesis of such cysts.

Clinical Abnormalities. Most of these cysts are discovered in the first and second decades of life and affect boys with

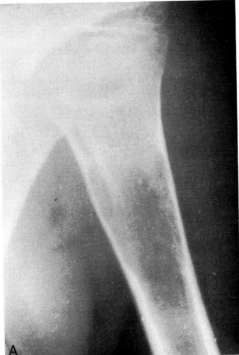

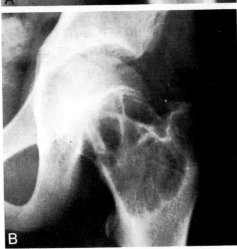

Figure 78–81. Simple (solitary or unicameral) bone cyst: Radiographic abnormalities—long tubular bones. A Humerus. A relatively well-defined, central osteolytic lesion in the proximal metaphysis of the humerus is virtually diagnostic of simple bone cyst. Note the elongated shape of the lesion and endosteal bone erosion. B Femur. A radiograph shows a well-marginated, osteolytic metaphyseal lesion juxtaposed to the physis.

In the osseous pelvis, it is the ilium (2 per cent) that usually is involved. Rare sites of localization are the ischium, pubic bone, ribs, patella, scapula, clavicle, and spine.

With regard to the long tubular bones, a metaphyseal location is the preferred site. Diaphyseal involvement is infrequent, and epiphyseal localization or extension is exceedingly rare. Simple bone cysts located in the metaphysis adjacent to the growth plate have been considered active because of their capacity for growth, whereas those that have "migrated" away from the plate have been considered latent. Examples of active cysts in the diaphysis are recorded, however. Such activity appears to correlate better with the age of the patient; the recurrence rate of these lesions is much greater in patients below the age of 10 years.

Radiographic Abnormalities. A centrally located radiolucent lesion with cortical thinning and mild osseous expansion is the radiographic hallmark of this lesion. Some cysts may possess a multilocular appearance. A thin, sclerotic margin is a frequent finding. In a tubular bone, additional radiographic features include a lesion mainly confined to the metaphysis, juxtaposed to the physis, and an elongated shape with the longitudinal axis of the lesion parallel to that of the parent bone (Fig. 78–81).

A pathologic fracture through a simple bone cyst is a common associated abnormality. Such a fracture may be accompanied by a vertical fragment within the cyst that migrates to a dependent portion of the lesion owing to its fluid content. This finding (Fig. 78–82), which has been designated the fallen fragment sign, virtually ensures the accurate analysis of the radiographs.

In some instances, diaphyseal lesions are large, multiloculated, and slightly expansile (Fig. 78–83), resembling the appearance of fibrous dysplasia, chondromyxoid fibroma, desmoplastic fibroma, and eosinophilic granuloma. Features of a

greater frequency than girls (ratio of 2 to 1). In those patients below the age of 20 years, cysts generally are observed in the tubular bones, particularly the proximal ends of the humerus and the femur. After the age of 20 years, cysts reveal predilection for the innominate bone and the calcaneus. In any site, simple bone cysts rarely are symptomatic unless a pathologic fracture has occurred.

Skeletal Location. The simple bone cyst is observed most frequently in a long tubular bone (approximately 90 to 95 per cent of cases). The humerus, the femur, and the tibia are involved most commonly, and lesions in the fibula, radius, and ulna are infrequent. With the exception of the calcaneus, which is affected in approximately 3 per cent of cases, simple bone cysts are rare in the small bones of the hand and foot.

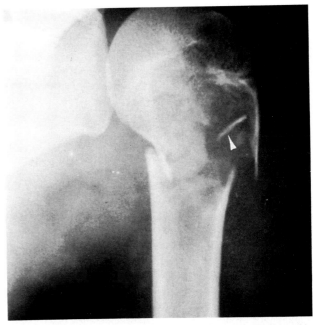

Figure 78–82. Simple (solitary or unicameral) bone cyst: Radiographic abnormalities—long tubular bones. A transverse pathologic fracture through a cystic lesion of the humerus is evident. Note the piece of cortex (arrowhead) that lies within the lesion. (Courtesy of D. Pate, D.C., San Diego, California.)

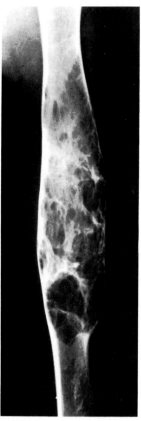

Figure 78–83. Multilocular bone cyst: Radiographic abnormalities—long tubular bones. Observe this multilobulated, expansile, osteolytic lesion in the diaphysis of the humerus. (Courtesy of A. D'Abreu, M.D., Porto Alegre, Brazil.)

simple bone cyst, including a central location, an elongated shape, and prominent radiolucency, usually allow its differentiation from these other processes. With epiphyseal involvement or extension, the cyst may produce radiographic abnormalities simulating those of chondromyxoid fibroma, chondroblastoma, or ischemic necrosis of bone.

In the calcaneus, the cyst is a well-defined and radiolucent lesion, invariably occurring in the base of the calcaneal neck just inferior to the anterior portion of the posterior facet (Fig. 78–84). Fracture of a simple cyst in the calcaneus is rare. The major differential diagnostic considerations are a lipoma and thinning of trabeculae that normally occurs in this portion of the calcaneus.

Simple cysts of the ilium are well defined and radiolucent, and they commonly possess a sclerotic margin (Fig. 78–85). Osseous expansion may be evident. Fibrous dysplasia is the primary differential diagnostic consideration. Simple bone cysts in the spine may localize in the vertebral body or posterior osseous elements.

Other Imaging Techniques. Computed tomography can be used to evaluate the extent of lesions in anatomically complex areas such as the spine or osseous pelvis. Computed tomographic analysis of simple bone cysts and other cystic lesions of bone has occasionally demonstrated intralesional gas (pneumatocyst) or gas-fluid levels. Magnetic resonance imaging can confirm the fluid content of a simple bone cyst,

documenting that the lesion has prolonged T1 and T2 relaxation times.

Pathologic Abnormalities. On macroscopic examination, the affected bone has an expanded cortex, resembling an eggshell, that is covered by an intact periosteum. The cyst usually contains fluid that is clear, yellow, orange, red, or brown, depending upon whether a previous fracture with hemorrhage has occurred. A membrane generally lines the cystic cavity.

Microscopically, the wall of the cyst is thin, consisting of well vascularized new bone produced by the overlying periosteum and of a loose network of trabeculae separated by dilated vascular channels. The membrane lining the cyst contains a fibrous stroma in which are located metaplastic bone or osteoid, multinucleated giant cells, hemosiderin pigment, and chronic inflammatory cells. Some cysts have an appearance that may be indistinguishable from an aneurysmal bone cyst.

Natural History. The natural history of simple bone cysts is not entirely clear. Aggressive growth potential and a higher frequency of recurrence after treatment appear to be characteristic of lesions that are discovered in children or adolescents; these features are less dependent on the precise anatomic location of the cyst within the bone. Although bone cysts may rarely undergo spontaneous regression, the usual approach to the management of simple bone cysts has been curettage and packing. An alternative method of treatment is the injection of steroid preparations (methylprednisolone acetate) directly into the simple cyst. This injection method has been reported to be effective in 70 to 95 per cent of cases of simple bone cysts, although recurrences of the lesion are evident in 10 to 20 per cent of cases. Radiographic signs of a favorable response include reduced size of the cystic cavity, increased radiodensity within the cyst, cortical thickening, and osseous remodeling.

Complications

Fracture. Fracture represents a significant sequela of simple bone cysts and one that generally results in the patient's seeking medical attention (Fig. 78–82). Complete fractures

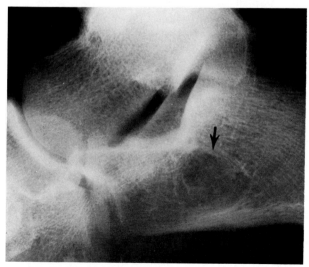

Figure 78–84. Simple (solitary or unicameral) bone cyst: Radiographic abnormalities—calcaneus. Note the typical appearance and location of this simple bone cyst (arrow).

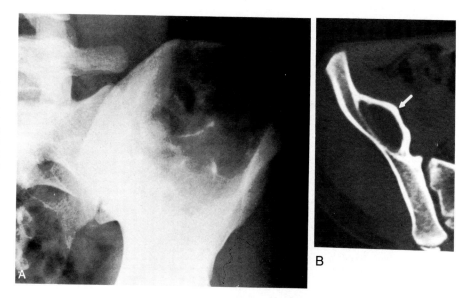

Figure 78–85. Simple (solitary or unicameral) bone cyst: Radiographic and computed tomographic abnormalities—ilium. A Radiography documents the large size, well-defined margins, and osteolytic nature of this cyst. B A transaxial computed tomographic scan in another patient reveals an eccentric location and an ossified shell (arrow), findings typical of a simple bone cyst at this site. (B, Courtesy of J. Healy, M.D., San Diego, California.)

are readily apparent on the radiographs and may be accompanied by the fallen fragment sign (see previous discussion). Complete healing of the fracture is expected after appropriate conservative management. Subsequent complications include refracture, articular or osseous deformity, and growth disturbance.

Cementoma. Acellular, amorphous, granular, fibrin-like material that is surrounded by osteoblasts has been identified histologically in approximately 10 to 15 per cent of simple bone cysts. In some instances, the term cementoma has been applied to lesions containing this material. The precise relationship of simple cysts and cementomas of bone is not entirely clear, however. Cementum-like bone production is most frequent in those simple bone cysts that develop in the proximal portion of the femur. Such lesions appear as radiolucent areas containing variable amounts of calcification or ossification. These radiographic findings are reminiscent of those of fibrous dysplasia and ossifying lipoma.

Malignant Transformation. There are rare reports of malignant tumors occurring in simple bone cysts. In some instances, irradiation had been employed in the treatment of the cyst, suggesting that the malignancy was a complication not of the cyst itself but of the therapeutic method.

Epidermoid Cyst

Epidermoid cysts of bone are uncommon. A history of blunt or penetrating trauma is evident in most affected patients, suggesting that such an injury may lead to intraosseous implantation of ectodermal tissue and the subsequent development of an epidermoid cyst. This concept is consistent with the typical localization of the lesion to superficially situated bones. Men are affected more frequently than women, and patients are usually in the second, third, or fourth decade of life. Clinical manifestations may include pain and swelling.

Intraosseous epidermoid cysts arise almost exclusively in the skull and phalanges of the hand. In the hands, the terminal phalanx is involved in almost all cases. The phalanges in the foot are involved occasionally. Rare sites of epidermoid

cysts are the tibia, ulna, femur, and sternum. Epidermoid cysts also are observed in the mandible and maxilla.

In the terminal phalanges of the fingers or toes, a well-defined, osteolytic lesion possessing a sclerotic margin is observed (Fig. 78–86). Soft tissue swelling can also be evident. The findings are not unlike those of an enchondroma, although the latter tumor rarely localizes in the terminal

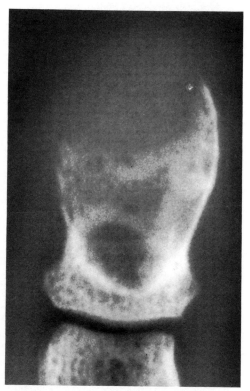

Figure 78–86. Epidermoid cyst: Radiographic abnormalities—terminal phalanx. A large, well-defined osteolytic lesion possesses a sclerotic margin. The distal cortex is incomplete.

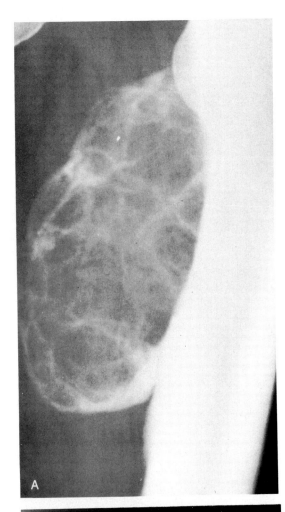

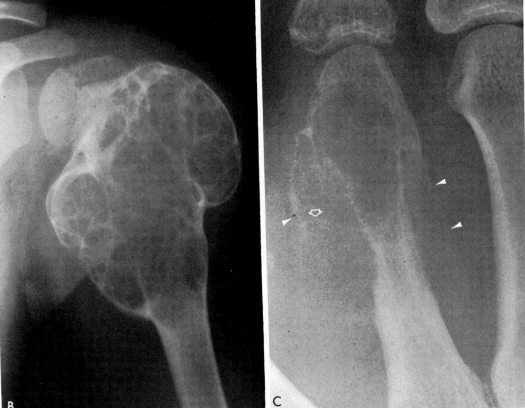

Figure 78–87. **Aneurysmal bone cyst: Radiographic abnormalities—spectrum of disease. A** Femur. An eccentric, heavily trabeculated lesion arises from the surface of the bone. **B** Humerus. Observe the expansile, osteolytic lesion of the proximal metaphysis and diaphysis of the humerus in a child. It is trabeculated and enclosed by a shell of bone. **C** Metacarpal bone. This aggressive lesion is associated with osteolysis and a soft tissue mass. A calcific shell (arrowheads) surrounds the mass, and faint horizontal trabeculae (open arrow) are evident. These features suggest the diagnosis of an aneurysmal bone cyst. (**C**, Courtesy of Regional Naval Medical Center, San Diego, California.)

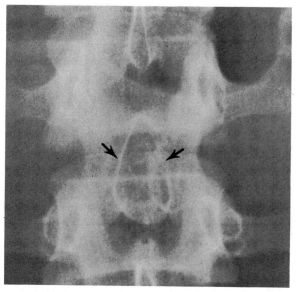

Figure 78–88. Aneurysmal bone cyst: Radiographic abnormalities—spine. Uniform enlargement of the spinous process of a lumbar vertebra is seen (arrows). (Courtesy of D. Pate, D.C., San Diego, California.)

phalanx. One other differential diagnostic consideration is a glomus tumor. In the skull, a well-marginated radiolucent lesion is seen. The characteristically sharp edge of an epidermoid cyst differs from the pattern of poorly defined osteolysis that accompanies skeletal infection or metastasis. Epidermoid cysts in the long tubular bones produce less diagnostic radiographic features.

Microscopically, sections of the cyst wall reveal stratified squamous epithelium supported by a dense fibrous tissue stroma. The contents of the cyst may rupture into the connective tissue stroma and elicit an intense inflammatory reaction to the liberated keratin. Cholesterol granulomas also may be present within this zone of reaction. Resulting accumulation of giant cells may at first suggest the diagnosis of a giant cell tumor or a giant cell reparative granuloma.

Aneurysmal Bone Cyst

An aneurysmal bone cyst is an expansile lesion containing thin-walled, blood-filled cystic cavities. It generally is regarded as nonneoplastic in nature. Trauma appears to be important in the pathogenesis of some aneurysmal bone cysts. This has led to speculation that local alterations of hemodynamics related to venous obstruction or arteriovenous fistulae that occur after an injury are important in the pathogenesis of an aneurysmal bone cyst. It is well documented that lesions resembling aneurysmal bone cysts accompany chondroblastoma, chondromyxoid fibroma, osteoblastoma, giant cell tumor, and fibrous dysplasia, and, less frequently, osteosarcoma, chondrosarcoma, and hemangioendothelioma. This phenomenon of "secondary" aneurysmal bone cysts assumes significance in clinical, radiologic, and pathologic analyses: rapidly developing clinical manifestations in a patient with a known primary disorder are consistent with the development or enlargement of an aneurysmal bone cyst; the radiographic

characteristics of the combination process (consisting of an aneurysmal bone cyst and another disorder) may be dominated by those of the coexisting lesion rather than the aneurysmal bone cyst; and histologic documentation of features of an aneurysmal bone cyst alone does not exclude the possibility of an associated malignancy.

Clinical Abnormalities. Aneurysmal bone cysts usually are observed in the first, second, or third decade of life. There appears to be a slight female predominance. Local findings include pain and swelling of weeks to years in duration. Aneurysmal bone cysts in the spine may be accompanied by neurologic abnormalities, those in the skull may be associated with moderate or severe headaches, lesions in the flat or irregular bones may lead to enlarging masses, and aneurysmal bone cysts in the tubular bones and the spine may result in pathologic fracture.

Skeletal Location. Aneurysmal bone cysts are most frequent in the long tubular bones and spine, which, together, account for approximately 60 to 70 per cent of cases. Typical sites of involvement include, in order of decreasing frequency, the tibia, vertebrae, femur, humerus, innominate bone, and fibula. The small bones in the feet and, less frequently, the hands are affected in approximately 10 to 14 per cent of cases.

Within the long tubular bones, aneurysmal bone cysts are seen almost exclusively in a metaphysis. Isolated or predominant involvement of the diaphysis occurs in about 8 per cent of cases. Epiphyseal extension of a metaphyseal aneurysmal bone cyst is rare.

In the spine, involvement of the thoracic, lumbar, cervical, or sacral level, in order of decreasing frequency, is seen. Vertebral aneurysmal bone cysts generally arise in the posterior osseous elements; the vertebral bodies are affected less frequently, and rarely does this occur without posterior osseous abnormalities.

Radiographic Abnormalities. Osteolysis and osseous expansion are the dominant radiographic abnormalities of aneurysmal bone cysts (Fig. 78–87).

Tubular Bones. An eccentric, osteolytic, occasionally trabeculated process centered in a metaphysis of a long tubular bone represents the classic appearance of an aneurysmal bone cyst (Fig. 78–87A,B). The inner margin of the lesion usually is well defined, and the cortical surface of the affected bone is expanded. The loss of cortical definition and the apparent extension of the lesion into the adjacent soft tissue are alarming features that simulate the appearance of a malignant tumor. Lifting of the periosteum results in bone formation that is important in the diagnosis of an aneurysmal bone cyst. Horizontally oriented trabeculae extending into the soft tissue component of the lesion from the parent bone and a partial or complete osseous shell at the margin of this component are features that are fundamental for precise analysis of the radiographs.

Although a more central location of an aneurysmal bone cyst leading to symmetric expansion of the entire metaphysis occasionally is evident in a long tubular bone, this pattern is more frequent in short tubular bones in the hands and feet. Cortical thinning, osseous expansion, trabeculation, periosteal reaction, pathologic fracture, and epiphyseal extension are all recognized features of aneurysmal bone cysts in these sites (Fig. 78–87C). The radiographic features may resemble those

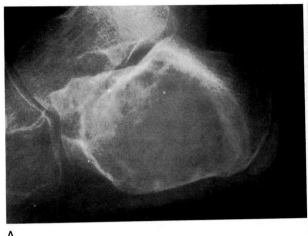

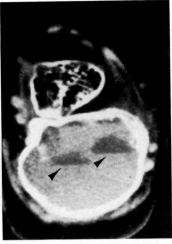

A

B

Figure 78–89. Aneurysmal bone cyst: Computed tomographic abnormalities—fluid level. The initial radiograph (A) shows an expansile trabeculated lesion of the calcaneus. Direct coronal computed tomographic scan (B) obtained with the patient supine and the knees flexed using soft tissue window settings reveals the expansile lesion with fluid levels (arrowheads). (Courtesy of T. Broderick, M.D., Orange, California.)

of a giant cell tumor, enchondroma, giant cell reparative granuloma, brown tumor of hyperparathyroidism, osteoblastoma and, rarely, infection.

Spine. The typical spinal lesion is osteolytic and expansile and involves either the posterior osseous elements (Fig. 78–88) or both the posterior elements and the vertebral body. When an aneurysmal bone cyst is confined to the spinous or transverse process in a child or adolescent, an accurate diagnosis generally is possible on the basis of the radiographic alterations, although osteoblastoma and even hemangioma represent reasonable alternative choices. In the vertebral body, however, the radiographic findings of an aneurysmal bone cyst are less specific. Involvement of adjacent vertebral bodies owing to violation of the intervening intervertebral disc, vertebral collapse, or extension into the spinal canal, ribs, and paraspinal soft tissues are findings of this lesion that resemble those of eosinophilic granuloma, malignant tumors, and infection.

Other Sites. In the innominate bone, osteolysis and bone expansion are present. Soft tissue extension in some aneurysmal bone cysts makes difficult their differentiation from a sarcoma. Similar difficulties are encountered during the interpretation of radiographs in patients with aneurysmal bone cysts of the ribs, scapula, and sternum. In the patella and in the tarsal and carpal regions, aneurysmal bone cysts may lead to osteolysis of an entire bone.

Other Imaging Techniques. During angiography, aneurysmal bone cysts usually are described as hypovascular lesions with localized regions of hypervascularity. These features may have diagnostic importance in differentiating aneurysmal bone cysts from more aggressive lesions, such as osteosarcoma and giant cell tumor, in which abundant tumor vessels are more characteristic.

Scintigraphy has only a limited role in the evaluation of aneurysmal bone cysts. The predominant pattern noted on the bone scan is accumulation of the radiopharmaceutical agent at the periphery of the lesion with little activity in its center. This scintigraphic pattern is evident also in giant cell tumors and chondrosarcomas.

Computed tomography is most useful in delineating the size and location of the intraosseous and extraosseous components of an aneurysmal bone cyst. The detection of fluid

levels in some aneurysmal bone cysts with computed tomography is of interest (Fig. 78–89). Such fluid levels also are apparent in giant cell tumors and chondroblastomas.

With magnetic resonance imaging of aneurysmal bone cysts, fluid levels have again been identified. Additional internal characteristics include prolonged relaxation times, complete delineation of the margin of the lesion by a rim of low intensity signal, and internal septations creating cystic cavities whose walls contain diverticulum-like projections (Fig. 78–90).

Pathologic Abnormalities. Aneurysmal bone cysts vary considerably in size. Although generally they are less than 10 cm in maximum dimension, some cysts, especially those in the ilium, scapula, or skull, measure 30 cm or more. The lesion may contain a single large cystic cavity or, more commonly, a meshwork of multiple cysts. The appearance is that of a blood-filled sponge.

Microscopically, cavernous blood-filled cysts are lined by fibroblasts and multinucleated osteoclast-type giant cells. Fibrous septa appear as incomplete strands that contain trabeculae of osteoid and woven or lamellar bone, multinucleated giant cells, histiocytes, and hemosiderin deposits. The solid portions of the lesion are composed predominantly of fibrous tissue that frequently contains numerous multinucleated giant cells. Three conditions, solitary bone cyst, giant cell tumor and, most importantly, telangiectatic osteosarcoma, pose significant diagnostic challenges to the pathologist interpreting these histologic findings.

Natural History. Aneurysmal bone cysts have a potential for rapid growth, considerable destruction of bone, and extension into adjacent soft tissue. Conventional therapeutic approach has consisted of either surgery or radiotherapy. One or more recurrences of an aneurysmal bone cyst are seen in approximately 10 to 20 per cent of patients.

Additional Types of Lesions. A solid variant of aneurysmal bone cyst has been identified. Boys and girls in the first or second decade of life usually are affected. There appears to be a preference for axial involvement by solid aneurysmal bone cysts compared with the distribution of the classic type of lesion. Radiographically, the solid variant of aneurysmal bone cyst is characterized either by abnormalities that are indistinguishable from those of a classic aneurysmal bone cyst

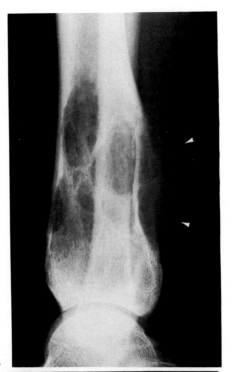

Figure 78–90. Aneurysmal bone cyst: Magnetic resonance imaging abnormalities. A Lateral radiograph reveals an elongated, slightly expansile, multiloculated osteolytic lesion involving the metaphysis and epiphysis in the distal portion of the tibia with extension to the subchondral bone. Observe a hazy soft tissue component of the lesion (arrowheads) containing faint trabeculae. **B** A T1 weighted sagittal magnetic resonance image (TE, 30 ms; TR, 0.5 s) shows the full extent of the lesion. Although it is predominantly of low signal intensity, this lesion reveals small cystic regions of higher signal intensity. **C** A T2 weighted sagittal magnetic resonance image (TE, 120 ms; TR, 2.0 s) reveals cystic regions with increased signal intensity within the lesion.

A

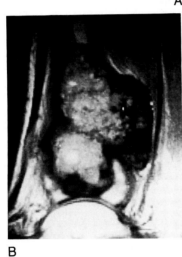

B

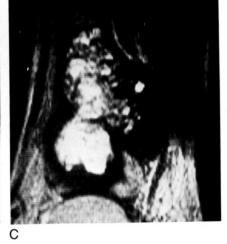

C

or by motheaten bone destruction, cortical violation, and soft tissue extension.

Aneurysmal bone cysts associated with other skeletal lesions have been designated secondary aneurysmal bone cysts. The associated osseous lesions have included chondroblastoma, chondromyxoid fibroma, fibrous dysplasia, giant cell tumor, osteoblastoma, simple bone cyst, hemangioma, brown tumor of hyperparathyroidism, telangiectatic osteosarcoma, hemangioendothelioma, giant cell reparative granuloma, and nonossifying fibroma. Estimates of the frequency of a precursor lesion in cases of aneurysmal bone cyst have varied from less than 1 per cent to greater than 30 per cent. The radiographic characteristics of the associated lesion, particularly when malignant, may obscure those of the aneurysmal bone cyst.

Locally Aggressive or Malignant Tumors
Adamantinoma (Angioblastoma)

Adamantinoma, an extremely rare, locally aggressive or malignant lesion, is composed of rows of epithelium-like cells in a dense fibrous stroma. The pathogenesis of adamantinoma is controversial. There is evidence to suggest that adamantinomas represent epithelial tumors. Furthermore, in some instances, adamantinoma contains Ewing's sarcoma-like tumor cells or tissue resembling that of fibrous dysplasia or ossifying fibroma. This latter phenomenon may explain the reported association of adamantinoma and fibrous dysplasia.

Clinical Abnormalities. Adamantinomas are slightly more common in men than in women. Most patients are in the second through fifth decade of life. A history of trauma is frequent, and many affected individuals describe local swelling with or without pain as the major clinical finding.

Skeletal Location. It is the striking predilection for the long tubular bones (97 per cent of cases) and, specifically, the tibia (80 to 85 per cent of cases) that represents the most characteristic feature of this tumor. Other bones that are involved, in order of decreasing frequency, include the humerus, ulna, femur, fibula, and radius, with rare localization to the innominate bone, ribs, and small bones of the hand

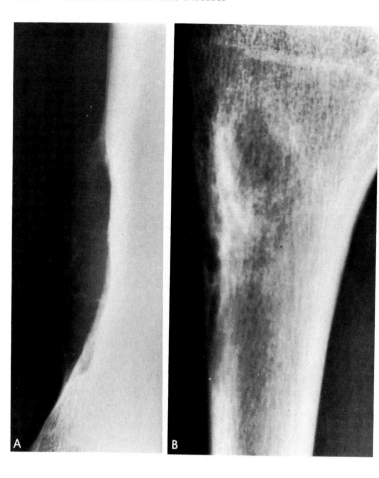

Figure 78–91 Adamantinoma (angioblastoma): Radiographic abnormalities. A A radiograph shows an expansile lesion arising from the distal tibial surface. The external portion of the cortex is eroded and trabeculae extend into the soft tissue component of the lesion. Minimal periostitis is seen. B In a different patient, an eccentric, predominantly osteolytic lesion involves the proximal metaphysis of the tibia. Bone sclerosis also is apparent, and periostitis is absent. (B, Courtesy of R. Freiberger, M.D., New York, New York.)

and foot. Multiple osseous sites of adamantinoma may represent synchronously or metachronously developing primary tumors or metastases.

Within a long tubular bone, diaphyseal localization predominates, although metaphyseal extension of lesions within the diaphysis or isolated involvement of a metaphysis is encountered occasionally. Epiphyseal abnormalities are uncommon.

Radiographic Abnormalities. In the tibia, adamantinoma usually is localized in the middle third of the bone and appears as a central or eccentric, multilocular, slightly expansile, sharply or poorly delineated osteolytic lesion (Fig. 78–91). Reactive bone sclerosis and small satellite radiolucent foci may be identified. In fact, lesions in the adjacent fibula may be seen. Periostitis usually is not apparent in the absence of a pathologic fracture. Occasionally, cortical destruction, exuberant periostitis, and a soft tissue mass are noted. Fibrous dysplasia, nonossifying or ossifying fibroma, aneurysmal or simple bone cyst, chondromyxoid fibroma, chondrosarcoma, hemangioendothelioma, and eosinophilic granuloma are reasonable alternative diagnoses in some cases.

The radiographic features of adamantinomas that are located in other tubular bones generally are similar to those of lesions in the tibia.

Pathologic Abnormalities. The lesions are between 3 and 15 cm in maximum dimension and may be located in the medullary or cortical bone. The microscopic pattern generally is one in which epithelium-like cells assuming a variety of forms reside within a fibrous stroma.

Natural History. Adamantinomas are a locally aggressive tumor with the potential to metastasize. Recurrence of tumor is frequent after inadequate therapy, and the behavior of the recurrent neoplasm resembles more and more that of a sarcoma. Some of these neoplasms may metastasize, even years after initial therapy.

Malignant Tumors
Ewing's Sarcoma

Ewing's sarcoma is a relatively common malignant tumor of unresolved histogenesis. It is now generally thought that the basic tumor cells are derived from either reticuloendothelial cells or undifferentiated mesenchymal cells of the bone marrow. Considerable difficulty in differential diagnosis results in distinguishing histologically between Ewing's sarcoma and other malignant small round cell tumors involving bone, including lymphomas and neuroblastoma (Table 78–4).

Clinical Abnormalities. Ewing's sarcoma usually is identified in patients in the first, second, or third decade of life; approximately 90 per cent of persons with this neoplasm are between the ages of 5 and 30 years at the time of clinical presentation. There is a slight male predilection and an overwhelming predominance of white patients (95 per cent). Localized pain and swelling may be combined with fever,

Table 78–4. DIFFERENTIAL DIAGNOSIS OF SMALL CELL TUMORS OF BONE IN CHILDREN

Ewing's Sarcoma	Non-Hodgkin's Lymphoma
Most common in second decade (but frequently occurs below 10 years of age)	No age or race predilection in children
Rare in blacks	Long bones most common (femur and tibia)
Pain is most common presenting symptom	Diffuse metaphyseal lesion, usually mixed osteolytic and osteosclerotic areas
Flat bones (ribs, scapula, pelvis) are common sites	Lymphadenopathy and splenomegaly may be present
Femur is most common site	Early diffuse bone marrow involvement in children
Metadiaphyseal lesion in long bones	Reticulum fibers demonstrable with special stain
Diffuse osteolytic lesion	Cell nuclei somewhat larger and rounder than in Ewing's sarcoma
Large soft tissue mass	
Positive PAS reaction for glycogen	Negative PAS reaction for glycogen
Negative reaction to reticulin stain	

Metastatic Neuroblastoma	Embryonal Rhabdomyosarcoma
Usually in children less than 5 years of age	Lesions of the trunk and extremity may frequently involve bone
Long bones frequently are symmetrically involved	Usually presents with soft tissue swelling rather than pain as the predominant symptom
Lytic lesions may be very extensive with a paucity of soft tissue mass	The soft tissue mass usually invades bone secondarily
Bone marrow aspiration may show cells in rosettes	Systemic symptoms are rare
Presence of primary tumor; abnormal intravenous pyelogram or paraspinal mass	Lesions in the head and neck area are usually primary, not metastatic
Urine may be positive for vanillylmandelic acid or catecholamine metabolites	Cells have a predominance of pink cytoplasm, and may exhibit striations on higher magnification

Modified from Rosen G: Management of malignant bone tumor in children and adolescents. Pediatr Clin North Am 23:183, 1976. Used with permission.

weight loss, anemia, and leukocytosis. Neurologic symptoms and signs or headaches may accompany a spinal or cranial lesion, a limp may indicate a tumor in the long or short tubular bones of the leg or foot, paresthesias may indicate a Ewing's sarcoma in the mandible and maxilla, and pleuritic manifestations are compatible with the diagnosis of involvement of the ribs.

Skeletal Location. Ewing's sarcoma affects principally the lower segment of the skeleton, with the sacrum, innominate bone, and bones in the lower extremity accounting for approximately two thirds of all cases. The most frequent sites of involvement, in order of decreasing frequency, are the femur, ilium, tibia, humerus, fibula, and ribs; Ewing's sarcoma is relatively uncommon in the vertebrae above the sacrum, scapula, bones of the forearm, hand and foot, mandible and maxilla, and clavicle, and it is rare in the skull, facial bones, and sternum.

In the long tubular bones, Ewing's sarcoma usually is metadiaphyseal or, less commonly, metaphyseal rather than purely diaphyseal. Although epiphyseal extension of Ewing's sarcoma may be observed in as many as 10 per cent of such cases, isolated involvement of the epiphysis is rare.

In the vertebral column, sacral involvement dominates, followed in order of decreasing frequency by the lumbar, thoracic, cervical, and coccygeal regions. The vertebral body is affected primarily, although the neoplasm not infrequently extends from this region to the posterior osseous elements of the vertebra.

Rare descriptions of Ewing's sarcoma in the soft tissues rather than in the bones exist, although the accuracy in interpretation of the precise site of origin in some of these reports is subject to question (see later discussion).

Radiographic Abnormalities. The fundamental radiographic findings in Ewing's sarcoma reflect the aggressive nature of this lesion and include osteolysis, cortical erosion or violation, periostitis, and a soft tissue mass. The bone destruction generally is permeative or motheaten in appearance; the periosteal response may consist of multiple layers of new bone (the laminated, onion-skin, or onion-peel pattern) or horizontally oriented osseous strands extending at right angles to the parent bone (the hair-on-end pattern). Although classically Ewing's sarcoma is a medullary lesion, changes in the cortex of the bone may be dominant, including longitudinal cortical striations and external cortical saucerization. Osteosclerosis is not uncommon and apparently results from reactive bone formation and osteoid deposition on foci of necrotic bone. Uncommon manifestations include pathologic fracture, osseous expansion, and cystic abnormality. Soft tissue calcification is rare.

Tubular Bones. A poorly defined, osteolytic, metadiaphyseal lesion in a long tubular bone accompanied by cortical erosion, periostitis, and a soft tissue mass is the classic description (Fig. 78–92). Bone sclerosis in some cases resembles that seen in an osteosarcoma. Similar abnormalities are observed in Ewing's sarcoma in the metacarpal and metatarsal bones and in the phalanges (Fig. 78–93). The major differential diagnostic considerations are osteosarcoma, lymphoma, and infection.

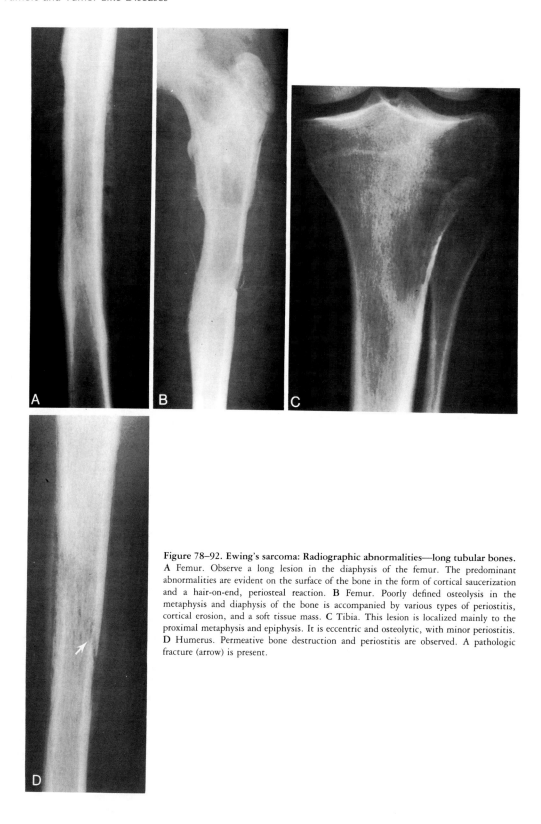

Figure 78–92. Ewing's sarcoma: Radiographic abnormalities—long tubular bones. **A** Femur. Observe a long lesion in the diaphysis of the femur. The predominant abnormalities are evident on the surface of the bone in the form of cortical saucerization and a hair-on-end, periosteal reaction. **B** Femur. Poorly defined osteolysis in the metaphysis and diaphysis of the bone is accompanied by various types of periostitis, cortical erosion, and a soft tissue mass. **C** Tibia. This lesion is localized mainly to the proximal metaphysis and epiphysis. It is eccentric and osteolytic, with minor periostitis. **D** Humerus. Permeative bone destruction and periostitis are observed. A pathologic fracture (arrow) is present.

Vertebral Column. A Ewing's sarcoma in a vertebral body leads to bone destruction, which may be followed by fracture and collapse (vertebra plana). Less frequently, osteosclerosis of a vertebral body or even a posterior osseous element is observed. Extension of the process into the paraspinal and intraspinal tissues is well described. In the sacrum, osteolysis, cortical destruction, and a soft tissue mass are encountered. The differential diagnosis of a Ewing's sarcoma in the vertebral

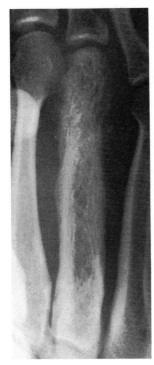

Figure 78–93. Ewing's sarcoma: Radiographic abnormalities—short tubular bones of the feet. Metatarsal bone. The distal two thirds of the bone is affected. Osteosclerosis, poorly defined osteolysis, and cortical permeation are evident.

column includes pyogenic or tuberculous osteomyelitis, lymphoma, leukemia, histiocytoses, and metastatic disease.

Innominate Bone. Although the radiographic abnormalities accompanying Ewing's sarcoma in any of the bones

constituting the innominate bone are similar to those occurring in other involved skeletal sites, a large soft tissue mass containing calcification may be evident (Fig. 78–94).

Other Sites. In the ribs (Fig. 78–95), Ewing's sarcomas produce lesions that are either predominantly osteolytic or osteosclerotic or reveal both osteolysis and osteosclerosis. Tumor growth may result in an extrapleural mass.

In the mandible or maxilla, permeative bone destruction, periosteal reaction, and an extraosseous soft tissue component are most typical.

Other Imaging Techniques. Scintigraphy using a bone-seeking radiopharmaceutical agent generally shows increased uptake of the radionuclide in foci of Ewing's sarcoma. Computed tomography (Fig. 78–96) is best used to define the extraosseous extent of a Ewing's sarcoma, especially in the skull, spine, ribs, and pelvis. Magnetic resonance imaging provides similar information to that obtainable with computed tomography (Fig. 78–96).

Pathologic Abnormalities. Ewing's sarcomas are relatively large at the time of initial clinical evaluation. An associated extraosseous neoplastic component is present in 80 to 100 per cent of cases. Pathologic fractures are evident in 2 to 15 per cent of cases.

Ewing's sarcoma is composed essentially of small, round, undifferentiated tumor cells, with little variation in either size or shape. Special stains indicate the relative absence of reticulin fibers within the tumor. Although Ewing's sarcomas usually are vascular, with frequent hemorrhagic areas, extensive necrosis is common. By light microscopy, PAS positivity for glycogen is found in 70 to 100 per cent of cases. Glycogen granules usually are absent in malignant lymphoma and metastatic neuroblastoma.

Natural History. Ewing's sarcoma is regarded as a highly aggressive tumor with the propensity to invade local tissues and disseminate throughout the body. It has been estimated

Figure 78–94. Ewing's sarcoma: Radiographic abnormalities—innominate bone. **A** Ilium. Subtle osteosclerosis is evident in the ilium adjacent to the sacroiliac joint. Note the large soft tissue mass, with displacement of the ureter. **B** Ilium. More prominent osteosclerosis is evident in a similar location.

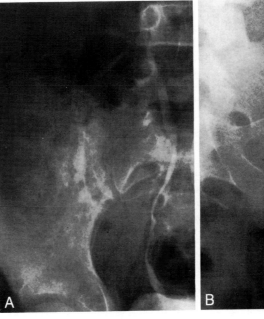
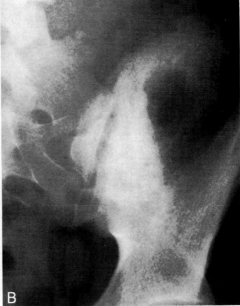

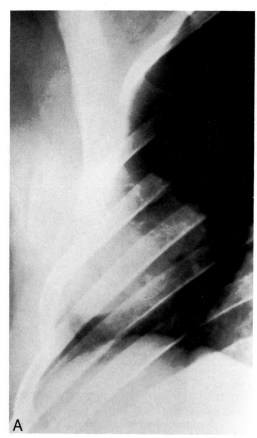

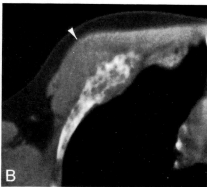

Figure 78–95. Ewing's sarcoma: Radiographic abnormalities—ribs. A radiograph (A) shows a mass as well as osteolysis involving the anterior portion of the right third rib. Computed tomography (B) reveals the extensive destruction of the rib with an anterior (arrowhead) and, to a lesser extent, posterior soft tissue mass.

that between 15 and 30 per cent of patients with Ewing's sarcoma have metastatic disease. The use of both radiation therapy and chemotherapy, sometimes in combination with surgery, in recent years has had a dramatic favorable impact on the prognosis of patients with this type of cancer. Radiographic changes suggesting healing include maturation of the periosteal response, reconstitution of the cortex, and increasing bone sclerosis. Tumor recurrences at or near the site of origin are frequent, however, with estimates ranging from 12 to 25 per cent.

Additional Types of Lesion. A large cell (atypical) type of Ewing's sarcoma represents approximately 6 to 13 per cent of all such sarcomas. The large cell sarcoma usually is observed in patients in the first or second decade of life and is more common in boys than in girls. The clinical and radiographic manifestations and behavior of this neoplasm appear to be identical to those of conventional Ewing's sarcoma.

A soft tissue neoplasm resembling Ewing's sarcoma (extraskeletal Ewing's sarcoma) has also been described. Common sites of involvement are the paravertebral region, pelvis, and lower extremity (Fig. 78–97). Although a soft tissue mass represents the hallmark of the lesion, osseous changes, including periosteal reaction, may be evident. It is not always clear in an individual case whether the tumor originated in an extraosseous, periosteal, or intraosseous site.

TUMORS OF DENTAL ORIGIN AND RELATED LESIONS

The accurate analysis of tumors and tumor-like lesions in the mandible or maxilla presents a unique challenge. These bones may be affected by many of the neoplastic and neoplastic-like disorders that have been described throughout this chapter. Furthermore, the mandible and maxilla and the adjacent soft tissues are the specific locations for a diverse group of odontogenic and nonodontogenic tumors and cysts. It is beyond the scope of this chapter to describe in detail the many tumors and tumor-like lesions that affect these bones and adjacent soft tissues. Rather, one tumor, the ameloblastoma, is emphasized owing to its relative frequency and characteristic radiographic abnormalities.

Locally Aggressive or Malignant Tumors
Ameloblastoma

An ameloblastoma is an invasive tumor of unknown origin that affects the mandible (in the region of the molar teeth and ramus or, less commonly, the symphysis) and, far less frequently, the maxilla (in the area of the maxillary sinus). Most patients with this tumor are adults. The lesion is seen with approximately equal frequency in men and women. Clinical findings include a gradually enlarging mass with or

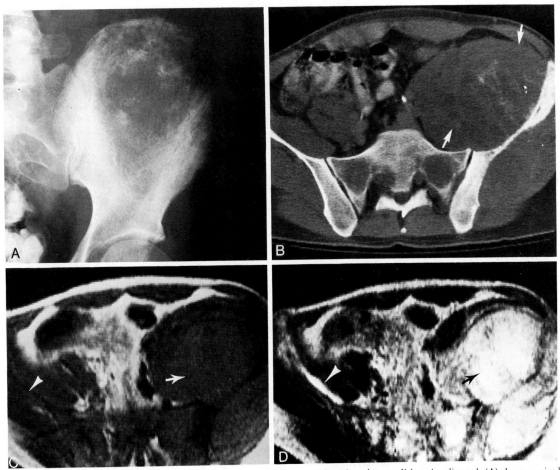

Figure 78–96. Ewing's sarcoma: Computed tomographic and magnetic resonance imaging abnormalities. A radiograph (**A**) shows a mixed osteolytic and osteosclerotic lesion involving the entire ilium. Although a soft tissue mass is observed extending into the pelvis, it is better seen (arrows) with computed tomography (**B**). Note the periosteal response and ossification in the intrapelvic soft tissue mass. In a T1 weighted transverse magnetic resonance image (TE, 32 ms; TR, 0.5 s) (**C**), the lesion reveals decreased signal intensity (arrow). In a T2 weighted transverse magnetic resonance image (TE, 120 ms; TR, 2.0 s) (**D**), a mass of high signal intensity is observed (arrow). In both **C** and **D**, the marrow in the opposite ilium appears to be replaced (arrowheads), presumably by tumor.

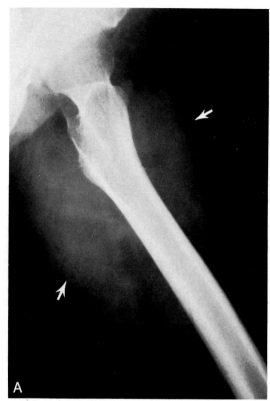

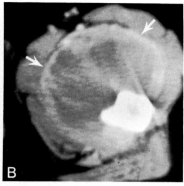

Figure 78–97. Ewing's sarcoma: Extraskeletal soft tissue origin. An oblique radiograph (A) shows the mass (arrows) containing poorly defined radiolucent areas. The femur appears normal. Computed tomography (B) after the introduction of intravenous contrast material reveals enhancement of the margin of the soft tissue tumor (arrows). At surgery, the bone was found to be uninvolved. (Courtesy of T. Broderick, M.D., Orange, California.)

without pain. Early diagnosis is important as invasion of surrounding structures, distant metastasis, and progressive facial deformity may occur.

A radiolucent, unilocular or multilocular cystic lesion with cortical expansion (Fig. 78–98) is typical. Resorption of the root or roots of neighboring teeth may be identified. Computed tomography may allow more precise delineation of the full extent of the primary or recurrent tumor (Fig. 78–98).

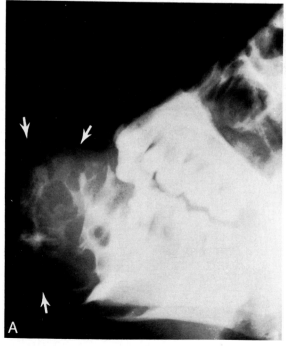

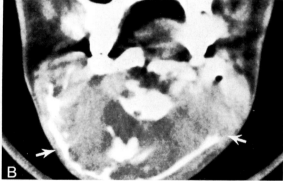

Figure 78–98. Ameloblastoma: Radiographic and computed tomographic abnormalities. Routine radiography (A) and a coronal computed tomographic scan (B) show a large, very expansile, trabeculated lesion (arrows).

FURTHER READING

Allman RA: RPC of the month from the AFIP. Radiology 93:167, 1969.

Arata MA, Peterson HA, Dahlin DC: Pathological fractures through nonossifying fibromas. Review of the Mayo Clinic experience. J Bone Joint Surg [Am] 63:980, 1981.

Azouz EM, Slomic AM, Marton D, Rigault P, Finidori G: The variable manifestations of dysplasia epiphysealis hemimelica. Pediatr Radiol 15:44, 1985.

Baker ND, Greenspan A, Neuwirth M: Symptomatic vertebral hemangiomas: A report of four cases. Skel Radiol 15:458, 1986.

Beggs IG, Stoker DJ: Chondromyxoid fibroma of bone. Clin Radiol 33:671, 1982.

Beltran J, Simon DC, Levy M, Herman L, Weiss L, Mueller CF: Aneurysmal bone cysts: MR imaging at 1.5T. Radiology 158:689, 1986.

Bertoni F, Boriani S, Laus M, Campanacci M: Periosteal chondrosarcoma and periosteal osteosarcoma. Two distinct entities. J Bone Joint Surg [Br] 64:370, 1982.

Bertoni F, Calderoni P, Bacchini P, Campanacci M: Desmoplastic fibroma of bone. A report of six cases. J Bone Joint Surg [Br] 66:265, 1984.

Bjorkengren AG, Resnick D, Haghighi P, Sartoris DJ: Intraosseous glomus tumor: Report of a case and review of the literature. AJR 147:739, 1986.

Blumberg ML: CT of iliac unicameral bone cysts. AJR 136:1231, 1981.

Bonakdarpour A, Levy WM, Aegerter E: Primary and secondary aneurysmal bone cyst: A radiological study of 75 cases. Radiology 126:75, 1978.

Boriani S, Bacchini P, Bertoni F, Campanacci M: Periosteal chondroma. A review of twenty cases. J Bone Joint Surg [Am] 65:205, 1983.

Boyko OB, Cory DA, Cohen MD, Provisor A, Mirkin D, DeRosa GP: MR imaging of osteogenic and Ewing's sarcoma. AJR 148:317, 1987.

Boyle WJ: Cystic angiomatosis of bone. A report of three cases and review of the literature. J Bone Joint Surg [Br] 54:626, 1972.

Broderick TW, Resnick D, Goergen TG, Alazraki N: Enostosis of the spine. Spine 3:167, 1978.

Brower AC, Culver JE Jr, Keats TE: Diffuse cystic angiomatosis of bone. Report of two cases. AJR 118:456, 1973.

Bucy PC, Capp CS: Primary hemangioma of bone with special reference to roentgenologic diagnosis. AJR 23:1, 1930.

Buirski G, Watt I: The radiological features of "solid" aneurysmal bone cysts. Br J Radiol 57:1057, 1984.

Buirski G, Ratliff AHC, Watt I: Cartilage-cell-containing tumours of the pelvis: A radiological review of 40 patients. Br J Radiol 59:197, 1986.

Byers P, Mantle J, Salm R: Epidermal cysts of phalanges. J Bone Joint Surg [Br] 48:577, 1966.

Caffey J: On fibrous defects in cortical walls of growing tubular bones: Their radiologic appearance, structure, prevalence, natural course, and diagnostic significance. Adv Pediatr 7:13, 1955.

Campanacci M, Cervellati G: Osteosarcoma. A review of 345 cases. Ital J Orthop Traumatol 1:5, 1975.

Campanacci M, Laus M: Osteofibrous dysplasia of the tibia and fibula. J Bone Joint Surg [Am] 63:367, 1981.

Campanacci M, Boriani S, Giunti A: Hemangioendothelioma of bone: A study of 29 cases. Cancer 46:804, 1980.

Campanacci M, Baldini N, Boriani S, Sudansese A: Giant-cell tumor of bone. J Bone Joint Surg [Am] 69:106, 1987.

Campanacci M, Picci P, Gherlinzoni F, Guerra A, Bertoni F, Neff JR: Parosteal osteosarcoma. J Bone Joint Surg [Br] 66:313, 1984.

Capanna R, Albisinni U, Caroli GC, Campanacci M: Contrast examination as a prognostic factor in the treatment of solitary bone cyst by cortisone injection. Skel Radiol 12:97, 1984.

Capanna R, Dal Monte A, Gitelis S, Campanacci M: The natural history of unicameral bone cyst after steroid injection. Clin Orthop 166:204, 1982.

Carlson DH, Wilkinson RH, Bhakkaviziam A: Aneurysmal bone cysts in children. AJR 116:644, 1972.

Cooper KL, Beabout JW, Dahlin DC: Giant cell tumor: Ossification in soft-tissue implants. Radiology 153:597, 1984.

Dahlin DC: Giant cell tumor of bone: Highlights of 407 cases. AJR 144:955, 1985.

Dahlin DC, Ivins JC: Benign chondroblastoma. A study of 125 cases. Cancer 30:401, 1972.

Dahlin DC, McLeod RA: Aneurysmal bone cyst and other nonneoplastic conditions. Skel Radiol 8:243, 1982.

Dahlin DC, Coventry MB, Scanlon PW: Ewing's sarcoma. A critical analysis of 165 cases. J Bone Joint Surg [Am] 43:185, 1961.

de Lange EE, Pope TL Jr, Fechner RE: Dedifferentiated chondrosarcoma: Radiographic features. Radiology 160:489, 1986.

Demos TC, Bruno E, Armin A, Dobozi WR: Parosteal lipoma with enlarging osteochondroma. AJR 143:365, 1984.

de Santos LA, Spjut HJ: Periosteal chondroma: A radiographic spectrum. Skel Radiol 6:15, 1981.

de Santos LA, Murray JA, Finklestein JB, Spjut HJ, Ayala AG: The radiographic spectrum of periosteal osteosarcoma. Radiology 127:123, 1978.

Destouet JM, Gilula LA, Murphy WA: Computed tomography of long-bone osteosarcoma. Radiology 131:439, 1979.

Destouet JM, Kyriakos M, Gilula LA: Fibrous histiocytoma (fibroxanthoma) of a cervical vertebra. A report with a review of the literature. Skel Radiol 5:241, 1980.

Dwyer AJ, Glaubiger DL, Ecker JG, Doppman JL, Prewitt JM, Plunkett J: The radiographic follow-up of patients with Ewing's sarcoma: A demonstration of a general method. Radiology 145:327, 1982.

Edeiken J, Farrell C, Ackerman LV, Spjut HJ: Parosteal sarcoma. AjR 111:579, 1971.

El-Khoury GY, Bassett GS: Symptomatic bursa formation with osteochondromas. AJR 133:895, 1979.

Enneking WF, Springfield DS: Osteosarcoma. Orthop Clin North Am 8:785, 1977.

Eversole LR, Rovin S: Differential radiographic diagnosis of lesions of the jawbones. Radiology 105:277, 1972.

Eyre-Brook AL, Price CHG: Fibrosarcoma of Bone. Review of fifty consecutive cases from the Bristol bone tumour registry. J Bone Joint Surg [Br] 51:20, 1969.

Feldman F, Norman D: Intra- and extraosseous malignant histiocytoma (malignant fibrous xanthoma). Radiology 104:497, 1972.

Feldman F, Hecht HL, Johnston AD: Chondromyxoid fibroma of bone. Radiology 94:249, 1970.

Fernbach SK, Blumenthal DH, Poznanski AK, Dias LS, Tachdjian MO: Radiographic changes in unicameral bone cysts following direct injection of steroids: A report on 14 cases. Radiology 140:689, 1981.

Firooznia H, Pinto RS, Lin JP, Baruch HH, Zausner J: Chordoma: Radiologic evaluation of 20 cases. AJR 127:797, 1976.

Freiberger RH, Loitman BS, Helpern M, Thompson TC: Osteoid osteoma: A report on 80 cases. AJR 82:194, 1959.

Friedman MM: Neurofibromatosis of bone. AJR 51:623, 1944.

Ginaldi S, de Santos LA: Computed tomography in the evaluation of small round cell tumors of bone. Radiology 134:441, 1980.

Glass TA, Mills SE, Fechner RE, Dyer R, Martin W III, Armstrong P: Giant-cell reparative granuloma of the hands and feet. Radiology 149:65, 1983.

Goergen TG, Dickman PS, Resnick D, Saltzstein SL, O'Dell CW, Akeson WH: Long bone ossifying fibromas. Cancer 39:2067, 1977.

Goldenberg RR, Campbell CJ, Bonfiglio M: Giant-cell tumor of bone. An analysis of two hundred and eighteen cases. J Bone Joint Surg [Am] 52:619, 1970.

Greenway G, Resnick D, Bookstein JJ: Popliteal pseudoaneurysm as a complication of an adjacent osteochondroma: Angiographic diagnosis. AJR 132:294, 1979.

Hart JAL: Intraosseous lipoma. J Bone Joint Surg [Br] 55:624, 1973.

Healey JH, Ghelman B: Osteoid osteoma and osteoblastoma. Current concepts and recent advances. Clin Orthop 204:76, 1986.

Henderson ED, Dahlin DC: Chondrosarcoma of bone—a study of two hundred and eight-eight cases. J Bone Joint Surg [Am] 45:1450, 1963.

Hudson TM: Fluid levels in aneurysmal bone cysts: A CT feature. AJR 141:1001, 1984.

Hudson TM, Chew FS, Manaster BJ: Scintigraphy of benign exostoses and exostotic chondrosarcoma. AJR 140:581, 1983.

Hudson TM, Hamlin DJ, Fitzsimmons JR: Magnetic resonance imaging of fluid levels in an aneurysmal bone cyst and in anticoagulated human blood. Skel Radiol 13:267, 1985.

Hudson TM, Schiebler M, Springfield DS, Enneking WF, Hawkins IF Jr, Spanier SS: Radiology of giant cell tumors of bone: Computed tomography, arthro-tomography, and scintigraphy. Skel Radiol 11:85, 1984.

Hudson TM, Springfield DS, Benjamin M, Bertoni F, Present DA: Computed tomography of parosteal osteosarcoma. AJR 144:961, 1985.

Huvos AG: Bone Tumors. Diagnosis, Treatment and Prognosis. Philadelphia, WB Saunders Co, 1979.

Huvos AG, Marcove RC: Adamantinoma of long bones. A clinicopathological study of fourteen cases with vascular origin suggested. J Bone Joint Surg [Am] 57:148, 1975.

Jacobs P: The diagnosis of osteoclastoma (giant-cell tumour): A radiological and pathological correlation. Br J Radiol 45:121, 1972.

Jaffe HL: Osteoid-osteoma of bone. Radiology 45:319, 1945.

Jaffe HL: Tumors and Tumorous Conditions of the Bones and Joints. Philadelphia, Lea & Febiger, 1958.

Jaffe HL, Lichtenstein L: Benign chondroblastoma of bone. A reinterpretation of the so-called calcifying or chondromatous giant cell tumor. Am J Pathol 18:969, 1942.

Jaffe HL, Lichtenstein L: Solitary unicameral bone cyst: With emphasis on the roentgen picture, the pathologic appearance and the pathogenesis. Arch Surg 44:1004, 1942.

Jaffe HL, Lichtenstein L: Chondromyxoid fibroma of bone: A distinctive benign tumor likely to be mistaken especially for chondrosarcoma. Arch Pathol 45:541, 1948.

Jaffe HL, Lichtenstein L, Portis RB: Giant cell tumor of bone. Its pathologic appearance, grading, supposed variants and treatment. Arch Pathol 30:993, 1940.

Jones SN, Stoker DJ: Radiology at your fingertips; lesions of the terminal phalanx. Clin Radiol 39:478, 1988.

Keats T: Dysplasia epiphysealis hemimelica. Radiology 68:558, 1957.

Kenney PJ, Gilula LA, Murphy WA: The use of computed tomography to distinguish osteochondroma and chondrosarcoma. Radiology 139:129, 1981.

Kumar R, David R, Cierney G: Clear cell chondrosarcoma. Radiology 154:45, 1985.

Kyriakos M, Land VJ, Penning L, Parker SG: Metastatic chondroblastoma. Report of a fatal case with a review of the literature on atypical, aggressive, and malignant chondroblastoma. Cancer 55:1770, 1985.

Landon GC, Johnson KA, Dahlin DC: Subungual exostoses. J Bone Joint Surg [Am] 61:256, 1979.

Laredo J-D, Reizine D, Bard M, Merland J-J: Vertebral hemangiomas: Radiologic evaluation. Radiology 161:183, 1986.

Lavallee G, Lemarbre L, Bouchard R, Beauregard CG, Dussault R: Ewing's sarcoma in adults. J Can Assoc Radiol 30:223, 1979.

Lee BS, Kaplan R: Turret exostosis of the phalanges. Clin Orthop 100:186, 1974.

Levy WM, Miller AS, Bonakdarpour A, Aegerter E: Aneurysmal bone cyst secondary to other osseous lesions. Report of 57 cases. Am J Clin Pathol 63:1, 1975.

Lichtenstein L: Aneurysmal bone cyst. A pathological entity commonly mistaken for giant-cell tumor and occasionally for hemangioma and osteogenic sarcoma. Cancer 3:279, 1950.

Lichtenstein L: Benign osteoblastoma: Category of osteoid- and bone-forming tumors other than classical osteoid osteoma, which may be mistaken for giant-cell tumor or osteogenic sarcoma. Cancer 9:1044, 1956.

Lindell MM Jr, Shirkhoda A, Raymond AK, Murray JA, Harle TS: Parosteal osteosarcoma: Radiologic-pathologic correlation with emphasis on CT. AJR 148:323, 1987.

Lodwick GS: The radiologist's role in the management of chondrosarcoma. Radiology 150:275, 1984.

Lorenzo JC, Dorfman HD: Giant-cell reparative granuloma of short tubular bones of the hands and feet. Am J Surg Pathol 4:551, 1980.

Manizer F, Minagi H, Steinbach HL: The variable manifestations of multiple enchondromatosis. Radiology 99:377, 1971.

Mathis WH Jr, Schulz MD: Roentgen diagnosis of glomus tumors. Radiology 51:71, 1948.

McFarland GB, Morden ML: Benign cartilaginous lesions. Orthop Clin North Am 8:737, 1977.

McInerney DP, Middlemiss JH: Giant-cell tumour of bone. Skel Radiol 2:195, 1978.

McIvor J: The radiological features of ameloblastoma. Clin Radiol 25:237, 1974.

McLeod RA, Dahlin DC, Beabout JW: The spectrum of osteoblastoma. AJR 126:321, 1976.

McLeod RA, Beabout JW: The roentgenographic features of chondroblastoma. AJR 118:464, 1973.

Meyer JE, Lepke RA, Lindfors KK, Pagani JJ, Hirschy JC, Hayman LA, Momose KJ, McGinnis B: Chordomas: Their CT appearance in the cervical thoracic and lumbar spine. Radiology 153:693, 1984.

Milgran JW: The origins of osteochondromas and enchondromas. A histopathologic study. Clin Orthop 174:264, 1983.

Mindell ER: Chordoma. J Bone Joint Surg [Am] 63:501, 1981.

Mirra JM, Marcove RC: Fibrosarcomatous dedifferentiation of primary and secondary chondrosarcoma. Review of five cases. J Bone Joint Surg [Am] 56:285, 1974.

Mirra JM, Gold RH, Rand F: Disseminated nonossifying fibromas in association with café-au-lait spots (Jaffe-Campanacci syndrome). Clin Orthop 168:192, 1982.

Mirra JM, Bernard GW, Bullough PG, Johnston W, Mink G: Cementum-like bone production in solitary bone cysts (so-called "cementoma" of long bones). Report of three cases. Electron microscopic observations supporting a synovial origin to the simple bone cyst. Clin Orthop 135:295, 1978.

Moseley JE, Starobin SG: Cystic angiomatosis of bone: Manifestation of a hamartomatous disease entity. AJR 91:1114, 1964.

Nakashima Y, Yamamuro T, Fujiwara Y, Kotoura Y, Mori E, Hamashima Y: Osteofibrous dysplasia (ossifying fibroma of long bones). A study of 12 cases. Cancer 52:909, 1983.

Norman A, Schiffman M: Simple bone cysts: Factors of age dependency. Radiology 124:779, 1977.

Norman A, Sissons HA: Radiographic hallmarks of peripheral chondrosarcoma. Radiology 151:589, 1984.

Ohno T, Abe M, Tateishi A, Kako K, Miki H, Sekine K, Ueyama H, Hasegawa O, Obara K: Osteogenic sarcoma. A study of one hundred and thirty cases. J Bone Joint Surg [Am] 57:397, 1975.

O'Neal LW, Ackerman LV: Chondrosarcoma of bone. Cancer 5:551, 1952.

Onitsuka H: Roentgenologic aspects of bone islands. Radiology 123:607, 1977.

Picci P, Baldini N, Boriani S, Campanacci M: Giant cell reparative granuloma and other giant cell lesions of the bones of the hands and feet. Skel Radiol 15:415, 1986.

Rambo VB, Davies NE: Giant ameloblastomas. JAMA 238:418, 1977.

Ramos A, Castello J, Sartoris DJ, Greenway GD, Resnick D, Haghighi P: Osseous lipoma: CT appearance. Radiology 157:615, 1985.

Reinus WR, Gilula LA, Shirley SK, Askin FB, Siegal GP: Radiographic appearance of Ewing sarcoma of the hands and feet: Report from the Intergroup Ewing Sarcoma Study. AJR 144:331, 1985.

Reinus WR, Gilula LA, the IESS Committee: Radiology of Ewing's sarcoma: Intergroup Ewing's Sarcoma Study (IESS). RadioGraphics 4:929, 1984.

Reiter FB, Ackerman LV, Staple TW: Central chondrosarcoma of the appendicular skeleton. Radiology 105:525, 1972.

Resnick D, Greenway G: Distal femoral cortical defects, irregularities, and excavations. A critical review of the literature with the addition of histologic and paleopathologic data. Radiology 143:345, 1982.

Reynolds J: The "fallen fragment sign" in the diagnosis of unicameral bone cysts. Radiology 92:949, 1969.

Ros PR, Viamonte M Jr, Rywlin AM: Malignant fibrous histiocytoma: Mesenchymal tumor of ubiquitous origin. AJR 142:753, 1984.

Rose JS, Hermann G, Mendelson DC, Ambinder EP: Extraskeletal Ewing sarcoma with computed tomography correlation. Skel Radiol 9:234, 1983.

Rosen RS, Schwinn CP: Adamantinoma of limb bone. Malignant angioblastoma. AJR 97:727, 1966.

Rosenthal DI, Schiller AL, Mankin HJ: Chondrosarcoma: Correlation of radiological and histological grade. Radiology 150:21, 1984.

Rosenthal DI, Scott JA, Mankin HJ, Wismer GL, Brady TJ: Sacrococcygeal chordoma: Magnetic resonance imaging and computed tomography. AJR 145:143, 1985.

Salvador AH, Beabout JW, Dahlin DC: Mesenchymal chondrosarcoma—observations on 30 new cases. Cancer 28:605, 1971.

Samter TG, Vellios F, Shafer WG: Neurilemmoma of bone. Report of 3 cases with a review of the literature. Radiology 75:215, 1960.

Schajowicz F: Juxtacortical chondrosarcoma. J Bone Joint Surg [Br] 59:473, 1977.

Schajowicz F: Tumors and Tumorlike Lesions of Bones and Joints. New York, Springer-Verlag, 1981.

Schajowicz F, Gallardo H: Epiphyseal chondroblastoma of bone. A clinicopathological study of sixty-nine cases. J Bone Joint Surg [Br] 52:205, 1970.

Schajowicz F, Lemos C: Osteoid osteoma and osteoblastoma: Closely related entities of osteoblastic derivation. Acta Orthop Scand 41:272, 1970.

Schwajowicz F, Aiello CL, Slullitel I: Cystic and pseudocystic lesions of the terminal phalanx with special reference to epidermoid cysts. Clin Orthop 68:84, 1970.

Seiss SW, Enzinger FM: Malignant fibrous histiocytoma: An analysis of 200 cases. Cancer 41:2250, 1978.

Sherman RS, Soong KY: Ewing's sarcoma: Its roentgen classification and diagnosis. Radiology 66:529, 1956.

Sherman RS, Soong KY: Aneurysmal bone cyst: Its roentgen diagnosis. Radiology 68:54, 1957.

Sherman RS, Wilner D: The roentgen diagnosis of hemangioma of bone. AJR 86:1146, 1961.

Sim FH, Dahlin DC, Beabout JW: Multicentric giant-cell tumor of bone. J Bone Joint Surg [Am] 59:1052, 1977.

Smith J, Ahuja SC, Huvos AG, Bullough PG: Parosteal (juxtacortical) osteogenic sarcoma. A roentgenological study of 30 patients. J Can Assoc Radiol 29:167, 1978.

Smith J, Heelan RT, Huvos AG, Caparros B, Rosen G, Urmacher C, Caravelli JF: Radiographic changes in primary osteogenic sarcoma following intensive chemotherapy. Radiological-pathological correlation in 63 patients. Radiology 143:355, 1982.

Smith RW, Smith CF: Solitary unicameral bone cyst of the calcaneus. A review of twenty cases. J Bone Joint Surg [Am] 56:49, 1974.

Snarr JW, Abell MR, Martel W: Lymphofollicular synovitis with osteoid osteoma. Radiology 106:557, 1973.

Spjut HJ, Dorfman HD, Fechner RE, Ackerman LV: Tumors of Bone and Cartilage. Atlas of Tumor Pathology. Second Series, Fascicle 5. Washington, DC, Armed Forces Institute of Pathology, 1971.

Steiner GM, Farman J, Lawson JP: Lymphangiomatosis of bone. Radiology 93:1093, 1969.

Sundaram M, McGuire MH, Herbold DR: Magnetic resonance imaging of osteosarcoma. Skel Radiol 16:23, 1987.

Swee RG, McLeod RA, Beabout JW: Osteoid osteoma. Detection, diagnosis, and localization. Radiology 130:117, 1979.

Taber DS, Libshitz HI, Cohen MA: Treated Ewing sarcoma: Radiographic appearance in response, recurrence, and new primaries. AJR 140:753, 1983.

Thayer C, Rogers LF: Unicentric osteosarcoma of bone with subsequent skeletal metastases. Skel Radiol 4:148, 1979.

Tonai M, Campbell CJ, Ahn GH, Schiller AL, Mankin HJ: Osteoblastoma: Classification and report of 16 patients. Clin Orthop 167:222, 1982.

Unni KK, Dahlin DC, Beabout JW, Sim FH: Chondrosarcoma: Clear-cell variant. J Bone Joint Surg [Am] 58:676, 1976.

Unni KK, Dahlin DC, McLeod RA, Pritchard DH: Intraosseous well-differentiated osteosarcoma. Cancer 40:1337, 1977.

Unni KK, Ivins JC, Beabout JW, Dahlin DC: Hemangioma, hemangiopericytoma, and hemangioendothelioma (angiosarcoma) of bone. Cancer 27:1403, 1971.

Utne JR, Pugh DG: The roentgenologic aspects of chordoma. AJR 74:593, 1955.

Vohra VG: Roentgen manifestations in Ewing's sarcoma. A study of 156 cases. Cancer 20:727, 1967.

Weiss SW, Dorfman HD: Adamantinoma of long bone. An analysis of nine new cases with emphasis on metastasizing lesions and fibrous dysplasia-like changes. Hum Pathol 8:141, 1977.

Wilner D: Radiology of Bone Tumors and Allied Disorders. Philadelphia, WB Saunders Co, 1982.

Wold LE, Unni KK, Beabout JW, Pritchard DJ: High-grade surface osteosarcoma. Am J Surg Pathol 8:181, 1984.

Wold LE, Unni KK, Cooper KL, Sim FH, Dahlin DC: Hemangiopericytoma of bone. Am J Surg Pathol 6:53, 1982.

Zimmer WD, Berquist TH, McLeod RA, Sim FH, Pritchard DJ, Shives TC, Wold LE, May GR: Magnetic resonance imaging of osteosarcomas. Comparison with computed tomography. Clin Orthop 208:289, 1986.

Chapter 79

Tumors and Tumor-Like Lesions in or About Joints

John E. Madewell, M.D.
Donald E. Sweet, M.D.

In this chapter the diverse nature of tumors and tumor-like lesions that occur in or about joints is emphasized. Such tumors usually have characteristic clinical, pathologic, and radiographic patterns. In most cases, careful evaluation of the clinical history and routine radiographs provides a single most likely diagnosis, although at times additional techniques, such as scintigraphy, sonography, arteriography, computed tomography, and magnetic resonance imaging, must be used.

Numerous tumors and tumor-like lesions of the soft tissues have been described. The soft tissue tumors may be benign or malignant and may vary greatly in size. In this chapter, those soft tissue tumors and tumor-like lesions that occur in or about the joint are discussed. Some of these lesions and the methods used to diagnose them are also discussed in Chapter 85.

BENIGN SOFT TISSUE TUMORS
Lipomatous Tumors

LIPOMAS. Lipomas arise from fatty tissue and are among the most common and widely distributed soft tissue tumors of mesenchymal origin. Lipomas may occur in any soft tissue that contains fat; those located deep within the limb grow within muscles (intramuscular type) or between muscles (intermuscular type). Lipomas most commonly occur in the extremities of women (Fig. 79–1). Lipomas are uncommon in children and rarely are congenital or familial. They may occasionally be associated with nerve paralysis, macrodactyly, osseous deformity, and carpal tunnel syndrome.

The lipomas, either subcutaneous or deep, are of special radiographic interest because of their fat density. When these fatty tumors are surrounded by tissues of water density, the radiograph shows a pathognomonic homogeneous radiolucent mass with sharp margins (Fig. 79–1). The intermuscular lipoma is a well-circumscribed, homogeneous, radiolucent mass with only occasional focal irregularity of the margin. Intramuscular lipomas frequently have an inhomogeneous radiolucent appearance because they may contain streaks of muscle bundles of higher density that traverse the mass (Fig. 79–2). Because the tumors are soft, muscular contraction may change the lipoma's shape.

The homogeneous radiolucency of lipomas may be disturbed by metaplastic bone or cartilage formation. The demonstration of bone and cartilage within the lipoma is not an indication of malignancy; however, bone and cartilage probably are more frequent in liposarcomas.

The nonhomogeneous fatty tumor always presents a bothersome pattern on radiography. An identical inhomogeneous pattern frequently is seen in liposarcomas. Arteriograms of the lipoma reveal displacement of normal vessels and absent neovascularity. Lipomas usually appear on computed tomography as homogeneous, sharply marginated, low density masses with attenuation numbers usually in the range of −50 to −60 Hounsfield units. These lesions are not enhanced on postcontrast computed tomographic scans. Magnetic resonance imaging also allows accurate diagnosis of a lipoma.

Synovial lipomas are rare and occur almost exclusively in the knee joint. They are solitary masses of mature fat, covered with synovium. On plain films, joint swelling and fat may be seen. Arthrography demonstrates a smooth, lobular synovial mass. This lesion is different from the more common lipoma arborescens, which also is monarticular and is found most commonly in the knee. Lipoma arborescens is characterized by numerous swollen synovial villous projections of fatty tissue and may be associated with degenerative joint disease, chronic rheumatoid arthritis, or posttraumatic conditions.

Lipomas originating in the periosteum also are rare (Fig. 79–3). The radiograph shows a radiolucent mass adjacent to

The opinions or assertions contained herein are the private views of the authors and are not to be construed as official or as reflecting the views of the United States Departments of the Army, Air Force, Navy, or Defense.

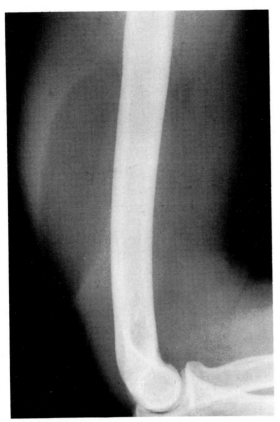

Figure 79–1. Intermuscular lipoma. Note a sharply circumscribed, homogeneous, radiolucent fatty mass. (Armed Forces Institute of Pathology Neg. No. 72-6580-2.)

Lipomatosis

Multiple lipomas (lipomatosis) usually are distributed randomly throughout the soft tissue. When symmetric, they are referred to as multiple symmetric lipomatosis. Affected patients reveal masses resembling overdeveloped and unusually located muscles. Some patients may have lipoma dolorosa, characterized by pain that develops in one lipoma after another.

DIFFUSE LIPOMATOSIS. Diffuse lipomatosis is a disorder of fat tissue in which part or all of a limb may be extensively infiltrated by adipose tissue. Diffuse lipomatosis is found most frequently in children. It is considered a congenital disorder and frequently presents clinically with overgrowth of the soft tissues and bone of the affected limb. The overgrowth is referred to as macrodystrophia lipomatosa (see Chapter 73).

LIPOBLASTOMATOSIS. Lipoblastomatosis is a rare type of embryonal fatty tumor. These tumors are mostly limited to the pediatric age group, especially in the first year of life. In most instances the tumor is located superficially in the extremities. It may be confused with liposarcoma histologically. Recurrence of the tumor after surgery is a particular problem.

bone, which frequently is associated with cortical hyperostosis. Calcifications may be present.

ANGIOLIPOMAS. The angiolipomas are rare benign fatty tumors composed of mature lipocytes with many areas of angiomatous elements. Most commonly the lesions are found in young adults. The tumors have been divided into (1) noninfiltrating and (2) infiltrating types. The noninfiltrating type is more common and usually is located in subcutaneous tissue. The infiltrating type of angiolipoma usually is found within the deep soft tissue and is less common than the noninfiltrating type. These tumors are poorly defined masses with infiltration of adjacent structures. Local invasion and recurrence are a problem.

Radiographically, the angiolipoma appears as a soft tissue mass with an inhomogeneous appearance and poorly defined margins. Ossification and phleboliths have been noted. Although they are benign, angiolipomas may be misdiagnosed as malignant on arteriography. Computed tomography demonstrates a poorly defined, heterogeneous mass with elements of both fat and water density and infiltration of the mass into adjacent tissue.

HIBERNOMAS. Hibernomas usually present in the 30 to 50 year old age group as a firm, movable, asymptomatic mass that occurs more frequently in women. Hibernomas are vascular and usually grow slowly. On plain films, the hibernoma resembles an inhomogeneous lipoma. Computed tomography also demonstrates this inhomogeneity.

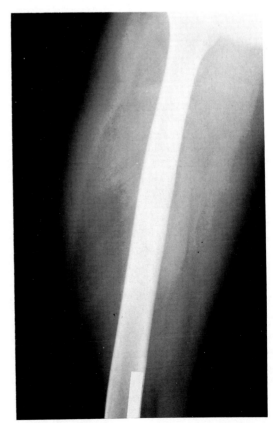

Figure 79–2. Intramuscular lipoma. Oblique radiograph demonstrates a well-circumscribed, nonhomogeneous fatty mass with oblique streaks of water density. (Armed Forces Institute of Pathology Neg. No. 69-5538.)

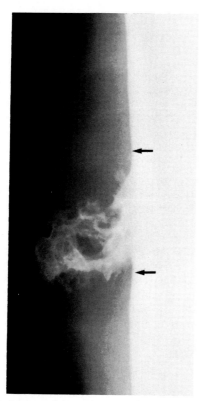

Figure 79–3. Lipoma of the periosteum of the femur. Anteroposterior radiograph of the proximal thigh shows a 9 × 4 cm, sharply marginated, radiolucent fatty mass with a central area of structured density. This dense area has both cortical margins and trabeculae, representing mature bone formation. Note its origin from the bone surface and secondary cortical scalloping (arrows). (Armed Forces Institute of Pathology Neg. No. 68-7665.)

Vascular Tumors

The most common vascular tumor is the hemangioma, which occurs in all tissues but is especially common in the skin. The majority of these cutaneous hemangiomas are asymptomatic and are infrequently studied radiographically. Deeper soft tissue hemangiomas do occur, however.

HEMANGIOMAS. The majority of deeper soft tissue hemangiomas are asymptomatic until late childhood or early adult life. The lesions frequently are associated with overlying skin abnormalities, such as reddish-blue discoloration, enlarged veins, or even cutaneous hemangiomas. Occasionally enlargement of the mass will occur in the dependent position, and rarely pulsations and bruits may be found. The deeper soft tissue hemangiomas may involve muscle, tendon, connective tissue, fatty tissue, synovium, bone, or combinations of these sites (Fig. 79–4). Hemangiomas are relatively common in skeletal muscle, with the highest frequency in the limbs and in young women.

Hemangiomas are associated with a variety of clinical problems, such as consumption coagulopathy, cardiac decompensation, gangrene, osteomalacia, varicose veins, massive osteolysis, Maffucci's syndrome, Klippel-Trenaunay-Weber syndrome, and Kasabach-Merritt syndrome (see Chapter 58). Growth discrepancies associated with vascular lesions also are not uncommon, frequently reflected by overgrowth and less commonly by shortening of the involved extremity.

Hemangiomas are benign lesions classically divided into capillary and cavernous types. Capillary hemangiomas are

composed of capillaries with a sparse fibrous stroma, whereas cavernous hemangiomas are composed of large, dilated, blood-filled spaces lined by flat endothelium. A spectrum of histologic composition may be evident in a single lesion, however.

Radiographically, hemangiomas appear as a nonhomogeneous mass of water density. The margin typically is poorly defined, but occasionally a sharp interface between the tumor and adjacent soft tissue is seen. Tortuous channels of water density representing the arterial supply and venous drainage of the tumor may occasionally be demonstrated radiographically within the adjacent subcutaneous fat. Calcification within the hemangioma is common. One relatively specific type of calcification is the phlebolith (Fig. 79–5). Phleboliths are rounded calcific masses frequently demonstrating a laminated structure. Occasionally, metaplastic ossification may be found in hemangiomas. Adjacent smooth bone erosions also can occur. Overgrowth of the bone and soft tissue of the extremity may be seen.

Arteriovenous malformations are composed of large tortuous arterial and venous vessels and thick-walled capillaries. Arteriographically, large vessels with densely opacified vascular spaces and early filling of draining veins are seen (Fig. 79–6). Venography may be required to evaluate venous malformations, which commonly are associated with lymphatic abnormalities as well.

SYNOVIAL HEMANGIOMAS. Hemangiomas of the synovium are uncommon tumors, occurring most frequently in the knee. They are invariably unilateral. Synovial hemangiomas usually occur in adolescent or young adult women and frequently are symptomatic. They commonly are associated with adjacent cutaneous and deeper soft tissue hemangiomas. Synovial proliferation accompanying diffuse synovial hemangioma can be quite similar to that seen in hemophilia.

The plain film radiographs usually show soft tissue swelling or a mass about the involved joint, occasionally with phle-

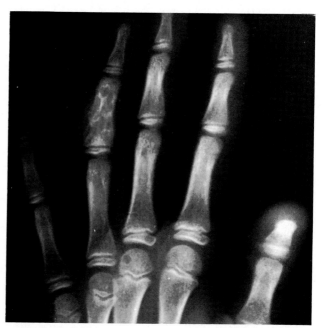

Figure 79–4. Hemangioma of soft tissue and bone of the ring finger. Oblique radiograph shows multiple, sharply circumscribed lytic lesions involving the middle phalanx, with sclerotic margins and extension into the adjacent soft tissue. (Armed Forces Institute of Pathology Neg. No. 78-6162-1.)

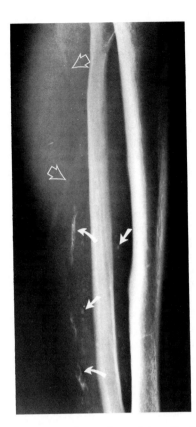

Figure 79–5. Intramuscular hemangioma of the calf with phleboliths. Lateral radiograph shows two patterns of calcification: small circular dense lesions (straight arrows) and linear dense areas with a central lucent core (curved arrows). The channels of water density (open arrows) result from dilated subcutaneous veins. Note the smooth pressure erosion of the tibia posteriorly. (Armed Forces Institute of Pathology Neg. No. 75-2058-3.)

boliths. Advanced maturity of the epiphysis, discrepancy in limb length, periosteal new bone, and articular destruction may be seen (see Chapter 58). Arthrography usually shows the intraarticular mass as multiple filling defects with a villous configuration (Fig. 79–7). The lesions are hypervascular on arteriography.

HEMANGIOPERICYTOMAS. Hemangiopericytomas are vascular tumors of the soft tissue that are believed to originate from the pericytes of Zimmerman, which surround the capillary wall. These slowly growing tumors most frequently present in adults and are located in the deep soft tissue of the thigh. The majority of hemangiopericytomas act in a benign fashion, although occasionally malignant lesions have been encountered.

The plain film radiograph shows a nonspecific soft tissue mass. The tumors may occasionally demonstrate calcification and bone erosion. Arteriography demonstrates an extremely hypervascular tumor.

LYMPHANGIOMAS. Lymphangiomas are rare tumors that are composed of multiple lymph-filled vessels and cystic spaces, with occasional foci of lymphoid tissue. They usually occur in the skin and subcutaneous tissue and frequently are noted at birth or by 1 year of age. Local invasion into adjacent tissues is common, and there is a high recurrence rate after local excision.

Cartilage Tumors

Chondromas may occur as cartilage proliferations of the soft tissue. They most commonly arise from synovium of joints and occasionally from a tendon sheath or bursa. In these sites they are referred to as (idiopathic) synovial (osteo)chondromatosis. Less commonly, chondromas of other soft parts are encountered.

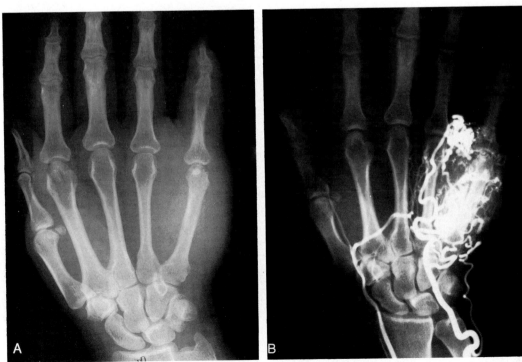

Figure 79–6. Arteriovenous malformation of the hand. A Frontal film shows diffuse soft tissue swelling about the fifth metacarpal bone and phalanges in association with erosions and osteoporosis of the underlying bone. **B** Arteriogram (arterial phase) demonstrates an enlarged ulnar artery and mass of tortuous vessels predominantly about the fifth metacarpal bone. (Armed Forces Institute of Pathology Neg. No. 78-8767-3, 78-8767-2.)

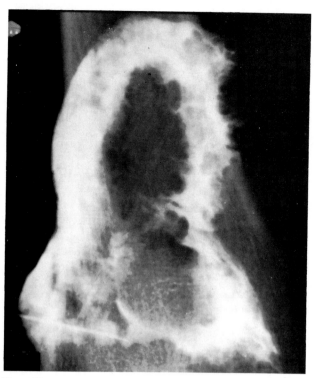

Figure 79–7. Hemangioma of the synovium of the knee. The arthrogram demonstrates a villonodular pattern. (Armed Forces Institute of Pathology Neg. No. 77-4645-6.)

show a nonspecific soft tissue mass, often with coarse specks of calcification. The mass can also cause extrinsic pressure erosion of the adjacent bone, with scalloping and a sclerotic margin.

Fibrous Tumors

Fibrous tumors of soft tissue represent a heterogeneous group of lesions. Benign forms of fibrous proliferative "tumors" have been termed "fibromatosis" to distinguish them from reparative scar tissue. Two principal groups of fibromatosis are recognized. In one group the disorder occurs as a congenital lesion or is diagnosed during childhood. From this group, some lesions can be differentiated by anatomic location and microscopic appearance into specific diagnoses, such as juvenile aponeurotic fibroma, infantile dermal fibromatosis, aggressive infantile fibromatosis, and congenital generalized fibromatosis. The other group of lesions is usually found in the adult.

JUVENILE APONEUROTIC FIBROMAS. Juvenile aponeurotic fibroma occurs in children or adolescents, with a male predominance. It usually arises in the aponeurotic tissue of the hands and feet and is manifested as a painless, firm soft tissue mass. The tumor grows slowly with infiltration and tends to calcify. Local recurrence is common.

INFANTILE DERMAL FIBROMATOSIS. Infantile dermal fibromatosis is a benign fibrous proliferative lesion that almost exclusively involves the extensor surfaces of fingers and

SYNOVIAL (OSTEO)CHONDROMATOSIS. Idiopathic synovial chondromatosis represents cartilage formation through a process of metaplasia of the synovial membrane. This disorder is almost invariably a monarticular disease with a chronic progressive course. The most common joints affected are the knee, hip, and elbow. The disorder is twice as common in men as in women and usually is found in the third to fifth decades of life. Clinically, patients show a several-year history of joint pain with limitation of motion. Intraarticular loose body formation is common. Focal recurrence after surgery is not uncommon. Synovial chondromatosis may rarely become malignant.

Radiographically, synovial chondromatosis commonly demonstrates multiple juxtaarticular radiodense shadows. They range in size from a few millimeters to several centimeters and show varying degrees of mineralization within each lesion. Some nodules may be of water density and seen only as soft tissue masses in or about the joint. The nodules may cause erosions of the adjacent bone and widening of the joint space (Fig. 79–8). Noncalcified lesions are best seen on arthrography (Fig. 79–9). In the late stages, many loose bodies will be found, and secondary osteoarthritis is common. The joint space at this time will be narrow, with eburnation and osteophyte formation consistent with secondary osteoarthritis.

SOFT TISSUE CHONDROMAS. Chondromas of the soft parts occur more frequently in men and are seen predominantly in the third and fourth decades of life. The tumors are slow-growing masses and almost invariably occur in the extremities, especially in the hands and feet. Radiographs

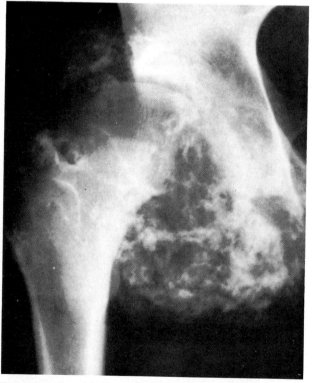

Figure 79–8. Synovial chondromatosis of the hip. Anteroposterior radiograph shows a large joint mass with stipples, rings, and arcs of calcification. The femoral head is displaced laterally and osteoarthritic changes are present. Bone erosions also are noted. (Armed Forces Institute of Pathology Neg. No. 74-12924-2.)

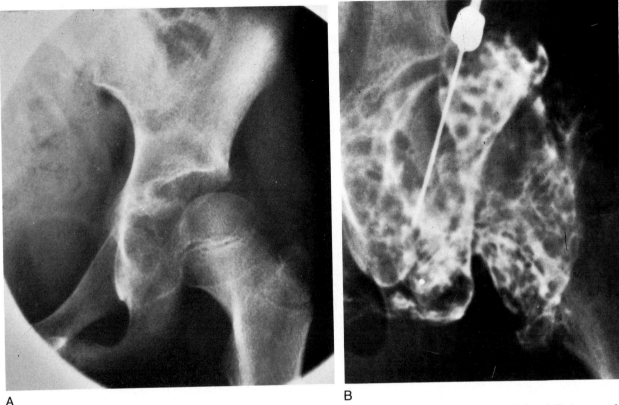

A

B

Figure 79–9. Synovial chondromatosis of the hip. A Anteroposterior radiograph of the hip shows a widened joint space with lateral displacement of the femoral head. There is no evidence of soft tissue calcification. **B** Arthrogram demonstrates multiple noncalcified nodules filling the joint. (Armed Forces Institute of Pathology Neg. Nos. 79-2001,2.)

toes. It appears within the first 2 years of life, particularly in boys. Classically, several digits are involved by multiple nodules, which are firmly attached to skin. They may also attach to the adjacent fascia or periosteum. Clinically, there may be a reddish appearance to the nodules. Recurrence is frequent after surgery.

Radiologically, multiple soft tissue masses are noted on the extensor surface of the digits. The fingers may be deformed with flexion contractures, and rarely bone erosions are found.

AGGRESSIVE INFANTILE FIBROMATOSIS. This lesion appears as painless soft tissue masses in the extremities, usually during the first 2 years of life (Fig. 79–10). The tumor rarely metastasizes; however, it is locally aggressive, infiltrating into muscles, vessels, nerves, fasciae, tendons, and subcutaneous fat. Histologic features make differentiation from fibrosarcoma difficult, and the lesions tend to recur after surgery. The radiographs demonstrate a soft tissue mass with occasional bone erosion.

INFANTILE MYOFIBROMATOSIS. Infantile myofibromatosis (also termed congenital generalized fibromatosis) is a disseminated disease that develops in utero and usually is fatal shortly after birth, if the infant is not stillborn. It consists of multiple nodular lesions of fibroblastic proliferation in superficial soft tissue, muscle, viscera, and bone. Familial occurrences have been noted. The radiograph shows soft tissue swelling or masses and frequently multiple lytic lesions in bone. When viscera are uninvolved, the prognosis is better (see Chapter 85).

Other Benign Soft Tissue Tumors

GANGLIONS. Ganglions are masses that are usually attached to tendon sheaths of the hands and feet. These lesions are characterized by cystic spaces with a myxoid matrix. The lesions rarely communicate with the synovium of a tendon sheath or a joint, and they are not lined by synovium. Radiographically, they appear as soft tissue masses, and if large enough, the fluid-filled space may be demonstrated by sonography or computed tomography. Angiography shows the mass to be avascular.

OTHER TUMORS. Other lesions occurring in soft tissue include histiocytoma, xanthomatosis, leiomyoma, myxoma, rhabdomyoma, and myoblastoma (see Chapter 85).

MALIGNANT SOFT TISSUE TUMORS
Malignant Fibrous Histiocytomas

Malignant fibrous histiocytoma is the most common soft tissue sarcoma occurring in late adult life. It is rare in children or in patients under 20 years of age. The tumor generally is regarded as arising from primitive mesenchymal cells that demonstrate partial histiocytic and fibroblastic differentiation. The lesion predominates in white men and is most frequent in the deep soft tissue of the extremities and retroperitoneum. Metastases are frequent, usually involving the lungs, lymph nodes, liver, and bones.

Radiologic evaluation shows a well-defined, homogeneous soft tissue mass that may calcify and, rarely, erode bone.

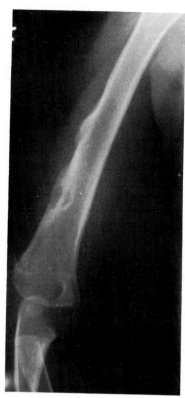

Figure 79–10. Aggressive infantile fibromatosis of the upper arm. Anteroposterior radiograph shows bony erosions with areas of cortical hyperostosis. (Armed Forces Institute of Pathology Neg. No. 67-6597-1.)

upper. The neoplasms generally arise adjacent to a joint, bursa, or tendon sheath. Fewer than 10 per cent are primarily located within the joint cavity, however. Synovial sarcomas occur at all ages but are most frequent in the young adult. The tumor usually grows slowly. Metastasis, when present, usually occurs to the lungs. Local recurrence after surgery is common and is associated with a poor prognosis.

Radiographically, a soft tissue mass possessing a smooth or indistinct margin usually is present. Spotty calcification occurs in about one third of lesions. The tumor can also cause adjacent bone destruction. Arteriography in synovial sarcoma usually demonstrates a hypervascular lesion. Computed tomography shows a soft tissue mass, which may infiltrate adjacent structures.

Rhabdomyosarcomas

Rhabdomyosarcoma is a common malignant soft tissue tumor of muscle origin, which has an exceedingly poor prognosis. In children, the mass is frequently found in the head and neck or genitourinary tract. Tumors in adult patients most commonly occur in the deep soft tissues of the extremities. Infiltration of local tissues is common and probably is responsible for the frequent recurrence after initial surgery. Distant spread to the lungs and occasionally lymph nodes also is common. There are three histologic types: embryonic, alveolar, and pleomorphic. The embryonic type is the most common type and typically occurs in children. The alveolar

Computed tomography demonstrates a mass with some areas that reveal enhancement and others that are nonenhancing, corresponding to sites of necrosis with cystic and hemorrhagic spaces. The malignant fibrous histiocytoma is usually hypervascular during angiography.

Liposarcomas

Liposarcoma is a common soft tissue malignancy. It is seen most frequently in adults but may occur at any age. The tumors usually are located in the buttock, thigh, lower leg, and retroperitoneum, and there is a slight male predominance. Clinically these lesions appear as masses that may recur after surgery. It is generally agreed that liposarcomas arise de novo rather than from benign lipomas. The most common sites for metastasis are the lungs, pleurae, and liver.

Radiographically, the liposarcoma usually presents as a nonhomogeneous, poorly defined mass that may calcify. The mass may be well circumscribed, however, with obvious fatty content on plain films. The latter finding is seen most frequently in the well-differentiated liposarcoma (Fig. 79–11). Computed tomography may demonstrate the fat-containing mass, with structures of water density and with poor margins. The portions of water density will usually show enhancement on computed tomography after intravenous injection of contrast medium.

Synovial Sarcomas

Synovial sarcoma is an uncommon malignant tumor, which is located most frequently in the soft tissue of the extremities (Fig. 79–12), the lower extremities more often than the

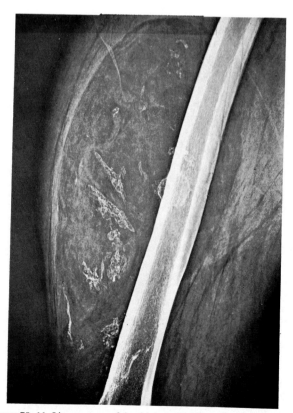

Figure 79–11. Liposarcoma of the thigh, well-differentiated type. Lateral xeroradiograph shows the sharply circumscribed, fatty mass with multiple calcifications. Some dense areas have a trabecular pattern and represent ossification. (Armed Forces Institute of Pathology Neg. No. 77-7859-4.)

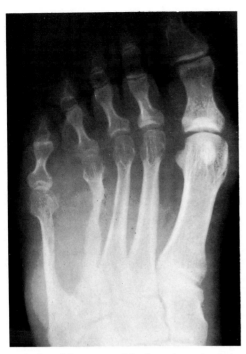

Figure 79–12. Synovial sarcoma of the foot. Aggressive destruction and infiltration of the fourth and fifth metatarsal bones are seen. (Armed Forces Institute of Pathology Neg. No. 74-12420-3.)

the joint; among these are malignant schwannoma, leiomyosarcoma, extraskeletal osteosarcoma, extraskeletal chondrosarcoma, mesenchymoma, and epithelioid sarcoma (see Chapter 85).

SOFT TISSUE TUMOR-LIKE LESIONS

Myositis Ossificans

Localized myositis ossificans is a tumor-like heterotopic formation of bone and cartilage in soft tissue, usually muscles, but also tendons, ligaments, fasciae, aponeuroses, and joint capsules. This lesion is discussed in Chapter 85.

Villonodular Synovitis

Villonodular synovitis is a proliferative disorder of the synovium. It is thought to arise in the synovial lining of joints, tendon sheaths, fascial planes, or ligamentous tissue. It usually involves young adults and is slightly more common in men.

A localized type of villonodular synovitis appears usually as a nonpainful soft tissue mass, frequently located in the digits of the hands and feet (Fig. 79–14). Other joints, especially the knees, and tendon sheaths can be involved. A monarticular distribution is the rule. The cause is unknown. A more diffuse pattern of pigmented villonodular synovitis is less common and usually involves the larger joints, especially the knee. Grossly, the lesion is brown, owing to extensive

type tends to affect older children and young adults and is frequently found in the extremities. The pleomorphic type is the least common and predominates in the skeletal muscles of adults. Radiographically, these tumors appear as poorly defined soft tissue masses. They tend to involve adjacent bone. Calcification within the tumor also may occur.

Fibrosarcomas

Fibrosarcoma arises in the fibrous supportive structures of muscles, tendons, ligaments, and fasciae. The tumor is most frequent in the extremities. Fibrosarcoma is found in both adults and children and has a male predominance. The tumor infiltrates the adjacent soft tissue, and therefore recurrence following surgery is frequent.

The fibrosarcoma appears as a nonspecific soft tissue mass on the plain film radiograph. Infiltration into adjacent bone with destruction and calcification, although not common, can be seen. Arteriography demonstrates hypervascularity with neovascularity. The more vascular tumors generally reflect a higher grade sarcoma and a poorer prognosis.

The fibrosarcomas in infants are unique. They usually occur within the first 2 years of life, frequently at birth, and have a better prognosis (Fig. 79–13). These tumors are more common in boys and chiefly affect the distal areas of the lower and upper extremities. Radiographically, a soft tissue mass is seen, and frequently severe deformity and marked erosions of adjacent bone are noted.

Other Malignant Soft Tissue Tumors

Other malignant soft tissue tumors may be considered in the differential diagnosis of soft tissue masses in and about

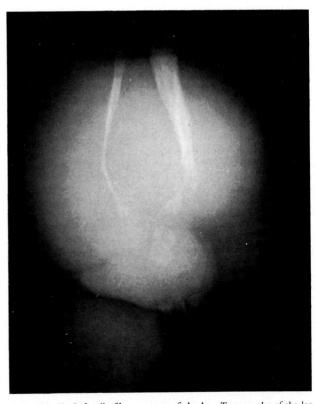

Figure 79–13. Infantile fibrosarcoma of the leg. Tomography of the leg shows a large mass of water density with displacement, deformity, and erosion of the tibia and fibula. (Armed Forces Institute of Pathology Neg. No. 77-477-9.)

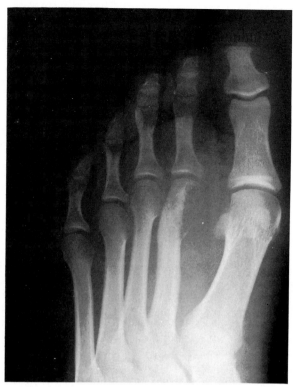

Figure 79–14. Villonodular synovitis of the foot. Radiograph shows a soft tissue mass widening the space between the first and second metatarsal bones and bone erosions. (Armed Forces Institute of Pathology Neg. No. 66-2598-1.)

hemosiderin deposition. It often is associated with hemorrhagic effusions.

On radiographs, localized villonodular synovitis appears as a soft tissue mass, frequently associated with bone erosions (Fig. 79–14). These erosions have well-defined sclerotic margins and are a sign of direct extension and pressure effect. Diffuse intraarticular pigmented villonodular synovitis produces a joint effusion. Usually, the joint space is normal in width and osteoporosis is absent or mild. Bone erosions can occur in juxtaarticular locations and are variable in size. Such osseous defects are more frequent in "tight" articulations, such as the hip, the elbow, and the wrist. Calcification is not typical. If hemosiderin deposition is extensive, it can be demonstrable on computed tomography as increased attenuation values or on magnetic resonance images as decreased signal intensity on T1 and T2 weighted images.

The differential diagnosis of the radiographic features of localized nodular synovitis includes other soft tissue tumors and tumor-like lesions. Diffuse pigmented villonodular synovitis must be differentiated from idiopathic synovial osteochondromatosis (in which calcification and ossification may appear), infection (in which osteoporosis, joint space loss, and poorly defined bone erosions may be seen), and other articular disorders.

Idiopathic Tumoral Calcinosis

Idiopathic tumoral calcinosis is a rare condition, consisting of calcium salt deposition in extracapsular soft tissues about joints. The masses occur most frequently in children and adolescents. An increased frequency in blacks and a familial

tendency are recognized. These lesions are found most commonly about the shoulders, hips, and elbows. Idiopathic tumoral calcinosis is discussed in Chapter 85.

Aneurysms

Popliteal artery aneurysm is the most common aneurysm found in the extremities. Patients usually first come to medical attention in the fifth or sixth decade of life with pain and claudication; however, ischemia and swelling in the lower leg and neurologic symptoms resulting from pressure on the sciatic nerve also can be noted. The aneurysm usually is palpated on physical examination.

Radiographically, the aneurysm appears as a pulsatile soft tissue mass in the popliteal space. Curvilinear calcification may be noted in its wall. The aneurysm also may erode adjacent bone, causing scalloping of the cortex. Arteriography is extremely helpful in evaluating the arterial and venous vascular beds and in demonstrating the vascular origin of the soft tissue mass.

Granulomatous Synovitis

Advanced granulomatous synovitis, especially tuberculous synovitis, may cause a soft tissue mass in or about the joint. The process is insidious and progressive, with ultimate destruction of the joint (see Chapter 61).

Synovial Cysts

A variety of cystic lesions may be found about a joint, especially the knee, including a synovial cyst, a distended bursa (with or without communication with the adjacent articulation), and a meniscal cyst. The term "synovial cyst" describes a continuation or herniation of the synovial membrane through the joint capsule. The common popliteal cyst results from a communication of the knee joint with the

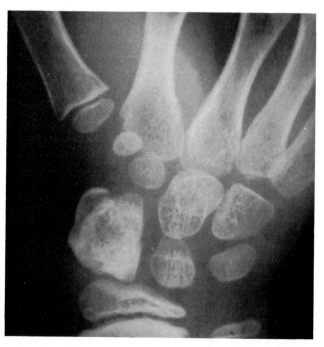

Figure 79–15. Trevor's disease. Note the asymmetric enlargement of the scaphoid. Histologically, the findings were virtually identical to those of an osteochondroma. More frequently, the bones about the knee or ankle are affected. (Courtesy of R. Freiberger, M.D., New York, New York.)

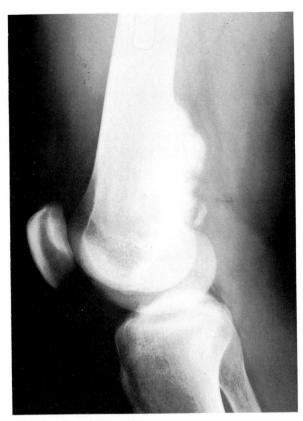

Figure 79–16. Parosteal osteosarcoma of the femur. Lateral radiograph shows a dense homogeneous mass with an irregular margin arising from the posterior surface of the distal femur. (Armed Forces Institute of Pathology Neg. No. 52-7554.)

gastrocnemiosemimembranosus bursa. Similar lesions at other locations can be seen but are less frequent. Synovial cysts commonly contain fluid and often are associated with traumatic, degenerative, or inflammatory processes in the joint. Rheumatoid arthritis is the most recognized cause of large synovial cysts.

Synovial cysts are of clinical significance because they may appear as a periarticular mass, cause pain or limitation of joint mobility, or compress adjacent neurovascular structures; they may also acutely rupture or dissect or become secondarily infected.

The identification of the fluid-filled cystic mass is best accomplished with arthrography (particularly if the cyst communicates with the nearby joint), sonography, computed tomography, and magnetic resonance imaging.

Small cysts about the knee may be associated with meniscal tears. These are referred to as meniscal cysts, and typically they involve the lateral aspect of the joint (see Chapter 14).

BONE TUMORS
Benign Bone Tumors

Benign tumors involving periarticular bone include osteochondroma, periosteal (juxtacortical) chondroma, articular chondroma (Trevor's disease) (Fig. 79–15), and osteoid osteoma. Occasionally benign intraosseous lesions such as giant cell tumor and chondroblastoma will extend beyond the confines of the bone cortex into the adjacent soft tissue. These lesions are described in Chapter 78.

Malignant Bone Tumors

Malignant bone tumors frequently extend into the adjacent soft tissue (see Chapter 78). This extension is commonly seen with primary skeletal malignancies, such as osteosarcoma, chondrosarcoma, and Ewing's tumor. The extraosseous extension can be evaluated by plain films, arteriography, and computed tomography and is easily differentiated from primary soft tissue lesions. Parosteal sarcoma, a malignant tumor developing from the periosteum, may be confused with soft tissue tumor, however. Radiographically, parosteal osteosarcoma usually shows a dense, homogeneous calcific mass on the cortical surface of the distal portion of the femur (Fig. 79–16). Calcification extends into the adjacent soft tissue, with an irregular margin. The tumor may occasionally grow into the adjacent medullary space.

FURTHER READING

Allen PW: The fibromatoses: A clinicopathologic classification based on 140 cases. Am J Surg Pathol 1:255, 1977.

Bliznak J, Staple TW: Radiology of angiodysplasias of the limb. Radiology 110:35, 1974.

Bouhoutsos J, Martin P: Popliteal aneurysm: A review of 116 cases. Br J Surg 61:469, 1974.

Burleson J, Bickel WH, Dahlin DC: Popliteal cyst. A clinicopathological survey. J Bone Joint Surg [Am] 38:1265, 1956.

Breimer CW, Freiberger RH: Bone lesions associated with villonodular synovitis. AJR 79:618, 1958.

Cavanagh RC: Tumors of the soft tissues of the extremities. Semin Roentgenol 8:73, 1973.

Cavanagh RC, Schwamm HA: Localized nodular synovitis. RPC of the month from the AFIP. Radiology 100:409, 1971.

Chung EB, Enzinger FM: Benign lipoblastomatosis. An analysis of 35 cases. Cancer 32:482, 1973.

Chung EB, Enzinger FM: Infantile fibrosarcoma. Cancer 38:729, 1976.

Chung EB, Enzinger FM: Chondroma of soft parts. Cancer 41:1414, 1978.

Chung SMK, Janes JM: Diffuse pigmented villonodular synovitis of the hip joint. Review of the literature and report of four cases. J Bone Joint Surg [Am] 47:293, 1965.

Condon VR, Allen RP: Congenital generalized fibromatosis. Case report with roentgen manifestations. Radiology 76:444, 1961.

Craig RM, Pugh DG, Soule EH: Roentgenologic manifestations of synovial sarcoma. Radiology 65:837, 1955.

Dahlin DC, Salvador AH: Cartilaginous tumor of the soft tissues of the hands and feet. Mayo Clin Proc 49:721, 1974.

Dionne GP, Seemayer TA: Infiltrating lipomas and angiolipomas revisited. Cancer 33:732, 1974.

Dooms GC, Hricak H, Sollitto RA, Higgins CB: Lipomatous tumors and tumors with fatty component: MR imaging potential and comparison of MR and CT results. Radiology 157:479, 1985.

Enzinger FM, Weiss SW: Soft Tissue Tumors. St Louis, CV Mosby Company, 1983.

Finberg HJ, Levin DC: Angiolipoma: A rare benign soft tissue tumor with a malignant arteriographic appearance. AJR 128:697, 1977.

Fischer HJ, Lois JF, Gomes AS, Mirra JM, Deutsch LS: Radiology and pathology of malignant fibrous histiocytomas of the soft tissues: A report of ten cases. Skel Radiol 13:202, 1985.

Fletcher AG Jr, Horn RC Jr: Giant cell tumors of tendon sheath origin. A consideration of bone involvement and report of two cases with extensive bone destruction. Ann Surg 133:374, 1951.

Goergen IG, Resnick D, Niwayama G: Localized nodular synovitis of the knee: A report of two cases with abnormal arthrograms. AJR 126:647, 1976.

Greenfield MM, Wallace KM: Pigmented villonodular synovitis. Radiology 54:350, 1950.

Hale DE: Synovioma with special reference to the clinical and roentgenologic aspects. AJR 65:769, 1951.

Heitzman ER, Jones JB: Roentgen characteristics of cavernous hemangioma of striated muscle. Radiology 74:420, 1960.

Horowitz AL, Resnick D, Watson RC: The roentgen features of synovial sarcoma. Clin Radiol 24:481, 1973.

Jacobs P: Parosteal lipoma with hyperostosis. Clin Radiol 23:196, 1972.

Jeffreys TE: Synovial chondromatosis. J Bone Joint Surg [Br] 49:530, 1967.

Kindblom LG, Angervall L, Stener B, Wickbom I: Intermuscular and intramuscular lipomas and hibernomas: A clinical, roentgenologic, histologic, and prognostic study of 46 cases. Cancer 33:754, 1974.

Kindblom LG, Gunterberg B: Pigmented villonodular synovitis involving bone. J Bone Joint Surg [Am] 60:830, 1978.

Levine E, Lee KR, Neff JR, Maklad NF, Robinson RG, Preston DF: Comparison of computed tomography and other imaging modalities in the evaluation of musculoskeletal tumors. Radiology 131:431, 1979.

Lewis RW: Roentgen recognition of synovioma. AJR 44:170, 1940.

Lichtenstein L: Tumors of synovial joints, bursae and tendon sheaths. Cancer 8:816, 1955.

MacKenzie DH: The Differential Diagnosis of Fibroblastic Disorders. Oxford, Blackwell Scientific Publications, 1970.

McMaster MJ, Soule EH, Ivins JC: Hemangiopericytoma. A clinico-pathologic study and long term follow-up of 60 patients. Cancer 36:2232, 1975.

Milgram JW: The classification of loose bodies in human joints. Clin Orthop 124:282, 1977.

Milgram JW: Synovial osteochondromatosis. A histopathological study of thirty cases. J Bone Joint Surg [Am] 59:792, 1977.

Moore O, Grossi C: Embryonal rhabdomyosarcoma of the head and neck. Cancer 12:69, 1959.

Pack GT, Pierson JC: Liposarcoma: A study of 105 cases. Surgery 36:687, 1954.

Piyachon C: Radiology of peripheral arteriovenous malformations. Australas Radiol 21:246, 1977.

Resnick D, Oliphant M: Hemophilia-like arthropathy of the knee associated with cutaneous and synovial hemangiomas. Report of 3 cases and review of the literature. Radiology 114:323, 1975.

Rosenthal DL: Computed tomography in bone and soft tissue neoplasm: application and pathologic correlation. CRC Crit Rev Diagn Imaging 18:243, 1982.

Sartoris DJ, Danzig L, Gilula L, Greenway G, Resnick D: Synovial cysts of the hip joint and iliopsoas bursitis: A spectrum of imaging abnormalities. Skel Radiol 14:85, 1985.

Shnitka TK, Asp DM, Horner RH: Congenital generalized fibromatosis. Cancer 11:627, 1958.

Smith JH, Pugh DG: Roentgenographic aspects of articular pigmented villonodular synovitis. AJR 87:1146, 1962.

Spjut HJ, Dorfman HD, Fechner RE, Ackerman LV: Tumors of Bone and Cartilage. Atlas of Tumor Pathology. Second Series, Fascicle 5. Washington, DC, Armed Forces Institute of Pathology, 1971.

Steinbach L, Hellman D, Petri M, Gillespy T, Genant H: Magnetic resonance imaging: a review of rheumatologic applications. Semin Arthritis Rheum 16:79, 1986.

Stout AP: Pathology and classification of tumors of the soft tissues. AJR 66:903, 1951.

Stout AP, Lattes R: Tumors of the Soft Tissues. Atlas of Tumor Pathology. Second Series, Fascicle 1. Washington DC, Armed Forces Institute of Pathology, 1967.

Trias A, Quintana O: Synovial chondrometaplasia: Review of world literature and a study of 18 Canadian cases. Can J Surg 19:151, 1976.

Weiss SW, Enzinger FM: Myxoid variant of malignant fibrous histiocytoma. Cancer 39:1672, 1977.

Weiss SW, Enzinger FM: Malignant fibrous histiocytoma: An analysis of 200 cases. Cancer 41:2250, 1978.

Zimmerman C, Sayegh V: Roentgen manifestations of synovial osteochondromatosis. AJR 83:680, 1960.

Zlatkin MB, Lander PH, Begin LR, Hadjipavlou A: Soft-tissue chondromas. AJR 144:1263, 1985.

Chapter 80

Skeletal Metastases

Donald Resnick, M.D.
Gen Niwayama, M.D.

Metastatic disease of the skeleton can arise from direct extension, lymphatic or hematogenous dissemination, or intraspinal spread of tumor. The osseous response to the neoplasm consists of bone resorption or bone formation, or both. Such metastases predominate in the bones of the axial skeleton, although atypical patterns of distribution are encountered. A variety of diagnostic techniques, including scintigraphy, computed tomography, and magnetic resonance imaging, can be used in addition to routine radiography in the initial detection and subsequent monitoring of the metastatic foci.

Any malignant neoplasm possesses the capacity to metastasize to the musculoskeletal system, although some do so more frequently than others. Furthermore, nonmalignant tumors can occasionally metastasize if, through the erosion of the wall of a blood vessel, neoplastic cells enter the vascular system. Of the potential pathways available for the dissemination of tumor, vascular channels are more important than lymphatic channels; extension of neoplastic cells through lymph vessels to regional lymph nodes generally is followed by entrance into the vascular system. Venous invasion is more common than arterial invasion as the arterial wall exhibits striking immunity to tumor penetration in the absence of associated infection.

GENERAL MECHANISMS OF SKELETAL METASTASIS

The skeleton is one of the most frequent sites of tumor metastasis and, as in other locations, successful metastatic implantation requires both the transport of viable tumor cells to the bone and the interaction of these cells with the osseous tissue.

Routes Allowing Spread of Tumor to Bone

Several distinct routes allow tumors to metastasize to bone: direct extension or invasion from adjacent tissues; lymphatic spread; hematogenous dissemination; and intraspinal spread.

DIRECT EXTENSION. Malignant neoplasms located in the soft tissues adjacent to a bone may subsequently penetrate that bone by direct extension. Examples include a squamous cell carcinoma of the skin that involves an underlying bone, a carcinoma at the apex of the lung (Pancoast tumor) that invades the ribs or cervical vertebrae (Fig. 80–1), a tumor of the nasopharynx that leads to destruction in the base of the skull, a carcinoma of the bladder or the rectum that involves the bones of the pelvis, or a pancreatic carcinoma that extends directly into the lower thoracic and lumbar vertebrae. In these instances, the intraosseous tumor is in direct continuity with the site of primary involvement. In other instances, contiguous spread of tumor into bone originates from a site that itself is distant from the primary tumor. Examples of this situation include carcinomas of the lung that extend into the mediastinum with subsequent involvement of the spine (Fig. 80–2), or a soft tissue metastatic deposit resulting from hematogenous or lymphatic dissemination that subsequently invades the adjacent osseous tissue.

In all of these situations, the resulting abnormalities typically consist of a soft tissue mass and osseous destruction. This combination of findings also is observed in infectious lesions of the skeleton and primary malignant tumors of the skeleton or soft tissues; a large soft tissue mass is an infrequent manifestation of skeletal metastasis arising from hematogenous dissemination of tumor.

LYMPHATIC SPREAD. Although the lymphatic system is relatively unimportant in the transportation of tumor cells to distant bones, metastatic deposits in regional draining lymph nodes can secondarily involve the adjacent osseous structures (Fig. 80–2). An important example of this phenomenon is the occurrence of vertebral destruction in cases of pelvic carcinomas arising in the prostate, bladder, cervix, and uterus. Imaging studies demonstrate a paravertebral soft tissue mass and scalloped erosions of one or more vertebral bodies. Similar abnormalities are observed in some patients with lymphoma and plasma cell myeloma, however. Furthermore, infectious lesions of the spine are accompanied by vertebral destruction and soft tissue masses.

HEMATOGENOUS DISSEMINATION. The blood stream is the major pathway allowing dissemination of malignant neoplasms to the skeleton. Two potential vascular routes exist, the arterial system and the venous system, particularly Batson's vertebral plexus. The predilection for metastases to affect the spine, and the presence of vertebral metastasis in the absence of pulmonary (or other organ) involvement are findings that support the significance of Batson's vertebral plexus in tumor spread (Fig. 80–3).

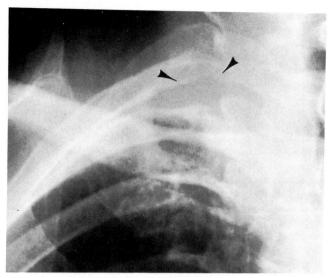

Figure 80–1. Routes of tumor spread to bone: Direct extension. Pancoast tumor. A carcinoma in the apex of the lung has led to destruction of the posterior portion of the second rib (arrowheads).

Reactive new bone occurs as a response to bone destruction and is similar to the callus that develops in fracture healing. This process is seen to variable extent in virtually all malignant neoplasms, but it may be a minor feature in highly anaplastic, rapidly growing tumors and in plasma cell myeloma, lymphomas, or leukemias.

GENERAL CLINICAL MANIFESTATIONS

Certain general clinical characteristics of skeletal metastasis deserve emphasis. Bone pain is a common abnormality that can relate to elevation of medullary pressure, stretching of the periosteal membrane, the occurrence of a pathologic fracture, or compression of adjacent neurologic structures. A soft tissue mass and deformity are additional possible manifestations.

Laboratory parameters of skeletal metastasis include elevation of the serum level of calcium. The hypercalcemia has a complex pathogenesis and is dependent on such factors as the degree of immobilization or bone resorption and destruction. Elevation of the serum level of alkaline phosphatase in patients with skeletal metastasis is less constant in persons with purely osteolytic lesions. Measurement of serum acid phosphatase is useful in the evaluation of patients with prostatic carcinoma.

FREQUENCY AND DISTRIBUTION OF SKELETAL METASTASIS

The estimated frequency of skeletal metastasis determined on the basis of radiographic examination obviously is low owing to the relatively insensitive nature of this diagnostic technique. Scintigraphy using bone-seeking radiopharmaceutical agents is a more sensitive method of analysis, although

INTRASPINAL SPREAD. The cerebrospinal fluid represents an additional pathway for tumor dissemination, allowing secondary deposits in the spinal canal to develop in patients with intracranial neoplasms. Children and adults are affected, and the types of tumors leading to subarachnoid spread (in children) are, in order of decreasing frequency, medulloblastoma, ependymoma, pineal neoplasms, astrocytoma, lymphoma, choroid plexus papilloma, and retinoblastoma. Although osteoblastic lesions of the vertebrae (as well as the pelvis and elsewhere), are seen occasionally, accurate diagnosis may require the use of myelography, computed tomography, and magnetic resonance imaging.

Osseous Response to Metastatic Tumor

The response of bone to secondary deposits of tumor can be classified broadly into two types: bone resorption and bone formation.

BONE RESORPTION. Osteoclast-mediated osteolysis is suggested as an early and quantitatively important mechanism of bone loss accompanying skeletal metastasis. A similar pattern of osteolysis is observed in patients with plasma cell myeloma and lymphoma, in which leukocytes produce an osteoclast activating factor. In carcinomas, the humoral substance promoting local bone loss may be a prostaglandin. Malignant cells themselves may secrete lytic enzymes responsible for the continued destruction of the bone.

BONE FORMATION. Two main mechanisms account for new bone formation associated with skeletal metastasis: stromal bone formation and reactive bone formation. Stromal new bone formation occurs only in those skeletal metastases that are associated with the development of fibrous stroma, particularly those arising from carcinoma of the prostate; highly cellular tumors possess little or no stroma and are not accompanied by this type of bone formation.

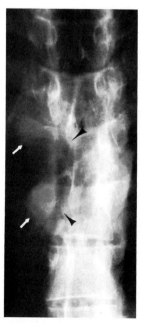

Figure 80–2. Routes of tumor spread to bone: Lymphatic spread with direct extension. A carcinoma of the lung has spread to paravertebral lymph nodes (arrows) with subsequent extension into several thoracic vertebrae (arrowheads). Note the pedicle destruction.

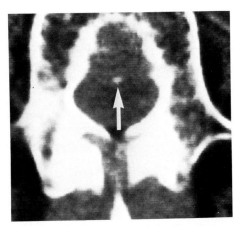

Figure 80–3. Routes of tumor spread to bone: Hematogenous dissemination via basivertebral veins. Renal cell carcinoma. A computed tomographic scan at the level of the third lumbar vertebra reveals involvement of the posterior portion of the vertebral body by the metastatic lesion. Observe tumor extension into the spinal canal with a small remnant of the posterior vertebral margin (arrow). (From Sartoris DJ, et al: Vertebral venous channels: CT appearance and differential considerations. Radiology 155:745, 1985. Used with permission.)

falsely negative examinations occur in some malignant tumors that are extremely aggressive in their behavior and in markedly debilitated patients. Pathologic inspection at the time of autopsy is potentially an accurate method of detecting osseous metastasis, but severe limitations of this technique also are encountered.

Most studies dealing with skeletal metastasis have confirmed the following observations:

1. The skeleton is a common site of metastasis in many types of primary malignant tumor.

2. Carcinomas of the breast, prostate, and lung, in decreasing order, are the common sources of skeletal metastases in a general population; in men, carcinomas of the prostate, lung, and bladder, in similar order, are the typical sources of such metastases, and in women, carcinomas of the breast and uterus are common causes of skeletal metastases.

3. On the basis of an equal number of various types of primary malignant tumors, carcinomas of the prostate, breast, kidney, lung, and thyroid gland, in order of decreasing frequency, metastasize to the skeleton.

4. The vast majority of metastatic lesions in the skeleton are encountered in middle-aged and elderly patients.

5. Typical causes of skeletal metastasis in children are neuroblastoma, Ewing's sarcoma, osteosarcoma, and malignant tumors of soft tissues.

6. In adults, carcinoma of the prostate, breast, kidney, and lung account for more than 75 per cent of cases of skeletal metastasis, carcinoma of the prostate is responsible for approximately 60 per cent of cases of such metastasis in men, and carcinoma of the breast accounts for approximately 70 per cent of cases of skeletal metastasis in women.

The predominance of skeletal metastasis in the axial skeleton, a region rich in red marrow, is well known. The vertebral column, the bones of the pelvis, the ribs, the sternum, the femoral and humeral shafts, and the skull, in

decreasing order, are the usual locations for skeletal metastasis. The frequency of metastasis is greatest in the lumbar region of the spine followed by the thoracic and cervical segments. Metastatic foci are more common in the vertebral bodies than in the posterior osseous elements, although pedicle destruction is more frequent in cases of skeletal metastasis than in those of plasma cell myeloma. Infrequent sites of skeletal metastasis are the mandible (a site more typically involved in plasma cell myeloma), the patella, and the bones of the extremities that are distal to the elbow and knee (Fig. 80–4). In unusual circumstances, metastasis develops at an osseous site that is already altered by disease (osteomyelitis and Paget's disease) or surgical manipulation.

RADIOGRAPHIC-PATHOLOGIC CORRELATION

The radiographic characteristics of skeletal metastases are highly variable and influenced by a number of factors, including the nature of the primary tumor, the age of the patient, the location of the metastatic lesion or lesions, and the timing of the radiographic examination.

Number of Lesions

Multiplicity is the general rule regarding sites of skeletal metastasis; however, solitary lesions certainly are encountered, especially in patients with carcinoma of the kidney or thyroid. Furthermore, in some instances, only one metastatic lesion is detected on routine radiographs at a time when scintigraphy indicates the presence of many such lesions.

Patterns of Bone Response

The radiographic appearance of skeletal metastases can be broadly classified as purely osteolytic, purely osteosclerotic, and mixed osteolytic-osteosclerotic. Purely osteolytic lesions typically arise from carcinoma of the thyroid, kidney, adrenal

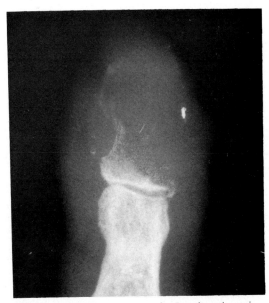

Figure 80–4. Skeletal metastasis: Hands. Bronchogenic carcinoma may metastasize to the phalanges of the hand and the foot. Extensive lysis of the terminal phalanx of the finger is associated with considerable soft tissue swelling. The articular space appears uninvolved.

Table 80–1. SITES OF SKELETAL METASTASES

Primary Focus	Type of Skeletal Lesion	Relative Frequency (Percentage) of Skeletal Lesion		
		X-ray	Bone Scan	Autopsy
Common Primary Cancer				
Breast	Lytic; also mixed; frequently blastic	30 to 50	52 to 67	57 to 73
Lung	Lytic; also mixed; occasionally blastic	14 to 25	54 to 64	19 to 32
Kidney	Invariably lytic	20 to 32	33 to 60	23 to 45
Thyroid	Invariably lytic	8	43	19 to 50
Prostate	Usually blastic; occasionally lytic	33 to 35	62 to 92	57 to 84
			44	
Head and Neck				
Upper respiratory and digestive tract				
Nasal fossa and nasopharynx	Lytic; occasionally blastic	4		
Oral cavity and oropharynx	Lytic	14 to 21		
Endolarynx and hypopharynx	Lytic	1 to 2		
Maxillary sinuses	Lytic	12		
Salivary glands	Lytic	5		
Other carcinomas of neck				28
Parathyroid	Lytic	<1		
Central nervous system				
Brain tumors	Lytic; infrequently blastic	<1		
Paragangliomas	Lytic	<1		
Chordoma	Lytic	15		
Neuroblastoma	Lytic or mixed; occasionally blastic	35 to 75		
Chest				
Pleura and pericardium				
Mesothelioma	Lytic	<1		
Mediastinum				
Thymoma	Lytic; frequently blastic	<1		
Teratoma	Lytic	<1		
Gastrointestinal Tract			41	
Esophagus	Lytic or mixed	3 to 5		1 to 2
Stomach	Lytic or mixed; occasionally blastic	0 to 2.6		2 to 17.5
Colon	Lytic or mixed; infrequently blastic	0.5 to 1	57	9 to 11
Rectum	Lytic or mixed; infrequently blastic	6 to 10	61	
Pancreas	Lytic or mixed; occasionally blastic	1.3 to 3.5		
Liver	Lytic or mixed	<1		
Gall bladder and bile ducts	Lytic or mixed	<1		
Genitourinary Tract			37	
Urinary bladder	Lytic; infrequently blastic	5 to 11	43	13 to 26
Adrenal	Lytic			44
Reproductive System			29	
Uterine cervix	Lytic or mixed; occasionally blastic	3 to 4	56	8 to 15
Uterine corpus	Lytic	6		22
Ovary	Lytic; rarely blastic	2 to 7		6
Testis	Lytic; occasionally blastic	6	8	10 to 20
Skin				
Squamous and basal cell carcinoma	Lytic	<1		
Malignant melanoma	Lytic	2 to 7	57	44 to 57
Primary Bone Tumors				
Osteosarcoma	Lytic or mixed; frequently blastic	4 to 14		
Chondrosarcoma	Lytic or mixed; occasionally blastic	2 to 18		
Fibrosarcoma	Lytic	2 to 23		
Malignant fibrous histiocytoma	Lytic	17		
Hemangioendothelial sarcoma	Lytic (frequently multifocal)	1 to 2		
Ewing's sarcoma	Lytic (permeative)	40 to 50		
Histiocytic lymphoma	Lytic (permeative)	49		
Primary Soft Tissue Tumors				
Fibrous histiocytoma, angiosarcoma, rhabdomyosarcoma	Lytic or mixed	10 or less	56	
Carcinoid Tumors				
Bronchial and abdominal carcinoids (other than appendix)	Blastic; frequently mixed, occasionally lytic	1 or less		

From Wilner D: Radiology of Bone Tumors and Allied Disorders. Philadelphia, WB Saunders Co, 1982, p 3646. Used with permission.

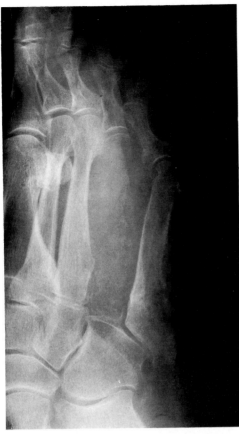

Figure 80–5. Skeletal metastasis: Purely osteolytic pattern. The entire fourth metatarsal bone reveals lytic destruction, and a similar lesion is present at the base of the fifth metatarsal bone. A poorly differentiated adenocarcinoma of unknown origin was responsible for the defects.

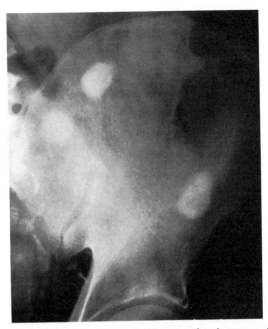

Figure 80–6. Skeletal metastasis: Purely osteosclerotic pattern. Carcinoma of the prostate resulted in multiple well-defined radiodense lesions of the ilium.

Bone Expansion

Metastatic lesions can occasionally lead to bone expansion. Carcinomas of the kidney or thyroid and hepatomas are among the primary malignant tumors that result in expansile, osteolytic skeletal foci. In some of these lesions, a distinctive

gland, uterus, and gastrointestinal tract; mixed osteolytic-osteosclerotic lesions generally occur in carcinomas of the lung, breast, and cervix, and in ovarian and testicular tumors; purely osteosclerotic lesions are encountered in carcinoma of the prostate, and, less constantly, in bronchial carcinoid tumor, bladder carcinoma involving the prostate, carcinomas of the nasopharynx and stomach, medulloblastoma, and neuroblastoma (Table 80–1). None of these patterns is without exception.

Osteolytic lesions (Fig. 80–5) may be well circumscribed (geographic bone destruction) or poorly defined (motheaten or permeative bone destruction). Osteosclerotic lesions (Fig. 80–6) may be focal or diffuse in distribution.

Periosteal Reaction

As a general rule, periosteal new bone is either absent or of limited extent in metastatic lesions, a characteristic that differs from the extensive degree of periostitis that commonly accompanies primary malignant tumors of the skeleton. In unusual circumstances, exuberant periosteal reaction is evident in cases of skeletal metastasis, especially those arising from prostatic carcinoma, gastrointestinal malignancies, retinoblastoma, and neuroblastoma.

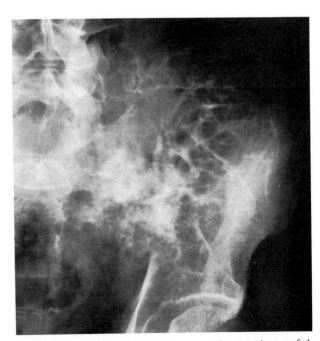

Figure 80–7. Skeletal metastasis: Bone expansion—carcinoma of the kidney. A large expansile, predominantly osteolytic lesion arises in the ilium. Note the septate appearance.

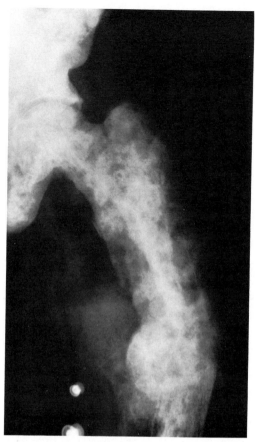

Figure 80–8. Skeletal metastasis: Bone expansion—carcinoma of the prostate. Exuberant new and abnormal bone cloaks the original femoral diaphysis in this patient with widespread osseous metastases. A previous pathologic fracture of the femoral shaft is apparent. The radiographic findings resemble those of Paget's disease.

carcinoma. Such ossification in the soft tissues adjacent to an area of bone destruction simulates the appearance of an osteosarcoma of osseous origin, whereas isolated soft tissue ossific collections in metastases resemble findings in posttraumatic heterotopic ossification, pseudomalignant osseous tumor of soft tissue, an osteosarcoma of soft tissue origin, and ossification following burns and neurologic injuries.

Pathologic Fracture

Metastatic lesions in the skeleton lead to osseous weakening and, frequently, to pathologic fracture (Fig. 80–9). This complication is well recognized in the spine, where compression or collapse of a tumor-containing vertebral body is seen. Pathologic fractures accompanying metastases in tubular bones are most commonly evident in the proximal portion of the femur. The likelihood of pathologic fracture in a tubular bone becomes greater with increasing degrees of cortical destruction.

SPECIFIC SITES OF OSSEOUS INVOLVEMENT
Skull

Single or multiple osteolytic lesions of variable size are evident. They typically possess irregular edges, without sclerotic margins, and involve the inner table, the outer table, or the diploic portion of the cranium alone or in combination. Rarely, a radiodense focus, the button sequestrum, exists in the center of the lesion (Fig. 80–10), although this finding is more typical of eosinophilic granuloma and is observed also in radiation necrosis, tuberculosis and other infections, fibrous dysplasia, multiple myeloma, Paget's disease, and dermoid and epidermoid tumors.

Other conditions that enter into the differential diagnosis of a solitary osteolytic metastatic lesion of the skull include

septate appearance accompanies the osseous expansion (Fig. 80–7). Expansile osteoblastic lesions, resembling Paget's disease, are evident in some patients with metastatic prostatic carcinoma (Fig. 80–8).

Soft Tissue Mass

As a general rule, prominent soft tissue masses are observed infrequently in association with skeletal metastasis, and the detection of such a mass favors the diagnosis of a primary malignant lesion of bone rather than a secondary deposit. Exceptions to this rule are encountered in certain locations and with certain types of neoplasms. In the ribs, extrapleural extension of metastatic lesions leads to soft tissue masses of variable size. Carcinoma of the colon may metastasize to the bones of the pelvis, producing soft tissue masses that occasionally contain calcification.

Soft Tissue Ossification

Ossification in sites of soft tissue metastases occurring with or without adjacent bone involvement has been identified, particularly with carcinoma of the colon, gastric carcinoma, other gastrointestinal malignancies, transitional cell carcinoma of the bladder, carcinoma of the breast, and bronchogenic

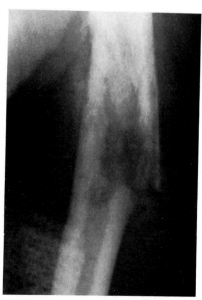

Figure 80–9. Skeletal metastasis: Pathologic fracture. Carcinoma of the lung. An oblique fracture has occurred through a motheaten region of bone destruction in the diaphysis of the humerus.

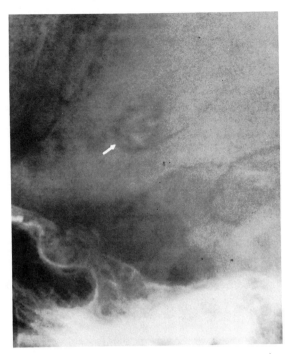

Figure 80–10. Skeletal metastasis: Skull—Button sequestrum. A metastasis from carcinoma of the breast has led to an osteolytic lesion (arrow) containing several small osseous spicules.

an epidermoid or dermoid tumor (which appears as a small, well-defined, round or oval radiolucent diploic focus with a sclerotic margin), hemangioma (which possesses a spiculated or reticular pattern), eosinophilic granuloma (which is an oval or lobulated lesion of the diploic portion of the cranium with differential involvement of the inner and outer tables that produces a beveled margin), fibrous dysplasia (which commonly has a ground-glass or sclerotic appearance, affecting the outer table to a greater degree than the inner table), the doughnut lesion (of unknown cause, which produces one or more radiolucent areas, each surrounded by a sclerotic margin of variable thickness), various infections, lymphomas, and sarcoidosis. Additional disorders that produce multiple osteolytic areas in the skull are multiple myeloma (in which uniformity of size and mandibular involvement are more characteristic), hyperparathyroidism (which produces the "salt and pepper" appearance), histiocytosis, radiation necrosis, prominent venous lakes, and arachnoid granulations.

Osteosclerotic metastatic lesions of the skull usually arise from carcinoma of the prostate. Osteosclerosis of the base of the skull is also a well-recognized manifestation of nasopharyngeal carcinoma. Additional causes of basal osteosclerosis include meningioma, fibrous dysplasia, and adjacent inflammatory processes; other disorders leading to multifocal or diffuse cranial osteosclerosis include Paget's disease, fibrous dysplasia, sarcoidosis, osteomas, syphilis, and a variety of congenital diseases.

Spine

The spine represents the most frequent site of skeletal metastasis. Involvement of the thoracic and lumbar levels

predominates, although the sacrum is often affected. Metastases occur more commonly in the vertebral bodies than in the posterior osseous elements. Of the malignant tumors that secondarily involve the spine, carcinomas of the lung, breast, and prostate (as well as lymphomas and plasma cell myeloma) are encountered most often.

The radiographic findings of spinal involvement in cases of metastatic disease also are variable, although some characteristic patterns emerge.

DESTRUCTION AND COLLAPSE OF VERTEBRAL BODY. Osteolysis of a vertebral body is difficult to detect with routine radiography until a large portion of the bone is destroyed. Preservation of discal height is remarkable in many cases of skeletal metastasis, serving as a useful diagnostic aid in differentiating tumor from infection.

Collapse of a vertebral body (or bodies) is an abnormality that occurs in skeletal metastasis; it is evident also in osteoporosis, osteomalacia, and plasma cell myeloma. Findings suggesting that a collapsed vertebral body has resulted from metastatic disease or other malignant tumors include involvement of the upper thoracic spine (a level of collapse infrequently observed in osteoporosis or osteomalacia); the presence of a soft tissue mass or pedicle destruction; and angular or irregular deformity of the vertebral endplates. As there is no specific pattern indicating vertebral metastasis, however, a biopsy is ultimately required for accurate diagnosis in many patients.

SCLEROSIS OF VERTEBRAL BODY. The detection of inhomogeneous or homogeneous sclerotic areas in one or more vertebral bodies in an elderly man is most compatible with a diagnosis of metastatic disease arising from carcinoma of the prostate, although other metastatic tumors as well as lymphomas and, rarely, chordoma or plasma cell myeloma must be considered. Additional causes of vertebral osteosclerosis include chronic osteomyelitis, mastocytosis, tuberous sclerosis, myelofibrosis, Paget's disease, discogenic abnormalities, renal osteodystrophy, compression fractures, primary bone sarcomas, enostosis, sarcoidosis, and a variety of congenital disorders. An entirely radiodense vertebral body (the ivory

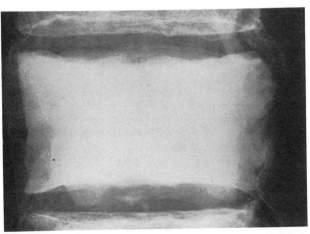

Figure 80–11. Skeletal metastasis: Spine—the ivory vertebral body (carcinoma of the prostate). Observe the uniformly increased radiodensity of the entire vertebral body in this radiograph of a spinal specimen.

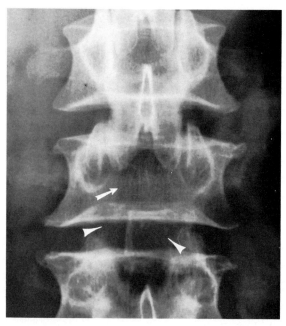

Figure 80–12. Skeletal metastasis: Spine—pedicle and lamina involvement. In this patient, osseous destruction (arrowheads) of a portion of the pedicles, the entire lamina, the inferior articulating processes, and the spinous process is seen. The appearance is that of an empty vertebral body (arrow).

vertebral body) also is observed in cases of skeletal metastasis (Fig. 80–11), particularly carcinoma of the prostate. An ivory vertebral body is a recognized manifestation of additional disorders, including lymphomas and, rarely, chordoma, plasmacytoma, and Paget's disease. It should be differentiated from the corduroy vertebral body (characterized by accentuated vertical striations) of a hemangioma, the rugger-jersey vertebral body (characterized by radiodense stripes at the top and the bottom of the vertebral body) of renal osteodystrophy, the picture-frame vertebral body (associated with condensation of bone along the margins of the vertebral body) of Paget's disease, and the sandwich vertebral body (accompanied by an extreme and uniform increase in radiodensity in the superior and inferior margins of the vertebral body) of osteopetrosis.

PEDICLE INVOLVEMENT. Destruction of one or both pedicles of a vertebra represents a well-known radiographic finding of skeletal metastasis (Fig. 80–12) that is rarely evident in plasma cell myeloma. It is best observed in the anteroposterior radiograph as an absence of one or both "eyes" of the vertebral body.

Pelvis

The bones of the pelvis are frequently involved in skeletal metastasis. Osteolytic, osteosclerotic, or mixed osteolytic-osteosclerotic lesions are seen. Diffuse osteosclerotic metastases (Fig. 80–13), especially from carcinoma of the prostate, should be differentiated from other disorders leading to sclerosis in the pelvic bones (and spine), such as Paget's disease, sickle cell anemia, lymphomas, myelofibrosis, mastocytosis, tuberous sclerosis, fluorosis, and a number of congenital diseases.

Long Tubular Bones

Of the long tubular bones, it is the femur and the humerus that are involved most commonly in cases of skeletal metastasis. Metaphyseal localization predominates, although diaphyseal or epiphyseal lesions are not infrequent. The medullary cavity typically is affected first with secondary involvement of the cortex in instances of hematogenous spread of tumor. Eccentrically located, scalloped erosions of the external surface of the cortex (cookie-bite sign) (Fig. 80–14), particularly in cases of bronchogenic carcinoma, may be observed, however. Features of a pathologic fracture, which may be evident in cases of skeletal metastasis, include an adjacent osteolytic lesion, fractures at certain sites, such as isolated avulsion of the lesser trochanter, and transversely oriented fracture lines.

Short Tubular and Irregular Bones

Metastatic lesions in the bones of the hands, wrists, and feet are infrequent. Bronchogenic, renal, and colonic carcinomas are the leading causes of such metastases (Fig. 80–4).

Sternum and Sacrum

These two bones are relatively common sites of metastasis. In both locations, routine radiographs often are suboptimal owing to overlying osseous and soft tissue structures, so that special techniques, including oblique projections and conventional or computed tomography, are required.

Chest Wall

Hematogenously derived rib metastases most typically produce osteolytic or osteosclerotic lesions without an accompanying soft tissue mass. Pathologic fractures are commonly seen with such rib lesions. With regard to contiguous spread of tumor, invasion of the chest wall occurs in approximately

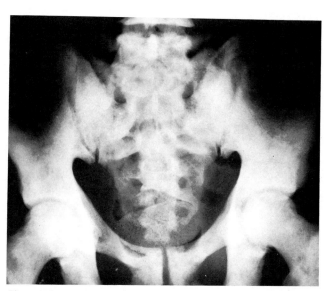

Figure 80–13. Skeletal metastasis: Pelvic bones. Osteosclerotic foci throughout the bones of the pelvis (as well as the spine and proximal portion of the femora) are related to metastases from carcinoma of the prostate.

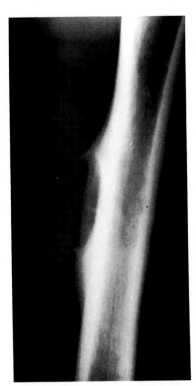

Figure 80–14. Skeletal metastasis: Long tubular bones—cookie-bite sign in bronchogenic carcinoma. A well-circumscribed erosion of the external surface of the diaphysis of the femur is associated with periosteal reaction. (Courtesy of W. Murphy, M.D., St. Louis, Missouri.)

10 per cent of patients with adjacent pulmonary malignancies. A soft tissue mass in these patients relates to the tumor itself or to pleural thickening.

SOME SPECIFIC TYPES OF TUMOR

Carcinoma of the Breast

A common cause of hematogenous skeletal metastasis, this tumor usually produces osteolytic or mixed osteolytic-osteosclerotic lesions or, rarely, osteoblastic lesions, predominating in the axial skeleton and ribs. Pathologic fractures are frequent.

Carcinoma of the Lung

Carcinoma of the lung, a common tumor, involves the skeleton owing to lymphatic spread to regional lymph nodes (mediastinal) with direct extension into bone, lymphatic spread through the diaphragm to regional lymph nodes (paraaortic) with direct osseous extension, and invasion of the pulmonary veins with dissemination via the arterial circulation. In squamous cell and anaplastic large cell carcinomas, osteolytic or mixed osteolytic-osteosclerotic lesions predominate; in small cell carcinoma and adenocarcinoma, osteoblastic lesions may be visible.

Characteristic patterns of skeletal involvement include rib erosion related to a peripheral tumor of the lung, destruction of vertebrae in association with tumor-containing mediastinal lymph nodes, destruction of ribs and cervical vertebrae in

response to a Pancoast tumor, and eccentric cookie-bite excavation of the external surface of the cortex.

Carcinoma of the Prostate

Carcinoma of the prostate is a common cause of osseous metastasis; potential routes allowing spread to the skeleton include Batson's venous plexus and extension from tumorous nodes in the pelvic and paraaortic regions. Osteoblastic metastases are characteristic, although not invariable (Fig. 80–15), and predominate in the axial skeleton.

Carcinoma of the Kidney

Renal cell carcinoma spreads principally in three ways: by direct extension; by involvement of lymphatic channels that ultimately drain into the paraaortic, hilar, paratracheal, and mediastinal regions; and by invasion of the renal veins with subsequent extension to the inferior vena cava, right atrium, and pulmonary vessels. Metastasis to the skeleton is common. Typical sites of involvement are the thoracolumbar spine, bones of the pelvis, ribs, and femora. Solitary osseous lesions are relatively frequent.

Osteolysis is the predominant radiographic finding (Fig. 80–7). Bone expansion, septation, a soft tissue mass, and a pathologic fracture are additional radiographic features of these metastases. Angiography reveals the hypervascular nature of the osseous lesions.

Wilms' Tumor

Skeletal metastasis in Wilms' tumor is regarded as infrequent. Bone metastases usually are osteolytic and have a widespread distribution in both the axial and the appendicular skeleton (Fig. 80–16). A honeycomb pattern of destruction is sometimes seen.

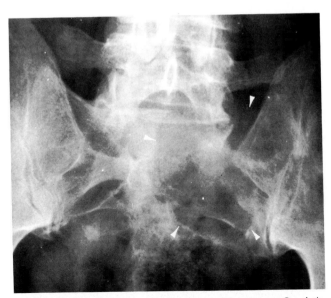

Figure 80–15. Skeletal metastasis: Carcinoma of the prostate. Osteolytic type. A large lesion of the sacrum (arrowheads) might be missed if comparison with the opposite side were not accomplished.

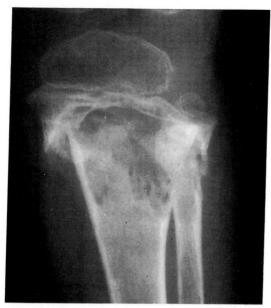

Figure 80–16. Skeletal metastasis: Wilms' tumor. Osteolytic lesions are observed in the tibia and fibula. Pathologic fractures are evident.

Carcinoma of the Thyroid

Hematogenous dissemination of thyroid carcinoma to the skeleton results in solitary or multiple osteolytic lesions predominating in the axial skeleton. An expansile nature, small calcific collections, a pathologic fracture, and a tendency to extend across articulations are features of thyroid metastases. Osteoblastic foci are exceedingly rare, except in instances of medullary carcinoma of the thyroid.

Carcinoma of the Bladder

Osseous lesions in carcinoma of the bladder arise either from direct extension from the primary neoplasm and tumorous lymph nodes or from hematogenous dissemination. They are relatively infrequent and typically affect the thoracolumbar spine and bones of the pelvis. Osteolytic changes are characteristic.

Malignant Melanoma

Skeletal metastasis from melanoma, arising as a result of hematogenous dissemination, is uncommon but not rare. Osteolytic lesions are observed, principally in the spine, ribs, and bones of the pelvis.

Intracranial Tumors

Osseous metastasis is a known manifestation of several different types of brain tumors. The typical pathway of spread in such neoplasms is along the leptomeninges and, occasionally, via the cerebrospinal fluid into the spinal canal. In some instances, ventricular shunts provide a pathway for extraneural dissemination of tumor, and in other circumstances, generally but not invariably after a craniotomy, dural disruption allows more widespread intravascular and perineural lymphatic dissemination.

Medulloblastomas appear to represent the intracranial tumor that is most likely to spread outside the central nervous system, and systemic metastases from this tumor are more frequent in children and adolescents than in adults. Skeletal involvement is characterized by osteosclerotic, osteolytic, or mixed osteolytic-osteosclerotic lesions. The vertebrae, pelvis, femora, and ribs are the typical sites of involvement (Fig. 80–17).

Other intracranial neoplasms, including astrocytomas, glioblastoma multiforme, and meningiomas, less commonly metastasize to the skeleton.

Neuroblastoma

Characteristics of skeletal metastasis from neuroblastoma include symmetric involvement, osteolysis with permeative bone destruction (Fig. 80–18), sutural widening, and collapse of vertebral bodies with adjacent soft tissue masses. Spinal cord compression is frequent.

Retinoblastoma

Retinoblastoma represents a common primary tumor of childhood. Patterns of tumor spread include direct extension beyond the orbit with destruction of the facial bones and sinuses, subdural and subarachnoid invasion with extension to the spinal canal, and hematogenous dissemination throughout the body with involvement of the skeleton. Osteolysis with a permeative pattern of bone destruction and periostitis are seen at one or more sites. These radiographic features resemble those of neuroblastoma and medulloblastoma.

Familial cases of bilateral retinoblastomas have been associated with secondary malignant tumors, particularly osteosarcoma and, less frequently, fibrosarcoma, angiosarcoma, Ewing's sarcoma, rhabdomyosarcoma, Wilms' tumor and other neoplasms.

Embryonal Rhabdomyosarcoma

Although rare, this neoplasm represents the most frequent soft tissue sarcoma of childhood. The tumor is extremely

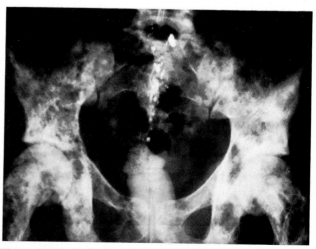

Figure 80–17. Skeletal metastasis: Medulloblastoma. Following the removal of a medulloblastoma, extensive osteoblastic metastases developed in the spine and, as shown here, throughout the pelvic bones and proximal portions of the femora.

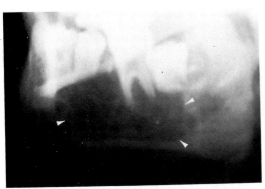

Figure 80–18. Skeletal metastasis: Neuroblastoma. Observe the osteolytic lesion (arrowheads) of the mandible in this 9 year old girl. Several teeth are partially destroyed and appear to be floating. The findings are similar to those of the histiocytoses.

malignant, with a tendency for local invasion, recurrence, and widespread dissemination to the lungs, liver, lymph nodes, and skeleton. Multiple lesions are common, and osteolysis with motheaten or permeative bone destruction predominates.

RADIOGRAPHIC MONITORING OF TUMOR RESPONSE TO TREATMENT

The initial manifestation of a healing response of a purely osteolytic lesion to chemotherapy or radiation therapy is the development of a faint sclerotic rim in its periphery. Continued healing is manifested as progressive bone sclerosis proceeding from the outside of the lesion toward its center, the conversion of the osteolytic focus to one that is uniformly or predominantly osteosclerotic, and the eventual shrinkage and disappearance of the osteosclerotic area. In some instances, a

successful response to therapy is manifested as sclerotic zones in regions of the bones that initially were radiographically normal, apparently owing to the presence of preexisting osteolytic destruction that was not detected on the radiographs. Signs of disease progression are an increase in the size of the osteolytic area, the development of new zones of osteolysis, or progressive osteolytic destruction in an osseous lesion that was responding to the therapy in a normal fashion.

With regard to a mixed osteolytic-osteosclerotic lesion, a successful response to chemotherapy or radiation therapy is its gradual conversion to a uniformly sclerotic area. Subsequent stages of the healing process are identical to those of purely osteolytic lesions. Radiographic signs of tumor progression include increasing osteolysis in sclerotic portions of the lesion and an increase in the overall size of the metastatic focus.

It is the response to therapy of a purely osteosclerotic lesion that is most complex and difficult to analyze. In general, a decrease in size or complete disappearance of an osteoblastic focus is a favorable prognostic sign, whereas increasing size of the osteosclerotic lesion and the development of osseous destruction within an osteosclerotic area are signs of tumor progression. The differentiation between osteolytic conversion of an osteosclerotic area (a sign of tumor progression) and

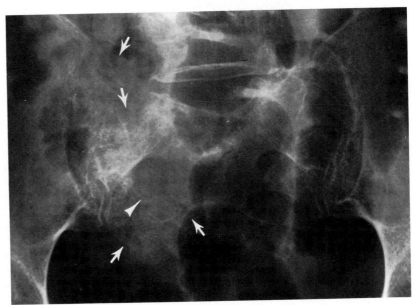

Figure 80–19. Skeletal metastasis: Conventional radiographic survey—problem area. Large lesions of the sacrum (arrows) are easily obscured by overlying structures. Distortion of the pelvic sacral foramina (arrowhead) is an important radiographic sign. Compare to the opposite (normal) side.

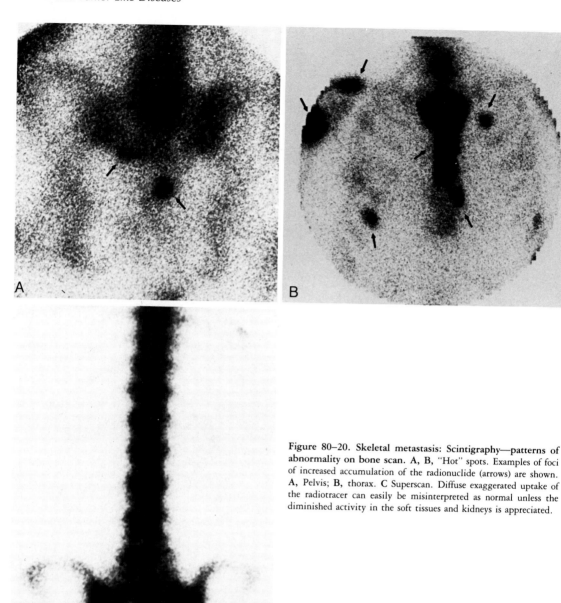

Figure 80–20. Skeletal metastasis: Scintigraphy—patterns of abnormality on bone scan. A, B, "Hot" spots. Examples of foci of increased accumulation of the radionuclide (arrows) are shown. A, Pelvis; B, thorax. C Superscan. Diffuse exaggerated uptake of the radiotracer can easily be misinterpreted as normal unless the diminished activity in the soft tissues and kidneys is appreciated.

fading of an osteosclerotic lesion (a sign of tumor response) is difficult. Furthermore, although an increase in the number of osteoblastic foci usually indicates progression of the disease, it also may signal a healing response of a preexisting lesion that was not initially identified on the radiographs.

Radiation therapy used in conjunction with skeletal metastasis is, in itself, associated with a number of osseous alterations that are discussed in Chapter 64.

OTHER DIAGNOSTIC TECHNIQUES
Conventional Radiographic Survey

The "metastatic bone survey" had long been a standard part of the radiographic protocols employed by most x-ray departments and is still in widespread use today. This survey was originally designed to detect, with a limited number of radiologic projections, the majority of metastatic foci in the skeleton. Owing to the propensity of such lesions to be located in the axial skeleton, this imaging strategy can be fulfilled with a series of radiographs (see Table 80–2). Currently a general consensus exists that, when used, the radiographic survey examination should be performed in conjunction with bone scintigraphy and that the latter examination is more appropriately obtained first so that its results can serve as a guide to the specific radiographic projections that are obtained subsequently. In certain tumors, such as carcinomas of the prostate, lung, and breast and lymphomas,

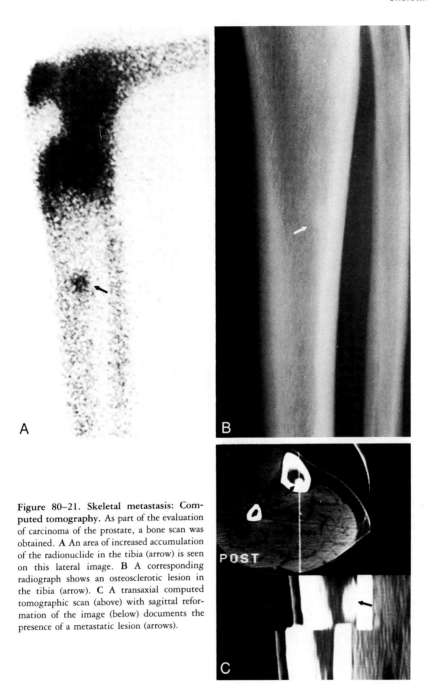

Figure 80–21. Skeletal metastasis: Computed tomography. As part of the evaluation of carcinoma of the prostate, a bone scan was obtained. **A** An area of increased accumulation of the radionuclide in the tibia (arrow) is seen on this lateral image. **B** A corresponding radiograph shows an osteosclerotic lesion in the tibia (arrow). **C** A transaxial computed tomographic scan (above) with sagittal reformation of the image (below) documents the presence of a metastatic lesion (arrows).

scintigraphy using bone-seeking radiopharmaceutical agents is a consistently sensitive means of detecting osseous sites of involvement; radiographic surveys of bones in these cases can be reasonably confined to areas of scintigraphic abnormality or, perhaps, to the pelvis when the bone scan is normal, in recognition of potential obscuration of a lesion in this region owing to radionuclide activity in the bladder. In other tumors, in which results of bone scans are less uniform, a standard skeletal survey supplemented with radiographs of scintigraphically abnormal areas is useful. Although diagnostic difficulties can be encountered during the interpretation of radiographs of any skeletal site, typical problem areas include the follow-

ing: lesions of the pelvic bones and sacrum that are partially obscured by adjacent soft tissues (Fig. 80–19); regions of rib or sternal destruction that are poorly visualized; and the differentiation of a vertebral body that is collapsed because of metastatic disease from one whose deformity is related to osteoporosis or trauma.

Scintigraphy

The sensitivity of the bone scan in detecting skeletal metastases (as well as other osseous lesions) can be attributed to its dependence on changes in regional blood flow and bone turnover that ensure the delivery of an abnormal amount of

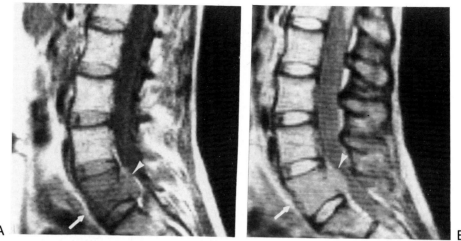

Figure 80–22. Skeletal metastasis: Magnetic resonance imaging. T1 weighted (**A**) and T2 weighted (**B**) sagittal images reveal tumorous replacement of the fifth lumbar vertebral body (arrows) related to metastasis from an adenocarcinoma of the breast. A prominent epidural mass is also evident (arrowheads). (Courtesy of M. Solomon, M.D., San Jose, California.)

the radiotracer to and its incorporation into sites of abnormality. The classic finding of skeletal metastasis is a focus (or foci) of increased accumulation of the radionuclide ("hot" spot) (Fig. 80–20). Modifications in the abnormalities of a positive bone scan include an area of diminished uptake of the radiotracer ("cold" spot), and an increased accumulation of the radiopharmaceutical agent diffusely throughout the skeleton ("superscan") (Fig. 80–20). Any neoplasm that is unaccompanied by ongoing new bone formation may lead to a "cold" region on the bone scan (if there is a great deal of bone destruction) or to an apparently normal examination; this situation is encountered most commonly in plasma cell myeloma, leukemia, and highly aggressive anaplastic carcinomas. Furthermore, a poor host response in debilitated individuals or in those who have undergone radiation therapy also accounts for falsely negative results in cases of skeletal metastasis. Falsely positive bone scans reflect the nonspecific nature of the scintigraphic examination.

The results of a bone scan certainly lack specificity. The presence of multiple and widespread focal areas of increased accumulation of the radionuclide on the bone scan in a patient with a known primary malignant tumor is a pattern most suggestive of metastases, but it is one that is occasionally simulated by other conditions. The identification of a superscan in a patient with prostatic carcinoma is not entirely pathognomonic for skeletal metastases, as a similar pattern may accompany hyperparathyroidism, osteomalacia, mastocytosis, and myelofibrosis.

The sequential evaluation of patients with skeletal metastasis who are receiving chemotherapy or radiation therapy has been accomplished with bone scintigraphy, although, as in the case of conventional radiography, difficulties in interpretation of the results arise. The beliefs that decreasing accumulation of a bone-seeking radionuclide implies tumor healing and that increasing accumulation of this radiotracer suggests tumor progression are both inaccurate. Aggressive behavior of a metastatic focus in the skeleton is accompanied by increasing bone destruction, which may be associated with little or no bone formation; the radionuclide manifestation of such tumor progression is a decrease in activity of the lesion on the bone scan. Conversely, an increase in the amount of accumulation of the bone-seeking radionuclide in a lesion, particularly during the early stages of therapy, may indicate tumor healing owing to the presence of the "flare" phenomenon. This phenomenon relates either to an increase in regional blood flow or to an accentuation of bone turnover, or both, at the site of metastasis. Fortunately, the more typical healing response of such metastases as observed on serial bone scans is a decrease in radionuclide accumulation. It has been suggested that the discovery of new lesions on serial bone scintigraphy is a more reliable sign of tumor progression than is an increase in radionuclide uptake at the site of old lesions.

Computed Tomography

Computed tomography may be used to further delineate the nature of a scintigraphically positive osseous region, especially if radiographs fail to document the existence of a metastatic focus. In the spine, computed tomography appears to be more sensitive than conventional radiography in the detection of metastatic lesions, and it may also be more specific, documenting findings characteristic of malignant neoplasm, including pediculate destruction, multiple osteolytic foci in the vertebral body, and paravertebral masses with adjacent bone erosion, or, alternately, abnormalities indicative of a non-neoplastic process. In the tubular bones of the appendicular skeleton, computed tomography is able to detect subtle changes in the attenuation coefficient of the marrow that may indicate tumor infiltration (a finding also evident in infection) or, more specifically, tumorous marrow deposits not apparent on conventional radiographs (Fig. 80–21).

Computed tomography represents an excellent means of defining the extent of any metastatic lesion, especially those located at sites that are difficult to evaluate with conventional imaging techniques, such as the vertebral column and pelvis. Paravertebral and intraspinal extension, transarticular spread, and soft tissue involvement with violation of neurovascular structures are examples of information that can be derived from the computed tomographic display.

Magnetic Resonance Imaging

Magnetic resonance imaging possesses certain advantages over computed tomography in the evaluation of patients with skeletal metastasis. Magnetic resonance imaging is better able to delineate the extent of tumor in the marrow (manifested as a decrease in signal intensity, especially on T1 weighted images, owing to replacement of marrow fat) and soft tissue, and direct sagittal and coronal images may be obtained; computed tomography is superior in the demonstration of calcific deposits and pathologic fractures. In the spine, magnetic resonance imaging documents with exquisite detail the relationship of an invasive tumor and the spinal cord (Fig. 80–22). After radiation therapy, this technique may allow differentiation of osseous changes related to the treatment itself from those associated with tumor recurrence.

Biopsy Techniques

As discussed in Chapter 17, skeletal biopsy procedures may provide a rapid and accurate diagnosis in some persons with solitary or multiple aggressive bone lesions in whom skeletal metastasis is suspected. As certain disseminated neoplasms are better controlled than others, the tissue removed during bone biopsy should be used as a guide for determining the need for further diagnostic studies; if the histologic diagnosis is one of adenocarcinoma or undifferentiated carcinoma, no additional diagnostic tests are required owing to the unlikelihood of identifying the site of the primary tumor and the expected short survival time of the patient. The recovery of tissue interpreted as clear cell carcinoma requires evaluation of the thyroid and kidney, whereas that diagnosed as squamous cell carcinoma should direct attention to the upper respiratory tract and lungs.

In the patient with a known primary tumor, single or multiple skeletal lesions discovered by conventional radiography, scintigraphy, or computed tomography, or any combination of the three, can be further evaluated with a bone biopsy, especially if the imaging features of the lesion(s) are not characteristic of metastasis. In this situation, the identification of a non-neoplastic cause for the osseous alterations may influence the subsequent treatment plan dramatically.

FURTHER READING

Abrams HL: Skeletal metastases in carcinoma. Radiology 55:534, 1950.

Amorosa JK, Weintraub S, Amorosa LF, Safer JN, Rafii M: Sacral destruction: Foraminal lines revisited. AJR 145:773, 1985.

Batson OV: The function of the vertebral veins and their role in the spread of metastases. Ann Surg 112:138, 1940.

Braunstein EM, Kuhns LR: Computed tomographic demonstration of spinal metastases. Spine 8:912, 1983.

Chinn D, Genant HK, Quivey JM, Carlsson A-M: Heterotopic-bone formation in metastatic tumor from transitional-cell carcinoma of the urinary bladder. A case report. J Bone Joint Surg [Am] 58:881, 1976.

Debnam JW, Staple TW: Osseous metastases from cerebellar medulloblastoma. Radiology 107:363, 1973.

Deutsch A, Resnick D: Eccentric cortical metastases to the skeleton from bronchogenic carcinoma. Radiology 137:49, 1980.

Eklof O, Mortensson W, Sandstedt B, Ahstrom L: Bone metastases in Wilms' tumor: Occurrence and radiological appearance. Ann Radiol 27:97, 1984.

Fisher MS: Lumbar spine metastasis in cervical carcinoma: A characteristic pattern. Radiology 134:631, 1980.

Forbes GS, McLeod RA, Hattery RR: Radiographic manifestations of bone metastases from renal carcinoma. AJR 129:61, 1977.

Fornasier VL, Czitrom AA: Collapsed vertebrae. A review of 659 autopsies. Clin Orthop 131:261, 1978.

Fornasier VL, Horne JG: Metastases to the vertebral column. Cancer 36:590, 1975.

Galasko CSB: The anatomy and pathways of skeletal metastasis. In L Weiss, HA Gilbert (Eds): Bone Metastasis. Boston, GK Hall, 1981, p 49.

Galasko CSB: Mechanisms of lytic and blastic metastatic disease of bone. Clin Orthop 169:20, 1982.

Goergen TG, Alazraki NP, Halpern SE, Health V, Ashburn WL: "Cold" bone lesions: A newly recognized phenomenon of bone imaging. J Nucl Med 15:1120, 1973.

Harbert JC, George FH, Kerner ML: Differentiation of rib fractures from metastases by bone scanning. Clin Nucl Med 6:359, 1981.

Kerin R: Metastatic tumors of the hand. A review of the literature. J Bone Joint Surg [Am] 65:1331, 1983.

Lehrer HZ, Maxfield WS, Nice CM: The periosteal "sunburst" pattern in metastatic bone tumors. AJR 108:154, 1970.

McNeil BJ: Value of bone scanning in neoplastic disease. Semin Nucl Med 14:277, 1984.

Mundy GR, Raisz LG, Cooper RA, Schechter G, Salmon SE: Evidence for the secretion of an osteoclast activating factor in myeloma. N Engl J Med 291:1041, 1974.

Pagani JJ, Libshitz HI: Imaging bone metastases. Radiol Clin North Am 20:545, 1982.

Pollen JJ, Reznek RH, Talner LB: Lysis of osteoblastic lesions in prostatic cancer: A sign of progression. AJR 142:1175, 1984.

Potter GD: Sclerosis of base of skull as a manifestation of nasopharyngeal carcinoma. Radiology 94:35, 1970.

Punt J, Pritchard J, Pincott JR, Till K: Neuroblastoma: A review of 21 cases presenting with spinal cord compression. Cancer 45:3095, 1980.

Ramsey RG, Zacharias CE: MR imaging of the spine after radiation therapy: Easily recognizable effects. AJR 144:1131, 1985.

Reed MH, Culham JAG: Skeletal metastases from retinoblastoma. J Can Assoc Radiol 26:249, 1975.

Resnik CS, Garver P, Resnick D: Bony expansion in skeletal metastasis from carcinoma of the prostate as seen by bone scintigraphy. South Med J 77:1331, 1984.

Rosen IW, Nadel HI: Button sequestrum of the skull. Radiology 92:969, 1969.

Sartoris DJ, Clopton P, Nemcek A, Dowd C, Resnick D: Vertebral-body collapse in focal and diffuse disease: Patterns of pathologic processes. Radiology 160:479, 1986.

Sim FH: Diagnosis and Management of Metastatic Bone Disease. A Multidisciplinary Approach. New York, Raven Press, 1988.

Springfield DS: Mechanisms of metastasis. Clin Orthop 169:15, 1982.

Stanley P, Senac MO Jr, Segali HD: Intraspinal seeding from intracranial tumors in children. AJR 144:157, 1985.

Steckel RJ, Kagan AR: Diagnostic persistence in working up metastatic cancer with an unknown primary site. Radiology 134:367, 1980.

Tofe AJ, Francis MD, Harvey WJ: Correlation of neoplasms with incidence and localization of skeletal metastases: An analysis of 1,355 diphosphonate bone scans. J Nucl Med 16:987, 1976.

Weiss L, Gilbert HA: Bone Metastasis. Boston, GK Hall, 1981.

Wilner D: Radiology of Bone Tumors and Allied Disorders. Philadelphia, WB Saunders Co, 1982.

MISCELLANEOUS DISEASES

LEVEL OF DIFFICULTY: 3

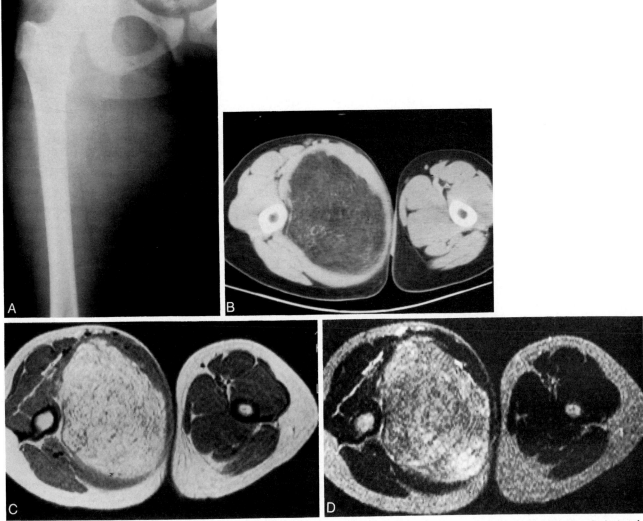

A 12 year old girl had a mass in the medial aspect of the thigh. The mass had been present for several years but had enlarged significantly during the previous few months. It was painless.

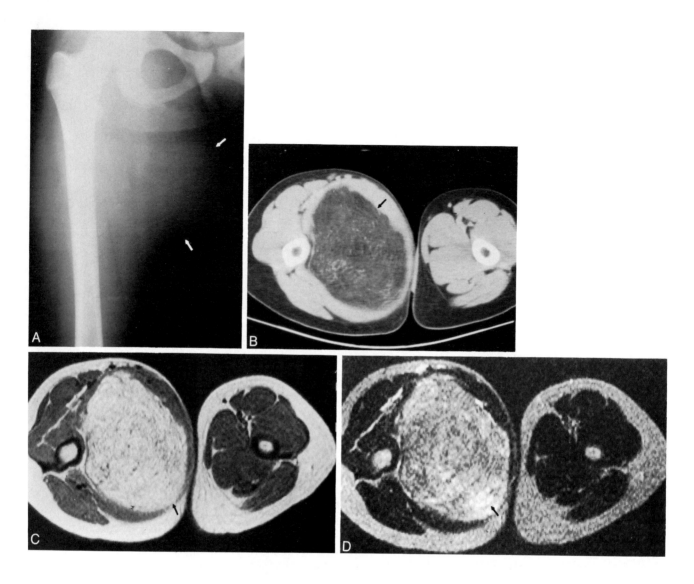

A frontal radiograph (*A*) shows a large mass (arrows) in the right thigh. The radiodensity in the mass is less than that of muscle, probably indicating that it contains fat. Transaxial computed tomography (*B*) reveals that the mass (arrow) is situated mainly in the adductor magnus muscle. It appears to be composed of fatty elements, although linear strands with increased attenuation are readily apparent. On a transaxial proton density magnetic resonance image (*C*), the signal intensity of the mass (arrow) is similar to that of fat, although linear regions of decreased intensity are evident. The mass is well circumscribed, with a smooth margin, and adjacent musculature is displaced. On a transaxial T2 weighted magnetic resonance image (*D*), the signal characteristics of the mass (arrow) are not uniform. In some regions, areas of intermediate signal intensity identical to the intensity of subcutaneous fat are seen. Elsewhere, regions of higher and lower signal intensity are evident.

The imaging abnormalities are those of a soft tissue neoplasm that contains fatty elements. The inhomogeneous nature of the lesion, as delineated by computed tomography and magnetic resonance imaging, suggests that a lipoma is unlikely, although intramuscular lipomas occasionally may contain muscle bundles that traverse the mass, leading to linear regions of increased attenuation on computed tomog-

raphy and decreased signal intensity on magnetic resonance imaging. A liposarcoma, representing a frequent malignant neoplasm that commonly localizes in the thigh, also must be considered as a diagnostic possibility. Liposarcomas are often large and bulky soft tissue tumors that may appear well circumscribed or poorly circumscribed depending on their degree of cellular differentiation. On routine radiographs, liposarcomas usually are nonhomogeneous and poorly defined fat-containing masses. With computed tomography, these tumors may show regions of fat density mixed with regions of water density. Similarly, with magnetic resonance imaging, portions of the neoplasm may reveal features typical of fat whereas other areas may not. Septations within the tumor may be apparent.

Although the imaging findings in the test case are compatible with the diagnosis of a low-grade or well-differentiated liposarcoma, two other diagnoses also must be considered. The first of these, angiolipoma, is a rare benign fatty tumor with distinctive cellular composition. Both infiltrating and noninfiltrating varieties of this neoplasm have been described. On radiographs, a soft tissue mass characterized by serpentine-like densities intermixed with fat, with or without pheboliths or ossification, may be evident. Computed tomography and magnetic resonance imaging may show a soft tissue mass, frequently in the extremities, with poorly defined margins and a heterogeneous mixture of fat and elements of water. The tumor may infiltrate adjacent tissues.

The final diagnostic consideration is lipoblastomatosis (lipoblastoma), a rare type of embryonal fatty tumor. This neoplasm predominates in children. Typically located superficially in the extremities, lipoblastomatosis may be circumscribed or diffuse in nature. Histologically, the neoplasm consists of lobulated immature adipose tissue composed of lipoblasts, a plexiform capillary pattern, and a richly myxoid stroma. The clinical course usually is favorable, with a very low rate of recurrence after complete surgical removal of the tumor.

The mass illustrated in case XV was biopsied and subsequently excised. Histologic examination confirmed the diagnosis of lipoblastomatosis.

FINAL DIAGNOSIS: Lipoblastomatosis (lipoblastoma).

FURTHER READING

Page 1183 and the following:

1. Chung EB, Enzinger FM: Benign lipoblastomatosis. An analysis of 34 cases. Cancer 32:482, 1973.
2. Gibbs MK, Soule EH, Hayles AB, Telander RL: Lipoblastomatosis: A tumor of children. Pediatrics 60:235, 1977.

(Case XV, courtesy of G. Greenway, M.D., Dallas, Texas.)

Chapter 81

Sarcoidosis

Donald Resnick, M.D.
Gen Niwayama, M.D.

Skeletal abnormalities in sarcoidosis are most frequently encountered in the hand; in this location, a coarsened trabecular pattern, cystic and marginal bone defects, and sclerosis are virtually diagnostic. Although findings can be encountered in other skeletal sites, such as the skull, facial bones, spine, and long tubular bones, as well as various joints, these alterations usually are not specific.

Sarcoidosis is a granulomatous disorder of unknown cause affecting multiple organ systems, especially in young adults, and leading principally to bilateral hilar adenopathy, pulmonary infiltrates, and skin or eye lesions. The diagnosis of the disease is substantiated by a combination of clinical, radiologic, and histologic features, the last consisting predominantly of widespread, noncaseating epithelioid cell granulomas. The course of the disease is variable, and it may be associated with significant musculoskeletal abnormalities. Its precise cause remains unknown.

CLINICAL ABNORMALITIES

Sarcoidosis has a worldwide distribution; in the United States, the highest concentration of cases occurs in the Southeast. The disease affects men and women equally. It usually becomes apparent between 20 and 40 years of age. Blacks are affected more frequently than whites.

The clinical manifestations are highly variable. In some patients, radiographic evidence of hilar adenopathy may appear in the absence of any symptoms and signs. In others, an acute or chronic form of the disease becomes evident. Pulmonary manifestations are frequent. Ocular abnormalities and skin nodules also are characteristic. Malaise, anorexia, weight loss, fever, hepatosplenomegaly, and lymphadenopathy are detected in many cases. Additional findings relate to involvement of other organs, including those of the central or peripheral nervous system, the heart, and the musculoskeletal system.

Laboratory analysis may indicate anemia, leukopenia, eosinophilia, a reduction in serum albumin concentration, an elevation of serum globulin level, and hypercalcemia. In 60 to 80 per cent of patients with sarcoidosis, an intradermal injection of 0.2 ml of a 10 per cent saline suspension of sarcoid tissue produces a nodule containing noncaseating granulomas. This represents a positive Kveim test.

GENERAL PATHOLOGIC ABNORMALITIES

The accurate diagnosis of sarcoidosis is made on the basis of compatible clinical and radiologic findings, the presence of supporting laboratory data, and the demonstration of typical noncaseating granulomas in the absence of other identifiable causes for such lesions. Granulomas can be apparent in almost any organ or tissue, including the bone marrow and muscle, but most often are present in the lung, lymph nodes, liver, and spleen.

MUSCULOSKELETAL ABNORMALITIES
Osseous Involvement

There has been much disagreement about the frequency of skeletal involvement in sarcoidosis. Indeed, the reported frequency of radiographic evidence of osseous involvement has varied from 1 to 13 per cent, averaging 5 per cent. As many of the skeletal lesions of sarcoidosis are asymptomatic, an accurate appraisal of the frequency of bone involvement in this disease is difficult. Osseous sarcoidosis is rarely detected in the absence of skin lesions. Furthermore, it has been estimated that 80 to 90 per cent of patients with sarcoidosis involving bone have radiographic evidence of pulmonary disease.

CLINICAL MANIFESTATIONS. Although bone changes often are entirely asymptomatic, clinical manifestations in some cases may be prominent. Soft tissue swelling and cutaneous lesions of the hands and feet can accompany osseous disease. Tenderness, stiffness, and restricted motion can be seen. Soft tissue swelling and deformity may be apparent also at other sites, including the nose, face and sinuses, skull, and extremities.

RADIOGRAPHIC MANIFESTATIONS. Osteoporosis has been observed in sarcoidosis. A coarsened, lacework trabecular pattern becomes evident. Localized cystic lesions may lead to a "punched-out" appearance; these cysts can be

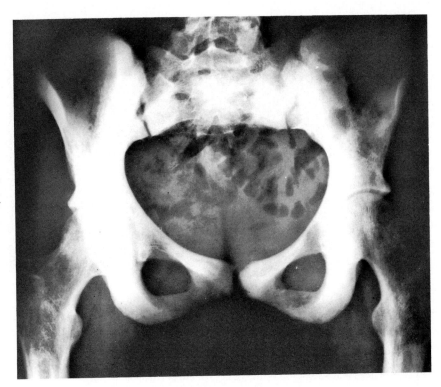

Figure 81–1. Sarcoidosis: Osteosclerosis. In the pelvis, there is uniform increased bone density, especially in the iliac bones, ischii, and superior pubic rami.

located centrally or eccentrically and may be sharply marginated and round or ovoid. At times, osseous destruction may be associated with a permeative pattern, cortical violation, and sequestration. Remarkably, periostitis is distinctly unusual.

Less typically, localized or generalized osteosclerosis is evident (Fig. 81–1). Nodular opacities can appear in the medullary cavities of the tubular bones of the hands and feet, or about the terminal phalanges (acroosteosclerosis). In unusual circumstances, a widespread increase in skeletal radiodensity may be seen, resembling changes in Paget's disease,

skeletal metastasis, lymphoma, myelofibrosis, mastocytosis, hemoglobinopathies, renal osteodystrophy, and fluorosis.

Hands and Feet. The hand is the predominant site of skeletal sarcoidosis. Unilateral or bilateral changes can be encountered. Abnormalities are found in the middle and distal phalanges and less often in the proximal phalanges and metacarpals. Several types of lesions are seen (Fig. 81–2). Diffuse trabecular alterations are especially characteristic, leading to a honeycomb or latticework configuration. More localized lytic lesions produce cystic defects that, as they heal, may become surrounded by a thin rim of sclerosis. These

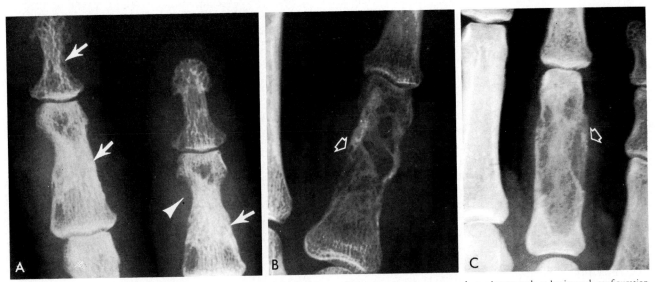

Figure 81–2. Sarcoidosis: Hand. A variety of radiographic changes can be seen. Trabecular alterations can produce a honeycomb or latticework configuration (solid arrows), more localized defects (open arrows), and marginal scalloping of bone (large arrowhead). (A, Courtesy of A. Brower, M.D., Washington, D.C.; B, courtesy of M. Dalinka, M.D., Philadelphia, Pennsylvania.)

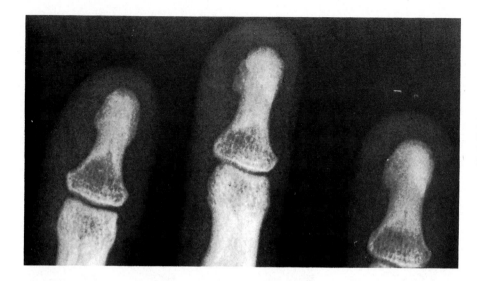

Figure 81–3. Sarcoidosis: Acroosteosclerosis. Observe widespread sclerosis of the terminal aspects of the phalanges. This appearance is not specific.

lesions can appear centrally in the spongiosa or eccentrically, leading to marginal scalloping of the bone. An entire phalanx can be affected in association with pathologic fracture, fragmentation, soft tissue swelling, and telescoping of a digit. In some instances, calcification of the lesion may simulate the appearance of one or more enchondromas. Periostitis is uncommon.

Acroosteosclerosis has been reported as a sign of sarcoidosis of the hands (Fig. 81–3). The finding is not specific, having been noted in scleroderma, rheumatoid arthritis, systemic lupus erythematosus, Hodgkin's disease, and hematologic disorders, and it also may occur in "normal" persons.

Changes in the wrist can include cystic or marginal lucent shadows, whereas those in the feet parallel the findings in the hand, with a coarsened trabecular pattern, localized lesions, and opaque areas.

Long Tubular Bones. Examples of destructive lesions of the long tubular bones of the extremities are rare (Fig. 81–4).

Skull and Face. Calvarial destruction in sarcoidosis is unusual. Osseous destruction of the facial bones can reflect the presence of granulomatous lesions in adjacent structures, such as the nasal skin, paranasal sinuses, nasal mucosa, optic nerve and canal, and lacrimal sac. Nasal bone destruction (Fig. 81–5) is especially characteristic.

Spine and Spinal Cord. Uncommonly in sarcoidosis, granulomas may localize within vertebral marrow. Clinical findings include pain, deformity, and neurologic dysfunction. On radiographs, bone lysis with marginal sclerosis can involve one or more vertebral bodies, with preservation of the intervening intervertebral disc spaces. Predilection for the lower thoracic and upper lumbar vertebrae is noted. Extension into the pedicles can be observed, and paraspinal swelling also is evident in some cases (Fig. 81–6).

Articular Involvement

Joint symptoms and signs appear in 10 to 35 per cent of patients with sarcoidosis. Two fundamental patterns of artic-

ular disease occur: acute polyarthritis and chronic polyarthritis.

ACUTE POLYARTHRITIS. Peripheral symmetric polyarthritis affects small and medium-sized joints, appearing early in the course of the disease in association with erythema nodosum, hilar lymph node enlargement, fever, uveitis, and typical skin lesions. This pattern of joint disease leads to soft tissue swelling, joint effusion, pain, tenderness, limitation of motion, and stiffness, findings that disappear in 4 to 6 weeks.

CHRONIC POLYARTHRITIS. A second variety of joint

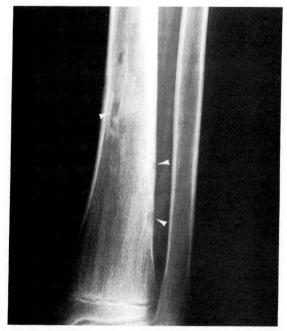

Figure 81–4. Sarcoidosis: Long tubular bones. Small, eccentric osteolytic lesions (arrowheads) in the tibia of a child are observed. They are sharply circumscribed, with minimal marginal sclerosis and no periostitis. (Courtesy of L. Cooperstein, M.D., Pittsburgh, Pennsylvania.)

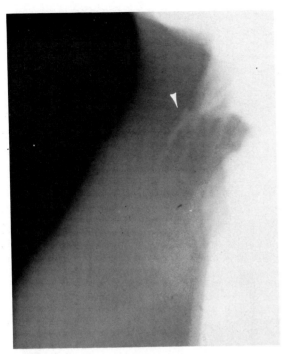

Figure 81–5. **Sarcoidosis: Face.** Soft tissue swelling and destruction of the nasal bones (arrowhead) are characteristic of the disease.

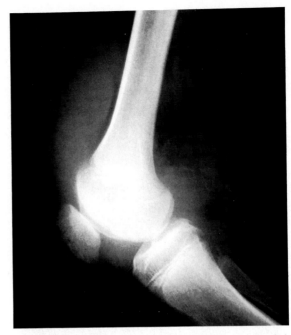

Figure 81–7. **Childhood sarcoidosis.** In this child, radiographic findings include osteopenia and a large effusion in the knee. (Courtesy of L. Cooperstein, M.D., Pittsburgh, Pennsylvania.)

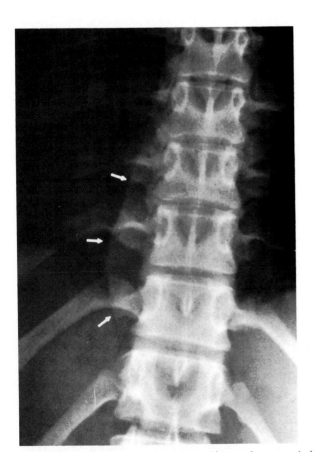

Figure 81–6. **Sarcoidosis: Paraspinal swelling.** Observe a large paraspinal mass (arrows) in the thoracic spine of this patient with sarcoidosis. Such a finding can accompany vertebral involvement or represent a manifestation of posterior lymphadenopathy.

disease, which occurs in cases of sarcoidosis that have persisted for months to years, is a chronic polyarthritis that subsides and recurs, and that may eventually lead to permanent disability and irreversible joint damage. The joints most typically affected are the ankles, knees, shoulders, wrists, and small joints of the hands. Cutaneous and pulmonary alterations are frequent. On radiographs, osseous sarcoidosis may or may not be present. Soft tissue swelling, periarticular osteoporosis, diffuse joint space loss, and erosive alterations can also be noted. Histologic examination of the synovium in either situation can indicate the presence of noncaseating granulomas.

OTHER PATTERNS. Sarcoid arthritis occurring in children has been emphasized. Although rare, articular abnormalities simulate those seen in some forms of juvenile chronic arthritis and usually are accompanied by both cutaneous and ocular involvement. Soft tissue enlargement and osteopenia

Table 81–1. MULTIPLE CYST-LIKE LESIONS OF THE METACARPAL BONES AND PHALANGES

Sarcoidosis
Gout
Rheumatoid arthritis
Xanthomatosis
Tuberous sclerosis
Fibrous dysplasia
Enchondromatosis (Ollier's disease)
Tuberculosis
Fungal disease
Metastasis (rare)
Plasma cell myeloma (rare)
Hyperparathyroidism (rare)
Basal cell nevus syndrome (rare)
Hemangiomas (rare)

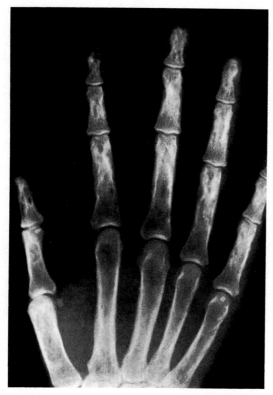

Figure 81–8. Tuberous sclerosis. Cyst-like lesions of variable size are evident in the phalanges and metacarpal bones. Periosteal apposition of bone has led to broadening of the phalanges and an irregular and nodular surface, especially in the metacarpal bones. (Courtesy of G. Greenway, M.D., Dallas, Texas.)

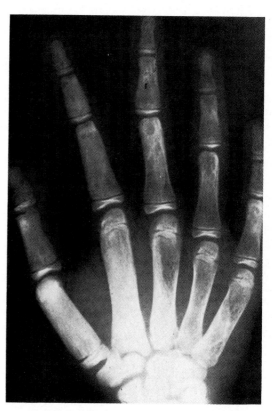

Figure 81–9. Fibrous dysplasia. In this child with polyostotic fibrous dysplasia, note the diffuse ground-glass appearance of the metacarpals and phalanges. Cortical thinning and osseous expansion are seen.

are the characteristic radiographic abnormalities; rarely, cartilaginous and osseous destruction is apparent (Fig. 81–7).

Differential Diagnosis

The skeletal alterations in sarcoidosis are sufficiently characteristic in most cases to allow an accurate radiographic diagnosis. Occasionally, the trabecular and cystic changes in the hand may be confused with abnormalities in other disorders (Table 81–1). In *tuberous sclerosis*, cyst-like foci in the phalanges and metacarpals are usually associated with a distinctive variety of periosteal proliferation, leading to nodular excrescences attached to the outer aspect of the bones (Fig. 81–8). *Fibrous dysplasia* can produce a widened medullary space of phalanges and metacarpals with a diffuse ground-glass appearance (Fig. 81–9). *Enchondromas* are benign tumors composed of cartilage that often are identified in the hands of asymptomatic persons. Although the appearance of a lucent lesion containing calcification in sarcoidosis can exactly simulate an enchondroma, other skeletal findings ensure accurate diagnosis.

Enchondromatosis or *Ollier's disease* is a syndrome of multiple enchondromas that produce soft tissue swelling in one or more extremities. Radiographs reveal multiple lucent and calcified lesions, although a more diffuse and bizarre appearance can be seen (Fig. 81–10).

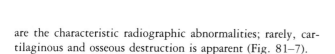
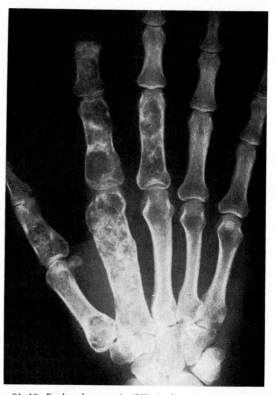

Figure 81–10. Enchondromatosis (Ollier's disease). Observe radiolucent foci containing calcification in the first, second, and third digits. Note endosteal scalloping, cortical diminution, and osseous expansion. The distal phalanx of the second finger had been removed surgically.

Multiple lucent lesions of phalanges, metacarpals, and metatarsals can also accompany tuberculosis and other granulomatous infections, hemangiomatosis, xanthomatosis, hyperparathyroidism, Gorlin's basal cell nevus syndrome, lipomatosis, plasma cell myeloma, and skeletal metastasis.

Nasal and facial bone destruction is encountered in sarcoidosis, syphilis, fungal and other infections, Wegener's granulomatosis, and neoplasms.

FURTHER READING

Berk RN, Brower TD: Vertebral sarcoidosis. Radiology 82:660, 1964.

Bonakdarpour A, Levy W, Aergerter EE: Osteosclerotic changes in sarcoidosis. AJR 113:646, 1971.

Boyd RE, Andrews BS: Sarcoidosis presenting as cutaneous ulceration, subcutaneous nodules and chronic arthritis. J Rheumatol 8:311, 1981.

Holt JF, Owens WI: The osseous lesions of sarcoidosis. Radiology 53:11, 1949.

James DG, Neville E, Carstairs LS: Bone and joint sarcoidosis. Semin Arthritis Rheum 6:53, 1976.

Kaplan H: Sarcoid arthritis: A review. Arch Intern Med 112:924, 1963.

Mayock RL, Bertrand P, Morrison CE, Scott JH: Manifestations of sarcoidosis: Analysis of 145 patients with a review of 9 series selected from the literature. Am J Med 35:67, 1963.

McBrine CS, Fisher MS: Acrosclerosis in sarcoidosis. Radiology 115:279, 1975.

Redman DS, McCarthy RE, Jimenez JF: Sarcoidosis in the long bones of a child. A case report and review of the literature. J Bone Joint Surg [Am] 65:1010, 1983.

Rosenberg AM, Yee EH, Mackenzie JW: Arthritis in childhood sarcoidosis. J Rheumatol 10:987, 1983.

Sartoris DJ, Resnick D, Resnik C, Yaghmai I: Musculoskeletal manifestations of sarcoidosis. Semin Roentgenol 20:376, 1985.

Stein GN, Israel HL, Sones M: A roentgenographic study of skeletal lesions in sarcoidosis. Arch Intern Med 97:532, 1956.

Toomey F, Bautista A: Rare manifestations of sarcoidosis in children. Radiology 94:569, 1970.

Yaghmai I: Radiographic, angiographic and radionuclide manifestations of osseous sarcoidosis. RadioGraphics 3:375, 1983.

Zimmerman R, Leeds NE: Calvarial and vertebral sarcoidosis. Case report and review of the literature. Radiology 119:384, 1976.

Chapter 82

Tuberous Sclerosis, Neurofibromatosis, and Fibrous Dysplasia

Frieda Feldman, M.D.

Tuberous sclerosis represents a widespread dysplasia of unknown pathogenesis. Its classic clinical triad consists of epileptic seizures, mental retardation, and skin lesions. Neurofibromatosis also is characterized by a classic clinical triad, consisting of cutaneous lesions, mental deficiency, and skeletal deformities. Fibrous dysplasia is a disorder of unknown causation in which the skeleton represents a prominent target tissue. A variety of endocrine abnormalities, including the McCune-Albright syndrome, may accompany the osseous abnormalities.

Tuberous sclerosis, neurofibromatosis, and polyostotic fibrous dysplasia involve multiple systems in multiple ways and may, therefore, be associated with a variety of seemingly unrelated radiographic stigmata. It is important to note, however, that these three conditions share certain common characteristics. Although they are grouped with the neuroectodermal and mesodermal dysplasias, all three germ layers may be involved in the development of each of these entities. Moreover, all have been associated with certain classic clinical triads, which are considered as aids in their identification. Although mutations do occur in these three disorders, the majority of cases are hereditary or familial.

TUBEROUS SCLEROSIS

Tuberous sclerosis or Bourneville's disease is a disorder of autosomal dominant inheritance. It has no known geographic, ethnic, or gender predilection. The disorder classically is characterized by a clinical triad of epileptic seizures, mental retardation, and skin lesions that have been regarded as hamartomas. Hamartomas also may occur in many organs with a variety of clinical manifestations. Their recognition is of prime importance as the components of the classic triad may not appear simultaneously or may not appear at all. Furthermore, seizures, although observed in the first decade of life, are nonspecific; mental retardation is difficult to evaluate at birth; and skin lesions may be subtle or absent in early life.

Cutaneous, Cranial, and Ocular Abnormalities

Almost all patients have cutaneous stigmata, four of which (adenoma sebaceum, shagreen patches, periungual fibromas,

and hypopigmented macules) are believed to be diagnostic. Lesions of the central nervous system are responsible for the epilepsy and mental retardation that constitute the remaining two components of the classic diagnostic triad. Almost all patients who are mentally retarded have epileptic seizures. Routine skull films may show patchy areas of calvarial sclerosis owing to hyperostosis of the inner table and prominent trabeculae in the diploic spaces (Fig. 82–1). Generalized thickening of both tables of the vault may also be noted. Evidence of raised intracranial pressure (i.e., sutural diastasis, sellar changes, increased convolutional markings) has been reported. Intracerebral calcifications occur in 50 to 80 per cent of cases (Fig. 82–1). They increase in frequency as the patient becomes older and commonly are undetectable on routine films of the very young. Calcifications may be single or multiple and are of variable size.

Brain lesions in tuberous sclerosis occur predominantly in three main loci: the ventricles, the white matter, and the cortex. The hamartomatous foci, which may or may not calcify, may be found in the cerebrum, cerebellum, medulla, and spinal cord. Most lie adjacent to cerebrospinal fluid pathways and are either subependymal nodules or cortical tubers located about the ventricles and arising within the basal ganglia. They may produce a candle guttering effect on the ventricular surface. Larger lesions near the foramen of Monro may result in obstructive hydrocephalus. Brain lesions are well shown with computed tomography and magnetic resonance imaging (Fig. 82–2).

Ocular abnormalities are seen at birth in 52 per cent of cases and may be evident as early as 3 months' gestation. Although many lesions have been described, only retinal hamartomas (i.e., phakomas) clearly are part of the syndrome.

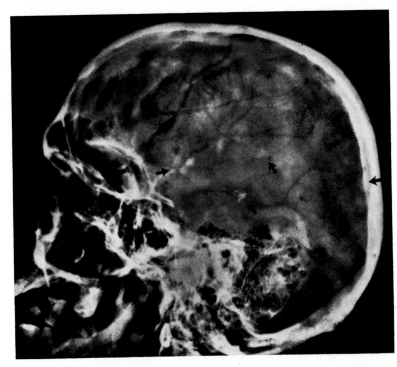

Figure 82–1. Tuberous sclerosis: Lateral view of the skull. Multiple intracerebral calcific deposits are noted, together with several scattered areas of calvarial sclerosis (arrows).

Extracranial Skeletal Abnormalities

In addition to the skull, the remainder of the skeleton may be involved focally or diffusely with medullary or cortical cyst-like radiolucent areas or dense sclerotic deposits. Cortical lesions in the form of nodules or depressions as well as irregular, subperiosteal new bone deposition that results in a undulating cortical contour most often involve the short tubular bones of the hands and feet (Figs. 82–3 and 82–4) and, occasionally, the long tubular bones.

The spine and pelvis are additional sites for osteoblastic deposits ranging from a few millimeters to centimeters in diameter (Figs. 82–5 and 82–6). Unusual prior to puberty, these lesions occur as later, asymptomatic manifestations.

Visceral Abnormalities

The viscera, as well as the skin, eyes, brain, and bones, serve as silent sites of tumor-like formations; the kidneys, heart, organs in the gastrointestinal tract, liver, lungs, and spleen may all be involved. Lesions may variously be identified as angiomyomas, angiofibromas, or myolipomas.

Approximately 50 per cent of patients with tuberous sclerosis have associated renal lesions, including cysts, angiomyolipomas, and aneurysms. Coarctation of the aorta and stenosis or aneurysms of the renal arteries have also been documented. In a patient with epilepsy and "cystic" renal enlargement, tuberous sclerosis is a serious diagnostic consideration, whereas a combination of renal cysts and angiomyolipomas is now thought to be pathognomonic of this disease.

The coincident occurrence of tuberous sclerosis of the brain and rhabdomyoma of the heart is reported in 30 to 50 per cent of patients with tuberous sclerosis. Although lack of symptoms does not exclude the presence of a cardiac rhab-

domyoma, most patients have circulatory difficulties leading to death in the first year of life.

Pulmonary lesions occur in approximately 1 per cent of patients with tuberous sclerosis. The lung in tuberous sclerosis

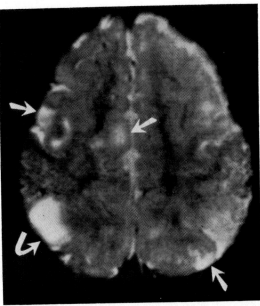

Figure 82–2. Tuberous sclerosis: Magnetic resonance image of the brain of a 22 month old girl clearly defines multiple tubers (arrows). Flat lesions (curved arrow) may fail to be appreciated grossly at surgery, although they are large and superficial. (Courtesy of J. Bello, M.D., New York, New York.)

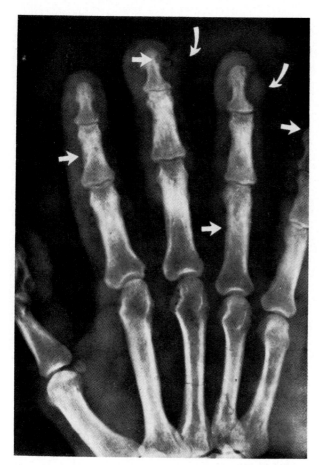

Figure 82–3. Tuberous sclerosis: Posteroanterior view of the hand. Numerous rounded intramedullary radiolucent lesions are seen in several phalanges of various digits, together with cortical pitting (straight arrows). Note neighboring periungual fibromas in the third and fourth digits (curved arrows).

typically demonstrates two findings: (1) a honeycomb of cystic spaces and small fibroleiomyomatous nodules, and (2) capillary angiomas. Thickened pulmonary arteries and pleural involvement have also been noted. Long-term prognosis in patients with tuberous sclerosis and pulmonary involvement is poor.

Endocrine Abnormalities

Hepatic, thyroid, and pancreatic adenomas have been noted in patients with tuberous sclerosis, as have pituitary, adrenal, and thyroid dysfunction and diabetes mellitus.

NEUROFIBROMATOSIS

Neurofibromatosis, which has an estimated frequency of 1 in 3000 births, is one of humanity's most common genetic disorders. It is inherited as an autosomal dominant trait with no sex predilection. At least 50 per cent of all index cases are thought to have resulted from mutations. This disorder remains of unknown cause.

Cutaneous and Ocular Abnormalities

Classically neurofibromatosis consists of a clinical triad that includes cutaneous lesions, mental deficiency, and skeletal deformities. In addition to its characteristic skin tumors, which histologically are neurofibromas, plexiform neurofibromas, and schwannomas, café-au-lait spots are common. The spots are age related and not uniformly present at birth, but they tend to increase in number, size, and pigmentation until the middle of the third decade of life, when they may begin to fade. The lesions of molluscum fibrosum are another cutaneous feature of neurofibromatosis.

The iris or Lisch nodule is a common ocular manifestation. The nodules may be superficial or deep within the iris stroma; they are usually bilateral, vary in number, and are most common after the age of 5 years.

A patient of any age with the three stigmata of café-au-lait spots, neurofibromas, and iris nodules is considered to have neurofibromatosis. Other ocular manifestations are of lesser diagnostic significance.

Osseous Abnormalities

CRANIUM. The orbit frequently displays a characteristic unilateral defect of the greater and lesser wings of the sphenoid bone (Fig. 82–7). The defect has been attributed to an underlying mesodermal dysplasia or complete absence of bone.

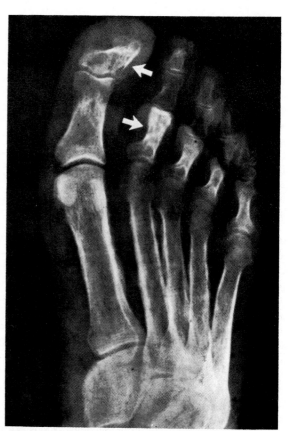

Figure 82–4. Tuberous sclerosis: Frontal view of the foot. A thickened, undulating cortex with well-defined external contours cloaks the first four metatarsal bones. Several small, rounded intramedullary radiolucent areas are seen in the distal phalanx of the first toe and the proximal phalanx of the second toe (arrows).

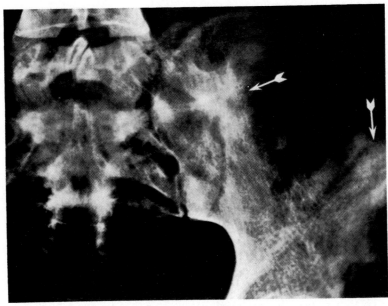

Figure 82-5. Tuberous sclerosis: Anteroposterior view of the left ilium. Irregular intramedullary osteosclerotic deposits are noted within both the ilium and the sacrum. Several are flame-shaped in configuration (arrows).

The deficient posterosuperior orbital wall may give rise to pulsating exophthalmos due to a temporal meningocele or temporal lobe herniation through the defect. Another bone defect tends to occur on the left side of the skull in the lambdoid suture (Fig. 82-8). Hypoplastic maxillary and ethmoid sinuses are also common. The mandible, maxilla, zygoma, and overlying soft tissues may be affected, with resultant facial deformity.

SPINE. Sixty per cent of patients with neurofibromatosis will have some abnormality of the spine. Scoliosis (with or without kyphosis) is the most common spinal manifestation. Scoliosis has two presenting patterns: one resembles an ordinary idiopathic spinal curve; the other is a dysplastic, sharply angulated, short segment kyphoscoliosis that commonly involves fewer than six middle or lower thoracic vertebrae, may be rapidly progressive, and is considered virtually diagnostic of neurofibromatosis (Fig. 82-9). The spinal deformity in neurofibromatosis is distinguished by the predominance of kyphosis over scoliosis. Rotation and lateral subluxation of vertebral bodies may be severe. Severe kyphoscoliosis and

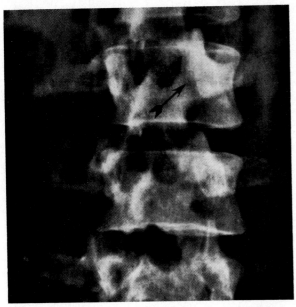

Figure 82-6. Tuberous sclerosis: Left oblique view of lumbar spine. The left pedicle and superior articular facet of a lumbar vertebra are homogeneously dense (arrow).

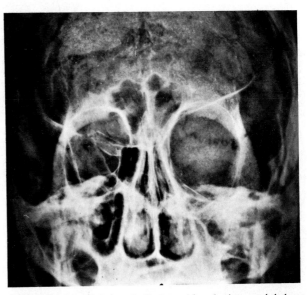

Figure 82-7. Neurofibromatosis: Patient with pulsating exophthalmos (posteroanterior view of the skull). The left orbit is enlarged and appears "empty" owing to loss of normal osseous landmarks that are present on the right. Note absence of both sphenoid wings and small ethmoid sinuses.

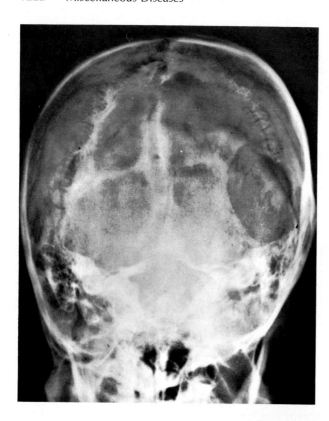

Figure 82–8. Neurofibromatosis: Posteroanterior (Towne) view of the skull. An oval calvarial defect involves the left lambdoid suture and extends toward the midline. This type of defect usually occurs on the left side.

Figure 82–9. Neurofibromatosis: Posteroanterior view of the chest. A moderate degree of thoracic spine scoliosis is associated with widened interpediculate distances of the thoracic vertebrae and deformed, widely spaced, overconstricted, and irregularly contoured ribs on the left side (arrows).

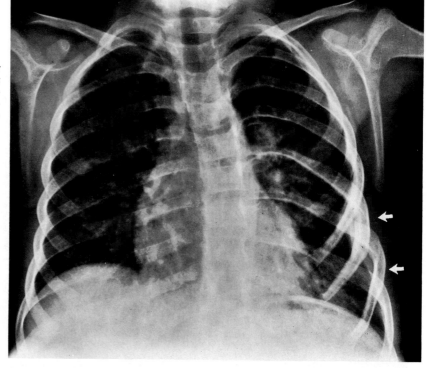

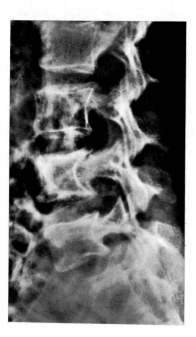

Figure 82–10. Neurofibromatosis. Marked posterior vertebral body scalloping is localized to the L3, L4, and L5 levels. There is no associated scoliosis and no change in the intervertebral disc spaces. Scalloping may result from the intrinsic dysplastic change within bone as well as from neighboring dural ectasia rather than from mechanical pressure exerted by a local neurofibroma.

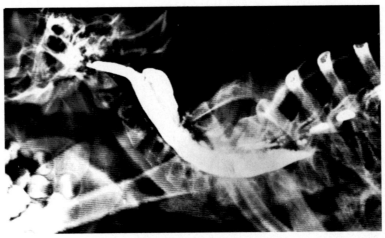

Figure 82–11. Neurofibromatosis. Prone cervical-thoracic myelogram demonstrates gross enlargement of the spinal canal with posterolateral dural ectasia.

many of the other spinal abnormalities (vertebral body wedging and scalloping, pedicle erosion, foraminal enlargement, and penciling and spindling of transverse processes and ribs) (Figs. 82–10 to 82–12) have been attributed to a primary mesodermal dysplasia.

Surgical results have been poor. The marked vertebral malalignment makes anterior access for both grafting and use of instruments difficult and mechanically ineffective in preventing progression of the spinal deformity.

OTHER SITES. In addition to the skull and spine, the ribs, pelvis, and long bones are sites of abnormal or deficient bone formation that reflects the basic mesodermal dysplasia (Figs. 82–13 to 82–16). Bowing, pathologic fracture, and pseudarthrosis of long bones occur, and callus formation and fracture healing may be defective. The tibia is affected most commonly. Anterolateral bowing of this bone, usually evident in the first years of life, is particularly characteristic and may be accompanied by a hypoplastic fibula.

When deformed or attenuated bones fracture in this disease, they frequently fail to reunite. Pseudarthroses may ultimately result, a finding that is most common in the tibia (Fig. 82–15). Pseudarthroses in this bone (or others) is usually evident during childhood and may be the sole manifestation of neurofibromatosis. Aberrations in normal growth lead to malalignment of joints and even dislocation (e.g., radial head).

The precise cause of defective fracture healing and pseudarthroses in neurofibromatosis is not clear. Neural tissue within the bone is not essential in the pathogenesis of pseudarthrosis.

Neural Tumors and Tumor-like Lesions

SPINAL NERVES. Two important manifestations of this disease are neurofibromas and, far more frequently, meningoceles. In fact, 70 to 80 per cent of all meningoceles occur in patients with neurofibromatosis and, in this disease, the meningoceles are commonly multiple and often asymptomatic. Radiographic differentiation of meningoceles and neurofibromas is difficult as both lesions may produce paraverte-

bral masses protruding laterally from enlarged neural foramina. Factors that may be responsible for meningoceles in neurofibromatosis include bone dysplasia (leading to weakened vertebrae that are susceptible to the normal pulsatile

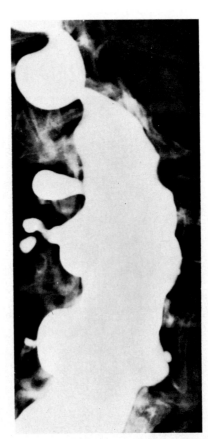

Figure 82–12. Neurofibromatosis: Lumbar myelogram. This patient had severe lumbar scoliosis and widespread vertebral body dysplasia. Note marked dural ectasia with involvement of multiple nerve root sleeves.

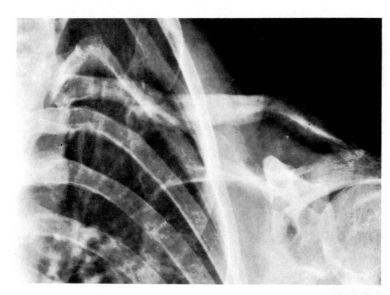

Figure 82–13. Neurofibromatosis: Left upper hemithorax. Typical appearing ribs are angulated and overconstricted. Some have wavy, undulating, ribbon-like configurations. The upper ribs are widely separated. A pseudarthrosis of the left clavicle is another associated abnormality.

Figure 82–14. Neurofibromatosis. There is marked pelvic asymmetry and hypertrophy accentuated by irregular mineralization and beak-like projections of the left inferior and superior iliac spines and proximal left femur. Note the elongated and partially detached right lesser tuberosity and deformed right pubis (small arrow) owing to previously fractured dysplastic bone. The involved acetabula still have a cup-like configuration. Note associated spinal involvement, relatively enlarged, flattened femoral heads, and the rounded, sharply circumscribed radiolucent area in the left femoral neck (large arrow).

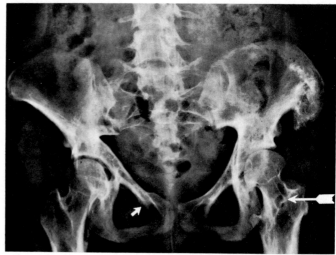

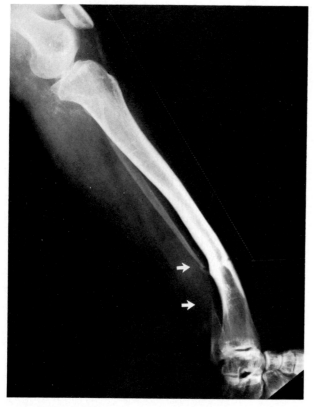

Figure 82–15. Neurofibromatosis: Lateral view of the tibia and fibula. Note pseudarthrosis of the most common site (i.e., junction of the middle and lower thirds of the tibia or fibula, or both, with attenuation and "penciling" of the neighboring fibular segments [arrows]), disuse osteoporosis distal to the pseudarthrosis, and secondary deformities of the talus and calcaneus. Anterior bowing of the leg is characteristic and is usually evident in the first years of life. Pseudarthrosis may develop spontaneously, after fracture, or after an osteotomy done to correct bowing.

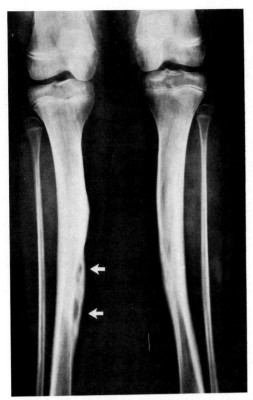

Figure 82–16. Neurofibromatosis: Anteroposterior view of tibiae and fibulae. Cortical thickening and hypertrophy have resulted in the development of two intracortical radiolucent lesions (arrows). These cyst-like, apparently intraosseous lesions may result from subperiosteal hemorrhage, with subsequent periosteal proliferation and repair, or from the incorporation or overgrowth of the periosteum around a previously external soft tissue lesion, such as a neurofibroma.

generally deformed and irregularly contoured ribs are more frequently due to dysplastic bone formation, however.

Neurologic sequelae, including paraplegia, may complicate severe kyphoscoliosis, bone dysplasia, or coexistent central nervous system lesions.

CRANIAL NERVES. Tumors of cranial nerves, usually schwannomas, are a recognized manifestation of neurofibromatosis. Acoustic neuromas, which are bilateral in 40 to 80 per cent of patients, are the most common type of associated tumor. Among the other tumors of the central nervous system that occur in patients with neurofibromatosis are opticochiasmatic gliomas and gliomas in the brain stem or supratentorial regions. In general, malignant gliomas are rare in this disease. Fifty per cent of all meningiomas are associated with neurofibromatosis (Fig. 82–19). Orbital tumors associated with neurofibromatosis include optic nerve gliomas and retrobulbar and palpebral plexiform neurofibromas.

Basilar impression, ventricular dilatation, and atlantoaxial dislocation have all been documented in neurofibromatosis. Macrocranium (increased skull size) and macrencephaly (increased brain size) also are associated with neurofibromatosis. Abnormalities (stenosis, aneurysms) of intracranial arteries occur in approximately one third of patients with neurofibromatosis.

PERIPHERAL NERVES. Peripheral nerve tumors in neurofibromatosis most frequently involve neural supporting tissues. The two most common benign forms are solitary or multiple neurofibromas and neurilemomas (schwannomas). Tumors of nerves may appear as focal enlargements or diffuse masses. Benign plexiform or cirsoid neurofibromas appear as bizarre soft tissue networks that recur after resection and have a potential for malignant transformation (Fig. 82–20).

Computed tomography and magnetic resonance imaging are far more sensitive than routine radiography in the detection of tumors of peripheral nerves. In general, both neurofibromas

pressure of the cerebrospinal fluid) and meningeal dysplasia (leading to ectatic, pulsatile dural sacs that may erode bone).

In the radiographic differentiation of meningoceles and neurofibromas, the presence of eccentric, unilateral spinal column scalloping has been said to favor the diagnosis of an adjacent nerve tumor, whereas central scalloping reputedly is more frequent with dural ectasia. This distinction is not absolute, however. Both lesions may assume a dumbbell or hourglass shape (Figs. 82–17 and 82–18). The presence of a scoliosis with the convex region directed toward the mass is a feature that favors the diagnosis of a meningocele, whereas calcification within a paraspinal mass rules against the presence of a meningocele. A posterior mediastinal lesion in a patient with neurofibromatosis or contrast material within an otherwise nonspecific mass of low density permits the diagnosis of meningocele.

Solid lesions in neurofibromatosis may occur in other than mediastinal or paraspinal locations. Intercostal neuromas may appear as extrapleural masses with or without erosion of adjacent ribs. Twisted, ribbon-like, notched, scalloped, or

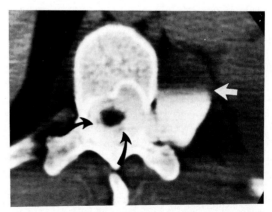

Figure 82–17. Neurofibromatosis: Computed tomogram of the T10 level following metrizamide myelogram. A dumbbell-shaped paravertebral mass on the left side, arising within the spinal canal, causes eccentric erosion of the left pedicle and posterior hemivertebra. Pooled contrast agent with a fluid level within the confines of the mass (white arrow) is indicative of a meningocele. Rounded radiolucent shadows represent intradural neurofibromas (black arrows).

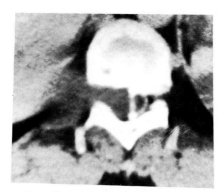

Figure 82–18. Neurofibromatosis: Computed tomogram following metrizamide myelogram in a patient with an asymptomatic neurofibroma. A low density, right paravertebral mass, with a dumbbell-shaped component in the spinal canal, enlarges the neural foramen, flattens the right hemivertebra focally, and displaces the cord markedly to the left. Contrast agent fails to enter the substance of the mass, which has no discernible fluid level.

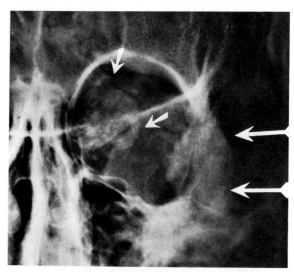

Figure 82–19. Neurofibromatosis with meningioma: Posteroanterior view of the orbit. Note intraorbital calcification and sclerosis and expansion of the left lesser sphenoid wing, which was the site of a meningioma (small arrows). Note also the dysplastic zygoma (large arrows).

and neurilemomas have lower attenuation coefficients on computed tomography than does muscle (Fig. 82–20). Some neurofibromas are isodense with muscle, however, and schwannomas may display densities as low as 5 to 10 Hounsfield units. Although the average values of 20 to 25 Hounsfield units in benign lesions have, with intravenous contrast material, been enhanced to 30 to 50 Hounsfield units, sarcomas also increase an average of 10 Hounsfield units or more after administration of the contrast agent.

MALIGNANT TRANSFORMATION. Estimates of malignant transformation of neurogenic tumors in patients with neurofibromatosis vary from 2 to 29 per cent, with 5 per cent representing an average estimate. The prognosis in patients with such sarcomas is poor. Although the vast majority of soft tissue sarcomas complicating neurofibromatosis are of nerve trunk origin and uniform composition (e.g., malignant schwannomas or neurofibrosarcomas) (Fig. 82–20), a second type of sarcoma showing pleomorphism also may occur, accounting for the occasional rhabdomyosarcoma, liposarcoma, or osteosarcoma occurring in the soft tissues in patients with this disease. Primary neurogenic, intraosseous tumors are extremely rare, and their malignant counterparts (i.e., primary neurogenic sarcomas arising in bone) are even rarer.

Miscellaneous Abnormalities

OTHER ASSOCIATED NEOPLASMS. Tumors other than those of neural supporting tissues occur much more frequently in patients with neurofibromatosis than in the general population. They include both lesions of neural crest origin (e.g., neuroblastoma, pheochromocytoma, medullary thyroid carcinoma, and melanoma) and lesions not clearly derived from the neural crest (e.g., Wilms' tumor, rhabdomyosarcoma, and leukemia).

ABERRATIONS IN GROWTH OF LIMBS. Skeletal aberrations frequently associated with neurofibromatosis may be attributable to deficient or premature cessation of growth as well as to overgrowth of bones and soft tissues. Elephantoid soft tissue hypertrophy of an entire limb, such as gigantism of a finger, may exist with normal-appearing bone structures or with hypertrophied or underdeveloped osseous elements.

Hemorrhage occurring in neurofibromatosis may be massive, recurrent, and fatal. Subperiosteal and soft tissue hemorrhage has been noted after comparatively minor insults (Fig. 82–16). An inherent abnormality of the periosteum or looseness in its adherence to the cortex has been incriminated.

CYSTIC LESIONS IN BONE. Two types of cystic lesions of bone, subperiosteal and intraosseous, have been noted. The subperiosteal form has been attributed to mechanical pressure from adjacent neurogenic tissue and to focal hemorrhage from poorly adherent, dysplastic periosteum. Intraosseous cystic lesions have been ascribed to direct invasion of the periosteum,

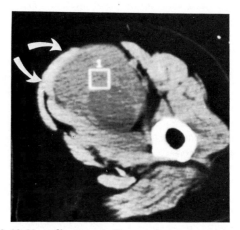

Figure 82–20. Neurofibromatosis: Computed tomogram of the proximal thigh—malignant schwannoma. A rounded, sharply marginated, inhomogeneous, low density mass compresses the relatively hyperdense adjacent muscles (curved arrows) and focally enlarges the medial aspect of the left thigh.

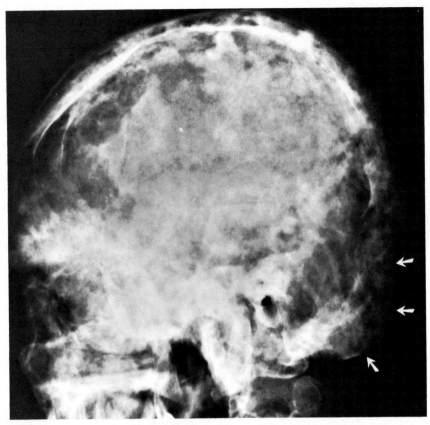

Figure 82–21. Fibrous dysplasia: woman with polyostotic fibrous dysplasia and McCune-Albright syndrome. Lateral view of the skull shows that the skull vault, base, and facial bones are extensively involved. Note involvement of less frequently affected sites, such as the temporal and occipital portions of the calvarium, with particularly marked thickening and expansion of the occipital outer table (arrows).

cortex, and haversian canals by neurofibromatous tissue. Most authorities believe bona fide intraosseous cystic lesions to be nonexistent or, at best, rare expressions of neurofibromatosis.

Reports have suggested that multiple nonossifying fibromas coexisting with brown skin patches might represent a forme fruste of neurofibromatosis (see Chapter 78). Most authors believe nonossifying fibromas to be a coincidental finding in this disorder, however.

VASCULAR LESIONS. Arterial abnormalities, including stenoses and aneurysms, may involve the genitourinary and gastrointestinal systems, spleen, endocrine glands, brain, heart, and great vessels. Renal artery stenosis constitutes a common underlying cause of hypertension in neurofibromatosis, although approximately 1 per cent of patients with neurofibromatosis have pheochromocytomas. Abdominal and thoracic aortic coarctations also have been described. Rib notching may, therefore, result from aortic coarctation as well as directly from bone dysplasia. Coarctation, however, most often is associated with focal depressions along the undersurfaces of ribs, whereas longer, generalized, ribbon-like deformities are more typical of dysplasia.

ENDOCRINE ABNORMALITIES. Associated endocrine abnormalities include hyperparathyroidism, osteomalacia, small bowel carcinoid tumors, multiple endocrine adenomatosis, and Sipple's syndrome (consisting of medullary thyroid carcinoma, pheochromocytoma, and multiple mucosal neuromas). Precocious sexual development, which is more frequently linked with fibrous dysplasia, has also been reported.

FIBROUS DYSPLASIA

Fibrous dysplasia is a skeletal developmental anomaly of bone-forming mesenchyme in which osteoblasts fail to undergo normal morphologic differentiation and maturation. It is of unknown cause and not hereditary, and it may affect one bone, a few bones, or many bones. The polyostotic variety and rarely the monostotic type, when associated with endocrine dysfunction—typically manifested by precocious female sexual development and cutaneous pigmentation—is known as the McCune-Albright syndrome.

Cutaneous and Mucosal Abnormalities

Abnormal cutaneous pigmentation is the most common extraskeletal manifestation of fibrous dysplasia. The pigmentation is evident in more than one half of patients with polyostotic disease and is almost always present in those with both multiple bone lesions and endocrine dysfunction. Although frequently paralleling the distribution of skeletal lesions, pigmentations often overlie the regions of the lower

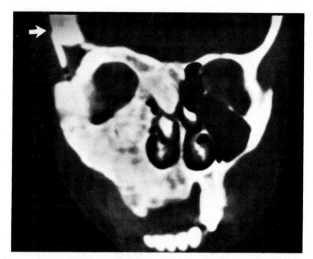

Figure 82–22. Fibrous dysplasia: Coronal computed tomogram. This scan defines the predominantly outward calvarial expansion (arrow) with an undisturbed inner table. The dappled, smoky appearance of the expanded bones rimming the right orbit and deforming the right maxilla and maxillary sinus results from their high fibrous and unmineralized osteoid content.

SKULL AND FACIAL BONES. Involvement of the skull and involvement of the facial bones occur with nearly equal frequency and are noted in approximately 10 to 25 per cent of patients with monostotic fibrous dysplasia and in 50 per cent of those with polyostotic involvement (Fig. 82–21). Common loci include the frontal, sphenoid, maxillary, and ethmoid bones. Hypertelorism, displacement of the globe, exophthalmos, diplopia, and visual impairment are related to associated alterations in orbital and periorbital bones (Fig. 82–22). Distortion of the sphenoid wing and temporal bone may similarly lead to tinnitus, vestibular dysfunction, and hearing loss, whereas involvement of the cribriform plate may produce hyposmia or anosmia.

Routine radiographs commonly reveal single or multiple, symmetric or asymmetric, radiolucent or sclerotic lesions in the skull or facial bones. Sclerosis tends to predominate in the skull and particularly affects the base and sphenoid wings, a stigma shared with Paget's disease. Concomitant involvement of the facial bones and prominence of the external occipital protuberance in fibrous dysplasia, however, are features that are less frequent in Paget's disease.

Hazy radiolucent lesions often are associated with widened

lumbar spine, sacrum, buttocks, upper back, neck, and shoulders. Pigmentation may, in fact, occasionally precede the development of skeletal or endocrine abnormalities. The café-au-lait spots of fibrous dysplasia, although brown and widely distributed as in neurofibromatosis, are usually fewer in number, more irregularly contoured, and darker in color.

Skeletal Abnormalities

Fibrous dysplasia may be associated with either solitary or multiple lesions in one or more bones. Approximately 70 to 80 per cent of cases are monostotic and 20 to 30 per cent are polyostotic; usually one or only a few bones are involved. Monostotic fibrous dysplasia is encountered most frequently in a rib, femur, tibia, gnathic bone, calvarium, and humerus, in order of decreasing frequency. Polyostotic fibrous dysplasia more frequently involves the skull and facial bones, pelvis, spine, and shoulder girdle.

Polyostotic fibrous dysplasia may affect several bones of a single limb or both limbs, with or without axial skeletal involvement. Extensive polyostotic disease commonly is associated with generalized and bilateral, albeit asymmetric, involvement. The severity and degree of osseous involvement are significantly more marked in polyostotic disease than in monostotic disease. Pain in an extremity associated with a limp or spontaneous fracture often constitutes the initial symptom. Conversely, monostotic lesions may be entirely asymptomatic for long periods until a fracture develops. Severe deformities also are unusual in monostotic disease.

Monostotic disease usually is recognized in the second and third decades of life. More severe manifestations of polyostotic fibrous dysplasia lead to earlier clinical and radiographic recognition; two thirds of patients are symptomatic before the age of 10 years.

The only significant laboratory abnormality associated with fibrous dysplasia has been an elevated serum alkaline phosphatase level.

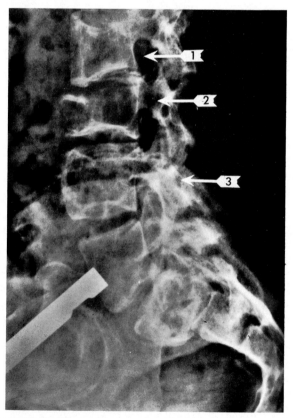

Figure 82–23. Fibrous dysplasia: Lateral view of the lumbar spine. Vertebral involvement may take the form of deformed vertebral bodies or posterior elements having a "ground glass" appearance (arrow 1) or clearer, purely radiolucent lesions having a "cystic" appearance. The latter most frequently contain a rubbery, fibrous tissue that does not weaken bone (arrow 3). Other cysts appear to relate to hemorrhage or ischemia and are more prone to compression and collapse (arrow 2).

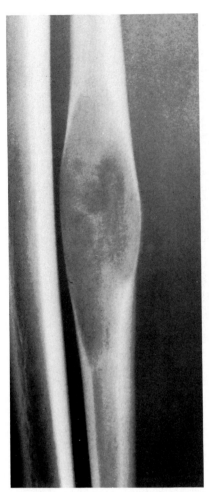

Figure 82–24. Fibrous dysplasia. A monostotic lesion in the diaphysis of the fibula is centrally located, hazy in appearance, well marginated, and slightly expansile, and it contains calcification. (Courtesy of G. Greenway, M.D., Dallas, Texas.)

described as a "ground glass" appearance (Fig. 82–24). The lesions usually are well defined and frequently are bordered by a zone of reactive sclerosis. More extensive modeling deformities may appear as areas of fusiform expansion of a long segment of bone. Focally calcified or ossified matrix contributes to radiographically appreciated intralesional opacities.

In polyostotic fibrous dysplasia, unilateral or asymmetric changes predominate. Weight-bearing bones become bowed and deformed. Pronounced curvature of the proximal portion of the femur commonly produces a severe coxa vara abnormality referred to as a "shepherd's crook" deformity (Fig. 82–25). Fractures frequently follow minor injuries. Stress (insufficiency) fractures also are encountered.

The radiographic features of fibrous dysplasia in metacarpal and metatarsal bones and phalanges are similar to those encountered in the long tubular bones (Fig. 82–26).

OTHER SKELETAL SITES. Fibrous dysplasia is the most frequently occurring benign lesion of the rib cage (Fig. 82–

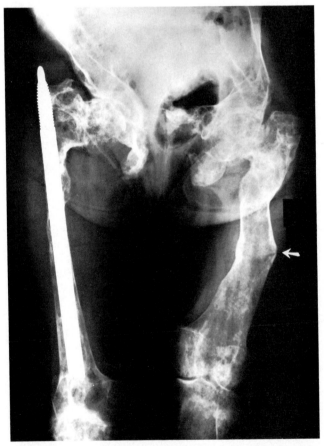

Figure 82–25. Fibrous dysplasia: Polyostotic involvement in a woman with McCune-Albright syndrome and a history of multiple fractures and surgical interventions. Note the severe pelvic distortion and bilateral proximal femoral varus deformities, the so-called shepherd's crook deformities. The femoral shafts are poorly modeled, with an intrinsic hazy, lucent appearance and little sclerosis or lesional calcification. The entire shafts, including the bone ends, are affected. There is an acute angulation at the site of a previously healed fracture (arrow).

diploic spaces and expansion in the skull and facial bones. The osseous expansion is almost always in an outward direction. Another radiographic pattern associated with fibrous dysplasia in the cranial vault is that of a varying sized but localized zone of relative radiolucency, which, when surrounded by a sclerotic rim, may take on a doughnut-shaped configuration.

SPINE. Involvement of the spine is infrequent in polyostotic fibrous dysplasia and rare in monostotic disease. Radiographic characteristics have included well-defined, expansile, radiolucent lesions with multiple internal septations that have involved the vertebral body and, occasionally, the pedicles and vertebral arch. Rarely associated sequelae have included paraspinal soft tissue extension and vertebral collapse, leading to angular deformity and spinal cord compression (Fig. 82–23).

TUBULAR BONES. Lesions in the long bones usually are intramedullary and predominantly diaphyseal in location. They are most often radiolucent, with a hazy quality classically

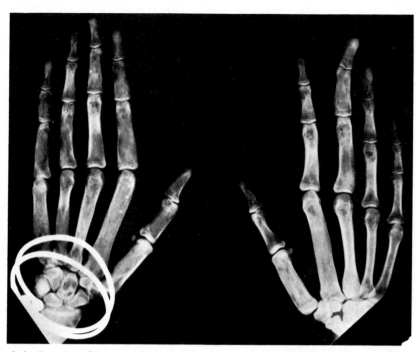

Figure 82–26. Fibrous dysplasia. Expansion of the spongiosa, cortical thinning, and alteration of bone texture are common findings in affected tubular bones. Several metacarpal bones and phalanges have rectangular or fusiform shapes, with a loss of definition between medullary and cortical bone. The hazy or "ground glass" appearance is particularly uniform in the second metacarpal bones. Localized radiolucent lesions with endosteal scalloping and areas of medullary sclerosis are also seen in several phalanges.

27). Rib involvement may be associated with expansion and deformity as well as with extraosseous extension of dysplastic tissue. A unilateral distribution, despite the presence of polyostotic involvement, serves as a means of distinction from hyperparathyroidism and skeletal metastases.

Unilateral or bilateral involvement of the innominate bones usually is associated with concomitant disease in the proximal portion of the femur (Fig. 82–28). Acetabular deformity and a markedly distorted triradiate pelvis often are evident.

NATURAL HISTORY. The prognosis in fibrous dysplasia generally depends on the extent and degree of initial skeletal involvement as well as on extraskeletal features. Monostotic involvement is not usually converted to polyostotic disease, and, in most instances, the size and number of skeletal lesions do not increase from those noted on the initial radiographic evaluation. Although both polyostotic and monostotic fibrous dysplasia generally become quiescent at puberty and remain so throughout life, in some instances progressive deformity supervenes. In such cases, fractures are common, deformity is severe, and ultimate prognosis is poor. Reactivation of skeletal lesions in fibrous dysplasia has also been noted during the course of pregnancy and estrogen therapy; in some instances, this may relate to the superimposition of an aneurysmal bone cyst.

MALIGNANT TRANSFORMATION. Malignant transformation of skeletal lesions is a rare complication of fibrous dysplasia. In many presumed examples, prior radiation to involved bones has complicated accurate determination of spontaneous malignant transformation. Osteosarcoma and fi-

brosarcoma are encountered most often. Although chondrosarcoma reputedly occurs, its recognition is particularly difficult in view of the intrinsic cartilaginous nodules that frequently coexist with fibrous dysplasia and that may lead to an erroneous diagnosis of low-grade chondrosarcoma. Clinically, pain and swelling accompanied by such radiographic changes as poorly defined areas of osteolysis, cortical destruction, and soft tissue masses in the vicinity of disrupted cortices have been regarded as highly suggestive of malignant transformation.

Endocrine Abnormalities

Fibrous dysplasia has no sexual predilection. The greater the number of polyostotic cases included in any review of the disease, the greater the likelihood of a female bias, however. Its characteristically associated endocrinopathy, the *McCune-Albright syndrome,* predominates in girls and classically consists of polyostotic fibrous dysplasia, cutaneous pigmentation, and precocious sexual development. Incomplete forms of the syndrome include sexual precocity and osseous lesions in the absence of cutaneous pigmentation. Sexual precocity in girls is characterized by the early appearance of vaginal bleeding, breast development, and axillary and pubic hair. In this syndrome, the possibility of increased sensitivity of target organs (i.e., gonads and breasts) to normal or minimally elevated prepubertal circulating pituitary hormones has been suggested. It is noteworthy that even in the absence of overt sexual precocity, apparent hormonal disturbances have been reflected in advanced skeletal maturation and accelerated linear

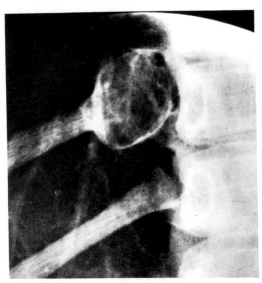

Figure 82–27. Fibrous dysplasia: Anteroposterior view of the rib. This solitary, expansile, multilocular-appearing lesion with an intact cortex was an incidental finding on a chest film.

growth, with or without subsequent premature closure of the physes.

Additional pluriglandular involvement has long been recognized in polyostotic fibrous dysplasia, including Cushing's disease, acromegaly, hyperthyroidism, hyperparathyroidism and extrainsular hypothalamic diabetes mellitus. Some of these clinical diagnoses must be regarded with caution because acromegalic facies, the exophthalmos of Graves' disease, and visual defects suggesting a pituitary tumor may all be mimicked by facial and skeletal involvement in fibrous dysplasia alone.

The association of endocrinopathies in fibrous dysplasia, with or without a concomitant McCune-Albright syndrome, continues to be explained by two major theories. One contends that congenital hypothalamic dysfunction with hypersecretion of releasing hormones results in increased stimulation of target organs. The other theory postulates an underlying form of multiple endocrine neoplasia with autonomous function of involved endocrine glands.

Other Abnormalities

Hypophosphatemic rickets and osteomalacia have been noted in patients with either monostotic or polyostotic fibrous dysplasia, both with and without the McCune-Albright syndrome. The findings are analogous to those seen when rickets and osteomalacia accompany neoplastic disorders of bone or soft tissue (see Chapter 48). In these instances, as well as in fibrous dysplasia, resection of the lesion may be followed by disappearance of the findings of rickets or osteomalacia. The synthesis of a phosphaturic hormone by a concomitant bone or soft tissue tumor or by benign fibrous lesions, such as fibrous dysplasia, has been one hypothesis developed to explain the associated metabolic disorder.

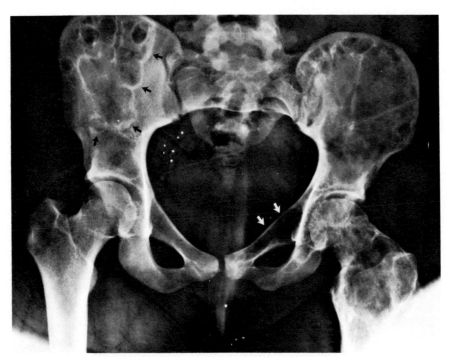

Figure 82–28. Fibrous dysplasia: Polyostotic fibrous dysplasia and McCune-Albright syndrome. The dysplasia has resulted in a thickened, foreshortened femoral neck and shaft held in varus position (a shepherd's crook deformity). Note the hazy, "ground glass" appearance of the involved left femur, with relative sparing of the femoral head. The left pubis and both ilia are also involved by roentgenographically typical lesions of fibrous dysplasia. The purely radiolucent pubic lesion is expansile and nonmineralized (white arrows). The central segments of the right iliac locus are hazy and smoky in appearance owing to a high proportion of osteoid and are well demarcated by an almost continuous curvilinear sclerotic rim (black arrows).

FURTHER READING

Albright F, Butler AM, Hampton AO, Smith P: Syndrome characterized by osteitis fibrosa disseminata, areas of pigmentation and endocrine dysfunction with precocious puberty in females. N Engl J Med 216:727, 1937.

Brown B: The radiologic features of bone changes in tuberous sclerosis with a case report. J Can Assoc Radiol 12:1, 1961.

Burrows EH: Bone changes in orbital neurofibromatosis. Br J Radiol 36:549, 1963.

Crawford AH Jr, Bogamery N: Osseous manifestations of neurofibromatosis in childhood. J Pediatr Orthop 6:72, 1986.

Drolshagen LF, Reynolds WA, Marcus NW: Fibrocartilaginous dysplasia of bone. Radiology 156:32, 1985.

Ducatman BS, Scheithauer BW, Dahlin DC: Malignant bone tumors associated with neurofibromatosis. Mayo Clin Proc 58:578, 1983.

Gibson MJ, Middlemiss JH: Fibrous dysplasia of bone. Br J Radiol 44:1, 1971.

Green GJ: The radiology of tuberous sclerosis. Clin Radiol 19:135, 1968.

Holt JF, Kuhns LR: Macrocranium and macrencephaly in neurofibromatosis. Skel Radiol 1:25, 1976.

Hunt JC, Pugh DG: Skeletal lesions in neurofibromatosis. Radiology 76:1, 1961.

Klatte EC, Franken EA, Smith JA: The radiographic spectrum in neurofibromatosis. Semin Roentgenol 11:17, 1976.

Komar NN, Gabrielsen TO, Holt JF: Roentgenographic appearance of lumbosacral spine and pelvis in tuberous sclerosis. Radiology 89:701, 1967.

Leeds N, Seaman WB: Fibrous dysplasia of the skull and its differential diagnosis. A clinical and roentgenographic study of 46 cases. Radiology 78:570, 1962.

Leeds NE, Jacobson HG: Spinal neurofibromatosis. AJR 126:617, 1976.

Lichtenstein L, Jaffe HL: Fibrous dysplasia of bone: A condition affecting one, several or many bones, the graver cases of which may present abnormal pigmentation of skin, premature sexual development, hyperthyroidism or still other extraskeletal abnormalities. Arch Pathol 33:777, 1942.

Mandell GA, Dalinka MK, Coleman BG: Fibrous lesions in the lower extremities in neurofibromatosis. AJR 133:1135, 1979.

Medley BE, McLeod RA, Houser OW: Tuberous sclerosis. Semin Roentgenol 11:35, 1976.

Pitt MJ, Mosher JF, Edeiken J: Abnormal periosteum and bone in neurofibromatosis. Radiology 103:143, 1972.

Riddell DH: Malignant change in fibrous dysplasia. J Bone Joint Surg [Br] 46:251, 1964.

Sack GH Jr: Malignant complications of neurofibromatosis. Clin Oncol 9:17, 1983.

Warrick CK: Polyostotic fibrous dysplasia—Albright's syndrome. A review of the literature and report of four male cases, two of which were associated with precocious puberty. J Bone Joint Surg [Br] 31:175, 1949.

Chapter 83

Enostosis, Hyperostosis, and Periostitis

Donald Resnick, M.D.
Gen Niwayama, M.D.

Numerous disorders are associated with localized or generalized cortical hyperostosis or periostitis. In these disorders, single or multiple areas of radiodensity commonly are detected on skeletal radiographs. They may appear as discrete foci within the spongiosa (enostosis) or on the surface of the cortex (osteoma), or as more widespread areas or cortical hyperostosis or periostitis. The changes must be distinguished from the periostitis that occurs as a response to an adjacent osseous process (neoplasm, infection, trauma) and from the hyperostosis that accompanies other congenital disorders. In some cases, these osseous changes may indicate the presence of a distant (and significant) extraskeletal lesion or an underlying systemic disorder.

Single or multiple areas of increased radiodensity commonly are detected on skeletal radiographs. These may appear as discrete foci within the spongiosa (enostosis) or on the surface of the cortex (osteoma), or as more diffuse and widespread areas of cortical hyperostosis or periostitis. In some cases, the detection of such osseous alterations indicates the presence of a distant (and significant) extraskeletal lesion or an underlying systemic disorder.

ENOSTOSIS (BONE ISLAND)

An enostosis, also designated a bone island, occurs frequently in all age groups; although any osseous site can be affected, the lesions have a predilection for the pelvis, proximal portion of the femur, and ribs. Enostoses appear radiographically as single or multiple intraosseous sclerotic areas with discrete margins in asymptomatic individuals. They are usually aligned with the long axis of the bone. Thorny, radiating bone spicules extend from the center of the lesion (Fig. 83–1), and the lesions do not protrude from the cortical surface of the involved bone. Their size is variable; some especially in the pelvis, may reach proportions greater than 40 by 40 mm.

They may increase or decrease in size or disappear completely. During periods of observation in adolescents, enostoses may appear for the first time and enlarge in proportion to bone growth. Even in adult patients, such enlargement can be encountered, simulating the appearance of an osteoblastic skeletal metastasis. Bone scintigraphy in cases of bone islands, however, usually yields normal results.

In the spine, enostoses may be apparent in 1 to 14 per cent of persons. At this location, they also have been termed endosteomas, and they create circular or triangular areas of increased density in the vertebral body that may reach 20 by 30 mm in size (Fig. 83–2).

The exact nature of enostoses is not clear. Histologically, they are composed of normal-appearing compact bone. Their pathologic characteristics can be differentiated readily from those associated with bone infarction, infection, or neoplasms, such as osteoid osteoma or osteosarcoma.

In addition to skeletal metastases, the differential diagnosis of enostoses includes osteomas, osteoid osteomas, enchondromas, bone infarcts, fibrous dysplasia, and osteopoikilosis (Table 83–1). Osteopoikilosis leads to formation of multiple radiodense foci, each one of which resembles an enostosis radiographically and histologically.

OSTEOMA

An osteoma is a protruding mass composed of abnormally dense but otherwise normal bone that is formed in the periosteum. Thus, the lesion is confined to areas of the bone that normally are produced by the periosteal membrane. Osteomas predominate in the skull and facial bones, although they may occasionally arise at other sites, including the tubular bones of the extremities. In the latter locations, osteochondromas containing cartilaginous caps are much more frequent and represent a different lesion.

Osteomas are very frequent in the sinuses, especially the frontal sinus. Osteomas also arise from the inner and outer tables of the cranial vault, the mandible, and the maxilla. They have been detected in persons of all ages, although the lesions predominate in patients in the fourth and fifth decades of life. Men are affected more commonly. Osteomas usually are asymptomatic.

On radiographs, the lesions appear as a single focus or as

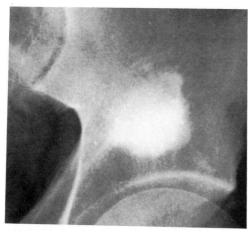

Figure 83–1. Enostosis: Pelvis. Note the homogeneous nature of the dense area and the radiating spicules extending into the adjacent bone.

multiple radiodense foci that protrude into a sinus or extend from the surface of a parent bone (Fig. 83–3). Their outline is smooth or lobular, and frequently they are homogeneous in appearance. Once discovered, osteomas usually remain unchanged on serial studies.

Multiple osteomas of the mandible, calvarium, or tubular bones can accompany *Gardner's syndrome* (Table 83–2). This is a familial autosomal dominant disease consisting of colonic polyposis, osteomatosis, and soft tissue tumors. The soft tissue tumors consist of epidermal or sebaceous cysts, subcutaneous fibromas and lipomas, and desmoid tumors. The osseous lesions frequently precede the appearance of clinical and radiographic evidence of intestinal polyposis. Osteomas are particularly frequent in the skull, sinuses, and mandible, but they may also be detected in the ribs and long bones. In the last-mentioned sites, however, the outgrowths may appear as wavy cortical thickening. Dental abnormalities in this syndrome include hypercementosis, supernumerary and unerupted teeth, odontomas, and dentigerous cysts. The major

differential diagnostic possibility is tuberous sclerosis (Fig. 83–4).

OSTEOPOIKILOSIS

Osteopoikilosis is an asymptomatic, uncommon osteosclerotic dysplasia. The disorder is seen in both men and women and may become evident at any age. Inherited and sporadic cases of osteopoikilosis have both been reported. Cutaneous lesions may be evident in approximately 25 per cent of cases.

Radiographic findings are diagnostic. Numerous small, circular or ovoid foci of increased radiodensity are clustered in periarticular osseous regions. A symmetric distribution is observed, with a predilection for the epiphyses and metaphyses of long tubular bones, carpus, tarsus, pelvis, and scapulae (Fig. 83–5). On serial radiographs, the radiopaque areas occasionally increase or decrease in size and number or disappear. Radionuclide examination with bone-seeking radiopharmaceutical agents usually reveals no evidence of increased activity about the skeletal lesions. The microscopic features of the lesion are identical to those encountered in bone islands.

The cause and pathogenesis of osteopoikilosis are not known. Some evidence suggests that a relationship exists between this condition and other osteosclerotic skeletal disorders, especially osteopathia striata and melorheostosis (Table 83–3). The resulting combination of abnormalities has been referred to as mixed sclerosing bone dystrophy (see later discussion).

The major differential diagnostic considerations in cases of widespread focal round or oval radiodense lesions are osteopoikilosis, osteoblastic metastases, mastocytosis, and tuberous sclerosis. The symmetric distribution, the propensity for epiphyseal and metaphyseal involvement, and the uniform size of the foci are features that suggest osteopoikilosis.

OSTEOPATHIA STRIATA

Osteopathia striata (Voorhoeve's disease) is an extremely rare disorder. Men and women of any age can be affected, and a genetic transmission, probably an autosomal dominant

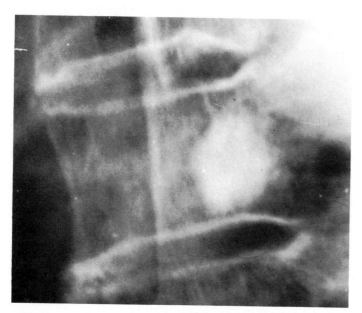

Figure 83–2. Enostosis: Spine. Note the homogeneous, well-defined circular lesion with radiating spicules. (From Broderick TW, et al: Enostosis of the spine. Spine 3:167, 1978. Used with permission.)

Table 83–1. LOCALIZED RADIODENSE LESIONS

Lesion	Location	Appearance
Enostosis (bone island)	Medullary	Round or oblong, thorny radiating spicules
Osteoma	Cortical protrusion	Homogeneous, smooth or lobular, extend from osseous surface
Osteochondroma	Cortical and medullary protrusion	Cortical and spongiosa are continuous with parent bone, calcified cap
Enchondroma	Medullary	Lucent, well-circumscribed, central calcifications
Bone infarct	Medullary	Lucent, well or poorly circumscribed, peripheral shell of calcification
Osteoid osteoma	Cortical, medullary, or subperiosteal	Cortical: Lucent with or without calcification surrounded by sclerotic bone
		Medullary: Lucent or calcified, with little sclerosis
		Subperiosteal: Scalloped excavation with or without calcification and sclerosis

one, has been suggested. Clinical manifestations are usually absent.

Radiography reveals linear, regular bands of increased radiodensity that extend from the metaphyses of tubular bones for variable distances into the diaphyses, and that are interspersed with areas of rarefaction (Fig. 83–6). In the ilium, a fan-like arrangement of radiodense striations radiates toward the iliac crests. The skeletal abnormalities usually are bilateral in distribution. Scintigraphy with bone-seeking radiopharmaceutical agents fails to reveal significant abnormalities.

Osteopathia striata may coexist with osteopoikilosis, melorheostosis, or osteopetrosis (Table 83–3). Metaphyseal flaring in some cases of osteopathia striata resembles the findings in Pyle's disease. A relationship between osteopathia striata and focal dermal hypoplasia (Goltz's syndrome) has been noted.

Osteopathia striata also has been associated with cranial sclerosis.

The cause and pathogenesis of osteopathia striata are not known. Its differential diagnosis includes prominent vertical trabecular formation that may be a normal variant; the adult form of osteopetrosis, in which linear striations of long bones

Table 83–2. MAJOR RADIOGRAPHIC ABNORMALITIES IN GARDNER'S SYNDROME

Colonic polyposis
Osteomas
Soft tissue tumors
Dental lesions

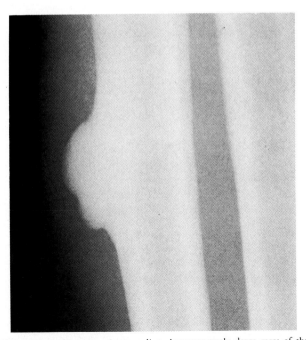

Figure 83–3. Osteoma. A protruding, homogeneously dense mass of the ulna is evident. It is of the same radiodensity and appearance as the underlying cortex. Note that there is no connection between the medullary bone of the ulna and the lesion.

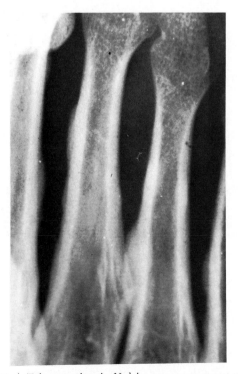

Figure 83–4. Tuberous sclerosis. Nodular osseous excrescences arise from the external cortex of the metatarsal bones. (Courtesy of V. Schiappacasse, M.D., Santiago, Chile.)

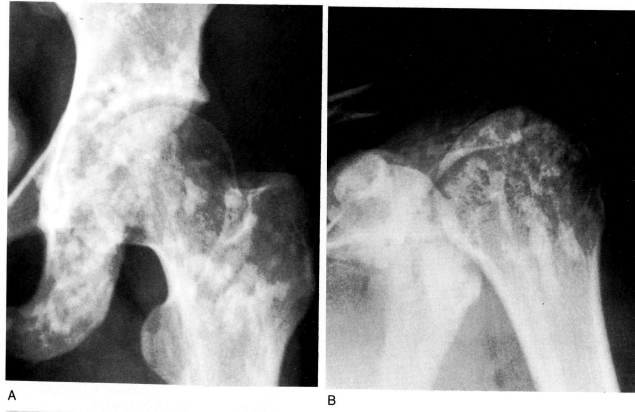

A

B

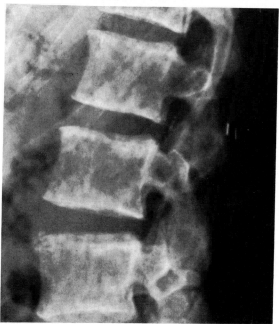

C

Figure 83–5. Osteopoikilosis. A Hip. Note the circular or ovoid radiodense foci of the femur and pelvis without abnormality of the intervening joint space. **B** Shoulder. The same radiographic characteristics are evident. **C** Spine. Observe radiodense foci in the margins of the vertebral bodies and in the posterior osseous elements. This patient has had a laminectomy. (C, Courtesy of A. Brower, M.D., Washington, D.C.)

and pelvis may be encountered; enchondromatosis (Ollier's disease), in which oval-shaped lesions may produce metaphyseal bands of diminished density; and osteopoikilosis, in which oval or circular radiodense foci are seen.

MELORHEOSTOSIS

Melorheostosis is a rare bone disorder that generally becomes manifest after early childhood. Men and women are affected equally, and no hereditary features have been established.

Initial clinical alterations of the disorder may include swelling of joints and pain. Subsequently, muscle contractures and tendon and ligament shortening may become evident. Growth disturbances can be severe and can lead to scoliosis, joint contracture and rigidity, and pes valgus, varus, or equinovarus. Soft tissue changes include erythematous skin, anomalous pigmentation, edema of subcutaneous tissues, fibrosis, atrophy of muscles, and linear scleroderma. Although life expectancy is not shortened, the disease can result in considerable deformity and disability.

Table 83–3. DISEASES ASSOCIATED WITH VARIOUS HYPEROSTOTIC LESIONS

Lesion	Possible Associated Diseases
Osteoma	Gardner's syndrome
Osteopoikilosis	Osteopathia striata Melorheostosis Hyperostosis frontalis interna
Osteopathia striata	Osteopoikilosis Melorheostosis Osteopetrosis Cranial sclerosis Focal dermal hypoplasia
Melorheostosis	Linear scleroderma Osteopoikilosis Osteopathia striata Neurofibromatosis Tuberous sclerosis Hemangiomas

Radiographic alterations are highly characteristic. Changes commonly are limited to a single limb. The lower extremity is involved more frequently than the upper extremity. Abnormalities may also be encountered in the skull and facial bones, ribs, and vertebrae. Peripherally located hyperostosis is evident in one bone or a series of bones (Figs. 83–7 and 83–8). The appearance of the osseous excrescences extending along the length of the bone simulates that of candle wax flowing down the side of a lit candle. A wavy and sclerotic bone contour is produced that may involve one side of the tubular bones of the upper or lower extremity, reaching the carpus and tarsus as well as the metacarpals, metatarsals, or phalanges. In the carpal and tarsal areas, more discrete round foci may resemble the findings of osteopoikilosis. Soft tissue calcification and ossification are not infrequent, having a predilection for paraarticular regions, and may lead to complete ankylosis of the joint (Fig. 83–9).

As opposed to the situation in osteopoikilosis and osteopathia striata, scintigraphy in cases of melorheostosis can reveal areas of increased skeletal accumulation of radionuclide, and the resulting scintigraphic image may simulate Paget's disease.

On pathologic examination, thickened and enlarged bone trabeculae are found to contain normal-appearing haversian systems that may be irregularly arranged.

Melorheostosis has been reported in association with other disorders (Table 83–3). Band-like linear scleroderma overlying osseous excrescences has been noted. The association of melorheostosis with osteopoikilosis and osteopathia striata also has been reported. In the axial skeleton, melorheostosis has been accompanied by fibrolipomatous lesions in adjacent areas.

As one of the most striking characteristics of the disease is a peculiar pattern of distribution, clues to the pathogenesis of melorheostosis may be uncovered by analyzing this characteristic. In many cases of melorheostosis, skeletal alterations correspond to a single sclerotome (a skeletal zone supplied by an individual spinal sensory nerve) or a part thereof, suggesting that the disease may represent the late result of a segmental sensory nerve lesion.

The radiographic abnormalities of melorheostosis are sufficiently characteristic to allow accurate diagnosis in most cases.

MIXED SCLEROSING BONE DYSTROPHY

Although osteopoikilosis, osteopathia striata, and melorheostosis each possess characteristic radiologic abnormalities, some patients demonstrate findings of more than one of these disorders and, occasionally, of all three (Fig. 83–10). This phenomenon is termed mixed sclerosing bone dystrophy. Four types of mixed sclerosing bone dystrophy have been identified: (1) osteopathia striata, melorheostosis, osteopoikilosis, and focal osteosclerosis; (2) osteopathia striata and cranial sclerosis with or without osteopoikilosis; (3) osteopathia striata, generalized cortical hyperostosis, and metadiaphyseal widening with or without cranial sclerosis and osteopoikilosis of the ribs; and (4) osteopoikilosis with diaphyseal periosteal proliferation. These types of mixed sclerosing bone dystrophy can be associated with lymphangiectasia, capillary hemangiomas, arteriovenous malformations, and Trevor's disease.

PRIMARY HYPERTROPHIC OSTEOARTHROPATHY (PACHYDERMOPERIOSTOSIS)

Hypertrophic osteoarthropathy represents a clinical syndrome consisting of clubbing of the digits of the hands and feet, enlargement of the extremities secondary to periarticular and osseous proliferation, and painful and swollen joints. The syndrome may be divided into two categories: primary (hereditary or idiopathic) and secondary. The primary form represents approximately 3 to 5 per cent of all cases of hypertrophic osteoarthropathy. Primary hypertrophic osteoarthropathy is also called pachydermoperiostosis.

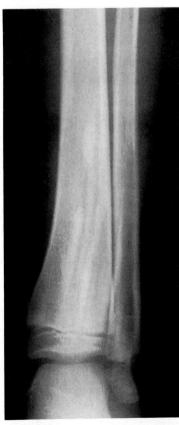

Figure 83–6. Osteopathia striata. Note linear radiodense areas principally in the metaphyses of the tibia. (Courtesy of R. Tobin, M.D., San Diego, California.)

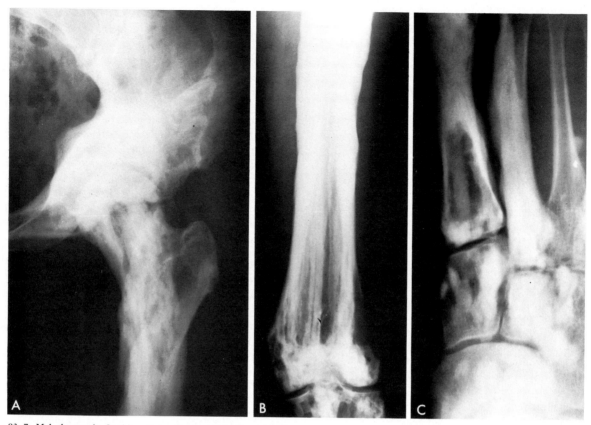

Figure 83–7. Melorheostosis. In this patient, characteristic radiographic abnormalities are evident throughout a single extremity. Note the hyperostosis of the left hemipelvis, paraacetabular region, and medial aspect of the proximal femur. In the distal portion of the femur, a peculiar linear radiodense pattern extends across the knee joint. Involvement of the medial rays of the foot is also seen. (Courtesy of R. Freiberger, M.D., New York, New York.)

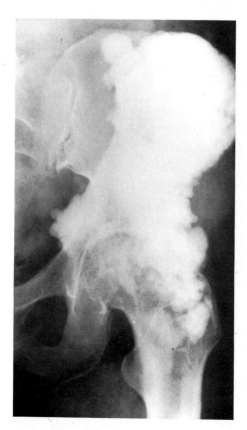

Figure 83–8. Melorheostosis. Osseous excrescences are observed in the lateral portion of the ilium, acetabular region, and femur, in combination with soft tissue ossification about the hip. (Courtesy of H. R. Fischer, M.D., Victoria, British Columbia, Canada.)

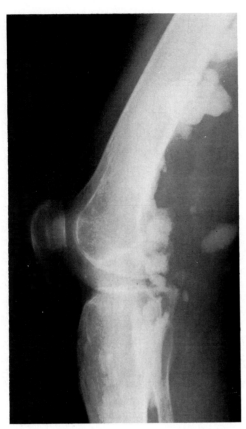

Figure 83–9. Melorheostosis. Prominent soft tissue calcification and ossification are noted along the posterior aspect of the thigh and the knee. Minor hyperostosis of the underlying cortex is evident.

Clinical Abnormalities

Pachydermoperiostosis demonstrates an autosomal dominant genetic transmission with marked variability of expression. It predominates in men and shows a predilection for blacks. An adolescent onset is typical. The clinical manifestations are somewhat variable, depending on whether the patient demonstrates the complete syndrome (pachydermia, periostitis, cutis verticis gyrata), the incomplete form (sparing of the scalp), or the forme fruste (pachydermia with minimal or absent periostitis).

There is an insidious onset of enlargement of the hands and feet, clubbing of the fingers and toes, and convexity of the nails. Coarsening of the skin of the face and scalp, excessive sweating, enlargement of the extremities, and vague pains in the bones and joints are also encountered. Pachydermoperiostosis generally progresses for approximately 10 years before arresting spontaneously. Chronic disabling complications may appear, however, with restricted motion, kyphosis, and neurologic manifestations. Life expectancy is normal.

Radiographic Abnormalities

The predominant radiographic feature of pachydermoperiostosis is periostitis (Fig. 83–11). Widespread and symmetric findings occur, although osseous thickening is most pronounced in the tubular bones of the extremities. Thickening of the calvarium and base of the skull can be detected.

Superficially, the periosteal proliferation of the tubular bones resembles that typically seen in secondary hypertrophic osteoarthropathy, but careful evaluation reveals significant differences (Table 83–4). Although the diaphyses and metaphyses can be affected in both conditions, periostitis commonly extends into the epiphyseal region in pachydermoperi-

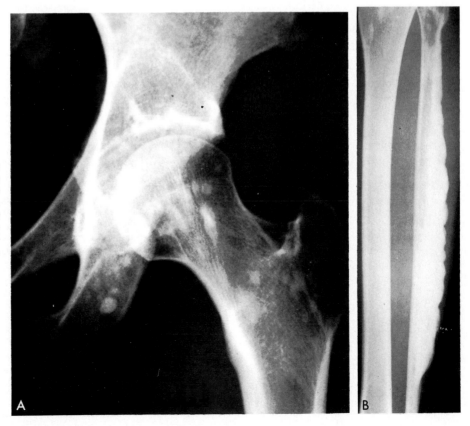

Figure 83–10. Mixed sclerosing bone dystrophy. A The changes in the hip are diagnostic of osteopoikilosis, although some of the foci are elongated or linear in shape. **B** Involvement of the fibula in the same patient consists of flowing, eccentrically located ossification, an appearance that is typical of melorheostosis. (Courtesy of A. Brower, M.D., Washington, D.C.)

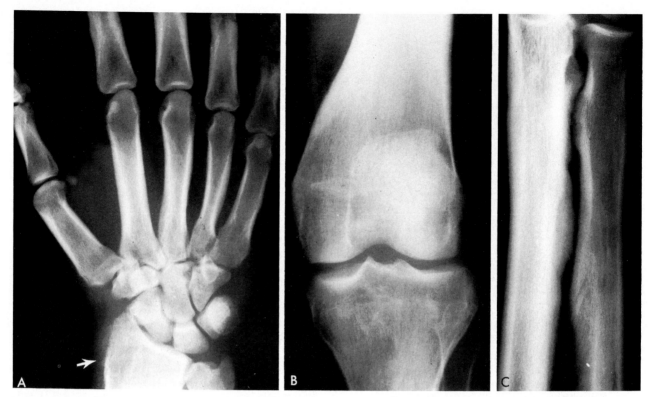

Figure 83–11. Primary hypertrophic osteoarthropathy (pachydermoperiostosis). A In addition to periosteal proliferation of the distal portion of the radius (arrow), note the widened metacarpals and phalanges. **B** An expanded contour of the distal portion of the femur is associated with cortical thickening. **C** Exuberant osseous proliferation is evident along apposing surfaces of radius and ulna.

Table 83–4. SOME CAUSES OF DIFFUSE PERIOSTITIS

Disease	Location	Characteristics
Primary hypertrophic osteoarthropathy (pachydermoperiostosis)	Tibia, fibula, radius, ulna (less commonly, femur, humerus, carpus, tarsus, metacarpals, metatarsals, phalanges, pelvis, ribs, clavicle)	Diaphyseal, metaphyseal, and epiphyseal involvement Shaggy, irregular excrescences Diaphyseal expansion Clubbing Ligamentous ossification Cranial and facial changes
Secondary hypertrophic osteoarthropathy	Tibia, fibula, radius, ulna (less commonly, femur, humerus, metacarpals, metatarsals, phalanges)	Diaphyseal and metaphyseal involvement Single or laminated, regular or irregular proliferation Clubbing Periarticular osteoporosis, soft tissue swelling Underlying primary lesion
Thyroid acropachy	Metacarpals, metatarsals, phalanges (less commonly, other tubular bones)	Diaphyseal involvement Radial side predilection Dense, solid, and spiculated proliferation Clubbing Soft tissue swelling Thyroid gland abnormalities
Venous stasis	Tibia, fibula, femur, metatarsals, phalanges	Diaphyseal and metaphyseal involvement Undulating osseous contour Cortical thickening Soft tissue swelling, ulceration, ossification Phleboliths
Hypervitaminosis A	Ulna, metatarsals, clavicle, tibia, fibula	Diaphyseal involvement Undulating contour Epiphyseal deformities Soft tissue nodules Intracranial hypertension
Infantile cortical hyperostosis (Caffey's disease)	Mandible, clavicle, scapula, ribs, tubular bones	Periostitis and cortical hyperostosis May become extreme Cranial destruction Soft tissue nodules Deformities

ostosis. Poorly defined bone outgrowths are especially characteristic of this disease, differing from the linear deposits that most typically accompany secondary hypertrophic osteoarthropathy. These outgrowths are also encountered in the pelvis, particularly about the ischium, symphysis pubis, acetabulum, and iliac crest. It should be emphasized, however, that differences in the pattern and distribution of periosteal proliferation in primary and secondary hypertrophic osteoarthropathy are related, at least in part, to the earlier age of onset and longer duration of the former disorder.

In more advanced cases of pachydermoperiostosis, expansion of the diaphyses of the tubular bones and sclerosis of the spongiosa in both appendicular and axial skeletal sites are evident. The skull may reveal prominent sinuses and enlargement of the mandible. Soft tissue prominence of the digits may be associated with tuftal osteolysis. Ligamentous calcification may appear in the calcaneus, the ulnar olecranon, the patella, and the interosseous regions between radius and ulna and between tibia and fibula.

Articular Abnormalities

Articular inflammation is less prominent in pachydermoperiostosis than in secondary hypertrophic osteoarthropathy. Pain and swelling are uncommon. Joint effusions may be encountered. In long-standing cases, limitation of joint motion reflects mechanical interference owing to periarticular osseous excrescences and intraarticular bone masses.

Etiology and Pathogenesis

A definite cause and pathogenesis of pachydermoperiostosis have not been unraveled. Measurements in patients with long-standing pachydermoperiostosis reveal diminished blood flow, although the significance of this finding is not clear.

Differential Diagnosis

The irregular periosteal deposits that appear about metaphyses and epiphyses of tubular bones as well as axial skeletal sites in this condition usually are not encountered in secondary hypertrophic osteoarthropathy. Some patients with congenital cyanotic heart disease and secondary hypertrophic osteoarthropathy have similar alterations, however. The early age of onset, a family history of disease, and the absence of significant joint pain are clinical characteristics of pachydermoperiostosis that differ from those of secondary hypertrophic osteoarthropathy. In thyroid acropachy, fluffy, spiculated periosteal bone is encountered in the hands and feet. It is rarely observed elsewhere, a fact that, taken in combination with typical clinical characteristics, such as exophthalmos and pretibial myxedema, ensures accurate diagnosis of thyroid acropachy. Some of the clinical and radiologic manifestations of acromegaly are observed in pachydermoperiostosis, but radiographic and laboratory signs of a pituitary tumor distinguish acromegaly from pachydermoperiostosis. Other disorders, such as Paget's disease, fibrous dysplasia, endosteal hyperostosis, diaphyseal dysplasia, and fluorosis, are easily differentiated from pachydermoperiostosis.

SECONDARY HYPERTROPHIC OSTEOARTHROPATHY

Hypertrophic osteoarthropathy may occur secondary to another process. It has been estimated that between 1 per cent and 12 per cent of patients with bronchogenic carcinoma develop hypertrophic osteoarthropathy. The disorder also is common in patients with pleural mesothelioma. Other intrathoracic diseases associated with this complication include pulmonary abscess, bronchiectasis, emphysema, Hodgkin's disease, diaphragmatic tumors, and metastasis (Table 83–5). Hypertrophic osteoarthropathy is rarely encountered in cases of pulmonary tuberculosis. Hypertrophic osteoarthropathy has also been associated with cyanotic congenital heart disease and many extrathoracic conditions (Table 83–5). In children, potential causes include pulmonary suppuration, cystic fibrosis, congenital cyanotic heart disease, Hodgkin's disease, metastasis, Crohn's disease, ulcerative colitis, biliary atresia, and primary pulmonary neoplasms.

Clinical Abnormalities

Digital clubbing is a frequent feature of hypertrophic osteoarthropathy; however, patients with diverse disorders can reveal clubbing without any associated findings of hypertrophic osteoarthropathy. Articular findings are apparent at some time in approximately 40 per cent of patients and may be the presenting manifestation of hypertrophic osteoarthropathy. The knees, ankles, wrists, elbows, and metacarpophalangeal joints are involved most commonly. Synovial effusions are frequent.

In cases of hypertrophic osteoarthropathy secondary to intrathoracic causes, thoracotomy frequently leads to prominent remission of the joint symptoms and signs within 24 hours. Even patients with nonresectable tumors may benefit from thoracotomy. Other surgical procedures that can lead to a regression of the clinical manifestations include hilar neurectomy, vagotomy, and ipsilateral occlusion of the pulmonary artery. Radiotherapy or chemotherapy may be associated with similar improvement. Regrowth of the neoplasm commonly is associated with exacerbation of the clinical and radiographic findings.

Table 83–5. SOME CAUSES OF SECONDARY HYPERTROPHIC OSTEOARTHROPATHY

Pulmonary	Bronchogenic carcinoma
	Abscess
	Bronchiectasis
	Emphysema
	Hodgkin's disease
	Metastasis
	Cystic fibrosis
Pleural, diaphragmatic	Mesothelioma
Cardiac	Cyanotic congenital heart disease
Abdominal	Portal or biliary cirrhosis
	Ulcerative colitis
	Crohn's disease
	Dysentery
	Gastrointestinal polyposis
	Neoplasms
	Biliary atresia
Miscellaneous	Nasopharyngeal carcinoma
	Esophageal carcinoma
	Infected aortic or axillary artery grafts

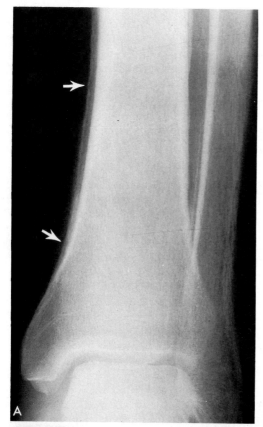

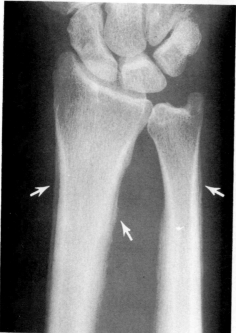

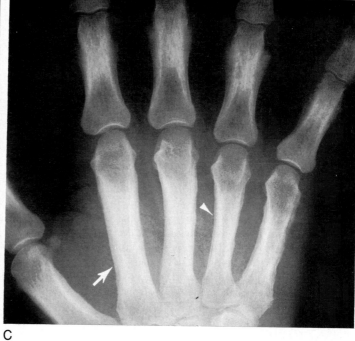

Figure 83–12. Secondary hypertrophic osteoarthropathy: Periostitis. A Distal portions of the tibia and fibula. Elevation of the periosteal membrane in the diaphyses of these bones has resulted in linear deposition of new bone (arrows). Involvement ends at the metaphyses. **B** Distal portions of the radius and ulna. In another classic location, observe linear periostitis of the diaphysis extending to the metaphysis of both bones (arrows). **C** Metacarpal bones and phalanges. Linear periostitis of the metacarpal bones has produced bone that is either separated from (arrowhead) or firmly merged with (arrow) the underlying osseous tissue. Bone proliferation at muscular insertions of the phalanges is also seen. Note some degree of periarticular osteoporosis.

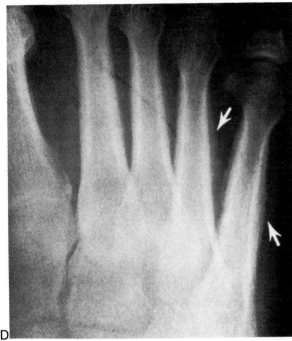
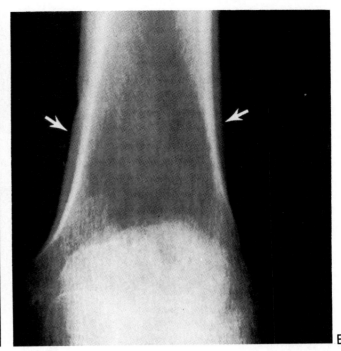

D

E

Figure 83–12 *Continued* **D** Metatarsal bones. New bone is evident along the diaphyses of multiple metatarsal bones (arrows). **E** Femur. Observe thick linear periosteal bone formation on the medial and lateral aspects of the femur (arrows). The endosteal surface of the cortex is not affected.

Radiographic Abnormalities

Periostitis is the hallmark of the disease. Periosteal bone deposition initially appears in the proximal and distal diaphyses of the tibiae, fibulae, radii, ulnae, and (less frequently) the femora, humeri, metacarpals, metatarsals, and phalanges (Fig. 83–12). With progression, periostitis becomes prominent in the metaphyseal regions as well as at musculotendinous insertions, but it does not usually extend into the epiphyses. Rarely, radiographic abnormalities may be detected in the scapulae, clavicles, ribs, spine, and even the cranium and facial bones.

Various types of periostitis are seen: simple elevation of the periosteum with a radiolucent area between the periosteal bone and subjacent cortex; laminated or "onion-skin" appearance, with smooth layers of new bone formation; irregular areas of periosteal elevation; irregular, solid areas of periosteal cloaking with a wavy contour; and cortical thickening, with application of the periosteal bone to the outer surface of the cortex.

Digital clubbing leading to radiographically detectable soft tissue swelling also is evident. The finding may be associated with focal areas of tuftal hypertrophy or resorption.

Articular Abnormalities

Pain and swelling about the knees, ankles, wrists, and even the fingers may be the presenting manifestation of hypertrophic osteoarthropathy, simulating the clinical presentation of rheumatoid arthritis. This clinical dilemma is accentuated by the presence of soft tissue swelling, joint effusions, and periarticular osteoporosis on radiographic examination. Considerable synovial inflammation is not a feature of hypertrophic osteoarthropathy, however. Articular space

narrowing and marginal and central erosions likewise are absent in persons with secondary hypertrophic osteoarthropathy.

Radionuclide Abnormalities

Radionuclide bone imaging represents a highly sensitive method of detecting abnormalities of primary or secondary hypertrophic osteoarthropathy. A diffuse, symmetric increased uptake in the diaphyses and metaphyses of tubular bones along their cortical margins · creates a distinctive "double stripe" or "parallel track" sign (Fig. 83–13). Associated synovitis can lead to increased radionuclide uptake in periarticular regions also. Unusual alterations include accumulation of radiopharmaceutical agents in the clavicles, scapulae, pelvis, and bones of the face, and digital accumulation related to clubbing.

The scintigraphic abnormalities frequently appear before the radiographic findings, correspond well with clinical manifestations, and decrease after appropriate therapeutic regimens. Recurrence of a tumor is followed by the return of an abnormal radionuclide pattern. Differentiation of the scintigraphic patterns in hypertrophic osteoarthropathy and in metastasis is not difficult. Asymmetry, focal areas of increased activity, and prominent involvement of the axial skeleton and medullary spaces characterize the radionuclide abnormalities of metastatic disease involving the skeleton.

Pathogenesis

Numerous theories have been proposed to explain the pathogenesis of the condition, none of which is entirely adequate. A neurogenic mechanism in this condition has gained increasing support from the observation that prompt

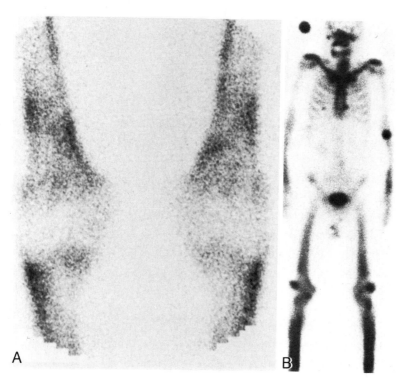

Figure 83–13. Secondary hypertrophic osteoarthropathy: Radionuclide abnormalities. A "Double stripe" or "parallel track" sign is present in the femora and tibiae. **B** Note diffuse uptake in both the appendicular and axial bones. (**B**, Courtesy of V. Vint, M.D., San Diego, California.)

relief of symptoms and signs can follow surgical disruption of the vagus nerve. It is postulated that neural impulses arise in the pulmonary or pleural lesion and pass as afferent impulses in the vagus nerve. The efferent pathways have not been delineated, however. The importance of increased blood flow in the pathogenesis of periostitis in hypertrophic osteoarthropathy also has been emphasized. It is indeed possible that several different mechanisms are responsible for secondary hypertrophic osteoarthropathy. A chemical substance, neurogenic mechanism, or hypervascularity working alone or in combination may be responsible in a specific situation or disease.

Differential Diagnosis

Periostitis (and clubbing) can also be observed in primary hypertrophic osteoarthropathy (pachydermoperiostosis) and thyroid acropachy (see Table 83–4) (Fig. 83–14). In the former condition, the osseous excrescences are more irregular and extend into the epiphyses of the tubular bones. In thyroid acropachy, periosteal proliferation has a predilection for the small bones of the hands and feet; significant or isolated abnormalities of the major tubular bones are distinctly unusual. Chronic venous stasis can produce periostitis, usually confined to the lower extremities (see discussion later in this chapter). Additional causes of diffuse periostitis or bone proliferation, such as hypervitaminosis A, infantile cortical hyperostosis, diffuse idiopathic skeletal hyperostosis, or fluorosis, are not usually confused with hypertrophic osteoarthropathy.

VASCULAR INSUFFICIENCY

Periosteal bone formation has been noted in association with chronic venous insufficiency. The lower extremities are affected almost exclusively (see Table 83–4). The diaphyseal

and metaphyseal segments are predominantly altered, and an undulating osseous contour is produced, with considerable new bone appearing on the outer aspect of the cortex (Fig. 83–15).

The frequency of periostitis increases with the severity and duration of the venous insufficiency. Infection is not fundamental to the appearance of periosteal proliferation. The pathogenesis of the periostitis may relate to hypoxia created by vascular stasis or hypertension.

Soft tissue edema and ossification represent radiographic findings that are commonly associated with venous insufficiency and periostitis (Fig. 83–16). Single or multiple phleboliths may be apparent, and in some cases a diffuse reticular ossific pattern is evident.

Arterial insufficiency also has been associated with periosteal bone proliferation. This may occur in polyarteritis nodosa or other arteritides (see Chapter 32).

INFANTILE CORTICAL HYPEROSTOSIS

Infantile cortical hyperostosis (Caffey's disease) is an uncommon disease, usually commencing in infancy, that affects predominantly the skeleton and adjacent fascial, muscular, and connective tissues. Infantile cortical hyperostosis affects boys and girls with approximately equal frequency.

Clinical Abnormalities

Almost without exception, the disease becomes evident in an infant less than 5 months of age; the average age of onset is 9 to 10 weeks. Familial instances (see later discussion) of the disease are recognized. Fever of abrupt onset, hyperirritability, and soft tissue swelling are typical. The swelling is especially prominent over the mandible but can also appear at other sites. Additional clinical features may include pallor, painful pseudoparalysis, and pleurisy. Laboratory analysis may

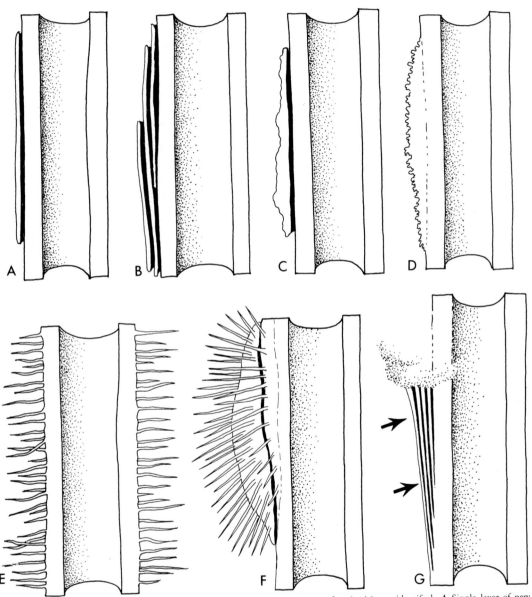

Figure 83-14. Differential diagnosis of periosteal new bone formation. Various types of periostitis are identified. **A** Single layer of new bone, which may be observed in benign or malignant tumors, infection, and secondary hypertrophic osteoarthropathy. **B** Multiple layers of new bone or "onion-skinning," which can be evident in infection, malignant tumors such as Ewing's sarcoma, hypertrophic osteoarthropathy, and other conditions. **C** A thick linear osseous deposit, which can be separate from (as indicated here) or mixed with the underlying bone. This pattern is common in hypertrophic osteoarthropathy and venous stasis. **D** An irregular osseous excrescence with spiculated contour that merges with the underlying cortex. This pattern can be observed in thyroid acropachy or primary hypertrophic osteoarthropathy (pachydermoperiostosis). **E** Thin, linear osseous deposits that extend in a direction perpendicular to the underlying cortex, a pattern that is highly characteristic of Ewing's sarcoma. **F** A sunburst pattern, in which linear deposits fan out from a single focus, an appearance that can be evident in osteosarcoma. **G** A Codman's triangle, consisting of triangular elevation of the periosteum with one or more layers of new bone (arrows), a pattern that is suggestive but not diagnostic of malignancy.

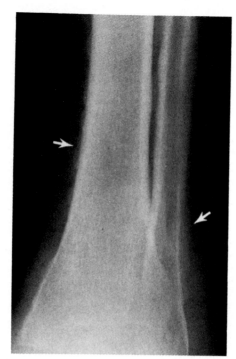

Figure 83–15. Chronic venous stasis: Periostitis. Observed undulating periosteal new bone in the diaphyses and metaphyses of the distal tibia and fibula (arrows). Soft tissue edema is present.

indicate an elevated erythrocyte sedimentation rate and an elevated serum level of alkaline phosphatase, a moderate leukocytosis, and anemia.

The clinical course is extremely variable. In many instances, clinical and radiographic features subside slowly over a period of a few months to a few years. Occasionally, active disease may persist, recurring intermittently for years. Thus, residua of the disease may be evident even in the third and fourth decades of life.

Radiographic Abnormalities

In any one patient, a single bone or many bones can be involved (see Table 83–4). Sequential involvement is typical. The mandible, clavicles, and ribs are involved most often (Fig. 83–17). Thoracic cage abnormalities may be combined with pleural effusions. The scapulae are altered in approximately 10 per cent of cases, and involvement at this site may be monostotic (Fig. 83–18). Changes in the ilia, cranial vault, and tubular bones also are encountered. In the tubular bones, asymmetry predominates, and the ulnae are involved most frequently (Fig. 83–19).

Cortical hyperostosis is the hallmark of the disease. New bone formation begins in the soft tissue swelling directly contiguous to the original cortex. The deposits of bone merge with the underlying osseous tissue. Predilection for the lateral arches of the ribs and the diaphyses and metaphyses of tubular bones is evident. Destructive lesions of the skull or, rarely, the tubular bones have been identified in some cases.

Radiographic improvement can occur in a period of weeks to months, to an extent that evidence of hyperostosis may be entirely lacking on follow-up examinations after 6 months to 1 year. Residual changes can be encountered, such as diaphy-

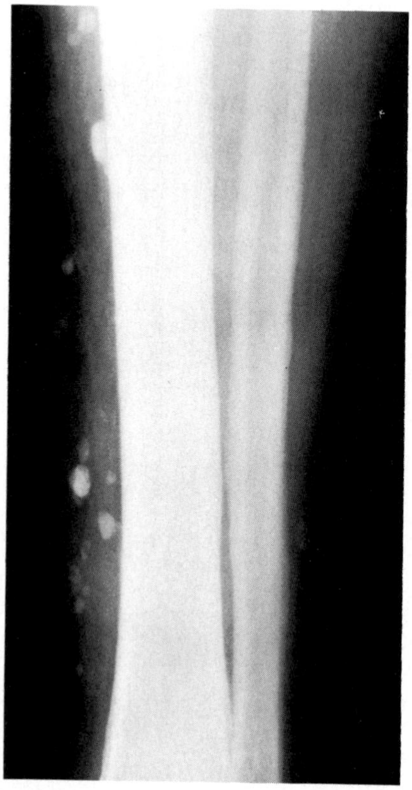

Figure 83–16. Chronic venous stasis: Soft tissue calcification. Note multiple phleboliths and periostitis.

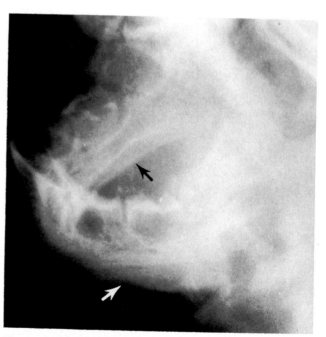

Figure 83–17. Infantile cortical hyperostosis: Mandible. Observe diffuse periosteal proliferation (arrows).

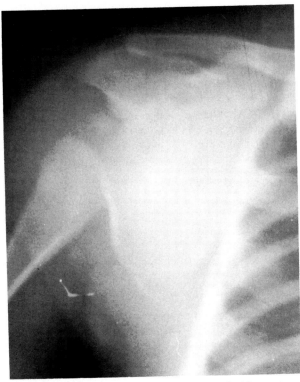

Figure 83–18. Infantile cortical hyperostosis: Scapula. Monostotic scapular disease has resulted in exuberant bone formation and considerable deformity and enlargement.

seal expansion; longitudinal overgrowth and bowing deformities; osseous bridging between adjacent bones such as the radius and ulna, tibia and fibula, and ribs; exophthalmos; and facial asymmetry.

Pathologic Abnormalities

In the early stage, acute inflammatory changes appear in the periosteal membrane. In the subacute phase, inflammatory changes diminish. Beneath the periosteum, a layer of immature, coarse-fibered trabeculae of variable thickness becomes identifiable. In the late phases, the peripheral bone is removed. Dilatation of the medullary cavity is seen, with subsequent remodeling and shrinkage of the dilated, thin-walled bone shaft.

Etiology and Pathogenesis

The cause of infantile cortical hyperostosis remains unknown. There are many clinical and pathologic features suggesting that an infectious agent is responsible for the disease. No bacterial or viral agents have yet been identified in the disease, however, and serologic tests for such agents have also been unsuccessful.

The appearance of infantile cortical hyperostosis in many members of a single family underscores the importance of genetic factors in the pathogenesis of the disease. An autosomal dominant pattern of inheritance with incomplete penetrance and variable expressivity is seen. Familial infantile cortical hyperostosis may represent the major pattern of disease that is evident today.

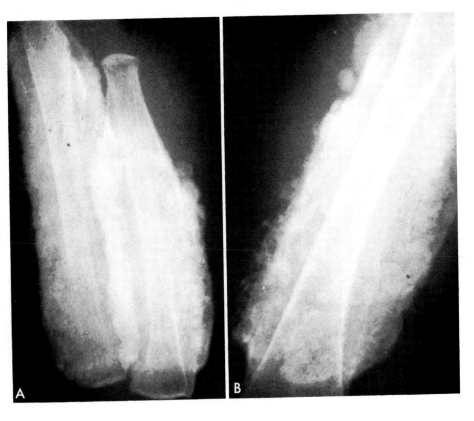

Figure 83–19. Infantile cortical hyperostosis: Tubular bones. Examples of radial and ulnar (A), and femoral (B) involvement are shown. The extent of new bone formation is remarkable. These deposits are initially evident in the soft tissues and later merge with the underlying bone.

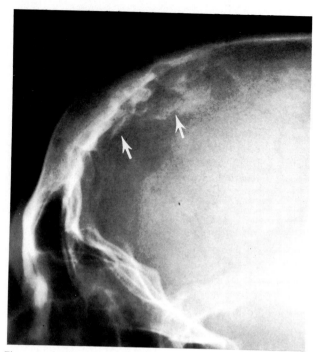

Figure 83–20. Hyperostosis frontalis interna. Note nodular hyperostosis of the inner table of the frontal bone (arrows).

outline (Fig. 83–20). The outer cranial contour generally is not altered. The radiographic findings are virtually diagnostic, although in some cases they may be misinterpreted as evidence of a meningioma, Paget's disease, skeletal metastasis, or acromegaly.

Hyperostosis similar to that seen in the frontal region in hyperostosis frontalis interna occurs in other areas of the cranial vault. These patterns, which are less common than hyperostosis of the frontal bones, are usually symmetric in distribution and affect the inner and outer tables as well as the diploë. The occipital bone is uninvolved.

OTHER DISORDERS

Numerous additional congenital disorders can lead to hyperostosis and increased skeletal density. These include osteopetrosis, pyknodysostosis, sclerosteosis, endosteal hyperostosis (van Buchem's disease, hyperostosis corticalis generalisata), hereditary hyperphosphatasia (juvenile Paget's disease), diaphyseal dysplasia (Camurati-Engelmann disease), and idiopathic hypercalcemia (Williams' syndrome).

Idiopathic Periosteal Hyperostosis with Dysproteinemia or Hyperphosphatemia

The combination of periostitis and dysproteinemia has been observed in some patients, and similar patterns of periosteal

Differential Diagnosis

Although periostitis and hyperostosis in an infant can also be observed in rickets and scurvy, the absence of epiphyseal or metaphyseal alterations and the resolution of clinical and radiographic features over a period of months in patients with infantile cortical hyperostosis allow its differentiation from these other disorders. Similarly, trauma, including that in the abused child, can lead to calcifying subperiosteal hematomas, but additional findings, such as microfractures and metaphyseal irregularity, are evident. In hypervitaminosis A, clinical and radiographic manifestations initially appear toward the end of the first year of life, metatarsal predilection is apparent, facial swelling and mandibular involvement are rare, and serologic testing indicates an elevation of vitamin A levels. The findings in osteomyelitis, leukemia, neuroblastoma, the kinky hair syndrome, and Camurati-Engelmann disease usually are not hard to differentiate from those of infantile cortical hyperostosis. The long-term administration of prostaglandin E_1 in infants with ductus-dependent cyanotic congenital heart disease is associated with periostitis and cortical hyperostosis (see Chapter 65).

HYPEROSTOSIS FRONTALIS INTERNA AND RELATED CONDITIONS

Hyperostosis frontalis interna is a descriptive term that is applied to hyperostosis involving predominantly the inner table of the frontal squama. It is usually observed in patients over the age of 40 years. Women predominate over men. In women, rhizomelic obesity, facial hirsutism, hypertension, headache, depression, anxiety, and historical evidence of menstrual irregularity are common but inconsistent findings.

Radiographically, the disorder leads to mild to moderate thickening of the inner table that is sessile or nodular in

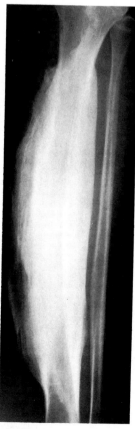

Figure 83–21. Neurofibromatosis. Exuberant subperiosteal bony deposition in the diaphysis of the tibia has resulted in an enlarged and bowed bone. (Courtesy of D. MacEwan, M.D., Winnipeg, Manitoba, Canada.)

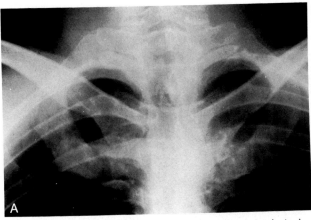
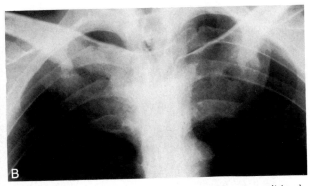

Figure 83–22. Sternocostoclavicular hyperostosis. Radiographs obtained over a 13 year period show progressive ossification involving the medial ends of the clavicles, upper portions of the sternum, and anterior aspect of the first ribs.

new bone formation have been accompanied by elevated serum levels of alkaline phosphatase and hyperphosphatemia. With regard to periostitis and hyperphosphatemia, children of both sexes are usually affected. Periosteal deposition typically is seen in the tubular bones. In some instances, periods of clinical activity, consisting of pain and fever, are followed after a few weeks by those of remission in which initial periosteal deposits are incorporated into the cortex. Biopsy shows vascular connective tissue, periosteal bone formation, and cellular infiltration. Although the cause of the syndrome is not clear, an infectious process is possible.

Hyperphosphatemia and periosteal bone formation have been identified in some children with tumoral calcinosis. Except for the presence of soft tissue calcification, clinical and radiologic features in these cases are similar to those in the reported patients with periostitis and hyperphosphatemia.

Fluorosis

Exuberant periosteal proliferation in the appendicular skeleton is encountered in patients with fluorosis, usually in combination with more well known axial skeletal alterations (see Chapter 65). These latter changes include osteosclerosis, osteophytosis, and ligamentous calcification and ossification.

Neurofibromatosis

Massive subperiosteal proliferation is seen in patients with neurofibromatosis. Involvement of the tubular bones of the lower extremity is characterized by bizarre, undulating periosteal deposits of varying size (Fig. 83–21). The pathogenesis of the changes is not clear (see Chapter 82).

Diffuse Idiopathic Skeletal Hyperostosis

Hyperostosis is a common manifestation of this disorder (see Chapter 37). Such hyperostosis affects spinal and extraspinal sites, leading to diagnostic flowing ossification of the spine, bone excrescences at sites of tendinous and ligamentous attachment, paraarticular osteophytes, and ligamentous calcification and ossification.

Sternocostoclavicular Hyperostosis

This disorder is characterized by distinctive hyperostosis and soft tissue ossification of the clavicle, anterior portion of

the upper ribs, and sternum. It is particularly frequent in Japan. Patients usually are in the fourth to sixth decades of life; men are affected more frequently than women. Bilateral alterations predominate. Clinical findings include pain, swelling, tenderness, and local heat in the anterior upper chest. Osseous overgrowth may lead to occlusion of the subclavian veins. A relationship of sternocostoclavicular hyperostosis and

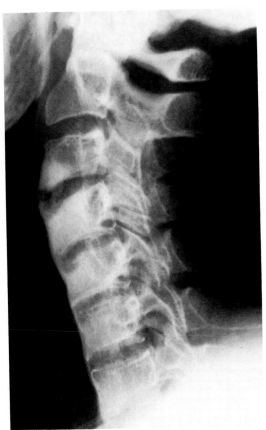

Figure 83–23. Sternocostoclavicular hyperostosis. Observe hyperostotic changes involving the anterior portion of the third to seventh cervical vertebral bodies and the development of syndesmophytes. (Courtesy of C. Resnik, M.D., Baltimore, Maryland.)

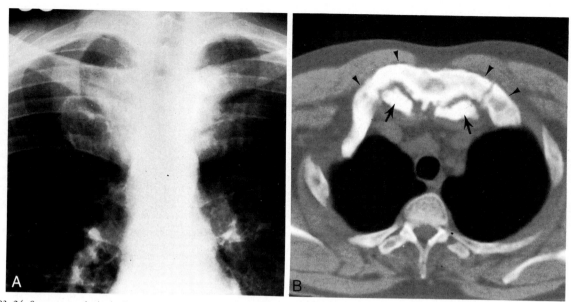

Figure 83–24. Sternocostoclavicular hyperostosis. A The frontal radiograph of the chest reveals the typical changes of this disease. **B** Computed tomography shows enlargement and irregularity of the medial ends of the clavicles (arrows) and ossification at the junction of the first rib and the sternum (arrowheads). Observe the increased radiodensity of the sternum, clavicles, and first ribs. (Courtesy of J. Schreiman, M.D., Omaha, Nebraska.)

a cutaneous disorder of the hands and feet, pustulosis palmaris et plantaris, is recognized.

The major radiographic abnormalities of sternocostoclavicular hyperostosis are seen in the anterior and upper portion of the chest wall. Ossification of varying degree involves the region of the costoclavicular ligament, inferior margin of the clavicle, and superior margin of the first rib (Fig. 83–22). Hyperostosis of the sternum, clavicle, and upper ribs is encountered and, in some cases, similar changes are evident at the manubriosternal junction. Additional changes occur in the vertebral column and resemble those of ankylosing spondylitis, diffuse idiopathic skeletal hyperostosis, or psoriatic spondylitis (Fig. 83–23). New bone formation in the cervical spine is occasionally exuberant. Abnormalities of the sacroiliac joint consist of either paraarticular osseous bridging and ligamentous calcification simulating degenerative joint disease or intraarticular bone erosions, sclerosis, and fusion simulating ankylosing spondylitis. Periosteal proliferation has been identified in some of the long tubular bones.

Computed tomography is useful in delineating the osseous nature of the thoracic mass, and scintigraphy with bone-seeking radiopharmaceutical agents documents abnormal skeletal accumulation of the radiotracers (Fig. 83–24).

The cause and pathogenesis of this progressive condition are not clear. In some respects, sternocostoclavicular hyperostosis resembles plasma cell osteomyelitis (recurrent multifocal osteomyelitis) (see Chapter 59): Both conditions are associated with pustulosis palmaris et plantaris and lead to hyperostosis of the clavicle. In other respects, it simulates Paget's disease, diffuse idiopathic skeletal hyperostosis, ankylosing spondylitis, and psoriatic spondylitis.

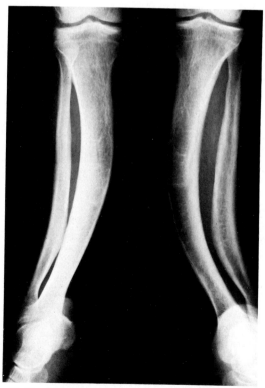

Figure 83–25. Weissmann-Netter-Stuhl syndrome. Observe bilateral bowing of the tibia and fibulae. Anterior and medial bowing is documented on the basis of this and other radiographs (not shown), and the femora were also affected. The fibulae are markedly enlarged, resembling the tibia. Cortical thickening is apparent. (Courtesy of A. Brower, M.D., Washington, D.C.)

Weismann-Netter-Stuhl Syndrome

This disorder, which is also termed toxopachyostéose diaphysaire tibiopéronière, affects both men and women of any age from infancy to the eighth or ninth decade of life. Short stature and delayed ambulation are early features, and mental retardation is sometimes apparent. A family history of this syndrome is an inconsistent feature.

The characteristic abnormality of the Weismann-Netter-Stuhl syndrome is bilateral bowing of the long tubular bones, principally the tibiae (Fig. 83–25). An anterior curvature of this bone is typical, and the posterior tibial cortex is usually thickened. The adjacent fibula commonly is bowed and enlarged. Additional sites of osseous bowing and deformity include the femur, the radius, the ulna, and the humerus.

Differential diagnostic considerations are syphilis, Paget's disease, rickets, and osteogenesis imperfecta.

FURTHER READING

Ali A, Tetalman MR, Fordham EW, Turner DA, Chiles JT, Patel SL, Schmidt KD: Distribution of hypertrophic pulmonary osteoarthropathy. AJR 134:771, 1980.

Amendola MA, Brower AC, Tisnado J: Weismann-Netter-Stuhl syndrome: Toxopachyostéose diaphysaire tibio-péronière. AJR 135:1211, 1980.

Azimi F, Bryan PJ: Weismann-Netter-Stuhl syndrome (toxopachyostéose diaphysaire tibio-péronière). Br J Radiol 47:618, 1974.

Beauvais P, Fauré C, Montagne JP, Chigot PL, Maroteaux P: Leri's melorheostosis: Three pediatric cases and a review of the literature. Pediatr Radiol 6:153, 1977.

Caffey J: On some late skeletal changes in chronic infantile cortical hyperostosis. Radiology 59:651, 1952.

Caffey J, Silverman WA: Infantile cortical hyperostoses. Preliminary report on a new syndrome. AJR 54:1, 1945.

Camp JD, Scanlan R: Chronic idiopathic hypertrophic osteoarthropathy. Radiology 50:581, 1948.

Chang CHJ, Piatt ED, Thomas KE, Watne AL: Bone abnormalities in Gardner's syndrome. AJR 103:645, 1968.

Clarke E, Swischuk LE, Hayden CK Jr: Tumoral calcinosis, diaphysitis, and hyperphosphatemia. Radiology 151:643, 1984.

DeKeyser J, Bruyland M, DeGreve J, Leemans J, Potvliege R, Six R, Ebinger G: Osteopathia striata with cranial sclerosis. Report of a case and review of the literature. Clin Neurol Neurosurg 85:41, 1983.

Dolan KD, Seibert J, Seibert RW: Gardner's syndrome. A model for correlative radiology. AJR 119:359, 1973.

Fairbank HAT: Osteopathia striata. J Bone Joint Surg [Br] 32:117, 1950.

Garver P, Resnick D, Haghighi P, Guerra J: Melorheostosis of the axial skeleton with associated fibrolipomatous lesions. Skel Radiol 9:41, 1982.

Gehweiler JA, Bland WR, Carden TS Jr, Daffner RH: Osteopathia striata—Voorhoeve's disease. Review of the roentgen manifestations. AJR 118:450, 1973.

Gershon-Cohen J, Schraer H, Blumberg N: Hyperostosis frontalis interna among the aged. AJR 73:396, 1955.

Goldbloom RB, Stein PB, Eisen A, McSheffrey JB, Brown BS, Wiglesworth FW: Idiopathic periosteal hyperostosis with dysproteinemia. A new clinical entity. N Engl J Med 274:873, 1966.

Greenfield GB, Schorsch HA, Shkolnik A: The various roentgen appearances of pulmonary hypertrophic osteoarthropathy. AJR 101:927, 1967.

Hall FM, Goldberg RP, Davies JAK, Fainsinger MH: Scintigraphic assessment of bone islands. Radiology 135:737, 1980.

Harbison JB, Nice CM Jr: Familial pachydermoperiostosis presenting as an acromegaly-like syndrome. AJR 112:532, 1971.

Joseph B, Chacko V: Acro-osteolysis associated with hypertrophic pulmonary osteoarthropathy and pachydermoperiostosis. Radiology 154:343, 1985.

Kay CJ, Rosenberg MA, Burd R: Hypertrophic osteoarthropathy and childhood Hodgkin's disease. Radiology 112:177, 1974.

Kim SK, Barry WF Jr: Bone island. AJR 92:1301, 1964.

Lagier R, Mbakop A, Bigler A: Osteopoikilosis: A radiological and pathological study. Skel Radiol 11:161, 1984.

Lippmann HI, Goldin RR: Subcutaneous ossification of the legs in chronic venous insufficiency. Radiology 74:279, 1960.

Martinez-Lavin M, Pineda C, Valdez T, Cajigas J-C, Weisman M, Gerber N, Steigler D: Primary hypertrophic osteoarthropathy. Semin Arth Rheum 17:156, 1988.

Melhem RE, Najjar SS, Knachadurian AK: Cortical hyperostosis with hyperphosphatemia: A new syndrome? J Pediatr 77:986, 1970.

Melnick JC: Osteopathia condensans disseminata (osteopoikilosis). Study of a family of 4 generations. AJR 82:229, 1959.

Murray RO, McCredie J: Melorheostosis and the sclerotomes: A radiological correlation. Skel Radiol 4:57, 1979.

Nathanson I, Riddlesberger MM Jr: Pulmonary hypertrophic osteoarthopathy in cystic fibrosis. Radiology 135:649, 1980.

Neiman HL, Gompels BM, Martel W: Pachydermoperiostosis with bone marrow failure and gross extramedullary hematopoiesis. Report of a case. Radiology 110:553, 1974.

Onitsuka H: Roentgenologic aspects of bone islands. Radiology 123:607, 1977.

Pitt MJ, Mosher JF, Edeiken J: Abnormal periosteum and bone in neurofibromatosis. Radiology 103:143, 1972.

Resnick D: Sternocostoclavicular hyperostosis. AJR 135:1278, 1980.

Resnick D, Vint V, Poteshman NL: Sternocostoclavicular hyperostosis. A report of three new cases. J Bone Joint Surg [Am] 63:1329, 1981.

Rosenthal L, Kirsh J: Observations on the radionuclide imaging in hypertrophic pulmonary osteoarthropathy. Radiology 120:359, 1976.

Sartoris DJ, Schreiman JS, Kerr R, Resnik CS, Resnick D: Sternocostoclavicular hyperostosis: A review and report of 11 cases. Radiology 158:125, 1986.

Saul RA, Lee WH, Stevenson RE: Caffey's disease revisited. Further evidence for autosomal dominant inheritance with incomplete penetrance. Am J Dis Child 136:56, 1982.

Silverman FN: Virus diseases of bone. Do they exist? AJR 126:677, 1976.

Smith J: Giant bone islands. Radiology 107:35, 1973.

Sonozaki H, Azuma A, Okai K, Nakamura K, Fukuoka S, Tateishi A, Kurosawa H, Mannoji T, Kabata K, Mitsui H, Seki H, Abe I, Furusawa S, Matsuura M, Kudo A, Hoshino T: Clinical features of 22 cases with "inter-sterno-costo-clavicular ossification." Arch Orthop Trauma Surg 95:13, 1979.

Sonozaki H, Kawashima M, Hongo O, Yaoita H, Ikeno M, Matsuura M, Okai K, Azuma A: Incidence of arthro-osteitis in patients with pustulosis palmaris et plantaris. Ann Rheum Dis 40:554, 1981.

Sonozaki H, Mitsui H, Miyanaga Y, Okitsu K, Igarashi M, Hayashi Y, Matsuura M, Azuma A, Okai K, Kawashima M: Clinical features of 53 cases with pustulosis arthro-osteitis. Ann Rheum Dis 40:547, 1981.

Swerdloff BA, Ozonoff MB, Gyepes MT: Late recurrence of infantile cortical hyperostosis (Caffey's disease). AJR 108:461, 1970.

Temple HL, Jaspin G: Hypertrophic osteoarthropathy. AJR 60:232, 1948.

Van Buskirk FW, Tampas JP, Peterson OS Jr: Infantile cortical hyperostosis: Inquiry into its familial aspects. AJR 85:613, 1961.

Vogl A, Goldfischer S: Pachydermoperiostosis. Primary or idiopathic hypertrophic osteoarthropathy. Am J Med 33:166, 1962.

Walter RD, Resnick D: Hypertrophic osteoarthropathy of a lower extremity in association with arterial graft sepsis. AJR 137:1059, 1981.

Whyte MP, Murphy WA, Fallon MD, Hahn TJ: Mixed-sclerosing-bone-dystrophy: Report of a case and review of the literature. Skel Radiol 6:95, 1981.

Wilcox LF: Osteopoikilosis. AJR 30:615, 1933.

Yaghmai I, Tafazoli M: Massive subperiosteal hemorrhage in neurofibromatosis. Radiology 122:439, 1977.

Chapter 84

Osteolysis and Chondrolysis

Donald Resnick, M.D.
Gen Niwayama, M.D.

A variety of disorders can lead to osteolysis and chondrolysis. In some, bone resorption is especially evident in the phalanges of the hand and foot and may be related to occupational or inherited factors. Posttraumatic osteolysis can be evident at many sites, particularly the distal end of the clavicle, pubic and ischial rami, and femoral neck. Massive osteolysis of Gorham can lead to regional destruction and disappearance of bone. Idiopathic multicentric osteolysis shows a predilection for the carpal and tarsal areas and must be differentiated from juvenile chronic arthritis. Chondrolysis of the hip can accompany a slipped capital femoral epiphysis or can appear on an idiopathic basis. It must be differentiated from juvenile chronic arthritis, infection, and regional osteoporosis.

Destruction of bone (osteolysis) or cartilage (chondrolysis) can become evident in innumerable neoplastic, infectious, metabolic, traumatic, vascular, congenital, and articular disorders that are discussed elsewhere in this book. There remains a group of heterogeneous conditions in which significant and severe osteolysis and chondrolysis may become manifest, and these are described in this chapter.

OSTEOLYSIS

Occupational Acroosteolysis

Routine radiographic surveys of persons in certain industrial plants have revealed that as many as 1 to 2 per cent of workers involved in the polymerization of vinyl chloride may develop acroosteolysis. Occasionally, exposure to vapors of other synthetic materials used in the manufacture of plastic products may produce similar abnormalities. Initial clinical manifestations include fatigue, asthenia, nervousness, and insomnia. A Raynaud's phenomenon–like disorder ensues, with digital pain, numbness, and tingling followed by the appearance of "drumstick" fingers and "watch-glass" nails. Further complications of vinyl chloride disease may include hepatic fibrosis or tumor, splenomegaly, portal hypertension, thrombocytopenia, and pulmonary changes.

The radiographic hallmark of the disorder is osteolysis that predominates in the terminal phalanges of the hands, although it may also affect other phalanges, the sacroiliac joints, the foot, and, rarely, additional skeletal structures, including the mandible. Band-like radiolucent areas across the waist of one or more terminal phalanges may be combined with tuftal resorption (Fig. 84–1). The thumb is affected more commonly than the other digits. If the exposure to polyvinylchloride is halted, the patient may reveal slow improvement of the radiographic abnormalities.

The cause and pathogenesis of the condition are unclear. The role of chemical or physical trauma would explain the predilection for involvement of the hand and the improvement in the clinical, radiographic, and scintigraphic alterations after cessation of the exposure to polyvinylchloride. A disturbance in circulation, especially in the small peripheral arteries of the hands, may be attributable to a toxic chemical substance. It also is possible that exposure to polyvinylchloride initiates an immune complex disease in predisposed individuals.

Band-like resorption of the terminal phalanges in this condition differs from the usual pattern of osteolysis that may accompany vasculitis, collagen disorders (e.g., scleroderma), psoriasis (Fig. 84–2A), epidermolysis bullosa, frostbite, thermal and electrical burns, hypertrophic osteoarthropathy, septic shock, multicentric reticulohistiocytosis (Fig. 84–2B), and neuroarthropathy. Similar band-like resorption can be seen in hyperparathyroidism and in certain familial conditions (see discussion later in this chapter).

Posttraumatic Osteolysis

Although some degree of bone loss is common after traumatic insult, particularly when complicated by fracture, there exist certain situations in which the degree of posttraumatic osteolysis may appear excessive (Table 84–1).

Posttraumatic osteolysis can lead to progressive resorption of the outer end of the clavicle. The process becomes apparent after single or repeated episodes of local trauma. Frequently, the traumatic insult is minor; in fact, a similar process has been related to chronic stress (as in weightlifters) without acute injury. The osteolytic process begins as early as 2 weeks and as late as several years after the injury. When untreated, it leads to pain and lysis of 0.5 to 3 cm of bone substance from the distal end of the clavicle over a period of 12 to 18 months, which may be associated with erosion and cupping of the acromion, soft tissue swelling, and dystrophic calcification (Fig. 84–3). After the lytic phase stabilizes, reparative changes occur over a period of 4 to 6 months. Eventually, the subchondral bone becomes reconstituted, although the

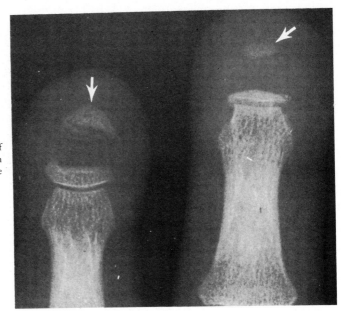

Figure 84–1. Occupational acroosteolysis. Note band-like resorption of the terminal phalanges of two digits, isolating small osseous fragments in the terminal tufts (arrows). Observe that the distal interphalangeal joints are intact.

acromioclavicular joint can remain permanently widened. Treatment with immobilization can shorten the course of the process. The pathogenesis of posttraumatic osteolysis of the clavicle is not certain.

The differential diagnosis of posttraumatic osteolysis about the acromioclavicular joint includes hyperparathyroidism, col-lagen disorders, infection, rheumatoid arthritis, and other articular processes.

Posttraumatic osteolysis can become prominent at other skeletal sites as well. In the pubic or ischial rami, exaggerated resorption of bone about a fracture, with or without associated sclerosis, can simulate the appearance of a malignant process (Fig. 84–4). Such fractures occur as a result of either direct trauma or, frequently, chronic stress in an osteopenic skeleton (insufficiency fractures). The cause of osteolysis about these ramus fractures is not known.

Prominent posttraumatic osteolysis has also been noted in the ulna, radius, and carpal bones. In the femoral neck, resorption and rotation at a fracture site can produce a radiographic picture that may be misinterpreted as a malignant process (Fig. 84–5). Osteolysis occurring after odontoid fracture can produce a separate bone at the tip of the dens, the os odontoideum.

Primary Osteolysis Syndromes

A diverse group of idiopathic disorders can lead to significant skeletal lysis. They differ in the presence or absence of genetic transmission, the associated clinical manifestations, and the major locations of osteolysis (Table 84–2).

ACROOSTEOLYSIS SYNDROME OF HAJDU AND CHENEY. This disorder may be familial, with a dominant

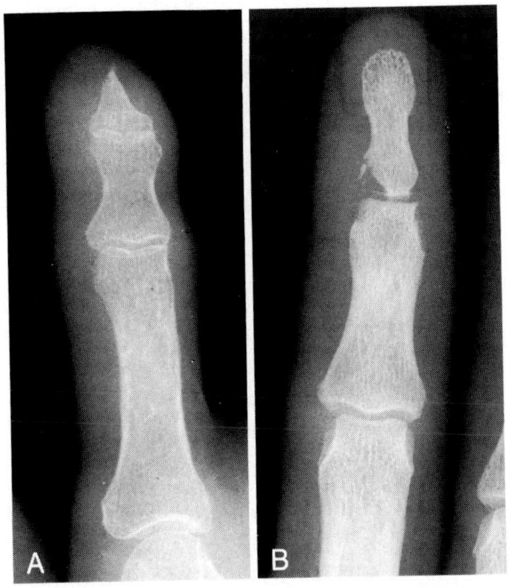

Figure 84–2. Other causes of acroosteolysis. A Psoriasis. Observe tapering of the terminal phalanx of the second finger with periarticular soft tissue prominence and deformity of the nail. (Courtesy of G. Greenway, M.D., Dallas, Texas.) B Multicentric reticulohistiocytosis. The extremely well-marginated osseous erosions in the phalangeal portions of the interphalangeal joint are typical of this disease. (Courtesy of M. Dalinka, M.D., Philadelphia, Pennsylvania.)

Table 84–1. COMMON SITES OF POSTTRAUMATIC OSTEOLYSIS

Distal portion of the clavicle
Pubic and ischial rami
Distal portion of ulna
Distal portion of radius
Carpus
Femoral neck

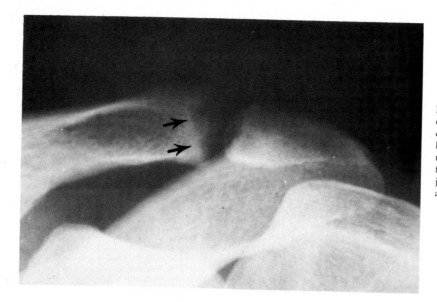

Figure 84–3. Posttraumatic osteolysis: Clavicle. Several weeks after local trauma, marked resorption of the distal end of the clavicle is seen (arrows). Similar but less extensive findings are evident in the acromion. The resulting radiographic picture, consisting of poorly defined osseous margins and a widened acromioclavicular joint, resembles that in septic arthritis, rheumatoid arthritis, and hyperparathyroidism.

mode of inheritance, or sporadic and is manifested by short stature, low-set ears, recessed mandible, malocclusion and early loss of teeth, coarse hairs, pseudoclubbing of the digits, joint laxity, conductive hearing loss, and speech impairment. Radiographic features include osteolysis of distal phalanges of the hands and feet; a dolichocephalic skull with basilar impression, delayed closure of cranial sutures, multiple wormian bones, hypoplastic frontal sinuses, prominent occipital ridge, and enlarged sella turcica; diminutive mandible and maxilla with poor dentition; generalized osteoporosis with vertebral compressions and fractures of tubular bones; valgus deformities of the knees; and hypoplasia and subluxation of the proximal radius. Renal function, which is altered in other osteolysis syndromes, is normal in this condition.

Osteolysis is especially characteristic (Fig. 84–6). Changes in the phalanges, which consist of resorption of tufts and band-like areas of lucency, simulate abnormalities in occupation-induced (polyvinylchloride) acroosteolysis, pyknodysostosis, Rothmund's syndrome, and collagen disorders. Osteolysis can also be apparent in the tubular bones, mandibular rami, and acromioclavicular joints. The pathogenesis is unknown.

MASSIVE OSTEOLYSIS OF GORHAM. This disease, which is also termed disappearing bone disease, vanishing bone disease, and Gorham's disease, can become evident in men and women of all ages, although most cases are discovered before the age of 40 years. A family history is not apparent. The process may affect either the axial or the appendicular skeleton. Some patients have an abrupt onset of pain and swelling, whereas others describe an insidious onset of painless soft tissue atrophy and limitation of motion. Some persons note the onset of the disorder after significant trauma.

The most dramatic aspect of massive osteolysis is its radiographic appearance (Fig. 84–7). Initially, radiolucent foci appear in the intramedullary or subcortical regions. Slowly progressive dissolution, fracture, fragmentation, and disappearance of a portion of the bone then occur. The process subsequently extends to contiguous bones. Thus, osteolysis of the ilium may be associated with resorption of the proximal portion of the femur, whereas changes in the scapula may

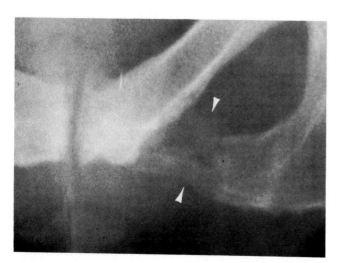

Figure 84–4. Posttraumatic osteolysis: Inferior pubic ramus. A radiograph obtained 4 weeks after a fracture reveals significant osteolysis about the fracture site (arrowheads). At this stage, the appearance resembles that of a pathologic fracture. Healing of the fracture occurred over the ensuing 4 weeks.

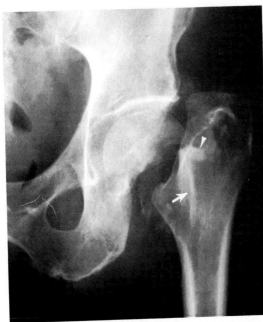

Figure 84–5. Posttraumatic osteolysis: Femoral neck. Observe the apparent disappearance of bone after an acute fracture, related both to true osteolysis and to rotation at the fracture site. A portion of the remaining femoral neck overlies the trochanteric region (arrow), and its superior margin can be identified (arrowhead).

later be combined with osteolysis of the proximal part of the humerus, clavicle, and ribs. Any bone may be involved, including the small tubular bones of the hands and feet, the spine, the skull, and the mandible. The degree of osseous destruction generally increases relentlessly over a period of years.

The exact nature of the process is unknown. In the early stages of the disorder, the pathologic features resemble those of skeletal hemangioma. In later stages, vascular fibrous tissue replaces the angiomatous tissue. These pathologic changes, coupled with the presence of soft tissue hemangiomatous or lymphangiomatous tissue, suggest that massive osteolysis represents a vascular derangement or a diffuse hemangiomatosis. The possibility that massive osteolysis may represent a neoplastic proliferation of hemangiomatous (or lymphangiomatous) tissue has also been suggested.

Although the degree of osseous deformity in the disease may become severe, serious complications are not frequent. Paraplegia may occur in cases of vertebral osteolysis. Death can result from thoracic cage, pulmonary, or pleural involvement.

IDIOPATHIC MULTICENTRIC OSTEOLYSIS (CARPAL-TARSAL OSTEOLYSIS). This rare disorder, which is associated with extensive osteolysis, usually in the carpal or tarsal areas, also has been designated essential osteolysis, familial osteolysis, hereditary osteolysis, and carpal and tarsal agenesis. Idiopathic multicentric osteolysis is further classified into two basic types: multicentric osteolysis with nephropathy and hereditary multicentric osteolysis. Not all cases fit neatly into one of these two categories, however.

Multicentric Osteolysis with Nephropathy. This entity is characterized by an early age of onset of osteolysis, associated with progressive renal failure that commonly is fatal by the third decade of life. There is no family history of either osteolysis or renal disease. Presenting clinical manifestations include swollen wrists with the presence or absence of foot deformities. Radiographs reveal progressive disappearance of the carpus and, less strikingly, the tarsus, with tapering of the adjacent tubular bones (Fig. 84–8). Osteolysis and sub-

Table 84–2. OSTEOLYSIS SYNDROMES

Syndrome	Age of Onset	Major Site of Osteolysis	Patterns of Inheritance	Associated Features
Acroosteolysis of Hajdu and Cheney	Second decade	Distal phalanges; rarely tubular bones, mandible, acromioclavicular joints	Dominant or sporadic	Generalized bone dysplasia, fractures, osteoporosis
Massive osteolysis of Gorham	Young adult	Variable; pelvic or shoulder girdles	Sporadic	Slowly progressive, extreme dissolution
Carpal-tarsal osteolysis: Multicentric osteolysis with nephropathy	Infant, child	Carpal and tarsal areas, elbows	Sporadic; occasionally dominant	Osteoporosis, deformity, hypertension, renal failure, death
Hereditary multicentric osteolysis	1–5 years	Carpal and tarsal areas, elbows, digits	Dominant; occasionally recessive or sporadic	Progressive deformity
Neurogenic osteolysis	Childhood	Phalanges	Dominant or recessive	Sensory neuropathy, skin ulcerations
Acroosteolysis of Joseph	Childhood	Distal phalanges	Recessive	Otherwise healthy
Acroosteolysis of Shinz	Second decade	Phalanges	Dominant	Skin ulcerations, no neurologic defect
Farber's disease	Infancy	Elbows, wrists, knees, ankles	Sporadic	Subcutaneous nodules
Winchester's syndrome	Infancy	Carpal and tarsal areas, elbows	Recessive	Osteoporosis, joint contractures, thick skin, corneal opacities
Osteolysis with detritic synovitis	Adulthood	Widespread	Sporadic	Progressive

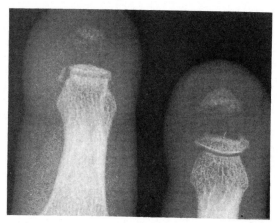

Figure 84–6. Acroosteolysis of Hajdu and Cheney. The typical pattern of osteolysis of the digits is demonstrated. Note that resorption occurs in a band-like fashion across the waist of the terminal phalanges, isolating one or more phalangeal fragments. Soft tissue swelling also is evident. The appearance is identical to that in occupational acroosteolysis. (Courtesy of M. Dalinka, M.D., Philadelphia, Pennsylvania.)

luxation about the elbow also can be apparent. Rarely, other sites are affected. Renal alterations accompany the onset of osteolysis and result in death in early adult life.

Hereditary Multicentric Osteolysis. This condition reveals a familial distribution, with most cases exhibiting a dominant mode of transmission. The onset of disease usually occurs at the age of 3 to 4 years, with articular complaints involving the wrists and ankles. After this, an asymptomatic period arises in adolescence in which a varying amount of

carpal and tarsal osteolysis is associated with progressive deformity. Radiographs outline dissolution of carpus and tarsus that, in most cases, is not associated with tapering of the adjacent tubular bones (Fig. 84–9). This latter characteristic, which differs from the "penciling" of tubular bones that is evident in multicentric osteolysis with nephropathy, is not constant. Rarely, osteolysis at additional sites can be encountered, including the elbows, shoulders, clavicles, hips, knees, ankles, feet, and ribs.

Pathology and Pathogenesis. The involved tissues in idiopathic multicentric osteolysis usually reveal an increased content of fibrous elements and increased vascularity, with little evidence of inflammation. Osteolysis is accompanied by osteoclastic activity. Bone formation appears normal. The pathogenesis of the process is unknown.

Differential Diagnosis. The major radiographic characteristic of the various forms of idiopathic multicentric osteolysis is the striking resorption of bone that predominates in the carpal and tarsal areas (and occasionally in the elbows). This distribution differs from that typically associated with occupational acroosteolysis (phalanges), posttraumatic osteolysis (distal end of the clavicle, pubic and ischial rami, femoral neck, ulna, radius), acroosteolysis syndrome of Hajdu and Cheney (phalanges), massive osteolysis of Gorham (variable distribution with predilection for pelvic and shoulder girdles), multicentric reticulohistiocytosis (hands, feet, wrists, ankles), acroosteolysis syndrome of Joseph or of Shinz (phalanges), and neurogenic acroosteolysis (phalanges). The changes may resemble those in juvenile chronic arthritis (Fig. 84–10) (see Chapter 23), Winchester's syndrome, Farber's disease, and neuroarthropathy in leprosy and diabetes mellitus.

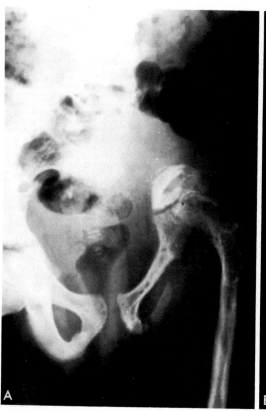

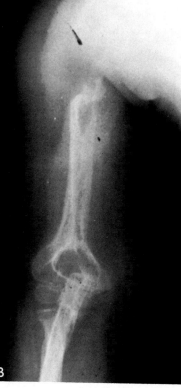

Figure 84–7. Massive osteolysis of Gorham. A In this 14 year old boy, observe the dissolution of most of the left hemipelvis and the narrowed and tapered left femur. Radiolucent foci and a coarsened trabecular patten are seen in the femur and pubic bone. **B** In a 6 year old girl, resorption of the proximal half of the humerus is evident. The remaining bone is osteoporotic, with lucent lesions.

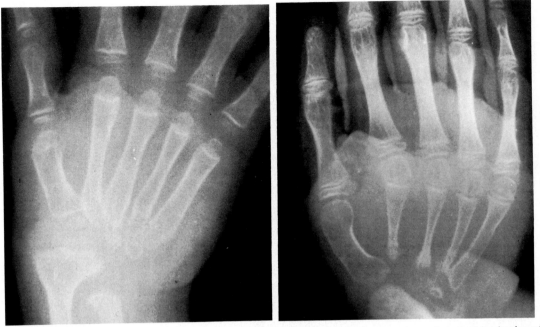

Figure 84–8. Multicentric osteolysis with nephropathy. A 14 year old boy developed progressive symmetric osteolysis involving hands, wrists, elbows, and feet, with associated renal failure and hypertension. **A** At approximately 4 years of age, a radiograph shows ulnar deviation of the hands on the wrists, principally due to shortening of the distal portion of the ulna. The two visible carpal bones are small and irregular, and the bases of the second, third, fourth, and fifth metacarpals are tapered. **B** At 14 years of age, progression of the osteolysis of the carpal bones, metacarpal bases, radius, and ulna is seen. The opposite side was similarly affected. (From MacPherson RI et al: Essential osteolysis with nephropathy. J Can Assoc Radiol 24:98, 1973. Used with permission.)

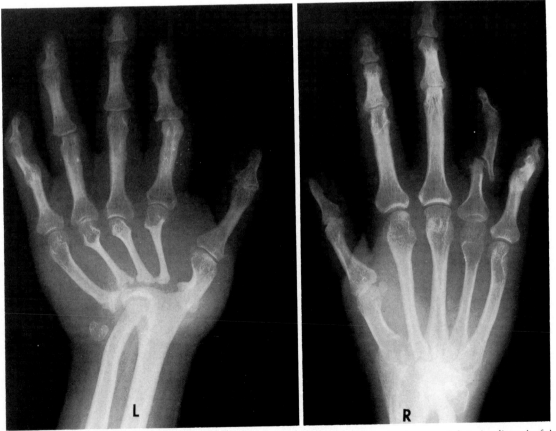

Figure 84–9. Hereditary multicentric osteolysis. This patient developed wrist symptoms and signs when he was an infant. A radiograph of the left wrist at age 40 years outlines absence of all but one of the carpal bones, hypoplasia of the metacarpal bones, and fusion of the fifth proximal interphalangeal joint. The right carpus is resorbed and fused, and there is destruction of the fourth proximal interphalangeal joint and fusion of the fifth. Osteolysis of portions of the metacarpal heads is evident. (From Whyte MP, et al: Idiopathic multicentric osteolysis. Report of an affected father and son. Arthritis Rheum 21:367, 1978. Used with permission.)

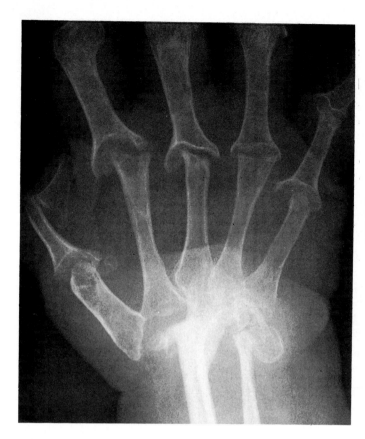

Figure 84–10. Still's disease. Observe the extreme destruction and resorption of carpus, radius, ulna, metacarpal bones, and phalanges. The findings are not unlike those of carpal-tarsal osteolysis syndromes. (Courtesy of V. Vint, M.D., La Jolla, California.)

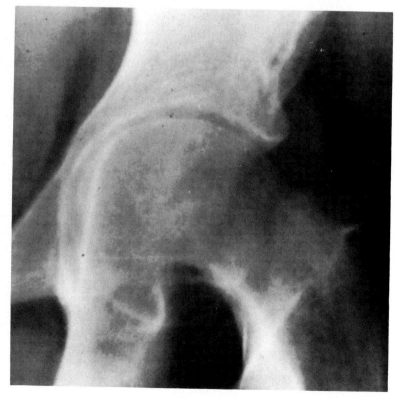

Figure 84–11. Chondrolysis after slipped capital femoral epiphysis: Radiographic abnormalities. Note osteoporosis, concentric joint space narrowing, protrusio acetabuli deformity, and an abnormal alignment of the femoral head and femoral neck.

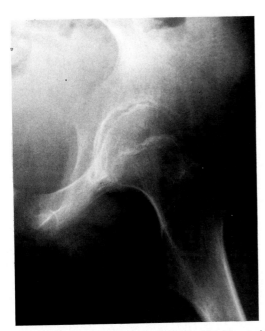

Figure 84–12. Idiopathic chondrolysis of the hip. This 10 year old black girl had a 7 month history of pain and deformity in her left hip. A radiograph demonstrates a joint contracture with the hip held in external rotation. Cartilage loss has occurred and diffuse osteoporosis is seen. (Courtesy of G. Greenway, M.D., Dallas, Texas.)

OTHER OSTEOLYSIS SYNDROMES. Other osteolysis syndromes are summarized in Table 84–2.

CHONDROLYSIS

Cartilage loss or destruction is an important complication of many articular disorders, including rheumatoid arthritis, seronegative spondyloarthropathies, septic arthritis, degenerative joint disease, and relapsing polychondritis. In addition, cartilage atrophy can appear after disuse, immobilization, or paralysis, perhaps related to interruption of normal patterns of chondral nutrition. Finally, chondrolysis may appear as a complication of a slipped capital femoral epiphysis or on an idiopathic basis.

Chondrolysis After Slipped Capital Femoral Epiphysis

Chondrolysis is recognized as a definite and important complication of slipping of the capital femoral epiphysis. The reported frequency of chondrolysis appearing in association with slipped femoral capital epiphysis varies from approximately 1 per cent to 40 per cent. Both men and women are affected. The age of the patient, the acuteness and extent of the epiphyseal separation, and the method of treatment probably are of minor importance in influencing the frequency of this complication.

Clinical manifestations of chondrolysis generally appear within a year of the epiphyseal separation. Pain, tenderness, limitation of motion, and flexion contracture are noted in the affected hip or, very rarely, in the hip that is contralateral to that with the slipped capital femoral epiphysis.

Three radiographic features of chondrolysis have been emphasized (Fig. 84–11). Initially, periarticular osteoporosis appears and may persist for variable amounts of time. The second finding is rapid narrowing of the joint space that most typically affects the entire joint or is isolated to the superior aspect. Superior joint space diminution is especially common when osteonecrosis is also present (7 to 25 per cent of cases). Third, thinning of the subchondral bone plate, osseous erosion, and flattening can be seen. Acetabular protrusion, subchondral cysts, and premature fusion of adjacent growth plates may be apparent.

The radiographic findings appear in a relatively short time and can subsequently stabilize, to be followed by changes of cartilaginous and osseous repair characterized by partial or complete "recovery" of the articular space, bone eburnation or sclerosis, and osteophytosis. At other times, especially in the presence of osteonecrosis, progressive deterioration of the joint is seen.

Pathologic alterations include thinning and pitting of articular cartilage, replacement of portions of the cartilaginous surface with fibrous tissue or fibrocartilage, and capsular thickening. The synovium initially undergoes proliferation with hypervascularity and is later replaced by fibrous tissue.

The cause and pathogenesis of chondrolysis in slipped capital femoral epiphyses are not clear.

The differential diagnosis of the radiographic features of chondrolysis accompanying slipped capital femoral epiphyses varies with the stage of the process. Initially, the osteoporosis observed in chondrolysis is identical to that seen in various inflammatory synovial disorders or in the reflex sympathetic dystrophy syndrome, transient osteoporosis of the hip, and regional migratory osteoporosis. At this stage, aspiration of joint contents is mandatory to exclude the possibility of infection. In the later stages of chondrolysis, findings simulate changes in infection, rheumatoid arthritis, and other inflammatory disorders. The absence of systemic symptoms, of elevation of the erythrocyte sedimentation rate, and of leukocytosis in chondrolysis is a clinical clue that helps to exclude a septic process. In advanced stages of chondrolysis, differential diagnosis includes pigmented villonodular synovitis and idiopathic synovial (osteo)chondromatosis.

Idiopathic Chondrolysis of the Hip

Chondrolysis of the hip joint may occur in adolescent girls, particularly blacks, who do not have slipped capital femoral epiphyses. Less commonly, boys and persons over the age of 20 years may be affected. Monarticular disease of the hip is typical, and clinical findings include pain, stiffness, restriction of motion, and the absence of a history of trauma. Radiographs outline periarticular osteoporosis, joint space narrowing, and erosion of the subchondral bone (Fig. 84–12). In addition, slight enlargement of the femoral head, an increase in width of the femoral neck, narrowing of the growth plate, and mild protrusio acetabuli may be evident. Joint aspiration usually confirms the absence of an effusion or organisms. Pathologic examination outlines changes in cartilage that are identical to those that occur in chondrolysis complicating slipped capital femoral epiphysis. The adjacent bone is osteoporotic.

Later stages of the process can be associated with obliteration of the articular space, cysts, osteophytes, and deformity.

Major alternatives in differential diagnosis include juvenile chronic arthritis, infection, transient osteoporosis of the hip, ischemic necrosis of the femoral head, primary protrusio acetabuli, and pigmented villonodular synovitis.

FURTHER READING

Amin PH, Evans ANW: Essential osteolysis of carpal and tarsal bones. Br J Radiol 51:539, 1978.

Cahill BR: Osteolysis of the distal part of the clavicle in male athletes. J Bone Joint Surg [Am] 64:1053, 1982.

Cannon SR: Massive osteolysis. A review of seven cases. J Bone Joint Surg [Br] 68:24, 1986.

Casey D, Mirra J, Staple TW: Parasymphyseal insufficiency fractures of the os pubis. AJR 142:581, 1984.

Cheney WD: Acro-osteolysis. AJR 94:595, 1965.

Duncan JW, Nasca R, Schrantz J: Idiopathic chondrolysis of the hip. J Bone Joint Surg [Am] 61:1024, 1979.

Elias AN, Pinals RS, Anderson HC, Gould LV, Streeten DHP: Hereditary osteodysplasia with acro-osteolysis (the Hajdu-Cheney syndrome). Am J Med 65:627, 1978.

El-Khoury GY, Mickelson MR: Chondrolysis following slipped capital femoral epiphysis. Radiology 123:327, 1977.

Gama C, Meira JBB: Occupational acro-osteolysis. J Bone Joint Surg [Am] 60:86, 1975.

Gilula LA, Bliznak J, Staple TW: Idiopathic nonfamilial acro-osteolysis with cortical defects and mandibular ramus osteolysis. Radiology 121:63, 1976.

Goergen TG, Resnick D, Riley RR: Post-traumatic abnormalities of the pubic bone simulating malignancy. Radiology 126:85, 1978.

Goldman AB, Schneider R, Martel W: Acute chondrolysis complicating slipped capital femoral epiphysis. AJR 130:945, 1978.

Gorham LW, Stout AP: Massive osteolysis (acute spontaneous absorption of bone, phantom bone, disappearing bone). J Bone Joint Surg [Am] 37:985, 1955.

Gorham LW, Wright AW, Shultz HH, Maxon FC Jr: Disappearing bones: A rare form of massive osteolysis. Report of two cases, one with autopsy findings. Am J Med 17:674, 1954.

Halaby FA, DiSalvo EI: Osteolysis: A complication of trauma. AJR 94:590, 1965.

Halliday DR, Dahlin DC, Pugh DG, Young HH: Massive osteolysis and angiomatosis. Radiology 82:637, 1964.

Hardegger F, Simpson LA, Segmueller G: The syndrome of idiopathic osteolysis. Classification, review, and case report. J Bone Joint Surg [Br] 67:89, 1985.

Ingram AJ, Clarke MS, Clark CS Jr, Marshall WR: Chondrolysis complicating slipped capital femoral epiphysis. Clin Orthop 165:99, 1982.

Kohler E, Babbit D, Huizenga B, Good TA: Hereditary osteolysis: A clinical, radiological and chemical study. Radiology 108:99, 1973.

Levine AH, Pais MJ, Schwartz EE: Posttraumatic osteolysis of the distal clavicle with emphasis on early radiologic changes. AJR 127:781, 1976.

Moule NJ, Golding JSR: Idiopathic chondrolysis of the hip. Clin Radiol 25:247, 1974.

Resnick D, Weisman M, Goergen TG, Feldman PS: Osteolysis with detritic synovitis. A new syndrome. Arch Intern Med 138:1003, 1978.

Roback DL: Posttraumatic osteolysis of the femoral neck. AJR 134:1243, 1980.

Swezey RL, Bjarnason DM, Alexander SJ, Forrester DB: Resorptive arthropathy and the opera-glass hand syndrome. Semin Arthritis Rheum 2:1972–1973.

Tuncbilek E, Besim A, Bakkaloglu A, Tuncer E, Secmeer G: Carpal-tarsal osteolysis. Pediatr Radiol 15:255, 1985.

Tyler T, Rosenbaum HD: Idiopathic multicentric osteolysis. AJR 126:23, 1976.

Wenger DR, Mickelson MR, Ponseti IV: Idiopathic chondrolysis of the hip. Report of two cases. J Bone Joint Surg [Am] 57:268, 1975.

Winchester P, Grossman H, Lim WN, Danes BS: A new acid mucopolysaccharidosis with skeletal deformities simulating rheumatoid arthritis. AJR 106:121, 1969.

Chapter 85

Soft Tissues

Donald Resnick, M.D.
Gen Niwayama, M.D.

The radiographic alterations in soft tissue disorders include masses, increased lucency, calcification or ossification, bands, contractures, foreign bodies, atrophy, hypertrophy, and edema. In most instances, the findings lack specificity, although at times, careful analysis may allow delineation of the benign or malignant nature of the process. Especially important is the differentiation of myositis ossificans trau-matica from various malignant tumors and the recognition that widespread skeletal abnormalities may accompany certain cutaneous syndromes. Use of other diagnostic imaging techniques may be required to supplement the radiographic evaluation and provide more accurate information regarding the extent of the soft tissue process and its relationship to adjacent structures.

There is no uniformly accepted definition of soft tissue. A broad definition could include the epithelium, fibrous tissue, fat, and voluntary muscles with inclusion also of the vessels and nerves that supply these structures. Abnormalities of the skin are much more amenable to clinical than radiologic examination and are the subject of an entire medical subspecialty, dermatology. Conversely, processes of the subcutaneous and muscular tissues are frequently better evaluated by radiography and related techniques than by palpation, percussion, or auscultation. Radiographic manifestations of such processes may include mass formation, alteration in radiodensity, including exaggerated lucency, calcification and ossification, and resorption and contracture.

SOFT TISSUE MASSES
Available Diagnostic Techniques

The causes of soft tissue masses are diverse. In many instances, local or distant clinical findings provide important diagnostic clues. Supplementary plain film radiography commonly adds useful information that indicates whether a neoplasm is present and, if so, whether that neoplasm is benign or malignant. *Low kilovoltage* (below 50 kVp), by exaggerating the differences in radiographic density of fat and muscle, can be useful (see Chapter 7). The role of *conventional tomography* in the evaluation of soft tissue masses is limited. *Xeroradiography*, with its edge contrast enhancement and great latitude, is better suited for delineating soft tissue changes than is conventional radiography (see Chapter 8).

Computed tomography has been emphasized as a useful technique in evaluating soft tissue masses (see Chapter 10). The ability of this technique to define the exact dimensions of a lesion, the relationship of the tumor to nearby bones, and the density characteristics of the affected tissue is important both in correct diagnosis and in proper therapy. Certain limitations in the application of computed tomography should be recognized. With the exception of a few types of masses, such as lipomas, the attenuation values do not allow a specific histologic diagnosis. Overestimation of tumor size on the basis of computed tomographic images is possible owing to adjacent soft tissue edema. The differentiation of actual invasion of neurovascular structures from simple distortion by the adjacent mass, even with the use of intravascular injection of contrast material, is difficult.

Classification of a soft tissue tumor as benign or malignant solely on the basis of the computed tomographic findings also is difficult, although certain criteria exist. Computed tomographic features of a benign process include a smooth, well-defined border, lack of involvement of multiple muscle groups, and absence of blurring of surrounding fat; features of a malignant process are poor margination, areas of diminished density, blurring of adjacent fat, involvement of multiple muscle groups, and invasion of bone. Locally aggressive but benign soft tissue neoplasms such as desmoid tumors can exhibit computed tomographic characteristics of a malignant process.

In some instances, a careful analysis of all of the computed tomographic features of a soft tissue lesion will allow the formulation of a likely diagnosis. Examples of this situation include a synovial cyst (periarticular mass, well-defined border, attenuation value close to that of water) (Fig. 85–1), heterotopic ossification or myositis ossificans (dense rim or shell of ossification), and a peripheral aneurysm (well-defined, round inhomogeneous mass, partial opacification after the intravenous injection of contrast material, and location in a neurovascular bundle) (Fig. 85–2).

Computed tomography can be used to monitor percutaneous needle biopsy of soft tissue masses (see Chapter 17); however, the use of computed tomography after complete or incomplete excisional biopsy of soft tissue sarcomas has met with varying success.

Ultrasonography has been used successfully to define the nature of certain soft tissue masses in both the axial and the

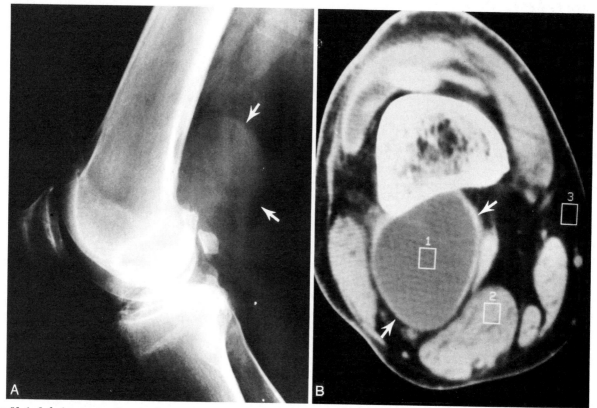

Figure 85–1. Soft tissue mass: Computed tomography—synovial (popliteal) cyst. A A portion of the mass is evident on the lateral radiograph (arrows). **B** After the administration of intravenous contrast material, a transaxial computed tomographic scan at the level of the mass shows a well-circumscribed, lucent cystic lesion (24 Hounsfield units) with an enhanced wall (arrows), displacing the adjacent soft tissues and muscles (semimembranosus, biceps femoris). (Courtesy of G. Greenway, M.D., Dallas, Texas.)

appendicular skeleton. Most notably, synovial cysts and aneurysms are well delineated with ultrasonography (see Chapter 12). A subcutaneous or intramuscular abscess may possess echogenic properties similar to those of a tumor, however.

Angiography may be used to define the extent and vascular supply of a tumor and to differentiate a benign from a malignant neoplasm (see Chapter 15). Differentiation of malignancy and hypervascular inflammatory masses may be more difficult, however.

Scintigraphy with technetium (or other radiopharmaceutical agents) may delineate the presence and extent of soft tissue tumors (see Chapter 16). The mechanism of isotopic uptake is incompletely understood, although increased blood flow, microcalcification, or a binding of the compounds by enzymes released in response to tissue damage may be important. Many of the tumors in which bone-seeking radioisotopes localize reveal radiographic or histologic evidence of calcification or ossification. The vast majority of malignant soft tissue neoplasms will accumulate the radiotracer; however, as many as 50 per cent of benign tumors will do the same. Although gallium was initially regarded as a tumor-localizing agent, it too may accumulate in inflamed or infarcted soft tissues. Positive gallium scans are more characteristic of malignant soft tissue tumors than benign ones.

Magnetic resonance imaging is at least equal and probably superior to computed tomography in defining the extent of a

soft tissue mass as well as the degree of osseous involvement (Fig. 85–3). Whether or not this technique has the ability to determine a specific histologic diagnosis in cases of soft tissue sarcomas is not yet known (Fig. 85–4). Furthermore, calcification, ossification, or gas formation in a soft tissue mass is not well delineated with magnetic resonance imaging.

Types of Tumors

Tumors of soft tissues can arise from the epidermis and the ectodermal structures of the skin, from the lymph nodes, and from two additional primitive tissue sources: the mesoderm and the neuroectodermal tissues of the peripheral nervous system. From the primitive mesenchyme are derived the supportive and reticuloendothelial tissues and their corresponding tumors; from the neuroectoderm are formed the Schwann sheath and possibly the endoneurium and perineurium and their corresponding tumors. The result is an overwhelming list of potential primary soft tissue neoplasms. The histologic characteristics of a neoplasm also may be altered through a process of differentiation or dedifferentiation of the primary cell type or as a result of proliferation of fibroblast cells owing to local tissue injury. Admixtures of various types of neoplastic cells therefore can result, typical examples of which are the malignant mesenchymoma, synovioma, and teratoma.

In general, benign tumors or tumor-like processes are far

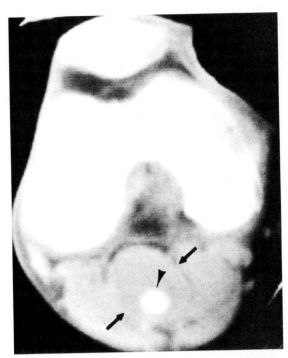

Figure 85–2. Soft tissue mass: Computed tomography—popliteal artery aneurysm. After an intravenous bolus injection of contrast material, a computed tomographic scan demonstrates the presence of an aneurysm (arrows) and its opacified lumen (arrowhead) in the popliteal fossa. The nonenhancing part of the mass represents atheroma or thrombus. (From Heikin JP, et al: CT of benign soft tissue masses of the extremities. AJR 142:575, 1984. Copyright 1984, American Roentgen Ray Society. Used with permisson.)

more frequent than malignant processes. Primary benign tumors can be classified as fibroblastic processes (fibroma, various forms of fibromatosis), myxomatoses, fibrous histiocytomas, lipomatoses, xanthomatoses, myomatoses, angiomatoses, lymphangiomatoses, and muscular types; primary malignant tumors can be regarded as fibrosarcomas, malignant histiocytomas, liposarcomas, lipomyosarcomas, rhabdomyosarcomas, angiosarcomatoses, lymphoid and reticuloendothelial tumors, extraskeletal osteosarcomas and chondrosarcomas, synovial sarcomas, malignant mesenchymomas, and miscellaneous types. If to this list are added the neurogenic tumors, metastatic deposits, and non-neoplastic masses, the diverse nature of soft tissue masses is readily apparent.

Of the primary malignant soft tissue tumors, liposarcoma, malignant fibrous histiocytoma and fibrosarcoma, rhabdomyosarcoma, unclassified sarcomas, leiomyosarcoma, and synovial sarcoma, in descending order of frequency, are encountered most commonly. Of the benign neoplasms, lipomas, fibrohistiocytic tumors, and hemangiomas are relatively common.

Tumors of Fat

Liposarcoma is a frequent malignant neoplasm of soft tissues that is usually encountered in middle-aged and elderly patients. It is common in the thigh, gluteal region, retroperitoneum, and leg (Fig. 85–5). Liposarcomas of the thigh predominate in the quadriceps muscle and the popliteal fossa. They rarely arise from a preexisting lipoma. On radiographs, a poorly defined mass of both water density and fat density may be observed. Although uncommon, calcification or ossification is encountered in well-differentiated liposarcomas. Computed tomography may reveal areas of low density in the mass. One type of lipoma, the *infiltrating angiolipoma*, is locally aggressive and is characterized radiographically by serpentine-like densities intermixed with fat.

Lipomas are common lesions that are typically encountered in patients who are 30 to 50 years of age. Women are affected more frequently, and solitary lesions predominate. The tumors show predilection for the subcutaneous tissues of the back, extremities, and thorax. A well-defined radiolucent mass is detected on the radiograph. Ossification in the tumor is occasionally observed (Fig. 85–6), and those lipomas located close to a bone may incite hyperostosis (Fig. 85–7). Computed tomography and magnetic resonance imaging reliably indicate

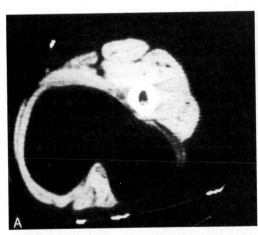
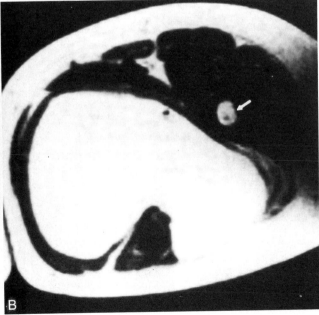

Figure 85–3. Soft tissue mass: Magnetic resonance imaging—lipoma. A computed tomographic scan (**A**) and a magnetic resonance image (**B**) reveal the characteristics of a lesion in the thigh. In **A**, note its smooth margin and lucent (−104 Hounsfield units) interior. In **B**, high signal intensity similar to that of the marrow fat (arrow) in the femur is seen. (Courtesy of K. Kortman, M.D., Los Angeles, California.)

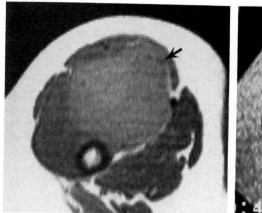
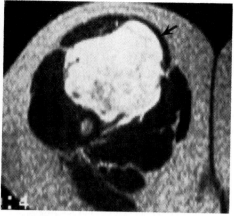

Figure 85–4. Soft tissue mass: Magnetic resonance imaging—malignant fibrous histiocytoma. On a T1 weighted transaxial magnetic resonance image (**A**), a mass in the thigh yields a low intensity signal (arrow). On a T2 weighted image (**B**), the mass displays areas of low and high signal intensity (arrow). (Courtesy of G. Greenway, M.D., Dallas, Texas.)

the fatty nature of the tumor. Histologically, the tumor tissue is similar to ordinary body fat.

Approximately 5 per cent of all patients with lipomas have multiple tumors. Additional varieties of fatty tumors are symmetric lipomatosis (in which diffuse and symmetric distribution of lipomas is recognized), hibernoma and lipoblas-

toma (which are rare embryonal fatty tumors), lipoma arborescens (in which fat collects beneath the synovial lining of the joint, especially the knee), macrodystrophia lipomatosa (which can lead to grotesque enlargement of a digit), and mesenchymoma (in which fatty, fibrous, vascular, smooth muscle, and osseous elements are evident).

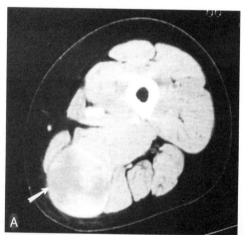

Figure 85–5. Liposarcoma. A After the intravenous injection of contrast material, a transaxial computed tomographic scan shows a large mass in the adductor musculature in which there are areas of enhancement as well as decreased attenuation (arrow). **B, C** T1 weighted (**B**) and T2 weighted (**C**) coronal magnetic resonance images show the lesion (arrows). In **B**, low signal intensity is apparent, whereas in **C**, homogeneous high signal intensity is evident. After excision, the mass was identified as a myxoid liposarcoma. (Courtesy of G. Greenway, M.D., Dallas, Texas.)

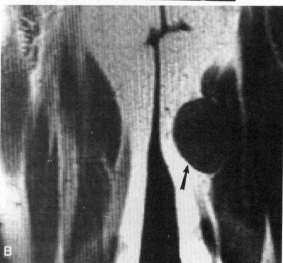
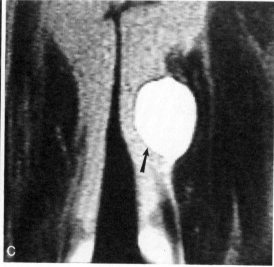

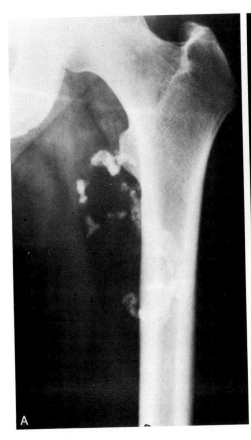

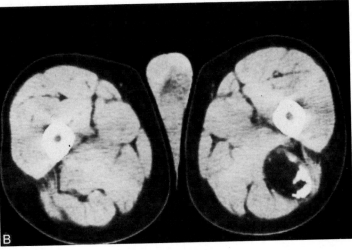

Figure 85–6. Lipoma: Soft tissue ossification. Conventional radiography (**A**) and computed tomography (**B**) show irregular ossification in a radiolucent mass. (Courtesy of G. Greenway, M.D., Dallas, Texas.)

Tumors of Fibrous Tissue

Fibrosarcomas occur in both adults and children, and they predominate in the external soft tissues. They are common in the region of the thigh and knee. The neoplasms lack any specific radiographic characteristics.

The classification of benign fibrous tumors is complicated (Table 85–1). Varieties of benign fibrous proliferation are termed *fibromatoses*. In this latter group is a *desmoid tumor*, which arises in the abdominal and extraabdominal musculature (especially the shoulder area) of men, women, and children and infiltrates the surrounding tissues. Recurrences are frequent.

Other types of fibromatoses are classified according to their location. *Recurring digital fibromas* of infancy represent a rare condition in which single or multiple fibromatous lesions arise from the fingers (and toes). They usually are painless. Their digital site of origin and their tendency to recur are characteristic features of this variety of fibromatosis. *Palmar* and *plantar fibromatoses* are terms applied to fibrous proliferations occurring in the palmar and plantar fasciae.

Juvenile aponeurotic fibroma is an aggressive variety of fibrous proliferation that arises in the aponeurotic tissues of the hands or feet of young children (Fig. 85–8). This lesion has a tendency to calcify, infiltrate adjacent tissues, and recur after incomplete excision.

Additional types of fibrous proliferation are indicated in Table 85–1. In one, *congenital generalized fibromatosis (infantile myofibromatosis)*, which affects infants, fibrous proliferation occurs not only in the superficial soft tissues but also in viscera and bones (Fig. 85–9). The condition may be familial and the tumors may disappear spontaneously.

Tumors of Muscle

Leiomyosarcomas are uncommon malignant neoplasms of soft tissues, affecting primarily adults. They may arise in the retroperitoneum, the peripheral soft tissues, or the major blood vessels. Those occurring in the retroperitoneal region

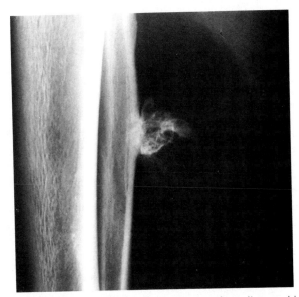

Figure 85–7. Lipoma: Hyperostosis. As demonstrated here, lipomas arising close to bone may lead to bizarre hyperostosis. (Courtesy of J. Castello, M.D., Madrid, Spain.)

Table 85–1. BENIGN FIBROUS PROLIFERATIONS AND FIBROMATOSES

Diagnosis	Typical Age of Presentation	Typical Location	Miscellaneous Data
Fibrous Proliferations of Infancy and Childhood			
Fibrous hamartoma	Infancy	Axillary, inguinal regions	Solitary, rarely recur
Congenital generalized fibromatosis (infantile myofibromatosis)	Infancy	Soft tissue, viscera, bone	Solitary or multiple, may regress, rarely recur
Infantile digital fibromatosis	Infancy	Fingers and toes	Solitary or multiple, may regress, commonly recur
Fibromatosis colli	Infancy	Sternocleidomastoid muscle	Solitary, rarely bilateral, may regress, rarely recur, associated torticollis
Juvenile aponeurotic fibroma	Infancy, childhood, or adolescence	Hands and feet	Solitary, may regress, commonly recur, may calcify
Juvenile hyaline fibromatosis	Childhood	Dermis and subcutis	Multiple, do not regress or recur
Infantile desmoid type fibromatosis	Infancy and childhood	Musculature	Solitary, commonly recur, no regression
Fibrous Proliferations of Adulthood			
Nodular fasciitis (pseudosarcomatous fasciitis)	Adulthood	Extremities	Solitary, may regress, rarely recur
Proliferative fasciitis	Adulthood	Extremities	Solitary
Proliferative myositis	Late adulthood	Trunk, shoulder girdle	Solitary
Elastofibroma	Late adulthood	Chest wall, scapula	Unilateral > bilateral
Keloid	Adolescence or adulthood	Face, shoulders, forearms, hands	Solitary or multiple, do not regress, common in blacks
Fibromatoses			
Palmar fibromatosis	Late adulthood	Hands	Unilateral or bilateral, associated Dupuytren's contracture
Plantar fibromatosis	Childhood or adulthood	Feet	Unilateral or bilateral, associated palmar fibromatosis
Peyronie's disease	Adulthood	Penis	May regress, associated palmar and plantar fibromatosis
Extraabdominal fibromatosis (desmoid tumors)	Adulthood	Musculature	Rarely regress, commonly recur
Abdominal fibromatosis (desmoid tumors)	Early adulthood	Musculature	Commonly recur, occur during or after pregnancy
Intraabdominal fibromatosis (pelvic fibromatosis, mesenteric fibromatosis, Gardner's syndrome)	Adulthood	Musculature, mesentery	May recur

Taken in part from Enzinger FM, Weiss SW: Soft Tissue Tumors. St Louis, CV Mosby, 1983, p 71. Used with permission.

are most common. *Leiomyomas* can be found in the skin and subcutaneous tissue. They arise at variable sites, are single or multiple, and may calcify.

Rhabdomyosarcoma is rare after the age of 45 or 50 years. In the pediatric age group, the tumors (juvenile rhabdomyosarcoma, embryonal rhabdomyosarcoma) predominate in the head, neck, and urogenital tract, and affect both boys and girls. On radiographic examination, soft tissue masses, which rarely calcify or invade neighboring bone, are noted. Skeletal metastasis can resemble neuroblastoma. In adult rhabdomyosarcoma (Fig. 85–10), many of the lesions are located in the deeper tissues of the extremities and torso.

The *rhabdomyoma* is an extremely rare benign tumor composed of striated muscle cells.

Myxomatoses

Neoplastic and non-neoplastic proliferation of myxoid tissue can be seen. The *ganglion* represents a cystic tumor-like lesion that usually is attached to a tendon sheath, particularly in the hands, wrists, and feet (Fig. 85–11). It also arises from tendons, muscles, and semilunar cartilages. Cystic swellings are observed. Radiographic evaluation may reveal a soft tissue mass, surface bone resorption, and periosteal new bone formation, and arthrography or tenography may outline the communication of the mass with the underlying articular or tendinous structure.

Ganglia arising about the proximal tibiofibular joint have been associated with compression of the common peroneal nerve. Those near articulations may communicate with subchondral cystic lesions, which are frequently interpreted as intraosseous ganglia. In the hip, a radiolucent paraacetabular soft tissue mass with subjacent bone erosion may be seen (Fig. 85–12).

The *myxoma* is a rare connective tissue tumor that may appear at any age. It demonstrates an invasive manner of growth and can recur.

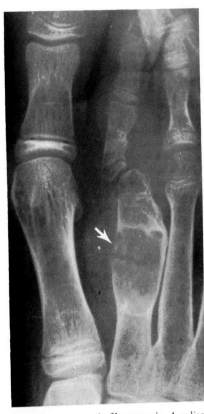

Figure 85–8. Juvenile aponeurotic fibromatosis. A radiograph reveals a soft tissue mass with adjacent osseous involvement and a pathologic fracture through a well-circumscribed lesion in the second metatarsal (arrow). There is displacement and deformity of the proximal phalanx in the same digit. (Courtesy of R. Freiberger, M.D., New York, New York, and J. Kaye, M.D., New York, New York.)

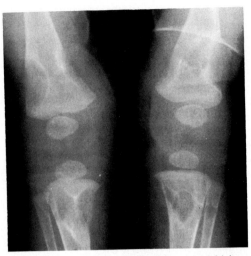

Figure 85–9. Congenital generalized fibromatosis. Multiple symmetrically distributed radiolucent foci, predominantly in the metaphyses of the tubular bones, represent sites of fibrous proliferation. (Courtesy of D. Weissberg, M.D., Orange County, California.)

Tumors of Histiocytic Composition

Malignant fibrous histiocytoma generally is evident in adult life, more frequently in men than in women; the lower extremity is the most common site of involvement (Fig. 85–13). The tumor typically involves deep fascia or skeletal muscle. It produces a mass of variable size with nonspecific radiologic features. Infrequently, metaplastic bone and cartilage formation occurs in the lesion. Erosion of bone, periosteal reaction, and pathologic fractures can be observed. Local recurrences and metastasis are encountered.

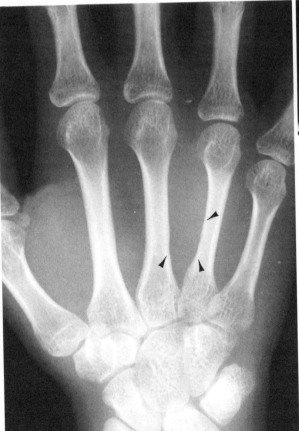

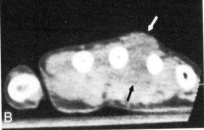

Figure 85–10. Rhabdomyosarcoma. A Observe erosion of both the third and the fourth metacarpals (arrowheads). B The computed tomographic scan shows the location of the mass (arrows). There is no evidence of calcification. (Courtesy of G. Greenway, M.D., Dallas, Texas.)

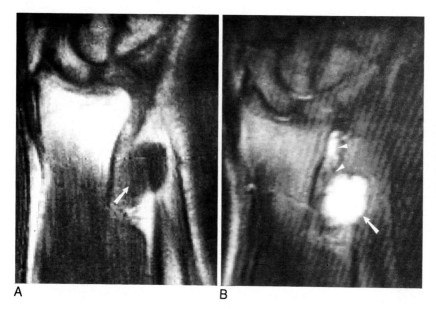

Figure 85–11. Ganglion. The T1 weighted coronal magnetic resonance image (**A**) reveals a lesion (arrow) with low signal intensity between the radius and ulna. The T2 weighted coronal magnetic resonance image (**B**) shows an increase in signal intensity (arrow) and communication with the inferior radioulnar joint (arrowheads). (Courtesy of G. Greenway, M.D., Dallas, Texas.)

A more benign variety, the *fibrous histiocytoma*, occurs in adults and children and can lead to painful soft tissue masses.

Xanthomatoses consist of a group of tumor-like proliferations characterized by the presence of a variable number of foam cells. Some of the tumors are associated with metabolic and endocrine disorders, such as hypercholesterolemia and diabetes mellitus (see Chapter 56). Many varieties are recognized. *Tendinous xanthomas* are common about the fingers, heel, elbow, and knee, where they may erode subjacent bone. Calcification appears in 20 to 25 per cent of cases. A *giant cell tumor of the tendon sheath* is detected in the hands and feet, attached to tendons, tendon sheaths, and fibrous capsules (Fig. 85–14) (see Chapter 79).

Angiomatoses

Angiomatoses are classified according to their tissue composition. A *capillary hemangioma* is composed solely of capillaries. This tumor is common, usually appearing early in life in the skin or subcutaneous tissue. If the capillaries are widely dilated, the tumor is called a *cavernous hemangioma*. If a vascular tumor has thicker walls and contains smooth muscle cells, it is called a *venous hemangioma*. This tumor is less frequent than the capillary hemangioma, and it predominates in children in the upper portion of the body. Capillary hemangiomas with prominent proliferation of the endothelial layer are called *benign hemangioendotheliomas*, whereas those with proliferation of pericytes are *benign hemangiopericytomas*. The most recognized variety of benign hemangiopericytomas is the *glomus tumor*. This uncommon tumor occurs with equal frequency in men and women and is usually detected in adults. It is typically located beneath the fingernail, leading to prominent symptoms. Radiographs may reveal an eccentric intraosseous lucent lesion or cortical erosion in the terminal phalanx (Fig. 85–15). Less frequent sites of involvement include the palm, wrist, forearm, foot, eyelid, and chest wall as well as intraosseous locations. Recurrence of the tumor is rare. Other benign types of angiomatoses are the *cirsoid aneurysm*, a vascular malformation consisting of arterial vessels; the *venous racemose aneurysm*, a malformation consisting of

venous structures; *diffuse angiomatosis* due to capillary proliferation; a *lymphangioma*, a proliferation of lymphatic vessels; and *lymphangiopericytomas*. Syndromes associated with some of these vascular lesions include the *Kasabach-Merritt syndrome* (see Chapter 58), the *blue rubber bleb nevus syndrome* (blue cutaneous cavernous hemangiomas commonly associated with hemangiomas of the gastrointestinal tract), and *Maffucci's syndrome* (multiple hemangiomas and enchondromas that may undergo malignant transformation).

Radiographs of hemangiomas and related lesions may reveal evidence of soft tissue masses containing circular calcified collections, termed phleboliths; in addition, osseous involvement, overgrowth, and articular abnormalities due to accompanying synovial lesions may be encountered (Fig. 85–16).

Angiosarcomatoses are much less frequent. These lesions are classified according to the dominant cell pattern. If endothelial cells predominate, a *malignant hemangioendothelioma* is present. With pericytic proliferation, a *malignant hemangiopericytoma* is found. A malignant tumor composed of lymphatic endothelioblasts is termed a *lymphangiosarcoma*. This

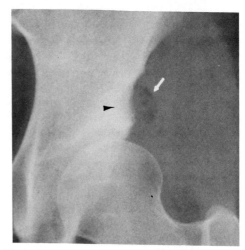

Figure 85–12. Ganglion. Observe a radiolucent soft tissue collection (arrow) with erosion and sclerosis of the adjacent bone (arrowhead). (Courtesy of G. Greenway, M.D., Dallas, Texas.)

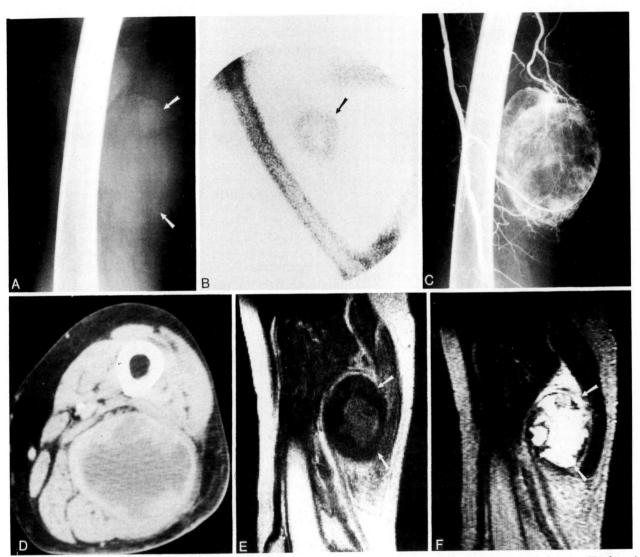

Figure 85–13. Malignant fibrous histiocytoma. A A large noncalcified soft tissue mass (arrows) is seen on a lateral radiograph of the leg. The femur is normal. **B** The bone scan reveals accumulation of the radionuclide in the periphery of the lesion (arrow) with a photopenic center. **C** Arteriography shows that the tumor is supplied by branches of the deep and superficial femoral arteries. A dense peripheral stain and arteriovenous shunting are observed. **D** On a transaxial computed tomographic scan at the level of the mass, note that it is moderately well defined, with decreased attenuation centrally. **E, F** T1 weighted **(E)** and T2 weighted **(F)** sagittal magnetic resonance images show the extent of the tumor (arrows) and its irregular bright signal in **F**. (Courtesy of G. Greenway, M.D., Dallas, Texas.)

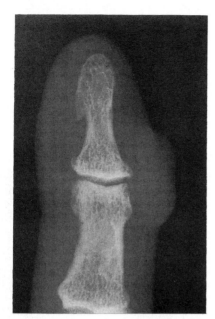

Figure 85–14. Giant cell tumor of tendon sheath. Note the noncalcified soft tissue mass about the distal interphalangeal joint.

tumor typically arises in women who have undergone radical mastectomies for carcinoma of the breast and who develop chronic and severe lymphedema.

Kaposi's sarcoma consists of both capillaries and fibrosarcoma-like cells. This lesion predominates in men, and is especially common in blacks in certain parts of Africa. Cutaneous nodules, frequently in the lower extremity, may lead to invasion of underlying bone (Fig. 85–17). Some patients also reveal evidence of an altered immunologic state, malignant lymphoma, lymphatic leukemia, diabetes mellitus, and varicosities.

Cartilaginous and Osseous Tumors

Soft tissue *chondromas* are rare. The tumors occur predominantly in the third and fourth decades of life, especially in the hands and feet. Radiographs reveal soft tissue masses frequently containing calcification (Fig. 85–18A). Although local recurrences can be seen, metastasis is not evident. Rarely, chondromas may arise within joints (Fig. 85–18B).

As extraskeletal chondromas commonly arise in close association with a tendon, tendon sheath, or joint capsule, the designation of *extraarticular synovial chondromatosis* or *tenosynovial chondromatosis* has been used to describe these lesions. Such chondromas should be differentiated from idiopathic (primary) synovial (osteo)chondromatosis (Fig. 85–19), in which metaplasia of the synovial lining in an articulation leads to numerous cartilaginous and osseous bodies (see Chapter 79). Tenosynovial chondromatosis is usually evident in the hand, wrist, foot, or, less frequently, knee. A slowly enlarging smooth or lobulated mass containing multiple small calcified or ossified densities, develops either near a joint or at some distance from it (Fig. 85–20).

Extraskeletal soft tissue *chondrosarcomas* also are very uncommon. These lesions are distinguished from those arising in a bone or in the periosteum and perichondrium. The soft tissues of the head and neck, extremities, shoulders, and buttocks are typically affected. A soft tissue mass with calcification and underlying osseous involvement can be detected radiographi-

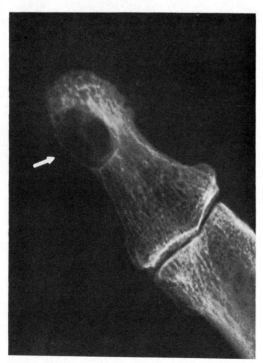

Figure 85–15. Glomus tumor. A well-defined cystic lesion of a terminal tuft is seen (arrow).

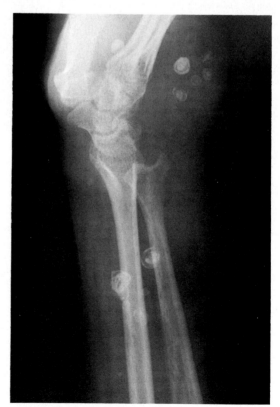

Figure 85–16. Hemangioma. Phleboliths of the forearm and hand are associated with soft tissue swelling and osseous involvement of the ulna, characterized by a coarsened trabecular pattern.

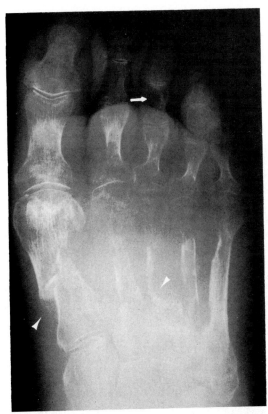

Figure 85–17. Kaposi's sarcoma. Note lytic destruction of the metatarsals and phalanges. Observe the eccentric location of many of the erosions (arrow) and pathologic fractures (arrowheads). (Courtesy of P. Ellenbogen, M.D., Dallas, Texas.)

cally (Fig. 85–21). The prognosis is variable; some lesions are highly aggressive, whereas others follow a more protracted course.

Osteomas of soft parts are rarely encountered. Soft tissue *osteosarcomas* likewise are rarely seen. These lesions are distinguished from medullary, periosteal, and parosteal osteosar-comas of bone. They are usually evident in middle-aged and elderly patients, in the deeper tissues of the extremities, thighs, or shoulder region.

Synovial Sarcomas

Synovial sarcomas are uncommon malignant neoplasms that can arise from within a joint but are more frequent in extraarticular locations. They are intimately related to tendons, tendon sheaths, bursal structures, and, less frequently, fasciae, ligaments, aponeuroses, and interosseous membranes. A distinct predilection exists for involvement of the thigh and lower extremity. Patients of all ages can be affected. Men are affected more frequently than women. On radiographs, a soft tissue mass is seen, which may reveal evidence of calcification in 20 to 30 per cent of cases and of osseous invasion in 5 to 20 per cent of cases (Fig. 85–22). Extensive bone destruction is rare, and reactive sclerosis is unusual. Recurrences are frequent and, in the majority of patients, sooner or later metastatic deposits appear, especially in the lungs.

Tumors of Peripheral Nerves

The most important benign tumors of peripheral nerves are the *neurofibroma* and the *neurilemoma*. The neurilemoma (benign schwannoma, neurinoma) is observed most commonly in men and women in the third to fifth decades of life. This tumor typically arises from the spinal nerve roots and the cervical, sympathetic, vagus, peroneal, and ulnar nerves, appearing in the head, neck, and flexor surfaces of the upper and lower extremities. It is predominantly a solitary, slowly growing lesion that, when large, leads to clinical manifestations that include pain, soft tissue prominence, and neurologic findings. Neurilemomas are benign in their behavior.

Although the discovery of a solitary neurofibroma should stimulate a thorough search for additional tumors as well as other manifestations of neurofibromatosis, its existence alone should not be regarded as synonymous with the diagnosis of von Recklinghausen's disease. Solitary neurofibromas predominate in young adult men and women. They affect all areas

Figure 85–18. Chondroma. A Soft tissue chondroma. Observe the calcified soft tissue mass adjacent to the base of the fifth metatarsal bone. **B** Intraarticular chondroma. A radiograph reveals a large calcified lesion in the infrapatellar fat pad, producing erosion of the patella and tibia.

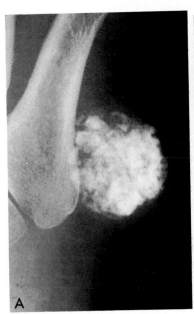

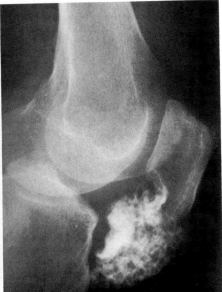

A   B

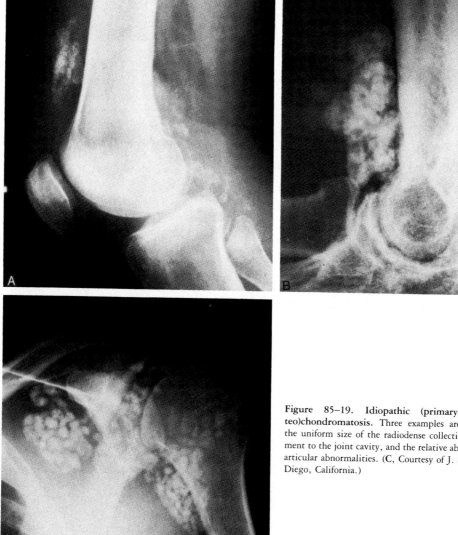

Figure 85–19. Idiopathic (primary) synovial (osteo)chondromatosis. Three examples are shown. Observe the uniform size of the radiodense collections, their confinement to the joint cavity, and the relative absence of additional articular abnormalities. (C, Courtesy of J. Slivka, M.D., San Diego, California.)

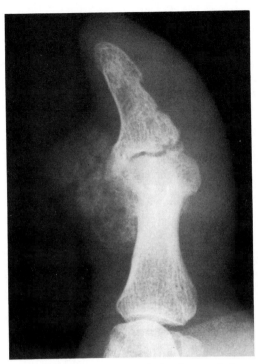

Figure 85–20. Extra-articular synovial chondromatosis (tenosynovial chondromatosis). Observe a large calcified or ossified mass arising on the dorsal aspect of the thumb, near the interphalangeal joint.

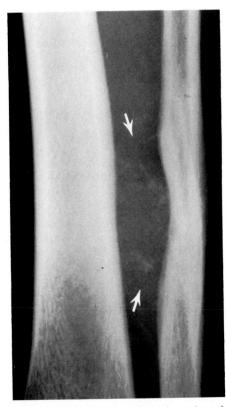

Figure 85–21. Chondrosarcoma. The radiograph reveals a soft tissue mass with calcification (arrows) between the tibia and fibula, with erosion of both bones. Note buttressing or thickening of the outer aspect of the fibula. The final diagnosis was mesenchymal chondrosarcoma. (Courtesy of R. Freiberger, M.D., New York, New York, and J. Kaye, M.D., New York, New York.)

of the body (Fig. 85–23), grow slowly, and rarely undergo malignant degeneration.

The detection of localized neurofibromas or neurilemomas by conventional radiography is difficult unless they are calcified or affect adjacent bones. The occurrence of a widened intervertebral foramen, however, is a well-recognized manifestation of dumbbell-shaped lesions extending between the spinal canal and posterior mediastinum (Fig. 85–24), but it is a finding that can relate also to a tortuous or enlarged vertebral artery, congenital absence of a pedicle, dermoids, teratomas, and hypertrophic interstitial polyneuritis (Déjèrine-Sottas syndrome). Computed tomography and magnetic resonance imaging represent more effective means of delineating the lesions (Fig. 85–25) and their relationship to surrounding structures. The tumors usually are well defined, with low attenuation values that may increase slightly after the administration of intravenous contrast material. A similar computed tomographic appearance may be evident in neurofibrosarcomas, however.

The *malignant schwannoma* is the major malignancy of the peripheral nerves. It may occur as an isolated phenomenon or, in less than 50 per cent of cases, with neurofibromatosis. Malignant schwannomas are seen in young and middle-aged men and women, appearing as enlarging masses, principally in the trunk and proximal portions of the extremities, in association with the sciatic nerve and brachial and sacral plexuses. Pain and neurologic manifestations are variable in frequency and intensity.

Other Tumors

Clear cell sarcomas are malignant neoplasms that arise in the vicinity of tendons and aponeuroses of the upper and lower extremities, especially in the region of the foot and ankle. Most patients are young adults. A slowly enlarging mass is typical. Radiographs reveal the mass, the usual absence of calcification, and, rarely, the presence of bone erosion. Frequent tumor recurrences and distant metastasis underscore the poor prognosis of this tumor.

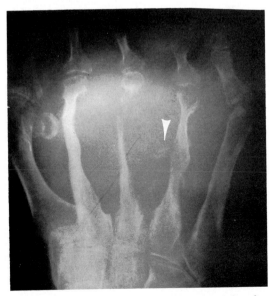

Figure 85–22. Synovial sarcoma. Observe the pressure erosion of multiple metatarsal shafts with fracture and soft tissue calcification (arrowhead).

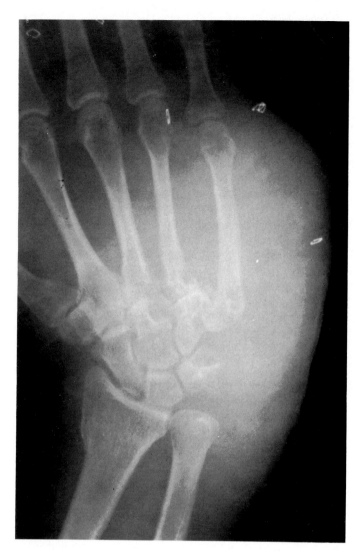

Figure 85–23. Neurofibroma. In this man with neurofibromatosis, a neurofibroma in the hand has led to an impressive soft tissue mass with erosion of the triquetrum, pisiform, hamate, capitate, and bases of the third to fifth metacarpals. Small osteolytic lesions are present in the distal portion of the radius. Soft tissue staples are also seen.

An *alveolar soft part sarcoma* (malignant granular cell myoblastoma) is usually found in muscles but may also appear in the orbit, retroperitoneum, and elsewhere, in both children and adults. The tumor grows slowly, may invade the underlying bone, and eventually may metastasize widely.

An *epithelioid sarcoma* is a rare neoplasm arising principally in the fingers, hands, and forearms of young adults. Malignant lymphoid and reticuloendothelial tumors such as *lymphoma, Ewing's sarcoma,* and *extraosseous plasmacytoma* rarely arise in the soft tissues. *Malignant melanoma* (melanosarcoma) can arise from the skin and produce local and distant osseous destruction (see Chapter 80).

Metastases

Soft tissue metastatic deposits can accompany a variety of primary malignant neoplasms. In general, a nonspecific soft tissue mass is produced. The underlying bone can be eroded.

Radiographic Approach

Considering the large number of soft tissue neoplasms, it is not surprising that the accurate preoperative radiographic diagnosis of the type of tumor is frequently impossible. Assessment of radiographic criteria, however, may allow differentiation of a neoplastic from a non-neoplastic disorder, and a benign from a malignant process (Table 85–2).

TUMOR SIZE AND RATE OF GROWTH. The actual size of a mass provides little information about its nature. There is a tendency, however, for malignant tumors to be larger than benign ones. More significantly, serial films will allow assessment of the rate of growth. Very rapid enlargement of a mass can indicate hemorrhage, inflammation, or perhaps a malignant neoplasm but is not characteristic of a benign tumor. Conversely, absent or slow growth is typical of benign neoplasm.

TUMOR SHAPE. As with tumor size, the amount of diagnostic information provided by the shape of the lesion is limited. Round masses more frequently are benign, whereas irregularly shaped masses more commonly are malignant.

TUMOR LOCATION AND NUMBER. Some of the characteristic tendencies of tumors to involve certain sites include the predilection of specific fibromatoses to involve the hands and the feet, of xanthomatoses to affect tendons about

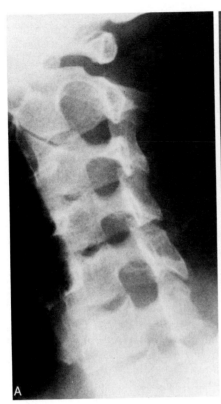

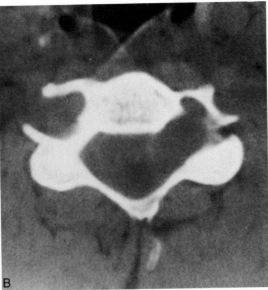

Figure 85–24. Neurofibromatosis. Enlargement of the neural foramina in the cervical spine is well shown by both conventional radiography (A) and computed tomography (B). (Courtesy of V. Vint, M.D., San Diego, California.)

the hands, elbows, and heels, and of synovial sarcomas to appear in the thighs or lower extremities. Deep masses more typically are malignant in nature.

Certain masses are frequently multiple, including neurofibromas and other neurogenic tumors, Kaposi's sarcomas, lipomas, and even metastases.

TUMOR RADIODENSITY. Lipomas produce radiolucent masses; liposarcomas are less radiolucent and, when poorly differentiated, may contain few if any lucent zones. Most of the other soft tissue neoplasms are of approximately the same radiodensity as the adjacent tissue unless they contain zones of calcification or ossification. The precise density of any such neoplasm is better delineated with computed tomography than with conventional radiography.

TUMOR CALCIFICATION OR OSSIFICATION. Calcification may appear in benign or malignant neoplasms as well as in non-neoplastic masses. Of the benign neoplasms, hemangiomas may reveal typical circular calcifications with lucent centers (phleboliths), whereas other tumors may be associated with circumscribed peripheral calcific collections (e.g., myxoma, xanthoma, hamartoma, lipoma) or foci of sand-like calcification (pilomatrixoma). Malignant neoplasms can lead to necrosis and hemorrhage, with secondary calcification. Such deposits are seen in synovial sarcomas, malignant histiocytomas, and rhabdomyosarcomas.

Extraskeletal chondrosarcomas or osteosarcomas may show irregular, poorly marginated calcific and ossific deposits that differ from the other patterns of calcification. The resulting deposits must be differentiated from non-neoplastic ossifying processes of soft tissue, such as myositis ossificans traumatica, and lipomas.

TUMOR INTERFACE (FIG. 85–26). Benign neoplasms characteristically are sharply demarcated, and the surrounding tissue planes are displaced but not obliterated. Malignant neoplasms can result in similar changes, however, although

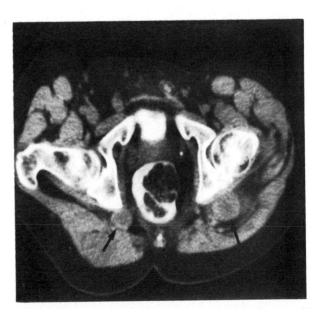

Figure 85–25. Neurofibromatosis. The transaxial computed tomographic scan reveals bilateral neurofibromas of the sciatic nerve (arrows). (From Lanzieri CF, Hilal SK: Computed tomography of the sacral plexus and sciatic nerve in the greater sciatic foramen. AJR 143:165, 1984, Copyright 1984, American Roentgen Ray Society. Used with permission.)

Table 85–2. RADIOGRAPHIC CHARACTERISTICS OF BENIGN AND MALIGNANT SOFT TISSUE TUMORS

	Benign Tumor	Malignant Tumor
Size	Variable	Variable
Rate of growth	Slow	Rapid*
Number	Single or multiple†	Single or multiple‡
Radiodensity	Vary from lucent (lipoma) to soft tissue density	Soft tissue density
Calcification or ossification	Possible§	Possible‖
Tumor interface	Sharply demarcated	Poorly or sharply demarcated¶
Osseous involvement	Smooth pressure erosion with or without sclerosis	Smooth pressure erosion without sclerosis; cortical osteolysis due to hyperemia; cortical invasion

*Rapid growth can also indicate hemorrhage or infection.
†Examples of multiple lesions are lipomas, fibromas, hemangiomas, neurogenic tumors.
‡Examples of multiple lesions are metastases, Kaposi's sarcomas.
§Examples of calcifying tumors are hemangiomas, xanthomas, myxomas, lipomas, pilomatrixomas, chondromas.
‖Examples of calcifying or ossifying tumors are synovial sarcomas, rhabdomyosarcomas, malignant histiocytomas, chondrosarcomas, osteosarcomas.
¶Infection can also produce indistinctness of mass outline.

distortion and blurring of part of the interface between neoplasm and soft tissues can be seen in some cases. In inflammatory conditions, the entire interface may be obscured owing to fluid infiltration into the adjacent soft tissues.

OSSEOUS INVOLVEMENT (FIG. 85–27). Smooth resorption of cortical bone is more indicative of the proximity of a soft tissue process to subjacent bone than of its nature. Thus, benign and malignant neoplasms arising near bone can both produce pressure scalloping of the periosteal surface. The presence of sclerosis about the osseous defect suggests a slowly evolving process and is more typical of benign neoplasm; the absence of such bone formation is suggestive but not diagnostic of malignancy. The presence of irregular

cortical destruction with or without medullary involvement is strongly indicative of a malignancy or infection.

Cortical hyperostosis subjacent to a soft tissue tumor usually implies a slow-growing process and should not be misinterpreted as bone invasion. The finding is most characteristic of lipomas but is observed in other neoplasms as well.

In the presence of a soft tissue mass and osseous abnormality, it may be difficult to differentiate a primary soft tissue tumor with osseous invasion from a bone tumor with soft tissue extension. In general, the site of more extensive abnormality (bone versus soft tissue) represents the initial focus of the process. Some osseous conditions, such as metastatic disease (thyroid, renal, bronchogenic, and prostatic

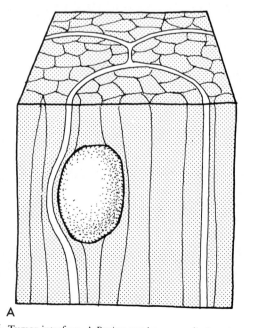 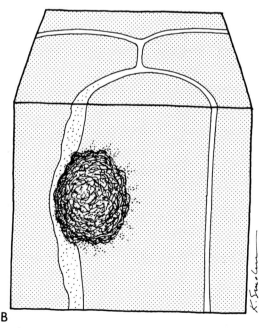

A   B

Figure 85–26. Tumor interface. A Benign neoplasms may displace tissue planes, but the planes are not obliterated. The tumors are frequently well defined or marginated. B Malignant neoplasms can distort and obscure portions of the tissue planes. A poorly defined or irregular tumor outline can be seen.

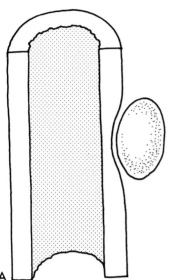
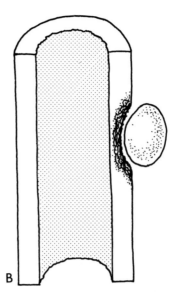
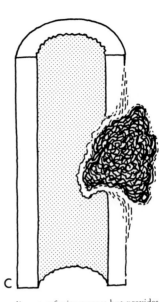

Figure 85–27. Osseous involvement. A Smooth resorption of the cortical surface of a bone indicates the presence of an adjacent soft tissue mass but provides little information regarding its benign or malignant nature. **B** Cortical resorption associated with reactive sclerosis suggests a slowly evolving process and is more compatible with a benign neoplasm. **C** Irregular cortical destruction with medullary involvement and periostitis is strongly indicative of a malignancy or infection.

carcinomas) and plasma cell myeloma, however, may produce extraordinary soft tissue components with minor bone destruction. The detection of a large soft tissue mass and resorption or destruction of more than one bone usually indicates the presence of a primary extraosseous neoplasm.

SOFT TISSUE CALCIFICATION AND OSSIFICATION

The radiographic detection of calcification and ossification in the soft tissues provides an important clue to proper diagnosis. Although it is certainly helpful to distinguish between calcific and ossific radiodense lesions, this is not always possible. The documentation of ossification depends on the recognition of a trabecular pattern within the dense areas, a pattern that is identified more easily when large ossific masses are encountered. Calcification appears as radiodense areas that do not possess trabecular or cortical structure.

Calcification

Conditions that lead to deposition of calcium within soft tissues can be classified into three types: metastatic calcification related to a disturbance in calcium or phosphorus metabolism; calcinosis due to the deposition of calcium in

Table 85–3. SOME CONDITIONS CAUSING CALCIFICATION OF SOFT TISSUES

Metastatic Calcification
   Hyperparathyroidism
   Hypoparathyroidism
   Renal osteodystrophy
   Hypervitaminosis D
   Milk-alkali syndrome
   Sarcoidosis
   Processes causing massive bone destruction (metastasis, plasma cell myeloma, leukemia)

Generalized Calcinosis
   Collagen disorders
   Idiopathic tumoral calcinosis
   Idiopathic calcinosis universalis

Dystrophic Calcification
   Neoplasms
   Inflammatory conditions
   Traumatic conditions

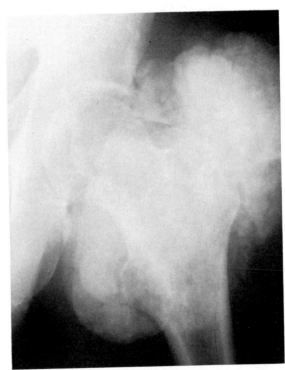

Figure 85–28. Metastatic soft tissue calcification. In renal osteodystrophy, massive periarticular calcified collections are encountered. (Courtesy of T. Broderick, M.D., Orange, California.)

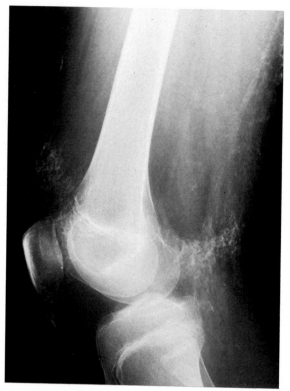

Figure 85–29. Generalized soft tissue calcinosis. A reticular pattern of soft tissue calcification is characteristic of dermatomyositis.

skin and subcutaneous tissue in the presence of normal calcium metabolism; and dystrophic calcification related to calcium deposits in damaged tissue in the absence of a generalized metabolic derangement. Table 85–3 lists common causes of each of these types. Figures 85–28 to 85–30 illustrate examples of soft tissue calcification in renal osteodystrophy, in dermatomyositis, and after trauma.

The terms calcinosis universalis, tumoral calcinosis, and calcinosis circumscripta should be regarded as descriptive designations for widespread, mass-like, or localized calcific deposits, respectively, not as a single disease entity. Thus, "universal," "tumoral," or "circumscribed" deposits can accompany several disorders or appear on an idiopathic basis.

In some conditions, the radiographic characteristics of the calcification are relatively diagnostic. Circular or elliptical calcific collections with radiolucent centers may represent the phleboliths in hemangiomas or varicosities (Fig. 85–31), the calcified fatty deposits in Ehlers-Danlos syndrome (Fig. 85–32), or cysticercosis. A reticulated pattern of calcification is frequent in dermatomyositis (Fig. 85–29).

The site of calcification also provides a clue to the correct diagnosis. Table 85–4 lists examples of typical sites of calcification in specific diseases.

Many of the disorders leading to calcific deposits in the soft tissue are described in other sections of the book. Two additional entities are noted here.

IDIOPATHIC CALCINOSIS UNIVERSALIS. This rare disorder of unknown cause affects infants and children. The

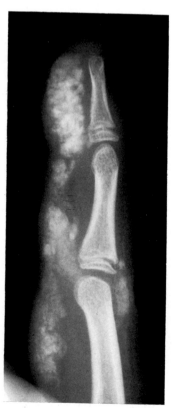

Figure 85–30. Dystrophic soft tissue calcification. Calcific deposits in the finger of this patient followed a local injury.

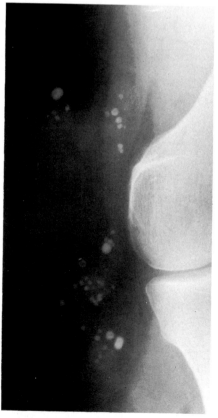

Figure 85–31. Hemangioma. Circular calcifications with lucent centers are typical of hemangiomas.

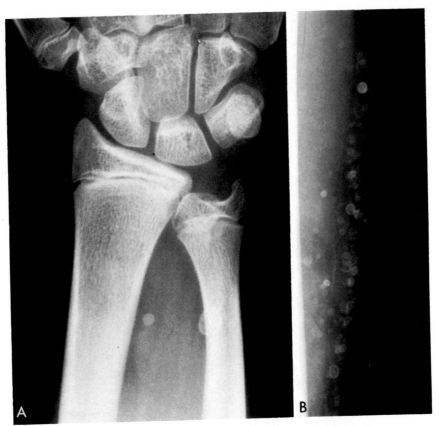

Figure 85–32. Ehlers-Danlos syndrome. Circular calcified fatty deposits with lucent centers can be seen in this syndrome. (Courtesy of M. Dalinka, M.D., Philadelphia, Pennsylvania.)

deposits initially appear in the subcutaneous fat of the extremities but subsequently involve muscles, ligaments, and tendons. Calcareous nodules coalesce, becoming large masses that may violate the skin. Internal organs are not affected. Serum calcium and phosphorus levels are normal. Radiographs reveal discrete conglomerations of calcium that are arranged in longitudinal bands (Fig. 85–33).

The major differential diagnoses are dermatomyositis, subcutaneous fat necrosis, extravasation of calcium gluconate injection solutions, and hyperparathyroidism.

IDIOPATHIC TUMORAL CALCINOSIS. Idiopathic tumoral calcinosis usually becomes manifest in the second and third decades of life. Men are affected more commonly than women, and blacks are especially susceptible. A family history is apparent in 30 to 40 per cent of cases. Firm, painless swellings are evident, especially about the hips, shoulders, and elbows.

Laboratory analysis usually indicates normal or slightly elevated levels of serum calcium and normal levels of alkaline phosphatase. The observation in some persons of slightly raised urinary levels of hydroxyproline and hyperphosphatemia has suggested that the disorder may be an inborn error of phosphorus metabolism.

Radiographs reveal well-demarcated masses of calcium about articulations (Fig. 85–34). Radiolucent linear bands separate the calcific foci. The individual lesions vary from 1 to 20 cm in diameter and may reveal fluid levels on erect, decubitus, or cross-table radiographs. These levels also are evident in other disorders associated with large soft tissue calcific collections. Radionuclide studies with technetium compounds may outline increased accumulation in areas of

Table 85–4. TYPICAL SITES OF SOFT TISSUE CALCIFICATION

Site	Diseases
Periarticular locations	Hyperparathyroidism Renal osteodystrophy Milk-alkali syndrome Hypervitaminosis D Collagen disorders
Tendons and bursae	Calcium hydroxyapatite crystal deposition disease Calcium pyrophosphate dihydrate crystal deposition disease
Lymph nodes	Granulomatous infections
Arteries	Renal osteodystrophy Diabetes mellitus Hypervitaminosis D
Nerves	Leprosy
Cartilage	Idiopathic calcium pyrophosphate dihydrate crystal deposition disease Hemochromatosis Hyperparathyroidism Other crystal deposition diseases
Intervertebral discs	Alkaptonuria Idiopathic calcium pyrophosphate dihydrate crystal deposition disease Hyperparathyroidism Immobilization Trauma
Fingertips	Scleroderma Other collagen disorders
Pinna of ear	Endocrine disorders Thermal or physical trauma Perichondritis

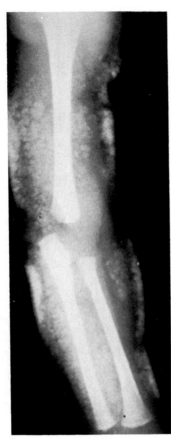

Figure 85–33. Calcinosis universalis (idiopathic). Longitudinal bands of calcification in the subcutaneous fat can be identified in this 3 month old male infant.

calcinosis. Analysis of the calcific material documents accumulations of calcium phosphate, calcium carbonate, or a mixture of these.

The diagnosis of idiopathic tumoral calcinosis is one of exclusion. Other processes, such as collagen disorders, hyper-

parathyroidism, hypervitaminosis D, milk-alkali syndrome, and chronic renal disease, must first be eliminated by clinical, laboratory, and radiologic examinations. The periarticular location of the calcifications in idiopathic tumoral calcinosis differs from the intraarticular radiodense deposits of idiopathic synovial (osteo)chondromatosis and calcium pyrophosphate dihydrate crystal deposition disease.

Ossification

The disorders leading to ossification of soft tissues are more limited in number than those producing soft tissue calcification (Table 85–5). Heterotopic ossification appears in association with neurologic disorders (see Chapter 68), thermal burns (see Chapter 63), and venous insufficiency (see Chapter 83). Ossification appearing in scars creates plaque-like radiodense areas, especially on abdominal radiographs. Osteosarcoma and other sarcomas of soft tissue represent additional causes of ossification. Metastases to soft tissues also may ossify.

Radiographs usually outline definite trabecular structure within the ossific collections, allowing differentiation of ossification from calcification. Serial radiographs may permit assessment of the maturity of the ossific deposit. Such an assessment is important, as removal of heterotopic bone prior to maturity in cases of burn or paraplegia may be followed by reaccumulation of the deposits. Serial radionuclide studies may be more accurate in this regard.

OSSIFICATION OF TENDONS AND LIGAMENTS. Although calcific tendinitis is common (see Chapters 40 and 41), ossification within tendons is relatively rare. Posttraumatic calcification and ossification of the medial collateral ligament of the knee (Pellegrini-Stieda syndrome) appears adjacent to the medial femoral condyle (Fig. 85–35). Ossification of the Achilles tendon has also been recognized. Calcification or ossification in the stylohyoid ligament is a frequent, incidental radiographic finding, although when excessive, a specific syndrome (termed the Eagle syndrome) may occur, leading to dysphagia, a "lump" in the throat, and pain.

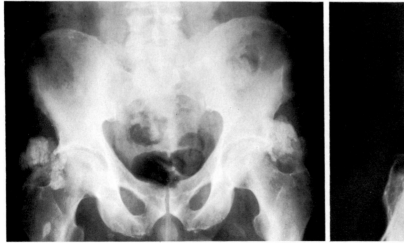
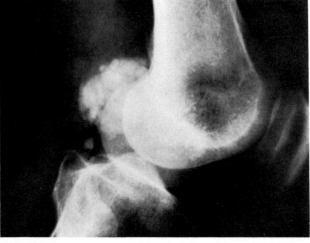

A   B

Figure 85–34. Tumoral calcinosis (idiopathic). Deposits of calcification are evident about the hips, the ischial tuberosities, and the knee. The joint spaces are normal. (From Brown ML, et al: Radiography and scintigraphy in tumoral calcinosis. Radiology 124:757, 1977. Used with permission.)

Table 85–5. SOME CAUSES OF SOFT TISSUE OSSIFICATION

Neurologic diseases
Physical and thermal injuries
Venous insufficiency
Neoplasms (e.g., parosteal osteosarcoma, extraskeletal
    osteosarcoma)
Pseudomalignant osseous tumor of soft tissue
Myositis (fibrodysplasia) ossificans progressiva
Melorheostosis
Surgical scars
Postoperative period

MYOSITIS OSSIFICANS TRAUMATICA. Sixty to 75 per cent of patients with localized soft tissue ossifications relate a clear history of trauma. The spontaneous cases are termed pseudomalignant osseous tumor of soft tissue (see discussion later in this chapter). The radiographic and pathologic features of myositis ossificans traumatica and pseudo-malignant osseous tumor of soft tissue are virtually identical. The designation "myositis ossificans" for these conditions, however, is not entirely accurate owing to the absence of inflammation as well as muscular involvement in some cases. Ossification may result from damage to the interstitium, not to the muscle.

Myositis ossificans traumatica usually appears in adolescents or young adults. The sites of localization are areas susceptible to injury, such as the elbow (Fig. 85–36), the thigh, the buttocks, and, less often, the shoulder and the calf. Shortly after injury, a soft tissue mass becomes apparent, which may be associated with periosteal reaction in 7 to 10 days. Flocculent dense lesions arise in the mass from 11 days to 6 weeks after the trauma. The calcific dense areas gradually enlarge, and at 6 to 8 weeks a lacy pattern of new bone is sharply circumscribed about the periphery of the mass. In some cases, an enlarging central cavity combined with peripheral ossification resembles an eggshell. Maturity is reached

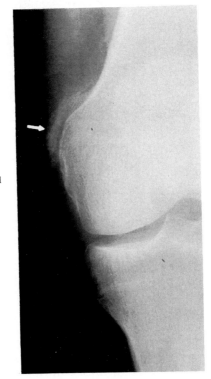

Figure 85–35. Pellegrini-Stieda syndrome. Note posttraumatic ossification (arrow) in the medial collateral ligament of the knee.

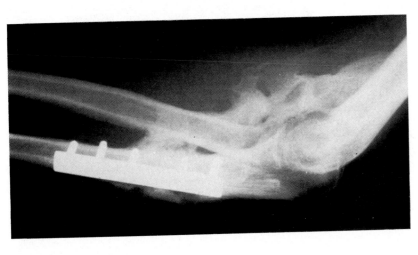

Figure 85–36. Myositis ossificans traumatica: Elbow. Heterotopic bone formation occurring after elbow injuries is a well-recognized finding.

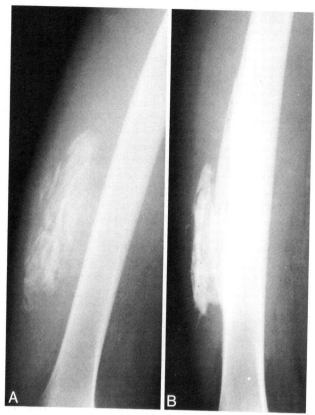

Figure 85–37. Myositis ossificans traumatica: Maturing ossification. Lateral radiographs of the femur 1 month (**A**) and 5 months (**B**) after an injury show maturation of the ossifying process. Initially separated from the bone, the process subsequently merges with the anterior femoral surface. (Courtesy of G. Greenway, M.D., Dallas, Texas.)

lignant" nature of the central portion of the lesion. Myositis ossificans must be differentiated from parosteal osteosarcoma, periosteal osteosarcoma, extraskeletal (soft tissue) osteosarcoma or chondrosarcoma, osteochondroma, and osteoma (see Chapter 78). *Parosteal osteosarcomas* arise in the metaphysis of tubular bones, especially along the posterior aspect of the distal part of the femur (Fig. 85–40). Although a lucent zone may exist between the tumor and underlying bone, the zone is usually incomplete. Furthermore, a parosteal osteosarcoma is more heavily calcified in its central portion and base of attachment; the periphery is less dense and poorly circumscribed. *Periosteal osteosarcomas* arise in the cortex of the diaphysis of a tubular bone and lead to cortical thickening and a spiculated osteoid matrix. An *osteochondroma* arises from and is connected to the subjacent bone. An *osteoma* is an osseous excrescence extending from the outer surface of the cortex.

PSEUDOMALIGNANT OSSEOUS TUMOR OF SOFT TISSUE. These lesions appear in men and women who do not relate a history of antecedent trauma. They are well circumscribed and compatible with long-term survival. Most patients are in the second and third decades of life and most lesions are located in the extremities or the gluteal regions (Fig. 85–41). Soft tissue swelling with or without pain precedes the appearance of calcification and ossification by a short interval of approximately 2 to 3 weeks. Radiographs reveal a well-circumscribed ossifying mass, with a dense periphery and lucent center. Periostitis may be identified. In some cases, the lesions have become smaller or disappeared. The histologic characteristics resemble those in myositis ossificans traumatica. The major significance of pseudomalignant osseous tumor of soft tissue is the fact that it must be distinguished from malignant processes.

in 5 to 6 months (Figs. 85–37 and 85–38), and the mass then shrinks.

The recognition of a peripheral rim of calcification and ossification about a more lucent center cannot be overemphasized as an important radiographic manifestation of myositis ossificans (Fig. 85–38). Furthermore, a radiolucent band or zone between the lesion and the subjacent cortex is also a very important finding, reflecting the lack of intimacy between the ossified mass and neighboring bone, and allowing differentiation of myositis ossificans from parosteal osteosarcoma (see discussion later in this chapter).

Histologically, the developing lesion demonstrates three distinct zones. The center of the lesion contains proliferating fibroblasts with areas of hemorrhage and necrosis. A middle zone contains osteoblasts with islands of immature bone. Biopsy of cellular inner and middle layers alone may result in an erroneous diagnosis of a sarcoma. It is the outer zone of the lesion that reveals the true benign nature of the process. In this region, mature trabeculae are clearly demarcated from the surrounding connective tissue. Thus, a peripheral shell of maturing bone exists about a soft cellular center, and maturation proceeds in a centrifugal fashion with the center layer being the last to ossify.

Identification of myositis ossificans is usually possible on the basis of the clinical and radiologic findings (Fig. 85–39). The pathologist, however, must be wary of the "pseudoma-

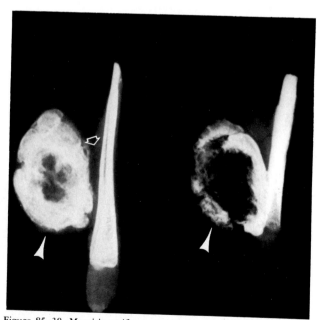

Figure 85–38. Myositis ossificans traumatica: Radiographic-pathologic correlation. Serial sections through a focus of myositis ossificans delineate a well-encapsulated lesion possessing a peripheral zone of ossification and a lucent center (arrowheads). Note the separation or clear zone (open arrow) between the lesion and the underlying bone. (Courtesy of A. Norman, M.D., New York, New York.)

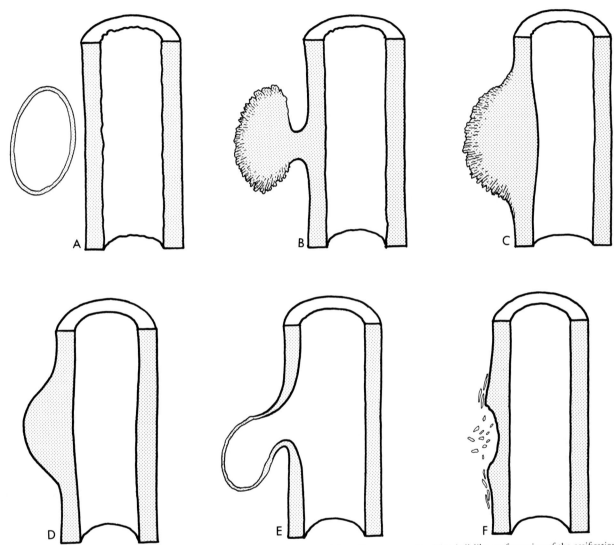

Figure 85–39. Myositis ossificans traumatica: Differential diagnosis. A Myositis ossificans traumatica. The shell-like configuration of the ossification with a clear zone between it and the underlying bone is typical of this condition. **B** Parosteal osteosarcoma. These lesions appear as central ossifying foci with irregular outlines and may be connected to the underlying bone by a stalk. **C** Periosteal osteosarcoma. These tumors arise in the cortex of the diaphysis of a tubular bone and produce cortical thickening and spiculated osteoid matrix. **D** Osteoma. Characteristic of this lesion is a localized excrescence that produces bulging of the cortical contour. **E** Osteochondroma. An exostosis protrudes from the cortical surface. Its medullary and cortical bone is continuous with that of the underlying osseous structure. **F** Juxtacortical (periosteal) chondroma. These periosteal lesions produce localized excavation of the cortex with periostitis. They may contain calcification.

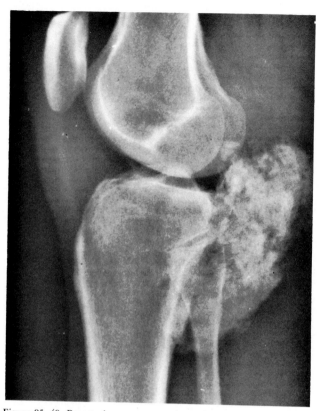

Figure 85–40. Parosteal osteosarcoma. An ossified rectangular mass arises from the posterior aspect of the proximal tibia. (Courtesy of J. Smith, M.D., New York, New York.)

FLORID REACTIVE PERIOSTITIS. This term is used to describe exuberant periosteal bone formation in the hands or, less commonly, the feet in association with local soft tissue swelling, pain, tenderness, or redness that is of weeks to years in duration. A history of trauma to the affected area may or may not be evident. Involvement of one of the proximal or middle phalanges predominates. A soft tissue mass containing calcification or ossification commonly dominates the radiographic findings and may occur prior to the development of osseous abnormality. The latter consists typically of periosteal reaction and, rarely, of cortical erosion or destruction (Fig. 85–42). These radiologic alterations are compatible with those of myositis ossificans or pseudomalignant osseous tumor of soft tissue. Although simulating in some respects a malignant neoplasm, the histologic features of reactive periostitis lack cellular pleomorphism or atypical mitotic figures. Local excision generally is adequate.

MYOSITIS OSSIFICANS PROGRESSIVA (FIBRO-DYSPLASIA OSSIFICANS PROGRESSIVA). Myositis ossificans progressiva is a rare disorder of mesodermal tissue in which inflammatory foci initially appear and proliferate in fibrous tissue. It is discussed in Chapter 73.

SOFT TISSUE BANDS AND CONTRACTURES

Amniotic (or Streeter's) constriction bands can affect any portion of a limb, but most frequently they involve the fingers. Their cause is debated, although it has been postulated that premature rupture of the fetal amnion without injury to the chorion can produce raw surfaces and strings that attach to and mechanically entrap the limb, leading to rings and

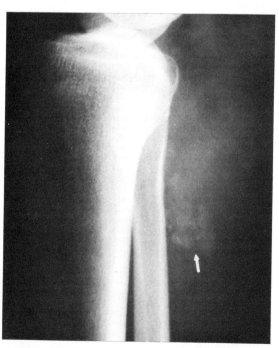

Figure 85–41. Pseudomalignant osseous tumor of soft tissue. Observe the mass containing peripheral ossification (arrow). (Courtesy of V. Vint, M.D., San Diego, California.)

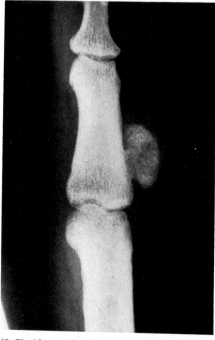

Figure 85–42. Florid reactive periostitis. Note a soft tissue mass containing considerable ossification. It appears to be attached to the phalanx by a stalk. (From Porter AR, et al: Florid reactive periostitis of the phalanges. AJR 144:617, 1985. Copyright 1985, American Roentgen Ray Society. Used with permission.)

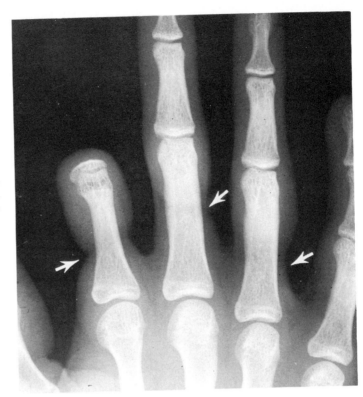

Figure 85–43. Amniotic (Streeter's) constriction bands. Soft tissue constrictions can be seen (arrows), and there has been an amputation of a portion of the second digit. (Courtesy of J. Slivka, M.D., San Diego, California.)

amputations. The frequency of such bands is variously recorded as 1 in 5000 to 1 in 45,000 births. The cases are sporadic, as no familial history has been noted. Many of the patients are products of first pregnancies and of young mothers with bleeding episodes in the third trimester of pregnancy. Common associated anomalies are clubbed feet and cleft lip and palate. On clinical examination, scarred rings are found to encircle a digit or limb. Symmetrically distributed lesions are typical. Radiographs delineate the soft tissue constrictions that may contact the subjacent bone. The underlying bones may be poorly developed, and distal to the lesions, calcification, lymphedema, or fatty accumulation may be encountered. Syndactyly or amputation can also be evident (Fig. 85–43).

Soft tissue contractures can accompany many congenital disorders, such as arthrogryposis multiplex congenita and contractural arachnodactyly; acquired conditions, such as Volkmann's ischemic contracture, thermal burns, and neurologic injury; and various rheumatologic diseases. Additional well-known examples in the hand are Dupuytren's contracture of the palmar fascia (Fig. 85–44); camptodactyly, in which a flexion contracture involves predominantly the proximal interphalangeal articulation of the fifth digit; clinodactyly, in which a curvature of a finger occurs in a mediolateral plane; and Kirner's deformity, in which palmar bending of the shaft of a terminal phalanx may be associated with epiphyseal separation. One additional example is the appearance of contracted and deformed soft tissues and bones associated with the former Chinese custom of binding women's feet. Another example is the popliteal pterygium syndrome, consisting of a popliteal web extending from the ischium to the heel, deformities of the foot and toes, toenail dysplasia, flexion contracture of the knee, and cleft palate.

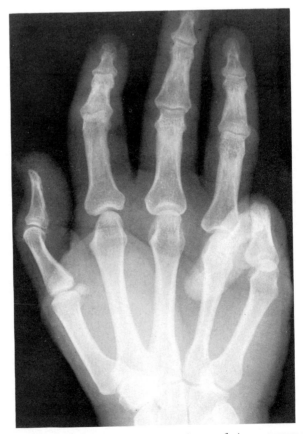

Figure 85–44. Dupuytren's contracture. A severe flexion contracture is evident in the fifth finger with minor changes in the other digits.

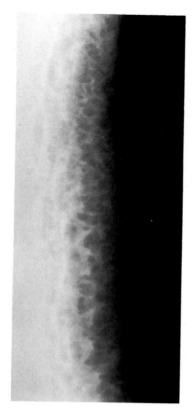

Figure 85–45. Lymphedema. A coned-down view delineates the reticular soft tissue pattern.

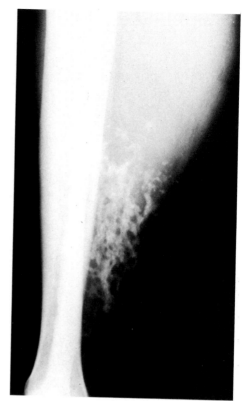

Figure 85–46. Edema: Soft tissue ossification. Venous insufficiency has produced a branching pattern of coarse ossification. (Courtesy of M. Nadel, M.D., Los Angeles, California.)

SOFT TISSUE EDEMA

Traumatic or inflammatory processes can lead to localized soft tissue edema. In addition, venous or lymphatic obstruction from many diverse causes may produce edema that is recognized radiographically as enlargement of the soft tissue contour, obliteration of the fascial planes, and a fine or coarsened reticular pattern (Fig. 85–45). Soft tissue calcifi-

cation or ossification may accompany the process (Fig. 85–46). Lymphedema may result from congenital disorders, trauma, infection (filariasis), irradiation, tumor, surgery, thyroid acropachy, melorheostosis, infantile cortical hyperostosis, and acromegaly. Lymphangiosarcomas may occur in areas of long-term lymphedema.

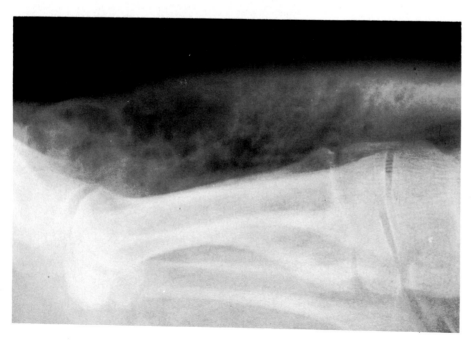

Figure 85–47. Soft tissue emphysema. Bubbly radiolucent soft tissue collections are not infrequent in diabetic patients with soft tissue infection.

SOFT TISSUE EMPHYSEMA

Collections of gas in the soft tissues can be caused by several mechanisms. Air can be introduced iatrogenically into the soft tissues or joints during puncture for diagnostic or therapeutic purposes. Air can also penetrate the soft tissues in cases of sinus tracts. Gas formation by bacteria such as Clostridium may lead to radiolucent streaks or bubbles in the subcutaneous or muscular tissues (see Chapters 59 and 61). This is not infrequent in diabetic patients (Fig. 85–47).

SOFT TISSUE FOREIGN BODIES

A variety of foreign bodies may become embedded or localize in the body's soft tissues owing to accidental or occupational trauma, surgical procedures (needles, sponges), or other causes. Metallic fragments resulting from various missiles are easily detected on routine radiographs. The identification of particles or fragments of glass or wood, two substances commonly associated with accidental injury, is more difficult.

Glass and Wood

The delineation of glass particles by conventional radiography depends on their size and orientation, their precise anatomic location (thick versus thin body parts), the nature of the surrounding tissue, and the specific radiographic technique (type of film, kilovoltage) that is employed (Fig. 85–48A). Furthermore, the radiopacity of some types of glass (beer and wine bottles) is greater than that of others (light bulbs). Xeroradiography, ultrasonography, and computed tomography can be helpful in defining small pieces of glass (as well as plastic) embedded in the soft tissues.

The difficulties encountered in the delineation of foreign bodies composed of wood with standard radiography are well recognized. Early detection is important, as sequelae of retained wood particles include granulomatous reactions and secondary infections. Of the additional diagnostic techniques that are available, computed tomography and ultrasonography have been most successful in detecting wood fragments.

Plant Thorns

An inflammatory reaction in the soft tissue, bone, or articular cavity is a potential complication of implantation of various types of foreign bodies, including surgical sponges, glass particles, Dacron threads, and some of the materials used in arthroplasties (see Chapter 20). The reaction may appear soon after the introduction of the foreign material or years later. Date palm, sentinel palm, blackthorn, hawthorn, box thorn, bougainvillea, rose thorn, mesquite, and yucca are among the plants capable of eliciting such a reaction. Children are affected more frequently than adults. The extremities are usually involved, especially the hands and feet. Pain and soft tissue swelling become evident soon after the injury. Subsequently, a period of improvement in these manifestations is common, followed by the reappearance of symptoms and signs. The elapsed time between the injury and the surgical removal of the foreign body commonly is weeks or months and occasionally may be years. Operative and pathologic findings include a foreign body granuloma with giant cells or an abscess.

The radiographic features vary according to the site of granuloma formation (Fig. 85–48B). Most frequently, an articulation, tendon sheath, or bursa is affected. Rarely, the bone is the primary site of involvement; a well-circumscribed osteolytic lesion with periostitis and soft tissue swelling is typical. Tenosynovitis or bursitis leads to soft tissue swelling and periosteal reaction. Vegetable material may be identified in synovial tissues.

Granulomatous reactions following the introduction of

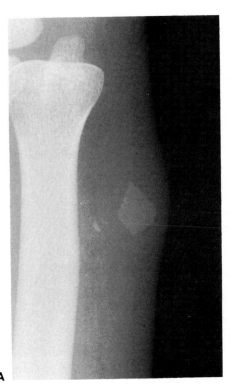
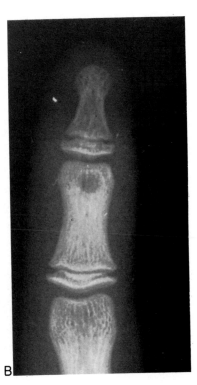

Figure 85–48. Foreign bodies. A Glass shards. Several radiopaque areas in the distal forearm represent pieces of glass. Note soft tissue swelling. B Plant thorn. Osteolytic lesions may relate to embedded plant thorns. (B, Courtesy of G. Greenway, M.D., Dallas, Texas.)

A

B

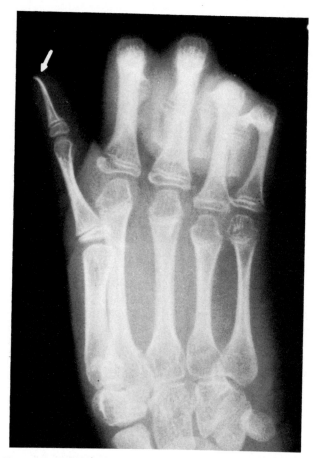

Figure 85–49. Epidermolysis bullosa. Observe contractures of the interphalangeal articulations, webbing between the digits, skin and bone atrophy, osteoporosis, epiphyseal deformity, and pointing of the terminal tufts of the phalanges, most evident in the thumb (arrow).

plant thorns appear to relate to a component of the thorn itself or a surface contaminant. Surgical removal of the thorn is required for reversal of the process.

A similar granulomatous reaction of the soft tissues, synovial membrane, or bone has been observed after puncture wounds by the spines of a variety of sea urchins.

SOFT TISSUE ATROPHY

Diffuse atrophy of soft tissue, including fat and muscle, is an accompaniment of chronic debilitating illnesses, lipoatrophic diabetes, and malnutrition. Localized atrophy of soft tissue is evident in many different types of disorders, including collagen diseases, prolonged disuse or immobilization of an extremity, thermal injury, and inflammatory or occlusive vascular processes.

Muscle atrophy (or rarely hypertrophy) occurs in certain neuromuscular disorders (see Chapter 68) and inflammatory conditions.

SOFT TISSUE HYPERTROPHY

Overgrowth of soft tissue alone or in combination with osseous enlargement may occur in a generalized or localized distribution. Generalized hypertrophy is a fundamental part of pituitary gigantism and acromegaly (see Chapter 50) but is also encountered in cerebral gigantism. Hemihypertrophy, representing overgrowth of one half or one side of the body, may occur on an idiopathic basis or in association with neurocutaneous syndromes (neurofibromatosis, tuberous sclerosis, Sturge-Weber disease, Lindau–von Hippel disease), the Beckwith-Weidemann syndrome, or skin and vascular abnormalities (angiodysplasias, lymphatic abnormalities, lipomatosis). Additional alterations associated with idiopathic congenital hemihypertrophy include a variety of tumors (especially Wilms' tumor, adrenocortical tumors, and hepatoblastoma) and renal abnormalities (nephromegaly and medullary sponge kidney).

Macrodactyly represents an increase in the size of all the structures (bones, tendons, nerves, vessels, subcutaneous fat, skin) in one or more digits of the hands and feet. It occurs on an idiopathic basis and in association with hemangiomas, lymphangiomas, arteriovenous malformations, neurofibromatosis, and macrodystrophia lipomatosa.

SPECIAL SYNDROMES OF SKIN AND SOFT TISSUE
Epidermolysis Bullosa

This is a rare, inherited chronic skin disorder that results from poor adherence of the epidermis to the dermis, as a

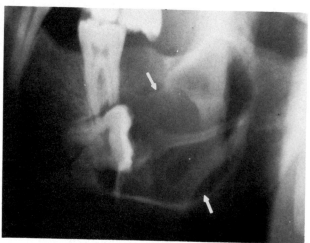

Figure 85–50. Nevoid basal cell carcinoma syndrome (Gorlin's syndrome): Mandibular abnormalities. Dentigerous cysts (arrows) are common in this syndrome.

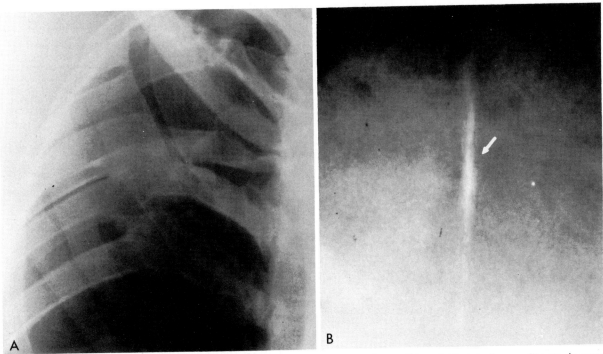

Figure 85–51. Nevoid basal cell carcinoma syndrome (Gorlin's syndrome): Other abnormalities. A Typical rib anomalies are demonstrated. **B** Calcification of the falx cerebri (arrow) is not unusual in this syndrome.

consequence of which vesicles, bullae, and ulcerations form either spontaneously or after minor traumatic insults. Radiographic findings vary with the type of disease that is present. Flexion contractures of the metacarpophalangeal and interphalangeal articulations, webbing between the fingers, and distal trophic changes can be encountered (Fig. 85–49). The terminal phalanges of the hands (and, less frequently, the feet) are pointed or wedged-shaped, resembling the findings in scleroderma. The combination of flexion deformities of the fingers and toes and webbing is important in the diagnosis of epidermolysis bullosa. Osteoporosis, slender diaphyses of the tubular bones, periapical abscesses, and esophageal strictures can be seen.

Nevoid Basal Cell Carcinoma Syndrome (Gorlin's Syndrome)

Nevoid basal cell carcinoma syndrome is an inherited disorder that is characterized by multiple basal cell carcinomas, palmar pits, odontogenic keratocysts, rib and spine anomalies, brachydactyly, and various neurologic and ophthalmologic abnormalities. The disorder is inherited in an autosomal dominant pattern and appears with equal frequency in both sexes.

Basal cell epitheliomas usually are seen near puberty; typically affected sites are the face and trunk. Dentigerous cysts of the mandible (Fig. 85–50) may antedate the appearance of the skin lesions. Swelling, pain, and spontaneous drainage are seen. Mandibular cysts can be single or multiple, are located predominantly at the angle of the jaw, and appear as radiolucent lesions with poorly defined margins.

The common rib anomalies are splaying, synostosis, and

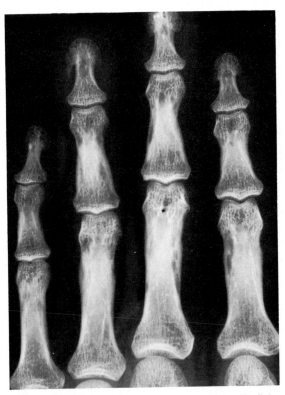

Figure 85–52. Nevoid basal cell carcinoma syndrome (Gorlin's syndrome): Cystic lesions of the hand. Note the flame-shaped configuration and eccentric location of many of the lucent lesions. (From Dunnick NR, et al: Nevoid basal cell carcinoma syndrome: Radiographic manifestations including cystlike lesions of the phalanges. Radiology 127:331, 1978. Used with permission.)

Table 85–6. CHARACTERISTICS OF THE VARYING PANNICULITIDES IN ADULTS

Condition	Clinical Features	Associated Conditions	Histopathologic Characteristics
Erythema nodosum	Tender erythematous nodules on lower extremities Fever Arthritis	Poststreptococcal infection Sarcoidosis Inflammatory bowel disease	Septal panniculitis (no vasculitis)
Subacute nodular migratory panniculitis	Painless nodules on lower leg Yellow centers Sclerodermoid changes	None	Septal panniculitis
Weber-Christian disease	Chronic, recurrent, tender, erythematous nodules Systemic symptoms of foot necrosis	Pancreatic disease Infections Autoimmune disorders	Lobular panniculitis Foam cells Fibrosis in late stages (no vasculitis)
Nodular vasculitis	Tender nodules or plaques on posterior aspect of lower legs	None	Lobular panniculitis with vasculitis
Erythema induratum	Nodules on posterior aspect of legs	Tuberculosis	Lobular panniculitis with vasculitis and caseation necrosis
Lupus panniculitis	Nodules on face, buttocks, arms Overlying scars	Discoid lupus erythematosus Systemic lupus erythematosus	Septal and lobular panniculitis
Connective tissue panniculitis	Erythematous, tender plaques and nodules Resolution with atrophy	Unclassified connective tissue disease	Lymphohistiocytic invasion of fat lobules with caseation (no vasculitis)
Cytophagic panniculitis	Erythematous, tender nodules Fever Oral ulcers Serositis	Lymphadenopathy Organomegaly Pancytopenia	Lobular panniculitis with fat necrosis and hemorrhage
Pancreatic panniculitis	Erythematous nodules	Pancreatitis Pancreatic malignancy	Lobular panniculitis with necrosis of lipocytes and ghost cells

From Thiers BH: Panniculitis. Dermatol Clinics North Am *1*:537, 1983. Used with permission.

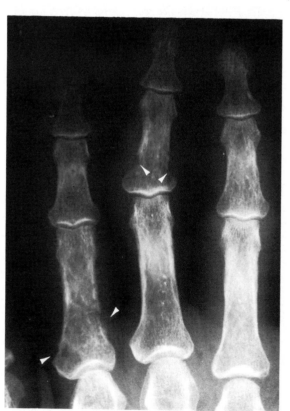

Figure 85–53. Pancreatic panniculitis. This man developed painful and tender erythematous soft tissue nodules as a result of pancreatic disease. The radiograph of one hand shows soft tissue swelling and osteolytic lesions with periostitis (arrowheads), consistent with fat necrosis. (Courtesy of R. Kerr, M.D., Los Angeles, California.)

bifid and cervical ribs (Fig. 85–51A). Shortening of the metacarpals, especially the fourth and fifth, is also a relatively common finding, similar to that which occurs in pseudohypoparathyroidism, multiple hereditary exostosis, and other conditions. Kyphoscoliosis, spina bifida occulta, block vertebrae, spondylolysis, spondylolisthesis, and hemivertebrae can be seen. Calcification of the falx cerebri (Fig. 85–51B), dura, tentorium, and choroid, partial agenesis of the corpus callosum, hypertelorism, and anosmia may occur. Mental retardation, congenital hydrocephalus, and ocular changes have been noted. Gonadal abnormalities include ovarian and uterine fibromas in the female and hypogonadism and cryptorchidism in the male.

Some reports have emphasized the occurrence of small, flame-shaped, cystic lucent areas in the phalanges and long tubular bones (Fig. 85–52). The lesions are multiple and frequently eccentric in location. The alterations may resemble those in sarcoidosis or tuberous sclerosis.

The presence of shortened metacarpals in as many as 50 per cent of patients with this syndrome, a finding that is also evident in pseudohypoparathyroidism and pseudopseudohypoparathyroidism, has raised the possibility of an association among these disorders.

Panniculitis and Related Syndromes

Panniculitides represent inflammatory disorders of subcutaneous fat. Although several distinct forms of panniculitis have been recognized (Table 85–6), clinical manifestations common to most forms include the presence of moderately tender nodules in the soft tissues. Some types of panniculitis may accompany inflammatory or neoplastic diseases of the pancreas (Fig. 85–53).

FURTHER READING

Abramowitz D, Zornoza J, Ayala AG, Romsdahl MM: Soft-tissue desmoid tumors: Radiographic bone changes. Radiology 146:11, 1983.

Alpert M: Roentgen manifestations of epidermolysis bullosa. AJR 78:66, 1957.

Barton DL, Reeves RJ: Tumoral calcinosis. Report of three cases and review of the literature. AJR 86:351, 1961.

Becker MH, Kopf AW, Lande A: Basal cell nevus syndrome: Its roentgenographic significance. Review of the literature and report of four cases. AJR 99:817, 1967.

Bliznak J, Staple TW: Radiology of angiodysplasias of the limb. Radiology 110:35, 1974.

Brinn LB, Khilnani MT: Epidermolysis bullosa with characteristic hard deformities. Radiology 89:272, 1967.

Brown ML, Thrall JH, Cooper RA, Kim YC: Radiography and scintigraphy in tumoral calcinosis. Radiology 124:757, 1977.

Carroll RE, Berman AT: Glomus tumors of the hand. Review of the literature and report on twenty-eight cases. J Bone Joint Surg [Am] 54:691, 1972.

Chew FS, Hudson TM, Enneking WF: Radionuclide imaging of soft tissue neoplasms. Semin Nucl Med 11:266, 1981.

Christopherson WM, Foote FW Jr, Stewart FW: Alveolar soft-part sarcomas. Structurally characteristic tumors of uncertain histogenesis. Cancer 5:100, 1952.

Demos TC, Bruno E, Armin A, Dabozi WR: Parosteal lipoma with enlarging osteochondroma. AJR 143:365, 1984.

Desai A, Eymontt M, Alavi A, Schaffer B, Dalinka MK: ^{99m}Tc-MDP uptake in nonosseous lesions. Radiology 135:181, 1980.

Drane WE: Myositis ossificans and the three-phase bone scan. AJR 142:179, 1984.

Dunnick NR, Head GL, Peck GL, Yoder FW: Nevoid basal cell carcinoma syndrome: Radiographic manifestations including cystlike lesions of the phalanges. Radiology 127:331, 1978.

Eagle WW: Elongated styloid process: Further observations and a new syndrome. Arch Otolaryngol 47:630, 1948.

Enzinger FM, Weiss SW: Soft Tissue Tumors. St Louis, CV Mosby Co, 1983.

Feldman F, Norman D: Intra- and extraosseous malignant histiocytoma (malignant fibrous xanthoma). Radiology 104:497, 1972.

Goldman AB: Myositis ossificans circumscripta: A benign lesion with a malignant differential diagnosis. AJR 126:32, 1976.

Gorlin RJ, Goltz RW: Multiple nevoid basal-cell epithelioma, jaw cysts, and bifid rib. A syndrome. N Engl J Med 262:908, 1960.

Greenfield GB, Rosado W, Rothbart F: Benign proliferative skin lesions causing destructive and resorptive bone changes. AJR 97:733, 1966.

Harris V, Ramamurphy RS, Pildes RS: Late onset of subcutaneous calcifications after intravenous injections of calcium gluconate. AJR 123:845, 1975.

Horowitz AL, Resnick D, Watson RC: The roentgen features of synovial sarcomas. Clin Radiol 24:481, 1973.

Kagan AR, Steckel RJ: Heterotopic new bone formation: Myositis ossificans versus malignant tumor. AJR 130:773, 1978.

Karasick D, O'Hara AE: Juvenile aponeurotic fibroma. A review and report of a case with osseous involvement. Radiology 123:725, 1977.

Karlin CA, De Smet AA, Neff J, Lin F, Horton W, Wertzberger JJ: The variable manifestations of extraarticular synovial chondromatosis. AJR 137:731, 1981.

Keller RB, Baez-Giangreco A: Juvenile aponeurotic fibroma. Report of three cases and a review of the literature. Clin Orthop 106:198, 1975.

Kolawole TM, Bohrer SP: Tumoral calcinosis with "fluid levels" in the tumoral masses. AJR 120:461, 1974.

Lagier R, Seigne JM, Mbakop A: Juxta-acetabular mucoid cyst in a patient with osteoarthritis of the hip secondary to dysplasia. Int Orthop (SICOT) 8:19, 1984.

Lile HA, Rogers JF, Gerald B: The basal cell nevus syndrome. AJR 103:214, 1968.

Mann SG: Kaposi's sarcoma. Experience with ten cases. AJR 121:793, 1974.

Martel W, Abell MR: Radiologic evaluation of soft tissue tumors. A retrospective study. Cancer 32:352, 1973.

McFarlane RM: The current status of Dupuytren's disease. J Hand Surg 8:703, 1983.

Moses JM, Flatt AE, Cooper RR: Annular constricting bands. J Bone Joint Surg [Am] 61:562, 1979.

Muheim G, Donath A, Rossier AB: Serial scintigrams in the course of ectopic bone formation in paraplegic patients. AJR 118:865, 1973.

Nakashima Y, Unni KK, Shives TC, Swee RG, Dahlin DC: Mesenchymal chondrosarcoma of bone and soft tissue. A review of 111 cases. Cancer 57:2444, 1986.

Norman A, Dorfman HD: Juxtacortical circumscribed myositis ossificans: Evolution and radiographic features. Radiology 96:301, 1970.

Ozonoff MB, Flynn FJ Jr: Roentgenologic features of dermatomyositis of childhood. AJR 118:206, 1973.

Petasnick JP, Turner DA, Charters JR, Gitelis S, Zacharias CE: Soft-tissue masses of the locomotor system: comparison of MR imaging with CT. Radiology 160:125, 1986.

Porter AR, Tristan TA, Rudy FR, Eshbach TB: Florid reactive periostitis of the phalanges. AJR 144:617, 1985.

Powers SK, Norman D, Edwards MSB: Computerized tomography of peripheral nerve lesions. J Neurosurg 59:131, 1983.

Poznanski AK, Pratt GB, Manson G, Weiss L: Clinodactyly, camptodactyly, Kirner's deformity and other crooked fingers. Radiology 93:573, 1969.

Radstone DJ, Revell PA, Mantell BS: Clear cell sarcoma of tendons and aponeuroses treated with bleomycin and vincristine. Br J Radiol 52:238, 1979.

Richman LS, Gumerman LW, Levine G, Sartiano GP, Boggs SS: Localization of Tc^{99m} polyphosphate in soft tissue malignancies. AJR 124:577, 1975.

Roberts WC: Radiographic characteristics of glass. AJR 115:636, 1972.

Ros PR, Viamonte M Jr, Rywlin AM: Malignant fibrous histiocytoma: Mesenchymal tumor of ubiquitous origin. AJR 142:753, 1984.

Schaffzin EA, Chung SMK, Kaye R: Congenital generalized fibromatosis with complete spontaneous regression. J Bone Joint Surg [Am] 54:657, 1972.

Shackelford GD, Barton LL, McAlister WH: Calcified subcutaneous fat necrosis in infancy. J Can Assoc Radiol 26:203, 1975.

Simmons M, Tucker AK: The radiology of bone changes in rhabdomyosarcoma. Clin Radiol 29:47, 1978.

Spjut HJ, Dorfman HD: Florid reactive periostitis of the tubular bones of the hands and feet. A benign lesion which may simulate osteosarcoma. Am J Surg Pathol 5:423, 1981.

Stout AP, Lattes R: Tumors of the Soft Tissues. Atlas of Tumor Pathology, Series 2, Fascicle 1. Bethesda, Md, Armed Forces Institute of Pathology, 1967.

Tanaka T, Rossier AB, Hussey RW, Ahnberg DS, Treves S: Quantitative assessment of para-osteo-arthropathy and its maturation on serial radionuclide bone images. Radiology 123:217, 1977.

Thiers BH: Panniculitis. Dermatol Clin North Am 1:537, 1983.

Tillotson JF, McDonald JR, Janes JM: Synovial sarcomata. J Bone Joint Surg [Am] 33:459, 1973.

Weiss SW, Enzinger FM: Malignant fibrous histiocytoma. An analysis of 200 cases. Cancer 41:2250, 1978.

Weston WJ: Thorn- and twig-induced pseudo-tumours of bone and soft tissues. Br J Radiol 36:323, 1963.

Yeh H-C, Rabinowitz JG: Ultrasonography of the extremities and pelvic girdle and correlation with computed tomography. Radiology 143:519, 1982.

Yousefzadeh DK, Jackson JH Jr: Organic foreign body reaction. Report of two cases of thorn-induced "granuloma" and review of literature. Skel Radiol 3:167, 1978.

Zlatkin MB, Lander PH, Begin LR, Hadjipavlou A: Soft-tissue chondromas. AJR 144:1263, 1985.

Index